NURSING CARE PLANS

ASSESSMENT TABLES

DIAGNOSTIC TEST AND PROCEDURE TABLES

Introductory Nursing Care of Adults

Introductory Nursing Care of Adults

ADRIANNE DILL LINTON, Ph.D., R.N.,C.

Assistant Professor
University of Texas Health Science Center at San Antonio
School of Nursing
San Antonio, Texas

MARY ANN MATTESON, Ph.D., R.N., F.A.A.N.

Associate Professor
Thelma and Joe Crow Endowed Professor
University of Texas Health Science Center at San Antonio
School of Nursing
San Antonio, Texas

NANCY K. MAEBIUS, Ph.D., R.N.

Instructor
The Health Institute of San Antonio
San Antonio, Texas

W.B. SAUNDERS COMPANY

A Division of Harcourt Brace & Company
Philadelphia London Toronto
Montreal Sydney Tokyo

W.B. SAUNDERS COMPANY
A Division of Harcourt Brace & Company

The Curtis Center
Independence Square West
Philadelphia, Pennsylvania 19106

Library of Congress Cataloging-in-Publication Data

Linton, Adrianne.
Introductory nursing care of adults / Adrianne Linton, Mary Ann Matteson, Nancy K. Maebius. — 1st ed.
p. cm.
ISBN 0–7216–3319–6
1. Nursing. I. Matteson, Mary Ann. II. Maebius, Nancy K.
[DNLM: 1. Nursing Care—in adulthood. 2. Nursing Process. WY 100 L761i 1995]
RT41.L735 1995
610.73—dc20
DNLM/DLC 94-36486

Unit Opening Photographs: Stephen Matteson, Jr.

INTRODUCTORY NURSING CARE OF ADULTS ISBN 0–7216–3319–6

Printed in the United States of America.

Last digit is the print number: 9 8 7 6 5 4 3

Adrianne Dill Linton
To Ken, Leigh, Mike, Gary, Ron, and Barry

Mary Ann Matteson
To Steve, Steve Jr., Sarah, Anne, Peter, and Katherine

Nancy K. Maebius
To Jed, Stephen, Elizabeth, Brian, and Andrew

Contributors

Irma G. Aguilar, M.A., M.S.N., R.N.
Assistant Professor of Nursing, Texas Tech Health Sciences Center; Consultant, Hospice of the Southwest, Inc., Odessa, Texas
The Nurse-Patient Relationship; Psychological Responses to Illness

Marge Balzer, Ph.D., R.N.
Assistant Professor, School of Nursing, University of Texas Health Science Center, San Antonio, Texas
Cerebrovascular Accident

J. Gail Barry, B.S.N., R.N.,C.
Instructor of Nursing, Odessa College, Odessa, Texas
The Nurse-Patient Relationship; Psychological Responses to Illness

Cheryl I. Bond, B.S.N., R.N.
Cedar Park, Texas
Acute Respiratory Disorders

Carol Boswell, M.S.N., R.N.
Assistant Professor of Nursing, Odessa College, Odessa; Quality Assurance Consultant, Permian General Hospital, Andrews, Texas
Peripheral Vascular Disorders

Gayle Dasher, M.S.N., R.N., C.C.R.N.
Clinical Nurse Specialist, Santa Rosa Northwest Hospital, San Antonio, Texas
Neurologic Disorders; Spinal Cord Injury

Edward P. Gruber, Ph.D., R.N., F.N.P.
Assistant Professor, School of Nursing, University of Texas Health Science Center, San Antonio, Texas
Inflammation and Infection; Patient Care Settings

Beverly F. Halter, M.S.N., R.N.
Nurse Manager, Intermediate Medical-Surgical Unit, Southwest Texas Methodist Hospital, San Antonio, Texas
Male Reproductive Disorders

J. Taylor Harden, Ph.D., R.N.,C.
Former Associate Professor, School of Nursing, University of Texas Health Science Center, San Antonio, Texas
The Older Patient

Mary L. Heye, Ph.D., R.N., C.S.
Assistant Professor, School of Nursing, University of Texas Health Science Center, San Antonio, Texas
Pain Management

Gayleen Ienatsch, M.S.N., R.N.
Acting Regional Dean and Instructor, Texas Tech University Health Sciences Center, School of Nursing in the Permian Basin, Odessa, Texas
Diabetes Mellitus and Hypoglycemia

Dorothy Greene Jackson, M.S.N., R.N., C.S.
Assistant Professor, School of Nursing, Texas Tech University Health Sciences Center; Vice-President, Seabury Nursing Care Unit, Odessa, Texas
Connective Tissue Disorders

Anne-Marie Jones, M.S.N., B.S.N., R.N., C.C.R.N.
Asheville, North Carolina
Immunity

Esperanza V. Joyce, Ed.D., R.N., C.N.S.
Assistant Professor, School of Nursing, University of Texas Health Science Center, San Antonio, Texas
Fluid and Electrolytes; Sexually Transmitted Diseases

Phyllis Karmels, M.S.N., M.A.Ed., R.N.,C.
Texas Tech University Health Sciences Center School of Nursing in the Permian Basin, Odessa, Texas
Diabetes Mellitus and Hypoglycemia

Sheila Kelly, Ph.D., M.S.N., R.N.
Former Assistant Professor, School of Nursing, University of Texas Health Science Center, San Antonio, Texas
Psychiatric Disorders

Kenn M. Kirksey, Ph.D., R.N., C.S., C.E.N., C.N.S.
Assistant Professor, School of Nursing, University of Texas Health Science Center; Clinical Associate, University Hospital Emergency Center, San Antonio, Texas
Fluid and Electrolytes; Sexually Transmitted Diseases

Pauline Lee, Ed.D., M.S.N., R.N.,C.
Assistant Professor, School of Nursing, and Interim Chair, Family Nursing Department, University of Texas Health Science Center, San Antonio, Texas
Female Reproductive Disorders

Adrianne Dill Linton, Ph.D., R.N.
Assistant Professor, School of Nursing, University of Texas Health Science Center, San Antonio, Texas
Chronic Respiratory Disorders; Digestive Tract Disorders; Disorders of the Liver, Gallbladder, and Pancreas; Ear and Hearing Disorders; Eye and Vision Disorders; First Aid and Emergency Care; Incontinence; Intravenous Therapy; Neurologic Disorders; Nose, Sinus, and Throat Disorders; The Ostomy Patient; The Patient with Cancer; Skin Disorders; Surgical Care; Thyroid and Parathyroid Disorders

Louis K. Linton, B.S., R.R.T., C.P.F.T.
Instructor of Respiratory Therapy, Respiratory Specialist Program, Brooke Army Medical Center, San Antonio, Texas
Chronic Respiratory Disorders

Lea Ann Loftis, B.S.N., R.N.
Instructor, Baptist School of Professional Nursing, San Antonio, Texas
Nutrition

Mary Ann Matteson, Ph.D., R.N., F.A.A.N.
Associate Professor, Thelma and Joe Crow Endowed Professor, School of Nursing, University of Texas Health Science Center, San Antonio, Texas
Acute Respiratory Disorders; Confusion; Cultural Aspects of Nursing Care; Developmental Processes; Falls; Fluid and Electrolytes; Fractures; Health and Illness; The Health Care System; Immobility; The Leadership Role of the Nurse; The Nursing Process; Nutrition

Joy M. Norton, Ed.D., R.N., C.S.
Assistant Professor, School of Nursing, University of Texas Health Science Center, San Antonio, Texas
Cardiac Disorders; Hypertension; Urologic Disorders

Kathleen Reeves, M.S.N., R.N.,C.
Clinical Instructor, School of Nursing, University of Texas Health Science Center; Medical-Surgical Clinical Nurse Specialist, Southwest Texas Methodist Hospital, San Antonio, Texas
Pain Management

Dianne Murray Rudolph, M.S.N., R.N., C.C.R.N.
Instructor, School of Nursing, University of Texas Health Science Center, San Antonio, Texas
Adrenal and Pituitary Disorders; Amputations

June Schneberger, M.S.N., R.N., C.S.
Clinical Supervisor, Santa Rosa Home Health, Mental Health, Santa Rosa Medical Center, San Antonio, Texas
Psychiatric Disorders; Substance Abuse

Cheryl Ross Staats, M.S.N., R.N.
Assistant Professor, School of Nursing, University of Texas Health Science Center; Relief Supervisor, Metropolitan Hospital, San Antonio, Texas
Loss, Death, and Dying

Stacey Young-McCaughan, M.S.N., R.N., O.C.N.
Oncology Clinical Nurse Specialist, Madigan Army Medical Center, Tacoma, Washington
Hematologic and Lymphatic Disorders

Reviewers

Lynda Allen, B.S.N., R.N., C.E.T.N.
Harris Methodist—Fort Worth
Fort Worth, Texas

Runice Ann Bauer, B.S., R.N.
School of Practical Nursing
Minnesota Riverland Technical College
Faribault, Minnesota

Annie L. Brown, M.S., B.S.N., R.N.
School of Vocational Nursing
St. Phillip's College
San Antonio, Texas

Gretchen Carrougher, M.N., R.N.
School of Nursing
University of Texas Health Science Center
San Antonio, Texas

Sharon E. Cowen, B.S., R.N.
School of Practical Nursing
Boonslick Area Vocational-Technical School
Boonville, Missouri

Carolann Mitchell Dallalis, B.S.N., R.N.
School of Nursing
St. Mary's Hospital
Richmond, Virginia

Michelle L. Dumpe, M.S.N., M.S., R.N.
Venango County Area Vocational-Technical School
Oil City, Pennsylvania

Mary M. Eimer, B.S.N., R.N.
School of Practical Nursing
Jefferson College
Hillsboro, Missouri

Judy M. Fair, M.Ed., R.N.
Sandusky School of Practical Nursing
Sandusky, Ohio

Janice Ray Finney, M.Ed., B.S., R.N.
School of Practical Nursing
John A. Logan College
Carterville, Illinois

Nancy Joan Girard, Ph.D., R.N., C.N.O.R., C.S.
School of Nursing
University of Texas Health Science Center
San Antonio, Texas

Leslie R. Goddard, Ph.D., R.N., C.N.R.N.
School of Nursing
University of Texas Health Science Center
San Antonio, Texas

Lillian Goodman, M.Ed., B.A., R.N.
School of Vocational Nursing
Los Angeles Unified School District
University of California, Los Angeles, Extension
Los Angeles, California

Teresa Jo Grooms, B.S.N., R.N.
School of Practical Nursing
Southern State Community College
Hillsboro, Ohio

Ruth Hall, M.A., R.N.
School for Practical Nursing
Augusta Technical Institute
Augusta, Georgia

Jo Anne Jacobson, B.S.N., R.N.
School of Practical Nursing
Southern State Community College
Hillsboro, Ohio

Martha J. Jett, R.N.
School of Practical Nursing
Southern State Community College
Hillsboro, Ohio

Glenda Kupferle, M.S.N., R.N., C.S., C.E.T.N.
Harris Methodist—Fort Worth
Fort Worth, Texas

Carolyn L. Lane, B.S.Ed., M.S.N., B.S.N., R.N.
School of Practical Nursing
Dodge City Community College
Dodge City, Kansas

Sharon Layton, M.S., B.S.N., R.N.
School of Practical Nursing
Lower Columbia College
Longview, Washington

Patricia B. Lisk, B.S., R.N.
School of Practical Nursing
Augusta Technical Institute
Augusta, Georgia

Tina K. Monlezun, B.S.N., R.N.
School of Practical Nursing
Jefferson Davis Technical Institute
Jennings, Louisiana

Mary Patricia Norrell, B.S.N., R.N.C.
School of Practical Nursing
Indiana Vocational-Technical College
Columbus, Indiana

Kay Patterson, B.S.N., R.N.,C., C.E.T.N., O.C.N.
Harris Methodist—Fort Worth
Fort Worth, Texas

Melba L. Perkins, B.S.N., C.R.N.I.
Southwest Texas Methodist Hospital
San Antonio, Texas

Dorie E. Pierce, M.S.N., R.N., C.N.S.
Metropolitan Hospital
San Antonio, Texas

Deborah L. Robinson, B.S.N., R.N.
Thompson School for Practical Nurses
Barre, Vermont

Edward L. Russell, Ph.D., R.N., C.S.
School of Nursing
University of Texas Health Science Center
San Antonio, Texas

Alice H. Sinclair, B.S.N., R.N.
School of Practical Nursing
Burlington County Vocational-Technical School
Medford, New Jersey

Barbara Talik, M.Ed., B.S.N., R.N.
Chairperson, Practical Nursing Program
Northwest Technical Institute
Springdale, Arkansas

Catherine Ann Ultrino, M.S., R.N., O.C.N.
Youville Hospital School of Practical Nursing
Cambridge, Massachusetts

Doris L. Walker, M.S.Ed., R.N.,C.
School of Practical Nursing
Lehigh County Community College
Schnecksville, Pennsylvania

Acknowledgments

We would like to acknowledge the people who have been helpful to us in developing this book. Dr. Patty Hawken, Dean of the School of Nursing at the University of Texas Health Science Center at San Antonio, and Dr. Helena McBride, Director of The Health Institutes of San Antonio, offered support and encouragement for this project. We called on Dr. Jo Ann Crow's critical eye and artistic sense as we sought illustrations that complemented our text. We were delighted with the photographs of Stephen Matteson, Jr., which fulfilled our hopes in their sensitive portrayal of nurses and patients. Melinda Bell was always willing to assist with any aspect of manuscript preparation and never lost her enthusiasm and positive outlook. Special thanks go to Linda Wienerman, Terri Wood, Sharon Roberts, Beverly Halter, and Lea Ann Loftis for their assistance and support in the production of the Instructor's Manual and the Study Guide.

A number of students contributed to this textbook in a variety of ways. Stephanie Appell, Suzanne DePoy, Edwin Learned, and Sheri Smith reviewed chapters and provided invaluable feedback from the student's viewpoint. Dr. Nancy Girard's perioperative nursing students and graduate student assistant served as subjects for many of the photographs we used. They included Carolyn Chase, Karen DuBose, Heather Feray, Janet Kawa, Edward Pastrano, Maria Patterson, Dora Reed, Herlinda Salazar, and Joyce Sears. Students of Dr. Nancy Maebius and Ms. Collette Strauss who allowed us to capture them in action included Charles Alva, Kevin Trainor, Yvette Velasquez, Nancy Michell, Elizabeth Navarro, Peggy Trainer, Lena Steen, Tracie Eddie, Loriann Romo, Adela Silva, and Jennifer Hammond. We are grateful to the nurses, patients, and families who consented to appear in the photographs as well.

We also thank the editorial team at W. B. Saunders, consisting of Tom Eoyang, Ilze Rader, Robin Richman, Paula Shargel-Green, Lee Ann Draud, Marie Thomas, Maura Connor, and Carolyn Naylor. We appreciate the patience and skill of the artists who worked with us to produce the fine illustrations. A special acknowledgment goes to Ilze Rader who guided, nurtured, supported, and critically analyzed our efforts and became a real friend in the process.

Preface

Introductory Nursing Care of Adults is a response to the evolving roles and opportunities for licensed practical nurses and vocational nurses today. As the population of elderly adults increases and as health care delivery systems change, nursing will be challenged to provide excellent care in more cost-efficient ways. To meet this challenge, the nurse's role in the next decade will include not only direct care in hospitals and in long-term care facilities but also in evolving ambulatory and community settings.

To help meet these challenges, we have built this text on four themes:

- Nursing care is given in a variety of settings.
- Learning is structured with the nursing process.
- Caring for the elderly is emphasized throughout.
- Greater depth and detail of information on disorders, treatments, and nursing care is given to prepare licensed practical nurses and vocational nurses for the complexity of care they will deliver.

NURSING CARE IN A VARIETY OF SETTINGS

Unit 1 introduces the changing health care system and the nurse's role in it. Chapter 2, "The Leadership Role of the Nurse," helps students recognize their responsibilities as part of the health care team and as leaders in a variety of health care settings. Chapter 17, "Patient Care Settings," introduces the student to these settings and discusses the nurse's role in many other settings.

Throughout the book, nursing care is presented as being *given in the hospital, in long-term care settings, and in other facilities.* Patient care scenarios in the 34 care plans are described for a variety of settings, including nursing homes, physicians' offices, emergency departments, patients' homes, and acute care hospitals.

LEARNING STRUCTURED THROUGH THE NURSING PROCESS

Consistent presentation of care in a nursing process format provides easier reading and learning for students. Every chapter from Chapter 25 through 52 presents disorders through the steps of *assessment, diagnosis, goals, interventions, and evaluation.*

In addition to text coverage of assessment, each chapter contains a summarizing assessment box to help students identify the key elements of assessment. Nursing diagnoses are clearly identified in bulleted lists. Goals and interventions are correlated with each diagnosis, in a clear, easy to understand fashion. In evaluation, the student is presented outcome criteria for judging the effects of interventions on achieving the goals of nursing care.

Thirty-four care plans, with patient stories, include assessment, goals and outcome criteria, and interventions to help students apply nursing process to real-life situations.

EMPHASIS ON CARING FOR THE ELDERLY

One of the greatest challenges for nurses in the coming decades is to provide care for the elderly—from health teaching and monitoring in the home to long-term care for the frailest, most vulnerable population. Chapter 7 introduces major concepts about gerontology, which are applied to specific disorders throughout the text. Major clinical problems are discussed in individual chapters, which include in-depth discussions about the causes of the problems and their prevention and treatments. Expected assessment findings in the older adult are noted, and modifications in medical and nursing care are emphasized. Unit 4 includes chapters on falls, immobility, confusion, and incontinence—all important problems in the nursing care of the aged. Separate chapters are also devoted to pain management, death and dying, and the ostomy patient.

GREATER DEPTH AND DETAIL ON DISORDERS AND NURSING CARE

Recognizing the increased acuity of patients in hospitals, the increased complexity of care, and the corresponding increased responsibilities of nurses, coverage of disorders and nursing care is comprehensive and detailed. Tables are included for the following:

- Diagnostic tests and procedures, including the nurse's role in preparation of the patient and care after the procedure
- Drug therapy, including side effects and nursing interventions for the particular drugs most commonly used in specific disorders

Careful attention has been given to long-term care considerations for chronic disorders and to rehabilitation.

USING THIS TEXT

The reader is encouraged to preview the Table of Contents to see the overall organization of the book.

The first five units provide a foundation for later chapters, and the reader will be referred back to these units at times. Therefore, the text is best approached by studying these initial chapters first. Subsequent units (Units 6 through 16) take a systems approach to disorders and are independent, so they can be studied in any order. Each unit begins with assessment, age-related changes, diagnostic tests and procedures, and common therapeutic measures related to the body system being studied. Units are divided into shorter chapters for easier reading.

Each chapter begins with a chapter outline, to help preview the chapter; objectives, so that the student is clear about what is to be learned; and a glossary of important terms with definitions; each concludes with numbered key concepts to help with recall.

Therapeutic procedures, nutrition boxes, and pharmacology "capsules" (important points to remember) are included in body systems chapters throughout to help the student recall and integrate learning from other courses.

A student **Study Guide** and an **Instructor's Manual** have been designed and written specifically for the text by Nancy Maebius. The Study Guide provides a detailed, clear method for the student to identify the most important material and helps students learn more efficiently. The Instructor's Manual provides more than 2000 multiple-choice questions for testing and a special section of exercises linked to the care plans in the text that is designed to promote critical thinking. The exercises provide the instructor with suggested questions to encourage student analysis of patient care situations presented in the care plans.

Also available to qualified adopters of the text is **a package of approximately 65 two-color transparencies** for classroom use.

TEXT ORGANIZATION

Unit 1 explores patient care concepts: the health care system, the role of the nurse, the nurse-patient relationship, culture, health and illness, developmental processes, the older patient, and the nursing process.

Units 2 and 3 include physiologic responses to illness and medical-surgical care. Both Units provide content basic to understanding many pathologic processes as well as medical and nursing interventions in subsequent chapters.

Unit 4 gives special attention to concepts related to long-term care, which is becoming the most critical part of the health care system in the United States.

Unit 5 introduces the reader to cancer and includes the characteristics of malignant cells, the metastatic process, diagnostic procedures, treatment options, and related nursing care. Early coverage of this content provides the reader with a foundation for approaching the study of various specific cancers in later chapters without requiring tedious repetition.

Units 6 through 15 cover specific disorders, including pathophysiology, signs and symptoms, complications, medical diagnosis and treatment, and nursing care. Each step of the nursing process is discussed thoroughly, and patient and family teaching are incorporated.

Unit 16 includes psychosocial responses to illness, psychiatric disorders, and substance abuse.

Brief Contents

Detailed Contents

CHAPTER 6

Mary Ann Matteson

CHAPTER 7

J. Taylor Harden

CHAPTER 8

Mary Ann Matteson

UNIT 2

CHAPTER 9

Edward P. Gruber

CHAPTER 10

Anne-Marie Jones

CHAPTER 11

Esperanza V. Joyce
Kenn M. Kirksey
Mary Ann Matteson

Fluid and Electrolytes 106

CHAPTER 12

Lea Ann Loftis
Mary Ann Matteson

Nutrition 122

UNIT 3

Medical-Surgical Care 143

CHAPTER 13

Adrianne Linton

First Aid and Emergency Care 145

CHAPTER 14

Adrianne Linton

Surgical Care 167

CHAPTER 15

Adrianne Linton

Intravenous Therapy 196

CHAPTER 16

Mary L. Heye
Kathleen Reeves

Pain Management 208

UNIT 4

Long-Term and Home Health Care 229

CHAPTER 17

Edward P. Gruber

Patient Care Settings 231

CHAPTER 18

Mary Ann Matteson

Falls 247

CHAPTER 19

Mary Ann Matteson

Immobility 255

CHAPTER 20

Mary Ann Matteson

Confusion 266

CHAPTER 21

Adrianne Linton

Incontinence 274

CHAPTER 22

Cheryl Ross Staats

Loss, Death, and Dying 293

UNIT 5

Cancer 309

CHAPTER 23

Adrianne Linton

The Patient with Cancer 311

CHAPTER 24

Adrianne Linton

The Ostomy Patient 334

UNIT 6

Neurologic Disorders 353

CHAPTER 25

Gayle Dasher
Adrianne Linton

Neurologic Disorders 355

CHAPTER 26

Marge Balzer

Cerebrovascular Accident 397

CHAPTER 27

Gayle Dasher

Spinal Cord Injury 421

UNIT 7

Respiratory Disorders 443

CHAPTER 28

Cheryl I. Bond
Mary Ann Matteson

Acute Respiratory Disorders 445

CHAPTER 29

Adrianne Linton
Louis K. Linton

Chronic Respiratory Disorders 487

UNIT 8

Cardiovascular Disorders 507

CHAPTER 30

Stacey Young-McCaughan

Hematologic and Lymphatic Disorders 509

CHAPTER 31

Joy M. Norton

Cardiac Disorders 537

CHAPTER 32

Carol Boswell

Peripheral Vascular Disorders 599

CHAPTER 33

Joy M. Norton

Hypertension 627

UNIT 9

Digestive Disorders 639

CHAPTER 34

Adrianne Linton

Digestive Tract Disorders 641

CHAPTER 35

Adrianne Linton

Disorders of the Liver, Gallbladder, and Pancreas 699

UNIT 10

Urologic Disorders 735

CHAPTER 36

Joy M. Norton

Urologic Disorders 737

UNIT 11

Musculoskeletal Disorders 779

CHAPTER 37

Dorothy Greene Jackson

Connective Tissue Disorders 781

CHAPTER 38

Mary Ann Matteson

Fractures 809

UNIT 13

Reproductive Disorders 917

CHAPTER 43

Pauline Lee

Female Reproductive Disorders 919

CHAPTER 44

Beverly F. Halter

Male Reproductive Disorders 965

CHAPTER 45

Kenn M. Kirksey
Esperanza V. Joyce

Sexually Transmitted Diseases 992

UNIT 14

Integumentary Disorders 1007

CHAPTER 46

Adrianne Linton

Skin Disorders 1009

UNIT 15

Disorders of the Eyes, Ears, Nose, and Throat 1039

CHAPTER 47

Adrianne Linton

Eye and Vision Disorders 1041

CHAPTER 48

Adrianne Linton

Ear and Hearing Disorders 1069

CHAPTER 49

Adrianne Linton

Nose, Sinus, and Throat Disorders 1088

UNIT 16

Mental Health and Illness 1113

CHAPTER 50

Irma G. Aguilar
J. Gail Barry

Psychological Responses to Illness 1115

CHAPTER 51

Sheila Kelly
June Schneberger

Psychiatric Disorders 1126

CHAPTER 52

June Schneberger

Substance Abuse 1140

GLOSSARY 1161
ABBREVIATIONS 1181
INDEX 1183

Color Plates

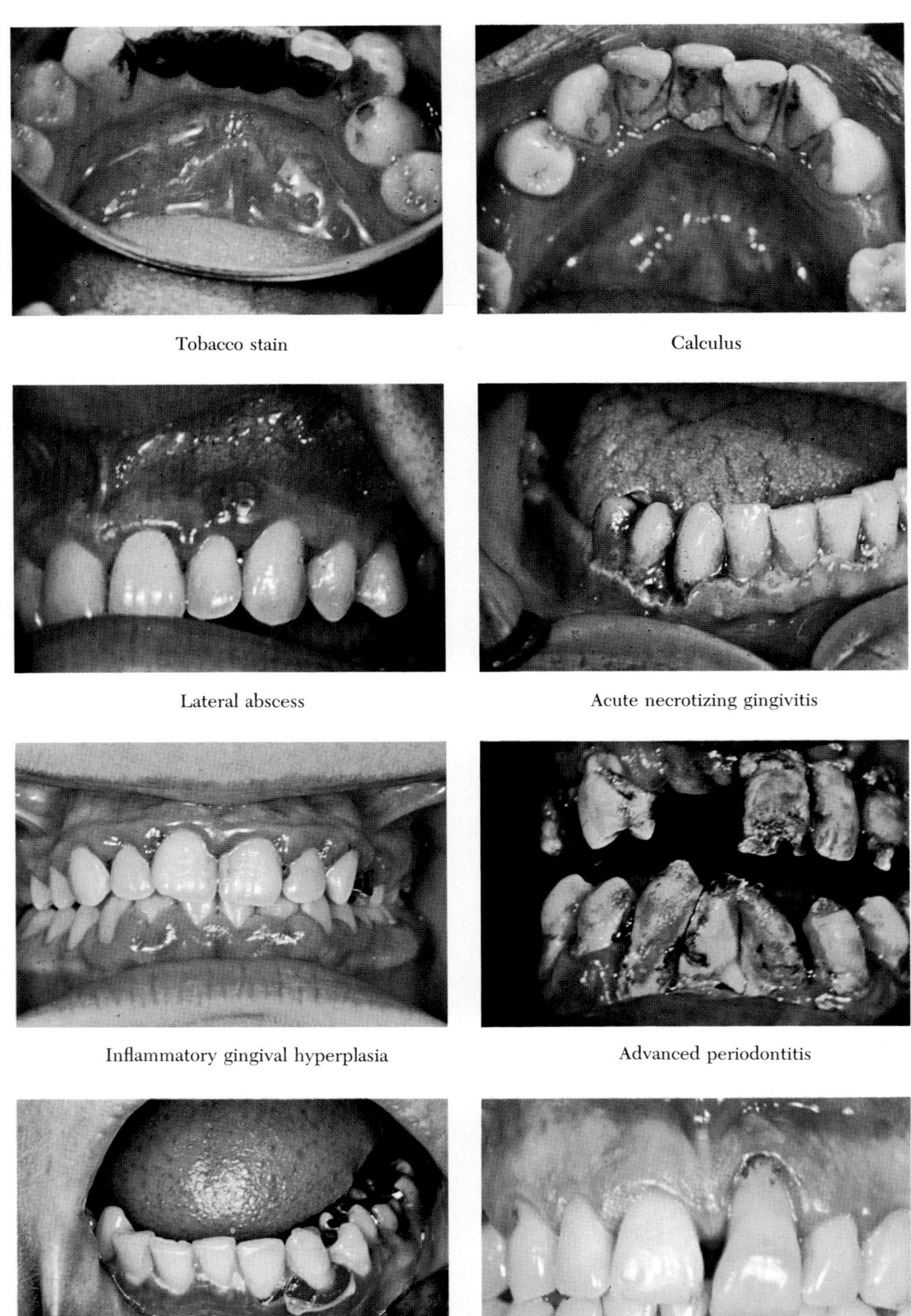

Tobacco stain

Calculus

Lateral abscess

Acute necrotizing gingivitis

Inflammatory gingival hyperplasia

Advanced periodontitis

Chronic desquamative gingivitis

Gingival recession

COLOR PLATE I

Oral conditions. (From Shafer, W. G., Hine, M. K., & Levy, B. M. [1983]. *Textbook of oral pathology* [4th ed., p. 767]. Philadelphia: W. B. Saunders.)

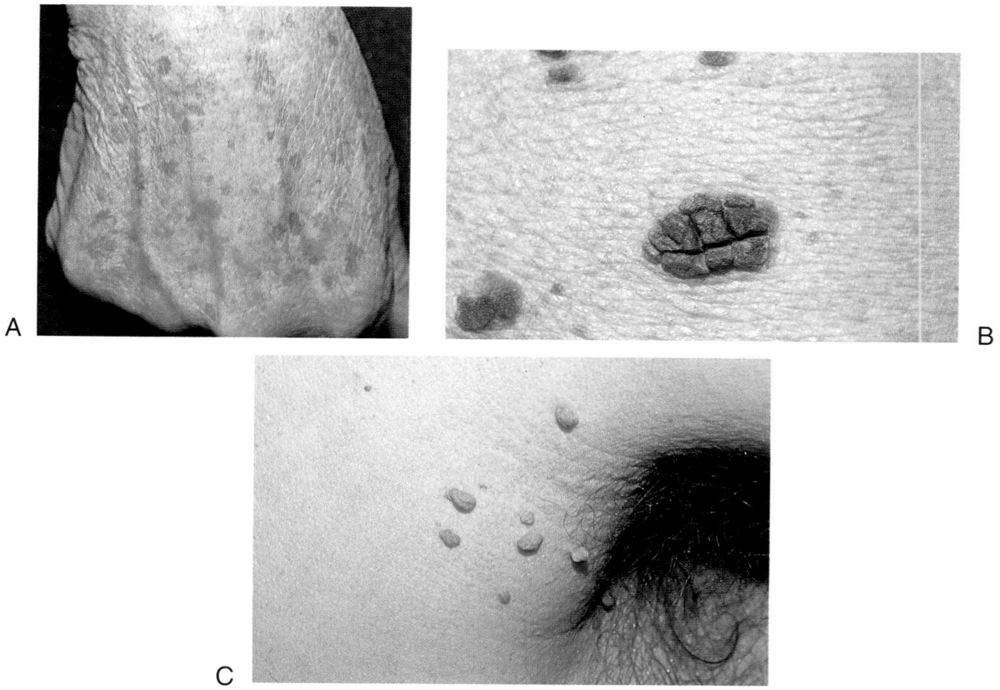

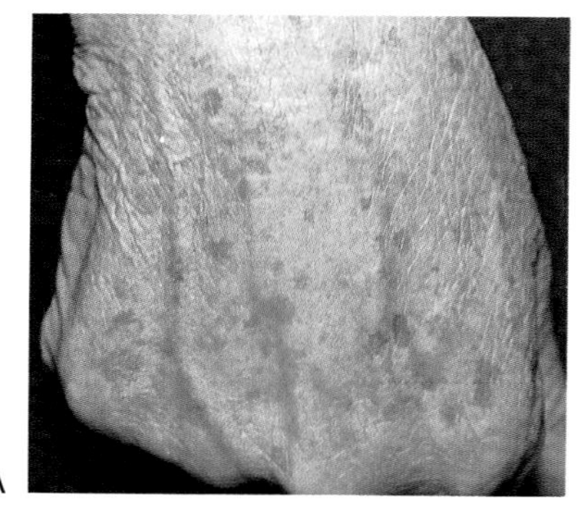

A

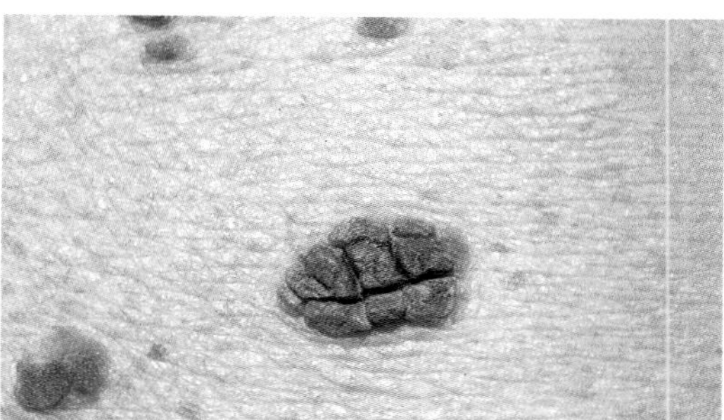

B

C

COLOR PLATE II

Common skin changes in the elderly. *A*, Lentigines; *B*, seborrheic keratoses; *C*, skin tags. (From Lookingbill, D. P., & Marks, J. G., Jr. [1993]. *Principles of dermatology* [2nd ed., pp. 89, 74, 75]. Philadelphia: W. B. Saunders.)

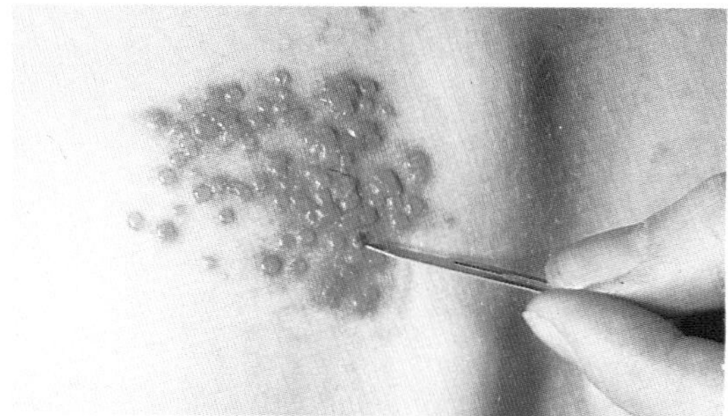

COLOR PLATE III

Herpes simplex lesions. (From Lookingbill, D. P., & Marks J. G., Jr. [1993]. *Principles of dermatology* [2nd ed., p. 162]. Philadelphia: W. B. Saunders.)

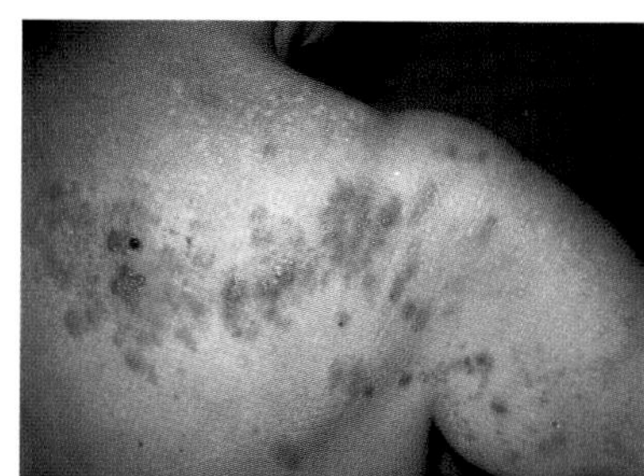

COLOR PLATE IV

Herpes zoster lesions ("shingles"). (From Lookingbill, D. P., & Marks, J. G., Jr. [1993]. *Principles of dermatology* [2nd ed., p. 166]. Philadelphia: W. B. Saunders.)

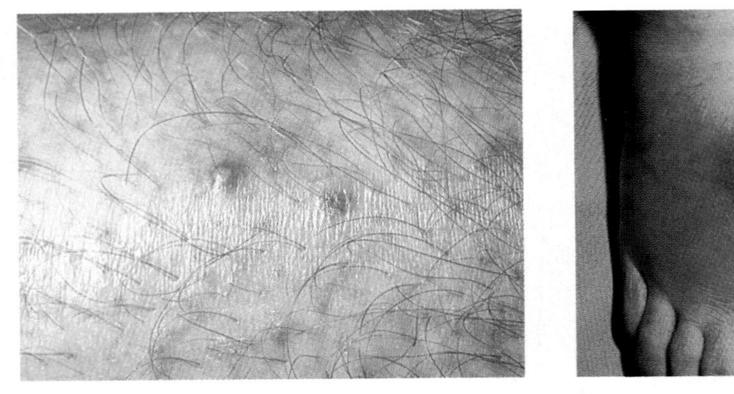

A

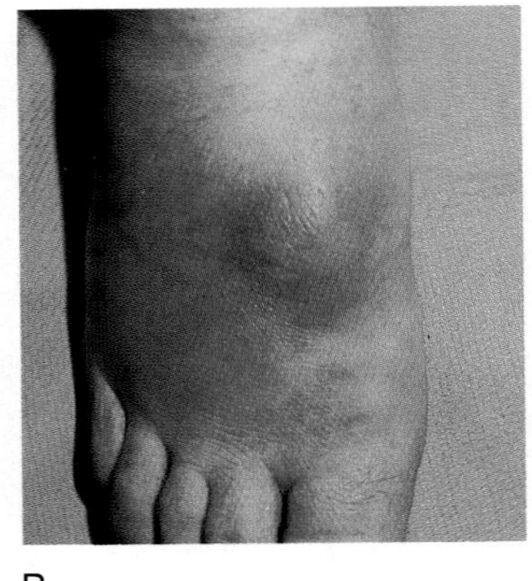

B

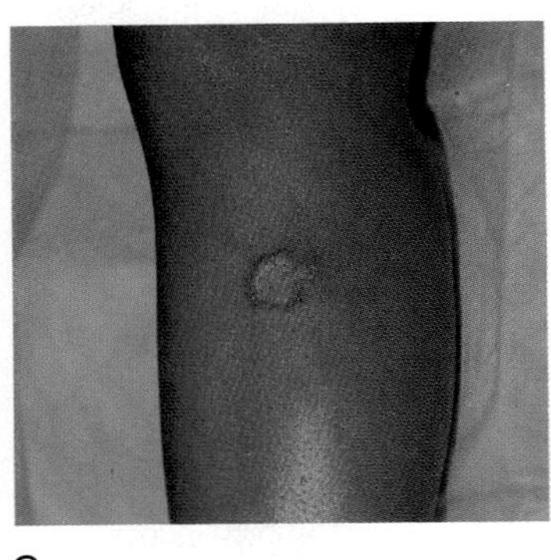

C

COLOR PLATE V

A, Folliculitis; *B*, furuncle and abscess; *C*, tinea corporis. (From Lookingbill, D. P., & Marks, J. G., Jr. [1993]. *Principles of dermatology* [2nd ed., pp. 196, 234, 144]. Philadelphia: W. B. Saunders.)

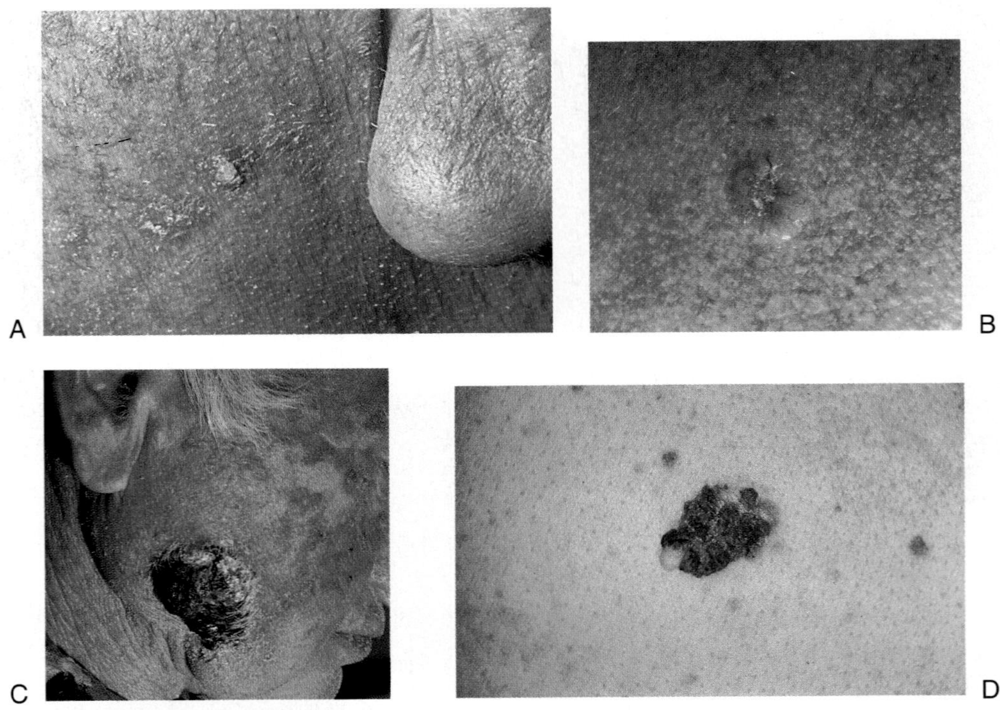

A B C D

COLOR PLATE VI

Skin cancers. *A*, Actinic keratosis (a premalignant lesion); *B*, basal cell carcinoma; *C*, squamous cell carcinoma; *D*, malignant melanoma. (*A*, *B*, and *C* from Lookingbill, D. P., & Marks, J. G., Jr. [1993]. *Principles of dermatology* [2nd ed., pp. 77, 81, 79]. Philadelphia: W. B. Saunders. *D* from Jarvis, C. [1992]. *Physical examination and health assessment* [p. 268]. Philadelphia: W. B. Saunders.)

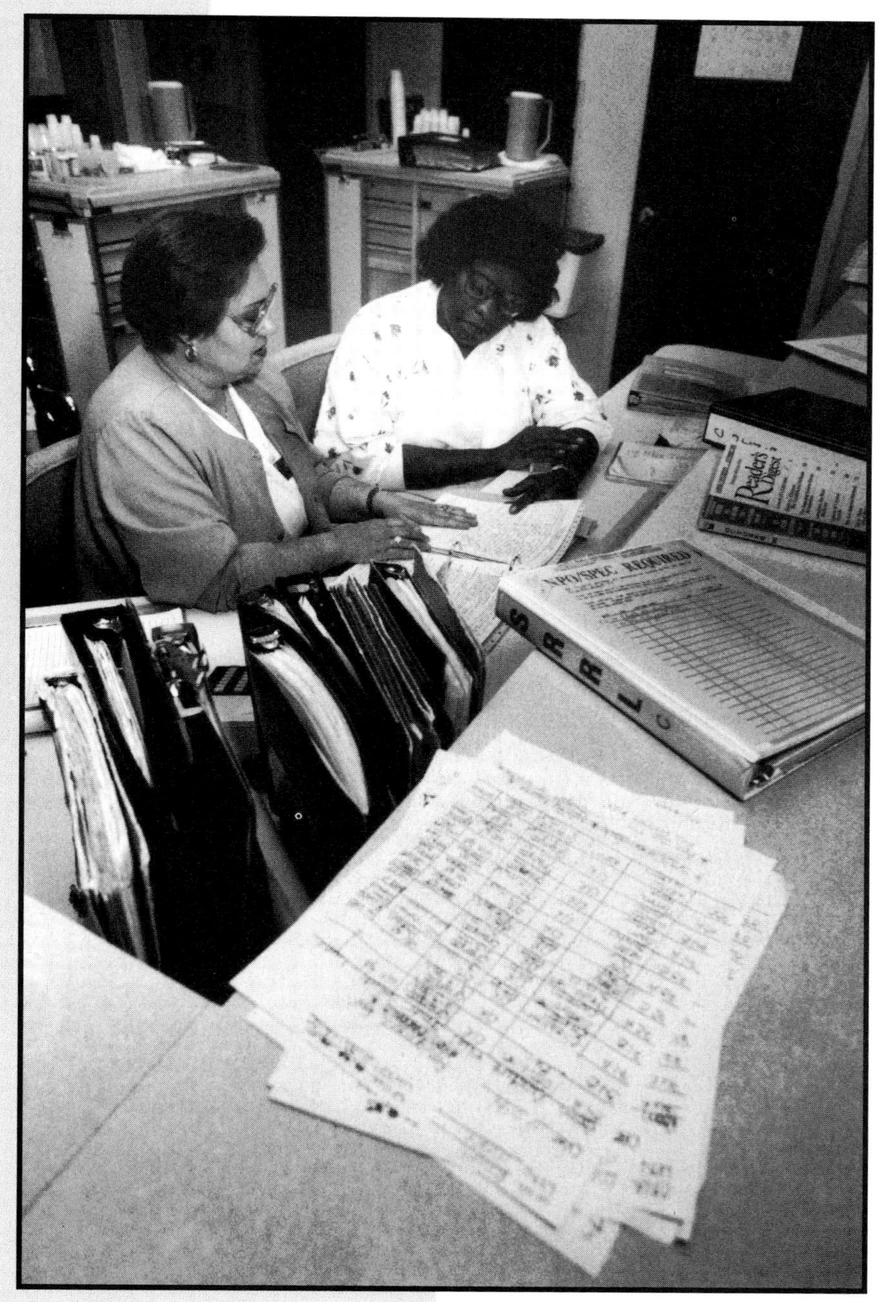

UNIT 1

Patient Care Concepts

Mary Ann Matteson

CHAPTER 1

The Health Care System

OBJECTIVES

1. Describe the organization of the health care system in the United States.
2. Describe the components of the health care system that provide both outpatient and inpatient care.

GLOSSARY

DIAGNOSIS RELATED GROUP (DRG) System enacted under Medicare that reimburses hospitals for patient care based on their medical diagnoses

HEALTH MAINTENANCE ORGANIZATION (HMO) Health care organization that provides care and services through group practice and prepayment plans

INTERMEDIATE CARE FACILITY Nursing homes that provide custodial care for people who are unable to care for themselves because of mental or physical infirmity

MEDICAID Program that provides health care services for needy, lower-income, and disabled individuals

MEDICARE Health insurance program administered by the federal government that is funded by Social Security payments

OLDER AMERICANS ACT Act passed in 1965 to ensure that elderly persons have an adequate income and suitable housing, physical and mental health services, community services, and the opportunity to pursue meaningful activities

PUBLIC HEALTH SERVICE Branch of the Department of Health and Human Services of the U.S. government whose chief purpose is to provide better health services for the American people

SKILLED NURSING FACILITY Type of nursing home that provides rehabilitative care for people who need nursing care that consists of observation during illness, administration of medications and treatments, bowel or bladder retraining, and changing of sterile dressings

The health care system in the United States today is a collection of complex political organizations that have gotten beyond anyone's control. With an increase in the elderly population and a resulting increase in the incidence of chronic illness, costs have risen beyond comprehension. Government officials, health care providers, and consumers are now faced with the hard issues of who is going to receive care and who is going to pay for it. Health care reform is a major issue for government officials and the American people, both of whom are interested in the provision of equitable health care to all Americans.

ORGANIZATION OF THE HEALTH CARE SYSTEM

The health care system is made up of individuals who provide health care services in a variety of settings. Many of the services available to individuals are funded with financial assistance from government or private agencies. Unfortunately, all citizens of the United States are not eligible for government funds or are unable or unwilling to obtain private insurance. In addition, government funding and private insurance frequently do not cover all the costs of health care. Therefore, many people are unable to pay for and receive the services that they so desperately need.

In addition to the problem of inadequate financing, there is an absence of an overall philosophy or plan for health care. At the present time, the emphasis is on crisis and illness rather than on the promotion of health and the prevention of disease. There are inadequate standards to ensure quality of care and little consumer participation in decision making. A lack of coordination of services and poor communication among providers of services also interfere with a comprehensive plan of health care provision.

ADMINISTRATION

In 1953, the Department of Health, Education, and Welfare was established to organize the various health and welfare agencies in the U.S. government. The department later became known as the Department of Health and Human Services when education became a separate department. The three primary branches of DHHS are Social and Rehabilitation Services, the Social Security Administration, and the Public Health Service.

The Public Health Service is of major concern to nursing, for its purpose is to provide better health services for the American people. Its major activities include (1) reviewing health care, particularly in relation to Medicare and Medicaid; (2) providing grants and conducting research to study health problems; (3) raising public awareness of serious health problems; (4) operating hospitals for national health problems, such as drug addiction, tuberculosis, and mental illness; (5) providing health science training grants to educational institutions; and (6) publishing vital statistics related to public health programs. The major agencies that carry out the activities of the Public Health Service are the National Institutes of Health, the Food and Drug Administration, the Health Services Administration, the Centers for Disease Control and Prevention, the Health Resources Administration, and the Alcohol, Drug Abuse, and Mental Health Administration.

FINANCING

Most health care agencies are funded through government funds or private insurance. Others are funded through out-of-pocket fees for service. The major means of government funding are Medicare and Medicaid (Table 1–1).

Medicare

Established in 1966, Medicare is a health insurance program administered by the U.S. government as part of the Social Security Act. It covers all people aged 65 and older as well as disabled individuals younger than 65 who qualify for Social Security benefits. A monthly premium is deducted from each worker's paycheck, and the funds are matched by the federal government.

Medicare insurance covers physician services, hospital expenses, home health care, and outpatient services. The list of services covered varies from time to time, depending on changing government regulations. Most of the coverage is for skilled care. Medicare benefits are geared toward acute, short-term care. They do not cover long-term care, such as nursing home care, over an extended period of time. If nursing home care is covered, it is usually for a period of less than 30 days.

Medicaid

Like Medicare, Medicaid was established in 1966 as part of the Social Security Act. Unlike Medicare, Medicaid is funded by federal, state, and local taxes. It is administered by both federal and state governments

TABLE 1–1
COMPARISONS BETWEEN MEDICARE AND MEDICAID

MEDICARE	MEDICAID
Funding Monthly premium from paycheck; funds matched by federal government	Federal, state, and local taxes
Eligibility All persons older than 65 years plus disabled persons younger than 65 who qualify for Social Security benefits	Needy, low-income, and disabled persons and their dependent children younger than 65 years
How Administered Federal government	Both federal and state governments
Benefits Physician services, hospital expenses, home health care, and outpatient services; geared toward acute, short-term care	Same health benefits as Medicare, plus nursing home care

(Medicare is administered only by the federal government) on a partnership basis. States develop and operate the Medicaid programs within federal guidelines. Thus, benefits vary from state to state.

Medicaid benefits are provided for needy, low-income, disabled individuals and their dependent children under age 65. Individuals older than 65 who are under a certain income level may also receive benefits, including services that Medicare does not cover. Services covered by Medicaid include inpatient and outpatient care, skilled nursing home care, physicians' fees, laboratory work, radiographs, and home health care. Medicaid is more likely to cover long-term care than Medicare.

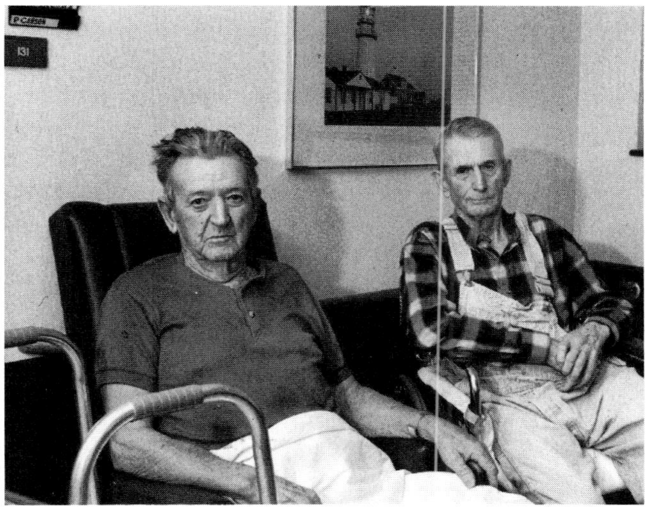

FIGURE 1-1
Outpatient clinics serve many people in the community. (From Matteson, M. A., & McConnell, E. S. [1988]. *Gerontological nursing* [p. 330]. Philadelphia: W. B. Saunders.)

COMPONENTS OF THE HEALTH CARE SYSTEM

Components of the health care system can be categorized into outpatient (ambulatory) care and inpatient care. Ambulatory care is provided for patients who do not require hospitalization. It may involve health promotion and disease prevention, diagnosis of disease, or treatment and follow-up of disease processes. Ambulatory care settings include physicians' offices; clinics; health maintenance organizations (HMOs); day surgery centers; daycare centers for the elderly, handicapped, or disabled; patients' homes; and hospices.

Inpatient settings include acute care hospitals, psychiatric hospitals, rehabilitation centers, and extended care facilities (nursing homes).

OUTPATIENT CARE

Physicians' Offices

Many people receive their primary medical care from physicians' offices, and this practice tends to increase with age. Older people have more office visits per year than younger people, especially since the enactment of Medicare and Medicaid. The cost of visits to physicians' offices is covered in part by some forms of private health insurance and Medicare, Part B. Physicians may practice in individual or group settings. A large number of group practices are made up of various medical specialties, so that clients may have all of their health care needs dealt with in one location. The focus of care is usually on the diagnosis and treatment of specific illnesses rather than on health promotion and other health services.

Clinics

Outpatient clinics may be associated with community hospitals, teaching hospitals, or public health departments (Fig. 1–1). They usually focus on care for the chronically ill, such as those with diabetes or heart disease, but people with acute illnesses also may be seen. The goal for care is to diagnose and treat the presenting illness.

Clinics offer many services, including physician services, nursing services, rehabilitative services, prenatal care, well baby checkups, immunizations, and laboratory and diagnostic services. In large hospitals, the clinics are usually organized according to medical subspecialties, such as urology, neurology, and orthopedics. For many people, especially the elderly, specialty clinics can be a problem because they have many chronic illnesses and are seen in many different clinics. This makes the coordination of care more difficult than if they were seen in a specific clinic with one set of health care providers.

Health Maintenance Organizations

Health maintenance organizations provide health care and services through group practice. They usually provide both outpatient and inpatient services. Individuals voluntarily join an HMO and pay a yearly fee on a prepayment plan. The fee covers all health care services, including acute and long-term medical care and health promotion and disease prevention programs. Depending on the plan, there are no further charges or there may be an additional small charge for services.

Because HMOs collect only a set fee from clients, they are invested in promoting health and maintaining wellness. Healthy clients do not need as many services as sick ones and are therefore less expensive to treat. HMOs employ physicians, nurses, and other health care providers and also have a broad group of specialists available for referral. Clients may use only the services of the physicians, other health care providers, and hospitals associated with the HMO.

In 1953, the federal government enacted the Health Maintenance Organization Act. Its purpose was to help private agencies to develop new methods of health care delivery in an effort to control the accessibility, quality, and cost of health care. This act helped to generate the development of HMOs throughout the United States.

The largest HMO in the country is the Kaiser-Permanente Medical Care Program. It provides services to more than 3 million people. The principles on which Kaiser-Permanente is based are typical of other HMOs. They include group practice with prepayment, voluntary enrollment, a combination of hospital and outpatient facilities, an emphasis on health promotion and prevention of illness, and physician responsibility for direction of patient care.

Day Surgery

One alternative to inpatient surgery is day surgery. People who need minor surgical procedures for cataracts, gynecologic problems, and the like may use day surgery. The procedures are carried out in hospitals, free-standing clinics, or physicians' offices. Most forms of insurance cover the expenses.

Day surgery is beneficial because it is less costly, and people are able to recover in the familiar surroundings of their own home. Patients usually have the preoperative assessments and laboratory tests performed on an outpatient basis several days ahead of the surgery and then arrive at the hospital or clinic early in the morning on the day of surgery. After the surgery they spend some time in a small recovery area and return home by the end of the day.

Daycare Centers

Daycare is a structured program designed to provide activities related to health and socialization for selected populations. The activities are most often directed toward the elderly and the mentally ill (Fig. 1–2). Daycare centers may be associated with hospitals or nursing homes, or they may function independently.

Older people can benefit from daycare services because they can continue to live in the community and have supervision during the day while family members work. The centers provide all kinds of health-related services, health promotion programs, nutritional meals, and social activities. Most services are provided on a sliding scale fee basis or without charge.

Many of the services provided at daycare centers are funded through the Older Americans Act, which was originally passed in 1965. The goals of the Older Americans Act are to ensure that elderly persons have adequate income and suitable housing, physical and mental health services, community services, and the opportunity to pursue meaningful activities.

Mental health services are also offered through daycare. People who need counseling, follow-up care after hospitalization, and rehabilitation related to chemical dependence may benefit from daycare programs. Most are covered by private insurance for a limited period of time.

Home Health Agencies

Home health services are provided to individuals and families in their homes to promote, maintain, or restore health or to minimize the effects of illness and disability (Fig. 1–3). The services include medical and dental care, nursing care, physical and occupational therapy, speech therapy, social work, nutrition counseling, home health aide, transportation, laboratory services, and medical equipment and supplies. Home health care is provided by hospitals, private profit-making and nonprofit agencies, and public agencies, such as public health and social service departments.

Home health agencies are regulated by the federal government and the individual states. Services are funded by individual payment, private insurance, Medicare and Medicaid. To be covered by Medicare, the agencies must adhere to regulations put forth by the federal government. Most nursing services that are paid for by Medicare must be "skilled" care with strict governmental guidelines that define the skilled care that must be provided. Regulations vary from state to state but are generally patterned after federal governmental regulations.

Hospices

Hospices provide care for terminally ill patients in the home and other specified facilities. Their purposes are to enable terminally ill patients to live as full a life as possible while managing the pain and discomfort as well

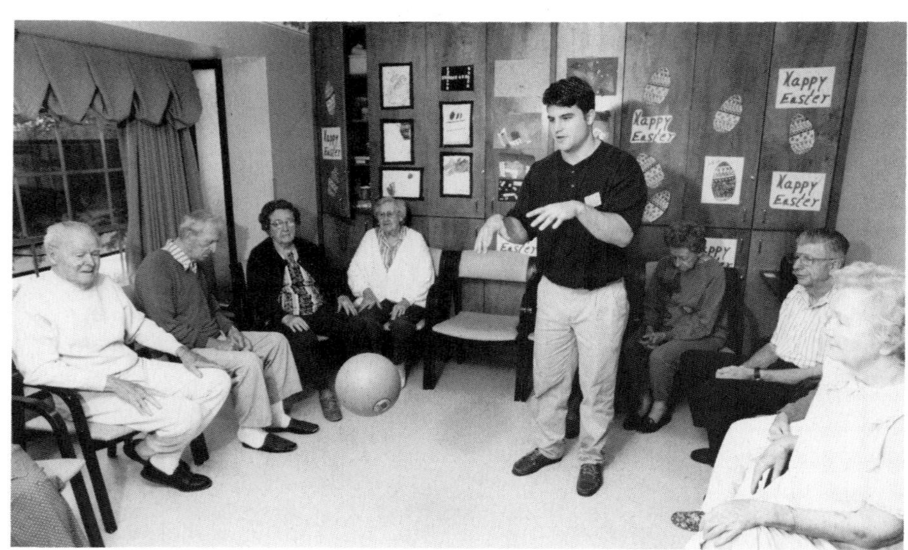

FIGURE 1-2
Daycare centers provide support for older adults in the community. (Photograph by Stephen Matteson, Jr.)

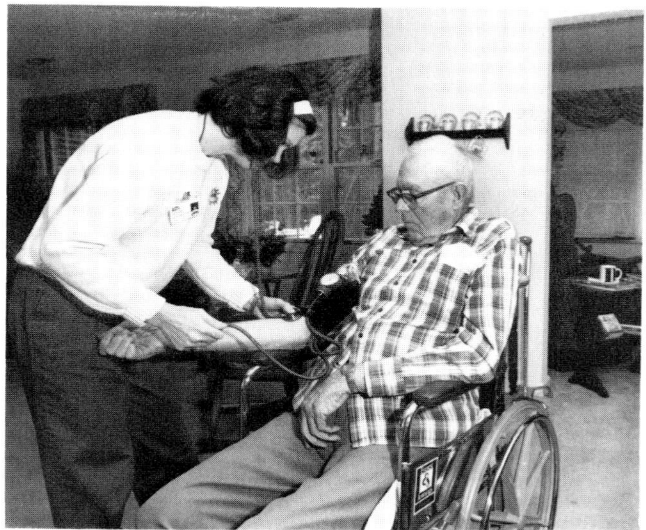

FIGURE 1-3
A nurse takes the blood pressure of a patient during a home visit. (Photograph by Stephen Matteson, Jr.)

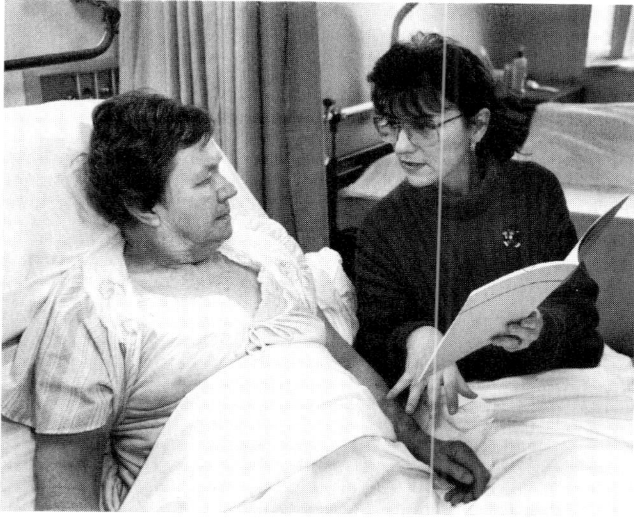

FIGURE 1-4
A large number of hospital patients are older adults. (From Matteson, M. A., & McConnell, E. S. [1988]. *Gerontological nursing* [p. 92]. Philadelphia: W. B. Saunders. Photograph by Stephen Matteson, Jr.)

as other symptoms associated with the illness. In addition they assist families during the bereavement process. Some hospices are associated with hospitals, whereas others are associated with home health agencies. Most are independent organizations in the community.

Patients who are cared for by hospices must be aware that they are terminally ill and have a life expectancy of less than 6 months. Most hospices require that a family member or close friend be involved in the care. Many of their services are funded by Medicare.

INPATIENT CARE

Hospitals

The size, shape, and organization of hospitals vary greatly throughout the United States. Some are small, 20-bed rural hospitals; others are large urban university medical centers. Some hospitals are public and financed by the local, state, or federal government; others are private and owned by churches, businesses, corporations, or charitable organizations. Many of the people who cannot pay for care go to public hospitals; those who go to private hospitals generally have insurance to cover expenses.

The number of older adults admitted to the hospital has increased steadily. Hospitals are major providers of health and related services to the elderly. Of all people older than 65 in the United States, one in five is admitted to the hospital each year. In addition, older people tend to have longer hospital stays than younger people (Fig. 1–4).

The predominant sources of payment for hospital services to the elderly are Medicare and private insurance. Medicare enacted a prospective payment system in 1983 called the diagnosis-related group (DRG) system. This system classifies patients according to their medical diagnosis. Under the DRG system, hospitals receive a fixed payment based on the patient's diagnosis and the DRG category placement.

The DRG system has had a great impact on hospital care and length of stay for older patients. Because hospitals only receive a fixed amount of money from Medicare, physicians are now discharging patients as early as possible to reduce costs. This means that admissions to nursing homes and home health agencies are increasing to care for older people who are not leaving the hospital as fully recovered as those who have had longer hospital stays. Therefore, the demand for "high-tech" services such as respirators and intravenous therapy at home and in nursing homes is increasing. In addition, many health care providers feel that there is now a "revolving door syndrome" with older clients; that is, older people frequently are coming back to the hospital for care after discharge because they were never fully able to recover at home.

Psychiatric Hospitals

Psychiatric patients may be treated in specialty areas of regular acute care hospitals, or separate hospitals may be designated specifically for mentally ill patients. These facilities provide inpatient and outpatient treatment for acute psychiatric illnesses with a focus on helping clients to control their behavior or to restore their behavior to what it was before entering the hospital.

Psychiatric hospitals may be private, nonprofit organizations that are sponsored by organized churches or ones that are operated by the local, state, or federal government. The cost of care is covered by most private insurance companies but only for 30 to 60 days.

Rehabilitation Centers

The aim of rehabilitation is either to restore individuals to their former level of functioning or to maintain or maximize remaining function (Fig. 1–5). Rehabilitation can and should be carried out in all health care settings by a variety of health care professionals with the active involvement of the patients and their families. Most formal rehabilitation centers are located either within the hospital or nursing home or in a free-standing residential institution.

Rehabilitation may focus on physical problems, such as those caused by stroke, spinal cord injury, or amputation, or on mental health problems, such as drug dependency or mental illness. To restore affected persons to their highest level of functioning, the rehabilitation process attempts to meet psychological, social, and physical needs. Therefore, the rehabilitation team is made up of many health professionals, including physicians, nurses, social workers, physical and occupational therapists, and speech therapists. It is very difficult to conduct a rehabilitation program without a team effort.

Extended Care Facilities

The term *extended care facility* was originally used to describe institutions that were attached to hospitals for the purpose of recovery from acute illness. The term is now used to describe several different kinds of institutions, such as nursing homes, convalescent homes, and some residential institutions whose primary purpose is to care for people with chronic illnesses and physical impairments. The focus of care is on those who do not require hospitalization but are unable to care for themselves.

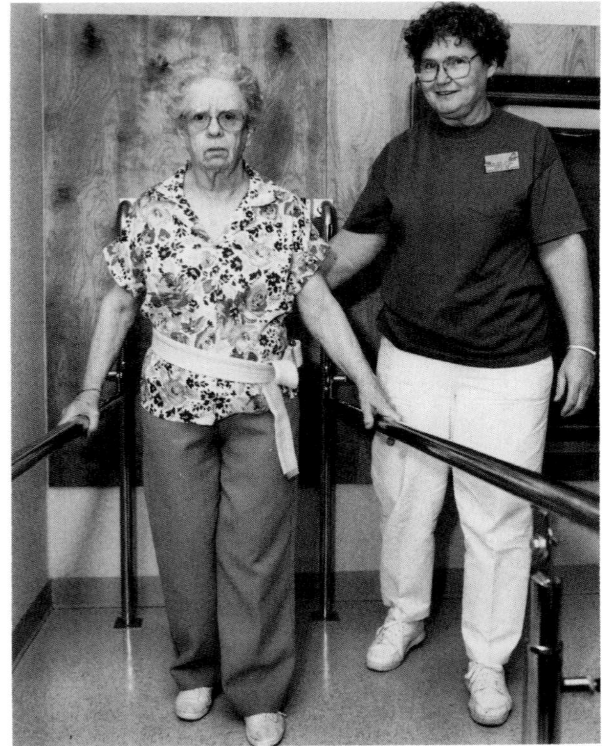

FIGURE 1-5
A patient is assisted with ambulation in a rehabilitation center. (Photograph by Stephen Matteson, Jr.)

Of the extended care facilities, nursing homes provide the highest level of care. There are two types of nursing homes: (1) skilled nursing facilities and (2) intermediate care facilities. Nineteen percent of nursing homes are certified by Medicare for skilled care, and 31% are certified by Medicaid for intermediate care. Approximately 24% of the homes are certified for both skilled and intermediate care, and 25% are not certified for either. Homes that are not certified by Medicare or Medicaid do not have to comply with the standards and regulations set by these programs.

The skilled nursing facility is designed to provide rehabilitative care for people who have the potential to regain function. Services include medical and nursing care; rehabilitation; pharmaceutical, dietary, and social services; dental care; and activities. To be admitted to a skilled nursing facility, residents must be in need of nursing care that consists of observation during an acute or unstable phase of an illness, administration of enteral (tube) feedings or intravenous fluids, bowel and bladder retraining (for a limited period of time), administration of intramuscular or intravenous medications, or changing of sterile dressings. Persons who do not fit into any of these categories are deemed to be in need of custodial care and thus are ineligible for skilled nursing care benefits under Medicare.

Intermediate care facilities are health-related nursing homes that provide custodial care for people who are unable to care for themselves because of mental or physical infirmity. The federal government does not consider intermediate care facilities to be medical facilities, so they are not given Medicare reimbursement. However, they do receive the bulk of their financing from Medicaid.

BIBLIOGRAPHY

Bocchino, C. (1991). Condition critical: The health care crisis and the American family. *Pediatric Nursing, 17,* 320.

Halamandaris, V. J. (1992). Uninsured and chronically ill Americans: The need for US health reform. *Caring, 11,* 4–7.

Kelly, L. S. (1991). Another look at the future of health care. *Nursing Outlook, 39,* 150–151.

Mallison, M. B. (1992). "Wait" is a four-letter word . . . access to health care is too crucial to have to wait for. *American Journal of Nursing, 92,* 7.

Merker, L. (1991). Meet the challenge: Health care in the 1990s. *Journal of Practical Nursing, 41,* 32–33.

Pender, N. J. (1992). Reforming health care: Future directions . . . from the AAN president. *Nursing Outlook, 40,* 8–9.

Ryan, S. A. (1990). A new decade of leadership: From vision to reality. *Nursing Clinics of North America, 25,* 597–604.

Strauss, A. (1990). A trajectory model for reorganizing the health care system. *NLN Publications, 41-2281,* 221–231.

Walker, D. (1991). Health care access: The social challenge of the 90's. *New Mexico Nursing, 36,* 1, 16.

Wright, J. E. (1991). Comprehensive health care: The Pepper Commission report to Congress. *Clinical Nurse Specialist, 5,* 63–64.

KEY CONCEPTS

1. The health care system is made up of individuals who provide health care services in a variety of settings.
2. An important problem in the health care system of the United States is that many people are unable to pay for and receive the services they need.
3. The emphasis of the health care system in the United States is on crisis and illness rather than on health promotion and disease prevention.
4. The Department of Health and Human Services is charged with organizing the various health and welfare agencies in the federal government.
5. The purpose of the Public Health Service is to provide better health services by reviewing health care, providing grants and conducting research, raising public awareness of health problems, operating hospitals for national health problems, providing health science training grants, and publishing vital statistics.
6. Most health care agencies are funded through government funds or private insurance.
7. Medicare is a federal health insurance program for people aged 65 and older and for disabled people that is geared toward acute, short-term care.
8. Medicaid provides health care benefits for needy, low-income, and disabled people and their children.
9. The health care system includes outpatient and inpatient services.
10. Outpatient services are provided in physicians' offices, clinics, health maintenance organizations, day surgery facilities, and daycare centers.
11. Inpatient services are provided in acute care hospitals, psychiatric hospitals, rehabilitation centers, and extended care facilities.
12. Extended care facilities, or nursing homes, include skilled nursing facilities designed to provide rehabilitative care, and intermediate care facilities that provide custodial care for people who are unable to care for themselves.

CHAPTER 2

Mary Ann Matteson

The Leadership Role of the Nurse

OBJECTIVES

1. Differentiate leadership from management.
2. Describe leadership styles and management theories.
3. Discuss the leadership process.
4. Describe the role of the licensed vocational nurse as a team leader.
5. Discuss leadership issues in relation to safe health care.

GLOSSARY

AUTOCRATIC LEADERSHIP Authoritarian, directive, or bureaucratic type of leadership

DEMOCRATIC LEADERSHIP Achievement of goals through participation by all group members

LAISSEZ-FAIRE LEADERSHIP Nondirective type of leadership

LEADERSHIP Guidance or showing the way to others; "inspiration"

MANAGEMENT Effective use of selected methods to achieve the goals; "perspiration"

PATIENT'S BILL OF RIGHTS Document issued by the American Hospital Association in 1973 that addresses the quality of care for patients

THEORY X Management by autocratic rule with little participation in decision making by workers

THEORY Y Democratic style of management with some participation in decision making by workers

THEORY Z Management with full participation in decision making by workers

With the rise in the older population and increase in the use of nursing home care, the demand for licensed practical/vocational nurses (LPN/LVNs) has increased. Most nursing homes are staffed primarily with LPN/LVNs and nursing assistants, who provide the majority of the "hands on" care. LPN/LVNs often find themselves in leadership or management positions in nursing homes, usually as team leaders. Therefore it is important to have a working knowledge of issues related to leadership, management, and safe health care delivery.

LEADERSHIP VERSUS MANAGEMENT

The terms *leadership* and *management* are sometimes used interchangeably, but, in fact, they have different meanings. Leadership is a difficult concept to define, but it generally means "guidance" or showing the way to others. Leaders inspire people to strive to accomplish particular goals. Management is the effective use of selected methods to accomplish goals. Management provides the means to achieve the goals. In other words, leadership may be thought of as the "inspiration," and management may be thought of as the "perspiration."

Both leaders and managers must have certain characteristics to be effective. First, they must be competent. They must have the respect of the people who work with them to accomplish their goals. Second, they must be able to communicate with others. People in leadership and management positions work with other people. Success or failure in interactions with others depends on their ability to communicate. Finally, leaders and managers must be able to motivate others. They must determine what motivates people, what other people consider important, and why they behave in certain ways. For example, some people are motivated by internal forces, such as needs or desires, and some are motivated by external forces, such as environmental or cultural influences.

Good leaders and managers seem to have certain characteristics in common, such as the ability to set realistic goals, to try out new ideas, and to be positive thinkers. Table 2–1 lists the characteristics of good leaders and managers.

TABLE 2-1
CHARACTERISTICS OF LEADERS

A LEADER

- is able to set realistic goals and work to achieve them
- seeks new ideas and methods; is willing to try them
- is a positive thinker
- is willing to make decisions even though they involve risks
- is competent in performing work
- is an effective communicator
- is assertive; refuses to be manipulated
- accepts responsibilities of leadership and delegation
- is emotionally mature; exercises self-control
- is committed to providing quality patient care
- recognizes worth of co-workers and welcomes suggestions; answers their questions
- is not selfish; is willing to share information with co-workers
- is able to use self-criticism; gives constructive criticism to others
- has a sense of humor; is able to laugh at self, never at others
- is loyal to co-workers
- is self-confident
- is never self-satisfied; recognizes the need for continued improvement
- is a facilitator

Adapted from Corona, D. F. (1982). Followership: The indispensable corollary to leadership. In E. C. Hein & M. J. Nicholson (Eds.), *Contemporary leadership behavior: Selected readings.* Boston: Little, Brown & Co.

LEADERSHIP STYLES

Many different leadership styles are used in various situations. The three basic types of leadership are (1) autocratic, (2) democratic, and (3) laissez-faire. They vary according to degrees of freedom and control, identity of the decision-makers, leader activity level, assumption of responsibility, output of the group, and efficiency (Table 2–2).

AUTOCRATIC LEADERSHIP

The autocratic type of leadership is also known as authoritarian, directive, or bureaucratic. Individuals who display this type of leadership achieve their goals by setting objectives and having them carried out without input or suggestions from others on how to do it. They believe that they have complete authority that should

TABLE 2-2
COMPARISON OF AUTHORITARIAN, DEMOCRATIC, AND LAISSEZ-FAIRE LEADERSHIP STYLES

	AUTHORITARIAN	DEMOCRATIC	LAISSEZ-FAIRE
Degree of freedom	Little freedom	Moderate freedom	Much freedom
Degree of control	High control	Moderate control	No control
Decision making	By the leader	Leader and group together	By the group or by no one
Leader activity level	High	High	Minimal
Assumption of responsibility	Primarily the leader	Shared	Abdicated
Output of the group	High quantity, good quality	Creative, high quality	Variable, may be poor quality
Efficiency	Very efficient	Less efficient than authoritarian	Inefficient

From Tappen, R. M. (1989). *Nursing leadership and management: Concepts and practice* (2nd ed.). Philadelphia: F. A. Davis.

not be questioned. Autocratic leaders do not encourage individual initiative or cooperation among members of the organization.

Autocratic leadership does not work well in many situations, but in some situations this type of leadership is necessary. One example is during an emergency when one person must take charge because there is no time for group conferences on the best plan of action. Autocratic leadership may also be justified when the leader obviously knows more or has more experience than anyone in the group. In this situation group members often need or want someone to tell them what to do and how to do it.

DEMOCRATIC LEADERSHIP

Democratic leaders achieve their goals through the participation of group members. People are encouraged to provide input into the problem-solving process, and decisions are often made through group consensus. Everyone in the group is informed of the goals and direction of the organization, so that input has a direct relationship to attaining the goals.

The primary role of the leader is to keep the group headed in the right direction. Democratic leaders lead by suggestion rather than by domination. They persuade and teach rather than rule. Most people who work with a democratic leader have a feeling of satisfaction because they have a part in managing their work situation.

LAISSEZ-FAIRE LEADERSHIP

The opposite of the autocratic leadership model is laissez-faire leadership. A laissez-faire leader provides little or no leadership. Individuals working in this situation are allowed to do anything they want with no direction from administration. The result is that people usually do not know or care about what they are supposed to do, and they lose all sense of initiative and desire for achievement. The organization then gradually disintegrates into a muddle of confusion.

CLASSICAL MANAGEMENT THEORIES

Management theories have emerged since the turn of the century to help explain what motivates people to work. Awareness of management theories helps nurses to determine the best management style for their work setting. The classical management theories are labeled X, Y, and Z.

THEORY X

In 1957, Douglas McGregor developed two theories to explain the nature of people and their relationship to the work environment, which he labeled theory X and theory Y. Theory X suggests that people in the work place

- find no pleasure in their work
- are naturally lazy and prefer to do nothing
- work mainly for the money
- work only because they fear being fired
- are basically childlike and like being told what to do
- do not want to think for themselves
- are not capable of making decisions for themselves

Because people have these general characteristics, they want to be directed and controlled. Leaders who adhere to the X theory of management usually have an autocratic style.

THEORY Y

According to theory Y, people are dynamic, flexible, and adaptive. It is assumed by believers in this theory that people

- are active and enjoy setting their own goals
- work for rewards other than money, such as doing the job well and working with others in the process
- are productive because of their own personal goals rather than because of goals set for them
- are mature and responsible
- are self-directed
- care about what they are doing
- are constantly striving to grow

People with these characteristics are thought to like their work when they know what is expected of them and when their work gives them satisfaction. Leaders who adhere to the Y theory of management usually have a democratic style.

THEORY Z

Theory Z originated in Japan and describes an organizational philosophy and structure. It grew out of the times when most employees were related to one another and worked together for the good of the company rather than for individual gains. The focus is on participative management based on mutual trust and loyalty.

This form of management involves all workers in every phase of the operation of the company, including planning, organizing, decision making, and problem solving (Figure 2–1). All members of the group have similar abilities and status, so they may be rotated to perform different duties. They have complete knowledge and understanding of their organizational objectives and methods of achieving them. It is thought that the Theory Z form of management results in greater efficiency and satisfaction among members of the work force. Leaders with a democratic management style often are able to fit into this type of management.

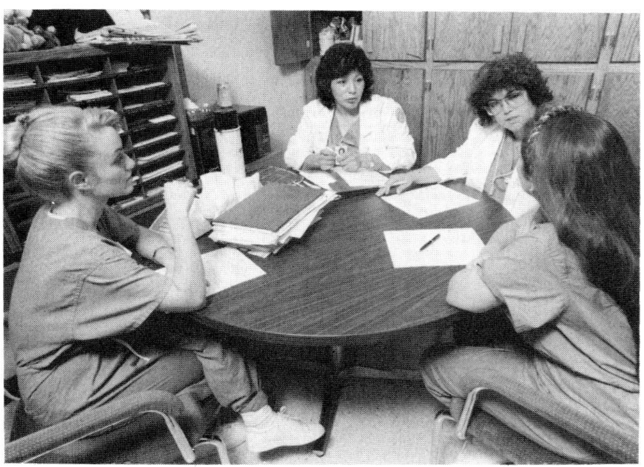

FIGURE 2-1
In the theory Z form of management, workers are involved in every phase of the operation of the organization. (Photograph by Stephen Matteson, Jr.)

FUNCTIONS IN THE MANAGEMENT PROCESS

The major functions of management are planning, organizing, directing, coordinating, and controlling.

PLANNING

Planning is the first step in the management process. Planning is deciding in advance what needs to be done and how to do it. To provide effective care for patients, a good plan for carrying out their care must be developed. Effective planning is as important for individual patient care as it is for a group of patients.

Two important components of planning are *decision making* and *problem solving*. Decision making is the process of selecting one course of action from alternatives. Problem solving is a part of the decision-making process.

The first step in the decision-making process is identifying a problem. Sometimes the problem is quite obvious, but at other times the existence of underlying issues make the real problem not so obvious. The nurse should go on a "fact-finding mission" to explore all aspects of the situation to identify the real problem. Answers to such questions as who, how, when, and why should be sought.

Once the real problem has been identified, all possible solutions should be explored. This is a creative process that can involve other people in the health care setting. Often brainstorming sessions are held to obtain input from a variety of sources.

The next step in the decision-making process involves choosing the most desirable action for solving the problem. In selecting the best solution, it is important to consider whether the action accomplishes the objectives of the organization. In addition, it is desirable to determine whether the action increases the effectiveness and efficiency of the organization and whether it is realistic to try to implement it.

After the decision has been made, it can be implemented. The decision should be communicated to other people who are involved in the organization to gain their support for carrying out the action. The communication should be expressed in such a way that other individuals become supportive of the decision rather than antagonistic toward it. Antagonism and negative feelings can be avoided in many cases when others are involved in the decision-making–problem-solving process from the beginning.

Evaluation of the results of the action is the final step in the decision-making process. There are many ways to carry out an evaluation. Written tools such as audits or checklists may be used, as well as verbal or written feedback from individuals in the organization or from patients who are receiving the care. If the solution to the problem is not satisfactory, another alternative can be selected and tried, followed by another evaluation. Table 2–3 lists the steps in the decision-making process.

ORGANIZING

Organizing is the second step in the management process. When the planning has been completed, there must be a formal structure or organization to ensure that individuals can carry out actions in the most efficient and effective manner possible. Organization also helps to develop order, promote cooperation among workers, and foster productivity.

Part of the process of organizing is developing objectives. Objectives help to guide the process of planning and organizing. Another part is establishing policies and procedures to provide guidelines for carrying out the objectives. The most qualified people should be assigned to carry out the specific activities and tasks that will best achieve the objectives. In nursing, the process of delegating responsibility for carrying out activities may involve the development of job descriptions, performance standards, and staffing patterns to provide the best patient care possible.

DIRECTING

Directing follows planning and organizing. Directing involves making assignments and directing people to

TABLE 2-3
STEPS IN THE DECISION-MAKING PROCESS

PROCESS	HOW TO ACCOMPLISH
Identify a problem	Go on fact-finding mission: Who, how, when, why
Explore possible solutions	Involve others: brainstorming
Choose most desirable action	Determine whether action is realistic and can accomplish objectives of the organization
Implement action	Communicate decision to others
Evaluate results	Use audits, verbal feedback

carry out the assignments. It also involves explaining what is to be done, how it is to be done, and why it is to be done.

In nursing, making assignments is related to patient care. Assignments should be made carefully, and an attempt should be made to match the skills of the personnel with patient needs. It is important to estimate the time needed to complete the care and the difficulty of the task. Help or additional instruction should be provided whenever necessary.

Only one person should be responsible for making assignments, especially with team nursing. Assignments should be specific and easily understood. They also should be posted where everyone can see them. Staff members should be helped to understand their assignments and the importance of each task.

Directing people to carry out their assignments requires good communication skills and assertive behavior. To give directions effectively, it is imperative that they be complete and understandable. It is also helpful to give directions in a clear, logical order and to limit the number given at any one time. Having written directions increases understanding and compliance.

The manner in which directions are given is also important. Usually directions are given in the form of a request, such as, "Will you help Mrs. Smith with her bath today?" Requesting that an individual carry out a task encourages cooperation and tends to ensure that more is accomplished. It implies that the individuals who are giving directions are "working with" people rather that having people "work for" them.

COORDINATING

Coordinating helps to pull together various activities to achieve a goal. It ensures that all important activities are being carried out and helps to identify overlap, duplication, and omissions. In nursing, coordinating involves personnel and services. The nurse wants to be sure that proper nursing care is given by the appropriate people.

The coordination process may be carried out in a specific nursing unit or among units and departments in a hospital, nursing home, or community agency. For example, the nurse may want to be sure that medications are being given by designated team members on a unit or that medications are being given in the same way throughout the nursing home.

Coordinating involves skill and experience in problem solving and decision making. It also requires good communication skills and an ability to help resolve conflicts within an organization. To be a good coordinator, a nurse should be able to assess what all individuals and groups in the organization are doing and recognize that it is important for all parts of the organization to function effectively for the good of the whole.

CONTROLLING

Controlling is the last step in the management process, and it is basically a form of evaluation. It is an ongoing process in which the activities of the organization are analyzed to make sure that the objectives are being carried out. Both the efficiency and the effectiveness of the organization are evaluated in the controlling process. The purposes of control in nursing service are to determine whether there are enough staff and supplies, whether the operation is economical, and whether the desired performance has been achieved.

Control has three basic steps:

1. Establishing standards and objectives
2. Measuring performance and comparing the results with the standards
3. Making corrections or adjustments to remedy the deficiencies in the caregiving operations

Continuous quality improvement (CQI) or *total quality management* (TQM) are terms that are frequently used in relation to control. The purpose of CQI is to ensure good nursing practice and quality care. The American Nurses' Association, the American Hospital Association, and the Joint Commission on Accreditation of Hospital Organizations are organizations that set standards for nursing practice and medical care. Most agencies also have CQI committees that set standards for care. Agencies are then evaluated to ensure that objectives and standards are being met and to make recommendations for necessary change.

THE LICENSED VOCATIONAL NURSE OR LICENSED PRACTICAL NURSE AS A LEADER

TEAM NURSING

Team nursing was introduced during the 1950s when there was a shortage of professional nurses and an abundance of auxiliary nursing staff. The purpose of the team concept is to use the skills and knowledge of the professional nurse to direct the care provided by a diverse staff through group action. All members of the team are expected to have input into the nursing care process by contributing suggestions and sharing ideas.

THE ROLE OF THE LICENSED PRACTICAL NURSE OR LICENSED VOCATIONAL NURSE AS A TEAM LEADER

The functions of the team leader are to plan, set priorities, supervise, and evaluate patient care. The role of the team leader traditionally is carried out by a registered nurse (RN) because it is thought that only registered nurses are prepared to plan nursing interventions, give supervision, make independent decisions, and evaluate nursing care or the work of team members. However, in many cases, an LPN or an LVN is assigned to the position of team leader, especially in nursing home settings. In these cases, the job description must be specific in differentiating between the practice of an RN team leader and an LPN or LVN team leader.

Team leaders are responsible for conducting an ongoing assessment of each patient and determining appropriate nursing interventions. They must be sure that medical orders and plans are carried out and documented. They are also responsible for keeping care plans up to date and documenting the nursing care provided. In addition, team leaders are responsible for planning and conducting team conferences. An LPN or LVN who assumes the position of team leader can help to carry out these responsibilities under the supervision and guidance of an RN.

ISSUES RELATED TO TEAM LEADERSHIP

Specific issues such as patients' rights, accident prevention and safety, and accountability concern the team leader.

PATIENTS' RIGHTS. Patients are the recipients of nursing care, and they are entitled to receive quality care provided in a safe, supportive, and nurturing environment. In 1973, the American Hospital Association issued a Patient's Bill of Rights (Table 2–4) that incorporates the components of quality care. No catalog of rights can guarantee for patients the kind of treatment they have a right to expect; however, hospitals, community agencies, and nursing homes, along with health care personnel, must provide the kind of care that demonstrates an overriding concern for patients and, above all, a recognition of their dignity as human beings.

ACCIDENT PREVENTION AND SAFETY. Every health care facility must meet minimal safety regulations established by law, in addition to those adopted by the agency to meet its unique needs. All staff members, particularly the team leader, should learn these regulations during orientation to the job. The team leader should know the regulations and be sure that staff members are aware of them. Everyone must understand procedures to follow in the case of disasters, such as fires, tornados, or hurricanes. In addition, everyday safety issues related to handling equipment, using proper procedures, and working with dangerous drugs must constantly be addressed to be sure that knowledge and skills are up to date.

TABLE 2-4
A PATIENT'S BILL OF RIGHTS

1. Considerate and respectful care.
2. Complete and current information concerning a patient's condition and care.
3. Necessary information in order to give an informed consent and the freedom to refuse treatment.
4. Right to an "advance directive" (e.g., a living will) concerning treatment and the naming of a surrogate decision maker.
5. Protection of privacy.
6. Protection of confidentiality.
7. Review of a patient's own medical records.
8. Response to reasonable requests for service.
9. Attainment of information regarding the hospital's relationship with other health and educational institutions.
10. Knowledge of any experimentation regarding a patient's care.
11. Reasonable continuity of care.
12. Explanation of the hospital bill and knowledge of hospital rules and regulations that will affect a patient's care.

Adapted from American Hospital Association. (1992). *A patient's bill of rights.* Reprinted with permission of the American Hospital Association, copyright 1992.

ACCOUNTABILITY. Team leaders must demonstrate accountability for their own actions, as well as that of the staff that they are directing. They are legally responsible for all nursing care and documentation. The team leader must ensure that proper and accurate charting is carried out for all nursing assessment, actions, and evaluation. Physicians' orders must be noted and followed precisely. Depending on the policy of the health care agency, nurses may take verbal orders from physicians. In the case of both written and verbal orders, the LVN or LPN should verify orders with an RN or the physician who wrote the orders.

Accountability also involves communicating patient needs to others through both verbal and written interactions. A common form of communication is the report given at the end (or beginning) of every shift. The LVN or LPN is usually responsible for reporting off to the RN in charge but may be only indirectly responsible for the report. Guidelines for clear and complete reporting are as follows:

1. Organize the report before beginning.
2. Give the patient's room number, name, age (if appropriate), diagnosis, and physician.
3. Provide a brief account of each patient's condition, including new or changed orders.
4. Refer to vital signs, temperature elevations, intravenous fluids, and intake and output as relevant.
5. Indicate the name of the patient's pain medication, the dosage and the number of times pain medications should be given, and the last time such medications were given.
6. Cover the necessary information concerning preoperative patients, including the chart in order, the preoperative teaching done, the time of preoperative medications, and the like.
7. Give information about postoperative patients, including time of arrival from operating or recovery room; general condition; vital signs; intravenous fluids required (e.g., kind, rate of flow, fluids to follow); dressings; voiding; diet; nature of breathing; coughing; and number, position, and patency of tubes.

The report may be given by means of a tape recording, a one-to-one discussion with another nurse, a summary in a group conference, or during walking rounds at the bedside. The key to good communication is to be clear, concise, and thorough.

CHARACTERISTICS OF A GOOD TEAM LEADER

Good team leaders must have skills in leadership, management, and supervisory techniques. They should be able to communicate effectively, both verbally and in writing. Good team leaders are able to work well with others and show that they value their input and suggestions regarding patient care. Figure 2–2 illustrates components of effective team leadership. The leader's pos-

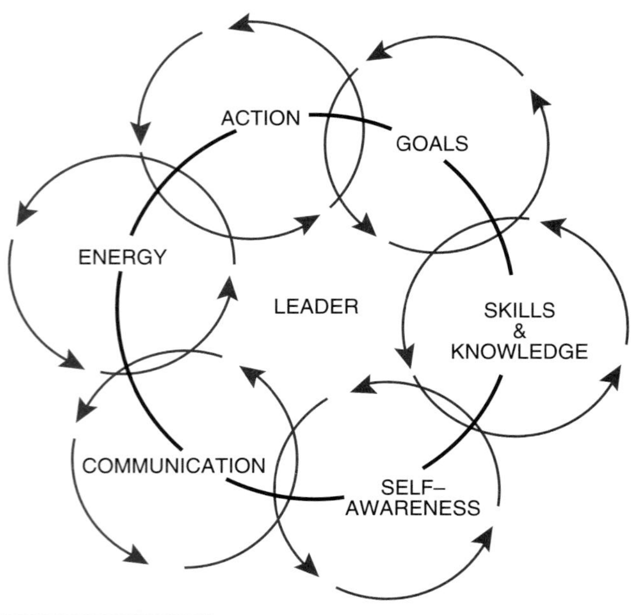

FIGURE 2-2

Components of effective team leadership. (From Tappen, R. M. [1989]. *Nursing leadership and management: Concepts and practice* [2nd ed., p. 58]. Philadelphia: F. A. Davis.)

session of these qualities leads to greater satisfaction among the staff and a higher quality of patient care.

BIBLIOGRAPHY

Bell, M. (1989). The expanding and contracting role of the LPN. *Florida Nurse, 37,* 7.

Brown, C. E. (1989). The law and your profession. *Journal of Practical Nursing, 39,* 14–15.

Corona, D. F. (1982). Followership: The indispensable corollary to leadership. In E. C. Hein & M. J. Nicholson (Eds.), *Contemporary leadership behavior: Selected readings.* Boston: Little, Brown & Co.

De Paola, B. (1992). Leadership skills—A growing need for LP/LVNs. *Journal of Practical Nursing, 42,* 37–38.

Merker, L. (1991). Meet the challenge: Health care in the 1990s. *Journal of Practical Nursing, 41,* 32–33.

Mitchell, M. E. (1989). Long-term care and licensed practical nursing—Working together to provide quality, cost-effective geriatric care. *Journal of Practical Nursing, 39,* 36–38.

Sullivan, E. J., & Decker, P. J. (1988). *Effective management in nursing* (2nd ed.). Menlo Park, CA: Addison-Wesley Publishing Co.

Tappen, R. M. (1989). *Nursing leadership and management: Concepts and practice* (2nd ed.). Philadelphia: F. A. Davis Co.

KEY CONCEPTS

1. Licensed practical and vocational nurses comprise the primary staffing and management of most nursing homes.
2. Leadership is defined as guidance, or showing the way to others.
3. Management is defined as the effective use of selected methods to accomplish goals.
4. Leaders and managers must be competent, must have the respect of the people they work with, and must be able to motivate others.
5. The three basic types of leadership are autocratic, democratic, and laissez-faire.
6. Autocratic leaders are authoritarian, meaning they act without input or suggestions from others.
7. Democratic leaders achieve their goals through participating, encouraging others to provide input, and making decisions through group consensus.
8. Laissez-faire leaders allow group members to do anything they want with no direction from administration.
9. Leadership styles are based on leaders' assumptions about workers' motivation.
10. The major functions of management are planning, organizing, coordinating, directing, and controlling.
11. Planning, the first step in the management process, involves decision making and problem solving.
12. Organizing provides a structure for carrying out the plan.
13. Directing involves making assignments and directing people to carry out the assignments.
14. Coordinating helps pull various activities together to achieve a goal.
15. Controlling includes establishing standards, measuring performance by the standards, and making corrections to remedy deficiencies.
16. Team nursing was designed to use the skills and knowledge of the professional nurse to direct the care provided by a diverse staff through group action.
17. Team leaders conduct ongoing assessments of patients and determine appropriate nursing interventions.
18. A good team leader has skill in leadership, management, and supervisory techniques.

Irma G. Aguilar
J. Gail Barry

CHAPTER 3

The Nurse-Patient Relationship

OBJECTIVES

1. Define holistic view of nursing.
2. Define the concept of *self*.
3. Discuss the use of self in the practice of nursing.
4. Compare the meaning of the terms *patient* and *client*.
5. List commonly held expectations of patients and families.
6. Describe guidelines for nurse-patient relationships.

GLOSSARY

ACTION Ability to respond to others with genuineness, warmth, sensitivity, and self-disclosure to promote their well-being

CARING A process characterized by understanding and action

CLIENT Denotes a feeling of partnership or working with someone

EMPATHY The ability to identify with and understand another person's situation, feelings, and motives

HOLISM A way of viewing people as whole individuals

PATIENT A person for whom the nurse provides care; denotes a feeling of doing to or for

SELF A term to describe one's personhood

UNDERSTANDING Ability to listen to others in order to perceive their feelings and the meaning of their words

Nursing means caring for persons. *Caring* is a process characterized by understanding and action. *Understanding* is the ability to listen to others in order to perceive their feelings and the meaning of their words. *Action* is the ability to respond to others with genuineness, warmth, sensitivity, and self-disclosure to promote their well-being.

In the caring process, a therapeutic relationship should develop between patients or clients and nurses. To develop a therapeutic relationship, nurses must value and accept patients and clients as unique individuals. In addition, nurses must be aware of themselves as individuals. Knowing how one's own attitudes, feelings, and beliefs affect the attitudes, feelings, and beliefs of others is vital to effective communication. An attitude of caring is essential to the practice of nursing.

A HOLISTIC VIEW OF NURSING CARE

Holism is a way of viewing people as whole individuals. According to the holistic theory, people are complex creatures made up of many parts. Each part interacts with the other, and the sum of the parts forms a unified whole.

Individuals are composed of mind, body, and spirit. It is not possible to care for one part without considering how the other parts are affected. Thus, in nursing, the physiologic, psychological, sociological, and spiritual influences on individual behaviors become integrated into a plan of care (Fig. 3–1). For example, patients who have had surgery may have physical needs, but the nurse must also consider their emotional needs and their feelings about the surgery. In addition, patients may have spiritual needs as they deal with the prospect of sickness and death.

USE OF THE SELF IN NURSING

Many tools are used in the tasks of nursing, including stethoscopes, sphygmomanometers, and thermometers; however, there is no more important tool that a nurse brings to each patient encounter than the use of self. *Self* is a term used to describe one's personhood: the knowledge, experience, values and beliefs, perceptions, strengths, and weaknesses that make each individual unique. The attitudes, beliefs, self-esteem, and feelings of the nurse become a part of the person's therapeutic environment, just as those of the person become a part of the nurse's environment. With the assistance of the nurse, individuals and their families may find meaning in their experience and may achieve a harmonious state of health.

VALUES, BELIEFS, AND ATTITUDES

Self-awareness involves knowing one's own values, beliefs, and attitudes. Nurses should be able to answer the questions Who am I? What do I believe? What is important to me? so that they can help others answer those questions. Almost every day, nurses encounter situations that require value judgments. They are required

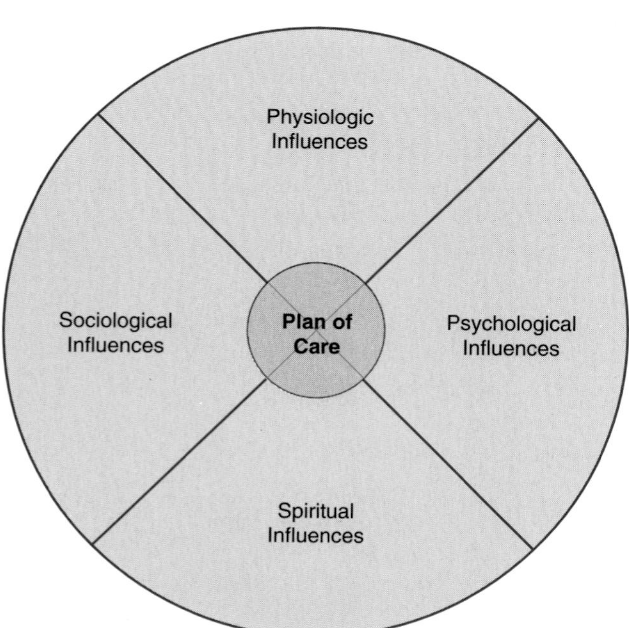

FIGURE 3-1
Physiologic, psychological, sociological, and spiritual influences on individual behaviors become integrated into a plan of care.

to make certain choices related to patient care, to respond to requests for help and guidance, and to provide emotional and spiritual support. The nurses' values, attitudes, and beliefs are outwardly expressed in their behavior as they interact with patients.

Values can be defined as principles or standards shared by members of a society that determine what is desirable or worthwhile. A *belief* is a conviction or opinion. *Attitudes* are reactions that flow from values and beliefs. An attitude indicates a feeling toward persons or things. Values and personal beliefs are developed in many ways. They may be acquired from religious education, from examples set by authority figures such as parents and teachers, or from peers.

Acquiring values and beliefs is a lifelong process that is affected by one's life experience. As people age, they generally have a fairly fixed set of values, but even older people are able to grow and change.

KNOWLEDGE

Knowledge is a component of self that is acquired through experience or study. The safe practice of nursing is dependent on one's knowledge base, and nursing school provides a basic introduction to the physical and social sciences. Nurses use their knowledge of physiology, psychology, and social science disciplines to give the best care possible to their patients. This knowledge is often shared with patients, families, and the community to promote health, prevent disease, and cope with illness. Nurses also share their knowledge with colleagues on the health care team.

The health care field is continually growing and changing. There is a greater emphasis on prevention of disease and promotion and maintenance of health. Nurses should act as models of good health care practices. It is important for nurses to continue to learn and expand their knowledge to benefit others as well as themselves.

SKILLS

Nursing is a skill-oriented field. Nursing care involves the use of many skills that require efficiency and safety. A nurse must master the technical skills that are required with sophisticated equipment as well as the skills required to carry out nursing interventions. A nurse's hands can be an instrument of healing when used with compassion, competence, and gentleness. A simple act of giving a bed bath or a back rub can be the best use of self that a nurse can offer a suffering patient.

Interpersonal skills are nursing actions that the nurse has learned to be able to communicate effectively with another person. They may be verbal and nonverbal. The nurse utilizes the skill of interpersonal communication to establish a caring relationship with the patient. It is through this relationship of caring that the nurse is able to build a therapeutic relationship with the patient. Factors necessary to develop skills for building a therapeutic nurse-patient relationship are the following:

- Formation of a humanistic system of values
- Ability to instill faith and hope
- Sensitivity to one's self and to others
- Ability to develop helping, trusting relationships
- Ability to express both positive and negative feelings
- Use of problem-solving methods for decision-making
- Promotion of interpersonal teaching and learning
- Provision of a supportive, protective, and corrective mental, physical, sociocultural, and spiritual environment
- Assistance with the gratification of human needs
- Allowance for the uniqueness of individuals and their experiences

THE PERSPECTIVE OF THE PATIENT

Should every surgeon have experienced surgery to know what it is like? Should every nurse have been a patient to gain a perspective of what being a patient means? Sometimes it is difficult to truly understand patienthood from the patient's perspective.

PATIENT VERSUS CLIENT

Nurses often use the term *client* rather than *patient*. This term evolved from a general belief or attitude about the nurse-patient relationship. The word *client* denotes a feeling of partnership or working with someone. The word *patient* has a connotation of doing to or for someone. Client seems to represent a more accurate view of the roles in the nurse-patient relationship, because the nurse values patients as individuals, honors their individuality, and helps them to achieve the highest level of wellness possible. However, because patient is also used and accepted by nurses and other health care professionals, and frequently by elderly people as well, *patient* and *client* are used interchangeably in this text.

PATIENTS' EXPECTATIONS

Respect the Patient

Even though human beings have many common needs, there are characteristics that make each person unique. The challenge to the nurse is to see and identify those characteristics that differentiate one patient or client from all others.

Each client enters the health care system with varying experiences, beliefs, values, and perceptions. The nurse must resist the tendency to prejudge the client according to preconceived characteristics of persons who share the client's culture, race, religion, or ethnicity. To do so is to form a nurse-patient relationship based on stereotypes and personal biases. Nurses need to be especially sensitive to clients who are members of ethnic or cultural minority groups.

Patients expect to be treated with courtesy and respect, and they want personalized care to meet their needs. Most surveys have revealed that patients care more about their interpersonal relationship with the nurse than about the nurse's skill and expertise.

A sensitive, caring nurse is one who approaches client care in an open, accepting, nonjudgmental manner. The nurse who is able to see the client as a unique human being is more apt to establish an effective, therapeutic nurse-client relationship based on trust and mutual respect.

Part of helping patients to retain their individuality is to speak and refer to them by name at all times. It is important to pronounce the name correctly and to introduce the patient by name to other health care providers. Patients should never be referred to by bed number or medical diagnosis.

Older patients, no matter what their state of mind, deserve to be treated with the same respect as younger patients. It is inappropriate for a nurse to call an older patient anything other than *Mr.* Smith or *Mrs.* Smith unless the patient has requested it. Terms such as "Pops," "Sweetie," "Gramps," or "Baby" are unprofessional and demeaning to older individuals (Fig. 3–2).

Explain the Care

The experience of illness and all the changes in a person's life that it precipitates, is, at best, very stressful. A method that the nurse can use to help reduce clients' stress and anxiety levels is to empower them to participate in their care. To do this, clients must be given the information that they need to be an active participant. They want to know what is going to be done to them, when, how, and why.

Clients need and are entitled to an explanation of the care to be given so that they know what to expect and what is expected of them. Clients who are knowledgeable about their care are more likely to be cooperative and less likely to be hostile and critical of the nurse's efforts. Explanation and teaching are often left to the nurse. Communication should take place in language that patients understand without talking down to them. Explanation of care is not only a therapeutic method to reduce the client's stress and fears, it is also a client's right. Patients who are not given an adequate explanation of what is to be done have been denied their rights as a human being.

Treat Patients as Partners in Care

The patient as a consumer of health care services is no longer willing to assume a passive role. Most clients not only want to assume more responsibility for their care but also expect to do so.

Clients who see themselves as partners in their care are more likely to accept responsibility for their care. Their sense of responsibility may serve to prevent needless complications resulting from noncompliance and risk factors that may otherwise prolong their care.

Some clients are more willing than others to accept the role of partner. Factors that may have an impact on clients' decisions to participate in their care are age, ethnicity, personality, social class, and educational level.

The client can assume an active role from the point of admission. The initial assessment is the nurse's first opportunity to set the tone for a relationship that encourages client participation. It is the nurse's role to help clients understand that their participation is not only wanted but needed. The nurse needs to assess clients to determine to what extent they wish to participate in their care. The nurse also needs to encourage the client's family to participate in the care whenever possible.

Accept Patient Behaviors

It is important to patients that nurses and health care providers accept their behavior. Illness is a stressful

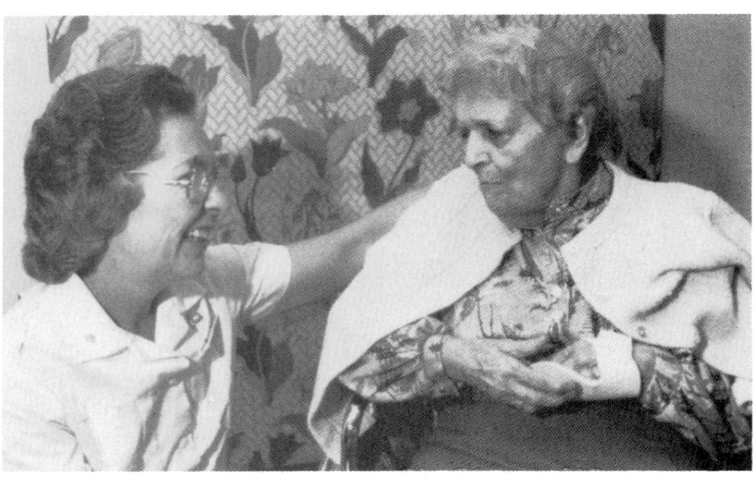

FIGURE 3-2
Older people should be treated with the same respect as younger people. (From Matteson, M. A., & McConnell, E. S. [1988]. *Gerontological nursing* [p. 809]. Philadelphia: W. B. Saunders.)

event and can cause people to react in unusual ways. In many cases, individuals behave differently than they would under normal circumstances.

For a nurse-patient relationship to be therapeutic, the nurse must be able to see the patients' experiences from their perspective. The nurse encourages them to feel free to share thoughts and feelings without fear of being judged. The nurse must be willing to accept unconditionally the client's values, beliefs, behaviors, and attitudes. This kind of a nurse-patient relationship is a special kind of caring in which the nurse has a high regard for the whole person. It conveys a sense of worth and dignity. Nurses are required to avoid imposing their own values and beliefs on the client, even if they differ from their own. Nurses should provide compassionate understanding of their patients' behavior and maintain a therapeutic, accepting environment.

Provide Safety and Security

Nurses have a high degree of responsibility for keeping their patients both physically and psychologically safe while in their care. Nurses must assess a situation quickly, make a decision, and act promptly to solve the problem. A patient needs to feel that a nurse can act quickly and decisively in a crisis to provide the best care possible.

Competence and consistency are two factors that can alleviate stress in patients. Nurses who appear confident and competent help patients to feel more secure. In addition, performing nursing procedures consistently can help reduce anxiety and build patients' confidence in the nurse. For example, changing dressings in the same step-by-step manner every time helps patients to know what to expect and to be reassured of the competence of each nurse who performs them.

The Role of the Family

Membership in a family has a tremendous influence on the individual through genetic endowment and the development of personal, social, moral, and cultural values. The family's major role is to protect and socialize its members. Among its many functions, of prime importance is that of providing emotional support and security to its members through love, acceptance, concern, and nurturing.

Families differ in their makeup and their patterns of interacting and relating. Many families today vary from the traditional pattern of mother, father, and children. More and more family units are composed of a single parent and children or parents and a combination of offspring from previous marriages. In addition, friends or partners of the same or opposite sex are now often considered family or extended family.

Families frequently provide support for patients. They may also need a great deal of support themselves during a loved one's illness. Nurses must consider the needs of family members, especially in cases of serious illness or threat of death. Families often need information and reassurance. Providing information can relieve anxiety and fear of the unknown (Fig. 3–3).

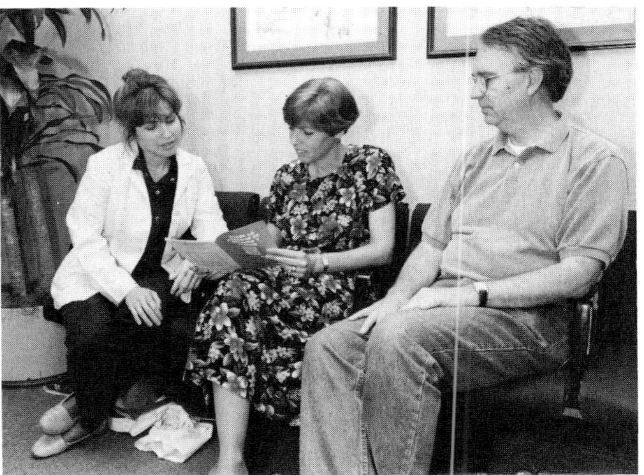

FIGURE 3-3
Family members need information and reassurance. (Photograph by Stephen Matteson, Jr.)

It is important to assess the relationships among the patient and other family members. Families can impose a number of burdens, provide considerable emotional support, or offer a mixed blessing. It should be determined whether family members are supportive or detrimental in the recovery process. Nurses must consider the family's influence on the individual as they assess, diagnose, plan, implement, and evaluate nursing care. The inclusion of family members in the client's care and the decision-making process helps maintain the self-esteem of both clients and families.

GUIDELINES FOR THE NURSE-PATIENT RELATIONSHIP

THE HELPER ROLE

A helping role occurs when one person reaches out to help another. The goal is to help another individual to grow, mature, cope, and function. A helping relationship is one in which there is genuine caring and compassion.

To assume the helper role, a nurse must have certain characteristics:

- Awareness of self and values
- Ability to analyze own feelings
- Ability to serve as a model to others
- Desire to help others
- Strong sense of ethics and high principles
- Sense of responsibility

Nurses act as helpers by administering direct care to clients, acting as advocates on behalf of clients, giving psychosocial support, and providing health education and counseling.

The role of helper obliges the nurse to maintain a therapeutic relationship. The nurse must provide an environment of trust. Trust occurs when the client experiences safety. Safety may include knowing that the nurse is honest and open, or it may mean confidence in the skill and knowledge of the nurse.

A helper in the professional sense cannot be a friend. The term *friend* connotes intimacy or affection. The nurse must transcend the role of friend to take on a caring role. In this way the nurse facilitates the health of the client. There is mutual responsibility between client and nurse—a partnership.

Just as nurses must be careful to avoid erring on the side of friendship, taking a strong authoritarian stance can likewise be damaging. Therapeutic communication is very much an art and a skill. It takes time and practice to be able to set firm limits with genuine warmth and honesty. Self disclosure refers to the ability to be open and honest about one's feelings. The nurse should not disclose personal information as one would do in a friend relationship. Table 3–1 notes comparisons between a helping person and a friend.

Touch can be used to show concern, inform a client of one's presence, or provide comfort. Giving a bedridden client a back rub before sleep can stimulate circulation, provide a caring moment, and promote relaxation. Some people are more comfortable with touching and being touched than others. Some clients may erroneously perceive touch as an invitation to intimacy. Perceptions differ from person to person. The judicious use of touch can convey warmth and caring.

COMMUNICATION

Communication skills are essential for carrying out the helper role. Communication is a process of exchanging ideas, beliefs, thoughts, and feelings between two or more people. It involves a message, a sender, and a receiver. The sender gives the message to the receiver.

TABLE 3-1
COMPARISON BETWEEN HELPING PERSON AND FRIEND

HELPING PERSON	FRIEND
Responsible to client	Relationship is for friendship or support
Objective of relationship is to meet client's needs	Individuals meet each other's needs
Relationship is goal directed	No plan involved
Attitude is nonjudgmental	Both individuals express feelings, attitudes, and opinions
Does not attempt to influence client to helper's way of thinking	Friends try to influence each other in discussing issues such as religion, politics, and personal philosophy
Does not keep secrets and explains in a direct manner the need to work with the treatment team	Friends may keep secrets
Discourages any sexual overtones in relationship	Sexual overtones or a sexual relationship may develop
Interacts with client in health care facility only	Friends meet in a variety of places
Relationship is time limited	Relationship may continue

There are two types of communication behavior: (1) verbal language, which conveys meanings through words, and (2) nonverbal language, which conveys meanings through symbols and actions other than words. Examples of nonverbal communication are body position, facial expression, gestures, moaning, crying, laughing, and smiling.

To communicate effectively, nurses must be able to recognize the meanings of both verbal and nonverbal language. Language is influenced by the cultural context in which it is used. To interpret the meaning of what is said or done without consideration of cultural context equals stereotyping.

Two essential parts of communication are *listening* and *observation*. Listening is an active process that involves trying to understand what is being said. The listener must display genuine interest and concentration to derive meaning from the words. A good listener can provide reassurance, lighten another person's burden, and clarify misunderstandings.

Observation of nonverbal language is as important to the communication process as listening is to verbal language. Nonverbal language can indicate a person's thoughts and feelings, as well as, if not better than, verbal language can. Nonverbal actions can be in conflict with the content of what is being said and thus can give clues to true feelings. For example, patients may claim that everything is all right but may be slumped over and wringing their hands. An astute nurse should recognize that something is indeed wrong even though patients deny it verbally.

Therapeutic communication is a skill that can be learned through study, observation, and practice. One must remember to be open, honest, and nonjudgmental. Self-awareness should be of primary concern. Nurses must actively seek to be cognizant of their own holistic dynamics. This implies that they have had the opportunity to self-explore and assess how the following areas may affect their ability to establish a therapeutic nurse-patient relationship:

- Ethnic, cultural, and socioeconomic background
- Attitudes, values, opinions, and beliefs
- Past unresolved experiences that are still emotionally laden
- Physical and psychological strengths and weaknesses

This self-awareness facilitates the therapeutic process. Behaviors that may help the nurse initiate a therapeutic interaction include the following:

- Focus attention on the client.
- Listen carefully.
- Ask the client to repeat information if necessary.
- Begin a mental assessment.

Questions that the nurse may ask, or use as an area of focus, to obtain a holistic assessment of the client may include the following:

1. What is the client's age?
2. What is the client's cultural background?
3. What is the client's perception of events?

4. Is the client using direct eye contact?
5. Is the client's body language open or closed?
6. What is the quality of the client's voice? Is it loud or soft?
7. Does the client use gestures?
8. Does the client's emotional tone (or affect) vary or does it remain constant (e.g., does the client appear sad, happy, or angry?)
9. Is the verbal message congruent with the client's body language, or is the client smiling while speaking of what would seem to be a sad event?

Listening is an active element of therapeutic communication. One must listen and attempt to understand what the client is saying. Understanding is the ability to listen to others to perceive their feelings and the meaning of their words. Some techniques used to facilitate communication are found in Table 3–2.

Other suggestions for therapeutic communication are the following:

- Use *I statements*. These are sentences that begin with the word *I* and indicate acceptance of responsibility for one's feelings and thoughts (e.g., "I felt angry when I heard I had cancer."). *You statements* generally are not as well accepted by the listener (e.g., "You ought to try getting more sleep.").
- Observe the client's gestures and nonverbal behavior. All behavior has meaning. Try to find the meaning in behavior.
- Use open-ended questions. Stay clear of questions that can be answered with a "yes" or a "no."
- Focus the client on pertinent issues.

Processing is the act of reviewing a therapeutic communication with a trusted teacher, supervisor, or colleague to evaluate content and themes as well as the techniques that are used. This tool enables the nurse to be critiqued and to learn new techniques. Communication is a complex process. "Helping" occurs regardless of one's experience if respect and authenticity are brought to each interaction.

EMPATHETIC RESPONSE

Effective communication requires an empathetic response from a nurse. *Empathy* is the ability to identify with and to understand another person's situation, feelings, and motives. An empathetic response requires compassion, understanding, and good therapeutic communication skills. Empathy differs from *sympathy*. When people sympathize with others, they understand another's feelings, but they also become immersed in the situation. Whatever affects one affects the other. The person who sympathizes can become as distressed as the person getting the sympathy. Empathy, in contrast, is an expression of understanding of another's thoughts and feelings without becoming overly emotionally involved or distressed.

Communicating empathy can be carried out through the simple use of verbal and nonverbal language. Nurses can communicate empathy by telling the patient what to expect, even when the patient is comatose or confused. Discussing plans for care, such as treatments or medications, and explaining laboratory studies can provide reassurance to patients who may be frightened. Nurses should also demonstrate their concern to patients and families by sharing their feelings. By sharing feelings, nurses show that they are human and can understand the difficulties of being ill or hospitalized.

Nurses can show sensitivity in nonverbal ways, such as respecting confidentiality, allowing the expression of feelings, and respecting patients' privacy. The use of touch provides an excellent means of communicating empathy. Holding a patient's hand during a period of anxiety or pain can provide effective relief and, in many cases, can be more effective than any verbal interaction. The judicious use of touch conveys the message that "I care what happens to you, and I will help you in every way that I can" (Fig. 3–4).

TABLE 3–2

TECHNIQUES FOR FACILITATING COMMUNICATION

TECHNIQUE	EXAMPLE OF USE
1. Silence	Fight the urge to fill quiet periods with conversation. It is more helpful to leave time for the client to think and respond.
2. Reflecting	Reflect back to clients what you have heard them say (e.g., "You say you're feeling better since your brother has returned?")
3. Summarizing	Review the subject matter that the client has discussed.
4. Restating	"I hear you say you're concerned about your son."
5. Clarification	"Do you mean sad when you say upset?"

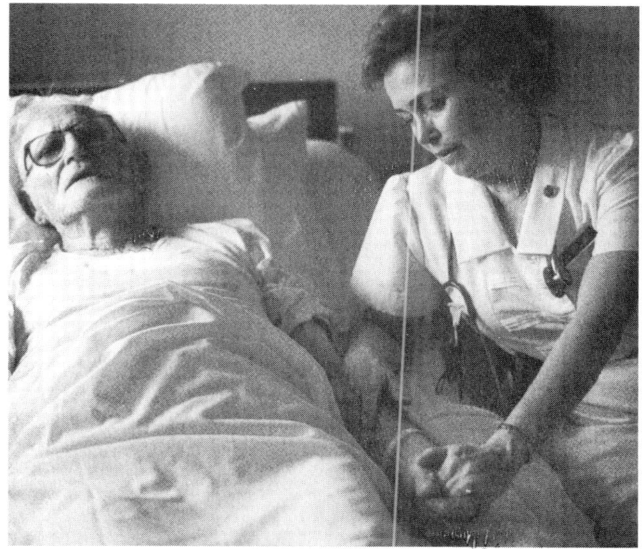

FIGURE 3–4

The judicious use of touch conveys the message that "I care what happens to you, and I will help you in every way I can." (From Matteson, M. A., & McConnell, E. S. [1988]. *Gerontological nursing*. Philadelphia: W.B. Saunders. Photograph by Stephen Matteson, Jr.)

When the nurse responds empathetically, she responds with genuineness, warmth, and sensitivity to promote well-being in the client. This is the essence of therapeutic communication.

BIBLIOGRAPHY

Allen, C. (1992). Ode to joy? . . . Nursing is an act of love. *Nursing Times, 88*(10), 24.

Alligood, M. R. (1992). Empathy: The importance of recognizing two types. *Journal of Psychosocial Nursing & Mental Health Services, 30*(3), 14–17, 33–34.

Andrews, J. (1992). Abuse of trust . . . Falling in love with your patient. *Nursing Times, 88*(43), 24.

Bishop, A. H., & Scudder, J. R., Jr. (1991). Nursing: The practice of caring. *NLN Publications*, 14–2442.

Bolstad, R. (1992). Building rapport . . . Communication skills in nursing. *New Zealand Nursing Journal, 85*(9), 17–19.

Brown, J. (1992). "Them" and "us" . . . Treat a patient as a fellow human being. *Nursing Times,* 88(6), 41.

Canis, P. (1992). Attending the spirit. *Nursing Times, 88*(32), 50.

Cochrane, D. A., Oberle, K., Nielsen, S., Sloan-Roseneck, J., Anderson, K., & Finlay, C. (1992). Do they really understand us? *American Journal of Nursing, 92*(7), 19–20.

Costa, P. (1992). Diamond in the rough . . . Sarah, a nursing assistant . . . cared for Bryan. *Nursing, 22*(7), 88.

Crowhurst, G. (1992). Gently does it . . . Working with people with challenging behavior. *Nursing Times, 88*(7), 65–66.

Davidhizar, R. (1991). The "how to's" of touch. *Advancing Clinical Care, 6*(6), 14–17.

Dubiel, D. (1992). Finding the right words. *Nursing, 22*(9), 74.

Easton, K. L. (1992). A lesson from Mr. C. . . . True rehabilitation nursing is the whole nurse treating the whole patient. *Rehabilitation Nursing, 17*(4), 199.

Fairlie, A. (1992). Nurse-patient communication barriers. *Senior Nurse, 12*(3), 40–43.

Fitzpatrick, J. J. (1992). Caring words. *Applied Nursing Research, 5*(1), 1.

Francis, B. (1992). John's best . . . Sometimes, comfort comes from those who need it most. *Nursing, 22*(5), 118.

Granger, B. (1992). Talking to Theresa. *Nursing, 22*(3), 120.

Green, D. B. (1992). Listening: An essential component of effective nursing care. *Virginia Nurse, 60*(2), 5–7.

Haybach, P. J. (1993). Suddenly seeing me. *American Journal of Nursing, 93*(1), 96.

Heath, I. (1992). Pain, hugs, PRN. *American Journal of Nursing, 92*(4), 120.

Heinrich, K. T. (1992). What to do when a patient becomes too special. *Nursing, 22*(11), 62–64.

Hodges, D. (1992). Can you hear me? *Nursing Times, 88*(27), 41.

Lister, G. (1992). Sometimes a rose is more than a rose . . . Caring skills. *RN, 55*(12), 21–22.

Manning, S. (1992). The nurses I'll never forget. *Nursing, 22*(8), 47.

McIntyre, R. C. (1992). The fifth sound . . . A call for comfort or human presence. *American Journal of Nursing, 92*(7), 84.

Sinclair, M. (1992). A special relationship. *Nursing Times, 88*(32), 49.

Smith, M., Skewes, A., & Darnell, J. D. (1992). In pursuit of nursing excellence. *American Journal of Nursing, 92*(11), 32–36.

Soper, S. (1992). Blessed reassurance. *Nursing Times, 88*(14), 49.

Strong, B. (1992). The view from the mattress: How to care more sensitively for your cancer patients. *Nursing, 22*(5), 46–49.

Sutton, S. (1992). Nurse as patient: Experiences from the other side of the bed. *New Zealand Nursing Journal, 85*(1), 12–13.

Walker, R. (1992). One from the heart . . . Human quality of being able to share feelings. *Nursing Times, 88*(1), 27.

Wilkinson, S. (1992). Confusions and challenges . . . Good communication between patient and nurse. *Nursing Times, 88*(35), 24–28.

Young-Mason, J. (1993). Mrs. Hammond speaks. *Clinical Nurse Specialist, 7*(1), 30–31.

KEY CONCEPTS

1. Caring is a process characterized by understanding and action.
2. Action is the ability to respond to others with genuineness, warmth, sensitivity, and self-disclosure to promote their well-being.
3. Holism views people as complex creatures made up of many parts that interact and form a unified whole.
4. The nurse incorporates physiologic, psychological, sociological, and spiritual influences into the plan of care.
5. Nurses must have awareness of their own values, beliefs, and attitudes and be willing to accept unconditionally the client's values, beliefs, and attitudes.
6. Nurses use their knowledge of physiology, psychology, and social sciences disciplines and their skills to give the best possible care to clients.
7. Nurses can reduce clients' stress and anxiety levels by empowering them to participate in their own care and by demonstrating competence and consistency.
8. The inclusion of family members in the client's care and the decision-making process helps maintain the self-esteem of both clients and families.
9. The role of a helper is to assist another to grow, mature, cope, and function.
10. Communication is basic to the helper role.
11. Empathy, genuineness, warmth, sensitivity, and self-disclosure are essentials of therapeutic communication.
12. Empathy is the ability to identify with and understand another person's situation, feelings, and motives.

Mary Ann Matteson

CHAPTER 4

Cultural Aspects of Nursing Care

OBJECTIVES

1. Describe cultural concepts related to nursing and health care.
2. Identify health habits and beliefs of major ethnic groups in the United States.
3. Explain cultural influences on interactions of patients and families with the health care system.
4. Discuss cultural influences and implications for nursing care.

GLOSSARY

CULTURAL DIVERSITY The existence of many cultures in a society

CULTURE Arts, beliefs, customs, institutions, and all other products of human work and thought created by a people or a group at a particular time

ENCULTURATION The process of learning to be part of a culture

SUBCULTURE A group of individuals within a culture whose members share different beliefs, values, and attitudes from those of the dominant culture

Nurses encounter people of many different backgrounds in their practice. The differences may stem from race, ethnicity, language, or religion. These diverse backgrounds can affect the ways in which individuals react to health and illness, hospitalization, and nursing care.

CULTURAL CONCEPTS

CHARACTERISTICS OF CULTURE

Culture is the arts, beliefs, customs, mores, institutions, and all other products of human work and thought created by a people or a group at a particular time. Culture represents the ideas, beliefs, values, and attitudes that a group of people possess. These values and beliefs guide individual behavior. They are the foundation for setting standards and rules of behavior that members of a society consider acceptable and proper.

Cultural diversity is a term used to describe the existence of many cultures in a society. The United States has a rich cultural diversity as result of the large number of immigrants that has entered the country over the past 200 years. America has been known as a "melting pot" as many immigrants sought to assimilate into their new society. Today, the term *salad bowl* is often used to describe the way in which new arrivals seek to maintain individual differences while acclimating to new surroundings. It is important to value and respect the differences among the various cultural groups within our society, for they provide unique contributions to art, science, politics, and health care.

Within certain cultures are groups of individuals who share different beliefs, values, and attitudes from those of the dominant culture. These groups are called *subcultures.* Examples of subcultures in the United States are members of various ethnic groups, such as African Americans, Latinos, Asians, and Native Americans (Fig. 4–1); homosexuals; the military; and religious groups, such as the Amish or Mormons.

Similarities

All cultures share certain basic characteristics: (1) Culture is learned; (2) culture is shared; and (3) culture is based on symbols. People *learn* to be a part of a culture as they are growing up. This process is known as *enculturation.* Cultural learning is passed down from

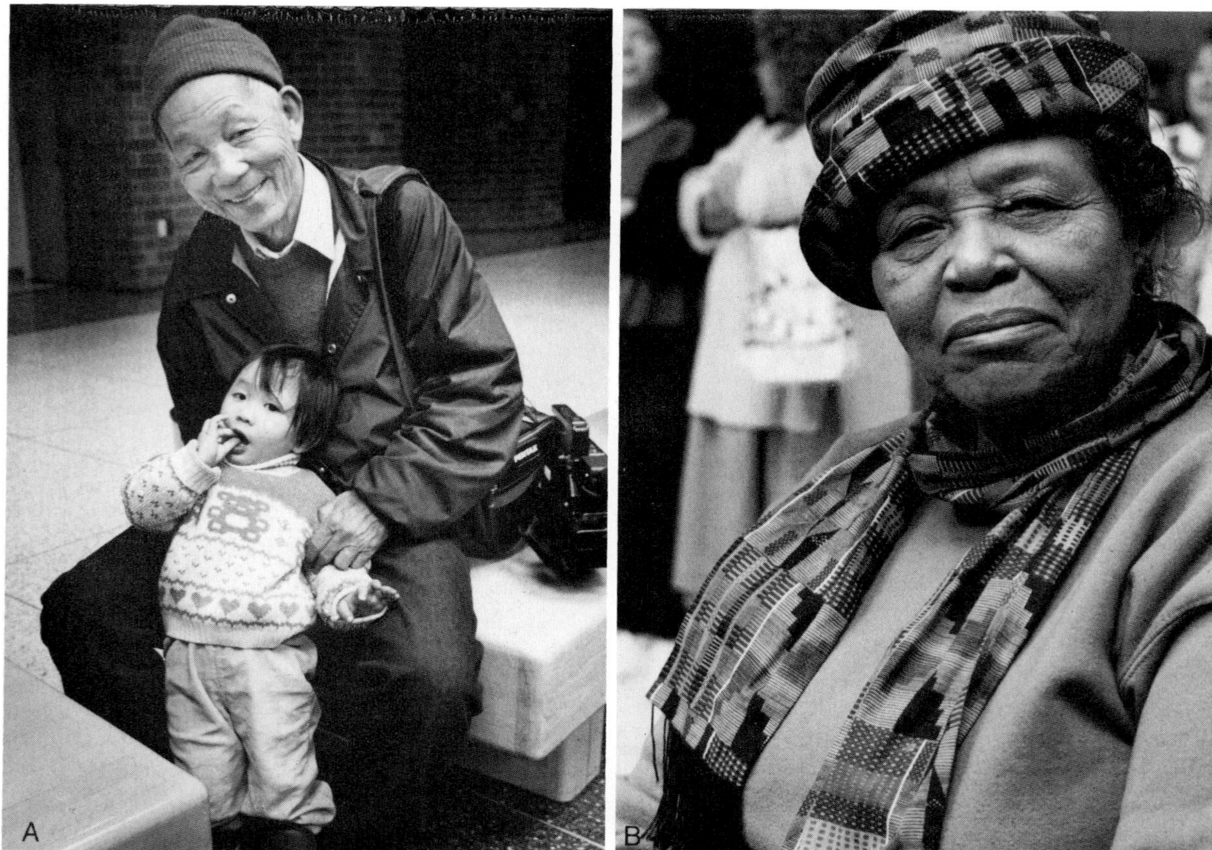

FIGURE 4-1

Many people living in the United States belong to a particular subculture. *A,* Asian; *B,* African American. (Photographs by Stephen Matteson, Jr.)

parent to child to grandchild, affecting the personality development of each generation. People learn what is expected of them and how they should behave, dress, and interact on particular occasions. For example, important life events are celebrated differently in different cultures. Weddings and funerals can be quiet, small occasions for introspection, or they can be robust, noisy celebrations with mobs of people in attendance.

Culture also is *shared*. Cultural beliefs, values, and behaviors are shared among individuals within a particular group. Individual behavior does not reflect a particular culture unless it is manifested by other people in the cultural group. From group behavior, behaviors of individuals then can be predicted.

Culture is based on *symbols*. Symbols represent means of communication, spiritual beliefs, economic interactions, and national origins, among other things. Examples of symbols are language (words), religious artifacts (crucifix, Star of David), money (economic interactions), and flags (national origin) (Fig. 4–2). Symbols help to convey the beliefs, values, and behaviors of a society or culture.

Differences

Cultural differences may occur among various groups in relation to family, religion, communication, educational background, social class, and economic level. Nurses should be aware of the differences in these areas and recognize how they affect the wellness, illness, and health care practices of their clients.

FAMILY. The family provides a major means for reproducing the population and rearing its children. The family unit is basic to every society. It is mainly through the family that cultural attitudes, values, and behaviors are transmitted.

The family structure may vary among and within cultures. The traditional nuclear family, consisting of a mother, a father, and children, is becoming less of a standard. The number of single-parent families has increased over the last several years to about 20% of all households in the United States. In addition, some cultural groups continue to have extended families living under the same roof (e.g., grandparents, parents, children, and other relatives). Some families have a strong patriarchal (male, father-dominated) influence, whereas others have strong matriarchal (female, mother-dominated) tendencies.

Culture can have an influence on the attitudes and beliefs of families in relation to health care. Behaviors related to health practices, hospitalization, and nursing home placement can vary among cultures. For example, Latinos are thought to have strong extended family units and family ties, and when a person is hospitalized, family members visit frequently. In addition, Latinos tend to care for their elders in a home setting rather than placing them in a nursing home. People from families of other cultural backgrounds may not visit relatives in the hospital as frequently or be as hesitant to place their elders in a nursing home. Nurses should become acquainted with the various cultural backgrounds of families and how they influence behavior rather than being judgmental about family behaviors.

RELIGION. Religious beliefs are culturally determined, and how individuals fulfill their spiritual needs stems from a lifetime of experience. Religious beliefs and practices can influence perceptions of health and illness, hospitalization, and death and dying. Some patients may observe specific dietary rules, and others may have particular practices regarding dress, modesty, daily living habits, or medical interventions. Religious differences also occur in relation to the observation of the sabbath, baptism, and last rites (Table 4–1).

Text continued on page 32

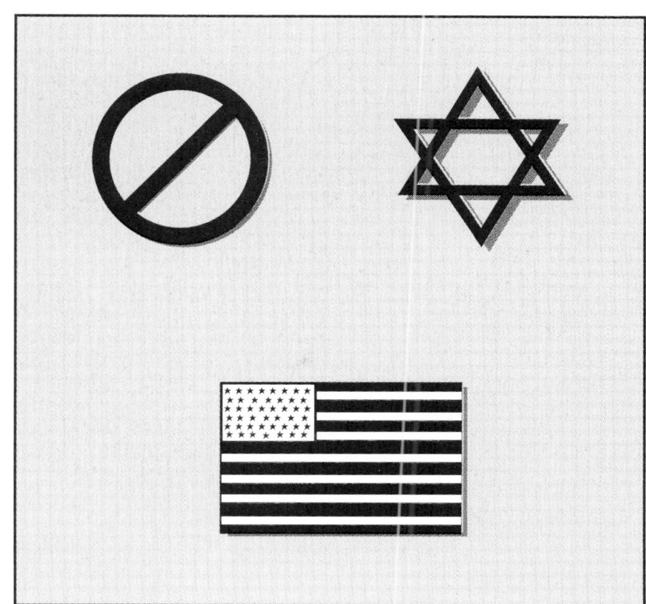

FIGURE 4–2

Examples of symbols. *A*, International sign for "no" (e.g., "No Smoking"). *B*, Jewish Star of David. *C*, Flag of the United States of America.

TABLE 4-1

RELIGIOUS BELIEFS AND PRACTICES AFFECTING HEALTH CARE

RELIGIOUS GROUP	BELIEFS AND PRACTICES
Western Religions *Judaism* Orthodox Jews and some Conservative Jewish groups	*Care of women:* A woman is considered to be in a ritual state of impurity whenever blood is coming from her uterus, such as during menstrual periods and after the birth of a child. During this time, her husband will not have physical contact with her. When this time is completed, she will bathe herself in a pool called a mikvah. Nurses need to be aware of this practice and be sensitive to the husband and wife because the husband will not touch his wife. He cannot assist her in moving in the bed, so the nurse will have to do this. An Orthodox Jewish man will not touch any women other than his wife, daughters, and mother. *Dietary rules:* (1) Kosher dietary laws include the following: No mixing of milk and meat at a meal; no consumption of food or any derivative thereof from animals not slaughtered in accordance with Jewish law; use of separate cooking utensils for milk and milk products; if a client requires milk and meat products for a meal, the dairy foods should be served first, followed later by the meat. (2) During Yom Kippur (Day of Atonement), a 24-hour fast is required, but exceptions are made for those who cannot fast because of medical reasons. (3) During Passover, no leavened products are eaten. (4) May say benediction of thanksgiving before meals and grace at the end of the meal. Time and a quiet environment should be provided for this. *Sabbath:* Observed from sunset Friday until sunset Saturday. Orthodox law prohibits riding in a car, smoking, turning lights on and off, handling money, and using television and telephone. Nurses need to be aware of this when caring for observant Jews at home and in the hospital. Medical or surgical treatments should be postponed if possible. *Death:* Judaism defines death as occurring when respiration and circulation are irreversibly stopped and no movement is apparent. (1) Euthanasia is strictly forbidden by Orthodox Jews, who advocate the strict use of life-support measures. (2) Prior to death, Jewish faith indicates that visiting of the person by family and friends is a religious duty. The Torah and Psalms may be read and prayers recited. A witness needs to be present when a person prays for health so that if death occurs God will protect the family and the spirit will be committed to God. Extraneous talking and conversation about death are not encouraged unless initiated by the client or visitors. In Judaism, the belief is that people should have someone with them when the soul leaves the body, so family and/or friends should be allowed to stay with clients. After death, the body should not be left alone until buried, usually within 24 hours. (3) When death occurs, the body should be untouched for 8 to 30 minutes. Medical personnel should not touch or wash the body but allow only an Orthodox person or the Jewish Burial Society to care for the body. Handling of a corpse on the Sabbath is forbidden to Jewish persons. If need be, the nursing staff may provide routine care of the body, wearing gloves. Water in the room should be emptied, and the family may request that mirrors be covered to symbolize that a death has occurred. (4) Orthodox Jews and some Conservative Jews do not approve of autopsies. If an autopsy must be done, all body parts must remain with the body. (5) For Orthodox Jews, the body must be buried within 24 hours. No flowers are permitted. A fetus must be buried. (6) A 7-day mourning period is required by the immediate family. They must stay at home except for Sabbath worship. (7) Organs or other body parts such as amputated limbs must be made available for burial for Orthodox Jews, because they believe that all of the body must be returned to earth. *Birth control and abortion:* Artificial methods of birth control are not encouraged. Vasectomy is not allowed. Abortion may be performed only to save the mother's life. *Organ transplant:* Donor organ transplants generally are not permitted by Orthodox Jews but may be allowed with rabbinical consent. *Shaving:* The beard is regarded as a mark of piety among observant Jews. For the very Orthodox, shaving should not be done with a razor but with scissors or electric razor, because a blade should not contact the skin. *Head covering:* Orthodox men wear skull caps at all times, and women cover their hair after marriage. Some Orthodox women wear wigs as a mark of piety. Conservative Jews cover their heads only during acts of worship and prayer. *Prayer:* Praying directly to God, including a prayer of confession, is required for Orthodox Jews. Nurses should provide quiet time for prayer.
Reform Jews	*Care of women:* Reform Jews do not observe the rules against touching. *Dietary rules:* Reform Jews usually do not observe kosher dietary restrictions. *Sabbath:* Usually worship in temples on Friday evenings. No strict rules. *Death:* Advocate use of life support without heroic measures. Allow for cremation but suggest that ashes be buried in a Jewish cemetery. *Organ transplants:* Donation or transplantation of organs allowed with permission of a rabbi. *Head coverings:* Generally pray without wearing skull caps.

TABLE 4-1
RELIGIOUS BELIEFS AND PRACTICES AFFECTING HEALTH CARE *Continued*

RELIGIOUS GROUP	BELIEFS AND PRACTICES
Christianity	
Roman Catholic	*Holy Eucharist:* For clients and health caregivers who are to receive communion, abstinence from solid food and alcohol is required for 15 minutes (if possible) prior to reception of the consecrated wafer. Medicine, water, and nonalcoholic drinks are permitted at any time. If a client is in danger of death, the fast is waived because the reception of the Eucharist at this time is very important. *Anointing of the sick:* The priest uses oil to anoint the forehead and hands and, if desired, the affected area. The rite may be performed on any who are ill and desire it. Clients receiving the sacrament seek complete healing, and strength to endure suffering. Prior to 1963, this sacrament was given only to clients at time of imminent death, so the nurse must be sensitive to the meaning this has for the client. If possible, the nurse calls a priest before the client is unconscious but may also call when there is sudden death, because the sacrament may also be given shortly after death. The nurse records on the care plan that this sacrament has been administered. *Dietary habits:* Obligatory fasting is excused during hospitalization. However, if there are no health restrictions, some Catholics may still observe the following guidelines: (1) Anyone 14 years or older must abstain from eating meat on Ash Wednesday and all Fridays during Lent. Some older Catholics may still abstain from meat on all Fridays of the year. (2) In addition to abstinence from meat, persons 21 to 59 years of age must limit themselves to one full meal and two light meals on Ash Wednesday and Good Friday. (3) Eastern Rite Catholics are stricter about fasting and fast more frequently then Western Rite Catholics, so it is important for the nurse to know if a client is Eastern or Western. *Death:* Each Roman Catholic should participate in the anointing of the sick as well as the Eucharist and penance before death. The body should not be shrouded until after these sacraments are performed. All body parts that retain human quality must be appropriately buried or cremated. *Birth control:* Prohibited except for abstinence or natural family planning. Referral to a priest for questions about this can be of great help. Nurses can teach the techniques of natural family planning if they are familiar with them; otherwise, this should be referred to the physician or to a support group of the church that instructs couples in this method of birth control. Sterilization is prohibited unless there is an overriding medical reason. *Organ donation:* Donation and transplantation of organs are acceptable as long as the donor is not harmed and is not deprived of life. *Religious objects:* Rosary prayers are said using rosary beads. Medals bearing the images of saints, relics, statues, and scapulars are important objects that may be pinned to a hospital gown or pillow or be at the bedside. Extreme care should be taken not to lose these objects, because they have special meaning to the client.
Eastern Orthodox	*Holy Eucharist:* The priest is notified if the client desires this sacrament. *Anointing of the sick:* The priest conducts this in the hospital room. *Dietary habits:* Fasting from meat and dairy products is required on Wednesday and Friday during Lent and on other holy days. Hospital clients are exempt if fasting is detrimental to health. *Special days:* Christmas is celebrated on January 7 and New Year's Day on January 14. This is important to the care of a client who is hospitalized on these days. *Death:* Last rites are obligatory. This is handled by an ordained priest who is notified by the nurse while the client is conscious. The Russian Orthodox Church does not encourage autopsy or organ donation. Euthanasia, even for the terminally ill, is discouraged, as is cremation. *Birth control:* This as well as abortion is not permitted.
Protestant	
Assemblies of God (Pentecostal)	*Holy Communion:* Notify clergy if the client desires. *Anointing of the sick:* Members believe in divine healing through prayer and the laying on of hands. Clergy is notified if client or family desires this. *Dietary habits:* Abstinence from alcohol, tobacco, and all illegal drugs is strongly encouraged. *Death:* No special practices. *Other practices:* Faith in God and in the health care providers is encouraged. Members pray for divine intervention in health matters. Nurses should encourage and allow time for prayer. Members may speak in "tongues" during prayer.
Baptist (over 27 different groups in the United States)	*Holy Communion:* Clergy should be notified if the client desires. *Dietary habits:* Total abstinence from alcohol is expected. *Death:* No general service is provided, but the clergy does minister through counseling, prayer, and Scripture as requested by the client or family, and the client is encouraged to believe in Jesus Christ as Savior and Lord. *Other practices:* The Bible is held to be the word of God, so the nurse should either allow quiet time for Scripture reading or offer to read to the client.

Table continued on following page

TABLE 4-1
RELIGIOUS BELIEFS AND PRACTICES AFFECTING HEALTH CARE *Continued*

RELIGIOUS GROUP	BELIEFS AND PRACTICES
Christian Church (Disciples of Christ)	*Holy Communion:* Open communion is celebrated each Sunday and is a central part of worship services. The nurse notifies the clergy if the client desires it, or the clergy may suggest it. *Death:* No special practices. *Other practices:* Church elders as well as clergy may be notified to assist with meeting the client's spiritual needs.
Church of the Brethren	*Holy Communion:* Usually received within church, but clergy will give it in the hospital when requested. *Anointing of the sick:* Practiced for physical healing as well as spiritual uplift and held in high regard by the church. The clergy is notified if the client or family desires. *Death:* The clergy is notified for counsel and prayer.
Church of the Nazarene	*Holy Communion:* Pastor will administer if the client wishes. *Dietary habits:* The use of alcohol and tobacco is forbidden. *Death:* Cremation is permitted, and term stillborn infants are buried. *Other practices:* Believe in divine healing but not to the exclusion of medical treatment. Clients may desire quiet time for prayer.
Episcopal (Anglican)	*Holy Communion:* The priest is notified if the client wishes to receive this sacrament. *Anointing of the sick:* Priest may administer this rite when death is imminent, but it is not considered mandatory. *Dietary habits:* Some clients may abstain from meat on Fridays. Others may fast before receiving the Eucharist, but fasting is not mandatory. *Death:* No special practices. *Other practices:* Confession of sins to a priest is optional; if the client desires this, the clergy should be notified.
Lutheran (18 different branches)	*Holy Communion:* Notify the clergy if the client desires this sacrament. Clergy may also inquire about the client's desire. *Anointing of the sick:* The client may request an anointing and blessing from the minister when the prognosis is poor. *Death:* A service of Commendation of the Dying is used at the client's or family's request.
Mennonite (12 different groups)	*Holy Communion:* Served twice a year, with foot washing as part of ceremony. *Dietary habits:* Abstinence from alcohol is urged for all. *Death:* Prayer is important at time of crisis, so contacting a minister is important. *Other practices:* Women may wear head coverings during hospitalization. Anointing with oil is administered in harmony with James 5:14 when requested.
Methodist (over 20 different groups)	*Holy Communion:* Notify the clergy if a client requests it prior to surgery or another health crisis. *Anointing of the sick:* If requested, the clergy will come to pray and sprinkle the client with olive oil. *Death:* Scripture reading and prayer are important at this time. *Other practices:* Donation of one's body or part of the body at death is encouraged.
Presbyterian (10 different groups)	*Holy Communion:* Given when appropriate and convenient, at the hospitalized client's request. *Death:* Notify a local pastor or elder for prayer and Scripture reading if desired by the family or client.
Quaker (Friends)	*Holy Communion:* Because Friends have no creed, there is a diversity of personal beliefs, one of which is that outward sacraments are usually not necessary because there is the ministry of the Spirit inwardly in such areas as baptism and communion. *Death:* Believe that the present life is part of God's kingdom and generally have no ceremony as a rite of passage from this life to the next. Personal beliefs and wishes need to be ascertained, and the nurse can then act on the client's wishes.
Salvation Army	*Holy Communion:* No particular ceremony. *Death:* Notify the local officer in charge of the Army Corps for any soldier (member) who needs assistance. *Other practices:* The Bible is seen as the only rule for one's faith, so the Scriptures should be made available to a client. The Army has many of its own social welfare centers, with hospitals and homes where unwed mothers are cared for and outpatient services provided. No medical or surgical procedures are opposed, except for abortion on demand.
Seventh-Day Adventist	*Holy Communion:* Although this is not required of hospitalized clients, the clergy are notified if the client desires. *Anointing of the sick:* The clergy are contacted for prayer and anointing with oil. *Dietary habits:* Because the body is viewed as the temple of the Holy Spirit, healthy living is essential. Therefore, the use of alcohol, tobacco, coffee, and tea and the promiscuous use of drugs are prohibited. Some are vegetarians, and most avoid pork.

TABLE 4-1
RELIGIOUS BELIEFS AND PRACTICES AFFECTING HEALTH CARE *Continued*

RELIGIOUS GROUP	BELIEFS AND PRACTICES
	Special days: The Sabbath is observed on Saturday. *Death:* No special procedures. *Other related practices:* Use of hypnotism is opposed by some. Persons of homosexual or lesbian orientation are ministered to in the hope of correction of these practices, which are believed to be wrong. A Bible should always be available for Scripture reading.
United Church of Christ	*Holy Communion:* Clergy are notified if the client desires to receive this sacrament. *Death:* If the client desires counsel or prayer, notify the clergy.
Other	
Christian Science	*Dietary habits:* Because alcohol and tobacco are considered drugs, they are not used. Coffee and tea are often declined. *Death:* Autopsy is usually declined unless required by law. Donation of organs is unlikely, but is an individual decision. *Other practices:* Do not normally seek medical care, because they approach health care in a different, primarily spiritual, framework. They commonly utilize the services of a surgeon to set a bone but decline drugs and, in general, other medical or surgical procedures. Hypnotism and psychotherapy are also declined. Family planning is left to the family. They seek exemption from vaccinations but obey legal requirements (e.g., report infectious diseases and obey public health quarantines). Nonmedical care facilities are maintained for those needing nursing assistance in the course of a healing. *The Christian Science Journal* lists available Christian Science nurses. When a Christian Science believer is in the hospital, the nurse should allow and encourage time for prayer and study. Clients may request that a Christian Science practitioner be notified to come.
Jehovah's Witnesses	*Dietary habits:* Use of alcohol and tobacco is discouraged, because these harm the physical body. *Death:* Autopsy is a private matter to be decided by the persons involved. Burial and cremation are acceptable. *Birth control and abortion:* Use of birth control is a personal decision. Abortion is opposed based on Exodus 21:22–23. *Organ transplants:* Use of organ transplant is a private decision and if used must be cleansed with a nonblood solution. *Blood transfusions:* Blood transfusions violate God's laws and are therefore not allowed. Clients do respect physicians and will accept alternatives to blood transfusions. These might include use of nonblood plasma expanders, careful surgical techniques to decrease blood loss, use of autologous transfusions, and autotransfusion through use of a heart-lung machine. Nurses should check unconscious patients for Medic Alert cards that state that the person does not want a transfusion. Since Jehovah's Witnesses are prepared to die rather than break God's law, nurses need to be sensitive to the spiritual as well as the physical needs of the client.
The Church of Jesus Christ of Latter-Day Saints	*Holy Communion:* A hospitalized client may desire to have a member of the church priesthood administer this sacrament. *Anointing of the sick:* Mormons frequently are anointed and given a blessing before going to the hospital and after admission by laying on of hands. *Dietary habits:* Abstinence from the use of tobacco; beverages with caffeine such as cola, coffee, and tea; alcohol and other substances considered injurious. Mormons eat meat but encourage the intake of fruits, grains, and herbs. *Death:* Prefer burial of the body. A church elder should be notified to assist the family. If need be, the elder will assist the funeral director in dressing the body in special clothes and will give other help as needed. *Birth control and abortion:* Abortion is opposed except when the life of the mother is in danger. Only natural means of birth control are recommended. Artificial means can be used when the health of the woman is at stake (including emotional health). *Personal care:* Cleanliness is very important to Mormons. A sacred undergarment may be worn at all times by Mormons and should only be removed in emergency situations. *Other practice:* Allowing quiet time for prayer and the reading of the sacred writings is important. The church maintains a welfare system to assist those in need. Families are of great importance, so visiting should be encouraged.
Unitarian Universalist Association	*Death:* Cremation is often preferred to burial. *Other practices:* Use of birth control is advocated as part of responsible parenting. Strong support for a woman's right to choice regarding abortion is maintained. Unitarian Universalists advocate donation of body parts for research and transplants.
Unification Church	*Baptism:* No baptism. *Special days:* Sunday mornings are used to honor Reverend and Mrs. Moon as the true parents, and members get up at 5:00 A.M., bow before a picture of the Moons three

Table continued on following page

TABLE 4-1
RELIGIOUS BELIEFS AND PRACTICES AFFECTING HEALTH CARE *Continued*

RELIGIOUS GROUP	BELIEFS AND PRACTICES
	times, and vow to do what is needed to help the Reverend accomplish his mission on earth.
	Death: Believe that after death one's place of destiny will depend on his or her spirit's quality of life and goodness while on earth. In the afterlife, one will have the same aspirations and feelings as before death. Hell is not a concern, because it will not be a place as heaven grows in size. Persons who leave the Unification Church are warned that Satan may try to possess them.
	Other practices: All marriages must be solemnized by Reverend Moon in order to be part of the perfect family and have salvation. The church supplies its faithful members with life's necessities. Members may use occult practices to have spiritual and psychic experiences.
Islam	*Dietary habits:* No pork is allowed, nor alcoholic beverages. All halal (permissible) meat must be blessed and killed in a special way. This is called zabihah (correctly slaughtered).
	Death: Prior to death, family members ask to be present so that they can read the Koran and pray with the client. An Imam may come if requested by the client or family but is not required. Clients must face Mecca and confess their sins and beg forgiveness in the presence of their family. If the family is unavailable, any praticing Muslim can provide support to the client. After death, Muslims prefer that the family wash, prepare, and place the body in a position facing Mecca. If necessary, the health care providers may perform these procedures as long as they wear gloves. Burial is performed as soon as possible. Cremation is forbidden. Autopsy is also prohibited except for legal reasons, and then no body part is to be removed. Donation of body parts or organs is not allowed, because according to culturally developed law persons do not own their body.
	Abortion and birth control: Abortion is forbidden, and many conservative Muslims do not encourage the use of contraceptives because this interferes with God's purpose. Others feel that a woman should only have as many children as her husband can afford. Contraception is permitted by Islamic law.
	Personal devotions: At prayer time, washing is required, even by those who are sick. A client on bed rest may require assistance with this task before prayer. Provision of privacy is important during prayer.
	Religious objects: The Koran must not be touched by anyone ritually unclean, and nothing should be placed on top of it. Some Muslims wear taviz, a black string on which words of the Koran are attached. These should not be removed and must remain dry. Certain items of jewelry such as bangles may have religious significance and should not be removed unnecessarily.
	Care of women: Because women are not allowed to sign consent forms or make a decision regarding family planning, the husband needs to be present. Women are very modest and frequently wear clothes that cover all of the body. During a medical examination, the woman's modesty should be respected as much as possible. Muslim women prefer female doctors. For 40 days after giving birth and also during menstruation, a woman is exempt from prayer because this is a time of cleansing for her.
American Muslim Mission	*Dietary habits:* In addition to refusing pork, many will not eat traditional black American foods such as corn bread and collard greens.

COMMUNICATION. Communication involves language. It is obvious that certain cultural or ethnic groups speak different languages, making communication almost impossible without an interpreter. However, there are also subtler forms of miscommunication that can arise because of group differences. The speed with which people speak and their tone and inflections vary according to cultural background.

Nonverbal communication also is culturally based. Personal space, eye contact, displays of emotions, and amount and meaning of touch may have different connotations in different cultures. Some cultures find emotional display more acceptable than others. Some are more comfortable with silence than others.

EDUCATIONAL BACKGROUND AND ECONOMIC LEVEL. There are wide differences in educational backgrounds within the United States. Approximately 60 million Americans have literacy skills below the eighth grade level. That means that one out of every three people has difficulty with reading and writing.

Educational level attained is strongly tied to ethnicity and economic background. School dropout rates appear to be higher among teenagers living in poverty areas. Because certain ethnic groups are found in large numbers in these areas, they tend to have high dropout rates. Examples include African Americans and Latinos.

Educational background and economic levels affect the ways in which people perceive the world, health and

TABLE 4-1
RELIGIOUS BELIEFS AND PRACTICES AFFECTING HEALTH CARE *Continued*

RELIGIOUS GROUP	BELIEFS AND PRACTICES
	Death: The family is contacted before any care of the deceased is performed. There are special procedures for washing and shrouding the body. *Other practices:* Quiet time is necessary to permit prayer. Members are encouraged to use black physicians for health care. Because these clients do not smoke, their request for a nonsmoking roommate should be honored.
Eastern Religions	
Hinduism	*Dietary habits:* Some sects are vegetarian, believing meats and intoxicants to be too stimulating to the senses. *Belief about illness:* View illnesses as a result of misuse of the body or a consequence of sins committed in a previous life. They do not oppose medical treatment, but view its effect as transitory. Believe that praying for health is the lowest form of prayer. *Death:* See death as a union with Brahman (God) achieved through prayers, ritual, purity, self-control, detachment, truth, nonviolence, charity, and compassion toward all creatures. Following death, one will be reborn (reincarnated) into a future life based on the behavior in this life. The record of behavior is called karma. Eventually, the process of rebirth stops which is called moksha. A priest may be called at the time of death, and may tie a thread around neck or waist as a blessing. The family washes the body, and it is cremated. *Other practices:* Offer daily worship at a shrine in the home. Daily offering to god, and morning and evening rites. Society is organized into castes, or strata. People are born into a caste, and the caste shapes one's entire life. Hindus practice a discipline of the mind and body, called yoga, to reach god. In the highest state, a meditating yogi does not see, hear, taste, feel, or smell. Beyond good and evil, time and space, he is one with god.
Buddhism	*Death:* Believe that salvation depends on one's own right living. Believe in reincarnation. Can speed the process toward Nirvana, the goal of all humanity's striving, through acts of merit. Meditation, worship, and prayer are some of the acts of merit. Buddhists may drive themselves into more and more ritual or contemplation in the hope that their last moments of consciousness may be filled with thoughts worthy enough to elevate them to a higher existence. Last rights of chanting may be performed at bedside. *Renunciation:* The most important Buddhist feasts. Young boys are taught to despise the world's vanity and the boy spends a night in a nearby monastery.
Taoism/Confucianism	*General beliefs:* Founded on ethical principles of Confucius. God is not clearly defined as in other religions. Taoism is a mixture of magic and religion. Believe that humans and nature are inseparable, and that if heaven is upset, earth does not prosper. This relationship is described as yang and yin, which are two interplaying forces. When yang and yin are in balance, good occurs. *Death:* The dead are remembered in all festivals. The fate of the dead in the afterworld depends not only on the life they led but also on being properly honored after death. Otherwise they may become demons. Graves are mounds like those dedicated to the gifts of the soil. Graves and houses must be in harmony with the universe, otherwise evil will befall the occupants.

From Black, J. M. & Matassarin-Jacobs, E. (1993). *Luckmann and Sorensen's medical-surgical nursing: A psychophysiologic approach* (4th ed.). Philadelphia: W. B. Saunders. Modified from Carson, V. B. (1989). *Spiritual dimensions of nursing practice.* Philadelphia: W. B. Saunders.

illness, and the health care system. Teaching about health becomes a challenge because many with low literacy levels have difficulty reading the materials presented and understanding health care jargon. In addition, people from economically deprived backgrounds may live in delapidated housing and have inadequate diets. Health promotion and disease prevention become difficult under these circumstances.

CULTURAL BELIEFS RELATED TO HEALTH AND ILLNESS

Health and illness have different meanings for different people and cultural groups. For some groups, illness is something that is expected as part of life and out of one's own control. For others, it is believed that illness can be prevented by taking action, such as eating a proper diet, getting exercise, or scheduling regular physical examinations.

Some groups attempt to attach meaning to illness to explain why illness occurs. They have developed many beliefs regarding the onset, course, and cure of disease, as well as the process of death and dying. For example, there is a belief in *divine punishment* as the cause of illness. Believers in divine punishment claim that illness is a result of punishment for a sin that an individual has committed. Another belief involves an individual's balance with nature. If a person maintains a proper balance, good health results; if a person is not in harmony with the environment, illness occurs.

The "hot" and "cold" theory is an ancient belief about health and illness that still is held widely in many cultures. According to the hot and cold theory, health and illness are influenced by four humors that regulate body functions. The four humors are phlegm, blood, black bile, and yellow bile. The humors are considered either hot (blood and yellow bile) or cold (phlegm and black bile), and an imbalance between the hot and the cold areas of the body causes illness. Examples of illnesses that are thought to be caused by cold entering the body are earaches, paralysis, stomach cramps, and arthritis. Examples of illnesses that are caused by heat include dysentery, sore throats, abscessed teeth, and kidney disease. Illnesses are treated with herbs, potions, and food that are considered to be either hot or cold, depending on their effects on the body.

Many ethnic groups engage in the use of healers who practice health care outside of the formal health care delivery system. The healers may be called *root doctors*, who often practice among urban African Americans, or *curanderos*, who are used by Latinos. They are contacted when mainstream health care is perceived as being too expensive, inconvenient, or unable to provide relief for the problem at hand. The healers provide psychosocial support and counseling in addition to helping with physiologic problems. They use a variety of potions and plants in their practice.

HEALTH HABITS AND BELIEFS OF MAJOR ETHNIC GROUPS IN THE UNITED STATES

Although it is not a good idea to stereotype particular groups, various ethnic groups in the United States tend to have distinguishing health habits and beliefs. Individuals may vary within a group, but as a whole, each ethnic group can be characterized in terms of ideas and practices regarding health promotion and disease prevention, attitudes and behaviors related to illness, and utilization of health care resources. In addition, people who are first- or second-generation Americans may have more characteristics associated with their ethnic group than people who have been in the United States for several generations and have become acculturated into U.S. society.

WHITES

Whites generally believe in the work ethic in which personal achievement, individualism, and competition are valued. Illness is viewed primarily as caused by germs in the environment or, in certain religious groups, by divine punishment; however, illness can be prevented by eating a proper diet, getting enough exercise, and allowing for adequate rest. White Americans often communicate directly, and tend to express feelings of pain during illness openly. Although members of this group tend to use the formal health care system for their medical and nursing needs, they may consult a spiritual adviser in times of illness.

AFRICAN AMERICANS

African Americans value family, community, religion, health, and work. Their many beliefs about the cause of illness include germs in the environment; divine punishment; and an imbalance among body, mind, and spirit. Prevention of illness is achieved through eating good food, living right, and keeping the system cleaned out. Communication may be direct or indirect, and expressions of pain during illness are displayed with varying degrees of stoicism or expressed as vocal outcries to God for assistance. African Americans tend to attempt self-care before consulting a health care professional when they are ill. They may also use folk medicine or consult a root doctor or spiritualist for help.

LATINOS

Latinos, particularly those who live in the southwestern United States, are family oriented and value harmony in interpersonal relationships. They believe that illness results from magical fright, divine punishment, imbalance of hot and cold, or environmental hazards. Prevention of illness is achieved through the use of charms, amulets, or crucifixes. Communication is usually indirect; however, expressions of pain are open and direct. Folk health specialists *(curanderos)* and family may be consulted along with the formal health care system in times of illness.

ASIANS

Asians value self-respect, self-control, respect for elders, family honor, loyalty, and pride. There is an emphasis on holistic health and harmony between the self and the universe. Asians in the United States favor health care that is provided by herbalists, acupuncturists, and other cultural healers, but many use the formal health care system in times of illness. Communication patterns tend to be indirect, and pain is expressed with varying degrees of stoicism.

NATIVE AMERICANS

There is considerable diversity among tribes and groups, so it is important to use caution when making generalizations about Native Americans. However, some general characteristics may be noted. Native Americans value family, respect for elders, generosity, and cooperation with others. They attempt to live in harmony with nature and have deep respect for the environment. Communication is usually indirect, with a great emphasis on nonverbal cues. Pain is usually dealt with stoically. Health practices are traditional, with emphasis on total healing, mental and spiritual renewal, and health maintenance. Ceremonial rituals guided by a medicine man are frequently used for treating illnesses before structured medical care is sought.

CULTURAL INFLUENCES ON PATIENT AND FAMILY INTERACTIONS WITH THE HEALTH CARE SYSTEM

In all health care settings, patients of different cultures may exhibit behavior that is not understood by health care providers. The culturally different patients may be labeled "noncomplaining," "difficult," "uncooperative," or "noncompliant," when in reality they are struggling to adapt to a culture that is foreign to them.

HOSPITAL HEALTH CARE

The hospital environment is often frightening even to people who are familiar with it. For individuals who may speak different languages, have different eating preferences, and maintain different attitudes towards health and illness, adapting to the hospital environment is a formidable task. Admission to the hospital may seem like traveling to a foreign country where an entirely different language is spoken. Hospital personnel become authority figures, and their permission is needed to carry out the most basic activities, such as toileting, eating, and dressing. Patients are stripped of their dignity when they are told to wear hospital gowns that barely cover private parts of the body. Modesty is often ignored, causing humiliation and anxiety.

People not only find themselves in a totally new environment but also must endure separation from their family and friends. Their support systems topple from under them as strict visiting rules are enforced. In some cultures, it is expected that families help with the nursing care, or at least sit with the patients to keep them company and provide support. Nurses and hospital personnel often are uncomfortable with this infringement on their territory.

Culture shock associated with hospitalization occurs in three phases. During the first phase, the patient asks questions regarding the hospital routine and the hospital's expectations of the patient. In the second phase, the patient becomes disenchanted with the whole situation and is frustrated, hostile, and then depressed and withdrawn. In the final phase, the patient begins to adapt to the new environment and is even able to maintain a sense of humor during interactions with others.

COMMUNITY HEALTH CARE

Settings in which culturally different individuals interact with the health care system include physicians' offices, outpatient clinics, community mental health centers, home health care, hospices, and daycare centers. As mentioned earlier, individuals who have different cultural backgrounds also may have their own network of health care, such as spiritualists, *curanderos*, or root doctors.

Many ethnic or cultural minorities have difficulty getting through the maze of health care services, either because of language differences or because of negative attitudes toward health care providers based on past experiences. Minority group members frequently are clinic patients who must wait hours for an appointment, only to receive a cursory assessment from the physician or nurse. Their questions about their condition may be left unanswered because of communication difficulties, which can result in inaccuracies in following directions for their care. These patients may be labeled "noncompliant" or "difficult," which only perpetuates the cycle of negative attitudes among patients and health care providers alike.

NURSING HOME HEALTH CARE

The majority of nursing home residents are white women. Some ethnic groups such as Latinos are extremely reluctant to admit older relatives to nursing homes and prefer to provide care at home. Others do not have the financial means to pay for nursing home care. Long-term care is largely paid for by Medicaid (80%); Medicare accounts for only 2% of nursing home funding, and the rest is through private pay. A large number of ethnic minorities must depend on Medicaid for nursing home care.

Many nursing home residents suffer from confusion, functional impairments (impaired ability to carry out activities of daily living such as bathing and dressing), and incontinence. Culturally diverse persons have the added strain of communication problems and extreme changes in lifestyle and food habits. These differences may contribute to further confusion, disability, and incontinence. For example, an older woman who speaks little English may have difficulty asking for help to the bathroom or a bedpan. Because older people tend to have very little time between the urge to void and the actual voiding experience, urinary incontinence can occur when a nurse has difficulty understanding their needs.

CULTURAL INFLUENCES AND IMPLICATIONS FOR NURSING CARE

When caring for a patient who is from another religious or ethnic background, the nurse should be sensitive to different cultural attitudes, beliefs, and behaviors. Patients may be labeled "difficult" or "uncooperative" because nurses do not understand their behavior. The more sensitive the nurse is to cultural differences, the more effective the nursing intervention. In addition, a nurse who provides care that is not culturally sensitive can cause additional stress and prolong recovery time in the patient.

It is important to gather information regarding the cultural background of a patient to provide sensitive care. For example, communication patterns, including the language spoken and the use of touching and gesturing, may differ among patients. Information regarding health beliefs, interpersonal relationships, the role of the family during illness, attitudes toward modesty, expressions of fear and pain, and food restrictions also should be obtained.

Sensitivity to cultural factors that affect behavior comes from cultural awareness. To develop cultural awareness, the nurse must make a conscious and consistent effort to study different cultural groups and their special cultural background.

THERAPEUTIC RELATIONSHIP

Because all nursing care takes place in the framework of the nurse-patient relationship, an environment of acceptance and respect for the beliefs and behaviors of culturally different patients should be established. Patients can develop a feeling of trust if they feel safe, respected, and accepted (Fig. 4–3).

The nurse should maintain an open and inquiring attitude regarding cultural differences. Patients of another culture, particularly a minority culture, initially may be quiet, polite, conforming, or shy. This behavior may reflect a guarded or cautious response because patients are not sure what is expected of them and how the interaction will go. It is a time to "size up" unfamiliar health care personnel without being too offensive or alarming. A good rule of thumb during an initial encounter with minority patients is to speak softly and in an unhurried manner to put them at ease. When nursing staff members are aggressive and demanding, patients tend to be silently angry and withdrawn. It is advisable to take the time to sit down with patients and their families, listen to their needs and concerns, and learn how they interact.

Culture serves as a guide to action and beliefs in times of crisis. Illness is a time of crisis. Therefore the nurse needs to know the patient's cultural patterns of thinking, feeling, and acting before a therapeutic plan of care can be developed. Once the nurse understands the lifestyle of the patient, the nursing care plan can be tailored to help the patient get through the crisis. The patient should be involved in the care plan, identifying familiar ways of coping with an illness or any other crisis.

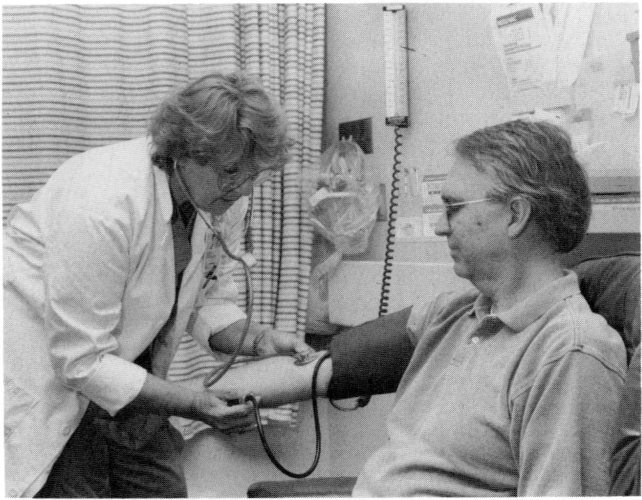

FIGURE 4–3

Patients can develop trust if they feel safe, respected, and accepted by the nurse. (Photograph by Stephen Matteson, Jr.)

Conflicts between the patient's health practices and beliefs and those of the health care system may arise. However, the cultural values of patients and families must be given full consideration. Patients are not likely to change their cultural values if they do not want to. It also is questionable whether it is within the rights of a health care professional to try to change a patient's belief system if he or she does not want it changed.

Changes in health patterns for many patients often require some major changes in lifestyle. If a patient does not respond well to prescribed changes in health practices or lifestyle, the patient may be labeled "uncooperative." The nurse must try to understand each situation from the viewpoint of the patient, family, and community. It is only then that effective modifications in health practices can take place.

BASIC BODILY NEEDS

Cultural attitudes may affect patients' perceptions of personal hygiene and the role of the nurse in assisting with caring for basic bodily needs. Some patients may not take baths routinely. Others may be extremely modest about disrobing in front of family and strangers. The nurse can show sensitivity to these feelings by knocking before entering the room and asking permission before touching the patient.

Most whites have cultural values of cleanliness that include daily bathing, tooth brushing, and application of deodorant. However, people of other cultures may not share these values. For example, Native Americans and Asians do not perspire often and seldom have body odor as a result of having fewer sweat glands. People of Nigeria value natural body odor and have difficulty understanding why Americans are preoccupied with bathing and the use of deodorants and colognes. The nurse should be careful to assess the cultural beliefs of others before assisting with daily hygiene to avoid the frustration caused by cultural differences.

During the bath, charms, crosses, medals, or other objects that a patient is wearing should not be removed. These objects usually have special meaning and cultural significance. Family members may assist with the bath, oral hygiene, bed making, ambulation, or other caregiving. The inclusion of significant others in caregiving helps to alleviate the stress and anxiety associated with entering the hospital environment and to fulfill cultural expectations for both patients and family members.

PATIENT TEACHING

Communication between the nurse and patients and families of different cultures may be especially difficult in the context of teaching. Patients and their families may not be able to understand written or spoken English even if they have some command of the language. Much of the language of health and illness is confusing and complicated and contains many new words that have not been heard before.

The first approach with people of other cultures is to be warm, understanding, and patient. It is important to establish a good interpersonal relationship to develop enough trust so that people feel free to ask questions. Many patients and their families nod their heads in agreement with everything that is taught even though little comprehension is taking place.

Using both verbal and written communication can help to reinforce what has been taught. Written communication in the native language of patients and families greatly aids in their understanding. Having them demonstrate what they have learned helps to ensure that learning has taken place. It may be helpful to seek assistance from staff members who are from the same or similar ethnic backgrounds to facilitate communication.

Knowledge of various cultural concepts of health and illness can promote learning in the teaching-learning process. For example, Latinos may believe that health and illness are controlled by God. Nurses must be aware of the role of religion and religious practitioners in the lives of Latinos. The role of the priest in the community may be used in planning and implementing health programs to make them more effective.

The timing of patient and family teaching needs to be considered in culturally diverse populations. Many cultural groups do not work by the clock and schedules. Time is used spontaneously, and life is regulated by human and bodily needs for many cultural groups, including Native Americans, Latinos, and African Americans. Some people from these groups may not appear for an appointment or may come several hours late. Rather than characterizing individuals as "lazy" or "undisciplined," it would be wiser to carry out patient teaching informally and spontaneously when the opportunity arises.

BIBLIOGRAPHY

ANA position statement on cultural diversity in nursing practice. (1991). *Prairie Rose, 60*(4), 13a–14a.

Bainbridge, W. (1991). Dying east, dying west. *Nursing Standard, 6*(6), 22–23.

Berg, J., & Berg, B. L. (1989). Compliance, diet and cultural factors among black Americans with end-stage renal disease. *Journal of National Black Nurses Association, 3*(2), 16–28.

Brink, P. J. (1989). Ethics across cultures. *Western Journal of Nursing Research, 11*(5), 518–519.

Bushy, A. (1992). Cultural considerations for primary health care: Where do self-care and folk medicine fit? *Holistic Nursing Practice, 6*(3), 10–18.

Campana, E. M. (1989). Cultural differences of the Hispanic patient. *Dimensions in Oncology Nursing, 3*(1), 21–24.

Campinha-Bacote, J. (1992). Voodoo illness. *Perspectives In Psychiatric Care, 28*(1), 11–19.

Campinha-Bacote, J., & Ferguson, S. (1991). Cultural considerations in child-rearing practices: A transcultural perspective. *Journal of National Black Nurses Association, 5*(1), 11–17.

Caralis, P. V. (1991). Hypertension in Hispanic-Americans: How ethnicity affects disease and therapy. *Consultant, 31*(7), 49–51, 54–56.

Charnes, L. S., & Moore, P. S. (1992). Meeting patients' spiritual needs: The Jewish perspective. *Holistic Nursing Practice, 6*(3), 64–72.

Chinn, P. L. (1992). Diversity: What does it mean? *Nursing Outlook, 40*(2), 54.

Cravener, P. (1992). Establishing therapeutic alliance across cultural barriers. *Journal of Psychosocial Nursing & Mental Health Services, 30*(12), 10–14, 37–38.

D'Avanzo, C. E. (1992). Bridging the cultural gap with Southeast Asians. *American Journal of Maternal Child Nursing, 17*(4), 204–208.

DeSantis, L. (1989). A profile of cultural diversity in nursing practice. *Florida Nurse, 37*(9), 15.

Doku, J. (1990). Approaches to cultural awareness. *Nursing Times, 86*(39), 69–70.

Fleming, J. (1989). Meeting the challenge of culturally diverse populations. *Pediatric Nursing, 15*(6), 566, 634, 648.

Germain, C. P. (1992). Cultural care: A bridge between sickness, illness, and disease. *Holistic Nursing Practice, 6*(3), 1–9.

Giger, J. N., & Davidhizar, R. (1990). Developing communication skills for use with black patients. *ABNF Journal, 1*(2), 33–35.

Giger, J. N., & Davidhizar, R. (1990). Culture and space. *Advancing Clinical Care, 5*(6), 8–11.

Green, J. (1989). Death with dignity: Judaism part 4. *Nursing Times, 85*(8), 64–65.

Haraldson, S. S. R. (1988). Health and health services among the Navajo Indians. *Journal of Community Health, 13*(3), 129–142.

Hoeman, S. P. (1989). Cultural assessment in rehabilitation nursing practice. *Nursing Clinics of North America, 24*(1), 277–289.

Lassiter, S. M. (1987). Coping as a function of culture and socio-economic status for Afro-Americans and Afro-West Indians. *Journal of the New York State Nurses Association, 18*(4), 18–30.

Leininger, M. M. (1991). Transcultural nursing: The study and practice field. *Imprint, 38*(2), 55, 57, 59–63.

Leininger, M. M. (1988). Transcultural eating patterns and nutrition: Transcultural nursing and anthropological perspectives. *Holistic Nursing Practice, 3*(1), 16–25.

Marshall, P. A. (1990). Cultural influences on perceived quality of life. *Seminars in Oncology Nursing, 6*(4), 278–284.

McNall, M. C. C., & Benner, P. (1989). Healing we cannot explain. *American Journal of Nursing, 89*(9), 1162–1163.

Meleis, A. I. (1991). Between two cultures: Identity, roles and health. *Health Care for Women International, 12*(4), 365–377.

Niederhauser, V. P. (1989). Health care of immigrant children: Incorporating culture into practice. *Pediatric Nursing, 15*(6), 569–574.

Panella, E. (1990). An insight into cultural and social influences on health and illness—A student's perspective. *Inforum, 11*, 37–39.

Reynolds, C. (1992). An administrative program to facilitate culturally appropriate care for the elderly. *Holistic Nursing Practice, 6*(3), 34–42.

Rosenbaum, J. N. (1991). A cultural assessment guide: Learning cultural sensitivity. *Canadian Nurse, 87*(4), 32–33.

Russell, K., & Jewell, N. (1992). Cultural impact of health-care access: Challenges for improving the health of African Americans. *Journal of Community Health Nursing, 9*(3), 161–169.

Schacht, R. (1989). Glimpses of China and Chinese elders. *Journal of Gerontological Nursing, 15*(1), 39–41.

Scholz, J. (1990). Cultural expressions affecting patient care. *Dimensions in Oncology Nursing, 4*(1), 16–26.

Siantz, M. L., Dee, V., & Ingram, C. A. (1991). How can we become more aware of culturally specific body language and use this awareness therapeutically? *Journal of Psychosocial Nursing & Mental Health Services, 29*(11), 38–41.

Smart, J. F., & Smart, D. W. (1992). Cultural issues in the rehabilitation of Hispanics. *Journal of Rehabilitation, 58*(2), 29–37.

Stone, L. (1992). Cultural influences in community participation in health. *Social Science & Medicine, 35*(4), 409–417.

Swaby-Ellis, D. (1990). Why worry about cultural differences? *Journal of Christian Nursing, 7*(3), 40, 31.

Uhl, J. E. (1991). Health promotion—A cultural affair. *Journal of Professional Nursing, 7*(5), 267.

Valente, S. M. (1989). Overcoming cultural barriers. *California Nurse, 85*(8), 4–5.

Wenger, A. F. Z. (1993). Cultural meaning of symptoms. *Holistic Nursing Practice, 7*(2), 22–35.

Westberg, J. (1989). Patient education for Hispanic Americans. *Patient Education & Counseling, 13*(2), 143–160.

KEY CONCEPTS

1. Culture is the arts, beliefs, customs, institutions, and all other products of human work and thought created by a people or group at a particular time.
2. Cultural diversity describes the existence of many cultures in a society.
3. Culture is learned, shared, and based on symbols.
4. Cultural differences may occur among various groups in relation to family, religion, communication, educational background, and economic level.
5. Health and illness have different meanings for different people and cultural groups, but the nurse must be careful not to stereotype people on the basis of their culture.
6. When caring for a patient who is from another religious or ethnic background, the nurse should be sensitive to different cultural attitudes, beliefs, and behavior.

Mary Ann Matteson

CHAPTER 5

Health and Illness

OBJECTIVES

1. Describe the health-illness continuum.
2. Discuss traditional and current views of health and illness.
3. List Maslow's five basic human needs.
4. Explain the four levels of adaptability to stress.
5. Discuss concepts related to health promotion, disease, prevention, and health maintenance.
6. Define acute and chronic illness.
7. Discuss illness behavior and the impact of illness on the family.
8. Describe nursing measures for health promotion, health maintenance, and illness.

GLOSSARY

ACUTE ILLNESS Illness or disease that has a relatively rapid onset and a short duration

CHRONIC ILLNESS Permanent impairment or disabilities that require long-term rehabilitation and medical or nursing treatment

COPING Any behavioral or cognitive activity used to deal with stress

HOMEOSTASIS A tendency of biologic systems to maintain stability of the internal environment while continuously adjusting to changes necessary for survival

PRIMARY PREVENTION Health promoting behaviors used to prevent or delay the onset of illness

SECONDARY PREVENTION Prevention of disease with an emphasis on screening for diseases already present in the body so that early diagnosis and treatment can be carried out

STRESS A physical and emotional state always present in individuals that is intensified when an internal or external environmental change or threat occurs to which they must respond

TERTIARY PREVENTION Rehabilitation and management of illness after the condition has stabilized and no further healing is expected

Human beings are complex organisms with interacting biologic, psychological, behavioral, and emotional systems. Systems within the human body are referred to as the internal environment. Systems outside the human body are known as the external environment. Health and illness are affected by both the internal and external environment.

The human body, mind, and spirit are parts of a living system. Human responses to actual or potential health problems include a myriad of reactions, many of them based on thoughts, emotions, and past experiences.

Because of cultural, educational, and social differences, individuals have very different concepts about what constitutes health and illness. People define health and illness depending on how they view themselves as a human being and as part of the surrounding environment. It is important to know how people view health and illness in order to help them achieve their personal goals for health and wellness.

THE HEALTH-ILLNESS CONTINUUM

TRADITIONAL VIEWS OF HEALTH AND ILLNESS

Traditionally, health and illness have been viewed as separate entities. People were either healthy, or they were ill. Health and illness were seen as physiologic phenomena. A typical dictionary definition of health is "soundness, especially of body or mind; freedom from disease or abnormality" (American Heritage Dictionary, 1992). In 1946, the World Health Organization defined health as "the state of complete physical, mental, and social well-being and not merely the absence of disease or infirmity."

Most definitions of health have not allowed for degrees of health nor illness and have failed to reflect the dynamic, ever-changing nature of health. Although the World Health Organization broadened the concept of health from that of a strictly physiologic entity to one that encompasses mental and social well-being, its definition is still seen today as a narrow view of health and illness.

CURRENT VIEWS OF HEALTH AND ILLNESS

Currently, health and illness are viewed as relative states along a continuum. Individuals have neither absolute health nor absolute illness but are in an ever-changing state of being, ranging from peak or high-level wellness to extreme poor health with death being imminent (Fig. 5–1).

Well-being or lack of well-being for individuals fluctuates along the continuum on a daily basis. Personal and environmental factors contribute to this state of flux. Unique internal factors within each individual influence how each person responds to external forces.

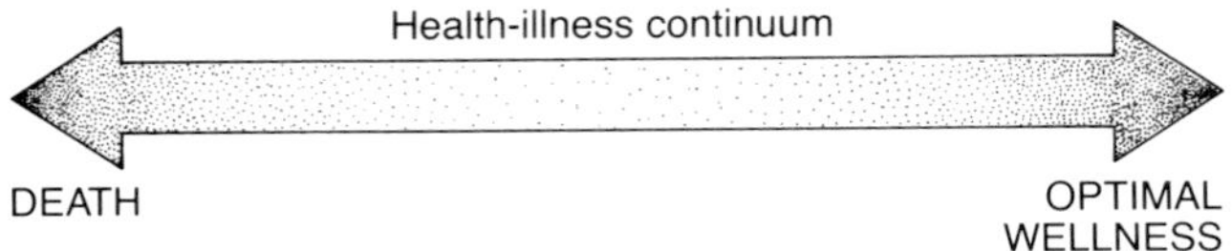

FIGURE 5-1
Common concept of health as a continuum ranging from optimal wellness at one end to illness culminating in death at the other end. (From Ignatavicius, D. D., & Bayne, M. V. [1991]. *Medical-surgical nursing: A nursing process approach* [p. 6]. Philadelphia: W. B. Saunders.)

These responses determine how individuals fulfill their needs and reach their highest health potential.

According to Dunn, who first used the term *high-level wellness*, people must accept responsibility for and take an active part in improving and maintaining their own state of wellness. Health and illness are viewed in relative terms. Each person's state of health depends on factors beyond biologic fitness. Personal, psychosocial, and spiritual values and beliefs influence how a person views health and illness.

This current view of health and illness is different from the traditional view in which health and illness were thought to be completely separate entities. An individual was considered either sick or well, with the focus of treatment on the physiologic aspects of the disease rather than on the person. Emphasis was on curing the disease or injury, not on helping individuals to maintain the highest quality of life possible when diseases are not curable. The focus of traditional health care has been on illness rather than on health promotion and disease prevention.

Keeping in mind the dynamic state of health and illness, Keane defined *health* as the ability to function well physically and mentally and to express the full range of one's potential within the environment in which one is living. A healthy person is able to adapt physically, mentally, emotionally, and socially to internal and external stimuli to maintain stability and comfort, according to Murray and Zentner.

Disease is a biologic or psychophysiologic malfunction, or both. It is a biomedical concept describing a condition of the patient that may be observed through objective means, such as temperature, presence of bacteria, or inability to perform social role tasks. Illness has a broader definition than disease. *Illness* refers to the ways the patient perceives and responds to not being well. It represents personal, interpersonal, and cultural reactions to disease.

BASIC HUMAN NEEDS

Key concepts in health and wellness include homeostasis, adaptation, the dynamic nature of the health-illness continuum, the influence of the internal and external environment, comfort, safety, social relationships, and prevention of disease and disability. To maintain the highest level of health and wellness, people must satisfy basic human needs. Three broad categories of human needs must be met: (1) physical, (2) libidinal (sensual and affectional), and (3) ego developmental.

Physiologic needs include oxygen, water, food, elimination, sleep, shelter, safety, and mobility. These needs must be met in order for individuals to survive. Libidinal needs refer to sensual-sexual and affectional-emotional needs. Sensual-sexual needs encompass the physiologic and psychological aspects of sexuality. Affectional-emotional needs are satisfied through love, security, approval, respect, support, and care. Ego-developmental needs refer to the need for cognitive, perceptual, and memory development. They are satisfied through education and training and enable individuals to attain motor coordination, independence, self-identity, social skills, communication skills, problem-solving skills, and moral development.

Abraham Maslow, a psychologist, organized human needs into a hierarchy (Fig. 5–2). Maslow's hierarchy of human needs has five levels: (1) physiologic, (2) safety and security, (3) belonging and love, (4) self-esteem, and (5) self-actualization. A person generally progresses up the hierarchy in an attempt to satisfy needs. Physiologic needs usually must be met first to progress to the satisfaction of safety and security needs, and safety and security needs must be satisfied before the needs of belonging and love can be met, and so on.

Physiologic needs include oxygen, fluid, nutrition, temperature, elimination, shelter, rest, and sex. Physiologic needs are the most fundamental because they sustain life. Individuals cannot continue to live without air, water, and food. Once the physical needs are satisfied, *safety* needs such as security, protection from harm, and freedom from anxiety and fear can be addressed. People need order and structure in their lives, and illness or disease can be very disruptive.

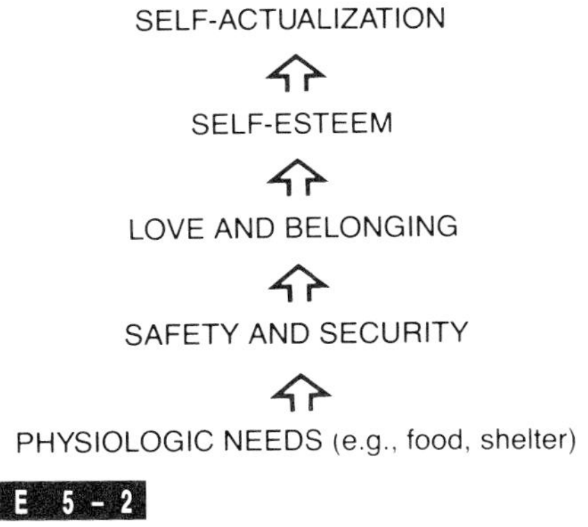

SELF-ACTUALIZATION

↑

SELF-ESTEEM

↑

LOVE AND BELONGING

↑

SAFETY AND SECURITY

↑

PHYSIOLOGIC NEEDS (e.g., food, shelter)

FIGURE 5–2

Maslow's needs hierarchy. Needs must be met in ascending order. For example, safety and security must be achieved before love and belonging. (From Ignatavicius, D. D., & Bayne, M. V. [1991]. *Medical-surgical nursing: A nursing process approach* [p. 29]. Philadelphia: W. B. Saunders.)

Love and belonging needs emerge after safety needs are met. They include feeling loved by one's family and friends and accepted by one's peers and community. Love and belonging are related to *self-esteem,* which is essential for carrying out health promoting behaviors. Self-esteem means feeling good about oneself and feeling that others hold one in high regard. Individuals with high self-esteem feel confident about themselves and confident that they are appreciated by others. People with low self-esteem may feel helpless and inferior.

Self-actualization, or self-fulfillment, is the highest level of Maslow's hierarchy. Self-actualized people are characterized by the following traits: (1) ability to solve problems, (2) willingness to accept suggestions and criticism from others, (3) broad interests, (4) good communication skills, (5) self-confidence and high self-esteem, (6) maturity, and (7) desire for new experiences and knowledge. Individuals rarely achieve self-actualization; rather, they spend most of their lives attempting to live more fully.

Although the hierarchy of needs is arranged in levels, the individual responds as a unified whole. Therefore, the needs cannot be isolated, nor can the focus of care be only on one level. In addition, individuals may move from one level to another under different conditions. However, priorities for nursing care can be based on the level of human needs, so that the physical needs must take priority over those for safety and security, and so on.

ADAPTATION TO STRESS

Human beings cannot go through life without stress. Stress is as much a part of life as breathing and eating. Stress can result from internal or external causes (Table 5–1). Environmental factors, life changes, and physiologic or emotional illness all contribute to stress.

Holmes and Ray identified life changes that caused stress for most people and ranked them according to the amount of stress that they produced. The top ten major stressors were the following:

1. Death of a spouse
2. Divorce
3. Marital separation from mate
4. Detention in jail or other institution
5. Death of a close family member
6. Major personal injury or illness
7. Marriage
8. Being fired at work
9. Marital reconciliation with mate
10. Retirement from work

Life changes can be positive or negative, but they require people to expend energy to adapt to the change. Many studies have found a significant relationship between life changes and development of physical and mental illness.

Hospitalization is a stressful event for most people. The hospital environment presents changes in the sights,

TABLE 5-1
STRESSORS: SOURCES AND EXAMPLES

SOURCES	EXAMPLES
Internal Stressors	
Physical	Overexertion or other imposed strains on body system; infections or allergens; physical trauma, e.g., surgery, accident; nutritional deficiency
Psychological	
Intrapsychic conflict	Feeling angry while fearing the consequences of expressing it
Perception of threat from events	Observing an angry person; illness of a loved one
Feelings of inadequacy, dependency, helplessness, powerlessness	Belief that life is impossible without the help and love of a significant other
Boredom	Isolated from friends and/or gratifying life experiences
External Stressors	
Conflictual relations	Marital conflict; incompatibility at work
Loss of relationship	Death of a loved one
Inability to relate, or so perceived	Language barrier
Socioeconomic	
Economic inadequacies	Unemployment, poor diet, poor housing, little recreation
Climatic extremes	Rain, clouds, little sun
Noxious stimuli	Noise, odors
Sensory deprivation	Isolation from things, people
Political climate	Repressive social system
Ethnic, religious, or national difference	Prejudice based on nationality, race, or creed

From Varcarolis, E. M. (1990). *Foundations of psychiatric mental health nursing* (p. 320). Philadelphia: W. B. Saunders.

sounds, smells, and usual routine of daily life. These changes amount to a major challenge to one's autonomy and control. Even people who are sick want to maintain a sense of control over their environment, and when they cannot, the loss of a sense of control becomes an additional stressor. Areas in which most people seek control even while they are sick include the following:

- Avoidance of pain and incapacitation
- The immediate hospital environment
- Treatments and procedures
- Relationships with hospital personnel
- Emotional balance
- A satisfactory self-image
- Relationships with family and friends
- Preparing for an uncertain future

THE STRESS RESPONSE

There are two types of stress response: (1) local adaptation syndrome and (2) general adaptation syndrome. Local adaptation syndrome is a short-term, localized response to a specific stressor that restores a body region or body part to homeostasis. Examples of this syndrome are blood clotting, wound healing, pain, and inflammation.

General adaptation syndrome is a physiologic response of the whole body to stress. It involves primarily the autonomic nervous system and the endocrine system; thus, it is often referred to as the *neuroendocrine response*. The general adaptation syndrome consists of three stages: (1) the alarm reaction, (2) the resistance stage, and (3) the exhaustion stage. The alarm reaction causes the body to respond to stress physiologically. Hormone levels, heart rate and cardiac output, respiratory rate, oxygen intake, and mental energy are increased. The pupils are dilated to allow for a larger visual field. These reactions together are called the *fight or flight response*, which helps the body to defend against stressors.

After the initial alarm stage, the body stabilizes, and physiologic processes return to normal levels. This resistance stage is characterized by adaption to the stressor. If the stressor can be overcome or the damage repaired, as in a short-term illness or injury, the body begins to heal. If the stressor is long term, such as one that accompanies a chronic physical or mental illness, an individual enters the third stage of adaptation, or the exhaustion stage. During the exhaustion stage, the body is drained of energy and can no longer defend itself against the stressor. Death may be the ultimate outcome.

There are several signs and symptoms of stress. These include cold hands and feet, tensed muscles, nervous movements, excessive sweating, tooth grinding, headaches, insomnia, and subjective complaints of feeling tense or nervous. When individuals do not cope well with stressors and are unable to adapt, they may withdraw and become depressed. Signs and symptoms of withdrawal and depression are slowed speech; lowered, hesitant speaking voice, decreased bodily movement; hunched-over, tired posture; insomnia; and subjective complaints of feeling blue, depressed, or unable to concentrate.

COPING

Coping is any behavioral or cognitive activity used to deal with stress. People cope with stress in different ways. They may use *problem-solving strategies,* which involve identifying the problem, generating alternatives, choosing the best alternative, and applying it to the problem.

Others may cope with stress by using *emotion-focused strategies.* Examples of emotion-focused strategies are distancing from the stress-provoking situation or denying its seriousness, self-isolation or withdrawal, blaming one's self or accepting responsibility for the problem, drawing strength from adversity, tension reduction, hostility, fatalism, social support, and faith. Common coping strategies and examples are listed in Table 5–2.

ADAPTATION

Adaptation to stress is essential to maintaining health. Through adaptation, individuals cope constructively with stressful conditions that are imposed either internally or externally. Adaptation is dependent on accurate appraisal of a stressful situation and effective coping. Adaptation can result in psychologic and psychological well-being.

TABLE 5-2

COMMON COPING STRATEGIES AND EXAMPLES

COPING STRATEGY	EXAMPLE
Event rehearsal	Mental and verbal preparation for an event or practice of coping strategies
Confrontation	Aggressive seeking of information, anger, refusal of treatments
Distancing or denial	Unwillingness or inability to talk about events, going on as if nothing has happened
Self-control	Stoicism, showing no feelings
Social support	Seeking out family, friends, or others in similar situations
Accepting responsibility	Verbally placing responsibility for situation on self
Faith	Praying, reading of religious material, seeking out clergy or religious guidance
Problem solving	Making plans, verbally outlining what will be done next
Positive reappraisal	Speaking of how situation has fostered growth
Event review	Discussing situations or coping that has occurred

From Ignatavicius, D. D., & Bayne, M. V. (1991). *Medical-surgical nursing: A nursing process approach* (p. 95). Philadelphia: W. B. Saunders.

A question is often raised regarding why some people adapt better than others to life circumstances. It is generally thought that adaptability is either an inborn personality trait or a characteristic that is acquired very early in childhood development. People who are able to adapt to stress usually live constructively and in relative harmony with others. They view stress as a challenge to be overcome, and they have a sense of control over their lives. Adaptable people do not feel helpless in the face of adversity but demonstrate a resilient nature in dealing with life's problems.

The nurse can help patients deal with stress by identifying their usual methods of coping or adapting to stress. These methods usually are based on the use of internal and external resources. Examples of internal resources are physiologic and psychological responses that occur when one is faced with a stressful situation such as smoking, drinking alcohol, eating, crying, and exercise. External responses include getting help from family, friends, service agencies in the community.

HOMEOSTASIS

Homeostasis is a term derived from Greek that describes a tendency of biologic systems to maintain stability of the internal environment while continually adjusting to changes necessary for survival. Although the suffix *-stasis* means "standing," this is quite the opposite of the meaning of homeostasis. Rather, the term means variation within the limits required by the body for optimal functioning. The variations take place in a predictable manner during every 24-hour period. Continuous adaptation and change must take place in the internal environment to be in harmony with the external environment.

HEALTH PROMOTION, DISEASE PREVENTION, AND HEALTH MAINTENANCE

Health promotion activities are directed toward maintaining or enhancing well-being as a protection against illness. Through consumer education, Americans increasingly have become health conscious and have begun to take responsibility for maintaining a healthy lifestyle.

The U.S. Department of Health and Human Services has developed a document outlining goals for the year 2000 called *Healthy People 2000,* and it offers a vision for the new century, characterized by significant reductions in preventable death and disability, enhanced quality of life, and greatly reduced disparities in the health status of populations within our society. The goals are as follows:

- Increase the span of healthy life for Americans
- Reduce health disparities among Americans
- Achieve access to disease prevention services for all Americans

Health promotion, health protection, and disease prevention services are activities targeted to meet these goals for all age groups (Table 5–3).

Specific activities that are generally thought to promote health are as follows:

- Adequate nutrition based on the "pyramid" concept (see Chapter 12). Foods should be eaten in moderation with emphasis on complex carbohydrates, followed by fruits and vegetables, proteins and dairy products, and a minimum amount of fats (no more than 30% of calories consumed) and simple sugars. Approximately 20 to 30 grams of dietary fiber should be taken in daily.
- Moderate exercise on a routine schedule. Twenty minutes of walking three times per week is considered ideal.
- Rest, approximately 7 to 8 hours of sleep every 24 hours.
- Healthy lifestyle, especially no smoking and limited consumption of alcohol.
- Balance of work and recreation.

These activities frequently are associated with high-level wellness.

Disease or illness prevention behavior is action taken by individuals to decrease the potential or actual threat of illness and its harmful consequences. Three levels of prevention are primary, secondary, and tertiary. *Primary prevention* includes the health promoting behaviors used to prevent or delay the onset of illness. The behaviors listed earlier, such as adequate nutrition, rest and exercise, and healthy lifestyle, are activities undertaken for primary prevention. The emphasis in *secondary prevention* is on screening for diseases that may be present in the body so that early diagnosis and treatment can be carried out. Examples of screening used for secondary prevention are mammograms, Papanicolaou smears, monthly breast examinations, and tests to detect glaucoma. *Tertiary prevention* involves rehabilitation and management of an illness after the condition has stabilized and no further healing is expected. The goal is to maintain an individual at the highest level of functioning and to prevent further disability. Examples of tertiary prevention are cardiac rehabilitation programs, rehabilitation programs for stroke, and diabetes management.

TABLE 5–3
***HEALTHY PEOPLE 2000* PRIORITY AREAS**

HEALTH PROMOTION

1. Physical activity and fitness
2. Nutrition
3. Tobacco
4. Alcohol and other drugs
5. Family planning
6. Mental health and mental disorders
7. Violent and abusive behavior
8. Educational and community-based programs

HEALTH PROTECTION

9. Unintentional injuries
10. Occupational safety and health
11. Environmental health
12. Food and drug safety
13. Oral health

PREVENTIVE SERVICES

14. Maternal and infant health
15. Heart disease and stroke
16. Cancer
17. Diabetes and chronic disabling conditions
18. Human immunodeficiency virus infection
19. Sexually transmitted diseases
20. Immunization and infectious diseases
21. Clinical preventive services

From U.S. Department of Health and Human Services (Public Health Service) (1990). *Healthy people 2000: National health promotion and disease prevention objectives* (DHHS Pub. No [PHS] 91-50212). Washington, DC: U.S. Government Printing Office.

THE CONCEPT OF ILLNESS

Illness in general is thought of as a deviation from a healthy state. However, illness may occur in the form of an acute episode or as a series of long-term events. Acute or chronic illnesses are experienced and viewed differently.

Acute illness is an illness or disease that has a relatively rapid onset and short duration. The condition usually responds to a specific treatment and ends in full recovery. Examples of acute illnesses are the common cold or influenza, appendicitis, and urinary tract infections.

Chronic illness usually involves permanent impairment or disability and requires long-term rehabilitation and medical or nursing treatment. Chronic illness is characterized by periods of remission, in which the disease seems to go away, alternating with episodes of exacerbation, in which acute symptoms flare up. Examples of chronic illnesses are rheumatoid arthritis, diabetes mellitus, and asthma.

ILLNESS BEHAVIOR

Reactions to illness vary among individuals. Some people take action, whereas others may do nothing. Those who take action may seek the help of health care providers, such as physicians, nurses, or dentists; others may seek help from friends or family members. In some sections of the United States, people may seek help from folk healers. The actions taken by individuals are influenced by the availability and affordability of health care, the client's perception of the problem, others' perception of the problem, or the failure or success of self-prescribed treatment.

People who take no action may wait to see whether the symptoms go away by themselves. Others may deny that something is wrong and are unwilling to admit that they are ill. People who take no action may be influenced by the same factors that affect those who take action.

Some individuals take counteraction in response to illness. They may engage in activities that should be avoided just to prove to themselves that the symptoms do not exist. For example, a person with symptoms of chronic bronchitis may continue to smoke regardless of the impaired breathing and choking that the smoke may cause. Patients who have a history of failure to follow proper health practices or treatment regimens are referred to as persons experiencing "altered health maintenance," which can have deleterious effects on health and self-esteem and can lead to death.

The Sick Role

When people become ill, they frequently adopt a "sick role." The sick role allows individuals time to recover from their disease. Because they cannot get well on their own, others must care for them. They are temporarily exempt from social responsibilities so that they can concentrate on getting well. It is assumed that people who are sick want to get well and therefore should seek the help of health professionals and cooperate with prescribed health care regimens (Table 5–4). However, some people derive other gains from the sick role, such as attention from family and health care professionals and avoidance of work. The sick role does not apply to individuals with minor illnesses, such as the common cold, or to those with terminal illnesses.

IMPACT OF ILLNESS ON THE FAMILY

Illness does not affect individuals in isolation; rather, it has an impact on the entire family. The illness may change the roles of the various family members, the daily activities carried out, or the economic stability of the family.

Three factors influence the effect of illness on the family. The first factor is the identity of the member of the family who is ill. For example, if the head of the household and chief breadwinner is sick, the financial resources may be threatened. If the person who normally cares for the home and children becomes ill, others have to pitch in to help. If an elderly member of the family becomes ill, grown children may have to provide care. The reversal in the parent-child roles may be difficult for both parents and children.

The second factor influencing the effect of illness on the family is the seriousness and duration of the disease. An acute illness certainly does not produce the long-term effects of a chronic disease. Family members are able to change roles temporarily to manage an acute illness, but during the long duration of a chronic illness, family relationships may become strained.

The third factor is the social and cultural customs of the family. Families of various cultures have different attitudes towards illness, caregiving, and changing family roles.

TABLE 5-4
SICK ROLE BEHAVIORS

1. Exemption from normal activities
2. Recognition that the sick person is not responsible for causing the condition
3. Expectation that the sick person wants to get well
4. Obligation to seek competent help

All of these factors can have an effect on family functioning. Feelings of frustration, anger, and grief must be dealt with so that all members of the family can function at their highest potential while providing care for the sick member.

IMPLICATIONS FOR NURSING CARE

PREVENT HEALTH PROBLEMS

Nurses can help clients to engage in healthier lifestyles to prevent disease. Nursing measures are geared toward helping clients to make informed decisions regarding their health care practices. Examples of nursing measures are the following:

- Inform clients of daily activities, such as the proper diet, exercise, and adequate sleep, that help maintain optimal health.
- Inform clients about the diseases for which they are at risk.
- Explain the consequences of the disease for which they are at risk.
- Give clients specific information about how they can reduce their risk for the disease.

It is important to keep in mind when counseling clients and their families that most health promotion and disease prevention measures require a change in lifestyle. Nurses should take into consideration the biophysical, psychological, sociocultural, and environmental dimensions of family life and structure and be realistic in their expectations for change.

HELP SATISFY PATIENT'S UNMET BASIC HUMAN NEEDS

For people to maintain the highest levels of health and wellness, basic human needs must be met. According to Henderson (1964), "The unique function of the nurse is to assist the individual, sick or well, in the performance of those activities contributing to health or its recovery (or to a peaceful death) that he would perform unaided if he had the necessary strength, will, or knowledge. And to do this in such a way as to help him gain independence as rapidly as possible."

Henderson identified 14 components of basic nursing care (Table 5–5). The needs are closely related to Maslow's hierarchy of human needs, in that components 1 through 8 address physical needs, component 9 refers to safety needs, 10 and 11 to belonging and love needs, and 12 through 14 to self-esteem and self-actualization needs.

INCREASE ADAPTABILITY

The first step in helping clients to increase adaptability is to determine what the client perceives as stressful and how stressful it is. One way to assess the degree

TABLE 5-5
COMPONENTS OF BASIC NURSING CARE

1. Breathe normally.
2. Eat and drink adequately.
3. Eliminate body wastes.
4. Move and maintain desirable posture.
5. Sleep and rest.
6. Select suitable clothing—dress and undress.
7. Maintain body temperature within the normal range by adjusting clothing and modifying the environment.
8. Keep the body clean and well-groomed and protect the integument.
9. Avoid dangers in the environment and avoid injuring others.
10. Communicate with others in expressing emotions, needs, fears, and opinions.
11. Worship according to one's faith.
12. Work in such a way that there is a sense of accomplishment.
13. Play or participate in various forms of recreation.
14. Learn, discover, or satisfy curiosity.

Reprinted with the permission of Simon & Schuster from Henderson, V. (1966). *The nature of nursing* (pp. 16–17). New York: Macmillan Co. Copyright © 1966 Virginia Henderson.

of stress is to ask clients to name the worst possible stressor and then compare the present stressor to that. The second step is to assess past methods of coping with stress that have been successful for the client. It is then helpful to apply past coping strategies to new situations. The nurse may assess internal coping strategies by asking, "What kinds of things do you do when you are stressed?" "Do you eat more or less?" "Do you drink alcohol?" "Do you smoke more?" "Do you sleep more or less?" Questions that help determine external coping strategies include, "Whom do you turn to when you are feeling stressed?" "Do you talk with others or do you keep things inside?" "Do you contact any professionals such as social workers, nurses, doctors, or social agencies when you have a problem?"

Elderly persons have particular difficulty coping with stress and adapting to new situations. When any type of stressor occurs, it takes longer and is much harder to get back to their previous level of functioning. Fortunately, people who have lived a long time have experienced many stresses throughout life and generally have developed a wide range of coping mechanisms and skills for adapting to change. Nursing interventions should be geared toward helping older clients to use past successful coping mechanisms to deal with new stressors. The emphasis should be on strengths rather than on limitations.

During hospitalization, the nurse can help clients and families adapt to a difficult situation by helping them to cope with the stress of a new environment, illness, and uncertainty. Some clients and families benefit from detailed information about the disease and the hospital procedures; others prefer not to know. Allowing patients to have as much control as possible helps to reduce stress. Even people who are very dependent on hospital personnel need to feel that they have some control over their lives. Other measures that may help to relieve stress and promote coping and adaptation are biofeedback, progressive muscle relaxation, meditation, and imagery. These strategies generally focus attention inward to the patient's own mind and body and reduce either physical or emotional tension.

FOSTER INDEPENDENCE

In acute illness, recovery is usually speedy, and people return quickly to their previous lifestyle. However, individuals with chronic illnesses must spend a lifetime managing symptoms. Many elderly persons have one or more chronic illnesses and may need some type of assistance in their daily lives. The goal is to maintain the highest level of independence possible and prevent further disability. The following tasks have been identified for chronically ill individuals: prevent and manage crises, carry out prescribed regimens, control symptoms, reorder time, adjust to changes in the course of the illness, prevent social isolation, and attempt to normalize social interactions.

PREVENT AND MANAGE CRISES. When symptoms flare up, a crisis situation may arise. Nurses can help clients and families to prevent and control a crisis situation. The client and family members must learn signs and symptoms of the onset of crisis and make a plan for how to deal with it.

CARRY OUT PRESCRIBED REGIMENS. Chronically ill individuals may need to take many medications, eat special foods, or be restricted in some activities. It is very difficult to have a restricted lifestyle day in and day out, especially when symptoms are not apparent. Nursing interventions include teaching clients about the necessity of carrying out regimens, providing moral support and encouragement, and finding ways to make carrying out regimens easier. Nurses may help increase patient compliance by forming "alliances" with patients, helping them to feel like an important participant in developing their own health regimen.

CONTROL SYMPTOMS. Chronically ill individuals must learn to control symptoms to continue desired activities. Nursing interventions should be geared to helping clients learn about the pattern of symptoms (typical onset, duration, and severity) and the limits of their abilities in controlling symptoms. Daily routines can be arranged so that the highest levels of activities are carried out when symptoms are lessened or absent, and periods of rest are taken when symptoms are most acute.

REORDER TIME. People with chronic illness may find they have either too much or too little available time. Forced retirement may increase the amount of free time; conversely, carrying out regimens to manage symptoms may be extremely time consuming for clients and caregivers. In both situations, the chronically ill and their family members may become frustrated and depressed. The nurse can help clients and caregivers to develop a daily schedule that allows time for desired activities while managing the regimens of the chronic illness.

ADJUST TO CHANGES IN THE COURSE OF THE DISEASE. Chronic illnesses often have unpredictable courses, and individuals must learn to live with the ups and downs of the disease. Nurses need to support chronically ill individuals to help them adjust to a life that is lived to their highest potential.

PREVENT SOCIAL ISOLATION. Chronically ill individuals and their families often become socially isolated. The ill person may withdraw from others, or others may feel uncomfortable and withdraw. Support groups are helpful for providing a social outlet with others in the same situation.

ATTEMPT TO NORMALIZE SOCIAL INTERACTIONS. Although chronically ill individuals may have to spend time and energy managing symptoms or they may look different because of disfigurement or the need to wear a special prosthesis, they need to maintain as normal a lifestyle as possible. They should be encouraged to live as independently as possible in spite of their illness.

It is important to assess the availability of support systems for the chronically ill. Families are the major support systems for persons with chronic illnesses and provide the day-to-day ongoing care. Formal support systems include social service agencies, health care providers, and community agencies. If family members are unavailable or unable to provide support, formal services may be needed.

ASSIST FAMILY MEMBERS IN DEALING WITH PATIENT'S ILLNESS

As noted earlier, families provide the bulk of support for the chronically ill. Because families provide the majority of the caregiving, the burden is heavy for them. They must assume an increased physical burden of work because of the need to assist with activities of daily living, deal with changes in the progress of the disease, cope with feelings of being psychologically and physically overwhelmed, and adapt to changes in their own social roles and identities as well as those of the family member because of the illness. In some cases, family caregivers also may have a chronic illness that must be managed, or they may develop a physical illness or disability as a result of the burdens of caregiving. This is especially true among elderly caregivers.

Health care providers need to assist clients and their family members in the development of a collaborative plan of care. In some cases, relief or respite can be obtained to ease the caregiving responsibility. Many communities have adult daycare centers for older adults or persons with particular chronic illnesses, which enable both the older or chronically ill individuals and their caregivers to assume a more "normal" lifestyle with social interaction and structure. Formal support services should be used whenever needed to assist families to take care of their chronically ill loved ones.

ASSIST TERMINALLY ILL PATIENTS TO A PEACEFUL DEATH

Unfortunately everyone must die. Nurses are often the health care providers who have the most intimate relationship with people who are terminally ill. When death comes accidentally or after an acute illness, there is little or no time to prepare for death. But when disease is chronic, patients and families often need to make difficult decisions regarding death.

In today's health care system with its sophisticated technology, terminally ill patients may be kept alive longer than has ever been possible before. Issues related to the setting in which the terminally ill are cared for, whether machines for artificial physiologic functioning are used, and when these machines are turned off must be faced on a daily basis. Families, more than anyone else, have to live with the memory of their loved ones and the events surrounding their death.

Nurses should be supportive of decisions made by clients and families. The dying patients and their loved ones should be informed of the options for care and their consequences. Open communication and acknowledgment of different attitudes toward terminal illness and death are extremely important. The nurse should have knowledge of the dying process and the needs of the dying person to provide compassionate care, promote comfort, and make the pain and physical treatment bearable. More detailed information on caring for terminally ill patients is found in Chapter 22.

BIBLIOGRAPHY

Abood, D. A., & Burkhead, E. J. (1988). Wellness: A valuable resource for persons with disabilities. *Health Education, 19*(2), 21–25.

Alford, D. M., & Futrell, M. (1992). Wellness and health promotion of the elderly. *Nursing Outlook, 40*(5), 221–226.

American heritage dictionary (3rd ed.). New York: Houghton Mifflin, 1992.

Benson, E. R., & McDevitt, J. Q. (1989). Home care and the older adult: Illness care versus wellness care. *Holistic Nursing Practice, 3*(2), 30–38.

Bestard, S., & Courtenay, M. (1990). Focusing on wellness. *Canadian Nurse, 86*(11), 24–25.

Cousins, N. (1989). Proving the power of laughter. *Psychology Today, 23*(10), 22–25.

deChesnay, M., & Magnuson, N. (1988). How healthy families cope with stress. *AAOHN Journal, 36*(9), 361–365.

DesRosier, M. B., Catanzaro, M., & Piller, J. (1992). Living with chronic illness: Social support and the well spouse perspective. *Rehabilitation Nursing, 17*(2), 87–91.

Edlin, G., & Golanty, E. (1992). *Health and wellness: A holistic approach* (4th ed.). Boston: Jones and Bartlett Publishers, Inc.

Faris, G. J. (1989). The power of positive thinking. *Clinical Management in Physical Therapy, 9*(6), 12–13, 15, 17–18.

Findlay, S., & Brownlee, S. (1990). The delicate dance of body and mind . . . The connection between emotions and health. *US News & World Report, 109*(1), 54.

Gorton, D. (1988). Holistic health techniques to increase individual coping and wellness. *Journal of Holistic Nursing, 6*(1), 25–30.

Henderson, V. (1964). The nature of nursing. *AJN, 64*, 64.

Hinds, C. (1992). Suffering: A relatively unexplored phenomenon among family caregivers of non-institutionalized patients with cancer. *Journal of Advanced Nursing, 17*(8), 918–925.

Holmes, T. H., & Rahe, R. H. (1967). The social readjustment rating scale. *Journal of Psychosomatic Research, 2*, 213–218.

Hull, M. M. (1992). Coping strategies of family caregivers in hospice homecare. *Oncology Nursing Forum, 19*(8), 1179–1187.

Ignatavicius, D. D., & Bayne, M. V. (1991). *Medical-surgical nursing: A nursing process approach.* Philadelphia: W. B. Saunders.

Jones, P. S. (1991). Adaptability: A personal resource for health . . . Including commentary by Hall, B. A. *Scholarly Inquiry For Nursing Practice, 5*(2), 95–112.

Kruger, S. (1992). Parents in crisis: Helping them cope with a seriously ill child. *Journal of Pediatric Nursing, 7*(2), 133–140.

Larsen, P., & Simons, N. (1993). Evaluating a federal health and fitness program: Indicators of improving health. *AAOHN Journal, 41*(3), 143–148.

Martin, P. (1990). A feeling that needs expressing: Helping patients manage their anxiety. *Professional Nurse, 5*(7), 374–375.

McHaffie, H. E. (1992). Coping: An essential element of Nursing. *Journal of Advanced Nursing, 17*(8), 933–940.

Monsen, R. B., Floyd, R. L., & Brookman, J. C. (1992). Stress-coping-adaptation: Concepts for nursing. *Nursing Forum, 27*(4), 27–32.

Morse, J. M., & Johnson, J. L. (1991). *The illness experience: Dimensions of suffering.* Sapaponack, NY: Sage Press, Inc.

Murray, R. B., & Zentner, J. P. (1989). *Nursing assessment and health promotion strategies through the life span* (4th ed.). Norwalk, CT: Appleton & Lange.

Paluszny, M. J., DeBeukelaer, M. M., & Rowane, W. A. (1991). Families coping with the multiple crises of chronic illness. *Loss, Grief & Care, 5*(1/2), 15–26.

Saltonstall, R. (1993). Healthy bodies, social bodies: Men's and women's concepts and practices of health in everyday life. *Social Science & Medicine, 36*(1), 7–14.

Selby, T. (1991). Wellness: Nurses lead the way to better health. *American Nurse, 23*(4), 1, 28.

Sheahan, S. L., & Garrity, T. F. (1992). Stress and tobacco addiction. *Journal of the American Academy of Nurse Practitioners, 4*(3), 111–116.

Smith, D. B. (1991). Two faces have I . . . The experience of cancer. *Oncology Nursing Forum, 18*(5), 835–839.

Snyder, R. (1992). Coping: You and your patient with cancer. *Clinical Management, 12*(4), 64–69.

Sutherland, J. E. (1991). The link between stress and illness: Do our coping methods influence our health? *Postgraduate Medicine, 89*(1), 159–164, 263–266.

Swinford, P. A., & Webster, J. A. (1989). *Promoting wellness: A nurse's handbook.* Germantown, MD: Aspen Publishers, Inc.

U.S. Department of Agriculture/U.S. Department of Health and Human Services, 1993.

U.S. Department of Health and Human Services (Public Health Service) (1990). *Healthy people 2000: National health promotion and disease prevention objectives* (DHHS Pub. No. [PHS] 91-50212). Washington, DC: U.S. Government Printing Office.

Varcarolis, E. M. (1990). *Foundations of psychiatric mental health nursing.* Philadelphia: W. B. Saunders.

Walker, S. N. (1992). Wellness for elders. *Holistic Nursing Practice, 7*(1), 38–45.

Wilson, L. M. (1988). The American revolution in health care. *AAOHN Journal, 36*(10), 402–407.

KEY CONCEPTS

1. Because of cultural, educational, and social differences, individuals have very different concepts about what constitutes health and illness.
2. Health and illness are viewed as relative states along a continuum that fluctuates on a daily basis.
3. Disease is a biologic or psychophysiologic malfunction, or both, and illness refers to how a person perceives and responds to not being well.
4. To maintain the highest level of health and wellness, people must satisfy basic human needs.
5. There are three broad categories of human needs: physical, libidinal, and ego developmental.
6. Stress is mental or emotional pressure resulting from internal or external causes.
7. Coping is any behavioral or cognitive activity used to deal with stress.
8. Homeostasis describes a tendency of biologic systems to maintain stability of the internal environment while continuously adjusting to changes necessary for survival.
9. Health promotion activities are directed toward maintaining or enhancing well-being as a protection against illness.
10. Illness is a deviation from a healthy state that may occur in the form of an acute episode or as a series of long-term events.
11. Reactions to illness vary among individuals.
12. When people become ill, they often assume a "sick role" that allows them time to recover from their disease.
13. The impact of illness on the family depends on which family member is ill, the seriousness of the illness, and the social and cultural customs of the family.
14. Nurses help people by striving to prevent disease, helping satisfy clients' unmet basic needs, helping clients increase adaptability, fostering independence, helping family members deal with patients' illnesses, and assisting terminally ill patients to a peaceful death.

Mary Ann Matteson

CHAPTER 6

Developmental Processes

OBJECTIVES

1. List the developmental tasks for successful adulthood.
2. Identify the health problems specific to the adult age groups.
3. Discuss the health care needs of young, middle-aged, and older adults.

GLOSSARY

BIOLOGIC AGE The functional capabilities of various organ systems in the body

PSYCHOLOGICAL AGE The behavioral capacity of a person to adapt to changing environmental demands

SOCIAL AGE The roles and habits of a person in relation to other members of society

Each stage of life has specific developmental processes that must be undertaken and mastered to go on to the next stage successfully. These developmental processes consist of physical, emotional, social, and psychological changes that present challenges to every living human being. In this chapter, we discuss the developmental processes associated with young adulthood, middle age, and older age.

YOUNG ADULTHOOD

Young adulthood comes at a time when physical growth ends and social expectations begin. It is considered to occur during a person's twenties, thirties, and forties; however, these decades are often divided by such terms as *young-young adult* (age 20–35) and *old-young adult* (age 35–45).

Young adulthood is a time for settling down to a job and raising a family and taking on new responsibilities. Most people in this age group are expected to leave their parents' home and to establish their own home. People in their twenties and early thirties must begin this process by establishing an intimate, lasting relationship with another person in which the physical satisfaction and psychological security of another are more important than their own. Without the development of an intimate relationship, the young adult can become isolated, lonely, and self-absorbed.

Many young people have extended their education and have prolonged the time in which they continue to live at home; or a job loss, divorce, or other stressor may precipitate a move back home. The entire family then has to adjust to a young adult living at home by redistributing roles and responsibilities, maintaining adequate communication, and reallocating budget and space. This may be a difficult time for parents, who had expected a new time of freedom and independence in their middle years. It is especially difficult if young grandchildren are included in the package.

DEVELOPMENTAL TASKS

The following developmental tasks must be achieved by young adults:

- Accept self and stabilize self-concept and body image.
- Establish independence from parental home and financial aid.
- Become established in a vocation or profession that provides personal satisfaction, economic independence, and a feeling of making a worthwhile contribution to society.
- Learn to appraise and express love responsibly through more than sexual contact.
- Establish an intimate bond with another, either through marriage or with a close friend.
- Establish and maintain a home and manage a time schedule and life stresses.
- Find a congenial social and friendship group.
- Decide whether to have a family and carry out tasks of parenting.
- Formulate a meaningful philosophy of life and reassess priorities and values.
- Become involved as a citizen in the community.

It is evident that these developmental tasks focus on marriage, childbearing, and work.

HEALTH PROBLEMS

Young adults, especially those in their twenties and early thirties have relatively few health problems. The four major causes of death in the young adult age group do not result from illness but from violence: (1) vehicular accidents, (2) other accidents, (3) suicide, and (4) homicide. As young adults progress into their late thirties and early forties, the primary causes of death are malignancies and heart disease, followed by accidents and infection with the human immunodeficiency (HIV) virus.

Typical health problems are related to stress on the job or in social interactions, lifestyle, and childbearing. They include depression; anxiety; complications of pregnancy; cervical and breast cancer; and back, hip, and limb injuries. In the quest for meaningful social relationships and a career that will gain them independence and success, young adults may experience tension and stress and may lack the time to attend to health promoting activities such as a proper diet and nutrition. They may work hard and party enthusiastically. Meals may be eaten on the run, and the diet may consist primarily of junk foods. Smoking and alcohol or drug abuse are common. These practices may have a direct bearing on health in the later years (Table 6–1).

As young adults enter their thirties and early forties, their focus is directed mainly toward raising a family and furthering a career (Fig. 6–1). It may be a time to reassess their lives and careers, and often major changes are made. Factors that contribute to health problems are stress related to work, marital problems, and stress related to managing a household. Couples who have postponed childbearing may have difficulties with conception and pregnancy.

HEALTH CARE NEEDS

Health care needs are related to promoting optimal health. It is a good idea to have at least one thorough physical examination during the twenties. A physical examination should include tests for sexually transmitted diseases, hypertension, and cholesterol level. A tetanus booster should be given if persons have not received one in the last 10 years. Young women should have a Papanicolaou smear every 3 years and should be taught breast self-examination. Young men should be taught to do a testicular examination.

Health counseling should focus on health promoting behaviors. Programs may be established to include topics such as nutrition; exercise and leisure; rest and sleep; human sexuality and family planning; and the effects of smoking, drugs, and alcohol.

TABLE 6-1

HARMFUL HEALTH PRACTICES, EFFECTS ON HEALTH IN THE LATER YEARS, AND PREVENTIVE MEASURES

HARMFUL HEALTH PRACTICE	POSSIBLE EFFECT ON HEALTH	PREVENTIVE MEASURES
Lack of physical activity and fitness	Diabetes, osteoporosis, heart disease, stroke, colon cancer, obesity, depression	Increase moderate daily physical activity and reduce sedentary lifestyle
Obesity	Heart disease, hypertension, atherosclerosis, cancer, stroke, non–insulin-dependent diabetes mellitus	Maintain ideal body weight; maintain low cholesterol, low-fat (<30%), nutritious diet with plenty of vegetables, fruits, and grain products
Cigarette smoking	Heart disease; cancers of the lung, larynx, pharynx, oral cavity, esophagus, pancreas, and bladder; chronic bronchitis and emphysema	Stop smoking or do not start smoking
Alcohol and drug abuse	Malnutrition, cirrhosis of the liver, brain damage, mental status changes, homicides, suicides, and motor vehicle fatalities	Limit alcohol intake and stop using drugs or do not start; participate in 12-step program for rehabilitation
Stress	Stress-related conditions such as hypertension and heart disease	Recognize and modify stressors; use a stress management program, such as exercise or biofeedback

Adapted from U.S. Department of Health and Human Services (Public Health Service). (1990). *Healthy people 2000: National health promotion and disease prevention objectives* (DHHS Publication No. [PHS] 91-50213). Washington, DC: U.S. Government Printing Office.

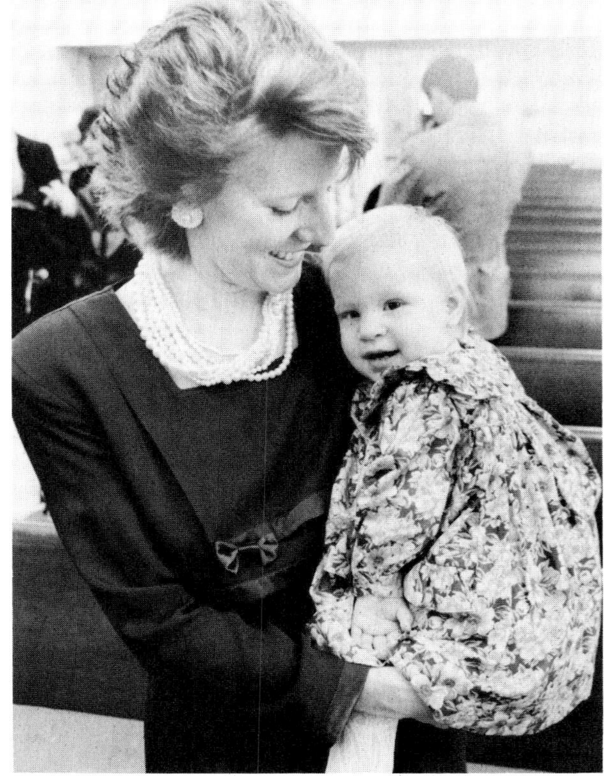

FIGURE 6-1
The focus of young adults is mainly on raising a family, furthering a career, or both. (Photograph by Stephen Matteson, Jr.)

In the years between 30 and 45, especially after age 35, young adults should begin to think about the prevention of chronic illness, particularly cancer and heart disease. They should have periodic physical examinations, usually recommended at age 30, age 35, and then every 3 years thereafter. The physical examination should include tests for hypertension, anemia, and cholesterol and a cervical Papanicolaou smear for women. Women should have a baseline mammogram at age 35. Monthly breast self-examinations for women and testicular self-examinations for men should be ongoing. It is suggested that people in this age group examine their skin and mouth periodically for precancerous lesions. Preventive dental checkups and treatment are usually recommended every 6 months to 2 years.

Health promotion and disease prevention programs have a similar focus to those for people in their twenties. Stress management, effective parenting, proper diet and nutrition, exercise, drug and alcohol awareness, and smoking cessation are appropriate topics for health teaching and counseling.

MIDDLE YEARS

The terms *middle years, middle age,* or *middle adulthood* usually refer to the ages between 45 and 65. However, other factors define middle age, particularly how a person acts and feels. Because life expectancy has increased so dramatically during the past 50 years, middle age is a relatively new concept. Previously, the majority of people did not live past their forties, so that what used to be old age is now middle age.

More than 40 million Americans, or one fourth of the U.S. population, are considered middle aged. They earn most of the money, pay most of the taxes, and have most of the power in business and government. Middle age is a time of relatively good health. People experience a new personal freedom and enjoy maximum command of themselves and influence over others.

Many people who are in their middle years belong to a group called the "sandwich generation." They may have teenagers and young adults at home and at the same time have ailing, elderly parents to care for. People who have put off pregnancy and childbearing may have even younger children at home.

Many of today's middle-aged women are working outside the home and have developed important careers. Work and family obligations together may require a balancing act for middle-aged women who are trying to maintain continued involvement both at work and at home. The result can be a great deal of stress and conflict.

DEVELOPMENTAL TASKS

The following developmental tasks should be accomplished by people in their middle years:

- Discover and develop new satisfaction with a mate or significant other by enjoying mutual activities, providing mutual support, and developing a deeper sense of unity and intimacy.
- Help growing and grown children to become happy and responsible adults.
- Create a pleasant, hospitable, and comfortable home, compatible with one's values, income, and resources.
- Balance work and other roles; prepare for retirement.
- Accept role reversal with aging parents; prepare emotionally for the eventual death of living parents.
- Achieve mature social and civic responsibilities and give time and resources to the community.
- Accept and adjust to the physical changes of middle age and maintain and establish a healthy lifestyle.
- Continue to formulate a philosophy of life and to grow spiritually.
- Develop satisfying leisure activities.
- Recognize the inevitability of death and prepare for one's own eventual death.

Middle-aged persons who successfully master developmental tasks begin to accept their age and gradually come to value the wisdom gained from living and experience rather than the physical power and strength that accompanies youth. Emotional and mental flexibility increases the ability to change and adapt to new situations and to be open to others. It is a time of "mellowing-out," of accepting what life has to offer.

HEALTH PROBLEMS

People in their middle years continue to be relatively healthy, and the same factors that contribute to the deterioration of health habits in the young adult apply to those in middle age. The major cause of death is cardiovascular disease, and the most common health problems, along with cardiovascular disease, are cancer, pulmonary disease, diabetes, obesity, alcoholism, anxiety, depression, and glaucoma. Respiratory conditions are a frequent cause for days absent from work in women; injuries are a frequent cause for men.

HEALTH CARE NEEDS

The health care goals for the middle aged are the same as those for the young. They are focused on health promotion and disease prevention to preserve and prolong the period of maximum energy and optimal mental and social activity.

During the middle years, regular assessment of health status is important for maintaining good health. Early diagnosis of illness helps prevent later complications. A complete physical examination is recommended at age 40 and every 3 years thereafter. Routine blood pressure screening and cholesterol and glucose testing are recommended.

Women should continue to conduct regular breast self-examinations and have a mammogram every 2 to 3 years during their mid to late forties and every year after age 50. Women usually enter menopause (permanent cessation of menstruation) between ages 45 and 50. Menopause is preceded by the perimenopausal period (approximately 5 years) in which there is a gradual decrease in estrogen accompanied by a gradual decrease in menstrual flow. During the menopausal years, women may experience symptoms such as hot flashes, dizziness, headaches, perspiration, palpitations, water retention, nausea, muscle cramps, fatigability, insomnia, or tingling of the fingers and toes. Many women take estrogen to relieve many of the symptoms of menopause.

Health promotion activities during middle age are the same as for young adulthood. The focus is on proper nutrition, exercise, stress management, and reduction or elimination of smoking, drug, and alcohol use.

OLDER ADULTS

Age 65 and older is frequently a marker of old age. However, many people in their sixties do not consider themselves old, and they continue to live healthy, productive lives. Other markers besides chronologic age may be more accurate in defining older age: (1) biologic age, (2) psychological age, and (3) social age. *Biologic age* focuses on the functional capabilities of various organ systems in the body. Many older people continue to function well, especially those who engage in exercise and other health promoting activities, whereas others seem to be prematurely ill and frail. *Psychological age* refers to the behavioral capacity of the person to adapt to changing environmental demands. The older person's ability to remember, learn, and exercise behavioral control are factors that affect psychological age. *Social age* refers to the roles and habits of a person in relation to other members of society, including such aspects as the person's type of dress, language, and social relationships.

During older age, men and women are required to make many adjustments to physiologic, psychological, and social changes. Declines in bodily function, particularly in vision and hearing, and physical strength and resiliency may have an effect on day-to-day functioning. Psychological changes are decreased short-term memory, slower performance on cognitive tasks, and longer learning time. Older people retain psychological skills, but they usually take longer to accomplish. Social changes include retirement, change in living conditions, and loss of spouse and significant others.

DEVELOPMENTAL TASKS

The following developmental tasks must be achieved by older adults:

- Recognize the aging process and adjust to decreasing physical strength and health changes.
- Adjust to retirement; adjust living standards to retirement income.
- Establish satisfactory living arrangements as a result of role changes.
- Maintain emotional satisfaction in relationships with spouse, children, grandchildren, and other living relatives.
- Establish an affiliation with members of own age group; maintain an interest in people outside the family and in the community.
- Maintain maximum level of health; learn to adjust to the loss of physical strength, illness, and the approach of one's death.
- Cope with the death of parents, spouses, and friends.
- Learn to combine new dependency needs with the continuing need for independence.

Developmental tasks in older age focus on the redirection of energy and talents to new roles and activities, the acceptance of life with its joys and limitations, and the development of a personal view of death in preparation for this final stage of life.

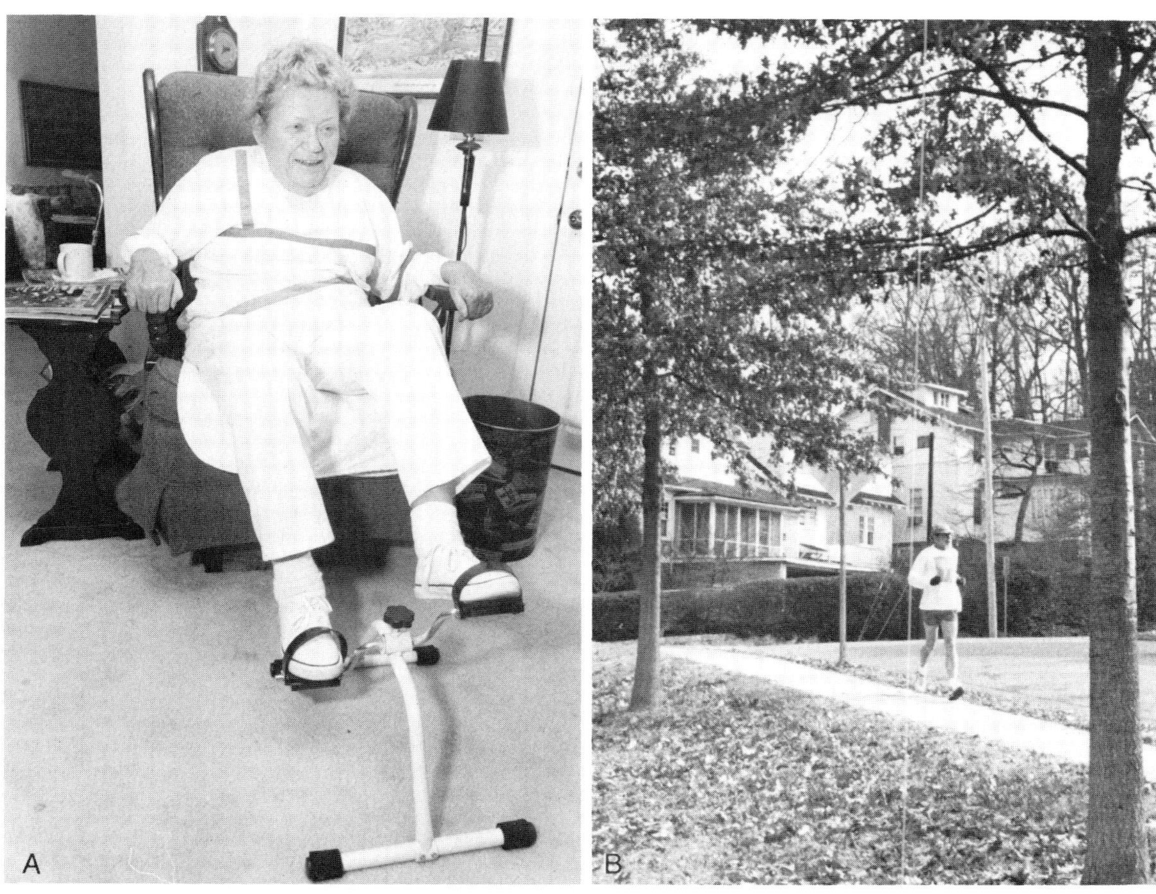

FIGURE 6-2
Exercise is beneficial for persons of any age and in any condition. (Photographs by Stephen Matteson, Jr.)

HEALTH PROBLEMS

The major causes of death in older age are related to chronic illness, specifically cardiovascular disease, cancer, and diabetes mellitus. Accidents, including falls, are the fourth leading cause of death in this age group. The most common illnesses are arthritis, gastrointestinal problems (peptic ulcer and constipation), acute and chronic respiratory diseases (influenza, pneumonia, emphysema), and gallbladder disease. Benign or malignant enlargement of the prostate is common in older men; breast cancer is common in older women.

HEALTH CARE NEEDS

The health care goals in the older age group are to manage chronic illnesses and to maintain and prolong the period of optimal physical, mental, and social activity. It is important to help older adults maintain their independence as long as possible in the face of one or more chronic illnesses.

Physical examinations should be done periodically and include the same assessment as indicated in the middle years. Dental examinations and treatment should also be continued into older age. As people age, periodic evaluation and treatment of the feet by a podiatrist is recommended to promote mobility. An influenza vaccination is recommended yearly for persons older than 65 years.

Health promotion activities should continue into older age. These activities can increase quality of life and in many cases, prevent many of the chronic illnesses that accompany the later years. Proper nutrition, especially a low fat, high fiber diet with a large amount of complex carbohydrates, helps to maintain energy, promote intestinal motility, and decrease the susceptibility to some chronic illnesses. Exercise can benefit older adults, even the very old who begin an exercise program for the first time. Walking is the ideal exercise, and 20 to 30 minutes three times a week is adequate to maintain weight, blood pressure, coordination, and mobility and to create a positive outlook on life (Fig. 6–2). Older people also can benefit from counseling for alcohol and drug abuse and smoking cessation. It is never too late to improve one's health habits.

Chapter 7 discusses health care issues related to the older adult in more depth.

BIBLIOGRAPHY

Erikson, E. (1963). *Childhood and society* (2nd ed.). New York: W. W. Norton.

Murray, R. B., & Zentner, J. P. (1989). *Nursing assessment and health promotion strategies through the life span* (4th ed.). East Norwalk, CT: Appleton & Lange.

U.S. Department of Health and Human Services (Public Health Service). (1990). *Healthy people 2000: National health promotion and disease prevention objectives* (DHHS Publication No. [PHS] 91-50213). Washington, DC: U.S. Government Printing Office.

KEY CONCEPTS

1. Developmental processes are changes that present challenges to human beings that must be undertaken and mastered to go on to the next stage successfully.
2. Developmental tasks for young adults center around acceptance of self, independence, intimacy, home and time management, social relationships, community involvement, and formulation of a meaningful philosophy of life.
3. Health problems of young adults are related to stress on the job or in social interactions, lifestyle, and childbearing.
4. Developmental tasks for middle-aged adults focus on interpersonal relationships, guidance of grown children, creation of a pleasant home, balanced roles, care of aging parents, civic responsibilities, adjustment of physical changes, satisfying leisure activities, formulation of a life philosophy, and recognition of death's inevitability.
5. Health problems of middle-aged adults include cardiovascular disease, cancer, pulmonary disease, diabetes, obesity, alcoholism, anxiety, depression, and glaucoma.
6. Developmental tasks for older adults include adjustment to aging and retirement, establishment of satisfactory living arrangements, maintenance of emotional satisfaction in relationships, affiliation with peers, maintenance of maximal level of health, coping with deaths of others, and learning to combine new dependency needs with the need for independence.
7. Health problems for older adults include cardiovascular disease, cancer, diabetes mellitus, accidents, arthritis, gastrointestinal problems, and respiratory diseases.

J. Taylor Harden

CHAPTER 7

The Older Patient

OBJECTIVES

1. Describe the roles of the gerontological nurse.
2. Compare the myths and stereotypes of the aging population with current statistical trends.
3. Describe biologic and physiologic factors associated with aging.
4. Explain psychosocial factors associated with aging.
5. Describe modifications needed for activities of daily living.
6. Identify various groups of drugs that need modification because of changes brought about by aging.

GLOSSARY

AGEISM A process of systematic stereotyping and discrimination against people because of their age; usually directed against older people

AGING The process of growing older or more mature

CATARACT Clouding or opacity of the normally transparent lens within the eye; causes blurred vision and objects to take on a yellowish hue

CONDUCTION DEAFNESS A hearing impairment due to a blockage of the ear canal caused by excessive wax buildup, abnormal structures, or infection

GERONTOLOGICAL NURSE Professional nurses and advanced level practitioners such as nurse practitioners, clinical specialists, and nurses holding national certification in the specialty of gerontological nursing

GERONTOLOGY The study of aging

GLAUCOMA Condition in which high pressure of the fluid in the eye causes damage to the optic nerve

PRESBYCUSIS The term for hearing loss associated with old age

PRESBYOPIA A visual impairment associated with older age in which the lens becomes more rigid and less able to change shape, resulting in a decreased ability to focus on near objects

SENSORINEURAL DEAFNESS A hearing impairment resulting from damage to the nerve centers within the brain as a result of exposure to loud noises, disease, and certain drugs

A Young Girl Still Dwells

What do you see nurse, what do you see?
Are you thinking when you look at me—
A crabbed old woman, not very wise,
Uncertain of habit with far away eyes,
Who dribbles her food and makes no reply
When you say in a loud voice—"I do wish you'd try."
Who seems not to notice the things that you do
And forever is losing a stocking or shoes,
Who resisting or not, lets you do as you will
With bathing and feeding, the long day to fill.
Is that what you're thinking is that what you see
Then open your eyes, nurse. You're not looking at me.

FOCUS ON THE FAMILY, 1985

Care, kindness, and knowledge are prerequisites for working effectively with the aged. Responding to the health challenges of a new century requires a clear understanding of the health-related threats and opportunities facing older adults. People who reach age 65 can now expect to live into their eighties. However, it is unlikely that all these years will be active and independent ones. Consequently, improving the functional independence of later life is an important element in promoting health for older adults.

DEFINITIONS OF OLD AGE

Older adults present many challenges to nurses who provide care. In many cases, the work is complex, time consuming, and oriented to caring for, not curing. It is often difficult to define what is meant by old age. A child or teenager may define "old people" as persons in their thirties, forties, or fifties, whereas people in their fifties may define old as, "at least 10 years older than I am." Age identification consists of much more than just recognition of chronologic age.

Most definitions of old age refer to "having lived or existed for a long time; far advanced in years of life." Aged is defined as "old or advanced in years." However, aging is defined as the process of growing older or more mature. We all experience the process of aging, but not all of us are old in years, roles, behaviors, health, or physical limitations.

Aging is an ongoing developmental process that begins at conception and ends in death. Most gerontologists agree that old age is not measured in years. Although the age of 65 is frequently used to indicate the onset of old age, this number is clearly arbitrary and a function of social policy.

Gerontology, the study of aging, can be dated to the early 1950s and includes aging research, education, and training activities. Geriatrics is the biomedical science of old age and the application of knowledge related to the biologic, biomedical, behavioral, and social aspects of aging to the prevention, diagnosis, treatment, and care of older persons. The term *geriatrics* was coined in recognition of the similarity to the field of pediatrics. Both gerontology and geriatrics are critical components of a young science with practitioners from many disciplines including nursing, medicine, dentistry, psychology, anthropology, and political science.

ROLES OF THE GERONTOLOGICAL NURSE

By the year 2000, the population of the United States will be older, continuing the aging trend of the past century. The projected 35 million people older than 65 will represent 13% of the population and will require regular primary health care services to help them maintain their health and prevent disabling and life-threatening diseases and conditions. Nurses have always been involved in the care of the aged. There is an ongoing need on the part of nurses for instruction in quality nursing care that takes into account changes brought about by aging. Gerontological nursing practice provides an appropriate theoretical perspective for competent care in an area still poorly understood in spite of increasing research in recent years.

Formal preparation for specialized care of the elderly occurs at the master's degree level, but there are also nursing personnel who have demonstrated competencies as a result of on-the-job training. At least 11 different levels of preparation exist for those providing care to the aged (Table 7–1), and the only consistent credentialing mechanism in the United States is the state licensing examination for registered nurses and licensed vocational or practical nurses. Licensed vocational or practical nurses are in a period of transition, moving from traditional hospital-bound positions to community-based nursing homes and home health care positions. The shift to more community-based sites should enhance the level of care in these settings.

The term *gerontological nurse* typically refers to professional nurses and advanced-level practitioners, such as nurse practitioners, clinical specialists, and nurses holding national certification in the specialty of gerontological nursing. According to Gunter and Estes, gerontological nursing is a health service that incorporates basic nursing methods and specialized knowledge about the aged to establish conditions within the client and within the environment that (1) increase healthy behaviors in the aged; (2) minimize and compensate for health-related losses and impairments of aging; (3) provide comfort and sustenance through the distressing and debilitating events of aging, including dying and death; and (4) facilitate the diagnosis, care, and treatment of disease in the aged.

AGEISM

Are old people more or less highly valued in our society today than they were a century or more ago? The pitfalls of trying to answer this question soon become apparent. Historical sociology is only approximately 35 years old, and evidence about the lives of older people in the past is sketchy. As if to make up for this deficiency in hard facts, an abundance of myths or stereotypes about the elderly masquerade as reality.

TABLE 7-1
LEVELS OF NURSING PRACTITIONERS INVOLVED IN CARE OF THE AGED

PRACTITIONER	FUNCTION	EDUCATION PREPARATION
Nursing assistant (also known as patient care assistants, nurses' aides, NAs, PCAs)	Assist professional nurse in patient care tasks	On the job training, sometimes certified through taking short courses at technical colleges or through inservice training.
Licensed practical nurse or licensed vocational nurse (LPN or LVN)	Assist professional nurse in patient care tasks	Technical college or vocational high school preparation, must pass licensure examination and maintain licensure to practice
Registered nurse (RN)	Practice professional nursing with patients and clients in any health care setting	Multiple levels of entry including: Associate degree (ADN) in 2-year program Diploma (3-year hospital-based program) Baccalaureate degree (BSN), 4-year university-based program Nursing doctorate (ND), 4-year program after college degree in another field State licensure required for all levels of entry
Nurse practitioner (NP) (sometimes also qualified by specialty area such as pediatric nurse practitioner: PNP; or family nurse practitioner: FNP	Performs "medical" acts, such as management of chronic disease, prescription of medicines, diagnosis of disease	Multiple levels of entry including: Certificate programs open to any RN regardless of level of preparation Master's level programs All are RNs certified jointly by state boards or nursing and medicine
Clinical specialist	Advanced practitioner of nursing, clinical teacher	Master's degree (MSN, MN) also are RNs
Nurse scientist	Nurse researcher, nurse educator, or both	Doctor of Nursing Science (DNSc) or Doctor of Philosophy (PhD) in nursing or other field (psychology, sociology, physiology, anthropology)

From Matteson, M. A., & McConnell, E. S. (1988). *Gerontological nursing: Concepts and practice.* Philadelphia: W. B. Saunders.

MYTHS AND STEREOTYPES

Ageism is a concept introduced by a well-known gerontologist, Dr. R. N. Butler, in 1969. Ageism is the process of systematic stereotyping and discrimination against people because of their age. It is usually directed against the elderly. Older people are ridiculed and labeled senile, rigid in thought, frigid in sexuality, and old-fashioned in morality. Ageism allows for separation and denial of the older person's humanness. It also allows those who practice ageism to distance themselves from their own aging. Ageism, like all other prejudices, influences the behavior of its victims. Some older people confront the problem, whereas others deny the problem with age-inappropriate behaviors (e.g., the 69-year-old blond who attempts to dress and act young in 3-inch heels and false breast supports).

Some of the myths associated with old age include unproductivity, disengagement, inflexibility, senility, inability to learn, retirement being a cause of death, and sexlessness. Myths are a poor substitute for scientific data. When older people are properly motivated, their intelligence does not wane. In fact, with better organizational skills borne of experience, the ability to organize thoughts efficiently may increase as one ages.

As one ages, the intelligence quotient (IQ) level does not plummet, and neither does the individual become senile. Less than 5% of persons older than 65 experience dementia. Senile dementia is often a consequence of disease, overmedication, neglect, and despair. Most of these conditions can be reversed.

Old age, like retirement, does not kill, nor does it render the older person sexless. According to researchers Masters and Johnson, people have reported sexual activity well into the ninth decade. Saying that older people are not interested in sex is another way of disguising the belief that older people should not be interested in sex. Sexual activity is a healthy expression of life and vitality. However, sexual dysfunction can occur at any age and is usually evidence of some illness or disease process. Knowledge of age-related biologic, physiologic, and psychosocial factors tends to negate many of the stereotypes of aging.

Other myths abound, but one must be shattered forever, and that is the conviction that older people are isolated, poor, ill, and disabled and live in nursing homes. Most older adults are members of multigenerational units and have extended family and support networks. Nurses must be careful not to generalize stereotypes to all older adults. Some older adults finally recognize the benefits of being independent of children and grandchildren and enjoy this solace. The basic facts are that people older than 65 are the wealthiest in today's economy. This collective group leads in buying power and disposable income. The majority of older adults are not disabled, and only about 12% of the older population live in nursing homes.

BIOLOGIC AND PHYSIOLOGIC FACTORS IN AGING

Immortality and the possibility of renewing youth have captured the imagination of humankind from before the time of recorded history. The ancient Greeks and Romans ascribed immortality to their gods and the few humans who became gods. Magical potions to fend off death have been sought by diverse cultures such as the Chinese, the ancient Hebrews, and the Europeans of the Middle Ages.

The theme of immortality surfaces in nearly every area of human experience. Medical science has made great strides in conquering many ills, but little has been achieved in extension of the life span. In modern times, the longest documented human life—recorded in Japan—lasted 120 years, and most experts believe that the human life span, the maximal attainable age, is approximately 115 to 120 years.

How and why do humans age? Why is individual aging so varied? Which of the many theories of aging are valid? Each of these questions represents a fascinating area for scientific exploration. However, despite intense interest in longevity by so many cultures, scientists do not agree on precisely why or how humans age. Much of what is now known comes from our increasing awareness of the growth in absolute numbers of older people and in the proportion of the population that is old. Knowledge of the underlying mechanisms of aging is critical for the development of a system that considers the special needs and health conditions of an aging population.

THEORIES OF AGING

Proposed theories of aging have ranged from the concept of purely genetic control of aging to the concept of environmental assaults to the organism that result in death (Table 7–2). Most experts now believe that aging is not explainable by a single theory but represents many processes working simultaneously. Therefore, several theories may be needed to explain all aging processes.

Most theories of aging can be divided into two general categories: error theories and programming theories. Error theories are based on the belief that the rate of aging is directly related to the organism's rate of living and that external events cause damage to the organism's cells. The damage from all causes accumulates over time, resulting in cellular, molecular, and organ malfunction or errors. Examples of these theories include Error Catastrophe, and Wear and Tear.

Programming theories are based on the belief that aging is an event that is programmed into the cell itself and is internal to the organism. These theories postulate that aging, like prenatal development and menopause, is the natural and expected result of a purposeful sequence of events written internally into gene structure. Examples of these theories include Programmed Senescence, and Immunologic Theory. It is important to remember that theories about aging continue to evolve and that little agreement exists on any one theory of aging.

TABLE 7–2

SELECTED THEORIES OF AGING: 1900 TO THE PRESENT

ERROR THEORY	PROPONENT SCIENTIST
Wear and tear theory	Pearl (1924)
Metabolic theory	Pearl (1928)
Somatic mutation theory	Sziliard (1959)
Error catastrophe theory	Orgel (1963)
Free radical theory	Harman (1955)
PROGRAMMING THEORY	
Collagen theory	Verzar (1957)
Programmed senescence theory	Hayflick (1961)
Cross-linking theory	Bjorkstein (1968)
Immunologic theory	Walford (1969)

Adapted from National Institute on Aging. *Answers about aging: New pieces to an old puzzle.* Washington, DC: U.S. Department of Health and Human Services.

PHYSIOLOGIC CHANGES IN BODY SYSTEMS

Aging occurs slowly and is a complex and dynamic process involving many internal and external influences. It is a process that affects virtually every system, organ, and cell in the body to varying degrees. With increasing age, the ability to meet challenges and to carry out physiologic activities is reduced. Shock summarized several physiologic changes associated with aging in a simple graph (Fig. 7–1).

The graph shows a decline in function in several physiologic processes. The changes vary from process to process. The conduction speed in the central nervous system shows only a slight decline with age, whereas the renal and respiratory processes show a marked decline with age. Consequently, an understanding of the age-related effects on body systems is an integral part of the scientific basis for nursing care of the aged. The effects of aging on principal systems of the body are discussed. The systems include the nervous system, the respiratory system, the cardiovascular system, the renal system, the integumentary system, the gastrointestinal system, the musculoskeletal system, and the sensory system.

Nervous System

Some of the most frequently discussed changes that occur with aging focus on the neural structures. However, it is essential that nurses know that in the absence of disease, most aged people remain alert, with functional intellectual capability, sound judgment, and creativity. Modest impairments in memory and learning are observed in most people after age 70 if individuals are relatively free from major disease.

There is a general impression that the brain size decreases with age, although evidence for this belief is not complete. Loss of neurons (brain cells) begins in the early thirties and continues progressively, although functional ability may not be affected significantly owing to the compensatory activity of reserve cells. In addition to the reduced number of cells, electrophysiologic changes such as a decrease in conduction speed and a diminished activity of the enzymes associated with synaptic transmission occur with aging. These changes may result in a progressive slowing of responses, impeded short-term memory, and altered learning.

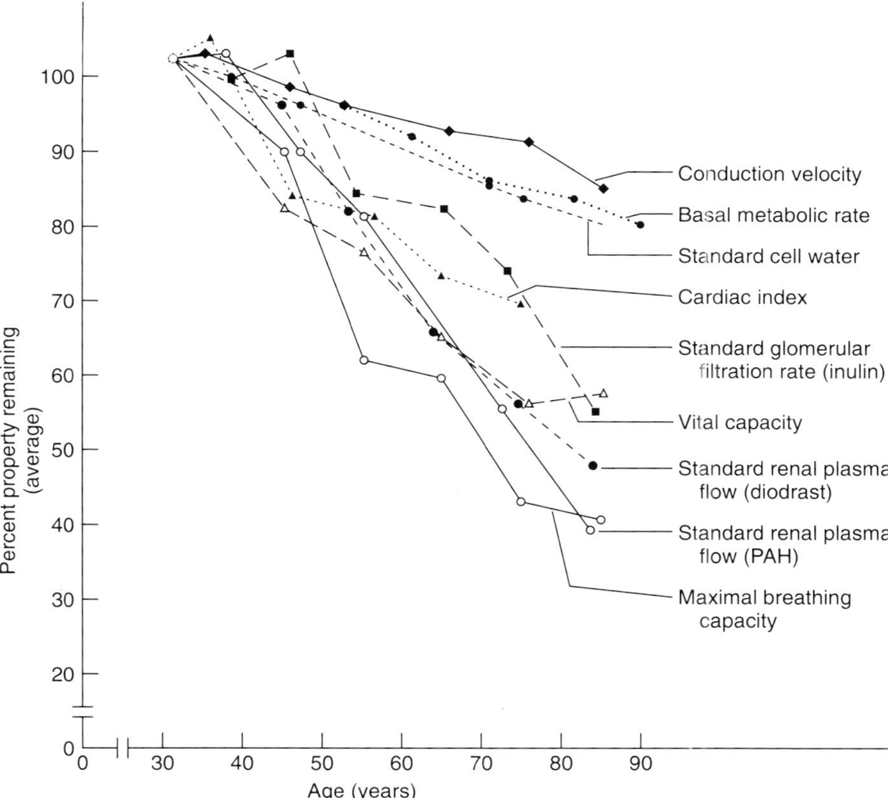

FIGURE 7-1

Summary of age changes in human physiologic functions. (From Shock, N. W. [1962]. The science of gerontology. In E. C. Jeffers [Ed.], *Proceedings of seminars 1959–61.* Durham, NC: North Carolina Council on Gerontology.)

Short-term memory loss is frequently a concern of the aged, although long-term memory may remain intact. Short-term memory is associated with a stimulus input into the neurons and is dependent on adequate tissue oxygenation. The aging brain may be considered to be in a chronic hypoxic state. The deficit in oxygen is related to atherosclerosis as well as decreased cellular respiration. Consequently, the aged person may experience difficulty remembering planned events for the day but may recall young adulthood experiences without difficulty. Using mnemonics, stringing together known and unknown information, and rehearsal memory training may improve memory performance for some older adults experiencing memory deficits. Further, some research indicates that long-term memory is not affected by chronic cerebral tissue hypoxia, but may be attributed to permanent changes in the structure of the neuron. If this is the case, then efforts to improve memory would most likely be managed with medications to prevent permanent neuron changes.

Other neurologic features that show age-related changes include temperature regulation, pain perception, and tactile sensation. The aged individual usually has a low tolerance for extremes in temperature, which may be related to deterioration in the vascular tone as well as changes in the hypothalamic temperature set-point. Pain and tactile sensation involve peripheral sensory receptors, a relay pathway, and cortical integration. A decrease in the number and sensitivity of sensory receptors, dermatomes, and neurons contributes to an overall dulling of these sensations.

The neurologic changes associated with aging occur gradually; thus, the aged person is able to compensate for these changes by modifying behavior. The person may avoid temperature extremes and accomplish tasks at a slower pace. Any stressor, such as an illness or a new environmental stressor, may seriously impair the person's ability to compensate and may contribute to confusion or disorientation.

Respiratory System

Tests of pulmonary physiology have shown a number of age-related alterations. Forced vital capacity, vital capacity, and maximum breathing capacity are thought to decrease progressively with aging. These alterations are related to atrophy and weakening of the respiratory muscles and to an increase in the anteroposterior diameter of the chest as a result of kyphosis, vertebral loss of calcium, and calcification of costal cartilage.

In addition, with aging there is a loss of elastic tissue surrounding alveoli and alterations in pulmonary circulation that result in decreased diffusion across the alveolar-capillary membrane. This physiologic alteration is reflected in arterial oxygen values that decrease progressively throughout aging to approximately 70 to 80 mm Hg by the age of 70.

Pulmonary blood flow in the aged person decreases owing to a reduction in cardiac output. Alterations in the pulmonary system associated with aging include a decreased number of capillaries, thickened capillary walls, and fewer capillaries surrounding the alveoli. The changes in the capillaries affect pulmonary diffusion so that gas exchange is impaired. With increasing age, alveolar dead space also occurs.

Despite the physiologic changes associated with aging, the ability of the aged to maintain adequate oxygenation is not seriously impaired under conditions of health and moderate activity. Problems arise when increased demands are placed on the body, for example, during periods of extreme exertion or respiratory illness. Exertional dyspnea is a frequent complaint with the aged. The ability to perform prolonged strenuous work decreases with aging.

Lung disease, acute or chronic, poses a threat to the aged client, and pulmonary secretions are handled less effectively. Ciliary action, responsible for the movement of secretions, is compromised owing to epithelial atrophy. The cough reflex is frequently diminished as a consequence of altered sensitivity to stimuli and decreased muscle tone. These factors in concert with impaired gas exchange are responsible for the devastating effects of respiratory problems in old age.

As a patient advocate, the nurse is concerned about environmental pollution and hazards associated with smoking. Assessment data should include baseline resting and exertional respiratory rates and pulmonary function test results, as appropriate. Deep breathing exercises and positioning to facilitate lung expansion and gas exchange are standard components of respiratory care for the older adult.

Cardiovascular System

An increase in resistance to blood flow occurs in many organs with increasing age. This increase in peripheral resistance has its greatest effect on splanchnic and renal areas and less effect on cerebral, coronary, and skeletal areas.

In the absence of cardiovascular disease, heart size remains unchanged or slightly decreased owing to shrinkage or loss of myocardial fibrils. Aging results in the development of whitish patches, fibrosis, and sclerosis in the endocardium that lines the heart cavities. As the heart becomes more rigid, myocardial contractility is compromised. Coronary blood flow in the aged person may be reduced by as much as 35% because of changes in the vessels. With advancing age, valvular rigidity and incomplete closure of the aortic and pulmonic valves may result in the presence of a murmur. Aging heart cells have a decreased capacity to utilize oxygen, which may be a factor in the aged person's reduced tolerance for physical work.

The blood vessels of the heart and the systemic circulation, particularly the arteries, are characterized by age-related changes that may begin as early as the teen years. Thickening and calcification of the intima layer is evident in the coronary arteries and aorta usually by age 20. Arterial dilation, vessel lengthening, and rigidity are in part due to changes in the structure of collagen. With aging, the pulse tends to increase in force, and the pulse pressure widens. By 70 years of age, the systolic blood pressure increases to approximately 150 mm Hg and the diastolic to 90 mm Hg for most people. These changes are due in part to decreased baroreceptor reflexes and inelasticity of the vessel walls.

Another change in the cardiovascular system caused by aging is noted in the resting cardiac output. The resting cardiac output, the amount of blood pumped by the heart each minute, decreases to 30 to 40% between the ages of 25 and 65 years. This reduced cardiac output reflects a decreased heart rate and a decreased stroke volume. Despite the diminished cardiac output, cerebral blood flow is maintained. However, other body systems, such as the liver and kidneys, receive a diminished blood supply. Even with this diminished blood supply, functional integrity of the organs is intact in part because of reduced functional requirements.

Anatomic and physiologic changes in the myocardium and blood vessels caused by aging are secondary to changes occurring at the molecular and cellular levels. It should be noted, however, that the changes mentioned earlier are not universal and may not be characterized as inevitable consequences of aging. It is nevertheless important that nurses be prepared to incorporate goals, plans, and actions related to nutrition, exercise, and behavior modification in providing care to aged clients with cardiovascular problems.

Renal System

The aging kidneys are characterized by a decrease in renal function, a decrease in cell mass, and an increase in extracellular fluid. By the seventh decade, the number of nephrons in each kidney is reduced by one half to two thirds, with corresponding changes in the glomeruli. Aging is accompanied by decreased filtration rate and plasma flow rate as well as decreased tubular reabsorption and secretion. The blood urea nitrogen measurement tends to increase.

The renal system participates in acid-base balance. The tubules of the aging kidneys have a diminished capacity for conserving base and ridding the body of excess hydrogen ions. In health, the aging kidneys are able to function appropriately; however, with the added burden of disease and chronic illness, the ability to maintain acid-base balance may be impaired significantly.

With advancing age, the ability to concentrate urine or dilute urine is hindered and is believed to be related to a deterioration in the pituitary release of antidiuretic hormone or an overresponsiveness to this hormone. Additional changes brought on by aging are noted in the ureters, bladder, and urethra as a result of deterioration in muscle tone. The bladder capacity may be reduced by half, resulting in frequent trips to the bathroom. Further, response to the stretch receptors in the bladder wall that signal the need to void may be delayed until the pressure is high and the capacity almost filled. This condition results in an urgency to urinate, which may be problematic for older adults with visual and motor limitations. Urge incontinence is a major health concern for older adults. Lax muscle tone and incomplete emptying of the bladder may lead to a residual amount of urine in the bladder. This residual volume may put the older person at risk for subsequent urinary tract infections. Other types of incontinence may appear as a symptom of upper or lower urinary tract dysfunction. For several of these conditions, conservative behavioral treatment is recommended as the first level of intervention. Behavioral treatments may include scheduled or prompted voiding, environmental adaptation, and pelvic muscle exercises (Kegel exercises). The renal system of the healthy older client is functionally adequate; however, in times of injury, disease, or disability, the additional function challenge may adversely affect the aging renal system.

Integumentary System

Skin changes caused by aging can be the most upsetting because they are so visible and readily apparent. They serve as a constant reminder that youth is fleeting. Changes related to aging of the skin include dryness, loss of elasticity, wrinkles, uneven pigmentation and brown spots, roughness, looseness, thinness, yellowing, and development of various skin lesions.

One of the first signs of aging is the development of wrinkles. Wrinkles occur when the deep layer of the skin loses moisture and elasticity. Tiny creases and folds are formed. The extent and timing of these wrinkles are determined by genetics and sun exposure. Persons in certain ethnic groups with thicker, oilier skin wrinkle at a slower rate and tend to maintain a youthful, wrinkle-free appearance longer. The same is true of older men because of their thicker and oilier skin.

Skin that is exposed to the sun most often, such as the face, hands, and back of the neck, wrinkles quickly. Older people are encouraged to use sunscreens to prevent excessive dryness and to prevent skin cancer, the third most common form of cancer in women over the age of 50.

Itching, another change caused by aging, becomes more common in later life and is due to loss of oils in the skin. Nurses might suggest to older persons that they take tepid baths; use moisturizers; and avoid overuse of antiperspirants, soaps, perfumes, and long hot baths. Furthermore, the older person needs to know that generalized itching may be a sign of illness such as diabetes, cancer, kidney disease, or liver disease. Persistent itching should be reported and appropriately assessed by the nurse and other members of the health care team.

Most older persons can expect some hair loss, hair thinning, and color changes in the hair and nails. Men tend to grow bald, and women experience thinning of the hair on the head and genitalia. The number of facial and nasal hairs may increase. Gray hair is caused by a slowing of pigment production in the hair follicles. Graying is determined by genetics and tends to be irreversible. Nails tend to become yellow and thicker. Routine visits to a podiatrist are encouraged for nail trimming and care of corns and callouses.

The most common benign lesions of aging are seborrheic dermatitis, acne, contact dermatitis, drug reactions, pressure ulcers, stasis ulcers, pruritus, herpes zoster, onychomycosis and tinea pedis, and impetigo. Routine skin assessments should be part of comprehensive nursing assessment for older adults.

Gastrointestinal System

Changes in gastrointestinal functions occur with normal aging. Changes in the oral cavity include a deterioration in the teeth and a decrease in the functional taste buds as well as a decrease in the secretion of saliva. Saliva tends to become more alkaline as the salivary glands secrete less ptyalin and amylase. The muscles associated with chewing weaken, peristalsis is slower, and the risk of formation of intestinal diverticula increases. These changes tend to interfere with the older person's ability and desire to eat a nutritious meal.

Further, gastric emptying is slower in older people than in the young. The gastric glands decrease their secretion with age; this includes the volume and concentration of hydrochloric acid, intrinsic factor, and pepsin. The amount of calcium absorbed with advanced age is reduced. Further, some reports indicate that bile tends to be thicker and that the gallbladder empties slowly.

Collectively, the changes in the gastrointestinal system caused by aging increase the older person's risk for anorexia, bloating, indigestion, gas, diarrhea, signs of pernicious anemia, and constipation. Constipation is one of the most frequent gastrointestinal complaints of older adults. Constipation may result from intestinal immotility, altered bacteria flora, a diet low in bulk and roughage, and lack of physical activity.

Because digestive complaints can be signs of more serious disorders, nurses must assess them completely. Symptoms that may suggest possible illness are decreased appetite, unexplained weight loss, excessive thirst, blood in the stool, or change in the usual pattern of bowel movements.

The nurse can assist older adults to maintain gastrointestional function by sharing information about the normal ranges for bowel activity. The usual frequency for a bowel movement may range from as many as three movements per day to as few as one bowel movement every seven days. The older adult should be educated about diet, activity, increased fluid intake, and avoidance of laxative abuse.

Musculoskeletal System

Of the multiple changes associated with an aging musculoskeletal system, changes related to mobility are most significant. Many people begin to feel old when they wake up with stiff joints. Other age-related changes include decreases in muscle strength, endurance, range of motion of joints, coordination, density of bone, and elasticity and flexibility of connective tissue.

Arthritis is the most prevalent chronic disease in men, is more severe in women, and is the leading cause of disability in old age. Osteoarthritis, the most common form of arthritis, is caused by damage to the inside surface of the joint. Age is the most obvious risk factor for arthritis, with heredity and obesity contributing to its development. The large weight-bearing joints of the body are most affected and include the knees, hips, and spine. *Kyphosis* is the term applied to the curvature of the thoracic spine and gives rise to the bent-over appearance of some older adults.

Assessment should include documentation of the range of motion in all joints, signs of inflammation, and complaints of pain associated with mobility. Muscle strength should be assessed bilaterally, and the typical amount, type, and frequency of exercise should be noted. In addition, the nurse should note any history of falls, hormonal therapy, or calcium supplementation.

Older adults should be taught the benefits of weight-bearing exercises. Walking, bicycling, and stair climbing help maintain bone and muscle mass. If necessary, assistive devices for walking and preventing falls should be utilized. Bedrest is to be avoided because of the detrimental effects of immobility.

Sensory System

Because we depend on our five senses in almost everything we do, any loss of sensory ability greatly affects the quality of life we live. Sensory changes in the older adult place them at risk for injury, weaken self-confidence, and can affect overall quality of life and general well-being.

Presbycusis is the term for hearing loss associated with old age. Older adults lose the ability to hear high-pitched sounds and the consonants *ch, f, g, s, sh, t, th,* and *z.* Twenty-five percent of older adults are hearing impaired. Older men tend to experience greater hearing loss, but nurses need to remember that not all older adults experience this loss and causes other than old age may be involved.

There are basically two types of hearing loss. Conduction deafness is a blockage of the ear canal caused by excessive wax buildup, abnormal structures, or infection. This type of loss is easily treated. The other type of hearing loss is sensorineural deafness. It results from damage to the nerve centers within the brain as a result of exposure to loud noises, disease, and certain drugs. Tinnitus, an annoying ringing or buzzing in the ear, is a sensorineural disorder. Some tinnitus is caused by the use of aspirin, certain antibiotics, diuretics, or the presence of tumors. Hearing aids may be used to correct both types of deafness.

Failing eyesight is not an inevitable consequence of age, but several eye diseases are associated with aging. The leading cause of new cases of blindness in older people is age-related macular degeneration, a disease that affects the macula, that part of the eye that is responsible for sharp central vision. Laser surgery is effective in preventing or delaying visual loss, and older adults should be informed of this as a treatment option.

Another serious eye disease that occurs with aging is cataract. Cataract is the development of clouding or opacity of the normal transparent lens within the eye. Cataracts are caused by changes in structural lens proteins, by damage to the lens as a result of high levels of blood sugar in people with diabetes, or by other means.

Cataract is treated by surgical removal of the clouded lens. Surgery is highly successful, and vision is usually restored in 90 to 95% of the cases. An artificial lens is placed in the eye after cataract removal. Eyeglasses may be prescribed after surgery to further improve vision.

A less serious age-related vision change is a condition called *presbyopia.* Presbyopia affects the shape of the lens. The shape of the lens is controlled by muscles in the eye. By changing its shape, the lens allows us to change focus when looking from objects that are near to objects that are far. With age, the lens becomes more rigid and less able to change shape. Consequently, reading and other types of close work become difficult. Presbyopia is easily corrected by reading glasses or bifocal lenses. Further, adapting to changes in lighting is also a function of the lenses. Maintaining bright lighting in the home, particularly in hallways and around walkways, can help to prevent falls and other accidents.

The leading cause of blindness in the United States is glaucoma. Glaucoma is characterized by high pressure of the fluid in the eye. The increased pressure causes damage to the optic nerve. The optic nerve carries visual impulses from the eye to the brain. Damage to the optic nerve can result in vision loss, which is characterized by "tunnel vision."

At present, glaucoma is not curable but is treatable with drugs or surgery. If glaucoma is detected early and treated effectively, the disease process can be halted or slowed and the remaining eyesight saved. Older adults should receive annual eye examinations and a test for glaucoma.

Disorders of the senses involving taste and smell are called *chemosensory disorders.* More than 10 million Americans are affected by this type of disorder. Most of these disorders occur after age 60 and involve the ability to smell. Men tend to be more affected than women, and many causes exist. Causes include nasal obstruction, allergies, and use of certain drugs. Some scientists believe that the decline in smell is due to the observed decrease in olfactory nerve fibers that occurs with advanced age.

A gradual loss in the number of taste buds begins around 50 to 60 years of age. In spite of this progressive loss, there is little perceptible change in taste sensitivity due to increased age alone. Major changes in the ability to taste are most often due to diseases or the side effects of certain drugs.

Dentures, hormonal changes, medications, and changes in chemicals needed to transmit taste are all potential causes of the older person's inability to taste. This loss can affect changes in appetite.

Sensory losses are more than a minor nuisance for older adults. Poor vision and hearing increase a person's risk for falls and other accidents, which are a leading cause of death and disability in people over the age of 65. Further, the inability to smell smoke, poisons, or other noxious odors endangers the lives of many older people. Decreased ability to taste food puts the older person at risk for malnutrition. Each of these sensory changes greatly reduces the quality of life. Nurses must assist older adults to control, correct, or compensate for sensory losses. Assessment is, of course, the first step.

In sum, physiologic changes associated with aging may reflect more the presence of age-related diseases than the fact of aging itself. The interrelationship between the process of normal aging and the effects of age-related disease has not yet been defined universally. Nurse scientists are actively engaged in this process as well as in other scientific endeavors to better understand and provide care to an enlarging segment of our population. Through research our knowledge of aging is rapidly expanding and changing. Conditions once thought to be the consequence of normal aging are now known to be the product of disease. Many of the diseases can be prevented or controlled by good health practices and competent nursing care.

PSYCHOSOCIAL FACTORS IN AGING

As with biologic aging, it is useful for nurses to consider important psychosocial changes associated with aging. The older adult shows cumulative developmental effects that produce unique personality styles, coping mechanisms, challenges, and growth, which occur in a societal context. Family, friends, and the community are influential factors in the aging process and are useful in the process of adapting to age-related changes.

The fact of survival is often used as an indicator of successful adaptation in old age. The survival of large numbers of relatively healthy older people is a new experience for humankind. By the year 2000, it is expected that those older than 65 will number more than 35 million. The vast majority of older people have adapted adequately. These individuals are able to function independently and maintain a sense of well-being. Only about 15% of the aged are unable to function independently and fail to maintain or sustain a sense of well-being.

Effective adaptation includes the individual's ability to meet environmental and functional needs and to obtain some sense of well-being in relation to the environment. Built into each developmental task of aging is the need for successfully coping and adapting to changes in the environment. Remember, environment refers to both internal and external realms.

Maturity is defined as an optimal psychological, social, and biologic adaptation achieved at some point during the midlife years arbitrarily set between 45 to 65 years of age. The years preceding the attainment of maturity are characterized as ascending and accelerating, and those thereafter are regarded as descending and decelerating. The dominant idea is that the realization of one's own vulnerability during the midyears provides, in part, the basis for the midlife crisis.

Eric Erikson developed one of the first personality theories in the area of aging. He viewed the entire process of human development as a series of stages a person goes through to develop the ego fully. Erikson describes eight stages of ego development from infancy to old age. Each of his stages represents a choice of crises in the ego. The tasks in adult life begin with intimacy versus isolation. In accomplishing this task, the person develops close relations with other people. If the person does not, then the crisis associated with isolation occurs and the person does not learn or experience love fully. The next task is generativity versus stagnation. In this developmental level, the challenge is to find a vocation or hobby in which the individual can help others or in some way contribute to society. Some examples include working as a nurse, raising a family in a responsible manner, or helping out in the case of a natural disaster.

The final developmental task identified by Erikson is ego-integrity versus despair, which is the one typically associated with old age. The developmental challenge is to review life and to gain a feeling of accomplishment and fulfillment. The older person is expected to be concerned with life in the face of death and to begin to experience the wisdom that he or she has gained. The opposite of ego-integrity relates to feelings of despair, in which the person feels bitter about the accomplishments of life and tends to regret life as he or she has lived it.

Old age involves much more than a psychological waiting station before death. It represents an important stage of development and coping that occurs between the high points and accomplishments of the midyears and the concerns that are involved as the end of life approaches. The poem *What It Means to Be Old* highlights some changes associated with the finite events of life and what it means to be old. In the final stage of development the older adult is faced with a variety of losses from internal and external environments that often require coping and adaptation using diminished biologic, psychological, and social resources. The challenge is to maintain performance in the face of adverse circumstances.

What It Means to Be Old

It means stepping down and stepping aside
It means more time alone
It means neglect
It means a back seat
It means less money
It means giving up things
It means loss
It means accepting help from others
It means the threat of illness or disability
It means being frightened
It means accepting past failures and realizing that much of the record of one's life is in
It means trying to figure out what one's life has meant
It means figuring out what you want to get done before you die
It means facing death.

ANONYMOUS

From Steffl, B. M. (1984). *Handbook of gerontological nursing.* New York: Van Nostrand Reinhold.

COPING AND ADAPTATION

Old age has been described as the season of losses, including loss of roles, statuses, physical abilities, and deep personal losses through death of friends and family networks. Loss, whether real, threatened, or imaginary, is a stressor that requires adaptation, flexibility, and resiliency if a person is to cope successfully and survive.

In most respects older people cope in much the same way as younger people. Differences are largely due to the different types of stressors experienced. Older people tend to experience more negative and irreversible types of stressors. Given the many losses associated with old age as potential stressors, the older person may cope with these losses with positive or negative adaptation. Positive adaptation might include rational action, perseverance, positive thinking (e.g., the lost loved one is now out of pain), intellectual denial (e.g., I don't want to think about it now), restraint, drawing strength from adversity, and humor.

Unfortunately, in nursing and health care we are most often confronted with those who are unable to cope effectively with their losses. Some older people respond to losses by losing their sense of personal identity and fulfillment and suffer from a deterioration in self-esteem, an altered self-concept, and a loss of meaningfulness in life. Many older people become seriously depressed and experience additional loss. Many lose motivation for working, playing, and living. Depression resulting from loss is associated with approximately two thirds of the suicides among older people.

Family

With an aging population and the need for support and assistance in positive coping and adaptation, kinship networks take on added importance and new shapes. Most of the aged in the United States occupy a variety of family roles and come from multigenerational units. It is not uncommon for a person at age 65 to be married, have at least one living adult child, have at least one living brother or sister, be a grandparent, and, most likely, also be a great-grandparent. The person over age 65 may also be a child of a much older parent. In addition, the kinship network can include cousins, nieces, and nephews. Of all of these roles and relationships, with the exception of marital relations, that of parent and child seems to be most important.

In an era when the old are frequently referred to as burdens, it is important to recognize that more financial support flows from the old to the young in the family than in the reverse direction. Although family responsibility appears to be an internalized value for most people, it is important to know that more than half of the states have legal statutes that can require children to provide financial support for needy parents. However, what is most needed and most often given is emotional support and help in times of illness and disability. Home health care for the frail elderly is most often given by a spouse or a child. Typically, the caregiver is a daughter. Three out of four caregivers are women, and almost half of these are raising children of their own simultaneously.

The combination of personal limitations, competing roles, and stresses generated by the care recipient's behavior and the physical demands created by various levels of emotional, physical, financial, and family strain places enormous stress on informal caregivers. Caregivers frequently report symptoms of depression, anxiety, helplessness, low morale, and emotional exhaustion. Nurses should be aware of the stressful impact of caregiving and should implement actions to minimize the stresses and burdens on both the caregiver and the care recipient.

In part, because of caregiver stress, more than 1 million aged persons are abused physically and psychologically or are neglected each year by their caregivers. Nurses are in an excellent position to assess caregiver–care recipient stress, depression, and abuse and to recommend interventions to alter these conditions. Education, learning, and positive adaptive behaviors can assist caregivers and care recipients. Caregivers who feel knowledgeable, useful, and productive are usually happier, less stressed, and less prone to abuse. Families must be part of the holistic approach in the assessment and care of the aged.

FUNCTIONAL ASSESSMENT

Assessment has become a key word in the fields of gerontology and geriatrics because of the numerous important roles that it plays in care planning and care delivery.

Functional assessment includes information about activities of daily living as well as environmental, financial, family, economic, and community resources. The functional assessment data may be used at several major stages: before illness, at the beginning of treatment, and following therapeutic intervention. Comparisons across these time points allow the nurse to plot the individual's functions that can serve to increase understanding of the aged person's problems and the effects of interventions.

Functional assessment is more than a diagnosis. A diagnosis alone cannot tell the nurse how sick an older person is or how much care is needed. For example, a medical diagnosis of coronary artery disease does not inform the nurse whether the older person is independent and controlled appropriately with medication or totally dependent on care and currently requiring intensive coronary care. For effective gerontological care, functional assessment is the crucial denominator in deciding care needs.

Functional status is more than a measure of activities of daily living. Knowing what activities the client performs alone, what activities require assistance, and what activities the person is totally unable to perform or to perform safely is essential for defining care needs. This information plus a diagnosis helps to inform the nurse regarding the cause of self-care problems and whether the problems are amenable to therapeutic intervention.

The older person's database should include two functional scales of basic and instrumental activities of daily living. The following areas are generally considered in an assessment of activities of daily living: grooming, bathing, dressing, eating, elimination, and mobility. Instrumental activities of daily living are less important in institutional settings but are prime determinants of potential discharge from nursing homes or institutions. Instrumental activities of daily living generally consider the older adult's ability to prepare a meal, shop for groceries, use the telephone, negotiate transportation, take medications, and maintain housekeeping and laundry tasks.

The Older Americans Research and Services (OARS) questionnaire is one example of a valid and reliable assessment guide for gathering information on the overall personal functional status and service use of adults. The OARS questionnaire has been used mainly with older adults and has two parts. The first part provides for assessment of the older adult in terms of social, economic, mental, and physical health and ability to perform activities of daily living. The second part provides for assessment of the older adult based on the need for 24 rather universal services. A content summary is provided in Table 7–3. A copy of the OARS questionnaire and training manuals may be obtained from OARS, Center for the Study of Aging and Human Development, Duke University Medical Center, Durham, NC 22710. In most instances, the nursing home minimum data set incorporates all components of a quality functional assessment. This comprehensive assessment tool is valid and reliable and currently used in multisite applied research.

TABLE 7-3

CONTENT AREAS OF THE OARS FUNCTIONAL ASSESSMENT QUESTIONNAIRE

PART A. FUNCTIONAL ASSESSMENT

Social	Physical
Contact with others	Prescribed medications used
Help from family and kin	Physical conditions with impairment levels
Economic	**Activities of Daily Living**
Amount of income and adequacy	Physical and instrumental activities of daily living
Home owership	
Mental	**Demographics and Administrative**
Mental and psychiatric status	Age, sex, race
Mental well-being	Location, length of interview
	Information source

PART B. SERVICES

Transportation	Medical	Financial
Social or recreational	Supportive devices	Food, groceries
Employment	Physical therapy	Housing
Sheltered employment	Continuous supervision	Coordination
Education	Checking	Information
Remedial training	Homemaker	Referral
Mental health	Meal preparation	
Psychotropic drugs	Legal and protective	
Personal care	Systematic evaluation	

Adapted from Older Americans Research and Services. (1978). Durham, NC: Center for the Study of Aging and Human Development, Duke University Medical Center.

DRUG THERAPY AND AGED ADULTS

ABSORPTION, DISTRIBUTION, METABOLISM, AND EXCRETION

The population group older than 65 years is the largest user of prescription medications. Approximately 20 to 25% of all prescription drugs are given to aged adults. Age-related changes influence patterns of drug use, consumption of drugs, and actions of medications on target organs (Table 7–4). The most important changes involve body composition, cardiovascular system, central nervous system, renal function, tissue sensitivity to drugs, and reduced blood pressure reflex sensitivity. The majority of age-related and disease-related changes in the elderly contribute to decreased ability to clear drugs through the liver and renal system.

With aging there is a reduction in body size, with a decrease in lean body mass and body water content (extracellular volume) and an increase in fat. The serum albumin concentration is lower, which tends to make available more free drug to tissues or to make available more drug to be eliminated from the body. A gradual decrease in blood flow to the internal organs in the abdomen reduces drug clearance through the liver or kidney. For example, a water-soluble drug may result in higher blood concentrations of that drug. However, a highly fat-soluble drug might bind to the increased fat in the aged body and may be stored longer before excretion. Diazepam (Valium) is a fat-soluble drug that has the potential for increased distribution in tissues and for delayed elimination. A 75-year-old woman was misdiagnosed as having progressive brain damage after she developed urinary incontinence, general mental deterioration, and inability to walk. She had taken 5 mg of nitrazepam for at least 1 year. After the drug was discontinued, the patient recovered in 3 days.

The liver prepares drugs for elimination in the urine or in feces. Age-related changes that have an impact on the inactivation of drugs by the liver include decreased liver size, reduced blood flow through the liver, and reduced liver enzyme activity on drugs. These changes have the overall effect of increasing drug concentrations

TABLE 7-4

ASSOCIATION BETWEEN AGE-RELATED PHYSIOLOGIC CHANGES AND PHARMACOKINETICS

AGE-RELATED CHANGES	DIRECTION OF CHANGE/PHARMACOKINETICS
Body fat	Increased/Storage
Body water	Decreased/Active concentration
Hepatic blood flow	Decreased/Clearance
Lean muscle mass	Decreased/Tissue concentration
Renal function	Decreased/Elimination
Serum albumin	Decreased/Concentration

in the blood and possibly increasing the amount of time it takes the body to get rid of the drug. Drugs that are principally eliminated in the urine may be given to older persons in reduced doses or less frequently to avoid accumulation and adverse effects.

Older persons tend to respond more vigorously to drugs that act on the central nervous system owing to a greater tissue sensitivity and altered physiologic changes as described earlier. Some of the potential adverse effects are postural imbalance, staggering, uncoordinated movements, respiratory depression, and changes in mental alertness. Drugs such as opiates, diazepam, and nifedipine may cause these effects.

ADVERSE DRUG REACTIONS

Adverse drug reactions are more common in older persons because older persons use more drugs. The risk factors for adverse drug reactions are age, gender, race (occurring most frequently in older white females), number of drugs consumed, dosage, duration of treatment, severity of illness, and client cooperation. The use of fewer drugs at lower doses usually increases client cooperation. Some of the common symptoms and signs of adverse drug reactions in the older person are restlessness, falls, depression, confusion, loss of memory, constipation, and urinary incontinence. Some drugs associated with adverse drug reactions are listed in Table 7–5.

Because the elderly have a greater number of drug reactions and interactions and are believed to be more sensitive to some medications, nurses must monitor their drug regimens carefully. It is helpful to assist clients to maintain a record of blood pressure, pulse, respiration, drug effect, and state of alertness in relation to current drug therapy. Such a record could be helpful in making necessary changes. Adverse reactions must be documented. It may be necessary to change a drug or reduce the dosage or lengthen the intervals between doses to minimize the risk of adverse drug reactions. Nurses are in key positions to provide appropriate assessment and competent care to minimize reactions.

TABLE 7-5

DRUGS COMMONLY ASSOCIATED WITH ADVERSE DRUG REACTIONS IN OLDER PERSONS

DRUG CLASS	EXAMPLE	PROBLEM
Analgesics	Aspirin	Bleeding
Antibiotics	Streptomycin	Nephrotoxicity
Anticoagulants	Warfarin	Hemorrhage
Antidepressants	Amitriptyline	Sedation
Antihypertensives	Verapamil	Hypotension
Antiparkinsonians	Levodopa	Extrapyramidal symptoms; dystonia
Antipsychotics	Haloperidol	Confusion
Diuretics	Diuril	Hypokalemia
Sedatives/hypnotics	Flurazepam	Drowsiness

Baseline and continual assessment should include the amount, frequency, and purpose of all medications taken; the older person's ability to take medications as recommended; the potential for drug interactions and adverse drug reactions; the effectiveness of the medication over time; and whether any of the drugs taken can be discontinued or decreased in dose.

This presentation of adverse drug reactions would not be complete without mentioning hazards associated with over-the-counter medications that may be contraindicated with the myriad prescription medications taken by older adults. Examples might include the use of aspirin with a prescribed anticoagulant or the use of large amounts of sodium bicarbonate with prescription sodium-based antacids. Further concern is raised in relation to the possibility of older adults mixing older prescription medications with newer ones and failing to discontinue and discard older prescriptions. Hoarding of medications may be viewed as future savings by the older adult. Nevertheless, nurses must recognize the inherent dangers in this situation and teach clients to review all medications, prescription and over-the-counter, with their primary nurse or other health care providers.

One of the greatest challenges for those working within health care is addressing the physiologic, psychosocial, behavioral, and mental well-being of older persons. This chapter presents information in each of these realms. The concept of *old age* is defined, the roles of gerontological nurses explored, the myths and stereotypes rebutted with scientific data, and the biophysiologic changes caused by aging delineated. Management and care of an aging population affects every sector of the nursing profession. Nurses at all levels of preparation are encouraged to meet this mandate with care, concern, and competence.

BIBLIOGRAPHY

Agency for Health Care Policy and Research. (1992). *Urinary incontinence in adults: Clinical practice guidelines.* Washington, DC: U.S. Government Printing Office.

Burggraf, V., & Stanley, M. (1989). *Nursing the elderly.* Philadelphia: J. B. Lippincott.

Gunter, L., & Estes, C. (1979). *Education for gerontic nursing.* New York: Springer Publishing Co.

Harper, M. S. (Ed.). *Management and care of the elderly: Psychosocial perspectives.* (1991). Newbury Park, CA: Sage Publications.

Matteson, M. A., & McConnell, E. S. (1988). *Gerontological nursing: Concepts and practice.* Philadelphia: W. B. Saunders.

Miller, C. A. (1990). *Nursing care of older adults: Theory and practice.* Glenview, IL: Scott, Foresman & Company.

Sayles-Cross, S. (1993). Perceptions of familial caregivers of elder adults. *Image: Journal of Nursing Scholarship. 25*(2), 88.

U.S. Department of Health and Human Services. (1990). *Healthy people 2000.* Washington, DC: U.S. Government Printing Office.

KEY CONCEPTS

1. Aging is an ongoing developmental process that begins at conception and ends at death.
2. Gerontology is the study of aging.
3. Geriatrics is the biomedical science of old age and the application of knowledge related to the biologic, biomedical, behavioral, and social aspects of aging to the prevention, diagnosis, treatment, and care of older persons.
4. Gerontological nursing aims to increase healthy behaviors in the aged, minimize and compensate for health-related losses and impairments of aging, provide comfort and sustenance through the events of aging, and facilitate the diagnosis, care, and treatment of disease in the aged.
5. Health care providers must recognize myths about the elderly and aging that result in stereotyping and discrimination against older people.
6. Aging occurs slowly and is a complex and dynamic process involving many internal and external influences.
7. Physiologic changes that are associated with aging may reflect more the presence of age-related diseases than the process of aging itself.
8. The older adult shows cumulative developmental effects that produce unique personality styles, coping mechanisms, challenges, and growth, which occur in a societal context.
9. Age-related changes contribute to a decreased ability to clear drugs through the liver and renal system.

CHAPTER 8

Mary Ann Matteson

The Nursing Process

OBJECTIVES

1. Describe the five components of the nursing process.
2. Explain the role of the licensed practical nurse or licensed vocational nurse in the nursing process.
3. Describe the proper documentation of the nursing process using a problem-oriented medical record format, nurses' notes, and flow sheets.

GLOSSARY

ASSESSMENT Collection of data about the health status of a patient or client

AUSCULTATION Listening to sounds produced by the body, such as heart, lung, and intestinal sounds

INSPECTION Purposeful observation or scrutiny of the person as a whole and then of each body system

NURSING DIAGNOSIS Actual or potential health problems derived from data gathered during the assessment of a patient or client

NURSING PROCESS Systematic, problem-solving approach to providing nursing care in an organized, scientific manner

OBJECTIVE DATA Information about the patient collected by the nurse or other members of the health care team

PALPATION Method of physical examination that uses the sense of touch to assess various parts of the body

PERCUSSION Tapping on the skin to assess the underlying tissues

PHYSICAL ASSESSMENT Physical examination that is a systematic, thorough way of obtaining objective data

PROBLEM-ORIENTED MEDICAL RECORD Method of record keeping that focuses on patient problems rather than on medical diagnoses

SUBJECTIVE DATA Information reported by patients or family members

The nursing process is a systematic method of providing care to patients. It is a problem-solving approach that enables the nurse to provide care in an organized, scientific manner. The goal of the nursing process is to alleviate, minimize, or prevent real or potential health problems. It enables the nurse to provide care in the areas of health maintenance and promotion, acute illness, chronic illness, and rehabilitation.

The nursing process can be applied in any interaction that involves a nurse and a patient or client. (As noted earlier, the terms *patient* and *client* are used interchangeably in this text.) The patient or client can be defined as an individual, a family, a group, a community, or a society. The process can take place in a variety of settings, including a hospital, community, or nursing home.

COMPONENTS OF THE NURSING PROCESS

There are five components or steps in the nursing process: (1) assessment (systematic collection of data relating to patients and their problems), (2) nursing diagnosis (interpretation of the data for problem identification), (3) planning (choice of solutions), (4) implementation or intervention (putting the plan into action), and (5) evaluation (assessing the effectiveness of the plan and changing the plan as indicated by current needs). Sometimes these steps are called *phases* or *stages*. Initially, the steps are followed in sequence (e.g., data collection and assessment first, then identification of the problems or nursing diagnoses, then planning care, and so forth). However, after the process has begun, it becomes continuous or cyclic. Each phase of the nursing process is dependent on the others, and there is a continuous interaction among the stages as information about the status of the patient changes. Evaluation and revision of the plan of care occur constantly. As problems are alleviated, new problems may arise, requiring new plans and actions.

The American Nurses Association has developed standards of care for nurses for each phase of the nursing process (Table 8–1). However, the role of the licensed practical nurse or licensed vocational nurse in the nursing process is not defined clearly at this time. Some questions remain about who is qualified to perform at what level. Most licensed practical nurses or licensed vocational nurses work in hospital, nursing home, or community settings in which the nursing process is used to achieve goals related to recovery from acute illness,

TABLE 8–1

AMERICAN NURSES ASSOCIATION STANDARDS OF CARE

STANDARD I. ASSESSMENT

THE NURSE COLLECTS CLIENT HEALTH DATA.

Measurement Criteria

1. The priority of data collection is determined by the client's immediate condition or needs.
2. Pertinent data are collected using appropriate assessment techniques.
3. Data collection involves the client, significant others, and health care providers when appropriate.
4. The data collection process is systematic and ongoing.
5. Relevant data are documented in a retrievable form.

STANDARD II. DIAGNOSIS

THE NURSE ANALYZES THE ASSESSMENT DATA IN DETERMINING DIAGNOSES.

Measurement Criteria

1. Diagnoses are derived from the assessment data.
2. Diagnoses are validated with the client, significant others, and health care providers, when possible.
3. Diagnoses are documented in a manner that facilitates the determination of expected outcomes and plan of care.

STANDARD III. OUTCOME IDENTIFICATION

THE NURSE IDENTIFIES EXPECTED OUTCOMES INDIVIDUALIZED TO THE CLIENT.

Measurement Criteria

1. Outcomes are derived from the diagnoses.
2. Outcomes are documented as measurable goals.
3. Outcomes are mutually formulated with the client and health care providers, when possible.
4. Outcomes are realistic in relation to the client's present and potential capabilities.
5. Outcomes are attainable in relation to resources available to the client.
6. Outcomes include a time estimate for attainment.
7. Outcomes provide direction for continuity of care.

STANDARD IV. PLANNING

THE NURSE DEVELOPS A PLAN OF CARE THAT PRESCRIBES INTERVENTIONS TO ATTAIN EXPECTED OUTCOMES.

Measurement Criteria

1. The plan is individualized to the client's condition or needs.
2. The plan is developed with the client, significant others, and health care providers, when appropriate.
3. The plan reflects current nursing practice.
4. The plan is documented.
5. The plan provides for continuity of care.

STANDARD V. IMPLEMENTATION

THE NURSE IMPLEMENTS THE INTERVENTIONS IDENTIFIED IN THE PLAN OF CARE.

Measurement Criteria

1. Interventions are consistent with the established plan of care.
2. Interventions are implemented in a safe and appropriate manner.
3. Interventions are documented.

STANDARD VI. EVALUATION

THE NURSE EVALUATES THE CLIENT'S PROGRESS TOWARD ATTAINMENT OF OUTCOMES.

Measurement Criteria

1. Evaluation is systematic and ongoing.
2. The client's responses to interventions are documented.
3. The effectiveness of interventions is evaluated in relation to outcomes.
4. Ongoing assessment data are used to revise diagnoses, outcomes, and the plan of care, as needed.
5. Revisions in diagnoses, outcomes, and the plan of care are documented.
6. The client, significant others, and health care providers are involved in the evaluation process, when appropriate.

From the Standards of Clinical Practice, © 1991, American Nurses Association, Washington, D.C. Used with permission.

health maintenance in chronic illness, or rehabilitation. Suggested roles for these nurses in relation to the nursing process are: (1) to contribute to an assessment database for patients by collecting information using a standardized form, performing basic psychosocial assessment, and taking objective measurements of body functions; (2) to assist with the development of nursing care plans and the implementation of the established plan of care; (3) to perform basic therapeutic and preventive nursing measures; and (4) to participate in the evaluation of the care given by reporting observed outcomes and making necessary changes according to the results of the evaluation.

ASSESSMENT

The assessment phase of the nursing process involves collection of data about the health status of the patient. The word *data* is the plural of *datum* and means information, especially information organized for analysis or decision making. There are two types of data: (1) subjective and (2) objective. *Subjective data* consist of information that is reported by the patient and family members in a health history in response to direct questioning or in spontaneous statement. Subjective data are usually documented in the patient's own words. *Objective data* are those that the nurse or other members of the health care team obtain through observation, physical examination, or diagnostic testing. Sources of subjective and objective data are the patient, the family and significant others, medical records, and consultation with other health care team members.

Health History

To gather subjective data, or health history, the nurse conducts an interview with the patient or family members or both. The manner in which the interview is conducted directly affects the accuracy and completeness of the information gained. Communication should be goal directed, orderly, and systematic. Some questions may be open ended to allow the patient or family to express their thoughts and feelings. By allowing expression of feelings, the nurse can establish a better working relationship with the patients and families.

The interview should be conducted in a quiet, private area to ensure patient comfort and confidentiality. The purpose of the interview should be explained to the patient and family members with the assurance that they can refuse to answer any questions and can add any pertinent information that is helpful. Usually the interview takes no longer than 20 to 30 minutes; however, some older patients may have difficulty hearing, and the length of time may be extended. Older patients may tire more easily than younger patients, so that several short interviews may be necessary.

Usually a nurse assessment form is used for the interview so that the nursing database is as complete as possible. The health history consists of the following components:

1. Biographical data
2. Reason for seeking care or "chief complaint"
3. Present health or history of present illness
4. Past history
5. Family history
6. Review of systems
7. Functional assessment or activities of daily living

Table 8–2 presents a description of each of these components.

When the interview is complete, the nurse should summarize the data with the patient or family members to be sure the information gathered is correct. The process of summarizing the data further strengthens the nurse-patient relationship because it demonstrates the nurse's interest in the patients and their needs. As the level of trust increases between patient and nurse, the patient may also think of additional information during this time that may have been omitted earlier.

Objective Data

Objective data are gained through physical assessment, diagnostic tests, and patient records. Observation is one of the most important means through which information is obtained. The nurse uses the senses of sight, hearing, smell, and touch to make observations. For example, a patient's disheveled appearance (sight) on admission may indicate an inability to carry out self-care activities at home. A patient's noisy and labored breathing (hearing) may suggest respiratory problems. A fruity mouth odor (smell) may be a sign of diabetic acidosis. Cold and clammy skin (touch) may signal that a patient is in shock.

When recording observational data, the nurse writes exactly what is observed. Words such as good, bad, better, or worse are avoided. For example, "The skin is warm and dry" is preferable to "The skin looks good."

PHYSICAL ASSESSMENT. Physical assessment or examination is a systematic, thorough way of obtaining objective data. Sometimes a complete head-to-toe examination is conducted, whereas at other times one system may be examined if symptoms arise that call for further assessment. Although some aspects of the physical examination require advanced training, the complete physical examination process is presented here.

There are four methods of examination: (1) inspection, (2) palpation, (3) auscultation, and (4) percussion.

Inspection. *Inspection* is purposeful observation or scrutiny of the person as a whole and then of each body system (Fig. 8–1). The observation begins as soon as the nurse meets the patient and is ongoing throughout the examination.

Palpation. *Palpation* uses the sense of touch to assess various parts of the body and helps to confirm things that are noted on inspection. The hands, especially the fingertips, are used to assess skin texture, moisture, and temperature or the presence of swelling, lumps, masses, tenderness, or pain (Fig. 8–2). The hands should be warmed before examination. Palpation should be light at first for surface characteristics and then deeper for abdominal contents. If any tender areas are noted, they

TABLE 8-2
THE HEALTH HISTORY

BIOGRAPHICAL DATA
Name, address, phone number, age, birthdate, birthplace, sex, marital status, race, ethnic origin, occupation, educational level

SOURCE OF HISTORY
Who furnishes information (patient, family); estimate of reliability of information

REASON FOR SEEKING CARE
Chief complaint; put in patient's own words

HISTORY OF PRESENT ILLNESS
Events leading up to chief complaint or reason for seeking care:
Location of symptoms or pain (e.g., pain in the chest radiating to the left arm)
Character or quality (e.g., burning, sharp or dull pain; sticky, dark, or coffee ground–colored blood)
Quantity or severity (severity of pain interrupted normal daily activities)
Timing (onset, duration, frequency); when symptoms appeared; how long they lasted; how often they occurred
Setting (what was happening when symptom occurred; what brought it on)
Aggravating or relieving factors (what makes symptoms worse; what makes them better)
Associated factors (what other symptoms are related, e.g., urinary frequency and burning associated with fever or chills)
Client's perception (meaning of symptoms to client; how they affect daily activities)

PAST HEALTH
Childhood illnesses
Accidents or injuries
Serious or chronic illnesses
Hospitalizations
Operations
Obstetric history
Immunizations
Last examination date
Allergies
Current medications

FAMILY HISTORY
Age, health, and cause of death of blood relatives
Family history of heart disease, high blood pressure, stroke, diabetes, blood disorders, cancer, sickle cell anemia, arthritis, allergies, obesity, alcoholism, mental illness, seizure disorders, kidney disease, and tuberculosis

REVIEW OF SYSTEMS
Evaluate past and present health state of each body system:
General overall health state (present weight, weight gain or loss, fatigue, weakness, fever, chills, night sweats)
Skin (history of skin disease; change in color, pigment, or mole; excessive dryness or moisture; itching; excessive bruising; rash or lesion)
Hair (recent loss, change in texture; change in shape, color, or brittleness of nails)
Head (history of head injury, headache, dizziness, or vertigo)
Eyes (difficulty with vision, including decreased acuity, blurring, blind spots; eye pain; double vision; redness or swelling; watering or discharge; glaucoma or cataracts)
Ears (earaches, infections, discharge, tinnitus or ringing in the ears)
Nose and sinuses (discharge; frequent or severe colds; sinus pain; nasal obstruction; nosebleeds; allergies or hayfever; change in sense of smell)
Mouth and throat (mouth pain, frequent sore throat, bleeding gums, toothache, difficulty swallowing, hoarseness, altered taste)
Neck (pain, limitation of movement, lumps or swelling, enlarged or tender nodes, goiter)
Gastrointestinal (history of abdominal diseases, e.g., ulcer, liver or gallbladder, jaundice, appendicitis, colitis; appetite; food intolerance; difficulty swallowing; heartburn; indigestion; abdominal pain; nausea and vomiting; vomiting blood; flatulence; type and frequency of bowel movement; rectal conditions, e.g., hemorrhoids, fistula)
Breast (pain, lump, nipple discharge, rash, history of breast disease or surgery)
Axilla (tenderness, lump or swelling, rash)
Musculoskeletal system (history of arthritis, gout, back pain or disk disease; pain, stiffness or swelling of joints; deformity; limitation of motion; noise with joint motion; muscle pain, cramps, or weakness; problems with gait or coordination; back pain, stiffness or limitation of motion)
Neurologic system (history of seizure disorder, stroke, fainting, or blackouts; weakness, tic, or tremor; paralysis or coordination problems; numbness or tingling; cognitive disorder; nervousness, mood changes, depression, or history of mental illness)
Respiratory system (lung diseases, e.g., asthma, emphysema, bronchitis, pneumonia, tuberculosis; chest pain with breathing; wheezing or noisy breathing; shortness of breath; cough; sputum; hemoptysis or coughing up blood)
Cardiovascular (chest pain, heart palpitation, cyanosis, dyspnea on exertion, orthopnea, nocturia, edema, heart murmur, hypertension, coronary artery disease, anemia)
Peripheral vascular (coldness, numbness and tingling of extremities; swelling of legs; discoloration of hands or feet; varicose veins; intermittent claudication or pain in legs on exertion; thrombophlebitis; leg ulcers)
Endocrine system (history of diabetes or diabetic symptoms, or thyroid disease; intolerance to heat and cold; change in skin pigmentation or texture; excessive sweating; relationship between appetite and weight; abnormal hair distribution; nervousness; tremors)
Urinary system (history of kidney disease, kidney stones, or urinary tract infections; frequency of urination; urgency; nocturia or number of times person awakens at night to urinate, painful or difficult urination; oliguria or polyuria; color of urine, e.g., cloudy, bloody, straw colored; incontinence; pain in the flank, groin, suprapubic region, or lower back)
Male genital system (penis or testicular pain; penile discharge; sores or lesions; lumps; hernia)
Female genital system (menstrual history, e.g., age at menarche, last menstrual period, cycle and duration, amenorrhea or absence of periods, or menometrorrhagia or bleeding between periods; premenstrual pain or dysmenorrhea or menstrual pain; vaginal itching; discharge and its characteristics; age at menopause; menopausal signs or symptoms; postmenopausal bleeding)

FUNCTIONAL ASSESSMENT
Self-care ability, including bathing, dressing, grooming, toileting, and transfer from bed to chair.

Adapted from Jarvis, C. (1992). *Physical examination and health assessment* (pp. 78–82). Philadelphia: W. B. Saunders.

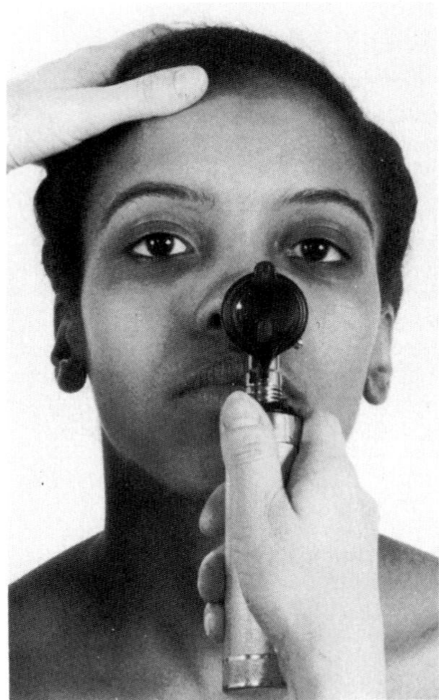

FIGURE 8-1
Inspection. (From Jarvis, C. [1992]. *Physical examination and health assessment* [p. 411]. Philadelphia: W. B. Saunders.)

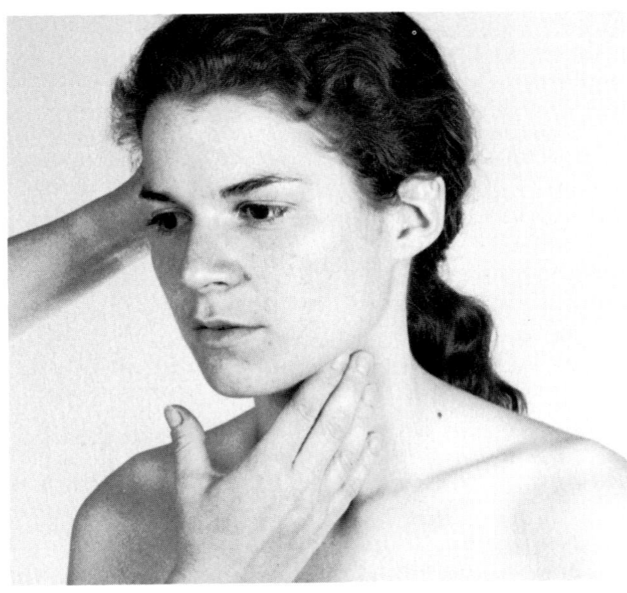

FIGURE 8-2
Palpation. (From Jarvis, C. [1992]. *Physical examination and health assessment* [p. 290]. Philadelphia: W. B. Saunders.)

should be palpated last. Deep palpation is usually done only by nurses with advanced skills.

Auscultation. *Auscultation* is listening to sounds produced by the body, such as heart, lung, and intestinal sounds. Auscultation is carried out through the use of a stethoscope (Fig. 8–3). The stethoscope should be in good working order and should contain both a bell and a diaphragm. The earpieces should fit snugly and point forward to the nose. The room should be quiet so that an accurate assessment of sounds can be made. The diaphragm of the stethoscope is most frequently used for assessment. The diaphragm should be warmed by rubbing it against the nurse's palm, and then placed lightly over the area that is being assessed. If the area is hairy, a crackling sound may be heard. To minimize the problem, it is helpful to wet the hair before examination.

Percussion. *Percussion* is tapping on the skin to assess the underlying tissues. The chest and abdomen are the most common areas for percussion. Short, sharp strokes elicit sounds and subtle vibrations that are characteristic of underlying organs and certain conditions. One hand lies flat on the skin over the area to be percussed. The middle finger of that hand is then lightly tapped by the tip of the middle finger of the other hand (Figs. 8–4, 8–5). It is tapped two times just behind the nailbed before moving on to the next area.

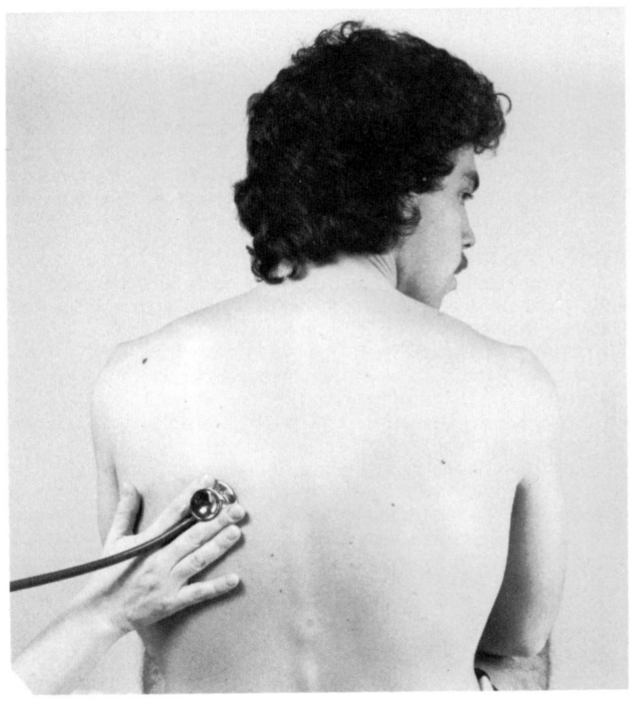

FIGURE 8-3
Auscultation. (From Jarvis, C. [1992]. *Physical examination and health assessment* [p. 499]. Philadelphia: W. B. Saunders.)

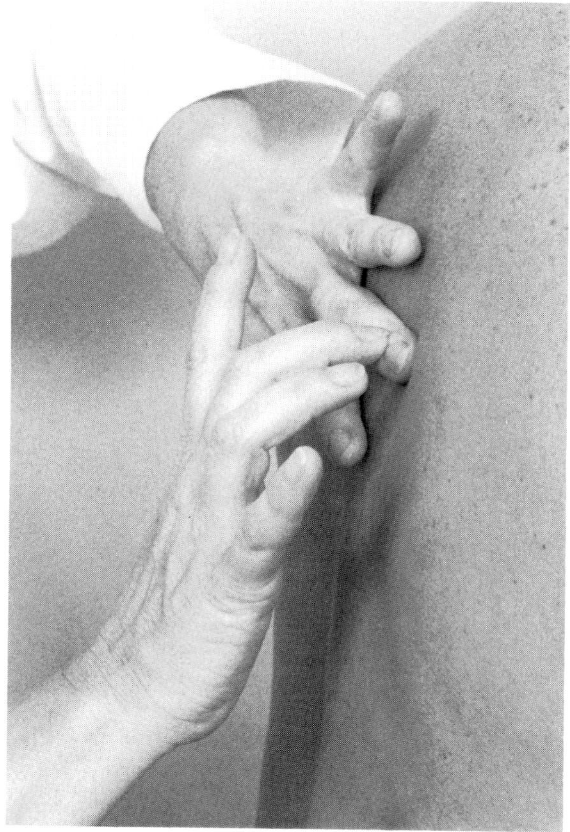

FIGURE 8-4
The stationary hand in percussion. (From Jarvis, C. [1992]. *Physical examination and health assessment* [p. 167]. Philadelphia: W. B. Saunders.)

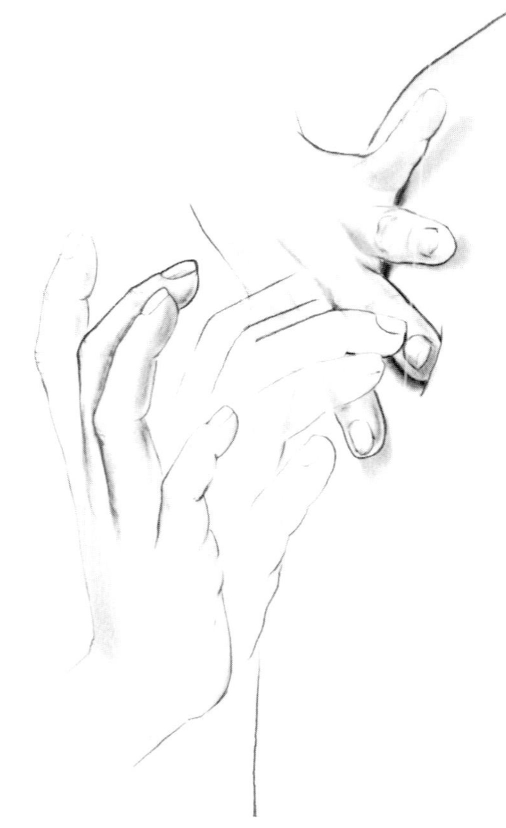

FIGURE 8-5
The striking hand in percussion. (From Jarvis, C. [1992]. *Physical examination and health assessment* [p. 167]. Philadelphia: W. B. Saunders.)

All four methods of examination require practice. Palpation, auscultation, and percussion may be awkward at first, but with time, the skills can be mastered.

The physical examination includes assessment of general appearance, height and weight, vital signs, and body systems. Table 8–3 presents an overview of the content of a complete physical examination.

DIAGNOSTIC TESTS. Diagnostics include radiographic examinations (x-rays), electrocardiograms, magnetic resonance imaging scans, computed tomography scans, ultrasound studies, laboratory blood and urine testing, and wound cultures. The information from these tests can be helpful to the nurse in identifying general areas in which a patient might have a health care problem or in validating a nursing diagnosis.

PATIENT RECORDS. Patient records provide a valuable source of information regarding the past medical history and illness patterns. They can confirm the subjective data and history that the patient and family give the nurse.

NURSING DIAGNOSIS

The nursing diagnosis is derived from data gathered during the assessment. Health problems or potential health problems are identified and formulated into nursing diagnoses. Nursing diagnoses provide a basis for planning nursing interventions that can help prevent, minimize, or alleviate specific health problems. They are then used to evaluate the response of the patient to the nursing interventions.

A nursing diagnosis is different from a medical diagnosis. The medical diagnosis is used to identify the etiology (cause) of the disease. The focus of the medical diagnosis is on the function and malfunction of a specific organ system. The nursing diagnosis focuses on the response of the whole person to the health problem.

The concept of nursing diagnosis has been discussed for many years. In 1973, the National Conference Group on the Classification of Nursing Diagnosis began meeting to develop standardized nursing diagnoses to be used in all health care settings. The group, now known as The North American Nursing Diagnosis Association

TABLE 8-3
THE PHYSICAL EXAMINATION

PHYSICAL APPEARANCE
Age, sex, level of consciousness, skin color, facial features, no signs of acute distress

BODY STRUCTURE
Stature, nutrition (normal weight for height and body build), symmetry, posture, body build (normal proportions), obvious physical deformities

MOBILITY
Gait, range of motion, no involuntary movement

BEHAVIOR
Facial expression, mood and affect, speech, dress, personal hygiene, hair, and makeup

MEASUREMENTS
Height, weight, vital signs

SKIN, HAIR, AND NAILS
Skin (color, general pigmentation, widespread color change, temperature, moisture, texture, thickness, edema, mobility and turgor, hygiene, vascularity or bruising, lesions)
Hair (color, texture, distribution, scalp lesions)
Nails (shape and contour, consistency, color)

HEAD AND NECK
Head (size and shape of skull, symmetry, and expression of face)
Neck (symmetry, range of motion, lymph nodes)

EYES
Central visual acuity, near and far vision, peripheral vision, extraocular muscle function (parallel alignment, nystagmus), external eye structures (eyebrows, eyelids and lashes, eyeballs, conjunctiva and sclera, lacrimal apparatus, cornea and lens, iris and pupils)

EARS
External ear (size and shape, skin condition, tenderness, the external auditory meatus), external canal, tympanic membrane, hearing acuity, vestibular apparatus

NOSE, MOUTH, AND THROAT
Nose (external nose, nasal cavity, sinus area)
Mouth (lips, teeth and gums, tongue, buccal mucosa, palate)
Throat (tonsils)

BREASTS AND REGIONAL LYMPHATICS
General appearance, skin, lymphatic drainage areas, nipple, axilla

THORAX AND LUNGS
Posterior chest (symmetric expansion, fremitus [palpable vibration], lung fields, breath sounds)
Anterior chest (shape and configuration of chest wall, level of consciousness, skin color and condition, quality of respirations, symmetric chest expansion, forced expiratory time [number of seconds to exhale])

HEART AND NECK VESSELS
Carotid artery pulse, jugular venous pulse, jugular venous pressure, anterior chest inspection, rate and rhythm, heart sounds, murmurs

ABDOMEN
Inspection (contour, symmetry, umbilicus, skin, pulsation or movement, hair distribution)
Auscultation (bowel sounds, vascular sounds)
Percussion (general tympany, liver span, splenic dullness)
Palpation (surface and deep areas, liver edge, spleen, kidneys)

PERIPHERAL VASCULAR SYSTEM
Pulses, capillary refill, skin color and temperature, edema, pain

MUSCULOSKELETAL SYSTEM
Inspection (size and contour of joint, skin and tissues surrounding joint), palpation (temperature, muscles, and bony articulations of joint) range of motion, muscle strength, functional assessment

NEUROLOGIC SYSTEM
Cranial nerves, motor system (muscles, cerebellar function), sensory system (pain, temperature, light touch, vibration, position), reflexes (stretch or deep tendon reflexes, superficial reflexes)

MALE GENITALIA
Penis, scrotum, hernia, inguinal lymph nodes

FEMALE GENITALIA
External genitalia (skin color, hair distribution, labia majora, labia minoris, clitoris, urethral opening, vaginal opening, perineum, anus)
Internal genitalia (cervix, vagina)

ANUS, RECTUM, AND PROSTATE
Perianal area, anus, rectum, stool

(NANDA), meets yearly to develop and revise nursing diagnoses. The current list (1992) of accepted nursing diagnoses and the 1994 Diagnoses in Progress are found in Table 8–4.

Nursing diagnoses are written in a format, called PES, developed by NANDA. *P* stands for the *problem*, *E* stands for the *etiology* or cause of the problem, and *S* stands for the *signs and symptoms* of the problem. The PES format helps to make the general nursing diagnosis fit a specific patient care problem. The following example using the general nursing diagnosis "Impaired skin integrity" for a specific patient situation is shown. An elderly woman has developed a 2-cm decubitus ulcer on her sacrum because she is bedridden and immobilized. Her specific nursing diagnosis would be written in the following manner:

> Impaired skin integrity (*P*) related to immobility (*E*) as evidenced by 2-cm decubitus ulcer on sacrum (*S*). The problem (*P*) or nursing diagnosis is "impaired skin integrity," the etiology (*E*) or cause is "immobility," and the signs or symptoms (*S*) are "2-cm decubitus ulcer on sacrum."

By using all of the components of the nursing diagnosis, the problem is clearly communicated to everyone involved in the patient's care.

Although NANDA is continually working to make the structure and content of nursing diagnoses consistent, they still are not universally used and accepted. It is difficult for nursing students to work and learn in an uncertain environment as nursing diagnoses are constantly evolving. However, nurses must work together to develop the most appropriate diagnoses to reflect current nursing practice.

The format for nursing diagnoses in this book presents the problem and the etiology to avoid repetitious lists of signs and symptoms. In an actual patient

TABLE 8-4

APPROVED NURSING DIAGNOSES, NORTH AMERICAN NURSING DIAGNOSIS ASSOCIATION, 1992

Activity Intolerance
Activity Intolerance, High Risk for
Adjustment, Impaired
Airway Clearance, Ineffective
Anxiety
Aspiration, High Risk for
Body Image Disturbance
Body Temperature, High Risk for Altered
Breastfeeding, Effective
Breastfeeding, Ineffective
Breastfeeding, Interrupted
Breathing Patterns, Ineffective
Caregiver Role Strain
Caregiver Role Strain, High Risk for
Communication, Impaired Verbal
Constipation
Constipation, Colonic
Constipation, Perceived
Decisional Conflict (Specify)
Decreased Cardiac Output
Defensive Coping
Denial, Ineffective
Diarrhea
Disuse Syndrome, High Risk for
Diversional Activity Deficit
Dysreflexia
Family Coping: Compromised, Ineffective
Family Coping: Disabling, Ineffective
Family Coping: Potential for Growth
Family Processes, Altered
Fatigue
Fear
Fluid Volume Deficit
Fluid Volume Deficit, High Risk for
Fluid Volume Excess
Gas Exchange, Impaired
Grieving, Anticipatory
Grieving, Dysfunctional
Growth and Development
Health Maintenance, Altered
Health-Seeking Behaviors (Specify)
Home Maintenance Management, Impaired
Hopelessness
Hyperthermia
Hypothermia
Incontinence, Bowel
Incontinence, Functional
Incontinence, Reflex
Incontinence, Stress
Incontinence, Total
Incontinence, Urge
Individual Coping, Ineffective
Infant Feeding Pattern, Ineffective
Infection, High Risk for
Injury, High Risk for
Knowledge Deficit (Specify)
Noncompliance (Specify)
Nutrition, Altered: Less Than Body Requirements
Nutrition, Altered: More Than Body Requirements
Nutrition, Altered: Potential for More Than Body Requirements
Oral Mucous Membrane, Altered
Pain
Pain, Chronic
Parental Role Conflict
Parenting, Altered
Parenting, High Risk for Altered
Peripheral Neurovascular Dysfunction, High Risk for
Personal Identity Disturbance
Physical Mobility, Impaired
Poisoning, High Risk for
Post-Trauma Response
Powerlessness
Protection, Altered
Rape Trauma Syndrome
Rape Trauma Syndrome: Compound Reaction
Rape Trauma Syndrome: Silent Reaction
Relocation Stress Syndrome
Role Performance, Altered
Self-Care Deficit
  Bathing/Hygiene
  Dressing/Grooming
  Feeding
  Toileting
Self-Esteem, Chronic Low
Self-Esteem, Situational Low
Self-Esteem Disturbance
Self-Mutilation, High Risk for
Sensory Perceptual Alterations (Specify) (visual, auditory, kinesthetic, gustatory, tactile, olfactory)
Sexual Dysfunction
Sexuality Patterns, Altered
Skin Integrity, Impaired
Skin Integrity, High Risk for Impaired
Sleep Pattern Disturbance
Social Interactions, Impaired
Social Isolation
Spiritual Distress
Suffocation, High Risk for
Swallowing, Impaired
Therapeutic Regimen, Ineffective Management of (Individuals)
Thermoregulation, Ineffective
Thought Processes, Altered
Tissue Integrity, Impaired
Tissue Perfusion, Altered (Specify Type) (renal, cerebral, cardiopulmonary, gastrointestinal, peripheral)
Trauma, High Risk for
Unilateral Neglect
Urinary Elimination, Altered
Urinary Retention
Ventilation, Inability to Sustain Spontaneous
Ventilatory Weaning Response, Dysfunctional
Violence, High Risk for: Self-directed or directed at others

From the North American Nursing Diagnosis Association. (1992). *Approved nursing diagnoses.* Philadelphia: Author.

care plan, the patient's specific signs and symptoms would be included.

PLANNING

The planning phase of the nursing process involves the development of a nursing care plan for the patient based on the nursing diagnoses. Nursing care plans are a form of communication to other health care professionals to ensure continuity of care, to prevent complications, and to provide for health teaching and discharge planning.

The steps in nursing care planning are (1) to determine priorities from the list of nursing diagnoses, (2) to set long-term and short-term goals to determine outcomes of care, (3) to develop objectives to reach the goals, and (4) to write nursing orders to direct care to meet the goals. *Priorities* are established according to the most immediate needs of the patient. They are usually based on Maslow's hierarchy of needs and what the patient perceives as important. *Goals* may be short term or long term, meaning that some may be achievable immediately whereas others will take a longer period of time. Goals should be stated in terms of observable patient outcomes. *Objectives* or "outcome criteria" are specific steps toward accomplishment of the goals. Using the patient previously mentioned with impaired skin integrity, the goal would be stated as "Restore skin integrity." The objective would be "Decubitus ulcer over sacrum healed within 2 weeks." *Nursing orders* are the actions for interventions prescribed to help achieve the stated goals and objectives. Nursing orders should include a specific description (what, where, when, how much, and how long) of how the order should be carried out. For example, "Keep off sacrum to promote healing; turn on each side q 2 hr. Get OOB (out of bed) twice a day; begin ambulating as tolerated."

INTERVENTION (IMPLEMENTATION)

Implementation is the actual performance of the nursing interventions identified in the plan of care. The interventions are coordinated with other members of the health care team and include direct patient care, health teaching, or carrying out ordered medical treatments such as medications or dressing changes.

Some interventions are unplanned because the nurse must respond to crises that demand immediate attention. Thus, the care plan must be flexible and reflect changes in the patient's health care needs. Nursing interventions and their results always should be documented in the patient's chart.

EVALUATION

Evaluation is an ongoing process in which the nurse determines what progress the patient has made in meeting the goals for care. The outcome criteria provide measures for determining outcomes of care. Using the previous example of impaired skin integrity, the outcome criteria would be "intact skin" and "absence of redness over bony prominences." In assessing outcomes of care, the nurse determines whether the goals have been met, partially met, or have not been met. If the goals have not been met, the nurse should reexamine the plan of care and modify it where necessary.

Evaluation helps to provide data regarding the quality of care in a health care institution. Quality assurance audits are conducted by the individual health care agencies as well as the Joint Commission on Accreditation of Healthcare Organizations (JCAHO), an organization that requires systematic review of hospitals and other health care organizations. Areas evaluated include the standards of nursing care used, the quality and effectiveness of nursing care, and the organization of the patient care system. Nursing audits are conducted by examining patient records as one method of gathering information to evaluate nursing performance. The American Nurses Association Standards of Care are used as a measure to determine whether nurses have carried out the nursing process as documented in the patient records.

NURSING PROCESS DOCUMENTATION

Documentation is an important component of nursing intervention. Patient assessments and observations and all nursing interventions should be charted as a permanent part of the patient's record. Documentation helps to achieve continuity of care because it provides for communication among caregivers as well as a record of the patient's progress. In addition, documentation provides a legal record of care provided and a verification of services rendered for insurance payments.

Nurses should document the following:

1. All treatments and care given, including medications
2. Diagnostic procedures performed at the bedside, on the unit, or inside or outside the facility
3. The patient's reaction to therapeutic and diagnostic procedures
4. Observations of the patient
5. Subjective and objective signs and symptoms experienced by the patient
6. Evidence of changes in the patient's physical, psychosocial, and spiritual needs and status
7. Any unusual incidents, such as falls or injuries, occurring during the patient's stay in the health care facility

Documentation should be clear, concise, complete, and accurate. All sheets should have the patient's name and the date and time information was entered. Writing should be legible, using proper grammar, punctuation, and spelling. All spaces must be filled with no empty lines left. Charting is carried out as soon after care is given as possible (never before care). Observations are objective and describe only what is seen, heard, felt, or smelled. Direct quotations from the patient regarding symptoms are very appropriate. Each time an entry is made, the nurse should sign with full name and title. Only permanent ink is used, and no erasures are made. If an error in charting is made, the entry should be crossed out and "error" written above it, followed by the nurse's initials.

FORMATS FOR DOCUMENTATION OF PATIENT CARE

Various formats are used for the documentation of patient care, including "nurses' notes," flow sheets, and problem-oriented medical records (POMR). Nurses' notes usually consist of pages of narrative recordings indicating the assessments, observations, and interventions carried out by the nurse. Flow sheets may be graphs of vital signs or tables in which nurses may check or initial boxes indicating activities or care provided.

The POMR is a method of record keeping that focuses on patient problems rather than on medical diagnoses. This method is popular in many clinical areas because it provides an excellent means of communication among the various disciplines who are providing care. Each health care provider involved in the care of the patient charts on the same progress notes in the same format.

The data from the history, physical examination, diagnostic tests, and medical diagnoses provide a foundation for problems formulated in the POMR. The problem list consists of active, inactive, potential, and resolved problems. The charting is done in a SOAPIER format. SOAPIER is an acronym for the components of the charting:

S *Subjective* information, or how the patient perceives the problem

O *Objective* information, or what the nurse observes about the patient

A *Assessment*, or why the patient has the problem

P *Plan*, or how the intervention is to be carried out

I *Intervention*, or what specific care is given

E *Evaluation*, or how effective was the plan or intervention

R *Revision*, or what changes should be made in the original plan of care

In *many* cases, the SOAPE form is used, omitting the intervention and revision sections. The intervention is closely related to the plan and can be a reiteration of the plan; a revision can be made in the plan by simply revising the original SOAPE notes.

An example of a SOAPE note using our previous example is as follows:

S Feels weak; does "not have the energy" to move around

O Does not turn self in bed; 2 cm, stage 2 decubitus ulcer on sacrum

A Decubitus ulcer on sacrum related to immobility

P Turn from side to side every 2 hr. Get out of bed at least twice a day. Begin ambulating as tolerated.

E Turned q 2 hr. OOB twice a day; taking 6 small steps to and from bed. Decubitus ulcer healing; now 1.5 cm.

A large amount of time is spent charting and keeping records, and many facilities are transforming their record keeping into more time-saving methods of documentation, such as computerized nursing care plans and nurses' notes. Nevertheless, regardless of the format, the essential data always should be recorded systematically.

BIBLIOGRAPHY

Alfaro R. (1990). *Applying nursing diagnosis and nursing process: A step by step guide* (2nd ed.). Philadelphia: J. B. Lippincott.

Atkinson, L. D., & Murray, M. E. (1990). *Understanding the nursing process: Fundamentals of care planning* (4th ed.). Tarrytown, NY: Pergamon Press.

Bleich, M. R. (1990). Clinical judgments: Essential elements of the nursing process. *Journal of Nursing Quality Assurance, 4*(4), 1–6.

Chana, C. H. (1992). Documenting the nursing process: A perioperative nursing care plan. *AORN Journal, 55*(5), 1231–1233, 1235.

Crouch, S. (1990). The nursing process. *Nursing, 4*(12), 16–18.

Doenges, M. E., Moorhouse, M. F., & McCoy, S. M. (1992). *Application of nursing process and nursing diagnosis: An interactive text.* Philadelphia: F. A. Davis.

Edelstein, J. (1990). A study of nursing documentation. *Nursing Management, 21*(11), 40–43, 46.

Exstrom, S., & Gollner, M. L. (1990). There is more than one use of SOAP. *Nursing Management, 21*(10), 12.

Fischbach, F. T. (1991). *Documenting care: Communication, the nursing process and documentation standards.* Philadelphia: F. A. Davis.

Fox, L., & Woods, P. (1991). Nursing process—evaluation of documentation. *Nursing Management*, *22*(1), 57–58.

Goldmann, R. C. (1990). Nursing process components as a framework for monitoring and evaluation activities. *Journal of Nursing Quality Assurance, 4*(4), 17–25.

Gross, D. L., & Andrea J. (1991). Development of a nursing process-based documentation system. *Journal of Emergency Nursing, 17*(3), 173–176.

Iyer, P. W., & Camp, N. H. (1991). *Nursing documentation: A nursing process approach.* St. Louis: Mosby-Year Book.

Kerr, S. D. (1992). A comparison of four nursing documentation systems. *Journal of Nursing Staff Development, 8*(1), 26–31.

Kobert, L., & Folan, M. (1990). Coming of age in nursing: Rethinking the philosophies behind holism and nursing process. *Nursing & Health Care, 11*(6), 308–312.

Langel, B. C., Brewer, S. G., & Olszewski, C. (1991). Developing quality documentation. *Nursing Management, 22*(11), 48–50, 52.

Leuner, J. D., Manton, A. K., Kelliher, D. B., Sullivan, S. P., & Doherty, M. (1990). *Mastering the nursing process: A case method approach.* Philadelphia: F. A. Davis.

McCloskey, J. C., Bulechek, G. M., Cohen, M. Z., Craft, M. J., Crossley, J. D., & Denehy, J. A. (1990). Classification of nursing interventions. *Journal of Professional Nursing, 6*(3), 151–157.

McHugh, M. K. (1991). Does the nursing process reflect quality care? *Holistic Nursing Practice, 5*(3), 22–28.

Moorhouse, M. F., & Doenges, M. E. (1990). *Nurse's clinical pocket manual: Nursing diagnoses, care planning, and documentation.* Philadelphia: F. A. Davis.

Ponder, P. M. (1990). The nursing process and computers. *Point of View, 27*(1), 14–15.

Rankin, S. H., & Stallings, K. D. *Patient education: Issues, principles, and practices* (2nd ed.). Philadelphia: J. B. Lippincott.

Ryan-Wenger, N. M. (1990). A nursing process methodology. *Nursing Outlook, 38*(4), 190–193.

Schroeder, P. (1990). From the editor . . . Assuring the use of the nursing process. *Journal of Nursing Quality Assurance, 4*(4), viii.

Weber, C. (1991). Making nursing diagnosis work for you and your client: A step-by-step approach. *Nursing & Health Care, 12*(8), 424–430.

Weber, M. (1991). Documentation: Short, simple, and meaningful. *Neonatal Network–Journal of Neonatal Nursing, 10*(1), 53–62.

Yura, H., & Walsh, M. B. (1988). *The nursing process: Assessing, planning, implementing, evaluating* (5th ed.). East Norwalk, CT: Appleton & Lange.

KEY CONCEPTS

1. The nursing process is a problem-solving approach that enables the nurse to provide care in an organized, scientific manner.
2. The steps of the nursing process are assessment, nursing diagnosis, planning, intervention, and evaluation.
3. Assessment involves collection of subjective and objective data about the client or patient from the client, family, significant others, medical records, and other care providers.
4. The health history includes biographical data, chief complaint and history of present illness, past medical history, family history, review of systems, and functional assessment.
5. The physical examination uses inspection, auscultation, palpation, and percussion to collect objective data about the patient.
6. The nursing diagnosis is a statement of a health problem or potential health problem derived from the assessment.
7. Nursing diagnoses differ from medical diagnoses in that they focus on the response of the whole person to the medical problem.
8. The planning phase of the nursing process involves the development of a nursing care plan for the patient based on the nursing diagnoses.
9. Planning includes priority setting, goal and objective statements, and nursing interventions to achieve the goals.
10. Intervention refers to the actual performance of the nursing interventions identified in the plan of care.
11. Evaluation is an ongoing process in which the nurse determines what progress has been made toward meeting the goals.
12. Documentation of assessments, interventions, and evaluation data is an essential aspect of nursing care.

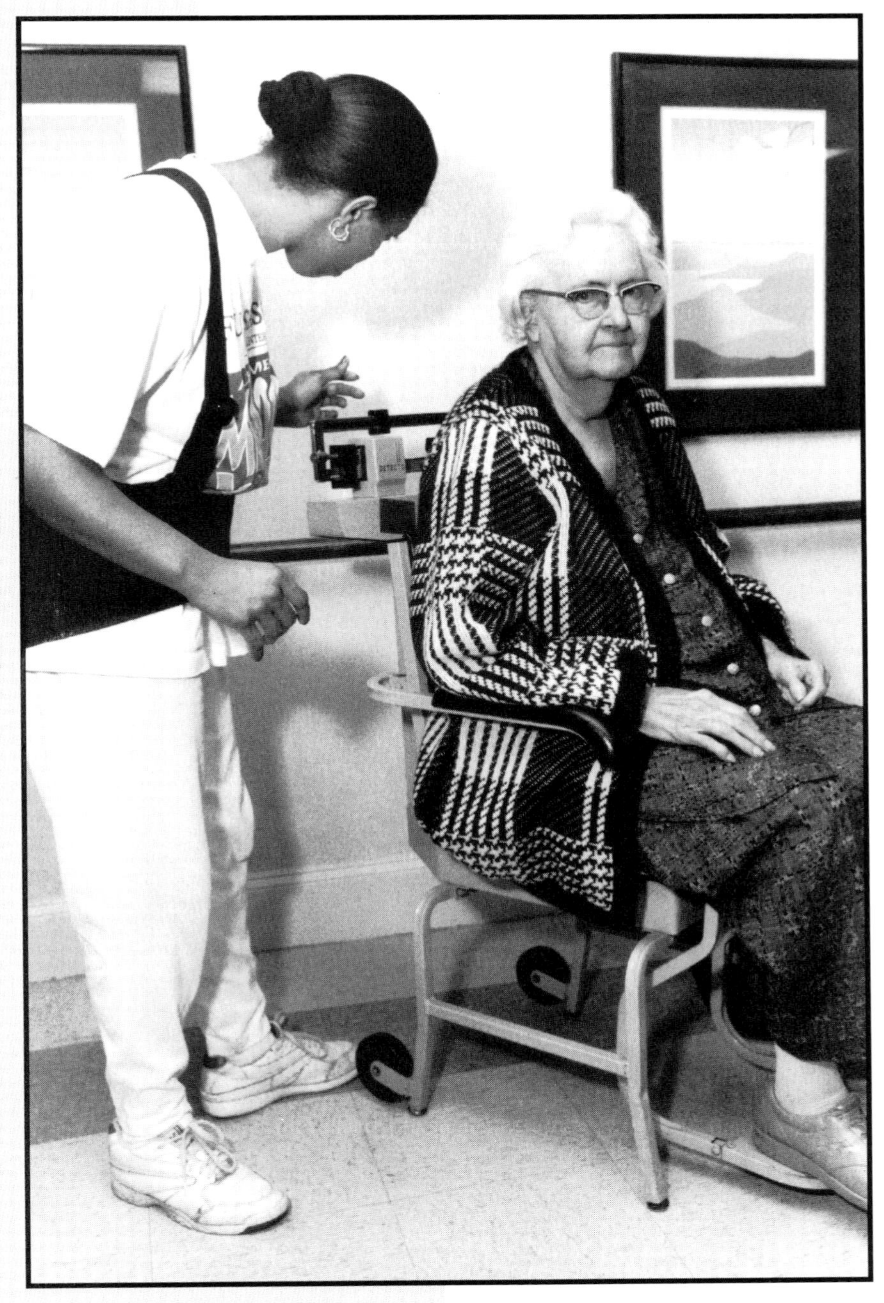

UNIT 2
Physiologic Responses to Illness

Edward P. Gruber

CHAPTER 9

Inflammation and Infection

OBJECTIVES

1. Explain the mechanisms of the protective structures of the body.
2. Describe the ways in which inflammatory changes act as bodily defense mechanisms.
3. Identify the signs and symptoms of inflammation.
4. Discuss the process of repair and healing.
5. Differentiate infection from inflammation.
6. Discuss the actions of commonly found infectious agents.
7. Describe the ways that infections are transmitted.
8. Identify the signs and symptoms of infection.
9. Compare community-acquired and nosocomial infections.
10. Discuss the nursing care of patients in isolation.
11. Discuss the nursing care of patients with infections.

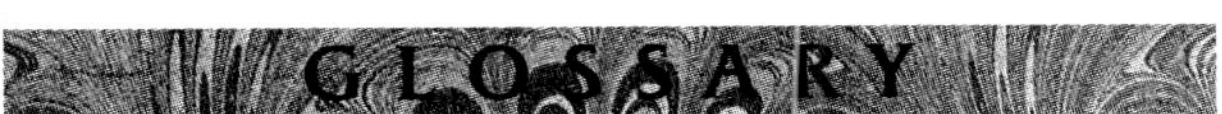

GLOSSARY

BACTERIA Several classifications of one-celled microorganisms that are capable of multiplying rapidly and causing illness

COMMUNITY-ACQUIRED INFECTIONS Infections that are acquired in day-to-day contact with the public

FUNGI Vegetable-like organisms that exist by feeding on organic matter and are capable of producing disease

HELMINTHS Worms that are parasites found in the soil and water and are transmitted to humans from hand to mouth

IATROGENIC INFECTIONS Infections caused by the caregiving process

ISOLATION TECHNIQUE Isolation of infected patients from other patients and health care workers

LEUKOCYTOSIS Part of the inflammatory process that causes an increase in white blood cells

MEDICAL ASEPSIS Limiting the spread of microorganisms, often called *clean technique*

MYCOPLASMAS Gram-negative organisms usually causing infections in the respiratory tract

NOSOCOMIAL INFECTIONS Hospital-acquired infections

PROTOZOA One-celled organisms capable of producing disease that is usually spread by contaminated food and water

Glossary continued

REGENERATION Replacement of damaged cells by cells of their own kind during the wound healing process

REPAIR Replacement of damaged cells by connective tissue and then eventually by scar tissue during the wound healing process

REVERSE ISOLATION Protection of severely compromised clients from other patients and health care workers

RICKETTSIAE Microorganisms that are usually transmitted to humans through flea and tick bites

SURGICAL ASEPSIS Elimination of microorganisms from any object that comes in contact with the patient, often called *sterile technique*

VIRUSES Microorganisms that cause illness by stimulating an antigen-antibody response in the tissues, producing inflammation and cell destruction

Suppose you were being attacked. How would you defend yourself? Perhaps you would shout or in some other way sound an alarm. You may even call in reinforcements to help you fight off the attacker, telling them the most direct route to your location. You would probably surround yourself with some sort of barrier either to shield yourself from further harm or to keep the attacker in the area so that it would not escape and harm someone else. Then, after the battle was over, you would likely enlist the help of some friends to clean up the debris and return your situation to normal.

It is quite remarkable to realize that, at a cellular level, the human body is protected in much the same way. The body relies on many effective barriers to protect itself from injury and disease. However, if these barriers are compromised, several sophisticated processes are triggered to isolate and eliminate the offender. In this chapter, we describe how the body defends itself from injury and disease and explain how the processes are helped along by good nursing care.

PROTECTIVE STRUCTURES AND MECHANISMS

The human body contains a number of protective structures designed to shield it from disease or injury. They include the skin, the gastrointestinal tract, the vagina, the liver, and various blood cells.

SKIN

The *skin* often has been called the body's first line of defense. This remarkable organ contains multiple layers of highly specialized cells that protect more delicate structures beneath it. The outer layer or *epidermis* contains several layers of different kinds of cells that vary in thickness depending on their location. The sole of the foot, for example, contains many more layers than the dorsum or top of the foot to protect it from more frequent exposure to injury during walking. The extreme outer layer of cells in the epidermis is shed regularly and replaced by newer cells. This intact surface protects the body from the invasion of microorganisms. This layer contains no nerves or blood vessels.

The inner layer or *dermis* contains nerves, blood vessels, hair follicles, and sweat glands. Some dermal structures project into the epidermis to allow the sensations of heat and cold and the excretion of salts and water. Hair follicles and sebaceous glands also reside in the dermis. Together the dermis and epidermis protect the body from penetrating and thermal injury that could permit the invasion of microorganisms.

The *mucous membranes* of the mouth and nose provide an additional barrier to invasion by injurious agents. Hair follicles in the nose filter out larger dust particles, and the mucous membrane surface provides a mechanical barrier that prevents smaller particles from reaching the smaller airways. In the respiratory tract, cilia in the lung trap and sweep out irritants. The moist membrane also serves to trap foreign material, keeping much of it out of the smaller airways.

GASTROINTESTINAL TRACT, VAGINA, AND LIVER

In the *gastrointestinal tract,* gastric secretions kill many bacteria unable to survive a strong acid environment, while a layer of mucous cells protects the stomach from chemical or bacterial injury.

In the *vagina* acidic secretions protect against the growth of bacteria and fungi.

The *liver* has many functions; however, some of the most important are its protective functions. The liver protects the body by detoxifying drugs, alcohol, and some environmental poisons.

BLOOD CELLS

Leukocytes are colorless blood cells that have the ability to phagocytize or ingest bacteria that can invade the body and cause infection. Two types of leukocytes (neutrophils and monocytes) are especially suited for this purpose. The measurement of these cells gives an indication of the severity of infection in the body.

Reticuloendothelial cells are found in the blood, connective tissue, liver, spleen, bone marrow, and lymph nodes. Some reticuloendothelial cells protect the body by their ability to digest and absorb foreign material, such as old red blood cells, bacteria, and colloidal particles. These cells may also be called *tissue macrophages.*

THE INFLAMMATORY PROCESS

The inflammatory process is a series of cellular changes that signal the body's response to injury or infection. This process has been identified since at least

1650 B.C. At that time the most common presentation of inflammation was infection. Although infection is still a common manifestation of inflammation, this complex phenomenon may be caused by trauma from (1) physical agents (excessive sunlight, x-rays), (2) chemical stimuli (insect venom, other chemicals), and (3) biologic agents (bacteria, viruses).

The word *inflammation* means literally "the fire within." This descriptive phrase illustrates the four classic observable signs of inflammation: (1) rubor (redness), (2) calor (heat), (3) tumor (swelling), and (4) dolor (pain). It is helpful to think about the appearance of a bee sting and recall the redness, warmth, swelling, and pain that it produces. These signs are the direct result of several related actions that occur when the inflammation process is initiated. The actions involve hemodynamic changes, increased permeability of membranes, chemical mediators, and hormonal factors.

ACTIONS IN THE INFLAMMATORY PROCESS

Hemodynamic Changes

The first of these actions are the *hemodynamic changes*. When the body senses a noxious stimulus, the small blood vessels (venules and arterioles) in the area become dilated. This dilation brings increased blood flow to the area. The increase in blood flow is at least partially responsible for the characteristic warmth and redness at the site of inflammation.

Increased Permeability

The second action is an *increase in permeability* (Fig. 9–1). After the increased blood flow brings leukocytes into the area, chemical mediators cause leukocytes to line the small blood vessel walls near the inflammatory site. This process is called *pavementing*. Gradually these cells pass through the vessel walls and inhabit the inflamed area. These cells, largely neutrophils and monocytes, are drawn to the site of injury or infection by chemotaxis where they ingest and carry away bacteria and other foreign particulates (phagocytosis). The permeability of these vessels causes protein-rich fluid to flow through the vessel walls into the interstitial space. Some red blood cells may pass through into this area as well. This collection of fluid is responsible for the swelling that is noted when the inflammation site is close to the surface of the skin. This swelling may also produce pain.

Chemical Mediators

The hemodynamic changes and vascular permeability occur with the help of several chemical mediators. These powerful substances occupy the cells and plasma and are liberated during the inflammatory process. *Vasoactive amines* such as histamine and serotonin, *acidic lipids* such as prostaglandins and slow-reacting substance of anaphylaxis, and *lysosomal enzymes* are all cellular substances responsible for vascular permeability and the chemotaxis of leukocytes. The *kinin system* produces bradykinin, which also mediates blood vessel dila-

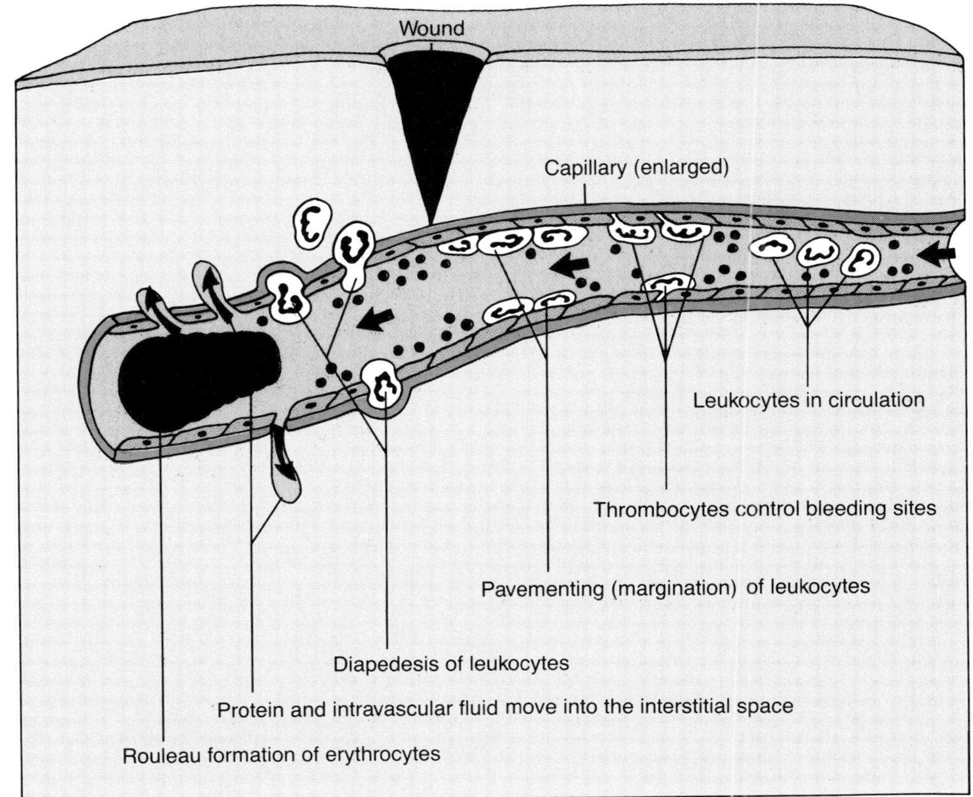

FIGURE 9–1
Neutrophils and phagocytosis. Neutrophils are attracted to the site of injury by chemical stimulation. The neutrophil leaves the blood vessel by sliding through holes in the vessel wall. The leukocytes also line the vessel wall, and the erythrocytes stack like coins to slow blood flow. (From Black, J. M., & Matassarin-Jacobs, E. [1993]. *Luckmann and Sorensen's medical-surgical nursing: A psychophysiologic approach* [4th ed., p. 378]. Philadelphia., W. B. Saunders.)

tion and permeability. It also produces pain, another classic sign of inflammation. Other mediators include the *complement system,* which is especially important in immunologically mediated reactions involving antigen-antibody complexes. These reactions cause a massive release of histamine and other substances that produce marked vasodilation, vascular permeability, and smooth muscle contraction. These cellular changes produce the classic sign of shock: hypotension, swelling, and bronchospasm.

Hormonal Factors

Some *hormonal factors* have an effect on inflammation. Cortisol, a hormone produced by the adrenal cortex, is an anti-inflammatory substance that slows the release of histamine, stabilizes lysosomal membranes, and prevents the chemotaxis of leukocytes. The end result of these actions is to impede the inflammatory process. Drugs that mimic this action (gluccocorticoids) are often used in the treatment of inflammatory conditions.

SIGNS AND SYMPTOMS OF INFLAMMATION

The *signs and symptoms of inflammation* vary depending on whether the reaction is local or systemic. Local inflammation generally produces the classic signs of heat, swelling, redness, pain, and loss of function, the loss of function being the result of the other four signs.

Systemic inflammation produces somewhat different reactions. Swelling, redness, and heat may not be visible; however, signs of the effects of the chemical mediators may be recognized in other ways. Fever is a common sign of systemic inflammation, probably caused by pyrogens (fever-producing substances) that are liberated during phagocytosis or by bacterial endotoxins, antigen-antibody complexes, and certain viruses. Other symptoms of systemic inflammation include headache, muscle aches, chills, and sweating.

Leukocytosis also is a frequent sign of systemic inflammation. This is probably a defensive reaction that provides abundant white blood cells for the inflammatory response. If infection is not present, inflammatory leukocytosis disappears within a few hours.

WOUND HEALING

Repair and regeneration of tissue is set in motion from the very beginning of the inflammatory process. The speed at which this process takes place depends on the type of tissue injured, the severity of the wound, the presence of infection, and the health of the host. At the outset, macrophage cells are produced to clean up inflammatory debris. Fibroblasts begin the repair process by laying down elastin and collagen at the edges of the wound that gradually migrate to the base forming granulation tissue. Capillaries are formed, providing circulation and nutrients to the new tissue. Epithelial cells migrate over the wound and under the scab (usually formed of dried blood and fibroblasts), eventually undercutting it. After a few days the scab falls off. Some tissue, such as connective tissue and smooth muscle, regenerates well. *Regeneration* means that damaged cells are replaced by cells of their own kind. Other tissue must undergo *repair,* which involves the replacement of injured cells by connective tissue and eventually a scar. In fact, most wounds manifest both types of tissue repair.

The age and general health of the person affect how rapidly the regeneration and repair process occurs. The healing process can be delayed in the elderly owing to a decreased blood supply to the tissues and a decrease in tissue elasticity. Also, a lack of vitamin C, zinc, and other important vitamins and minerals can delay the regeneration and repair process.

Occasionally a wound becomes infected or ulcerated, and there is tissue loss. Granulation tissue and capillary buds form at the margins of the wound, and it is eventually filled with granulation tissue. Sometimes the wound is too large for the granulation tissue to fill. In this case the wound is usually cleaned and débrided. When infection is no longer present, the wound is sutured closed. This is called *delayed primary closure.*

INFECTION

Infection is a process involving the invasion of body tissues by microorganisms, the multiplication of the invading organisms, and the subsequent tissue damage. Infection is different from inflammation in that inflammation is the nonspecific reaction by the body to tissue injury, whereas infection refers to a specific process that produces tissue injury. Infection nearly always results in inflammation, but inflammation may be caused by processes other than infection. Infection may be caused by a wide variety of microorganisms.

INFECTIOUS AGENTS

The major infectious agents are bacteria, viruses, fungi, protozoa, rickettsiae, helminths, and mycoplasmas.

Bacteria

Bacteria are one-celled microorganisms capable of multiplying rapidly within a susceptible host. These organisms have a rigid, three-layer cell wall and a gelatinous capsule protecting it from phagocytosis. Several antibiotics fight infection by interfering with the formation of the bacterial cell wall. Bacteria are classified as either *gram-positive* or *gram-negative* depending on their ability to take up and retain a violet-colored solution. Gram-positive bacteria retain the stain, whereas gram-negative bacteria can be decolorized and counterstained pink.

Bacteria are also classified according to shape. Round bacteria are called *cocci,* and they are further classified according to how they group or cluster together. Groups of two are called *diplococci,* and clusters of cocci are called *staphylococci.* Chains of these microorganisms are called *streptococci.*

Rod-shaped organisms, however, are called *bacilli.* These may be further subdivided into *fusiform* (with tapered ends) or *spirochetes* (spirals).

Bacteria may also be classified according to their ability to grow in the presence of oxygen. Those that do are classified as *aerobes;* those that do not are labeled *anaerobes.*

These classifications have a very important purpose. Each classification highlights a characteristic of a microorganism that is considered in the design of an antimicrobial drug to kill or retard the growth of the organism. For example, gram-positive bacteria are labeled as such because of their inclination to take up the violet-colored stain. This happens because of a thick polypeptide and peptoglycan covering. Antibiotics synthesized to fight these microorganisms interfere with the formation of that covering, causing the cell wall to be destroyed. Similarly, other antibiotics rely on the ability of a bacterial cell to take up oxygen to produce their effects.

Viruses

Viruses are very small microorganisms that cause significant morbidity in humans and include everything from the common cold to acquired immunodeficiency syndrome (AIDS). Many childhood illnesses (e.g., measles, chickenpox) as well as several forms of hepatitis are caused by viruses. These microorganisms cannot be seen with ordinary microscopes but are visible with electron microscopy. They contain a strand of genetic material and are surrounded by a protein capsule but have no cell wall. Viruses cannot replicate on their own but depend on the resources of the host cell.

Viruses produce their damage by stimulating the antigen-antibody response in the tissues that causes inflammation and cell destruction. Because replication of the virus occurs within the host cell, it is seldom possible to kill the virus without harming the host cell. This explains why there are so few antiviral drugs available. Prevention (immunizations, hygiene) is still the best way to combat viral illness.

Fungi

Fungi are vegetable-like organisms that exist by feeding on organic matter. Mushrooms and molds are examples of fungal organisms. A few species of fungi are capable of producing disease in humans. Ringworm (tinea corporis) and athlete's foot (tinea pedis) are two examples. Many of these infections are superficial skin infections that rarely produce serious illness. Systemic fungal infections caused by *Cryptococcus* and *Aspergillus* species, however, can be life threatening. Patients who have conditions that affect their immune systems (e.g., AIDS) are at especially high risk of acquiring opportunistic fungal infections.

Protozoa

Protozoa make up a large group of one-celled organisms. Ones that produce disease in humans include the *Plasmodium* species (malaria), *Entamoeba histolytica* (amoebic dysentery), *Giardia lamblia* (diarrhea), and *Trypanosoma gambiense* (sleeping sickness). Infections are often spread by food or water that is contaminated by human or animal feces. *Pneumocystis carinii* is another protozoal infection that was relatively rare before the onset of the AIDS epidemic. Lowered immunity in the AIDS patient is responsible for the dramatic rise in pneumocystic pneumonia.

Rickettsiae

Rickettsiae are microorganisms that are between bacteria and viruses in size. They may appear as rods, cocci, or pleomorphic (varied) shapes. These organisms multiply in the cells of animal hosts such as rats and squirrels and are transmitted to humans through the bites of fleas and ticks. Diseases produced by these microorganisms include Rocky Mountain spotted fever and typhus. Diseases caused by rickettsiae tend to be more prevalent in areas in which sanitation is poor and rodent and insect populations are not well controlled.

Helminths

Helminths are worms. These parasites are found in soil and water and are generally transmitted from hand to mouth. Infections occur commonly in the gastrointestinal tract and may produce mild abdominal pain and bloating, or they may be asymptomatic. Pinworms are most common, especially in children, and often produce rectal irritation. Tapeworms are found in the gastrointestinal tract and may produce malnutrition and weight loss as well as abdominal pain and bloating. Hookworms often enter an individual through the soles of the feet and migrate through the body. Symptoms initially may be respiratory in origin, but these parasites can also produce abdominal pain, diarrhea, and anemia.

Mycoplasmas

Mycoplasmas are gram-negative, multishaped organisms without cell walls that are responsible for several infections in humans. They are sometimes called pleuropneumonia-like organisms. Mycoplasma infections are responsible for a primary atypical pneumonia and have been linked to urethritis and pharyngitis in humans. Infections are usually found in the upper respiratory tract and most often affect children and young adults. Mycoplasma infections respond well to erythromycin.

TRANSMISSION OF INFECTION

Infection, or the invasion of the body by microorganisms, is only possible when several factors are present. These factors must occur in sequence for human infectious disease to occur. They include (1) a causative agent, (2) a reservoir, (3) a portal of exit, (4) a mode of transfer, (5) a portal of entry, and (6) susceptible host.

CAUSATIVE AGENT. Certain agents cause infections. *Causative agents* are the microorganisms (e.g., bacteria, viruses, protozoa) that are present in sufficient number and virulence to damage human tissue.

RESERVOIR. Areas in which organisms can pool and reproduce are called *reservoirs.* Reservoirs may be human or animal tissues as well as any substance such as soil or animal feces in which microorganisms can pool and multiply. When a reservoir of microorganisms occurs in the tissues of humans or animals, the human or animal is called a *host.*

PORTAL OF EXIT. A *portal of exit* refers to the route by which the infectious agent leaves one host and travels to another. A common route is the gastrointestinal tract through which bacteria or viruses may escape an infected host. The nose and mouth also are common portals of exit for organisms spread by droplet contamination through sneezing or coughing. Fecal-oral transmission of hepatitis A is common.

MODE OF TRANSFER. *Mode of transfer* refers to the means by which a microorganism is transported to a host. *Person-to-person* transfer may take place in either a direct or an indirect manner. Direct contact refers to the transfer of microorganisms directly, as seen in sexually transmitted diseases. Indirect contact occurs when pathogens are spread through droplets expelled during a sneeze or a cough or inanimate objects (eating utenils on which microorganisms can be transported [fomites]).

Common vehicle transmission occurs when water, food, blood or air currents contaminated with a pathogen are shared by a number of people. Air currents, for example, are often the common vehicle for transmission of *Legionella,* the organism responsible for legionnaires' disease. *Vector* transmission occurs when microorganisms are transported to a host by a living organism such as a fly or mosquito.

PORTAL OF ENTRY. Areas through which infectious agents can enter the body are referred to as *portals of entry.* Flu and cold viruses often enter the body through the mucous membranes of the nose and mouth. Worms and bacteria that cause food poisoning enter the gastrointestinal tract through the mouth. Open wounds can also be portals for entry for bacteria.

SUSCEPTIBLE HOST. To produce tissue damage, microorganisms must become implanted in a *susceptible host.* Not all people exposed to disease-producing microorganisms become ill. Populations adequately immunized against rubella, for example, are not susceptible to measles. Similarly, individuals who have had chickenpox have developed immunity to the virus and, if exposed a second time, do not become ill.

SIGNS AND SYMPTOMS OF INFECTION

Once an individual becomes infected with a pathogen, symptoms may or may not be apparent. Often there is a period of subclinical infection or an incubation period during which there are few, if any, symptoms. During this period, persons who are infected may be more contagious than those who are exhibiting symptoms. This is true of people infected with such viruses as measles and many cold viruses. Persons who have some sexually-transmitted diseases such as AIDS remain infected permanently. Persons who have illnesses such as tuberculosis may remain relatively well and can come in contact with many other people. Still other persons may remain contagious throughout their convalescence. Asymptomatic carriers, such as patients recovering from typhoid, may go back to their communities and infect others.

Symptoms of *localized infections,* such as bacterial infection of a wound, are similar to the symptoms of inflammation. Redness, pain, warmth, and swelling are common. In addition, pus may form.

Generalized infections may not show all the signs that are apparent in localized infections. Redness, for example, may not be visible. Pain may be moderate to severe, depending on the location of the infection. Swelling of infected tissues may produce symptoms ranging from mild to severe depending on its location. Swelling in a large organ, such as the liver, may produce a dull ache, whereas swelling in a small structure, such as an infected appendix, may produce severe discomfort. Warmth is generally expressed as fever in a generalized infection as pyrogens are produced as part of the inflammatory process. Other symptoms that often are present in generalized infections include malaise, anorexia, and prostration.

In some cases, infections in the extremities such as the hands or feet exhibit a faint red line as infection extends upward along the lymphatic channels. Lymph nodes in this chain also are swollen and tender. Prompt antibiotic treatment is necessary in these cases.

TYPES OF INFECTIONS

Two type of infections are (1) community acquired and (2) hospital acquired.

Community-Acquired Infections

Community-acquired infections are acquired in day-to-day contact with the public. Many viral infections are pervasive in society and occur at predictable times of the year. Childhood illnesses are common in September when children bring back to school all the new viruses they were exposed to during the summer. This "sharing" of microorganisms is made easier when 20 to 40 children occupy the same classroom. During the fall and winter people share more indoor activities, thus increasing the likelihood that they will share microorganisms with one another. Poverty, low immunization rates, overcrowding, and unsanitary living conditions are at least partially responsible for the increase in infectious diseases that were once well controlled.

The recent resurgence of tuberculosis is an example. Before 1984, tuberculosis had been on the decline in the United States. In the past 6 years, however, the number of reported cases has increased by at least 18%. This rise has been attributed to poverty, the AIDS epidemic, an increase in the number of infected immigrants, and declining resources for public health programs. This bleak picture is further complicated by the emergence of strains of bacteria that are resistant to multiple drug therapy. It now becomes necessary to give at least two drugs to which a particular tuberculosis bacillus is susceptible. However, health care providers must often provide treatment without having information on susceptibility. That is why the Centers for Disease Control and Prevention now recommends that therapy with four drugs (isoniazid, rifampin, pyrazinamide and either ethambutol or streptomycin) rather than two be considered. Health care providers can help ensure the success of drug therapy by insisting on directly observing patients take their medications. These Direct Observation Therapy programs are important for all patients because it is impossible to tell who takes medicine regularly and who does not.

Food-borne illness is a common community-acquired infectious disease. It is more common in the summer when picnics and hot weather bring the possibility of food poisoning from *Staphylococcus* and *Salmonella* organisms. Periodic outbreaks of hepatitis A are possible any time of the year and are due to poor hygiene by food handlers.

Sexually transmitted diseases such as gonorrhea, syphilis, and AIDS also are acquired in the community. These diseases and many others are required to be reported to public health authorities. The reports are important for several reasons:

- They facilitate disease control.
- They make possible the evaluation of control programs.
- They keep track of emerging disease patterns.

A list of reportable diseases can be found in Table 9–1.

PREVENTION AND CONTROL. Prevention and control of communicable diseases are possible in a number of ways. Childhood infectious disease can be prevented by ensuring childhood immunizations. Indifferent attitudes toward childhood immunizations have resulted in the reemergence of several childhood diseases that were once well controlled. Measles and pertussis (whooping cough) are occurring at an increasing rate. Although state laws that require certain immunizations before a child starts school have improved the picture somewhat, large groups of children from 2 to 5 years of age remain susceptible to serious illness. In addition, repeat vaccinations of older school children may be required to prevent illnesses such as measles.

Although the solutions to this problem defy easy answers, at least part of the problem includes barriers in the health care system that result in missed opportunities to immunize those who are most susceptible. Barriers include such things as rigid fee schedules; giving immunizations only during regular working hours Monday through Friday; and only giving immunizations at official, fixed sites such as health departments. It is important for health professionals to take advantage of all possible opportunities to immunize. Schools, doctors' offices, shopping malls, and large neighborhood health fairs are places where large numbers of children and parents may present themselves for immunization.

Transmission of infectious agents can be interrupted in a number of ways. First, education of food handlers regarding the importance of hand washing and proper food handling and refrigeration techniques decreases the spread of food-borne disease. Second, diseases such as tuberculosis can be detected through screening and treated early to prevent their spread. Isolation separates the infected individual from the public, thereby breaking the chain of infection. Other measures aimed at interrupting transmission include control of vectors (spraying for mosquitos), medications such as antibiotics to prevent traveler's diarrhea, or prompt treatment of streptococcal pharyngitis (strep throat). Sanitation of water supplies helps to prevent the occurrence of water-borne diseases. Cooking meat, eggs, and poultry until well done kills bacteria that can cause serious illness and, in some cases, death.

Personal measures to control the spread of communicable disease include the use of personal barriers such as condoms and good hygiene such as hand washing. Deciding to stay home when symptoms of an infectious disease are present also can break the chain of infection.

TABLE 9–1
REPORTABLE DISEASES

Reportable Diseases
Acquired immunodeficiency syndrome
Amebiasis
Anthrax
Aseptic meningitis
Botulism
Brucellosis
Chancroid
Cholera
Diphtheria
Encephalitis
Gonorrhea
Granuloma inguinale
Hansen's disease (leprosy)
Hepatitis (all types)
Legionellosis
Leptospirosis
Lyme disease
Lymphogranuloma venereum
Malaria
Measles (rubeola)
Meningococcal infections
Mumps
Pertussis (whooping cough)
Plague
Poliomyelitis
Psittacosis
Rubella (German measles)
Rabies
Rheumatic fever
Rocky Mountain spotted fever
Salmonellosis
Shigellosis
Syphilis
Tetanus
Toxic shock syndrome
Trichinosis
Tuberculosis
Tularemia
Typhoid fever
Typhus
Yellow fever

Hospital-Acquired Infections

Hospital-acquired or nosocomial infections are an important cause of increased morbidity, prolonged hospitalization, and higher health care costs. Nosocomial infections occur within a health care facility and may affect both the patient and the health care worker. These infections are much more serious than those acquired in the community because strains of bacteria in the hospital are usually more virulent and are often resistant to antibiotics.

Resistant bacterial strains develop for a number of reasons. Bacterial cells normally develop mutations. As antibiotics suppress normal forms of the bacteria, the mutations are allowed to grow. Chromosomal mutation also causes the bacteria to produce an enzyme that deactivates the antibiotic. Finally, mutation alters bacterial cell membranes, making antibiotic penetration more difficult. Newer antibiotics are then developed to counteract the most resistant strains. With frequent use of the newer antibiotics, resistance again develops and the cycle is repeated. This cycle can be slowed by the practice of culturing wound drainage, collecting urine and blood for laboratory analysis, and identifying specific pathogens and their sensitivities to specific antibiotics. This allows for more specific therapy and delays the onset of resistant strains.

Nosocomial infections are more serious for the hospitalized patient because many are at higher risk for infection. Patients with compromised immune systems are much more susceptible to hospital-acquired infections. These groups include patients with AIDS and cancer patients who are receiving chemotherapy. Common sites for nosocomial infections in hospitalized patients include surgical wounds, the urinary tract, and the respiratory tract. Health care workers are also at higher risk for hospital-acquired infections. Hepatitis B, for example, may be transmitted through needle sticks. Small open wounds on the upper extremities may come in contact with resistant strains of *Staphylococcus* or *Pseudomonas*, causing infection and delayed healing. In addition, health care workers and patients have developed legionnaires' disease when *Legionella* was spread through the facility on air currents.

Iatrogenic infections are those caused through the process of caregiving. Occasionally a patient who has had a Foley catheter inserted develops a urinary tract infection because of improper technique during insertion. If the infection is caused by the caregiving process, it is called an iatrogenic infection. Other examples include septicemia following the insertion of peripheral or central venous access lines. Scrupulous aseptic technique can prevent many iatrogenic infections.

Another form of iatrogenic infection can be caused by the treatment of a primary infection. Antibiotic therapy for one microorganism can cause the overgrowth of a second microorganism that can also cause illness. The term for this process is *superinfection*. It is especially common with treatment using broad-spectrum antibiotics. An example of this phenomenon is the occurrence of a bowel infection following treatment with oral broad-spectrum antibiotics. The organism *Clostridium difficile* resides in the gastrointestinal tract of many individuals. It is kept in check by the normal bacterial flora of the gastrointestinal tract. Broad-spectrum antibiotics can kill enough of the normal flora to allow the *C. difficile* to grow out of control, producing the colitis.

NURSING CARE OF THE PATIENT IN ISOLATION

Just as controls must be instituted to stop the spread of infections acquired in the community, so must there be a process to keep hospitalized patients from acquiring a nosocomial infection. The key to preventing the spread of infection in the hospital is good medical and surgical asepsis.

MEDICAL ASEPSIS

Medical asepsis means limiting the spread of microorganisms as much as possible. This is often called *clean technique* and refers to practices such as changing bed linen, sanitizing bedpans, using individual medication cups for each patient and for each medication administration, and washing one's hands frequently.

Hand Washing

The most basic and effective method of preventing cross-contamination is hand washing (Fig. 9–2). Soiled hands are the primary cause of nosocomial infections. Although everyone agrees in principle with the need for frequent hand washing, problems arise when the nurse is busy. For example, suppose the nurse is passing medications and is asked by a patient with pulmonary secretions to hand her the box of tissues. At the same time,

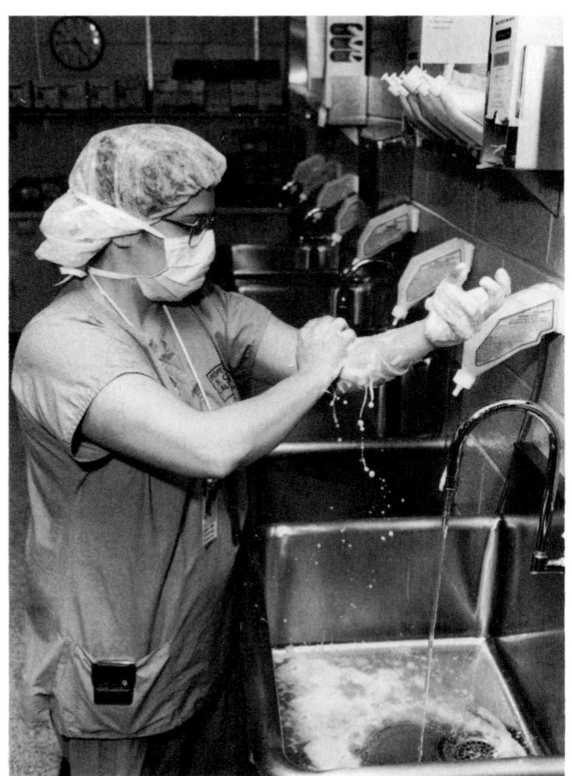

FIGURE 9–2
Hand washing is the most basic and effective method of preventing cross-contamination. (Photograph by Stephen Matteson, Jr.)

the patient's roommate asks the nurse to fill her water glass. After doing this, the nurse hurries out of the room to assist a physician with a dressing change. This example illustrates how a chain of infection begins. Unless the nurse interrupts the chain with good hand washing technique, infection is easily spread from one patient to another.

Good hand washing technique includes the use of running water, soap, and friction. The rubbing together of lathered hands should last for at least 15 seconds or longer if the nurse works in a high-risk area. The use of antimicrobial soaps is also recommended when working with patients who are more susceptible to infection, such as premature infants or immunocompromised patients.

SURGICAL ASEPSIS

Surgical asepsis, or *sterile technique,* refers to the elimination of microorganisms from any object that comes in contact with the patient. This includes care techniques that prevent unsterile surfaces from coming in contact with the patient, such as dressing changes using sterile gloves and forceps.

ISOLATION TECHNIQUES

To prevent the spread of infection in a health care facility, infected patients are sometimes isolated from other patients. The extent of the isolation depends on the type of infection. Highly virulent microorganisms that are spread easily by air or direct contact require strict precautions. Microorganisms that are less easily spread require less stringent precautions. Complete guidelines are provided by the Centers for Disease Control and Prevention (see Category-Specific Isolation Precautions).

STRICT ISOLATION. *Strict isolation* often is employed for more virulent infections that are spread easily, such as diphtheria or chickenpox (varicella). Patients are kept in a private room with the door closed. Gown, gloves, and mask are required by all persons entering the room. Visitors are restricted to avoid transmitting the infection.

CONTACT ISOLATION. *Contact isolation* is indicated when infection can be spread by coming into direct contact with infected surfaces. Examples include children with impetigo. Gowns and gloves may be worn if it is likely that the nurse will come in contact with infected material, such as when giving a bath or changing bed linen.

RESPIRATORY ISOLATION. *Respiratory isolation* is necessary when there is danger of microorganisms being spread by droplets. Measles, mumps, and pneumonia are common illnesses spread by droplet infection. Masks are indicated if individuals come in close contact with the patient.

ENTERIC PRECAUTIONS. Patients with infections that reside primarily in the gastrointestinal tract are cared for using *enteric precautions.* Hepatitis A and gastroenteritis caused by a virulent organism are examples of diseases requiring this type of isolation.

TUBERCULOSIS ISOLATION. *Tuberculosis isolation* is carried out for patients with active pulmonary tuberculosis. Usually these patients have positive sputum cultures or a pulmonary lesion that is visible on radiograph. A private room is required. Also recommended is a ventilation system that prevents contaminated air from being vented outside the room. Strict adherence to hospital isolation policy is essential to limit the development of multiple drug–resistant strains of tuberculosis.

DRAINAGE AND SECRETION PRECAUTIONS. *Drainage and secretion precautions* are necessary for patients with infected wounds. Extensive burns and surgical wounds sometimes become infected and produce significant amounts of drainage. Wound dressings, clothing, and bed linens are frequently contaminated with infected material. Gowns and gloves are worn whenever contact with wound drainage is likely.

UNIVERSAL BLOOD AND BODY FLUID PRECAUTIONS. With the advent of AIDS and a greater appreciation of the morbidity caused by hepatitis B and other blood-borne pathogens, the Centers for Disease Control and Prevention has recommended the use of *universal blood and body fluid precautions* on all clients, especially those cared for in settings in which exposure to blood is common. Universal precautions means that health care workers assume that everyone with whom they come in contact carries the human immunodeficiency virus (HIV). Specific recommendations by the Centers for Disease Control and Prevention are included in Table 9–2.

TABLE 9–2
BLOOD AND BODY FLUID PRECAUTIONS

These precautions are to be used with all clients to protect health care providers from blood-borne communicable diseases.

Gloves should be worn for contact with blood and body fluids, nonintact skin, and mucous membranes of all clients; for handling surfaces or items that are soiled with blood and body fluids; and for performing venipuncture and other vascular access procedures. Gloves should be changed after each client contact.

Masks or protective goggles should be worn during procedures that are likely to cause splashes of blood or body fluids.

Gowns or aprons should be worn during procedures that are likely to result in splashes of blood or body fluids.

Hand washing should be done immediately on contact with blood or other body fluids. One should wash hands as soon as gloves are removed.

Needles and sharp instruments should be placed in puncture-resistant containers for disposal to prevent injuries from needles or other sharp items. Needles should not be recapped, bent, or removed from the syringe.

Mouth-to-mouth resuscitation should be performed using mouthpieces or other ventilation devices.

Based on Centers for Disease Control and Prevention. (1987). Recommendations for prevention of HIV transmission in health-care settings. *Morbidity and Mortality Weekly Report, 36*(2S), 3–17.

BOX 9-1 SPECIFIC ISOLATION PRECAUTIONS

Strict Isolation

Strict isolation is an isolation category designed to prevent transmission of highly contagious or virulent infections that may be spread by both air and contact.

Specifications for Strict Isolation

1. Private room is indicated; door should be kept closed. In general, clients infected with the same organism may share a room.
2. Masks are indicated for everyone entering the room.
3. Gowns are indicated for everyone entering the room.
4. Gloves are indicated for everyone entering the room.
5. Hands must be washed after touching the client or potentially contaminated articles and before taking care of another client.
6. Articles contaminated with infective material should be discarded or bagged and labeled before being sent for decontamination and reprocessing.

Diseases Requiring Strict Isolation

Diphtheria, pharyngeal
Lassa fever and other viral hemorrhagic fevers, such as Marburg virus disease (A private room with special ventilation is indicated.)
Plague, pneumonia
Smallpox (A private room with special ventilation is indicated.)
Varicella (chickenpox)
Zoster, localized in immunocompromised client or disseminated

Contact Isolation

Contact isolation is designed to prevent transmission of highly transmissible or epidermiologically important infections (or colonization) that do not warrant strict isolation.

All diseases or conditions included in this category are spread primarily by close or direct contact. Thus, masks, gowns, and gloves are recommended for anyone in close or direct contact with any client who has an infection (or colonization) that is included in this category. For individual diseases or conditions, however, one or more of these three barriers may not be indicated. For example, masks and gowns are not generally indicated for care of infants and young children with acute viral respiratory infections; gowns are not generally indicated for gonococcal conjunctivitis in newborns; and masks are not generally indicated for clients infected with multiply resistant microorganisms, except those with pneumonia. Therefore, some degree of "overisolation" may occur in this category.

Specifications for Contact Isolation

1. Private room is indicated. In general, clients infected with the same organism may share a room. During outbreaks, infants and young children with the same respiratory clinical syndrome may share a room.
2. Masks are indicated for those who come close to the client.
3. Gowns are indicated if soiling is likely.
4. Gloves are indicated for touching infective material.
5. Hands must be washed after touching the client or potentially contaminated articles and before taking care of another client.
6. Articles contaminated with infective material should be discarded or bagged and labeled before being sent for decontamination and reprocessing.

Diseases or Conditions Requiring Contact Isolation

Acute respiratory infections in infants and young children including croup, colds, bronchitis, and bronchiolitis caused by respiratory syncytial virus, adenovirus, coronavirus, influenza viruses, parainfluenza viruses, and rhinovirus
Conjunctivitis, gonococcal in newborns
Diphtheria, cutaneous
Endometritis, group A streptococcus
Furunculosis, staphylococcal in newborns
Herpes simplex, disseminated, severe primary or neonatal
Impetigo
Influenza, in infants and young children
Multiply resistant bacteria, infection, or colonization (any site) with any of the following:

1. Gram-negative bacilli resistant to all aminoglycosides that are tested. (In general, such organisms should be resistant to gentamicin, tobramycin, and amikacin for these special precautions to be indicated.)
2. *Staphylococcus aureus* resistant to methicillin (or nafcillin or oxacillin if they are used instead of methicillin for testing).
3. *Pneumococcus* resistant to penicillin.
4. *Haemophilus influenzae* resistant to ampicillin (beta-lactamase–positive) and chloramphenicol.
5. Other resistant bacteria may be included if they are judged by the infection control team to be of special clinical and epidemiologic significance.

Pediculosis
Pharyngitis, infectious, in infants and young children
Pneumonia, viral, in infants and young children
Pneumonia, *Staphylococcus aureus* or group A streptococcus
Rabies

BOX 9-1 SPECIFIC ISOLATION PRECAUTIONS (Continued)

Rubella, congenital and other
Scabies
Scalded skin syndrome, staphylococcal (Ritter's disease)
Skin wound or burn infection, major (draining and not covered by dressing or dressing does not adequately contain the purulent material) including those infected with *Staphylococcus aureus* or group A streptococcus
Vaccinia (generalized and progressive eczema vaccinatum)

Respiratory Isolation

Respiratory isolation is designed to prevent transmission of infectious diseases primarily over short distances through the air (droplet transmission). Direct and indirect contact transmission occurs with some infections in this isolation category but is infrequent.

Specifications for Respiratory Isolation

1. Private room is indicated. In general, clients infected with the same organism may share a room.
2. Masks are indicated for those who come close to the client.
3. Gowns are not indicated.
4. Gloves are not indicated.
5. Hands must be washed after touching the client or potentially contaminated articles and before taking care of another client.
6. Articles contaminated with infective material should be discarded or bagged and labeled before being sent for decontamination and reprocessing.

Diseases Requiring Respiratory Isolation

Epiglottitis, *Haemophilus influenzae*
Erythema infectiosum
Measles
Meningitis
Haemophilus influenzae, known or suspected
Meningococcal, known or suspected
Meningococcal pneumonia
Meningococcemia
Mumps
Pertussis (whooping cough)
Pneumonia, *Haemophilus influenzae,* in children (any age)

Tuberculosis Isolation *(AFB Isolation)*

Tuberculosis isolation (AFB isolation) is an isolation category for clients with pulmonary tuberculosis who have a positive sputum smear or a chest film that strongly suggests current (active) tuberculosis. Laryngeal tuberculosis is also included in this isolation category. In general, infants and young children with pulmonary tuberculosis do not require isolation precautions because they rarely cough, and their bronchial secretions contain few AFB, compared with adults with pulmonary tuberculosis. On the instruction card, this category is called AFB (for acid-fast bacilli) isolation to protect the client's privacy.

Specifications for Tuberculosis Isolation (AFB Isolation)

1. Private room and special ventilation is indicated; door should be kept closed. In general, clients infected with the same organism may share a room.
2. Masks are indicated only if the client is coughing and does not reliably cover mouth.
3. Gowns are indicated only if needed to prevent gross contamination of clothing.
4. Gloves are not indicated.
5. Hands must be washed after touching the client or potentially contaminated articles and before taking care of another client.
6. Articles are rarely involved in transmission of tuberculosis. However, articles should be thoroughly cleaned and disinfected or discarded.

Enteric Precautions

Enteric precautions are designed to prevent infections that are transmitted by direct or indirect contact with feces. Hepatitis A is included in this category because it is spread through feces, although the disease is much less likely to be transmitted after the onset of jaundice. Most infections in this category primarily cause gastrointestinal symptoms, but some do not. For example, feces from clients infected with "poliovirus" and coxsackieviruses are infective, but those infections do not usually cause prominent gastrointestinal symptoms.

Specifications for Enteric Precautions

1. Private room is indicated if client's hygiene is poor. A client with poor hygiene does not wash hands after touching infective material, contaminates the environment with infective material, or shares contaminated articles with other clients. In general, clients infected with the same organism may share a room.
2. Masks are not indicated.
3. Gowns are indicated if soiling is likely.
4. Gloves are indicated for touching infective material.
5. Hands must be washed after touching the client or potentially contaminated articles and before taking care of another client.
6. Articles contaminated with infective material should be discarded or bagged and labeled before being sent for decontamination or reprocessing.

Box continued on following page

BOX 9-1 SPECIFIC ISOLATION PRECAUTIONS *(Continued)*

Diseases Requiring Enteric Precautions

Amebic dysentery
Cholera
Coxsackievirus disease
Diarrhea, acute illness with suspected infectious etiology
Echovirus disease
Encephalitis (unless known not to be caused by enteroviruses)
Enterocolitis caused by *Clostridium difficile* or *Staphylococcus aureus*
Enteroviral infection
Gastroenteritis caused by
- *Campylobacter* species
- *Cryptosporidium* species
- *Dientamoeba* fragilis
- *Escherichia coli* (enterotoxic, enteropathogenic, or enteroinvasive)
- *Giardia lamblia*
- *Salmonella* species
- *Shigella* species
- *Vibrio parahaemolyticus*
- Viruses—including Norwalk agent and rotavirus
- *Yersinia enterocolitica*
- Unknown etiology but presumed to be an infectious agent

Hand, foot, mouth disease
Hepatitis, viral, type A
Herpangina
Meningitis, viral (unless known not to be caused by enteroviruses)
Necrotizing enterocolitis
Pleurodynia
Poliomyelitis
Typhoid fever *(Salmonella typhi)*
Viral pericarditis, myocarditis, or meningitis (unless known not to be caused by enteroviruses)

Drainage/Secretion Precautions

Drainage/secretion precautions are designed to prevent infections that are transmitted by direct or indirect contact with purulent material or drainage from an infected body site. This newly created isolation category includes many infections formerly included in wound and skin precautions, discharge (lesion), and secretion (oral) precautions, which have been discontinued. Infectious diseases included in this category are those that result in the production of infective purulent material, drainage, or secretions, unless the disease is included in another isolation category that requires more rigorous precautions. For example, minor limited skin, wound, or burn infections are included in this category, but major skin, wound, or burn infections are included in contact isolation.

Specifications for Drainage/Secretion Precautions

1. Private room is not indicated.
2. Masks are not indicated.
3. Gowns are indicated if soiling is likely.
4. Gloves are indicated for touching infective material.
5. Hands must be washed after touching the clli-ent or potentially contaminated articles and before taking care of another client.
6. Articles contaminated with infective material should be discarded or bagged and labeled before being sent for decontamination and reprocessing.

Diseases Requiring Drainage/Secretion Precautions

The following infections are examples of those included in this category provided they are not (1) caused by multiple resistant microorganisms; (2) major drainage (and not covered by a dressing or dressing does not adequately contain the drainage) skin, wound, or burn infections, including those caused by *Staphylococcus aureus* or group A streptococcus; or (3) gonococcal eye infections in newborns. See contact isolation if the infection is one of these three.

Abscess, minor limited
Burn infection, minor limited
Conjunctivitis
Decubitus ulcer, infected, minor or limiited
Skin infection, minor or limited
Wound infection, minor or limited

Centers for Disease Control and Prevention (1983). *CDC guidelines for isolation precautions in hospitals.* HHS publication number CDC 83-8314. Atlanta: The Center.

CARE OF SEVERELY COMPROMISED PATIENTS. This category was previously called "reverse" isolation. It is designed to protect patients who have decreased immunity to infection. Patients on chemotherapy and other patients with low white blood cell counts are at increased risk of infection. Leukemia and aplastic anemia are two examples. A private room is indicated for these patients. Gowns and gloves are required for all people coming into the room. Masks are worn if one is coming into close contact with the patient.

NURSING CARE OF PATIENTS WITH INFECTION

Patients with generalized infections easily become dehydrated because of fever and anorexia. Fluid intake should be at least 2 liters per day to replace fluids lost through perspiration. Fluid intake is also important in the transportation of nutrients to the cells to fight infection. Nutrition is also important. A well-balanced diet with adequate amounts of vitamin C is important in proper wound healing and the prevention of future infections. Patients with poor appetites may benefit from a consultation with a dietician.

If a patient's infection does require isolation, the nurse should be aware that effective isolation techniques may also isolate the patient from normal human stimulation. Nurses may be tempted to hasten their work to minimize their chance of becoming infected. This forced seclusion can cause patients, particularly children, to feel lonely, rejected, and depressed. Nurses should engage the patient in conversation while giving direct care. Topics about things other than the patient's disease may lessen feeling of being unclean or rejected. Patients should be encouraged to move about as much as possible to increase stimulation.

Antibiotic drug therapy is the cornerstone of treatment for many infections. Early hospital discharges mean that patients are frequently discharged on oral antibiotics. Studies have demonstrated that many people fail to take antibiotics once they begin to feel better. It is important to instruct the patient to continue with therapy until specifically ordered by their physician to stop.

Early discharges also mean that substantial therapy may continue in the home after discharge. Home health care is frequently ordered for infected patients for a number of reasons. The patient is exposed to fewer nosocomial infections, fewer opportunities arise for infection to be spread to other hospitalized patients, and patients often do better in their own surroundings. If therapy is to be continued at home, it is important to teach the patient and other family members how to manage the remaining part of the care. Close coordination between the hospital nurse and the home health nurse is important to ensure good continuity of care.

BIBLIOGRAPHY

Benenson, A. (1990). *Control of communicable diseases in man* (15th ed.). Washington, D.C.: American Public Health Association.

Black, J. M., & Matassarin-Jacobs, E. (1993). *Luckmann and Sorensen's medical-surgical nursing: A psychophysiologic approach* (4th ed.). Philadelphia: W. B. Saunders.

Ignatavicius, D. D., & Bayne, M. V. (1991). *Medical surgical nursing: A nursing process approach.* Philadelphia: W. B. Saunders.

Potter, P., & Perry, A. (1989). *Fundamentals of nursing: Concepts, process and practice.* St. Louis: C. V. Mosby.

Swanson, J. M., & Albrecht, M. (1993). *Community health nursing: Promoting the health of aggregates.* Philadelphia: W. B. Saunders.

KEY CONCEPTS

1. Protective structures that shield the body from disease or injury include the skin, the gastrointestinal tract, the vagina, the liver, and various blood cells.
2. Neutrophils and monocytes are two types of leukocytes that are measured to indicate the severity of infection in the body.
3. Reticuloendothelial cells, found in the blood, connective tissue, liver, spleen, bone marrow and lymph nodes, protect the body by digesting and absorbing foreign material such as old red blood cells, bacteria, and colloidal particles.
4. Four signs of inflammation and infection are rubor (redness), calor (heat), tumor (swelling), and dolor (pain).
5. The onset of wound healing occurs at the same time that the inflammatory process begins.
6. The process of wound healing includes the production of macrophage cells to clean up inflammatory debris, the initiation of the repair process by fibroblasts, the formation of capillaries to provide circulation and nutrients to the new tissue, and the migration of epithelial cells under the scab to form a scar.
7. Age and general health affect how rapidly wound healing occurs, particularly in the elderly who heal more slowly as a result of a decreased blood supply to the tissues and a decrease in tissue elasticity.
8. The major infectious agents are bacteria, viruses, fungi, protozoa, rickettsiae, helminths, and mycoplasmas.
9. Infection, or the invasion of the body by microorganisms, is only possible when there is a causative agent, a reservoir, a portal of exit, a mode of transfer, a portal of entry, and a susceptible host.
10. Signs and symptoms of generalized infections are moderate to severe pain, swelling, fever, malaise, anorexia, and prostration.
11. Two types of infections are (1) community-acquired through daily contact with the public and (2) hospital acquired, or nosocomial infections.
12. The most basic and effective method of preventing cross-contamination is hand washing.
13. The Centers for Disease Control and Prevention recommends the use of universal blood and body fluid precautions (assumes that everyone carries the human immunodeficiency virus) for all patients, especially those cared for in settings in which exposure to blood is common.

CHAPTER 10

Anne-Marie Jones

Immunity

OBJECTIVES

1. Describe the two major types of immunity: natural and acquired.
2. Identify blood cells involved in immunity.
3. Identify organs involved in immunity.
4. Identify nonspecific defense mechanisms.
5. Describe the nonspecific defense mechanisms.
6. Differentiate between humoral and cell-mediated immunity.
7. Describe the three types of disorders of the immune system.
8. Give examples of each type of immune system disorder.
9. Develop a nursing care plan for the patient with an immune system disorder.

GLOSSARY

ACQUIRED IMMUNITY Immunity acquired after birth as a result of the body's natural immune responses to antigens

ACTIVE ACQUIRED IMMUNITY Immunity developed after direct contact with an antigen through illness or vaccination

ALLERGEN An antigen that causes a hypersensitive reaction

ANTIBODY (IMMUNOGLOBULIN) A protein that is created in response to a specific antigen

ANTIGEN Any substance that invades the body and is capable of stimulating a response from the immune system

AUTOIMMUNITY A condition in which the body is unable to distinguish self from nonself causing the immune system to react and destroy its own tissues

CELL-MEDIATED IMMUNITY A delayed response to injury or infection involving T cells and the production of substances that enhance the immune response and influence the destruction of antigens

COMPLEMENT A series of proteins that enhance the inflammatory process and immune response

HUMORAL IMMUNITY An immediate response to specific antigens involving B lymphocytes and the production of antibodies

IMMUNODEFICIENCY A condition in which the immune system is unable to defend the body against a foreign invasion of antigens

INTERFERON A substance produced in viral infections that inhibits the replication of viruses

LEUKOCYTES White blood cells that play a key role in immune responses toward infectious organisms and other antigens

NATURAL IMMUNITY Immunity that is present at birth

PASSIVE ACQUIRED IMMUNITY Temporary immunity acquired after receiving antibodies or lymphocytes produced by another individual

PHAGOCYTES The clean-up cells of the body that engulf and destroy microorganisms and cellular debris through a process known as *phagocytosis*

PYROGEN A substance released in inflammation that causes body temperature to increase

The immune system is the body's defense network against infection. Immunity provides the body with resistance to invading organisms and enables it to fight off invaders once they have gained access. The body is constantly exposed to microorganisms capable of causing disease. If the immune system is intact and functioning properly, it is able to provide adequate protection from most infections and diseases in a healthy individual. When the immune system is not functioning properly, the potential for overwhelming infection exists. Many factors can compromise the immune system, such as disease states, congenital defects, aging, stress, and therapeutic interventions. It is important for nurses to understand the normal immune response and to be familiar with common immune system disorders so that they can assess patients at risk for infection and provide appropriate interventions.

ANTIGENS AND ANTIBODIES

Any substance that is capable of stimulating a response from the immune system is called an *antigen.* In most cases, the antigen is foreign to the body, and the body recognizes the antigen because it is different from itself *(nonself).* Antigens can be microorganisms (bacteria, viruses, fungi, or parasites), abnormal or mutated body cells, transplanted cells (from blood transfusions or organ transplants), noninfectious substances from the environment (pollens, insect venom, foods), or foreign molecules from drugs such as penicillin. When healthy, the body protects what it recognizes as self and attempts to destroy that which is nonself. Tissue that is normally recognized as self may be seen as nonself by the immune system if it undergoes change (mutation), is in an abnormal location, or changes structure. Once the body recognizes a substance as an antigen, natural and acquired defenses are put into action to destroy the invader and prevent disease.

Antibodies, also known as *immunoglobulins,* are proteins that are created in response to specific antigens. The formation and function of antibodies are discussed later in this chapter under humoral immunity.

NATURAL VERSUS ACQUIRED IMMUNITY

Natural immunity is present in the body at birth and is not dependent on a specific immune response or a previous contact with an infectious agent. It may be specific to a species of animal, a race, or an individual. For instance, humans are not as susceptible to distemper as animals such as dogs and cats are. Factors such as nutritional status, stress, and environment may influence natural immunity. Nonspecific defense mechanisms that include physical and chemical barriers to infection, phagocytosis (the process of enveloping and destroying foreign matter), and the inflammatory process contribute to natural immunity.

An individual develops *acquired immunity* after birth as a result of the body's natural immune responses to antigens. Acquired immunity depends on the proper development and functioning of B and T lymphocytes, which are white blood cells (WBCs) that fight infection.

Active acquired immunity is developed after direct contact with an antigen through illness or vaccination. Vaccinations may be prepared by three methods: (1) using dead organisms that can no longer cause disease, as in the diphtheria and pertussis vaccines; (2) destroying bacterial toxins that act as antigens, as in the tetanus toxoid vaccine; and (3) altering the structure of live organisms so that they are unable to cause disease yet maintain their antigenic properties to prevent many viral diseases, such as measles and poliomyelitis. Once the body has been exposed to an antigen through illness or vaccination, antibodies develop and retain memory for the antigen. If the body is exposed to the same antigen later, the antibodies can react quickly to fight off disease.

When people are injected with *immune globulin* or antiserum (made from human or animal blood) that contains antibodies to a specific agent, such as for emergency treatment for snakebite, rabies, or exposure to hepatitis, they receive antibodies or lymphocytes that were produced by another individual. This type of immunity, *passive acquired immunity,* is temporary and is the kind of immunity newborns receive from their mothers through the placenta or through ingestion of breast milk (especially colostrum).

Both natural and acquired immunity are necessary for a healthy individual to have protection from disease.

CELLS AND ORGANS INVOLVED IN IMMUNITY

WHITE BLOOD CELLS (LEUKOCYTES)

A variety of cells work together to provide the body with an adequate defense against injury or disease. *Leukocytes,* or WBCs, play a key role in immune responses toward infectious organisms and other antigens. There are two categories of WBCs: (1) granulocytes (also known as polymorphonuclear leukocytes and (2) nongranulocytes.

Granulocytes (Polymorphonuclear Leukocytes)

Granulocytes consist of neutrophils, eosinophils, and basophils. *Neutrophils* migrate to areas of inflammation or bacterial invasion, where they ingest and kill invading organisms. They go to a part of the body that has been injured or invaded by bacteria, attracted by chemicals released from inflamed tissue.

Nature's cleanup is accomplished by *phagocytosis.* Microorganisms and cellular debris are engulfed and destroyed by lysosomal enzymes within phagocytes, the cleanup cells of the body (Fig. 10–1).

Eosinophils are phagocytes that migrate to infected or inflamed areas, where they engulf and destroy antigens. They also are important in allergic reactions and autoimmune diseases. *Basophils* are not phagocytes but participate in inflammatory and allergic responses by releasing substances such as histamine, heparin, and serotonin.

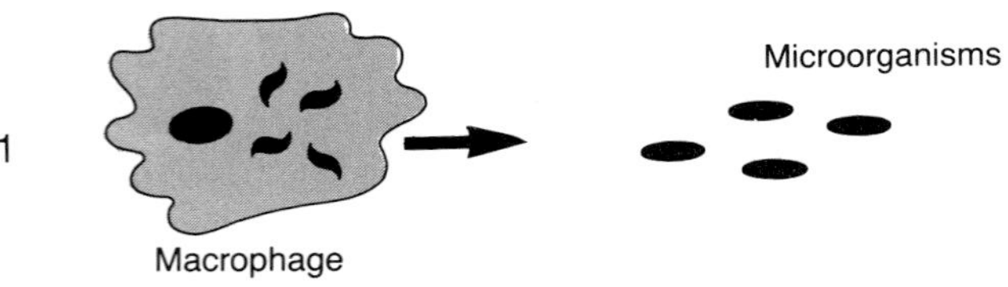

Chemotaxis to inflammatory site

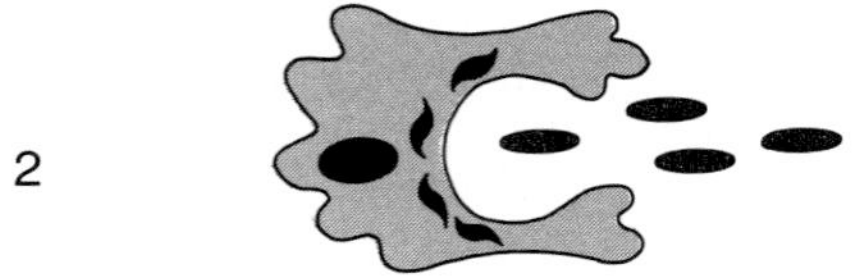

Formation of phagosome

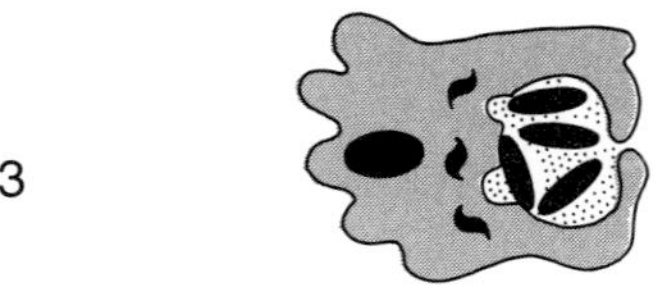

Release of lysosomal enzymes

FIGURE 10–1

Phagocytosis. (1) Macrophages migrate to an inflammatory site by chemotaxis. (2) Macrophages engulf the microorganisms. A phagosome or phagocytic vacuole forms around the microorganisms. (3) Lysosomes attach to the phagosome and release their enzymes, which destroy the microorganisms. (From Black, J. M., & Matassarin-Jacobs, E. [1993]. *Luckmann and Sorensen's medical-surgical nursing: A psychophysiologic approach* [4th ed., p. 533]. Philadelphia: W. B. Saunders.)

Nongranular Leukocytes

Nongranular leukocytes include monocytes and lymphocytes. *Monocytes* are the largest of the WBCs. When released into the blood stream, they become *macrophages,* powerful phagocytes that operate as "seek and destroy" scavengers. Macrophages are capable of ingesting large foreign particles, cell fragments, necrotic (dead) tissue, or other debris in the circulation. They also migrate and reside in specific tissues, such as the liver and lung, where they work. Macrophages begin specific immune responses by recognizing and processing antigens and secreting chemicals.

Lymphocytes also are involved with specific immune responses and are vital in the body's defense against microorganisms. Lymphocytes participate in the surveillance of abnormal cell growth, allergic reactions, autoimmune diseases, and rejection of foreign tissue. Table 10–1 highlights the values and functions of WBCs.

ORGANS INVOLVED IN IMMUNITY

Although all parts of the body work together as a whole to resist and fight off disease, several organs are vital to a functional immune system. They include the thymus, bone marrow, lymph nodes, spleen, and liver (Fig. 10–2). The thymus and bone marrow participate in the formation and maturation of immune system cells. Located throughout the body, the lymph nodes attack antigens and debris in the interstitial fluid and produce and circulate lymphocytes. The spleen acts as a filter to remove dead cells, debris, and foreign molecules from the blood. The liver filters the blood and plays a part in the production of specific immunoglobulins and other chemicals involved in the immune response.

TABLE 10–1

TYPES OF WHITE BLOOD CELLS (WBCs)

TYPE	% OF TOTAL WBC	FUNCTION
Neutrophils Bands (immature) Segmented (mature)	40–75	Phagocytosis
Eosinophils	2–5	Phagocytosis Allergy Suppresses inflammation Decreases granulocyte migration
Basophils	0.2–0.5	Inflammatory response by release of substances
Monocytes (macrophages)	2–6	Phagocytosis
Lymphocytes	20–35	Immunity

Modified from Black, J. M., & Matassarin-Jacobs, E. (1993). *Luckmann and Sorensen's medical-surgical nursing: A psychophysiologic approach* (4th ed., p. 531). Philadelphia: W. B. Saunders.

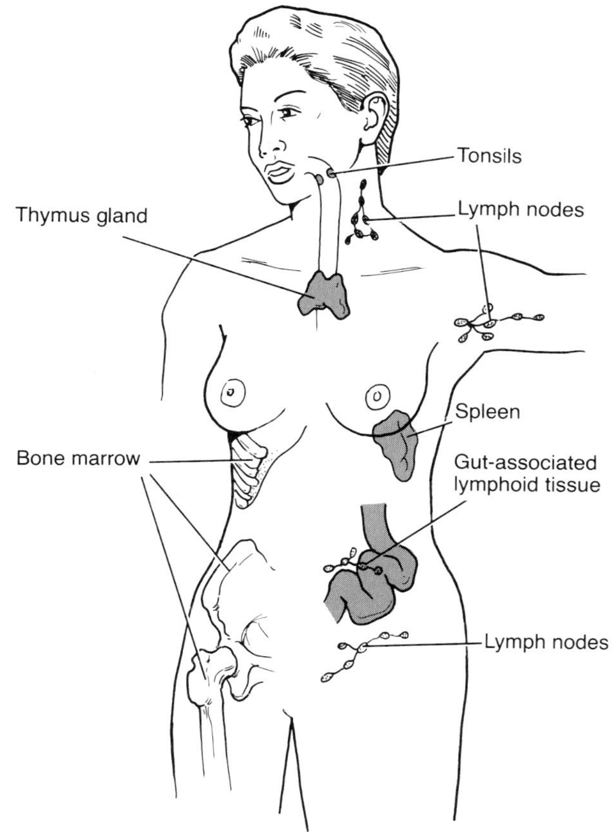

FIGURE 10-2
Organs involved in immunity.

NONSPECIFIC DEFENSES AGAINST INFECTION

As discussed earlier, natural immunity is present at birth and consists of physical and chemical barriers to invasion of the body as well as processes and substances that protect and repair tissues and stimulate the body to fight off disease. These are *nonspecific defenses* against infection.

PHYSICAL AND CHEMICAL BARRIERS

The skin and mucous membranes are the body's first line of defense. They act as a protective covering and secrete substances that inhibit the growth of microorganisms. The sweat glands secrete lysozyme, an antimicrobial enzyme. Sebaceous glands secrete sebum, which has antimicrobial and antifungal properties. Secretions from the skin and the mucosa of the gastrointestinal and genitourinary systems are acidic, which inhibit the growth of many pathogenic organisms. Secretions from the mammary glands and the respiratory and gastrointestinal tracts contain the antibody IgA, as well as cleanup phagocytes. Also, skin and mucous membrane surfaces are colonized by "normal" bacterial flora, which prevent pathogens (disease-causing microorganisms) from attaching and gaining access to the body. The cilia in the respiratory tract, the motility of the gastrointestinal tract, and the sloughing of dead skin cells all work to distribute and remove microorganisms, preventing their overgrowth and invasion.

INFLAMMATION AND PHAGOCYTOSIS

The second line of defense comprises two processes: (1) inflammation and (2) phagocytosis. Inflammation is necessary for tissue repair but can be harmful if uncontrolled. When injury to tissue occurs, special substances (chemical mediators) are released. These chemical regulators increase blood flow to the injured area, dilate the blood vessels, and increase the permeability of the capillaries so that cells and substances can more readily pass in and out of the circulation. Mediators also enhance chemotaxis (chemical stimulation of cell migration) and phagocytosis by neutrophils. The signs and symptoms of inflammation—heat, tenderness, redness, and swelling—are caused by these responses. Phagocytosis helps to rid the body of invading microorganisms and debris.

OTHER NONSPECIFIC DEFENSES

Other substances that are manufactured by the body to protect against disease include complement, pyrogen, and interferon. *Complement* is a series of proteins that enhance the inflammatory process and the immune response. Chemotaxis, phagocytosis, and the activity of antibodies are stimulated by complement. *Pyrogen* is a substance released in inflammation that causes body temperature to increase. Fever is thought to inhibit the growth of pathogens and slow enzymatic reactions that occur in infectious processes. Another substance, *interferon,* is produced in viral infections and acts to inhibit the replication of viruses. Interferon also affects the function of T lymphocytes and is used in the treatment of selected malignancies.

SPECIFIC DEFENSES AGAINST INFECTION—THE IMMUNE RESPONSE

The immune response is the process by which antigens are recognized as foreign, processed, and destroyed. The two types of immunity—humoral and cell-mediated—function interdependently to provide the immune response.

HUMORAL (IMMEDIATE) IMMUNITY

Humoral immunity is immediate. This first-line defense involves B lymphocytes and the production of antibodies in response to specific antigens. The humoral immune response is initiated when an antigen binds to a special receptor on a B lymphocyte. This results in the production of antibodies that seek out and "stick to" specific antigens in the body. This combination forms antigen-antibody complexes (Fig. 10–3), which are then

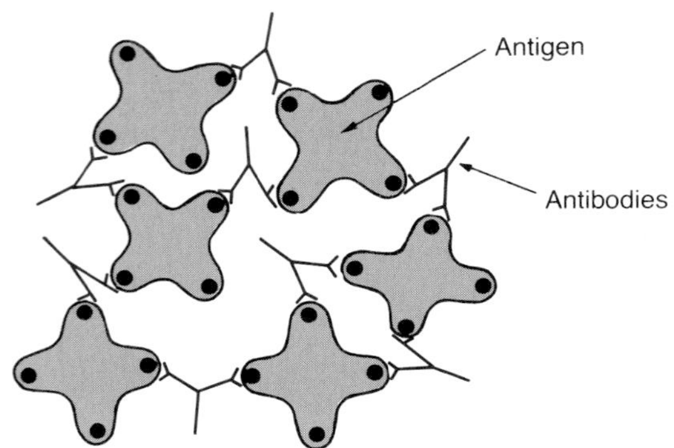

FIGURE 10-3

Binding of antigens and antibodies. (From Guyton, A. C. [1991]. *Textbook of medical physiology* [8th ed., p. 378]. Philadelphia: W. B. Saunders.

targeted for cleanup by neutrophils and macrophages. Formation of these complexes activates complement and intensifies T-lymphocyte activity. Since circulating antibodies bind with antigens as soon as they are recognized, the chemical process is triggered immediately.

Antibodies (immunoglobulins) are divided into five classes: IgG, IgM, IgA, IgE, and IgD. IgG is the most abundant immunoglobulin; it crosses the placenta to provide passive immunity for the newborn. IgE is important in allergic reactions and in parasitic infections. Immunoglobulins and their functions are summarized in Table 10–2.

CELL-MEDIATED (DELAYED) IMMUNITY

Cell-mediated immunity is a delayed response to injury or infection. Cellular immunity is delayed because of the time involved for the migration of *T cells*, as well as for the production of substances that enhance the immune response and influence the destruction of antigens.

T cells include helper cells, suppressor cells, and killer cells. *Helper T cells* enhance humoral immunity; *Suppressor T cells* help "turn off" the humoral response. Disease may occur when the normal ratio of helper to suppressor cells (2:1) is altered. In acquired immunodeficiency syndrome (AIDS), for instance, the number of helper T cells is diminished. When the number of suppressor T cells is too high, infections, allergy, or immune disease develops. *Killer T cells* directly destroy antigens.

Cellular immunity fights most viral or bacterial infections and hinders the growth of malignant cells. This process also launches an attack on transplanted tissue or organs in the body.

TABLE 10-2

ANTIBODIES (IMMUNOGLOBULINS)

ANTIBODY (IMMUNOGLOBULIN)	COMMENTS
IgG	Most abundant antibody Crosses placenta Coats microorganisms to enhance phagocytosis Activates complement
IgM	First antibody produced in response to antigen Activates complement
IgA	Called *secretory IgA*—present in many body secretions: saliva, sweat, tears, mucus Protects epithelial surfaces Passes to breastfeeding newborn through colostrum Activates complement
IgE	Active in allergic and inflammatory responses, parasitic infections
IgD	Function not well understood

Adapted from Jones, A. M. (1993). Hematology/immunology. In J. Hartshorn, M. Lamborn, & M. L. Noll (Eds.), *Introduction to critical care nursing* (p. 372). Philadelphia: W. B. Saunders.

DISORDERS OF THE IMMUNE SYSTEM

IMMUNODEFICIENCY

Etiology and Risk Factors

When the body's self-defenses against foreign invasion fail to function normally, a state of immune deficiency (immunodeficiency) exists. In this state, the body is unable to launch an adequate immune response and is at great risk for infection. The primary clinical clue to immunodeficiency, whatever the cause, is the tendency to develop recurrent infections. Immune deficiencies can be congenital or, more commonly, acquired and can result from problems with humoral immunity, cell-mediated immunity, vital mediators such as complement, or the process of phagocytosis.

In *congenital* immunodeficiencies, some part of the immune system fails to develop properly. The result is a defect in the B or T lymphocytes, phagocytes, or complement.

Acquired immunodeficiencies result from factors outside the immune system that render a previously functional immune system inadequate. Some causes of acquired deficiencies are infections, malignancies, autoimmune diseases (systemic lupus erythematosus, rheumatoid arthritis), chronic diseases (diabetes mellitus, renal disease), drugs, aging, stress, and malnutrition.

The very young and the very old are at risk for infection. Newborns are protected only for several weeks or months by the passive immunity they receive from their mothers. Infants do not develop a competent immune system of their own until they are between 1 and 2 years of age. Aging diminishes the immune response, and elderly patients have an increased incidence of infection, as well as autoimmune disease and malignancy.

Stress, whether physical or emotional, alters the body's response to disease. Although the mechanism is not fully understood, the release of hormones plays a part. Stressors include such things as serious illness, job loss, and divorce; even noise and cold play a part.

The nutritional state of the patient also affects immunity. The malnourished patient is much more susceptible to infection, especially when a protein deficiency exists. People with chronic conditions such as diabetes and renal disease usually are debilitated and are unable to fully defend themselves against infection. Trauma victims, especially those with burns, have diminished immune responses. Many malignant disorders alter the functioning of the immune system. Infectious diseases also cause immunodeficiencies, especially acute viral infections.

Many treatments and interventions aimed at helping patients cause immunodeficiency. Medications often place patients at risk for infection: antibiotics, steroids, chemotherapeutics, anticonvulsants, and immunosuppressive drugs (used for transplant recipients) are a few.

Surgery, anesthesia, and irradiation for cancer also can alter immune function. In addition, invasive procedures such as urinary catheterization and venipuncture for intravenous therapy or bloodwork bypass the patient's first line of defense. In the hospitalized patient, all of these factors come into play: disease, stress, nutritional alterations, medications, and procedures—all set the patient up for infection.

Medical Treatment

Congenital immunodeficiencies usually are treated with replacement therapy of the deficient immune component. Bone marrow transplants or fetal thymus tissue transplants may be used in some cases. Treating an acquired immunodeficiency lies in the correction of the underlying condition that is causing the problem, such as reducing stressors, correcting malnutrition, and discontinuing medications that alter immunity.

Nursing Care of the Immunodeficient Patient

The primary nursing responsibility in cases of immunodeficiency is to prevent infection. Proper hand washing by personnel and visitors is the single most important measure in prevention. Avoiding breaks in the patient's skin and the use of urinary catheters are important also. Frequent vital signs and assessments should be performed.

In an immunodeficient patient, signs and symptoms of infection are often atypical, masked, or absent. The nurse should be aware that a small increase in body temperature can be significant and should be reported. Rectal thermometers should be avoided if possible because of the potential for damage to the rectal mucosa. Adequate nutritional intake should be encouraged. Good skin, mouth, perineal, wound and intravenous site care with continuous assessment for signs of infection must be performed. Patients should be encouraged to turn, cough, and breathe deeply if they are not ambulatory. Protective isolation may be necessary. Flowers or plants may be prohibited because they provide a reservoir for bacterial growth. Fresh produce may be eliminated from the diet if the WBC count is too low.

Patient education concerning the risks for and signs of infection should be reinforced. The nurse should provide a supportive listening environment, as these patients may have anxiety as well as a high stress level, and often feelings of powerlessness are overwhelming.

ACQUIRED IMMUNODEFICIENCY SYNDROME

At present, AIDS remains a fatal disease that has reached epidemic proportions in the United States and is seen in all health care settings. Although AIDS was first recognized in the United States as a disease that affected mainly homosexuals and drug abusers, it now is rapidly growing in the heterosexual community, especially in women and among teenagers.

In 1981 AIDS was identified by the Centers for Disease Control and Prevention when the incidence of a rare pneumonia and cancer increased in the male homosexual population. By 1982, hemophiliacs were noted to have similar symptoms. In 1984, the causative organism was isolated, although it was not until 1987 that it received the name *human immunodeficiency virus (HIV)*.

The human immunodeficiency virus is a highly infectious virus that is transmitted through intimate sexual contact or contact with contaminated blood or blood products. Sexual intercourse with an infected person, use of contaminated intravenous drug equipment, transfusion with contaminated blood products, and accidental needle sticks or blood contact with broken skin can spread the virus. In addition, a mother can infect her fetus in utero or during childbirth; an infant can be infected through breast milk (Table 10–3).

Although HIV has been isolated from other body fluids such as tears or saliva, no known transmission through these fluids has occurred. The incubation of the virus and the appearance of symptoms varies greatly, but an infected individual can transmit HIV despite a negative HIV antibody laboratory test. Depending on the route of exposure, it may take anywhere from 4 weeks to 14 months for infected individuals to develop antibodies to HIV. Infected individuals may be totally without symptoms (asymptomatic) for several years.

TABLE 10–3
RISK FACTORS FOR TRANSMISSION OF HIV

Frequent rectal or vaginal intercourse with multiple partners
Intravenous drug abuse with sharing of needles
Recipient of contaminated blood or blood products as the result of transfusion
HIV-positive mother transmits virus to fetus during gestation or childbirth; to newborn during breastfeeding
Occupational exposure to infected blood or body fluids through needle sticks or sharp instruments

HIV, Human immunodeficiency virus.

From Jones, A. M. (1993). Hematology/immunology. In J. Hartshorn, M. Lamborn, & M. L. Noll (Eds.), *Introduction to critical care nursing* (p. 379). Philadelphia: W. B. Saunders.

TABLE 10–4
SYMPTOMS OF HIV INFECTION AND AIDS

Fever
Night sweats
Fatigue, weakness
Generalized lymph node disease
Malaise
Anorexia
Weight loss
Diarrhea
Dementia
Peripheral neuropathy
Malignancies: Kaposi's sarcoma lymphoma
Opportunistic infections

HIV, Human immunodeficiency virus; AIDS, acquired immunodeficiency syndrome.

Modified from Jones, A. M. (1993). Hematology/immunology. In J. Hartshorn, M. Lamborn, & M. L. Noll (Eds.), *Introduction to critical care nursing* (p. 380). Philadelphia: W. B. Saunders.

The human immunodeficiency virus infects and knocks out helper T cells. The ratio of helper T to suppressor T cells plunges, resulting in a dysfunctional immune response that leaves the infected person susceptible to disease, especially infections.

Acute infection with HIV occurs with mild flu-like symptoms such as fatigue, fever, and muscle aches. A late manifestation of HIV infection, AIDS shows itself by the presence of recurrent opportunistic infections (pathogens that cause disease when the immune response is disrupted), rare malignancies, or both. Weight loss and wasting are common. Neurologic symptoms such as personality changes, apathy, memory and cognition problems (AIDS dementia), and even psychosis may result. Table 10–4 lists symptoms of HIV infection and AIDS. Laboratory work may document immunodeficiency by a decreased WBC count (especially lymphocytes) and an abnormal helper T- to suppressor T- ratio, as well as a positive HIV antibody test.

The most common opportunistic infection seen in AIDS is *Pneumocystis carinii* pneumonia. Candidiasis (thrush or yeast infection) also is common. Kaposi's sarcoma is the most frequent malignancy seen in AIDS, which usually appears as a purplish-brown lesion on the skin of the extremities.

Medical Treatment

Medical management of AIDS is aimed at the early detection and treatment of opportunistic infections and malignancies. The use of antiviral medications is the primary form of treatment for AIDS. Antiviral medications are given to prevent viral replication to protect cells that are not yet infected. The most widely used antiviral is azidothymidine (AZT) now called zidovudine. Although other drugs have the approval of the U.S. Food and Drug Administration for AIDS treatment, research continues to produce new drugs because HIV quickly becomes resistant to drugs used in therapy. Development of a vaccine has not yet been possible, mainly because HIV mutates quickly and exists in many antigenic forms.

Another approach to treatment has been to "boost" the immune system through injection of immune mediators such as interferon or interleukin-2, transfusions with healthy WBCs, or even bone marrow transplants. However, the virus quickly infects the new cells.

Other medical interventions in AIDS depend on the specific illnesses seen. Pneumonia caused by *P. carinii* is treated with the drugs trimethoprim and sulfamethoxazole (Bactrim, Septra), pentamidine isethionate (Pentam 300), or both. Kaposi's sarcoma and other malignant disorders may be treated with chemotherapy.

Nursing Care of the Patient with AIDS

Nursing care of the patient with AIDS includes prevention of infection, maintenance of adequate hydration and nutritional status, maintenance of skin and mucous membrane integrity, maintenance of optimal gas exchange, relief of pain, and promotion of rest and comfort. Psychosocial interventions include providing a caring, supportive atmosphere, as these patients often are anxious, not coping effectively, and engaging in anticipatory grieving. Table 10–5 lists nursing diagnoses in AIDS. In addition, nurses are responsible for using universal precautions to protect themselves and other patients from the spread of HIV. *Universal precautions* suggested by the Centers for Disease Control and Prevention are listed in Chapter 9.

HYPERSENSITIVITY AND ALLERGY

Etiology and Risk Factors

When a normally inoffensive foreign substance stimulates an atypical immune response, *allergy* or *hypersensitivity* occurs. Immunity is beneficial, but hypersensitivity can be harmful, sometimes producing deadly symptoms. It is estimated that 20 to 25% of the U.S. population suffers from allergies of some sort, with allergic rhinitis (hay fever) and asthma occurring most

TABLE 10–5
NURSING DIAGNOSES IN AIDS

High risk for infection related to immunodeficient state
High risk for impaired gas exchange related to respiratory infection
High risk for impaired skin and mucous membrane integrity related to infectious lesions, immobility
Altered nutrition: less than body requirements related to anorexia
Diarrhea
High risk for fluid volume deficit related to diarrhea, profuse sweating
Anxiety
Pain related to disease processes, interventions
Altered self-concept
Social isolation

AIDS, Acquired immunodeficiency syndrome.

Modified from Jones, A. M. (1993). Hematology/immunology. In J. Hartshorn, M. Lamborn, & M. L. Noll (Eds.), *Introduction to critical care nursing* (p. 382). Philadelphia: W. B. Saunders.

TABLE 10–6

COMMON ALLERGIES AND THEIR CAUSES

ALLERGIC REACTION	STIMULUS
Asthma	Pollens, dust, molds, cigarette smoke, air pollutants, animal dander
Allergic rhinitis	Pollens, dust, molds, animal dander
Anaphylaxis	Antibiotics (penicillin)
	Insect venom (bee, wasp stings)
	Blood transfusions
Urticaria (hives)	Food, drugs
Atopic dermatitis (eczema)	Soaps, cosmetics, chemicals, fabrics
Allergic contact dermatitis	Plants (poison ivy)
	Metals (nickel)
	Chemicals, cosmetics
	Latex gloves
Gastrointestinal allergies	Foods, drugs

often. Other allergies include allergic contact dermatitis, angioedema (localized swelling), atopic dermatitis, anaphylaxis (severe allergic reaction), gastrointestinal allergies, and urticaria (hives). The tendency to develop an allergy is inherited, although the type of allergy may vary. Someone who is prone to allergies may be referred to as *atopic.*

An antigen that causes a hypersensitive reaction is called an *allergen.* Any substance can act as an allergen to a susceptible person, but some of the more common ones are house dust, animal dander, pollens, molds, foods, pharmacologic agents, cigarette smoke, feathers, and insect venoms. Table 10–6 lists common allergens.

The allergic response begins with *sensitization.* The first encounter with a specific allergen results in only a small amount of antibody production. With subsequent exposure, however, the body steps up its defense by producing large amounts of antibodies, which circulate in the blood stream and travel to the affected tissues. This sets off the release of histamine and other chemical agents. Neutrophils arrive at the scene to engulf and destroy the antigens. A multitude of reactions occur that produce the symptoms typical of an allergic response, although they vary depending on the area affected (Fig. 10–4).

Medical Treatment

Medical treatment of allergic patients varies depending on the specific allergy. In general, antihistamines are used to reduce the symptoms caused by histamine release. Many people suffer side effects from antihistamines, such as dry mouth, nausea, blurred vision, diz-

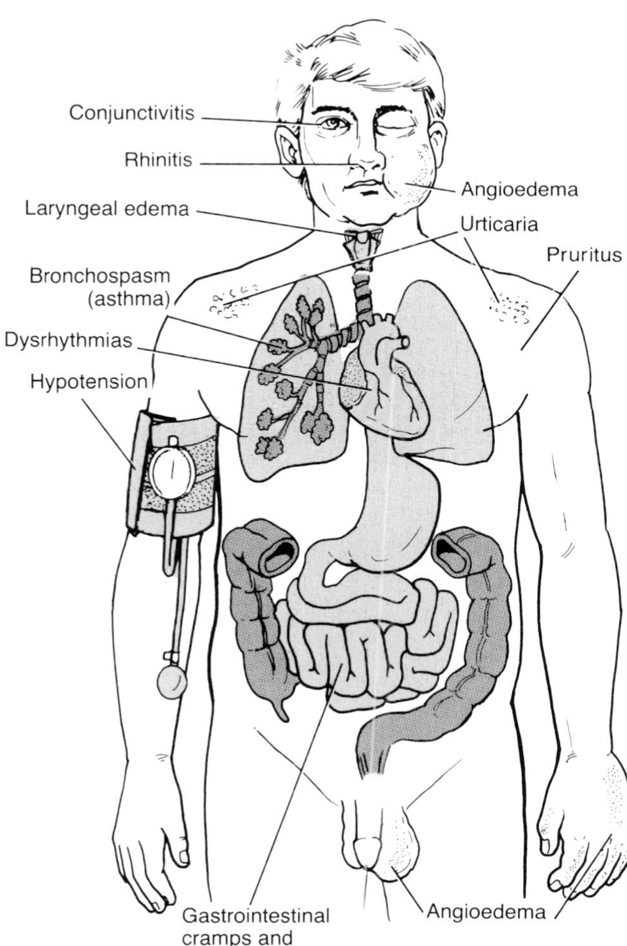

FIGURE 10–4

Local manifestations of allergic reactions.

ziness, and drowsiness. For asthma sufferers, bronchodilators, steroids, or both, may be prescribed to improve air movement and to decrease inflammation in the lungs; oxygen and breathing treatments may also be ordered. Besides antihistamines, topical lotions and ointments may be prescribed to relieve itching associated with urticaria, atopic dermatitis, or allergic contact dermatitis.

Long-term medical treatment of allergies involves testing to determine specific allergens. Testing is performed by injecting small amounts of allergen under the skin (intradermally) or by pricking the surface of the patient's skin and monitoring for the degree of wheal and flare reaction. After determining the specific agents, the patient may be desensitized by injections of minute quantities of the allergen, gradually increasing the dosage over a prolonged period of time. Desensitization is aimed at increasing tolerance to the offending agent and decreasing the severity of the allergic response.

Nursing Care of the Patient with Allergies

When dealing with the hospitalized allergic patient, the most important nursing intervention is to document *all* allergies, the symptoms they cause, and any treatment currently used. Allergies should be posted on the front of the patient's chart, on all medication records, and on the nursing care plan. Never administer any drug that the patient reports a previous allergic reaction to until you consult the physician.

The pharmacy and dietary departments should be alerted to drug and food allergies, and the physician should be notified of any allergies that may determine which medications to avoid. For instance, an asthmatic patient should not receive beta-blocking drugs such as propranolol, because severe bronchospasm may result. The nurse must also make sure that the patient continues to receive necessary allergy medication while hospitalized, such as routine inhaler treatments.

Patient education is important for all patients with allergies. This includes knowledge of specific allergens, limiting exposure to or avoiding allergens, the proper use of medications such as inhaled bronchodilators, and the actions and side effects of drugs. Patients who are at risk for life-threatening (anaphylactic) reactions should wear a MedicAlert bracelet that identifies their allergy. Individuals with insect sting allergies should obtain an emergency sting kit and should be taught how to self-inject epinephrine. This kit should be kept readily available at all times.

Nurses should avoid the overuse of perfumes and scented cosmetics while working with patients. Live plants and flowers should not be allowed in the allergic patient's room.

ANAPHYLAXIS

When an allergen enters the blood stream, allergic reactions can occur throughout the body within minutes. This is *anaphylaxis*, a life-threatening situation that can quickly deteriorate into shock, coma, and death. Histamine released in anaphylaxis causes bronchospasm, vasodilation, and increased vascular permeability throughout the body, which causes fluid to leave the circulation and enter the tissues, causing shock from hypovolemia and edema. Signs and symptoms of anaphylaxis include anxiety, wheezing and difficulty breathing, bluish skin color (cyanosis), hives, facial edema, joint pain (arthralgia), and low blood pressure (hypotension).

Anaphylaxis is an emergency situation, and the patient's life depends on rapid intervention. The most common cause of anaphylaxis is the use of antibiotics, especially penicillin. Other causes include medicines or serum from animal sources, insect venom (especially bees and wasps), iodinated radioactive contrast media, local anesthesia, and blood products.

Medical Treatment

In anaphylaxis, oxygen, epinephrine, aminophylline, diphenhydramine, and corticosteroids may be administered intravenously, and other drugs such as dopamine may be necessary to raise the patient's blood pressure.

Nursing Care of the Patient with Anaphylaxis

The most vital component of all nursing care is prompt recognition of the situation. Nursing interventions are aimed at minimizing the patient's anxiety, ensuring adequate hydration to combat hypovolemia, and assisting the patient with breathing and oxygenation.

The patient should be monitored for difficulty breathing, dyspnea, tachypnea, or a change in respiratory rate, as well as for development of cyanosis.

AUTOIMMUNE DISEASES

Etiology and Risk Factors

The body's ability to determine self from nonself is called *tolerance.* When tolerance is disrupted, the immune system reacts against and destroys its own tissues. This breakdown in tolerance and subsequent damage to self is termed *autoimmunity.* An autoimmune process may be initiated when there is injury to tissues, infection, or malignancy. The exact causes and pathology of most autoimmune diseases are poorly understood, but many of these disorders cause severe illness and death.

There appear to be genetic factors involved, as autoimmune diseases tend to be familial. Some autoimmune disorders have apparent causes, such as drug-induced anemia or low platelet count (thrombocytopenia). Infection often is present before the onset of an autoimmune disease, leading to the conclusion that the disease results as a complication (sequelae) of the infection. Autoimmune diseases cause injury in three ways: (1) the effect of antibodies on cell surfaces; (2) the deposit of antigen-antibody complexes (particularly in capillaries, joints, and renal tissue), and (3) the action of sensitized T cells.

Autoimmunity can involve any tissue or organ system. In multiple sclerosis, the white matter of the brain and

TABLE 10–7
AUTOIMMUNE DISORDERS AND THEIR TARGETS

DISORDER	TISSUE AFFECTED
Endocrine system	
Hyperthyroidism (Graves' disease)	Thyroid
Autoimmune thyroiditis	Thyroid
Insulin-dependent diabetes mellitus	Pancreas
Addison's disease	Adrenal gland
Central nervous system	
Multiple sclerosis	Brain and spinal cord
Myasthenia gravis	Neuromuscular junctions
Cardiovascular system	
Rheumatic fever	Heart
Cardiomyopathy	Heart
Gastrointestinal system	
Ulcerative colitis	Colon
Crohn's disease	Ileum
Connective tissue	
Rheumatoid arthritis	Joints
Systemic lupus erythematosus	Multiple tissues
Scleroderma	Multiple tissues
Hematologic system	
Autoimmune hemolytic anemia	Red blood cells
Autoimmune thrombocytopenic purpura	Platelets
Idiopathic neutropenia	Neutrophils
Idiopathic lymphopenia	Lymphocytes
Respiratory and Renal	
Goodpasture's disease	Lung, kidney
Skin	
Pemphigus vulgaris	Skin
Psoriasis	Skin

Adapted from McCance, K. L., & Huether, S. E. (1994). *Pathophysiology: The biologic basis for disease in adults and children* (2nd ed., pp. 270–271). St. Louis: C. V. Mosby.

spinal cord is affected, and the myelin sheath that protects nerve fibers is destroyed. Rheumatoid arthritis affects the lining of the joints. In insulin-dependent diabetes mellitus, the pancreatic cells that secrete insulin are attacked. Table 10–7 lists some of the more common autoimmune diseases and the tissues they affect. Probably the most infamous of the autoimmune disorders is systemic lupus erythematosus (SLE), which affects multiple organs.

Medical Treatment

Medical interventions vary depending on the specific autoimmune disease and the tissues affected, as well as the symptoms. In general, corticosteroids and nonsteroidal anti-inflammatory drugs are used to treat inflammation. Immunosuppressive therapies may be tried to moderate the autoimmune response.

Nursing Care of the Patient with an Autoimmune Disorder

Although nursing interventions vary according to the specific disorder, multiple nursing diagnoses may apply to any patient with an autoimmune disease. They include high risk for activity intolerance, activity intolerance, anxiety, impaired skin integrity, ineffective breathing pattern, impaired gas exchange, knowledge deficit, pain, fear, fatigue, self-care deficit, ineffective individual coping, high risk for infection related to chronic disease and immunosuppressive therapy, and altered nutritional status: less than body requirements. Adequate rest, maintenance of optimal hydration and nutritional status, and prevention of infection are vital in preventing complications in these patients. In addition, a supportive, caring atmosphere is important to enhance coping skills and promote emotional health.

SYSTEMIC LUPUS ERYTHEMATOSUS

Systemic lupus erythematosus is a chronic inflammatory disease that eventually affects almost every organ, especially the kidneys. Antibodies are produced against a variety of host tissues. Systemic lupus erythematosus and most other autoimmune diseases occur more frequently in women, aged 20 to 40 years, with blacks affected more often than whites.

Symptoms of SLE generally begin in early adulthood. Because symptoms vary greatly and tend to "come and go," SLE is very difficult to diagnose. Diagnosis is usually made on the basis of the presence of several clinical manifestations. These include facial rashes, arthralgias, hair loss, anemia, low platelet count (thrombocytopenia), renal disease (as evidenced by excessive protein in the urine), inflammation of the sac containing the heart (pericarditis), and neurologic symptoms such as seizures or psychoses. Bloodwork may show antinuclear antibody (ANA titer).

Medical Treatment

Traditionally, treatment of SLE has been aimed at depressing the inflammatory response through the administration of nonsteroidal anti-inflammatory drugs (NSAIDs) and corticosteroids. The NSAIDs, such as aspirin or indomethacin (Indocin), often cause gastrointestinal problems, from nausea to ulcers and bleeding. Corticosteroids, especially if used long term, can cause several adverse reactions. Antimalarial drugs may be used, although the reason they are helpful in SLE is unclear. If the patient has life-threatening complications, plasmapheresis (taking blood from the patient, separating components, and retransfusing the remainder back into the patient) may be performed to remove the circulating immune complexes that exacerbate problems. Cytotoxic drugs may be used to depress the immune response.

Nursing Care of the Patient with Systemic Lupus Erythematosus

In SLE, fatigue and joint stiffness are common problems. Nurses should encourage patients with SLE to get adequate rest and moderate exercise to maintain joint mobility and flexibility. A diet high in protein, vitamins, and iron is important for optimal nutritional status and for combating anemia. Monitoring for side effects from medications is vital, as is patient education concerning the disease and its management. Specific nursing interventions are designed to maintain skin integrity; promote rest, comfort, and pain relief; maintain optimal nutritional status and adequate hydration; reduce stress; alleviate anxiety; and promote healthy coping skills.

TRANSPLANTATION, IMMUNOSUPPRESSION, AND TISSUE REJECTION

When an organ is irreversibly damaged and unable to function yet is necessary to sustain life, a transplant is a desirable option. However, transplanted tissue is at risk for destruction by the immune response because it can be recognized as nonself. T lymphocytes and cell-mediated immunity are especially responsible. Because of this, donor tissue needs to be matched closely to that of the recipient, much like blood is before transfusion. Immunosuppressive drugs are used to minimize the immune response against transplanted tissue. Great advances in immunosuppressive therapy have been made in the last decade, enhancing the survival and quality of life for transplant recipients. However, because these drugs suppress the immune system, the patient is at risk for developing infections. Transplant patients must be monitored closely for any signs or symptoms of both organ rejection and infection.

BIBLIOGRAPHY

Anastasi, J. K., & Rivera, J. (1994). Understanding prophylactic therapy for HIV infections. *American Journal of Nursing, 94*(2), 36–41.

Anonymous. (1992). A.I.D.S. precautions: Sharing concerns. *Nursing, 22*(4), 14, 17.

Anonymous. (1993). AIDS update. *Nursing, 23*(3), 21, 23.

Black, J. M., & Matassarin-Jacobs, E. (1993). *Luckmann and Sorensen's medical-surgical nursing: A psychophysiologic approach* (4th ed.). Philadelphia: W. B. Saunders.

Davis, M. (1993). Dropping the barriers between Jim and us. *Nursing, 23*(11), 62–64.

Erlen, J. A., Lebeda, M., & Tamenne, C. J. (1993). Respect for persons: The patient with AIDS. *Orthopaedic Nursing, 12*(4), 7–10.

Guyton, A. C. (1991). *Textbook of medical physiology* (8th ed.). Philadelphia: W. B. Saunders.

Haddad, A. (1993). A young postop patient with AIDS is given a regular bed among patients: What would you do? *RN, 56*(9), 21–22, 24.

Halloran J. (1993). Taking the risk to care. *American Journal of Nursing, 93*(7), 20.

Jackson, S. A. (1991). The immune system: Basic concepts for understanding transplantation. *Critical Care Nursing Quarterly, 13*(4), 83–88.

Jennings, B. M. (1991). The hematologic system. In J. G. Alspach (Ed.), *Core curriculum for critical care nursing* (pp. 495–561). Philadelphia: W. B. Saunders.

Jones, A. M. (1993). Hematology/immunology. In J. Hartshorn, M. Lamborn, & M. L. Noll (Eds.), *Introduction to critical care nursing* (pp. 348–385). Philadelphia: W. B. Saunders.

Killeen, M. E. (1993). Getting through our grief: For caregivers of persons with AIDS. *American Journal of Hospice & Palliative Care, 10*(5), 18–19, 23–24.

Lippert, J. (1990). How your immune system works. *Ladies Home Journal, 107*(10), 118, 120, 124.

McCance, K. L., & Huether, S. E. (1994). *Pathophysiology: The biologic basis for disease in adults and children* (2nd ed.). St. Louis: C. V. Mosby.

Nguyen, T. V., & McHugh, M. K. (1991). Psychosocial nursing and immunocompetence. *Holistic Nursing Practice, 5*(4), 1–72.

Patten, B. C. & Holt, J. A. (1992). When your patient is allergic. *American Journal of Nursing, 92*(9), 58–61.

Rote, N. S. (1990). Alterations in immunity and inflammation. In K. L. McCance & S. E. Huether (Eds.), *Pathophysiology: The biologic basis for disease in adults and children* (pp. 249–278). St. Louis: C. V. Mosby.

Scherer, P. (1990). How AIDS attacks the brain. *American Journal of Nursing, 90*(1), 44–52.

Ufema, J. (1993). A.I.D.S. patient: Finding contentment. *Nursing, 23*(11), 22.

KEY CONCEPTS

1. The immune system is the body's defense network against infection; it provides the body with resistance to invading organisms and enables it to fight off invaders once they have gained access.
2. Antigens are substances that stimulate a response from the immune system, whereas antibodies, also known as immunoglobulins, are proteins that are created in response to specific antigens.
3. Natural immunity is present in the body at birth, whereas acquired immunity develops after birth as a result of the body's natural immune responses to antigens.
4. Acquired immunity depends on the proper development and functioning of B and T lymphocytes, which are white blood cells that fight infection.
5. Many types of leukocytes act as nature's cleanup mechanism by migrating to infected or inflamed areas and engulfing and destroying antigens through a process known as *phagocytosis.*
6. Body organs that are vital to a functional immune system include the thymus, bone marrow, lymph nodes, spleen, and liver.
7. Two types of immunity—humoral and cell-mediated—function interdependently to provide the immune response.

8. Humoral immunity is the first line of defense and involves B lymphocytes and the production of antibodies in response to specific antigens.

9. Cell-mediated immunity is a delayed response to injury or infection that involves T cells.

10. Immunodeficiency occurs when the body is unable to launch an adequate immune response, resulting in risk for infection.

11. Immunodeficiencies may be congenital or acquired through infections, malignancies, autoimmune diseases, chronic diseases, drugs, aging, stress, and malnutrition.

12. When a normally inoffensive foreign substance stimulates an atypical immune response, allergy or hypersensitivity occurs.

13. Autoimmunity occurs when the body fails to recognize itself, and the immune system reacts by destroying the body's own tissues.

CHAPTER 11

Fluid and Electrolytes

Esperanza V. Joyce
Kenn M. Kirksey
Mary Ann Matteson

OBJECTIVES

1. Describe extracellular, intracellular, and transcellular fluid compartments.
2. Describe the composition of extracellular and intracellular body fluid.
3. Discuss the mechanisms of fluid transport and fluid balance.
4. Identify the causes, signs and symptoms, and treatment of fluid imbalance.
5. Describe the major functions of the major electrolytes: sodium, potassium, calcium, and magnesium.
6. Identify the causes, signs and symptoms, and treatment of electrolyte imbalances.
7. Discuss the nursing management of persons with fluid and electrolyte imbalances.
8. Describe the major considerations in relation to fluid and electrolyte balance in the elderly.
9. List the four types of acid-base imbalances.
10. Identify the major causes of each acid-base imbalance.

GLOSSARY

ACID A solution containing a high number of hydrogen ions

ACID-BASE BALANCE The homeostasis of the hydrogen ion (H^+) concentration in the body fluids

ACTIVE TRANSPORT Movement of solutes across membranes using greater energy or force

ALKALINE OR BASE A solution containing a low number of hydrogen ions

DIFFUSION The random movement of particles in all directions through a solution

ELECTROLYTE A substance that develops an electrical charge when dissolved in water

EXTRACELLULAR FLUID Fluid outside the cell

FILTRATION Transfer of water and solutes through a membrane from a region of high pressure to a region of low pressure

FLUID VOLUME DEFICIT A decrease in extracellular fluid

FLUID VOLUME EXCESS An increase in extracellular fluid

HOMEOSTASIS A tendency of biologic systems to maintain stability of the internal environment while continuously adjusting to changes necessary for survival

INTRACELLULAR FLUID Fluid within the cell

OSMOLALITY Measurement of the ratio of water to solutes in a solution

OSMOSIS Movement of water across a membrane from a less concentrated solution to a more concentrated solution

pH The symbol used to indicate hydrogen ion balance. A solution with a low pH (<7) is an acid; a solution with a high pH (>7) is alkaline or base. A pH of 7 is neutral. The normal pH of body fluids is between 7.35 and 7.45.

SELECTIVELY PERMEABLE MEMBRANE Membranes that separate fluid compartments of the body that permit movement of water and certain solutes from one compartment to another

Many disease processes and medical interventions pose actual or potential threat to patients' fluid and electrolyte balance. Even patients who are only mildly ill can rapidly develop critical imbalances. Therefore, the nurse must understand the basic principles of fluid and electrolyte balance to detect imbalances and to maintain or restore balance.

HOMEOSTASIS

Approximately 50 to 60% of the human body is composed of water. To maintain internal balance, the body must be able to regulate the fluids within it. The ability to maintain internal balance is called *homeostasis.* All organs and structures of the body are involved in the maintenance of homeostasis.

Homeostasis is necessary for cells to be able to carry out their work. Body fluids are in constant motion, maintaining healthy living conditions for body cells. The process of homeostasis involves the delivery of nutrients such as oxygen and glucose to the cells and removal of wastes such as carbon dioxide from the cells. When the body does not maintain homeostasis, the cells do not work well, and illness results.

BODY FLUID COMPARTMENTS

Body fluids are divided into two portions: (1) intracellular fluid, and (2) extracellular fluid. *Intracellular fluid* is fluid within a cell, and *extracellular fluid* is fluid outside the cell. Most of the body's fluids are found within the cell. Table 11–1 shows the distribution of total body fluids in adult males, adult females, and infants.

TABLE 11-1
TOTAL BODY FLUIDS

	ADULT MALE (%)	ADULT FEMALE (%)	INFANT (%)
Intracellular	40	36	40
Extracellular	20	18	35
Total body fluids	60	54	75

Extracellular fluids are found in the blood vessels in the form of plasma or serum (called *intravascular fluids*); in the fluid surrounding the cells (called *interstitial fluid*), including lymph fluid; and in other areas such as digestive secretions, sweat, and cerebrospinal fluid. Extracellular fluid is mainly responsible for the transport of nutrients and wastes throughout the body.

COMPOSITION OF BODY FLUIDS

WATER

As noted earlier, water makes up the largest portion of the body. The percentage of body weight that is water is affected by age, gender, and amount of body fat. Body water usually decreases with advancing age. In addition, females have a lower percentage of body water than males, because women have more fat than men and fat cells contain less water than other cells. Obese people have a lower percentage of body water owing to a higher number of fat cells.

SOLUTES

In addition to water, body fluids contain dissolved substances known as *solutes,* such as electrolytes and nonelectrolytes.

Electrolytes

An *electrolyte* is defined as a substance that develops an electrical charge when dissolved in water. Examples of electrolytes are sodium, potassium, calcium, chloride, bicarbonate, and magnesium. When these substances are dissolved in water, they break up into small particles called *ions,* which have either a positive (+) or a negative (−) charge. Ions that have a positive electrical charge are called *cations.* Examples are the ions of sodium (Na^+), potassium (K^+), calcium (Ca^{++}), and magnesium (Mg^{++}). Ions that have a negative charge are called *anions.* Examples are the ions of chloride (Cl^-), bicarbonate (HCO_3^-), and phosphate (HPO_4^{--}).

Electrolytes maintain a balance between positive and negative charges. For every positively charged cation, there is a negatively charged anion. In every fluid compartment of the body, the cations and anions combine to balance one another out. This process keeps the body in homeostasis.

The concentration of an electrolyte in a solution or body fluid compartment is measured in milliequivalents (mEq). Milliequivalents indicate the chemical activity or combining power of ions. Hydrogen is used as a standard for comparing chemical activities of electrolytes. One mEq of an electrolyte has the same chemical combining power of 1 mEq of hydrogen.

Electrolytes move freely from one fluid compartment to another. However, they are concentrated in either extracellular or intracellular compartments. Concentrations of electrolytes in extracellular and intracellular fluid compartments are shown in Table 11–2.

Nonelectrolytes

Although the majority of the solutes in the body are electrolytes, other substances are dissolved in the body fluids. Examples are urea, protein, glucose, creatinine, and bilirubin. These solutes do not carry an electrical charge and are measured in weight per solution (mg/dl).

AGE-RELATED CHANGES

No studies indicate that electrolytes change as the result of aging. When changes in serum electrolytes occur in older adults, they are considered abnormalities caused by an underlying illness. The cause should always be evaluated and treated to reduce the risk of life-threatening illnesses.

Overall fluid volume decreases in the elderly. However, the decline is found primarily in intracellular compartments, not in the extracellular compartments.

TRANSPORT OF WATER AND ELECTROLYTES

MEMBRANES

The fluid compartments of the body are separated by *selectively permeable membranes* that permit movement of water and certain solutes. Some solutes cross membranes more easily than others. For example, small molecules and water move freely across membranes, whereas larger molecules such as protein move less readily. The purpose of selective permeability is to maintain the unique composition of each compartment of the body while allowing for the transport of nutrients and wastes to and from cells. For example, selectively permeable membranes surround cells to separate fluid in the cells from fluid in the tissues.

TABLE 11-2
COMPOSITION OF EXTRACELLULAR AND INTRACELLULAR FLUIDS

MAJOR EXTRACELLULAR FLUID	MAJOR INTRACELLULAR FLUID
Sodium Na^+ (130–145 mEq/L)	Potassium K^+ (3.8–4.4 mEq/L)
Chloride Cl^- (100–110 mEq/L)	Phosphate HPO_4^{--} (2 mEq/L)
Calcium Ca^{++} (5 mEq/L)	Magnesium Mg^{++} (2.5–3.5 mEq/L)
Bicarbonate HCO_3^- (24 mEq/L)	

TRANSPORT PROCESSES

Water is transported between intracellular and extracellular fluid compartments by one or more of the following processes: (1) diffusion, (2) active transport, (3) filtration, and (4) osmosis.

DIFFUSION. *Diffusion* is the random movement of particles in all directions through a solution. The natural tendency is for a substance to move from an area of higher concentration to an area of lower concentration. One example is the movement of oxygen from the alveoli (lung cells) to the pulmonary capillaries. The concentration of oxygen in the alveoli is greater, enabling the oxygen to go into the capillaries and then through the blood stream to other parts of the body. Another example is the movement of water. If a fluid compartment has less water and more sodium, water from another compartment moves to the more concentrated compartment to create a better fluid balance.

ACTIVE TRANSPORT. When conditions are not favorable for movement across membranes, solutes require greater energy or force. This process is called *active transport.* Many solutes, such as sodium, potassium, glucose, and hydrogen are actively transported across cell membranes.

FILTRATION. *Filtration* is the transfer of water and solutes through a membrane from an area of high pressure to an area of low pressure. This pressure is known as *hydraulic pressure* and is a combination of pressures from the force of gravity on the fluid and the pump action of the heart. Filtration is a necessary process for directing fluid out of the capillaries into the arteries and for filtering plasma through the kidneys.

OSMOSIS. *Osmosis* is the movement of water across a membrane from a less concentrated solution to a more concentrated solution. It involves the movement of water only, but sometimes the force of movement across the membrane carries some solutes along.

OSMOLALITY

Osmolality controls water movement and distribution in body fluid compartments by regulating the concentration of fluid in each compartment. When solutes such as electrolytes are added to water, the volume is expanded to include both the weight of the water and the solutes. Osmolality is a measurement of the ratio of the water to the solutes. It is determined by the number of dissolved particles per kilogram of water. A higher osmolality means that there is a higher concentration of salt or any other solute in water because the solution contains less water (Fig. 11–1).

The osmolality of intracellular fluid and extracellular fluid tends to equalize because there is constant shifting of water. A change in osmolality of intracellular fluid affects the osmolality of extracellular fluid and vice

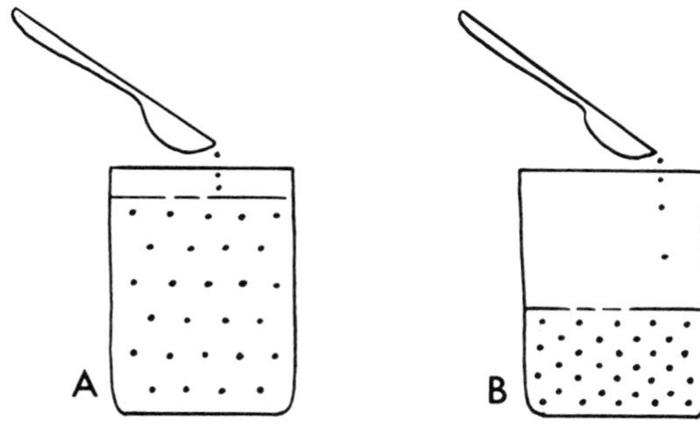

FIGURE 11-1

Although the actual salt content in both glasses is the same, glass B has a higher osmolality (concentration of salt in water) because it contains less water. Therefore, osmolality can be influenced by both water and sodium. (From Black, J. M., & Matassarin-Jacobs, E. [1993]. *Luckmann and Sorensen's medical-surgical nursing: A Psychophysiologic approach* [4th ed., p. 262]. Philadelphia: W. B. Saunders.)

versa. The osmolality of intracellular fluid is maintained primarily by potassium, and the osmolality of the extracellular fluid is maintained primarily by sodium. The normal range of osmolality of the body fluids is between 280 and 294 milliosmoles (mOsm) per kg.

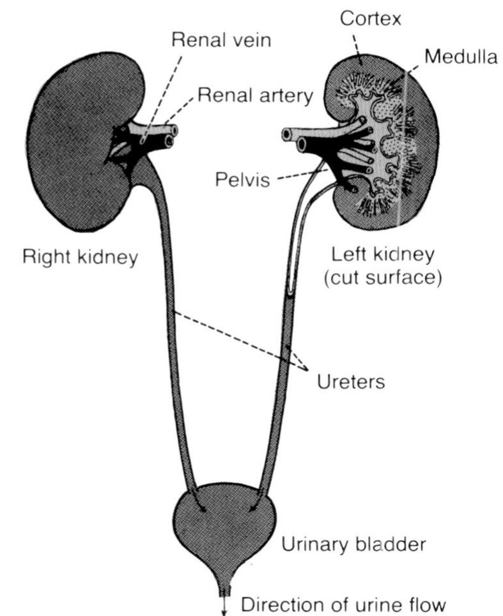

FIGURE 11-2

The general organizational plan of the urinary system. (From Guyton, A. C. [1991]. *Textbook of medical physiology* [8th ed., p. 287]. Philadelphia: W. B. Saunders.)

REGULATORY MECHANISMS

Regulation of fluid balance requires the constant adjustment of fluid redistribution, composition, and elimination. This process is accomplished by the kidneys and circulatory system, which are influenced by the action of specific hormones.

KIDNEYS

The kidneys are the main monitors of fluid balance. They control extracellular fluid by regulating the concentration of specific electrolytes, osmolality of body fluids, volume of extracellular fluid, blood, volume, and pH. Kidney function is delicately controlled by hormones and other coordinating mechanisms.

The kidneys, shaped like kidney beans, are located outside of the perineal cavity along the posterior abdominal wall. There are two kidneys, one on either side of the vertebral column. The upper portions of the kidney are located beneath the twelfth rib. An adrenal gland rests at the top of each kidney and secretes hormones that affect renal function. The kidney is composed of two parts: (1) the medulla, or inner part, and (2) the cortex, or outer part (Fig. 11–2).

Blood flows to the kidneys from the renal artery and leaves through the renal vein. Each kidney has a ureter that extends down to the urinary bladder. The ureters transport urine to the bladder from the kidney.

The nephron is the functioning unit of the kidney. There are more than a million nephrons in each kidney. Most nephrons are located in the cortex. Each nephron is made up of a glomerulus and tubules. The glomerulus is the filtering portion of the nephron, and the tubule is responsible for reabsorption. The nephrons conduct the work of the kidney through the processes of filtration, reabsorption, and secretion.

FILTRATION. A primary activity of the kidney is *filtration.* Blood plasma entering the kidney is delivered to the glomerulus and filtered. About 20% of the plasma is filtered; most of the remaining plasma leaves the kidney through the renal vein. The filtered plasma, or filtrate, then moves through the tubules where it undergoes many changes until it becomes urine and is transported through the ureters to the bladder.

REABSORPTION. *Reabsorption* is a process that occurs in the kidney tubules. Before the unfiltered plasma leaves the kidney, much of it goes into the renal capillaries. Water and solutes move from the capillaries into the tubules and act as a balance for the filtered plasma that is already there. Tubular reabsorption is important for adjusting the volume and composition of the filtrate and for preventing excessive fluid loss through the kidneys.

SECRETION. *Secretion* is the last phase in the work of the kidneys. During this phase, the filtrate is transformed to urine. Urine secretion is dependent on the reabsorption of potassium and hydrogen ions in the glomerulus and the extent to which they are secreted into the tubules.

HORMONES

Two hormones that have a major effect on fluid balance are aldosterone and antidiuretic hormone. *Aldosterone* is released by the adrenal glands. This hormone acts on the kidney tubules to increase the reabsorption of sodium (and water) and decrease the reabsorption of potassium. Because the retention of sodium causes water retention, aldosterone acts as a volume regulator. The release of aldosterone from the adrenal gland is stimulated by many factors, including increased potassium levels and decreased sodium levels in the blood.

Antidiuretic hormone is produced by the hypothalamus and is secreted into the general circulation by the posterior pituitary gland. It causes the kidney tubules to reabsorb more water, so that urine is more concentrated and there is less volume excreted in urination. An increase in plasma osmolality (less fluid in the plasma) stimulates the release of antidiuretic hormone into the blood stream to replenish needed fluid in the body. Other factors that stimulate the release of antidiuretic hormone are related to situations in which there may be less fluid volume in the blood stream such as hypotension, pain, stress, surgery, and certain medications.

THIRST

An additional regulatory mechanism is *thirst,* which regulates fluid intake. Increased plasma osmolality stimulates osmoreceptors in the hypothalamus to give the sensation of thirst. In other words, more sodium and less water in the body makes a person thirsty. The kidneys are alerted in this situation to conserve water and return it to the body.

FLUID GAINS AND LOSSES

In a healthy adult, the 24-hour fluid intake and output are approximately equal (Table 11–3). Fluids are gained by drinking and eating and are lost through the kidneys, skin, lungs, and gastrointestinal tract. The usual adult urine volume is between 1 and 2 liters per day, or 1 ml per kg of body weight per hour.

Water and electrolyte (Na^+, Cl^-, K^+) losses through the skin occur by sweating. Water loss through the lungs occurs by evaporation at a rate of 300 to 400 ml per day. Water loss via the skin and lungs increases in a hot, dry environment. In addition, increased respiratory rate, fever, or skin injury, such as burns, causes an increase in water loss.

In the kidneys, water loss varies largely with the amount of solute excreted and with the level of antidiuretic hormone. In the gastrointestinal tract, the usual loss of fluid is about 100 to 200 ml per day. The bulk of fluid is reabsorbed in the small intestine.

TABLE 11-3
24-HOUR INTAKE AND OUTPUT OF BODY FLUIDS

GAINS		LOSSES	
Liquids	1000 ml	Lungs	400 ml
Food (solid)	1200 ml	Skin	400 ml
H_2O of oxidation	300 ml	Kidneys (urine)	1500 ml
Daily total intake	2500 ml	Intestines (feces)	200 ml
		Daily total output	2500 ml

FLUID BALANCE

FLUID VOLUME DEFICIT. A decrease in extracellular fluid is called *fluid volume deficit,* or hypovolemia. A fluid volume deficit may result from decreased intake, abnormal fluid losses, or both. Examples of abnormal fluid losses are the loss of water through the skin as a result of severe burns, excessive bleeding, and certain conditions, such as severe vomiting and diarrhea. Hypovolemia can result in severe dehydration. The body attempts to compensate for fluid volume deficits by increasing the heart rate to pump more fluid to other parts of the body or to conserve water in the kidneys by increasing reabsorption and decreasing the secretion of urine.

FLUID VOLUME EXCESS. An increase in extracellular fluid is called *fluid volume excess,* or hypervolemia. A fluid volume excess may result from excessive sodium and water intake, conditions that would cause the kidneys to save sodium and water, increased production of antidiuretic hormone, or abnormal renal function. Severe hypervolemia can result in heart failure and pulmonary edema. The body attempts to compensate for fluid volume excess by increasing the filtration and excretion of sodium and water by the kidneys and decreasing the production of antidiuretic hormone. Figure 11–3 diagrams the regulation of body fluid volume.

ELECTROLYTE BALANCE

The kidneys are the primary regulators of electrolytes in the serum. The major electrolytes include sodium, potassium, chloride, and calcium.

Sodium

Sodium (Na^+) is the most abundant electrolyte in the body, and is the primary electrolyte in the extracellular fluid. It plays a major role in the regulation of body fluid volumes, muscular activity, nerve impulse conditions, and acid-base balance. Sodium in the body comes primarily from the diet.

A lower than normal concentration of sodium in the blood stream is known as *hyponatremia.* Hyponatremia occurs when there is a loss of sodium or an excess of body water. A deficiency in sodium ions in the extracellular fluid results. The body attempts to compensate by increasing the amount of water excreted from the kidneys.

A greater than normal concentration of sodium in the blood stream is known as *hypernatremia.* Hypernatremia may result from an increased intake of sodium or a decrease in body water. The body attempts to correct

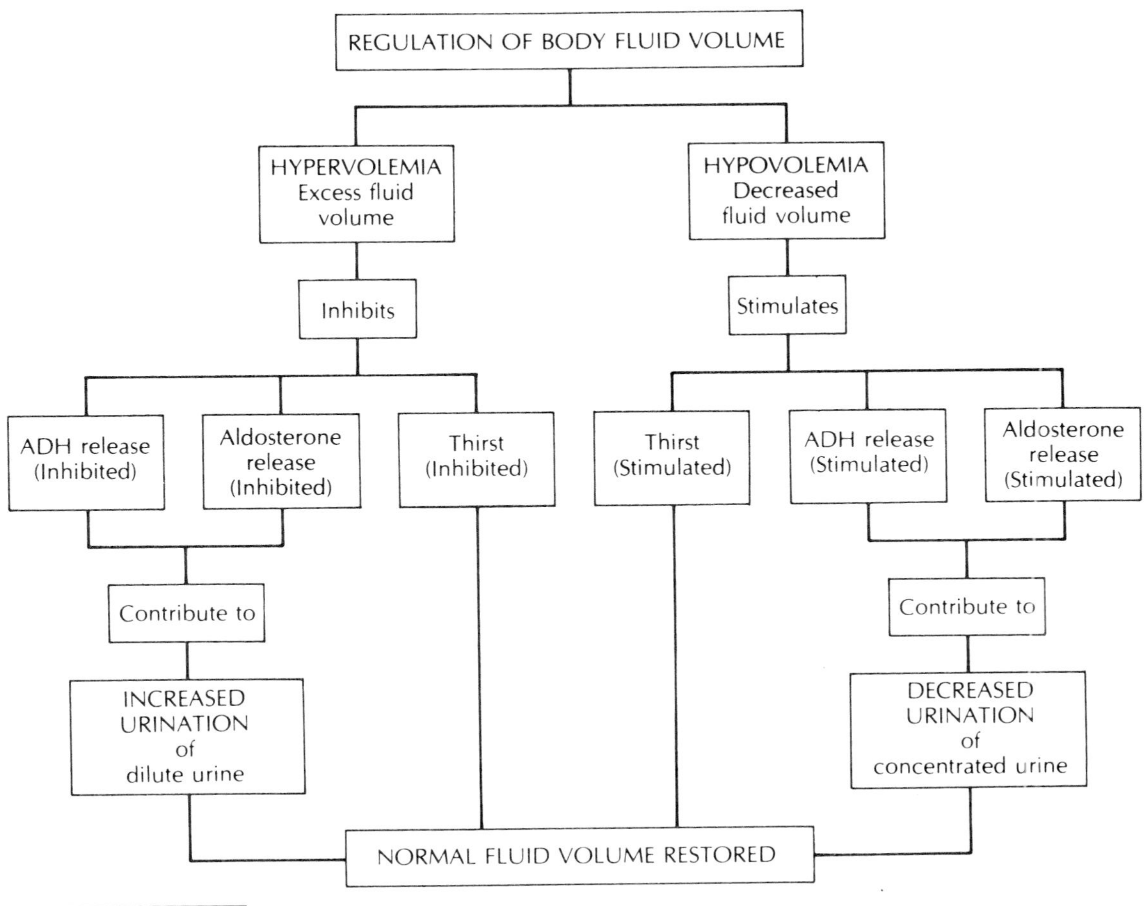

FIGURE 11-3
Regulation of body fluid volume depends on aldosterone (ADH) and thirst. (From Bolander, V. [1994]. *Sorensen and Luckmann's basic nursing* [3rd ed., p. 1016]. Philadelphia: W. B. Saunders.)

the imbalance of sodium and water by reabsorbing more water in the kidneys.

Potassium

Potassium (K^+) is found mainly in the intracellular fluid and is the major intracellular cation. Like sodium, it comes primarily from the diet. Potassium is excreted from the kidneys, so that any condition that causes a decrease in urine output causes an increase in the retention of potassium.

An abnormally low serum level of potassium is called *hypokalemia*. It usually occurs when the kidneys excrete too much potassium, even when the body needs it. Cell injury or medications such as diuretics can cause hypokalemia.

Hyperkalemia occurs when there is too much potassium in the blood stream. Hyperkalemia results from renal disease or damage, limiting the ability of the kidneys to excrete potassium.

Potassium plays a major role in nerve stimulus conduction and muscle activity. Abnormally high or low levels of potassium can result in dangerous cardiac arrhythmias and death.

Chloride

Chloride is an extracellular anion that is usually bound with other ions, especially sodium or potassium. Its major functions are to regulate osmotic pressure between fluid compartments and to assist in regulating acid-base balance. Because chloride is usually bound with other electrolytes, imbalances are in conjunction with the other electrolyte imbalances.

High serum chloride, known as *hyperchloremia*, usually is associated with metabolic acidosis. Low serum chloride, known as *hypochloremia*, usually occurs when sodium is lost because chloride is most frequently bound with sodium. Hypochloremia may be caused by vomiting and uncontrolled diabetes.

Serum Calcium

Calcium is usually combined with phosphorus to form the mineral salts of the bones and teeth. Ninety-nine percent of the body's calcium is concentrated in the bones and teeth, and 1% is in the extracellular fluid. Calcium is ingested through the diet and absorbed through the intestine.

In addition to maintaining strong teeth and bones, calcium promotes normal transmission of nerve impulses and helps to regulate normal muscle contraction and relaxation. Constant regulation of calcium levels takes place in the body. If more calcium is needed in the blood stream, it is either taken from the bones or reabsorbed through the kidneys. If more is needed in the bones, it is taken from the blood stream as well as reabsorbed through the kidneys.

A low serum (blood) level of calcium is called *hypocalcemia.* Hypocalcemia results from diarrhea, inadequate dietary intake of calcium or vitamin D, and infusions of too much citrated blood (citrates bind to the calcium), in addition to some diseases.

Hypercalcemia occurs with increased serum levels of calcium. A high calcium or vitamin D intake can cause hypercalcemia. In addition, immobility, which causes stores of calcium in the bone to enter the blood stream, can result in hypercalcemia.

Serum Magnesium

Magnesium is a cation that is found in bone (50–60%), intracellular fluid (39–49%), and extracellular fluid (1%). Next to potassium, magnesium is the most abundant cation in intracellular fluid, so it is vital to cellular function. It plays a role in metabolism of carbohydrates and proteins, storage and use of intracellular energy, and neural transmission. Magnesium is important in the functioning of the heart, nerves, and muscles.

About 30 to 40% of magnesium ingested through the diet is absorbed in the body, mainly through the small intestine. Magnesium is excreted through the kidneys, and the rate of excretion is regulated by sodium and calcium excretion, extracellular fluid volume, and the parathyroid hormone.

A lower than normal concentration of magnesium in the blood stream is known as *hypomagnesemia.* Hypomagnesemia results from decreased gastrointestinal absorption or excessive gastrointestinal loss (usually from vomiting and diarrhea) or from increased urinary loss. Hypomagnesemia is frequently associated with hypocalcemia and hypokalemia.

A higher than normal concentration of magnesium in the blood stream is known as *hypermagnesemia.* It occurs most frequently with excessive use of magnesium-containing medications or intravenous solutions in patients with renal failure or preeclampsia in pregnancy.

NURSING CARE TO MAINTAIN OR RESTORE FLUID AND ELECTROLYTE BALANCE

ASSESSMENT

Because electrolyte disturbances produce nonspecific symptoms, they can be confirmed only with laboratory tests. Some disease or trauma states that have great potential for altering fluid balance are kidney diseases, diabetes, salicylate poisoning, burns, congestive heart failure, cerebral injuries, ulcerative colitis, and hormonal imbalances. Vomiting and diarrhea also have potential for causing fluid and electrolyte imbalances.

In the assessment process, the nurse should obtain a good health history to determine whether patients have any conditions that may contribute to fluid or electrolyte imbalances. In addition, a good physical assessment should be carried out. Measurement of vital signs, intake and output, and body weight are basic to the physical assessment of fluid and electrolyte balance, as are observation of the skin and mucous membranes for appearance and turgor.

VITAL SIGNS. Assessment of pulse, respiration, temperature, and blood pressure can indicate changes in both fluid and electrolyte balance (Table 11–4). For example, an increase in temperature signals that a fever is present, and fever is responsible for increased metabolism and resulting fluid loss. Or an increased pulse rate can signal an excess in sodium ions, whereas a decreased pulse rate can be a sign of magnesium excess.

INTAKE AND OUTPUT. It is essential to maintain a careful intake and output to be confident that the patient's intake is equal to output (Table 11–5). All fluids entering or leaving the body should be noted.

BODY WEIGHT. Measurement of body weight is a good indicator of fluid loss or retention (Table 11–6). Excessive weight gain (a weight gain of 2.2 lb or 1 kg) equals 1 liter of fluid retention. A patient can accumulate up to 10 pounds (4.5 kg) of fluid before pitting edema is evident. The patient should be weighed daily

TABLE 11–4
ASSESSMENT OF VITAL SIGNS

PULSE	Increased pulse indicates sodium excess or magnesium deficit. Decreased pulse indicates magnesium excess. Weak, irregular, and rapid pulse suggests severe potassium excess or sodium deficit. Bounding pulse occurs in volume excess and often results in circulatory overload.
RESPIRATION	Changes in respiratory function are noted with electrolyte imbalances. Slow, shallow respirations with intermittent periods of apnea occur in severe metabolic alkalosis. Deep, fast respirations indicate metabolic acidosis.
TEMPERATURE	Fever increases metabolism causing fluid loss. It also increases the respiratory rate, which results in loss of water vapor from the lungs.
BLOOD PRESSURE	A fall in systolic pressure greater than 10 mm Hg from the lying to the standing or the lying to the sitting position usually indicates fluid volume deficit.

TABLE 11-5
ASSESSMENT OF INTAKE AND OUTPUT

INTAKE AND OUTPUT
Many serious balance problems can be averted by maintaining careful intake and output.
If the total intake is substantially less than the total output, it is obvious that the patient is in danger of fluid volume deficit.
If the total intake is substantially more than the total output, the patient is in danger of fluid volume excess.
Intake should include all fluids taken into the body: oral fluids, foods that are liquid at room temperature, intravenous fluids, subcutaneous fluids, fluids instilled into drainage tubes or irritants, tube feeding solutions, water given through feeding tubes, enema solutions.
Output measures include urine, vomitus, diarrhea, drainage from fistulas, drainage from suction machines, estimated perspiration, and drainage from excisions; normal adult urine output is 40–80 ml/hr.

TABLE 11-6
ASSESSMENT OF BODY WEIGHT

BODY WEIGHT

The use of body weight as an accurate index of fluid balance is based on the assumption that the patient's dry weight remains relatively stable. Even under starvation conditions, an individual loses no more than 1/3 to 1/2 lb dry weight a day.

A rapid loss of body weight occurs when the total fluid intake is less than the total fluid output.

A rapid gain of body weight occurs when total fluid intake is *more* than the total fluid output.

	MILD	MODERATE	SEVERE
Rapid loss	2%	5%	8% = deficit
Rapid gain	2%	5%	8% = excess

Rapid gain or loss of 1 kg (2.2 lb) of body weight is approximately equivalent to the gain or loss of 1 L of fluid.

on the same scale, at the same time of day, and wearing the same number of clothes.

SKIN

Skin Appearance. Dry, flushed skin is associated with dehydration. Pale, cool, and clammy skin is associated with the severe fluid volume deficit that occurs with shock.

Facial Appearance. The patient who is severely dehydrated usually has a pinched, drawn facial expression. Soft, sunken eyes accompany a fluid volume deficit of 10% body weight, which causes decreased intraocular pressure. Tearing and salivation may be absent. Puffy eyeballs and fuller cheeks suggest fluid volume excess.

Skin Turgor. Skin turgor is best measured by pinching the skin over the sternum, the inner aspects of the thighs, or the forehead. In patients who are dehydrated, skin flattens more slowly after the pinch is released. Older people generally have a slower return to normal, so assessment should include other indicators such as moisture in the mucous membranes.

Edema. Edema reflects sodium retention, which can result from excessive reabsorption or inadequate secretion due to failing kidney function. The skin should be inspected and palpated for edema. Edema is described as *pitting* if a depression remains in the tissue after pressure is applied with a fingertip. Edema is tested by pressing the skin that lies over the tibia, fibula, sacrum, or sternum. Pitting edema is evaluated on a four-point scale, ranging from 1+ edema (barely detectable pit) to 4+ edema (deep and persistent pit that is approximately 1 inch or 2.54 cm deep).

Edema can be so severe that pitting is not possible. The tissue becomes so full that fluid cannot be displaced. The edematous tissue feels hard and may be referred to as *brawny edema.* Brawny edema commonly occurs after a radical mastectomy because axillary nodes have been removed, and fluid accumulates in the affected arm.

MUCOUS MEMBRANES

Tongue Turgor. In a normal person, the tongue has one longitudinal furrow. A person with fluid volume deficit has additional longitudinal furrows, and the tongue is smaller owing to fluid loss. Sodium excess causes the tongue to appear red and swollen.

Moisture of the Oral Cavity. A dry mouth may be the result of fluid volume deficit or mouth breathing. The examiner can run a finger along the area where the cheek and the gum meet. Dryness in this area indicates a true fluid volume deficit.

VEINS. Observations of the jugular veins in the neck and the veins in the hands can be indicators of either a fluid volume deficit or a fluid volume excess.

Neck Vein Distention. Distention of the jugular neck vein can indicate fluid volume excess. Inspection of the neck veins for fluid volume excess is carried out by having the patient sit at the head of the bed elevated at a 30- to 45-degree angle. If the jugular veins can be seen more than 3 cm above the sternal angle, then fluid volume excess is most likely present.

Fluid volume deficit is determined by examining the jugular neck veins in a lying down position. If no distention occurs, then fluid volume deficit is most likely present.

Hand Veins. Observation of hand veins also can be helpful in evaluating the patient's fluid volume. When the hands are elevated, the veins usually empty in 3 to 5 seconds. When the hands are placed in a dependent position, the veins usually fill in 3 to 5 seconds. If the volume is decreased, veins take longer than 3 to 5 seconds to fill. When the fluid volume is increased, veins take longer than 3 to 5 seconds to empty.

TABLE 11-7

NORMAL VALUES OF FLUID AND ELECTROLYTES

URINE	BLOOD
Urine pH: 4.6–8.0	Hematocrit: males 44; females 40
Urine specific gravity; 1.001–1.035	Blood urea nitrogen: 8–20 mg/dl
Urine osmolality: 48–1350 mOsm/kg	Serum osmolality: 280–294 mOsm/kg
Urine creatinine clearance: 100–120 ml/min for 1.73 m² of body surface area	Serum sodium: 136–145 mEq/L
Urine sodium: 40–220 mmol/24 hr	Serum potassium: 3.5–5.0 mEq/L
Urine potassium: 30–90 mmol/24 hr	Serum chloride: 98–106 mEq/L
	Serum calcium: 9.0–11.0 mEq/L
	Serum magnesium: 1.5–2.5 mEq/L

DIAGNOSTIC TESTS AND PROCEDURES

A variety of laboratory tests may be performed to assess fluid and electrolyte status. Normal values are found in Table 11–7.

Urine Studies

URINE pH. The kidneys can change the acidity or alkalinity of the urine by excreting hydrogen (H^+) ions. Urine pH is a measure of hydrogen ions in the urine. It is useful for determining whether the kidneys are responding appropriately to metabolic acid-base imbalances. The normal range is 4.6 to 8.0; however, fresh urine is usually acidic (about 6.0). A urine specimen that is not tested within 4 hours of collection may become alkaline. Therefore, urine pH should be measured within 1 to 2 hours of collection.

URINE SPECIFIC GRAVITY. Urine specific gravity (SpGr) measures the kidney's ability to conserve water or concentrate urine. In most instances, normal urine specific gravity is between 1.001 and 1.035 in adults.

Specific gravity is a good indicator of fluid balance. A high specific gravity indicates that the urine is highly concentrated, usually as a result of fluid volume deficit. A low specific gravity indicates that the urine contains a large amount of water, usually as a result of fluid volume excess.

URINE OSMOLALITY. Osmolality measures the number of dissolved particles in a solution. This provides a more precise measurement of the kidney's ability to concentrate urine than the specific gravity. The normal urine osmolality range is 48 to 1350 mOsm per kg.

URINE CREATININE CLEARANCE. Urine creatinine clearance tests are used to detect glomerular damage in the kidney. A 24-hour specimen is required. The patient is instructed to void, discard the specimen, record the time, and start collecting for 24 hours. The specimen must be refrigerated. During the specimen collection period, the patient should not engage in vigorous exercise and should avoid high-protein diet, coffee, tea, or cola drinks. The normal creatinine clearance is 100 to 200 ml per minute per 1.73 m^2 of body surface area.

URINE SODIUM. Urine sodium reflects sodium intake and fluid volume status. A high sodium intake results in a decreased sodium excretion in the urine. A high fluid volume results in a decreased sodium excretion in the urine. The normal urine sodium is 50 to 130 mEq per liter. If collected over a period of 24 hours, the normal range is 40 to 220 mmol per 24 hours.

URINE POTASSIUM. Urine potassium is a measure of renal tubular function. It requires the collection of a 24-hour specimen. The normal value is 30 to 90 mmol per 24 hours.

Blood Studies

SERUM HEMATOCRIT. The hematocrit measures the percentage of blood volume that is composed of red blood cells. Increased hematocrit is related to fluid volume deficit and dehydration. The normal hematocrit is 44 for adult males and 40 for adult females.

BLOOD UREA NITROGEN. Blood urea nitrogen (BUN) provides a measure of renal function. Normal is 8 to 20 mg per dl. A high BUN is associated with fluid volume deficit and dehydration; conversely, a low BUN is associated with fluid volume excess. When a patient has an elevated BUN, the hematocrit should be monitored because a high BUN can cause breakdown of red blood cells. Patients with an elevated BUN may be confused and disoriented.

SERUM OSMOLALITY. Serum osmolality is a measure of blood concentration. High serum osmolality is related to fluid volume deficit, and low serum osmolality is related to fluid volume excess. The normal range is 280 to 294 mOsm per kg.

SERUM ELECTROLYTES. Normal values for serum sodium, potassium, chloride, and calcium are shown in Table 11–7.

NURSING CARE OF THE PATIENT WITH A FLUID VOLUME DEFICIT

ASSESSMENT

The severity and speed with which a fluid volume deficit develops affect the kinds of signs and symptoms observed. Symptoms are not as apparent with deficits that are mild and have a gradual onset, but the symptoms are quite dramatic when the onset is severe and abrupt. In adults, diarrhea is an example of a mild fluid volume deficit, and acute hemorrhage is an example of a severe fluid volume deficit.

General signs and symptoms of fluid volume deficit (or dehydration) are dizziness, weakness, fatigue, syncope (fainting), nausea or vomiting, anorexia, thirst, confusion, and sparse urine output (oliguria). Assessment of vital signs is important to detect postural hypotension and increased temperature and heart rate. Inspection of skin and tissue turgor, as well as neck veins, is also important.

INTERVENTION

The primary intervention for fluid volume deficit is fluid replacement. Intravenous therapy is the first line of treatment, with care being taken to give fluids rapidly enough and in sufficient quantity to ensure adequate tissue perfusion without overloading the cardiovascular system. Intravenous fluids are administered as ordered by the physician. It is the nurse's responsibility to monitor intake and output closely (at least hourly) and to look for signs of fluid volume overload. Intake should exceed output during therapy for a fluid volume deficit.

AGE-RELATED CHANGES

The aging kidney is slower to adjust to changes in acid-base, fluid, and electrolyte balance. These balances, however, are not impaired by age alone. Older adults frequently have a reduced sense of thirst and therefore are chronically in a state of poor hydration. Poor hydration frequently has an adverse effect on functional abilities. Severe dehydration, whether related to blood loss or fluid loss, should be treated appropriately.

Some of the contributors to inadequate hydration are traumatic illness, infections, fevers, flu or colds, and drug therapies (diuretics, antidepressants, and sedating drugs). Among the chronic conditions that may contribute to dehydration in the elderly are mental deficits, Parkinson's disease, and a gradual decrease in the physical ability to get fluids (people with severe arthritis who cannot ambulate or grasp containers easily).

The nurse needs to evaluate hydration in the elderly and be alert to the consequences of poor hydration. Deterioration of mental status, disorientation, confusion, constipation, and abnormal readings in blood tests (increased hematocrit, BUN, sodium) are some common signs of dehydration. Unless contraindicated by other fluid imbalance problems, fluid requirements for older adults, based on ideal body weight are 30 ml per kg in persons aged 55 to 65 and 25 ml per kg in persons aged 65 and over. The average person needs 1500 to 2000 ml of fluid per day for adequate hydration.

Data collected should include a report of fluid intake patterns, medications, mental status, and recent weight loss. The physical examination for hydration includes measurement of vital signs (temperature, blood pressure lying and standing) and observation of changes in mental status and tissue and skin turgor (use sternum or forehead for better accuracy). In addition, the nurse should monitor laboratory values, such as serum sodium and BUN-creatinine. Urine is evaluated for color and specific gravity, and daily fluid intake and output records should be kept.

NURSING CARE OF THE PATIENT WITH A FLUID VOLUME EXCESS

ASSESSMENT

As with fluid volume deficit, the severity of the symptoms in fluid volume excess depends on how quickly the condition develops. A major cause of severe fluid volume excess is an overload of intravenous fluids, which can be administered too rapidly. Signs and symptoms of fluid volume excess are shortness of breath, edema, weight gain, elevated blood pressure, bounding pulses, tachycardia, wheezing and crackling lung sounds, and moist skin. Vital signs, examination of the lungs and skin, and daily weight measurements are cornerstones for the assessment of fluid volume excess. Intake and output are monitored hourly, and urine output should be at least 30 to 60 ml per hour.

INTERVENTION

Treatment of fluid volume excess is aimed at eliminating the cause of the problem and returning to normal fluid balance. Restriction of sodium and water and administration of diuretics are the major therapeutic measures. Salt substitutes may be used in the diet if there are no concerns about increased potassium intake. Low-salt diets are encouraged, and foods high in sodium such as bouillon, cheese, condiments (pickles, mustard, olives, sauerkraut), high-salt snack foods, and preserved meats should be avoided (Table 11–8). Limiting fluids may be difficult for some patients, but the nurse can help by offering ice chips. Good oral hygiene is important for dry mouth.

When breathing problems occur, patients should be kept in an upright position. The head of the bed can be elevated 30 degrees, and restrictive clothing should be avoided. Oxygen may be ordered by the physician.

If pitting edema is present, the risk of skin and tissue breakdown increases. Patients should be turned and repositioned at least every 2 hours, and the skin over the ankles and bony prominences should be examined. An egg crate or an air mattress may be used to decrease pressure on sensitive skin. Pressure sores are treated according to the institutional protocol.

Patients should be observed for dehydration in the event that treatment results in overcorrection of the fluid volume excess.

Table 11–9 lists and decribes nursing assessment and interventions for fluid volume deficit and fluid volume excess.

TABLE 11-8
COMMON FOOD SOURCES OF SODIUM

FOODS HIGH IN SODIUM (APPROXIMATELY 250 mg PER SERVING)

Grains
- Cold cereal, 1 oz
- Corn chips, 14 chips
- Instant hot cereal, ½ cup
- Potato chips, 14 chips

Cheeses
- Natural cheese, 1 oz
- Processed cheese, 1 oz
- Creamed cheese, ½ cup

Meats
- Sausage, 1 oz
- Luncheon meats, 1 oz
- Frankfurters, 1 oz
- Cooked bacon, 2 slices
- Ham, 1 oz

Convenience foods
- Pizza, 2 to 3 slices
- Pot pies, 8 oz
- Ravioli, canned, 8 oz
- Soups (canned or dehydrated), 1 cup

FOODS LOW IN SODIUM (LESS THAN 50 mg PER SERVING)

Fruits and vegetables
- Fresh fruits or canned, ½ cup
- Fresh, frozen, ½ cup

Grains
- Unsalted pastas, ½ cup
- Oatmeal, cooked, 1 cup
- Popcorn (unsalted), 1 oz
- Puffed rice, 1 cup
- Shredded wheat, 1 biscuit

Meats
- Fresh meat, 1 oz
- Fresh chicken, 1 oz
- Fresh fish, 1 oz

Beverages

Data from Laquarta, I., & Gerlach, M. (1990). *Nutrition in clinical nursing.* Albany, NY: Delmar Publishers; and Burtis, G., et al. (1988). *Applied nutrition and diet therapy.* Philadelphia: W. B. Saunders. From Black, J. M., & Matassarin-Jacobs, E. (1993). *Luckmann and Sorensen's medical-surgical nursing: A psychophysiologic approach* (4th ed., p. 275). Philadelphia: W. B. Saunders.

NURSING CARE OF THE PATIENT WITH AN ELECTROLYTE IMBALANCE

The two electrolytes that cause the majority of problems when there is an imbalance are sodium (Na^+) and potassium (K^+).

HYPONATREMIA (SODIUM DEFICIT)

ASSESSMENT. If hyponatremia is suspected, the patient should be monitored for signs and symptoms that include headache, muscle weakness, fatigue, apathy, confusion, abdominal cramps, and postural hypotension. Blood pressures are taken lying or sitting and then standing to determine whether there is a significant

TABLE 11-9
NURSING ASSESSMENT AND INTERVENTION FOR FLUID VOLUME DEFICIT AND FLUID VOLUME EXCESS

	FLUID VOLUME DEFICIT	FLUID VOLUME EXCESS
CLINICAL SIGNS	Vomiting, diarrhea, weight loss, decreased skin turgor, polyuria, fever, excess sweat, rapid pulse, dry mucous membranes, urine output below 30 ml/hr, postural hypotension, flat neck veins, ↓ BP Lab: High BUN, Hct, SpGr	Weight gain, peripheral edema, distended neck and peripheral veins, SOB, polyuria, ascites, pleural effusion, bounding pulse, pulmonary edema, ↑ BP Lab: Low BUN, Hct, SpGr
INTERVENTION	Measure I&O q 8 hr *Monitor:* daily weight, postural hypotension (drop of more than 10 mm Hg systolic BP), tachycardia, skin and tongue turgor, mucous membranes, urine concentration, body temperature, sensorium. Give oral fluids, medications. Explain need for fluid replacement. Lab: High BUN	Measure I&O q 8 hr; daily weights, watch for acute gain. Assess breath sounds, edema, vein distention. Provide low Na^+ diet. Encourage rest, head of bed elevated 30 degrees if dyspnea or orthopnea is present. Lab: Low BUN, Hct
EVALUATION	Balanced electrolyte levels, adherence to medical regimen.	Balanced electrolyte levels, adherence to prescribed care

BP, Blood pressure; BUN, blood urea nitrogen; Hct, hematocrit; SpGr, specific gravity; SOB, shortness of breath; I&O, input and output; Na^+, sodium.

drop (drop in systolic blood pressure >20 mm Hg). Patients who are taking diuretics should be observed for sodium depletion.

INTERVENTION. The usual treatment for hyponatremia is to provide oral sodium supplements, encourage dietary sources of salt, and avoid giving water to drink. To prevent hyponatremia in patients with feeding tubes, normal saline (rather than water) should be used for irrigation. Patients may need assistance with ambulation if their blood pressure is low or they have postural hypotension.

HYPERNATREMIA (SODIUM EXCESS)

ASSESSMENT. Signs and symptoms of hypernatremia are thirst, flushed skin, dry mucous membranes, low urine output, restlessness, increased heart rate, and convulsions. Assessment consists of checking for low-grade fever, flushed skin, edema, and postural hypotension.

INTERVENTION. Patients with hypernatremia are encouraged to drink water for hydration. Intravenous lines are closely monitored, especially when the patient's cardiac or renal function is abnormal. A low-sodium diet is often prescribed.

Patient education is important. A nurse should teach the patient with hypernatremia about tracking daily intake and output and recognizing the signs and symptoms of fluid retention or depletion. Patients are advised that dietary restrictions are part of the treatment. High levels of sodium (Na^+) are found in catsup, monosodium glutamate (Accent), mustard, pickles, olives, ham, most canned foods, artificial sweeteners, laxatives, cough medications, and antacids. Salt substitutes cannot be used if potassium (K^+) is restricted. Patients also can learn to take their own blood pressure, especially if they have renal conditions.

HYPOKALEMIA (POTASSIUM DEFICIT)

ASSESSMENT. Signs and symptoms of hypokalemia are muscle weakness, anorexia, nausea and vomiting, lethargy, arrhythmias, and decreased ability to concentrate urine. Assessment consists of observations for decreased bowel sounds, weak and irregular pulse, decreased reflexes, and decreased muscle tone. Patients with nasogastric tubes are at high risk for hypokalemia, so ongoing assessment for signs and symptoms is important. In addition, the heart rate of patients on digitalis should be closely watched, because hypokalemia can cause digitalis toxicity. Cardiac monitors may be used to detect arrythmias.

INTERVENTION. Oral potassium supplements are administered as prescribed. They should be given with a full glass of water or fruit juice to avoid gastrointestinal irritation. Patients should be instructed to sip slowly. Dietary sources of potassium, particularly fruits and vegetables, such as bananas and oranges or orange juice are encouraged (Table 11–10).

TABLE 11-10
COMMON FOOD SOURCES OF POTASSIUM

HIGH IN POTASSIUM (AVERAGE 7 mEq PER SERVING)
Vegetables ($\frac{1}{2}$ cup cooked or 1 cup raw)
Artichokes
Broccoli
Brussels sprouts
Cabbage
Carrots
Celery
Collards
Cucumber
Mushrooms
Spinach
Tomatoes
Fruits
Apricots, fresh, 4 medium
Apricots, canned, 4 halves
Apricots, dried, 7 halves
Banana, 7 inches
Cantaloupe, $\frac{1}{4}$ small
Guava, 1 medium
Honeydew melon, $\frac{1}{8}$ medium
Nectarine, $\frac{1}{2}$
Orange, 1 small
Prunes, 3 medium
Strawberries, $1\frac{1}{4}$ cup
Tangerine, 2 medium
Watermelon, $1\frac{1}{4}$ cup
Beverages
Brewed coffee
Tomato juice
Vegetable juice cocktail, unsalted
LOW IN POTASSIUM (AVERAGE 3 mEq PER SERVING)
Vegetables
Corn, $\frac{1}{3}$ cup
Sweet potato, yams, $\frac{1}{4}$ cup
Lima beans, $\frac{1}{3}$ cup
French fried potatoes, 10
Fruit
Apple, 1 small
Apple juice, $\frac{1}{2}$ cup
Applesauce, $\frac{1}{2}$ cup
Blueberries, $\frac{3}{4}$ cup
Cranberries, $1\frac{1}{4}$ cup
Beverages
Coffee, instant
Cola
Cranberry juice cocktail, $\frac{1}{3}$ cup
Ginger ale
Noncarbonated soft drinks
Root beer
Lemon-lime soda

Data from Mahan, K. L., & Arlin, M. (1992). *Food, nutrition and diet therapy* (8th ed.). Philadelphia: W. B. Saunders. From Black, J. M., & Matassarin-Jacobs, E. (1993). *Luckmann and Sorensen's medical-surgical nursing: A psychophysiologic approach* (4th ed., p. 283). Philadelphia: W. B. Saunders.

Intravenous potassium is administered as ordered. Potassium is always diluted and never given in concentrated form. A central rather than peripheral line is used because intravenous potassium can cause irritation of the veins, phlebitis, or both. Potassium is never given by intravenous push.

The patient's urine output should be checked before starting an intravenous infusion of potassium. Urinary output should be no less than 30 ml per hour. If it is less than 30 ml per hour, for 2 consecutive hours, the nurse should alert the physician, who may stop the infusion.

HYPERKALEMIA (POTASSIUM EXCESS)

ASSESSMENT. Patients who are taking potassium supplements or diuretics must be monitored carefully for signs and symptoms of hyperkalemia. They include nausea and vomiting, diarrhea, irritability, anxiety, abdominal cramps, weakness, cardiac dysrhythmias, and decreased urine output. An irregular pulse rate is a cardinal sign. Because decreased renal function can cause hyperkalemia, intake and output should be monitored.

INTERVENTION. Serum potassium levels greater than 5.0 mEq/L can cause cardiac arrest. A physician should be notified if this situation occurs, and patients are usually placed on cardiac monitors.

The first line of treatment for hyperkalemia is restriction of potassium intake (see Table 11–10), including potassium penicillin. Calcium may be given to counteract the effects of excessive potassium in the heart. Sodium bicarbonate and glucose-insulin infusions may be administered to shift extracellular potassium into the cells, and sodium polystyrene sulfonate (Kayexalate) may be given to increase potassium loss by way of the gastrointestinal tract. Patients should be taught to look for signs and symptoms of abnormal potassium levels and to understand why frequent blood tests are required to monitor potassium levels.

ACID-BASE DISTURBANCES

Acid-base balance is the homeostasis of the hydrogen ion (H^+) concentration in the body fluids. A solution containing a higher number of hydrogen ions is an acid, and a solution containing a lower number of hydrogen ions is an alkaline or base. The symbol used to indicate hydrogen ion balance is pH. There is an inverse relationship between pH levels and the number of hydrogen ions. As the number of hydrogen ions increases, the acidity increases and the pH decreases. Conversely, as the number of hydrogen ions decreases, the alkalinity decreases and the pH increases. A pH less than 7.35 is acid; a pH greater than 7.45 is alkaline. When the solution is between 7.35 and 7.45, it is neutral.

Hydrogen ion concentration is indicated by the pH of the blood. The normal pH of blood is between 7.35 and 7.45, or neutral. When the blood is below 7.35, *acidosis* is present; when it is above 7.45, *alkalosis* is present.

The normal acid-base balance is maintained by three primary, complex mechanisms: (1) blood buffers, (2) respiratory control of carbon dioxide (CO_2), and (3) renal regulation of bicarbonate (HCO_3^-). To maintain a neutral environment, the blood buffers circulate throughout the body in pairs, acting as sponges to soak up hydrogen ions. One of the buffers takes away a hydrogen ion if a fluid is too acid, and one of the buffers gives an ion if the fluid is too alkaline.

The lungs and kidneys are the next line of defense after the blood buffers for maintaining acid-base balance. The lungs are primarily responsible for the regulation of carbon dioxide, which is influenced by the rate and depth of respirations. The respiratory system regulates the pH by removing carbon dioxide from the blood. If the pH of the blood becomes too high or too low, the respiratory center in the brain sends signals to the lungs to increase or decrease respirations to "blow off" or retain the appropriate amount of carbon dioxide.

The kidneys are the metabolic regulators of the pH by excreting acids or bases as needed. Renal regulation of HCO_3^- and secretion of H^+ are the chief means of regulating acid-base control through the kidneys. HCO_3^- is a major acid buffer in the blood, and it is through the kidneys that HCO_3^- is reabsorbed and produced.

If acid-base imbalances exist, there is an imbalance in the functioning of the lungs, kidneys, or both. The four major types of acid-base imbalances are (1) respiratory acidosis, (2) respiratory alkalosis, (3) metabolic acidosis, and (4) metabolic alkalosis.

RESPIRATORY ACIDOSIS

Respiratory acidosis occurs when the respiratory system fails to eliminate the appropriate amount of carbon dioxide to maintain the normal acid-base balance. Retention of carbon dioxide occurs, with a resultant increase of carbonic acid in the blood. The respiratory rate increases, and respirations are shallow as the body attempts to eliminate the excessive carbon dioxide in the lungs. The kidneys attempt to help by reabsorbing more HCO_3^- to balance the amount of carbonic acid in the blood.

Acute respiratory acidosis is caused by respiratory diseases such as pneumonia, drug overdose, head injuries or injury to the chest wall, obesity, asphyxiation, drowning, or acute respiratory failure. Common clinical signs and symptoms include rapid heart and respiratory rates, headache, sweating, lethargy, and confusion.

ASSESSMENT. Assessment of carbon dioxide levels is done by measuring partial pressure carbon dioxide ($Paco_2$) levels in arterial blood. The $Paco_2$ levels directly reflect the carbon dioxide levels and the degree of respiratory dysfunction. In addition, patients should be observed for signs of respiratory distress, including restlessness, anxiety, confusion and rapid breathing (>20 breaths/min). It is important to note frequently the rate, depth, and rhythm of respirations. Assessment of level of consciousness, including orientation to person, place, and time, should be carried out to note changes in mental status.

INTERVENTION. Interventions for respiratory acidosis are geared toward improving ventilation, which in turn restores the $Paco_2$ to normal. Underlying respiratory conditions are treated to eliminate the cause of respiratory acidosis. Antibiotics, bronchodilators, and specific breathing treatments such as intermittent positive-pressure breathing often are used. Fluid intake (0.5–2.0 L/day) is encouraged to loosen secretions and keep mucous membranes moist. Patients are positioned upright at a 30-degree angle to promote comfort and ensure optimal gas enchange. Confused patients should be observed frequently. Because confused patients may fall as they try to get to the bathroom, they should be assisted to the bathroom every 2 hours, especially if fluids are increased. Constant reassurance and reorientation are helpful.

RESPIRATORY ALKALOSIS

The most common cause of respiratory alkalosis is hyperventilation. Hyperventilation is another term for rapid or deep respirations, or both. Excessive amounts of carbon dioxide are lost through the lungs with a resulting decrease in $Paco_2$ levels and an increase in pH in the blood.

The major cause of hyperventilation leading to respiratory alkalosis is anxiety. Other causes are conditions that result in decreased oxygen in the blood such as pneumonia, anemia, severe blood loss due to trauma, and congestive heart failure. Fever, pain, drugs (aspirin overdose), head trauma, and gram-negative septicemia also may contribute to respiratory alkalosis.

ASSESSMENT. Clinical signs and symptoms include increased respiratory and heart rates, anxious appearance, irritability, dizziness, lightheadedness, muscle weakness, and numbness of the fingers. In extreme respiratory alkalosis, confusion, fainting, and seizures may occur. Assessment of the rate and depth of respirations is the key observation for this condition.

INTERVENTION. The major goal of therapy is to treat the underlying cause of the condition. In addition, sedation and constant reassurance are provided to relieve anxiety. Patients should be encouraged to breathe slowly to retain carbon dioxide in the body. Having patients breathe slowly into a paper bag helps them to rebreathe exhaled carbon dioxide. When breathing stabilizes, patients need time for uninterrupted rest because hyperventilation can result in fatigue.

METABOLIC ACIDOSIS

Metabolic acidosis occurs when the body retains too many hydrogen ions or loses too many HCO_3^- ions. With too many acids and too few bases, the pH of the blood rises. Metabolic acidosis leads to hyperventilation, because the lungs try to compensate by blowing off carbon dioxide and lowering $Paco_2$ levels.

Causes of metabolic acidosis are starvation, dehydration, diarrhea, shock, renal failure, and diabetic ketoacidosis. Signs and symptoms vary according to the underlying cause and the severity of the acid-base disturbance. However, patients may experience changing levels of consciousness, ranging from fatigue and confusion to stupor and coma, headache, vomiting and diarrhea, anorexia, muscle weakness, and cardiac dysrhythmias.

ASSESSMENT. Vital signs are important in the assessment because patients with metabolic acidosis may experience decreased blood pressure, abnormal heart rates, and rapid breathing. The temperature and appearance of the skin should be noted. With acidosis the skin is cold and clammy.

INTERVENTION. Acidosis is usually treated with intravenous infusion of sodium bicarbonate. Mechanical ventilation may be necessary, especially in patients who are comatose. Other interventions are geared toward treating underlying disorders such as ketoacidosis, diarrhea, drug toxicity, and acute renal failure. Nursing care is directed toward helping confused patients to be reassured and oriented. Abnormal breathing patterns may result in dry mouth, so that good mouth care is essential.

METABOLIC ALKALOSIS

Metabolic alkalosis is the opposite of metabolic acidosis. It results from an increase in HCO_3^- levels or a loss of hydrogen ions. Loss of hydrogen ions may be due to prolonged nasogastric suctioning, excessive vomiting, diuretics, and electrolyte disturbances. Retention of HCO_3^- may result from the administration of bicarbonate or massive blood transfusions. Common clinical signs and symptoms are headache; irritability; lethargy; changes in level of consciousness; confusion; changes in heart rate; slow, shallow respirations with periods of apnea; nausea and vomiting; hyperactive reflexes; and numbness of the extremities.

ASSESSMENT. Vital signs and daily weight measurements are essential for monitoring heart rate, respirations, and fluid gains and losses. Accurate intake and output records should be kept, including the amount of fluid removed by suction.

INTERVENTION. As with other acid-base imbalances, treatment depends on the underlying cause and severity of the condition. Nurses should monitor laboratory values, especially pH and serum HCO_3^-. Isotonic saline solutions rather than water should be used for irrigating nasogastric tubes because the use of water for irrigation can result in a loss of electrolytes. Reassurance and comfort measures should be provided to promote safety and well-being.

Mechanisms of respiratory and metabolic acidosis and alkalosis are found in Table 11–11.

TABLE 11-11
MECHANISMS OF RESPIRATORY AND METABOLIC ACIDOSIS AND ALKALOSIS

CONDITION	CAUSE	pH	H^+	HCO_3^-	$Paco_2$
Respiratory acidosis	Hypoventilation	↓	↑	↑	↑
Respiratory alkalosis	Hyperventilation	↑	↓	↓	↓
Metabolic acidosis	Diabetic ketoacidosis Lactic acidosis Diarrhea Renal insufficiency	↓	↑	↓	↑
Metabolic alkalosis	Vomiting HCO_3 retention Volume depletion K^+ depletion	↑	↓	↑	↓

BIBLIOGRAPHY

Bilezikian, J. (1992). Management of acute hypercalcemia. *New England Journal of Medicine, 326,* 1196–1203.

Horne, M., Easterday-Heitz, U., & Swearingen, P. (1991). *Fluid, electrolyte, and acid-base balance: A case study approach.* St. Louis: Mosby-Year Book.

Kuhn, M. M. (1991). Colloids vs crystalloids. *Critical Care Nurse, 11,* 37–51.

Levinsky, N. G. (1991). Acidosis and alkalosis. In J. D. Wilson, E. Braunwald, & K. J. Isselbacher (Eds.), *Harrison's principles of internal medicine* (12th ed., pp. 289–295). Philadelphia: W. B. Saunders.

Metheny, N. (1987). *Fluid and electrolyte balance: Nursing considerations.* Philadelphia: J. B. Lippincott.

Pagana, K. D., & Pagona, T. J. (1992). *Mosby's diagnostic and laboratory test reference.* St. Louis: Mosby-Year Book.

Thompson, J., McFarland, G. I., Hirsch, J. E., & Tucker, S. M. (1993). *Mosby's clinical nursing.* St. Louis: Mosby-Year Book.

KEY CONCEPTS

1. Approximately 50 to 60% of the human body is composed of water, and to maintain homeostasis, the body must be able to regulate the fluids within it.
2. The process of homeostasis involves delivery of nutrients such as oxygen and glucose to the cells and removal of wastes such as carbon dioxide from the cells.
3. Body fluids are divided into two portions: (1) intracellular fluid (fluid within the cell) and (2) extracellular fluid (fluid outside the cell). Most of the body's fluids are found within the cell.
4. Extracellular fluid is mainly responsible for transport of nutrients and wastes throughout the body.
5. Electrolytes, which are substances that develop an electrical charge when dissolved in water, maintain a balance between positive and negative charges to keep the body in homeostasis.
6. Overall fluid volume decreases in the elderly; however, the decline is found primarily in intracellular fluid compartments, not in the extracellular compartments.
7. The fluid compartments of the body are separated by selectively permeable membranes that permit movement of water and certain solutes.
8. Water is transported between intracellular and extracellular fluid compartments by one or more of the following processes: (1) diffusion, (2) active transport, (3) filtration, and (4) osmosis.
9. The kidneys are the primary regulators of fluid balance in the body, and the nephrons conduct the work of the kidney through the processes of filtration, reabsorption, and secretion.
10. Two hormones that have a major effect on fluid balance are aldosterone, released by the adrenal glands, and antidiuretic hormone, produced by the hypothalamus and secreted into the general circulation by the posterior pituitary gland.
11. An additional regulatory mechanism is thirst, which regulates fluid intake.
12. In a healthy adult, the 24-hour fluid intake and output are approximately equal.
13. The body attempts to compensate for fluid volume deficits by increasing the heart rate to pump more fluid to other parts of the body or to conserve water in the kidneys by increasing reabsorption and decreasing excretion of urine.
14. The body attempts to compensate for fluid volume excess by increasing the filtration and ex-

cretion of sodium and water by the kidneys and decreasing the production of antidiuretic hormone.

15. The kidneys are the primary regulators of electrolytes in the blood, and two electrolytes that cause the majority of problems when there is an imbalance are sodium (Na^+) and potassium (K^+).
16. Measurement of body weight is a good indicator of fluid loss or retention.
17. Edema reflects sodium retention, which can result from excessive reabsorption or inadequate secretion due to failing kidney function.
18. Older adults frequently have a reduced sense of thirst and therefore may be chronically poorly hydrated.
19. Acid-base balance is the homeostasis of the hydrogen ion (H^+) concentration in the body fluids.
20. Mechanisms that maintain acid-base balance are blood buffers, respiratory control of carbon dioxide, and renal regulation of bicarbonate (HCO_3^-).
21. If acid-base imbalances exist, there is an imbalance in the functioning of the lungs, kidneys, or both.
22. The four major types of acid-base imbalance are (1) respiratory acidosis, (2) respiratory alkalosis, (3) metabolic acidosis, and (4) metabolic alkalosis.

CHAPTER 12

Lea Ann Loftis
Mary Ann Matteson

Nutrition

OBJECTIVES

1. Discuss the role of the alimentary system in the digestion of food.
2. Discuss the digestion and absorption of food.
3. List the functions of each of the six classes of essential nutrients.
4. List the functions of proteins, carbohydrates, and fats.
5. List the food sources of proteins, carbohydrates, and fats.
6. List the food sources of dietary fiber.
7. List the possible health benefits of dietary fiber.
8. List the food sources of each of the vitamins and minerals.
9. Discuss the changes in nutrient needs as the individual ages.
10. Distinguish between anorexia nervosa and bulimia.
11. Discuss the different types of nutritional support.
12. Identify guidelines for the nutritional assessment.

GLOSSARY

AMINO ACIDS A group of 22 substances that can be bonded in different ways to make a variety of proteins. The body can manufacture sufficient amounts of these provided the nine essential amino acids are derived from the diet

BASAL METABOLIC RATE Measurement of energy expenditure taken in the morning after awakening and approximately 10 to 12 hours after the last meal

CALORIE Standard unit for measuring energy; the amount of heat needed to raise the temperature of 1 ml of water at a standard temperature by 1 degree centigrade

COMPLEMENTARY PROTEIN Combination of incomplete proteins that provide all nine essential amino acids when consumed together

COMPLETE PROTEIN Protein containing all nine essential amino acids; usually of animal origin (e.g., meat, eggs)

INCOMPLETE PROTEIN Plant protein lacking one or more essential amino acids

INSOLUBLE FIBER Indigestible roughage found in plant cells; aids in stool formation and elimination

LIPIDS Fats in solid or liquid form; store energy, carry fat-soluble vitamins, maintain healthy skin and hair; supply essential fatty acids and promote a feeling of fullness (satiety)

LIPOPROTEINS Lipid-wrapped proteins carried into the blood stream; includes high-density and low-density lipoproteins, which carry cholesterol

MINERALS Small amounts of metals (calcium, sodium and potassium) and nonmetals (chloride, phosphate) that are essential to the body; can build up

PROTEINS Large organic compounds made of various combinations of amino acids; found in meat, milk, fish, and eggs

RESTING METABOLIC RATE Measurement of energy expenditure taken at any time of the day and 3 to 4 hours after the last meal

SATURATED FATTY ACIDS Compounds that come chiefly from animal sources and are usually solid at room temperature; also coconut and palm oils

TRIGLYCERIDES Neutral fats found in plant and animal food sources

UNSATURATED FATTY ACIDS Compounds that come from plants or fish and are generally liquid at room temperature; can be monounsaturated (olive, peanut, canola, and avocado oils) or polyunsaturated (corn, safflower, and sesame oils)

VITAMINS Organic compounds supplied by food that the body requires for normal growth and development

Nutrition is the cornerstone of the healing process. To support and maintain life or fight disease the body must be supplied with the proper nutrients.

ANATOMY AND PHYSIOLOGY OF THE GASTROINTESTINAL SYSTEM

The gastrointestinal system (GI tract or "gut"), also known as the alimentary system, is used for receiving food, transporting food to the area where nutrients are absorbed, and transporting waste products out of the body. The mouth receives food and reduces it to particle size by chewing, as digestion begins. As the food is chewed, it is lubricated with saliva for passage through the esophagus. The mixture is then transported through the esophagus to the stomach. The stomach provides temporary storage for the mixture, and digestion continues. As the food is broken down in the stomach, it moves into the small intestine, where the secretions of the pancreas and liver are added to help further aid the digestive process. After movement through the small intestine, food moves into the large intestine and the rectum, where water, electrolytes, and some of the final products of digestion are absorbed. The large intestine, also known as the *colon*, and rectum provide temporary storage for waste products that serve as a medium for bacterial synthesis of some vitamins. The anus controls defecation.

DIGESTION AND ABSORPTION

Normally 92 to 97% of the mixed American diet is digested and absorbed. Most substances such as water, simple sugars, vitamins, minerals, and alcohol are absorbed in their original form. However, substances such as lipids, proteins, and complex sugars must be converted to simple forms before they are absorbed.

The digestion of food is made possible by hydrolysis, a process through which a complex molecule splits into smaller units by the addition of water. The process works under the direction of enzymes along with cofactors such as bile and hydrochloric acid. During the digestive process, enzymes help to break down food particles to their simplest form so that the nutrients can be absorbed by the body. Enzymes are secreted throughout the intestinal tract, except in the large intestine, because digestion and absorption already have been completed by the time the food mixture reaches the colon. Only water, salt, vitamins, and minerals are absorbed in the colon.

REGULATORS OF GASTROINTESTINAL ACTIVITY

Regulation of the gastrointestinal system requires two mechanisms: (1) neural control and (2) secretion of hormones. Neural control is accomplished through the enteric nervous system, which is located in the gut wall, and an external system of nerve fibers from the autonomic nervous system. The enteric nervous system consists of receptors in the gastric mucosa that are sensitive to the acidity of the gastrointestinal tract and the feeling of fullness.

Autonomic innervation is supplied by sympathetic nerve fibers that run along blood vessels and by parasympathetic fibers in the vagus nerve. The parasympathetic nerves generally stimulate digestive activity, whereas the sympathetic nerves inhibit activity. The vagus nerve stimulates acid secretion in the stomach in response to the sight or smell of food.

Hormones are secreted into the gastrointestinal tract to help regulate the process of digestion. They help to regulate gastric pH, gastric motility, and appetite, and they stimulate the pancreas to secrete insulin and enzymes.

DIGESTIVE PROCESS

Digestion of food occurs in three areas of the gastrointestinal system: (1) the mouth, (2) the stomach, and (3) the small intestine. When food is placed into the mouth, the teeth grind and crush the food into small particles. The food forms into a mass that is moistened and lubricated by saliva. While still in the mouth, a secretion containing an enzyme known as *ptyalin* begins to digest any starch that is present. The mass, or bolus, is then passed to the pharynx and through the esophagus by the process of swallowing. Peristalsis moves the food rapidly through the esophagus into the stomach.

In the stomach, the mass is mixed with gastric secretions. Active chemical digestion is accomplished by the secretion of gastric juice. The stomach produces an average of 2000 to 2500 ml of gastric juice daily. The juice contains hydrochloric acid, enzymes, mucus, and the gastrointestinal hormone gastrin. The juice aids in the digestive process by converting the mass to a semiliquid substance called *chyme*.

The stomach is normally emptied in 1 to 4 hours, depending on the amount and kinds of foods eaten. When eaten alone, carbohydrates leave the stomach most rapidly, followed by protein, and then by fat. However, in a mixed diet, emptying of the stomach is prolonged.

Valves (sphincters), located at the entrance (cardiac sphincter) and exit (pyloric sphincter) of the stomach, prevent the backflow of the food mass from the stomach into the pharynx and from the duodenum into the stomach. The valves can become stimulated during emotional upsets and go into spasm, causing excruciating pain.

The small intestine is divided into the duodenum, the jejunum, and the ileum. Most of the digestive process is completed in the duodenum, and the jejunum and ileum function mostly in the absorption of the nutrients.

Mechanisms of Absorption

The primary organ of absorption is the small intestine. It is 22 feet in length and is arranged in folds. The folds are covered with finger-like projections called *villi*. The villi absorb the nutrients into the blood and lymph vessels that support them. Each day the small intestine absorbs several hundred grams of carbohydrate, 100 grams or more of fat, 50 to 100 grams of amino acids, 50 to 100 grams of ions, and 7 to 8 liters of water.

Absorption is accomplished by the combination of the processes of diffusion and active transport. *Diffusion* involves the movement of particles from an area of higher concentration to an area of lower concentration. *Active transport* requires the input of energy for the movement of particles across a membrane against an energy gradient. This movement requires a carrier protein. The best-known carrier is the *intrinsic factor*, which is responsible for the absorption of vitamin B_{12}.

NUTRIENTS

Food contains many nutrients, including carbohydrates, proteins, lipids, vitamins, minerals, and fluids. Each of these nutrients is digested and absorbed differently.

Carbohydrates

Carbohydrate digestion, as discussed earlier, is begun in the mouth where the enzyme amylase is released. When carbohydrates reach the stomach, the activity of amylase is halted when it comes in contact with hydrochloric acid. If the carbohydrates remain in the stomach long enough, the hydrochloric acid reduces most of them to their simplest form. The stomach generally empties into the small intestine before this occurs so most of the digestion of carbohydrates occurs within the small intestine. In the small intestine, pancreatic amylase is released to continue digestion. After the carbohydrates have been broken down, they pass through the villi into the blood stream, where they are carried by the portal vein to the liver and absorbed. Some forms of carbohydrate, particularly fiber, cannot be digested by humans and are excreted unchanged in the feces.

Protein

Digestion of protein does not begin until it reaches the stomach. There proteins are split into smaller molecules. Most protein digestion occurs in the duodenum, not in the stomach. Almost all of the protein is absorbed by the time it reaches the end of the jejunum. Only 1% of ingested protein is found in the feces.

Fat

Digestion of fat also begins in the stomach. Gastric lipase, an enzyme, breaks down the triglycerides that make up fat into fatty acids and glycerol. The major portion of fat digestion takes place in the small intestine. The peristaltic action of the small intestine, along with bile that has been secreted by the liver, breaks down the larger fat globules into smaller particles.

Fluids, Vitamins, and Minerals

Fluids, vitamins, and minerals are absorbed through the intestinal mucosa. Each day about 8 liters of fluid from the body pass back and forth across the membrane of the gut to keep the nutrients in solution. Vitamins and water pass unchanged from the small intestine into the blood by passive diffusion. Mineral absorption is a more active, complex process that takes place in several stages.

FACTORS AFFECTING DIGESTION

Factors that affect the digestion of food include psychological state, bacterial action, and food processing.

PSYCHOLOGICAL STATE. The look, smell, and taste of food have an impact on digestion as does the emotional climate surrounding eating. When humans see, smell, taste, and even think of food, secretions of saliva and stomach juices of the gastrointestinal tract increase. The emotions of fear, anger, and worry can cause the hypothalamus to stimulate the autonomic nervous system, which inhibits peristalsis, depresses the gastric secretions, and slows the movement of food through the gut.

BACTERIAL ACTION. The second factor that affects digestion of food is related to bacterial action in the gastrointestinal tract. The gut is made up of a complex community of bacteria that has about 100 different species. A healthy person frequently is not disturbed by these bacteria because they dwell in the gastrointestinal tract as normal flora. Very little bacterial action occurs in the stomach, because the hydrochloric acid acts as a germicidal agent. Bacterial action is most intense in the large intestine. Colonic bacteria contribute to the formation of gases, acids, and various toxic substances, many of which contribute to the odor of feces.

FOOD PROCESSING. The last factor that affects digestion is food processing. Cooked foods generally are more digestible than raw foods. The manner in which the food was cooked can also affect digestion. Frying foods at excessive temperatures retards the flow of digestive juices, whereas adding meat extracts stimulates digestion. Personal makeup or allergies may account for differences in the way various people react to certain foods, their preparation, and additives in the foods.

ENERGY

Energy is defined as the capacity to do work. In the context of nutrition, energy refers to the way in which the body makes use of the energy received through the food that is eaten.

ENERGY EXPENDITURE

To understand the concept of energy, it is important to examine energy expenditure. The largest portion of energy expenditure is during rest. When the body is at rest, energy is used in the mechanical activities needed to sustain life processes. Activities include respiration and circulation, maintenance of body temperature, and movement of ions across membranes.

Measurement by Metabolic Rate

Energy expenditure is measured by the *basal metabolic rate* (BMR) or the *resting metabolic rate* (RMR). The measures are carried out when the body is at complete physical and mental rest, relaxed but not asleep, several hours after any strenuous exercise or activity, and in a comfortable temperature and environment. Measurements of BMR and RMR are considered interchangeable and differ only in the time of day when the test is administered and the length of time elapsed since the last meal. The BMR is measured in the morning after the subject awakens and is in the postabsorptive state (10 to 12 hours after the last meal). The RMR may be measured at any time of day and 3 to 4 hours after the last meal. Factors that can cause the metabolic rate to vary among individuals include body size and composition, periods of growth, secretion of hormones, temperature, and menstrual cycle.

Body surface area is closely related to the metabolic rate and the maintenance of body temperature. The metabolic rate is affected significantly by the amount of heat lost to the atmosphere by evaporation from the skin, which is directly related to the body surface area. The metabolic rate is determined primarily by the extent of fat-free mass or lean body mass, which is measured most accurately by underwater weighing. Estimates of metabolic rate are based on body weight or body surface area. Sex and age do not significantly affect the estimate. The metabolic rate is highest during the periods of rapid growth, mostly during the first and second years, and reaches a lesser peak during adolescence.

The secretions of the endocrine glands, particularly thyroxine and norepinephrine, are the principal regulators of the metabolic rate. Disorders of the thyroid gland can affect the secretion of thyroxine and thus affect the BMR. Other hormones that have an effect on the BMR include cortisol, growth hormone, and insulin.

Other factors that affect the BMR are sleep, fever, environmental temperature, the menstrual cycle, and pregnancy. The BMR of a sleeping person is approximately 10% below the level of an awake and alert person as a result of muscle relaxation and decreased activity of the sympathetic nervous system. A fever can increase the BMR by 7% for each degree above 98.6° Fahrenheit. In addition, environmental temperature affects the BMR in response to the amount of an individual's exercise and sweating. The BMR rises and falls in response to the hormonal levels of the female body during the menstrual cycle and pregnancy.

As noted earlier, physical activity can affect the BMR. The expenditure of energy associated with exercise can vary considerably depending on body size and efficiency of a person's habits of motion. The level of fitness can indirectly affect the energy output. Physically fit people frequently have larger amounts of muscle mass, and the greater the muscle mass, the greater the increase in the BMR with exercise. Although students might disagree, it has been found that mental activity does not affect energy requirements appreciably.

Eating is another activity that can affect the BMR. Consumption of carbohydrates or fat increases the metabolic rate by about 5% of the total calories consumed. If the food intake consists solely of protein, the increase may be as much as 25%.

ENERGY MEASUREMENTS AND CALCULATIONS. The standard unit for measuring energy is the *calorie.* A calorie is the amount of heat energy required to raise the temperature of 1 ml of water at a standard initial temperature by 1°C. A kilocalorie (kcal), which is equal to 1000 calories, is the measurement used most often in nutritional guidelines. Most people refer to a kilocalorie as a calorie with a capital "c."

CARBOHYDRATES

DEFINITION AND COMPOSITION OF CARBOHYDRATES

Most of the energy needed to move, perform activities, and live is consumed in the form of carbohydrates. These are organic compounds that consist of carbon, hydrogen, and oxygen. Carbohydrates vary from simple to complex depending on the amount of carbon sugars they contain. All of the sugars and starches that people eat and most types of fibers are carbohydrates.

Plants manufacture and store carbohydrates as their chief source of energy. The plants gather carbon dioxide from the air and water from the soil, and with chlorophyll found inside the plant, they use the energy of sunlight to form glucose. When animals consume plants, the glucose furnishes the energy needed to live. Glucose is the main sugar in the blood and the body's basic fuel; it serves as the primary source of energy.

CLASSIFICATION AND FOOD SOURCES OF CARBOHYDRATES

There are two general types of carbohydrates: (1) simple and (2) complex. Simple carbohydrates are sugars that include glucose and fructose from fruit and vegetables, lactose from milk, and sucrose from cane or beet sugar. Complex carbohydrates are actually large chains of glucose molecules. They consist primarily of starches as well as cellulose or fiber that exists in all plant foods.

Carbohydrates are classified according to the number of simple sugars or saccharides: (1) monosaccharides, (2) disaccharides, (3) oligosaccharides, and (4) polysaccharides. *Monosaccharides* (one saccharide) are the simplest form of carbohydrate. Examples of monosaccharides are glucose, fructose, and galactose. Major food sources are fruits, vegetables, and honey. *Disaccharides* (two saccharides) contain two monosaccharide molecules, and *oligosaccharides* contain three to 10 monosaccharide molecules. Examples are sucrose, lactose, and maltose. They usually are found in sugars and maple or corn syrups (sucrose), milk (lactose), and malt products (maltose).

Polysaccharides have 10 to 10,000 or more molecules. They are usually insoluble (indigestible) and include fibers such as cellulose. Major food sources include stalks and leaves of vegetables, outer coverings of fruits and seeds, and beans. Some soluble (digestible) polysaccharides are starch and glycogen. Starch is found in grains and vegetables, and glycogen is in meat products and seafood. Table 12–1 shows the carbohydrate content of certain foods.

CARBOHYDRATE METABOLISM

Carbohydrates are converted primarily to glucose for immediate use by the body's cells. When too many carbohydrates are taken in, they are converted to glycogen and stored in the liver until they are needed. At that time, they are converted to glucose through a process called *glucogenesis.* The amount of glucose produced depends on how much the body needs for energy. Each gram of carbohydrate yields about four calories of energy.

The glucose level is maintained within normal limits through release of glucose from liver glycogen. Normal blood glucose levels are 70 to 100 mg per 100 ml. After a meal, the blood sugar level may rise to 120 to 130 mg per 100 ml but will return to normal within 2 to 3 hours. As the glucose in the blood is used by the cells

TABLE 12–1
CARBOHYDRATE CONTENT OF FOODS

SUGAR	CARBOHYDRATE (%)	STARCH	CARBOHYDRATE (%)
Concentrated Sweets		**Grain Products**	
Sugar: Cane, beet, powdered,	99.5	Starches: Corn, tapioca, arrowroot	86–88
brown, maple	90–96	Cereals (dry): Corn, wheat, oat, bran	68–85
Candies	70–95	Flour: Corn, wheat (sifted)	70–80
Honey (extracted)	82	Popcorn (popped)	77
Syrup: Table blends, molasses	55–75	Cookies: Plain, assorted	71
Jams, jellies, marmalades	70	Crackers, saltines	72
Carbonated, sweetened beverages	10–12	Cakes: Plain, without icing	56
Fruits		Bread: White, rye, whole wheat	48–52
Prunes, apricots, figs (cooked, unsweet)	12–31	Macaroni, spaghetti, noodles, rice (cooked)	23–30
Bananas, grapes, cherries, apples, pears	15–23	Cereals (cooked): Oat, wheat, grits	10–16
Fresh: Pineapples, grapefruits, oranges, apricots, strawberries	8–14	**Vegetables**	
		Boiled: Corn, white and sweet potatoes, lima, dried beans, peas	15–26
Milk		Beets, carrots, onions, tomatoes	5–7
Skim	6	Leafy: Lettuce, asparagus, cabbage, greens, spinach	3–4
Whole	5		

From Mahan, L. K., & Arlin, M. (1992). *Krause's food, nutrition & diet therapy* (8th ed., p. 42). Philadelphia: W. B. Saunders.

of the body, the glycogen in the liver is constantly converted to glucose to maintain a safe level in the blood. When sufficient glucose is not available, such as during long periods of fasting or prolonged exercise, amino acids are converted to glucose.

A number of hormones are involved in the regulation of blood glucose levels. They include insulin, glucagon, epinephrine, glucocorticoids, and growth hormone. These hormones and their actions are summarized in Table 12–2.

DIETARY FIBER

Fiber (or roughage) is a group of polysaccharides that act differently from other carbohydrates because they pass through the digestive tract without being completely broken down or absorbed. They are found only in plant foods and are resistant to human digestive enzymes. Their major role is to help form a soft, firm stool and to aid in the process of elimination.

There are two types of fiber: (1) insoluble and (2) soluble. *Insoluble fiber* acts like a sponge to absorb many times its weight in water, swelling up within the intestine. It helps to provide a full feeling long after eating. *Soluble fiber* helps to produce a softer stool but does less to help the passage of food. Instead, soluble fiber works chemically to prevent or reduce the absorption of certain substances in the blood stream.

TABLE 12-2

HORMONES INVOLVED WITH THE REGULATION OF BLOOD SUGAR

HORMONE	SITE OR PRODUCTION	EFFECTS
Insulin	Beta cells of the islets of Langerhans in the pancreas	Increases the rate of glucose utilization for oxidation, glycogenesis, and lipogenesis
Glucagon	Alpha cells in the islets of Langerhans in the pancreas	Raises the amount of sugar in the blood by increasing glycogenolysis and gluconeogenesis; it also stimulates the release of insulin from the pancreas
Epinephrine	Adrenal gland	Causes the breakdown of liver and muscle glycogen to yield blood glucose; also decreases the release of insulin from the pancreas
Glucocorticoids	Adrenal cortex	Stimulates gluconeogenesis, reduces glucose utilization, and increases the rate at which glycogen is converted into glucose
Growth hormone	Anterior pituitary gland	Increases amino acid uptake and protein synthesis by all cells, the uptake of glucose, and the mobilization of fat for energy

RECOMMENDED DIETARY ALLOWANCE

There is no recommended dietary allowance for carbohydrates. However, diets without at least 50 to 100 grams of carbohydrates per day are likely to lead to ketosis. *Ketosis* is a condition that causes an excessive breakdown of tissue protein, loss of sodium and other cations, and involuntary dehydration.

In addition, although many nutritionists speak about the need for fiber in the diet, no specific recommendations have been established for what amount should be consumed daily. Several groups have recommended that Americans should increase their intake of dietary fiber and that this increase should come from a wide variety of whole-grain products, fruits, vegetables, and legumes. Table 12–3 lists the dietary fiber content of foods.

Fiber intake should consist of equal amounts of soluble and insoluble fiber. The mean fiber intake for adults in the United States is estimated to be about 11 to 13 grams per day or about 6 grams per 1000 kcal.

LIPIDS

Butter, margarine, and salad dressing are all more than half fat. Fat is a vital part of the diet, but most Americans eat far too much of it. Technically, fats in the diet should actually be called lipids. *Lipids* are similar to carbohydrates and contain the same three elements: (1) carbon, (2) hydrogen, and (3) oxygen. Fat metabolism utilizes more oxygen and releases more energy than either carbohydrate or protein metabolism. The structure of lipids also allows them to be stored compactly with little or no water. Proteins and carbohydrates generally require more space for storing the same number of calories.

Lipids come in solid or liquid (oil) form. They are insoluble in water. Although carbohydrates are the body's main source of food energy, fats are the most concentrated source, supplying 9 calories per gram, whereas carbohydrates and protein supply only 4 calories per gram. The functions of lipids include (1) storing energy, (2) maintaining healthy skin and hair, (3) carrying fat-soluble vitamins, (4) supplying essential fatty acids, and (5) promoting satiety.

Triglycerides, also called neutral fats, are the most common fat found in foods of both animal and plant origin. Triglycerides consist of three fatty acids attached to a glycerol molecule. These fatty acids vary in length and in degree of saturation of hydrogen atoms, and it is these variations that determine the properties of different fats.

All fats are combinations of *saturated* and *unsaturated* fatty acids. Fats containing mainly saturated fatty acids are described as "highly saturated," whereas fats that are primarily polyunsaturated or monounsaturated are described as "highly unsaturated." Saturated fatty acids are loaded with all the hydrogen atoms they can carry. Fats that are largely saturated come chiefly from animal

TABLE 12-3
DIETARY FIBER CONTENT OF FOODS IN COMMONLY SERVED PORTIONS

FOOD GROUP	LOW AMOUNTS (<1 gm)	MODERATE AMOUNTS (1–4 gm)	HIGH AMOUNTS (4 gm+)
Breads (1 slice)	Bagel, white, French	Whole wheat, bran muffin (1)	
Cereals (1 oz)	Rice Krispies, Special K, Cornflakes	Wheaties, Shredded Wheat, Most, Honey Bran	Bran Chex, 40% Bran Flakes, Raisin Bran, Corn Bran, All-Bran, Bran Buds, 100% Bran
Pasta (1 cup)		Macaroni, spaghetti, whole-wheat spaghetti	Lima beans, dried peas, kidney beans, baked beans, navy beans
Rice (½ cup)	White	Brown	
Legumes (½ cup cooked)		Lentils	
Vegetables (½ cup cooked unless stated)	Cucumber, lettuce (1 cup), green pepper	Asparagus, green beans, cabbage, cauliflower, potato (w/o skin, 1), celery, broccoli, Brussels sprouts, carrots, corn, potato (w/skin, 1), spinach, peas	
Fruits (1 medium fruit unless stated)	Grapes (20), watermelon (1 cup)	Apricots (3), grapefruit (½), peach w/skin, pineapple (½ cup), apple w/o skin, banana, orange, apple w/ skin, pear w/skin, raspberries (½ cup)	

Adapted with permission from Slavin, J. L. (1987). Dietary fiber: Classification, chemical analyses, and food sources. *Journal of the American Dietetic Association, 87,* 1164. Copyright The American Dietetic Association.

sources and include butter, milk fat, and the fat in meats; two vegetable oils—coconut and palm oils—also are highly saturated. Highly saturated fats are usually solid at room temperature and keep well.

Unsaturated fatty acids do not have all the hydrogen atoms they can carry. Depending on the number of missing hydrogen atoms, these fatty acids are called either monounsaturated (olive, peanut, canola, and avocado oils are largely monounsaturated) or polyunsaturated (corn, safflower, and sesame oils). The important dietary unsaturated fats come from plants and fish. They are generally liquid at room temperature and may become rancid quickly because the absence of hydrogen makes the carbon atoms very reactive.

LIPID TRANSPORT AND STORAGE

Most of the lipids taken into the body are absorbed from the intestinal mucosa into the lymphatic system. Energy reserves of lipids are stored in adipose tissue (fat). Most human adipose cells are in the form of white fat, which accumulates in subcutaneous tissue (50%), around the internal organs in the abdominal cavity (45%), and in the intramuscular tissue (5%). These fat cells can store up to 95% of their volume as triglycerides.

Brown fat is much less abundant and is located primarily in the interscapular region and on the back of the neck. The amount of this fat is higher in the neonate and decreases with age, but it can increase with extended exposure to cold.

LIPID METABOLISM

Lipids are a major source of energy for muscle tissue, even when glucose is available. Most lipids are carried to the liver where they can be converted to energy or used in the synthesis of new triglycerides. The liver is a major center of lipid metabolism and is largely responsible for the regulation of lipid levels in the body.

For fat to be digested, it must be emulsified, or pulled into suspension with digestive juices. Bile, a secretion of the liver, is necessary to emulsify fat. Bile is stored in the gallbladder and dispensed into the duodenum when fat is present. Once emulsified, fats can be broken down and absorbed. Fat may be used for various functions mentioned previously or may be used for energy. Excess dietary fat is stored as adipose tissue.

After absorption, lipids are carried in the blood stream in packages called *lipoproteins.* Simply stated, lipoproteins are lipids wrapped in protein. Types of lipoproteins include chylomicrons, high-density lipoproteins (HDL), low-density lipoproteins (LDL), and very low density lipoproteins (VLDL). Of particular interest in cardiovascular disease are the HDLs and the LDLs. Both lipoproteins carry cholesterol in the blood stream; however, it appears that the cholesterol found in the LDLs increases the risk of atherosclerosis by contributing to plaque buildup on the artery walls. In contrast, HDL cholesterol seems to have the opposite effect. It appears that the HDLs carry cholesterol from the blood stream to the liver to be degraded and excreted. The LDLs are sometimes referred to as carrying the "bad" cholesterol, whereas the HDLs carry the "good" cholesterol.

RECOMMENDED DIETARY ALLOWANCE

Most nutritionists are recommending that people limit their fat intake to 30% or below of their daily caloric intake. People also should try to eat unsaturated fats rather than saturated fats to minimize the risk of heart disease. There has been a trend in the United States to limit fat in the diet, particularly saturated fat.

FOOD SOURCES OF FAT

Animal products are the major source of saturated fats in the American diet. They include beef, dairy products, and eggs. Interestingly, many manufacturers are making fat-free products such as nonfat milk, cheese, and ice cream. In addition, cattle and pigs are being bred to yield beef and pork lower in saturated fat. Sources of unsaturated fats are vegetable oils, including corn oil, cottonseed oil, and safflower oil. Fruits, vegetables, and cereal grains are relatively low in fat. Refer to Table 12–4 for more sources of dietary fat.

TABLE 12-4

FAT CONTENT OF SOME COMMON FOODS

Food
0 Grams of Fat
Most fruits and vegetables
Nonfat milk
Nonfat yogurt
Plain pasta and rice
Angel food cake
Popcorn, air-popped, unbuttered
Soft drinks
Jam, jelly
1–3 Grams of Fat
Popcorn, oil-popped, unbuttered, 1 cup
Low-calorie salad dressing, 1 T
Baked beans, ½ cup
Soup, chicken noodle, canned, 1 cup
Whole wheat bread, 1 slice
Dinner roll, 1
Waffle, frozen, 4 inch, 1
Coleslaw, ½ cup
Flounder or sole, baked, 3 oz
Chicken, without skin, roasted, 3 oz
Tuna, canned in water, 3 oz
Cheese, cottage, 2% fat, ½ cup
Ice milk, soft serve, ½ cup
4–6 Grams of Fat
Low-fat yogurt, 1 cup
Cheese, mozarella, part-skim, 1 oz
Chicken, roasted with skin, 3 oz
Egg, scrambled, 1
Turkey, roasted, 3 oz
Granola, 1 oz
Muffin, bran, 1 small
Pizza, cheese, ¼ of 12-inch pie
Burrito, bean, 1
Brownie, with nuts, 1 small
Margarine or butter, 1 tsp
Popcorn, oil popped, buttered, 1 cup
French dressing, regular, 1 T
7–10 Grams of Fat
Cheese, cheddar, 1 oz
Milk, whole, 1 cup
Bologna, beef, 1 slice
Sausage, 1 patty
Steak, sirloin, broiled, 3 oz
Potatoes, French fried, 10
Chow mein, chicken, 1 cup
Chocolate candy bar, 1 oz
Corn chips, 1 oz
Doughnut, cake type, plain, 1
Mayonnaise, 1 T
15 Grams of Fat
Hot dog, beef, 2 oz
McDonald's Chicken McNuggets, 6 pieces
Peanut butter, 2 T
Pork chop, broiled, 3 oz
Sunflower seeds, dry roasted, ¼ cup
Avocado, ½ medium
Chop suey, beef and pork, 1 cup
Cinnamon roll, 1
20 Grams of Fat
Cheesecake, 1/12 cake
Lasagna with meat, 1 medium piece
Macaroni with cheese, homemade, 1 cup
Peanuts, dry roasted, ¼ cup
Ground beef, broiled, 3 oz
25+ Grams of Fat
Polish sausage, 3 oz
Cheeseburger, large
Pie, pecan, ⅛ 9-inch pie
Chicken pot pie, frozen, baked, 1 pie
Quiche, bacon, ⅛ pie

T, Tablespoon.

Data from Healthy Dividends, Rosemont, IL, National Dairy Council, 1990. From Mahan, K. L., & Arlin, M. (1992). *Krause's food, nutrition & diet therapy* (8th ed., p. 53). Philadelphia: W. B. Saunders.

PROTEINS

DEFINITION AND COMPOSITION OF PROTEINS

The word *protein* is derived from a Greek root meaning "of first importance," and protein—which constitutes about one fifth of an adult's body weight—is the basic material of life. Proteins also contain carbon, hydrogen, and oxygen. They are unique because they also contain about 16% nitrogen, along with sulfur and sometimes other elements such as phosphorus, iron, and cobalt. Just as "energy balance" is measured by weight gain or weight loss, protein "balance" is most accurately measured by nitrogen.

Protein is not a single, simple substance but a multitude of chemical combinations. The basic structure of protein is actually a chain of *amino acids* that can form many different configurations and can combine with other substances. The possible arrangements can be almost infinite, and tens of thousands of different proteins have been identified.

Food proteins can be classified as either complete or incomplete. A *complete protein* contains all nine essential amino acids in sufficient quantity and ratio for the body's needs. Complete proteins are generally of animal origin and are found in foods such as meat, poultry, fish, milk, cheese, and eggs.

Incomplete proteins are lacking in one or more of the essential amino acids. Incomplete proteins are of plant origin. This includes the protein in grains, legumes, nuts, and seeds. For the body to use protein for functions other than energy, all nine essential amino acids must be present at the same time. When various incomplete proteins are consumed at the same time, the body can use them together to obtain a balance of the essential amino acids. Incomplete proteins consumed together are called *complementary proteins*.

Amino Acids

There are 22 common amino acids, and they can be bonded in a variety of ways to form different proteins. The body uses all 22 amino acids, but only nine of them are considered essential amino acids. The nine essential amino acids must be obtained from the diet. The body can manufacture adequate amounts of the other amino acids from the essential amino acids.

PROTEIN METABOLISM

When food containing protein is eaten, the small intestine breaks down the protein to the constituent amino acids. The acids then travel through the blood to the cells where they are synthesized into tissue protein. It is important to note that if one or more of the essential amino acids is in short supply or not available at all, nonessential amino acids that may be on hand cannot be used to form a protein. That is why it is important to eat a diet that contains all of the essential amino acids, plus enough additional amino acids to allow for synthesis of the nonessential amino acids.

PROTEIN DEFICIENCY

The body cannot store protein, so it needs to be eaten in the diet each day. Low protein intakes can be tolerated by both children and adults up to a point, depending on the quality of the protein ingested and the level of energy intake. Nitrogen in the urine is a good indicator of protein levels in the body. Low levels of nitrogen indicate that the body is attempting to compensate for the lack of protein. But there is a critical point at which the body can no longer adapt, and the signs of protein deficiency become evident. These signs include edema, wasting of body tissues, fatty liver, dermatosis, diminished immune response, weakness, and loss of vigor.

EVALUATION OF PROTEIN QUALITY

Protein deficiency is not a problem in the healthy American population. The average person eating a normal balanced diet consumes about 100 grams of protein per day, nearly twice as much as the recommended daily allowance. Children under the age of 18 need some additional protein to allow for growth, and the younger they are, the more protein they need per pound of body weight. Preschoolers and adolescent males tend to have intakes close to twice the recommended daily allowance.

The protein content, by weight, of cooked meat, fish, poultry, and milk solids is between 15 and 40%. The protein content of cooked cereals, beans, and lentils ranges from 3 to 10%. Ingesting a diet high in animal protein is not necessary and may be too high in fat. Most people tend to eat a mixture of foods in a meal, and when available in sufficient quantity, the various proteins tend to complement or supplement each other by providing a total mixture containing all of the essential amino acids.

More total protein is required in a vegetable protein diet than in a diet of mixed vegetable and animal proteins because more of the lower-quality protein is needed to meet the minimum requirements for amino acids and nitrogen. Because of their lower digestibility values, vegetable proteins are less available. Table 12–5 gives the protein content of typical foods in the American diet.

TABLE 12–5
PROTEIN CONTENT OF SOME FOODS

0–1 gram
Butter, margarine, 1 tsp
Pear, 1 medium
Cake, 1 piece
2–3 grams
Milk chocolate, 1 oz
Cereal, refined, 1 oz
Bread, 1 slice
Corn, canned, ½ cup
Chicken noodle soup, 1 cup
French fries, 1 regular serving
4–6 grams
Cereal, bran, 1 oz
Baked potato, 1 large
Peas, ½ cup
7–8 grams
Navy beans, cooked, ½ cup
Egg, 1 medium
Cheese, 1 oz
Tuna, 1 oz
Tofu, 3½ oz
Milk, 1 cup
9–10 grams
Peanuts, roasted, 1 oz
Macaroni and cheese, ¾ cup
Pizza, cheese, ⅛ of a 12-inch pie
12–15 grams
Taco, 1
Hamburger, 1
Chili with meat, 1 cup
22–26 grams
Meat, lean, 3 oz
Big Mac, 1

From Mahan, K. L., & Arlin, M. (1992). *Krause's food, nutrition & diet therapy* (8th ed., p. 67). Philadelphia: W. B. Saunders.

VITAMINS

Vitamins are organic compounds that the body requires for normal growth and development. They help regulate metabolic functions within cells; however, only tiny amounts are needed to carry out these functions. The body cannot manufacture vitamins, so they are mainly supplied in the diet. Vitamins are usually designated by letters and are classified into two groups on the basis of solubility: (1) fat-soluble vitamins, or those that can be dissolved in fat, and (2) water-soluble vitamins, or those that can be dissolved in water.

FAT-SOLUBLE VITAMINS

Fat-soluble vitamins include vitamins A, D, E, and K. Because they are fat soluble, they are usually absorbed in the body with other lipids. Like lipids, fat-soluble vitamins need bile and pancreatic juices for absorption. After entering the body, fat-soluble vitamins attach to lipoproteins and are transported to the liver. If the amount of a vitamin taken in exceeds that which is needed, the extra amount is stored in the fat cells of the body. As stores build up serious problems can develop. Therefore, it is recommended that people *not* take excessive amounts of these vitamins.

WATER-SOLUBLE VITAMINS

Water-soluble vitamins include the B complex group (thiamine, riboflavin, niacin, B_6, folate, B_{12}, pantothenic acid, and biotin) and vitamin C (ascorbic acid). Excessive amounts of these vitamins are not as toxic as those of fat-soluble vitamins because water-soluble vitamins are readily excreted from the body and do not build up to such dangerous levels. If taken in very large doses, some can have "bad" effects, but such doses are unlikely when food is the major source of these vitamins.

Most of the water-soluble vitamins are components of essential enzyme systems. Many are involved in the reactions that support energy metabolism. They have an essential role in the metabolic processes of living cells, both plant and animal. Table 12–6 gives more information about the sources and functions of vitamins.

MINERALS

Minerals, like vitamins, are needed in small amounts for good health. Like vitamins, they play many roles in the body. As in the case of the fat-soluble vitamins, the body may not be able to rid itself of a high dose, so minerals can build up in the body and cause serious problems.

Minerals occur in the body and in food chiefly in their ionic form. Metals such as sodium, potassium, and calcium form *positive ions* (cations); nonmetals such as chloride, phosphate, and sulfate form *negative ions* (anions). Minerals represent about 4 to 5% of body weight. About half is made up of calcium, and another quarter is phosphorus. The remaining 25% is made up of all the other minerals. Food sources and functions of each of the minerals are presented in Table 12–7.

WATER

Water is the largest component of the body and body tissues and is essential to all life processes in the body.

TABLE 12–6
SUMMARY OF INFORMATION ON VITAMINS

NAME	SOURCES	COMMENTS
Fat-Soluble Vitamins		
Vitamin A	Liver, kidney, milk fat, fortified margarine, egg yolk, yellow and dark leafy vegetables, apricots, cantaloupe, peaches	Essential for normal growth, development, and maintenance of epithelial tissue. Essential to the integrity of night vision. Helps provide for normal bone development and influences normal tooth formation. Toxic in large quantities.
Vitamin D	Vitamin D milk, irradiated foods, some in milk fat, liver, egg yolk, salmon, tuna fish, sardines	Essential for normal growth and development; important for formation of normal bones and teeth. Influences absorption and metabolism of phosphorus and calcium. Toxic in large quantities.
Vitamin E	Wheat germ, vegetable oils, green leafy vegetables, milk fat, egg yolk, nuts	Is a strong antioxidant. May help prevent oxidation of unsaturated fatty acids and vitamin A in intestinal tract and body tissues. Protects red blood cells from hemolysis.
Vitamin K	Liver, soybean oil, other vegetable oils, green leafy vegetables, wheat bran. Synthesized in intestinal tract.	Aids in production of prothrombin, a compound required for normal clotting of blood. Toxic in large amounts.
Water-Soluble Vitamins		
Thiamine	Pork, liver, organ meats, legumes, whole-grain and enriched cereals and breads, wheat germ, potatoes. Synthesized in intestinal tract.	Aids in removal of CO_2 from alpha-keto acids during oxidation of carbohydrates. Essential for growth, normal appetite, digestion, and healthy nerves.
Riboflavin	Milk and dairy foods, organ meats, green leafy vegetables, enriched cereals and breads, eggs	Essential for growth. Plays enzymatic role in tissue respiration and acts as a transporter of hydrogen atoms.
Niacin	Fish, liver, meat, poultry, many grains, eggs, peanuts, milk, legumes, enriched grains. Synthesized by intestinal bacteria.	Aids in transfer of hydrogen and acts in metabolism of carbohydrates and amino acids. Involved in glycolysis, fat synthesis, and tissue respiration.
Vitamin B_6	Pork, glandular meats, cereal bran and germ, milk, egg yolk, oatmeal, and legumes. Synthesized by intestinal bacteria.	Aids in the synthesis and breakdown of amino acids and in the synthesis of unsaturated fatty acids from essential fatty acids. Essential for normal growth.
Folate	Green leafy vegetables, organ meats (liver), lean beef, wheat, eggs, fish, dry beans, lentils, cowpeas, asparagus, broccoli, collards, yeast. Synthesized in intestinal tract.	Essential for normal maturation of red blood cells.
Vitamin B_{12}	Liver, kidney, milk and dairy foods, meat, eggs. Vegans require supplement.	Role in metabolism of nervous tissue. Involved with folate metabolism. Related to growth.
Vitamin C (ascorbic acid)	Acerola (West Indian cherry-like fruit), citrus fruit, tomato, melon, peppers, greens, raw cabbage, guava, strawberries, pineapple, potato	Important in immune responses, wound healing, and allergic reactions. Increases absorption of iron.

Adapted from Mahan, L. K., & Arlin, M. (1992). *Krause's food, nutrition & diet therapy* (8th ed., pp. 105–106). Philadelphia: W. B. Saunders.

TABLE 12-7
MINERALS IN HUMAN NUTRITION

MINERAL	LOCATION IN BODY AND SOME BIOLOGIC FUNCTIONS	FOOD SOURCES
Calcium	99% in bones and teeth. Ionic calcium in body fluids essential for ion transport across cell membranes.	Milk and milk products, sardines, clams, oysters, kale, turnip greens, mustard greens, tofu
Phosphorus	About 80% in inorganic portion of bones and teeth. Phosphorus is a component of every cell and of highly important metabolites, including DNA, RNA, ATP (high energy compound), and phospholipids. Important to pH regulation.	Cheese, egg yolk, milk, meat, fish, poultry, whole-grain cereals, legumes, nuts
Magnesium	About 50% in bone. Remaining 50% is almost entirely inside body cells with only about 1% in extracellular fluid. Ionic Mg functions as an activator of many enzymes and thus influences almost all processes.	Whole-grain cereals, tofu, nuts, meat, milk, green vegetables, legumes, chocolate
Sodium	30 to 45% in bone. Major cation of extracellular fluid, and only a small amount is inside cell. Regulates body fluid osmolarity, pH, and body fluid volume.	Common table salt, seafoods, animal foods, milk, eggs. Abundant in most foods except fruit.
Chloride	Major anion of extracellular fluid, functioning in combination with sodium. Serves as a buffer, enzyme activator; component of gastric hydrochloric acid. Mostly present in extracellular fluid; less than 15% inside cells.	Common table salt, seafoods, milk, meat, eggs
Potassium	Major cation of intracellular fluid, with only small amounts in extracellular fluid. Functions in regulating pH and osmolarity and cell membrane transfer. Iron is necessary for carbohydrate and protein metabolism.	Fruits, milk, meat, cereals, vegetables, legumes
Sulfur	Bulk of dietary sulfur is present in sulfur-containing amino acids needed for synthesis of essential metabolites.	Protein foods such as meat, fish, poultry, eggs, milk, cheese, legumes, nuts
Iron	About 70% is in hemoglobin; about 26% stored in liver, spleen, and bone. Iron is a component of hemoglobin important in oxygen transfer.	Liver, meat, egg yolk, legumes, whole or enriched grains, dark green vegetables, dark molasses, shrimp, oysters
Zinc	Present in most tissues, with higher amounts in liver, voluntary muscle, and bone. Constituent of many enzymes and insulin.	Oysters, shellfish, herring, liver, legumes, milk, wheat bran
Copper	Found in all body tissues; larger amounts in liver, brain, heart, and kidney	Liver, shellfish, whole grains, cherries, legumes, kidney, poultry, oysters, chocolate, nuts
Iodine	Constituent of throxine and related compounds synthesized by thyroid gland. Thyroxine functions in control of reactions involving cellular energy.	Iodized table salt, seafoods, water, and vegetables in nongoiterous regions
Manganese	Highest concentration is in bone; also relatively high concentrations in pituitary, liver, pancreas, and gastrointestinal tissue.	Beet greens, blueberries, whole grains, nuts, legumes, fruit, tea
Fluoride	Present in bone and teeth. In optimal amounts in water and diet; reduces dental caries, and may minimize bone loss.	Drinking water (1 ppm), tea, coffee, rice, soybeans, spinach, gelatin, onions, lettuce

Adapted from Mahan, L. K., & Arlin, M. (1992). *Krause's food, nutrition & diet therapy* (8th ed., pp. 137–138). Philadelphia: W. B. Saunders.

It provides form and structure to cells and tissues; is essential to the digestion, absorption, and excretion of metabolic and indigestible wastes; is a transport medium for nutrients and all body substances; maintains physical and chemical constancy of intracellular and extracellular fluids; and regulates body temperature through the process of evaporation of perspiration.

The intake of water is controlled by thirst. The sensation of thirst serves as a signal to seek fluids. Water is also ingested through food. The breakdown of food in the body produces water as an end product. Water is lost from the body through the kidneys as urine, through the intestines as part of feces, through the lungs with air expired, and through the skin as evaporated sweat. When an imbalance of the amount of water taken in versus the amount of water lost occurs, various organs in the body, especially the kidneys, compensate by conserving more water and excreting less. The amount of water taken in daily should be equivalent to the amount of water lost.

There is no way the body can store water. It is essential that all living things replenish water daily to maintain health and efficiency. The longest period of time that people can go without water and sustain life is 4 days. Adults generally should take in about 2500 ml, or 2 to 3 quarts, of water per day.

AGE-RELATED CHANGES

Healthy eating is a lifelong commitment that pays particular benefits in the later years of life. Maintaining

TABLE 12-8
NUTRITION-RELATED SYSTEM CHANGES IN THE OLDER ADULT

SYSTEM	CHANGES SEEN
Sensory	Senses of taste, smell, sight, hearing, and touch are diminished; there is a decreased number of taste buds, decreased sensitivity to sweet and salty tastes; may experience glossodynia (pain in the tongue), decreased olfactory sense.
Gastrointestinal	Changes in appetite response contribute to anorexia; ill-fitting dentures and periodontal disease make eating painful; decreased salivary secretion, which decreases the ability to masticate and swallow foods; decreased acid secretion causes an overgrowth of the bacteria of the gut; lack of the intrinsic factor, which leads to decreased absorption of vitamin B_{12}; increased incidence of gallbladder disease; decreased mobility of the intestines leads to constipation.
Metabolic	Decreased tolerance to glucose leads to an increase in plasma glucose levels; basal metabolic rate decreases by 20% due to decrease in lean body mass.
Cardiovascular	Blood vessels become less elastic; total peripheral resistance increases; there is an increased risk for hypertension.
Renal	Kidney function diminishes; acid-base response to metabolic challenges is slowed; there is increased difficulty in handling excessive amounts of protein waste products.
Musculoskeletal	Progressive replacement of lean body mass by fat and connective tissue; body protein decreased by 30–40%; more fat is deposited on the trunk and around visceral organs; bone density is diminished, and there is shortening of the spinal column.
Immunocompetence	The immune function declines with age; there is a diminished ability to fight infection.
Psychosocial	Many experience depression as a result of a sense of loss—loss of loved ones, productivity, a sense of worth, mobility, income, and body image.

a good diet can help middle-aged and older people to maintain a high level of function and reduce the risks of chronic disease. There are many functional changes that naturally occur in humans as they age. Table 12–8 summarizes these changes in terms of the effects on the nutritional status of the older adult.

Energy

Because of the normal decline in metabolism and physical activity, energy needs are lower with age. This leads to a reduction in the amount of kcal taken in per day. The recommended daily allowance in 1989 included a reduction of 600 kcal per day for older men and 300 kcal per day for older women. However, according to recent research findings, lifestyle and health status of older adults vary widely, and these figures may need adjustments for each individual. Nutrients previously discussed in this chapter, including proteins, carbohydrates, lipids, vitamins, minerals, and water may need adjustment as people age (Table 12–9).

TABLE 12-9
CHANGES IN THE NUTRITIONAL REQUIREMENTS FOR THE OLDER ADULT

NUTRIENT	CHANGES IN NEEDS	SPECIAL PROBLEMS
Protein	Experience a decreased need unless ill	Protein-calorie undernutrition may be a special problem for older males who live alone
Carbohydrate	Reduced glucose tolerance, diminished lactose secretion	Insulin sensitivity, lactose intolerance
Lipid	Remains at not more than 30% of the total kcal	Serum cholesterol levels in men tend to peak during middle age and then drop slightly; levels in women continue to rise with increasing age
Minerals	The need for trace elements is reduced owing to decreased lean body mass; continued calcium intake of 800 mg/day for women 51 years of age and over	Hypertension is common, which results in the need to decrease sodium and increase potassium and magnesium for those taking diuretics
Vitamins	Vitamin A is not insufficient in the older adult owing to stores in the liver; vitamin D may be low owing to lack of exposure to sunlight and may require supplement; vitamin C may be low in the older adult; vitamin B_6 and folacin are maintained with diet; vitamin B_{12} may be a problem owing to loss of the intrinsic factor	A maintenance level multivitamin and mineral supplement may be required; must be monitored closely for overdose
Water	30 to 35 ml/kg of ideal body weight	Dehydration is the most common cause of fluid and electrolyte disturbance; must be monitored closely

Nutritional Care of the Older Adult

DIETARY PLANNING. Dietary planning for the older adult is no different from planning for a younger adult. Meals need to be appealing, taking into consideration individual likes and dislikes, and should be tasteful and filling. Planning may be different for older adults with special needs. Many may prefer four to five small meals over three large ones. In addition, problems such as difficulty swallowing, dentures that do not fit properly, and arthritis, which makes using utensils uncomfortable, must be considered.

The diet should include all of the food groups. Counseling the older adult about substitutions for any of the food groups is important to ensure adequacy of nutrients.

NUTRITION PROGRAMS. Many community-based programs for the older adult, administered by both public and private agencies, provide hot, nutritious meals to older adults. The meals are served either in a group setting or in the home. Special regulations and conditions must be met to qualify for these programs.

NUTRITIONAL NEEDS DURING PROLONGED ILLNESS. All people have increased nutritional needs during periods of illness. Older adults with chronic diseases such as emphysema and bronchitis, cancer, organic brain disease, cirrhosis, and maldigestion or malabsorption syndromes have an increased risk for protein deficiency and negative nitrogen balance. Individuals at risk need to be watched very carefully for this condition, which can be prevented by increasing nutritional support. Nasogastric tube feedings or parenteral nutrition may be required to meet these increased needs.

NUTRITIONAL CARE IN INSTITUTIONAL SETTINGS. Older adults in institutional settings such as nursing homes may have special nutritional needs. These needs may change over a period of time, depending on the aging process, chronic and acute disease, use of medication, and emotional and mental state. Periodic reassessment of nutritional status is critical to avoid imposing unnecessary diet restrictions or missing important nutritional needs.

GUIDELINES FOR DIETARY PLANNING

THE FOOD GUIDE PYRAMID

A number of guidelines have been established in the United States to help in planning for optimal nutrition. Until July 1992, the basic four food groups were considered the standard food guide. At that time, the U.S. Department of Agriculture established the food guide pyramid. The food guide pyramid expanded the basic four food groups of milk, meat, fruits and vegetables, and grains and added a fats, oils, and sweets group. This pyramid shows the ideal natural grouping for the way the American public should eat (Fig. 12–1).

RECOMMENDED DAILY ALLOWANCE

Recommended daily allowances are guidelines for the amounts of nutrients that healthy people should consume daily. Nutrient requirements vary among individuals, so that these recommended amounts tend to be high.

Food Labeling

With the increase in public awareness of health and nutrition, people have expressed an increased need to be informed about what they are eating. Many more foods are now labeled so the average person can make determinations about the quality and quantity of the nutrients they are consuming. Because of the lack of space available on a package label, the table is abbreviated to include essential information to describe the number of nutrients per serving (Fig. 12–2).

NATIONAL GUIDELINES FOR DIET PLANNING

Also because of the increased public awareness of the importance of health and good nutrition, much research has been done on the connection between nutrition and disease. As a result, many current guidelines are available concerning proper nutrition to maintain health and prevent disease. The task of planning a proper diet that includes recommendations from the various guidelines is sometimes a difficult one. Table 12–10 presents a composite of the dietary guidelines from the Surgeon General's Report on Nutrition and Health (1988) that can be used as a basis for dietary planning.

NURSING ASSESSMENT OF NUTRITIONAL STATUS

The first step in determining the nutritional status of any person is assessment. The areas covered in a nutritional assessment include appearance, diet history, food intake, height and weight measurements, and body composition.

Observation of physical appearance includes looking for signs of malnutrition, obesity, and other factors that may indicate nutritional deficits. Things to look for are shiny and healthy looking hair, bright and clear eyes, a face with smooth skin and good color, smooth lips and tongue, and healthy teeth and gums. People who are malnourished may have dull, thin, and sparse hair, pale conjunctiva around the eyes, a swollen or pale face, swollen lips and tongue, teeth with cavities or missing teeth, and bleeding or receding gums.

The diet history includes areas that influence nutritional intake, such as economic situation, physical activity, ethnic or cultural background, appetite, and medications. Table 12–11 highlights information to obtain when taking a dietary history.

FOOD GUIDE PYRAMID

A Guide to Daily Food Choices

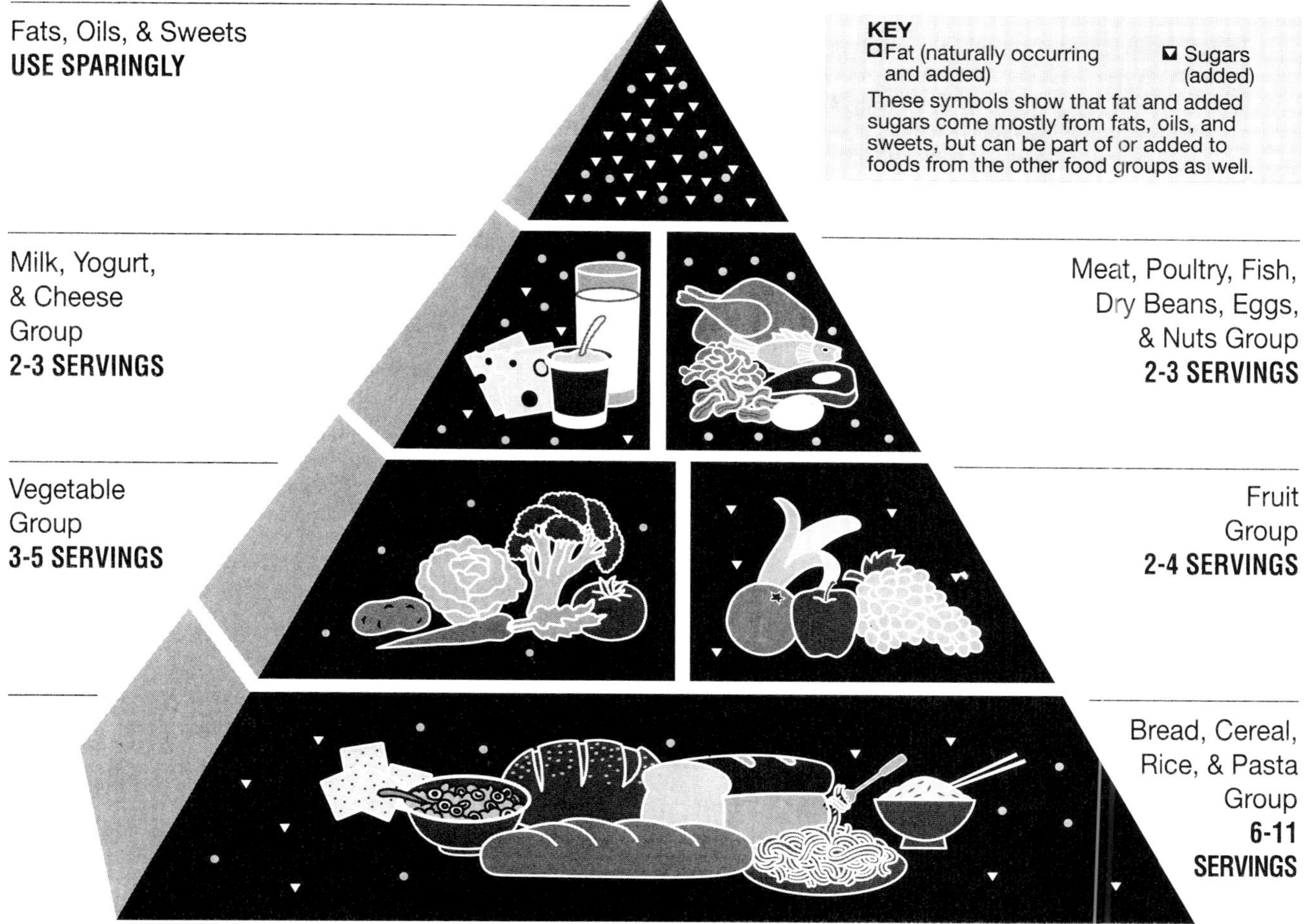

The amount of food that counts as 1 serving is listed below. If you eat a larger portion, count it as more than 1 serving. For example, a dinner portion of spaghetti would count as 2 or 3 servings of pasta.

Be sure to eat at least the lowest number of servings from the five major food groups listed below. You need them for the vitamins, minerals, carbohydrates, and protein they provide. Try to pick the lowest fat choices from the food groups. No specific serving size is given for the fats, oils, and sweets group because they should be used SPARINGLY.

Vegetable

1 cup of raw leafy vegetables	1/2 cup of other vegetables, cooked or chopped raw	3/4 cup of vegetable juice

Milk, Yogurt, and Cheese

1 cup of milk or yogurt	1½ ounces of natural cheese	2 ounces of process cheese

Fruit

1 medium apple, banana, orange	1/2 cup of chopped, cooked, or canned fruit	3/4 cup of fruit juice

Meat, Poultry, Fish, Dry Beans, Eggs, and Nuts

2–3 ounces of cooked lean meat, poultry, or fish	1/2 cup of cooked dry beans, 1 egg, or 2 tablespoons of peanut butter count as 1 ounce of lean meat

Bread, Cereal, Rice, and Pasta

1 slice of bread	1 ounce of ready-to-eat cereal	1/2 cup of cooked cereal, rice, or pasta

FIGURE 12-1

The food guide pyramid with examples from each food group. (Adapted from Monahan, F. D., Drake, T., & Neighbors, M. [1994]. *Nursing care of adults*. Philadelphia: W. B. Saunders).

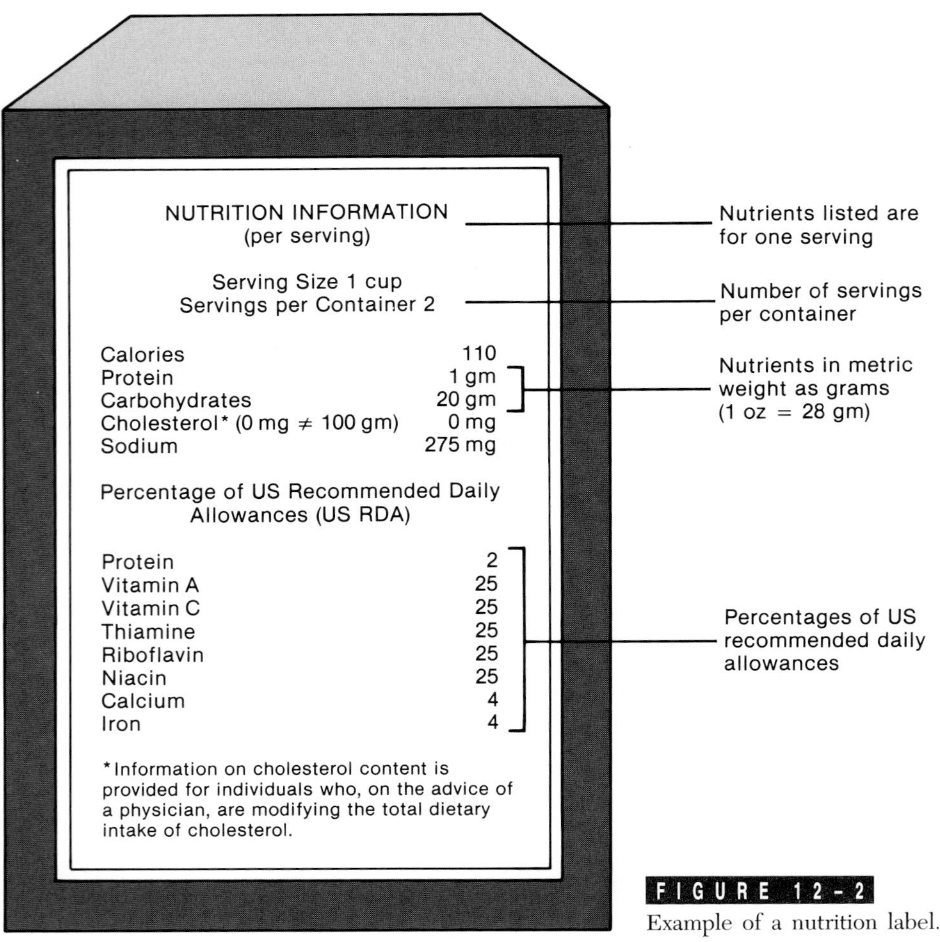

FIGURE 12-2
Example of a nutrition label.

TABLE 12-10
COMPOSITE OF SELECTED DIETARY GUIDELINES

GENERAL	SPECIFIC	INSTRUCTION
Reduce consumption of fat (especially saturated fat) and cholesterol.	Reduce total fat intake to 30% or less of calories. Reduce saturated fat intake to less than 10% of calories and the intake of cholesterol to less than 300 mg/day.	Substitute extra lean ("select") beef and pork, skinless chicken and turkey, fish and shellfish (except shrimp) for high-fat meats. Eat a maximum of 7 oz animal protein daily. Use cottage, pot, ricotta, and other low-fat cheeses in place of hard cheeses as much as possible. Maximal use of legumes, whole grains, vegetables, and fruits. Minimal use of butter, margarine, mayonnaise, salad dressings, peanut butter, rich sauces, and gravies. Use reduced fat versions if possible. Use no more than 3 to 4 egg yolks per week.
Increase consumption of carbohydrates, especially complex carbohydrates and fiber.	Increase carbohydrate consumption to at least 55% of total calories. Limit intake of refined sugars to 10% of calories.	Every day, eat at least 5 servings of fruits and vegetables, including potatoes and those high in vitamins A (orange-yellow and dark green) and C. Eat at least 6 servings of whole-grain breads, cereals, or pasta each day. Eat less of sugar-rich foods (jams, jellies, syrups, candies, rich desserts, baked goods).

TABLE 12-10
COMPOSITE OF SELECTED DIETARY GUIDELINES *Continued*

GENERAL	SPECIFIC	INSTRUCTION
Maintain protein at moderate levels.	Do not exceed two times the RDA for protein, or approximately 100 gm for an adult woman and 125 gm for an adult man.	Eat moderate portions of high-protein foods. Limit meat servings to 7 oz/day. (A 3-oz serving is about the size of a deck of cards and contains around 20 gm of protein.) Limit dairy products to a total of 3 or 4 servings daily. One cup of milk or 1 oz of hard cheese contains 8 gm of protein.
Limit intake of salt (sodium chloride.)	Limit daily salt intake to 6 gm (1 level tsp) or less.	Do not add salt to food at the table; use only small amounts during cooking and serving. Minimal use of salty foods (chips, crackers, other salted snack foods, French fries), processed foods (canned soups, frozen entrees), salt-preserved and salt-pickled foods.
Maintain adequate calcium intake.	Meet daily RDA, particularly for adolescents and young women up to 25 years of age (1200 mg)	Increase daily intake of nonfat or low-fat milk or dairy products to at least 2 to 3 servings (1 cup milk or equivalent). Eat tofu (calcium sulfate processed), vegetable greens, broccoli, or calcium-fortified orange juice frequently.
Emphasize dietary cancer prevention.	Reduce fat consumption to 30% of calories and use foods high in vitamins A and C (see earlier). Include cruciferous vegetables in the diet. Avoid potential dietary carcinogens.	Include broccoli, Brussels sprouts, cauliflower, cabbage, kale, turnips, and rutabagas frequently. Avoid charcoal-broiled meats or eat them infrequently. Reduce fat intake as described earlier.
Children, adolescents, and women of childbearing age should consume foods that are good sources of iron.		Eat lean red meats, fish, beans, whole-grain products, and daily servings of iron-enriched cereals.
Community water systems should contain fluoride at optimal levels for prevention of tooth decay.		Drink water containing fluoride at the level of approximately 1 ppm. When fluoridated water is not available, use supplementary fluoride.
Avoid taking dietary supplements in excess of the RDA in any 1 day.		Do not take vitamins and minerals indiscriminately just because they are available.
If you do drink, do so in moderation. Pregnant women should avoid alcoholic beverages.	Limit consumption to the equivalent of less than 1 oz of pure alcohol in a single day.	Limit daily intake to two cans of beer or two small glasses of wine or two 1½ oz jiggers of distilled spirits, each of which contains 1 oz of alcohol.
Balance food intake and physical activity to achieve and maintain appropriate body weight.	Appropriate weight is 15–18% body fat for men and 20–24% body fat for women. Overweight is 120% of desirable weight or body mass index above 25.	Reduce weight slowly to appropriate level when necessary. Exercise aerobically at least three times per week.

RDA, Recommended daily allowance.
From Mahan, K. L., & Arlin, M. (1992). *Krause's food, nutrition & diet therapy* (8th ed., p. 288). Philadelphia: W. B. Saunders.

Food intake should be assessed for a 24-hour period to note any patterns. Patients can be asked to recall exactly what they ate during the past 24 hours, usually from the time of awakening until the next morning. Everything that enters the mouth should be noted, including meals, snacks, drinks (especially water), and seasonings (especially salt). From this 24-hour assessment, the nurse can determine dietary deficits and excesses.

Height and weight measurements should be performed correctly to complete an accurate assessment of the patient. Table 12–12 gives guidelines on the proper way to perform these measurements.

Body composition is related to the ratio of fat to lean muscle mass. Determining a person's body composition requires taking several measurements. These measurements include skinfold thickness and hydrostatic weighing. Skinfold thickness is measured by means of calipers that pinch skin over areas of the body that seem to reflect best the fat content of the subcutaneous tissue. These sites include areas over the triceps, biceps, below the scapula, above the iliac crest, and upper thigh (Fig. 12–3).

Hydrostatic weighing is done underwater. The advantage of weighing underwater is that it provides a good

TABLE 12-11

DIETARY HISTORY INFORMATION

Economics
Income—frequency and steadiness of employment
Amount of money for food each week or month and individual's perception of its adequacy for meeting food needs
Eligibility for food stamps and cost of stamps
Public aid recipient?

Physical Activity
Occupation—type, hours/week, shift, energy expenditure
Exercise—type, amount, frequency (seasonal?)
Sleep—hours/day (uninterrupted?)
Handicaps

Ethnic or Cultural Background
Influence on eating habits
Religion
Education

Home Life and Meal Patterns
Number in household (eat together?)
Person who does shopping
Person who does cooking
Food storage and cooking facilities (stove, refrigerator)
Type of housing (home, apartment, room, etc.)
Ability to shop and prepare food

Appetite
Good, poor, any changes
Factors that affect appetite
Taste and smell perception and any changes

Attitude Toward Food and Eating
Disinterest in food
Irrational ideas about food, eating, and body weight
Parental interest in child's eating

Allergies, Intolerances, or Food Avoidances
Foods avoided and reason
Length of time of avoidance
Description of problems caused by foods

Dental and Oral Health
Problems with eating
Foods that cannot be eaten
Problems with swallowing, salivation, food sticking

Gastrointestinal
Problems with heartburn, bloating, gas, diarrhea, vomiting, constipation, distention
Frequency of problems
Home remedies
Antacid, laxative, or other drug use

Chronic Disease
Treatment
Length of time of treatment
Dietary modification—physician prescription?, date of modification, education, compliance with diet

Medication
Vitamin and/or mineral supplements—frequency, type, amount
Medications—type, amount, frequency, length of time on medication

Recent Weight Change
Loss or gain
How many pounds, over what length of time
Intentional or nonvolitional

Dietary or Nutritional Problems (as Perceived by Patient)

From Mahan, K. L., & Arlin, M. (1992). *Krause's food, nutrition & diet therapy* (8th ed., p. 300). Philadelphia: W. B. Saunders.

TABLE 12-12

RECOMMENDATIONS FOR THE MEASUREMENT OF HEIGHT AND WEIGHT

HEIGHT	WEIGHT
• Height should be measured without shoes.	• Use a beam balance scale, not a spring scale, whenever possible.
• Feet should be together with the heels against the wall or measuring board.	• Periodically calibrate the scale for accuracy, using known weights.
• The subject should stand erect, neither slumped nor stretching, looking straight ahead, without tipping the head up or down. The top of the ear and outer corner of the eye should be in a line parallel to the floor.	• Weigh the subject in light clothing without shoes.
• A horizontal bar, a rectangular block of wood, or the top of the statiometer should be lowered to rest flat on the top of the head.	• Record weight to the nearest ½ lb or 0.2 kg. Measurements above the 90th or below the 10th percentiles warrant further evaluation.
• Height should be read to the nearest ¼ inch or 0.5 cm.	

estimate of body density as a person is submerged, indicating the amount of adipose tissue or percentage of body fat.

WEIGHT MANAGEMENT AND EATING DISORDERS

Most Americans today are on some form of "diet." People feel an increasing dissatisfaction with their appearance and a constant need to change that appearance. Dieting is rarely fun. It takes motivation, hard work, and a willingness to control behavior over a long period of time. Most adults have the ability to maintain a constant weight, but to do so, they must keep up consistent food and exercise patterns on a daily basis.

Overweight individuals are considered obese if their weight is 20% or more above ideal body weight. Obesity is associated with coronary artery disease, lipid disorders, and type II diabetes mellitus (non–insulin-dependent diabetes mellitus). It is also considered a risk factor for some kinds of cancer and is associated with joint disease, gallstones, and respiratory problems.

The underweight person is one whose weight is 15 to 20% or more below accepted weight standards. This

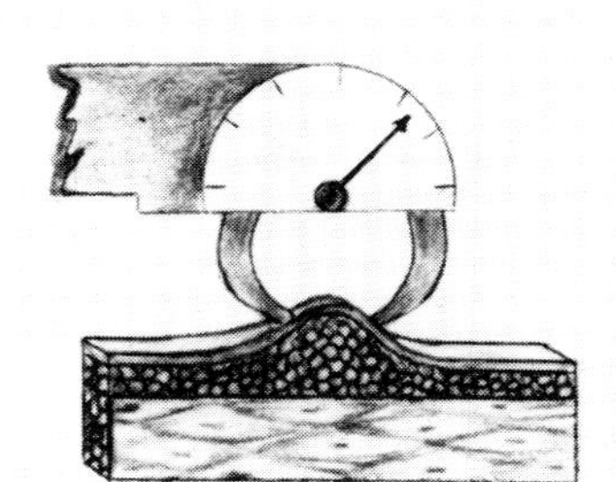

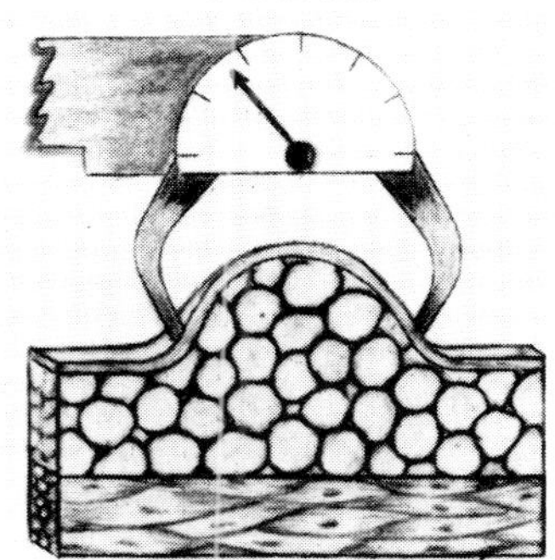

FIGURE 12-3
Skinfold calipers measure in millimeters the thickness of the subcutaneous fat tissue, which gives a rough measurement of adiposity. (Diagram courtesy of Dorice Czajka-Narins, Ph.D. From Mahan, L. K., & Arlin, M. [1992]. *Krause's food, nutrition & diet therapy* [8th ed., p. 308]. Philadelphia: W. B. Saunders.)

may be caused by an insufficient food intake to meet activity needs, excessive activity, poor absorption and utilization of food consumed, a wasting disease, or psychological or emotional stress.

Eating disorders are becoming more common among teenaged girls and young women. Puberty brings with it hormonal changes and the emergence of sexual characteristics. Some teenagers, particularly girls, resist these changes and turn to inappropriate dieting. Two eating disorders, anorexia nervosa and bulimia, may begin in adolescence. Young women may develop these disorders when attempting to achieve the "perfect" body.

ANOREXIA NERVOSA

Anorexia nervosa is an eating disorder characterized by self-imposed starvation. Certain features are common in individuals with this disorder. They are generally women in their midteens, although young adult women and men sometimes develop the disorder. Often they are high achievers from educated, middle-class families. The young person with anorexia nervosa is frequently a perfectionist who uses food and exercise as a means of controlling the body.

People with anorexia nervosa become obsessed with weight loss and soon develop a distorted body image, seeing themselves as fat even when their weight is much less than average for their height and age. They experience personality changes, depression, and apathy. Death may occur in as many as 20% of those with anorexia nervosa. Psychiatric treatment is usually recommended (see Chapter 51).

BULIMIA

Bulimia is an eating disorder characterized by periods of binge eating followed by purging. This behavior may be alternated with periods of fasting as well. The cycle may go something like this: The person may binge several times a week. The episode may last 2 hours or more, and the person will consume large amounts of easily ingested kilocalorie-dense foods such as ice cream, candies, cakes, breads, and pastries. The binge often is followed by self-induced vomiting or the use of laxatives, diuretics, or a combination of these.

Bulimia occurs more frequently than anorexia nervosa and is seen most often in young women. People with bulimia are usually of normal weight or even overweight. Most are aware that their eating patterns are abnormal. They may experience fear of not being able to stop eating and depression, guilt, and remorse after a binge. Clinical symptoms of bulimia may include tooth erosion, calloused knuckles, stomach lacerations, and esophageal infections from excessive vomiting. Electrolyte imbalances may occur, leading to abnormal heart rhythms and injury to the kidneys. Repeated infections of the bladder and kidney may lead to renal failure.

METHODS OF NUTRITIONAL SUPPORT

SUPPLEMENTAL FEEDINGS

The preferred method of meeting nutritional requirements is, of course, through eating a balanced diet. This is not always possible, however, and there are times when a person's nutritional needs cannot be met by oral feeding. At these times a person's needs must be met with some type of nutritional supplement. These supplements can be formulated using fluid or powdered milk, powdered whole eggs, and powdered egg albumin as concentrated protein sources. Liquid feedings meet the nutritional requirements of patients who are unable to take solid food. Table 12–13 summarizes the situations that might require artificial feeding.

Enteral Tube Feedings

Patients who are unable to take in supplemental liquid feedings orally may require enteral tube feedings. Conditions that interfere with taking in liquids orally include oral surgery, gastrointestinal surgery, dysphagia (difficulty swallowing), unconsciousness, anorexia, or esophageal obstruction. The tubes enter the body through the nose, esophagus, stomach, or jejunum (Fig. 12–4).

Enteral tube feedings may cause complications such as nausea or vomiting, diarrhea, gastrointestinal bleeding, aspiration pneumonia, hyperkalemia (excessive po-

TABLE 12-13
SITUATIONS REQUIRING ARTIFICIAL FEEDING TECHNIQUES

PHYSIOLOGIC PROBLEM	RECOMMENDED FEEDING	CLINICAL SITUATION OR DISORDER
Inability to ingest food	Liquid feedings: whole food or milk-based formula Route of administration: Tube Nasogastric Gastrostomy Jejunostomy Oral	Carcinoma of esophagus or stomach Dental or oral surgery Inflammatory disease of esophagus Coma
Inability to digest food	Chemically defined diet Route of administration: Oral Tube	Pancreatitis Biliary tract disease
Decreased ability or inability to absorb food	Chemically defined diet Route of administration: Oral Tube Peripheral vein nutritional support Total parenteral nutrition	Radiation therapy Sprue Inflammatory bowel disease Short-bowel syndrome
Inability to handle colonic residue	Chemically defined diet Route of administration: Oral Tube Peripheral vein nutritional support Total parenteral nutrition	Inflammatory bowel disease Presurgical preparation Ileostomy, colostomy Draining fistula
Inability to meet nutritional requirements fully with normal foods	Liquid feeding Oral supplement Tube feeding Peripheral vein nutritional support Central vein nutritional supplementation	Major surgery Burns Trauma Extended fever Anorexia of chronic illness Anorexia nervosa

From Mahan, K. L., & Arlin, M. (1992). *Krause's food, nutrition & diet therapy* (8th ed., p. 508). Philadelphia: W. B. Saunders.

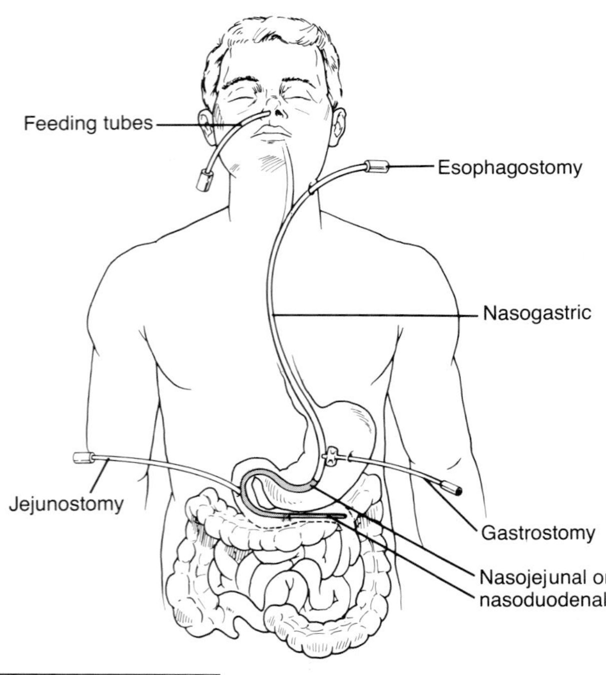

FIGURE 12-4
Diagram of the placement of enteral feeding tubes. (From Mahan, L. K., & Arlin, M. [1992]. *Krause's food, nutrition & diet therapy* [8th ed., p. 509]. Philadelphia: W. B. Saunders.)

tassium), hyponatremia (sodium deficit), hyperglycemia, or nutritional deficiencies. They are caused either by problems with the liquid supplement or by mechanical difficulties with the tube feeding, such as misplacement of the tube or too rapid administration of the feeding.

Parenteral Nutrition

Another method of administering nutrients is through parenteral nutrition. This method is used for nutrition only if the gastrointestinal tract cannot be used, and it can be lifesaving. The two major types of parenteral nutrition are (1) peripheral parenteral nutrition (PPN) and (2) central parenteral nutrition (CPN) or total parenteral nutrition (TPN). Peripheral parenteral nutrition is given through the peripheral veins in the arms and legs; CPN or TPN is given through a central vein, usually the superior vena cava.

PERIPHERAL PARENTERAL NUTRITION. Peripheral parenteral nutrition is the standard intravenous therapy that is usually a 5% glucose solution. Vitamins, minerals, and electrolytes may be added. Total nutritional requirements usually are not met with PPN therapy, and at most it supplies 1800 kcal per day.

TOTAL PARENTERAL NUTRITION. Central parenteral nutrition or TPN feedings are used for patients who are unable to obtain adequate nutrition enterally or with PPN. They are usually debilitated and malnourished with a weight loss of 10% of the body weight or more. Patients with short-bowel syndrome, bowel fistulas or obstruction, inflammatory bowel disease, or hypermetabolic states in which the gastrointestinal tract is completely or partially unusable benefit from this form of nutritional support.

Total parenteral nutrition can meet the high energy and protein needs of burn patients. It can also be used for the cancer patient who has become malnourished owing to oncologic treatments. Total parenteral nutrition can supply up to 4000 kcal per day. This is possible because the solution is administered through a Hickman or Broviac-type catheter inserted into the superior vena cava, where the hypertonic solution can be diluted rapidly by the large, fast-flowing volume of blood.

Patients who are being fed parenterally should be monitored closely for any signs of complications. Frequently occurring complications include pulmonary complications, injury to the veins and arteries surrounding the TPN site, air embolism, infection, electrolyte imbalance, mineral deficiencies, and rebound hypoglycemia if treatment is ended suddenly.

Transitional Feeding

When patients are ready to be changed from one of these methods to another, they are ready for transitional feeding. Transitional feeding can be from parenteral nutrition to enteral tube feeding or oral intake, from enteral tube feeding to oral formula or food, or a combination of these.

It is important that this transitional feeding be done gradually and with specific principles in mind. If patients who have been without food for an extended period of time are given food too quickly, they may develop nutritional recovery syndrome. This syndrome causes hypophosphatemia (deficiency of phosphates in the blood) from the shift of phosphorus from the plasma to the intracellular compartment. This shift may also affect potassium as it moves into cells with the glucose during refeeding.

Refeeding of the malnourished patient disrupts the adaptive state of starvation and therefore must proceed slowly with close patient monitoring. The ideal early feeding appears to be moderate in carbohydrates, low in sodium, lactose-free, and supplemented with phosphorus and potassium.

When moving from parenteral to enteral feeding, it is important to continue the parenteral feeding. This allows for maintenance of adequate nutrient and fluid intake as tolerance of enteral feedings is assessed. As the patient is able to tolerate the enteral feedings, the parenteral feedings can be tapered off.

When moving from parenteral to oral intake, it is again important to maintain parenteral support until the oral intake is assessed for tolerance. As the patient's tolerance and intake of formula or foods increase, the parenteral feeding can be tapered off.

When moving from enteral to oral feedings, the patient may complain of a poor appetite. In making this transition it may be helpful to change the enteral feeding from a continuous drip to an intermittent feeding. This way the patient has a chance to get hungry between feedings, and desire for food may increase.

B I B L I O G R A P H Y

Cerrato, P. L. (1992). Goodbye four food groups. *RN, 55,* 61–62.

Davis, J., & Sherer, K. (1994). *Applied nutrition and diet therapy for nurses* (2nd ed.). Philadelphia: W. B. Saunders.

Johnson, K., & Kligman, E. W. (1992). Preventive nutrition: An "optimal" diet for older adults. *Geriatrics, 47* (10), 56–60.

Mahan, L. K., & Arlin, M. (1992). *Krause's food, nutrition, and diet therapy* (8th ed.) Philadelphia: W. B. Saunders.

Newbern, V. (1992). Failure to thrive, a growing concern in the elderly. *Journal of Gerontological Nursing, 18,* 21–25.

Walker, S. N. (1992). Well for elders. *Holistic Nurse Practice,* 7(1), 38–45.

KEY CONCEPTS

1. Nutrition is the cornerstone of the healing process, and to support and maintain life or fight disease the body must be supplied with the proper nutrients.
2. During the digestive process, enzymes help to break food particles down to their simplest form so that the nutrients can be absorbed by the body.
3. Regulation of the gastrointestinal system involves neural control and the secretion of hormones.
4. Parasympathetic nerves generally stimulate digestive activity, and sympathetic nerves inhibit activity.
5. The stomach is normally emptied in 1 to 4 hours, depending on the amount and kinds of foods eaten.
6. The primary organ of absorption is the small intestine.
7. Fluids, vitamins, and minerals are absorbed through the intestinal mucosa.
8. The body makes use of the energy received through the food that is eaten, and the largest portion of energy expenditure occurs during rest to carry out the mechanical activities needed to sustain life processes.
9. Most of the energy needed to move, perform activities, and live is consumed in the form of carbohydrates, which are converted primarily to glucose for immediate use by the body's cells.

KEY CONCEPTS *(continued)*

10. Although carbohydrates are the body's main source of food energy, fats are the most concentrated source, supplying 9 calories per gram, whereas carbohydrates and protein supply only 4 calories per gram.
11. Lipids are a major source of energy for muscle tissue, even when glucose is available.
12. People should try to limit their fat intake to 30% or less of their daily caloric intake and should try to eat unsaturated fats rather than saturated fats.
13. Proteins are made of smaller units called amino acids.
14. Vitamins and minerals are needed in small amounts for good health.
15. Water is the largest component of the body and body tissues and is essential to all life processes in the body.
16. Maintaining a good diet can help middle-aged and older adults to maintain a high level of function and reduce the risks of chronic disease; however, because of the normal decline in metabolism and physical activity, energy needs lessen with age.
17. Most adults have the ability to maintain a constant weight, but to do so, they must keep up consistent food and exercise patterns on a daily basis.
18. Anorexia nervosa and bulimia are eating disorders that often begin in adolescence, especially in young women who are attempting to achieve the "perfect" body.

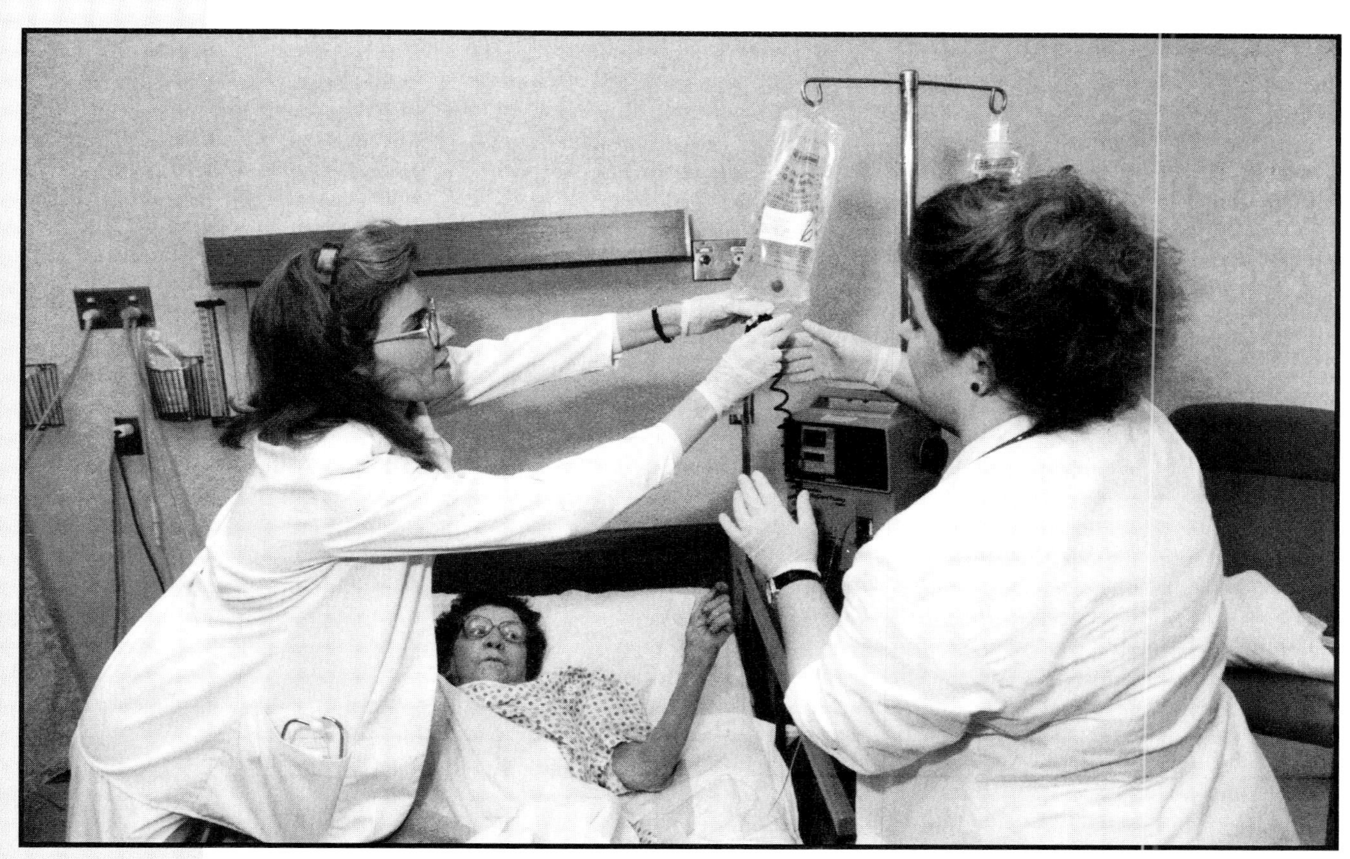

UNIT 3
Medical-Surgical Care

Adrianne Linton

CHAPTER 13

First Aid and Emergency Care

OBJECTIVES

1. List the principles of emergency and first aid care.
2. List the steps of the initial assessment and interventions for the person requiring emergency care.
3. Describe the components of the nursing assessment of the person requiring emergency care.
4. Outline the steps of the nursing process for emergency or first aid treatment of victims of cardiopulmonary arrest, choking, shock, hemorrhage, traumatic injury, burns, heat or cold exposure, poisoning, bites, and stings.
5. Explain the legal implications of administering first aid in emergency situations.

GLOSSARY

ANAPHYLACTIC SHOCK A severe, potentially fatal, allergic reaction characterized by hypotension and bronchial constriction

AVULSION Tearing away of tissue

CARDIOPULMONARY ARREST Absence of heartbeat and breathing

EPISTAXIS Nosebleed

EVISCERATION Protrusion of internal organs through a wound

HEMORRHAGE Loss of a large amount of blood

HEMOTHORAX Presence of blood in the pleural cavity causing the lung on the affected side to collapse

HYPERTHERMIA Elevation of body core temperature above 99°F

HYPOTHERMIA Decrease in body core temperature below 95°F

POISON Any substance that, in small quantities, is capable of causing illness or harm following ingestion, inhalation, injection, or contact with the skin

Glossary continued

PNEUMOTHORAX Presence of air in the pleural cavity that causes the lung on the affected side to collapse

RESPIRATORY ARREST Absence of breathing

SHOCK Inadequate circulation caused by falling blood pressure

SPRAIN An injury to a ligament

STRAIN An injury to muscle tissue or the tendons that attach them to bones, or both

In the inpatient setting, the nurse is often the first on the scene when accidents or emergencies occur. Nurses also need to be prepared to act in emergency situations away from health care facilities. Knowledge of first aid can make the difference between life and death in many situations. This chapter addresses first aid interventions for common emergencies. Some emergency conditions that require further medical attention are covered in greater detail elsewhere in this book.

GENERAL PRINCIPLES OF EMERGENCY CARE

When accidents or emergencies occur, the victim and any observers are often understandably frightened. It can be very reassuring to them to know that a nurse is present, but the nurse must remember a cardinal rule: remain calm.

The nursing process is used in emergencies, just as it is in other nursing situations. The important difference is that assessment and intervention must be done *very* quickly and *very* efficiently to identify and treat priority needs immediately.

While approaching the victim, the nurse tries to determine the nature of the emergency. Has there been an automobile accident, a fall, a diving accident, or an electrocution? The nurse must also recognize any hazards to the victim and the rescuer. For example, is the victim in a burning vehicle or lying in the middle of the highway? Failure to recognize such dangers may result in injuries to the rescuer and additional injuries to the victim.

Initial assessment and immediate intervention proceed in the following sequence:

1. Assess the ABC's: airway, breathing, circulation.
2. Initiate cardiopulmonary resuscitation or rescue breathing as needed.
3. Look for uncontrolled bleeding, identify the source, and apply pressure to the source.
4. Systematically assess for injuries from the head to the feet.
5. Look for a medical alert tag, usually a necklace or a bracelet.

GUIDELINES FOR FIRST AID TREATMENT

General guidelines for first aid treatment of emergency patients are the following:

1. Splint injured parts in the position they are found.
2. Prevent chilling, but do not add excessive heat.
3. Do not remove penetrating objects.
4. Do not try to give anything by mouth to an unconscious person or to one who appears to need surgical intervention.
5. Stay with the injured person until medical care or transport arrives.

NURSING ASSESSMENT IN EMERGENCIES

Patient emergencies can occur in every setting. Sometimes nurses observe the events and know what has happened, but at other times evidence at the scene must give clues as to the circumstances. It is difficult to intervene appropriately in emergencies that cannot be immediately understood. The nurse must be prepared to do a quick assessment and then act promptly to provide appropriate care that may save a life. The health history and physical examination are presented separately here but in fact may be done almost simultaneously in emergencies.

HEALTH HISTORY

If the victim is able to speak or a witness is available, a brief history is obtained. Data are limited in emergency situations and should include the chief complaint, the treatment given, and the relevant medical history.

Chief Complaint

To describe the chief complaint, the nurse determines the nature of the problem, the signs and symptoms, and the circumstances under which the injury or illness occurred. If the victim is or has been unconscious, the length of time unconscious is noted.

Medical Treatment

The nurse notes what treatment, if any, has been given and the effect of the treatment. In the event of an injury, it is significant to note whether the victim has been moved.

Past Medical History

If information about known health problems can be obtained, it may provide important clues to the immediate problem or influence the care provided. Current health problems that should be recognized include diabetes and cardiac and pulmonary diseases. Especially when a victim is unconscious, a quick check for a medical alert tag may yield essential information. Current medications and known allergies are identified if possible.

PHARMACOLOGY CAPSULE

The medical alert tag can provide clues about medical emergencies and alert rescuers to known allergies.

PHYSICAL EXAMINATION

The nurse begins to collect objective data as soon as the victim is seen. All the senses are used in the assessment process. The first assessment priorities must be airway, breathing, and circulation. The nurse watches the victim's chest for rhythmic breathing and listens near the patient's mouth and nose for air movement. Carotid and peripheral pulses are palpated. Once the adequacy of respiration and circulation has been established, the nurse assesses for uncontrolled bleeding and shock. If there is no evidence of uncontrolled bleeding or shock, the next step is a systematic head-to-toe assessment. At each step, the nurse looks for obvious injury, bleeding, swelling, bruising, and drainage. Skin color, warmth, and temperature are also assessed at each step.

The systematic assessment begins with inspection of the head. The nurse speaks to the victim and evaluates the response to assess level of consciousness (alert, disoriented, unresponsive). Comprehension can be evaluated by asking the patient to follow simple commands like opening and closing the eyes. The eyes are inspected with particular attention to pupil size, equality, and reaction to light. The alert victim is asked about neck pain or stiffness, and ability to swallow. The chest is inspected for symmetry of the chest wall movement. Respiratory effort, dyspnea, and abnormal sounds associated with respirations are assessed. The contour of the abdomen is examined to detect distention. Light palpation may detect areas of pain or tenderness. The extremities are inspected for deformity, injury, and movement. Peripheral pulses, warmth, and sensation are assessed.

Initial assessment of the patient requiring first aid or emergency care is summarized in Table 13–1.

TABLE 13-1
ASSESSMENT OF THE PATIENT WHO REQUIRES FIRST AID OR EMERGENCY CARE

HEALTH HISTORY

Chief complaint: nature of illness or injury, signs and symptoms, circumstances of illness or injury, how long unconscious
Treatment: what has been done, effects, whether moved after injury
Past medical history: current health problems, current medications, allergies

PHYSICAL EXAMINATION

ABC's: airway, breathing, circulation
Skin: color, temperature, obvious injury
Head: level of consciousness
Eyes: opening, pupil size, equality, response to light
Neck: stiffness, pain, ability to swallow
Chest: symmetry of movement, dyspnea, respiratory rate and effort
Abdomen: contour, rigidity, distention, pain, tenderness
Extremities: deformity, movement, sensation, peripheral pulses

SPECIFIC EMERGENCIES

CARDIOPULMONARY ARREST

When the heart stops beating, a person is in cardiac arrest. When respirations cease, the person is in respiratory or pulmonary arrest. The cardiac and respiratory systems are so dependent on each other that when one fails, the other quickly fails as well. Cardiopulmonary arrest is the absence of a heartbeat and respirations.

Nerve tissue is so susceptible to hypoxia (low levels of oxygen) that in most circumstances the brain begins to die after 4 minutes without oxygen. Unless circulation and oxygenation are restored very quickly after cardiopulmonary arrest, permanent brain damage results. Prompt recognition and treatment of cardiopulmonary arrest can maintain the oxygen supply to the brain until circulation and respiration are restored.

Cardiopulmonary resuscitation (CPR) can be part of basic life support or advanced life support. Basic life support is the immediate care given to maintain oxygenation of the brain until advanced medical support is available. This chapter focuses on basic life support outside the health care setting. Key points are emphasized, but literature published by the American Heart Association or the American Red Cross provides additional, more specific information. Advanced life support is covered in Chapter 31.

Causes

Examples of causes of cardiopulmonary arrest are myocardial infarction, heart failure, electrocution, drowning, drug overdose, anaphylaxis, and asphyxiation.

Signs and Symptoms

Victims of cardiopulmonary arrest collapse and quickly lose consciousness. There is no pulse or respiration.

Nursing Assessment

In cardiopulmonary arrest, assessment and interventions are quickly interwoven. The steps of CPR therefore include assessment and intervention and are presented in sequence below. Only CPR for adults is addressed here.

Nursing Diagnoses and Goals

Cardiopulmonary arrest is a medical rather than a nursing diagnosis. Nursing diagnoses that may be appropriate are altered tissue perfusion and ineffective breathing patterns. The goal of CPR is maintenance of oxygenation until the heartbeat and respirations are restored.

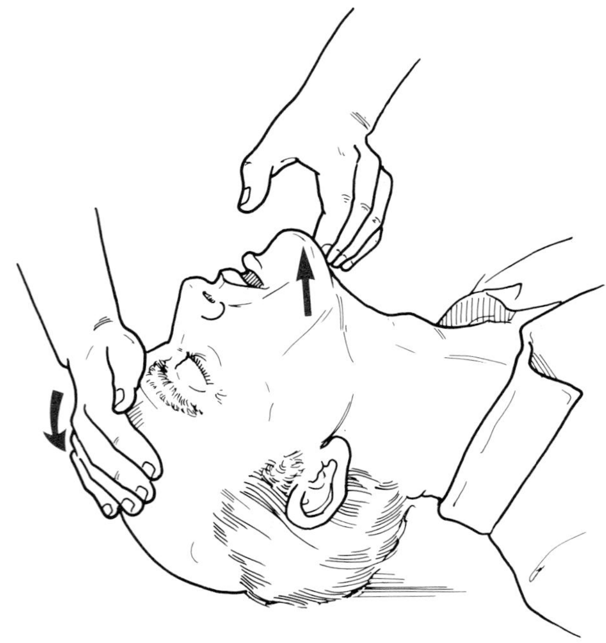

FIGURE 13-1
To open the airway, apply pressure to the forehead with one hand and use the other hand to lift the chin forward.

Interventions

The reader should refer to the latest American Heart Association guidelines for CPR because they are revised at intervals.

1. When cardiopulmonary arrest is suspected, tap the victim urgently and ask "Are you okay?"
2. If there is no response, call for someone to contact the emergency medical service.
3. Place the victim supine on a firm, flat surface.
4. If no neck injury is suspected, open the airway by applying pressure to the forehead with one hand and using the other hand to lift the chin forward (Fig. 13–1).
5. If a neck injury is suspected, use the jaw-thrust method of opening the airway. The jaw-thrust is done by lifting the lower jaw with both hands (Fig. 13–2).
6. Put your ear near the victim's nose and mouth to listen for breathing for 3 to 5 seconds. Watch to see if the chest rises and falls.
7. If the victim is not breathing, give 2 slow breaths at a rate of 1.5 to 2.0 seconds per breath. To do this, first pinch the nostrils shut (Fig. 13–3). Take a deep breath, seal your mouth around the victim's and breathe into the victim's mouth. Watch the victim's chest. If it rises, ventilation is effective. If not, treat for airway obstruction as described later. Various masks and airways are available to avoid direct mouth-to-mouth contact, but these are often not on hand in emergency situations.
8. Check for cardiac arrest by palpating the carotid artery on the side of the neck nearest you.
9. If there is no pulse, begin cardiac compressions to restore circulation (Fig. 13–4).
   a. Locate the proper place to compress. Run the middle finger along the lower rib margin to the notch where the rib meets the sternum.
   b. Place the index finger next to the middle finger on the lower part of the sternum.
   c. Place the heel of the other hand next to the index finger.
   d. Place the hand used to locate the tip of the sternum over the other hand and keep fingers off the victim's chest.
   e. Lean over the victim so that your shoulders are above your hands and your arms are straight.
   f. Apply pressure to depress the sternum 1½ to 2 inches, counting "one and two and three and four" for 15 compressions.
   g. Keep your hands in contact with the chest at all times.
   h. At the completion of 15 compressions, ventilate the victim twice.
10. Perform four cycles of 15 compressions and two

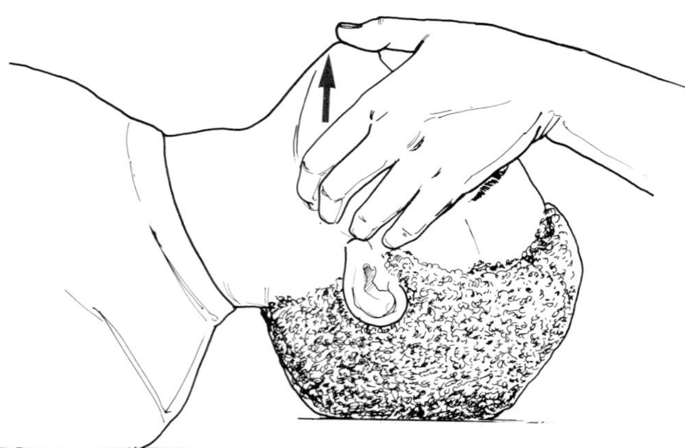

FIGURE 13-2
To open the airway when a neck injury is suspected, lift the lower jaw with both hands.

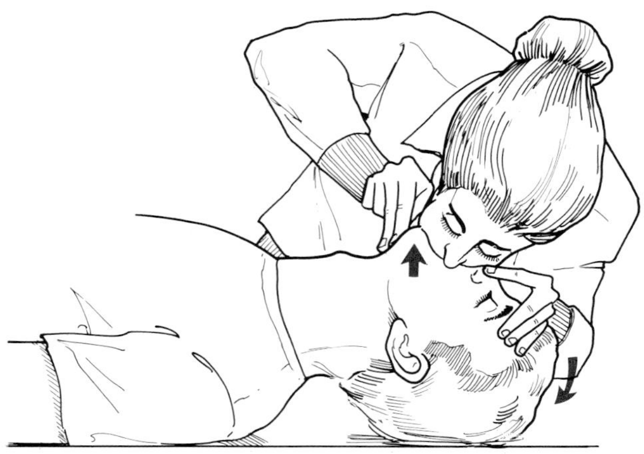

FIGURE 13-3
To ventilate the victim, pinch the nostrils shut, take a deep breath, seal your mouth over the victim's, and breathe into the victim's mouth.

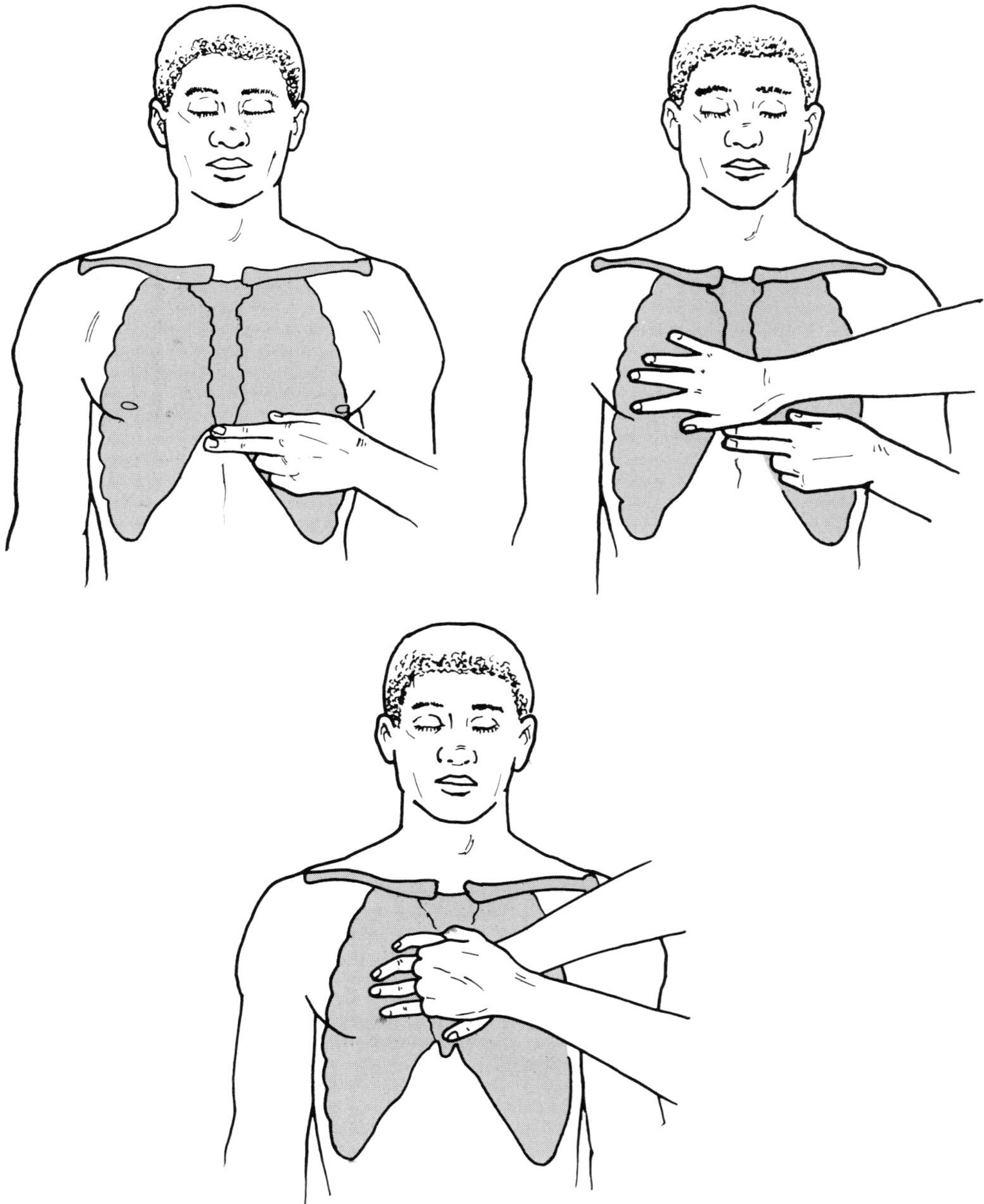

FIGURE 13-4

The proper place for compression is located two finger widths above the tip of the sternum.

ventilations and then reassess circulation at the carotid artery for 5 seconds.

11. If no carotid pulse, resume CPR with 15 compressions followed by two ventilations until help arrives or until you are exhausted.

TWO-RESCUER CPR. Two-rescuer CPR is taught only to health care providers. If two trained people are present to perform CPR, one rescuer compresses the chest five times, then pauses briefly for the second rescuer to ventilate the victim once. The cycle is repeated until the compressor tires. The compressor calls for a switch and trades places with the ventilator at the end of a cycle.

RECOVERY POSITION. The unresponsive victim who is breathing should be log-rolled to one side (the "recovery position") if no cervical trauma is suspected.

Evaluation

The criteria for successful intervention are restoration of heartbeat and spontaneous breathing.

CHOKING OR AIRWAY OBSTRUCTION

Choking is airway obstruction caused by a foreign body that enters the airway.

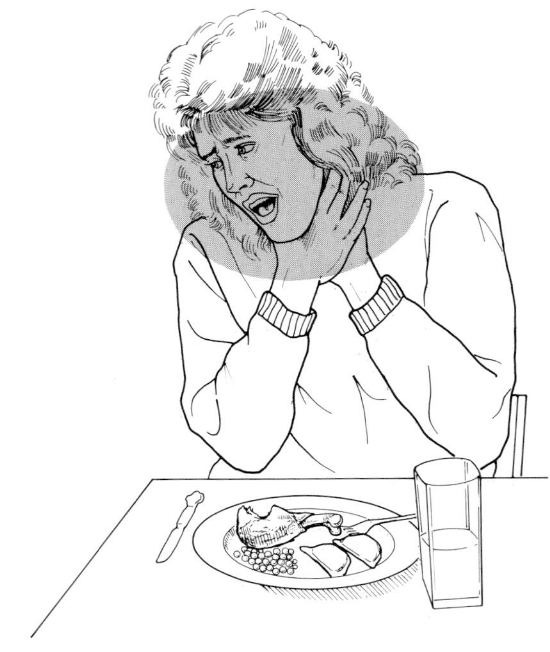

FIGURE 13-5
The universal choking sign.

Assessment

The universal sign for choking is grabbing the throat with one or both hands (Fig. 13–5). Fear of suffocation is terrifying, and the victim may look panicky. The rescuer first determines whether the airway is completely blocked. If the victim is able to speak, breathe, or cough with good air exchange, the rescuer should do nothing. If the victim is unable to speak, breathe, or cough with good air exchange, the rescuer must act quickly to prevent suffocation.

Nursing Diagnosis and Goal

The primary nursing diagnosis for the choking victim is ineffective airway clearance related to obstruction. The goal for treatment is a patent airway with normal respirations.

Interventions

If the choking victim is conscious, the rescuer performs the Heimlich maneuver, a "bear hug" procedure named for the physician who first described and prescribed it. The rescuer stands behind the victim and reaches around the victim slightly above the umbilicus and below the xiphoid process (Fig. 13–6). One of the rescuer's hands is held in a fist with the other hand pressing the fist against the victim. The rescuer tightens the arms around the victim and performs quick upward thrusts into the victim's abdomen. This motion exerts pressure upward on the diaphragm, forcing air out of the lungs. If effective, the air expels the foreign body from the airway. If not, the maneuver is repeated until the object is expelled or the victim loses consciousness.

If the victim is unconscious or loses consciousness, the rescuer positions the victim on his or her back and calls for help. Three measures are then employed:

1. Lift the jaw and sweep a finger through the mouth to try to remove the object.
2. Tilt the head back, lift the chin, pinch the nostrils, and try to ventilate the victim by breathing into the mouth once. If the airway is still obstructed, attempts at ventilation will fail.
3. Straddle the victim's thighs, place one hand on top of the other and give up to five abdominal thrusts in the same area described for the Heimlich maneuver (Fig. 13–7).

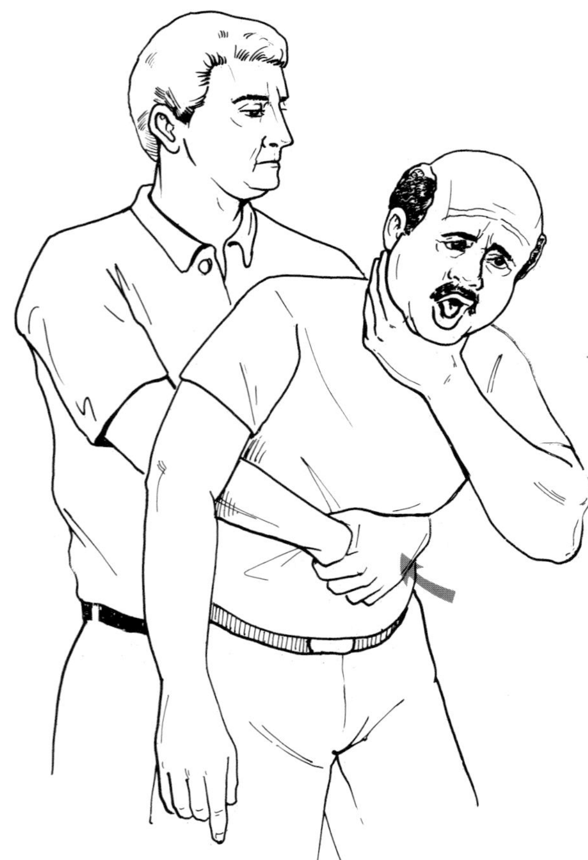

FIGURE 13-6
The Heimlich maneuver for the conscious choking victim.

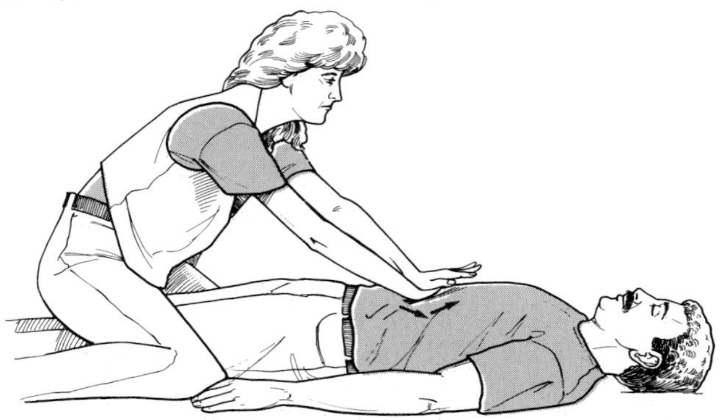

FIGURE 13-7
The Heimlich maneuver for the unconscious choking victim.

Repeat these three steps until the airway is clear. Once the airway is open, CPR may be necessary to restore cardiac and respiratory function. Even if the obstruction is removed, the victim should see a physician as soon as possible.

Evaluation

Evidence of effective treatment of choking includes expulsion of the obstructing object, spontaneous respirations, normal skin color, and decreased anxiety.

Prevention

Most choking deaths are preventable. Nurses can teach people to reduce the risk of choking by cutting food into small pieces, eating slowly, and chewing thoroughly. People should be reminded not to laugh and talk while chewing and swallowing. Finally, people should be taught how to perform the Heimlich maneuver. It is quite simple to perform and can save a life.

SHOCK

Shock results from acute circulatory failure. Conditions that may lead to shock include blood loss, heart failure, overwhelming infection, severe allergic reactions, and extreme pain or fright. Various types of shock are discussed in other sections of this book. This section covers common first aid measures for shock.

Nursing Assessment

Assessment of the victim in shock may detect the following signs and symptoms:

- **Pulse:** rapid and weak, "thready," imperceptible
- **Respirations:** air hunger initially, then increased rate; shallow
- **Blood pressure:** decreased
- **Skin:** cool and moist; cyanosis of lips and nailbeds
- **Urine output:** decreased
- **Mental status:** restless, then listless; unconscious
- **Thirst:** increased

Nursing Diagnosis

Nursing diagnoses vary with the cause of shock. Possible diagnoses include the following:

- **Decreased Cardiac Output** related to low arterial blood pressure, decreased venous return, hypovolemia
- **Altered Cerebral Tissue Perfusion** related to hypovolemia, pump failure
- **Fear** related to the possibility of death

Goals

Goals for first aid treatment of the patient in shock are increased cardiac output, improved cerebral blood flow, and reduced fear.

Interventions

For the patient in shock, the first priority is to maintain blood flow to the brain. The patient is positioned flat and kept still and quiet. The legs may be elevated unless the shock is caused by heart failure, the head or neck is bleeding, spinal injury is possible, intracranial pressure is increased, or the patient has dyspnea.

The patient should be protected from cold but not overheated. The skin feels cool because blood has been shunted to vital internal organs. This is a protective response to falling blood pressure. Warming the patient causes blood vessels in the skin to dilate, bringing blood away from vital organs. Excessive warming also may cause perspiration, which further reduces the volume of body fluid. Even if the patient complains of thirst, oral fluids are usually not given in case surgical intervention is needed.

The nurse attempts to identify and treat the underlying cause of shock. Measures are taken to treat pain and reduce fear. The nurse reassures victims by telling them what is being done and that someone will stay with them. Measures to control bleeding are discussed next.

Evaluation

Criteria for evaluating nursing interventions for the patient in shock are an increase in pulse strength, a rise in blood pressure, an increase in alertness, a patient statement of reduced fear, and a more relaxed expression on the part of the patient.

HEMORRHAGE

Hemorrhage is the loss of a large amount of blood. The loss of more than 1 liter of blood in an adult may lead to hypovolemic shock. Continued bleeding, of course, results in death. Bleeding may be external or internal. Internal bleeding is suspected if a trauma victim shows signs of shock but no external bleeding.

Assessment

The nurse assesses for signs and symptoms of hemorrhage that may include obvious bleeding and early or late signs of shock. If bleeding is internal, the victim may have other symptoms, such as abdominal distention, hematemesis, or dyspnea depending on the site of the bleeding.

Nursing Diagnosis

Nursing diagnoses for the person who is hemorrhaging include the following:

- **Decreased Cardiac Output** related to hypovolemia
- **Fear** related to possible impending death

Goals

The goals of nursing care for the patient who is hemorrhaging are increased cardiac output and reduced fear.

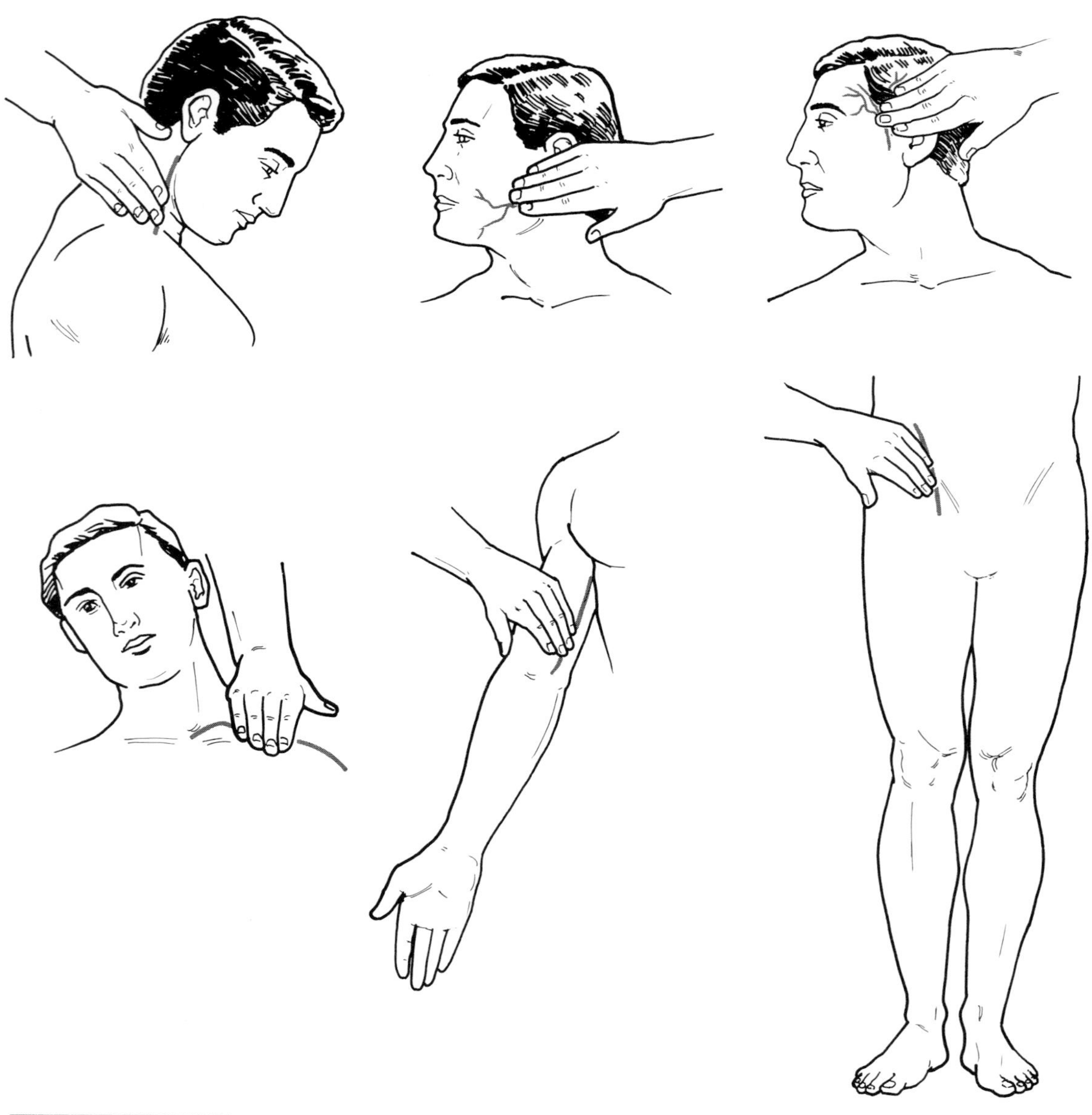

FIGURE 13-8
Major arterial pressure points.

Interventions

The immediate treatment for external bleeding is direct, continuous pressure. Ideally, a sterile dressing is placed over the wound. If sterile supplies are unavailable, a clean cloth can be used. The injured part is elevated (unless fracture is suspected) and immobilized. Elevation decreases blood flow to the area; immobilization prevents dislodging clots that have formed. After bleeding stops, a large dressing, if available, is secured over the wound. The nurse reinforces the dressing, but does not change it.

If direct wound pressure and elevation fail to control bleeding, pressure is applied to the main artery that supplies the area. Figure 13–8 depicts the major arterial pressure points.

The use of a tourniquet to control severe bleeding in an extremity is controversial. Some sources do not recommend it under any circumstances. Others indicate it should be used only as a last resort when a limb is mangled, crushed, or amputated. The least dangerous tourniquet is an pneumatic one like a blood pressure cuff that allows the nurse to control pressure. The cuff is inflated above the victim's systolic blood pressure. If the victim's blood pressure cannot be measured, the cuff is inflated until the bleeding stops. Once the cuff is inflated, only a physician should remove it.

Unfortunately, modern equipment often is not available in emergencies outside the hospital. A makeshift tourniquet can be made using a long strap such as a tie or belt, a folded cloth pad, and a stick. The pad is

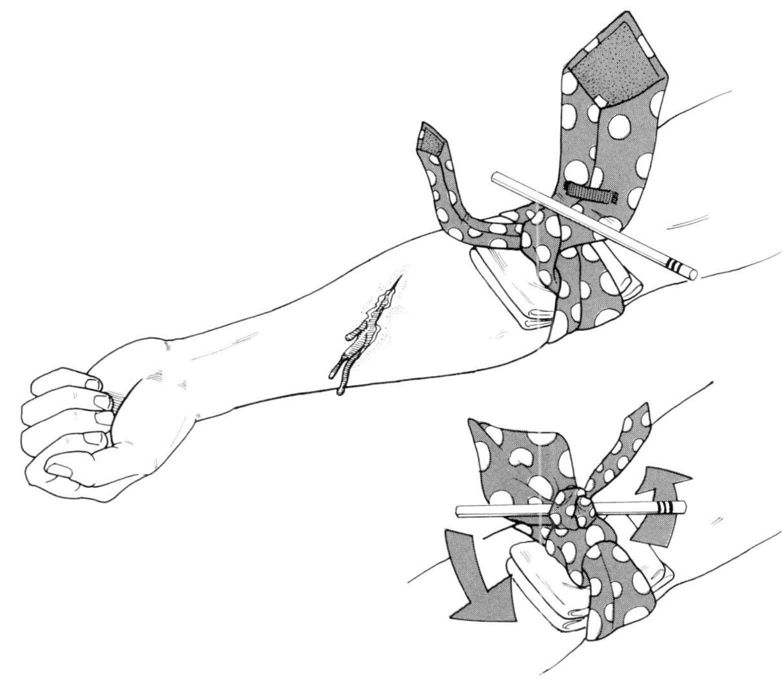

FIGURE 13-9
A makeshift tourniquet.

placed on the inner surface of the limb. The strap is wrapped twice around the limb and over the pad. The stick is inserted into the strap and tied as illustrated in Figure 13–9. Pressure is applied by twisting the stick. Once the bleeding stops, the tourniquet is stabilized and not disturbed until medical help is available. When a victim with a tourniquet is transferred, it is very important for the receiving caregiver to know a tourniquet is in place.

EPISTAXIS. One type of bleeding that requires special intervention is epistaxis (nosebleed). Blood may come from the anterior or the posterior portion of the nose. Most anterior nosebleeds respond to pressure. The patient is instructed to sit down and lean the head forward. The nostrils are pinched shut as shown in Figure 13–10 for at least 10 minutes. In most cases, this stops the bleeding. Afterward, the patient is advised not to blow or pick at the nose for several hours. Continued bleeding or bleeding from the posterior area of the nose requires medical treatment as described in Chapter 49.

Evaluation

Criteria for evaluating the success of interventions for hemorrhage are improved pulse quality, cessation of bleeding, patient's statement of reduced anxiety, and calm appearance.

TRAUMATIC INJURY

Traumatic injuries result from a variety of events. Sports injuries, motor vehicle accidents, falls, and acts of violence often require emergency treatment at the scene of the injury.

Fractures

A fracture is a break in a bone. A fracture may be described as simple or compound, open or closed, complete or incomplete. A simple (closed) fracture does not break the skin. A compound (open) fracture is one in which the ends of the broken bone protrude through the skin. In a complete fracture, the broken ends are separated. The bone ends in an incomplete fracture are not separated. Other types of fractures are discussed in Chapter 38.

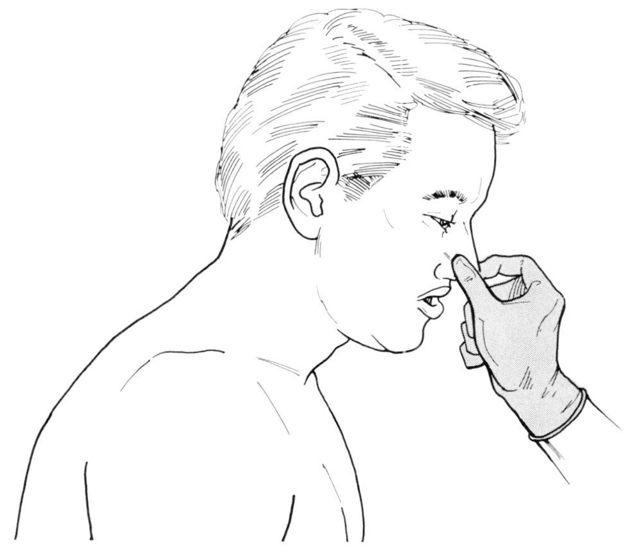

FIGURE 13-10
Epistaxis may be controlled by having the patient sit up, lean forward slightly, and pinch the nostrils.

ASSESSMENT. The nurse assesses the victim of traumatic injury for signs and symptoms of fractures. The primary symptom of fracture is pain, although some people, especially the elderly, do not always have severe pain with fractures. Numbness and tingling may be present as a result of injury to nerves and blood vessels. Objective signs of fracture include deformity, swelling, discoloration, decreased function, and bone fragments protruding through the skin. Suspected fractures should be treated as such until they are ruled out by the physician.

NURSING DIAGNOSIS. Nursing diagnoses for the emergency treatment of the person with a suspected fracture are the following:

- **High Risk for Trauma** related to movement of unstable fractures
- **Pain** related to tissue trauma

GOALS. Goals of emergency nursing intervention are avoidance of additional trauma and pain.

INTERVENTIONS. The key to emergency management of fractures is immobilization. The nurse immobilizes the injured part including joints above and below the injury to avoid further trauma to the bone and surrounding soft tissue. The nurse does not attempt to straighten a broken bone but splints it in the position that it was found. Boards, sticks, magazines, and strips of cloth can all be used to immobilize an injured limb. A cool pack may be applied to reduce swelling.

Severe bleeding may be present with compound fractures. In such cases, the nurse applies direct pressure to the artery above the injury. The victim is given nothing by mouth and is transported for medical care as soon as possible.

EVALUATION. The primary criterion for evaluating emergency care of the patient with a suspected fracture is immobilization of injured parts without evidence of additional injury or pain.

Strains and Sprains

Strains are injuries to muscles or to the tendons that attach them to bones, or to both. Sprains are injuries to ligaments. Ligaments are bands of tissue that hold bones in position in the joints. These injuries are painful, and swelling may be present. Emergency treatment for both is immobilization and elevation. The victim should see a physician for further evaluation.

Head Injury

Head injury is not always apparent immediately after an accident. It should be suspected with any type of blow to the head or unexplained loss of consciousness. An important complication of head injury is increased intracranial pressure caused by bleeding or swelling associated with trauma. Increased intracranial pressure progressively impairs brain function and may lead to cessation of breathing.

Elderly people are at special risk for head injuries because they are more likely to have sensory deficits, unstable gait, or circulatory disorders. Head injuries may be overlooked if the nurse attributes confusion to age without finding out the person's usual level of mental function.

ASSESSMENT. When the nurse suspects head injury, assessment includes inspection and palpation of the head and evaluation for signs and symptoms of increased intracranial pressure. Signs of increased intracranial pressure are the following:

- Change in behavior, agitation, confusion
- Decreasing level of consciousness
- Pupil dilation or constriction, inequality, slow or no response to light
- Impaired sensory or motor function
- Increasing blood pressure with widening pulse pressure
- Decreasing pulse and respiratory rates

The nurse is also alert for the leakage of cerebrospinal fluid that occurs with basilar skull fractures. Cerebrospinal fluid leakage is usually seen as clear, colorless fluid draining from the nose or ear. If the fluid drains onto a white cloth, it appears as a yellowish stain. If there is blood in the fluid, it produces a pink "halo" around the yellow center.

NURSING DIAGNOSIS. The following are nursing diagnoses that might apply to the patient with a head injury during the emergency phase of treatment:

- **Ineffective Breathing Patterns** related to neurologic trauma
- **High Risk for Injury** related to increasing intracranial pressure, improper movement after spinal fracture

GOALS. The goals of emergency nursing care of the patient with a head injury are adequate ventilation and absence of further injury.

INTERVENTIONS. The victim of a head injury must be assessed by a physician as soon as possible. Because head injuries often accompany spinal injuries, one must always treat the victim as if there were a spinal injury until it is ruled out. This is especially important when the victim is unconscious or when no history can be obtained. The victim is kept flat with proper alignment of the neck and head. A backboard is used for transporting the victim.

Even if the head injury seems to be minor, the physician may admit the victim to the hospital for observation as a precaution. This is because bleeding and swelling are sometimes so slow that signs and symptoms of increased intracranial pressure may not appear until hours or even weeks after the initial injury. Detailed neurologic assessment and care of the hospitalized patient with a head injury are covered in Chapter 25.

EVALUATION. Criteria for evaluating the achievement of nursing goals for the emergency care of the head injury patient are normal respiratory rate and depth, normal pulse rate, and stable neurologic status with secure spinal immobilization.

Neck and Spinal Injuries

The nurse suspects neck and spinal injuries with head injuries, especially if the victim has had a diving or motor vehicle accident. The victim should not be moved during the initial assessment unless absolutely necessary. Improper movement of the patient with a spinal injury may damage the spinal cord, causing permanent paralysis. After a diving injury, efforts are made to immobilize the neck and back while removing the victim from the water.

ASSESSMENT. When there is a neck or spinal injury, breathing and circulation are assessed first, and resuscitation is begun if needed. The nurse then assesses the victim's movement and sensation in all extremities.

NURSING DIAGNOSIS AND GOAL. The priority nursing diagnosis for the person with a neck or spinal injury is high risk for trauma related to improper movement of the fractured spine. The goal is absence of additional injury.

INTERVENTIONS. An expert emergency team is summoned immediately when neck or spinal injury is suspected. A professional team has the equipment and the expertise to immobilize and transport the victim properly. In remote or life-threatening settings, the victim may have to be moved. If so, a rolled towel or article of clothing can be used as a collar to support the neck. The victim can then be moved by log-rolling to one side and then rolling back onto a board, keeping the spine as straight as possible. Throughout the movement, one rescuer supports the head while two others support the shoulders, hips, and legs.

EVALUATION. Successful nursing intervention is based on continuous immobilization of the back and spine and transport for medical care.

Eye Injury

Eye conditions that warrant immediate attention include foreign bodies, chemical contact, perforation of the globe, and eyelid trauma.

ASSESSMENT. After an injury, the nurse inspects the lid for trauma and the eye for redness, foreign bodies, or penetrating objects. To inspect for foreign bodies, the nurse everts the lids as shown in Figure 13–11. If the eye has been exposed to an irritant, the nurse attempts to determine what the substance was.

NURSING DIAGNOSIS. Nursing diagnoses for the patient with an eye injury include the following:

- **High Risk for Injury** related to foreign body in the eye
- **Impaired Tissue Integrity** related to chemical trauma

GOAL. The goal of emergency nursing care for an eye injury is minimized risk for injury.

INTERVENTIONS

Foreign Bodies. Foreign bodies that are not embedded can be removed by irrigation or by gently touching the object with the corner of a clean cloth or gauze pad.

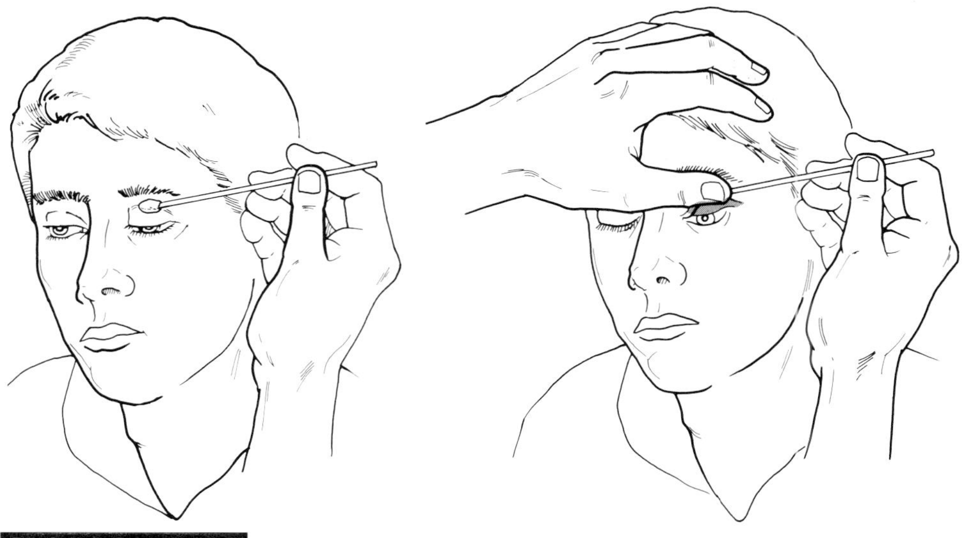

FIGURE 13-11

Eversion of the upper eyelid for inspection. *A*, Gently hold a cotton-tipped applicator against the closed lid. *B*, Use your thumb to evert the lid over the applicator.

Embedded foreign bodies should be removed *only* by a physician.

Chemical Contact. When chemicals come in contact with the eye, it should be flushed immediately. Ideally, sterile normal saline or water is used to irrigate the eye for 30 minutes. Tap water may be used if sterile water is not available. Irrigating fluid should flow from the inner canthus to the outer canthus of the eye. Even if the flushing seems to relieve all symptoms, the patient should see a physician to assess the eye for injury.

Perforation of the Globe. If an object perforates the eye, the nurse should *not* attempt to remove it. To do so may cause greater harm. The important thing is to limit movement of the object and the eye and to transport the victim for immediate medical care. The injured eye can be protected by covering it with a shield that does not touch the object. Sometimes an inverted paper cup can be taped over the eye. Since the eyes move together, the unaffected eye is patched as well. This limits movement in both eyes. The patient should be told why both eyes need to be covered.

Eyelid Trauma. Eyelid trauma requires medical evaluation because there is always a chance that the globe might have been injured as well. Direct pressure should *not* be applied to a bleeding eyelid. If the globe has been injured, pressure could cause greater harm. A loose dressing should be applied and the victim transported for medical care.

Ear Trauma

The position and structure of the external ear make it vulnerable to traumatic injury. The most serious injury to the external ear is avulsion. Avulsion means that all or part of the auricle is torn loose.

ASSESSMENT. The nurse assesses the extent of the injury, whether any tissue is fully separated, and the severity of bleeding. Direct pressure is applied to the site of the injury to control bleeding if necessary.

NURSING DIAGNOSIS AND GOAL. If bleeding is under control, the priority nursing diagnosis for a traumatic injury to the auricle is impaired tissue integrity related to mechanical destruction. The goal is preservation of the tissue to maximize successful repair.

INTERVENTIONS. If the injured part is actually separated, reattachment may be possible. The tissue is retrieved, wrapped in plastic, kept cool, and transported with the victim.

EVALUATION. Criteria for successful nursing intervention are recovery, protection, and transport of avulsed tissue with the patient.

Chest Injury

Injuries to the chest can result in serious impairment of respiratory function. Chest injuries are open or closed. The most critical injuries are open pneumothorax, flail chest, massive hemothorax, and cardiac tamponade. Any injury at or below the nipple line may cause both chest and abdominal injuries.

ASSESSMENT. When there is a chest injury, assessment of respiratory status always takes first priority. The nurse observes the rate and character of the victim's respirations. Other important aspects of assessment are the skin color, the pulse rate and rhythm, the symmetry of the chest wall movement, and the presence of any apparent injuries to the chest. Signs and symptoms of chest injuries that impair respirations are dyspnea, tachycardia, restlessness, cyanosis, asymmetric or other abnormal chest wall movement, and abnormal sounds associated with breathing. The nurse also notes the patient's mental state and level of consciousness.

NURSING DIAGNOSIS AND GOAL. The primary nursing diagnosis for chest injury is impaired gas exchange related to altered anatomic structure. The goal is adequate oxygenation.

INTERVENTIONS. Specific interventions for emergency management of specific injuries are described here. Care of the patient with chest wounds is covered in greater detail in Chapter 28.

Pneumothorax. Open chest wounds that penetrate the pleural cavity allow air to enter (pneumothorax). This causes collapse of the lung on the affected side. Signs and symptoms of pneumothorax include dyspnea and asymmetric chest wall movement. A "sucking" sound may be heard as air moves in and out of the wound with respirations. The wound should be covered immediately with a vented dressing. A vented dressing is taped on three sides and left loose on the fourth side. This allows air to escape but not to enter the chest wound (Mitchell, 1992). An occlusive dressing is not used because air from the lung continues to escape into the pleural cavity. If the air had no outlet, pressure would build up and eventually a tension pneumothorax could develop.

Flail Chest. Flail chest is the term used when several adjacent ribs are broken in more than one place. The fractures cause a loss of support in the affected section of the chest wall. The affected section moves inward instead of outward on inspiration. On expiration, it moves outward instead of inward (Fig. 13–12). The abnormal chest wall movement is called *paradoxical motion*, and it causes impaired gas exchange. Flail chest is treated by providing support for the injured area. A small pad or pillow can be held or taped over the injury to splint the ribs.

Hemothorax and Cardiac Tamponade. Hemothorax is the accumulation of blood in the pleural cavity that causes the lung or lungs to collapse. Cardiac tamponade is the presence of blood in the pericardial sac that causes decreased cardiac output. If a trauma victim has increasing respiratory or circulatory failure, one or both

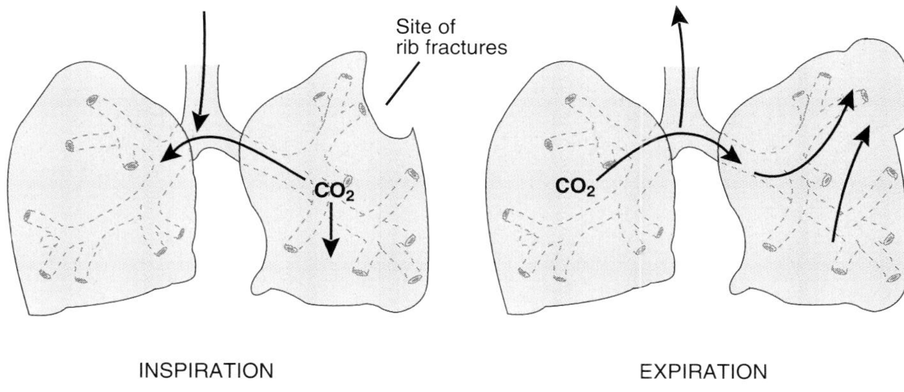

FIGURE 13-12
Paradoxical motion caused by loss of chest wall support.

of these complications may be present. These conditions cannot be diagnosed directly or treated by the first aid care provider. The victim requires prompt treatment in a medical facility.

EVALUATION. Criteria for evaluating nursing care of the patient with a chest injury are absence of dyspnea, normal pulse and respiratory rates, and normal skin color.

Abdominal Injury

ASSESSMENT. The nurse assesses the abdomen for evidence of injury. In addition to asking the patient about abdominal symptoms, the nurse inspects the abdomen for abnormalities. Internal abdominal injuries are suspected when the victim complains of abdominal pain or the abdomen shows evidence of trauma or distention. The protrusion of internal organs through a wound is called evisceration. Eviscerated organs are subject to trauma and drying.

NURSING DIAGNOSIS. Nursing diagnoses for the patient who has an abdominal injury are the following:

- **Impaired Tissue Integrity** related to mechanical destruction
- **High Risk for Infection** related to break in skin, possible injury to intestinal tract

GOALS. The goals of nursing intervention are protection of injured tissue and decreased risk of infection.

INTERVENTIONS. Possible internal injuries require medical evaluation. The patient is given nothing by mouth while being prepared for transport. The nurse does not attempt to replace eviscerated organs in the abdomen as this may cause additional harm. Eviscerated organs are covered with some material such as plastic wrap or foil to conserve moisture and warmth. A saline-soaked sterile dressing is ideal, but is not likely to be available on the scene of an accident. The wound is then covered with a clean cloth and the patient transported to a hospital.

EVALUATION. The main criterion for evaluating emergency nursing care of the patient with an abdominal wound is protection of the wound.

BURNS

Care of the burn patient is discussed in detail in Chapter 46. This chapter addresses only emergency measures. When a burn accident occurs, the immediate concern is to stop the burning process. A victim whose clothing is burning should drop to the ground and roll to extinguish the flames. Rescuers can smother the flames with coats or blankets or extinguish the flames with water. Burning materials should be removed from the victim.

Assessment

The nurse first determines the type of burn that has occurred. If the victim has had a flame burn or has been in a closed, smoke-filled area, the nurse begins with assessment of respirations. Attention then turns to determining the extent and depth of the burns. The skin is inspected for color, blisters, and tissue destruction. Superficial burns are typically pink or red and painful. Deeper burns may be red, white, or black, and may destroy not only the skin but the underlying tissues as well. The deepest burns are not painful because nerves are destroyed. Because the depth of a burn is often not uniform, however, patients with deep burns often have pain.

Electrical burns are difficult to assess initially because the full extent of tissue damage may not be apparent for several days. In the event of chemical burns, the presence of any remaining chemical is noted and immediately removed.

Nursing Diagnosis

Depending on the severity and type of the burn, nursing diagnoses for the burn victim immediately following the injury may include the following:

- **Impaired Gas Exchange** related to inhalation or thermal injury, edema of airway tissues
- **Impaired Skin or Tissue Integrity,** or both, related to thermal destruction, chemical injury
- **Pain** related to thermal injury

Goals

Goals of first aid nursing care for the burn victim are adequate oxygenation, limited extent of injury, and reduced pain.

Interventions

The first concern is to ensure a patent airway and respirations. If the burns were caused by flames, fumes, or chemicals, the victim may have inhaled substances that cause respiratory impairment. Rescue breathing, if needed, is described with cardiopulmonary resuscitation. Other interventions are addressed for each of the major types of burns.

MINOR BURNS. Superficial burns usually do not require medical care. The first aid for minor superficial burns is to immerse the injured body part in cool water for 2 to 5 minutes. The old remedy of applying butter to the burn is not recommended.

SUNBURN. Sunburn is quite painful, especially when large areas of skin are affected. Topical preparations that contain benzocaine may be soothing. Many people believe that aloe vera is very effective in treating minor burns, but this treatment is still being studied. Children and elderly people with extensive sunburn sometimes require hospitalization for dehydration.

The public needs to be educated about the potential harm of excessive sun exposure. The long-term effects include premature aging of the skin and skin cancers. Measures to reduce sun exposure are recommended, including the use of sunscreens on exposed body surfaces.

EXTENSIVE BURNS. When a large body surface area is burned or any area is severely burned, the burn should be covered with a clean, dry dressing or cloth. Medications and absorbent materials are *not* placed on the burn. Burned fingers and toes are wrapped separately to keep them from sticking together. The victim must be transported for medical care immediately.

PHARMACOLOGY CAPSULE

Topical medications should not be applied to an extensive burn as a first aid measure.

CHEMICAL BURNS. Many chemicals are capable of causing injury to the skin and mucous membranes. The main goal of treatment of chemical burns is to dilute and remove the chemical as quickly as possible. Once a chemical has burned into the skin, it can continue to burn even after being flushed with water.

Contaminated clothing is removed. Liquid chemicals are flushed from the skin with running water for at least 30 minutes. Powdered chemicals are thoroughly dusted from the skin, then flushed with water for 30 minutes. If the dry chemical is not removed before flushing, the water may cause the chemical to become caustic, resulting in additional injury. A dressing or covering is then applied, and the victim transported for medical care.

Evaluation

Evaluation of emergency care of the burn victim is based on the absence of symptoms of respiratory distress (dyspnea, confusion, cyanosis) or respiratory arrest, the skin surfaces free of burning materials with burned surfaces protected as recommended, and the patient's statement of pain reduction.

HEAT AND COLD EXPOSURE

A number of mechanisms work to maintain body temperature within a fairly narrow range. If the body temperature is lowered or raised excessively, vital functions begin to fail. Infants and the elderly are less able to adapt to temperature extremes than other people. This places them at greater risk for excessive alterations in body temperature.

Extreme heat or cold may have local or systemic effects. Local thermal injuries are discussed elsewhere in this chapter under Burns. This section addresses systemic responses to heat and cold exposure and local cold injuries.

Heat Exposure

Excessive heat exposure may cause hyperthermia, a condition in which body temperature rises above 37.2°C (99°F). Heat edema and heat cramps are mild degrees of hyperthermia. Heat exhaustion and heat stroke are more serious.

HEAT EXHAUSTION. Heat exhaustion is most likely to develop when a person loses an excessive amount of fluid and is exposed to high environmental temperature and humidity. As the body temperature rises, so does the metabolic rate. This increases the demand for oxygen by body tissues. Cardiac output and heart rate increase at first, then fall. The loss of fluids causes hypovolemia (low blood volume) and electrolyte imbalances.

Assessment. The nurse assesses for signs and symptoms of heat exhaustion, including dizziness, headache, muscle cramps, nausea and vomiting, and sometimes collapse. The skin is usually pale and damp. The rectal temperature is elevated and may be as high as 41.1°C (106°F).

Nursing Diagnosis. Nursing diagnoses for the victim of heat exhaustion are the following:

- **Hyperthermia** related to exposure to heat, dehydration, and inappropriate clothing
- **High Risk for Fluid Volume Deficit** related to excessive fluid loss

Goals. The goals of nursing care for the patient with heat exhaustion are reduced body temperature and improved hydration.

Interventions. Heat exhaustion is treated by cooling and hydrating the victim. The person is moved to a cooler environment, preferably one that is air-conditioned, and clothing is loosened. Cool water can be splashed on the skin. Commercially prepared electrolyte drinks, if available, can be offered if the victim is alert.

Evaluation. Criteria for evaluating the outcomes of immediate nursing care of the patient with heat exhaustion are lowered body temperature, reduction of symptoms associated with heat exhaustion, intake and retention of fluids, and normal pulse rate and quality.

Prevention. Nurses can teach people how to prevent heat exhaustion. Points to emphasize are the following:

- Avoid strenuous activities outdoors when it is very hot
- Increase fluid intake to replace excessive fluid loss

HEATSTROKE. Heatstroke is defined as a body core temperature of 41.1°C (106°F) or greater. It is more serious than heat exhaustion. Heatstroke occurs when the mechanisms in the brain that regulate temperature fail. It is most often associated with strenuous activity in hot, humid weather. Some drugs such as diuretics and anticholinergics increase the risk of heatstroke by affecting the body's heat-reducing defenses.

When the body temperature reaches 41.1°C (106°F), the functions of the heart, kidneys, and central nervous system are depressed. The victim is unable to sweat and will die if the temperature is not lowered.

Assessment. When a person appears to have been affected by excessive heat, the nurse attempts to determine the severity of the condition. At first, heatstroke appears similar to heat exhaustion. The victim becomes dizzy, weak, and nauseated. As the condition worsens, the skin appears red and feels hot and dry. *Perspiration is noticeably absent.* If the condition is not reversed, the victim may collapse and have seizures. The body temperature may reach as high as 43.3°C (110°F).

Nursing Diagnosis. Nursing diagnoses for the patient experiencing heatstroke include the following:

- **Hyperthermia** related to heat, dehydration, and inappropriate clothing
- **High Risk for Injury** related to seizures secondary to hyperthermia

Goals. The goals of immediate nursing care for the victim of heatstroke are reduced body temperature and absence of complications of heatstroke.

Interventions. It is critical to cool the person quickly. Immediate transport for medical care is recommended. Anyone who cannot be transported immediately should be moved into the shade or to an air-conditioned area if possible. Wet, cool towels can be applied to the trunk and the extremities. Ice packs can be placed on the forehead and axilla. If a tub is available, the victim can be placed in a cool bath. Cooling measures are continued until the body temperature falls below 30.3°C (101°F).

Evaluation. Criteria for evaluating the outcomes of nursing measures in the immediate treatment of the victim of heatstroke are a cooler skin, a body temperature below 30.3°C (101°F), and an absence of seizures or associated injuries.

Cold Exposure

FROSTNIP AND FROSTBITE. Mild tissue damage caused by cold is called *frostnip.* The term *frostbite* is used for more serious injury. When the body is exposed to extreme cold, blood vessels in the skin and in the extremities constrict. Blood clots form, and circulation to the affected areas decreases. Circulatory impairment deprives tissues of oxygen and nutrients, causing cell injury and death. Ice crystals form in cells causing them to swell and rupture.

Assessment. When cold injury is suspected, the nurse assesses the presence of significant symptoms and the sites affected. Cold injury is painful at first; it then causes tingling followed by numbness. Sites most often affected are the nose, cheeks, fingers, and toes.

Nursing Diagnosis and Goal. The priority nursing diagnosis for the victim of frostbite is high risk for impaired skin integrity related to vascular changes caused by extreme cold exposure. The primary goal of nursing care for the victim of cold injury is minimal injury to affected tissue.

Interventions. The immediate treatment of mild cold injury is rapid rewarming. Cold hands can be warmed by placing them in the axillae or between the thighs.

Victims of more serious cold injuries require additional treatment and should be transported for medical care as soon as possible. If the victim is in a remote area, the rescuer seeks a setting where warm water is available. One should not attempt to thaw the tissue unless warmth can be maintained. The best way to rewarm frostbitten extremities is to immerse them in a warm water bath of 37.7 to 40.5°C (100–105°F). The affected areas should be handled very gently to avoid additional tissue trauma. *Do not* rub, massage, or apply cold to the tissue. As the tissue warms, the skin turns bright pink and blisters. Rewarming is very painful. If the procedure is done in a medical facility, analgesics are administered as ordered before the rewarming begins.

After warming the extremities, the nurse pats them dry and wraps them in sterile dressings. Each finger or toe is wrapped separately to prevent injured tissue from sticking together. The affected parts are immobilized and elevated. With severe or deep frostbite, thawed tissue dies and eventually has to be surgically débrided (removed).

Evaluation. The criterion for effective first aid care for the victim of cold injury is increased warmth of affected body areas.

HYPOTHERMIA. Hypothermia is a decrease in body core temperature below 36°C (95°F). It may be caused by prolonged exposure to cold, extremely cold temperatures, or immersion in cold water. Hypothermia causes depression of vital functions and, if not corrected, death results from cardiac arrhythmias.

Elderly people are susceptible to hypothermia because of loss of subcutaneous fat, diminished circulation, and reduced neural control over circulation. They are unable to conserve heat effectively. It has been found that confusion in some older people is caused by hypothermia. It may be helpful, therefore, to evaluate the temperature of confused patients. Additional warmth may result in improved function for some of them.

Assessment. The nursing assessment includes temperature measurement (if a thermometer is available) and observation for signs and symptoms of hypothermia. A rectal temperature lower than 36°C (95°F) is considered evidence of hypothermia. Shivering and impaired performance are present with mild hypothermia. Progressive chilling causes heart and respiratory rates and blood pressure to fall. Heart and breathing patterns become irregular, and cardiopulmonary arrest follows if the hypothermia is not treated.

Nursing Diagnosis. Nursing diagnoses for the patient with hypothermia include the following:

- Severe **Hypothermia** related to exposure to cold, inadequate clothing
- **Impaired Tissue Perfusion** related to hypothermia
- **Decreased Cardiac Output** related to dysrhythmias associated with rewarming

Goals. Goals of emergency nursing care for the patient with hypothermia are increased body temperature, improved tissue perfusion, and absence of cardiac complications of rewarming.

Interventions. Mild hypothermia is treated by wrapping the victim in warm, dry clothing and blankets. Victims of severe hypothermia should be transported immediately for treatment. They must be rewarmed aggressively, but it must be done gradually. Rewarming too rapidly sends lactic acid and cold blood from the extremities to the heart, possibly triggering cardiac dysrhythmias.

The torso is warmed first. It may be wrapped in blankets or immersed in tepid water. Once the body temperature reaches 36°C (95°F), attention can be turned to warming the extremities also. The physician may order internal rewarming when the patient reaches a medical facility. Internal rewarming measures include the use of warmed oxygen and intravenous fluids, peritoneal lavage, and extracorporeal blood warming.

Evaluation. Criteria for evaluating the effects of intervention for the hypothermia victim are temperature above 36°C (95°F), improved color and warmth of affected tissues, and normal cardiac rate (60–100 bpm) with regular rhythm.

POISONING

A poison is any substance that, in small quantities, is capable of causing illness or harm following ingestion, inhalation, injection, or contact with the skin. Large quantities of most chemicals, including all medications, can act as poisons. Even common drugs like aspirin, acetaminophen, and vitamins can be poisonous if taken in excessive amounts.

PHARMACOLOGY CAPSULE

Common drugs such as aspirin, acetaminophen, and vitamins can be poisonous if taken in excessive amounts.

Carbon Monoxide Poisoning

Carbon monoxide is an odorless, invisible gas emitted by automobile engines, gas stoves and furnaces, and burning charcoal as well as other burning materials. When carbon monoxide is inhaled, it enters the blood stream and promptly binds with hemoglobin. Carbon monoxide binds to hemoglobin much more readily than oxygen. Therefore, it soon occupies many of the sites on the hemoglobin needed to transport oxygen to the cells. The patient becomes hypoxemic and can die.

ASSESSMENT. The nurse assesses for signs and symptoms of carbon monoxide poisoning. Symptoms of early carbon monoxide poisoning are headache and shortness of breath with mild exertion. Dizziness, nausea, vomiting, and mental changes appear next. As the amount of carbon monoxide in the blood stream rises, the victim loses consciousness and develops cardiac and respiratory irregularities. A victim usually dies when the carbon monoxide bound with hemoglobin exceeds 70%. A clear indicator of carbon monoxide poisoning is a cherry red skin color; however, skin color is often pale or bluish with reddish mucous membranes.

NURSING DIAGNOSIS. The primary nursing diagnosis for the victim of carbon monoxide poisoning is impaired gas exchange related to carbon monoxide poisoning.

GOAL. The goal of nursing care for the emergency treatment of the victim of carbon monoxide poisoning is normal oxygenation.

INTERVENTIONS. The victim of carbon monoxide poisoning is removed immediately to fresh air. If the person is not breathing, rescue breathing is started. Emergency medical assistance is sought immediately. Oxygen should be given as soon as it is available. At the hospital the patient may be placed in a hyperbaric chamber. A hyperbaric chamber uses pressure to force oxygen into the blood and tissues.

EVALUATION. Criteria for evaluating the effects of nursing interventions are regular pulse with a rate of 60 to 100 beats per minute, regular respirations with a rate of 12 to 20 per minute, and mental alertness.

PREVENTION. Because carbon monoxide poisoning is usually accidental, measures must be taken to prevent poisoning additional victims from the same circumstances. Instructions that may prevent such poisoning include the following:

1. Keep gas furnaces and stoves in proper repair.
2. Burners that use gas must be vented to the outside.
3. Do not use charcoal or wood-burning devices in a closed area without ventilation.
4. Never let an automobile engine run in a closed garage.

Drug or Chemical Poisoning

Poisoning by drugs or chemicals can result from accumulation, excessive dosage, drug interactions, and ingestion of inappropriate substances.

ASSESSMENT. In situations that suggest poisoning, the nurse collects data about relevant signs and symptoms. The signs and symptoms vary with the type of poison. The history is an important part of the assessment of a poisoning victim and should include the following:

1. Name of the drug or chemical involved. If the victim cannot provide the information, look for clues. Save the container.
2. Amount of substance consumed.
3. Length of time since the substance was taken.
4. Last food consumed: amount, time.
5. Signs and symptoms that may be caused by poisons.
6. Victim's age and approximate weight.

NURSING DIAGNOSIS AND GOAL. The primary nursing diagnosis for the victim of drug or chemical poisoning is potential for injury related to poison. The general goal of nursing intervention for a poisoning victim is decreased or minimized injury caused by the poisoning agent.

INTERVENTIONS. Specific interventions depend on the exact poison. The product label often provides guidelines for appropriate treatment measures. Some general guidelines for treatment are as follows:

1. Give water to dilute ingested poisons.
2. Contact the local poison control center for information about proper treatment.
3. Induce vomiting *except:*
   a. with caustic substances or petroleum products.
   b. if the victim is already vomiting.
   c. if the victim is unconscious.
   d. if the victim is having seizures.

   Syrup of ipecac can be used to induce vomiting. The usual adult dose of syrup of ipecac is 15–30 ml taken with a large amount of water. If vomiting has not occurred after 20 minutes a second dose of 15 to 30 ml may be given.
4. Save urine and emesis (vomited material) for analysis.
5. Seek medical attention promptly.
6. If the victim is unconscious, position on the side and maintain an open airway. Do not try to give oral fluids or drugs.

PHARMACOLOGY CAPSULE

Syrup of ipecac can be used to stimulate vomiting in poisoning cases unless the victim has consumed caustic substances or petroleum products, the victim is already vomiting, or the victim is unconscious or having seizures.

Once the patient reaches an emergency facility, additional measures may be ordered. Gastric lavage and cathartics may be used to remove the remaining poison from the digestive tract. Activated charcoal may be ordered because it binds to many poisons, thus preventing their absorption.

Many drugs and chemicals have antidotes. Antidotes are substances that block or reverse the effects of other substances. If the poisonous substance is known, an antidote may be ordered.

EVALUATION. The criterion for evaluating successful intervention for drug or chemical poisoning is the absence of ill effects from the substance.

Food Poisoning

Food poisoning is caused by ingesting contaminated food. Contaminants can be bacteria, chemicals, or natural toxins. Bacteria most often associated with food poisoning are *Clostridium botulinum, Clostridium perfringens, Staphylococcus aureus,* and *Salmonella* spp. Table 13–2 summarizes the important features of each type of food poisoning.

ASSESSMENT. Victims of food poisoning often recognize the relationship between their symptoms and the ingestion of food. The most common symptoms of food poisoning are nausea, vomiting, abdominal cramps, and diarrhea. Botulism caused by *C. botulinum* has neurotoxic effects, including difficulty breathing, seeing, and swallowing. An important clue that food poisoning is causing the victim's symptoms is that all who consumed a certain food become ill.

NURSING DIAGNOSIS AND GOAL. The primary nursing diagnosis for the victim of food poisoning is potential for injury related to poisoning. The specific type of injury depends on the action of the contaminant. The goal of nursing care for the victim of food poisoning is the absence or reduction of ill effects from the poison.

INTERVENTIONS. In general, the treatment of food poisoning aims to identify the poison and decrease the symptoms. Analyses of vomited material and stool samples may be ordered.

Medical care is necessary if symptoms are severe or persist, especially in children and the elderly. The physician may order antiemetics and antidiarrheals, but sometimes vomiting and diarrhea are allowed to continue within limits to eliminate the offending substances. Intravenous fluids may be prescribed with severe vomiting and diarrhea. Patients with botulism may require ventilatory support.

EVALUATION. The criterion for evaluating the effects of intervention for food poisoning is diminished symptoms (e.g., decreased pain, respiratory rate of 12–20, depending on the poison).

PREVENTION. Most cases of food poisoning can be attributed to improper storage or preparation of perishable foods. People need to be taught the importance of cleanliness when handling and cooking food as well as the means of preparing food for storage.

BITES AND STINGS

Snakes, ticks, bees, wasps, household pets, and even humans are capable of causing serious harm by their bites or stings. The most serious effects of bites are anaphylaxis, infection, and tissue destruction.

TABLE 13–2
FOOD POISONING

ORGANISM	SOURCE	SIGNS AND SYMPTOMS	TREATMENT	PREVENTION
Clostridium botulinum	Improper home canning	Onset 18–36 hr after ingestion: nausea and vomiting, headache, dry throat and mouth, dysphagia, diplopia; 4–5 days after ingestion: descending paralysis affecting speech, breathing, and swallowing; can be fatal	Gastric lavage, IV fluids, trivalent botulism antitoxin (ABE), mechanical ventilation if needed	Discard food containers that are swollen or have broken seals; spores are not destroyed by boiling; do not depend on taste or odor to detect *C. botulinum*
Staphylococcus aureus	Poor hygiene of food handlers; inadequate refrigeration of food, especially milk products and mayonnaise	Onset within 6 hr: weakness, nausea and vomiting, diarrhea, abdominal cramps; rarely fatal	IV fluids, antiemetics, sedation	Proper refrigeration of food; good hygiene
Clostridium perfringens	Improper canning; inadequately cooked meat or poultry	Onset 6–12 hr after ingestion: abdominal cramps, diarrhea	Antidiarrheals	Thorough cooking
Salmonella spp.	Contaminated food; poorly cooked meat or eggs	Abdominal cramps, diarrhea, nausea and vomiting	Antidiarrheals, antiemetics, IV fluids	Thorough washing and cooking

IV, Intravenous.

Assessment

In the assessment, the nurse tries to determine the type of bite the patient has received. The bite wound is inspected to identify the characteristics of the actual bite site and the changes in surrounding tissue. The nurse asks about any symptoms that developed after the bite such as pain, edema, numbness, tingling, nausea, fever, dizziness, and dyspnea.

Nursing Diagnosis

Nursing diagnoses for the patient who has been bitten include the following:

- **High Risk for Infection** related to (human, animal, insect) bite
- **High Risk for Injury** related to exposure to allergens or toxins

Goals

Goals of nursing care for the emergency treatment of bite victims include wound cleanliness and absence of allergic reaction or toxic effects.

Interventions for Specific Bites

SNAKEBITE. The poisonous snakes commonly found in the United States are the rattlesnake, copperhead, cottonmouth water moccasin, and coral snake. Unfortunately, people are often so alarmed at being bitten that they may not be able to provide a good description of the snake. It is helpful to describe the shape of the head and the color to assist in identification. If the snake has been captured or killed, it should be taken with the victim to the hospital.

Signs and Symptoms. The site of a snakebite is examined for characteristic findings. The bites of poisonous snakes usually leave two distinct fang marks, although a finger or a toe may be pierced by only one fang. Venom is injected through the fangs into the victim. Venom may act by affecting the nervous system or the blood and blood vessels.

Venom that affects the nervous system is neurotoxic. Neurotoxic venom can cause nausea and vomiting, dizziness, tachycardia, muscular twitching, and respiratory distress.

Local effects include discoloration, pain, and mild to severe edema.

Interventions. The immediate objective of treatment is to limit absorption of the venom. The part where the bite is located should be immobilized and kept at or below the level of the heart.

A wide, constricting band can be applied 2 to 4 inches above the bite. The band should be just tight enough to stop lymph and venous blood flow but not tight enough to stop arterial blood flow. The nurse should be able to detect the pulse below the band.

At one time people were advised to cut the bite wound and suck out the venom. This procedure is controversial as an inexperienced person may cause serious injury. In general, it is not recommended unless medical help will not be available for several hours. To be useful, incision and suction must be done within 30 minutes after the bite.

When incision and suction are appropriate, small side-by-side incisions (⅛ to ¼ inch long and ⅛ inch deep) are made over each fang mark. The incisions should *not* cross each other. Suction is then applied to remove venom from the bite. The type of suction cup supplied in snakebite kits is ideal. If it is not available, the mouth can be used if the oral tissues are healthy and intact.

The application of ice or cold packs is no longer recommended. This practice has been found to contribute to local tissue injury.

The victim should be transported to a medical facility as soon as possible. The physician may order antivenom to counteract the effects of the venom. Some tissue around the bite often becomes necrotic and must be removed surgically.

INSECT BITE OR STING. Insect bites and stings are potentially fatal for those who are very sensitive to their venom. The venom of bees, wasps, hornets, and ants causes severe allergic reactions in some people. The most serious type of allergic reaction is anaphylactic shock.

Signs and Symptoms. For most people, bites simply cause local itching, edema, and erythema. People who have serious allergies react with systemic symptoms of urticaria (hives), edema, and possibly anaphylaxis. Anaphylaxis is a severe, potentially fatal, allergic reaction. Bronchial constriction causes tightness in the chest with progressive difficulty breathing. Peripheral blood vessels dilate and fluid leaks from the capillaries causing a decrease in blood volume. The victim's blood pressure falls. If the process is not reversed, the victim quickly loses consciousness and dies. The nurse should especially anticipate anaphylaxis in victims who develop systemic symptoms rapidly. If anaphylaxis is going to develop, it usually happens within 30 minutes after the bite.

Interventions. Mild bite reactions are painful and annoying but not dangerous. Local discomfort may be relieved somewhat by applying calamine lotion or a paste of baking soda or meat tenderizer.

Only the honeybee leaves its stinger in the victim. The stinger continues to inject venom after it detaches from the bee. It should be promptly removed with a scraping motion rather than by grasping and pulling on it. Pinching the stinger to grasp it injects more venom.

People who know they are severely allergic to insect venom should carry emergency epinephrine. Aqueous epinephrine 1:1000 is given subcutaneously after a bite or sting to prevent anaphylaxis. The usual adult dose is 0.1 to 0.5 ml. This dose can be repeated after 20 minutes if needed.

PHARMACOLOGY CAPSULE

Severe allergic responses are treated with 0.1 to 0.5 ml of 1:1000 aqueous epinephrine administered subcutaneously to prevent anaphylaxis.

A band can also be applied above the bite if it is on an extremity to slow the absorption of venom. The band should not be tight enough to cut off arterial circulation.

The patient with severe allergies should be taken to a medical facility. In addition to epinephrine, drugs used to prevent or treat anaphylaxis are diphenhydramine chloride (Benadryl), aminophylline, and hydrocortisone.

TICK BITES. Tick bites require attention because ticks carry organisms that cause several serious diseases including Rocky Mountain spotted fever and Lyme disease.

People usually discover they have been bitten when they find ticks attached to the skin. Because victims may be unaware of the presence of ticks at first, people who have been in wooded areas need to check themselves carefully for ticks. They can easily be missed on hairy parts of the body and in body folds.

Once the tick is discovered, it needs to be removed promptly. The problem is that the insect burrows part of the head in the skin. The nurse attempts to remove the tick intact, without leaving the embedded part in the skin or crushing the tick. Sources disagree on the best way to remove ticks. The Centers for Disease Control and Prevention recommends grasping the tick near the victim's skin with tweezers and using a firm, steady motion to pull the tick loose. Others suggest covering it with mineral oil or petroleum jelly and waiting until the insect loosens its attachment to the skin. Apparently the oily substance interferes with the tick's breathing, causing it to release its hold. There is concern that these interventions may cause the tick to deposit infectious material in the bite wound.

After the tick has been removed, it is inspected to see if it is intact. The site is washed with soap and water, and an antiseptic is applied. The patient is instructed to have a blood test for Lyme disease approximately 2 months later. Lyme disease causes flu-like symptoms. Neurologic and joint problems develop in some people. If Lyme disease is diagnosed, it is treated with antibiotics.

In addition to Lyme disease, tick bites may infect the victim with the parasites that cause Rocky Mountain spotted fever. Symptoms of Rocky Mountain spotted fever appear 3 to 10 days after the bite and include chills, fever, headache, pain behind the eyes, joint and muscle pain, and a rash. The rash begins on the wrists and ankles and spreads to the extremities, the trunk, and sometimes the face. Tetracycline and chloramphenicol are effective treatments for Rocky Mountain spotted fever. If not treated, the infection can be fatal.

SPIDER BITES. Most spider bites cause only local tissue reactions that do not require medical care. The bites of the black widow and brown recluse spiders can be very serious.

The black widow is easily recognizable because of the red hourglass on its abdomen. The venom is neurotoxic and causes pain, nausea and vomiting, fever, weakness, muscle cramps, and headache. More serious effects include respiratory distress, hypertension, seizures, and shock. The site of the sting should be washed, a cool compress applied, and the victim transported for medical care. Antivenin is available for black widow spider bites. Constricting bands have not been found to reduce the effects of the venom.

The brown recluse spider is light brown in color with a fiddle-shaped dark brown mark on the thorax. The bite is not especially painful, but within a few hours the area usually swells. Initially, a bluish ring appears around the bite. Later the bite appears to be surrounded by a white ring encircled by a red "halo."

Some people experience nausea and vomiting, fever, and joint pain. Severe cardiac, renal, and neurologic reactions are uncommon. Three to 4 days after a brown recluse spider bite, the affected tissue becomes necrotic. Eventually the tissue sloughs off or needs to be débrided. The injury can be so extensive that reconstructive surgery is needed. Medical attention should be sought for these bites, but there is no specific antivenin to counteract the venom.

ANIMAL BITES. Animal bites should be cleaned thoroughly and a bulky dressing applied. The patient is advised to have a tetanus booster if immunizations are not current. Animal bites are treated very seriously because of the risk of rabies and other infections. Untreated rabies is almost always fatal.

The animal should be held for observation if possible. Pet owners should be asked to show proof of rabies vaccinations. Most cities have ordinances regarding handling of animals that have bitten people. The caregiver may be required to report the bite to the police or to the health department. The usual pattern is to require the animal to be quarantined and observed for 10 days. If there is no evidence of disease, no rabies treatment is needed. If the animal shows signs of rabies or cannot be located, the victim should be given prophylactic (preventive) rabies vaccines. There are several types of rabies vaccine. The newer vaccine is given in five doses over a 1-month period. This is much less distressing than the daily injections required with older forms of the vaccine.

HUMAN BITES. Human bites are potentially very dangerous because of the risk of infection. The most common site is the hand or fingers, caused by hitting a person in the mouth. Human bite wounds should be cleaned thoroughly and dressed. The victim should seek medical attention.

Evaluation

Criteria for evaluating care of a victim of a bite include a wound that is free of debris, a patient who is alert without dyspnea, and an absence of specific toxic effects.

Prevention

People who are very sensitive to venom should be taught how to avoid and treat bites. The following points should be made in the teaching plan:

1. Wear a medical alert tag stating "Allergic to insect bites."
2. Obtain an emergency allergy treatment kit. Learn to use it. Teach a family member to use it. Carry it with you at all times.
3. Avoid perfumes, hair spray, and bright colors when working outside. Insects are drawn to strong scents and bright colors.
4. Wear long pants and sleeves, shoes and socks, and gloves when gardening.
5. Keep the car windows closed when driving.
6. Consider desensitizing injections if recommended by a physician. These injections gradually reduce sensitivity to venom.

LEGAL ASPECTS OF EMERGENCY CARE

In the first aid treatment of emergencies outside the hospital, the nurse is expected to demonstrate the same skill, knowledge, and care that would be provided by other nurses in the same community with the same credentials. Good Samaritan laws in most states limit liability and provide protection against malpractice claims when health care providers render first aid at the scene of an emergency. These laws do not protect the nurse in the event of gross negligence or willful misconduct.

BIBLIOGRAPHY

Alexander, J., Marshall, E., & Hambright, F. D. (1991). Would you recognize this emergency? *RN, 54*(1), 26–31.

American Heart Association. (1988). *Health care provider's manual for basic life support.* Dallas, TX: Author.

American Heart Association. (1994). *Instructor's manual for basic life support.* Dallas, TX: Author.

Arendt, D. L., & Arendt, D. B. (1992). Rescue operations for snakebite. *American Journal of Nursing, 92*(7), 26–30.

Aumick, J. E. (1991). Head trauma. *RN, 54*(4), 27–32.

Boyd-Monk, H. (1989). Eye trauma. *RN, 52*(12), 22–29.

Calistro, A. M. (1993). Burn care basics and beyond. *RN, 56*(3), 26–33.

Chandra, N. C. (1992). Interim training guidelines for basic life support. *Currents, 3*(4). American Heart Association and the Citizen CPR Foundation, Inc.

Cuzzell, J. Z., & Rodriquez, L. A. (1989). How to use a bag-valve-mask device for artificial ventilation. *American Journal of Nursing, 89*(7), 932–933.

Deglin, J. H., Vallerand, A. H., & Russin, M. M. (1991). *Davis's drug guide for nurses* (2nd ed.). Philadelphia: F. A. Davis.

Doenges, M. E., & Moorhouse, M. F. (1991). *Nursing diagnoses with interventions* (3rd ed.). Philadelphia: W. B. Saunders.

Hefti, D. (1991). Chest trauma. *RN, 54*(5), 28–32.

Hodgson, B. B., Kizior, R. J., & Kingdon, R. T. (1993). *Nurse's drug handbook.* Philadelphia: W. B. Saunders.

Howell, E., Widra, L., & Hill, M. G. (1988). *Comprehensive trauma nursing.* Glenview, IL: Scott, Foresman, and Co.

Huston, C. J. (1993). Assessing a spider bite. *Nursing 93, 23*(2), 33.

Ignatavicius, D. D., & Bayne, M. V. (1991). *Medical-surgical nursing: A nursing process approach.* Philadelphia: W. B. Saunders.

Jackson, S. (1991). Assessing a femoral fracture. *Nursing 91, 21*(11), 57.

Jackson, S. (1992). Assessing a head injury. *Nursing 92, 22*(9), 49.

JAMA. (1992). *Guidelines for cardiopulmonary resuscitation and emergency cardiac care.* Chicago: Author.

Jarvis, C. (1992). *Physical examination and health assessment.* Philadelphia: W. B. Saunders.

Jepson, D. L. (1992). Lightning injury. *American Journal of Nursing, 92*(8), 39–42.

Klein, D. M. (1991). Shock. *Nursing 91, 21*(11), 74–76.

Lancaster, M. J. (1990). Botulism: North to Alaska. *American Journal of Nursing, 90*(1), 60–62.

Mitchell, J. T. (1992). Nursing role in management: Lower respiratory problems. In S. M. Lewis & I. C. Collier (Eds.). *Medical-surgical nursing* (3rd ed., pp. 500–566). St. Louis: Mosby Year Book.

Moore, K. (1992). Do you know these new emergency protocols? *RN, 55*(11), 34–35.

O'Toole, M. (Ed.). (1992). *Miller-Keane encyclopedia and dictionary of medicine, nursing, and allied health* (5th ed.). Philadelphia: W. B. Saunders.

Paparone, P. (1990). The summer scourge of Lyme disease. *American Journal of Nursing, 90*(6), 44–47.

Potter, P. A., & Perry, A. G. (1992). *Fundamentals of nursing* (3rd ed.). St. Louis: C. V. Mosby.

Ratko, J. E. (1991). Pesticide poisoning. *Nursing 91, 21*(5), 33.

Rhoads, J. (1992). Nursing role in management: Selected emergency situations. In S. M. Lewis & I. C. Collier (Eds.). *Medical-surgical nursing* (3rd ed., pp. 1762–1778). St. Louis: Mosby Year Book.

Rich, J. (1993). 13 ways to protect your practice. *Nursing 93, 23*(2), 60–61.

Shlafer, M. (1993). *The nurse, pharmacology, and drug therapy* (2nd ed.). Redwood City, CA: Addison-Wesley Publishing Co.

Shovein, J. T., Land, L. P., & Richter, G. (1989). Near drowning. *American Journal of Nursing, 89*(5), 680–686.

Sidebottom, J. (1992). When it's hot enough to kill. *RN, 55*(8), 30–34.

Sullivan, S. A. (1992). How severe is this frostbite? *American Journal of Nursing, 92*(2), 59–64.

Walhout, M. E. (1992). Treat for hypothermia. *RN, 55*(4), 50–55.

Willens, J. S. (1991). B.C.L.S. forecast. *Nursing 91, 21*(11), 53–56.

Willens, J. S., & Copel, L. C. (1989). Performing CPR on adults. *Nursing 89, 19*(1), 34–43.

Adrianne Linton

CHAPTER 14

Surgical Care

OBJECTIVES

1. State the purpose of each type of surgery: diagnostic, exploratory, curative, palliative, and cosmetic.
2. List data to be included in the nursing assessment of the preoperative patient.
3. Identify the nursing diagnoses, goals, and interventions during the preoperative phase of the surgical experience.
4. Outline a preoperative teaching plan.
5. List the responsibilities of each member of the surgical team.
6. Explain the nursing implications of each type of anesthesia.
7. Explain how the nurse can help prevent postoperative complications.
8. List data to be included in the nursing assessment of the postoperative patient.
9. Identify nursing diagnoses, goals, and interventions for the postoperative patient.
10. Explain patient needs to be considered in discharge planning.

GLOSSARY

ANESTHESIOLOGIST A physician who specializes in the administration of anesthetics and monitors the patient while under anesthesia

ANESTHETIC An agent that abolishes the pain sensation

DEHISCENCE Separation of previously joined edges; reopening of a surgical wound

EVISCERATION Protrusion of body organs through an open wound

HYPOTHERMIA Reduction in body temperature

NURSE ANESTHETIST A registered nurse who specializes in the administration of anesthetics and monitors the condition of patients receiving anesthetics

OXIMETER A device that uses a photoelectric sensor to measure the oxygen saturation of the blood

PALLIATIVE Relieves symptoms or improves function without correcting the basic problem

SANGUINEOUS Bloody

SEROSANGUINEOUS Made up of blood and serum

SEROUS Containing serum

Surgical treatments have been performed since primitive times. Until quite recently, however, surgery was considered the last resort to be performed only when more conservative measures had failed. Advances in technology and science during the twentieth century brought antibiotics, safe anesthesia, and improved diagnosis and treatment of illness and injury. Surgery became safer and now is almost commonplace (Fig. 14–1).

Surgical procedures are performed in physicians' offices, clinics, ambulatory surgery centers, and full service hospitals. In all of these settings, nurses often play important roles. Nurses who care for patients before, during, and after surgery are called *perioperative nurses.* They admit surgical patients, do initial assessments, prepare them for surgery, assist in the procedures, and provide postoperative care.

PURPOSES OF SURGERY

Surgery may be done for a variety of reasons. Surgical procedures classified by purpose include diagnostic, exploratory, curative, palliative, and cosmetic.

DIAGNOSTIC SURGERY. Diagnostic surgery involves the removal and study of tissue to make an accurate diagnosis. An example is a biopsy of a skin lesion or a lump in breast tissue.

EXPLORATORY SURGERY. Exploratory surgery is a more extensive procedure than a biopsy. It usually requires opening a body cavity to diagnose and find out the extent of a disease process. A common example is an exploratory laparotomy in which the abdomen is opened to find the cause of unexplained pain. Some exploratory surgery can be done using specialized scopes inserted into the body through small incisions.

CURATIVE SURGERY. Curative surgery is done to remove diseased tissue or to correct defects. Removal of an inflamed appendix, for example, is curative for appendicitis. The term *ablation* refers to removal of tissue. Defects that can be corrected include cleft lip, arthritic joints, and hernias. The repair of damaged tissue is a reconstructive procedure, whereas a constructive procedure repairs congenitally malformed structures.

PALLIATIVE SURGERY. Palliative surgery relieves symptoms or improves function without correcting the basic problem. For example, palliative surgery may be done to remove a malignant tumor obstructing the intestine even though the cancer is widespread.

COSMETIC SURGERY. Cosmetic surgery can be done to correct serious defects that affect appearance but is often done simply because the patient wants to change a physical feature. Common cosmetic procedures are performed to change the shape of facial features, remove wrinkles, flatten the abdomen, and change the size or shape of the breasts.

VARIABLES AFFECTING SURGICAL OUTCOMES

Among the variables that must be considered when caring for surgical patients are age, nutritional status, fluid and electrolyte balance, medical diagnoses, drugs, and habits.

AGE

Health care providers and the elderly themselves often believe that surgery is dangerous for older people. This is unfortunate because modern surgical techniques

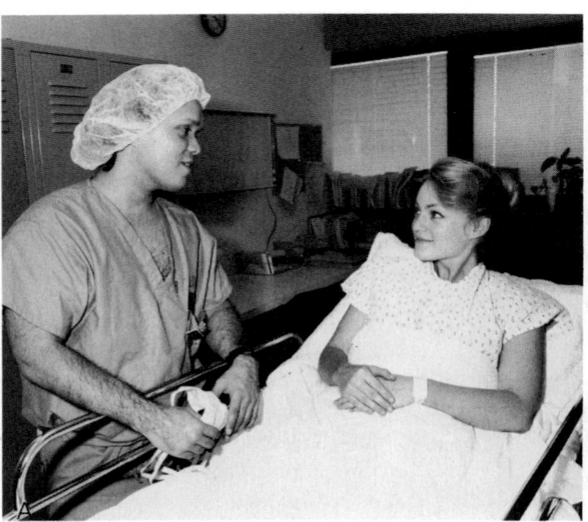

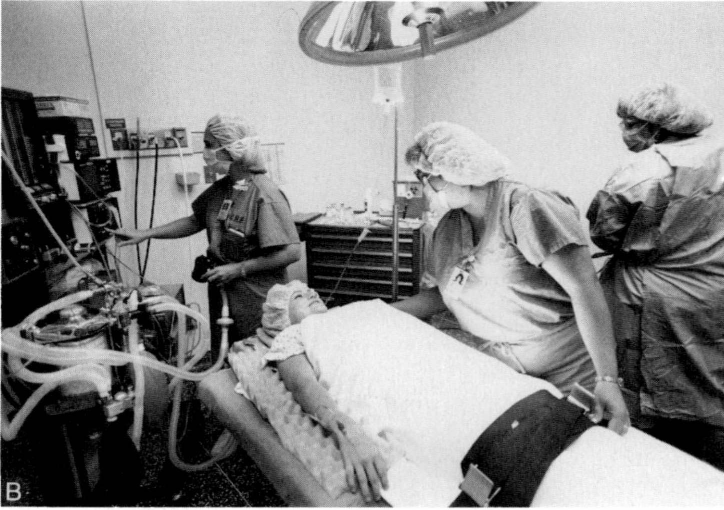

FIGURE 14-1
The nurse provides continuity of care for the surgical patient. (Photographs by Stephen Matteson, Jr.)

can restore many lost functions and often greatly improve the patient's quality of life. Elderly people who are in good health are likely to do just as well in surgery as younger people.

The older person, however, is often at greater risk for surgical complications for several reasons. Chronic health problems are more common among the elderly. These include high blood pressure, diabetes mellitus, heart failure, and arthritis. Hospitalization and surgery may disrupt control of these conditions, leading to impaired healing and recovery.

As a general rule, inactivity is not good for anyone. It is especially bad for the older person who takes longer to regain strength. One other important consideration is that older people may respond differently to drugs owing to changes in liver and kidney function and drug interactions.

Surgical risks for the elderly person can be greatly reduced if chronic conditions are well controlled, drug therapy is carefully evaluated, and the patient is well hydrated and nourished before surgery. For that reason emergency procedures carry greater risks for older patients than scheduled procedures.

NUTRITIONAL STATUS

Patients who are overweight or underweight present special problems. The patient who is malnourished is at risk for poor wound healing and infection. Obese patients are generally in surgery longer and are more likely to have postoperative respiratory and wound complications. Effective deep breathing exercises are limited by the excess weight. Because adipose tissue has poor blood supply, the healing process is slower. The obese patient also takes longer to recover from anesthesia because the drug tends to remain longer in adipose tissue.

FLUID BALANCE

Fluid and electrolyte status can have significant bearing on the outcome of surgery. Adequate fluids are necessary to maintain blood volume and urine output. Excess body fluid can overload the heart, aggravating the stress of surgery. Electrolyte imbalances may predispose the patient to dangerous cardiac arrhythmias. Physicians usually order laboratory tests to measure serum electrolytes before surgery. Fluid and electrolyte imbalances can then be corrected preoperatively.

MEDICAL DIAGNOSES

A number of medical conditions increase surgical risks or require special attention in the perioperative period. Patients with bleeding disorders are at risk for excessive bleeding and must be closely monitored. People with heart disease are at risk for cardiac complications related to anesthesia and to the stress of surgery. Chronic respiratory disease increases the risk of pulmonary complications as a result of anesthesia or hypoventilation. A patient who has liver disease may have impaired wound healing and may experience drug toxicity due to the inability to metabolize drugs effectively. Patients with diabetes mellitus also heal more slowly and are at greater risk for infection. In addition, the control of chronic conditions may be disrupted by surgery, which may require adjustments in therapy.

DRUGS

Many drugs, including cardiac drugs, antibiotics, antiarrhythmics, and anticonvulsants, have the potential to interact with anesthetic agents. Serious adverse effects may result. In addition, long-term drugs may require dosage adjustments owing to the effects of surgery or additional drugs.

HABITS

Habits that alert the nurse to the possibility of specific perioperative complications are smoking and alcohol use. Smoking increases the risk of pulmonary complications because secretions are more copious and tenacious and ciliary activity is less effective. Alcohol interacts with many drugs. In addition, patients who use alcohol excessively may have liver damage, which affects the metabolism of drugs including anesthetic agents.

THE PREOPERATIVE PHASE

The preoperative phase begins when a decision is made to perform a surgical procedure. It ends when the patient enters the operating room. During the preoperative phase the goals of nursing care are to prepare the patient for what to expect, to reduce patient anxiety, and to decrease the risk of complications during and after surgery.

PREOPERATIVE NURSING CARE

Assessment

When nonemergency surgery is scheduled, a thorough assessment is made, which starts with the physician's health history and physical examination. This is usually done before admission to the nursing care unit. Laboratory studies of blood and urine, a chest radiograph, and an electrocardiogram (ECG) may be done. Often these and other procedures are done on an outpatient basis before admission.

Most surgical facilities have standardized forms for assessing the newly admitted patient. The nursing assessment should obtain important data needed to plan preoperative, intraoperative, and postoperative care. It also provides baseline data for monitoring the patient's status (Table 14–1).

HEALTH HISTORY

Identifying Data. Identifying data are recorded, including the patient's age.

History of Present Illness. The history of the present illness describes the problem that is being treated surgically.

TABLE 14-1
PREOPERATIVE NURSING ASSESSMENT

HEALTH HISTORY
- Identifying data: age, marital status
- History of present illness: problem being treated surgically
- Past medical history: acute and chronic conditions, previous hospitalizations and surgeries, allergies, recent and current medications
- Review of systems: disabilities and limitations: hearing or vision loss, paralysis, stiffness, weakness, cognitive impairment; any current health deviations
- Functional assessment: occupation, roles, responsibilities, diet and fluid intake, exercise, tobacco and alcohol use, sources of stress and support, coping strategies, expectations of surgery

PHYSICAL EXAMINATION
- General survey: emotional state, ability to communicate, response to directions
- Height and weight
- Vital signs
- Skin: color, lesions, bruises, warmth, turgor, moisture
- Thorax: respiratory pattern and effort, breath sounds, apical pulse
- Abdomen: distention, scars, bowel sounds
- Extremities: color, hair distribution, lesions, deformities, range of motion, crepitus, pain, weakness
- Prostheses: hearing aids, eyeglasses, contact lenses, dentures, artificial limbs, other devices

Past Medical History. The patient's past medical history includes acute and chronic conditions, hospitalizations, surgeries, allergies, and drug history. All chronic health problems such as diabetes, heart failure, pulmonary disease, or kidney disease are recorded.

Any known allergies (food, drug, tape, chemical) are recorded according to agency policy. An allergy alert bracelet is commonly placed on the patient's wrist if there are any allergies. A number of drugs are routinely given to surgical patients. During and immediately after surgery, the patient is unable to report allergies. If an emergency should arise, the presence of allergies can be determined promptly.

A complete list is compiled of medications the patient is taking or has recently taken. Knowledge of the patient's drug history enables the nurse to anticipate possible effects of drug interactions.

PHARMACOLOGY

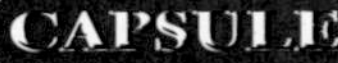

Long-term drug therapy such as anticoagulants and hypoglycemic agents may require adjustment before and after surgery.

REVIEW OF SYSTEMS. The nurse assesses each body system, noting any abnormalities. Any disabilities or limitations are recorded. The presence of acute problems including a cold or a bout of diarrhea could necessitate delay of a surgical procedure. In addition to the conditions identified in the past medical history, the nurse documents problems that may be significant during the surgical experience such as vision or hearing loss, partial paralysis or stiffness, weakness, or cognitive impairment.

FUNCTIONAL ASSESSMENT. The patient's usual activity pattern is described, including occupation, roles, and responsibilities. Usual diet and fluid intake are determined as well as use of tobacco and alcohol. Exercise and rest patterns are noted. The nurse asks about sources of stress and support, usual coping mechanisms, and specific fears or concerns about this surgery.

PHYSICAL EXAMINATION. Throughout the physical examination, the nurse assesses the patient's emotional state, ability to communicate, and ability to understand directions.

Height and Weight. The patient's height and weight are measured. Unless the patient is very ill or malnourished, the admission weight provides a goal weight to be maintained after surgery.

Vital Signs. Vital signs measured shortly after admission provide a baseline for evaluating readings following surgery. If the patient's pulse and blood pressure are slightly higher than expected on admission, it may be due to anxiety. After allowing the patient to rest, the nurse should retake the vital signs. If they remain abnormal the physician should be notified.

Skin. The skin is inspected for color, lesions, and bruises. The nurse palpates to assess texture, warmth, turgor, and moisture.

Thorax. The patient's respiratory rate, pattern, and effort are observed. Lungs are auscultated to assess breath sounds. The apical heart beat is assessed for rate and rhythm.

Abdomen. The abdomen is inspected for distention and scars, and bowel sounds are auscultated.

Extremities. Extremities are inspected for skin color, hair distribution, lesions, and deformities. Range of motion is assessed while listening for crepitus and noting pain or weakness.

Prostheses. The nurse notes the presence of any prosthetic devices including hearing aids, contact lenses, eyeglasses, dentures, artificial limbs, or other devices used to maintain appearance or function.

Nursing Diagnosis

Some of the nursing diagnoses that might be made during the preoperative phase are listed in what follows.

- **Anxiety** related to uncertain outcome of surgery, anticipated pain, potential disfigurement, or loss of function
- **Knowledge Deficit** of the surgical experience

More specific diagnoses are made based on individual patient data and specific surgical procedures.

Goals

Goals of preoperative nursing care for the general diagnoses presented are reduced anxiety and patient's knowledge about the surgical experience.

Interventions

ANXIETY. Most patients are somewhat anxious about surgery. The nurse determines the level and presence of anxiety, the contributing factors, and the need for intervention. It is especially important to find out the patient's previous experiences, if any, with hospitalization and surgery. If a patient admitted for heart surgery had an acquaintance who died after similar surgery, the patient might understandably be frightened. However, if previous experiences have been positive, the patient is more likely to expect this procedure to go well. If the nurse thinks the patient is excessively nervous or fearful about the surgery, it should be reported to the surgeon or to the anesthesia personnel. Extreme fear is associated with surgical complications, so it should be controlled with preoperative medication and other therapeutic interventions. Sometimes surgery is postponed until anxiety is reduced.

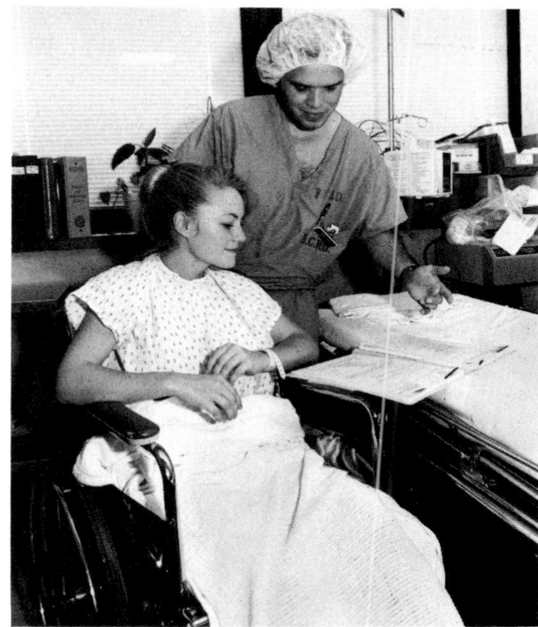

FIGURE 14-2
Preoperative teaching prepares the patient for the surgical experience. (Photograph by Stephen Matteson, Jr.)

KNOWLEDGE DEFICIT. Patient teaching may be done in the physician's office, the clinic, during the preadmission work-up, or after admission to the hospital. Ideally, it is not left until the evening before surgery when many activities are scheduled and the patient may be distracted. A cost-saving trend is to admit patients very early on the morning of surgery. In this case, the burden of preoperative teaching rests heavily on the physician, the office nurse, the admission nurse, or the clinic nurse.

Preoperative teaching should include the patient and those who will be with the patient during the recovery period. An attentive family member or companion can reinforce instructions and help reassure the patient. Telling the patient and family or friends what to expect in the immediate postoperative phase can prevent unnecessary stress. An appropriate teaching plan is based on an assessment of what the patient already knows, wants to know, and needs to know (Fig. 14–2).

Teaching Methods. The teaching methods selected depend on the situation. Direct patient teaching by the nurse is probably used most often. This has advantages in that the teaching plan can be individualized and the patient can ask questions freely. The main disadvantage of one-to-one instruction is that it is time consuming.

Some hospitals have group classes for all preoperative patients. The main advantage of group classes is economy of time. Also, some people like talking to others who are having similar procedures. Group classes have several disadvantages. The scheduled times may conflict with other preoperative procedures. Some patients are less likely to ask questions or express fears in a group setting. Also, information presented to mixed groups of patients is necessarily rather general.

Whatever approach is used for patient teaching, it may be supplemented with audiovisual materials. Books, pamphlets, audiotapes, and videotapes are available for patient use. Ideally, they are used along with other teaching strategies. The nurse can provide the materials for the patient's use and return later to answer questions and assess understanding of the material. Unfortunately, many patient teaching materials are appropriate for a limited audience. The reading level may be above the patient's ability, or too many technical terms may be used. Nurses sometimes forget how they felt the first time they encountered medical terminology. In the United States many people do not speak or read English well enough to learn from these materials. So although audiovisual materials can be very helpful, they should not be depended on completely for patient teaching.

Content. The patient needs to know what is done in preparation for surgery; what to expect in the operating and postanesthesia care unit (commonly called the PACU or recovery room); what tubes, dressings, or equipment may be in place after surgery; and how patient participation can promote postoperative recovery. The importance of turning, coughing, deep breathing, and performing leg exercises in the postoperative period is stressed. These procedures are described under postoperative care but should be taught in the preoperative phase if possible. In addition, the nurse encourages the patient to report pain and assures that measures will be taken to provide pain relief. The nurse determines how much detail is appropriate for each patient.

Most people need basic information and simple explanations without technical details. The family will probably want to know the expected time of surgery, where to wait for the patient, and how they will be informed when the procedure is over.

PREPARATION FOR SURGERY. Preparation of the patient for surgery starts before or shortly after admission. Patients admitted for emergency surgery may not have the benefit of preoperative teaching.

INFORMED CONSENT. Before surgery a patient must sign a legal document called a *consent form* (Fig. 14–3). It states that the patient has been informed about the procedure to be done, the alternative treatments, and the risks involved and that the patient agrees to the procedure. It is the physician's responsibility to explain the procedure and risks to the patient, but the nurse may obtain and witness the patient's signature on the form if agency policy allows. If the patient has questions or seems to be in doubt, the physician is contacted.

Because the consent form is a legal document, the patient must be fully alert and aware of what it contains when signing it. If the patient is a minor, a parent or guardian must sign the form. The age at which a person is considered an adult varies from state to state. Nurses should know the laws in the states in which they practice.

A patient who is confused, mentally incompetent, or under the influence of drugs cannot give informed consent. For that reason, the consent form is always signed before the patient is given preoperative medications.

The patient should sign the consent form in the presence of a witness who also signs the form. The witness's signature confirms that the patient was observed signing the form. The consent form becomes part of the patient's record.

PREPARATION OF THE DIGESTIVE TRACT. The extent of bowel preparation, if any, depends on the type of anesthesia and the type of surgery planned. For surgery on the abdomen or the digestive tract, laxatives and enemas are generally given to empty the bowel. Sometimes patients are instructed to do this at home before being admitted to the hospital.

Bowel cleansing serves three purposes. First, it reduces the risk of contamination from fecal matter during the operation. Second, it helps prevent postoperative distention until normal bowel function returns. Third, it avoids constipation and straining in the postoperative period. Straining can cause pressure on the surgical wound. Surgery may be canceled if bowel preparation is inadequate.

FOOD AND FLUID RESTRICTION. Even if bowel cleansing is not ordered, oral fluids and foods are restricted for a specific period of time. The evening meal before the day of surgery may be restricted to fluids. Typically, adult patients are given nothing by mouth (NPO) from midnight before the scheduled surgery. This reduces the risk of vomiting and aspiration during or after anesthesia. Occasionally the physician makes an exception and orders a shorter NPO period, especially for pediatric and geriatric patients. If a patient's medication is considered essential, it may be ordered early on the morning of surgery with a few sips of water or given parenterally.

SKIN PREPARATION. When an incision is made in the skin, microorganisms can enter the wound. Skin preparation is intended to reduce the number of organisms near the incision site. It usually includes scrubbing and removing hair from a wide margin around the planned surgical site. The exact skin preparation is ordered by the physician or outlined in a procedure manual (Fig. 14–4).

A typical procedure requires the patient (if able) to shower and wash with an antiseptic soap the evening before the surgery and again the next morning. The perioperative nurse or operating room technician scrubs the operative site and gently removes hair in the area shortly before surgery.

Hair can be removed by shaving or using a depilatory cream. The nurse should test for allergy before using depilatory cream on a patient. Current thinking is that shaving causes tiny nicks in the skin that shelter organisms. Therefore, shaving is often delayed until shortly before surgery to allow less time for organisms to multiply.

DRESS AND GROOMING. On the morning of surgery, the patient is provided a clean gown and instructed to remove all undergarments. Jewelry should be removed. If a ring cannot be removed or the patient refuses to remove it, it can be taped in place or secured with a loop of gauze slipped through the ring and tied to the wrist. The gauze must not be too tight to prevent circulatory impairment. Since jewelry often has considerable sentimental as well as monetary value, it must be handled carefully. The patient may leave jewelry with a relative or friend. It should not be left at the bedside or accepted by the nurse for safekeeping. Most hospitals have a process for valuables to be collected, signed for, and stored in a safe until the patient asks for them to be returned. The disposition of jewelry is documented in the patient's chart.

Long hair is braided or secured with a rubber band. Hair pins or clips must be removed. A cap is provided to cover the hair. Traditionally, dentures have been removed and placed in a denture cup and stored in a safe place. Many anesthesiologists and nurse anesthetists today prefer that dentures be left in. Institutional policies should be specific about this.

Nail polish is removed to permit assessment of nailbeds for circulation. If the patient has acrylic nails, consult with the anesthesiologist or perioperative nurse about the need to remove them. At least one acrylic nail is usually removed so the pulse oximeter can be used. Makeup, including mascara, is also removed.

A patient identification band is usually placed on the patient's wrist on admission. Other wrist bands are placed to indicate allergies and blood type. Before surgery, the nurse checks to be sure all bands are in place.

NORTHWEST HOSPITAL CENTER

REQUEST AND AUTHORIZATION FOR MEDICAL AND/OR SURGICAL TREATMENT

1. I HEREBY REQUEST AND AUTHORIZE DR.____________________ AND/OR HIS ASSOCIATES AND WHOMEVER THEY MAY DESIGNATE AS THEIR ASSISTANTS, TO ADMINISTER SUCH TREATMENT AS IS NECESSARY, AND TO PERFORM THE FOLLOWING OPERATION____________________ ____________________ AND SUCH ADDITIONAL OPERATIONS OR PROCEDURES AS ARE CONSIDERED NECESSARY ON THE BASIS OF CONDITIONS THAT MAY BE REVEALED DURING THE COURSE OF SAID OPERATION OR TREATMENT.

2. I REQUEST AND AUTHORIZE THE ADMINISTRATION OF SUCH ANESTHETICS AND/OR OTHER MEDICATIONS AS ARE NECESSARY.

3. FINAL DISPOSITION OF ANY TISSUES OR PARTS SURGICALLY REMOVED IS TO BE HANDLED IN ACCORDANCE WITH THE CUSTOMARY PRACTICES OF THE HOSPITAL.

4. REASONS WHY THE ABOVE NAMED SURGERY AND/OR TREATMENT IS CONSIDERED NECESSARY, ITS ADVANTAGES, PROBABILITY OF SUCCESS, POSSIBLE COMPLICATIONS, AND RISKS, AS WELL AS POSSIBLE ALTERNATIVE MODES OF TREATMENT WERE EXPLAINED TO ME BY DR. ____________________.

5. I AM AWARE THAT THE PRACTICE OF MEDICINE AND SURGERY IS NOT AN EXACT SCIENCE AND I ACKNOWLEDGE THAT NO GUARANTEES HAVE BEEN MADE TO ME CONCERNING THE RESULTS OF THE OPERATION OR PROCEDURE.

6. I HEREBY ACKNOWLEDGE THAT I HAVE READ AND FULLY UNDERSTAND THE ABOVE REQUEST AND AUTHORIZATION FOR MEDICAL AND/OR SURGICAL TREATMENT.

DATE:____________________ TIME: ____________________

SIGNED: ____________________
Patient

OR: ____________________
Legal Representative

____
Relationship (if any)

____
WITNESS

/PL/2736N
702/1019-E-R-5/90 40-1331

FIGURE 14-3

Surgical consent form. (From Ignatavicius, D. D., & Bayne, M. V. [1991]. *Medical-surgical nursing: A nursing process approach* [p. 440]. Philadelphia: W. B. Saunders. Courtesy of Northwest Hospital Center, Randallstown, MD.)

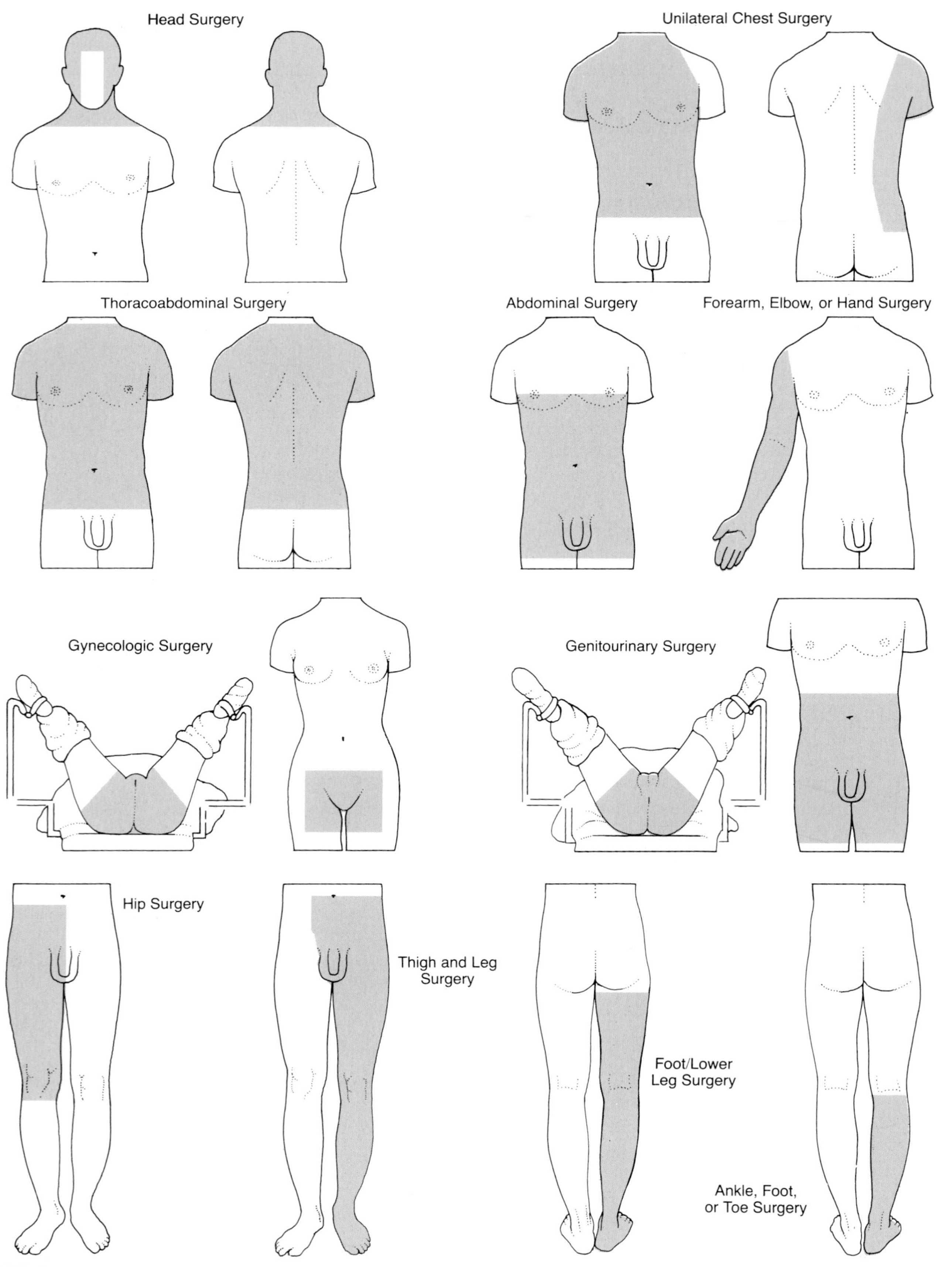

FIGURE 14-4
Skin preparation of common surgical sites. (From Ignatavicius, D. D., & Bayne, M. V. [1991]. *Medical-surgical nursing: A nursing process approach* [p. 442]. Philadelphia: W. B. Saunders.)

PHARMACOLOGY CAPSULE

Allergies must be clearly identified on a wrist band because the anesthetized patient cannot report them to the surgical staff.

PROSTHESES. Prostheses are usually removed, marked, and secured before surgery to prevent their being lost or damaged or causing injury during anesthesia. The nurse should be sure that the devices are returned to the patient when needed. A hearing-impaired patient without a hearing aid may seem uncooperative with postoperative instructions. If the patient is very stressed at having to go to surgery without the prosthesis, the nurse should consult with the perioperative nurses about making an exception to the rule.

PREOPERATIVE MEDICATIONS. Physicians' orders for the surgical patient often include a preoperative medication to be given shortly before the patient is transported to surgery. If the drug is ordered "on call," the nurse is notified by operating room personnel when it should be given. If the exact time of surgery is known, the order may specify that the drug be given at a certain time.

Preoperative medication may include a narcotic, an antiemetic (to control nausea and vomiting), and an anticholinergic drug to decrease secretions. Examples are listed in Table 14–2.

PHARMACOLOGY CAPSULE

Preoperative medications usually consist of a narcotic, an antiemetic, and an anticholinergic drug.

Preoperative medications must be given at the time they are ordered, because they interact with the anesthesia.

For safety reasons, the patient is asked to void immediately before the preoperative medication is given. Following administration of the medications, the patient is told to expect to feel drowsy and to have a dry mouth. Side rails are then raised, the call bell is placed within reach, and the patient is instructed to remain in bed.

PREOPERATIVE CHECKLIST. Most agencies have a preoperative checklist that must be completed and signed before the patient leaves the unit. The nurse must check to be sure that all laboratory and radiology reports are on the chart; that jewelry, prostheses, and nail polish have been removed; that the patient has

TABLE 14-2
PREOPERATIVE MEDICATIONS

DRUG	USE/ACTION	SIDE EFFECTS	NURSING INTERVENTIONS
		Tranquilizers	
Chlorpromazine (Thorazine)	Anticholinergic Sedative Antiemetic	Hypotension, dizziness and fainting, with parenteral route Dry mouth, blurred vision, urinary retention, constipation, or diarrhea Extrapyramidal symptoms: akathesia, parkinsonism, dystonias	Keep patient in bed after parenteral administration Intramuscular (IM) dose: inject slowly, deeply; massage site Contraindicated with severe central nervous system (CNS) depression Monitor blood pressure Take safety measures for drowsiness
Diazepam (Valium)	CNS depressant Skeletal muscle relaxation	Intravenous (IV) route: respiratory depression, arrhythmias, thrombophlebitis Drowsiness, ataxia, orthostatic hypotension, headache, blurred vision, confusion	Do not mix parenteral form with other drugs. IM injection—deep deltoid site IV route should use large vein; not administered faster than 5 mg/min Monitor pulse and respirations Contraindicated with acute narrow angle glaucoma or acute alcohol intoxication Keep in bed after parenteral administration
Hydroxyzine hydrochloride (Vistaril, Atarax)	CNS depressant Anticholinergic	Tissue damage with IM route Drowsiness, dry mouth, pain at injection site, dizziness, ataxia	IM dose should be given deep in large muscle mass using Z technique Maintain oral hygiene Take safety measures for drowsiness

Table continued on following page

TABLE 14-2
PREOPERATIVE MEDICATIONS *Continued*

DRUG	USE/ACTION	SIDE EFFECTS	NURSING INTERVENTIONS
Tranquilizers			
Promethazine hydrochloride (Phenergan)	Sedative Antihistamine Anticholinergic Antimotion sickness	Drowsiness, disorientation, hypotension, confusion Fainting in elderly Dry mouth, urinary retention, thickening of bronchial secretions Paradoxical reaction: excitation	IM dose must be deep IV dose given through IV infusion tube at 25 mg/min Contraindicated with CNS depression, acute asthma attack, Reye's syndrome Monitor pulse and blood pressure Maintain oral hygiene Take safety precautions for drowsiness
Narcotic Analgesics			
Meperidine hydrochloride (Demerol)	Analgesic Decreases response to CO_2 Decreases gastrointestinal (GI) secretions	Sedation, nausea, vomiting, light-headedness, dizziness, sweating Respiratory depression with overdose Tolerance and physical dependence with repeated use	Slow parenteral injection Monitor pulse, blood pressure, and respirations Withhold if respiratory rate less than 12/min Take safety precautions for drowsiness Contraindicated with monoamine oxidase (MAO) inhibitors
Morphine sulfate (MS Contin, Duramorph)	Analgesic Decreases response to increased CO_2 Decreases GI secretions	Circulatory collapse, cardiac arrest with rapid IV administration Dizziness, hypotension, nausea and vomiting Shallow breathing Occasional: sedation, vomiting, flushing, urinary retention	Administer parenteral forms slowly; rotate sites Dose should be reduced in elderly Monitor respirations and blood pressure Take safety precautions if drowsy Contraindicated with surgical anastomosis, after biliary tract surgery
Anticholinergics			
Atropine sulfate Glycopyrrolate (Robinul)	Decreases secretions Decreases GI and urinary motility Mydriatic Reduces salivation, respiratory and GI secretions	Dry mouth, decreased sweating, constipation, blurred vision, drowsiness, urinary retention Tachycardia, palpitations, tachypnea with overdose	Oral hygiene Monitor vital signs; record bowel movements and urine output Take safety precautions if drowsy Numerous contraindications
Sedatives and Hypnotics			
Pentobarbital sodium (Nembutal sodium) and Secobarbital sodium (Seconal Sodium)	Produces sedation	Drowsiness, sedation, lethargy, irritability, nausea, anorexia, muscle aches and pain, gastric distress Severe CNS depression with overdose Tolerance/dependence with prolonged use	Deep IM injection in large muscle Monitor vital signs before and after IV administration Administer IV at prescribed rate Take safety precautions if drowsy Dosage should be reduced for elderly
Chloral hydrate (Noctec)	CNS depression	Occasional nausea, vomiting, flatulence, diarrhea, disorientation Somnolence, confusion, respiratory depression, coma with overdose	Monitor pulse, blood pressure, and respirations

voided; that premedication has been given; that vital signs have been recorded, and that the consent form has been signed (Fig. 14–5).

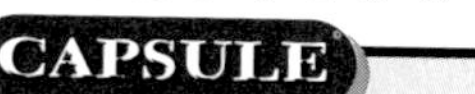

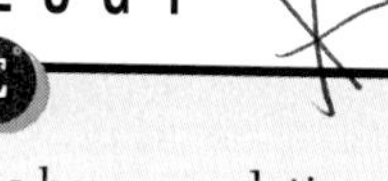

Because preoperative medications have a sedative effect, the surgical consent form should be signed before the medications are given. After the medications are given, the patient is instructed to remain in bed.

Evaluation

Criteria for the achievement of goals in the preoperative phase are the patient's statement of reduced anxiety and calm appearance and the patient's descriptions of what to expect before and after surgery and of the patient's role in promoting recovery from surgery.

THE INTRAOPERATIVE PHASE

Operating room personnel transfer the patient from the nursing unit to the surgical suite. They assist the patient onto a gurney (stretcher) and take the patient and the chart to the surgical area.

The patient may be taken directly to an operating room or may go to a holding room first. In the holding room, skin preparation may be done and intravenous fluids started, if these procedures were not done earlier. In some settings, preoperative medications are not given until the patient is received in the holding area. The patient who has been told earlier what to expect will feel more secure in the surgical area.

When moved into the operating room, the patient can expect to see many pieces of equipment, bright lights, and various people. The patient is helped to move to the operating room table and positioned in a specific way for the type of surgery being done. Safety straps are applied carefully because there is a risk of impaired circulation or nerve damage caused by pressure. Comfort and alignment are confirmed while the patient is awake. Anesthesia is then administered and is maintained throughout the procedure (Fig. 14–6).

THE SURGICAL TEAM

On arrival in the surgical suite, the patient is greeted by the nurse, the physician, the anesthesiologist, or the nurse anesthetist. A number of people participate in the intraoperative period. They include the following:

- The surgeon who actually performs the procedure.
- An assistant surgeon, a nurse first assistant, or a physician assistant who assists the surgeon in the procedure.
- The registered nurse who circulates. This nurse is responsible for assessing the patient, planning intraoperative nursing care, and maintaining patient safety. This person is in charge of the operating room. Responsibilities include setting up the room, monitoring aseptic technique, assisting in positioning and monitoring the patient, preparing the skin, and providing needed supplies and equipment (Fig. 14–7).
- A registered nurse or technician who scrubs and handles instruments within the sterile field during the procedure.
- The nurse anesthetist or anesthesiologist who administers anesthetics and monitors the patient's status throughout the procedure. A nurse anesthetist is a registered nurse with special training in anesthesia. An anesthesiologist is a physician who specializes in anesthesia.
- Other technical personnel with specialized jobs. For example, a perfusionist operates the heart bypass machine during open heart surgery.

Near the end of procedures done under general anesthesia, the anesthetist or anesthesiologist administers drugs to reverse the effects of the anesthetic. When the procedure is completed, a member of the surgical team escorts the patient to the postanesthesia care unit, where careful monitoring can be done until the patient recovers from the anesthesia.

ANESTHESIA

Although surgery has been done since prehistoric times, anesthesia has been used only for approximately 150 years. Anesthetic agents are used to alter sensation so that surgical procedures can be done painlessly and safely. Agents used for anesthesia include general and local anesthetics.

Regional Anesthesia

Regional anesthesia is performed by using local anesthetics that block the conduction of nerve impulses in a specific area. These anesthetics do not cause the patient to lose consciousness. For some procedures, intravenous sedatives are given in addition to the local anesthetic.

Examples of local anesthetics are lidocaine hydrochloride (Xylocaine), bupivacaine hydrochloride (Marcaine HCl), and dibucaine hydrochloride (Nupercaine). They are commonly used for dental procedures, eye surgery, cosmetic surgery on the face, repair of lacerations, childbirth, and other procedures in which general anesthesia is not needed or desired by the patient. Local anesthetics are often the agents of choice for elderly patients because of other medical conditions.

Local anesthetics may be administered topically, by local infiltration, and by nerve blocking techniques. Topical anesthetics are applied directly to the area to be anesthetized. For local infiltration, the anesthetic agent is injected into and under the skin around the area of treatment. A nerve block is done by injecting an anesthetic agent in or around a nerve to block the transmission of impulses. Epidural anesthesia and subarachnoid anesthesia are examples of regional nerve blocks. Both are achieved by injecting the anesthetic agent into the

Preoperative Checklist

Allergies: **Date of Surgery** ____________ **Addressograph Plate**

CLINICAL DATA:	**Yes**	**No**	**Comments**
Authorization for surgical treatment completed			
Height and weight charted			
History and physical			
Chest x-ray			
ECG report			
Urine report			
Blood sugar within acceptable range (50–300 mg/dL)			
Hematocrit within acceptable range (30–50 mL/dL)			
Potassium within acceptable range (3.5–6 mEq/L)			
Unacceptable test results reported to Dr.		Time	By
CLIENT PREPARATION:	**Yes**	**No**	**Comments**
Jewelry removed			
Hairpiece, wig, hairpins, barrettes, beads, rubber bands removed			
Loose teeth or caps noted			
Dentures removed			

Preoperative Checklist *Continued*

Allergies: **Date of Surgery** ____________ **Addressograph Plate**

CLINICAL DATA:	**Yes**	**No**	**Comments**
Artificial eye, contact lenses, glasses removed			
Any prosthetic appliance removed			
Voided or catheterized — I&O sheet on chart			
Identification bracelet in place			
Parenteral fluids patent and infusing at mL/h			
B/P, T.P.R. charted			
Premedication given as ordered			
Side rails up — care data and care plan on chart			
COMMUNICATION ASSESSMENT:	**Normal**	**Abnormal**	**Comments**
Vision			
Hearing			
Mental			
Speech			
Other			
Client's preferred name:			

NURSE TO NURSE REFERRAL

Limb for burial _____ **Yes** _____ **No at** ____________ **Funeral home**

FIGURE 14-5

The preoperative checklist must be completed before the patient goes to surgery. (From Ignatavicius, D. D., & Bayne, M. V. [1991]. *Medical-surgical nursing: A nursing process approach* [pp. 448–449]. Philadelphia: W. B. Saunders. Courtesy of Northwest Hospital Center, Randallstown, MD.)

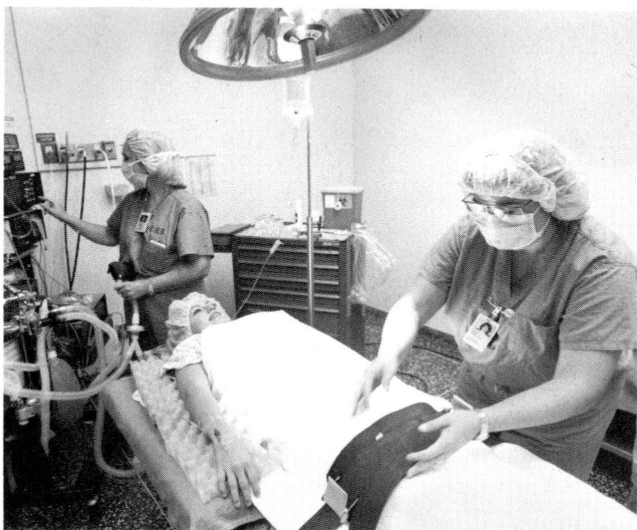

FIGURE 14-6

The nurse ensures the patient's safety on the operating table (Photograph by Stephen Matteson, Jr.)

area around the spinal nerves. Motor and sensory functions are blocked above and below the level of the anesthetic administration. This anesthesia is especially useful for surgical procedures of the lower abdomen and legs. The level of anesthesia is controlled by the amount of the drug injected and the position of the patient on the operating table.

As a rule, spinal and epidural anesthesia poses less risk for respiratory, cardiac, and gastrointestinal complications than general anesthesia. If the level of spinal or epidural anesthetic agent rises higher than intended, there is a risk of respiratory and cardiovascular depression.

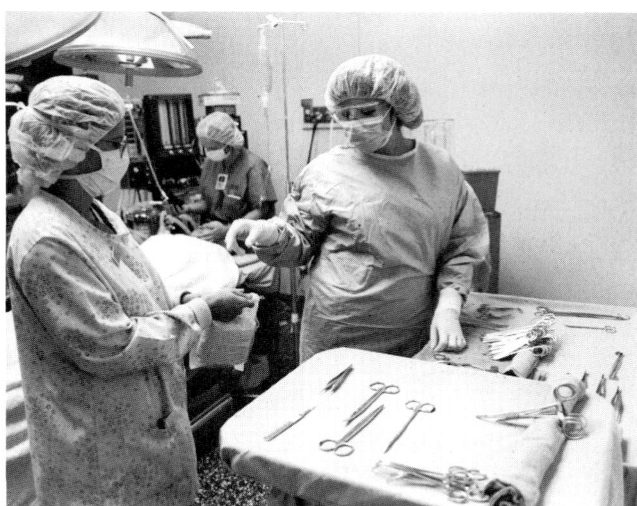

FIGURE 14-7

The nurse sets up the operating room. (Photograph by Stephen Matteson, Jr.)

One complication of spinal anesthesia is postspinal headache. It is caused by the leaking of cerebrospinal fluid at the puncture site. Postspinal headache can be severe and may last for several weeks. It is relieved by lying flat. It is more common in women, especially postpartum women. Keeping the patient flat after spinal anesthesia has *not* been found to prevent the headache. The nurse should always check the postoperative orders, however, for any positioning or activity restrictions. Forcing fluids in the postoperative period, if allowed, may help.

Severe spinal headache is sometimes treated by injecting a small amount of the patient's blood into the epidural space at the site of the previous subarachnoid puncture. The blood clots, forming a "blood patch" that prevents further leaking. The procedure can be repeated if it is unsuccessful the first time. A successful patch relieves the headache immediately. Postanesthesia headache does not occur with epidural anesthesia.

As the effect of a regional anesthetic wears off, the patient often reports that the affected limbs feel numb and heavy. The nurse should provide reassurance that this is normal and that movement and sensation gradually return to normal. It is vital to do passive range of motion until motility returns to prevent thrombus (clot) formation.

Complications of local anesthesia include toxicity caused by overdose, local tissue damage, and allergic responses. Signs and symptoms of toxicity are initially excitement and central nervous system stimulation and then depression of the central nervous system and the cardiovascular system. Local tissue effects may be inflammation and edema. Abscesses and necrosis sometimes develop at the injection site. This is thought to be caused by poor technique rather than by the anesthetic agent.

General Anesthesia

General anesthesia acts on the central nervous system causing loss of sensation, reflexes, and consciousness. General anesthetic agents can be given by inhalation, intravenous infusion, intramuscular injection, or rectal administration. Although the intramuscular and rectal routes can be used to administer anesthetic agents, the use of those routes is uncommon.

INHALATION AGENTS. Inhalation agents include halothane (Fluothane), isoflurane (Forane), enflurane (Ethrane), desflurane (Suprane), and nitrous oxide. For most procedures using inhalation agents, the patient is first induced with a short-acting intravenous agent. Then an endotracheal tube is inserted into the patient's trachea to permit administration of the maintenance inhalation anesthesia and to control mechanical ventilation. A cuff on the endotracheal tube prevents leakage during mechanical ventilation and aspiration of gastric contents while the patient is unconscious (Fig. 14–8).

INTRAVENOUS AGENTS. Intravenous agents include thiopental sodium (Pentothal), methohexital sodium (Brevital Sodium), propofol (Diprivan), midazolam

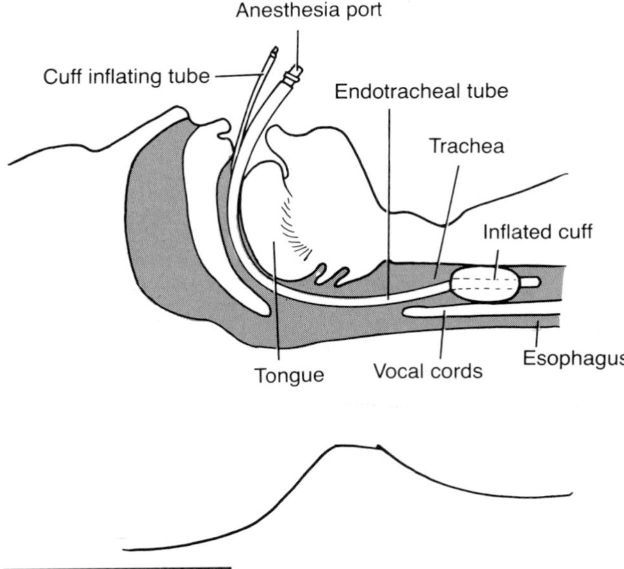

FIGURE 14-8
Inhalation anesthesia is given through an endotracheal tube. (From Ignatavicius, D. D., & Bayne, M. V. [1991]. *Medical-surgical nursing: A nursing process approach.* Philadelphia: W. B. Saunders.)

(Versed), a combination of fentanyl and droperidol (Innovar), and ketamine hydrochloride (Ketalar).

OTHER AGENTS. Muscle relaxants and opioids are often given with the anesthetic agents. Muscle relaxants prevent movement of muscles during the surgical procedure.

COMPLICATIONS. Inhalation anesthetic agents and the endotracheal tube itself can cause irritation of the respiratory tract and the larynx. Individual agents may have serious adverse effects such as cardiac arrhythmias, seizures, liver toxicity, nausea and vomiting, and death.

Malignant hyperthermia, although rare, is life threatening. It is characterized by increasing body temperature and metabolic rate, tachycardia, hypotension, cyanosis, and muscle rigidity. When malignant hyperthermia occurs, the surgery is interrupted and measures taken to cool the patient (e.g., iced intravenous solutions, ice packs). One hundred percent oxygen is administered, and the patient is given steroids, diuretics, and dantrolene sodium.

HYPOTHERMIA. Hypothermia refers to a condition in which the body temperature is lower than normal. For some surgical procedures, the body temperature is deliberately lowered to reduce the metabolic rate and the need for oxygen. Cooling or freezing of a local area to block pain impulses is called *cryoanesthesia.*

INTRAOPERATIVE NURSING CARE

Intraoperative nursing care is a specialty and is beyond the scope of this chapter. Only potential nursing diagnoses and goals are listed here.

Nursing Diagnosis

During the intraoperative phase of the surgical experience, nursing diagnoses may include the following:

- **High Risk for Injury** related to the effects of anesthesia, positioning, and use of restraints
- **Impaired Gas Exchange** related to the effects of anesthesia and immobility
- **Altered Tissue Perfusion (Peripheral)** related to immobility and restraints
- **Decreased Cardiac Output** related to drug effects or blood loss
- **High Risk for Fluid Volume Deficit** related to blood loss, insensible loss of water, or NPO status

Goals

Goals of nursing care in the intraoperative phase are the absence of physical injury, adequate oxygenation, normal pulse and blood pressure, normal color of extremities and normal peripheral pulses, and balanced fluid intake and output.

THE POSTOPERATIVE PHASE

When the surgical procedure is completed, the patient is usually transferred to the postanesthesia care unit (recovery room) or the intensive care unit before returning to the nursing unit. Exceptions are patients who have had minor procedures with only local anesthesia.

SURGICAL COMPLICATIONS

The patient who has surgery is at risk for a number of complications. These complications may be related to the surgical procedure itself, to the drugs used before and during the procedure, or to immobility after the surgery. The types of postoperative complications vary depending on the length of time since the surgical procedure. For example, shock and hypoxia are most likely to occur in the immediate recovery period. Wound infection, however, does not appear for several days after surgery. Complications in the immediate and later postoperative periods are described in Table 14–3. Prevention, recognition, and nursing implications are discussed in the section on nursing care.

Shock

Shock is most likely to occur as an effect of anesthesia or loss of blood. If narcotic analgesics are given before the anesthesia wears off, they may contribute to a drop in blood pressure.

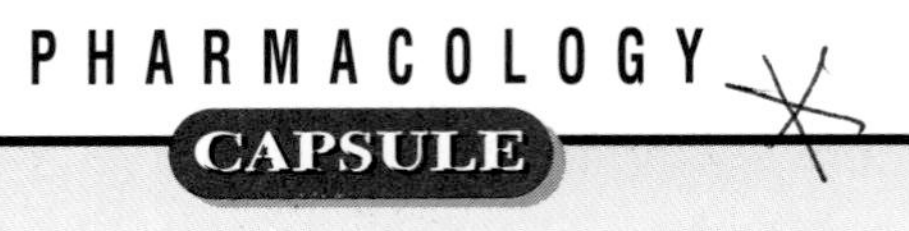

Narcotic analgesics given before the effects of general anesthesia wear off may cause a drop in blood pressure.

TABLE 14-3
SURGICAL COMPLICATIONS

COMPLICATIONS	PREVENTION	TREATMENT
Shock	Assess wound dressing. Report excessive drainage or bleeding. Monitor vital signs every 15 minutes till stable. Note early changes in vital signs. Report tachycardia, tachypnea, hypotension. Monitor input and output. Keep intravenous fluid rate on schedule. Assess respirations before giving narcotics.	Fluid or blood replacement. Vasopressors (drugs to raise blood pressure) as ordered. Additional surgery may be needed to control bleeding.
Hypoxia	Airway in place till patient awakens. Position unconscious patient on side if not contraindicated. Suction as necessary. Monitor vital signs every 15 minutes till stable. Encourage deep breathing.	Position to promote effective ventilation. Suction as necessary. Administer oxygen. Encourage deep breathing and coughing.
Impaired wound healing Dehiscence Evisceration Infection	Adequate fluids and nutrition. Splint incision during activity, coughing, and deep breathing. Good handwashing. Sterile technique for wound care.	Cover the open wound with a sterile dressing. If organs protrude, saturate the dressing with normal saline. Notify physician. Keep patient still and quiet.
Inadequate oxygenation Pneumonia Atelectasis	Change position at least every 2 hr. Assist to cough and deep breathe hourly. Incentive spirometry.	Rest. Oxygen and antibiotics as ordered.
Digestive disturbances Nausea and vomiting	Withhold oral fluids until nausea subsides. Give antiemetics to prevent vomiting as soon as nausea is reported.	Antiemetic drugs as ordered.
Altered elimination Urine retention Kidney failure Abdominal distention "Gas" pains Constipation	Provide privacy. Offer warm bedpan. Position comfortably. Take to bathroom or bedside commode chair if allowed. Pour warm water over the perineum. Let tap water run. Promptly report urine output of less than 30 ml/h. Nothing by mouth till bowel sounds return. Encourage ambulation as allowed. Encourage fluids, food, and ambulation as ordered. Use stool softeners as ordered.	Catheterization as ordered. Rectal tube, heat to abdomen, bisacodyl suppositories as ordered. Position on right side. Nasogastric intubation with suction as ordered. Ambulate frequently when permitted. Laxatives or enemas, or both, as ordered.
Thrombophlebitis	Avoid pressure on blood vessels. Leg exercises every 1–2 h. Early, frequent ambulation as ordered. Elastic or automatic compression stockings.	Bedrest. Anticoagulant therapy as ordered.
Fluid and electrolyte imbalances	Monitor intravenous fluid rate. Provide a variety of oral fluids when permitted. Treat vomiting. Recognize signs of imbalances (see Chapter 11).	Give intravenous fluids as ordered. Encourage oral intake when allowed.

Shock may also result from low blood volume (hypovolemic shock). Bleeding is an obvious cause of low blood volume, but other factors may contribute as well. Dehydration without adequate fluid replacement or fluid losses through wounds and suction can explain low blood volume.

Hypoxia

Hypoxia refers to inadequate oxygenation of body tissues. The patient is at risk for hypoxia in the immediate postoperative phase for several reasons. First, general anesthetics depress respirations so that the patient's breathing efforts may be inadequate initially. Second, when the patient is unconscious the tongue may fall back and block the airway. Third, anesthesia depresses the cough and swallowing reflexes. Until these reflexes return, vomitus and saliva can enter the airway. A fourth reason that hypoxia may occur in the immediate postoperative period is the risk of laryngospasm or bronchospasm. Spasm of the larynx or bronchi narrows the airway and obstructs air flow.

Injury

Immediately after surgery, the patient is at risk for injury because of the decreased level of consciousness associated with general anesthesia or other sedatives. If the patient has had regional anesthesia, the affected body part may be injured because it lacks sensation and movement.

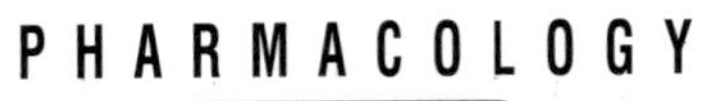

PHARMACOLOGY CAPSULE

Regional anesthesia blocks sensation and movement so the affected body part is at risk for injury.

Pneumonia and Atelectasis

Drug effects and immobility place the surgical patient at risk for pneumonia and atelectasis. Patients who are most prone to these complications are the elderly, the obese, those with chronic pulmonary disease, and those having chest or abdominal surgery. General anesthetics and narcotic analgesics depress respiratory function. Anticholinergics cause pulmonary secretions to be drier and thicker.

PHARMACOLOGY CAPSULE

General anesthetics and narcotic analgesics depress respirations.

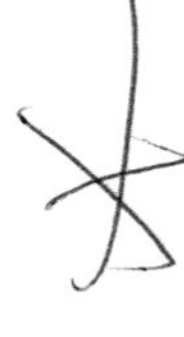

Immobility limits lung expansion and allows fluids to pool in the lungs. Fluid provides a medium for infectious organisms to grow. An infection of the lungs due to immobility is called *hypostatic pneumonia*.

As secretions accumulate, they begin to block off branches of the respiratory tree. When gases can no longer enter or leave the affected alveoli, they collapse. *Atelectasis* is the term used to describe collapse of a portion or all of a lung. Because atelectasis impairs the exchange of gases, it can be very serious.

Wound Complications

Complications in wound healing include dehiscence, evisceration, and infection. All are, to some extent, preventable.

DEHISCENCE AND EVISCERATION. *Dehiscence* is the reopening of the surgical wound. It involves one or more layers of tissue. Dehiscence is most likely to happen when strain on the suture line is excessive. Factors that increase the risk of dehiscence include wound infection, malnutrition, obesity, dehydration, and extensive abdominal wounds or injuries. Dehiscence is most likely to occur between the fifth and twelfth postoperative days. *Evisceration* is the term used when body organs protrude through the open wound. Dehiscence and evisceration are illustrated in Figure 14–9.

INFECTION. The risk of wound infection is greatest in cases of traumatic injuries, wounds that were not treated promptly, and wounds that were infected before surgery.

Gastrointestinal Disturbances

The primary gastrointestinal problems that follow surgery are nausea, vomiting, impaired peristalsis, and constipation. Nausea and vomiting are most common in the early postoperative period. Causative factors include anesthesia, pain, narcotics, decreased peristalsis, and resuming oral intake too soon.

Several factors cause peristalsis to be impaired after surgery. They include anesthesia, immobility, narcotic analgesics, and handling of the bowel during surgery. Patients who develop metabolic imbalances, respiratory problems, or shock are also at risk for gastrointestinal disturbances.

The effects of slowed peristalsis can be mild or severe. Gas normally forms in the digestive tract. When peristalsis is slow, the gas builds up and causes cramping pain and distention. Mild effects are generally seen as gas pains that typically occur on the second or third postoperative day. Constipation is also related to slow peristalsis.

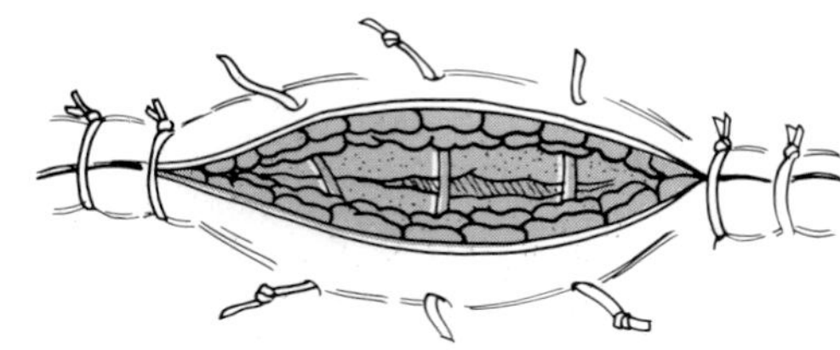

A Dehiscence

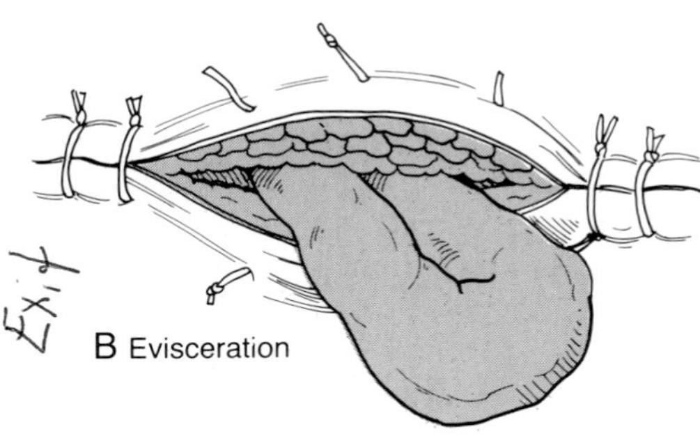

B Evisceration

FIGURE 14-9

Complications of wound healing: *A*, Dehiscence; *B*, evisceration. (From Ignatavicius, D. D., & Bayne, M. V. [1991]. *Medical-surgical nursing: A nursing process approach.* Philadelphia: W. B. Saunders.)

If peristalsis stops completely, the patient is said to have a paralytic ileus. The patient with a paralytic ileus has abdominal distention that may be severe enough to impair lung expansion and decrease blood return from the legs, causing cardiac output to fall. Distention also causes strain on an abdominal incision.

Urinary Retention and Renal Failure

With urinary retention, the kidneys produce urine but the patient is unable to empty the bladder. Urinary retention can be caused by the effects of anesthesia or narcotics, trauma to the urinary tract, or anxiety about voiding. Urine output may also be decreased owing to dehydration or blood loss.

With kidney failure, the kidneys are unable to produce enough urine to remove wastes from the body. Urine output falls dangerously low.

Thrombophlebitis

The risk of hemorrhage and shock decreases after the immediate postoperative period. A more common circulatory problem in the later period is thrombophlebitis. Thrombophlebitis is the inflammation of veins with the formation of blood clots. It occurs most often in the legs following a period of immobility. Patients who have very lengthy surgical procedures or who must be immobilized are most likely to develop thrombophlebitis.

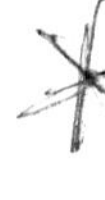

Clots that cling to the walls of blood vessels are called thrombi. Thrombi that break loose and flow with the venous blood are called emboli. Emboli formed in the legs are most likely to pass through the heart and lodge in the pulmonary circulation. If they are large enough to seriously impair pulmonary blood flow, the patient develops severe respiratory distress and may even die.

POSTOPERATIVE NURSING CARE

Assessment

When the patient is admitted to the postanesthesia care unit, the nurse determines the medical diagnosis and the surgical procedure. The patient's status (level of consciousness, vital signs) is promptly assessed and the wound or dressing inspected. Equipment, such as suction devices, oxygen, urinary drainage, and intravenous lines, is checked and set up as needed. When the patient returns to the nursing unit, more complete assessments are done. The complete assessment is discussed here.

HEALTH HISTORY. The nurse reviews the patient's preoperative assessment (outlined in Table 14–1), noting long-term conditions, disabilities, prostheses, drugs, and allergies. When the patient is able to respond, the nurse asks about significant symptoms including pain, nausea, and altered sensations.

PHYSICAL EXAMINATION

Vital Signs. Vital signs are taken, and the results are compared with the preoperative readings. The respiratory rate, depth, and effort are assessed. The pulse is taken, noting rate, rhythm, and quality. Blood pressure is recorded. Measurements are usually repeated every 15 minutes until they stabilize.

Neurologic Status. The assessment of neurologic status includes level of consciousness and pupil size, equality, and reaction to light. Sensation is evaluated in affected body areas. Spontaneous movements are noted, and the patient's ability to move affected parts on command may be assessed. For example, when a cast has been applied to a fractured arm, the nurse may test the patient's ability to move fingers.

Integument. The skin is inspected for color and palpated for temperature. The surgical area is inspected. If the wound is visible, the nurse assesses the incision for intactness of the wound margins, drainage, and excessive redness or swelling. If a dressing covers the incision, the dressing is inspected for bleeding or other drainage. If closed drains are in place, the nurse observes the amount and appearance of the drainage.

Thorax. Chest expansion is observed with respirations. Chest movement should be symmetric. Breath sounds are auscultated to detect atelectasis, crackles, and wheezes.

Heart. The apical pulse may be taken if the peripheral pulse is weak or irregular or if the patient has heart disease.

Abdomen. The abdomen is inspected for distention and auscultated for bowel sounds. Light palpation may also be done to assess bowel and bladder distention and tenderness. The patency of gastrointestinal tubes is checked.

Extremities. The nurse assesses the color and capillary refill of nailbeds and the presence and quality of peripheral pulses in affected extremities. The presence of edema or excessive warmth or redness is also noted. The color and temperature of both arms or legs are assessed simultaneously to detect differences. The foot is dorsiflexed to assess for pain in the calf, a finding called a positive Homans's sign. This finding is suggestive of thrombophlebitis.

The postoperative nursing assessment is summarized in Table 14–4.

Nursing Diagnosis for the Immediate Postoperative Phase

Specific nursing diagnoses vary with the type of surgery and the individual patient. Nursing diagnoses and interventions for the immediate and later postoperative periods are presented separately. The following nursing diagnoses take priority in the immediate postoperative phase when the patient is recovering from anesthesia and is being stabilized:

- **Decreased Cardiac Output** related to excessive loss of blood and other body fluids or the effects of drugs

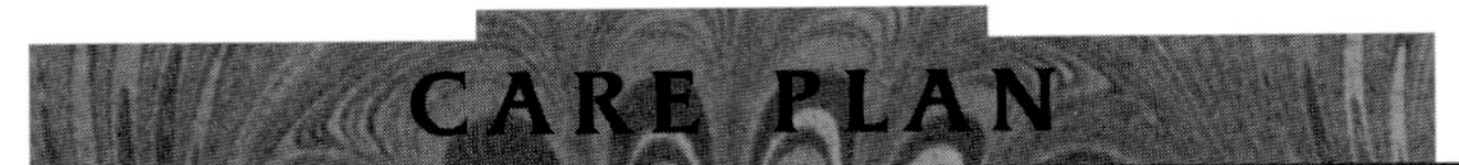

Care of the Postoperative Patient

ASSESSMENT

Health History: 27-year-old Hispanic female admitted for abdominal pain. Is a secretary, married, and the mother of a 3-year-old child. Is one day postappendectomy. Complains of moderate abdominal and incisional pain. Has been out of bed three times since surgery. Ambulated well with assistance. Catheterized once previous evening but has since voided twice (300 ml, 230 ml) Intravenous fluids infusing at 100 ml/hr. No nausea, but nothing by mouth (NPO) until noon when 550 ml clear liquids were taken and retained.

Physical Examination: Alert and oriented. Vital signs: blood pressure, 130/86; pulse, 90; respiration 16; temperature, 99.4°F orally. (Admission vital signs were blood pressure, 126/82; pulse, 94; respiration, 20; temperature, 99°F orally.) Breath sounds clear to auscultation. Abdomen soft. Wound covered with dry dressing. Bowel sounds present but hypoactive.

NURSING DIAGNOSIS	GOALS AND OUTCOME CRITERIA	INTERVENTIONS
Acute pain related to tissue trauma.	Patient will report pain relief and appear more relaxed.	Assess nature, location, and severity of pain. Medicate with meperidine 75 mg intramuscularly every 3 to 4 hours as needed and evaluate effectiveness. Assure patient that narcotics can be taken safely for acute pain for a limited time. Assist to change positions. Give backrub. Coach in relaxation exercises and mental imagery. Assess anxiety and explore causes. Be available. Reassure.
Impaired tissue integrity related to surgical incision.	Patient's wound edges will remain clean and closed until discharge.	Check dressing hourly for bleeding first 24 hours, then twice each shift. Report bleeding to physician. Protect wound by supporting during respiratory exercises. Treat nausea promptly.
High risk for infection related to break in skin, invasive devices, and procedures.	Patient will remain free of infection as evidenced by oral temperature less than 100°F, decreasing redness of incision, no purulent drainage, clear breath sounds, no dysuria, no phlebitis.	Monitor vital signs every 4 hours. Report increasing temperature. Assess wound for increasing redness, edema, or drainage. Inspect for purulent drainage. Exercise good handwashing. Use sterile gloves for wound care. Monitor and encourage fluid intake. Collect specimens for culture if ordered. Teach patient how to care for wound after discharge.
Impaired gas exchange related to stasis of pulmonary secretions, thrombosis, emboli.	Patient's breath sounds will remain clear and respiratory rate will be between 12 and 20 without dyspnea.	Help patient support incision and turn, cough, and deep breathe or use incentive spirometry at least every 2 hours. Auscultate breath sounds for rales or atelectasis. Encourage fluid intake.
Urinary retention related to effects of anesthesia.	Patient's urine output will be approximately equal to fluid intake; no bladder distention.	Measure all fluid intake and output. Palpate for distended bladder. Provide privacy and try to stimulate voiding. Catheterize using sterile technique as ordered if patient is unable to void.
Colonic constipation related to effects of drugs, immobility, bowel manipulation during surgery.	Patient will have bowel sounds and pass flatus prior to discharge.	Assess bowel sounds and ask patient to report passage of flatus ("gas"). Encourage frequent ambulation as allowed. Position the patient on the right side. Report distention.

Care of the Postoperative Patient *(Continued)*

NURSING DIAGNOSIS	GOALS AND OUTCOME CRITERIA	INTERVENTIONS
High risk for fluid volume deficit related to wound drainage, NPO status.	Patient's fluid intake and output will be approximately equal, and serum electrolytes will remain within normal limits.	Measure fluid intake and output. Assess fluid status: tissue turgor, mucous membranes, pulse quality. Administer antiemetics promptly for nausea or vomiting. Offer fluids as prescribed.
Impaired physical mobility related to weakness, tissue trauma.	Patient will gradually increase activity and assume more self-care.	Assist out of bed until patient can safely do so alone. Teach patient importance of ambulation to promote healing and prevent complications.
Body image disturbance related to change in body appearance.	Patient will state any concerns about appearance of wound.	Observe the patient's reaction to the incision. Ask if there are any questions or concerns. Answer questions honestly or refer to surgeon. Tell the patient the incision will fade and the edema will diminish.
Knowledge deficit related to postoperative routines, self-care.	Patient will correctly describe postoperative routines and self-care during hospitalization and after discharge.	Reinforce physician's instructions for wound care and activity limitations. Encourage consideration of adaptations needed in work or home roles and responsibilities. Stress need for good nutrition. Explain any drugs that are being prescribed: dosage, schedule, side effects, and adverse effects that should be reported to the physician. Include husband in teaching.

- **Ineffective Breathing Patterns** and/or **Ineffective Airway Clearance** related to the effects of anesthesia or pain
- **Pain** related to tissue trauma or to positioning during surgical procedures
- **Altered Thought Processes** related to the effects of anesthetic agents
- **High Risk for Injury** related to decreased level of consciousness or loss of sensation and movement related to the effects of anesthesia.

Goals

The goals of nursing care in the immediate postoperative phase of the surgical experience are adequate circulation, adequate oxygenation, pain control, mental orientation, and freedom from injury.

Interventions

DECREASED CARDIAC OUTPUT. The nurse is alert to the possibility of shock. To detect impending shock, the patient's vital signs are usually checked every 15 minutes in the postanesthesia care unit. Signs and symptoms of impending shock include rapid, thready pulse; restlessness; decreasing blood pressure; and decreasing urine output. The patient's preoperative vital signs are used to evaluate whether postoperative vital signs are normal. An increasing pulse usually precedes a fall in blood pressure. Intravenous fluid intake and urinary output are monitored. When blood volume is low (hypovolemia), the kidneys reduce urine production. Continuous cardiac monitoring is often done to identify

TABLE 14-4

POSTOPERATIVE NURSING ASSESSMENT

HEALTH HISTORY

Reason for surgery, name of procedure, medical diagnosis, disabilities, prostheses, drugs, allergies. Presence of pain, nausea, altered sensations.

PHYSICAL EXAMINATION

Vital Signs

Neurologic status: Level of consciousness; pupil size, equality, response to light; sensation; spontaneous movement, response to commands.

Integument: Color, temperature, incision or dressing appearance, amount and appearance of drainage.

Thorax: Chest expansion, symmetry, breath sounds.

Heart: Apical pulse.

Abdomen: Contour, bowel sounds, bladder distention, tenderness.

Extremities: Color, capillary refill, pulses, edema, warmth, redness, Homans's sign.

early signs of hypovolemia or potentially dangerous changes in cardiac rhythm.

Measures to reduce the risk of shock include prompt recognition and treatment of bleeding, replacement of lost fluids, and cautious use of narcotic analgesics. Wound dressings and drains are checked frequently for the color and the amount of drainage. The amount of bleeding expected varies with different surgical procedures.

An open intravenous route must be maintained during the early postoperative period. This permits the infusion of fluids, blood, and emergency medications if needed. The nurse therefore checks the venipuncture site to be sure the fluid is infusing properly. The intravenous fluid infusion rate is ordered by the physician, but the nurse regulates the rate. If the rate falls behind, the patient may not receive adequate fluids to replace losses during surgery. If given too rapidly, intravenous fluids can overload the circulatory system, causing heart failure.

INEFFECTIVE BREATHING PATTERNS. To detect early signs of hypoxia, the nurse in the postanesthesia care unit monitors the patient's respiratory status. Respiratory depth, rate, and effort are assessed. The nurse listens for abnormal breath sounds that suggest breathing difficulty. Changes in the pulse rate must also be watched as an increasing pulse rate is often an early indicator of poor oxygenation. An oximeter is used to monitor the oxygenation of the blood. The oximeter is a device with a wire that clips to a finger or an earlobe.

The patient's color, especially in the nailbeds and lips, provides a clue to oxygenation. Because cyanosis is a late sign of hypoxia, however, one should detect problems long before color changes develop.

Measures must be taken to reduce the risk of hypoxia during the immediate postoperative period. An airway is inserted to keep the air passages open until the patient begins to awaken. The unconscious patient can be positioned on one side to reduce the risk of aspirated fluids. Suctioning is done if necessary to remove secretions or vomitus.

PAIN. Decisions to medicate for pain in the early postoperative phase are based on physician's orders and nursing judgment. If narcotic analgesics are given too early, their effects combined with the effects of the anesthesia may lead to shock. Severe pain may also cause shock, however.

ALTERED THOUGHT PROCESSES. As patients begin to regain consciousness, they may move around and touch dressings and drains. The nurse can tell them where they are, that the surgery is over, and what is happening. Simple explanations and gentle reminders are often sufficient to calm and reassure them. The amnesic effects of anesthetics may cause the patient to forget what the nurse has said, making it necessary to repeat information.

HIGH RISK FOR INJURY. Patients who have had local anesthesia may be sent to the postanesthesia care unit postoperatively, or they may be returned directly to the nursing unit or the ambulatory surgery unit. In the immediate postoperative period they are usually drowsy because preoperative and intraoperative sedatives typically have been given.

When regional block anesthesia is used, the nurse must remember that sensation in the area is impaired. Caution must be taken, therefore, to prevent injury to the anesthetized body region.

Following spinal anesthesia the patient regains the ability to move the legs before sensation returns. The times that the patient regains movement and sensation should both be charted. The bladder should be assessed for distention because the patient is unable to feel pressure.

In the past, as was previously noted, patients were often kept flat for a specific period of time to prevent spinal headache. This practice has not been found to make a difference and is less common now.

Evaluation

Criteria for evaluating the outcomes of goals of nursing care in the immediate postoperative phase are pulse and blood pressure similar to patient's norms; respiratory rate between 12 and 20, clear breath sounds, and normal skin color; absence of patient complaint of pain, patient calmness; patient verbalizes understanding of physical location; and, patient suffers no injuries during the immediate postoperative phase.

The Patient's Family

The time between the patient's leaving the nursing unit and returning can be 3 or 4 hours even for relatively simple procedures. This may seem like a very long time for family and friends who are waiting. Most hospitals have some system for communicating the patient's status to those who wait. These visitors are usually relieved to know when the patient is in the recovery room. Many surgeons take time to speak with the visitors shortly after the surgery is completed. When problems arise, it is thoughtful to offer visitors privacy and the services of a patient representative or a spiritual counselor.

Discharge from the Postanesthesia Care Unit

The patient's progress in the postanesthesia care unit is carefully monitored. Several systems of scoring have been used to determine when recovery is adequate and the patient can be transferred. In general, the patient can be moved from the recovery room when the following five conditions, noted by Allison and Love (1992), are met:

1. Vital signs are stable.
2. Respiratory and circulatory functions are adequate.
3. The effects of anesthesia have been reversed.
4. The patient is awake or can be awakened easily.
5. Complications are absent or are under control.

Most patients remain in the postanesthesia care unit for 1 to 2 hours, although the time varies considerably. Patients who are unstable or who require very close observation may be transferred to an intensive care unit.

Postoperative Care on the Nursing Unit

When the patient is transferred to the nursing unit, the postanesthesia care unit nurse reports on the patient to the nurse who will be caring for that patient. Several people are usually required to move the patient safely from the gurney to the bed. Caution is needed to prevent pulling or dislodging tubes and to prevent shearing force on the skin. Intravenous fluids must be hung and set at the ordered rate. Nasogastric suction tubes must be connected to suction equipment. Drains should be identified and arranged to avoid obstruction. Safety precautions include raising the side rails, lowering the bed, placing the call button within reach, and instructing the patient not to get up without assistance.

A nursing assessment should be done promptly as described earlier and summarized in Table 14–4. Critical elements of the assessment are the level of consciousness, the respiratory and circulatory status, the wound condition, the urinary function, and the gastrointestinal function.

Nursing Diagnosis

Once the immediate postoperative phase has passed, the type of potential complications changes somewhat. The risks of shock and hypoxia lessen. The nurse's attention turns toward other nursing diagnoses, which include the following:

- **Pain** related to tissue trauma
- **Impaired Tissue Integrity** related to poor wound healing
- **High Risk for Infection** related to break in skin or invasive devices and procedures
- **Impaired Gas Exchange** related to stasis of pulmonary secretions, thrombosis, or emboli
- **Urinary Retention** related to the effects of anesthesia or restricted position
- **Colonic Constipation** related to the effects of drugs, immobility, or bowel manipulation during surgery
- **High Risk for Fluid Volume Deficit** related to wound drainage, inadequate intake, vomiting, or gastrointestinal decompression
- **Altered Nutrition: Less than Body Requirements** related to nausea and vomiting or medical restriction of intake
- **Impaired Physical Mobility** related to weakness, tissue trauma, or medical activity restrictions
- **Body Image Disturbance** related to change in body appearance and function
- **Knowledge Deficit** of postoperative routines or self-care

Goals

Goals of nursing care after recovery from anesthesia are pain relief, wound healing, absence of infection, adequate oxygenation, lack of vascular inflammation, normal urine output, normal gastrointestinal function, normal hydration, adequate nutrition to meet metabolic demands, increase in physical endurance, adaptation to changes in body image, and patient's understanding of routines and self-care activities (see Care Plan: Care of the Postoperative Patient).

Interventions

PAIN. Pain is expected in the early postoperative phase. Pain receptors are stimulated because tissues are cut and stretched during surgery. Muscle spasms in the area around the incision add to the patient's discomfort. The pain is usually most severe during the first 48 hours after surgery. During that time narcotic analgesics such as meperidine or morphine are most appropriate. The physician may order doses to be given at 3- to 4-hour intervals when needed, or patient-controlled anesthesia may be used. Patient-controlled anesthesia is discussed in Chapter 16. By the third postoperative day most patients require less medication for pain relief. The dosage or frequency may be reduced, or the order may be changed to an oral analgesic such as acetaminophen with codeine.

When postoperative patients complain of pain, the nurse determines the exact nature of the complaint. Where is the pain located? It is easy to assume that the pain is incisional when, in fact, the patient may have a headache or a backache. Chest pain, leg pain, or gas pain requires additional assessment and interventions. How severe is the pain? The patient can be asked to rate the severity of the pain on a scale of 1 to 10 with 1 being mild pain and 10 being the worst pain imaginable. This provides a system for evaluating response to comfort measures.

During the first few days after surgery, the patient is medicated promptly for pain. Pain is controlled better if it is treated before it becomes severe. Pain medication can also be given before activities that normally cause pain. Some patients are afraid that they will become addicted to narcotics. They can be assured that the short-term use of narcotics for acute pain generally has not been associated with addiction.

A patient whose pain is controlled adequately is better able to participate in the exercises necessary to prevent postoperative complications. Turning, coughing, deep breathing, and even walking can be scheduled to take advantage of periods when the patient is most comfortable. Of course, a medicated patient must be closely supervised when out of bed.

Although drugs are the mainstay of pain management in the early postoperative phase, other nursing measures can be used to help reduce pain. Position changes and backrubs can be very soothing. Relaxation exercises and mental imagery are often very effective alone or in combination with other nursing measures.

One source of discomfort in the postoperative patient is singultus, commonly known as hiccups. Hiccups are caused by intermittent spasms of the diaphragm. They are uncomfortable, may put stress on the incision, disrupt rest, and interfere with the intake of food and fluids. If hiccups persist, the physician should be notified.

Anxiety seems to intensify discomfort. Measures to decrease anxiety may therefore enhance the effects of pain relief measures. The nurse should recognize when the patient is tense and try to discover the source of the anxiety. Patients need to feel safe and need reassurance about what is happening to them.

IMPAIRED TISSUE INTEGRITY. Various techniques are used to close the wound after surgery. The patient's incision may be closed with sutures, staples, or tape as shown in Figure 14–10. When the patient returns to the nursing unit, a dressing probably covers the wound. Following some procedures such as rectal, vaginal, nasal, or ear surgery, the operative site may be packed with gauze. In some situations wounds are left open and covered with a dressing.

In healthy people surgical wounds begin to heal immediately. By the third or fourth day, the healing is stronger. Although the wound appears to be healed after about 10 days, complete healing may take as long as a year.

Clean sutured incisions heal by first intention. Because the wound edges are closed, tissue bonds with little scarring. An infected wound is left open to heal from the bottom up. This is called healing by second intention. Some sources refer to healing by third intention. This term may be used when the wound is initially left open and later closed. Figure 14–11 illustrates these three types of healing.

The physician usually does the first dressing change, inspects the wound, and orders specific wound care. For the first 24 hours the nurse checks the dressing hourly for bleeding or drainage. If dressings become saturated, the nurse reinforces them using aseptic technique. Depending on physician preference and agency policy, reinforcement may be done several ways. The nurse may

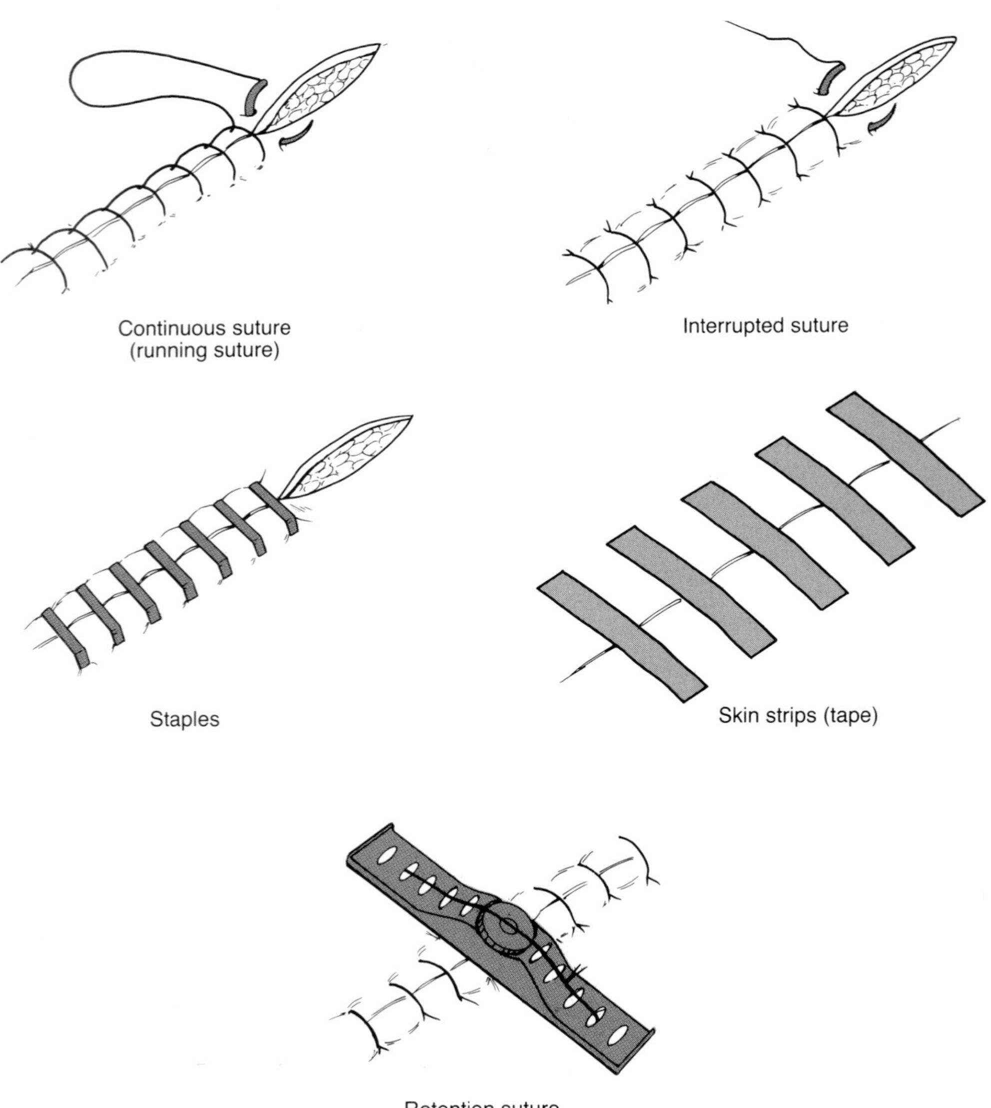

FIGURE 14–10

Methods of wound closure. (From Ignatavicius, D. D., & Bayne, M. V. [1991]. *Medical-surgical nursing: A nursing process approach.* Philadelphia: W. B. Saunders.)

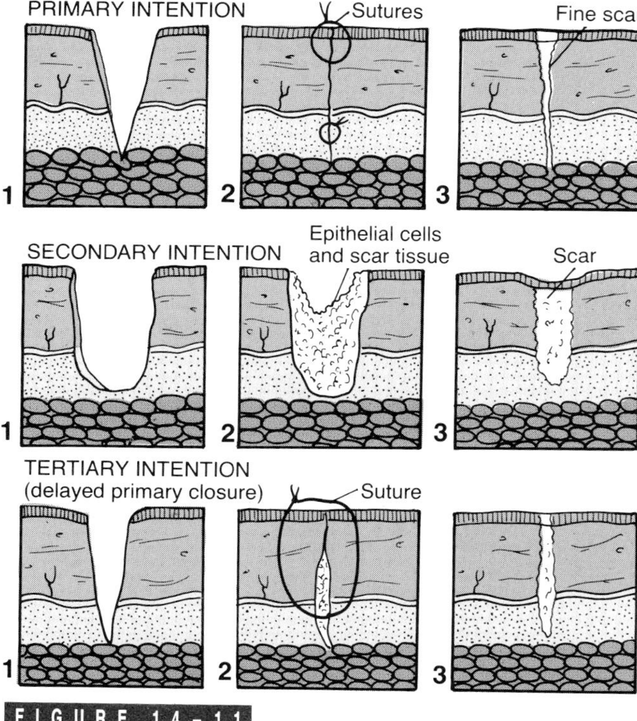

FIGURE 14-11
Wound healing.

simply place dry dressings over the wet ones. Another method is to remove bulky outer layers of the wet dressing and replace them with dry dressings. After the first 24 hours the dressing is checked once or twice each shift. Bleeding should be minimal and should stop within a few hours after the wound is closed. Continued or excessive bleeding is reported to the physician.

Some wounds have drains in a "stab" wound close to the incision (Fig. 14–12). Drains remove fluids from the operative site. Fluid accumulation in a wound interferes with healing. A Penrose drain is a soft tube that permits passive movement of fluids from the wound. The drainage is absorbed by the wound dressing.

Other types of drains are attached to collection devices that create suction to draw fluid from the wound. This type of drain is called an *active drain.* Examples of low-suction active drains are the Hemovac and the Jackson-Pratt. Both create negative pressure when they are compressed. As they fill with fluid, the collection devices expand. They must be emptied and recompressed ("recharged") to maintain their effectiveness. The frequency of emptying depends on the amount of drainage and the physician's orders. Wound drains may also be connected to sump drains. Drainage is measured and recorded as output.

In the immediate postoperative phase, wound drainage is often bright red (sanguineous). As the amount of blood in the drainage decreases, the fluid becomes pinkish (serosanguineous). It should become progressively lighter in color and thinner until it is straw colored and clear (serous). At the same time that the color is changing, the amount of drainage should steadily decrease.

The nurse takes care to reduce the risk of wound complications: dehiscence, evisceration, and infection. Although dehiscence is not expected in a clean wound, measures should always be taken to avoid strain on the suture line. The patient is taught to support the incision during coughing and when getting in and out of bed (Fig. 14–13). Patients who have had abdominal surgery should not use trapeze bars to move themselves. Nausea should be treated promptly to avoid the stress of retching and vomiting. Because many surgical patients go home in less than a week, they need instructions about safe activities. The exact type of surgery determines the restrictions. The nurse consults with the physician about correct instructions.

Wounds that are healing normally are unlikely to undergo dehiscence. If infection develops under surgical sutures, the sutures dissolve too soon. Fluid accumulates in the wound, and the wound dehisces. A sudden increase in wound drainage may precede wound dehiscence. When the suture line ruptures, the patient may feel like the wound is "pulling apart."

If dehiscence occurs, the patient is kept in bed and in a position to decrease strain on the wound and decrease the risk of evisceration. The wound is covered with a sterile dressing and the physician notified. If evisceration also occurs, the usual practice is to cover the wound with sterile dressings saturated with normal saline. The saline is thought to prevent damage from drying of the exposed organs. Some are concerned, however, that moisture increases the risk of wound contamination by promoting bacterial movement through the dressings. Covering the saline-soaked gauze with a dry dressing may prevent this complication.

INFECTION. The patient is continuously assessed for indications of infection. Signs and symptoms of wound infection usually do not develop until the third to fifth day after the operation. They may appear as late as a week after surgery. The classic signs and symptoms of wound infection include pain, fever, redness, swelling, and purulent drainage. Surgical pain should decrease as the days go by. Continued or increasing pain suggests the possibility of infection. A low-grade fever is common during the first 2 postoperative days because of the normal inflammation stage of healing. If the temperature is higher than 38°C (100.4°F) or lasts more than 2 days, however, it may be due to infection. Early signs of infection are sometimes hard to detect in elderly surgical patients because they typically do not develop high fevers even with serious infections. Some redness is expected at the wound suture line and around the sutures or staples. Increasing redness or redness that spreads to surrounding tissue is not normal.

Prevention of wound infection requires decreasing the exposure to microorganisms and maintaining the patient's resistance to infection. Good handwashing, use of sterile gloves, aseptic dressing changes, and diligent wound care prevent the introduction of infectious organisms. Good hydration and nutrition support the patient's healing and resistance to infection.

If infection is suspected, a culture of any drainage may identify the infectious organism or organisms. The

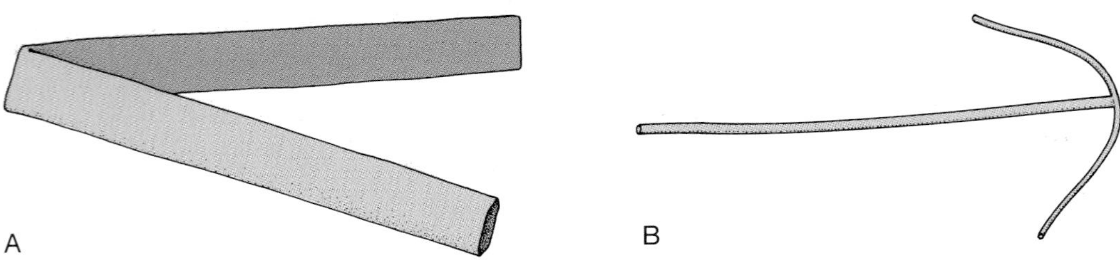

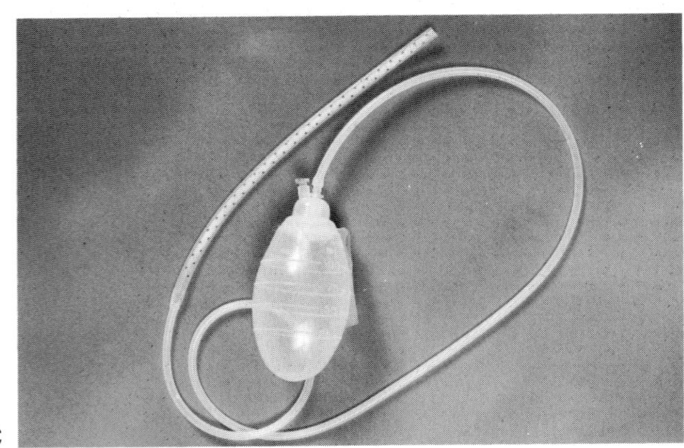

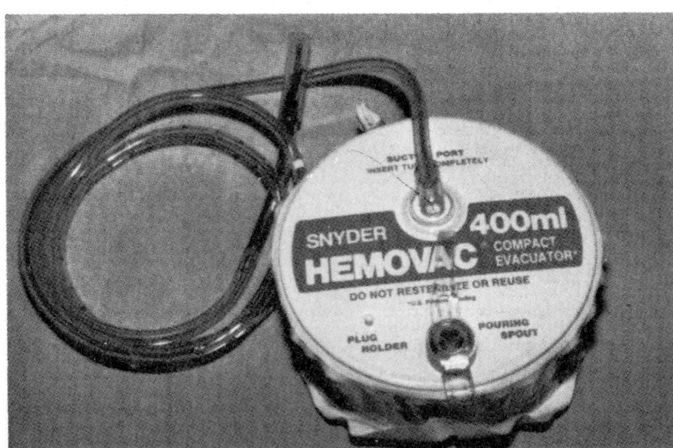

FIGURE 14-12

Types of surgical drains used to remove fluid from wounds. Passive or gravity drains include the Penrose *(A)* and the T-tube *(B)*. Drains that work by creating negative pressure when the receptacle is compressed are the Jackson-Pratt *(C)* and the Hemovac *(D)*. *(A, B,* and *D* from Ignatavicius, D. D., & Bayne M. V. [1991]. *Medical-surgical nursing: A nursing process approach* [p. 480]. Philadelphia: W. B. Saunders. *C* from Bolander, V. B. [1994]. *Sorensen and Luckmann's basic nursing* [3rd ed.]. Philadelphia: W. B. Saunders. Courtesy Deknatel, Inc., Fall River, MA.)

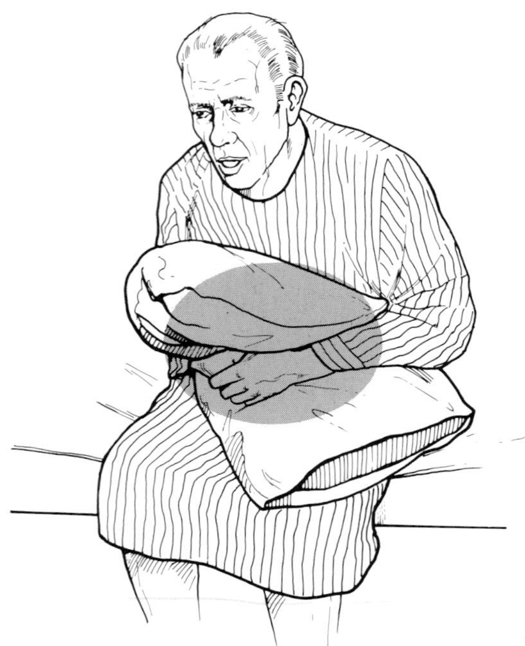

FIGURE 14-13

Splinting supports the incision during coughing.

antibiotics that are most likely to be effective can then be prescribed. The culture specimen should be taken before antibiotic therapy is begun. While awaiting results of the culture and sensitivity test, the physician often orders a broad-spectrum antibiotic. Various cleansing procedures may also be ordered. The patient may need to be isolated from other patients to prevent transfer of the organisms. The presence of highly contagious organisms such as methicillin-resistant *Staphylococcus aureus* requires patient isolation.

Because infection may develop after the patient is discharged, patient teaching should include signs and symptoms of infection that should be reported to the physician. The patient also should know whether the wound requires any special treatment. If wound care is needed at home, the nurse must make sure the patient or a family member is able to do it before the patient leaves the hospital.

IMPAIRED GAS EXCHANGE. The nurse assesses the patient's respiratory status every hour for the first 24 hours and once or twice a shift after that. Signs and symptoms of pneumonia include dyspnea, fatigue, fever, cough, purulent or bloody sputum, and "wet" breath sounds. When gas exchange is impaired, as with pneumonia or atelectasis, the pulse rate generally increases. Breath sounds are absent in areas of atelectasis.

The most important nursing measures to prevent pneumonia and atelectasis are frequent position changes and coughing and deep breathing exercises. Initially, the patient must be assisted to turn at least every 2 hours. Patients are often assisted out of bed on the day of surgery. They are usually ambulated several times daily beginning the second day. Early ambulation has been found to reduce the respiratory complications of surgery greatly.

Deep breathing inflates the lungs fully, and coughing removes secretions. The nurse helps the patient cough and deep breathe every hour. The patient is instructed to take in a deep breath through the nose and gradually blow out through the mouth, After taking several deep breaths, a cough should be attempted to bring up secretions.

The incentive spirometer is a device used to promote lung expansion (Fig. 14–14). It consists of a tube through which air is inhaled and a cylinder containing a ball. The ball rises in the cylinder as the patient inhales through the tube. The more air taken in, the higher the ball moves. Markings on the cylinder indicate the volume of air taken in. This gives the patient a measurable goal to work for while using the spirometer.

Deep breathing and coughing are painful for the patient who has had abdominal or chest surgery. The nurse can reduce discomfort by coordinating the exercises with analgesics and by splinting the incision. The patient can splint by holding a pillow firmly over the surgical area while coughing.

It is best to teach turning, deep breathing, coughing, and use of the incentive spirometer before surgery. A patient in pain or drowsy from anesthesia is not in the best condition for learning. There are a few instances in which coughing is contraindicated. They include surgeries for hernias and cataracts, as well as brain surgery.

If the patient develops pneumonia, it is treated with rest, oxygen, and antibiotics. Care of the patient with pneumonia is discussed in Chapter 28.

Another factor that may cause severe, sometimes fatal, respiratory complications is pulmonary emboli. Pulmonary emboli usually arise from thrombi that develop in veins, especially the veins of the legs and pelvis. Measures to prevent thrombophlebitis and related pulmonary emboli include leg exercises, early ambulation, and frequent position changes within the limits of any restrictions imposed by the physician. Antiembolic stockings may be ordered. Signs and symptoms that alert the nurse to possible pulmonary emboli are dyspnea, tachypnea, chest pain, and hemoptysis. If the embolus is very large, the patient may become cyanotic and go into shock. Emboli may be treated with heparin, thrombolytic agents, or both (Fig. 14–15).

URINARY RETENTION. Urinary output must be monitored carefully following surgery. In the first 24 hours, urinary output is typically reduced because of the stress response. The nurse is aware, however, of the possibilities of urine retention or kidney failure in the early postoperative phase. Urinary function is monitored by measuring intake and output and by checking for bladder distention.

PHARMACOLOGY CAPSULE

Anesthesia, narcotic analgesics, and anticholinergics can contribute to urinary retention.

Patients who have had perineal or abdominal surgery are most likely to have difficulty voiding. They often have indwelling catheters inserted before or during sur-

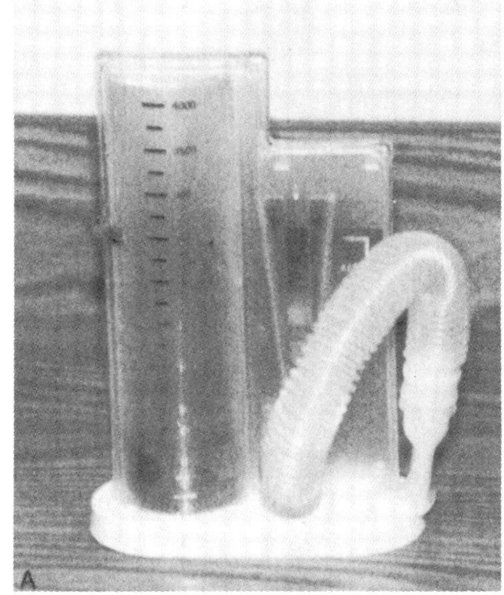

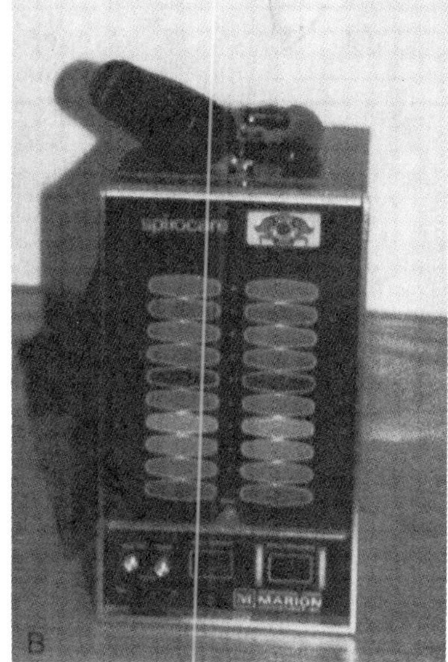

FIGURE 14-14

The incentive spirometer is used to promote lung expansion. (From Ignatavicius, D. D., & Bayne, M. V. [1991]. *Medical-surgical nursing: A nursing process approach* [p. 446]. Philadelphia: W. B. Saunders.)

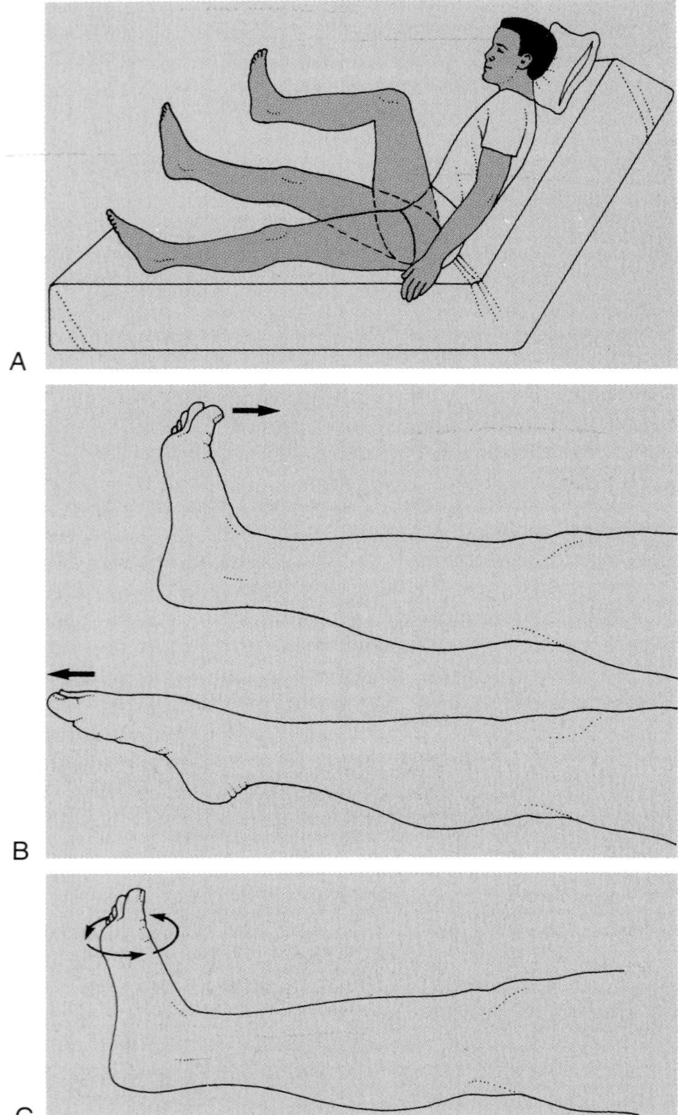

FIGURE 14-15

Postoperative leg exercises promote venous return. (Modified from Ignatavicius, D. D., & Bayne, M. V. [1991]. *Medical-surgical nursing: A nursing process approach* [p. 447]. Philadelphia: W. B. Saunders.)

gery. The patient with a urine retention problem usually reports feelings of fullness and pressure over the lower abdomen. Some patients are unable to void at all. When a patient passes small amounts of urine frequently without feeling relief of the fullness, the nurse suspects retention with overflow. The bladder releases just enough urine to reduce the pressure but without complete emptying. Gentle palpation of the lower abdomen usually reveals the smooth, rounded, full bladder.

If the patient is unable to void, catheterization is necessary. Because catheterization can cause urinary infection, it should be done only if other interventions fail. Interventions must take the physician's activity orders into consideration. The patient should be granted privacy while attempting to void. The toilet is preferred if the patient can go to the bathroom. If a bedpan has to be used, it should be warmed first. The head of the bed should be raised, if permitted, to create a normal position for voiding. Men who need to stand to void should be assisted to do so if not contraindicated.

Sensory stimuli help some people overcome difficulty voiding. The sound of running water or the sensation of warm water poured over the perineum or hands may encourage voiding. The water should be measured so it can be subtracted from the urine output.

If all independent measures fail, a physician's order is required for catheterization. There is usually an "as necessary" order to empty the bladder with a catheter if the patient does not void within 6 to 8 hours after surgery.

Some agencies have policies that limit the amount of urine that can be drained from a full bladder at one time. These limits are usually 750 to 1000 ml. After the removal of the allowed amount of urine, the catheter may be clamped for a specified period of time before the bladder is drained again. This procedure is referred to as *bladder decompression*. Research in this area has raised some question as to whether draining the bladder completely is, in fact, dangerous.

If the patient has to be catheterized several times, the physician may order the insertion of an indwelling catheter. Catheterization and the care of the patient with a catheter are discussed in Chapter 36.

If there are no signs of bladder distention but little or no urine output, the patient may be in kidney failure. Thirty ml per hour is considered the minimal urine output. Failure to produce at least 30 ml in an hour should be reported promptly to the physician. The diagnosis and treatment of kidney failure is discussed in Chapter 36.

COLONIC CONSTIPATION. Gastrointestinal function is disrupted by surgery. Postoperatively, the nurse inspects and palpates for abdominal distention and auscultates for bowel sounds. The passage of flatus and the first bowel movement are documented. The patient may not realize the signficance of passing flatus and may wonder why the nurse asks about it. The nurse can explain that passing flatus means the digestive tract is beginning to function again. Most patients pass flatus about 48 hours postoperatively.

Early, frequent ambulation is the best way to prevent gastrointestinal discomfort. The intake of oral fluids and a normal diet also help to stimulate peristalsis. Oral intake is usually withheld, however, until bowel sounds return (normally 24–48 hours after surgery).

Measures to promote the passage of flatus may be ordered, including early ambulation, insertion of a rectal tube for 20 minutes every 2 to 3 hours, application of heat to the abdomen, positioning the patient prone or on the right side, and insertion of bisacodyl suppositories.

If gastrointestinal function does not resume, the patient has a paralytic ileus manifested by abdominal pain, distention, tenderness, and absence of bowel sounds. Other signs and symptoms of paralytic ileus are nausea, vomiting, and not passing flatus or feces.

Severe abdominal distention develops if normal bowel activity does not resume within a few days. In that case, a nasogastric tube may be ordered to permit decompression of the intestines. If the surgical procedure is one that often causes gastrointestinal problems, the nasogastric tube may be inserted during surgery to prevent problems.

The patient should have a bowel movement within a few days after resuming the intake of solid foods. Sometimes a suppository or an enema is necessary to stimulate emptying of the bowel.

FLUID VOLUME DEFICIT AND ALTERED NUTRITION. Depending on the type of surgery done, fluid and nutrition needs are met in a variety of ways. Some patients are given regular diets the evening of surgery. Others receive nothing by mouth for several days. Most patients return from the postanesthesia care unit with intravenous infusions. Patients are usually given liquids at first. If liquids are retained, the diet is "advanced" to include soft foods, then regular foods.

When the patient is able to tolerate liquids well, the intravenous infusion is usually discontinued unless it is needed for the administration of medication. The nurse monitors the flow rate and the patient response. Nursing care of the patient receiving intravenous fluids is discussed in Chapter 15. Alternative methods of feeding may be used if the patient is unable to resume oral intake for a long time. These methods are discussed in Chapter 34.

Fluid intake and output are usually measured for several days after surgery. In addition, laboratory studies of serum electrolytes are often ordered.

Nausea and vomiting interfere with the intake of food and fluids and can cause considerable fluid loss. Antiemetics (drugs used to control nausea and vomiting) are usually ordered as necessary. General nursing measures for the patient with nausea and vomiting are discussed in Chapter 34.

PHARMACOLOGY CAPSULE

Antiemetic drugs control postoperative nausea and vomiting.

IMPAIRED PHYSICAL MOBILITY. After general anesthesia and invasive surgical procedures, patients are usually weak and tire quickly. The physician prescribes measures to increase the patient's activity level, progressive ambulation in most cases. The patient should be assisted out of bed the first few times until the nurse is sure the patient can get up alone safely. The nurse helps the patient sit on the bedside, press the feet on the floor, stand, and then walk increasingly greater distances. The patient is monitored for weakness and dizziness. The nurse emphasizes the physical benefits of early ambulation to the patient.

BODY IMAGE DISTURBANCE. The effects of surgery (scars, loss of body organs, altered physical functions) can be very traumatic. A sense of loss can be demonstrated by anger, depression, or even denial. The nurse should understand and accept these responses. Nursing care of the grieving patient is discussed in detail in Chapter 22. Surgery can also produce positive changes in body image when it serves to improve appearance or function or to relieve symptoms.

KNOWLEDGE DEFICIT. Patient teaching in the postoperative phase emphasizes recovery from the surgical experience and preparation for return to maximum possible function. Discharge planning should be started when the patient is admitted for surgery and revised as needed during the course of hospitalization. Topics to include in the discharge teaching plan are shown in Table 14–5.

TABLE 14-5

POSTOPERATIVE PATIENT TEACHING

1. Drug therapy: New medications, instructions about dosage and schedule, management of side effects, adverse effects to report to the physician.
2. Wound care: Proper cleansing technique, care of drains, dressing procedure, signs and symptoms (infection, impaired healing) that should be reported to the physician.
3. Activity: When regular activities can be resumed, how much weight can be lifted, recommended activity to promote recovery, need for assistance, referral to community services if needed.
4. Fluids and nutrition: Special diet, fluid needs.
5. Equipment and supplies: How to obtain and use assistive devices, special equipment, and supplies.
6. Home environment: Any adaptations needed.
7. Follow-up care: Importance of keeping medical appointments.

PHARMACOLOGY CAPSULE

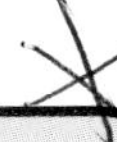

Discharge teaching includes information about drug therapy.

Evaluation

Criteria for evaluating the outcomes of the identified nursing goals are patient's statement of pain relief, relaxed expression; intact wound margins; absence of fever, purulent wound drainage, excessive redness or edema; absence of redness and tenderness in legs; absence of chest pain and dyspnea; urine output consistent with fluid intake; presence of bowel sounds, passage of flatus; approximately equal fluid intake and output, normal serum electrolytes; retention of oral fluids and food, absence of nausea and vomiting; gradual increase in mobility to maximal level; patient's expression of acceptance of physical changes; and patient's statement of postoperative routines and self-care after discharge.

NUTRITION CONCEPTS

- Surgery is accompanied by a stress response and an increase in metabolic rate that may lead to nutritional deficiency.
- Nutritional deficits may impair surgical wound healing.
- Intravenous fluids do not supply sufficient kilocalories and most nutrients needed for wound healing and should not be the only source of nutrition for more than 7 to 10 days after surgery.
- After the immediate postoperative recovery period, patients should be encouraged to eat a diet high in kilocalories and protein for 6 to 12 weeks.
- Dietary supplements such as Sustacal or Ensure may be needed for patients whose intake of regular foods is inadequate for healing.

BIBLIOGRAPHY

Allison, J. F., & Love, C. W. (1992). Nursing role in management: Postoperative client. In S. M. Lewis & I. C. Collier (Eds.), *Medical surgical nursing* (3rd ed., pp. 276–301). St. Louis: Mosby Year Book.

Boyle, K., Nance, J., & Passau-Buck, S. (1992). Post-hospitalization concerns of medical-surgical patients. *Applied Nursing Research, 5*(3), 122–126.

Caldwell, L. M. (1991). The influence of preference for information on preoperative stress and coping in surgical outpatients. *Applied Nursing Research, 4*(4), 177–183.

Campbell, A., & Johnston, C. A. (1991). OR/PACU reports: What they should tell you about your postoperative patient. *Nursing 91, 21*(10), 49–51.

Cerrato, P. L. (1991). Surgery, stress, and metabolism. *RN, 54*(8), 63–65.

Cushing, M. (1991). Demystifying informed consent. *American Journal of Nursing, 91*(11), 17–19.

Deglin, J. H., Vallerand, A. H., & Russin, M. M. (1991). *Davis's drug guide for nurses* (2nd ed.). Philadelphia: F. A. Davis.

Doenges, M. E., & Moorhouse, M. F. (1991). *Nursing diagnoses with interventions* (3rd ed.). Philadelphia: W. B. Saunders.

Fromm, C. G., & Metzler, D. (1993). Preparing your older patient for surgery. *RN, 56*(1), 38–44.

Howell, E. E., & Eldridge, J. E. (1989). The nurse's role in informed consent. *The Journal of Practical Nursing, 39*(3), 28–31.

Howie, J. N. (1989). How and when should I respond to post-op fever? *American Journal of Nursing, 89*(7), 984–986.

Ignatavicius, D. D., & Bayne, M. V. (1991). *Medical-surgical nursing: A nursing process approach.* Philadelphia: W. B. Saunders.

Jarvis, C. (1992). *Physical examination and health assessment.* Philadelphia: W. B. Saunders.

Lawler, M. (1991). Managing other complications. *Nursing 91, 21*(11), 40–46.

Leckrone, L. (1991). Preparing your patient for surgery. *Nursing 91, 21*(7), 47–49.

Lewis, S. M., & Collier, I. C. (1992). *Medical-surgical nursing* (3rd ed.). St. Louis: Mosby Year Book.

Litwak, K. (1991). What you need to know about administering preoperative medications. *Nursing 91, 21*(8), 44–47.

Litwak, K. (1991). Managing postanesthetic emergencies. *Nursing 91, 21*(9), 49–51.

Marshall, M. (1993). Postoperative confusion: Helping your patient emerge from the shadows. *Nursing 93, 23*(1), 44–47.

McConnell, E. A. (1991). Minimizing respiratory problems. *Nursing 91, 21*(11), 35–39.

O'Toole, M. (Ed.). (1992). *Miller-Keane encyclopedia and dictionary of medicine, nursing, and allied health* (5th ed.). Philadelphia: W. B. Saunders.

Peden, L. (1992). Helping postop patients sleep. *RN, 55*(4), 24–26.

Potter, P. A., & Perry, A. G. (1992). *Fundamentals of nursing* (3rd ed.). St. Louis: C. V. Mosby.

Rowland, M. A. (1990). Myths—and facts—about postop discomfort. *American Journal of Nursing, 90*(5), 60–64.

Shlafer, M. (1993). *The nurse, pharmacology, and drug therapy* (2nd ed.). Redwood City, CA: Addison-Wesley Publishing.

Sweeney, M. J. (1991). Your role in informed consent. *RN, 54*(8), 55–60.

Walsh, J. (1993). Postop effects of OR positioning. *RN, 56*(2), 50–57.

Wild, L., & Coyne, C. (1992). Epidural anesthesia: The basics and beyond. *American Journal of Nursing, 92*(4), 26–36.

KEY CONCEPTS

1. Surgical procedures classified by purpose are diagnostic, exploratory, curative, palliative, and cosmetic.
2. Variables that affect surgical outcomes are age, nutritional status, fluid and electrolyte balance, medical diagnoses, drugs, and habits such as use of tobacco and alcohol.
3. The phases of the surgical experience are preoperative, intraoperative, and postoperative.
4. Nursing measures to reduce patient anxiety and increase knowledge about the surgical experience may actually decrease complications.
5. Preoperative teaching should include surgical preparation; what to expect in the surgical suite and postanesthesia care unit; what tubes, dressings, or equipment may be in place after surgery; and how patient participation can promote recovery.
6. Before surgery, the patient or legal guardian must sign a legal consent form.
7. Preparation for surgery may involve bowel cleansing, food and fluid restriction, skin scrubbing and shaving, securing and covering hair, and administering preoperative medications as ordered. Clothing, jewelry, nail polish, and prostheses are usually removed.
8. After preoperative medications are given, the patient should remain in bed.
9. The surgical team consists of nurses who circulate, nurses who scrub, one or more surgeons, an anesthesiologist or a nurse anesthetist, and other technical personnel.
10. Anesthetic agents are used to alter sensation so that surgical procedures can be done painlessly and safely.
11. The nursing goals in the intraoperative phase are absence of physical injury, adequate oxygenation, normal pulse and blood pressure, adequate peripheral circulation, and balanced fluid intake and output.
12. Postoperative surgical complications may include shock, hypoxia, wound infection, wound dehiscence and evisceration, injury, pneumonia, atelectasis, nausea and vomiting, impaired peristalsis, urinary retention, renal failure, and thrombophlebitis.
13. Goals of nursing care in the immediate postoperative period are adequate circulation and oxygenation, pain relief, mental orientation, and freedom from injury.
14. Visitors need to be advised where to wait and how they will be informed of the patient's status.
15. Goals of nursing care after recovery from anesthesia are pain relief, wound healing, absence of infection, adequate oxygenation, lack of vascular inflammation, normal urine output and gastrointestinal function, good hydration, adequate nutrition, restoration of physical endurance, adaptation to changes in body image, and patient understanding and participation in self-care activities.
16. Patient teaching for discharge emphasizes drug therapy, wound care, activity limitations, fluid and nutrition needs, equipment and supplies needed, adaptation for the home environment, and the importance of follow-up care.

CHAPTER 15

Adrianne Linton

Intravenous Therapy

OBJECTIVES

1. Identify the indications for intravenous fluid therapy.
2. Describe the types of fluids used for intravenous fluid therapy.
3. Describe the types of venous access devices used for intravenous therapy.
4. Given the prescribed hourly flow rate, calculate the correct drop rate for an intravenous fluid.
5. Explain the causes, signs and symptoms, and nursing implications of the complications of intravenous fluid or drug therapy.
6. Explain the nursing responsibilities when a patient is receiving intravenous therapy.

GLOSSARY

CANNULA A tube that can be inserted into a body cavity or duct; needle or catheter employed for intravenous therapy

EMBOLISM An obstruction of a blood vessel created by a trapped blood clot or other substance

EMBOLUS (*pl.* EMBOLI) An unattached blood clot or other substance in the circulatory system

EXTRAVASATION Escape of fluid or blood from a blood vessel into body tissue

HYPERTONIC A term used to describe a solution that has a higher concentration of electrolytes than normal body fluids

HYPOTONIC A term used to describe a solution that has a lower concentration of electrolytes than normal body fluids

INFILTRATION A collection of infused fluid in tissues surrounding a cannula inserted for intravenous therapy

ISOTONIC A term used to describe a solution that has the same concentration of electrolytes as normal body fluids

PHLEBITIS Inflammation of a blood vessel

SOLUTION A liquid containing one or more dissolved substances

THROMBUS (*pl.* THROMBI) Stationary blood clot

TONICITY A measure of the concentration of electrolytes in a fluid.

Intravenous therapy is the administration of fluids directly into a vein. Most hospitalized patients receive some form of intravenous therapy.

INDICATIONS FOR INTRAVENOUS THERAPY

Intravenous therapy is used to administer drugs, fluids, and blood or blood components. Intravenous drugs may be ordered when a rapid drug effect is needed, when the drug is not available in an oral form, or when the patient is unable to take oral drugs. The intravenous route is also recommended when a drug must be maintained at a certain level in the blood.

In addition to drugs, intravenous fluids can provide water, electrolytes, amino acids, lipids, vitamins, and glucose. Intravenous lines may also be used to provide continuous venous access for intermittent drug administration and emergency drug administration.

Whole blood or blood components are also given intravenously. Blood components include packed red blood cells, frozen red blood cells, platelets, or plasma proteins. Blood transfusions are discussed in Chapter 30.

TYPES OF INTRAVENOUS FLUIDS

By definition, a fluid is any liquid or gas. A solution is a liquid containing one or more dissolved substances. The terms *fluid* and *solution* are often used interchangeably in relation to intravenous therapy.

TONICITY

Fluids can be classified by tonicity, a measure of the concentration of electrolytes in the fluid. The normal concentration of electrolytes in body fluids is about 310 mEq per liter. Other fluids with the same concentration are called *isotonic* fluids. When the concentration is greater than 375 mEq per liter, the fluid is said to be *hypertonic. Hypotonic* fluids have a concentration of less than 250 mEq per liter. The tonicity of fluids is important because it affects blood volume.

COMPONENTS

Many types of fluids are available for intravenous use. The physician selects the appropriate fluid to meet the patient's fluid and electrolyte needs. The most commonly used intravenous solutions are specific combinations of water, sugar (in the form of dextrose), sodium chloride, and other electrolytes.

In most intravenous solutions, dextrose is the only source of calories. The patient receives 34 calories for each 1% of dextrose in a liter of fluid; thus, 1 liter of 5% dextrose provides 170 calories ($34 \times 5 = 170$). Dextrose fluids given in a peripheral vein are 2.5%, 5.0%, or 10.0% dextrose. Fluids infused into a larger (central) vein may have a much higher percentage of dextrose.

Sodium chloride solutions are also commonly used. An isotonic solution is 0.9% sodium chloride and is called *normal saline.* It is used to supply balanced amounts of water and sodium chloride. A hypotonic solution of 0.45% sodium chloride may be ordered if the patient's body fluids are concentrated owing to excessive water loss. More concentrated hypertonic solutions are needed when the patient has had excessive losses of sodium and chloride.

Dextrose, sodium chloride, and other electrolytes are available in numerous combinations. Some commonly used combined electrolyte solutions are Plasma-Lyte and lactated Ringer's.

When a patient needs long-term or aggressive intravenous therapy for nutrition, total parenteral nutrition may be indicated. A catheter is placed in a large vein, usually the subclavian, for administering total parenteral nutrition fluids. These fluids provide dextrose, water, amino acids, electrolytes, vitamins, and minerals. Fat emulsions can also be given intravenously. Total parenteral nutrition is discussed in greater detail in Chapter 12.

VENOUS ACCESS DEVICES

Intravenous fluid is delivered by various types of venous access devices (Fig. 15–1). These include needles, over-the-needle catheters, inside needle catheters, subcutaneous infusion ports, and subcutaneously implanted pumps. The term *cannula* is used to describe both a needle and a catheter.

The administration of intravenous fluids requires placement of the venous access device into a peripheral or central vein. Peripheral veins are those located in the extremities (and the scalp of an infant). They are used for short-term therapy, when a patient has healthy veins, and when relatively nonirritating fluids are given. Figure 15–2 shows common peripheral infusion sites for intravenous fluids.

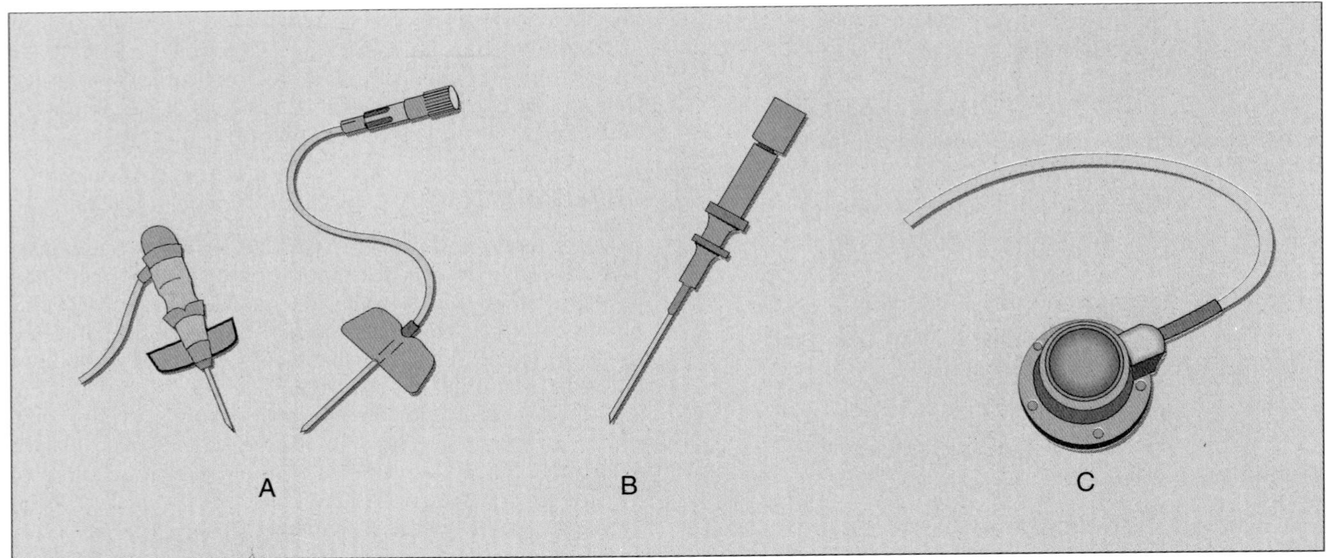

FIGURE 15-1

Venous access devices. *A*, Winged infusion needles; *B*, catheter; *C*, infusion port; *D*, infusion pump. (*D* Courtesy of Pharmacia/Deltec, Inc., St. Paul, MN.)

Central veins, located in large vessels close to the heart, are used when long-term therapy is required, when the patient has poor peripheral veins, and when irritating fluids are to be administered. Central lines are inserted into the subclavian or jugular vein or into the superior vena cava. The line may be placed through a peripheral vein and advanced to the desired location or may be inserted through a skin incision and tunneled under the skin and into the large vessel. The central line threaded through a peripheral vein is called a peripherally inserted central (PIC) catheter. Examples of tunneled catheters are the Hickman, Broviac, and Hickman-Broviac. Other examples of central access devices are the implanted pump and the port-A-Cath, an implanted subcutaneous port. Central lines can be left in place much longer than peripheral lines.

NEEDLES

One type of needle used is a winged infusion needle, a short needle with two plastic wings that are held during insertion. A winged infusion needle is useful in infants when a scalp vein is used for intravenous therapy. It is also used at times for adults who have very poor veins, for in-and-out therapy, and for therapy of short duration. Some institutions routinely use winged infusion needles for peripheral intravenous therapy.

CATHETERS

A catheter is a small plastic tube that fits over or inside a needle. After insertion into the vein, the needle

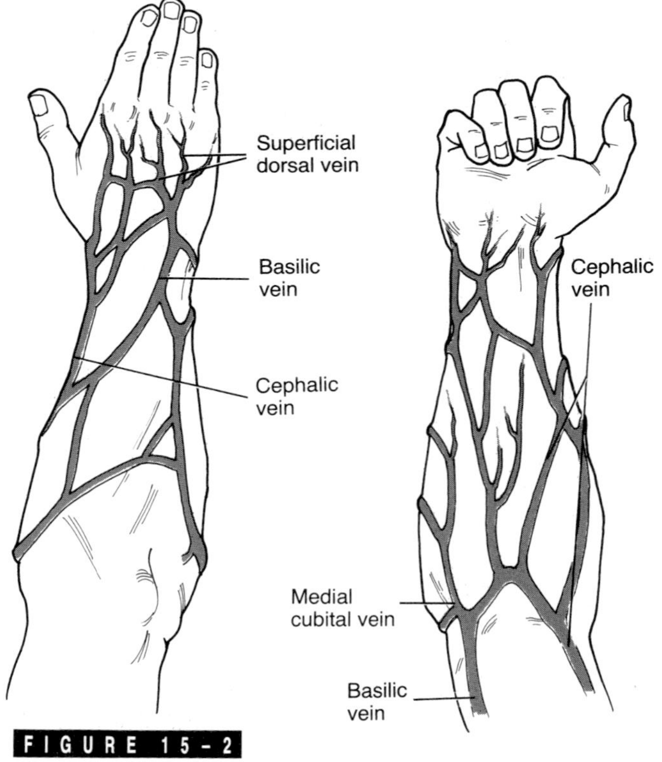

FIGURE 15-2

Common peripheral intravenous infusion sites.

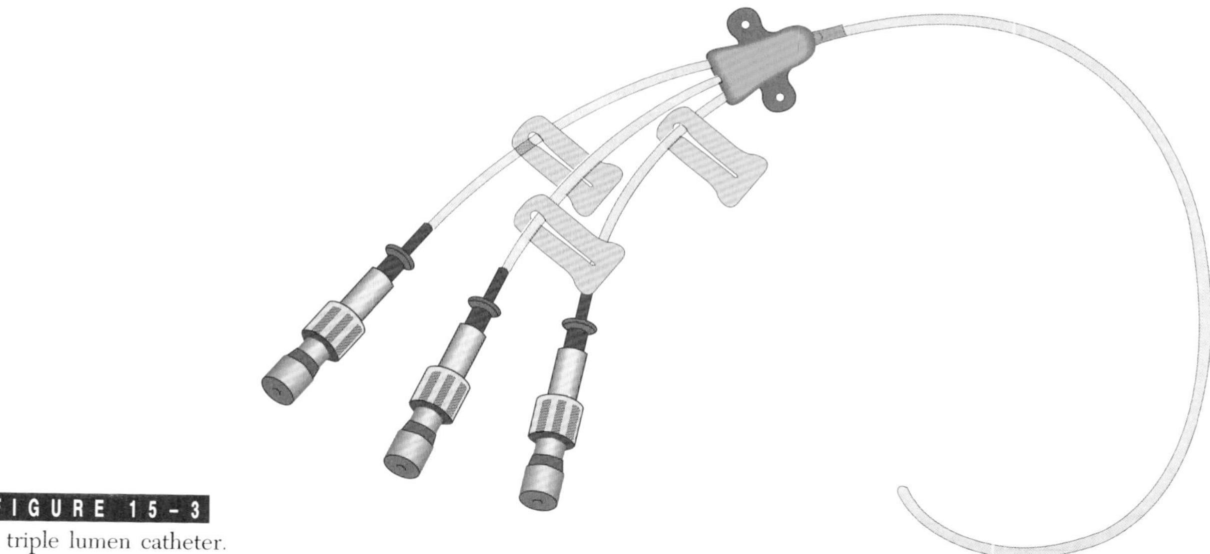

FIGURE 15-3
A triple lumen catheter.

is withdrawn. The plastic catheter is then connected to tubing to deliver the fluid. Catheters are less likely than needles to puncture the vein once they are in place. They come in a variety of lengths. Nurses generally insert only short (1¼–2 inch) catheters.

Tunneled catheters are inserted only by the physician. Some special catheters may be inserted at the patient's bedside, but the Hickman-Broviac catheter requires a surgical procedure.

One type of subclavian catheter is the triple lumen catheter (Fig. 15–3). It is essentially one catheter with three separate channels. Each channel has a port through which blood can be drawn. One port is used to measure central venous pressure. The other two ports can be used to give drugs, fluids, or blood.

A central catheter that can be inserted by trained nurses is the PIC catheter (Fig. 15–4). The PIC catheter is inserted into a vein in the antecubital space and

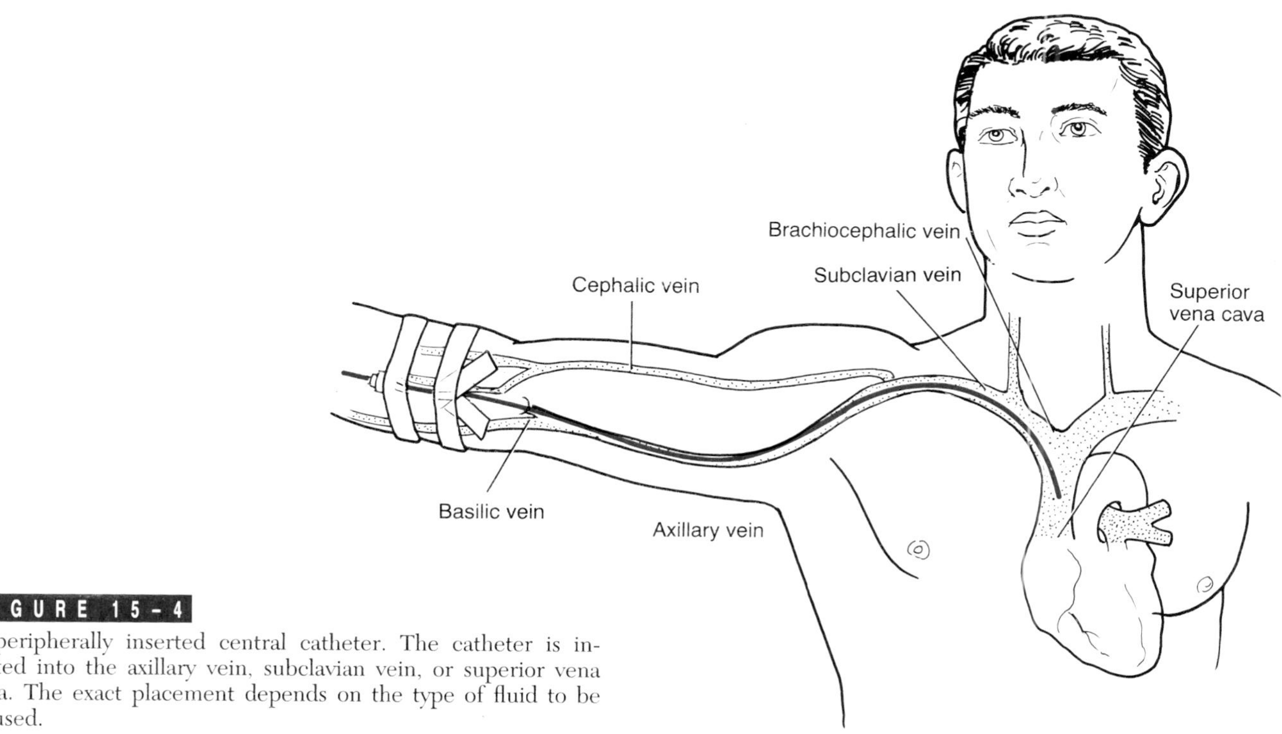

FIGURE 15-4
A peripherally inserted central catheter. The catheter is inserted into the axillary vein, subclavian vein, or superior vena cava. The exact placement depends on the type of fluid to be infused.

advanced into the axillary, subclavian, or brachiocephalic vein or the superior vena cava. Advantages of the PIC catheter over other central catheters include easier insertion, cost savings, and reduced risk of pneumothorax, hemothorax, or air embolism. When compared with peripheral cannulas, PIC catheters can be left in place longer, do not restrict arm movement, and are less traumatic to the vein.

IMPLANTED DEVICES

Some devices can be implanted to allow immediate access to a vein without repeated, painful venipunctures. They include infusion ports and pumps that are implanted under the skin and external infusion pumps. Infusion ports consist of a catheter and a chamber into which fluids can be injected directly into a vein or an artery. They are also used for intraspinal infusions. The chamber is easily felt directly under the skin. Infusion pumps are filled using a special needle that is inserted through the skin into the port. They dispense the fluid into the vein at a very slow rate. The rate of infusion is sometimes affected by body temperature, with fever increasing the delivery rate. The infusion rate of some infusion pumps can be set electronically by passing a wand over the pump. Infusion pumps are often used to administer chemotherapy drugs for cancer.

INTERMITTENT INFUSION DEVICES

Many patients need intravenous medications at specific intervals such as every 4 or every 6 hours. Such drugs are often given "piggyback," that is, the drug is given through an injection port in the tubing of a continuous infusion.

PHARMACOLOGY CAPSULE

> A drug given "piggyback" is administered through an injection port in the tubing of a continuous infusion.

If the patient does not need continuous fluids, however, an intermittent infusion device can be used to give the medication.

PHARMACOLOGY CAPSULE

> An intermittent infusion device can be used to administer intravenous medications when continuous fluids are not needed.

Any intravenous cannula (needle or catheter) can be made intermittent by attaching a resealable cap or an extension with a cap.

A heparin lock is a short cannula with an attached injection port. It is taped in place, and medications are injected when needed through the port. It is called a heparin lock because it is usually flushed with a dilute heparin solution after each use to keep clots from forming and blocking the catheter. Current research suggests that flushing with normal saline may be just as effective as and less expensive than using heparin. Also, heparin prolongs the time required for blood to clot, whereas saline does not. The nurse should know the agency's procedure for flushing these devices.

INITIATION OF INTRAVENOUS THERAPY

Nurse practice acts and agency policies determine which nurses can perform venipunctures, hang intravenous fluids, and give intravenous medications.

EQUIPMENT

The nurse responsible for starting intravenous fluids gathers the equipment needed to start the infusion: cannula, tourniquet, skin cleansing solution, tape, dressing supplies, gloves, tubing, and solution container. The smallest possible cannula should be used, although blood and some fluids require larger cannulas. The product literature is read to identify any special requirements such as a filter. The prescribed solution or drug is obtained using the "five rights": right solution or drug, right dose or strength, right patient, right route, and right time. Tubing is attached to the solution container, and air is cleared from the tubing by allowing some fluid to run through it.

SITE SELECTION

The nurse then selects the venipuncture site for the infusion. The site chosen should be the least restrictive (i.e., not over a joint or on the hand). It should have a large vein that is in good condition. A new device called a Vein Light may facilitate locating a vein. The preferred site is usually the patient's nondominant arm. Venipuncture should not be done in an arm that has impaired circulation or poor lymphatic drainage, as in the patient who has had a radical mastectomy.

PROCEDURE

A tourniquet is applied above the venipuncture site to distend the vein. The tourniquet should be at least ½-inch wide and should not obstruct arterial blood flow. The venipuncture site is gently cleansed. The venipuncture is done using universal precautions. The cannula is inserted through the skin carefully and guided into the vein in the direction of blood flow. If the first attempt is unsuccessful, the nurse selects another site, changes cannulas, and tries again. After two unsuccessful attempts, most nurses call on a more experienced nurse to start the infusion. When the cannula has been threaded into the vein successfully, it is taped securely but without restricting circulation. The site is dressed and the dressing changed according to agency policy. Some use a clear occlusive dressing that allows inspection of the insertion site.

The cannula and the tubing are usually changed every 48 hours in accordance with standards of the Intravenous Nurses' Society. Seventy-two hours is the maximum time between cannula changes; there is controversy about the maximum time between tubing changes. Research is in progress to determine whether complications increase when cannulas remain in place for 72 hours. Dressings on central lines are changed every 48 hours. An intravenous fluid container should not be used for more than 24 hours. Agency policies are generally quite specific about the schedule.

DOCUMENTATION

The date and time that the cannula was inserted is written on the site dressing as well as the length and gauge of the cannula and the nurse's initials. Every bag of fluid and tubing is labeled with the date and time that it was hung and the fluid's expiration date.

MAINTENANCE OF INTRAVENOUS THERAPY

The physician orders the type of fluid and the rate at which it is to be given. The nurse is responsible for maintaining the correct rate of flow and for monitoring the patient's response to the infusion. Intravenous fluids can be allowed to flow by gravity or can be regulated by an electronic infusion control device. When gravity flow is used, the rate is determined by adjusting a clamp on the tubing.

The infusion rate should be checked hourly even if an infusion control device is used. If the fluid is running too slowly, it should be adjusted. No attempt should be made to "catch up" by administering extra fluid rapidly. If the fluid is running too quickly, the rate should be slowed and the patient assessed for signs of fluid volume excess.

If the patient is ambulatory, an intravenous line attached to a pole with wheels is provided, and the patient is told how to protect the infusion.

FACTORS AFFECTING INFUSION RATE

Even after the nurse sets the infusion rate, many factors can alter that rate. The main determinants of the infusion rate are the following:

1. The height of the fluid container over the patient's heart. When the container is raised, the fluid flows faster. Lowering the container causes the fluid to run more slowly.
2. The volume of fluid in the container. A full container causes the fluid to run faster. As the container empties, the rate slows down.
3. Viscosity of the fluid. Thin fluids such as normal saline flow more quickly than thick fluids such as blood.
4. Needle diameter. Fluid flows more quickly through a large needle than through a small needle.
5. Venting of the fluid container. Plastic bags collapse as they empty, but glass containers cannot do that. Therefore, glass containers must be vented to allow air to enter as fluid leaves. Without proper venting, the fluid does not flow.
6. Position of the extremity. With peripheral lines, certain movements or positions may interfere with the flow of fluid. If that happens, the nurse may need to splint the extremity to limit movement or advise the patient to avoid certain movements or positions.

CALCULATION OF INFUSION RATE

The nurse should know how to calculate infusion rates even if infusion control devices are used routinely. To calculate the infusion rate, the nurse must first know (1) the ordered fluid volume per hour and (2) the number of drops equal to 1 ml in the delivery set used (called the drop factor). To set the rate of flow, the nurse needs to count the number of drops per minute.

The physician's order specifies the amount of fluid to be administered in a specific period of time. The instructions on the delivery set package state how many drops equal 1 ml using that set. Standard delivery sets (sometimes called macrodrip sets) deliver 10, 15, or 20 drops per milliliter. Microdrip sets deliver 60 drops per milliliter, they are used in pediatrics and when small volumes of fluid are being given.

EXAMPLE

Physician's order: 1000 ml 5% dextrose in 0.45% normal saline every 8 hours. Delivery set: 20 drops = 1 ml.

STEP 1: Calculate how many milliliters should be given in 1 hour. Divide the total number of milliliters to be given by the prescribed number of hours.

$$1000 \text{ ml} \div 8 \text{ hr} = 125 \text{ ml per hr}$$

STEP 2: Calculate how many drops should be given in 1 hour. Multiply the number of milliliters to be given each hour times the number of drops in 1 ml using the specific delivery set.

$$125 \text{ ml} \times 20 = 2500 \text{ drops per hr}$$

STEP 3: Calculate how many drops should be given in 1 minute. Divide the number of drops per hour by 60 to find out how many drops should be given in 1 minute.

$$2500 \text{ drops} \div 60 \text{ min} = 41.6 \text{ or } 42 \text{ drops per min}$$

Some people prefer to use a formula to calculate the drop rate. The formula is:

$$\frac{\text{Fluid volume to be infused} \times \text{Number of drops per ml with selected infusion set}}{\text{Time in minutes}} = \text{drops per minute}$$

Once the infusion rate per minute is known, the nurse adjusts the flow rate until the correct number of

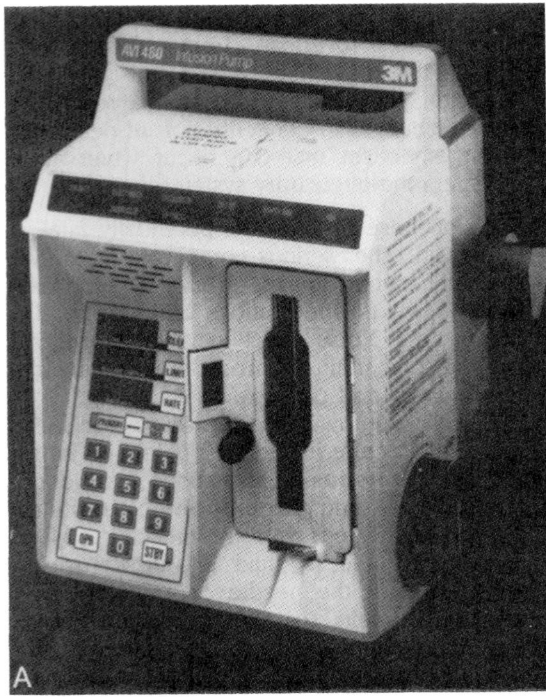

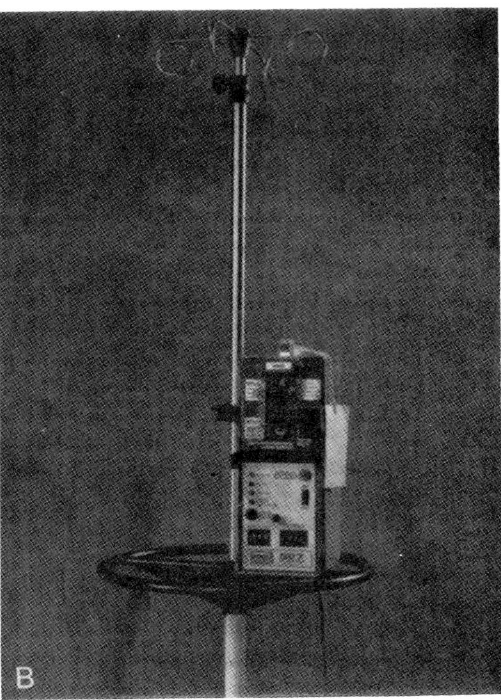

FIGURE 15–5
Electronic infusion pumps. *A*, The AVI 480 infusion pump (Courtesy of 3M Co., St. Paul, MN.) *B*, The IMED 927 infusion pump attached to an intravenous line pole. (From Bolander, V. B. [1994]. *Sorensen and Luckmann's basic nursing: A psychophysiologic approach* [3rd ed., p. 1325]. Philadelphia: W. B. Saunders.)

drops per minute are falling. The rate should be rechecked hourly. Common practice is to put a timed tape on the fluid container that shows where the fluid level should be each hour. This allows a quick assessment of whether the fluid is running on schedule.

INFUSION CONTROL DEVICES

Electronic infusion control devices maintain an infusion rate set by the nurse. The most commonly used types also have alarms that sound when the fluid bag is empty, when there is air in the line, or when there is resistance to infusion. A variety of infusion control devices are available (Fig. 15–5). The nurse must become familiar with the type used in the work setting. Infusion control devices save time and should prevent accidental delivery of large amounts of fluid. They do not excuse the nurse, however, from monitoring the flow rate at intervals and assessing the catheter or needle insertion site.

INTRAVENOUS MEDICATIONS

Agency policies usually dictate what medications the nurse may give by piggyback or by direct injection through a cannula into the vein (IV push). When giving such medications, the nurse should know how the medication must be diluted and the correct rate of infusion. Improper administration of intravenous medications can be extremely dangerous.

TERMINATION OF INTRAVENOUS THERAPY

To discontinue intravenous therapy, the flow of fluid is stopped, the tape and dressing are loosened or removed, and the cannula is removed gently. Gloves are worn and the needle or catheter is disposed of according to universal precaution guidelines. Pressure is applied to the puncture site for 1 or 2 minutes to prevent bleeding. Once bleeding has stopped, a sterile dry dressing is applied to the puncture site.

PRECAUTIONS

When performing a venipuncture or handling used needles or catheters, the nurse must always be aware of the risk of exposure to blood-borne pathogens. The most serious infections that can be transmitted by this route are the human immunodeficiency virus and hepatitis B.

A number of new products for venipuncture and intravenous therapy that reduce the risk of needle sticks or other exposure to blood are appearing on the market. Unfortunately, nurses tend to resist using new products and may need encouragement to learn to use new devices. In this situation, use of safer equipment may be lifesaving. Every nurse should be familiar with the agency needle stick and body fluid exposure guidelines.

Most policies require blood specimens to be drawn from the nurse and the patient to test for blood-borne infections. Drug therapy may be advised if the patient has an infectious disease. Documentation of the incident and the health status of the nurse at the time of the exposure may be very important if the nurse becomes ill as a result of the exposure.

COMPLICATIONS OF INTRAVENOUS THERAPY

Intravenous therapy is so widely used that it is easy to take it for granted. Several potential complications of intravenous therapy can be very serious, however. Complications include tissue trauma, infiltration, inflammation, infection, fluid volume excess, bleeding, and embolism.

TISSUE TRAUMA

The insertion of a cannula is traumatic to the skin and underlying tissues. Tape may irritate or tear the skin.

INFILTRATION

Infiltration is the collection of infused fluid in tissue surrounding the cannula. *Extravasation* is another term that is often used interchangeably with infiltration. Infiltration can be caused by leakage at the point where the cannula enters the vein or by puncture of a second site in the vein by the cannula. When the infusion is infiltrated, the patient may report pain or a burning sensation in the area. On inspection, the site may be pale and puffy. If a lot of fluid is in the tissue, it may feel hard and cool. Drugs that are especially toxic to subcutaneous tissues are called *vesicants*. Common vesicants are vasopressors, potassium chloride, and antineoplastic agents.

PHLEBITIS

Inflammation of the vein is called phlebitis. With intravenous fluid therapy, phlebitis may be due to irritation by the cannula or by medications.

PHARMACOLOGY CAPSULE

Drugs that are toxic to body tissues are called vesicants. They can cause phlebitis or tissue necrosis.

Redness, warmth, and tenderness near the insertion site suggest phlebitis. The inflammation may be mild or severe and carries the possibility of the formation of blood clots in the vein (thrombophlebitis).

INFECTION

Infection of a venipuncture site can be caused by contamination of the site itself, by the intravenous fluid, or by the tubing used to deliver the fluid. The infected site is red and warm and may have purulent drainage.

FLUID VOLUME EXCESS

The patient's blood volume may become excessive when fluid is delivered directly to the blood stream. This is most likely to happen when large volumes of fluid are infused, especially in patients who have impaired renal or cardiac function.

PHARMACOLOGY CAPSULE

Rapid intravenous administration of drugs or fluids may cause serious adverse effects.

Early signs and symptoms of fluid volume excess include rising blood pressure, bounding pulse, and edema. Severe fluid volume excess produces congestive heart failure and pulmonary edema (discussed in Chapter 31).

BLOOD LOSS

Bleeding may occur if the cannula is moved excessively after insertion. Even more serious bleeding is possible if the tubing becomes disconnected from the cannula allowing blood to flow freely from the vein.

EMBOLISM

An embolus is an unattached blood clot or other substance in the circulatory system. With intravenous therapy, there are risks of emboli from blood clots, air, and broken catheters. An embolus can have serious, even life-threatening, effects if it lodges and obstructs blood flow in a critical blood vessel. The obstruction created by a trapped embolus is called an *embolism*.

Blood clots (thrombi) can develop in intravenous needles or catheters. Air can enter the blood stream if the infusion system is opened. As little as 10 cc of air can cause serious complications. The risk of air embolism with peripheral lines has been greatly reduced by the use of plastic rather than glass fluid containers. The danger is greatest with central venous lines such as the subclavian, Hickman-Broviac, and triple lumen catheters mentioned earlier. If a port is disconnected, air may be drawn into the blood stream. The patient experiences shortness of breath, hypotension, and possibly shock and cardiac arrest.

A rare occurrence is a catheter embolus. This occurs when a piece of the catheter breaks off in the vein. Broken catheters may be due to defects in the catheter, reintroduction of the needle into the catheter, accidental cutting with scissors, and pulling catheters through needles.

THE OLDER PATIENT AND INTRAVENOUS THERAPY

The elderly patient requires special consideration during intravenous therapy. When performing the venipuncture, the nurse may be able to distend the vessel by simply pressing the vein. If a tourniquet is needed, fragile skin can be protected by wrapping a washcloth under the tourniquet. Special adhesives or dressings may be needed to prevent damage to the skin. Because older people have less subcutaneous tissue, infiltrated fluid may drain away from the cannula insertion site. For example, if the hand is elevated, fluid may collect in the elbow area. Monitoring for fluid volume excess is especially important as older people often have less efficient cardiac and renal function.

NURSING CARE DURING INTRAVENOUS THERAPY

ASSESSMENT

When a patient is receiving intravenous therapy, the nurse's assessment is done to ensure that the correct fluid is infusing at the correct rate and that the patient is not suffering any complications from this therapy.

The nurse checks the physician's order to be sure the correct intravenous solution is infusing. The prescribed rate of flow is determined, and the actual flow rate is assessed. The infusion site is inspected for edema, pallor or redness, bleeding, and drainage. The infusion site is palpated for edema and assessed for warmth or coolness. The patient is asked if the infusion site is painful.

Many people believe that the infusion is not infiltrating if blood flows into the tubing when the fluid container is lowered. This is not an accurate sign, as blood may return even when fluid is escaping into the tissue. Interestingly, the lack of blood return does not necessarily mean the needle is out of the vein either. Therefore, this time-honored test for needle placement is not reliable. Inspection and palpation of the infusion site remain the best means of evaluating for infiltration.

The nurse takes the patient's vital signs and compares the readings with previous findings to detect increased pulse and blood pressure. The fluid intake and output are measured and recorded, and the patient's breath sounds are auscultated for rales.

NURSING DIAGNOSIS

When a patient is receiving intravenous therapy, nursing diagnoses address the risk for complications, the need for assistance with activities of daily living, and the need for patient teaching. Specific nursing diagnoses are the following:

- **High Risk for Injury** related to trauma, inflammation
- **High Risk for Infection** related to disruption of skin integrity or the presence of a cannula in a vein
- **Fluid Volume Excess** related to rapid fluid infusion
- **Decreased Cardiac Output** related to blood loss
- **Altered Tissue Perfusion** related to the obstruction of blood flow by an embolus
- **Self-Care Deficit** (feeding, hygiene, dressing, toileting) related to restricted movement of infusion site and connection to fluid delivery system
- **Knowledge Deficit** of the management of intravenous therapy

GOALS

The goals of nursing care when a patient receives intravenous therapy are minimal trauma; absence of infiltration, infection, and inflammation; normal fluid balance; unobstructed blood flow; patient's performance of self-care activities; and patient's knowledge of own role in intravenous therapy.

INTERVENTIONS

Trauma

Gentle technique when performing the venipuncture and anchoring the cannula reduces tissue trauma.

Infiltration

Frequent assessments for signs and symptoms of infiltration are necessary. When there is evidence of infiltration (edema, coolness, pain), the infusion should be stopped and restarted in a different vein. Otherwise, the patient may not be receiving the drug or fluid as intended. Tissue that is edematous with infiltrated fluid is fragile and should be handled gently. Elevating the affected arm on a pillow promotes reabsorption of excess fluid.

Because many medications harm subcutaneous tissue, the physician should be notified if solutions containing toxic drugs infiltrate. When administering vesicants, it is especially important to select a large, soft vein; use a small cannula; ensure cannula placement before giving the vesicant; and flush the cannula after the vesicant is given.

Inflammation and Infection

Strict aseptic technique is used when starting and handling intravenous infusions. Agency policy describes specific site care, including the frequency of dressing changes.

If the infusion site appears to be inflamed or infected, the infusion should be stopped and restarted in another site. Inflammation and infection are characterized by redness, swelling, and warmth. In addition, an infected site may have purulent drainage, and the patient might have a fever. If agency policy permits, a warm compress can be applied to the inflamed site. If there is evidence of infection, the physician should be notified. Antibiotic therapy may be ordered.

Fluid Volume Excess

The nurse reduces the risk of fluid volume excess by controlling the rate of fluid infusion. If the infusion falls

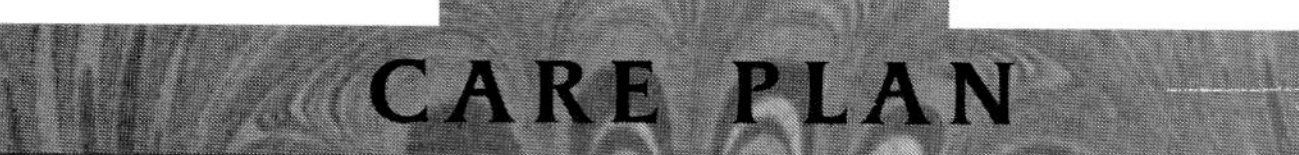

Care of the Patient Receiving Intravenous Therapy

ASSESSMENT

Health History: 67-year-old white female admitted for nausea and vomiting for 3 days. Reports fluid intake of only water and cola for last 2 days. Complains of dizziness and fatigue. Intravenous fluids infusing at 150 ml/hr via 21-gauge cannula.

Physical Examination: Lethargic but oriented. Vital signs: blood pressure, 96/58; pulse, 102; respirations, 22; temperature, 101.6°F orally. Mucous membranes dry and sticky. Urine dark yellow. Intravenous infusion site: no swelling or redness.

NURSING DIAGNOSIS	GOALS AND OUTCOME CRITERIA	INTERVENTIONS
High risk for injury related to trauma, infiltration.	The patient will experience minimal trauma as evidenced by absence of bruising, bleeding, swelling, or pallor.	Use gentle technique to start the infusion. Inspect the infusion site for redness, swelling, and bleeding. Palpate for warmth or coolness. Anchor the tubing securely. Exercise caution to prevent movement of the cannula. Stop the infusion if there are signs of infiltration (swelling near infusion site, pain, slow infusion rate) and restart it.
High risk for inflammation and infection related to disruption of skin integrity, presence of cannula in vein.	The patient will remain free of infection at infusion site as evidenced by absence of redness, swelling, edema, drainage.	Use strict aseptic technique when starting the infusion and handling the site. Assess for signs of inflammation and infection: redness, swelling, warmth, purulent drainage, fever. Report signs to physician. Administer antibiotics and apply warm compress to inflamed site as ordered.
Fluid volume excess related to rapid fluid infusion.	The patient's fluid status will be normal as evidenced by normal vital signs and fluid intake approximately equal to output.	Monitor rate of fluid infusion and maintain correct rate of flow. Measure all fluid intake and output. Assess for signs and symptoms of fluid volume excess (hypervolemia): increasing blood pressure, bounding pulse, dyspnea. If patient is hypervolemic, slow infusion rate, elevate patient's head, and notify physician.
Decreased cardiac output related to blood loss.	The patient will have no bleeding at infusion site or tubing connections.	Check connections to be sure they are secure. Tape tubing to prevent accidental dislodgment.
Altered tissue perfusion related to obstruction of blood flow by embolus.	The patient will maintain normal circulation as evidenced by usual skin color and absence of respiratory distress.	Do not irrigate obstructed cannula. Assess and report any signs of respiratory distress.
Self-care deficit (feeding, dressing, hygiene, toileting) related to restricted movement of infusion site and connection to fluid delivery system.	The patient will accomplish self-care activities without disruption of intravenous therapy.	Provide assistance with meals, hygiene, dressing, and toileting as needed. Provide gown that unfastens at the shoulder. Assure the patient that she can move with the infusion.
Knowledge deficit of management of intravenous therapy.	The patient will demonstrate ability to protect and manage the infusion.	Tell the patient the purpose of the infusion and what symptoms should be reported: pain, bleeding, swelling. Assure the patient that movement is possible with the infusion as long as it is protected and the tubing is not disconnected.

behind schedule, the rate is corrected as noted previously, but is not increased to make up for the slow infusion. Normally, fluid intake and output are approximately equal. When the heart or kidneys are unable to handle excess blood volume, heart failure may develop. Young children and elderly adults are monitored closely for fluid volume excess because they do not adapt to fluid changes as readily as a young adult. If indications of fluid volume excess (increasing blood pressure, bounding pulse, dyspnea) appear, the infusion rate is slowed, the patient's head is elevated, and the physician is notified.

Bleeding

To prevent bleeding, the nurse makes sure all connections in the infusion set are secure. Tubing is taped so that it is not pulled loose easily. The infusion site and tubing are protected when the patient moves. If a large amount of blood is lost, the nurse takes the patient's vital signs and notifies the physician. Emergency measures are instituted if the patient is in shock.

Embolism

When the cannula seems to be obstructed, blood clots may have formed in it. Irrigation of the cannula is not recommended as it may force clots into the blood stream.

Signs of circulatory obstruction may be due to an embolism and should be reported to the physician immediately. If a catheter breaks in a peripheral vein, pressure and then a tourniquet are placed a few inches above the intravenous insertion site. The patient is kept quiet with the head elevated. The physician is notified. A radiograph is ordered to locate the broken catheter. The fragment may be removed surgically or by using angiography.

The nurse exercises extra caution when a patient has a central line to prevent an air embolism. The infusion set must remain closed. When hanging new bags of fluid, the catheter port is clamped to prevent air from entering the blood stream. When a central catheter is inserted or removed, the patient is instructed to take a deep breath and bear down. This helps prevent air from entering the blood stream. If air accidentally enters the line, the leak is closed immediately. The patient is turned on the left side with the head lowered. This position traps the air in the right atrium where it can be absorbed gradually. Air in the blood stream is an emergency situation in which cardiac arrest is possible, so close monitoring is vital. The physician is notified, and the crash cart must be kept close at hand. One hundred percent oxygen may be administered with a nonrebreather mask.

Self-Care

The nurse provides assistance as needed with eating, dressing, toileting, and hygiene. Dressing may be easier if the patient is provided with a gown or shirt that unfastens at the shoulder. They are simpler to remove than garments that must be removed over the arm. Some patients are fearful of moving with an intravenous infusion. The nurse explains what restrictions are needed, if any, to protect the infusion.

Patient Teaching

When intravenous therapy is ordered, the nurse explains what will be done and why. With long-term therapy, it is especially important to teach the patient (and family if appropriate) how to care for the infusion site, administer fluids or drugs, and recognize signs that should be reported to the physician. If infusion ports are to be flushed at intervals, the nurse teaches the patient how to do this as well. Patients who go home with central lines or implanted infusion ports need instruction in their care. Teaching should begin well before discharge so the patient's ability to do the care can be assessed.

EVALUATION

Criteria for evaluating nursing care include absence of bruising or bleeding; absence of edema, pallor, redness, and drainage at the infusion site; normal vital signs and fluid output equal to intake; normal circulation as evidenced by usual skin color and absence of respiratory distress; patient's completion of activities of daily living without disruption of intravenous therapy; and patient's demonstration of correct technique in self-administered therapy.

Intravenous therapy is frequently prescribed for hospitalized patients. It is being used more commonly outside the hospital setting as well. Therefore, nurses must be skilled in managing intravenous lines and in teaching patients and their families to manage them. Nurses must also be knowledgeable about recognizing and preventing complications.

BIBLIOGRAPHY

Dick, M. J., Maree, S. M., & Gray, S. (1993). How to boost the odds of a painless IV start. *American Journal of Nursing, 92*(6), 49–50.

Hendrickson, M. L. (1993). How to access an implanted port. *Nursing 93, 23*(1), 50–53.

Hennessey, B., Fitzgerald, A., & Graham, D. (1993). Venous air embolism. *American Journal of Nursing, 93*(11), 54–56.

Holder, C., & Alexander, J. (1990). A new and improved guide to IV therapy. *American Journal of Nursing, 90*(2), 43–47.

Howard, M. P., Eisenberg, P. G., & Gianino, S. (1992). Dressing a central venous catheter: A better way. *Nursing 92, 22*(3), 60–61.

Ignatavicius, D. D., & Bayne, M. V. (1991). *Medical-surgical nursing: A nursing process approach.* Philadelphia: W. B. Saunders.

Meares, C. (1992). P.I.C.C. and M.L.C. lines: Options worth exploring. *Nursing 92, 22*(10), 52–55.

Millam, D. A. (1992). Starting IV's: How to develop your venipuncture expertise. *Nursing 92, 22*(9), 33–47.

Negron, S. B. (1989). A smart way to secure an IV. *American Journal of Nursing, 89*(5), 687.

Potter, P. A., & Perry, A. G. (1992). *Fundamentals of nursing* (3rd ed.). St. Louis: C. V. Mosby.

Rountree, D. (1991). The PIC catheter: A different approach. *American Journal of Nursing, 91*(8), 22–28.

Scharnweber, K. S. (1992). Intravenous Nurses' Society. *RN, 55*(2), 97–99.

Sieh, A., & Brentin, L. (1993). A little light makes venipuncture easier. *RN, 56*(3), 40–43.

Teplitz, L. (1992). Responding to an air embolism. *Nursing 92, 22*(7), 33.

Thomason, S. S. (1991). Using a Groshong central venous catheter. *Nursing 91, 21*(10), 58–60.

Tuten, S. H., & Gueldner, S. H. (1991). Efficacy of sodium chloride versus dilute heparin for maintenance of peripheral intermittent intravenous devices. *Applied Nursing Research, 4*(2), 63–71.

Whitney, R. G. (1991). Comparing long-term central venous catheters. *Nursing 91, 21*(4), 70–71.

Wood, L. S., & Gullo, S. M. (1993). IV vesicants: How to avoid extravasation. *American Journal of Nursing, 93*(4), 42–46.

Yucha, C. B., Hasting-Tolsma, M., Szeverenyi, N. M., Tompkins, J., & Robson, L. (1991). Characterization of intravenous infiltrates. *Applied Nursing Research, 4*(4), 184–186.

CHAPTER

16

Pain Management

Mary L. Heye
Kathleen Reeves

OBJECTIVES

1. Define pain.
2. Explain the physiologic basis for pain.
3. Identify situations in which patients are likely to experience pain.
4. Explain the relationships between past pain experiences, anticipation, culture, anxiety, activity, and a patient's response to pain.
5. Identify differences in duration and patient response with acute and chronic pain.
6. Explain the special needs of the elderly patient who has pain.
7. List the data to be collected in assessing pain.
8. Describe interventions used in the management of pain.
9. Describe nursing care of patients receiving opioid and nonopioid analgesics for pain.
10. List the factors that should be considered when pain is not relieved with analgesic medications.

GLOSSARY

ACUTE PAIN Pain that lasts less than 6 months, has an identifiable cause, and goes away as healing occurs

ADDICTION Behavioral pattern of compulsive drug use characterized by craving for an opioid and obtaining and using the drug for effects other than pain relief

ANALGESIC Drug that acts on the nervous system to relieve or reduce the suffering or intensity of pain

CHRONIC PAIN Pain that lasts longer than 6 months

NOCICEPTION Process of pain transmission; usually related to pain sensation resulting from stimulation of pain receptors and transmission of stimuli to pain fibers, spinal cord, and brain

PAIN Unpleasant sensory and emotional experience associated with actual or potential tissue damage existing whenever the person says it does; a unique, private experience involving the holistic person in a time dimension of past, present, and future and influenced by internal and external environment

PAIN THRESHOLD Level of intensity that causes the sensation or feeling of pain

PAIN TOLERANCE Amount of pain a person is willing to endure before taking action to relieve pain

PHYSICAL DEPENDENCE Physiologic adaptation of the body to an opioid so a person exhibits withdrawal symptoms when the opioid is stopped abruptly after repeated administration

TOLERANCE A physiologic result of repeated doses of an opioid where the same dose is no longer effective in achieving the same analgesic effect; a larger dose of opioids is required to achieve the same analgesic effect

Pain is one of the most complex experiences to understand and treat. It is also the most common problem that nurses encounter. Research about pain mechanisms and pathways, analgesics, and the mind-body influence is just beginning to filter down to nursing practice. Still, many questions about pain remain unanswered.

Pain is influenced by many variables: the individual experiencing it, the cause of the pain, and the environment. Pain may arise from a new source, occur from an old injury, or result from nerve injury. Sometimes the cause is unknown. Pain relief rests primarily with the nurse, who must assess the patient and implement appropriate interventions.

Nurses have many categories of pain-relieving interventions to choose from, yet they frequently choose to administer just analgesics. Most nurses believe pain is easily managed with analgesic drugs. Patients, however, often report that pain remains moderate to severe despite these medications. Research indicates that nurses fail to assess pain, tend to undermedicate for pain, and have inadequate knowledge about pain relief measures.

The purpose of this chapter is to provide information to enable the nurse to understand pain and to provide the most effective interventions for pain relief.

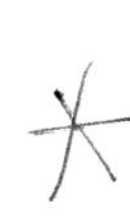

Pain is defined in many ways. The International Association for the Study of Pain defines it as an unpleasant sensory and emotional experience associated with actual or potential tissue damage. McCaffery, a nurse and leader in the pain management field, has a more useful definition for nurses. She says, "Pain is whatever the person experiencing it says it is and exists whenever he says it does." Graffam, a nursing scientist, says pain is a unique, private experience involving the holistic person in a time dimension of past, present, and future and is influenced by internal and external environments.

PHYSIOLOGY OF PAIN

Pain consists of various sensory experiences such as time, space, emotion, and cognition. The perception of pain involves afferent pathways, the central nervous system, and efferent pathways. Afferent pathways carry messages to the brain, where the messages are interpreted, and efferent pathways carry messages away from the brain, through the spinal cord, and to the rest of the body.

Afferent pathways are composed of pain receptors called nociceptors. These pain receptors are unevenly distributed within muscles, tendons, subcutaneous tissue, and the skin. This may explain why parts of the body are more sensitive to pain than other parts. Pain receptors are sensitive to chemical changes, temperature, mechanical stimuli, and tissue damage. Some receptors are sensitive to more than one type of stimuli. Pain receptors are unable to adapt to repeated stimuli and thus continue to react until the stimuli are removed.

When pain receptors are stimulated, impulses are transmitted through small-diameter nerve fibers to an area in the spinal cord called the substantia gelatinosa. The impulses then travel up the spinal cord to the brain. The brain perceives the painful sensation, and then the thalamus and cortex identify the location and qualities of the pain. Other structures involved in the interpretation of pain signals are the limbic system, reticular formation, and hypothalamus. These structures produce the unpleasant qualities associated with pain and activate the stress response. Endorphins are also released in response to pain and stress.

Endorphins are the body's natural opioid-like substances that lock into opioid receptors in the brain and spinal cord. Endorphins block the transmission of painful impulses to the brain. Differences in the amount of endorphins in individuals may explain differences in individual pain perception. Research suggests that prolonged stress and pain, as well as prolonged use of morphine and alcohol, decrease endorphins. Factors that increase endorphins include brief stress and pain, laughter, exercise, placebos, acupuncture, transcutaneous electrical nerve stimulation (TENS), massive trauma, and sexual activity.

GATE-CONTROL THEORY

Although many theories have been proposed to explain pain, none fully describe the pain experience. One of the best known theories is Melzack and Wall's gate-control theory. It is based on the belief that the pain experience reflects both physiologic and psychological variables. As mentioned previously, painful impulses are transmitted to the spinal cord through small-diameter fibers. When these small-diameter fibers are stimulated, the gate opens, which facilitates the transmission of impulses and enhances pain perception. Factors that cause the gate to open include tissue damage, a monotonous environment, and fear of pain. These small-diameter fibers end in the substantia gelatinosa in the spinal cord along with large-diameter fibers. The stimulation of large-diameter fibers can close the gate so that impulses are decreased or not transmitted from the spinal cord to the brain or from the brain to the spinal cord, and this causes diminished pain perception. Large-diameter nerve fiber stimulation includes cutaneous (skin) stimulation through massage, position change, and heat or cold applications. Sensory input such as distraction, guided imagery, and preparatory information also may close the gate. Figure 16–1 shows the structures and mechanisms described in the gate-control theory.

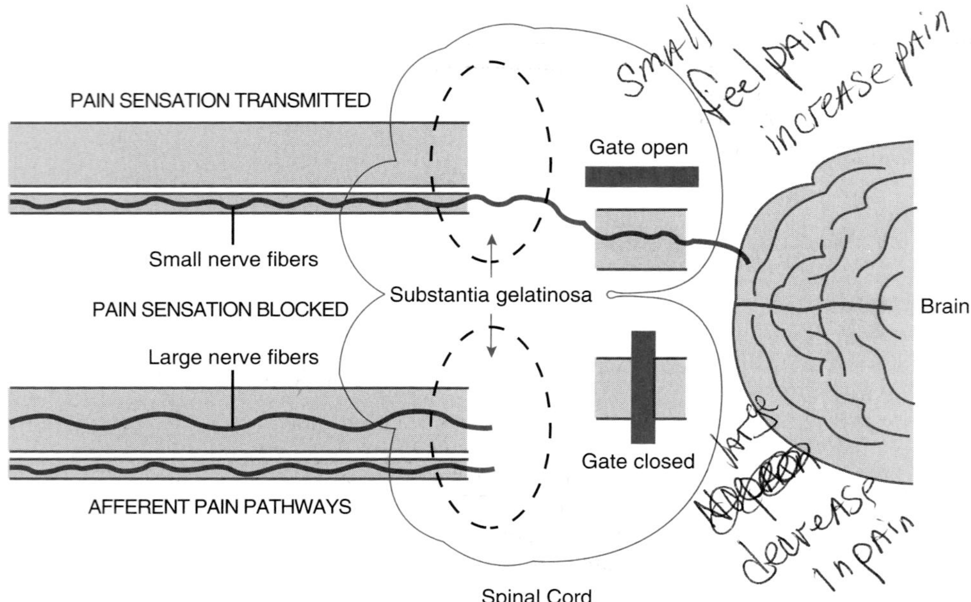

FIGURE 16-1
The gate-control theory of pain.

FACTORS INFLUENCING RESPONSE TO PAIN

Consider the following example: Miss Smith and Mrs. Johnson are roommates in Room 200. Miss Smith, age 19 underwent a cholecystectomy the previous day, as did Mrs. Johnson, age 67. The nurses discussed the difference in behavior of each patient: "Miss Smith is constantly on the call light wanting more pain medication. She moans and groans all the time. She won't even turn, cough, and deep breathe for more than 10 seconds. She rarely rates her pain at less than a 9 or 10 on the pain scale. On the other hand, look at Mrs. Johnson. She's already ambulating. She rarely rates her pain as more than a 5 or 6 on the pain scale. She usually just complains of aching, and she sure doesn't ask for as much pain medication as Miss Smith. You'd never guess they had undergone the same procedure."

This example illustrates that although people may experience the same injury or insult (in this case surgery), they may react and respond differently. This is because numerous physical and psychosocial factors affect response to pain. It is important for health professionals to be nonjudgmental and to avoid comparing one individual in pain with another individual in pain.

PHYSICAL FACTORS

Although the following list is not exhaustive, some physical factors influencing response to pain include pain threshold, pain tolerance, age, physical activity, nervous system integrity, and, in cases of surgery, the type of surgery performed, and the type of anesthesia used.

Pain Threshold

Pain threshold is that point at which a stimulus causes the sensation or feeling of pain. Anger, fatigue, anxiety, insomnia, depression, and uncontrolled pain all lower the pain threshold; that is, the person experiences pain sensation more readily with less stimuli. During hospitalization or illness, a patient may experience anxiety, fatigue, or loss of sleep, which can lower pain threshold or cause the patient to experience pain more easily.

Pain Tolerance

Pain tolerance, or the intensity of pain that a person will endure, is another factor influencing response to pain. Pain tolerance varies between patients and varies for an individual patient depending on the situation. As a patient experiences more pain or prolonged pain, pain tolerance may be lowered because the patient thinks the pain may not be relieved, thus causing increased anxiety and fear. Low pain tolerance or high pain tolerance must be respected and must not interfere with adequate pain management.

Age

Age may also influence response to pain. At times, older patients do not report their pain or they report their pain as much less severe than it really is. Some do not report pain because they are stoic or they have erroneously been told that pain is a normal part of aging. Some older patients may not want to "bother" the nurse, or they may fear rejection from the caregiver. Pain is *not* a normal part of aging, although elderly persons often suffer from chronic conditions such as arthritis, cancer, and bone fractures that are associated with pain.

Physical Activity and Nervous System Integrity

Physical activity and the integrity of the nervous system also can influence reaction to pain. Physical activity may aggravate or precipitate pain. However, with some patients, physical activity may be used as a measure to relieve pain. Because pain is perceived and interpreted within the nervous system, the integrity of the system affects response to pain. For example, patients with certain diseases like diabetic neuropathy lose sensation in the extremities and may not feel pain there.

Surgery and Anesthesia

Two other factors, the type of surgery performed and the type of anesthesia used, can influence response to pain. Surgery performed to the upper abdominal region of the body is thought to be the most painful type because of the numerous tissues traumatized during the procedure. Within this group are cardiac, pulmonary, gastric, and gallbladder surgeries. The type of anesthetic agent used can influence postoperative pain. For example, nitrous oxide has analgesic properties. Some anesthetic agents injected at the operative site may prolong analgesia for 12 to 24 hours after surgery. When these types of agents are used, patients may experience much less pain after surgery compared with those who do not receive these anesthetic agents.

Surgery or invasive procedures may be performed to relieve pain that is intractable or severely debilitating. Surgery such as rhizotomy or cordotomy interrupts the pain pathways through destruction of nerve tissue or a portion of the spinal cord that transmits nerve impulses. These surgeries leave the patient with some neurologic deficit; for example, the patient may be unaware that a body area is painful and how to protect that area from harm. Pain relief from these procedures may not be permanent because nerve tissue regenerates. Nerve blocks are procedures that involve destruction or anesthesia of a nerve root with injection of a chemical to achieve pain relief in a specific body area. For example, intercostal anesthetic nerve blocks may be performed with cardiac surgery to reduce postoperative pain in the thoracic area. Acupuncture is another invasive technique that produces anesthesia or analgesia. It is an ancient Chinese practice whereby tiny needles are inserted into the skin or subcutaneous tissues at specific points on the body. This technique may be used to relieve pain and provide anesthesia during diagnostic, surgical, and labor and delivery procedures.

Along with a variety of physical factors, several psychological factors can influence response to pain, including culture, religion, past experiences with pain, anxiety, and situational factors.

PSYCHOLOGICAL FACTORS

Culture and Ethnicity

Although studies have been conducted to determine the effect of culture and ethnicity on reaction to pain, it is critical to avoid making judgments based on how the nurse thinks a person should react or behave. Some persons may deny pain, remain calm and unemotional, or withdraw. Other persons may be quite demonstrative; they may cry, moan and groan, and involve their families in the painful experience. The nurse must be aware of the different ways to express pain and respect individual variations in the response to pain.

Religious Beliefs

Religious beliefs also may have an impact on reaction to pain. Some patients may pray and believe that divine intervention will help them to endure the pain. Others may view pain as a punishment for sins. Some individuals believe that penance is required before pain relief can be obtained.

Past Experiences and Anxiety

Past experiences and anxiety may affect a person's response to current pain. A person may have developed positive and adaptive coping strategies to deal with previous painful experiences that can help him or her with the current situation. If, however, previous coping strategies have been unsuccessful, anxiety related to enduring another painful experience may be viewed as an overwhelming threat to the patient.

Situational Factors

Finally, situational factors may influence response to pain. If the pain is associated with a serious illness such as cancer, the pain may have an impact on mood and activity more so than if the pain is associated with a less serious condition. The pain associated with childbirth is relatively short-lived and usually results in a beautiful outcome, whereas cancer pain may be chronic and increasing and may be associated with progression of the disease.

RESPONSES TO PAIN

AUTONOMIC NERVOUS SYSTEM

The pain signal is interpreted by the brain as a stressor, and the brain dictates the response to the stressor. The fight or flight response may occur when the autonomic nervous system is activated and certain physiologic responses are initiated. Table 16–1 indicates some of the sympathetic and parasympathetic responses that occur and the associated symptoms. The patient in pain may respond with these physiologic responses and with behaviors such as grimacing, moaning, and verbalizing

TABLE 16–1
AUTONOMIC NERVOUS SYSTEM RESPONSES TO PAIN

SYMPATHETIC	PARASYMPATHETIC
↑ Blood pressure	Constipation
↑ Pulse rate	Urinary retention
↑ Respiratory rate	
Dilated pupils	
Perspiration	
Pallor	

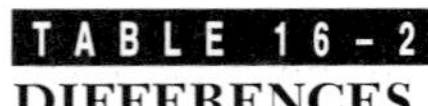

TABLE 16-2

DIFFERENCES IN ACUTE AND CHRONIC PAIN

CHARACTERISTIC	ACUTE	CHRONIC
Time	Limited, short duration	Lasts 6 mo, longer duration
Purpose	Sign of tissue injury	No purpose
Verbal	Reports pain, focuses on pain	No report of pain unless questioned
Behavioral	Restless, thrashing, rubbing body part, pacing, grimacing, and other facial expressions of pain	Tired-looking, minimal facial expression, quiet, sleeps, rests, attention on other things
Physiologic	Increased heart rate, blood pressure, respiratory rate	Normal heart rate, blood pressure, respiratory rate
Interventions	Responds to analgesics	Less responsive to analgesics
	Standard doses effective	Higher doses needed for pain relief
	Parenteral or oral route used	Oral route preferred
	Additional drugs seldom needed to manage pain	Additional drugs (adjuvant) often needed to manage pain

pain or withdrawing and being noncommunicative. The nervous system responses can be identified and measured—for example, increased heart rate, respiratory rate, and blood pressure. These are predictable responses to acute pain; however, the responses in pain behavior may vary from individual to individual. There is also a difference in response depending on whether the pain is acute or chronic. Table 16–2 shows differences in acute and chronic pain characteristics.

ACUTE PAIN

Most pain experiences in the hospital fall into the category of acute pain, such as postoperative pain from incisions, renal colic pain from kidney stones, and labor pain in childbirth. Acute pain is temporary, and its cause is known and treatable. It serves as a warning of tissue damage and subsides when healing takes place. Nurses observe behavioral and physiologic signs of acute pain when the patient guards or rubs a body part, wrinkles the brow, bites the lip, and has changes in heart rate, blood pressure, and respiratory rate. These responses may be absent or sharply modified in chronic pain.

CHRONIC PAIN

Chronic pain is usually defined as pain that persists or recurs for more than 6 months, and it may last a lifetime. The cause of the pain may be unknown, and treatment may or may not be helpful in relieving the pain. There are several types of chronic pain. Classifications of chronic pain and examples are included in Table 16–3. Chronic pain is associated with a variety of diagnoses, including cancer, arthritis, peripheral vascular diseases, and traumatic injuries.

Chronic benign pain is pain that cannot be explained or that persists after healing has taken place. It usually occurs daily and is not life threatening, and treatments may or may not be successful in relieving the pain. Many of these conditions affect the older adult. Phantom limb pain is an example of chronic benign pain that can be extremely debilitating if it is not recognized and treated early. It may occur in any related body part that has been amputated or traumatized. Phantom limb pain is associated with interruption or abnormal function of sensory nerves. A number of therapies may be used to reduce this type of pain (e.g., analgesic opioids, antidepressants, nerve block, surgical revision, and physical therapy).

Phantom limb pain is also classified as neuropathic pain. This is a new term that encompasses some puzzling and challenging pain syndromes classified as chronic pain. Neuropathic pain results from nerve damage due to a wide variety of anatomic and physiologic conditions and underlying diseases. It includes unusual sensations such as burning, shooting pain and abnormal sensations or increased reaction to a stimulus.

COMPARISON OF ACUTE AND CHRONIC PAIN

In contrast to acute pain, chronic pain serves no useful purpose, and it can have a debilitating and destructive effect on a person's life. Chronic pain can lead to depression, marital difficulties, loss of self-esteem, immobility, and isolation. The patient in chronic pain often does not report pain and shows little facial expression or physical signs of pain. When pain is chronic, adaptation may occur. The sympathetic nervous system responses may be diminished or absent as the person learns to cope with the pain. The heart rate, blood pressure, and respiratory rate may not be elevated, and the patient may rest, sleep, or turn attention to other activities.

The nurse may underestimate pain severity or undermedicate the patient with chronic pain. Nursing assessment of pain is essential to identify (1) the type and amount of pain, (2) whether the pain is chronic or acute, and (3) whether the patient has both acute pain and chronic pain at the same time. When the patient says that he or she is in pain but shows no physical symptoms, this does not mean that the patient is not experiencing pain. It may simply mean that he or she has learned other ways to deal with the pain, or the

TABLE 16-3

CHRONIC PAIN

CLASSIFICATION	EXAMPLES
Recurrent acute episodes	Neuralgia (herpes zoster) Migraine headaches Sickle cell crisis
Chronic malignant	Cancer pain syndromes
Chronic nonmalignant or benign	Low back pain Rheumatoid arthritis Phantom limb pain

patient may be on medication that blocks the response of the sympathetic nervous system to pain (e.g., alpha and beta blockers such as terazosin [Hytrin] and propranolol [Inderal]). In order to manage the patient's pain, the nurse must first complete an accurate assessment.

NURSING CARE OF THE PATIENT IN PAIN

Pain management continues to be a challenge for every nurse. As discussed, every individual experiences pain differently and reacts to pain with a variety of physiologic and behavioral responses. On the basis of an accurate assessment of pain, the nurse provides nonpharmacologic and pharmacologic measures together to provide pain relief. The nurse plays a key role by assessing, intervening, and evaluating the patient in pain. Figure 16–2 shows these steps and the variety of interventions nurses can use to relieve pain.

ASSESSMENT

Assessment is the first step in pain management because it provides information that influences how the nurse will act to relieve pain. Assessment of pain should begin early and be ongoing during the pain experience. A baseline assessment should be made on admission to the unit, and frequent and regular assessments should follow any medical treatment or nursing intervention for pain relief. Nurses should anticipate pain as a result of procedures, surgery, or progression of a disease. For example, it is convenient to perform a pain assessment with each set of vital signs. The data should be accurately recorded and compared with previous information so that the pattern of pain or the effectiveness of an intervention can be evaluated.

Serious barriers to pain assessment can exist, especially in the older adult. Visual, verbal, hearing, and motor impairments may limit the ability of older patients to communicate pain or to use scales to rate pain. Patients with cognitive impairment may be unable to report pain or recall pain sensations. Pain can also cause confusion, irritation, and depression in older adults. These aspects should be considered as the nurse performs pain assessments with the older adult.

The assessment described in this section focuses on the patient who can communicate verbally. When the patient cannot do this, he or she may be able to point to or direct your attention to a location on a body chart or pain intensity scale. The nurse may also have to use family observations and patient behaviors to assess pain and pain relief in this type of situation.

The six steps in pain assessment are listed in Table 16–4.

Accept the Patient's Report

The first step in pain assessment is to establish rapport with the patient and accept what the patient says about his or her pain. All the information about pain should be obtained directly from the patient when possible. The person in pain is the only authority on the pain; no one else can really know what the pain feels like. The report should be accepted in a nonjudgmental

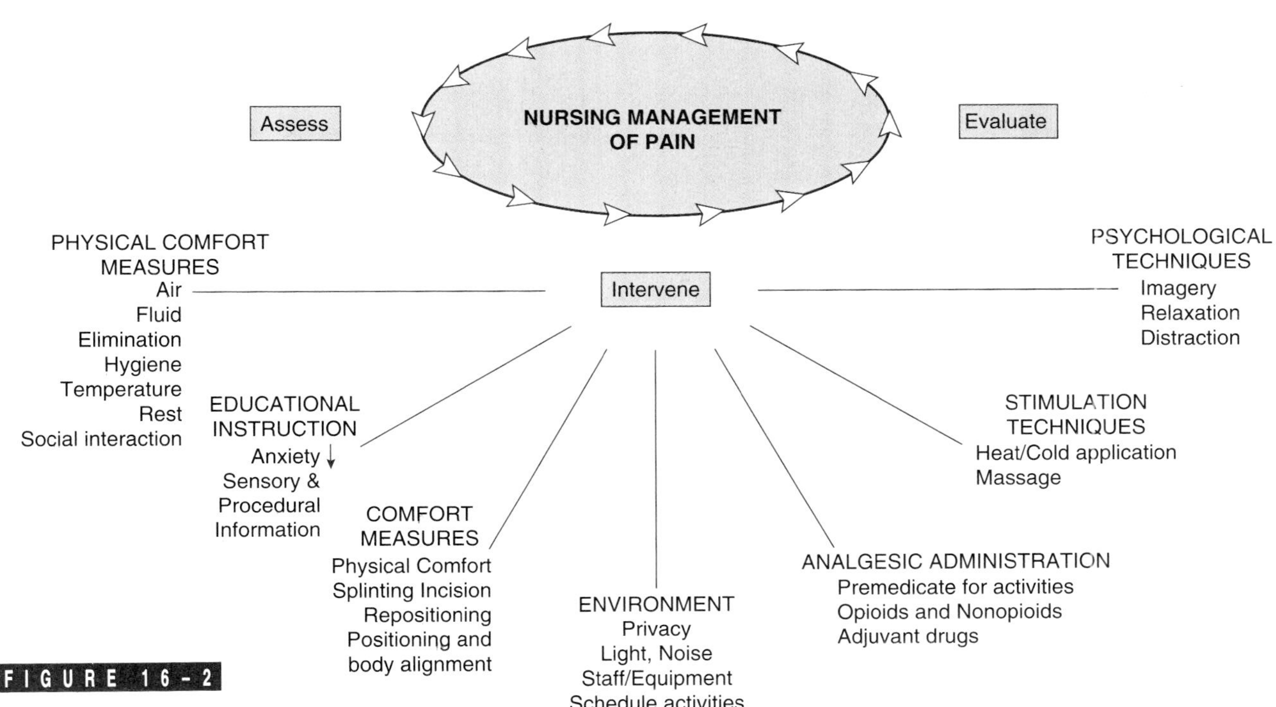

FIGURE 16–2

TABLE 16-4
SIX STEPS IN PAIN ASSESSMENT

1. Accept the patient's report
2. Determine status of pain
3. Describe pain
   a. Location
   b. Quality
   c. Intensity
   d. Aggravating and alleviating factors
4. Examine site
5. Identify coping methods
6. Record assessment findings and evaluation of interventions

and caring manner. Specific details about the pain should be obtained, and the nurse should respond positively that action will be taken to obtain relief.

The assessment of pain requires using therapeutic communication skills at their best. Important attitudes are conveyed through verbal and nonverbal behaviors. Listening patiently without interruption, using eye contact, touching the patient, and repeating and clarifying information in an unhurried manner are helpful to establishing rapport and obtaining information. The nurse should *not compare* one patient's report of pain with another's report because pain is an individual experience.

Determine Status of Pain

The second step in pain assessment is to determine whether the pain is a new occurrence or has been experienced before. The nurse can ask the patient if he or she has had this pain before, and if it was diagnosed by a physician. On the basis of the patient's responses and history, the nurse may judge the pain to be of a chronic nature or acute pain that needs immediate treatment. For example, a patient who is recovering from a prostatectomy may describe indigestion-like discomfort that is not associated with the surgery or incision. The patient identifies this discomfort as the typical angina pain for which medication has been given previously. A similar patient with substernal chest pain and no previous cardiac history should be seen by a physician immediately because this is a new pain that the patient has not had before. Although both patients need to be evaluated by a physician, an accurate nursing assessment is essential to determine the difference between these two types of pain and consequently the action to be taken.

Describe Pain

The third step in pain assessment is to describe the pain in terms of its location, quality, intensity, and aggravating and alleviating factors.

LOCATION. The nurse asks the patient to describe where the pain is and to point to the exact location with one finger. If there is more than one location of pain, a body chart, as shown on Figure 16–3, should be used, having the patient shade in or mark an X at the locations of pain. The various locations can then be numbered on the body chart so that, when charting, the nurse can refer to the number and does not have to write the exact location each time it is assessed. The nurse also determines whether the pain is confined to one area or whether it starts at one place and moves to another.

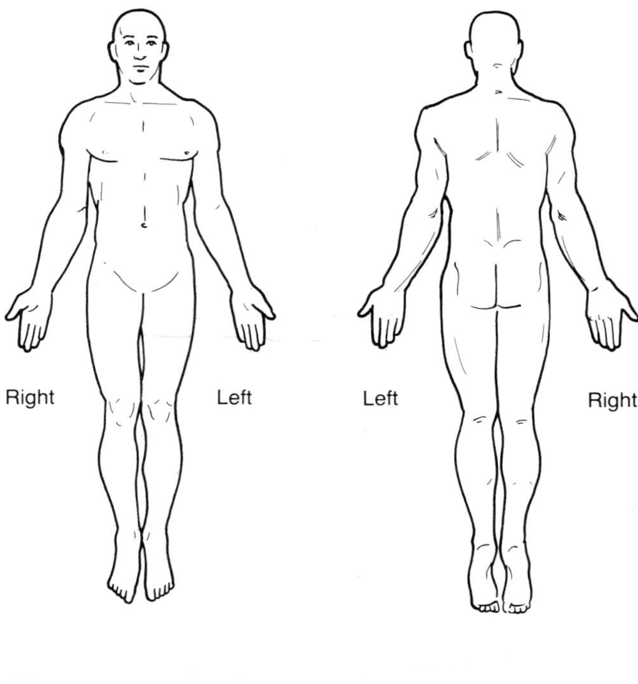

FIGURE 16-3
Body chart.

The location identified as painful does not always correspond with the disease or surgical site. For example, patients may experience back and neck spasm after surgical procedures. Another example is referred pain. Referred pain is often experienced in a location different from its source (Fig. 16–4). For example, pain from appendicitis is usually felt around the umbilicus and is of the aching, cramping type. The pain impulses come from an inflamed appendix in the right lower quadrant of the abdomen, where there may also be a sharp type of pain. Angina pain is another type of referred pain. It is caused by the lack of blood flow to the heart muscle and may be experienced as pain in the jaw, arm, and neck area as well as in the chest.

QUALITY. The nurse asks the patient, "What words do you use to describe your pain?" or "What would you do to me to have me feel the pain you have?" If the patient has difficulty describing the pain, the nurse can

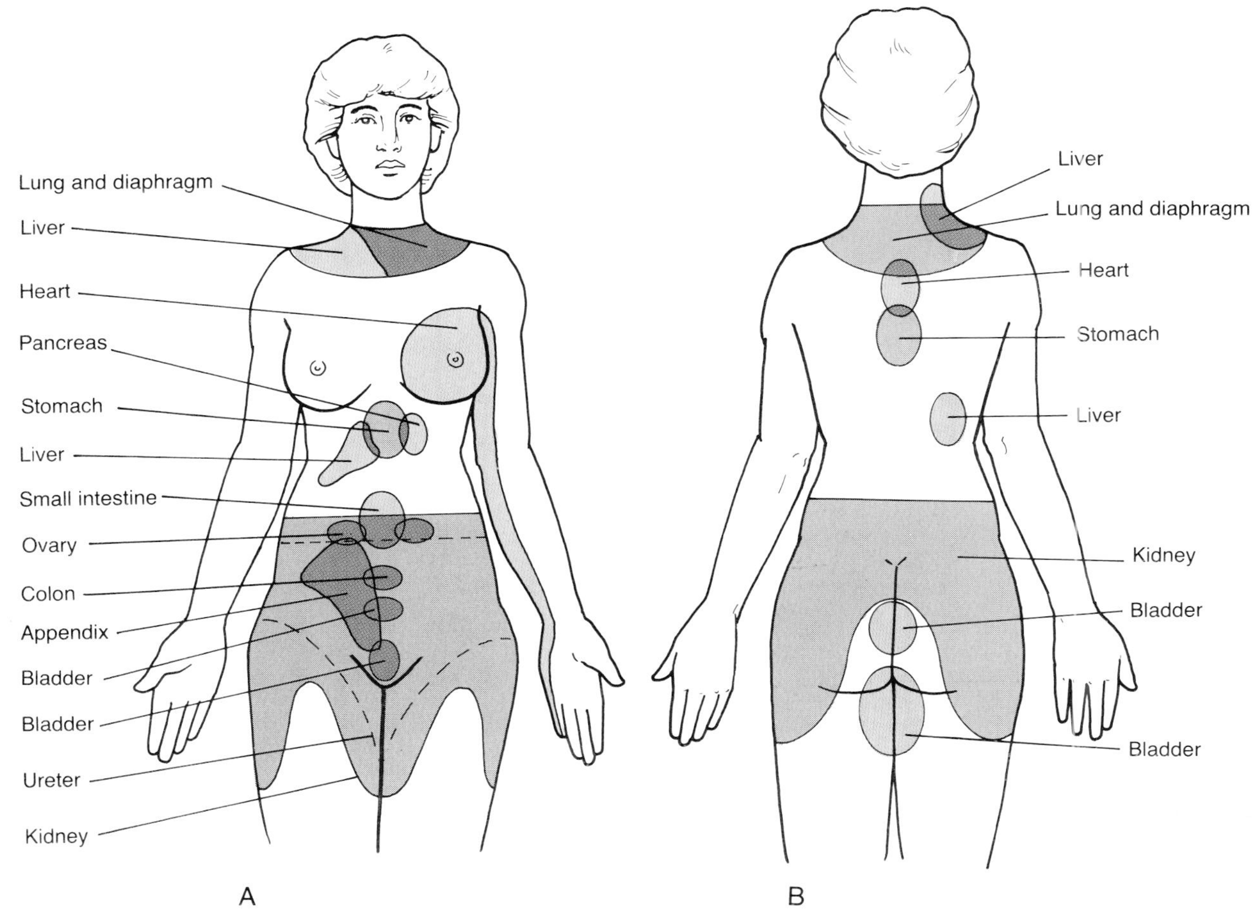

FIGURE 16-4

Anterior and posterior referred pain sites. (Redrawn from Ignatavicius, D. D., & Bayne, M. V. [1991]. *Medical-surgical nursing: A nursing process approach* [p. 110]. Philadelphia: W. B. Saunders.)

suggest words. Commonly used words are sharp, dull, cramping, aching, gnawing, burning, heavy, tender, and throbbing. However, it is best to allow the patient to use his or her own words, and these should be recorded in the chart.

INTENSITY. Because pain is a subjective experience, nurses must have some way to measure the strength or severity of pain. The purpose of asking about intensity is to put the patient's description into an objective term or number. To determine intensity, the nurse can use one of the several scales shown in Figure 16–5. A simple descriptive scale uses words of varying intensity—for example, mild, moderate, or severe. Some patients have difficulty with these words, and it may be better to use a scale with words such as "a little pain," "a lot of pain," or "too much pain." A numeric scale can be 0 to 10 or 0 to 5, with 0 meaning "no pain" and the highest number meaning the "worst pain experienced." The visual analogue scale (or VAS) allows the patient to mark an X anywhere on a line that shows intensity of pain at one end as "no pain" and at the other end as "pain as bad as it could be."

Once the use of the scale is explained to the patient, the nurse asks, "Where would you rate your pain right now?" The scale used should make sense to the patient, be easy to use, and be consistently used with the same words or numbers. It is important to explain the scale to the patient each time pain intensity is assessed. The advantage of using a scale is that it provides a personal measure for the patient's pain and allows the nurse to evaluate pain relief using a consistent measure. A scale that is meaningful to the patient and that can be used repeatedly by the nurse requires less effort for the patient in pain.

For example, a 42-year-old male with multiple fractures in the right arm used the numeric scale from 1 to 10 for rating pain. The patient complained of throbbing in his right arm and a backache. He rated the intensity of both pains at 7 on the scale at 8:00 P.M. The nurse applied heat to the lower back as ordered, massaged his back, and administered 10 mg of morphine intramuscularly. At 9:00 P.M., the patient rated intensity of both pains at 2 and stated that the pain was slowly going away. The nurse recorded this information and identified that the interventions were effective in relieving the

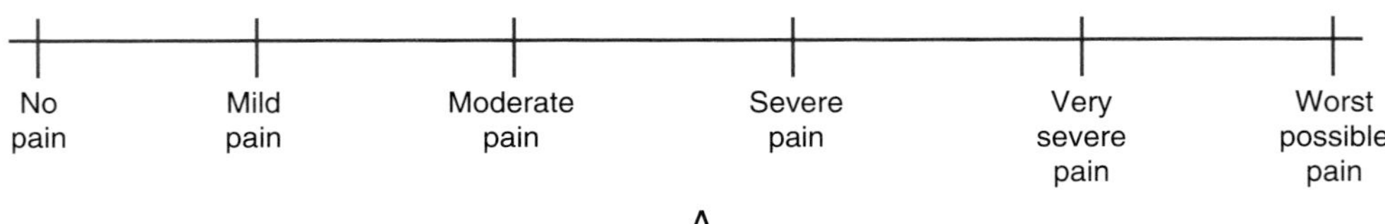

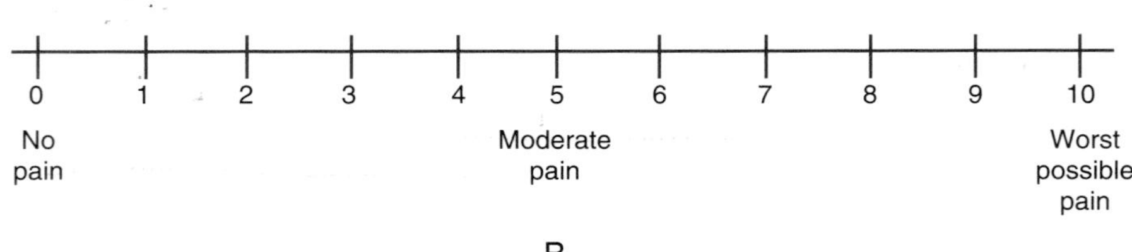

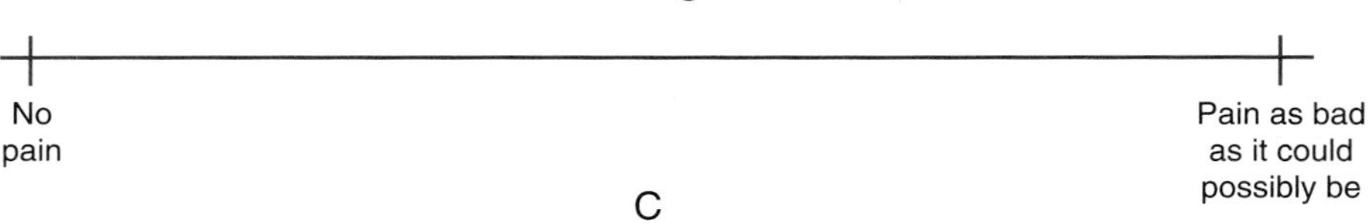

[1]If used as a graphic rating scale, a 10 cm baseline is recommended.
[2]A 10 cm baseline is recommended for VAS scales.

FIGURE 16-5
Examples of pain intensity scales. *A*, Simple descriptive pain intensity scale; *B*, 0–10 numeric pain intensity scale; *C*, visual analog scale (VAS). (From Acute Pain Management Guidelines Panel. [1991]. Acute Pain Management [DHHS Publication No. 92-0052, p. 116, D1]. Rockville, MD: Agency for Health Care Policy and Research, Public Health Service, U.S. Department of Health and Human Services.)

pain because the pain intensity had decreased from 7 to 2 on the 0 to 10 scale.

AGGRAVATING AND ALLEVIATING FACTORS. The nurse asks if any event or activity causes the pain or makes it better or worse. The nurse should ask, "What were you doing when the pain occurred?" Aggravating factors make the pain worse. Certain positions, temperatures, or times of day or night may cause the pain to be more severe. Likewise, alleviating factors might include specific positions, application of heat, cold, or menthol, or physical activities that reduce pain in specific areas.

Patients can usually identify the things that aggravate or reduce pain and what specific pain relief methods have worked in the past. For example, four patients with arthritic pain of the right shoulder had four different means of reducing the pain. The first patient obtained relief with elevation and rest of the right arm. The second applied an analgesic balm, a menthol ointment. The third patient used a heating pad to the area, and the fourth increased the anti-inflammatory drug dose as prescribed by the physician.

Examine Site of Pain

The fourth step in the assessment of pain is to examine the location that the patient states is painful. The area should be examined for signs of heat, redness, swelling, tenderness, abnormal position, or other factors that may be causing local irritation.

Patients may identify a location of pain that is not expected as part of their medical problem. This pain location may be due to a complication or an injury that was sustained during a procedure or hospitalization. For example, one patient who had orthopedic surgery on the ankle also sustained a large burn on his back at some point during the procedure. When the nurse examined the pain location, the burn was discovered.

Another example is a patient who had abdominal surgery and complained of pain in the right calf. Examination of the right calf revealed a red, firm, tender area that was reported to the physician and diagnosed as thrombophlebitis. By examining the exact location of pain, the nurse may identify the correct cause of the pain.

Identify Coping Methods

The fifth step in pain assessment is the identification of coping methods. People develop coping methods to increase control over pain or to relieve pain. Nurses should identify the methods patients use to cope with pain and should support the coping method. Some patients actively deal with pain—for example, they may complain and get up and move around or do some other activity. Some patients cope by staying quiet, praying, sleeping, or withdrawing.

Nurses must emphasize to patients and their families that their cooperation and information is a critical factor in achieving pain relief. Some patients expect nurses to know that they are experiencing pain and to know what to do about it. The nurse can confirm how the patient copes with pain by discussing observations of the patient's behavior with him or her. The nurse can also advise the patient of other coping methods that could be used to relieve pain (e.g., changing positions, imagery, and distraction).

Record Assessment Findings and Evaluate Interventions

The sixth and last step in the pain assessment is to write the information in the patient's chart so that this information can be conveyed to nurses on other shifts and to other health professionals. The location, quality, and intensity of the pain, related factors, and how the patient copes with pain should be identified. After interventions, the intensity of pain should be recorded again, and the record should include whether the pain relief intervention was effective. If the nursing intervention was not effective, the nurse should record what was done about the pain.

NURSING DIAGNOSIS AND GOALS

Nursing diagnoses are formulated after assessing the patient. A nursing diagnosis statement includes the possible cause of pain along with the patient's specific signs and symptoms. Nursing diagnoses directly related to patients in pain are the following:

- Potential or actual **Pain**
- **Chronic Pain**

An example of a nursing diagnosis may be pain (acute) related to surgery as evidenced by reports of discomfort at surgical incision.

The nurse may also use the following diagnoses to identify other problems that often accompany pain:

- **Activity Intolerance**
- **Anxiety**
- **Fatigue**
- **Self-Care Deficit**
- **Sleep Pattern Disturbance**

Once the diagnosis is made, the nurse begins to plan interventions to relieve pain.

INTERVENTIONS

Nonpharmacologic Interventions

Nonpharmacologic interventions include a wide range of physical and psychological interventions for pain relief (Table 16–5). Physical interventions usually involve comfort measures, control of environmental factors, and cutaneous application techniques such as heat or cold. Psychological interventions include providing unconditional acceptance of the patient's report; preparatory information about pain, analgesics, and procedures or psychological strategies such as relaxation and imagery. These types of interventions should be initiated and used along with appropriate analgesic administration to obtain optimal pain relief.

PHYSICAL INTERVENTIONS

Physical Comfort Measures. These nursing interventions focus on the patient and the environment. When the patient is comfortable, pain tolerance may be increased and the patient may experience less pain. Attention to adequate air, food and fluid, elimination, mobility, hygiene, temperature, and rest and sleep is essential to comfort. The nurse should monitor these

TABLE 16–5
NONPHARMACOLOGIC INTERVENTIONS

INTERVENTION	COMMENTS
Physical	
Heat, Cold, Massage, TENS	Increase pain threshold, reduce muscle spasm, and decrease congestion in injured area. Effective in reducing pain and improving physical function. Require skilled personnel and special equipment. May be useful as adjunct to drug therapy.
Psychological	
Relaxation	
Jaw relaxation Progressive muscle relaxation	Effective in reducing mild to moderate pain and as an adjunct to analgesic drugs for severe pain.
Simple imagery	Use when patients express an interest in relaxation. Requires 3–5 min of staff time for instructions.
Music	Both patient-preferred and "easy listening" music are effective in reducing mild to moderate pain.
Imagery	Effective for reduction of mild to moderate pain. Requires skilled personnel.
Educational instruction	Effective for reduction of pain. Should include sensory and procedural information and be aimed at reducing activity-related pain. Requires 5–15 min of staff time.

Adapted from Acute Pain Management Guidelines Panel. (1992). *Acute pain management: Operative and medical procedures and trauma. Clinical practice guidelines* (AHCPR Publication No. 92-0032). Rockville, MD: Agency for Health Care Policy and Research, Public Health Service, U.S. Department of Health and Human Services.

areas for potential problems. For example, patients who are sleep deprived or fatigued may have increased pain. Therefore, providing for uninterrupted sleep and periods of rest can enhance pain relief.

For the patient in pain, progressive exercise or immobility may be prescribed as a treatment for pain depending on the underlying problem. The patient with an injury or incision should be moved carefully so that further trauma is avoided. Turning the patient carefully from side to side or supporting an affected extremity during activity can reduce pain. Usually the patient can tell the nurse which movements or positions increase or decrease the pain. Telling the patient what activities are expected after surgery allows the patient to anticipate and recognize normal postoperative events.

Administering analgesic medications prior to activities or procedures is important to reduce the pain intensity and anxiety associated with the event. Aggressive treatment of pain, nausea, vomiting, appetite suppression, constipation, and other problems is important. Nurses should assist and teach patients how to splint abdominal and thoracic wounds externally to minimize pain when deep breathing, coughing, and ambulating. A change of bed linen and sheets free of wrinkles can be refreshing and reduce irritation of the skin. Applying ointment to cracked lips or providing ice chips for a dry mouth are examples of other comfort measures. Any tubes or equipment attached to the patient should be secure but not produce tension on the skin. Correct body alignment and frequent changes of position will relieve monotony, increase circulation, and prevent muscle contractures and spasms.

PHARMACOLOGY CAPSULE

Analgesics can be administered before painful activities or procedures to reduce the pain intensity and anxiety associated with the event.

Environmental Control. Each patient has individual preferences and should be asked about areas that enhance comfort. This is especially true when the nurse attempts to control the environment. Some patients prefer an active environment in which they can be distracted from pain. Listening to tapes or music, watching television, working with their hands, walking around, or visiting with others allows a person to focus attention on stimuli other than the pain sensation. Distraction or diversion allows one to focus on the five senses for input, which can lessen attention to painful stimuli. The hospital environment, with its lights, noise, and constant activity, often causes sensory overload for the patient in pain. This can increase pain. When this occurs, the nurse should coordinate with staff to promote a quiet environment with nonglaring lights and scheduled rest and activity periods that meet the patient's needs.

Stimulation Techniques. Stimulation to the skin and underlying tissues produces pain relief. Various types of skin or cutaneous stimulation can be applied, and each has variable effects. These techniques are not curative; rather, they can decrease the intensity of pain or change the sensation so that it is more acceptable. The exact mechanism for pain relief is unknown, but it is thought that superficial stimulation may act on large fibers, blocking transmission of pain impulses to the brain. The applications of heat, cold, massage, and TENS are discussed here as examples of cutaneous stimulation. These tend to be most effective for mild to moderate pain, well-localized pain, and acute and chronic pain. The effects of these therapies last as long or slightly longer than the application. These therapies may have relaxing or distracting effects, and they allow the patient to participate in the therapy.

The physician may prescribe heat or cold application for pain. Applications of heat or cold are used to reduce muscle spasm and decrease congestion or swelling in an injured area. Either therapy may be applied to the painful site, at a location beyond the site, between the site and the brain, or on the opposite side of the body. These therapies should be applied intermittently, not continuously. Heat and cold may be alternated. Both therapies should be applied at a comfortable level of intensity for the patient, and the patient should be monitored frequently.

Cold may be applied with ice packs or cooling pads to decrease initial tissue injury and swelling (e.g., with musculoskeletal sprains or orthopedic procedures). Cold is contraindicated for patients with peripheral vascular disease or heart disease because it may cause further vasoconstriction of blood vessels and thus decrease circulation. The application of cold should be limited to 15 minutes per session to avoid tissue injury or frostbite.

Moist or dry heat can be applied with heating pads, hot-water bottles, towels, gel packs, or warm tub baths or showers. Superficial heat has been shown to be effective for gastrointestinal cramps and muscle and joint pain. Treatment should be limited to 30 minutes to avoid tissue injury and burn. Heat should not be applied to a malignancy site, to areas of decreased sensation or circulation, or to patients who cannot communicate their discomfort.

Massage involves rubbing, kneading, manipulating, and applying pressure and friction to the body. Rubbing or massaging an area is a natural response when one has an injury or ache. Massage may be used to promote relaxation and relieve muscle cramps. Massage is commonly applied to the back, neck, and large leg muscles; however, massage of the hands and feet is more accessible and acceptable and perhaps more effective. Massage should not be applied to areas with injury, phlebitis, or skin lesions or to patients with bleeding problems.

Cold, heat, and massage are easy to apply, inexpensive, effective, and simple for the patient or family to learn. For each therapy, the nurse should give the patient a choice, evaluate whether the method or location of application is effective, and monitor for any side effects.

Compared with the above therapies, TENS is much more expensive and less widely available. It requires a physician's order, and often the physical therapy department handles the equipment. The therapy involves external electrical stimulation of the skin and underlying tissues through electrodes attached to a small unit that the patient can carry around. The electrodes are placed over, above, or below painful sites and attached to a battery-operated device that delivers low-voltage electrical currents. The electrical current is adjusted through a dial on the unit. The patient should feel a mild tingling or vibrating or prickly sensation over the area of application. Nursing responsibilities with TENS include the following:

1. Applying electrodes in the correct locations and with good contact with the skin.
2. Checking that all connections are secure from skin electrodes to unit.
3. Adjusting the current to the patient's level of comfort.
4. Documenting and evaluating pain relief.

The major disadvantage of TENS is irritation of the skin under the electrodes. The electrodes should be changed daily, the sites rotated, and the skin inspected. Figure 16–6 shows the application of electrodes and a TENS unit.

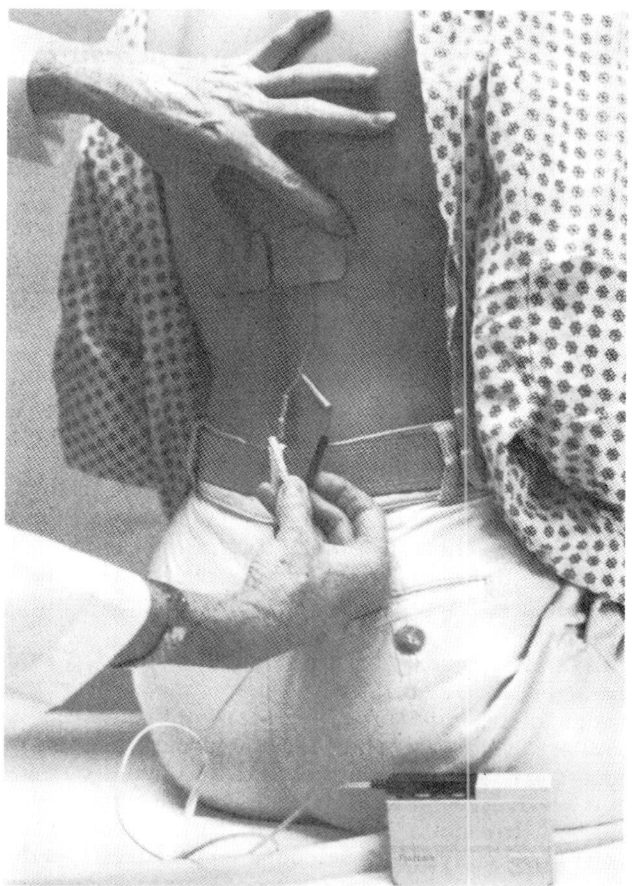

FIGURE 16-6
Application of a TENS Unit. (From Ignatavicius, D. D., & Bayne, M. V. [1991]. *Medical-surgical nursing: A nursing process approach.* Philadelphia: W. B. Saunders.)

PSYCHOLOGICAL INTERVENTIONS

Anxiety Reduction. Anxiety, fear of the unknown, and feelings of loss of control may be directly related to the level of pain experienced. The patient who is anxious and uncertain will tend to rate pain high. If the nurse can increase predictability and control of painful stimuli, pain may be reduced. An important aspect of relieving anxiety associated with pain is the relationship between the nurse and the patient. The nurse can be with the patient, assure the patient that everything possible is being done, and provide timely and appropriate interventions for pain relief.

Several strategies are used to decrease anxiety and increase control. Telling the patient about events and providing descriptions of the sensations or feelings that may accompany the event can reduce anxiety; however, some patients may prefer not to know this information, and their wishes should be respected. Allowing the patient to choose physical comfort measures and the time for treatments or to rearrange items in the room also provides control.

When teaching patients preoperatively about pain, it is also important to teach skills to cope with their pain —for example, breathing, relaxation, or imagery techniques. By providing strategies to cope with pain and anxiety, the nurse is also providing the patient with a sense of control. Table 16–5 describes such psychological interventions used for pain relief.

Distraction. Distraction refers to focusing on stimuli other than pain. Distraction may help the patient have a sense of control as well as increase pain tolerance, decrease pain intensity, and alter the quality of pain, but it does not eliminate pain. Because the pain is not eliminated, the patient will usually require analgesics and other methods of pain relief. A patient using distraction may not appear or behave as if in pain and may cause other people to doubt that the pain exists. After a patient has used a distraction technique, he or she may once again focus on the pain and experience a heightened awareness of pain.

Distraction techniques are often most helpful with mild to moderate pain or during brief periods of pain associated with procedures such as dressing changes, intramuscular injections, and venipunctures. Although the following list is not exhaustive, examples of distraction methods include rhythmic breathing, listening to music, laughing, counting, watching television, reading, exercising, resting, talking on the phone, and visiting with others. Elderly persons may find reminiscing (relating past experiences) to be a beneficial distraction technique. It is helpful to include several distraction techniques in the plan of care so that the patient can utilize the methods most effective for his or her individual pain relief.

Relaxation. Patients should be aware that the use of relaxation is one of the options for pain relief. Patients may already come to the hospital using this technique or may be taught relaxation techniques while hospitalized. The nurse should be aware that the patient is using relaxation, know the rationale for using relaxation, and know the effects of relaxation.

Relaxation is a cognitive approach to pain management. It is a self-hypnotic technique that may, but does not always, produce the relaxation response. The relaxation response, which counteracts the stress response, is characterized by decreased muscle tension, decreased heart rate, decreased respiratory rate, and normal or decreased blood pressure. Relaxation decreases mental stress and physical tension; this is helpful because pain is often accompanied by increased anxiety and muscle tension. Relaxation is usually most effective for mild to moderate pain rather than severe pain.

Rhythmic breathing is a relaxation technique that focuses on just breathing, as described in Table 16–6. Relaxation techniques that focus on total body relaxation require the patient's active participation. Each part of the body is deliberately relaxed, usually in an orderly sequence such as head to toe or vice versa. Relaxation often involves breathing exercises combined with a variety of methods to promote freedom from anxiety and muscle tension. Methods may include yoga, meditation, and music.

In the clinical setting, the patient may be taught to utilize relaxation through the use of a script or a taped relaxation exercise. To promote mental and physical relaxation, a relaxation technique should include the following:

1. A quiet, private environment free from interruptions.
2. A comfortable position in which extremities are not crossed.
3. A mental device such as rhythmic breathing.
4. A passive attitude.
5. Patient control.
6. Practice.
7. Coaching by means of a script or taped exercise.

Although most patients benefit from relaxation, not all patients are appropriate candidates for this technique. Patients who may not be good candidates for relaxation include those with severe asthma (because of the rhythmic breathing), cardiac dysrhythmias (because of stimulation of the vagus nerve), a psychiatric history involving delusions and hallucinations (because of the introspective nature of some exercises), and depression (because of the potential for further withdrawal). Elderly patients may respond better to simple relaxation techniques such as jaw relaxation rather than lengthy relaxation exercises.

When teaching patients relaxation, it is best to delay teaching if the patient is experiencing severe pain. The patient in severe pain may not be able to concentrate on or be receptive to relaxation techniques. In addition, relaxation is usually not effective for severe pain, although the techniques can help reduce the anxiety and tension associated with pain.

It is also important to stress to patients that the use of relaxation does not indicate that the pain is thought to be psychological or that the patient must substitute relaxation for analgesics. Relaxation can be viewed as a technique that can be used in addition to analgesics to enhance pain control.

Imagery. Imagery is another cognitive approach to pain control that encourages physical and mental relaxation. Imagery uses a person's imagination to help control pain. Besides promoting relaxation, imagery may be used for distraction or may help the patient imagine pain relief.

Patients are asked to describe the quality of pain they are experiencing. On the basis of this description, imagery can be used to modify the patient's experience. For example, if the pain is described as "burning," an image of something cool may help reduce pain intensity. As with relaxation, the use of imagery does not mean that the pain is viewed as being imaginary. In both relaxation and imagery, the nurse may read a script or use a prerecorded tape to guide the patient through the experiences. The nurse should encourage the patient to practice relaxation or imagery, or both, in order to evaluate potential effectiveness.

TABLE 16–6

SAMPLE RELAXATION EXERCISE: SLOW RHYTHMIC BREATHING

1. Breathe in slowly and deeply.
2. As you breathe out slowly, feel yourself beginning to relax; feel the tension leaving your body.
3. Now breathe in and out slowly and regularly at whatever rate is comfortable for you. You may wish to try abdominal breathing. If you do not know how to do abdominal breathing, ask your nurse for help.
4. To help you focus on your breathing and to breathe slowly and rhythmically, do the following:
   a. Breathe in as you say silently to yourself, "in, two, three."
   b. Breathe out as you say silently to yourself, "out, two, three."
   c. Each time you breathe out, say silently to yourself a word such as "peace" or "relax."
5. You may imagine that you are doing this in a place you have found very calming and relaxing, such as lying in the sun at the beach.
6. Do steps 1 through 4 only once, or repeat steps 3 and 4 for up to 20 min.
7. End with a slow, deep breath. As you breathe out, say to yourself, "I feel alert and relaxed."

ADDITIONAL POINTS

If you intend to do this for more than a few seconds, try to get in a comfortable position in a quiet environment. You may close your eyes or focus on an object. This technique has the advantage of being very adaptable in that it may be used for only a few seconds or for up to 20 min.

Adapted with permission from McCaffery, M., & Beebe, A. (1989). *Pain: Clinical manual for nursing practice.* St. Louis: C. V. Mosby.

Pharmacologic Interventions

Drug therapy continues to be the mainstay of pain management. Although the physician orders specific analgesics, it is the nurse's responsibility to assess the pain, to decide which analgesic and how much to administer, and to evaluate the drug's effectiveness.

When administering analgesics, the nurse should keep in mind that it is critical to use a preventative approach to pain management. When pain is predictable, such as with postoperative pain and cancer pain, analgesics are more effective when given around-the-clock (ATC) rather than as needed (PRN). With an ATC schedule, therapeutic blood levels of the analgesics are maintained. With a PRN schedule, the patient may have frequent periods of unrelieved pain and may also have more significant and frequent side effects such as sedation. Even when a physician orders analgesics PRN, the nurse can administer the analgesics on an ATC schedule. The ATC schedule is usually based on how long the drug lasts or the duration of its effect; thus, when the order says every 3 to 4 hours, the analgesic should be administered every 3 to 4 hours to maintain the analgesic effect.

When pain is unpredictable, it may be appropriate to administer analgesics on a PRN basis. In these situations, the patient must be instructed to request medication as soon as the pain begins rather than waiting for the pain to become more severe. Patients often report that they wait to call for analgesics, thinking that the pain will decrease with time. Unfortunately, waiting often results in pain reaching an intensity level that is difficult to control.

The three categories of drugs that are used to relieve pain are: (1) nonopioid analgesics, (2) opioid analgesics, and (3) adjuvant drugs.

NONOPIOID ANALGESICS. Nonopioid analgesics include aspirin, acetaminophen, and nonsteroidal anti-inflammatory drugs (NSAIDs), such as ibuprofen. The nonopioids are generally the initial treatment choice for mild pain. These analgesics may also be combined with opioids to control moderate to severe pain.

Nonopioid analgesics act on the peripheral nervous system and are used for pains such as arthritic pain, backache, headache, dysmenorrhea, postoperative pain, cancer pain, and bone pain. Nonopioids may have one or all of the following properties: antipyretic (reduces fever), analgesic (reduces pain), and anti-inflammatory (reduces inflammation). This range of actions makes them especially useful for many conditions.

Most of the nonopioids are oral preparations, but a few are available for rectal administration. A parenteral NSAID, ketorolac (Toradol), also is available and is generally used for the short-term management of postoperative pain. It has been found that 30 mg of ketorolac given intramuscularly provides the same amount of pain relief as 12 mg of morphine or 100 mg of meperidine (Demerol) given intramusculary. Ketorolac has a longer duration of action than many of the opioid analgesics and has side effects similar to those of other NSAIDs.

The nonopioids, unlike the opioids, have a ceiling effect on analgesia. This means that, beyond a certain dosage, improved analgesia will *not* occur. However, these drugs do have side effects, including stomach irritation, fluid retention, and increased bleeding time. Therefore, they are usually not recommended for patients with liver or kidney disorders, thrombocytopenia, or neutropenia. (Thrombocytopenia is a deficiency of platelets in the blood. Neutropenia is a decreased percentage of neutrophils [white blood cells that respond to inflammation]). Some nonopioids should be used cautiously in patients with congestive heart failure or hypertension because the side effect of fluid retention may aggravate these conditions. Because nonopioids have many side effects, the nurse should assess the patient's history and present condition before administering prescribed analgesics.

Table 16–7 identifies commonly used NSAIDS and some considerations when administering these drugs. Older adults may be more sensitive to NSAIDs and experience a greater number of side effects. The nurse should carefully monitor each patient's reaction to the analgesic. For example, older adults should be monitored for signs of increased bleeding, gastrointestinal irritation, and unusual drug reactions such as confusion, constipation, and headaches.

Many nurses forget to administer nonopioids because they fail to recognize the importance of using these drugs for the types of mild to moderate pain mentioned previously. Nurses should recognize that the nonopioids can be administered along with opioids and may be as effective as lower doses of opioids. For instance, 650 mg of oral aspirin or acetaminophen provides the same amount of analgesia as 32 mg of oral codeine or 50 mg of oral meperidine. Nonopioids tend to block pain transmission peripherally, whereas opioids block pain transmission at the central nervous system. It is advantageous to administer both for pain relief.

PHARMACOLOGY CAPSULE

Adverse effects of nonopioid analgesics include stomach irritation, fluid retention, and increased bleeding time.

OPIOID ANALGESICS. This group of analgesics is generally used for moderate to severe acute pain, chronic cancer pain, and specific instances of chronic pain unrelated to cancer. These drugs reduce pain by acting on the central nervous system. Opioids vary in potency and duration of action.

There are currently two types of opioid analgesics:

- Opioid agonists—examples include codeine, methadone (Dolophine), hydromorphone (Dilaudid), meperidine (Demerol), morphine, and fentanyl.
- Opioid agonist-antagonists—examples include buprenorphine (Buprenex), nalbuphine (Nubain), butorphanol (Stadol), and pentazocine (Talwin).

TABLE 16-7
NONOPIOID ANALGESICS: COMMONLY USED NSAIDS

DRUGS	USUAL ADULT DOSE*	COMMENTS
Oral NSAIDs		
Acetaminophen	650–975 mg q 4 hr	Lacks the peripheral anti-inflammatory activity of other NSAIDs.
Aspirin[†]	650–975 mg q 4 hr	The standard against which other NSAIDs are compared. Inhibits platelet aggregaton; may cause postoperative bleeding.
Choline magnesium trisalicylate (Trilisate)	1000–1500 mg bid	May have minimal antiplatelet activity; also available as oral liquid.
Diflunisal (Dolobid)	1000 mg initial dose followed by 500 mg q 12 hr	
Etodolac (Lodine)	200–400 mg q 6–8 hr	
Fenoprofen calcium (Nalfon)	200 mg q 4–6 hr	
Ibuprofen (Motrin, others)	400 mg q 4–6 hr	Available as several brand names and as generic; also available as oral suspension.
Ketoprofen (Orudis)	25–75 mg q 6–8 hr	
Magnesium salicylate	650 mg q 4 hr	Many brands and generic forms available.
Meclofenamate sodium (Meclomen)	50 mg q 4–6 hr	
Mefenamic acid (Ponstel)	250 mg q 6 hr	
Naproxen (Naprosyn)	500 mg initial dose followed by 250 mg q 6–8 hr	Also available as oral liquid.
Naproxen sodium (Anaprox)	550 mg initial dose followed by 275 mg q 6–8 hr	
Salsalate (Disalcid, others)	500 mg q 4 hr	May have minimal antiplatelet activity.
Sodium salicylate	325–650 mg q 3–4 hr	Available in generic form from several distributors.
Parenteral NSAID		
Ketorolac	30 or 60 mg IM initial dose followed by 15 or 30 mg q 6 hr Oral dose following IM dosage: 10 mg q 6–8 hr	IM dose not to exceed 5 days.

Adapted from Acute Pain Management Guidelines Panel (1992). *Acute pain management: Operative and medical procedures and trauma. Clinical practice guidelines* (AHCPR Publication No. 92-0032). Rockville, MD: Agency for Health Care Policy and Research, Public Health Service, U.S. Department of Health and Human Services.

Note: Only the above NSAIDs have U.S. Food and Drug Administration approval for use as simple analgesics, but clinical experience has been gained with other drugs as well.

* Drug recommendations are limited to NSAIDs where pediatric dosing experience is available.

[†] Contraindicated in presence of fever or other evidence of viral illness.

NSAIDs, Nonsteroidal anti-inflammatory drugs; q, every; bid, twice a day; IM, intramuscularly, intramuscular.

Both types of opioids relieve pain at the level of the central nervous system. The agonist-antagonists, however, block some of the side effects of the pure opioid agonists much the same way that naloxone (Narcan) acts as an opioid antagonist to block the effects of opioids. Thus, a patient receiving pure opioid agonists should not be given opioid agonist-antagonists because this can precipitate withdrawal symptoms and increase pain.

Older adults are generally more sensitive to the analgesic effects of opioids. They may require smaller doses because serum drug levels tend to remain higher than in young patients. The higher serum levels may be attributed to the delayed excretion and slower metabolism of the older adult. Also, side effects may be more pronounced in older adults. Thus, it is important to titrate analgesic dosages on an individual basis to provide optimum pain control with minimal or no side effects.

It is important to refer to an equianalgesic (approximately equal analgesia) table when changing to a new opioid or a different route. Table 16–8 shows such a table with approximate equianalgesic oral and parenteral doses. The information in the table helps to estimate the new dose, which should then be modified based on the specific patient reaction and drug. An equianalgesic table shows that oral doses are two to six times higher than parenteral doses of the same drug. This is because oral opioids must pass through the liver after absorption, which reduces the amount of medication absorbed. Therefore, higher doses of oral opioids must be ordered to provide the same amount of analgesia as parenteral opioids. For example, a patient receives 10 mg of morphine intramuscularly for pain relief and the order is

TABLE 16–8

OPIOID ANALGESICS: DOSING DATA

DRUG	APPROXIMATE EQUIANALGESIC ORAL DOSE	APPROXIMATE EQUIANALGESIC PARENTERAL DOSE	RECOMMENDED STARTING DOSE (ADULTS > 50 KG BODY WEIGHT)		RECOMMENDED STARTING DOSE (CHILDREN AND ADULTS < 50 KG BODY WEIGHT)*	
			Oral	Parenteral	Oral	Parenteral
Opioid Agonist						
Morphine†	30 mg q 3–4 hr (around-the-clock dosing) 60 mg q 3–4 hr (single dose or intermittent dosing)	10 mg q 3–4 hr	30 mg q 3–4 hr	10 mg q 3–4 hr	0.3 mg/kg q 3–4 hr	0.1 mg/kg q 3–4 hr
Codeine‡	130 mg q 3–4 hr	75 mg q 3–4 hr	60 mg q 3–4 hr	60 mg q 2 hr (intramuscular/ subcutaneous)	1 mg/kg q 3–4 hr§	Not recommended
Hydromorphone† (Dilaudid)	7.5 mg q 3–4 hr	1.5 mg q 3–4 hr	6 mg q 3–4 hr	1.5 mg q 3–4 hr	0.06 mg/kg q 3–4 hr	0.015 mg/kg q 3–4 hr
Hydrocodone (in Lorcet, Lortab, Vicodin, others)	30 mg q 3–4 hr	Not available	10 mg q 3–4 hr	Not available	0.2 mg/kg q 3–4 hr§	Not available
Levorphanol (Levo-Dromoran)	4 mg q 6–8 hr	2 mg q 6–8 hr	4 mg q 6–8 hr	2 mg q 6–8 hr	0.04 mg/kg q 6–8 hr	0.02 mg/kg q 6–8 hr
Meperidine (Demerol)	300 mg q 2–3 hr	100 mg q 3 hr	Not recommended	100 mg q 3 hr	Not recommended	0.75 mg/kg q 2–3 hr
Methadone (Dolophine, others)	20 mg q 6–8 hr	10 mg q 6–8 hr	20 mg q 6–8 hr	10 mg q 6–8 hr	0.2 mg/kg q 6–8 hr	0.1 mg/kg q 6–8 hr
Oxycodone (Roxicodone, also in Percocet, Percodan, Tylox, others)	30 mg q 3–4 hr	Not available	10 mg q 3–4 hr	Not available	0.2 mg/kg q 3–4 hr§	Not available
Oxymorphone† (Numorphan)	Not available	1 mg q 3–4 hr	Not available	1 mg q 3–4 hr	Not recommended	Not recommended
Opioid Agonist-Antagonist and Partial Agonist						
Buprenorphine (Buprenex)	Not available	0.3–0.4 mg q 6–8 hr	Not available	0.4 mg q 6–8 hr	Not available	0.004 mg/kg q 6–8 hr
Butorphanol (Stadol)	Not available	2 mg q 3–4 hr	Not available	2 mg q 3–4 hr	Not available	Not recommended
Nalbuphine (Nubain)	Not available	10 mg q 3–4 hr	Not available	10 mg q 3–4 hr	Not available	0.1 mg/kg q 3–4 hr
Pentazocine (Talwin, others)	150 mg q 3–4 hr	60 mg q 3–4 hr	50 mg q 4–6 hr	Not recommended	Not recommended	Not recommended

Adapted from Acute Pain Management Guidelines Panel. (1992). *Acute pain management: Operative and medical procedures and trauma. Clinical practice guidelines* (AHCPR Publication No. 92-0032). Rockville, MD: Agency for Health Care Policy and Research, Public Health Service, U.S. Department of Health and Human Services.

Note: Published tables vary in the suggested doses that are equianalgesic to morphine. Clinical response is the criterion that must be applied for each patient; titration to clinical response is necessary. Because there is not complete cross tolerance among these drugs, it is usually necessary to use a lower than equianalgesic dose when changing drugs and to retitrate to response.

Caution: Recommended doses do not apply to patients with renal or hepatic insufficiency or other conditions affecting drug metabolism and kinetics.

* *Caution:* Doses listed for patients with body weight less than 50 kg cannot be used as initial starting doses in babies less than 6 months of age. Consult the *Clinical Practice Guideline for Acute Pain Management: Operative or Medical Procedures and Trauma* section on management of pain in neonates for recommendations.

† For morphine, hydromorphone, and oxymorphone, rectal administration is an alternate route for patients unable to take oral medications, but equianalgesic doses may differ from oral and parenteral doses because of pharmacokinetic differences.

‡ *Caution:* Codeine doses above 65 mg often are not appropriate due to diminishing incremental analgesia with increasing doses but continually increasing constipation and other side effects.

§ *Caution:* Doses of aspirin and acetaminophen in combination with opioid/NSAID preparations must also be adjusted to the patient's body weight.

changed to oral morphine. To receive an equianalgesic dose of morphine, the patient should be given 30 mg of morphine orally.

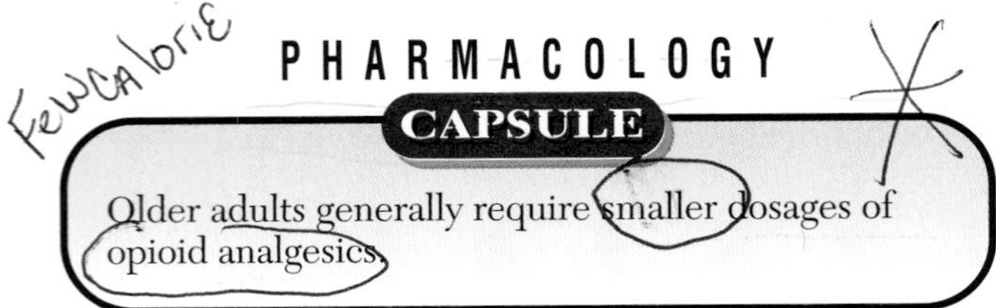

Misconceptions about Opioid Analgesics. When discussing opioid analgesics, it is critical to review a few terms that are often misunderstood and result in undertreatment of pain. Patients, families, nurses, and physicians have misconceptions about addiction; therefore, the term must be defined and differentiated from the terms tolerance and physical dependence. Table 16–9 contains information about these terms. When patients take opioids over a period of time or for chronic pain, physiologic adaptation may occur, resulting in tolerance and physical dependence. The patient who is tolerant requires higher doses of a drug to achieve an analgesic effect. The patient who is physically dependent on an opioid will experience unpleasant withdrawal symptoms when the opioid is stopped. The nurse should recognize both tolerance and physical dependence as normal responses to continued opioid administration for pain relief; they do not lead to a craving for the drug for its mind-altering effects. Fear of addiction is greatly exaggerated, and addiction rarely occurs (<1%) in the patient taking opioids for pain relief.

Routes of Administration. The opioids can be administered through various routes depending on the needs of the patient. If tolerated, the oral route is preferred, especially for patients with chronic pain. Oral opioids can control severe pain when given in adequate dosages.

The intramuscular route is commonly used to administer opioids postoperatively. The nurse should consider the type and amount of drug being administered when selecting appropriate needle-gauge size and administration site. The intramuscular route is not indicated for chronic pain. Absorption is often unpredictable with intramuscular injections, particularly with the older adult who has reduced muscle mass. This route is also painful. An accessible and appropriate site for intramuscular analgesics is the ventral gluteal muscle, especially for the older adult.

A limited number of opioids, such as morphine, hydromorphone, and oxymorphone, may be administered rectally. This route is useful when the patient is nauseated or has difficulty swallowing. The rectal route should not be used in patients with neutropenia, thrombocytopenia, or diarrhea.

Opioids may also be administered subcutaneously. Intermittent bolus injections, continuous infusions, or patient-controlled analgesia (PCA) are methods of administering medications subcutaneously. This method may be used in patients who are unable to utilize the oral and rectal routes and who also have poor intravenous access.

The intravenous route is another method of administering opioids. Intravenous PCA is commonly used postoperatively. With PCA, the patient is able to self-administer doses of analgesics in order to control his or her pain. Opioids, when administered intravenously, have a rapid onset but shorter duration of action than when given by any other route. Although the registered nurse is usually responsible for the PCA, the practical nurse may be responsible for monitoring the patient's response and the effectiveness of the medication. Side effects should be reported to the registered nurse.

Opioids can also be administered via the spinal route epidurally (in the epidural space) or intrathecally (in the subarachnoid space). Conditions in which these routes may be utilized to provide pain control are postoperative pain and chronic cancer pain. The practical nurse may participate in monitoring the patient. Side effects such as itching, hypotension, nausea, urinary retention, sedation, and respiratory depression may occur more frequently in patients receiving opioids epidurally or intrathecally than by other routes of administration. The older adult with a spinal opioid infusion is at increased risk for respiratory depression. If anesthetics such as bupivacaine are used with spinal opioids, the nurse must be alert for side effects of sensory loss and motor weakness. Side effects, as well as any adverse effects, should be reported promptly. A sedation assessment scale should be used with patients receiving spinal opioid infusions.

Other routes of administration of opioids also are available. Morphine may be administered sublingually. Fentanyl lollipops are being investigated as to the effectiveness of that delivery method. Duragesic transdermal patches are being used for both acute and chronic pain. Intranasal butorphanol is available and usually used preoperatively and postoperatively for analgesia. Package inserts should be reviewed regarding dosing, precautions, and administration guidelines.

TABLE 16-9

CHARACTERISTICS OF TOLERANCE, PHYSICAL DEPENDENCE, AND ADDICTION

Tolerance
Physiologic changes that occur from repeated doses of opioids.
Result: The need for higher doses to achieve pain relief.

Physical Dependency
Physiologic changes that occur from repeated doses of opioids.
Result: Withdrawal symptoms may occur if the opioid is stopped abruptly (e.g., irritability, chills, sweating, nausea).

Addiction
Psychological dependence characterized by continued craving for opioid for other than pain relief.
Result: Compulsive obtaining and use of drug for psychic effects.
Note: Risk of addiction is not a concern in treating acute or cancer pain.

PHARMACOLOGY CAPSULE

Oral analgesics are preferred for treatment of chronic pain.

Side Effects. Regardless of the route of administration, opioid analgesics have specific side effects. A common side effect is constipation. Tolerance to this side effect does not develop. The nurse must assess the patient for abdominal distention, cramping, and abdominal pain. The use of laxatives, along with encouragement to increase fluid, exercise, and bulk-containing foods, may prevent this side effect.

Opioids may also cause nausea with or without vomiting. Some patients develop a tolerance to nausea but may require antiemetic therapy until tolerance to nausea develops. At times, the order may need to be changed to a different opioid to relieve this problem.

Sedation is another side effect that may occur initially with opioids, but it usually subsides in a few days. In patients who have had unrelieved pain for some time and have been sleep deprived, the control of pain may allow the patient to rest, which may be misinterpreted as sedation. When sedation is noted, however, the dose of the opioid may need to be titrated to a level that does not cause sedation but does provide pain relief. The nurse should be aware that drugs such as promethazine (Phenergan), which are sometimes ordered to be given with opioids, may also contribute to sedation. Promethazine does not potentiate or increase the analgesic effects of opioids but does potentiate sedation, respiratory depression, and hypotension. If sedated, the patient may benefit from having separate orders for the opioid and for the promethazine. The nurse and patient may then work together to achieve the most effective pain relief.

Respiratory depression can occur but does not occur as frequently as commonly thought. If a patient is easily arousable, it is highly unlikely that respiratory depression has occurred.

Other side effects may be noted with the use of opioid analgesics. These include confusion, hypotension (especially orthostatic), dizziness, itching, and urinary retention.

Meperidine. One opioid worth mentioning when discussing side effects is meperidine. The nurse must be aware of the side effects mentioned previously but must also be alert to the signs of toxicity associated with meperidine administration. One of the products of meperidine metabolism is normeperidine. Normeperidine is a central nervous system stimulant. When this metabolite accumulates in the body, the patient may exhibit the following: anxiety, twitching, tremors, muscle jerking, and generalized seizures. Therefore, meperidine is generally not used for chronic pain, nor is it the analgesic of choice for older adults or patients with renal dysfunction because the risk for toxicity is high.

PHARMACOLOGY CAPSULE

Adverse effects of opioid analgesics include constipation, nausea, sedation, respiratory depression, confusion, hypotension, dizziness, itching, and urinary retention.

ADJUVANT ANALGESICS AND MEDICATIONS. Drugs that are usually not classified as analgesics may relieve pain in certain situations. For instance, a patient who has had back surgery may complain more about muscle spasms than incisional pain. The use of a muscle relaxant may be more effective in relieving his or her pain than the use of an opioid alone. It is important that patients, families, nurses, and physicians be aware that specific pain syndromes may be controlled with drugs other than the commonly known analgesics. Table 16–10 lists adjuvant drugs and the conditions they effectively treat.

PROBLEM SOLVING WITH PAIN MEDICATION. Nurses are often faced with patients whose prescribed analgesic drugs do not relieve pain. In these situations, the nurse must use all of the information presented here. By asking questions about the analgesic drug and the "five rights" (right dose, right patient, right time,

TABLE 16–10
ADJUVANT ANALGESICS AND MEDICATIONS

DRUG CLASSIFICATION	TYPE OF PAIN OR PROBLEM ASSOCIATED WITH PAIN
Antidepressants Amitriptyline (Elavil) Doxepin (Sinequan)	Neuropathic pain, dull, aching pain Pain associated with herpes zoster (shingles) Sleep disturbances
Muscle relaxants Methocarbamol (Robaxin) Cyclobenzaprine (Flexeril)	Muscle spasms and anxiety
Benzodiazepines Alprazolam (Xanax) Lorazepam (Ativan)	Muscle spasms and anxiety
Antihistamines Hydroxyzine (Vistaril, Atarax)	Nausea, anxiety
Corticosteroids Prednisone (Deltasone) Dexamethasone (Decadron)	Spinal cord or nerve compression Bone pain
Anticonvulsants Carbamazepine (Tegretol) Phenytoin (Dilantin)	Neuropathic pain, stabbing pain Trigeminal neuralgia Pain associated with herpes zoster (shingles) Other nerve pain

TABLE 16-11

SOUTHWEST TEXAS METHODIST HOSPITAL NURSING PLAN OF CARE: ALTERATION IN COMFORT

NURSING DIAGNOSIS/PATIENT PROBLEM

Alteration in comfort/pain (acute/chronic) related to:

Date/Initials

_____ Disease processes/illness
_____ Surgery
_____ Injury/trauma
_____ Diagnostic procedures
_____ ______________________
_____ ______________________

As Evidenced by:

_____ Verbalization of pain/discomfort
_____ Verbalization of spasms (specify bladder, back, muscle) __________
____
_____ Facial grimacing
_____ Tense body posture
_____ Rubbing/guarding of body parts
_____ Inability to concentrate
_____ Increased vital signs
_____ Restlessness/difficulty sleeping
_____ Crying, moaning
_____ Withdrawal
_____ Change in appetite
_____ Decreased activity
_____ ______________________
_____ ______________________

STANDARD OF CARE/EXPECTED OUTCOME

Patient will verbalize/demonstrate minimal discomfort or absence of pain AEB:

_____ Statements of pain relief and effectiveness of pain medications and/or other interventions
_____ Decreased need for pain medication
_____ Relaxed facial expression and body part
_____ Increase in voluntary movement, ambulation, and ADL
_____ Increased ability to concentrate
_____ Stable vital signs
_____ Statements or demonstrations of coping behaviors and/or factors which reduce or eliminate discomfort or pain
_____ Able to sleep/rest
_____ Increased appetite
_____ ______________________
_____ ______________________

STANDARDS OF PRACTICE/GUIDELINES FOR CARE

_____ Accept patient's level/tolerance of pain
_____ Assess pain characteristics to include location, intensity, duration, type, precipitating factors
_____ Provide the patient with prescribed medication as ordered
_____ Provide and teach alternative methods of pain relief based on individual needs and/or physician orders:
  _____ Positioning
  _____ Back rub
  _____ Massage
  _____ Application of heat
  _____ Application of cold
  _____ Diversion/distraction
  _____ Relaxation/imagery
  _____ Exercise/ambulation
  _____ Range of motion
  _____ Other:
  _____ Consults: ______________
  ____
_____ Teach patient and/or significant other pain management strategies:
  _____ Use of PCA
  _____ Medications
_____ Explain procedures to decrease/relieve anxiety
_____ Validate patient's understanding/coping
_____ Evaluate effectiveness of interventions and reintervene as necessary

From Southwest Texas Methodist Hospital, San Antonio, Texas.
ADL, Activities of daily living; ROM, range of motion; OOB, out of bed; PCA, patient-controlled analgesia; PRN, as needed; q, every.

right route, right analgesic), the nurse may identify the reason the patient is not getting adequate pain relief. Table 16–11 provides a nursing plan of care checklist. Administration of analgesics is simply one intervention in the nursing care of a patient in pain. Table 16–12 provides a method for problem solving when analgesic drugs do not work to provide effective pain relief. This includes the expected patient outcomes and guidelines for nursing care that are important for the nurse to utilize in managing the patient in pain.

BIBLIOGRAPHY

Acute Pain Management Guidelines Panel. (1992). *Acute pain management in adults: Operative procedures. Quick reference guide for clinicians* (AHCPR Publication No. 92-0019). Rockville, MD: Agency for Health Care Policy and Research, Public Health Service, U.S. Department of Health and Human Services.

Acute Pain Management Guidelines Panel. (1992). *Acute pain management: Operative and medical procedures and trauma. Clinical practice guidelines* (AHCPR Publication

TABLE 16-12

PROBLEM SOLVING WITH PAIN MEDICATION

When the analgesic medication prescribed for pain is not effective in relieving pain, the nurse should take the following steps to solve the problem:

1. Check the analgesic order.
   a. **Right dose:** Is the dose prescribed a recommended starting dose for analgesia, or is the dose prescribed less? If a range of medication is prescribed, has the maximum dose been administered? If the order states morphine 10–20 mg IM PRN for pain, and 10 mg morphine is ineffective for pain relief, has 20 mg been administered? *Solution:* Adjust the dose up as ordered until pain is relieved.
   b. **Right patient:** Is the patient experiencing side effects of the analgesic at the present dose? Can the patient tolerate the increase in dose with few side effects?
   c. **Right time:** What is the onset, peak, and duration of the analgesic? Is the analgesic administered around-the-clock based on the duration or properties of the drug? *Solution:* Evaluate pain intensity periodically to see if correct timing of drug is more effective in relieving pain.

If the patient's pain is still not relieved, the following steps should be taken:

2. Consider an alternative prescription.
   a. **Right patient:** What is the diagnosis or source of pain, and what analgesic is most effective for this type of pain? What are patient characteristics to consider (e.g., age, liver or renal problems, NPO status)?
   b. **Right route:** Which route is most appropriate for the patient condition, severity of pain, and medication prescribed (e.g., IV, IM, PO, or topical administration)?
   c. **Right analgesic:** Which analgesic is best for this type of pain? Which analgesic has proven effective for the patient in the past or in a similar condition?
   d. **Right dose:** What is the suggested starting dose for the analgesic? What is the equianalgesic dose to administer when switching from one analgesic to another?
   e. **Right time:** What is the time interval at which the analgesic should be administered or evaluated given its duration of action?
3. Collaborate with patient, physician, nurses and family.
   a. Collect information.
   b. Establish credibility with facts about the patient, analgesics, and written references (articles or drug guides).
   c. Anticipate questions.
   d. Be assertive and keep trying.
   e. Always use other nursing interventions in addition to the analgesic to relieve pain.

IM, Intramuscularly; PRN, as needed; NPO, nothing by mouth; IV, intravenously; PO, orally.

No. 92-0032). Rockville, MD: Agency for Health Care Policy and Research, Public Health Service, U.S. Department of Health and Human Services.

American Pain Society. (1992). *Principles of analgesic use in the treatment of acute pain and chronic cancer pain: A concise guide to medial practice* (3rd ed.). Skokie, IL: Author.

Bonica, J. (Ed.). (1990). *The management of pain* (Vols. I and II, 2nd ed.). Philadelphia: Lea & Febiger.

Ferrell, B. A. (1991). Pain management in elderly people. *Journal of the American Geriatric Society, 39,* 64–73.

Graffam, S. (1989). Pain in the elderly. In V. Burggraf & M. Stanley (Eds.), *Nursing the elderly: A care plan approach.* Philadelphia: J. B. Lippincott, pp. 356–368.

Lindley, C. M., Dalton, J. A., & Fields, S. M. (1990). Narcotic analgesics: Clinical pharmacology and therapeutics. *Cancer Nursing, 3*(1), 28–38.

McCaffery, M., & Beebe, A. (1989). *Pain: Clinical manual for nursing practice.* St. Louis: C. V. Mosby.

McGuire, L. (1990). Administering analgesics: Which drugs are right for your patient. *Nursing, 20*(4), 34–41.

Meinhart, N. T., & McCaffery, M. (1983). *Pain: A nursing approach to assessment and analysis.* Norwalk, CT: Appleton-Century-Crofts.

Puntillo, K. (Ed.). (1991). *Pain in the critically ill: Assessment and management.* Gaithersburg, MD: Aspen Publishers.

Titlebaum, H. (1988). Relaxation. In Zahourek, R. P. (Ed.), *Relaxation and imagery: Tools for therapeutic communication and intervention.* Philadelphia: W. B. Saunders, pp. 28–52.

Wall, P. D., & Melzack, R. (Eds.). (1989). *Textbook of pain* (2nd ed.). New York: Churchill Livingstone.

Watt-Watson, J., & Donovan, M. (1992). *Pain management: Nursing perspective.* St. Louis: Mosby Year Book.

Zahourek, R. P. (1988). *Relaxation and imagery: Tools for therapeutic communication and intervention.* Philadelphia: W. B. Saunders.

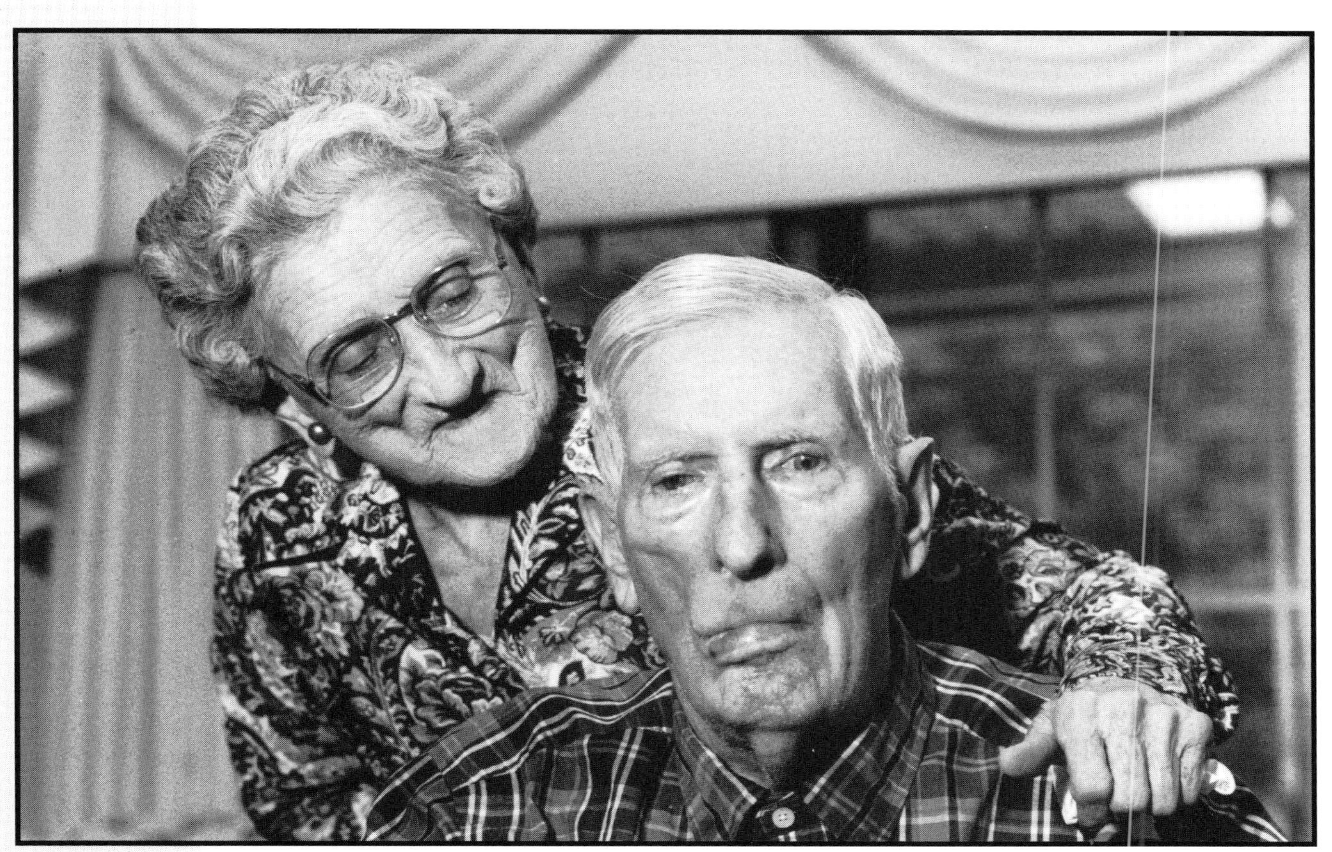

UNIT 4
Long-Term and Home Health Care

Edward P. Gruber

CHAPTER 17

Patient Care Settings

OBJECTIVES

1. Describe the principles of rehabilitation.
2. List the four levels of disability.
3. Discuss legislation passed to protect the rights of the disabled.
4. Identify the goals of rehabilitation.
5. Name the members of the rehabilitation team.
6. Compare the differences and similarities between home health nursing and community health nursing.
7. Describe the three levels of prevention.
8. Name the five criteria for Medicare home health nursing reimbursement.
9. Discuss the criteria for admission to hospice care.
10. List the four levels of modern nursing home care.
11. Discuss the effects of institutionalization on the elderly client.
12. Describe the principles of nursing home care.

GLOSSARY

DISABILITY Quantifiable loss of function, usually for the purpose of indicating a diminished capacity for work (see *handicap*)

HANDICAP Inability to perform one or more normal daily activities because of mental or physical disability (see *disability*)

IMPAIRMENT Physical or psychological disturbance in functioning

PRIMARY PREVENTION Steps taken to increase health of individual by strengthening body systems and preventing disease or injury

REHABILITATION Process of restoring individuals to best possible health and functioning following physical or mental impairment

SECONDARY PREVENTION Steps taken to find disease early and begin treatment as soon as possible

SKILLED OBSERVATION AND ASSESSMENT Used to determine adequacy of home environment, knowledge level of the patient and family regarding care procedures, side effects of treatment, and family's level of comfort in performing specific procedures

SKILLED PROCEDURES Certain nursing procedures, such as dressing changes, Foley catheter insertions, and venipuncture

TERTIARY PREVENTION Steps taken to prevent disease recurrence or complications

The acute phase of many illnesses is often followed by a prolonged chronic phase. This phase may run from days to years and usually involves the delivery of a number of health care services in a variety of settings, such as rehabilitation centers, nursing homes, outpatient facilities, group homes, and, increasingly, the patient's own home. Many people think only of elderly persons in nursing homes when they think of long-term care settings. Long-term care services, however, are required by people of all ages who struggle to return to a level of independent functioning. Thus, long-term care refers to a range of services that address the health, personal care, and social needs of all people who lack some capacity for self-care.

REHABILITATION

PRINCIPLES OF REHABILITATION

Rehabilitation Is a Process of Restoration

Rehabilitation is the process of restoring an individual to the best possible health and functioning following a physical or mental impairment. The type of assistance provided allows people to care for themselves. Inherent in this process is a commitment by the caregiver to provide the care and support that fosters the independence of the client.

Impairment Is a Disturbance in Functioning

Impairment refers to a disturbance in functioning that may be either physical or psychological. For example, a physical impairment may be the paralysis of an arm or leg as the result of a brain hemorrhage, whereas a mental impairment such as loss of memory may occur as a result of Alzheimer's disease. In either case there is a loss of function.

Disability Is a Quantifiable Loss of Function

The term *disability* generally refers to a quantifiable loss of function, usually for the purpose of indicating a diminished capacity for work. For example, individuals with an injured back may be classified as 50% disabled, meaning that they are incapable of doing 50% of their job. This type of quantifiable loss of function allows for specific reductions in work responsibility or may indicate how much compensation a worker may be entitled to.

Handicap Is an Inability to Perform Daily Activities

Handicap means that an individual is not able to perform one or more normal daily activities because of a mental or physical disability. For example, the person who experienced a brain hemorrhage may be handicapped in driving a car because of the paralysis.

It is important to remember that disability and handicap are not the same thing. A person can be moderately disabled but still manage to perform routine daily activities. People who were born without arms are often able to perform all essential activities of daily living (ADL) by using their feet and certain assistive devices. It can be said that, although these people are disabled, they are not handicapped. Impairments and their resulting disabilities may not be reversible, but handicaps can often be prevented or reduced with environmental modification and a community attitude that seeks to promote the abilities of the disabled.

LEVELS OF DISABILITY

A disability is often classified into levels to determine its degree of impact on an individual's quality of life and appropriate levels of compensation:

- Level I: Slight limitation in one or more ADL, usually able to work.
- Level II: Moderate limitation in one or more ADL, able to work but workplace may need modifications.
- Level III: Severe limitation in one or more ADL, unable to work.
- Level IV: Total disability characterized by near complete dependence on others for assistance with ADL, unable to work.

GOALS OF REHABILITATION

The goals of rehabilitation are to return the disabled individual to a maximum state of functioning and to prevent further disability.

Return of Function

The goal of return of function includes the restoration of as much function as possible in the traditional ADL, such as bathing, dressing, eating, toileting, and walking. Ideal functioning includes independence in the instrumental activities of daily living (IADL) as well, such as preparing meals, shopping, doing laundry, and using the telephone. The ultimate goal of rehabilitation is to live independently. Full independence implies a return to employment status.

Prevention of Further Disability

Rehabilitation also involves the prevention of further disability (secondary disability) that may potentially be caused by the patient's primary disability. Examples include prevention of problems in stroke patients such as pneumonia, decubitus ulcers, and limb contractures, which are often caused by lack of mobility. The nurse plays an important role in the prevention of secondary disability.

Rehabilitation is a long-term process requiring the commitment of both the patient and the family. The process is often difficult and marked by areas of progress followed by occasional relapses in functional ability. These relapses can be frustrating to everyone involved and require determination on the part of the family as well as patience and understanding by the nurse. The rehabilitation process can place additional burdens on family members when roles once fulfilled by the disabled family member are redistributed to other members. Attention is frequently focused on the disabled member, leaving other family members feeling neglected. Ongoing family problems may intensify during this time, making the rehabilitation process even more difficult.

It is important for the nurse caring for a disabled patient to be aware of the attitudes and behaviors of all family members. Often families can be assisted in adjusting to role changes that occur during the rehabilitation process. The more consistently patients and family are involved in the process, the more likely success will occur. Involvement in goal setting and a clear explanation of patient and family roles in daily rehabilitation activities help families to understand better the challenges of the process. This gives a sense of control and increases family strength.

LEGISLATION

Public attitudes toward people with disabilities play a significant role in the degree of handicap experienced by the disabled. Lack of knowledge about a disability often causes the public to react negatively to people who appear disabled. Individuals who are blind are sometimes treated as though they are deaf as well. People with conditions such as cerebral palsy that affect speech and muscle control are often treated as though they have decreased intelligence. Employers are reluctant to hire disabled workers, fearing an increase in insurance rates or negative reactions from their customers.

The federal government has passed laws over the years to protect the rights of the disabled. The first law passed to aid the rehabilitation of World War I servicemen was the Vocational Rehabilitation Act of 1920. This law provided job training for injured veterans. The Social Security Act of 1935 provided additional aid to states for both direct relief and vocational rehabilitation. It was the Rehabilitation Act of 1973, however, that provided a comprehensive approach to problems experienced by the disabled. The act not only expanded available resources for vocational training but defined services to be included in rehabilitation programs. It also began affirmative action programs to assist in the employment of the disabled and prohibited discrimination against the disabled in programs receiving federal funds. In 1990, the Americans With Disabilities Act was passed. This law extended the protection given to the disabled in the public sector by the Rehabilitation Act of 1973 to the private sector as well. It was designed to give the disabled full access to housing, employment, transportation, and communications. As a result of this law, any business endeavor designed to serve the public must ensure that its services are accessible to the disabled. In many cases, this involves the installation of wheelchair ramps, the construction of restrooms that can accommodate wheelchairs, and the provision for communication services for the hearing and speech impaired. Public transportation authorities must ensure that buses, train cars, and concession shops are all accessible to the disabled.

To date, there has been somewhat less than full implementation of this statute. Businesses with fewer than 25 employees are currently exempt from many of the law's provisions. By 1995, however, only businesses with fewer than 15 employees will be exempt. Full implementation of this law will go a long way toward improving the quality of life of many disabled people.

THE REHABILITATION TEAM

Nurses who care for disabled clients must consider the whole patient when planning interventions. Difficulties in physical functioning may affect many aspects of a person's life and require the coordinated services of a number of health care professionals in order for the individual to stay well and avoid complications or injuries.

The case of Mr. Thompson, who has had a recent stroke and resulting right-sided paralysis, provides a good example of the kinds of expertise and the number of services that may be required during rehabilitation.

> Mr. Thompson, age 72, suffered a left-sided brain hemorrhage 3 weeks ago. Because of this, he was unable to speak or use his right arm or leg. He was also incontinent of urine and exhibited some right-sided facial paralysis. After 5 days in the hospital, it was determined that Mr. Thompson's condition had stabilized, and he was transferred to a rehabilitation facility to continue the rehabilitation process. At this time, his speech had returned but was slurred and halting. He had minimal movement in his right arm and leg but was still unable to walk or feed himself. The incontinence of urine persisted, and he had several reddened areas on his right hip and coccyx. Mr. Thompson lives alone with his wife of 50 years, who also is in ill health. They have no family living in the state, and she is quite concerned about how she will care for him once he is sent home.

When trying to comprehend all that is involved in helping Mr. Thompson return to full functioning (if that is possible), it is helpful first to imagine a typical day in the Thompson household and to identify all the ADL and IADL competencies required to get through the day. Next, the types of people and services that may be necessary to prevent further injury and to increase functioning should be considered. At a minimum, the rehabilitation team will consist of the patient's wife, personal physician, rehabilitation physician, and rehabilitation nurse. Other likely members include the physical therapist, who assists the patient in all aspects of mobility from regaining strength and function in the extremities to the use of assistive devices such as crutches and walkers; the occupational therapist, who assists the patient with regaining fine motor skills necessary for dressing, eating, and grooming; the speech therapist, who assists the patient in regaining swallowing or speaking functions; and the social worker, who may assist with coordinating resources for placement in the home or a convalescent facility after discharge. Other members of the team may include a clinical nurse specialist in rehabilitation nursing, a psychologist, a recreational therapist, and a vocational counselor.

The nurse's concern at this time should be with becoming an effective member of the rehabilitation team. The successful resolution of rehabilitation problems often depends on the ability of health care workers to consider how the individual functions within the family and to work closely with other health professionals toward a common goal. If this goal is to be successful, good communication skills are essential. These entail clear, specific documentation of the patient's functional deficits and abilities and active participation in multidisciplinary conferences to resolve patient problems.

REHABILITATION FACILITIES

It has been said that good rehabilitation commences immediately after the injury and continues until the patient returns to maximum functioning. If this is true, the settings for rehabilitation activities can be many and varied. The most common are rehabilitation services within acute care hospitals and freestanding rehabilitation hospitals. Large hospitals frequently have rehabilitation teams that begin working with disabled individuals early in their hospital course and continue to offer services such as physical therapy and occupational therapy on an outpatient basis following discharge. Rehabilitation hospitals provide intensive, focused rehabilitation services for a period of time ranging from weeks to months.

Home health agencies also deliver rehabilitation services, often providing and coordinating the services of a large number of health care professionals (Fig. 17–1).

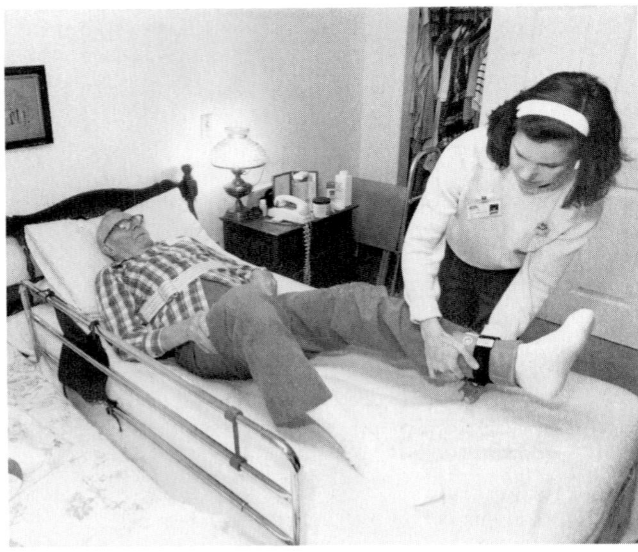

FIGURE 17–1
Home health agencies deliver the rehabilitation services of a variety of professionals. (Photograph by Stephen Matteson, Jr.)

Independent living centers also are important facilities for disabled individuals. These centers provide living space that promotes independent living for the disabled. Usually, several people live together in these settings with the help of a common caregiver. The advantage of independent living centers is that they provide sufficient support to allow the person to live outside of an institution at a relatively reasonable cost.

Other settings for delivering services to the handicapped exist where need is demonstrated and funding is available. These include, among others, burn centers and psychiatric rehabilitation centers.

APPROACHES TO REHABILITATION PATIENTS

Perhaps the most important concept in the successful rehabilitation of a disabled person is independence. This fact is sometimes forgotten when a caregiver sees the slow, agonizing attempts to move an arm or a leg. The tendency is to do for patients what is difficult for them to accomplish. There are times when patients should be helped to complete a task, especially when they become increasingly frustrated. However, caregivers who intervene too soon encourage dependence and delay rehabilitation. Rehabilitation patients should be cheerfully encouraged to do as much as possible for themselves. Praise for accomplishing a task should be given promptly, and caregivers should reflect continuing optimism about the patient's progress.

Health professionals frequently plan comprehensive programs of rehabilitation without much thought as to how the program will be implemented once the patient returns home. To be effective, the program should include involvement of the patient and family from the outset. Failure to involve the family in establishing goals and strategies often produces family dependence just as doing too many things for the patient produces individual dependence.

Rehabilitation nurses perform a number of roles all designed to assist the patient and family in returning to a high level of functioning. These roles include care planner, teacher, caregiver, counselor, coordinator, and advocate.

In the home setting, nurses can best assist patients and families by helping them adjust their activities to accommodate the disability. Even though families may have been taught care routines in a previous setting, routines must often be adapted to the new setting and prioritized differently. In this role, the nurse is an expert caregiver and teacher. Problem-solving sessions often identify ways in which care routines can be adapted to the realities of the home setting. Caregivers may not have thought through changes in sleeping arrangements, how they will transport the patient for follow-up office visits, or how to plan for periodic relief from their caregiver role. Nurses can help families anticipate these predictable stress points and plan realistically for how they will handle them.

Nurses should also be prepared to handle a wide range of patient and family emotions, ranging from extreme optimism to depression. At these times, families need a great deal of support and may need the assistance of outside community support systems. Local support groups can often be very effective in helping families respond appropriately to the stresses of a disabled family member. Professional organizations such as the Rehabilitation Nurses' Association can be an invaluable resource to nurses working in the rehabilitation field.

COMMUNITY AND HOME HEALTH NURSING

Community health nursing and home health nursing are specialized areas of nursing practice that are often thought of as being similar. This probably comes from defining community health nursing as anything that occurs outside of the hospital setting. These two practice areas, although sharing common historic roots, have significant differences.

COMMUNITY HEALTH NURSING

Community health nursing is the synthesis of public health concepts and nursing practice. In public health, the focus of attention is on improving the health of communities and aggregates (collections of people). The main goal of public health intervention is to protect and improve the health of populations at risk in the community and to prevent disease and disability. Community health nursing, therefore, is the application of the nursing process to communities or aggregates. Community health nurses work with individuals and groups to improve the health of the entire community.

The focus of community health nursing intervention is usually directed to the three levels of prevention: primary, secondary, and tertiary (Table 17–1).

PRIMARY PREVENTION. In primary prevention, the aim is to increase the health of the individual by strengthening body systems and preventing disease or injury. Exercise programs to increase strength and cardiovascular fitness are examples of health promotion. Campaigns in schools to prevent children from smoking and efforts to educate people to wear seat belts are examples of primary prevention.

SECONDARY PREVENTION. In secondary prevention, the assumption is that disease may have already occurred. The focus at this level is to find the disease early in its course and to begin treatment as soon as possible. Providing Papanicolaou smears and mammograms at reduced cost is an example of secondary prevention.

TERTIARY PREVENTION. Tertiary prevention is aimed at the prevention of disease recurrences or complications. The use of physical therapy to prevent contractures in a stroke patient and teaching a diabetic proper diet and foot care are examples of this third form of prevention.

Community Health Nursing Activity

The following example of community health nursing activity demonstrates several levels of prevention and typical community nursing roles in a long-term care setting.

> A community health nurse notices a rise in blood pressure, an increase in weight, and a general lack of fitness in members of a senior citizen high-rise in her district. Her assessment shows that there are no recreational facilities nearby, the meals served at the high-rise tend to be high in fat, and there seems to be a general lack of social activity at the facility. On the positive side, she notes that a residents' organization exists, although it has never been very active. By working with the residents' organization and a local church, the nurse initiates a group exercise program to improve the strength, cardiovascular fitness, and weight control of the elderly residents. By working with the management of the high-rise and the residents' association, the nurse gets the building manager to serve low-fat, low-cholesterol meals. The nurse also asks a local school of nursing to hold a monthly blood pressure and health education clinic for the residents.

In this example, the community health nurse not only gave direct service to individual clients but worked with three existing community groups to provide a number of services designed to increase the health of the senior citizen group. Community health nurses often work with many different individuals and groups to create or modify systems of care to improve the health of a defined group. This requires the nurse to assume a number of roles to accomplish care goals. The roles listed in the example include case finder, care manager, teacher, advocate, and coalition builder. Table 17–2 lists many of the roles assumed by the community health nurse. Most

TABLE 17-1
LEVELS OF PREVENTION

Primary Prevention
Health promotion: exercise, diet
Prevention: smoking cessation, seat belts

Secondary Prevention
Early diagnosis and treatment: Papanicolaou smears

Tertiary Prevention
Rehabilitation: physical therapy after cerebrovascular accident

TABLE 17-2
COMMUNITY HEALTH NURSING ROLES

Advocate	Group leader
Caregiver	Health planner
Care manager	Home visitor
Case finder	Occupational health nurse
Clinic nurse	Researcher
Coalition builder	School nurse
Counselor	Supervisor
Epidemiologist	Teacher

of these roles require at least a bachelor's degree in nursing to perform all aspects of the role.

HOME HEALTH NURSING

Home health nursing is the synthesis of direct nursing care and community health nursing. The main difference between home health nursing and traditional public health nursing is the increased focus on direct care to patients. The main difference between home health nursing and nursing in an institution is the increased emphasis on the family and the environment.

Home health nursing requires careful consideration of the family and its role in the care of the ill member. Although giving direct care to an individual is frequently a part of home health care, a more important nursing role is to teach the patient and family to care for themselves (Fig. 17–2). This important role is similar to that of the rehabilitation nurse, for whom the goal is the independent functioning of the patient and family.

The environment in which home health nursing is practiced is very different from that of the hospital. Homes often contain a fraction of the resources of the hospital. Small bedrooms, low beds, inadequate climate control, and lack of space are common conditions. Often families are overwhelmed by the task of caring for loved ones. They need instruction not only in the care of the patient but also in how to perform the care within the context of daily family activities in a home often poorly designed for the purpose.

Nurses must perform a complete assessment of the patient, the family, and the environment and use that information to modify care procedures accordingly. Concerns about dressing changes include not only wound care technique but also who will do it, where materials can be obtained, how to dispose of soiled dressings, and what should be done if something goes wrong.

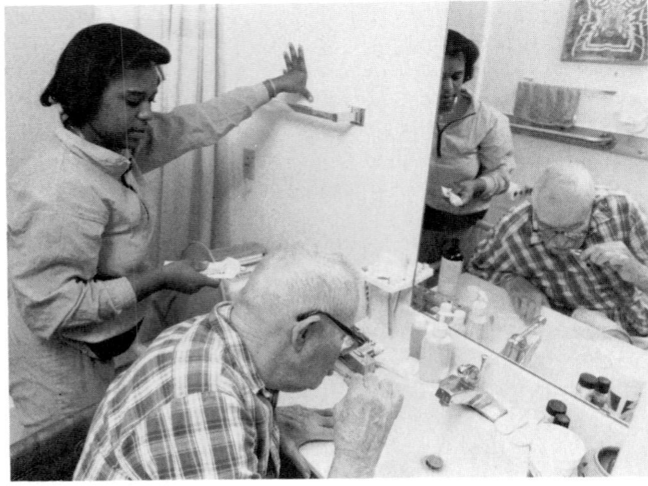

FIGURE 17-2
An important nursing role in home health care is to teach patients to care for themselves. (Photograph by Stephen Matteson, Jr.)

Home care nurses also need good clinical judgment skills. The frequency of visits varies widely. Visits can be made daily, several times a week, or monthly. The primary nurse is often the only health professional who sees the patient for several weeks. If, for example, a slight weight gain and edema in the ankles are missed in a patient with a history of congestive hearth failure, it may not be noticed for several days until more serious symptoms are present. Unlike the hospital setting, there is no "second shift" to follow up what was not done.

History of Home Health Nursing

Home health nursing has a long and distinguished history. St. Vincent de Paul organized the Daughters of Charity in 1617. Members often went from house to house bringing food, education, and health care to the sick in their homes. This was one of the first organized groups to speak of providing health education to the poor to help people help themselves.

In the mid-1800s, William Rathbone, a wealthy English businessman, was impressed with the skill of the nurses who cared for his dying mother at home. Convinced that visiting nurses could help the poor and ill of Liverpool, he organized the first district nursing organization. This experiment was so successful that, in 1859, he opened the first training school for visiting nurses. Because he was the first to employ the district nursing concept, he is often called the Father of the Visiting Nurses Association.

In the United States, Lillian Wald is considered to be the predecessor to modern public health nursing. She came from a wealthy family and studied nursing at New York Hospital in 1891. Her experiences teaching bedside nursing to women in the poor sections of New York City had a profound impact on her and led to the foundation of the Henry Street Settlement House in 1893. The facility was a place where the poor could come for care and was supported by funds from the wealthy. Lillian Wald believed that all people had the right to direct access to the services of a nurse. She also maintained that nurses should live in the area where their patients lived to gain insight into the complexity of health care problems and their probable causes. Many of Lillian Wald's beliefs about people and nursing are finding expression today in Nursing's Agenda for Health Care Reform, in which community-based services and access to care are key issues.

Types of Agencies

Historically, home health nursing in the United States has been delivered by many different types of agencies.

VOLUNTARY AGENCIES. Voluntary agencies were the first to deliver nursing care in the home. They were usually financed by wealthy philanthropists in the community, and their mission was to care for the sick poor. Today the Visiting Nurses Associations are the most common example of voluntary agencies. They are usually governed by a community board of directors that determines service delivery policies and assists with fund raising. Because board members are drawn from different areas and social strata within the community, services often reflect community needs. Funding for voluntary agencies usually comes from a variety of sources, including Medicare, Medicaid, United Way, private insurance, endowments, donations, and patients themselves.

Once the primary provider of home care services, visiting nurses associations have seen their share of the home care market dwindle with the growth of proprietary (for profit) agencies.

OFFICIAL AGENCIES. Official agencies are those supported by tax dollars and are authorized by law to deliver services to a defined area or community. Traditionally, state, regional, and local health departments have been assigned the responsibility of providing health promotion and disease prevention services as well as communicable disease investigation and environmental health protection. The nursing divisions of state, regional, and local health departments are usually tasked with delivering nursing services to populations at risk. In most states, this includes maternal and child services, sexually transmitted disease clinics, tuberculosis surveillance and treatment, and other health services as funds permit.

Thirty years ago, home health services were often delivered by local health departments as well as voluntary agencies. As the concept of public health became more defined, caring for the sick in the home was no longer seen as a public health role. Gradually, more and more health departments dropped home health services. By the 1980s, competition from proprietary and hospital home health agencies had reduced the number of official home health agencies to a handful.

PROPRIETARY AGENCIES. Proprietary agencies are organized to make a profit on their operation. They may or may not participate in Medicare, but most do. Proprietary agencies may be owned by individuals or corporate chains. Often their sources of revenue come from private insurance, private pay clients, Medicare, and Medicaid.

Changes in hospital funding in the early 1980s caused hospitals to discharge patients more quickly than ever before. For years hospitals were able to bill Medicare for their costs *after* they incurred them. Under this system there was little incentive to save money. In 1983, however, the system changed and hospitals were reimbursed *prospectively* for the amount of resources the average patient with a certain condition would be expected to use. This financing process grouped patients according to diagnoses that accounted for similar amounts of resources and was called *diagnosis-related groups*. Under the new system, hospitals were reimbursed a flat fee for a specified number of days. If the patient got better faster, the hospital made money. If the patient required a longer stay, the hospital lost money. This abrupt change in Medicare financing caused the early discharge of thousands of patients.

This practice contributed substantially to the growth of home health care. Much of this growth has been in the number of proprietary and hospital-based home health agencies. The increasing number of sick elderly and policy changes in how the Medicare home health benefit is administered have expanded the profitability of proprietary agencies.

HOSPITAL-BASED AGENCIES. Institution-based home health agencies also have increased in number since the 1980s. Hospitals that found that they were losing money under the prospective payment system saw the opportunity to recoup lost profits by opening home health agencies. These agencies are usually separate departments within the hospital, although they are typically governed by the hospital board of directors. The hospital-based agency usually gets most of its referrals from the hospital itself. Philosophy and policies are usually consistent with those of the parent institution.

Reimbursement Realities

Medicare, though not the sole source of home health care funding, is probably the most important. This fact makes home health nursing considerably different from nursing care in the hospital. Reimbursement by the Medicare program depends on documentation in the patient record that five basic criteria have been met: (1) care must be skilled; (2) care must be reasonable and necessary; (3) the patient must be homebound; (4) the physician must authorize a plan of care; and (5) care must be intermittent.

CARE MUST BE SKILLED. Medicare reimburses nursing care in the home provided that the care given is "skilled." This means that the care delivered must be of a type such that only a nurse trained in that care could be expected to do it. Just because the care is done by a nurse does not mean that it qualifies as being skilled. An example might be an injection of regular insulin. In most instances, simply injecting insulin is not considered skilled because most diabetics give their own insulin. Teaching the skill of drawing up the insulin and injecting it properly, however, is considered skilled because teaching is considered a skilled activity. Once the injection skill is learned, it is no longer skilled by the Medicare definition.

Nursing is one of three primary home health care services considered to be skilled. The others are physical therapy and speech therapy. Occupational therapy is sometimes considered skilled depending on the complexity of the patient's problems. Social work and home health aide services are not considered skilled in themselves but, rather, may be reimbursed only after the patient has qualified under one of the three primary services. These home care services are discussed in more detail later in this chapter.

Remember that the preceding definition and examples of what constitutes skilled care are interpretations of the Medicare law. Other nursing activities not listed above require the skill of a nurse but may not be recognized as skilled under Medicare. Medicare law does not prevent nurses from giving the care they judge necessary. It only defines what care is *reimbursable* under that law.

CARE MUST BE REASONABLE AND NECESSARY. To meet this criterion, objective clinical evidence clearly justifying the type and frequency of services is required. The nurse must provide clear documentation of functional losses and goals for care. Periodically, progress or lack of progress toward treatment goals must be documented in the record. Failure to do this not only jeopardizes patient care but often results in denial of the institution's claim for payment because the documentation did not prove that the care given was "reasonable and necessary." It is clear that in home care, inadequate charting has serious financial as well as legal and clinical consequences.

THE PATIENT MUST BE HOMEBOUND. This criterion does not mean that the patient must be bedridden. It does mean, however, that when the patient leaves the home, it requires considerable effort to do so. Medicare also requires that absences be infrequent and of short duration. According to Medicare regulations, if patients are well enough to leave home frequently, they are able to visit the doctor's office for treatment and, therefore, are not in need of home care.

THE PHYSICIAN MUST AUTHORIZE A PLAN OF CARE. All home care treatment must be authorized by a physician. A plan of care must include pertinent diagnoses, mental status, types of services, supplies and equipment ordered, frequency of visits, prognosis, rehabilitation potential, functional limitations, nutritional requirements, medications, and treatments. This plan must also include safety measures to protect against injury and plans for discharge.

In practice, the initial referral usually includes the patient's name, address, and telephone number, the major diagnoses, and a list of medications and treatments—not unlike physician's orders in a hospital. On the first visit, the admitting nurse usually formulates the plan of care, adding all other required elements. This plan is sent to the physician for his or her review and signature. It should be remembered that care in the home is predominately *nursing* care, so it is not surprising that the nurse has a major role in developing the plan of care.

CARE MUST BE INTERMITTENT. The fifth criterion for Medicare reimbursement requires that the visits be intermittent in nature. This means that visits occur periodically and do not usually exceed 28 hours per week. Under normal circumstances, the patient is not seen daily. Situations exist, however, in which daily visits are justified. In these situations, there is usually the need for family members to be trained in daily procedure such as diabetic care or dressing changes. Under these circumstances, Medicare will reimburse daily visits for 2 or 3 weeks. These are considered special cases, and reimbursement depends on clear and accurate documentation of the need for daily visits. Otherwise, visiting frequency can range from three to four times per week to monthly. Visits may continue indefinitely as long as all five Medicare criteria are met.

Types of Home Health Services

As mentioned earlier, there are three primary skilled services in home health care: (1) nursing, (2) physical therapy, and (3) speech therapy. Secondary services include occupational therapy (may be primary under certain conditions), social work services, and home health aide services.

SKILLED NURSING. According to Medicare regulations, skilled nursing includes skilled observation and assessment, teaching, and performing skilled procedures.

Skilled Observation and Assessment. The phrase skilled observation and assessment implies that the skills of a nurse are required to observe patient progress, to assess the importance of signs and symptoms, and to decide on a course of action. For example, good assessment and judgment skills are required to detect the signs and symptoms of congestive heart failure early enough to prevent rehospitalization.

Teaching. Teaching is considered a skilled task because to do it effectively the nurse must identify the patient's and family's current level of knowledge, discern their learning style, relay information at a pace they can handle, and evaluate the results of the teaching.

Performing Skilled Procedures. Performing skilled procedures includes changing dressings, inserting Foley catheters, and performing venipuncture. However, after certain nursing procedures are taught to the family, they are no longer "skilled" and cannot be reimbursed under Medicare. Also, procedures such as enemas, administration of eye drops, changing of unsterile dressings, and cleansing of small wounds are usually not considered skilled because they can be performed safely by most people.

PHYSICAL THERAPY. Home health patients recovering from health problems affecting mobility, such as hip fractures and strokes, are common candidates for physical therapy. Physical therapists assess for assistive devices such as walkers, wheelchairs, and grab bars and work with patients and their families on therapies to regain strength and mobility. To receive these services in the home, it is necessary for the patient to be homebound.

SPEECH THERAPY. Speech therapists work with patients who have speech or swallowing disorders. A common indication for speech therapy is the stroke patient who is aphasic. As with all home health services, to receive speech therapy in the home that is reimbursed by Medicare, it is necessary to meet all of the five Medicare criteria.

OCCUPATIONAL THERAPY. Patients who have conditions impairing movement of the upper extremities are prime occupational therapy candidates. People with arthritis or strokes may benefit from assistive devices for dressing and other daily household activities. Occupational therapists also provide muscle re-education, splinting, and improved control of fine motor movement. Timely occupational therapy interventions can help the patient become more safe and independent in the home setting.

SOCIAL WORK SERVICES. Social workers can provide valuable assistance to families trying to manage chronic illness in the home. Typically, social workers work with families to identify problems in the management of their illness in the home and recommend referrals to community resources. They may also provide information about financial assistance and help families with applications for community services such as Meals on Wheels and respite care.

HOME HEALTH AIDE. The home health aide is a valuable member of the home care team. Home health aides provide personal care for the patient in the home, such as bathing, ambulating, transferring, skin care, and oral hygiene. They may also take and record vital signs and do other basic, nonskilled tasks. Incidental homemaking such as making the bed and picking up the sick room are also common home health aide tasks. General house cleaning, shopping, and laundry are inappropriate tasks for home health aides. Patients qualify for home health aide services if they already have one of the three primary skilled services.

HOMEMAKERS. Homemakers are usually provided by families or state and local assistance programs. Their duties include common household chores such as cooking, light housekeeping, laundry, shopping, and picking up medications.

ENTEROSTOMAL THERAPISTS. Enterostomal therapists are common in many larger home health agencies. They are specialists in the care of all types of wounds, such as decubitus ulcers, surgical wounds, and ostomies. They provide care to patients and consultation to nurses on how to manage wounds. They also have extensive knowledge of skin care products and ostomy appliances.

OTHER HOME HEALTH SERVICES. Sometimes dietitians, nurse practitioners, and psychologists deliver services in the home.

Specialty Home Care

Prospective payment systems and the use of diagnosis-related groups have provided a stimulus for the development of specialty care in the home, especially for patients with terminal, pediatric, or psychiatric diseases. In addition, insurance companies, faced with rising costs of intravenous and ventilator therapies in the hospital setting, have recognized the potential cost savings of delivering these therapies in the home. In the last few years, the number of high-technology cases in the home has increased dramatically. The most common of these have been patients requiring intravenous therapy and ventilator-dependent patients.

INTRAVENOUS THERAPY. Rising hospital costs and the development of a number of reliable intravenous pumps have stimulated the growth of intravenous therapy in the home (see Fig. 17–1). The most common intravenous therapies used in the home are hydration, antibiotics, pain control, hyperalimentation, and chemotherapy. Treatments are administered through either peripheral or central lines. The use of a heparin lock and butterfly needle is most common. Peripherally inserted central catheter (PICC) lines provide a longer access time for therapy. However, many different types of lines may be used. Nurses should be familiar with the most commonly used devices in their area. Pain-control medications and chemotherapy drugs are almost always given through central lines such as the Hickman-Broviac catheter or the port-A-Cath.

High-technology therapies bring an increased level of complexity to the home environment. Their use may be more cost-effective than a hospital stay, but it also significantly increases the risk to the client and the liability of the home health agency. Agency policies and procedures should be current and specific enough to guide the nurse in managing the provision of intravenous therapy in the home. These policies serve to protect not only the agency and the patient but the nurse as well.

The successful provision of any high-technology therapy in the home depends on the commitment of everyone involved. Families must be capable of understanding what is required and have the time to participate fully in the patient's care. Nurses delivering this type of care must be thoroughly trained in the procedures and use of equipment involved in these therapies. Agencies must have appropriate staff to provide care at any time if needed, including days, evenings, nights, and weekends. The pharmacy or intravenous therapy company must provide high-quality products and support to both the nurse and the family. Finally, physicians must be closely involved and available to the nurse or family, or both, to respond to emergent problems.

The nurse's role in the delivery of high-technology care in the home includes skilled observation and assessment, the ability to perform skilled procedures, and teaching. Skilled observation and assessment in the delivery of intravenous therapy include determining the adequacy of the home environment and the knowledge level of the patient and family regarding care procedures. Also necessary is assessment of the intravenous site for signs of erythema, swelling, and redness, any side effects of the treatment, and the family's level of comfort with performing specific procedures.

Skilled procedures include changing site dressings and performing venipunctures. Because home care nurses are not instantly available 24 hours a day, some procedures must be taught to the family.

Teaching is arguably the most important skill in home care. Much of what is done in the home must be done by the patient and caregiver. Good patient teaching begins in the hospital setting, but most often newly arrived home care patients need considerable teaching to manage their care at home. When high-technology therapies are involved, teaching is doubly important.

Families often have difficulty understanding broad, high-technology concepts and are easily intimidated by technology when answers to their questions are not readily available. Skilled nurses understand this problem and ensure that their teaching is thorough and addresses precisely what the family needs to know to care successfully for their loved one at home. To do this, the nurse must identify the exact nature of the problem. A family member's difficulty in performing a heparin flush may arise from a lack of knowledge of the procedure, a fear of needles, an inability to read the markings on the syringe, or a denial of the disease process. Identifying the specific learning need is critical to successful patient teaching. In teaching high-technology care, it is especially important to keep instructions as simple and specific as possible. Each step in the procedure should be written and reviewed with the patient. The skill should be demonstrated several times, asking the family caregiver to cue the nurse for each step. After this is done a few times, the caregiver should perform a return demonstration of the skill.

Family caregivers must understand exactly what should be done in an emergency. Any questions about the family's ability to manage their portion of the care should be immediately referred to the home care nurse responsible for establishing the care plan and managing the case.

VENTILATOR THERAPY. Ventilator-dependent patients are increasingly being cared for in the home setting. This type of care is complex and should be done only by nurses and caregivers specifically trained in the use of necessary equipment and procedures. Often the care of ventilator-dependent patients in the home is coordinated by the respiratory therapist. The home care nurse seeing the patient should be aware of policies and procedures followed by the respiratory therapy company, be familiar with respiratory therapy equipment, and be certified in cardiopulmonary resuscitation.

Initial assessment of the home environment includes all the factors important in other high-technology therapies with the addition of an assessment of the electrical and structural condition of the home. This is important to ensure proper functioning of the equipment and necessary backup systems. As with intravenous therapy, there must be committed family members or other caregivers available. In this case, the commitment is for around-the-clock observation. Physicians and respiratory therapists must be on call for any problems.

HOSPICE CARE. Hospice is a concept of caring that traces its origin to fifteenth-century Europe, where travelers were provided places of respite and comfort. Later, this concept was extended to the dying in both hospitals and home settings. Families and hospital personnel collaborated on providing palliative care to dying family members.

During the early part of the twentieth century, the dying experience in the United States gradually shifted from the home to hospitals. Instead of being surrounded by family and friends in familiar settings, the dying found themselves in unfamiliar settings and being largely cared for by strangers. The first hospice in America was established in Connecticut in 1974 and provided both home care and inpatient care. Today, many more freestanding and hospital-based hospices all over the country deliver around-the-clock services to the dying.

Hospice services may be delivered in the home, acute care hospital, or extended care facility. Requirements for admission to hospice care include the following:

- A diagnosis of a terminal illness
- A prognosis of less than 6 months
- Informed consent by the patient to elect hospice care
- A physician's order

The hospice philosophy of care contains several basic elements: quality of life, comprehensiveness, a team approach, utilization of volunteers, and Medicare benefit coverage.

Quality of Life. Hospice workers concentrate on providing the best quality of life rather than focusing on extending life. The hospice team is skilled in the ability to manage symptoms and control pain so that the terminally ill client can get the most out of his or her remaining days. Only assessments and interventions that relate to the control of pain or relief of symptoms are used. A new hospice nurse may find this concept disturbing. Nurses are usually trained to fight disease. Nursing interventions in acute care hospitals are typically directed at preserving life and halting the spread of disease. In hospice care, death is the expected outcome. Interventions are aimed at controlling uncomfortable physical symptoms and creating a climate in which the patient and family can enjoy whatever life is left. This may mean not performing routine vital signs or not insisting that the patient remain hydrated. In these cases, the family is in control, and nurses must learn to work closely with family caregivers on what approaches to use.

Comprehensive Care. Hospice care includes not only the physical aspects of care but the social, psychological, and spiritual aspects as well. All patients and family needs are considered. Care is also given on a 24-hour basis and is delivered by a wide variety of providers. This wide scope of service highlights the importance of continuity of care.

Team Approach. Hospice care is provided by nurses, doctors, social workers, ministers, therapists, and aides all working together on making the dying family member more comfortable. The hospice nurse is often the coordinator and planner for the team. The nurse makes the initial visit and establishes the plan of care, bringing in as many services as necessary. Team conferences are scheduled to evaluate the care and suggest new approaches.

Utilization of Volunteers. The hospice movement has always made use of volunteers to provide services such as visiting, shopping, and meal preparation. Volunteers may be from any walk of life and are a traditional and important part of the hospice philosophy.

Medicare Hospice Benefit. Hospice services are provided by the Medicare statute. Under law, hospice services are granted for a total of 210 days. If the patient elects hospice services, he or she must waive the traditional home care services. All the criteria for the home care benefit must be met except for the homebound requirement. In return, the client is eligible for the following services:

- Nursing, home health aide, social worker, and therapist visits as determined by the team
- Other services, including pastoral care, dietary counseling, and respite care
- Prescription drugs related to symptom management and pain control
- Durable medical equipment as required

Hospice care is a worthwhile alternative for the terminally ill that provides a more natural and humane approach to the dying process. The team method is used to meet a variety of physical, psychological, social, and spiritual problems encountered by the terminally ill and their families. A multidisciplinary team of professionals and volunteers contribute their collective efforts to provide a better quality of life for the dying and their families.

PEDIATRIC HOME CARE. Since the late 1980s, there has been a rise in the care of ill children in the home. This is largely due to advancements in technology that have enabled the medical community to save many newborns who otherwise would not have survived. These same technologic advancements have produced the equipment necessary to provide adequate care in the home environment. Small, compact pumps, ventilators, and monitors have enabled children with cancer, respiratory disease, and cerebral palsy to live more normal lives at home.

Pediatric home care provides a better quality of life for young patients, but it also contributes to strain and role overload on parents and other caregivers. More and more home health agencies are providing a wide array of pediatric services in the home. Many of these services are funded by Medicaid and state crippled children's services. Private insurance companies are showing a growing interest in funding pediatric home care because of the potential cost savings over hospital treatment.

MENTAL HEALTH HOME CARE. A new and growing area of home care is the delivery of mental health services in the home. Nurses in this role have advanced training in psychiatric disease; they provide medication monitoring and teaching and perform mental status examinations and suicide assessments. They often provide consultation to other home care nurses on mental health problems that arise in patients with nonpsychiatric problems.

Communication between Home Health Care Team Members

It is not possible to overemphasize the importance of the team concept in home health care. In many instances, quality home care is the result of the collaboration of several disciplines. These disciplines most often deliver their services in the home at different times. This means that if effective collaboration is to occur, interdisciplinary communication is a must. This communication is accomplished through clear, detailed documentation and case conferences.

DOCUMENTATION. In any interdisciplinary work, it is important to grasp the fact that the actions of one discipline often depend on the actions of another. A nursing assessment that discovers an unused walker in the corner of a room may prompt the physical therapist to recommend strengthening exercises and gait training. A social worker's attempts to find funding for a patients medications may reveal a fear of taking pain medications that can be addressed by the nurse. If these concerns are not communicated, however, they will not be addressed. Most quality of care problems in home health can be attributed to a failure to communicate patient care problems. Most of the time, the failure lies with either incomplete documentation or failure to keep the nursing case manager informed.

As mentioned earlier, reimbursement for home health nursing visits depends on clear documentation of homebound status, the skilled nature of the services, and the medical necessity of the services. Failure to do this often results in a denial of reimbursement by the Medicare fiscal intermediary. These denials have serious consequences for the home health agency and, when excessive, have resulted in agencies going out of business.

CASE CONFERENCES. Clear documentation of interdisciplinary case conferences can go a long way in preventing denials that are based on lack of medical necessity. These conferences often provide detailed information about the complexity of problems that justifies increased visit numbers.

Usually, a home health nurse must report to a case manager for each patient. This individual is usually responsible for admitting the patient, establishing the plan of care including visit frequencies, and coordinating the efforts of other disciplines. The case manager schedules periodic, formal case conferences in which all disciplines attend and work together to solve clinical problems. The details of these conferences are recorded in the patient record.

In addition to these regularly scheduled conferences, it is important to keep the case manager informed of any changes in the response of the patient or family to the plan of care as they happen. Changes in vital signs, weight, and wound parameters are important physiologic indications for a call to the case manager. A change in the home environment such as an absence of family caregivers, deterioration in sanitation, or signs of patient neglect or abuse would also prompt a call to the case manager.

Communication by the case manager also is important. Field nurses have the right to expect clear and current information regarding recent changes in physician's orders, current laboratory information, and availability of documentation by other nurses and disciplines. High-quality patient care cannot be accomplished without meticulous communication from all disciplines involved in the care of the patient.

NURSING HOME CARE

Nursing home care dates back to at least the turn of the century, when the ill and elderly with no families to care for them were housed in publicly funded homes or boarding homes. The care provided was largely custodial and included housing, food, and personal care. These homes were not licensed, and standards were few. Quality depended on the good graces of those providing the care. Later, nursing home care became tied to the medical care system, and the nursing home increasingly became a place for patients needing skilled nursing and social services.

It may be a surprise to many that only 5% of elderly live in institutions. Many live with extended families or by themselves. Unfortunately, a large number of elderly living alone are poor and exist in inadequate housing, often without adequate heat, ventilation, food, or telephones. Eventually, problems with mobility and mental functioning force many elderly into nursing homes.

RISKS FOR INSTITUTIONALIZATION

Government statistics indicate that only 1% of people aged 65 to 74 reside in nursing homes. This figure rises to 6% for ages 75 to 84 and 20% for those 85 and over. The main reason for institutionalization, however, is not simply age. The best indicator of who will need nursing home placement is ADL dependency. Only about 12% of those with one or two ADL limitations live in nursing homes, whereas 50% of elderly with five or six ADL limitations reside there. These statistics highlight the fact that if home care services were available to assist elderly in meeting more ADL needs, costly institutionalization could be delayed.

Other factors bearing on who requires nursing home placement include such things as financial resources, whether the person lives alone or with family, presence of mental illness, type of disease process, and degree of social support.

LEVELS OF CARE

Modern nursing home care consists of four levels: (1) domiciliary care, (2) sheltered housing, (3) intermediate care, and (4) skilled care. Often one type of facility will offer more than one level of care (usually skilled and intermediate); however, in most states, institutions must have approval for whatever levels of care they plan to provide.

Domiciliary Care

Facilities providing basic room, board, and supervision are sometimes called domiciliary care facilities. In this arrangement, 24-hour care is not provided. Residents usually come and go as they please.

Sheltered Housing

Similar to domiciliary care facilities, sheltered housing settings contain some modification to provide care for the frail elderly and usually include community dining facilities. Twenty-four hour care, however, is not provided.

Intermediate Care

Intermediate care facilities provide custodial care at a level usually associated with nursing homes. Patients at this level often need assistance with two to three ADL (Fig. 17–3). Facilities offering this level of care must have personnel available 24 hours a day. They are not considered by the government to be medical facilities and thus receive no reimbursement under Medicare. Many do, however, receive the bulk of their financing under Medicaid. Federal regulations require a registered nurse to serve as director of nursing and a licensed nurse to be on duty at least 8 hours a day.

Skilled Care

Skilled nursing facilities must have skilled health professionals present around the clock. The care of patients

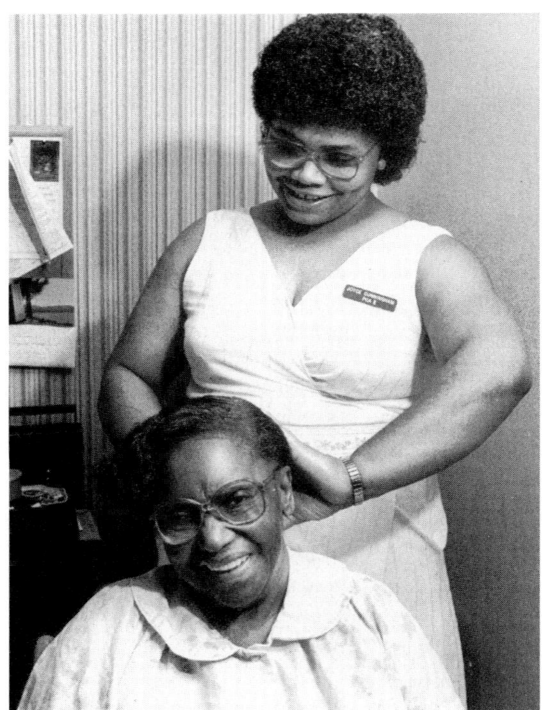

FIGURE 17-3

Patients in intermediate care facilities often need assistance with activities of daily living. (From Matteson, M. A., & McConnell, E. S. [1988]. *Gerontological nursing* [p. 650]. Philadelphia: W. B. Saunders. Photograph by Stephen Matteson, Jr.)

in skilled nursing facilities must be supervised by a physician and requires the services of a registered nurse, physical therapist, or speech pathologist.

IMPACT OF RELOCATION

The decision to place a relative in a nursing home is never easy. In the best of circumstances, families and health professionals are aware that such a decision is pending. In ideal cases, families seek help from extended family members and professionals in making the decision for nursing home placement, and funding has been set aside for the purpose. In reality, however, the situation is usually somewhat different. Often a crisis situation precipitates the decision. A sole caregiver may become ill, leaving the care of the disabled elder to the hands of extended family members who may be either unable or unwilling to continue care. Frequently, family members feel guilty for considering nursing home care. Few know very much about modern nursing homes and have not investigated potential placement sites.

In this situation, home health nurses, social workers, and other health professionals must work closely with the family to diffuse the crisis situation and provide realistic options from which the family may choose. This is a time when families need the utmost support and acceptance. Simply clarifying the situation, affirming the family's previous caring and concern, and pointing out realistic options will often return a family to effective functioning.

If nursing home placement is the only logical choice, the patient and family must be prepared for the relocation. Research has shown that the more prepared the patient, the better the adjustment to nursing home living. This includes providing as much choice as possible for the elderly family member. If possible, choices of facility, room location, types of personal belongings, and room decor are helpful, as are tours of the facility prior to entering. It is also helpful if professional staff check on the new patient frequently during the first few weeks. Questions should be encouraged. It is also helpful to introduce patients to other residents with like interests.

EFFECTS OF INSTITUTIONALIZATION

The effects of institutionalization are predictable and must be considered in helping the new nursing home patient adjust to the surroundings. Frequently observed effects are depersonalization, indignity, redefinition of "normal," regression, and social withdrawal.

Depersonalization

Depersonalization plays a major part in institutional life. Caregivers often know little of a patient's life history and therefore treat individual patients in light of their diagnosis or dysfunctional behavior patterns. The story about Herman and Kristina (see box) illustrates this point.

CASE STUDY

I don't think I truly understood what depersonalization was until I met Herman. Herman and his wife Kristina lived alone in a small house in a northwestern city. Herman was 62 years old and had Alzheimer's disease. I met them while working as a home health nurse. I was asked to look into respite services to help relieve Kristina of the strain of caring for Herman. I remember my first impression of Herman formed after reading his chart and talking to the staff nurse about his care problems. He was starting to neglect his personal appearance and was becoming a safety hazard in the home. The staff nurse said he often put soup on the stove for lunch, then went out into the garden to tend his flowers, forgetting about the soup. This and other images of his functioning created in me a picture of an incompetent and helpless old man.

Over a period of weeks, Kristina shared many stories with me about who this man was, what he cared about, how they met, and her deep devotion to her husband of 35 years. Gradually, I was able to see the distorted image I held. In his youth, Herman was an Olympic gold medal skier from Austria who came to this country as a young man. He held several jobs as a ski instructor and repaired ski equipment until he met and married Kristina and moved to the northwestern United States to become owner and manager of a small ski resort. He was tall and muscular with an easy smile and a kind word for everyone. He was admired by many in the community for his skill as a skier and his friendliness. He was a good father and family man who was known as "the rock" because all his family and friends relied on him for advice and assistance.

Over a period of 5 years, Herman became more and more forgetful, less talkative, and often preoccupied with household tasks that he would start but not complete. He also failed to recognize many of his close friends and, at times, would wander off downtown without knowing why or where he was going. Throughout this, Kristina remained fiercely devoted to Herman, though the strain of the caregiver role was beginning to affect her health. "He cared for us for so many years. Now it is my turn to care for him."

I was surprised at how different was my previous view of Herman. I saw him as dependent, helpless, and a burden to his small and frail wife—a view created by my observations of his behavior and what I knew of the Alzheimer's disease process, and a view that changed radically once I knew more about Herman. I doubt I will ever again minimize the importance of learning about the whole patient.

One way to help see the nursing home resident as a whole person with past relationships, accomplishments, and interests is to ask family members to bring in photographs. The photographs may have been taken on significant occasions, such as graduation or wedding days, or may be simple family pictures that depict the older person's place in the family or community. The photographs can be mounted on poster board or placed on a bulletin board in the resident's room. This effort helps caregivers to see more than a frail, weak older person and can open up conversation that encourages reminiscing, which is a very therapeutic means of dealing with one's past life and preparing for death.

Indignity

Indignity is another effect of institutionalization. Routine activities such as toileting and obtaining food and drink must be requested. At times, the prompt fulfillment of the request depends on the relationship between the patient and the caregiver. Nursing home residents may be exposed unnecessarily, especially when caregivers enter rooms without knocking. Nurses should think to themselves, "How would I want to be treated if I were weak and frail and could not do the things that I can do for myself now?"

Redefinition of "Normal"

Behaviors that were considered normal at home may be labeled as abnormal or unacceptable in an institution. Watching television at 3:00 A.M., loud singing, or sexual activity may not be permitted, depending on institutional rules. Although consideration of others is important, it is also important to give nursing home residents some flexibility and some measure of control in their daily lives.

Regression

Over a period of time, a resident's physical, mental, and social abilities may be lost because of disuse. If people are left in bed a greater part of the day, it soon becomes impossible for them to walk. If visits from friends and relatives are few, the skill of conversation also may be lost. It is important to encourage independence and social interaction as much as possible.

Social Withdrawal

If a resident never leaves the nursing home, or if family visits are few and include little discussion of the outside world, the institution can become a barrier, cutting off interest and participation in the outside world. If this is allowed to continue, life in the nursing home becomes, for many patients, their entire world. They tend to withdraw into the boundaries of their own room.

PRINCIPLES OF NURSING HOME CARE

Nursing home care has been called custodial care. This term invokes passive images such as maintenance, warehousing, or waiting to die. Some people have called nursing homes "heaven's waiting rooms." Abuses by some nursing homes in the 1970s are at least partly responsible for these negative stereotypes of nursing home care. Nursing homes, however, have changed substantially since the 1970s. Although some nursing homes continue to give care of questionable quality, many excellent facilities exist.

Modern nursing homes care for patients with a wide array of medical and surgical problems. In many communities, the nursing home has become a convalescent hospital for elderly patients with recent surgical procedures such as fractured hip repairs. These acute cases often strain already insufficient resources.

Not all patients are admitted for permanent stays in the nursing home. Many are admitted for short stays that may be prompted by care demands that temporarily overwhelm the family. Illness of a family caregiver can also result in a nursing home admission. When the home situation is stabilized, these patients often return home. Increasingly, those admitted for long stays are elderly and suffer from mental health problems. In these cases, the family has exhausted most of their physical, emotional, and financial resources and home care is no longer feasible.

When the patient is admitted to a nursing home, the care delivered is based on three principles: (1) promotion of independence, (2) maintenance of function, and (3) maintenance of autonomy.

Promotion of Independence

Successful relocation to a nursing home depends in part on the ability of patients to do things for themselves and the involvement of families to keep the elderly family member in contact with the outside world. It may be tempting for institutional caregivers to feed a patient rather than to take the time to encourage residents to feed themselves. When the workday is a never-ending series of tasks, doing things quickly often takes priority over promoting independence. Professional personnel should watch for this type of behavior and try to restructure assignments of nonprofessional personnel to reward the promotion of independence. This can be accomplished by setting specific goals for each patient that encourage independent functioning. The nurse then explains to the nonprofessional staff members how their efforts can contribute to the goal. Involvement of staff in this way often produces results.

Maintenance of Function

Often the circumstance that prevents an elderly person from staying at home is a loss of function. Health professionals who are disease oriented often concentrate on the disease process at the expense of a functional assessment. An incontinent patient may be incorrectly perceived as having a complication of the aging process. The behavior that stems from this type of thought process is usually one of maintenance, leading to efforts to prevent skin breakdown by frequent clothes and linen changes. A more thorough assessment begins with the determination of possible causes for the incontinence. A functional assessment asks what factors might be responsible for the incontinence. Mobility of the elder may be the root cause. Questions to ask include, Is the patient normally mobile? If so, is there a light in the room allowing him or her to find his way to the bathroom? Are the siderails normally up or down? Viewing this problem as a functional problem may lead to simple solutions such as placing a light in the room at night or a urinal next to the bed. Interventions, whenever possible, should be focused on restoring and preserving function.

Maintenance of Autonomy

Most people value control over their lives. Successful relocation to a nursing home depends on the preservation of as much autonomy as possible. Research shows that elders who are allowed to participate in picking a nursing home adjust better than those who have no choice in the matter.

It is also important to allow as much flexibility as possible in establishing a routine for the new nursing home resident. Choices in activities, such as when to have a bath or how late to watch television, go a long way in preserving the autonomy and self-esteem of the elderly resident. As much as possible, the resident should be allowed to assist in establishing care goals. Frequency and duration of exercise and numbers of pounds of weight to be lost are all areas for potential resident autonomy. Mutually established goals are more likely to be achieved than those selected for the resident.

Families also have a role in maintaining autonomy in the elderly member. Autonomy depends on knowing one's place in the world and what roles one still holds in the family structure. Families who relate to their elder members by reinforcing their importance in the family and keeping them up to date on family happenings and decisions reinforce one very important idea: the elder remains a valued family member who simply resides at another address.

BIBLIOGRAPHY

Anderson, C., & Hughes, E. (1933). Implementing modular nursing in a long term care facility. *Journal of Nursing Administration, 23*(6), 29–35.

Bernstein, L. (1992). Functional facts: A public health approach to functional assessment. *Caring, 9*(12), 32–38.

Clemen-Stone, S., Eigsti, D., & McGuire, S. (1991). *Comprehensive family and community health nursing* (3rd ed.). New York: McGraw-Hill.

Dittmar, S. (1989). *Rehabilitation nursing: Process and application.* St. Louis: C. V. Mosby.

Eng, M. (1993). The hospice interdisciplinary team: A synergisitic approach to the care of dying patients and their families. *Holistic Nursing Practice, 7*(4), 49–56.

Fraley, A. (1992). *Nursing and the disabled: Across the lifespan.* Boston: Jones & Bartlett.

Gale, B., & Steffl, B. (1992). The long-term care dilemma: What nurses need to know about medicare. *Nursing & Health Care, 13*(1), 34–41.

Humphrey, C., & Milone-Nuzzo, P. (1991). *Home care nursing: An orientation to practice.* East Norwalk, CT: Appleton & Lange.

Martinson, I., & Widmar, A. (1989). *Home health care nursing.* Philadelphia: W. B. Saunders.

Rice, R. (1992). *Home health nursing practice: Concepts and application.* St. Louis: Mosby Year Book.

Stanhope, M., & Lancaster, J. (1992). *Community health nursing: Process and practice for promoting health* (3rd ed.). St. Louis: C. V. Mosby.

Stephany, T. (1993). In praise of the hospice team. *Home Healthcare Nurse, 11*(3), 66.

Van Auken, E. (1991). Crisis intervention: Elders awaiting placement in an acute care facility. *Journal of Gerontological Nursing, 17*(11), 30–33.

Weight, B. (1993). Behavior diagnosis by a multidisciplinary team. *Geriatric Nursing, 14*(1), 30–35.

KEY CONCEPTS

1. Care of chronically ill patients usually involves the delivery of a number of health care services in a variety of settings such as rehabilitation centers, nursing homes, outpatient facilities, group homes, and, increasingly, the patient's own home.
2. Long-term care refers to a range of services that address the health, personal care, and social needs of all people who lack some capacity for self-care.
3. Rehabilitation is the process of restoring an individual to the best possible health and functioning following a physical or mental impairment and to prevent further disability.
4. Caring for disabled clients requires coordinated services of a number of health care professionals to help clients stay well and avoid complications or injuries.
5. As an effective member of a multidisciplinary rehabilitation team, the nurse is a care planner, teacher, caregiver, counselor, coordinator, and advocate.
6. Health care workers must consider how a disabled individual functions within the family, and the patient and family should be involved from the outset in determining the plan of care.
7. Community health nurses work with individuals and groups to protect and improve the health of populations at risk in the community and to prevent disease and disability.
8. The focus of community health nursing intervention is usually directed to the three levels of prevention: primary, secondary, and tertiary.
9. The aim of primary prevention is to increase the health of an individual by strengthening body systems and preventing disease or injury.

10. The focus of secondary prevention is to find a disease early in its course and to begin treatment as soon as possible.
11. The aim of tertiary prevention is to prevent disease recurrences or complications.
12. Home health nursing is the synthesis of community health nursing and direct patient care.
13. A major nursing function in home health care is teaching the patient and family to care for themselves to promote independent functioning.
14. Medicare is a major source of home health care funding.
15. To receive Medicare reimbursement, five basic criteria must be met: (1) care must be skilled; (2) care must be reasonable and necessary; (3) the patient must be homebound; (4) the physician must authorize a plan of care; and (5) care must be intermittent.
16. Specialty home care services include high-technology interventions (intravenous therapy and ventilator therapy), hospice services, pediatric care, and mental health care.
17. Government statistics indicate that only 1% of people aged 65 to 74, 6% of people aged 75 to 84, and 20% of people aged 85 and over reside in nursing homes.
18. Dependence in activities of daily living is the best indicator of who will need nursing home placement.
19. Modern nursing home care consists of four levels: (1) domiciliary care, (2) sheltered housing, (3) intermediate care, and (4) skilled care.
20. Care delivered in a nursing home is derived from three principles: (1) promotion of independence, (2) maintenance of function, and (3) maintenance of autonomy.

Mary Ann Matteson

CHAPTER 18

Falls

OBJECTIVES

1. Define falls.
2. List the incidence of falls.
3. Describe predisposing factors related to falls.
4. Discuss the relationship among restraint use and falls, types of restraints, and regulations for restraint use.
5. Demonstrate knowledge of fall-prevention techniques.
6. Describe nursing interventions to be used when a fall occurs.

GLOSSARY

CHEMICAL RESTRAINTS Psychotropic medications given to subdue agitated or confused patients

EXTRINSIC FACTORS Factors in the environment that can cause falls

FALL Circumstance in which one unintentionally falls to the ground or hits an object such as a chair or stair

INTRINSIC FACTORS Factors related to the internal functioning of an individual, such as the aging process or physical illness

OMNIBUS RECONCILIATION ACT (OBRA) Law enacted in 1987 to protect patients in nursing homes

PHYSICAL RESTRAINT Anything that restricts movement

If one were to ask a group of people whether or not they had fallen in the last 6 months, the chances are that many would say, "Yes!" The chances are even better that those who had fallen, particularly the young and healthy ones, had not sustained a significant injury. Although falls do not necessarily result in serious physical injuries or death, many older people who have fallen become less confident in their ability to function independently. Because they fear falling, they tend to restrict their physical and social activities, become more dependent, and have an increased need for long-term care. In addition, nurses tend to restrict older persons' activity for fear that ill or frail people who have been weakened from sickness, hospitalization, or aging may fall and injure themselves.

DEFINITION OF FALLS

Definitions of falls vary from "unexpected displacement" to "an unintentional change in position" to "inadvertent events in which the subject comes to rest unintentionally on the ground." A useful definition that seems more descriptive of an actual fall is "a circumstance in which one unintentionally falls to the ground or hits an object such as a chair or stair."

INCIDENCE AND RISK FACTORS

Although falls and fall-related injuries occur at every age, the greater severity of injuries in old age combined with longer recovery periods makes a fall a particularly serious threat to the health and functioning of older people. One in three persons aged 65 or older falls in a given year. There appears to be a steady increase in the number of falls among those aged 75 and older. Older women residing in community and long-term care facilities also appear to be at higher risk of falling than older men. However, it has been found that older men seem to be more likely to fall in a hospital setting.

The risk of injury from falls is highest in people over age 65, and falls are the most frequent cause of accidental injury and death among the elderly. The elderly constitute only 11% of the total U.S. population; however, they account for 72% of total deaths due to falls. The rate of death from falls increases from 5 in 100,000 between ages 45 and 64 to 200 in 100,000 for people older than 85.

The U.S. Public Health Service has estimated that two thirds of the deaths due to falls are preventable. Potentially avoidable environmental factors are the cause of 40 to 50% of fatal falls. In addition, they estimate that adequate medical evaluation and treatment for underlying medical conditions could probably prevent most of the remaining 50 to 60% of fatal falls.

The elderly are at particular risk for accidents because of changes brought about by aging, greater potential for injury, and poorer clinical outcomes. Falls occur because of two major factors: (1) *intrinsic factors*, or factors related to the functioning of the individual such as the aging process or physical illness, and (2) *extrinsic factors*, or environmental factors. Intrinsic factors enhance the possibility of falling, whereas extrinsic factors enhance the opportunity to fall.

Intrinsic factors related to falls include age-related sensory changes such as in vision and hearing; age-related changes in posture and gait; confusion or depression; lack of exercise leading to weakness and decline in physical vigor; multiple medications related to the increased incidence of chronic illness in the elderly; diseases affecting the central nervous system that may affect balance by causing dizziness and gait disorders; and overestimation of abilities.

Extrinsic factors may differ according to setting. For example, potential hazards in the home environment include low-lying and poorly visible tables, trailing electrical wires, pets, steep and unlit stairs, loose carpeting, unsafe walking aids, and inconvenient bathroom or kitchen arrangements. Falls occurring in the institutional setting as a result of excessive environmental demand are often related to changes in position, such as transferring to and from a bed or chair, toileting procedures, and unstable and defective equipment (nonfunctioning brake locks on wheelchairs, wet or excessively waxed floors, and improper placement of food trays in the hallway). Falls often occur during periods of high activity when the staff is busy. In addition, falls may result from imposed immobility. Patients may be confined to a bed or chair or be physically restrained, resulting in weakness or problems with balance.

In about 65 to 75% of all reported falls, no injuries occur. Contusions, cuts, or lacerations occur in about 25 to 30% of all reported falls, and deep tissue damage or concussion occurs in about 5%. Fractures result in about 1 to 4% of all reported falls.

People who are at greatest risk for injury are those with the following:

- A history of previous falls
- Osteoporosis (especially white women over age 75)
- Post stroke with hemiparesis (weakness or paralysis of one side of the body) or sensory impairment (vision or hearing deficits)
- Anticoagulation therapy
- Parkinson's disease
- Diabetes with peripheral neuropathies (decreased circulation and feeling in the lower extremities) and poor healing
- Falls associated with loss of consciousness or on a hard surface

RESTRAINTS

Restraints are frequently used as a preventive measure against falls. Restraints restrict individuals' movement and are classified as either physical or chemical. Physical restraints consist of vest, waist, wrist, or ankle ties. Wrist and ankle restraints may be made of soft material or leather. Anything that restricts movement, such as geriatric chairs or siderails, is considered a physical restraint. If patients are able to apply or release a safety device themselves, it is not considered a restraint. Chemical restraints are chiefly psychotropic medications that are given to subdue patients who are agitated or confused.

PHYSICAL RESTRAINTS

Older patients are more likely to be physically restrained than younger patients, probably because of their greater likelihood of falling and confusion. The most common reasons given for using "protective" restraints with elderly patients in hospitals or nursing homes are protection of the patient, equipment, or others from harm; prevention of falls from bed or chair; and prevention of wandering. The most common precipitating incidents for the use of restraints involve attempts to get out of bed or resistance to treatment while confused or disoriented.

Restraints seldom eliminate the risk of injury, however, and may actually cause or worsen problems. Patients are often able to untie their restraints and wriggle out of them, resulting in falls from wheelchairs and beds. In addition, accidental strangulation can occur when some forms of physical restraint, particularly a restraint vest, are used.

Restraints may have damaging psychological effects on older patients. Patients have described feelings of anger, discomfort, resistance, and fear in response to physical restraint. Other behaviors noted include loss of self-image, growing dependency, increased confusion and disorientation, regressive behavior, and withdrawal.

Because the use of physical restraint can be counterproductive to good nursing care, it is becoming evident that policies and alternatives for use must be developed. The Omnibus Reconciliation Act (OBRA) of 1987 was enacted to protect patients from unnecessary restraint in nursing homes. The law specifies that nursing home residents have the right to be free from any physical restraints imposed and any psychoactive drug administered for the purposes of discipline or convenience and not required to treat residents' medical symptoms. Additionally, a physician's order is required for restraint use, and the order must specify the duration and the circumstances under which the restraint may be used.

According to OBRA regulations, the only people who are considered restrainable are those who

- Have a history of severe falls or are at extremely high risk of taking a fall that is *life threatening*.
- Are neurologically, orthopedically, or muscularly impaired and need postural support for safety or comfort, or both.
- Experience any of a number of mental dysfunctions that may cause patients to be a *serious hazard* to themselves, objects, or others.
- Have medical symptoms that are life threatening, and a restraint is used *temporarily* to provide necessary treatment.

TABLE 18-1

ALTERNATIVES TO PHYSICAL RESTRAINT

1. Provide general comfort measures.
2. Position with pillows, recliners, etc.
3. Change forms of treatment contributing to restraint use; e.g., substitute oral feedings for intravenous or nasogastric tubes and remove catheters or external urinary drains.
4. Provide companionship and supervision by involving staff, family, friends, or volunteers, especially at night.
5. Use therapeutic touch when appropriate.
6. Distract attention with television, radio, tape player, or other activities.
7. Use a circular or semicircular room arrangement around nursing station for maximal visibility.
8. Redesign furniture; e.g., lower beds or put mattress on floor or remove wheels from furniture.
9. Manipulate environment to provide easy access to nurse and equipment; e.g., call bell accessible, bedside commode accessible, bedrails in down position, adequate lighting.
10. Provide a policy for a restraint-free environment that is supported by administration and staff.

Data from Strumpf, N. E., Evans, L. K., & Schwartz, D. (1991). Physical restraint of the elderly. In W. C. Chenitz, J. T. Stone, & S. A. Salisbury (Eds.), *Clinical gerontological nursing* (pp. 340–341). Philadelphia: W. B. Saunders.

If a physical restraint is used, the least restrictive device is best. For example, a mitt is preferable to a wrist restraint that limits movement. The patient should be checked frequently, at least every 15 to 30 minutes. A patient who is agitated or combative must be monitored continuously. The nurse should make sure that the patient's condition is good and that the restraint is used properly and is providing adequate protection and comfort for the patient. Physical restraints should be removed and released *every 2 hours* for 10 minutes to provide for range of motion, toileting, nourishment, and restorative activities such as physical therapy, ambulation, and cognitive activities.

Identification of patients at risk for restraint may reduce the use of these devices by concentrating surveillance and prevention on this group. Several alternatives to physical restraint include physical therapy, sitting and talking with patients for short periods of time, and asking staff to be responsible for wanderers in small blocks of time (Table 18–1). In addition, it has been suggested that after being apprised of the risks and benefits, patients or family members, or both, rather than nurses should decide whether or not to use physical restraint.

CHEMICAL RESTRAINTS

The same guidelines that apply to the use of physical restraints apply to chemical restraints. Psychoactive drugs should never be used for the purposes of discipline or convenience; rather, they should be used only for extreme potential for self-injury or injury to others. The administration of a psychoactive drug requires a written physician's order that specifies the duration and circumstance under which the medication is to be used.

Many psychoactive drugs are used, but the most commonly prescribed are haloperidol (Haldol), thioridazine (Mellaril), and lorazepam (Ativan). All have the potential for causing side effects and even untoward effects, such as greater confusion, agitation, and an increased number of falls.

PHARMACOLOGY CAPSULE

Psychotropic drugs, especially neuroleptics, antidepressants, and sedatives, commonly cause orthostatic hypotension, which may result in falls. Also, some antihypertensives and diuretics may produce orthostatic hypotension, leading to falls.

If at all possible, the use of psychoactive drugs should be avoided. The same alternatives to physical restraints apply to chemical restraints (see Table 18–1).

NURSING ASSESSMENT AND INTERVENTION

FALL PREVENTION

The most important intervention for falls is prevention. The best preventive method is to educate patients and caregivers about ways to prevent falls. Prevention is aimed toward minimizing both the intrinsic and the extrinsic factors causing falls and the potential for injury.

The first step in preventing falls and injury is to determine who is at greatest risk (see Care Plan: The Patient with a History of Falls). People who are at greatest risk for falls and injury are those who have fallen before and those who have multiple intrinsic risk factors. Table 18–2 lists intrinsic risk factors for falling and possible interventions.

TABLE 18-2

INTRINSIC RISK FACTORS FOR FALLING AND POSSIBLE INTERVENTIONS

RISK FACTORS	INTERVENTIONS
Impaired Vision	
Reduced visual acuity	Be sure individual wears glasses, if appropriate. Keep glasses clean. Encourage regular eye examinations.
Impaired dark adaptation	Maintain adequate lighting; reduce glare from shiny floors and allow time to adjust to light levels—e.g., from a dark room to outside. Use night light in bedroom and bathroom.
Impaired color perception	Use bright colors as markers, especially oranges, yellows, and reds.
Impaired Hearing	
Impacted cerumen (ear wax)	Remove ear wax.
Presbycusis	Speak slowly; use low voice; decrease background noise. Encourage use of hearing aid.
Balance and Gait Problems	
Musculoskeletal disorders	Encourage balance and gait training and muscle-strengthening exercises.
Balance disorders	Encourage balance exercises.
Peripheral neuropathy	Use correctly sized footwear with firm soles.
Foot Disorders	Trim toenails. Use appropriate footwear.
Cardiovascular Disease	
Postural hypotension	Encourage dorsiflexion exercises. Use pressure-graded stockings (TEDs). Elevate head of bed. Teach individual to get up from chair or bed slowly. Individual should avoid tipping head backward.
Neurologic Disease	
Stroke	Call bell in visual field and within reach of arm that has use. Anticipate needs for toileting, dressing, eating, and bathing. Assist with transfer. Provide passive range of motion exercises to improve functional ability.

Data from Chenitz, W. C., Kussman, H. L., & Stone, J. T. (1991). Preventing falls. In W. C. Chenitz, J. T. Stone, & S. A. Salisbury (Eds.), *Clinical gerontological nursing* (p. 316). Philadelphia: W. B. Saunders.

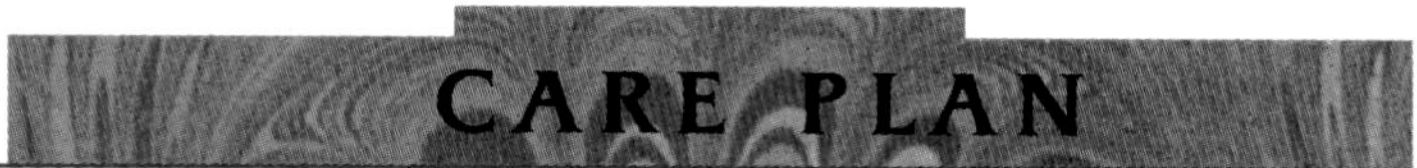

The Patient with a History of Falls

ASSESSMENT

Health History: A 75-year-old female was confined to a nursing home because of chronic health problems including emphysema, dementia, and a history of several falls at home. She has had several fractures as a result of these falls in the past. The nursing staff has used several methods to prevent her from falling, such as restraints, sedation, and sitters, but she is continuing to have problems. When she is restrained, the staff has noted that she becomes very agitated, and they are unable to calm her without administering sedatives.

Physical Examination: Vital signs: blood pressure, 144/76; pulse, 92; respiration, 22; temperature, 97°F. Height, 5′1″; weight, 98 lb. Her skin is warm and dry. Wheezing is noted on expiration. The patient is not oriented to time and place; she is oriented to person.

NURSING DIAGNOSIS	GOALS AND OUTCOME CRITERIA	INTERVENTIONS
Injury, high risk for related to confusion.	Patient will remain free from fall-related injury due to confusion.	Approach patient in a calm manner. Assess patient and environment for possible hazards and remove. Orient patient frequently to person, place, and time. Keep bed at lowest level, wheelchair brakes on. Have patient wear glasses or hearing aid when appropriate. Have someone familiar stay with patient to monitor as frequently as possible. Provide restraints only as a last resort to maintain safety, use type that are least restrictive, monitor frequently while on patient, remove at least every 2 hours for 10 minutes for range of motion, toileting, nourishment, and restorative activities. Get patient up and out of room as tolerated.

Fall-prevention strategies are carried out in the home and institutional environments. Fall-prevention guidelines for the home are listed in Table 18–3 and for institutional settings in Table 18–4.

In summary, basic strategies for reducing all types of falls include the following:

- Increase physical activities that enhance and maintain muscular strength, endurance, and flexibility.
- Increase regular, moderate physical exercise.
- Reduce visual impairments.
- Increase provider review of prescribed and over-the-counter medications.
- Increase provider screening and referral for alcohol and drug problems.
- Modify the environment to reduce or eliminate environmental factors that can cause falls or to minimize injury if a fall occurs.

WHEN A FALL OCCURS

Falls occur no matter what precautions may be taken. In some societies, such as in Great Britain, falls are indicators of greater activity and independence. Health care providers accept a high number of falls as an inevitable risk that is outweighed by the benefits of physical activity and rehabilitation.

When a fall occurs in a hospital or nursing home, nurses should assess the circumstances of the fall and any injuries sustained, and, of course, they should report the fall according to the protocol of the institution. It is important to note what the patient was doing at the time of the fall, the patient's mental and emotional status, and environmental factors that may have contributed to the fall. When the cause of the fall is determined, steps should be taken to remove or correct the cause. Ambulation should begin as soon after the fall as possible and at least several times a day in order to prevent hazards of bedrest and fear of falling again. It is tempting to apply restraints after a fall, but this procedure should be avoided at all costs.

Dealing with falls in the home requires the cooperation of the faller and family and possibly of neighbors. A plan of action for when a fall occurs should include information about getting up and seeking help.

There are several ways to get up after a fall in the home (Table 18–5). These techniques should be practiced by the potential faller to ensure confidence in managing the problem. If none of the methods is possi-

TABLE 18-3
FALL-PREVENTION GUIDELINES FOR THE HOME

Lights and Lighting

1. Eyes tire quickly in improper lighting. Illuminate reading material or the object worked on. Illuminate steps, entranceways, and rooms before entering. Use 70- or 100-watt bulbs, not 60-watt bulbs.
2. Avoid glaring light caused by highly polished floors or large expanses of uncovered glass. Use sunglasses to avoid the glare of highway driving, but use light tints or photoray lenses.
3. Allow more time to adjust to changes in light levels. When going from a dark to a light room or vice versa, allow a minute or two for the eyes to accommodate to the change in light before proceeding.
4. Dirty glasses or outgrown prescription lenses inhibit vision. Keep glasses clean. Have regular eye examinations to identify changes and to get new glasses when needed. If possible, do not use bifocals when walking because you cannot see the ground clearly.
5. Ability to see up, down, and sideways decreases with age. Observe the "lay of the land"; learn to look ahead at the ground to spot and avoid hazards such as cracks in the sidewalks. Use canes, walking sticks, and walkers that are prescribed.
6. At night, keep a nightlight on in your bedroom and bathroom. When getting out of bed at night, put the light on and wait a minute or two for the eyes to adjust before getting up. Have a telephone in the bedroom so you don't have to get out of bed to answer the phone. Before you go out in the evening or late afternoon, turn a light on for your return.

Activity

1. Get up from a chair slowly.
2. When getting out of bed, sit up, then wait a minute or two. Move to the side of the bed and wait another minute. Rest after you have sat for a few minutes.
3. If you are dizzy, sit down immediately. Sit on a step or a chair, or ease yourself to the sidewalk if you are outdoors.
4. Avoid tipping the head backward (extending the neck). Activities to avoid that extend the neck are washing windows, hanging clothes, and getting things from high shelves.
5. Use shelves at eye level. Avoid rapid turning of the head.
6. If weather is rainy and windy, avoid going out.
7. Use alcohol and tranquilizers with caution.
8. Exercise programs keep bodies limber. Consult your physician and then enroll in a senior exercise program.
9. Shoes and slippers should be flat and rubber-soled. Avoid clothing such as long robes and loose-fitting garments that may catch on furniture or door knobs.

Around the House

1. Avoid scatter rugs and small bathroom mats that can slide. Repair loose, torn, wrinkled, or worn carpet.
2. Avoid slick, high polish on floors.
3. Put things in easy reach, and avoid reaching to high shelves.
4. Use nonskid treads on stairs and nonskid mats in tub.
5. You may wish to install a grab rail in the bath, shower, and also by the toilet.
6. Install handrails on both sides of the stairs. Paint stair edge in bright contrasting color.
7. Remove door thresholds.
8. Remove low-lying objects, such as coffee tables and extension cords.
9. Wipe up spills immediately.
10. Watch for pets underfoot and scattered pet food.
11. Check for even, nonglare lighting in every room, with easily accessible light switches.
12. Avoid floor coverings with complex patterns.
13. Avoid clutter in living areas.
14. Select furniture that provides stability and support, such as chairs with arms.
15. Check walking aids routinely, such as rubber tips on canes and screws on walkers.

From Chenitz, W. C., Stone, J. T., & Salisbury, S. A. (Eds.). (1991). *Clinical gerontological nursing* (p. 310). Philadelphia: W. B. Saunders.

TABLE 18-4
FALL-PREVENTION TECHNIQUES USED IN HOSPITALS AND NURSING HOMES

Patient-Oriented

Exercise to strengthen muscles and prevent weakness
Electronic alarm devices, such as Bed-Check Ambularm

Medications

Note hypnotic or sedative drugs given at night, especially to elderly or postoperative patients
Note diuretics and laxatives given at night

Activities of Daily Living

Assist patient to void every 4 hrs
Check for proper slippers and footwear (nonskid footwear)
Keep patient's belongings close to bed
Provide rehabilitation training to improve functional ability

Environment-Oriented

Relocation of patient with high fall risk to room close to nurses' station or in hallway
Nurse call light system in place, e.g., pinned to pillow within reach
Teach patient and family about use of call light system, bed controls, bathroom facility, and movable furniture
Bed rails up when in bed
Bed in low position
Room light on, light bright and even
Place TV controls within reach
Clutter-free rooms and hallways
Carpet all hard surfaces
Nonskid wax
Clean up spills, including urine
Lock all equipment with wheels
Keep equipment on one side of hallway
Maintain equipment in good repair
Night lights in rooms
Safety (grab) bars in bathroom and hall
Higher-seated lounge chairs and toilets
Use bedside commodes
Remove wheels from bedside commodes
Safety posters in room to encourage asking for help

Patient Education

Hand out safety brochure to patient and family on admission
Teach patient about safety and equipment
Encourage patient to request help
Encourage use of bathroom and corridor handrails
Teach transfer from bed to chair

Nursing Assessment

Perform assessment at admission and throughout hospital stay
Assign safety risk
Frequent rounds/checks/observations

Other

Monitor falls, watch for trends, and conduct in-service when trend emerges
Have staff move slowly around ambulatory, unsteady patients

Adapted from Chenitz, W. C., Kussman, H. L., & Stone, J. T. (1991). Preventing falls. In W. C. Chenitz, J. T. Stone, & S. A. Salisbury (Eds.), *Clinical gerontological nursing* (pp. 309–328). Philadelphia: W. B. Saunders.

TABLE 18-5

METHODS FOR GETTING UP AFTER A FALL

The Roll

1. Roll onto the right side
2. Bend the right knee
3. Lever upward to the kneeling position by pressing down on the right forearm
4. Reach out with the left arm to a nearby chair or bed
5. With a twist of the trunk, pull into a sitting position
6. Sit on the chair or bed to recover

The Crawl

1. Roll to a prone position
2. Get up on all fours
3. Crawl to a sturdy couch, chair, or bed and place hands on it
4. Bring one foot forward, putting the foot flat on the floor
5. Pull up to a standing position
6. Sit on chair or bed to recover

The Shuffle

1. Pull to a sitting position on the floor
2. Shuffle on the buttocks to a nearby piece of furniture
3. Pull up onto the knees directly in front of the furniture
4. Stand up

The Stair Shuffle

1. Pull to a sitting position on the floor
2. Shuffle on the buttocks to the stairs
3. Gradually move up and backward to a stair height suitable for standing
4. Grab onto the handrail and pull up

Data from Chenitz, W. C., Kussman, H. L., & Stone, J. T. (1991). Preventing falls. In W. C. Chenitz, J. T. Stone, & S. A. Salisbury (Eds.), *Clinical gerontological nursing* (pp. 321–322). Philadelphia: W. B. Saunders.

ble, a person who is at risk for falling would be wise to have a call system to obtain help from others. Devices worn around the neck that can send signals to a control center are very effective and provide a feeling of well-being for the potential faller. Additionally, having a person or agency call every day can provide reassurance.

BIBLIOGRAPHY

Benner, Z., Longello, C. A., Lowery, K., Moyer, J., & Zapf, R. (1992). Falls, fractures and finances. *Nursing Management, 23*(9), 150.

Carbary, L. J. (1991). How to help prevent falls. *Journal of Practical Nursing, 41*(2), 13–14.

Chrisman, L., & Bonnel, W. B. (1992). Planning and implementing a housewide fall prevention program. *Journal of Nursing Staff Development, 8*(4), 187–188.

Christenson, M. A. (1990). Enhancing independence in the home setting. *Physical & Occupational Therapy in Geriatrics, 8*(3/4), 49–65.

Cohen, L., & Guin, P. (1991). Implementation of a patient fall prevention program. *Journal of Neuroscience Nursing, 23*(5), 315–319.

Craighead, J., Fletcher, R., & Maxwell, J. (1991). Seven steps for fall prevention. *Dimensions in Health Service, 68*(4), 25–26.

Croft, W., & Foraker, S. (1992). Working together to prevent falls. *RN, 55*(11), 17–18, 20.

Cutchins, C. H. (1991). Blueprint for restraint-free care. *American Journal of Nursing, 91*(7), 36–44.

Evans, L. K., & Strumpf, N. E. (1989). Tying down the elderly: A review of the literature on physical restraint. *Journal of the American Geriatrics Society, 37*, 65–74.

Evans, L. K., & Strumpf, N. E. (1990). About elder restraint. *Image: Journal of Nursing Scholarship, 22*, 124–128.

Foxwell, L. G. (1992). Minimizing risk in the nursing home. *Nursing Homes, 41*(1), 13–15.

Ginter, S. F., & Mion, L. C. (1992). Falls in the nursing home: Preventable or inevitable? *Journal of Gerontological Nursing, 18*(11), 43–48, 57–58.

Jech, A. O. (1992). Preventing falls in the elderly. *Geriatric Nursing, 13*(1), 43–44.

Jones, W. J., Simpson, J. A., & Pieroni, R. E. (1991). Preventing falls in hospitals: The roles of patient age and diagnostic status in predicting falls. *Hospital Topics, 69*(3), 30–33.

Kallmann, S. L., Denine-Flynn, M., & Blackburn, D. M. (1992). Comfort, safety, and independence: Restraint release and its challenges. *Geriatric Nursing, 13*(3), 142–148.

Mion, L. C., & Mercurio, A. T. (1992). Methods to reduce restraints: Process, outcomes, and future directions. *Journal of Gerontological Nursing, 18*(11), 5–11.

Morse, J. M., & McHutchion, E. (1991). Releasing restraints: Providing safe care for the elderly. *Research In Nursing & Health, 14*(3), 187–196.

Redford, J. B. (1991). Preventing falls in the elderly. *Hospital Medicine, 27*(2), 57–58, 60, 62.

Ross, J. E. R. (1991). Iatrogenesis in the elderly: Contributors to falls. *Journal of Gerontological Nursing, 17*(9), 19–23.

Schmid, N. A. (1990). Reducing patient falls: A research-based comprehensive fall prevention program. *Military Medicine, 155*(5), 202–207.

Strumpf, N. E., & Evans, L. (1988). Physical restraint of the hospitalized elderly: Perceptions of patients and nurses. *Nursing Research, 37*, 132–137.

Strumpf, N. E., Evans, L., & Schwartz, D. (1990). Restraint-free care: from dream to reality. *Geriatric Nursing, 11*, 122–124.

Walker, J. E., & Howland, J. (1991). Falls and fear of falling among elderly persons living in the community: Occupational therapy interventions. *American Journal of Occupational Therapy, 45*(2), 119–122.

White, D. (1991). Old age is not a reason to fall. *Nursing Standard, 6*(8), 20–21.

Wood, L., & Cunningham, G. (1992). Fall risk protocol and nursing care plan. *Geriatric Nursing, 13*(4), 205–206.

KEY CONCEPTS

1. The risk of injury from falls is highest in people over age 65, and falls are the most frequent cause of accidental injury and death among the elderly.
2. The U.S. Public Health Service estimates that two thirds of the deaths due to falls are preventable.
3. Falls occur in the elderly because of intrinsic factors, or factors related to the functioning of the individual such as the aging process or physical illness, and extrinsic factors, or environmental factors.
4. In an institutional setting, falls often occur during periods of high activity when the staff is busy.
5. In about 65 to 75% of all reported falls, no injuries occur; fractures result in about 1 to 4% of all reported falls.
6. People who are at greatest risk for falls and injury are those who have fallen before and those who have multiple intrinsic risk factors.
7. Older patients are more likely to be physically restrained than younger patients, probably because of their greater likelihood of falling and confusion.
8. Restraints seldom eliminate the risk of injury and may actually cause or worsen problems.
9. The Omnibus Reconciliation Act (OBRA) of 1987 was enacted to protect patients from unnecessary restraint in nursing homes.
10. A physician's order is required for restraint use, and the order must specify the duration and the circumstances under which the restraint may be used.
11. Several alternatives to physical restraint include physical therapy, sitting and talking with patients for short periods of time, and asking staff to be responsible for wanderers in small blocks of time.
12. The most important intervention for falls is prevention, and the first step in preventing falls and injury is to determine who is at greatest risk.
13. When a fall occurs in a hospital or nursing home, nurses should assess the circumstances of the fall and any injuries sustained and report the fall according to the protocol of the institution.
14. When the cause of a fall is determined, steps should be taken to remove or correct the cause.

Mary Ann Matteson

CHAPTER 19

Immobility

OBJECTIVES

1. Describe common problems associated with immobility.
2. Discuss the impact of exercise and positioning on preventing complications related to immobility.
3. Identify risk factors of pressure ulcers.
4. Describe the stages of pressure ulcers.
5. Provide methods of preventing and treating pressure ulcers.
6. Discuss the impact of immobility on respiratory status, nutrition, and elimination.

GLOSSARY

ACTIVE EXERCISE Exercise carried out by the patient

CONTRACTURE Shortening of the muscles and tendons

ERYTHEMA Redness of the skin; usually a sign that capillaries have become congested because of impaired blood flow

IMMOBILITY The inability to move; imposed restriction on entire body

ISOMETRIC EXERCISE Muscle contraction without movement used to maintain muscle tone

PASSIVE EXERCISE Exercise of the patient that is carried out by the therapist or nurse without the assistance of the patient

PRESSURE ULCER An open wound caused by pressure on a bony prominence; also called a "pressure sore"

RANGE-OF-MOTION EXERCISE Exercise in which each joint is moved in various directions to the farthest possible extreme

SHEARING FORCES Two contacting parts slide on each other

Immobility, or the inability to move, is an imposed restriction on the entire body. People become immobilized for various reasons, including hospitalization, chronic illness, pain, and the effects of aging. Therapeutic reasons for rest and immobility include (1) relief from pain and further injury of a part, as in a fractured bone; (2) reduction of the workload of the heart in a cardiac or renal condition; (3) promotion of healing and repair; and (4) reversal of the effects of gravity, as in abdominal hernias and prolapsed organs.

Immobility can have a profound impact on both the mind and the body. Psychological effects include depression, fear, anxiety, social withdrawal, apathy, loss of financial and personal independence, and lack of meaningful existence. Almost every body system can be affected by immobility, depending on the extent and time of immobilization. Physiologic effects of immobility are described in Table 19–1.

The elderly are particularly vulnerable to the effects of immobility, because often the same changes that occur with immobility also occur with aging. Examples of changes that accompany aging are loss of flexibility and strength and changes in posture and gait. In addition, the elderly tend to have one or more chronic illnesses that increase the likelihood of immobilization. Pain associated with chronic disease may also be a factor leading to immobility in the elderly.

The impact of immobilization on an individual is proportionally related to the duration, degree, and type of limitation on mobility. Immobility begins a vicious cycle that can lead to an ever-increasing loss of independence for patients. As they become less able to move, they become more dependent, and as they become more dependent, they are less able to care for themselves—which in turn leads to an increasing number of adverse effects from immobility.

Whatever the reason for resting a part or all of the body, some effort must be made to prevent as much as possible the adverse effects of immobility. It is the nurse's responsibility to prevent the vicious cycle of events from beginning by helping patients to maintain normal functioning of each bodily system as much and for as long as possible (see Care Plan: Preventing Falls). If preventive measures have not been taken and patients have begun to suffer the ill effects of immobility, a therapeutic program of interventions should be planned. The nurse needs to work cooperatively with the physician and other members of the health care team to develop a plan of care so that preventive and therapeutic measures are carried out according to patients' individual needs.

TABLE 19-1

CONSEQUENCES OF IMMOBILITY ON BODY SYSTEMS

BODY SYSTEM	CONSEQUENCES
Musculosketetal	Thickening of joint capsule; loss of smoothness of cartilage surface; decreased flexibility of connective tissues; changes similar to osteoarthritis—joint contractures, demineralization of bone, bone loss; atrophy and shortening of muscle; decrease in muscle strength; decreased muscle oxidative capacity; decline in aerobic capacity
Pulmonary	Arterial oxygen desaturation; increased hypostatic pooling; increased risk of atelectasis and infection
Cardiovascular	Decreased cardiac output and stroke volume; increased peripheral resistance; net loss of total body water and total blood volume
Integumentary	Pressure ulcers
Gastrointestinal	General weakening of muscles, causing altered colonic motility, constipation
Urinary	Increased nitrogen, phosphorus, total sulfur, sodium, potassium, and calcium excretion; renal insufficiency; decreased glomerular filtration rate; loss of ability to concentrate urine; lower creatinine tolerance
Metabolic	Decreased basal metabolic rate; increased storage of fat or carbohydrate; negative nitrogen and calcium metabolic balance due to decreased absorption of protein and calcium intake; decreased glucose tolerance; metabolic alkalosis
Sensory	Decreased sensory stimulation (kinesthetic, visual, auditory, tactile); decreased social interaction; changes in affect, cognition, and perception

Modified from Chenitz, W. C., Stone, J. T., & Salisbury, S. A. (1991). *Clinical gerontological nursing* (p. 234). Philadelphia: W. B. Saunders.

NURSING ASSESSMENT AND INTERVENTION

Before carrying out any interventions, nurses should assess the patients' needs and limitations. Physicians may write specific orders that address the problems associated with immobility, or it may be up to the nurse to carry out measures independently to prevent side effects of immobility. Nursing interventions include promoting exercise, and maintaining proper positioning, adequate respiratory status, adequate food and fluid intake, proper elimination, and skin integrity (see Case Study).

EXERCISE

Exercise is the best medicine for immobility. Exercise can be done anywhere. A well individual of any age can walk, participate in aerobic exercises, swim, engage in sports activities, garden, or do housework. Those who are ill or disabled can carry out modified exercise regardless of the acuity of their disease. For example, patients with fractures can tighten and relax muscles in an immobilized extremity; debilitated patients can gradually increase their range of movement, number of movements, or resistance against movement; and patients in pain can move slowly and smoothly while breathing deeply to ease pain and anxiety.

Exercises may be *active*—that is, carried out by the patient—or *passive*—that is, carried out by the thera-

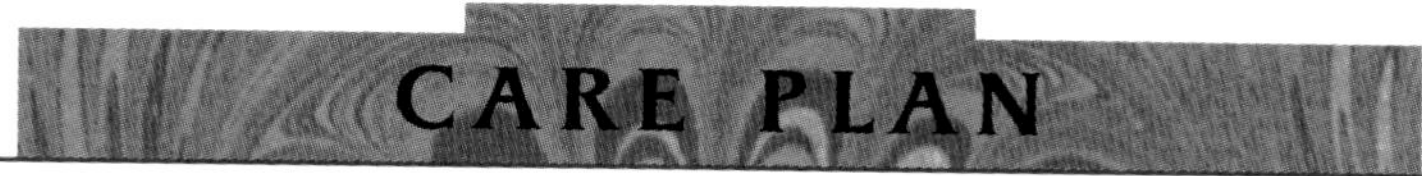

CARE PLAN

Preventing Falls

ASSESSMENT

Health History: An 84-year-old woman has been living in a nursing home for the past 2 years after falling and breaking a wrist, which interfered with her ability to shop, cook, and dress herself. While living in the nursing home, she continued to fall many times and preferred to keep to herself in her room. She stayed in her bed or in a chair most of the time and became so weak that she had to move about by means of a wheelchair. She also was incontinent of urine and mildly confused.

Physical Examination: Blood pressure, 130/78; pulse, 96; respiration, 26; temperature, 96.7°F. Height, 5′3″; weight 126 lb. Unable to hold urine long enough to void in the bathroom. Appears quiet, sad, and depressed. Does not interact with others. Daughter visits 2 to 3 times a week.

NURSING DIAGNOSIS	GOALS AND OUTCOME CRITERIA	INTERVENTIONS
Injury, high risk for, related to weakness.	The patient will remain free of injury due to weakness.	Walk with patient 3 times daily, gradually increasing distance as tolerated. Teach isometric exercises that can be done while lying and sitting to increase strength. Teach and assist in active range-of-motion exercises. Carry out exercises while assisting with daily care.
Incontinence, functional, related to immobility.	The patient will maintain continence as evidenced by lack of soiling of underwear and clothes.	Place on a schedule for toileting. Remind patient often to go to the bathroom to urinate.
Social isolation related to declining health.	The patient will demonstrate social interaction as evidenced by attendance at functions and visits and phone calls by significant others.	Encourage patient to attend activities that are offered. Have the patient go to the bathroom immediately before activity to decrease the possibility of accidents. Encourage family members and friendly visitors to make short, periodic visits. Visit with patient at least once per shift for at least 10 minutes. Encourage patient to listen to favorite radio and television shows.

pist or nurse without assistance from the patient. Active and passive exercises may be done lying down in bed, sitting in a chair, or standing upright. The exercises do not have to be done as a separate part of care. They can easily be carried out while giving care such as during a bed bath or other activities. Examples of bed and chair exercises are listed in Table 19–2.

Range-of-Motion Exercises

Range-of-motion exercises are effective in preventing disabilities of the musculoskeletal system as well as other systems. Each of the joints of the body has a range of motion—that is, extremes to which the joint may be moved in various directions. Muscular activity maintains that range of motion by allowing the joint to remain flexible and functional. When there is little or no motion of the joint, its structures change. The muscles lose their elasticity and become shorter. Normal tissue is replaced by fibrous tissue. This adaptive shortening of the muscles and tendons is called a *contracture*. A contracture can severely and permanently limit joint movement.

The purpose of range-of-motion exercises is to put each joint that is at risk for loss of motion through its full range of motion to the highest degree possible. The major motions are rotation, flexion, extension, abduction, and adduction. The exercises may be active or passive. Range-of-motion exercises should be initiated in

CASE STUDY

Mrs. Smith is an 84-year-old white woman who has resided in an intermediate care nursing home for the past 2 years. She was admitted to the nursing home because she had been living at home alone and had become unable to shop and cook for herself or to dress herself after sustaining a broken wrist from a fall. She was incontinent of urine and was mildly confused.

Mrs. Smith had previously been quite active in the community, but in the nursing home she remained confined to her room and was not interested in interacting with other people. Her daughter came to visit her approximately two to three times a week.

Because Mrs. Smith preferred to stay in bed or in a chair most of the time, the nurses and other members of the interdisciplinary team were concerned about the consequences of her immobility. She had fallen many times, usually on the way to the dining room to eat. It had gotten to the point where she stayed in a wheelchair most of the time because she had become too weak to walk.

The team held a case conference and identified problems associated with her immobility: (1) continued falling, (2) incontinence, and (3) isolation and perhaps depression. They formulated a plan to get her up and moving while at the same time avoiding falls. Every day the nurses walked with Mrs. Smith three times a day. The first week they walked around the bed. The second week they walked to the door and back. The third week they walked a few feet outside the door to her room. As the weeks progressed, Mrs. Smith was able to walk to the dining room at the end of the hall without falling. The nurses encouraged the in bed and in chair exercises to further build up her strength.

Eventually, Mrs. Smith was able to walk to the bathroom independently. The nurses worked with her to develop a regular schedule of toileting so that the number of "accidents" decreased. Because she was a little bit confused and disoriented, the nurses provided gentle reminders for her to go to the bathroom. After a meal, they would guide her back to her room to use the bathroom. Other times they would stop by her room, look in, and suggest that she go to the bathroom.

With all of the increased activity, Mrs. Smith became more outgoing and involved in activities. She sat with the same group at meals and developed friendships with others around her. The nurses found that taking small steps with a walking program can have many benefits for a person of any age in almost any condition.

TABLE 19-2
SAMPLE EXERCISES

IN BED EXERCISES	IN CHAIR EXERCISES
• Deep breathing (slow inhalation and full exhalation)	• Deep breathing
• Neck rolls (neck forward flex, backward extend, lateral flex, rotate)	• Head rolls (neck forward flex, backward extend, lateral flex, rotate)
• Knee to chest (on back or side, bring one knee to chest, wrap arms around hold and breathe, straighten leg slowly)	• Knee to chest
• Pelvic tilts (on back, knees bent, feet flat, tuck in tummy, relax)	• Head to knees
• Bridging (on back, feet flat on bed, raise hips, lower slowly)	• Shoulder rolls (forward and back)
• Head raising in prone and supine	• Weight shifts (hip to hip)
• Unilateral leg lifts	• Hands on head, elbows out-and-in, lateral trunk flex-extension, trunk rotation)
• Foot dorsiflexion	• Leg lifts
• Rolling	• Ankle rotation and dorsiflexion
• Prone lying	• Ankle on knee (external hip rotation, put ankle on opposite knee and lower the bent leg)
• Arms straight over head of bed in supine	• Push through legs as to stand, lean forward, weight bear
• Arms out to sides, palms up, in supine	
• Hands behind head, elbows bent	
• Hands at lower back	

From Giduz, B. H., Snow, T. L., Wildman, D. L., & McConnell, E. S. (1986). *Geriatric first aid kit* (p. 5). Chapel Hill, NC: Program on Aging, University of North Carolina.

immobile patients immediately on admission to the hospital to prevent contractures.

Isometric Exercises

Isometric exercises are performed to maintain muscle tone without moving the joint. In these exercises, the muscle is contracted and held in that position for several seconds. The muscle is then relaxed for a few seconds and contracted again. As noted earlier, this type of exercise is especially helpful in maintaining muscle strength after a fracture.

POSITIONING

Proper positioning in a bed or chair is extremely important for preventing many of the side effects of immobility. The position of the patient should be changed at least every 2 hours to prevent undue pressure on the skin while maintaining joints in their functional positions so that they are not abnormally flexed or extended.

Position maintenance for patients lying in bed can be accomplished by using a foot board that keeps the feet at right angles to the legs so that foot drop is avoided, by splinting limbs so that they are kept straight, by using a bed board to prevent curvature of the spine, and by placing a firm splint in the hands to keep the fingers from drawing up into a tight fist. The patient also should not be positioned with pillow and mattress supports that cause the knees and hips to remain flexed. It is helpful to picture persons standing and try to achieve that position while they are lying down.

SKIN INTEGRITY

When positioning, it is important to keep people off of pressure points on the skin that tend to break down and form *pressure ulcers*, the preferred term of the National Pressure Ulcer Advisory Panel for what are commonly called "bed sores." Pressure ulcers are localized areas of tissue necrosis that tend to develop when soft tissue is compressed between a bony prominence and an external surface for a prolonged period. They are found over bony prominences such as the elbows, hips, shoulders, and sacrum (Fig. 19–1). The most frequent sites of skin breakdown are the sacrum (35%), ischial tuberosities (16%), heels (11%), trochanters (7%), ankles (3%), and scapulae (2%).

Pressure ulcers have been called pressure sores because they result from pressure against the blood vessels that supply the affected area of the skin. Another term that was previously used is *decubitus ulcer*. The word *decubitus* means "lying down," and an ulcer is a lesion produced by the sloughing of necrotic, inflammatory tissue (Fig. 19–2). Thus, a decubitus ulcer is an open wound that is associated with lying in bed; however, skin breakdown can develop in patients who are in a sitting position for a long period of time as a result of the pressure against the blood vessels. Again, the preferred term is *pressure ulcer*.

Development of Pressure Ulcers

An area of *erythema* (redness) is the beginning of a pressure ulcer and is a sign that capillaries in the area have become congested because of impaired blood flow.

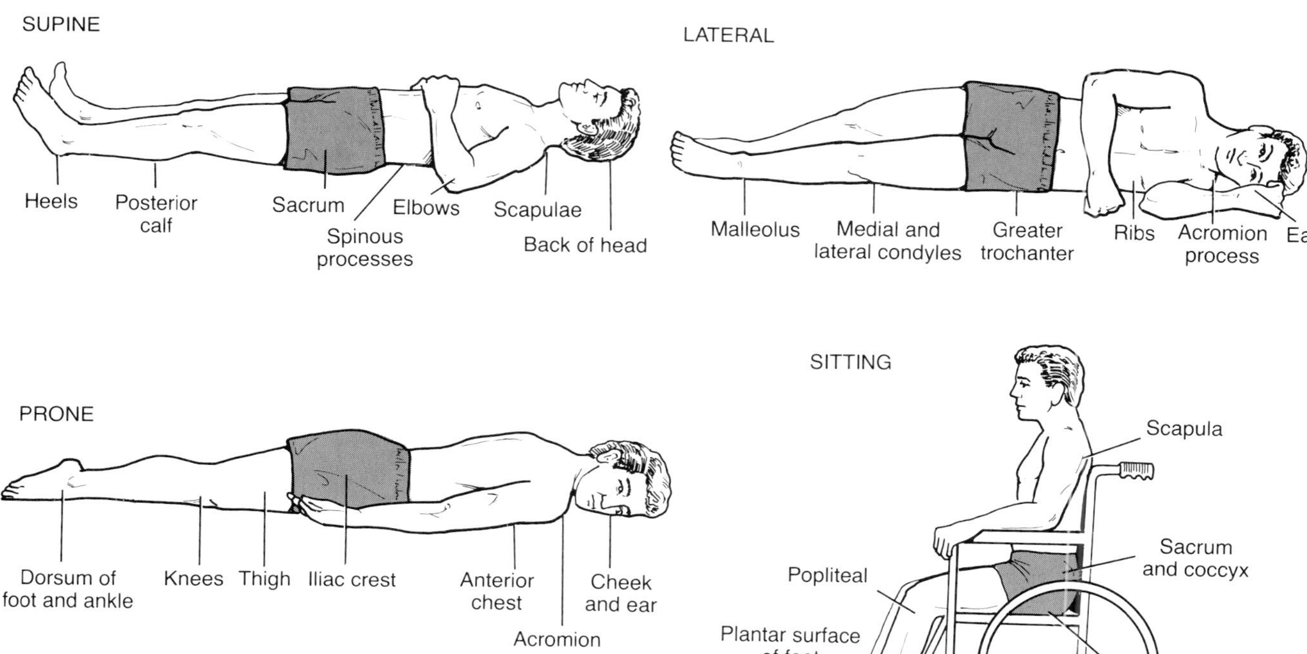

FIGURE 19-1
Possible locations of pressure ulcers.

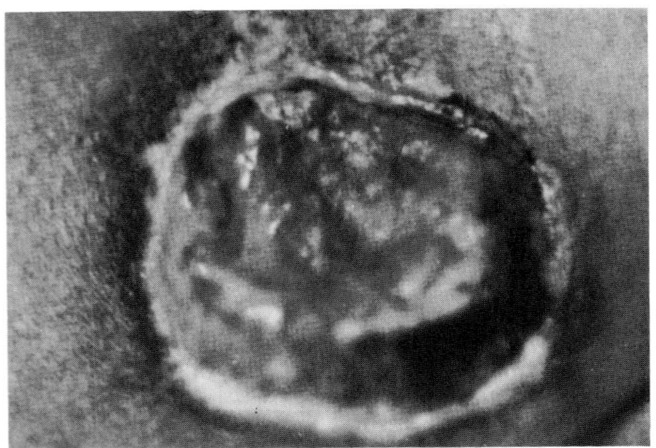

FIGURE 19-2

Stage IV pressure ulcer, with full thickness of all soft tissue. (From Bolander, V. [1994]. *Sorensen and Luckmann's basic nursing* [3rd ed., p. 1346]. Philadelphia: W. B. Saunders.)

The reddened area can occur within an hour or two in a person with healthy skin and adequate circulation. It is even more likely to develop and to progress rapidly to an ulcerated stage in persons who are malnourished, obese, aged, or suffering from circulatory disease.

Factors in addition to immobility that contribute to the development of pressure ulcers are shearing forces, the presence of chemical irritants such as urine, and sedation. *Shearing forces* exert a downward and forward pressure on tissues underlying the skin. Shearing action occurs when a patient slumps down while sitting in bed or in a chair.

Pressure ulcers are expensive to treat, result in longer hospital stays, increase the likelihood of nursing home placement, and increase mortality. Therefore, it is important to prevent their development whenever possible, keeping in mind that *nursing care is a major factor in pressure ulcer prevention.*

Prevention of Pressure Ulcers

The first step in prevention is to assess patients who are at risk for the development of pressure ulcers. The Norton scale is a useful instrument for identifying those at risk (Fig. 19–3). The scores for all five categories are added. If the score is greater than 14, there is little risk of pressure ulcer development. If the score is less than 14, there is significant risk for pressure ulcer development. Any patient with a score under 14 needs a formal pressure ulcer prevention program started as soon as the risk is noted.

A pressure ulcer prevention protocol consists of the following:

1. Turn at least every 2 hours (or change position if wheelchair bound).
2. Keep bed linens dry, smooth, and free of wrinkles. Keep skin and clothing clean and dry.
3. Avoid friction when moving patients in bed to prevent damage to the uppermost layers of the skin.
4. Use a special mattress or bed designed to reduce pressure such as an egg crate foam (minimum 2 inches thick), static air, alternating air, gel, or water mattress (Fig. 19–4).
5. Apply sheepskin to prevent shearing forces, especially around the heels.
6. Take measures that enhance patient mobility, such as trapeze bars.
7. Instruct patient and family about risk factors and strategies for preventing pressure ulcers.

Remember that the best preventive measure is frequent position change. Massage is *not* recommended for pressure points. It is thought that any kind of massage around or on a reddened area of skin causes fragile capillaries to be more likely to break down. In addition, rubber rings and doughnuts should *not* be used to keep heels or sacral areas elevated. Rings and doughnuts cause a concentrated area of pressure that puts patients at higher risk for developing pressure ulcers. *Remember: No massage and no rings or doughnuts!*

NORTON SCALE

		PHYSICAL CONDITION	MENTAL CONDITION	ACTIVITY	MOBILITY	INCONTINENT	
		Good 4 Fair 3 Poor 2 Very bad 1	Alert 4 Apathetic 3 Confused 2 Stupor 1	Ambulant 4 Walk/help 3 Chairbound 2 Bedrest 1	Full 4 Slightly limited 3 Very limited 2 Immobile 1	Not 4 Occasional 3 Usually/urine 2 Doubly 1	TOTAL SCORE
Name	Date						

FIGURE 19-3

Norton scale for identification of those at risk for development of pressure ulcers. (From Norton, D., McLaren, R., & Eston-Smith, A. N. [1962]. *An investigation of geriatric nursing problems in the hospital.* London: National Corporation for the Care of Old People [now the Centre for Policy on Ageing].)

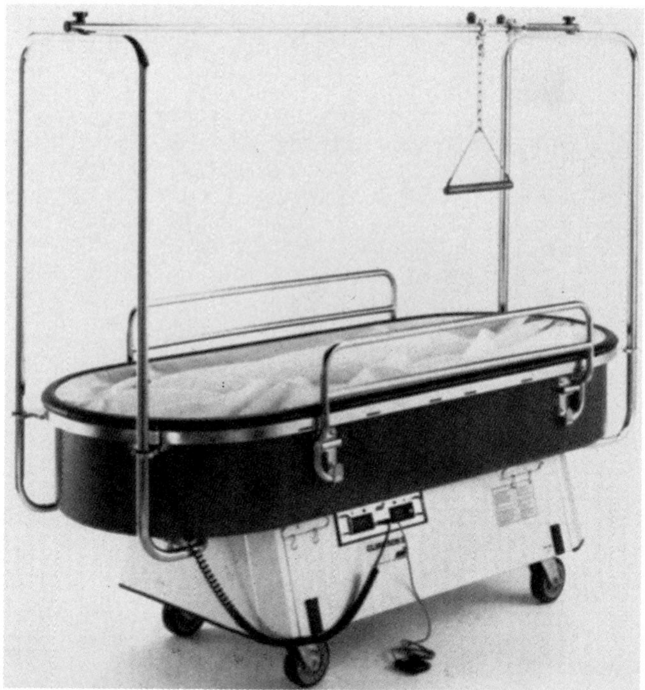

FIGURE 19-4
CLINITRON Air Fluidized Therapy Unit. (Courtesy of Support Systems International, Inc., Charleston, SC.)

In spite of all preventive measures, pressure ulcers may develop or they may be present on admission. It is useful to assess the stage of ulceration and document accurately. Proper documentation can show that an ulcer was present on admission and can be helpful in evaluating the effectiveness of treatment and progress toward healing and repair. Pressure ulcers are classified into four stages (Fig. 19–5).

Stages of Pressure Ulcers

STAGE I. The major characteristic of this stage is nonblanchable erythema. Before stage I begins, a finger pressed on a reddened area causes temporary blanching (whiteness at the point of pressure), followed by a return of the erythema when the finger is removed. In stage I, the redness does not fade when the finger is removed. The color ranges from red to the dusky blue that is seen with cyanosis. The area of pressure is irregular and ill-defined and reflects the shape of the object creating the pressure or the bony prominence underlying the skin. Pain and tenderness may be present, with swelling and hardening of the tissue and associated heat. At this stage there is little destruction of tissue, and the condition is reversible.

STAGE II. In stage II, there is some skin loss in the epidermis and dermis. A shallow ulcer develops and appears blistered, cracked, or abraded. The ulcer is surrounded by a broad and indistinct painful, reddened area that is hot or warmer than normal.

STAGE III. This stage is characterized by full-thickness skin loss involving damage or necrosis of the dermis and subcutaneous tissue. There is a crater-like sore with a distinct outer margin formed as the epidermis thickens and rolls over the edge toward the ulcer base. The wound may be infected, and it is usually open and draining with a loss of fluid and protein. The patient may have fever, dehydration, anemia, and leukocytosis (increase in the number of white blood cells in the blood).

STAGE IV. There is full-thickness skin loss with extensive destruction of the deeper underlying muscle and possibly bone tissue. The ulcer is usually extensively infected and may appear black with exudation, foul odor, and purulent drainage.

The first step in treatment of pressure ulcers is to continue all preventive measures. No treatment can heal a pressure ulcer unless measures to relieve the pressure that initially caused it are taken. There are numerous treatments used to promote wound healing that vary from institution to institution; however, no conclusive studies support one method of treatment over another.

In general, in treating stage I and II pressure ulcers, it is advisable to clean the wound with mild soap and water or normal saline. Pastes, creams, ointments, and powder should not be used because they may promote infection in the ulcer. Alcohol, antiseptics, disinfectants, topical and oral antibiotics, and massaging should be avoided because their effectiveness has not been proved, and they may actually cause harm. The use of a heat lamp is not recommended because a rise in temperature increases the metabolic demands of the skin and places additional stress on the affected area.

The most effective dressing for a stage I or II pressure ulcer is one that provides a moist environment and maintains a temperature close to body temperature. All wound covers should be permeable to allow the tissues adequate access to oxygen. Wound healing is enhanced when the ulcer and surrounding tissues can freely take up oxygen and expel carbon dioxide.

Stage III and IV pressure ulcers require more extensive treatment and supportive care. The wound usually requires débridement to promote granulation of new, healthy tissue. Wet to dry dressings are used for smaller amounts of débridement; further débridement is carried out by whirlpool baths. Surgery is preferred for very advanced cases. Débridement is sufficient when the ulcer bed appears pink, indicating healthy granulation tissue. Supportive care consists of measures to treat anemia, dehydration, protein depletion, and infection. Nutritional intervention consists of oral supplements high in protein and vitamins, nasogastric feedings, or parenteral nutrition to provide the additional nutrients necessary for healing.

In summary, in addition to preventive measures, the three major principles of wound management should be followed in the treatment of pressure ulcers:

1. Clean the area
2. Promote formation of granulation tissue
3. Ensure adequate nutritional intake for wound healing.

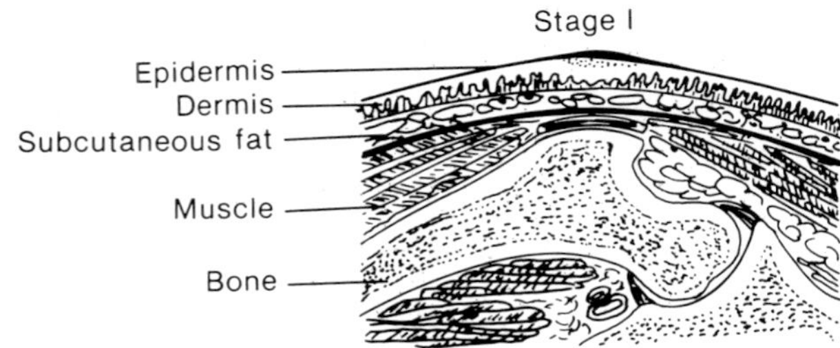

Non-blanching erythema of intact skin; the heralding lesion of skin ulceration.

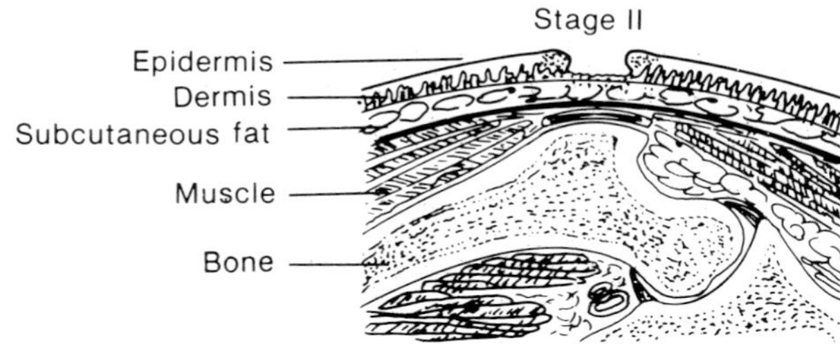

Partial-thickness skin loss involving epidermis and/or dermis. The ulcer is superficial and presents clinically as an abrasion, blister, or shallow crater.

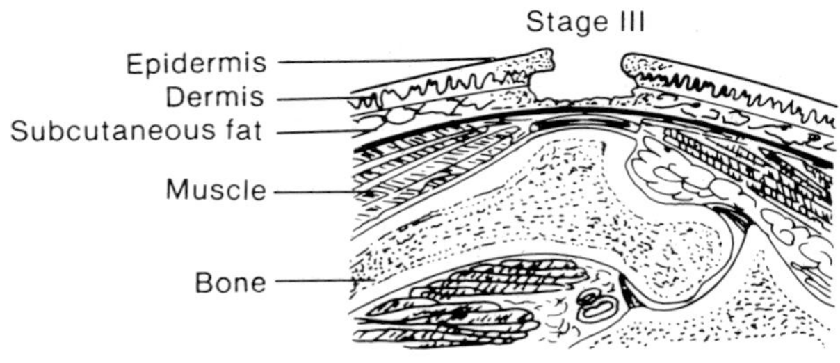

Full-thickness skin loss involving damage or necrosis of subcutaneous tissue, which may extend down to, but not through, underlying fascia. The ulcer presents clinically as a deep crater with or without undermining of adjacent tissue.

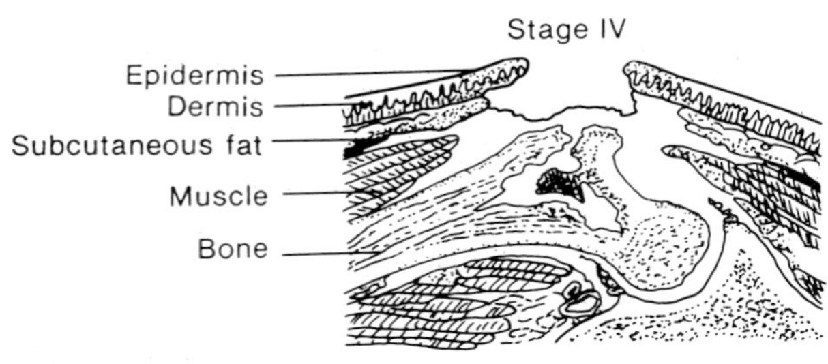

Full-thickness skin loss with extensive destruction, tissue necrosis, or damage to muscle, bone, or supporting structures (e.g., tendon, joint capsule, etc.).

FIGURE 19-5

Classification of pressure ulcers. (From Chenitz, W. C., Stone, J. T., & Salisbury, S. A. [1991]. *Clinical gerontological nursing* [p. 254]. Philadelphia: W. B. Saunders [based on the National Pressure Ulcer Advisory Panel, 1989].)

RESPIRATORY STATUS

Immobility can interfere with the normal exchange of oxygen and carbon dioxide in the lungs. For this exchange to take place, the mucous membrane that lines the airway passages and the alveoli must be thin and moist. Most healthy people take about six to eight deep, sighing breaths every hour. The breaths help keep the lungs expanded and move secretions upward along the air passages. When a person remains immobile or does not take deep breaths, there is an accumulation of thick secretions, which have a tendency to pool in the lower respiratory structures. These secretions interfere with the normal exchange of gases (oxygen and carbon dioxide).

Individuals who are at risk for impaired breathing capacity related to immobility are those who have been given drugs such as general anesthesia, narcotics, or sedatives; who have tight binders or bandages that would limit chest expansion; who have abdominal distention from gas, fluid, or feces; and who lie in one position for extended periods of time. Older adults are also at high risk for respiratory problems related to immobility because of changes that occur with aging that tend to reduce lung expansion and breathing capacity.

Nursing interventions for patients at risk for respiratory complications include frequent turning and position change and coughing and deep breathing exercises. These interventions must be carried out every 2 hours to be effective. Coughing and deep breathing exercises are done at the same time during the day to allow for periods of rest and to obtain the best results.

Effective coughing may be difficult for patients, especially those who are in pain from a surgical incision or those who have chronic coughs and are worried that the coughing may trigger a long, exhaustive coughing experience. Patients should be taught that the objective of coughing is to gradually move the secretions upward and to cough them out a little at a time. They should avoid a very large, explosive cough that can be painful or cause exhaustion.

Deep breathing is achieved by expanding the lower chest and using the abdominal muscles and diaphragm to improve aeration of the lungs. Patients should concentrate on exhaling the air slowly while pursing their lips. They should focus on the *volume* of air being exhaled rather than the force with which they exhale it.

The most effective technique for clearing secretions from the lower parts of the air passages is taking a single deep breath and following it with three consecutive coughs, trying to clear all the air from the lungs with each cough. This is most effective when the patient is in a sitting position while doing the coughing and deep breathing. Discomfort can be minimized by supporting the abdomen while the procedures are being carried out, especially if there is a surgical incision and sutures.

FOOD AND FLUID INTAKE

The most common problem associated with immobility in relation to food and fluid intake is anorexia (loss of appetite). Factors that contribute to anorexia are worry, depression, anxiety about dependence on others, and decreased metabolic needs due to inactivity. *Hypoproteinemia*, or protein deficiency can develop in immobilized patients.

Patients who are immobilized also may have inadequate fluid intake. Getting up for a drink of water may be too difficult and time-consuming for inactive individuals, or they may not think to drink liquids regularly. Older people are particularly prone to developing dehydration from an inadequate fluid intake, resulting in complications such as confusion, constipation, or urinary tract infection.

Nurses should keep accurate records of patients' dietary and fluid intakes. Small, frequent meals are usually more effective than three large meals for anorectic patients. Dietary supplements with high protein content may also be encouraged. Fluids, even small sips of water, juice, or other liquids, should be offered at least every hour. fluids need to be within reach so the patients may have easy access to them if they are able to drink without help. Family members also could offer fluids while they are visiting.

ELIMINATION

Constipation

One of the most common disorders associated with inactivity and immobility is constipation. Factors contributing to constipation in relation to immobility are change in usual routine and environment, inability to defecate on a bedpan because of embarrassment or discomfort, and weakened muscle tone. Constipated individuals may strain to defecate, causing an increase in intra-abdominal pressure. This is called the *Valsalva maneuver* or vasovagal reflex, which can lead to cardiovascular alterations, and, ultimately, to lightheadedness and fainting. The vasovagal reflex can be especially problematic in older persons whose circulation may be somewhat impaired.

Unconscious or confused patients may ignore the normal urge to have a bowel movement. If the impulse is ignored for a considerable time, the natural urge to defecate can diminish and eventually disappear.

Long-standing constipation can result in a fecal impaction. A *fecal impaction* is the presence of either hardened or putty-like feces in the rectum and sigmoid colon. If the condition is not relieved, intestinal obstruction can occur. Symptoms of a fecal impaction include painful defecation, feeling of fullness in the rectum, abdominal distention, and sometimes cramps and watery stool. The presence of diarrheic stools does not mean that a fecal impaction has been removed; the liquid fecal material may bypass the hardened mass.

When an impaction develops, the mass of feces must be broken up with a gloved finger (a doctor's order usually is needed). Before digital removal of the mass, it may be helpful to give an oil retention enema to soften the mass. In addition, an analgesic may be given 1 hour before digital removal of an impaction.

Inactivity, decreased fluid intake, and lack of adequate fiber in the diet can combine to cause constipation. The vicious cycle of immobility promotes inactivity, decreased fluid intake, and poor appetite, so that patients become weaker and more immobile and less likely to eat and drink adequately. The combined measures of encouraging proper foods with adequate roughage, fluids, and as much activity as possible can help to prevent or relieve constipation. Whenever possible, patients should use a bedside commode or be taken to the bathroom to defecate to avoid the difficulties of using a bedpan. Laxatives should be used sparingly; however, stool softeners may be helpful if the stools are hard and difficult to pass.

Urinary Incontinence

The urinary system functions best when it is upright. Urine flows from the kidney downward much like the pull of gravity. When the body is in a reclining position, the kidney must force urine into the ureters against the pull of gravity. Urine is continually being formed in the kidney, but the peristaltic action of the kidney and ureters is insufficient to maintain a constant flow of urine. If the body remains in a supine (lying down) position even for a few days, the flow becomes sluggish and the urine pools. This sets the stage for the development of a urinary tract infection.

Lying in bed can also cause a loss of control of the urinary sphincter muscles and result in incontinence. Without the downward pressure of the full bladder against the sphincter muscles, there is less awareness of the need to void. The result is bladder distention and an overflow or a dribbling of urine without the patient's awareness of it.

Elderly individuals who have problems with mobility may have forced incontinence because they are unable to respond to the urge to void in time. The bladder is usually more full when the urge to void occurs, so there is less time to get to the bathroom. In addition, their bodies may not be able to move quickly enough because of the slowed reflexes and responses associated with older age or infirmities associated with chronic illness.

The most effective way to prevent urinary incontinence associated with immobility is to set up a toileting program. Patients should have scheduled toiletings with adjustments in schedule based on patient's voiding patterns. If voiding patterns are not able to be assessed, patients should at the very least be taken to the bathroom or commode or offered a bedpan every 2 hours during the waking hours. Some individuals restrict fluids at certain times of the day, especially after dinner and through the night to avoid nighttime incontinence. However, studies have been inconclusive regarding the effectiveness of limiting fluids.

BIBLIOGRAPHY

Alterescu, V., & Alterescu, K. B. (1992). Pressure ulcers: Assessment and treatment. *Orthopedic Nursing, 11*(2), 37–49.

Blaylock, B. (1991). Mobility and ambulation: Not easy tasks for all older adults. *Advancing Clinical Care, 6*(6), 20–21, 41.

Goodridge, D. M. (1993). Pressure ulcer risk assessment tools: What's new for gerontological nurses. *Journal of Gerontological Nursing, 19*(1), 23–27.

How to predict and prevent pressure ulcers . . . clinical practice guideline released by the Agency for Health Care Policy and Research. (1992). *American Journal of Nursing, 92*(7), 52, 54–56, 58–60.

Kelley, L. S., & Mobily, P. R. (1991). Iatrogenesis in the elderly: Impaired skin integrity. *Journal of Gerontological Nursing, 17*(9), 24–29.

Krasner, D. (1992). The 12 commandments of wound care. *Nursing, 22*(12), 34–42.

Malone, C. (1992). Intensive pressures . . . reduce the incidence of pressure sores. *Nursing Times, 88*(36 Wound Care), 57–58, 60, 62.

Marklebust, J., & Magnan, M. A. (1992). Approaches to patient and family education for pressure ulcer management. *Decubitus, 5*(4), 18–20, 24, 26.

Mobily, P. R., & Kelley, L. S. (1991). Iatrogenesis in the elderly: Factors of immobility. *Journal of Gerontological Nursing, 17*(9), 5–11.

National Pressure Ulcer Advisory Panel. (1992). *Statement on pressure ulcer prevention.* Buffalo, New York.

Norman, G. M., & Gibbs, J. A. (1991). Why walk when you can ride? Clinical ambulation incentives for the immobile elderly. *Journal of Gerontological Nursing, 17*(8), 28–33.

Olson, E. V., Johnson, B. J., & Thompson, L. F. (1990). The hazards of immobility. *American Journal of Nursing, 90*(3), 43–44, 46–48.

Ouellet, L. L., & Rush, K. L. (1992). A synthesis of selected literature on mobility: A basis for studying impaired mobility. *Nursing Diagnosis, 3*(2), 72–80.

Pressure ulcers in adults: Prediction and prevention. (1992). *Decubitus, 5*(3), 26–30.

Preventing pressure ulcers: A patient's guide. (1992). *Decubitus, 5*(3), 34–35, 38, 40.

Public Health Service, Agency for Health Care Policy and Research. (1992). *Pressure ulcers in adults: Prediction and prevention* (DHHS Clinical Practice Guideline No. 3). Rockville, MD: U.S. government Printing Office.

Thomas-Hess, C. (1992). Pressure ulcers: Current treatment trends. *Nursing Homes, 41*(5), 37–40.

Thompson, R., & Murray, S. (1992). Pressure ulcers: Developing a program of care. *Journal of ET Nursing, 19*(6), 213–215.

Vernon, D. (1991). Pressure sore success. *Nursing Times, 87*(49 Wound Care), 62, 64, 66.

Winman, G., & Ashley, L. (1992). Prevention is better than cure: A survey of the use of Pegasus Airway. *Professional Nurse, 8*(3), 158–161.

KEY CONCEPTS

1. Psychological effects of immobility include depression, fear, anxiety, social withdrawal, apathy, loss of financial and personal independence, and lack of meaningful existence.
2. Some of the most problematic physiologic side effects of immobility are pressure ulcers, respiratory problems, impaired nutrition, constipation, and urinary incontinence.
3. Exercise is the best medicine for immobility.
4. Exercises may be active—that is, carried out by the patient—or passive—that is, carried out by the therapist or nurse without assistance from the patient.
5. Pressure ulcers are expensive to treat, result in longer hospital stays, increase the likelihood of nursing home placement, and increase mortality.
6. Pressure ulcers should be prevented whenever possible, keeping in mind that nursing care is a major factor in pressure ulcer prevention.
7. The best preventive measure for pressure ulcers is frequent position change.
8. In addition to preventive measures, the three major principles of pressure ulcer wound management are the following: (1) clean the area, (2) promote formation of granulation tissue, and (3) ensure adequate nutritional intake for wound healing.

9. Immobility can promote respiratory problems in older adults; patients who have been given drugs such as general anesthesia, narcotics, or sedatives; patients who have tight binders or bandages that limit chest expansion; patients with abdominal distention from gas, fluid, or feces; and patients who lie in one position for extended periods of time.
10. Nursing interventions for patients at risk for respiratory complications include frequent turning and position change, and coughing and deep breathing exercises.
11. The most common problem associated with immobility in relation to nutrition is anorexia (loss of appetite).
12. Immobility causes constipation by causing a change in the usual routine and environment, an inability to defecate on a bedpan because of embarrassment or discomfort, and a weakening of muscle tone.
13. Immobility can promote a loss of control of the urinary sphincter muscles, resulting in incontinence.
14. The most effective way to prevent urinary incontinence associated with immobility is to set up a toileting program.

CHAPTER 20

Confusion

Mary Ann Matteson

OBJECTIVES

1. Define delirium and dementia.
2. Identify the causes of acute confusion.
3. Describe the differences between delirium and dementia.
4. Discuss nursing assessment and interventions related to delirium and dementia.

GLOSSARY

DELIRIUM An acute organic disorder usually caused by some underlying illness that is characterized by disturbances in attention, thinking, perception, orientation, short-term memory, and sleep

DEMENTIA A clinical syndrome or collection of symptoms that is chronic in nature and is characterized by impairment of intellectual function, problem-solving ability, judgment, memory, orientation, and appropriate behavior

Confusion is a symptom experienced by various patients under varying circumstances. Older people often experience confusion as a first symptom of disease; others may experience confusion in the intensive care unit or in the recovery room after surgery. Confusion may be acute, transient, or permanent. It has many causes, names, and expressions and can be very difficult to manage.

The collection of symptoms associated with confusion falls into two categories: (1) acute confusional states, or delirium, and (2) chronic confusion, or dementia. *Delirium* is a short-term confusional state that has an acute onset and is often reversible. It is more prevalent in children and the elderly. *Dementia* is an organic mental syndrome that is often chronic and irreversible. It is more prevalent in the elderly. Delirium and dementia have been called *organic brain syndrome, acute brain syndrome, chronic brain syndrome, senile dementia,* or *senility.* Elderly individuals are the most susceptible to confusion related to delirium or dementia.

DELIRIUM

Delirium is an organic disorder characterized by disturbances in attention, thinking, perception, orientation, short-term memory, and sleep. A delirious person may alternate between hyperactivity or hypoactivity. The level of consciousness may fluctuate from drowsiness to stupor or coma, or the individual may be hyperalert. Speech may be slurred and disjointed, with aimless repetitions. Other symptoms include anxiety, depression, irritability, anger, apathy, or euphoria.

Delirium is usually caused by some underlying illness such as neurologic, pulmonary, or cardiovascular disease; cancer; diabetes mellitus; and thyroid disease or by conditions such as infection, dehydration, constipation with fecal impaction, nutritional imbalances, sensory impairment, overmedication, and alcohol or drug abuse.

PHARMACOLOGY CAPSULE

Withdrawal from central nervous system depressants including alcohol may cause agitation and confusion.

Almost any kind of over-the-counter or prescription medicine can cause delirium in the elderly. Table 20–1 lists systemic and central nervous system causes of delirium.

Acute confusion begins abruptly, and usually lasts a short period of time—usually 1 week, rarely more than a month. However, if the underlying cause is not identified and treated, delirium can become a permanent condition, especially in older adults. The symptoms tend to fluctuate and often become worse at night.

TABLE 20–1
SYSTEMIC AND CENTRAL NERVOUS SYSTEM CAUSES OF DELIRIUM

SYSTEMIC CAUSES	
Cardiovascular disease	Neoplasm
Congestive heart failure	Postoperative state
Arrhythmias	Substance abuse and poisons
Cardiac infarction	Alcohol
Hypovolemia	Amphetamines
Aortic stenosis	Sedatives/hypnotics
Infections	Heavy metals
Pneumonia	Solvents
Urinary tract infection	Pesticides
Bacteremia	Carbon monoxide
Septicemia	Trauma
Medications	Head injury
Analgesics	Burns
Anticholinergics	Hip fracture
Antidepressants	
Antihistamines	
Antiparkinsonian agents	
Cimetidine	
Digitalis glycosides	
Diuretics	
Neuroleptics	
Sedatives/hypnotics	
Metabolic	
Electrolyte and fluid imbalance	
Hepatic, renal, or pulmonary failure	
Diabetes, hyper- or hypothroidism, and other endocrinopathies	
Nutritional deficiencies	
Hypothermia and heat stroke	
CENTRAL NERVOUS SYSTEM CAUSES	
Infections	Vascular disorder
Meningitis	Transient ischemic episodes
Encephalitis	Stroke
Septic emboli	Chronic subdural hematoma
Neurosyphilis	Vasculitis
Brain abscess	Arteriosclerosis
Neoplasm	Hypertensive encephalopathy
Primary intracranial	Subarachnoid hemorrhage
Metastatic (bronchogenic, breast)	Seizure
Trauma	Ictal and postictal states
Subdural hematoma	
Extradural hematoma	
Contusion	

From Zisook, S., & Braff, D. L. (1986). Delirium: Recognition and management in the older patient. *Geriatrics, 41*(6), 67–78. Reprinted by permission.

DEMENTIA

Dementia is a clinical syndrome characterized by impairment of intellectual function, problem-solving ability, judgment, memory, orientation, and appropriate behavior (Table 20–2). There are several types of dementia with various causes and symptoms: (1) senile dementia, Alzheimer's type (Alzheimer's disease); (2) vascular de-

TABLE 20-2

DSM-IV DIAGNOSTIC CRITERIA FOR DEMENTIA

A. The development of multiple cognitive deficits manifested by both
   1. memory impairment (impaired ability to learn new information or to recall previously learned information)
   2. one (or more) of the following cognitive disturbances:
      a. aphasia (language disturbance)
      b. apraxia (impaired ability to carry out motor activities despite intact motor function
      c. agnosia (failure to recognize or identify objects despite intact sensory function)
      d. disturbance in executive functioning (i.e. planning, organizing, sequencing, abstracting)

B. The cognitive deficits in Criteria A1 and A2 each cause significant impairment in social or occupational functioning and represent a significant decline from a previous level of functioning.

C. The deficits do not occur exclusively during the course of a delirium.

FEATURES OF SPECIFIC DEMENTIAS

Dementia of the Alzheimer's Type

The course is characterized by gradual onset and continuing cognitive decline.

The cognitive deficits in Criteria A1 and A2 are not due to any of the following:

1. other central nervous system conditions that cause progressive deficits in memory and cognition (e.g., cerebrovascular disease, Parkinson's disease, Huntington's disease, subdural hematoma, normal-pressure hydrocephalus, brain tumor)
2. systemic conditions that are known to cause dementia (e.g., hypothyroidism, vitamin B_{12} or folic acid deficiency, niacin deficiency, hypercalcemia, neurosyphilis, human immunodeficiency virus [HIV] infection)
3. substance-induced conditions

Vascular Dementia

Focal neurologic signs and symptoms (e.g., exaggeration of deep tendon reflexes extensor plantar response, pseudobulbar palsy, gait abnormalities, weakness of an extremity) or laboratory evidence indicative of cerebrovascular disease (e.g., multiple infarctions involving cortex and underlying white matter) that is judged to be etiologically related to the disturbance.

Dementia Due to Other General Medical Conditions

There is evidence from the history, physical examination, or laboratory findings that the disturbance is the direct physiologic consequence of one of the following medical conditions: dementia due to HIV disease, dementia due to head trauma, dementia due to Parkinson's disease, dementia due to Huntington's disease, dementia due to Pick's disease, dementia due to Creutzfeldt-Jakob disease, dementia due to normal pressure hydrocephalus, etc.

Substance-Induced Persisting Dementia

There is evidence from the history, physical examination, or laboratory findings that the deficits are etiologically related to the persisting effects of substance use (e.g., a drug of abuse, a medication)

Modified with permission from American Psychiatric Association (1994). *Diagnostic and statistical manual of mental disorders* (4th ed., pp. 142, 143, 146, 151, 152, 154, 155). Washington, DC: American Psychiatric Association.

mentia; (3) Pick's disease; (4) Huntington's disease; (5) Creutzfeldt-Jakob disease; and (6) Parkinson's disease. Other conditions are associated with dementia, including normal pressure hydrocephalus, subdural hematoma, brain tumors, neurosyphilis (dementia paralytica) and acquired immunodeficiency syndrome. All of these diseases and conditions are types of dementia. Dementia is not a disease entity itself but a clinical syndrome—a collection of symptoms that can be characteristic of many types of diseases. The two most prevalent types of dementia are Alzheimer's disease that affects the neurons in the brain and vascular dementia that affects the blood vessels in the brain and causes multiple small strokes.

NURSING ASSESSMENT AND INTERVENTION

ASSESSMENT

The first step in assessing a confusional state is to observe the patient's behavior, orientation, memory, and sleep habits. The nurse should try to determine how long the symptoms of confusion have been present and how and when they started. It is helpful to find out what medications (including home remedies and over-the-counter medications) the patient has been taking.

Family members often provide helpful information if the patient is too confused or disoriented. These assessment data help the physician to determine whether the patient is suffering from delirium or dementia. Some major differences between the clinical features of delirium and dementia are described in Table 20–3.

PHARMACOLOGY CAPSULE

Drugs that most often cause confusion include anticholinergics, digoxin, H-2 receptor blockers, benzodiazepines, nonsteroidal anti-inflammatory drugs, and many antiarrhythmics and antihypertensives.

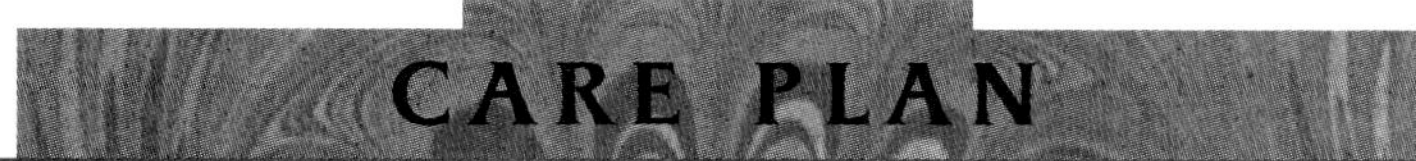

The Patient with Delirium

ASSESSMENT

Health History: An 81-year-old male was admitted for hip replacement surgery 2 days ago. Before his surgery he lived alone and cared for himself. He was active, alert, and independent. However, since his surgery he has been confused and at times combative with the nurses. His physician believes that he is suffering from delirium related to the anesthesia from surgery and that it should resolve within a few days.

Physical Examination: Blood pressure, 165/95; pulse, 98 with slight irregularity; respiration, 20; temperature, 97.4°F orally. Height, 5′7″; weight, 178 lb.
Alert, disoriented to time, place, and sometimes person; combative. Awakens during the night. Dark circles around eyes. Refuses food or fluids.

NURSING DIAGNOSIS	GOALS AND OUTCOME CRITERIA	INTERVENTIONS
Sensory-perceptual alterations related to anesthesia during surgery.	The patient will have improved sensory perceptions as evidenced by orientation to time, place, and person and absence of combative behavior.	Place in a private room with minimal stimuli, soft lighting. Request a family member to stay with patient. Maintain consistency with the nursing staff caring for the patient. Approach and communicate with the patient in a calm, reassuring manner. Have patient use hearing aid or glasses if used previously. Reorient patient frequently and consistently. Place familiar objects in the room: pictures, clock, calendar.
Sleep pattern disturbance related to agitation and mood alterations.	The patient will have adequate sleep and rest as evidenced by fewer awakenings during the night, absence of dark circles around the eyes, and no complaints of fatigue.	Provide a back rub or offer milk at bedtime. Engage in soothing conversation to relax the patient. Plan activities for long periods (at least 2–4 hr) of uninterrupted sleep.
Nutrition, altered: less than body requirements related to confused state and inability to feed self.	The patient will have adequate fluid and food intake as evidenced by eating meals as offered and maintenance of normal body weight.	Assist the patient with feeding. Offer small light meals more frequently. Stay with the patient during meals to monitor and provide safety.

INTERVENTION

Caring for Patients with Delirium

Interventions for delirium and dementia differ somewhat (see Care Plan: The Patient with Delirium). When managing delirium, the physician first attempts to treat the cause of the problem while maintaining a physiologic balance with adequate hydration, nutrition, electrolytes, and oxygenation. During the confusion episode, the nurse should focus attention on supporting the patient to provide safety and comfort.

PHARMACOLOGY CAPSULE

Nursing care can be more effective than drugs in managing confusion.

Patients with delirium usually require hospitalization. If possible they should be in a private room with continuous supervision. The first priority for nursing interventions is to maintain life. Basic physiologic needs must be met, including nutrition and fluid balance. Adequate sleep is important to avoid further disorientation and confusion that can result from sleep deprivation. Nursing measures such as a back rub, a glass of warm milk,

TABLE 20-3

CLINICAL FEATURES IN DELIRIUM AND DEMENTIA

	DELIRIUM	DEMENTIA
Duration	Few weeks to 3 months	In progress at least 1 to 2 yr
Paranoid states	Prominent while cognitive impairment is mild or variable	More consistent with degree of impairment; less prominent paranoia
Fluctuations	Marked contrasts in levels of awareness	Not seen in such contrast Progressive decline
Persecutory delusions	Ordered and cohesive	Vague, random, contradictory
General intellectual powers	Preserved during lucid intervals	Consistent loss and decline
Affect	Intermittent fear, perplexity, or bewilderment	Flat or indifferent affect
Perceptual disturbances	Hallucinations are often disturbing and very clearly defined	Hallucinations vague, fleeting, ill-defined, and in many cases it is difficult to make a clear judgment that they exist

From Chenitz, W. C., Stone, J. T., & Salisbury, S. A. (1991). *Clinical gerontological nursing.* Philadelphia: W. B. Saunders.

and soothing conversation may help the patient relax and fall asleep. Medications or treatments should be scheduled at times that do no interrupt nighttime sleep. The presence of a family member may help to calm an agitated and confused patient (Fig. 20–1).

The room should be kept quiet and uncluttered to avoid agitation caused by extraneous stimuli. Lighting should be soft and diffuse to avoid shadows that may be misinterpreted and add to the patient's fears. Familiar objects such as pictures, a clock, and a large calendar placed in the room can help orient to place and person. Patients who normally wear hearing aids and glasses should be allowed to use them (Fig. 20–2).

Communication with a confused patient should be simple and direct. Anyone dealing with a delirious patient should be calm, warm, and reassuring. It is helpful if the same personnel are assigned to care for the patient. Rough excessive handling of the patient during procedures or turning should be avoided.

Patients with delirium may have hallucinations that can be frightening to them. They may lash out, cry, or scream in response to a hallucination. The best response is to orient the patient to the reality of being sick and hospitalized rather than to acknowledge the reality of the hallucinations. The nurse might say, "You are sick in the hospital, and what you are seeing is part of the illness." Hallucinating patients in a delirious state require one-to-one nursing observation and repeated verbal reorientation. They need to be assured that the medical and nursing staff are helping them and keeping

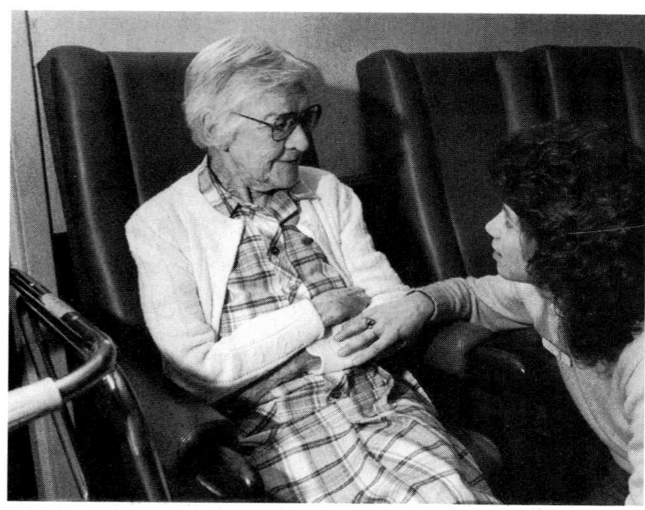

FIGURE 20-1

The presence of a family member may help to calm a confused patient. (From Matteson, M. A., & McConnell, E. S. [1988]. *Gerontological nursing* [p. 122]. Philadelphia: W.B. Saunders. Photograph by Stephen Matteson, Jr.)

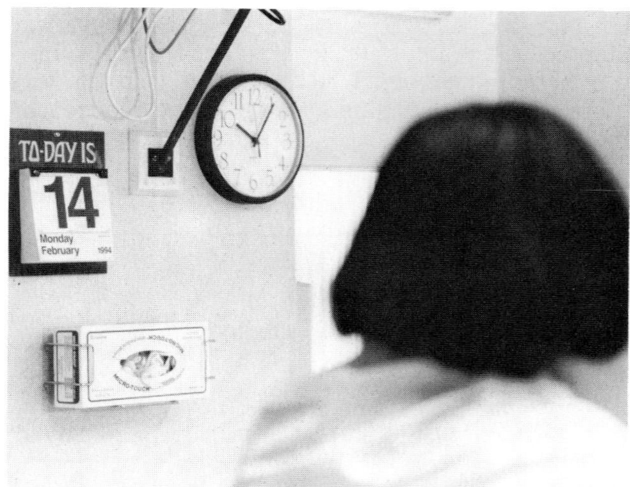

FIGURE 20-2

A clock and calendar may help to orient a patient with delirium; however, they must be in a place where they can be seen easily. In addition, patients with visual impairments should wear their glasses if possible. (Photograph by Stephen Matteson, Jr.)

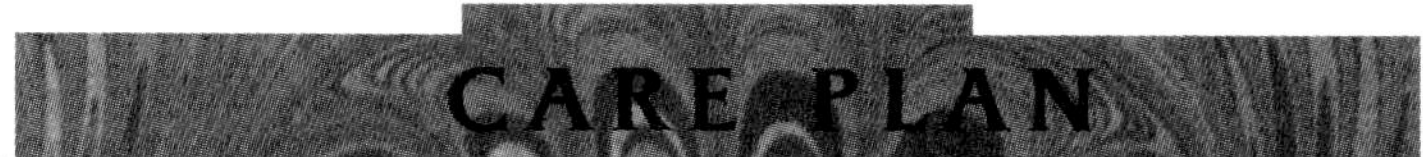

The Patient with Dementia

ASSESSMENT

Health History: A 75-year-old woman is admitted to a nursing home by her daughter because she has been unsafe living alone at home. Her daughter reports that the patient has been in good health, but during the past 5 years she has gradually had more and more problems with her memory, and during the past year, she has refused to take a bath or to change her clothes. Lately, she has had times that she has not even known her daughter. At times she has been unable to find the bathroom and has been incontinent of urine. She often forgets to eat, and when she does eat, prefers only junk foods. Recently she has begun "wandering." She was found at a local park not knowing who she was or where she lived. Her physician has diagnosed her with Alzheimer's disease.

Physical Examination: Blood pressure, 170/95; pulse, 88; respiration, 22; temperature, 98.2°F. Height, 5′3″; weight, 126 lb.
Inability to bathe and dress self. Disoriented to time, place, and person.

NURSING DIAGNOSIS	GOALS AND OUTCOME CRITERIA	INTERVENTIONS
Self-care deficit syndrome related to nervous system disorder.	The patient will perform activities of daily living (ADLs) as independently as possible as evidenced by ability to participate in bathing and dressing with the assistance of the nurse.	Assess the patient's ability to perform own ADLs. Allow the patient to perform as many of own ADLs as possible. Remain with the patient while performing ADLs to maintain safety. Work out a routine toileting schedule and encourage patient to go to bathroom at regular intervals.
Nutrition, altered: less than body requirements related to nervous system disorder.	The patient will maintain adequate nutrition as evidenced by keeping within 5 pounds of ideal weight.	Cut the food into small portions. Offer finger foods. Offer foods high in protein and carbohydrates. Offer small, frequent meals and snacks. Offer fluids frequently. Stay with the patient while eating to maintain safety.
Sensory-perceptual alterations due to neurologic changes.	The patient will remain free of combative behavior as evidenced by a calm, cooperative manner during times when nursing care is performed.	Speak to patient in a calm, reassuring manner. Avoid confrontations with patient. Break tasks down into individual steps to be done one at a time. Provide consistency in nursing care.

them safe. The use of physical restraints should be avoided because they tend to increase anxiety and agitation in confused patients.

Frequent orientation to the surroundings and the situation is important for patients with delirium. Orienting phrases such as "here in the hospital" or "now that it is evening" can be woven into the conversation. Choices should be kept at a minimum. Simple, direct statements ("Now it is time to take your bath") are better than questions ("When would you like to take a bath?"). All communication and nursing care should be carried out in a way that conveys respect and preserves the patient's dignity.

Caring for Patients with Dementia

Most people with a dementia have the misfortune of suffering from a chronic, debilitating illness with little hope for recovery. The goal for dementia patients is to maintain the highest level of functioning possible as their abilities gradually diminish (see Care Plan: The Patient with Dementia).

As with patients who have delirium, the first priority for dementia patients is to have their basic needs met. Adequate nutrition, fluid and electrolyte balance, sleep, elimination, and hygiene must be maintained. Patients with dementia have varying levels of competence when it comes to carrying out these functions. The nurse should assess the patient to determine the level of functioning that exists and then assist at whatever level is needed. When patients resist activities such as bathing or dressing, confrontations should be avoided. Confrontations only provoke agitation and possible violence; it is better to come back at another time. Tasks should be broken down into individual steps done one at a time.

Sleep and awakening are often reversed in dementia patients. It is helpful to try to keep them awake during the day and to get them to sleep at night. Tests and treatments can be scheduled during the morning and early afternoon to allow the patients time to wind down by bedtime. Some nurses have found that a quiet hour in the afternoon with soft music playing promotes sleep at night. Patients who awaken during the night and become confused and agitated should be reassured in a soft, soothing manner to avoid precipitating extreme agitation and loss of control.

People with dementia may eventually need help with eating. Assistance with mealtimes may mean cutting food or total feeding. Finger foods high in protein and carbohydrates allow patients to feed themselves more easily. Small, frequent meals are less confusing to the patients. Fluids should be offered frequently during the day.

Dementia patients may be incontinent of urine and feces. Frequent, routine toileting helps to prevent unwanted voiding and soiling. The nurse should observe for signs of constipation. Laxatives should be avoided; instead, high fiber foods in the diet are more effective for promoting regular bowel movements.

A safe, structured environment is essential for a person with dementia. Nothing should be left around that could harm the patient. Falls and injuries may be prevented with careful observation, muscle strengthening, and a fall prevention program. A consistent schedule of care given by the ·ame caregivers provides security for a dementia patient.

NUTRITION CONCEPTS

1. Confused people may forget to eat food, so it is helpful to offer small meals and snacks consisting of nutritious finger foods approximately six times a day.
2. Confused people may forget to drink liquids, so fluids should be offered frequently, especially nutritious drinks, such as orange juice, and water.
3. People with dementia may be overwhelmed by too many choices at mealtime, so one type of food at a time should be served.

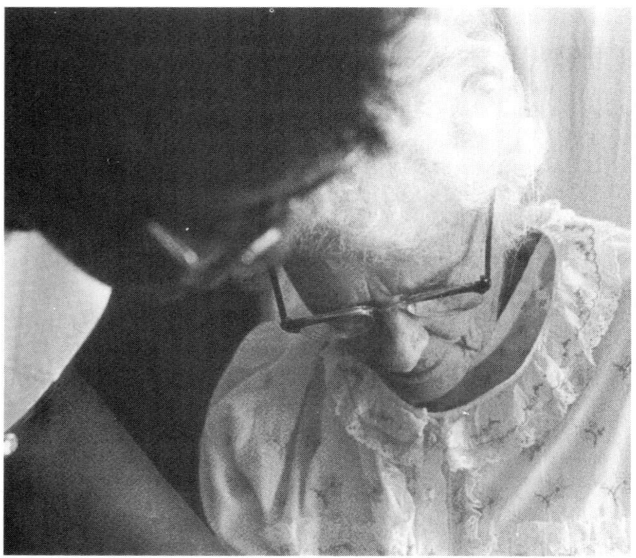

FIGURE 20-3
It is best to calmly divert the attention of confused, agitated patients somewhere else by gently guiding them to another activity. (From Matteson, M. A., & McConnell, E. S. [1988]. *Gerontological nursing.* Philadelphia: W.B. Saunders. Photograph by Stephen Matteson, Jr.)

Communication usually becomes increasingly difficult. Dementia patients are disoriented and have impaired thinking ability. They are confused by what is going on around them. Communication should be simple and direct. Patients must be approached gently, calmly, and quietly. They tend to copy the behavior of people around them, so a nurse who is anxious or upset can easily convey these feelings to a patient. Nonverbal communication is extremely important. The nurse should look for cues from patients' actions and facial expressions because they frequently are not able to express their needs verbally.

Whereas constant reality orientation is helpful for the patient with delirium, such orientation is controversial for the patient with dementia. Clocks, calendars, constant mention of the date and time, and other such orientation reminders used to be a staple of care for demented patients. However, it is now thought that reality orientation tends to agitate people with dementia by pointing out to them their forgetfulness and confusion. It is better to assist them in a nonconfrontational manner without constantly reminding them of their deficits.

It is helpful to keep in mind two important concepts when taking care of patients with dementia: (1) they usually forget things relatively quickly and (2) they are usually unable to learn new things. For example, if persons with dementia start to become very restless, anxious, or agitated and are becoming more so by the minute, it is best to divert their attention somewhere else. They may be gently guided to another activity, and within a relatively short period of time they will forget what was bothering them in the first place and focus on the new activity (Fig. 20–3). The caregiver may take advantage of the fact that dementia patients are usually unable to learn new things by putting new locks on the doors in new places for wandering patients. Nurses can be very creative in their care of dementia patients by using these two concepts as a basis for their care.

BIBLIOGRAPHY

Anderson, K. H., Hobson, A., Steiner, P., & Rodel, B. (1992). Patients with dementia: Involving families to maximize nursing care. *Journal of Gerontological Nursing, 18*(7), 19–25.

Bostrom, A. C. (1992). Early identification of confusion in hospitalized elderly patients. *Michigan Nurse, 65*(3), 11–12.

Brower, H. T. (1993). Special care units for dementia. *Journal of Gerontological Nursing, 19*(2), 3, 6.

Davis, L. E. (1991). Aiding the Alzheimer's dementia patient to live in safety and security. *Caring, 10*(12), 36–42.

Feil, N. (1990). Validation therapy helps staff reach confused residents. *Provider, 16*(12), 33–34.

Harvis, K. A. (1990). Care plan approach to dementia. *Geriatric Nursing, 11*(2), 76–80.

Jubeck, M. E. (1992). Are you sensitive to the cognitive needs of the elderly? *Home Healthcare Nurse, 10*(5), 20–25.

Kettl, P. A. (1993). 10 Basic rules for managing dementia. *Patient Care, 27*(1), 79–81, 84, 86.

Marr, J. (1992). Acute confusion. *Nursing Times, 88*(21), 31–32.

Marshall, M. (1993). Postoperative confusion: Helping your patient emerge from the shadows. *Nursing, 23*(1), 44–47.

Matteson, M. A., & McConnell, E. S. (1988). *Gerontological nursing: Concepts and practice.* Philadelphia: W. B. Saunders.

Mattice, M., & Mitchell, G. J. (1990). Caring for confused elders. *Canadian Nurse, 86*(11), 16–18.

McConnell, E. A. (1991). Assessing confusion in an elderly patient. *Nursing, 21*(3), 95, 97, 99.

Neelon, V. J. (1990). Postoperative confusion. *Critical Care Nursing Clinics of North America, 2*(4), 579–587.

Norton, D. (1991). Investigating the sundown syndrome. *Nursing Standard, 5*(47), 26–29.

O'Brien, L. A., Grisso, J. A., Maislin, G., Chiu, G. Y., & Evans, L. (1993). Hospitalized elders: Risk of confusion with hip fracture. *Journal of Gerontological Nursing, 19*(2), 25–33.

Palmieri, D. T. (1991). Clearing up the confusion: Adverse effects of medications in the elderly. *Journal of Gerontological Nursing, 17*(10), 32–35, 40–41.

Rasin, J. H. (1990). Confusion. *Nursing Clinics of North America, 25*(4), 909–918.

Roper, J. M., Shapira, J., & Chang, B. L. (1991). Agitation in the demented patient: A framework for management. *Journal of Gerontological Nursing, 17*(3), 17–21, 35–37.

Sloane, P. D., & Matthew, L. J. (1991). An assessment and care planning strategy for nursing home residents with dementia. *Gerontologist, 31*(1), 128–131.

Tess, M. M. (1991). Acute confusional states in critically ill patients: A review. *Journal of Neuroscience Nursing, 23*(6), 398–402.

KEY CONCEPTS

1. The two major types of confusion are (1) acute confusional states, or delirium, and (2) chronic confusion, or dementia.
2. Elderly individuals are the most susceptible to confusion associated with delirium or dementia.
3. Delirium is a short-term confusional state that usually appears within hours or days and is often reversible.
4. Delirium is characterized by disturbances in attention, thinking, perception, orientation, short-term memory, and sleep.
5. Delirium is usually caused by some underlying illness such as neurologic, pulmonary, or cardiovascular disease or conditions such as infection, dehydration, and overmedication.
6. Dementia is an organic mental syndrome that is often chronic and irreversible.
7. Dementia is characterized by impairment of intellectual function, problem-solving ability, judgment, memory, orientation, and appropriate behavior.
8. Dementia is not a disease entity itself, but a clinical syndrome—a collection of symptoms that can be characteristic of many types of diseases, including Alzheimer's disease, vascular dementia, Huntington's disease, and Parkinson's disease.
9. The first step in assessing a confusional state is to observe the patient's behavior, orientation, memory, and sleep habits.
10. The nurse should try to determine how long the symptoms of confusion have been present and how and when they started.
11. In caring for a patient with delirium, the nurse should provide safety and comfort and provide frequent orientation to the surroundings and the situation.
12. The goal for dementia patients is to maintain the highest level of functioning possible as their abilities gradually diminish.
13. A safe, structured environment is essential for patients with dementia, and tasks should be broken down into individual steps that can be performed one at a time.
14. When patients with dementia resist activities such as bathing or dressing, it is best to avoid confrontations and divert their attention elsewhere.

CHAPTER 21

Adrianne Linton

Incontinence

OBJECTIVES

1. Identify types of urinary and fecal incontinence.
2. Explain the pathophysiology and treatment of specific types of incontinence.
3. Identify common therapeutic measures used for the incontinent patient.
4. List nursing assessment data needed to assist in the evaluation and treatment of incontinence.
5. Specify nursing goals, diagnoses, interventions, and evaluation criteria for the patient with incontinence.

GLOSSARY

ANORECTAL INCONTINENCE Fecal incontinence caused by weak perineal muscles, loss of anal reflexes, loss of anal sphincter tone, or rectal prolapse

CREDÉ'S TECHNIQUE Expression of urine from the bladder by applying pressure over the lower abdomen

FECAL INCONTINENCE The inability to control the passage of feces

FUNCTIONAL INCONTINENCE Inappropriate voiding in the presence of normal bladder and urethral function

MICTURITION Urination

NEUROGENIC BLADDER Condition in which the bladder does not function normally because of some disorder affecting the nerves of the bladder

NEUROGENIC INCONTINENCE Reflexive uncontrolled bowel movement, usually seen with dementia

OVERFLOW INCONTINENCE (FECAL) Uncontrolled passage of stool associated with constipation

OVERFLOW INCONTINENCE (URINE) Involuntary loss of urine associated with a full bladder

STRESS INCONTINENCE Involuntary loss of urine during physical exertion

SYMPTOMATIC INCONTINENCE Incontinence associated with colorectal disease

TRANSIENT INCONTINENCE Temporary loss of control over voiding

URGE INCONTINENCE Involuntary loss of urine, usually shortly after a strong urge to void

URINARY INCONTINENCE The inability to control the passage of urine

VOID Urinate

Incontinence is the term used to describe the inability to control the passage of urine (urinary incontinence) or feces (fecal incontinence). Many conditions and situations can cause either temporary or permanent incontinence. Incontinence deserves special attention because of the toll it takes on the individual. The person who is troubled by incontinence faces physical, psychosocial, and financial burdens. The management of incontinence also requires many hours of nursing care.

The goals of treatment for the incontinent person include restoration or improvement of control for treatable incontinence, management of irreversible incontinence, and prevention of complications.

URINARY INCONTINENCE

The Department of Health and Human Services estimates more than 10 million Americans suffer from urinary incontinence. Exact figures are difficult to obtain because people often do not report the problem to health care providers. The figures most often quoted are based on studies of elderly people in institutions, approximately 50% of whom are reportedly incontinent. It has been estimated that 15 to 30% of people living outside of institutions have some problem with urinary incontinence as well. The problem is twice as common among women as it is among men. Even though it is more common in older people, urinary incontinence should not be considered normal. It can usually be improved or cured, no matter how old the patient is.

The cost of managing the incontinence of institutionalized elderly people in the United States is estimated to be more than $10 billion each year. Health care providers need to recognize the economic and personal value of treating incontinence aggressively. Nurses play an important role in educating people about the need for evaluation and treatment.

PHYSIOLOGY OF URINATION

The passage of urine is called *urination* or *micturition*. Nurses and physicians more commonly refer to the process of urinating as voiding. For that reason, the terms *void* and *voiding* are used in this chapter.

Normal controlled voiding requires healthy bladder muscles (detrusor muscles), a patent (open) urethra, normal transmission of nerve impulses, and mental alertness. Alterations in any of these factors may produce incontinence.

The urinary bladder receives urine continuously from the kidney. The function of the bladder is to store urine until it can be eliminated. The walls of the bladder are muscular and capable of stretching. When 200 to 250 ml of urine collect in the bladder, stretch and tension receptors are stimulated. The bladder contracts, and the internal sphincter relaxes. A message is sent to the brain, making the person aware of the need to void. Because the act of voiding is normally voluntary, it can be delayed until an appropriate time. Then the external sphincter can be relaxed, permitting urine to flow out through the urethra (Fig. 21–1).

There is, of course, a limit to the amount of urine the bladder can hold. When the limit is exceeded, pressure causes the bladder to contract and force urine out involuntarily. If the bladder cannot be emptied, urine backs up into the kidneys (a condition called hydronephrosis) and can cause kidney damage.

DIAGNOSTIC TESTS AND PROCEDURES

The presence and specific type of urinary incontinence is diagnosed on the basis of the patient's history and physical examination and the results of a number of diagnostic tests and procedures. Diagnostic studies may include laboratory tests, measurement of urine volumes, radiographic studies, endoscopy, stress tests, and urodynamic studies.

LABORATORY TESTS

A clean-catch urinalysis with a culture and sensitivity test is usually ordered. The specimen is studied for bacteria, red blood cells, white blood cells, and glucose. If the patient cannot cooperate with the clean-catch procedure, catheterization may be necessary. A blood sample may be collected to measure blood urea nitrogen (BUN) and creatinine.

POSTVOID RESIDUAL

It is useful to know whether the patient is emptying the bladder completely. The amount of urine remaining in the bladder after voiding is called the *postvoid residual*. Several methods are used to determine the postvoid residual. One method is to catheterize the patient immediately after voiding and measure the amount of urine obtained by catheterization. A second method is

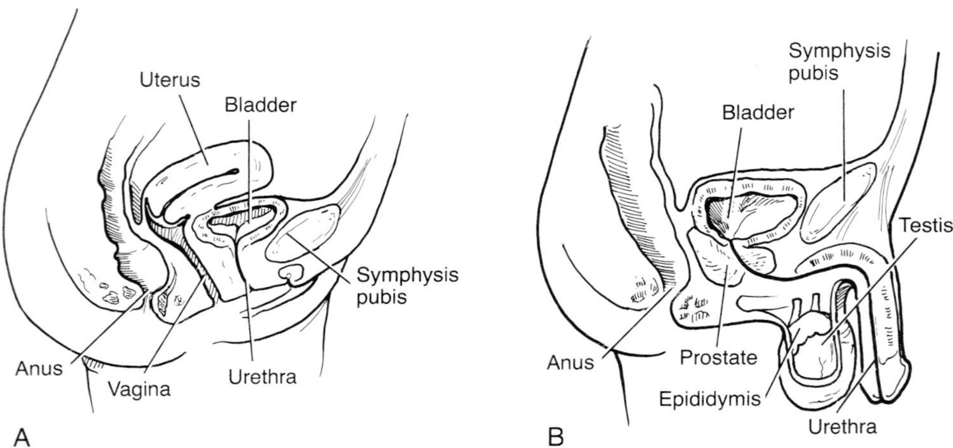

FIGURE 21-1

The bladder, urethra, and external urethral sphincter. *A*, Female; *B*, male. (Modified from Jacob, S. W., et al. [1982]. *Structure and function in man* (5th ed.). Philadelphia: W. B. Saunders.)

to use an ultrasound device to estimate the amount of urine remaining in the bladder after voiding. Some physicians estimate postvoid residual by abdominal palpation and percussion. Normally less than 50 ml of urine remain after voiding. An amount greater than 199 ml reflects inadequate emptying.

UROFLOWMETRY

Uroflowmetry measures voiding duration and the amount and rate of urine voided. The patient voids into the funnel of the flowmeter. Sometimes serial measurements are made over 2 to 3 days. The patient is advised to void before defecating and not to allow stool or bathroom tissue to enter the funnel. The patient's position for each voiding is recorded. Fluid intake is measured during the testing period. Additional urodynamic tests are discussed in Chapter 36.

PROVOCATIVE STRESS TESTING

Provocative stress testing is done to detect involuntary passage of urine when abdominal pressure increases. The patient may be positioned in a standing or lithotomy position. The physician encourages the patient to relax and then to cough vigorously. The examiner observes for urine loss during coughing.

CYSTOMETRY

Cystometry is used to evaluate the neuromuscular function of the bladder. Signed consent is obtained before beginning the procedure. The patient voids into a flowmeter, after which a catheter is inserted and postvoid residual is measured. Fluid or air, or both, is instilled into the bladder, and the patient's sensations and bladder response are determined. The bladder is filled until the patient feels uncomfortable or it is apparent that the patient is unable to sense the pressure. The bladder is then drained, or the patient is permitted to void. The physician may administer a drug that stimulates bladder tone and repeat the test. After the test, the patient should force fluids if not contraindicated. The nurse advises the patient to report difficulty voiding or signs of infection (fever, burning during urination, chills, pain, blood in urine).

CYSTOSCOPY

Cystoscopy is covered in Chapter 36. Briefly, it employs a scope inserted through the urethra to visualize the urethra and bladder. Signed consent is required, and the procedure may be done under local or general anesthesia. Postprocedure care includes monitoring urine output and encouraging fluid ingestion (if not contraindicated). The patient is advised to report difficulty voiding, continued blood in urine (it is normally pink-tinged at first), and fever, chills, or pain that may indicate infection.

IMAGING PROCEDURES

Imaging procedures such as computed tomography or magnetic resonance imaging may be ordered to create images of the urinary structures. Imaging procedures for the urinary tract are discussed in Chapter 36.

COMMON THERAPEUTIC MEASURES

Depending on the type of urinary incontinence, a number of therapeutic measures may be prescribed. These are generally classified as behavioral, pharmacologic, or surgical treatments.

BEHAVIORAL TECHNIQUES

Behavioral techniques include bladder training or retraining, habit training, prompted voiding, and pelvic muscle exercises. These techniques are low risk and are often effective in decreasing the frequency of incontinent episodes.

BLADDER TRAINING. Bladder training uses patient education, scheduled voiding, and positive reinforcement. The teaching plan includes information about normal urinary anatomy and physiology and the bladder training program. With scheduled voiding, the patient is encouraged to delay voiding and void only at specific times. Initially, voiding is usually scheduled every 2 to 3 hours while awake. The length of time between voidings is gradually increased. If the patient voids ahead of schedule, the next voiding may be rescheduled at the prescribed interval. Another approach is to ignore the unscheduled voiding and have the patient void again at the previously scheduled time. The patient's efforts and improvement are positively reinforced throughout the treatment period, which usually lasts several months.

HABIT TRAINING. Habit training is also called timed voiding. It is similar to bladder training in that the patient is encouraged to void at scheduled intervals. The difference is that the patient is not advised to resist the urge and delay voiding. The voiding schedule is based on the patient's usual pattern.

PROMPTED VOIDING. Prompted voiding is often used with habit training for people who are dependent or cognitively impaired. The caregiver checks the patient for wetness at regular intervals and asks the patient to state whether wet or dry. The caregiver then encourages the patient to try to use the toilet. The caregiver praises the patient for trying to use the toilet and for remaining dry. This process is intended to help the patient recognize incontinence and to ask caregivers for help with toileting.

PELVIC MUSCLE EXERCISES. Pelvic muscle exercises are commonly called Kegel exercises. They actively exercise the pubococcygeus muscle, which helps close the urethra and strengthen muscles of the pelvic floor. The patient is taught to contract the muscle that inhibits voiding. The contraction should be held for up to 10 seconds, and then relaxed for the same period of time. The exercise is repeated 30 to 80 times a day for a minimum of 6 weeks, and may be needed indefinitely.

Sometimes vaginal cones are used with pelvic muscle training in women. The cones are ceramic devices of increasing weight that are inserted into the vagina. The patient begins with the lightest cone, inserts it, and tries to retain it for up to 15 minutes twice daily. When the lightest cone is successfully retained, the heavier cones are used in succession. The use of the weighted vaginal cones is relatively new and the effectiveness with various patients and types of incontinence is being studied.

BIOFEEDBACK. Biofeedback may be used in conjunction with other behavioral treatment techniques. Electronic or mechanical sensors are used to give the patient feedback about the physiologic activity involved in bladder control.

REFLEX TRAINING

Reflex training is sometimes employed by people with spinal cord injury. This technique uses the Valsalva maneuver with rectal stretching to force urine from the bladder. The Valsalva maneuver is performed by taking a deep breath, holding it, and bearing down. At the same time the rectum is stretched by inserting a gloved finger into the rectum and pulling toward the back. This creates pressure on the urinary sphincter and relaxes the pelvic floor allowing urine to flow. Patients who use this method of emptying the bladder should be checked for residual volume at times. Ideally, the residual volume will be less than 100 ml. Patients who learn to use this method successfully may no longer need catheterization.

DRUG THERAPY

The use of drug therapy to treat urinary incontinence is being studied. Classifications of drugs that are being used include anticholinergics, smooth muscle relaxants, calcium channel blockers, tricyclic antidepressant agents, nonsteroidal anti-inflammatory drugs, alpha-adrenergic agonists, and estrogen supplements. Examples of these drugs, their side effects, and nursing considerations are presented in Table 21–1.

PHARMACOLOGY CAPSULE

Anticholinergic drugs often relieve urge incontinence but have bothersome side effects, including constipation and dry mouth.

In addition to drugs used to control incontinence, a variety of creams and sprays are available to coat and protect the skin of the perineum and buttocks of the incontinent patient. A light dusting powder can be used to absorb moisture. Cornstarch is not recommended because it promotes the development of yeast infections. Talc and lotion should not be used on the same area because the combination creates an abrasive paste.

URINE COLLECTION DEVICES

EXTERNAL DEVICES. External urine collection devices are useful for males. These latex sheaths, sometimes called condom catheters or Texas catheters, drain urine into a bag that is usually secured to the leg. These are quite effective in maintaining dryness, but the adhesive may cause skin irritation on the penis. The directions for applying a condom catheter must be followed

TABLE 21-1
DRUGS USED TO TREAT URINARY INCONTINENCE

DRUG	USE	ACTION	NURSING INTERVENTIONS
Cholinergics Bethanecol chloride (Urecholine)	Atonic bladder (overflow incontinence)	Bladder contraction	Common side effects: sweating, flushing, GI distress, headache, visual disturbances Toxicity: nausea, dyspnea, irregular pulse, headache Antidote: atropine Contraindications: bladder or intestinal obstruction, asthma, hyperthyroidism, ulcer, cardiac disease, parkinsonism Works quickly: 15–30 min after SC route, 1 hr after PO route; be sure bedpan or toilet is accessible *Warning:* dosages are very different for SC and PO routes; check drug references
Anticholinergics Propantheline bromide (Pro-Banthīne) Oxybutynin chloride (Ditropan)	Urge incontinence	Bladder relaxation and sphincter contraction Delayed desire to void	Common side effects: constipation, dry mouth, blurred vision (pupil dilation), fatigue tachycardia Contraindicated with glaucoma, severe coronary artery disease, some GI disorders Use cautiously in the elderly
Alpha Adrenergics Ephedrine Phenylpropanolamine (PPA)	Stress incontinence Enuresis (with atropine)	Sphincter contraction	Common side effects: cardiac arrhythmias, nervousness, palpitations Contraindications: severe hypotension, narrow angle glaucoma Elderly people are more likely to have hallucinations, convulsions, CNS depression, insomnia, and urinary retention
Alpha-Adrenergic Blockers Prazosin hydrochloride (Minipress) Phenoxybenzamine hydrochloride (Dibenzyline)	Overflow incontinence	Relaxation of internal sphincter	Side effects: postural hypotension (especially in the elderly), tachycardia, headache, dizziness, nasal congestion After the first dose, the patient should lie down for 2 hours to prevent fainting; elastic stockings may help During dosage adjustment, monitor blood pressure; most side effects decrease over time
Beta-Adrenergic Blockers Propanolol hydrochloride (Inderal)	Stress incontinence	Improved sphincter tone	Side effects: cardiac depression Contraindicated in asthmatics

GI, Gastrointestinal; SC, subcutaneous; PO, by mouth; CNS, central nervous system.

carefully. The nurse makes sure the patient and all caregivers know not to encircle the penis with tape. To do so can restrict circulation. There is no external device for women in common use at this time although several are being tested.

INDWELLING CATHETERS. An indwelling catheter may be ordered to control urinary incontinence. This is usually done when all other measures have failed and skin integrity is endangered. A catheter may also be needed temporarily if urine is coming in contact with a wound. Care of the patient with an indwelling catheter is covered in Chapter 36.

INTERMITTENT SELF-CATHETERIZATION. Some patients are quite successful using intermittent self-catheterization. Of course, this requires dexterity, adequate vision, and ability and motivation to learn. Clean technique rather than sterile is usually taught for use in the home setting. Initially the bladder is drained every 4 hours. If more than 500 ml of urine is obtained, the time interval is shortened. If less than 200 ml is obtained, the time is extended. Most people produce more urine at certain times of day. Individual schedules can be adjusted to accommodate this variation.

GARMENTS AND PADS FOR INCONTINENCE

A variety of incontinence products are available that help maintain dryness. Disposable briefs and pads are found in most pharmacies and grocery stores. Some elderly women wear perineal pads to absorb urine.

"Geri pads" are used in many nursing homes. These are washable waterproof briefs with absorbent cotton liners. Another style has a stretchy brief with a perineal pouch through which absorbent pads can be changed. The best product is one that draws urine away from the skin through a liner that remains dry. These products do not, however, protect the skin against feces.

Those who discourage the use of incontinence briefs and pads say it encourages patients to void in their clothing. This may be true at times, but there is a place for these items. It may give a person the confidence to be socially active without the risk of an embarrassing accident. When trying to restore control, it is best to use briefs that can be removed easily for toileting. For patients who will never be continent, these products may be an acceptable management tool.

For the immobile patient, an absorbent pad with a waterproof backing may be used instead of briefs. These pads can also be placed under the buttocks of a bedridden patient wearing briefs in case leakage occurs. One factor to remember is that multiple layers of padding interfere with special beds or mattresses designed to prevent decubitus ulcers. Some paper pads stick to the skin and become lumpy when wet. The patient should never be placed directly on a plastic surface as this keeps the skin wet from perspiration as well as urine.

PENILE CLAMP

The penile clamp is a device that is applied to the penis. It compresses the urethra, preventing the passage of urine. To prevent circulatory impairment and pressure sores, the clamp must be removed and repositioned frequently. The use of the penile clamp is controversial (Fig. 21–2).

SURGICAL TREATMENT

Surgical intervention may be recommended for some conditions that cause urinary incontinence. Specific surgical procedures may be done to remove obstructions, treat severe bladder instability, implant an artificial sphincter, reposition the sphincter unit, implant electrodes that inhibit the micturition reflex, improve perineal support, and inject substances that increase urethral compression. Nursing care of the patient having surgery on the urinary tract is described in Chapter 36.

The artificial sphincter illustrated in Figure 21–3 consists of an inflatable cuff, a reservoir of fluid that fills the cuff, and a pump. The cuff is positioned around the urethra or bladder neck. The reservoir is placed in the abdomen and the pump in the scrotum or labia. Fluid fills the cuff, applying pressure to the urethra to prevent urine passage. To void, the patient compresses the pump, which deflates the cuff by transferring fluid from the cuff to the reservoir and allowing urine to pass through the urethra.

TYPES OF URINARY INCONTINENCE

There are six basic types of urinary incontinence. They are urge, overflow, reflex, stress, functional, and total incontinence (Table 21–2). It is possible for a patient to have more than one type at the same time (mixed incontinence). Urinary incontinence may be transient or persistent. Transient incontinence is caused by reversible conditions and is often corrected by treatment of the underlying problem.

URGE INCONTINENCE

DESCRIPTION. Urge incontinence is the involuntary loss of urine shortly after a strong, abrupt urge to urinate. It most often results from involuntary detrusor contractions called detrusor overactivity or hyperreflexia. Detrusor overactivity may be associated with neurologic disorders like stroke, multiple sclerosis, and spinal cord

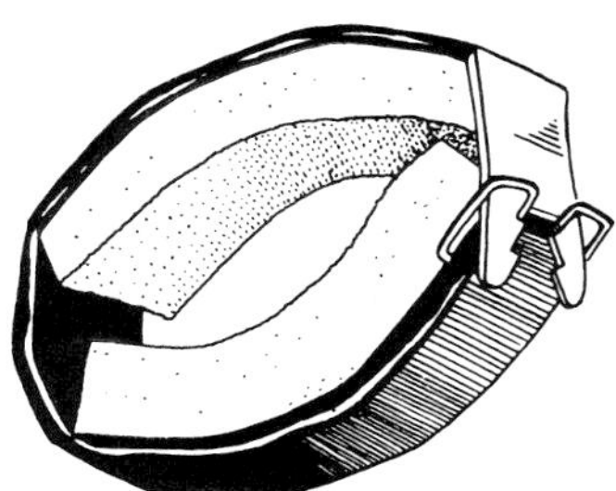

FIGURE 21-2

A penile clamp for urinary incontinence. (From Black, J. M., & Matassarin-Jacobs, E. [1993]. *Luckmann and Sorensen's medical-surgical nursing: A psychophysiologic approach* [4th ed.]. Philadelphia: W. B. Saunders.)

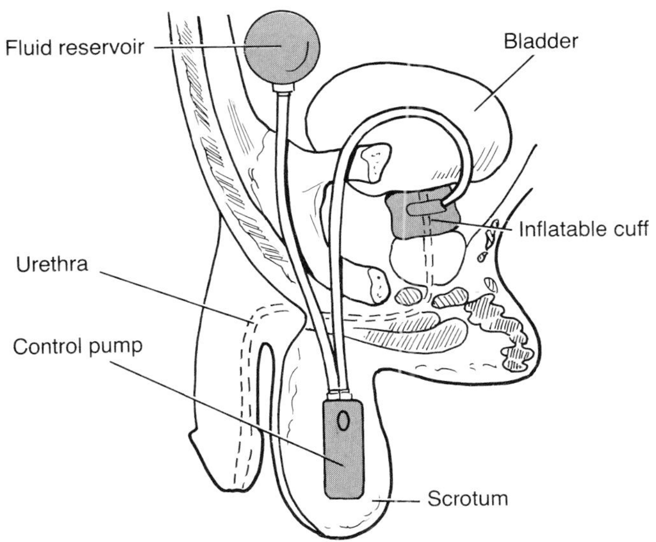

FIGURE 21-3

An artificial urinary sphincter in place. (Modified from Black, J. M., & Matassarin-Jacobs, E. [1993]. *Luckmann and Sorensen's medical-surgical nursing: A psychophysiologic approach* [4th ed.]. Philadelphia: W. B. Saunders.)

TABLE 21-2
TYPES OF URINARY INCONTINENCE

TYPE	DESCRIPTION	CAUSES	NURSING CARE	TREATMENT
Urge	Loss of urine that usually follows a strong desire to void	Nervous system disorders Urinary tract infection Bladder obstruction	Keep incontinence record Scheduled toileting Limit fluids 2 hr before bedtime Administer drugs as ordered to control bladder contractions (see Table 21–1)	Behavior modification Drug therapy Anticholinergics Surgical procedures to increase bladder capacity or decrease bladder contractions
Overflow	Loss of urine associated with a full bladder Frequent voiding Volume usually small	Urethral obstruction Disorders of bladder, nerves, or muscles Spinal cord injury Postanesthesia	Catheterize as ordered; teach self-catheterization as appropriate Administer drugs as ordered to stimulate the bladder and relax the internal sphincter (see Table 21–1)	Surgery to relieve obstruction Drug therapy to stimulate the bladder and relax the sphincters Catheterization
Reflex	Loss of urine due to reflexive contraction	Spinal cord injury above T12	Cutaneous triggers; teach stimulation techniques	Catheterize as necessary
Stress	Loss of urine during physical exertion	Relaxation of pelvic floor muscles Urethral trauma Sphincter injury	Teach Kegel exercises Advise patient to void frequently Administer drugs as ordered to stimulate sphincter (see Table 21–1)	Surgical correction Bladder suspension Artificial sphincter Drug therapy to improve sphincter contraction
Functional	Bladder functions normally but patient voids inappropriately	Dementia Head injury Cardiovascular accident (stroke)	Scheduled toileting Reinforce appropriate behavior Remove environmental barriers	
Total	Loss of urine when other types of incontinence have been ruled out	May be unclear; possibly neurologic, or bladder sphincter injury	Timed voiding Incontinence briefs	Catheterization

lesions. Inability to control the passage of urine owing to injury to the spinal cord above the twelfth thoracic vertebra is called reflex incontinence.

If no neurologic disorder is found, the patient is said to have an unstable bladder or detrusor instability. Some patients with urge incontinence have involuntary urethral relaxation in addition to abnormal detrusor activity. Urinary tract infection and fecal impaction sometimes cause temporary urge incontinence.

MEDICAL TREATMENT. Treatment of urge incontinence is aimed at correcting the cause, if possible: antibiotics for infection, removal of impaction. When the problem is not related to reversible conditions, behavioral techniques, drug therapy, or surgical intervention may be employed. Bladder training with scheduled voiding and positive reinforcement may be effective. Pelvic muscle exercises may be prescribed to supplement bladder training. Anticholinergics are the drugs most commonly used for urge incontinence. The nurse is aware that anticholinergics may cause confusion and agitation that could be mistaken for dementia in the elderly.

If behavioral techniques, drugs, or both do not work, some surgical procedures may be recommended. These include stretching the bladder, cutting some of the bladder nerves, and enlarging the bladder surgically.

It is essential to maintain bladder drainage in the patient with reflex incontinence. If the bladder becomes overdistended, the patient with reflex incontinence may have a very serious reaction called *autonomic dysreflexia*. The blood pressure rises to life-threatening levels. This can be prevented by emptying the bladder often enough to prevent overdistention. Among the techniques that may be used to stimulate the bladder to empty in patients with reflex incontinence are cutaneous triggering methods and include tapping the suprapubic area and stroking the inner thigh. These techniques and others are more fully described in texts on rehabilitation. Nurses know that Credé's method is *not* used for patients with reflex incontinence. Chapter 27 discusses care of the patient with spinal cord injury in detail.

OVERFLOW INCONTINENCE

DESCRIPTION. Overflow incontinence is the involuntary loss of urine associated with an overdistended bladder. Small amounts of urine are lost either continuously or at frequent intervals. Patients who have normal sensation usually feel uncomfortable due to bladder distention.

Factors that contribute to overflow incontinence are obstruction to urine flow, underactive detrusor muscle, or impaired transmission of nerve impulses. In addition, some females have overflow incontinence after anti-incontinence surgery. Patients with certain types of spinal cord injuries have neurogenic bladders. These patients are not aware of bladder fullness, and the bladder becomes overdistended. Urinary retention with overflow is also fairly common after general anesthesia or childbirth or following removal of an indwelling catheter. Drugs that may cause retention include antihistamines, epinephrine, anticholinergics, and theophylline (Table 21–3).

MEDICAL TREATMENT. The medical treatment of overflow incontinence depends on the cause. The physician may prescribe drugs to stimulate the bladder (bethanecol chloride) and relax the internal sphincter (prazosin). A common reason for obstruction in males is prostate enlargement. Surgical removal of all or part of the gland often restores normal bladder emptying.

In some cases intermittent or indwelling catheterization is necessary. Postoperative and postpartum patients usually require intermittent catheterization only once or twice before normal bladder function returns. Other techniques that may be used to empty the bladder are Credé's method, the Valsalva maneuver, and the anal stretch maneuver. Credé's technique involves using the open hand to gently press the abdomen over the bladder and promote urine passage. The physician should be asked about the safety of this procedure for individual patients. These techniques and others are described more fully in rehabilitation texts. The indwelling catheter is considered the measure of last resort in the management of overflow incontinence. Self-catheterization using clean technique may be taught to patients who are able to do it in the home setting. This technique works very well for many patients.

TABLE 21-3

DRUGS THAT CAUSE URINARY RETENTION OR INCONTINENCE

Drugs that can cause urinary retention:
- Anticholinergics: atropine sulfate
- Antihistamines: diphenhydramine hydrochloride (Benadryl)
- Sympathomimetics: epinephrine hydrochloride (Adrenalin Chloride)
- Xanthine: theophylline (Theo-Dur)

Drugs that may contribute to incontinence:
- Alpha-adrenergic blockers: prazosin hydrochloride (Minipress)
- Anticholinergics: atropine sulfate
- Antihistamines: diphenhydramine hydrochloride (Benadryl)
- Antiparkinson agents: levodopa (Dopar), trihexyphenidyl hydrochloride (Artane)
- Antipsychotics: chlorpromazine (Thorazine)
- High ceiling diuretics: furosemide (Lasix)
- Opiate agonist: morphine sulfate (Epimorph)
- Sedatives or hypnotics: phenobarbital sodium (Luminal Sodium), diazepam (Valium)
- Sympathomimetics: phenylephrine hydrochloride (Neo-Synephrine), isoproterenol hydrochloride (Isuprel)

STRESS INCONTINENCE

DESCRIPTION. Stress incontinence is the involuntary loss of small amounts of urine during physical activity that increases abdominal pressure. Coughing, laughing, sneezing, and lifting are examples of activities that often result in urine loss. In women it is usually due to relaxation of the pelvic floor muscles as a result of pregnancy, childbirth, obesity, and aging. Urethral trauma, sphincter injury, congenital sphincter weakness, urinary infection, neurologic disorders, and stress can cause stress incontinence in men and women. It may occur after prostatectomy or radiation therapy.

MEDICAL TREATMENT. Sometimes stress incontinence is successfully treated with behavioral methods such as scheduled voiding and pelvic muscle exercises. In addition, the patient is advised to maintain a fluid intake of at least 2000 ml a day. Fluids that have a diuretic effect (tea, coffee, cola) should be avoided. The drug phenylpropanolamine may be prescribed to stimulate the urinary sphincter. The most common surgical intervention is bladder suspension.

FUNCTIONAL INCONTINENCE

DESCRIPTION. Functional incontinence is the term used when a person voids inappropriately because of inability to get to the toilet. The problem could be due to confusion, immobility, or barriers in the environment.

MEDICAL TREATMENT. The treatment of functional incontinence depends on the cause. The environment should be arranged to permit independent toileting. Assistive devices that enable the immobile patient to void appropriately are provided. The confused patient may respond well to scheduled or timed voiding and efforts to improve orientation to toilet facilities. In long-term care facilities, it is important to promote the attitude that incontinence can usually be improved even in physically and cognitively impaired patients.

TOTAL INCONTINENCE

DESCRIPTION. Some sources use the term *total incontinence* to describe urine loss when all other types of incontinence have been ruled out. Total incontinence may be demonstrated by constant dribbling or just occasional events of urine loss. Causes may include injury to bladder sphincters and some neurologic disorders.

MEDICAL TREATMENT. Timed voiding may help these patients empty the bladder often enough to avoid incontinence. For some, the use of a catheter or incontinence briefs is necessary.

NURSING ASSESSMENT OF THE PATIENT WITH URINARY INCONTINENCE

HEALTH HISTORY

The nurse's assessment helps in the identification of the type of incontinence, the possible causes, and the patient response to treatment.

Chief Complaint

A thorough description of the chief complaint is essential. Assessment includes awareness of the need to void and ability to hold the urine once aware of the need to void. The nurse determines the pattern of incontinent voiding, urine volume, and related symptoms.

PATTERN. The patient is asked to describe the frequency of incontinent episodes and whether they occur during any particular activities, such as sneezing or laughing. A voiding diary is a helpful tool in identifying the pattern of urinary incontinence. Many patients are able to keep their own diaries. If the patient is unable to maintain an accurate record, the nurse or other caregiver must do it.

VOLUME. If a patient is incontinent, measurements of urine can only be estimated, but the patient can probably describe the amount voided as being large, moderate, or small. If pads or briefs are used, the number used and the degree of saturation can be recorded. When assessing the patient in the long-term care facility or a hospital, the amount of urine passed with continent voiding is measured and recorded as well.

RELATED SYMPTOMS. The nurse assesses the presence of dysuria (painful voiding) or pain in the suprapubic area (the lower abdomen where the bladder is located).

Past Medical History

Past problems that might be related to incontinence include urologic, gynecologic, neurologic, and endocrine conditions. The nurse specifically asks if the patient has diabetes mellitus. People who have diabetes may develop neurologic problems that affect the bladder. Also, if their diabetes is poorly controlled, they may produce large volumes of urine that quickly fill the bladder.

All abdominal disorders, surgeries, and trauma are documented. The number of pregnancies and types of deliveries are recorded. The nurse inquires about current and recent medications because many drugs can affect kidney or bladder function in some way. Drugs that might contribute to urinary incontinence are high-ceiling (loop) diuretics, major tranquilizers, anticholinergics, antihistamines, decongestants, some sedatives or hypnotics, and antiparkinsonian drugs. Other drugs that can disrupt normal voiding are epinephrine, theophylline, isoproterenol, and prazosin.

PHARMACOLOGY CAPSULE

When urinary incontinence develops suddenly, check the patient's drug profile for drugs known to contribute to incontinence.

Review of Systems

The review of systems may detect clues to conditions that contribute to incontinence. For example, the patient with severe arthritis in the hands or severely impaired vision may have difficulty managing toileting independently.

Functional Assessment

The functional assessment documents the patient's usual activities and habits. Of special interest when assessing incontinence are usual fluid intake and consumption of alcohol.

PHYSICAL EXAMINATION

The physical examination begins with the measurement of vital signs and height and weight. The nurse is alert for fever, tachycardia, and weight gain. The patient's level of awareness and appropriateness of responses are assessed. The skin is inspected for edema.

Sometimes incontinence is first recognized when the nurse detects an odor of urine during the assessment or when providing care. When assessing the incontinent patient, the nurse palpates the abdomen for masses, tenderness, fullness, or distention. A distended bladder or abdominal distention associated with constipation are important findings. Examination of the male genitalia includes inspection for abnormalities of the foreskin, glans penis, and perineal skin. The female perineum is inspected for redness or irritation. The physician or nurse practitioner performs a pelvic examination on the female patient to inspect for prolapse of abdominal organs and to evaluate perineal muscle tone. A rectal examination is done to determine sensation, sphincter tone, and presence of fecal impaction. In males, the prostate is palpated for contour and consistency.

Assessment of the patient with urinary incontinence is outlined in Table 21–4. The environment must also be assessed, including toilet accessibility, grab bars, lighting, and availability of toileting options (urinals, commode chairs) (see Care Plan: Patient with Stress Incontinence).

NURSING DIAGNOSIS

Nursing diagnoses for the patient with urinary incontinence may include the following:

- **Knowledge Deficit** of causes of incontinence and corrective measures
- **Functional Incontinence** related to physical, cognitive, or environmental barriers

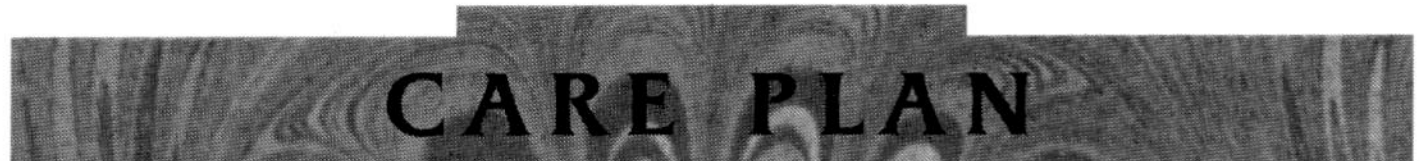

The Patient with Stress Incontinence

ASSESSMENT

Health History: Mrs. Seigel is an 80-year-old white nursing home resident. She complains of having trouble "holding my urine." Is unable to control urination if she strains, coughs, or laughs. She is the mother of five children, all born at home. Reports no other physical complaints except for arthritis in her hips and knees and hypertension. Her medications are acetaminophen, 325 mg qid, and hydrochlorothiazide, 25 mg daily. Fear of losing control of her urine has caused her to avoid leaving her room except for meals. She is wearing perineal pads to keep her clothing dry.

Physical Examination: Vital Signs: temperature, 98°F orally; pulse, 72; respiration, 20; blood pressure, 130/86. Height, 5'3"; weight, 179 lb. Heart and breath sounds normal. Abdomen obese and soft. No bladder distention. Faint urine odor present. Rises with some difficulty. Walks slowly with walker. Limited range of motion in knees and hips.

NURSING DIAGNOSIS	GOALS AND OUTCOME CRITERIA	INTERVENTIONS
Stress incontinence related to weak pelvic muscles and high intra-abdominal pressure.	The patient will report fewer incidents of stress incontinence.	Explain to the patient how weak perineal muscles cause stress incontinence. Instruct her how to do Kegel perineal exercises: contract the perineal muscles and hold the contraction for 4 seconds; repeat the contraction three more times; repeat the set of four contractions four times a day. Advise the patient to empty her bladder every 2 hours while awake. Encourage intake of normal amounts of fluid but discourage liquids with diuretic effects: coffee, tea, and alcohol. Explain that obesity increases intra-abdominal pressure and contributes to stress incontinence. Explore interest in weight loss and consult with physician and dietitian if patient agrees.
High risk for impaired skin integrity related to prolonged contact of urine with skin.	The patient's skin will remain intact and free of excessive redness.	Inspect the perineal area and buttocks and report signs of irritation: redness, breaks in the skin. Apply skin protectants as ordered or per agency protocol. Teach the patient the importance of good perineal care to remove urine from the skin. Encourage her to cleanse the area with mild soap, rinse, and gently dry twice daily. Perineal pads or other incontinence pads should be changed promptly if they are wet.
Social isolation related to fear of embarrassment due to incontinence.	The patient will report resumption of previous activities and participation in social activities.	Identify activities that patient would like to resume. Discuss strategies to decrease embarrassment about incontinent episodes: 1. Empty bladder before leaving room. 2. Wear perineal pads or special incontinence pads to absorb urine and protect clothing and furniture. Avoid any comments that could humiliate the patient such as references to "diapers" and avoid discussing her problem in front of others.

TABLE 21-4

ASSESSMENT OF THE PATIENT WITH URINARY INCONTINENCE

HEALTH HISTORY

Chief Complaint: pattern of continent and incontinent voiding, behaviors or activities associated with incontinent voiding, amount of urine passed with continent and incontinent voiding, awareness of need to void, ability to hold urine once aware of need to void, dysuria

Past medical history: urologic, gynecologic, neurologic, and endocrine problems; abdominal surgeries, trauma, disorders; mental confusion; current and recent medications

Review of systems: disorders that might contribute to incontinence: diabetes mellitus, CVA, paralysis

Functional assessment: usual activities, fluid intake, alcohol consumption

PHYSICAL EXAMINATION

Vital signs: fever, tachycardia
Height and weight: weight gain
Level of consciousness: orientation
Odor of urine
Abdomen: masses, tenderness, fullness, or distention
Male genitalia: abnormalities of foreskin, glans penis, perineal skin
Female genitalia: redness, irritation
Rectal examination: sensation, sphincter tone, fecal impaction

- **Reflex Incontinence** related to neurologic impairment
- **Stress Incontinence** related to weak pelvic structures, increased intra-abdominal pressure
- **Total Incontinence** related to neurologic dysfunction
- **Urge Incontinence** related to decreased bladder capacity or bladder spasms
- **Social Isolation** related to fear of embarrassment
- **Situational Low Self-Esteem** related to loss of control over voiding
- **High Risk for Impaired Skin Integrity** related to the presence of urine on the skin
- **High Risk for Infection** related to chronic bladder distention or catheterization

GOALS

Goals for nursing care of the patient with urinary incontinence may be patient's understanding of incontinence and its treatment, continent voiding with appropriate support, decreased episodes of involuntary voiding due to full bladder, decreased episodes of voiding associated with increased abdominal pressure, adequate management of irreversible incontinence to prevent spillage, ability to hold increased volume of urine, absence of social isolation, improved self-esteem, absence of skin breakdown due to urine, and absence of urinary tract infection.

INTERVENTIONS

KNOWLEDGE DEFICIT

Patient and caregiver education are key elements in the management of urinary incontinence. Often the nurse must overcome the assumption that the condition is not treatable, especially in frail, elderly people. The nurse stresses that improvement or correction is possible for most people. The patient who has been incontinent may be very discouraged and unwilling to try retraining techniques. The nurse must be positive and encouraging and praise attempts and successes. Many people believe that patients try harder if they are dressed in street clothes and are not wearing incontinence garments.

The teaching plan usually includes an overview of normal urination, explanation of the type of incontinence the patient is experiencing, and detailed explanations of the prescribed treatment. Verbal information should be supplemented with written material. The patient is told that improvement takes time—immediate results are not expected. The nurse praises the patient's interest in working toward continence, adherence to the prescribed treatment, and successful voiding. Specific methods of improving continence were identified under Common Therapeutic Measures. The appropriate methods for managing various types of incontinence are emphasized in the next section.

INCONTINENCE

Nursing interventions for various types of incontinence overlap. Therefore, interventions are discussed in general terms here. Table 21–2 summarizes the treatments for each type of incontinence.

Bladder Training or Retraining

Bladder training or retraining may be recommended for stress and urge incontinence. The nurse teaches the patient (and caregiver if appropriate) the basic principles of bladder training. A schedule for voiding every 2 to 3 hours is established. The patient is not usually asked to get up during the night, so pads or an external collection device may be needed during sleep. The nurse emphasizes the importance of the patient trying to delay voiding until the scheduled time. The nurse praises the patient's efforts and encourages the caregiver to do so as well.

Habit Training

If habit training is prescribed, the nurse may initiate an incontinence record to help establish the schedule for timed voiding (Fig. 21–4). The nurse or other caregiver must then remind the patient to try to void at the scheduled times. It might be argued that the nurse rather than the patient is being trained. This is true to some extent, but in many cases the patient is able to take responsibility for toileting on the prescribed schedule and remain continent.

If the patient has difficulty voiding at the scheduled time, the nurse tries to stimulate voiding. Measures to promote voiding include comfortable position, privacy, and use of specific stimuli. Stimuli that may encourage voiding include stroking the inner thigh, pouring warm water over the perineum, and drinking water while on the toilet.

INCONTINENCE MONITORING RECORD

INSTRUCTIONS: EACH TIME THE PATIENT IS CHECKED:
1) Mark *one* of the circles in the BLADDER section at the hour closest to the time the patient is checked.
2) Make an X in the BOWEL section if the patient has had an incontinent or normal bowel movement.

● = Incontinent, small amount ∅ = Dry X = Incontinent BOWEL
● = Incontinent, large amount △ = Voided correctly X = Normal BOWEL

PATIENT NAME ____________________ ROOM # __________ DATE __________

	BLADDER			BOWEL			
	INCONTINENT OF URINE	DRY	VOIDED CORRECTLY	INCONTINENT X	NORMAL X	INITIALS	COMMENTS
12 am	● ●	○	△ cc ____				
1	● ●	○	△ cc ____				
2	● ●	○	△ cc ____				
3	● ●	○	△ cc ____				
4	● ●	○	△ cc ____				
5	● ●	○	△ cc ____				
6	● ●	○	△ cc ____				
7	● ●	○	△ cc ____				
8	● ●	○	△ cc ____				
9	● ●	○	△ cc ____				
10	● ●	○	△ cc ____				
11	● ●	○	△ cc ____				
12 pm	● ●	○	△ cc ____				
1	● ●	○	△ cc ____				
2	● ●	○	△ cc ____				
3	● ●	○	△ cc ____				
4	● ●	○	△ cc ____				
5	● ●	○	△ cc ____				
6	● ●	○	△ cc ____				
7	● ●	○	△ cc ____				
8	● ●	○	△ cc ____				
9	● ●	○	△ cc ____				
10	● ●	○	△ cc ____				
11	● ●	○	△ cc ____				
TOTALS:							

FIGURE 21-4

An incontinence record. (From Greengold, B. A., & Ouslander, J. [1986]. Bladder retraining. *Journal of Gerontological Nursing, 12*[6], 31–35.)

Fluid intake may be spaced at 2-hour intervals to provide regular filling of the bladder. Nighttime wetness can be reduced by limiting fluids after 7 P.M. Patients or their caregivers sometime decrease fluid intake to reduce urinary incontinence. This makes it harder to schedule toileting and can lead to other problems (urinary tract infection, urinary calculi). Most references recommend 2000 to 3000 ml of fluid daily unless contraindicated. If a patient has cardiovascular or renal disease, the physician is consulted about the ideal fluid intake. Fluid intake is increased gradually for older patients as they often do not adapt well to rapid changes in blood volume.

SOCIAL ISOLATION

The person with urinary incontinence may curtail social activities out of fear of embarrassing accidents. Also, access to toilets in public places is often limited, so patients who cannot delay voiding may be afraid to venture far from home. If continence is unlikely or not yet established, a variety of incontinence products are available that may permit the patient to venture out without fear of wetness or odor. Specially designed pads and undergarments as well as some external urine collection devices may be used. As was mentioned earlier, external collection devices are more readily available and more satisfactory for men than for women. The patient can also be encouraged to maintain the voiding schedule during the social outing. If the patient has an incontinent episode, the nurse is careful not to express disapproval.

SITUATIONAL LOW SELF-ESTEEM

The ability to control elimination is an important childhood accomplishment. Adults who are incontinent may be so embarrassed that they are reluctant to tell anyone about it. Nurses often discover that a newly admitted patient has concealed incontinence from family and physician. Some older people do not seek help for incontinence because they think it is caused by old age and cannot be corrected.

The nurse helps patients learn to manage incontinence and to see that it is not a barrier to achieving a full life. The nurse's attitude toward the patient and toward incontinence influences how the patient deals with the change in body function. Caregivers must be commmited to efforts to help patients avoid incontinence. The situation described below should not be allowed to happen:

> A partially paralyzed nursing home patient called out, "I need to go to the bathroom!" A busy nursing staff member rushed by, patted her on the hand, and said, "That's all right. You have a diaper on. Go ahead and pee."

The nurse encourages the patient to attend to dress and grooming to promote a more positive self-image. By taking an active role in carrying out the treatment plan, the patient may feel less helpless and better able to cope with incontinence. Caregivers are also advised not to refer to incontinence pads and undergarments as "diapers" because of that term's association with infants.

IMPAIRED SKIN INTEGRITY

A major problem for the incontinent patient is the risk of skin breakdown. Urine and feces, if left in contact with the skin, cause a rash. Continuous moisture causes the skin to lose its oily protective barrier. Skin breakdown may follow. The key to preventing breakdown is to keep the skin clean, dry, and free of urine or feces. If a patient is incontinent and unable to report voiding, the nurse checks hourly for wetness. Wet garments and linens are removed immediately. The skin is washed with soap and warm water, rinsed, and gently patted dry. The genitals, perineum, thighs, and buttocks are inspected for redness and skin breakdown. Protective creams may be applied as ordered or according to agency policy. If breakdown does occur, the nurse notifies the physician and provides treatment as ordered or according to agency policy.

HIGH RISK FOR INFECTION

The patient who is incontinent of urine is at risk for urinary tract infection and urinary calculi (stones). These complications are most likely to occur in patients who retain urine and in those who restrict their fluids. Retained urine is a good medium for bacterial growth, and the overstretched bladder wall is susceptible to infection. Patients may restrict fluid intake to try to reduce the frequency of incontinence. Concentrated urine is a risk factor for infections and calculi. Patients with indwelling catheters are at even greater risk for urinary tract infections.

The risk of urinary tract infection can be reduced by emptying the bladder as scheduled, providing adequate fluids, and using strict aseptic technique during catheterization. The perineal area must also be kept clean. The nurse encourages the intake of 2000 to 3000 ml of fluid daily unless contraindicated. Details of catheter care are covered in Chapter 36.

EVALUATION

Successful nursing outcomes are determined by patient's description of condition and participation in treatment plan, decreased episodes of incontinent voiding (for reversible incontinence), satisfactory management of irreversible incontinence (for irreversible incontinence), patient's participation in usual social activities, patient's demonstration of positive self-image (confidence, pride in appearance), intact skin without redness or breakdown, and normal body temperature and white blood cell count.

FECAL INCONTINENCE

Fecal incontinence is less common than urinary incontinence, but it can be very distressing for patients who are affected by it.

PHYSIOLOGY OF DEFECATION

The structures that maintain bowel control are the internal and external sphincters and the puborectal muscle. The muscles of the pelvic floor and the external sphincter are under voluntary control (Fig. 21–5). The bowel has its own nerve network that stimulates peristalsis when it is distended. Therefore, disorders of the central nervous system and spinal cord do not impair bowel control as much as they do bladder control.

The fecal mass enters the rectum by mass movement. The presence of feces in the rectum creates a desire to defecate. Defecation occurs when the anal sphincter

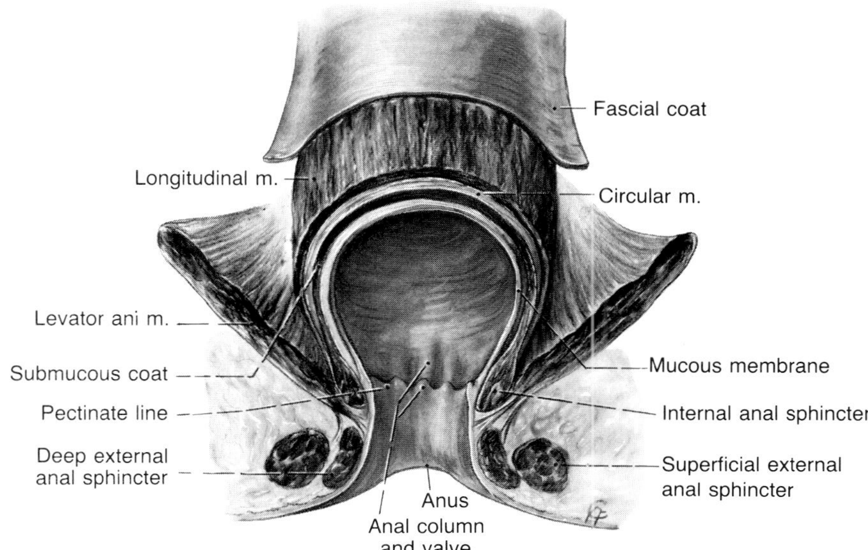

FIGURE 21-5

The anal sphincters and musculature. (Modified from Jacob, S. W., & Francone, C. A. [1989]. *Elements of anatomy and physiology* [2nd ed.]. Philadelphia: W. B. Saunders.)

relaxes and the rectum contracts. Tightening of the diaphragm and abdominal muscles promotes defecation by increasing pressure in the abdomen. If defecation does not occur soon after this pressure is felt, the sensation of needing to defecate soon fades. People who often ignore or delay defecation tend to become constipated.

DIAGNOSTIC TESTS AND PROCEDURES

Evaluation of fecal incontinence may include assessment of rectal sphincter tone, laboratory examination of a stool specimen for blood or pathogens, and endoscopic or radiologic procedures to detect underlying problems. Diagnostic tests and procedures for the gastrointestinal system are presented in detail in Chapter 34.

COMMON THERAPEUTIC MEASURES

ENEMAS

Enemas may be necessary to stimulate emptying of the bowel. Various types of enemas and nursing considerations are discussed in Chapter 34. In general, frequent use of large-volume enemas is not advised because it overstretches the bowel and contributes to loss of muscle tone. Sometimes, however, enemas are necessary. The patient with poor rectal sphincter tone may have difficulty retaining enema solutions. An adapter can be placed on the enema tubing and inserted into the anus. The nipple-like adapter helps the patient retain the solution.

POUCHES

Plastic pouches, much like ostomy bags, may be applied to the perianal area and held in place with adhesive. They are helpful for patients who have frequent stools. Because they are bulky and uncomfortable, they are not usually used on ambulatory patients. Another disadvantage is the skin irritation caused by the adhesive. When the pouch is changed, meticulous skin care should be provided. An alternative to the pouch is an adult incontinent brief or (for bed patients) linen protectors.

DRUG THERAPY

Types of drugs employed to treat fecal incontinence include laxatives, stool softeners, and antidiarrheal drugs. These drugs are discussed in Chapter 34.

BIOFEEDBACK

Patients who are motivated and able to follow directions and whose external anal sphincter is capable of responding to rectal distention may achieve bowel control with biofeedback. A balloon is inserted into the rectum and inflated. A manometer creates a tracing of the normal response of the sphincter to rectal pressure. The patient tries to consciously reproduce the pattern by contracting the muscles that delay defecation. The size of the balloon is progressively decreased to help the patient recognize and respond to the amount of rectal distention expected with normal stool volume. Biofeedback has been effective for many patients but has not proved useful for patients with fecal incontinence associated with diabetes, spinal cord injury, rectal trauma, or radiation injury.

TYPES OF FECAL INCONTINENCE

There are four types of fecal incontinence: overflow, anorectal, neurogenic, and symptomatic. Table 21–5 summarizes the features of each type.

OVERFLOW INCONTINENCE

DESCRIPTION. Fecal overflow incontinence is caused by constipation in which the rectum is constantly distended. The fecal mass backs up until the entire colon is full. There may or may not be a fecal impaction. The patient passes semisolid stools frequently. This condition may be related to a long-standing dependence on laxatives or enemas.

MEDICAL TREATMENT. Medical management of fecal overflow incontinence is concerned with the immediate relief of the constipation and the long-term control of the problem. The first step is to cleanse the colon. Phosphate enemas and suppositories may be ordered to empty the rectum. Daily enemas for 7 to 10 days are then needed to empty the entire colon. Instead of the enemas, the physician may order oral laxatives such as bisacodyl or mannitol. If hard masses of stool are present, they can be softened with oil retention enemas and then removed digitally.

Once the colon has been cleansed, regular evacuation is essential. Increased fluids and fiber may be helpful, but some patients require regular aids to elimination. The physician may order enemas or suppositories twice a week or daily laxatives. For elderly patients, senna or lactulose is preferred by many geriatric specialists. Mineral oil should be avoided because it interferes with absorption of fat-soluble vitamins and because it may be aspirated, causing lipid pneumonia. Phenolphthalein is also not recommended for long-term therapy because it can cause fluid and electrolyte disturbances (hypokalemia, hypocalcemia, metabolic acidosis, or metabolic alkalosis).

NEUROGENIC INCONTINENCE

DESCRIPTION. Many people report having a bowel movement shortly after the first meal of the day. This is due to the gastrocolic reflex. When food enters the stomach, it stimulates activity throughout the digestive tract and causes the movement of the fecal mass into the rectum. Patients who do not voluntarily delay defecation are said to have neurogenic incontinence. This occurs most often in dementia patients. These patients usually have one or two formed stools daily after meals.

MEDICAL TREATMENT. Neurogenic incontinence is usually treated with scheduled toileting based on the patient's usual time of defecation. If this is not successful, some physicians order a constipating drug (such as codeine) each morning and a laxative (senna or milk of magnesia) each night. This routine results in a controlled bowel movement each morning and avoids later accidents. It does not, however, correct the underlying problem.

SYMPTOMATIC INCONTINENCE

DESCRIPTION. Symptomatic incontinence is the result of colorectal disease. These patients usually have incontinence with diarrhea. Blood or mucus may be seen in the stool.

MEDICAL TREATMENT. When a patient has symptomatic incontinence, medical care should be sought to identify and treat the cause.

TABLE 21–5
TYPES OF FECAL INCONTINENCE

TYPE	DESCRIPTION	CAUSES	NURSING CARE
Overflow	Uncontrolled, frequent passage of small semisoft stools Fecal impaction may be present	Constipation in which entire colon is full of fecal matter	Administer laxatives and enemas as ordered Increase fluids and fiber as appropriate
Anorectal	Uncontrolled passage of stool several times a day	Weak pelvic muscles Loss of anal reflexes Poor rectal sphincter tone Rectal prolapse	Teach Kegel exercises Prepare for surgery, if planned
Neurogenic	Formed stools are passed after meals Usually seen in dementia patients	Gastrocolic reflex stimulates defecation Patient does not delay until appropriate time	Scheduled toileting
Symptomatic	Incontinent stools, usually diarrhea Not related to other types of fecal incontinence	Colon or rectal disease	Comfort measures; skin care Prepare for diagnostic tests and procedures

ANORECTAL INCONTINENCE

DESCRIPTION. Anorectal incontinence is associated with nerve damage that causes the muscles of the pelvic floor to be weak. There may be rectal abnormalities including loss of anal reflex and loss of anal sphincter tone. Patients typically have several incontinent stools a day.

MEDICAL TREATMENT. Anorectal incontinence is treated with pelvic muscle exercises and sometimes biofeedback. If these techniques are ineffective, surgical repair may be advised, most commonly postanal repair.

NURSING ASSESSMENT OF THE PATIENT WITH FECAL INCONTINENCE

A thorough nursing assessment can help diagnose the type and cause of fecal incontinence and guide the selection of treatment.

HEALTH HISTORY

CHIEF COMPLAINT. When a patient has fecal incontinence, the nurse assesses usual bowel pattern, changes, stool characteristics, and related symptoms such as pain or cramping.

BOWEL PATTERN. Bowel patterns are usually well established in the adult. The frequency of bowel movements may range from several times daily to several times a week. The nurse documents the patient's usual frequency of bowel movements. In relation to incontinent episodes, the nurse asks if the patient is aware of the need to defecate. For dementia patients, a caregiver may be able to detect clues that the patient is about to have a bowel movement. If the patient is confused, the nurse may need to initiate a record of times and circumstances when defecation occurs.

CHARACTERISTICS OF STOOLS. The nurse assesses the consistency, color, and constituents of the patient's stools. Terms used to describe consistency include liquid, watery, pasty, tarry, semiformed, formed, and hard. Most of these terms are self-explanatory. Tarry is used to describe stools that are shiny, sticky, and black. Stool is normally brown in color. Abnormal colors are black, red, green, and white. Abnormal stool constituents might include blood, mucus, or undigested food.

PAST MEDICAL HISTORY. The nurse documents chronic illnessses, past acute illnesses, and surgeries or trauma to the abdomen or rectum. Neurologic conditions including stroke, spinal cord injury, and dementia are significant. Recent current medications and all allergies are listed. It is especially important to determine the use of laxatives, enemas, or suppositories. Because these are often purchased without a prescription, the patient may not mention them when reporting medications. An obstetric history is recorded, including number of pregnancies, types of deliveries, and complications of childbirth.

REVIEW OF SYSTEMS. The review of systems identifies problems that may be related to fecal incontinence such as motor, sensory, or cognitive impairments.

FUNCTIONAL ASSESSMENT. The functional assessment focuses on habits that may be related to bowel function, including diet, fluid intake, and exercise or activity pattern. Recent travel to other countries may be significant, as travelers sometimes acquire uncommon intestinal infections.

PHYSICAL EXAMINATION

The nurse inspects and palpates the abdomen for distention and auscultates for bowel sounds. The perianal area is inspected for irritation or breakdown. The physician or nurse practitioner may perform a rectal examination and test the strength of the rectal sphincter.

Assessment of the patient with fecal incontinence is outlined in Table 21–6.

NURSING DIAGNOSIS AND GOALS

Nursing diagnoses for the patient with fecal incontinence may include the following:

- **Bowel Incontinence** related to impaction, cognitive impairment, neurologic impairment, environmental barriers, or impaired mobility
- **Impaired Skin Integrity** related to contact of feces with skin
- **Situational Low Self-Esteem** related to loss of control over elimination

TABLE 21-6
ASSESSMENT OF THE PATIENT WITH FECAL INCONTINENCE

HEALTH HISTORY

Chief complaint: bowel pattern changes, stool characteristics (consistency, color, constituents), awareness of need to defecate, symptoms associated with passage of incontinent stool

Past medical history: chronic illnesses, past acute illnesses, abdominal or rectal trauma or surgery, abdominal radiotherapy, recent and current medications, allergies

Review of systems: motor, sensory, or cognitive dysfunction that could affect continence

Functional assessment: diet, fluid intake, exercise or activity pattern, foreign travel

PHYSICAL EXAMINATION

Abdomen: distention, bowel sounds

Perianal area: irritation, breakdown

Goals for nursing care of the patient with fecal incontinence are controlled bowel elimination, absence of skin breakdown, and improved self-esteem.

INTERVENTIONS

BOWEL INCONTINENCE

Continued assessment is an essential part of the nurse's role in caring for the patient with incontinence. Documentation of the patient's usual bowel pattern provides a guideline for scheduled elimination and for setting realistic goals. To establish a bowel program, the patient is taken to the toilet at the usual time of defecation, usually 30 minutes after eating. If suppositories or enemas are ordered, the nurse administers them and documents the results.

When enemas or laxatives are prescribed on a routine basis for overflow incontinence, the nurse may fear creating laxative or enema dependency. For these patients, however, normal bowel function may not be a realistic goal. They may do better with a program that promotes regular bowel evacuation. It is far better than the miserable process of emptying a full colon every few weeks.

The nurse explains normal bowel physiology and interventions for incontinence to the patient. The patient is advised to consume adequate fluids and fiber to prevent constipation and impaction. A fluid intake of 2000 ml per day is recommended if not contraindicated. Fluids are increased gradually in the elderly patient because fluid overload can lead to heart failure. The nurse and dietician teach the patient that fresh fruits and vegetables provide bulk and fiber that keep the stool moist and soft. Ambulation is encouraged if the patient is able to walk. If perineal exercises are prescribed, the nurse advises the patient to practice contracting the muscles that control defecation. The contraction should be held up to 10 seconds and repeated several times each day.

IMPAIRED SKIN INTEGRITY

After each incontinent stool, the patient's perianal area is cleaned thoroughly. Protective creams or ointments may be applied as ordered or per agency policy. Incontinence undergarments may be needed to prevent soiling and embarrassment, but they must be checked frequently so that stool does not remain in contact with the skin. Fecal pouches may be used, but the adhesive and plastic can irritate the skin, so that good skin care is still a priority.

SITUATIONAL LOW SELF-ESTEEM

Loss of bowel control can be devastating for the patient. The nurse expresses understanding of the patient's distress and encourages the patient to strive for as much improvement as possible. The patient is praised for participation in the treatment program and for decreased frequency of incontinent stools. The nurse encourages the patient to practice good grooming and to resume social activities. The social schedule can be coordinated with the patient's bowel program.

EVALUATION

Criteria for goal achievement for the patient with fecal incontinence are regular bowel evacuation of soft to formed stool, intact skin without redness or breakdown, and patient's comments and behaviors reflecting a positive view of self.

BIBLIOGRAPHY

Brandeis, G. H., Valla, S. V., & Resnick, N. M. (1992). In E. Calkins, et al. (Eds.), *Practice of geriatrics* (2nd ed., pp. 220–228). Philadelphia: W. B. Saunders.

Brocklehurst, J. C. (1990). Disorders of the lower bowel. In W. B. Abrams & R. Berkow (Eds.), *The Merck manual of geriatrics* (pp. 505–521). Rahway, NJ: Merck Sharp & Dohme Research Laboratories.

Campbell, E. B., Knight, M., Benson, M., & Colling, J. (1991). Effect of an incontinence training program on nursing home staff's knowledge, attitudes, and behavior. *The Gerontologist, 31*(6), 788–794.

Hogstel, M. O., & Nelson, M. (1992). Anticipation and early detection can reduce bowel elimination complications. *Geriatric Nursing, 13*(1), 28–33.

Ignatavicius, D. D., & Bayne, M. V. (1991). *Medical-surgical nursing: A nursing process approach.* Philadelphia: W. B. Saunders.

Lyder, C. H., McCray, G., & Singh, M. K. (1992). Efficacy of condom catheters in controlling incontinence odor. *Applied Nursing Research, 5*(4).

Newman, D. K., Lynch, K., Smith, D. A., & Cell, P. (1991). Restoring urinary continence. *American Journal of Nursing, 91*(1), 28–34.

Palmer, M. H., Bone, L. R., Fahey, M., Mamom, J., & Steinwachs, D. (1992). Detecting urinary incontinence in older adults during hospitalization. *Applied Nursing Research, 5*(4).

Powers, I., & Williams, D. (1992). Urinary incontinence: Helping a patient regain control. *Nursing 92, 22*(12), 46–47.

Richter, J. E. (1990). Functional disorders of the gastrointestinal tract. In W. B. Abrams & R. Berkow (Eds.), *The Merck manual of geriatrics* (pp. 475–486). Rahway, NJ: Merck Sharp & Dohme Research Laboratories.

Scheve, A., Engle, B., McCormick, K., & Leahy, E. G. (1991). Exercise in continence. *Geriatric Nursing, 12*(3), 124.

Shlafer, M. (1993). *The nurse, pharmacology, and drug therapy* (2nd ed.). Redwood City, CA: Addison-Wesley.

U.S. Dept. of Health and Human Services (1992). *Urinary incontinence in adults.* AHCPR Publication No. 92-0038. Rockville, MD: Author.

Williams, S. G., & DePalma, J. A. (1992). Medication-induced digestive system injury in the elderly. *Geriatric Nursing, 13*(1), 39–42.

KEY CONCEPTS

1. Incontinence is the inability to control the passage of urine or feces.
2. Normal controlled voiding requires healthy bladder muscles, a patent urethra, normal transmission of nerve impulses, and mental alertness.
3. Assessment of urinary incontinence includes recording the voiding pattern, urine volume, associated signs and symptoms, medications, past medical history, and physical findings.
4. The types of urinary incontinence are transient, urge, stress, overflow, reflex, functional, and total.
5. Transient incontinence is caused by reversible conditions and is often corrected by treatment of the underlying problem.
6. Urge incontinence, involuntary loss of urine after a strong urge to void, may be corrected by treating the cause by using behavior modification and drug therapy.
7. Overflow incontinence, involuntary loss of urine associated with a full bladder, may be corrected by treating the cause (enlarged prostate) or by using drugs that stimulate the bladder and relax the internal sphincter.
8. Stress incontinence, the involuntary loss of urine during physical exertion, may be improved by strengthening the perineal muscles, by surgical intervention, or by placing an artificial sphincter.
9. Functional incontinence is inappropriate voiding despite normal urinary function.
10. Assessment of fecal incontinence includes recording the usual bowel pattern, stool characteristics, related symptoms, activity, diet, fluid intake, medications, and use of aids to elimination as well as performing an abdominal assessment.
11. Types of fecal incontinence include overflow, anorectal, neurogenic, and symptomatic.
12. Fecal overflow incontinence is caused by constipation in which the rectum is constantly distended and is treated by relieving the constipation and preventing future episodes.
13. Anorectal incontinence is caused by abnormalities in the pelvic muscle, anus, or rectum and may require pelvic floor muscle exercises or surgery.
14. Neurogenic incontinence is automatic defecation seen in people (such as dementia patients) who do not voluntarily delay defecation; it may be corrected by scheduled toileting.
15. Symptomatic incontinence results from colorectal disease and requires correction of the basic problem.
16. Nursing care of the patient who is incontinent may address measures to correct the specific type of incontinence, to maintain skin integrity, to improve situational low self-esteem, and to improve knowledge of management.
17. Techniques to restore bladder control include bladder retraining using scheduled toileting, Credé's technique for emptying the bladder, Kegel exercises to strengthen pelvic floor muscles, and reflex training.
18. Bowel training may be accomplished by scheduled toileting, stimulation techniques, or both.

Cheryl Ross Staats

CHAPTER 22

Loss, Death, and Dying

OBJECTIVES

1. Describe beliefs and practices related to death and dying.
2. Describe responses of patients and their families to terminal illness and death.
3. Identify nursing diagnoses that are appropriate for the terminally ill.
4. Identify nursing goals that are appropriate for the terminally ill.
5. Identify nursing interventions to meet the needs of terminally ill and dying patients.
6. Discuss the needs of the terminally ill patient's significant others.
7. Discuss the ways nurses can intervene to meet the needs of the terminally ill patient's significant others.
8. Explore the responses of the nurse who works with the terminally ill.
9. Explore the needs of the nurse who works with terminally ill patients.
10. Identify issues related to caring for the dying patient including advance directives, do not resuscitate decisions, brain death, organ donations, and pronouncement of death.

GLOSSARY

ADVANCE DIRECTIVE Written statement of a person's wishes regarding medical treatment

ALGOR MORTIS Cooling of the body after death

AUTOPSY Examination of a body after death to determine or confirm the cause of death

CEREBRAL DEATH Absence of cerebral cortex functioning

DENIAL A defense mechanism in which the individual thinks and behaves as if not aware of an unpleasant reality

GRIEF An emotional response to a loss

LIVOR MORTIS Discoloration of the body after death

LOSS A real or potential absence of someone or something that is valued

RIGOR MORTIS Stiffening of the body after death

SHROUD A wrap in which the body is placed after death for transport to the morgue or mortuary

A time to be born and a time to die . . .
ECCLESIASTES 3:2

Throughout history life and death have intrigued humankind. Artists, writers, philosophers, scientists, religious leaders, and ordinary people have questioned and pondered the meaning of life and death.

Human mortality and the death experience have not been a priority in American society. American society tends to be a youth- and beauty-oriented culture, generally approaching the life cycle in an unrealistic way. Death is a real part of life, just as birth and aging are.

The concepts of death and dying were studied rarely before the 1960s. Many times patients who were not expected to survive were placed in isolated hospital areas and were given less than quality care. Many patients who were dying went without appropriate care and technically could have been termed *abandoned* by the medical profession. Family members, church associates, or both more often than not were the care providers.

Today, with the reality of the "graying of America" and the increasing number of persons with acquired immunodeficiency syndrome (AIDS), the aging process, terminal illness, and dying are not viewed as the taboo topics that they once were. The specialized needs of the dying and the terminally ill are no longer ignored nor are they denied. The processes associated with dying and death are researched by scientists, health care professionals, theologians, and lay persons. Information concerning death and dying can be found in popular literature and in open discussions, as well as in professional literature.

This chapter presents information concerning the death process in persons for whom death is imminent. The grieving process for the dying person and the person's friends and family is presented with a special emphasis on nursing care.

CONCEPT OF LOSS

Death, like birth, is a natural part of the life cycle. Death favors no age, social, religious, economic, or racial groups. It is inevitable for everyone. People in general experience similar feelings and thoughts related to loss, whether the loss is real or potential.

Loss may be defined as a real or potential absence of someone or something that is valued. Real losses occur when something actually happens so that valued people or articles no longer are available. Potential losses relate to an individual's perceptions of what might occur if a valued person or object were lost permanently. Anxiety, fear, and grief are common with both real and potential losses. An example of a potential loss is a 45-year-old woman, pregnant for the first time, who is concerned that her infant may be born with congenital disabilities.

TYPES OF LOSSES

Loss is experienced in many ways. Changes in self-image, developmental changes, loss of possessions, and loss of significant others are common types of loss.

Change in Self-Image

In addition to a perception of self, within each individual's life, ideas about personal worth, usefulness, roles, and beliefs are created. Each aspect of the person may be subject to change. Some change is planned. Some change is beyond the individual's control. Situations that lead to a perceived change in body image, such as pregnancy, hair loss, disability, or radical surgery can alter a person's self-concept. New parenthood and forced retirement often lead to lifestyle changes. These changes include uncertainty about roles, functions, and usual patterns of productivity. The uncertainties and insecurities in role changes result in perceived loss in terms of former roles.

Developmental Changes

Within the life cycle, changes or milestones take place. Insecurities, fears, and feelings of loss result. During infancy and childhood, parents experience a loss of control over their children as children gain independence and self-control. Examples of increasingly independent function are weaning, toileting, walking, talking, and attending school.

As maturation progresses, additional changes take place. As they grow into adulthood, individuals may relate loss to changes in routines that were previously secure and dependable. These changes include moving away from parents, getting a job, and a general loss of dependence and innocence.

Multiple losses can occur throughout the life span. Frequently the losses associated with old age happen rapidly. Age-related physical and body function changes and return to dependence lead to a loss of self-concept in addition to the developmental loss. Dying and death at any age challenge the individual with multiple, successive losses.

Loss of Possessions

Loss of valued possessions may affect the individual. Generally, a possession has a perceived value to the owner, and its value may not be readily apparent to others. An object may be irreplaceable because of the memories associated with it, or it may be valuable from a monetary standpoint. Loss of an appointment calendar may be as tragic as the loss of a family heirloom. The loss of a pet can affect the owner as significantly as the loss of a family member.

For aged persons, the loss of a lifetime's accumulation of possessions through placement into housing for the elderly can be devastating. When a significant object is lost or left behind, the individual loses a part of his or her identity.

Loss of Significant Others

Loss of significant others occurs through death but may also occur through separation, growth of children, change of residence, divorce, or lack of communication.

Separation from significant others may be related to actual distance, or it may be emotional in nature. Children leaving their parents to go to school or to start their own families can produce feelings of loss for all concerned. Placement of a family member in an institution for long-term care or acute care can lead to prolonged separation and feelings of loss.

Emotional aspects of loss of significant others may be related to a lack of fulfillment of expected roles. Feelings of disappointment for persons who have remained unmarried or who have not had children can lead to perceptions of loss. Communication breakdowns or barriers can divide significant others as completely as changing their place of residence.

The loss of a loved one through death is a permanent loss. In nonindustrialized societies death is looked on as a natural, normal event. In American society death is frequently seen as a negative and unacceptable event. This society values preserving and prolonging life. Americans expect to live into old age, even if old age is not considered as attractive as youth.

A death by accident or by unexpected illness is related to a specific situation. Loss that occurs during normal development can be anticipated and possibly prepared for, such as children leaving home or retirement and death of aging friends and family members.

No matter who or what is lost, those left behind react to the event. Not all people react in the same fashion to similar situations.

GRIEF

Grief is a normal, natural response to a loss. It is an emotional reaction that is necessary to maintain quality in both emotional and physical well-being. The grieving process involves a total individual experience associated with thoughts, feelings, and behaviors. The grief process is usually most profound when the loss experienced is death. In particular, grieving during a death loss is a complex and intense emotional experience.

In conjunction with grief, significant others who survive respond to the loss of the loved one through bereavement. Bereavement is the individualized response to the loss of a significant person.

The grief process or working through the grief process helps the dying person and the significant others adapt to the loss. Grief that is helpful or that assists the person in accepting the reality of death is called *adaptive grief*. Grief that is prolonged, unresolved, or disruptive to the experiencing person may be termed *maladaptive* or *dysfunctional grief*.

Adaptive grief is a healthy response. It may be associated with grieving before a death actually occurs or when the reality that death is inevitable is known. This adaptive response is termed *anticipatory grief*. Anticipatory grief is usually related to a loss or death. It may be a healthy or an unhealthy response to the grief process. Both the patient and the family members can experience anticipatory grieving. After an actual loss or a death occurs, the grief is considered to be reactive. That is, with *reactive grief* the loss has already happened.

Grief that is delayed or exaggerated may be identified as dysfunctional. Dysfunctional grieving may relate to a real loss or a perceived loss. It may occur in the absence of anticipatory grief, when grief is not resolved from a prior experience, or when the expression of grief is blocked in some way. Within dysfunctional grief, feelings and behaviors may become exaggerated and disruptive to a person's typical lifestyle.

Specific behaviors are associated with dysfunctional grief. Many times there are expressions of distress at the loss. Unresolved issues may be identified and past experiences reviewed. Emotions such as anger, sadness, guilt, and denial may be present in all types of grief. Some people have difficulty expressing these feelings. The person experiencing grief may show signs of changes in eating, sleeping, and other activities of daily living.

THE GRIEVING PROCESS

People experiencing the inevitability of the final loss, death, are in need of caregivers who are knowledgeable about personal attitudes that affect the experience. The attitudes of the dying person, those of the significant others, and the nurse's own attitudes affect the death experience.

The nurse must be able to understand various aspects of the dying person's life to provide appropriate care. An adequate understanding of cultural, religious, familial, and developmental influences is beneficial in focusing on the dying person's needs, wants, and fears. Although there may be influences from culture, religion, family, and stages of development, the uniqueness of each person causes responses to vary.

Culture, religious beliefs, and age affect a person's understanding and reaction to death or loss. Frequently, beliefs and attitudes are interrelated between culture and religion. The American work ethic is closely related to the Protestant ethic, which tends to believe in independence, self-reliance, hard work, and rugged individualism. With these attitudes, many people believe that privacy is imperative. Death and dying tend to be private matters shared only with significant others. Oftentimes, feelings are repressed or internalized. People who believe in "toughing it out" or "being strong" may not express themselves when they have experienced a tragic loss.

Some cultural groups such as African Americans and Latinos may express their feelings more easily. In some predominantly African American churches, expressing emotions plays an important role. Kinship tends to be very strong within the Latino culture. Family members, both immediate and extended, provide support for one another. Expressing feelings of loss is encouraged and accepted easily.

Religious beliefs influence a person's reaction to loss and death. Most religious groups have common practices related to dying and death. Practices and beliefs vary from group to group regarding dying and the care of the body after death. Specific information should be obtained from the family concerning religious preferences.

Family beliefs and practices and family members' stages of development are responsible for attitudes surrounding death and dying. Past experience with facing the death of a loved one provides a frame of reference for members of the family. The past abilities of persons to adapt and accept losses can help them adapt to the death of a loved one.

The age or stage of development affects a person's reactions to death and dying. Through experience with other losses, a generalized acceptance of dying can take place. Maturity contributes toward understanding and accepting death. Table 22–1 presents some common age-related attitudes associated with death.

Children have a different understanding of loss and death from that of adults. Some adults believe that children should be protected from the pain associated with the death of a loved one. Oftentimes, however, children who are "protected" may feel abandoned, frightened, and alone with their feelings. A child who loses a loved one to death may regress or be delayed in emotional development until the grief can be resolved.

Adults generally become experienced in accepting the inevitability of death. During adulthood, people must come to terms with the death of their parents and other older family members. Coping with the death of one's parents is often identified as a developmental crisis. During adulthood people have to confront their own mortality.

For elderly adults, the impact from the death of a spouse is profound. Elderly adults may also outlive their children. Loss of one's child at any age is an especially traumatic event. With the increase in the elderly population, it stands to reason that the majority of deaths are among the elderly. Richter pointed to what seems to be an increase in health problems for widowed persons during the first year of widowhood. Elderly adults comprise the largest group of people requiring health care services, so it is imperative that nurses be sensitive to their individual needs concerning loss.

STAGES OF GRIEVING

Many researchers have identified stages of grief. Among them are Kübler-Ross and Martocchio.

TABLE 22–1
AGE-RELATED BELIEFS TOWARD DEATH

AGE RANGE	BELIEFS
Infancy to 5 yr (preschool)	• Little or no understanding of death • Death is temporary and reversible like sleep
6 to 9 yr (school age)	• Death is final • Own death can be avoided • Death is related to violence • Wishing or hoping for death can make it happen
10 to 12 yr (preadolescent)	• Death is an inevitable end to life • Grasps own mortality by discussing fear of death or life after death • Expresses feelings of death based on adult attitudes
13 to 18 yr (adolescent)	• Afraid of prolonged death • May act out defiance for death through dangerous or self-destructive acts • Has a philosophic or religious approach to death • Seldom thinks about death
19 to 45 yr (young adulthood)	• Cultural and religious beliefs influence attitudes • Death is seen as a future event
46 to 65 yr (middle adulthood)	• Accepts own mortality as inevitable • Faces death of parents and peers • May experience death anxiety
65 yr and older (older adulthood)	• Afraid of prolonged health problems • Faces death of family members and peers • Sees death as inevitable • Examines death as it relates to various meanings, such as freedom from discomfort

Kübler-Ross

One of the most prominent and popular authors is Kübler-Ross, who in 1969 identified five stages of grieving. The five stages are denial, anger, bargaining, depression, and acceptance. The stages represent a series of responses to an anticipated or actual loss. Kübler-Ross identified specific behaviors for each stage.

DENIAL. The person refuses to acknowledge the loss and may put forth a cheerful appearance to prolong the denial of the loss. Denial serves to protect the patient, family, or both from the reality of the loss.

ANGER. The patient or family members may become angry or outraged with situations. The anger and resentment may be a result of a comparison between their sadness and the happiness of others. The anger may be directed toward the nurse, the staff, or the institution as well as toward significant others.

BARGAINING. In the bargaining stage, the person wishes for more time to avoid the loss. The individual may express feelings that the loss is occurring as a punishment for past actions and may try to bargain with a higher power to gain time.

DEPRESSION. The patient may speak openly or may withdraw from feelings concerning past losses. The patient needs to review his or her life. In this stage, the person realizes that the loss is final and that the situation cannot be altered.

ACCEPTANCE. The patient identifies the loss as inevitable and may want to make plans. Acceptance can involve peaceful acknowledgment of the loss. There is a sense of inner resolution of the loss.

The stages may alternate with the individual and the situation. Not all people experience all stages, and there is no predictable timetable for the stages to occur.

Martocchio

In 1985 Martocchio presented five clusters of grief. These five clusters include shock and disbelief; yearning and protest; anguish, disorganization, and despair; identification in bereavement; and reorganization and restitution.

SHOCK AND DISBELIEF. Persons may feel numb. Feelings of anger, sadness, or guilt may be expressed. Denial may be present.

YEARNING AND PROTEST. Anger may be directed toward God, health care providers, survivors, and even toward the deceased for dying. Surviving loved ones may withdraw into themselves, not wishing to share their feelings.

ANGUISH, DISORGANIZATION, AND DESPAIR. There may be a decreased interest in the future. Decision making is difficult. Survivors may express a general lack of purpose for living. Crying at this stage is common.

IDENTIFICATION IN BEREAVEMENT. Behaviors unique to the deceased such as habits, traits, or goals may be imitated by the survivors.

REORGANIZATION AND RESTITUTION. Grieving does not simply stop all at once. Typical patterns of life gradually return. No timetable can be set for the process of grieving. Some people seem to recover from grief quickly, whereas others may experience recurrent grief throughout their lives.

A comparison of Kübler-Ross's stages of grief and Martocchio's clusters of grief is found in Table 22–2.

TABLE 22-2
COMPARISON OF STAGES OF GRIEVING

KÜBLER-ROSS (1969)	MARTOCCHIO (1985)
Denial	Shock and disbelief
Anger/Bargaining	Yearning and protest
Depression	Anguish, disorganization, and despair
	Identification of bereavement
Acceptance	Reorganization and restitution

COMMON SIGNS AND SYMPTOMS OF GRIEF

Common signs and symptoms of grief are shared by the terminally ill person and those who lose a significant other. Knowledge of the signs and symptoms enables the nurse to better communicate with everyone involved.

Physical symptoms are experienced during the grief process. The physical symptoms are a reaction to stress. Some symptoms include tightness in the chest, sensations of shortness of breath, suffocation, generalized weakness, intense tightening in the abdomen, and emptiness or churning in the stomach. These symptoms may fluctuate throughout the grief process. Generally, they may occur with the initial acknowledgment of death as the outcome. The patient and the family members may experience the symptoms of a stress reaction.

The nurse should be aware that the stress reaction is a very real experience. Nursing intervention may be needed to assist a person in regaining a sense of physical function.

Awareness of Terminal Illness

Awareness of terminal illness and impending death affects the dying person and the family emotionally and physiologically. Strauss and Glaser have identified three states of awareness: closed awareness, mutual pretense, and open awareness.

CLOSED AWARENESS. When closed awareness occurs, the family and the patient recognize that the patient is ill. They may not understand the severity of the illness. There is a lack of awareness related to impending death.

MUTUAL PRETENSE. With mutual pretense, the patient, the loved ones, and the care providers know of the terminal prognosis. No one discusses the issue openly and may make every effort to avoid the subject. Frequently the patient avoids the subject to protect the family and the caregivers from discomfort.

OPEN AWARENESS. Most health care providers prefer open awareness in most situations. With open awareness, the patient and others involved freely discuss the impending death. The discussions may be difficult, but they allow the patient and the family to become comfortable with the topic. The patient can participate in making final arrangements for personal business. Open awareness is not necessarily appropriate for all people. Some people are unable emotionally to cope with an open, honest discussion of death.

Generally, honesty is the best choice in dealing with death. Many times ethical dilemmas occur over whether to "tell" the patient about the terminal illness and impending death. At times the physician may decide not to tell the patient about the expected outcome of the illness or disease. The decision may be the physician's alone or it may be based on family wishes. More often than not, the patient knows the prognosis even if he or she is not told directly. If such is the case, the patient may feel distrustful and suspicious of the care providers and the family. This suspicion can be a source of great discomfort for the patient.

Honesty in most cases provides patients with the opportunity to accept their fate. Through understanding of the illness and participation in their own care, patients can work through and take control of their grief.

FEARS ASSOCIATED WITH TERMINAL ILLNESS AND DEATH

Fear is a typical feeling associated with dying. The nurse is frequently called on to deal with the dying person's fears. Williams identified three specific fears associated with dying. They are fear of pain, fear of loneliness, and fear of meaninglessness.

Fear of Pain

There is a tendency to associate death with pain. Common sayings such as "on pain of death" or "a violent death" have colored the way we perceive death. A dying person who has lost a loved one to a painful death may expect the same type of experience. Subsequently many people assume that pain always accompanies death.

Physiologically, there is no absolute indication that death is always painful. Psychologically, pain may occur based on the anxieties and separations related to the loss through dying.

Terminally ill patients who do experience physical pain should have medication available when it is needed. The patient and family need assurance that medication is available and will be given promptly when it is needed. Patients can participate in their own pain relief by discussing pain relief measures and their effects. Most patients want their pain relieved without the side effects of grogginess or sleepiness. Pain relief measures such as medication need not deprive the patient of the ability to interact with others.

Prevention of pain and relief from discomfort should be handled with compassion. Pain control must be consistent. It is necessary to provide constant relief rather than to wait until the pain is unbearable and then try to relieve it. Addiction to narcotics is of little concern when dealing with the terminally ill patient. When death is inevitable, nursing interventions are aimed at maintaining comfort rather than promoting wellness. Pain management is discussed in Chapter 16.

PHARMACOLOGY CAPSULE

The terminally ill patient should not be denied pain relief measures. Pain relief is best achieved by scheduled administration of analgesics rather than administration as necessary.

Fear of Loneliness

Most terminally ill and dying people do not want to be alone. Many are afraid that they will be abandoned by loved ones who cannot cope with imminent death. Dying patients typically want someone that they know and trust to stay with them. It may be a loved one or a caregiver. The simple presence of someone provides support and comfort. Neither words nor actions are necessary unless the patient requires something. Holding hands, touching, and listening are quality nursing responses. Simply providing companionship allows the dying person a sense of security.

Fear of Meaninglessness

During the dying process most people review their lives. They review their intentions during life, examining actions and expressing regrets about what might have been. Patients need to look at positive aspects of their lives. Relatives can help patients to review their lives. The worth of the dying person needs to be expressed.

Nurses can assist patients and families by pointing out positive qualities of the patient's life. Prayers, thoughts, and feelings may provide comfort for the patient. While remaining nonjudgmental during interventions, the nurse can respect and accept the practices and rituals associated with the patient's life review.

CLINICAL SIGNS OF IMPENDING DEATH

Death occurs when all vital organs and systems cease to function. During the death process, systems and organs slow and lose their ability to maintain life. There is a general loss of muscle tone, a decrease in the cardiovascular system, a decrease in respiratory function, and decreases in sensory abilities. All systems are involved.

LOSS OF MUSCLE TONE

The muscular system weakens gradually. Body movements slow. Facial muscles lose tone, and the jaw may sag. Speech may be difficult because of decreased muscle coordination. Swallowing becomes increasingly difficult, and the gag reflex is eventually lost. The functions of the gastrointestinal and the genitourinary systems slow down. Peristalsis diminishes, which can lead to constipation, gas accumulation, distention, and nausea. Pain medications may enhance the gastrointestinal slowing. Loss of sphincter control may produce fecal and urinary incontinence.

CIRCULATORY AND RESPIRATORY CHANGES

Vital signs provide valuable information related to cardiovascular and respiratory changes that precede death. The pulse slows and weakens. Blood pressure drops. Temperature may be elevated. Respirations may be rapid, shallow, and irregular, or they may be very slow. Breathing may sound wet and noisy. The noisy, wet-sounding respirations, termed the death rattle, are a response based on mouth breathing and accumulation of mucus in the upper airways. Cheyne-Stokes respirations are irregular with periods of apnea and develop as a person nears death.

Decreased circulation causes the skin to become fragile. The extremities become mottled and cyanotic. The skin feels cool to the touch, first in the feet and legs, then progressing to the hands and arms. It is important to remember that the patient may feel warm because of an elevated temperature.

SENSORY CHANGES

Sensation decreases. Sensory changes include decreasing pain and touch perception, blurred vision, and decreasing sense of taste and smell. The blink reflex is lost eventually, and the patient appears to stare. Lubrication of the eyes with liquid tears may be ordered by the physician.

The sense of touch deereases first in the lower extremities in response to circulatory changes. Hearing is commonly believed to be the last sense to remain intact during the death process. The nurse should assume that the patient can hear and understand. Speaking slowly and clearly may increase the patient's understanding. The nurse must explain to the patient's family and visitors that the patient may still be able to hear. Family members should be encouraged to talk to the patient.

During the death process, the body gradually relaxes until all function ends. Generally, the respirations cease first. The heart stops beating within a few minutes. The physician is responsible for ordering discontinuation of life support if it is in use. The physician is also responsible for pronouncement of death in most situations.

In 1968, a committee of the Harvard Medical School faculty developed the Harvard Criteria for determining a permanently nonfunctioning brain. The criteria deal with specific functions that must be evaluated before a physician can determine death. According to the Harvard Criteria the following must occur:

1. Unresponsiveness to external stimulation that would normally be painful
2. A complete absence of spontaneous movement and breathing
3. A total lack of reflexes that are normally found with a neurologic examination, particularly the reaction of the pupils to light
4. A flat electroencephalogram (EEG) for 24 hours, which indicates that there is no electrical activity in the brain
5. The lack of circulation to the brain for 24 hours as identified by technology

Usually the first three criteria are enough for a pronouncement of death by the physician. The EEG and other technology are generally used when life support equipment is in use. The Harvard Committee recommended that if the final two criteria are used that the tests be repeated 24 hours later.

Another definition associated with the diagnosis of death is cerebral death. Cerebral death occurs when the cerebral cortex stops functioning or is irreversibly destroyed. The cerebral cortex or the higher brain is responsible for voluntary movement and actions as well as for thought. Many people believe that cerebral cortex function *is* the individual.

Since technology has been developed that assists in supporting life, many controversies have arisen. Questions and discussions have developed around whether brain death occurs when the whole brain (cortex and brain stem) ceases activity or when cortical function alone stops. Currently legal and medical standards require that all brain function must cease for death to be pronounced.

PHYSICAL CHANGES AFTER DEATH

After death, many changes take place in the body rapidly. After body functions cease, decomposition takes place. Three specific changes are rigor mortis, algor mortis, and livor mortis.

Immediately following death, some involuntary jerking movements may take place. Within 2 to 4 hours the body stiffens, a condition referred to as *rigor mortis.* Rigor mortis is caused by chemical changes within the body's cells that prevent muscle relaxation.

After death the body begins to cool gradually. This is known as *algor mortis.* Body temperature falls until it reaches room temperature in approximately 24 hours. As the body cools, the skin tends to lose elasticity and can be broken easily.

The breakdown of red blood cells after death causes a discoloration in the skin, which is called *livor mortis.* The skin may appear bruised. Generally, the blood settles in the dependent parts of the body. It is most obvious in the back and the buttocks.

Decomposition of the body happens faster in warmer temperatures because of bacterial growth. To slow decomposition, the body must be kept cool. Embalming reverses the process of decomposition by replacing the body's fluids with chemicals that prevent further growth of the bacteria that cause decomposition.

NURSING CARE OF TERMINALLY ILL AND DYING PATIENTS

Nursing care of terminally ill and dying patients deals with the psychological and physical aspects of care. Nursing care focuses on the grieving process as well as the physical changes that are associated with dying. The patient and the family need to be the focus of nursing care. Respect, dignity, and comfort are important for the patient and for the family. In addition, nurses and other care providers must recognize their own needs when dealing with grief and dying.

ASSESSMENT

Assessment of the terminally ill or dying patient varies with the patient's condition. In general, the assessment is limited to essential data.

The nurse documents the specific event or change that brought the patient into the health care facility. The patient's medical diagnoses, medication profile, and allergies are recorded. If the patient is alert, the nurse briefly reviews the body systems to detect important signs and symptoms. Discomfort such as pain or nausea are documented for prompt intervention.

The functional assessment of activities of daily living elicits information about the patient's abilities, food and fluid intake, patterns of sleep and rest, and response to the stress of terminal illness. The nurse determines how the patient (if able to communicate) and family are coping. Inferences can be made about the stage of grief and coping mechanisms based on statements reflecting sorrow, anger, guilt, or denial.

The physical assessment is abbreviated and detects changes that accompany terminal illness. The frequency of assessment depends on the patient's stability but is done at least every 8 hours. As changes occur, documentation is done more frequently.

Neurologic assessment is especially important and includes level of consciousness, reflexes, and pupil responses. Evaluation of vital signs, skin color, and temperature indicates changes in circulation. The nurse monitors respiratory status and describes the character and pattern of respirations and the characteristics of breath sounds. Renal and gastrointestinal functions are assessed by monitoring nutritional and fluid intake, urinary output, and bowel function. Skin condition must also be monitored, as skin becomes very fragile and may break down. Detailed assessment of the immobile patient is covered in Chapter 19.

To reemphasize, it is important for the nurse to be sensitive and not to impose repeated, unnecessary assessments on the dying patient. If health history data are available in the chart, the nurse should use that resource rather than tiring the patient with an interview. However, the nurse checks on the patient frequently so the patient does not feel abandoned.

NURSING DIAGNOSIS

The nursing diagnoses frequently used during the grieving process are the following:

- **Anticipatory Grieving** related to terminal illness
- **Dysfunctional Grieving** related to the inability to adapt to the loss

Additional diagnoses for the dying patient and family may be pain, fear, impaired skin integrity, altered nutrition: less than body requirements, ineffective airway clearance, spiritual distress, hopelessness, powerlessness, and ineffective individual or family coping. The reader is referred to Chapter 19 for specific nursing diagnoses and interventions for the immobile patient and to Chapter 16 for pain management.

GOALS

Resolution of grief is the primary goal for diagnoses of anticipatory and dysfunctional grieving. Goals and interventions are similar to these two types of grieving, and therefore they are addressed together. Specific goals are formulated for the stage of the grief process or the specific feelings expressed by the patient. Examples of goals for anticipatory and dysfunctional grief are patient expression of feelings related to grief, acknowledgment of the impending loss, and demonstration of behaviors that reflect progress in grief resolution.

INTERVENTIONS

Nurses need to be aware of how grief affects them personally. The nurse who is responsible for the care of terminally ill or dying patients is not immune to feelings of loss. It is common for nurses to feel helpless and powerless when dealing with death. Their feelings of sorrow, guilt, and frustration need to be expressed. Nurses must also remember that there are many interventions that help to ease physical and emotional suffering. It is necessary for nurses to recognize and acknowledge what they can and cannot control. The basic recognition of the nurse's own feelings allows an openness with the patient and family in exchanging feelings. The nurse must realize that it is okay to cry with the patient or family during the grief process. It is okay to be human.

Priority interventions for anticipatory and dysfunctional grief must focus on providing an environment that allows the patient to express feelings. Open discussion of feelings helps the patient and family work toward resolution of the grief process. The patient should be free to express feelings of anger, fear, or guilt without judgment on the part of the nurse. The patient and family need to know that the grief reaction is normal.

Respect for the patient's privacy and need or desire to talk (or not to talk) is important. Honesty in answering questions and giving information is necessary.

Families and patients need encouragement to continue their usual activities as much as possible. They need to discuss their activities and maintain some control over their lives. At times, it helps to discuss what can and cannot change.

Grieving relatives, friends, and significant others can provide emotional support for one another. Health care providers need to be sensitive to the importance of significant others who are not necessarily relatives. Resources such as community counseling and local support may assist some people in working through their grief. Generally, simply allowing the involved people to express their feelings helps to resolve the grief.

It is useful to identify the stage of grief (denial, anger, bargaining, depression, acceptance) that the person is experiencing. Awareness of the stage permits the nurse to react according to individual needs. Respect for the person's right to privacy, right to have emotions, and right to talk when he or she chooses is necessary for developing the nurse-patient relationship. Assistance with planning for the future or for the funeral may be needed based on the patient's or family's coping abilities.

Anger is a common and normal response to grief. It is important for the nurse to understand that the grieving person cannot be forced to accept the loss. The nurse must acknowledge and encourage the expression of feelings but at the same time realize how difficult it is to come to terms with grief. Nurses are sometimes the target of the anger, and they must understand what is happening and not react on a personal level.

Feelings of hopelessness and powerlessness are common in terminal illness and during grief. Realistic hope should be encouraged within the limits of the situation. The patient and the family should be allowed to identify and to deal with what is within their control and to recognize what is beyond their control. Patient-identified goals can be encouraged to restore some sense of power.

During terminal illness and after death physical care is important. Nursing care during the last stages of life involves comfort measures and physical maintenance care.

Meeting the patient's physiologic needs and needs for safety are the priorities. Physical requirements for oxygen, nutrition, pain relief, mobility, elimination, and skin care remain throughout the life cycle. Physical care should be maintained and monitored. People who are dying deserve and require the same physical care as people who are expected to recover.

EVALUATION

Evaluation of patient-centered goals focuses on specific coping skills learned and expressed by the patient or the significant others. Criteria for goal achievement include verbalization of specific feelings related to the grief process, expression that the loss is real, and identification of specific progress in the resolution of grief. The criteria are evaluated based on specific behaviors and verbalizations exhibited by the patient or the significant others.

CARE OF THE BODY AFTER DEATH

Following death the body must be prepared for transfer to the morgue or the funeral home. Nurses are responsible for the care and preparation of the body.

Legal and moral issues may affect the care required for the disposition of the body. In certain instances an autopsy may be required. An autopsy is a postmortem examination of the deceased. An autopsy may be requested by the next of kin, suggested by the physician, or required by law. Consent for an autopsy must be signed before the procedure can be performed unless the procedure is required by law.

Each state has its own laws regarding autopsy. Under the law in most states, an autopsy is required if a person expires by suicide, homicide, within 24 hours of admission to a health care facility, or from unknown causes. In such cases the coroner or the medical examiner must be notified.

During an autopsy, organ specimens and samples may be removed for examination. Body parts that are removed are either disposed of or preserved for burial depending on the situation and the family's wishes. Signs of an autopsy are not apparent following embalming.

Typically, the family wants to view the body before it is transported to the mortuary or the morgue. The nurse must make the environment as comfortable for the family as possible. It is the nurse's responsibility to prepare the body for viewing before the transfer.

Normally, following death the body is placed in the supine position with the arms placed at the sides or with the hands across the abdomen. Identification bands should remain in place. A single pillow is placed under the head and shoulders to prevent discoloration of the face from pooling of the blood. Large overstuffed pillows should be avoided.

Gently holding the eyelids closed for a few seconds helps them to remain closed. If the eyelids do not remain closed after a few seconds, the application of moist cotton balls for a few minutes may help.

Dentures may be inserted gently to maintain the normal facial appearance. If the dentures cannot be inserted easily, do not force them. Dentures that are not in place should be stored in a denture container, marked with identification, and sent with the body to the mortuary. The mouth is closed. A rolled towel placed under the chin helps hold the mouth closed.

Areas of the body that are soiled should be washed. Linen savers are placed under the buttocks to absorb urine or feces that may be released as the sphincters relax. A clean gown is applied, and the hair is combed.

Tubes that are present in the body may be removed unless an autopsy is required. Some agencies require that tubes remain in place or that they be trimmed to approximately 1 inch and taped in place. It is important to review state and agency requirements.

Jewelry is generally removed except for the wedding band, which may be taped to the finger. If rings cannot be removed easily, they should be taped in place. An inventory of the deceased's possessions and valuables is done with the family. Each valuable is listed and signed for by the family. If no family is available, the inventory of valuables is listed and signed for by the funeral director. The disposition of possessions is documented in the medical record.

Following the positioning and preparation of the body, the top linens are straightened and pulled up to the shoulder level. The family may view the body after the nurse has finished the preparation.

Many times the family needs the nurse's emotional support while viewing the body. If only one family member is present, it is wise for a nurse to accompany the person while viewing the body. The door may be closed to allow for privacy. The family should be allowed as much time as desired.

When the family leaves, the nurse applies additional identification tags to the wrist and ankle or toe of the deceased. The gown is removed, and the body may be wrapped in a shroud. The shroud may be a large square or rectangle of cloth or plastic material. An identification tag is placed on the outside of the shroud. Additional identification markings may be required if the deceased had a communicable disease. The body is then transported to the morgue or removed by the mortician. Agency policy regarding the transport of a body from the room may vary. Some agencies require that all patient doors be closed before transport and that service elevators be used.

ISSUES RELATED TO TERMINAL ILLNESS AND DEATH

Patients and families struggle with many emotional decisions during the terminal illness and dying experience. The decisions often focus on physical and emotional comfort. Many people decide that the outcomes should be based on their own wishes. The decisions may involve the choice for advance directives or living wills, organ donations, and resuscitation.

ORGAN DONATION

Organ donation may be made by any person who is legally competent. Any part or the entire body may be donated. The decision to donate organs or to provide anatomic gifts may be made by a person before death. The decision may be made by immediate family members following death.

Many people carry donor cards. Some states allow for organ donation to be marked on drivers' licenses. The physician should be notified immediately when organ donation is intended since some tissues must be used within hours after death.

CARDIOPULMONARY RESUSCITATION

In the past 30 years it has become common practice in health care for cardiopulmonary resuscitation (CPR) to be practiced. Patients who suffered respiratory or cardiac arrest were given CPR unless a do not resuscitate (DNR) order was given by the physician. Many times patients and families have had no choice as to whether CPR was used.

In recent years much has been written concerning the right to die and the right to choose. Many people believe that the patient or the patient's family has the right to decide whether CPR will be used. It is no longer the sole decision of the physician.

In 1991 the Omnibus Reconciliation Act of 1990 became effective. It is frequently known as the Patient Self-Determination Act. This act requires that all institutions that participate with Medicare must provide written information to patients concerning their rights to accept or refuse treatment. The information must include information about the right to initiate advance directives. Advance directives are written statements of a person's wishes regarding medical care (Fig. 22–1). The first advance directive was developed by the Euthanasia Education Council in 1974. It was called the Living Will.

Most states have replaced the idea of living wills with natural death acts. Within many of these acts are specific aspects related to the individual's wishes and for durable powers of attorney for health care. Directives to physicians may be included. Under the natural death acts an individual can tell the physician exactly what is desired.

Special forms for durable power of attorney and directives for physicians can be obtained from local medical associations. Specific details as to withholding or withdrawing treatments must be included (Fig. 22–2). What is to be done and what is not to be done must be included in very clear terms.

A person may write a durable power of attorney or directive to physicians without special forms. Verbal directives may be given to physicians with specific instructions in the presence of two witnesses. Attorneys and notaries are not necessarily required.

In the event that the person is not capable of communicating his or her wishes, the family and the physician can agree on what measures will or will not be taken. The physician should document the family's decision.

Several different types of CPR decisions may be made. Complete and total heroic measures, which may include CPR, medications, and mechanical ventilation, can be referred to as a full code. Some people choose variations of the full code. A chemical code involves the use of medications for resuscitation without the use of CPR. A no code or a DNR order allows the person to die without the interference of technology.

Another option is the durable power of attorney for health care. This document allows individuals to select someone to make health care decisions for them if they are unable to do so for themselves. The power of attorney can be used only if the physician certifies in writing

ADVANCE DIRECTIVE
Living Will and Health Care Proxy

Death is a part of life. It is a reality like birth, growth and aging. I am using this advance directive to convey my wishes about medical care to my doctors and other people looking after me at the end of my life. It is called an advance directive because it gives instructions in advance about what I want to happen to me in the future. It expresses my wishes about medical treatment that might keep me alive. I want this to be legally binding.

If I cannot make or communicate decisions about my medical care, those around me should rely on this document for instructions about measures that could keep me alive.

I do not want medical treatment (including feeding and water by tube) that will keep me alive if:
- I am unconscious and there is no reasonable prospect that I will ever be conscious again (even if I am not going to die soon in my medical condition), or
- I am near death from an illness or injury with no reasonable prospect of recovery.

I do want medicine and other care to make me more comfortable and to take care of pain and suffering. I want this even if the pain medicine makes me die sooner.

I want to give some extra instructions: *[Here list any special instructions, e.g., some people fear being kept alive after a debilitating stroke. If you have wishes about this, or any other conditions, please write them here.]*

The legal language in the box that follows is a health care proxy.
It gives another person the power to make medical decisions for me.

I name ________________________________, who lives at ________________________________

________________________________, phone number ________________________________,

to make medical decisions for me if I cannot make them myself. This person is called a health care "surrogate," "agent," "proxy," or "attorney in fact." This power of attorney shall become effective when I become incapable of making or communicating decisions about my medical care. This means that this document stays legal when and if I lose the power to speak for myself, for instance, if I am in a coma or have Alzheimer's disease.

My health care proxy has power to tell others what my advance directive means. This person also has power to make decisions for me, based either on what I would have wanted, or, if this is not known, on what he or she thinks is best for me.

If my first choice health care proxy cannot or decides not to act for me, I name ________________________

________________________, address ____,

phone number ________________________, as my second choice.

(over, please)

FIGURE 22-1

Sample advance directive (Living Will and Health Care Proxy). (Reprinted by permission of Choice in Dying Inc. [formerly Concern for Dying/Society for the Right to Die], 200 Varick Street, New York, NY 10014-4810.)

Illustration continued on following page

I have discussed my wishes with my health care proxy, and with my second choice if I have chosen to appoint a second person. My proxy(ies) has(have) agreed to act for me.

I have thought about this advance directive carefully. I know what it means and want to sign it. I have chosen two witnesses, neither of whom is a member of my family, nor will inherit from me when I die. My witnesses are not the same people as those I named as my health care proxies. I understand that this form should be notarized if I use the box to name (a) health care proxy(ies).

Signature ______________________________

Date ______________________________

Address ______________________________

Witness' signature ______________________________

Witness' printed name ______________________________

Address ______________________________

Witness' signature ______________________________

Witness' printed name ______________________________

Address ______________________________

Notary [to be used if proxy is appointed] ______________________________

Drafted and Distributed by Choice In Dying, Inc.—the National Council for the right to Die. Choice In Dying is a National not-for-profit organization which works for the rights of patients at the end of life. In addition to this generic advance directive, Choice In Dying distributes advance directives that conform to each state's specific legal requirements and maintains a national Living Will Registry for completed documents.

CHOICE IN DYING INC.—
the national council for the right to die
(formerly Concern for Dying/Society for the Right to Die)
200 Varick Street, New York, NY 10014 (212) 366-5540

5/92

FIGURE 22-1
Continued

March 1993

Artificial Nutrition and Hydration in Living Will Statutes

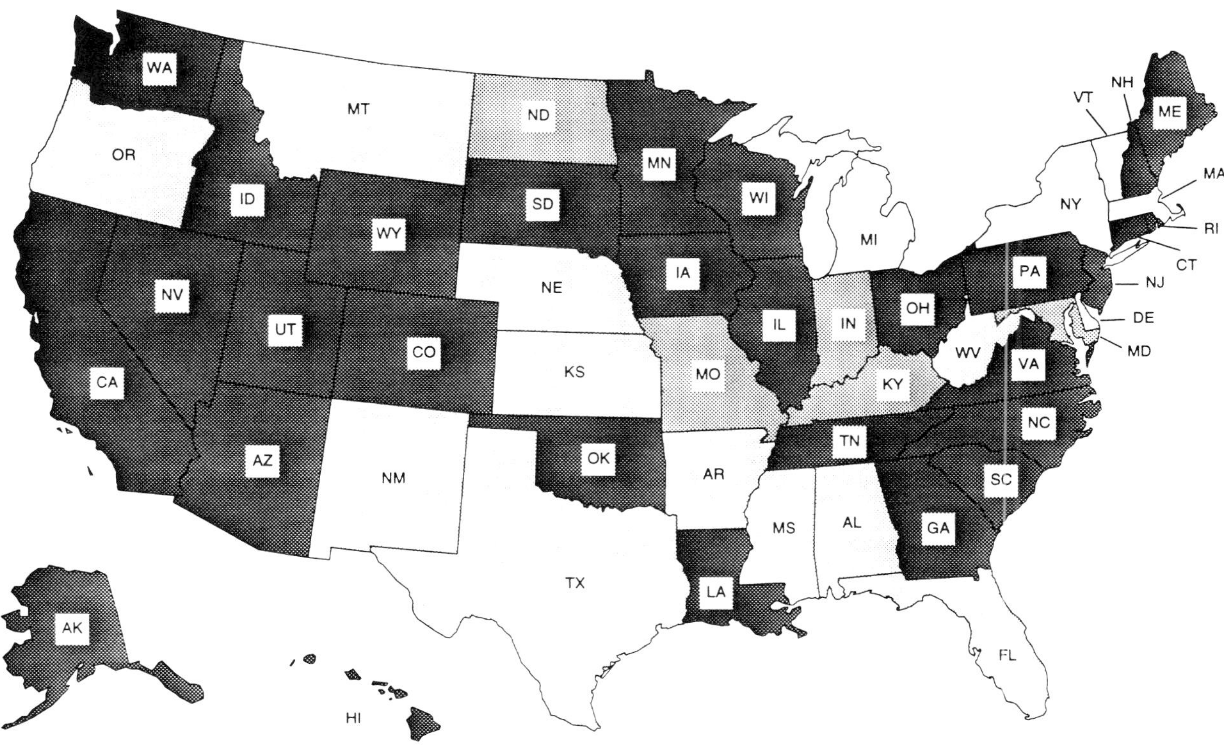

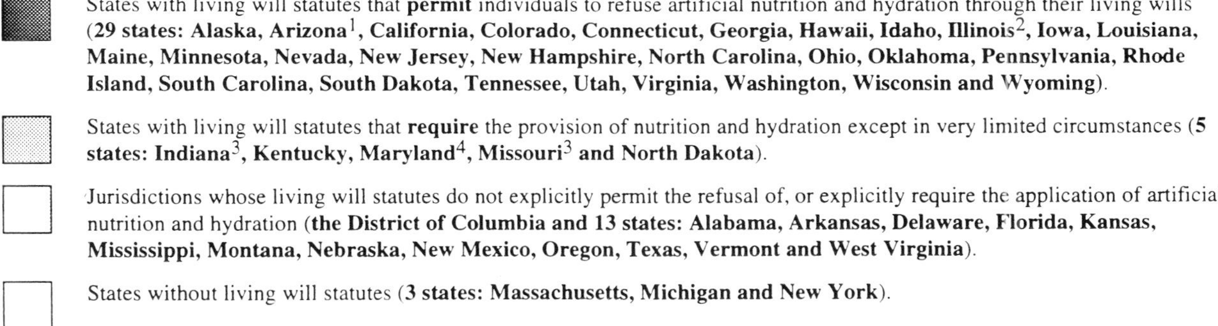

States with living will statutes that **permit** individuals to refuse artificial nutrition and hydration through their living wills (**29 states: Alaska, Arizona**[1]**, California, Colorado, Connecticut, Georgia, Hawaii, Idaho, Illinois**[2]**, Iowa, Louisiana, Maine, Minnesota, Nevada, New Jersey, New Hampshire, North Carolina, Ohio, Oklahoma, Pennsylvania, Rhode Island, South Carolina, South Dakota, Tennessee, Utah, Virginia, Washington, Wisconsin and Wyoming**).

States with living will statutes that **require** the provision of nutrition and hydration except in very limited circumstances (**5 states: Indiana**[3]**, Kentucky, Maryland**[4]**, Missouri**[3] **and North Dakota**).

Jurisdictions whose living will statutes do not explicitly permit the refusal of, or explicitly require the application of artificial nutrition and hydration (**the District of Columbia and 13 states: Alabama, Arkansas, Delaware, Florida, Kansas, Mississippi, Montana, Nebraska, New Mexico, Oregon, Texas, Vermont and West Virginia**).

States without living will statutes (**3 states: Massachusetts, Michigan and New York**).

[1] The authority to withhold or withdraw artificial nutrition and hydration is only explicitly mentioned in the sample document.
[2] Artificial nutrition and hydration cannot be withheld or withdrawn if the resulting death is due to starvation or dehydration.
[3] The medical power of attorney statutes in Indiana and Missouri permit appointed agents to refuse artificial nutrition and hydration on behalf of the principal.
[4] Although the act requires the "administration of food and water," a Maryland Attorney General's Opinion has stated that artificial nutrition and hydration may be refused through a living will.

Produced by **Choice In Dying, Inc.** (formerly Concern for Dying/Society for the Right to Die)
200 Varick Street, 10th Floor New York, NY 10014 212-366-5540

FIGURE 22-2
Artificial nutrition and hydration in Living Will statutes, by state. (Reproduced by permission of Choice in Dying Inc., March 1993.)

that the person is incapable of making decisions. Until the physician does this, the individual remains in control of his or her own decisions.

The nurse needs to be aware of legal issues and the wishes of the patient. Advance directives and organ donor information should be located in the medical record and identified on the Kardex or the nursing care plan. All caregivers responsible for the patient need to know the patient's wishes.

Terminal illness and dying are very personal events that affect the patient, the family, and the caregivers. Grief is experienced by everyone differently but with similar patterns of behavior. The dying process and death require specific physical, emotional, spiritual, and legal nursing interventions. Caring for the terminally ill and dying is a challenging and rewarding experience.

BIBLIOGRAPHY

Aber, C. S. (1992). Spousal death, a threat to women's health. *Image, 24*(2), 95–99.

Ad Hoc Committee of the Harvard Medical School to Examine the Definition of Irreversible Coma. (1968). *Journal of the American Medical Association, 261,* 2205–2210.

Annas, G. J. (1991). The health care proxy and the living will. *New England Journal of Medicine, 324,* 1211.

Billings, J. A. (1985). Comfort measures for the terminally ill. *Journal of the American Gerontological Society, 33,* 808–810.

Carpenito, L. J. (1989). *Nursing diagnoses: Application to clinical nursing practice* (3rd ed.). Philadelphia: J. B. Lippincott.

Carter, S. L. (1989). Themes of grief. *Nursing Research, 38*(8), 354–358.

Cassel, C. K. (1991–1992). Cassel confronts aging issues. *The Chronicle of the Center for Health Research, 5.*

Clark, M. D. (1984). Healthy and unhealthy grief behaviors. *Occupational Health Nursing, 32*(12), 633–635.

Davitz, L., Sameshima, Y., & Davitz, J., et al. (1976). Suffering as viewed in six different cultures. *American Journal of Nursing, 76*(8), 1296–1297.

Demi, A. S., & Miles, M. S. (1986). Bereavement. *Annual Review of Nursing Research, 4,* 105–123.

Doenges, M. E., & Moorhouse, M. F. (1991). *Nurse's pocket guide: Nursing diagnoses with interventions* (3rd ed.). Philadelphia: F. A. Davis.

Ebersole, P., & Hess, P. (1990). *Toward healthy aging.* St. Louis: Mosby Year Book.

Fetsch, S. H. (1984). The 7 to 10 year old child's conceptualization of death. *Oncology Nurse's Forum, 11*(6), 52–56.

Field, D. (1984). "We didn't want him to die on his own"—nurse's accounts of nursing dying patients. *Journal of Advanced Nursing, 1,* 59–70.

Flarey, D. (1991). Advance directives: In search of self-determination. *Journal of Nursing Administration, 21*(11), 16–21.

Hoff, I. A. (1984). *People in crisis.* Menlo Park, CA: Addison-Wesley.

Kellmer, D. (1986). No code orders: Guidelines for policy. *Nursing Outlook, 34*(4), 179–183.

Kübler-Ross, E. (1974). *Questions and answers on death and dying.* New York: Macmillan.

Kübler-Ross, E. (1975). *Death, the final stage of growth.* Englewood Cliffs, NJ: Prentice-Hall.

Kübler-Ross, E. (1978). *To live until we say goodbye.* Englewood Cliffs, NJ: Prentice-Hall.

Kübler-Ross, E. (1981). *Living with death and dying.* New York: Macmillan.

Kübler-Ross, E. (1983). *On children and death.* New York: Macmillan.

MacKay, S. (1992). Durable power of attorney for health care. *Geriatric Nursing, 13*(2), 99–108.

Mandel, H. R. (1981). Nurses feelings about working with the dying. *American Journal of Nursing, 81*(6), 1194–1197.

Martocchio, B. C. (1985). Grief and bereavement healing through hurt. *Nursing Clinics of North America, 20*(6), 327–341.

Matteson, M. A., & McConnell, E. S. (1988). *Gerontological Nursing.* Philadelphia: W. B. Saunders.

Morris, E. (1988). A pain of separation—How can nurses best assist the dying and the bereaved? *Nursing Times, 84*(10), 54–56.

Moss, M. S., & Moss, S. Z. (1983–1984). The impact of parental death on middle aged children. *Omega, 14*(1), 65–75.

Omnibus Reconciliation Act. (1990). Title IV. Section 4206. *Congressional Record.* October 26, 1990, 12638.

Peretz, D. (1970). Development, object relationship, and loss. In B. Schoenberg, et al. (Eds.), *Loss and grief: Psychosocial management in medical practice.* New York: Columbia University Press.

Richter, J. M. (1984). Crisis of mate loss in the elderly. *American Nursing Society, 6*(4), 45–54.

Schultz, R. (1978). *The psychology of death, dying, and bereavement.* Reading, MA: Addison-Wesley.

Strauss, A. L., & Glaser, B. G. (1970). Awareness of dying. In B. Schoenberg, et al. (Eds.), *Loss and grief: Psychosocial management in medical practice.* New York: Columbia University Press.

Tittle, M. B., Moody, L., & Becker, M. P. (1991). Preliminary development of two predictive models for DNR patients in intensive care. *Image, 23*(3), 140–144.

Vernale, C., & Packard, S. (1990). Organ donation and gift exchange. *Image, 22*(4), 239–242.

Waltman, R. E. (1992). When a patient's spouse dies. *Nursing 92, 22*(7), 48–51.

Williams, J. C. (1976). Allaying common fears. In *Dealing with death and dying. Nursing 77 skillbook series.* Horsham, PA: Intermed Communications, pp. 27–32.

Williams, J. C. (1976). Stages of bereavement. In *Dealing with death and dying. Nursing 77 skillbook series.* Horsham, PA: Intermed Communications, pp. 73–76.

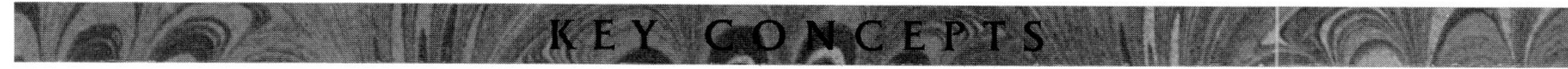

KEY CONCEPTS

1. Terminal illness and dying are no longer viewed as the taboo topics they once were, and health care providers are more sensitive to the special needs of people who are terminally ill and dying.
2. Loss is the real or potential absence of someone or something that is valued.
3. People experience loss when faced with changes in self-image, developmental changes, loss of possessions, and loss of significant others through death or other means.
4. The response to loss, called grief, is similar regardless of the nature of the loss but is usually most profound when the loss experienced is death.
5. Adaptive grief is a healthy response to loss; dysfunctional grief is a delayed or an exaggerated response.
6. Anticipatory grieving is the response to a loss before it happens.
7. Culture, religion, and age affect a person's understanding and reaction to death or loss.
8. Kübler-Ross's stages of grieving are denial, anger, bargaining, depression, and acceptance.
9. Martocchio's five clusters of grief are shock and disbelief; yearning and protest; anguish, disorganization, and despair; identification in bereavement; and reorganization and restitution.
10. The stages of awareness of terminal illness are closed awareness, mutual pretense, and open awareness.
11. Common fears associated with terminal illness and dying are fear of pain, fear of loneliness, and fear of meaninglessness.
12. Clinical signs of impending death are loss of muscle tone, bradycardia, hypotension, abnormal respiratory pattern, abnormal breath sounds, cyanosis, cool skin, blurred vision, and sensory changes.
13. Current legal and medical standards require that all brain function must cease for death to be pronounced.
14. Changes in the body after death are rigor mortis, algor mortis, and livor mortis.
15. Assessment of the terminally ill or dying person varies with the person's condition but is often limited to essential data.
16. Nursing diagnoses for the patient who is terminally ill or dying may include anticipatory grieving, dysfunctional grieving, pain, fear, impaired skin integrity, altered nutrition, ineffective airway clearance, spiritual distress, hopelessness, powerlessness, and ineffective individual coping.
17. The nurse is responsible for the care and preparation of the body after death.
18. An autopsy is a postmortem examination of the body that requires family consent unless the procedure is required by law.
19. Decisions that terminally ill patients and their families may record in advance directives include desired medical interventions and organ donations.

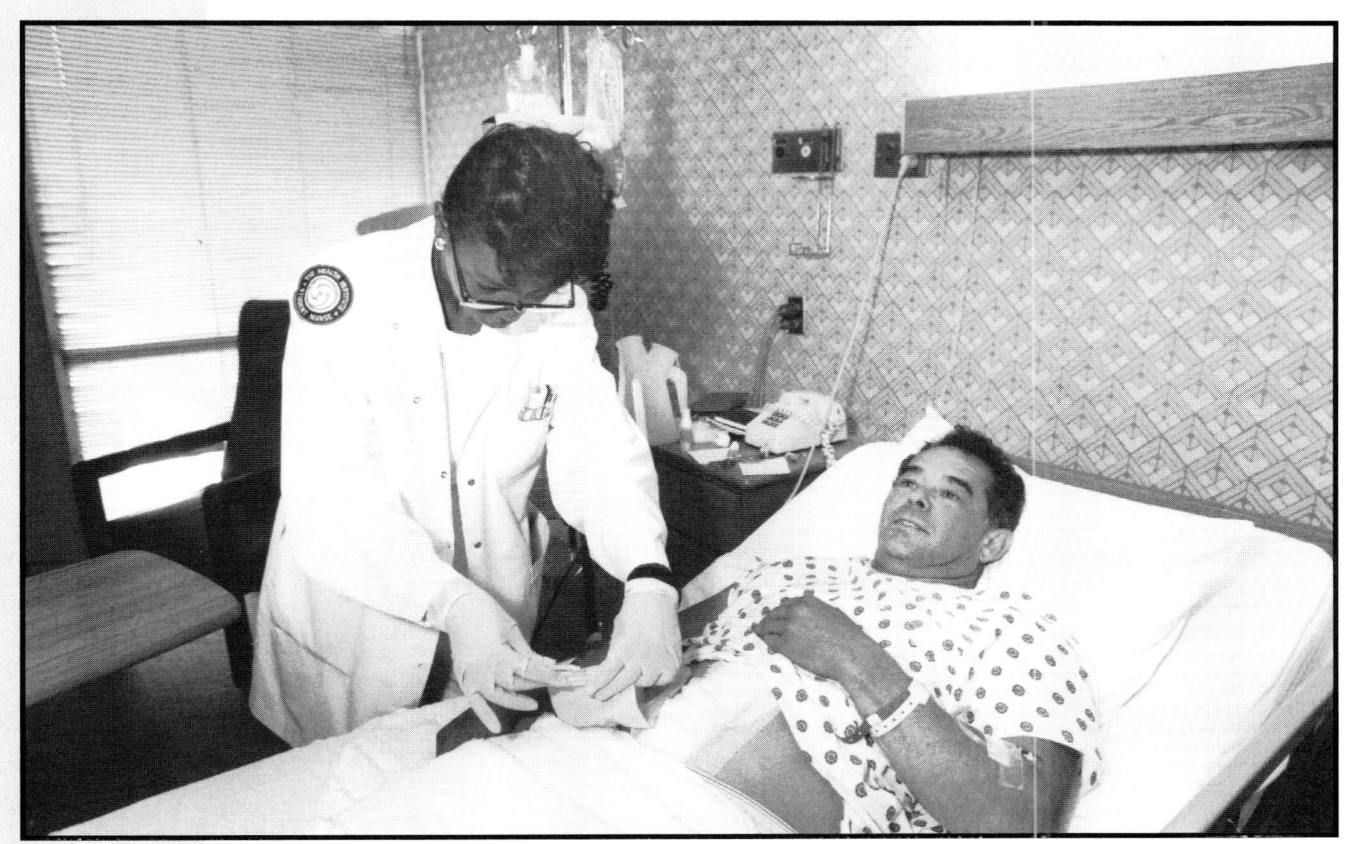

UNIT 5
Cancer

Adrianne Linton

CHAPTER 23

The Patient with Cancer

OBJECTIVES

1. Explain the differences between benign and malignant tumors.
2. List the most common sites of cancer in men and women.
3. Describe measures to reduce the risk of cancer.
4. Define terms used to name and classify cancer.
5. List nursing responsibilities in the care of patients having diagnostic tests to detect possible cancer.
6. Explain the nursing care of patients undergoing each type of cancer therapy: surgery, radiation, chemotherapy, biological response modifiers.
7. Identify nursing needs of the terminally ill cancer patient and the family.

GLOSSARY

ALOPECIA Loss of hair

ANTINEOPLASTIC An agent that inhibits the maturation or reproduction of malignant cells

BENIGN Not malignant

CARCINOGEN A substance that can cause cancer

CHEMOTHERAPY Use of chemicals to treat illness

MALIGNANT Tending to progress in virulence; has the characteristics of becoming increasingly undifferentiated, invasive of surrounding tissues, and colonizing distant sites

METASTASIS The transfer of cells from a primary site to a distant site

NEOPLASM New growth; may be benign or malignant

ONCOFETAL ANTIGEN A gene product that is normally suppressed in adult tissues but reappears in the presence of some types of cancer

RADIOTHERAPY The use of radiation in the treatment of cancer and other diseases

WHY STUDY CANCER?

Specific cancers are discussed with almost every body system in this book. Why, then, is a separate chapter devoted to the subject? The American Cancer Society defines cancer as "a large group of diseases characterized by uncontrolled growth and spread of abnormal cells." More than 200 diseases are classified as cancer. They share some common characteristics, progress in similar ways, and respond to similar types of treatments. This chapter addresses the common features of those diseases known as cancer.

When looking at health statistics, all types of cancer are often grouped together. Not surprisingly, cancer is listed as the second most common cause of death in the United States. Almost everyone has been touched by cancer. It is estimated that one in four Americans will have cancer at some time. The most common sites of cancer in males and in females are shown in Figure 23–1. Because so many die of cancer, many people assume that a diagnosis of cancer is a death sentence. In reality, more than 6 million Americans who have had cancer are alive today.

Some cancers can be prevented by avoidance of causative agents. Early diagnosis has been found to make a significant difference in survival with many types of cancer. Advances in treatment have prolonged the lives of many cancer patients.

Nurses play roles in the prevention and detection of cancer. They also care for patients undergoing diagnostic procedures and treatments for cancer. In almost any specialty, nurses work with patients who are being treated for cancer.

Leading Sites of Cancer Incidence and Death—1994 Estimates

Cancer Incidence by Site and Sex*		Cancer Deaths by Site and Sex	
Male	**Female**	**Male**	**Female**
Prostate 200,000	Breast 182,000	Lung 94,000	Lung 59,000
Lung 100,000	Colon & Rectum 74,000	Prostate 38,000	Breast 46,000
Colon & Rectum 75,000	Lung 72,000	Colon & Rectum 27,800	Colon & Rectum 28,200
Bladder 38,000	Uterus 46,000	Pancreas 12,400	Ovary 13,600
Lymphoma 29,400	Ovary 24,000	Lymphoma 12,100	Pancreas 13,500
Oral 19,800	Lymphoma 23,500	Leukemia 10,500	Lymphoma 10,650
Melanoma of the Skin 17,000	Melanoma of the Skin 15,000	Stomach 8,400	Uterus 10,500
Kidney 17,000	Pancreas 14,000	Esophagus 7,800	Leukemia 8,600
Leukemia 16,200	Bladder 13,200	Liver 7,200	Liver 6,000
Stomach 15,000	Leukemia 12,400	Bladder 7,000	Brain 5,800
Pancreas 13,000	Kidney 10,600	Brain 6,800	Stomach 5,600
Larynx 9,800	Oral 9,800	Kidney 6,800	Multiple Myeloma 4,800
All Sites 632,000	All Sites 576,000	All Sites 283,000	All Sites 255,000

*Excluding basal and squamous cell skin cancer and carcinoma in situ.

Source: American Cancer Society, *Cancer Facts & Figures—1994.*

FIGURE 23-1

Leading sites of cancer incidence and deaths—1993 estimates. (From American Cancer Society. [1994]. *Cancer facts and figures—1994.* Atlanta GA: Author. Used by permission. © 1994 Cancer Facts and Figures—1994. American Cancer Society, Inc.)

WHAT IS CANCER?

BENIGN TUMORS

In the human body, cells are continuously regenerating themselves. Normal cells divide to produce additional identical cells. Cells that reproduce abnormally and in an uncontrolled manner form neoplasms (new tissue) or tumors. Such cells may be benign or malignant. Benign tumors are relatively harmless, largely because they do not spread to other parts of the body. Benign tumors present problems, however, if they create pressure on or obstruct body organs. Because of this, surgical removal of benign tumors is often recommended.

MALIGNANT TUMORS

The presence of malignant cells is the basis for a diagnosis of cancer. As they grow, malignant tumors cause some of the same problems as benign tumors. They press on normal tissues and compete with normal cells for nutrients. Malignant growths are more threatening, however, because they can invade nearby tissues or disperse cells to colonize in distant parts of the body. *Regional invasion* is the term used to describe the movement of cancer cells into adjoining tissue. The process by which cancer spreads to distant sites is called *metastasis*. Tumors found away from the original site of malignant cells are called metastatic growths. The most common sites of metastasis are the liver, the brain, bone, and the lungs. Once metastasis has occurred, cancer treatment is more difficult and less likely to be curative.

A comparison of the features of benign and malignant cells is presented in Table 23–1.

TABLE 23-1
A COMPARISON OF BENIGN AND MALIGNANT TUMORS

CHARACTERISTIC	BENIGN	MALIGNANT
Growth rate	Usually slow	Usually rapid, but may be slow
Growth mode	Enlarges and expands	Invades surrounding tissue
Cell structure and differentiation	Cells closely resemble those of tissue of origin	Tissue of origin not readily identifiable
Recurrence after removal	Unlikely	Common
Metastasis	No	Yes
Tissue destruction	Usually none unless compression or obstruction occurs	Can cause necrosis, ulceration, perforation, tissue sloughing; effects can be fatal

CLASSIFICATION OF TUMORS

Tumors are classified by anatomic site, stage, and cell appearance and differentiation.

Anatomic Site

The suffix *-oma* means tumor. Technically, a tumor is a swelling. The word is most commonly used, however, to refer to a malignant or benign neoplasm. Tumors are named according to the type of tissue from which they developed originally. Common benign growths are fibromas, lipomas, and leiomyomas. Fibromas develop from fibrous connective tissue, lipomas from fat tissue, and leiomyomas from smooth muscle tissue.

Malignant tumors are classified as carcinomas, sarcomas, melanomas, leukemias, and lymphomas. Carcinomas originate from tissues in the skin, glands, and linings of the digestive, urinary, and respiratory tracts. Sarcomas originate from bone, muscle, and other connective tissue. Melanomas develop from the pigment cells in the skin. Leukemias and lymphomas arise from the blood-forming tissues, which include lymphoid tissue, plasma cells, and bone marrow.

Additional prefixes may be used to designate the exact type of malignant tissue. For example, a sarcoma could be an osteosarcoma or a chondrosarcoma. An osteosarcoma is a tumor of the bone, whereas a chondrosarcoma is a cartilage tumor. Many other combinations of terms are used to describe tumors precisely by origin and location.

Staging System for Cancer

Because cancers tend to grow and spread in predictable ways, their progress can be described in stages. There are specific stages for all types of cancer. One method of describing the extent of cancer is the TNM staging system. T stands for the primary tumor. It is staged T0, Tis, T1, T2, T3, or T4. T0 means there is no evidence of the primary tumor. Tis refers to carcinoma in situ. T1 through T4 classifications reflect increasing size and extension of the tumor.

N stands for regional lymph nodes. N0 means there is no involvement of regional lymph nodes. If regional lymph nodes are involved, they are staged N1, N2, or N3 to reflect increasing involvement. M represents distant metastasis. M0 means there is no distant metastasis. M1 indicates the presence of distant metastasis. An example of staging with the TNM system is as follows: a patient whose primary tumor has grown and spread to regional lymph nodes but not to distant sites would be staged T2, N1, M0.

Staging is done at the time of diagnosis and at intervals during and after treatment. Such staging is helpful in planning treatments and in predicting long-term survival.

Another example of a common staging classification is shown in Table 23–2.

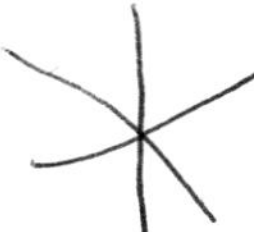

TABLE 23-2
STAGING CLASSIFICATION FOR CANCER

STAGE	DESCRIPTION
Stage I	The malignant cells are confined to the tissue of origin. There is no invasion of other tissues.
Stage II	There is limited spread of the cancer in the local area, usually to nearby lymph nodes.
Stage III	The tumor is larger or has spread from the site of origin into nearby tissues, or both. Regional lymph nodes are likely to be involved.
Stage IV	The cancer has metastasized to distant parts of the body.

RISK FACTORS

A single, exact cause of cancer has not been identified. Both genetic and environmental factors appear to increase the risk of developing cancer. Cancer-causing agents, called *carcinogens*, include a variety of chemicals, radiation, and viruses. Other factors thought to be associated with cancer development are heredity and hormones. Table 23–3 is a partial list of carcinogens. Carcinogens such as cigarette smoke, asbestos, and nitrites are commonly found in the environment. Drugs that may act as carcinogens include diethylstilbestrol (DES), androgenic steroids, high-dose unopposed synthetic estrogens, and phenacetin.

TABLE 23-3
COMMON CARCINOGENS

Viruses

Chemicals
- Tar
- Soot
- Asphalt
- Aniline dyes
- Hydrocarbons
- Crude paraffin oils
- Nickel
- Arsenic
- Benzene
- Cadmium

Physical agents
- Radiation
- Asbestos
- Tobacco smoke

Hormones
- Synthetic estrogens
- Androgenic anabolic steroids

Immunosuppressants
- Corticosteroids
- Antimetabolites
- Alkylating agents
- Antilymphocyte serum

Cytotoxic drugs
- Phenylalanine mustard
- Cyclophosphamide

PHARMACOLOGY CAPSULE

Some drugs are carcinogenic, meaning they can cause cancer. Examples are diethylstilbestrol, androgenic steroids, high-dose unopposed synthetic estrogens, and phenacetin.

It seems that carcinogens stimulate the initial change of normal cells, making them susceptible to malignant changes. Other factors also play a part in promoting the cells to become malignant. Examples of factors that promote cancer growth are increasing age, diet, hormones, and chronic irritation. A person's general emotional and physical health may also be a factor in promoting or slowing the growth of cancer cells.

SEVEN WARNING SIGNS

The signs and symptoms of cancer vary with the location and severity of the disease. The American Cancer Society has identified seven warning signs that are associated with many common types of cancer. They can serve to guide the nurse and the public in identifying problems that require medical evaluation. The first letters of the signs spell out CAUTION, making it easier to remember them (see Box).

PREVENTION AND EARLY DETECTION

A number of things can be done to reduce the risk of developing cancer or to detect it in the early stages. They include (1) general measures to promote health, (2) avoidance of known carcinogens, (3) identification of high-risk people, and (4) cancer screening.

Health Promotion

Many behaviors associated with good health may reduce the risk of some cancers. The recommended diet is high in fiber and low in fat, calories, and preservatives. A balanced program of activity and rest and stress management may enable the body to resist diseases, including cancer.

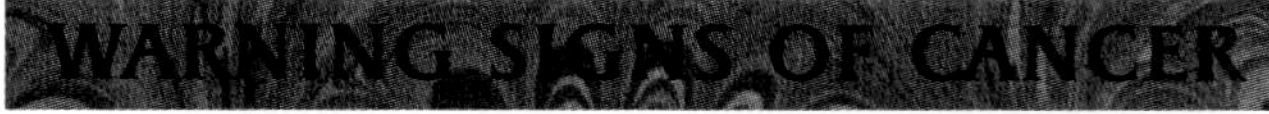

Change in bowel or bladder habits
A sore that does not heal
Unusual bleeding or discharge
Thickening or lump in a breast or elsewhere
Indigestion or difficulty in swallowing
Obvious change in a wart or a mole
Nagging cough or hoarseness

Avoidance of Carcinogens

Some specific carcinogens were mentioned earlier. They include cigarette smoke, alcohol, a variety of chemicals and drugs, and even excessive sunlight. Public education has focused attention on carcinogens, and people are becoming more aware of the need to avoid them.

For example, smoking tobacco has long been known as a risk factor for cancers of the lung, bladder, head and neck, mouth, and stomach. Only in the last few years, however, have antismoking programs had a real impact. Although the percentage of physicians who smoke had dropped dramatically by the late 1980s, nurses continued to smoke at a rate higher than that of other women. The fact that 1 million people quit smoking each year demonstrates that public education is making a difference. On a broader scale, legal restrictions on public smoking are reducing the exposure of nonsmokers. Not only is smoking tobacco harmful, but use of smokeless tobacco increases the risk of oral cancers.

Alcohol consumption also increases the risk of cancers of the mouth, head and neck, and stomach. Many industrial products are carcinogens as well. Their use is regulated by the Occupational Safety and Health Administration guidelines for the safety of workers and consumers. Avoidance of excessive sunlight is beginning to receive attention as people are encouraged to use sunscreens to protect themselves.

Identification of High-Risk People

Identifying people at risk for developing specific cancers serves several purposes. It helps researchers recognize factors that may contribute to the development of various cancers. Also, people who are known to fall into high-risk categories can be monitored closely to detect cancer early. Examples of people at risk for specific cancers are those with familial rectal polyposis, those with family histories of breast cancer, and those with Down's syndrome, who are at increased risk for leukemia.

Screening for Cancer

When cancer does occur, the best hope for a cure is early diagnosis and treatment. Public education should emphasize the following:

- The value of early detection and treatment
- The seven warning signs of cancer
- How to do self examinations (breast, skin, testicular)
- The importance of periodic examinations for common cancers

The American Cancer Society recommends specific examinations or procedures to detect cancers of the colon, prostate, cervix, endometrium, and breast. The recommendations are summarized in Table 23–4.

TABLE 23-4

AMERICAN CANCER SOCIETY RECOMMENDATIONS FOR EARLY CANCER DETECTION IN AYSMPTOMATIC PERSONS

CANCER SITE	TEST OR PROCEDURE	SEX	AGE	FREQUENCY
Colon, rectum	Sigmoidoscopy	M & F	50 and over	Annually for 2 yr; if normal, every 3–5 yr thereafter
	Fecal occult blood test	M & F	50 and over	Every yr
	Digital rectal examination	M & F	40 and over	Every yr
Prostate	Prostate examination and prostate-specific antigen blood test	M	50 and over	Every yr
Cervix	Papanicolaou test and pelvic examination	F	18–40 yr plus younger sexually active females	Annually for 3 yr; if normal, every 1–3 yr thereafter
			Over 40	Every yr
Endometrium	Endometrial biopsy	F	At menopause *if* at high risk*	At menopause *if* at high risk and on physician's advice
Breast	Self-examination	F	20 and over	Every month
	Professional examination		20–40 yr	Every 3 yr
			Over 40	Every yr
	Mammography		40–49 yr	Every 1–2 yr
			50 and over	Every yr
Thyroid, testicles, ovaries, lymph nodes, mouth, skin	Counseling and checkup	M & F	Over 20	Every 3 yr
			Over 40	Every yr

* Obesity, failure to ovulate, abnormal uterine bleeding, unopposed estrogen or tamoxifen therapy.

From Mettlia, C., et al. (1993). Defining and updating the American Cancer Society guidelines for cancer-related checkup: Prostate and endometrial. *CA-Cancer Journal for Clinicians, 43*(1), 45.

DIAGNOSIS OF CANCER

The health history and physical examination often provide the first clues to the presence of cancer. Diagnostic procedures may be used when cancer is suspected, when high-risk persons are screened or when determining the extent of known disease. Diagnostic procedures employ tissue examinations, radiologic studies, endoscopic procedures, magnetic resonance imaging, and laboratory tests. Combinations of procedures may be indicated for cancers that are difficult to locate or to determine whether there is more than one growth.

TISSUE EXAMINATIONS

Direct examination of tissue is used to identify the presence of malignant cells. Cells can be obtained for cytologic examinations. The Papanicolaou smear is one example of a cytologic examination. It is used to detect cancer cells in the cervix. Cells can also be obtained from some body fluids and from the digestive and respiratory tracts. The leukemias and lymphomas are detected by microscopic examination of blood cells.

Another way to obtain cells for study is by biopsy. Biopsy is the removal of cells from living tissue for microscopic examination. Tissue may be obtained by removing the entire growth, cutting a sample from the growth, or drawing cells out of the growth with a needle.

Findings of tissue examinations are usually not reported for several days. Sometimes, however, specimens are removed during surgery and sent for an immediate study, called a frozen section. The tissue is quickly frozen, sliced, dyed, and examined by the pathologist. Results are reported to the surgeon who uses the findings in deciding how to proceed with the surgery.

RADIOLOGIC STUDIES

Plain and Contrast Radiographs

Radiologic studies include a variety of radiographs useful in detecting cancer, especially in bones and hollow organs. Plain films such as routine chest radiographs may reveal suspicious changes in the lungs. Mammography is a low dose radiograph of breast tissue used to detect potentially malignant calcifications before they can be felt.

Other radiographs use contrast media administered orally or intravenously to outline hollow organs. This permits the radiologist to see shadows of abnormal structures. Examples of radiographs with contrast media are the barium enema and the intravenous pyelogram. Specific diagnostic radiographs are discussed with related conditions.

Computed Tomography

Computed tomography, commonly called a CT scan, is useful in diagnosing tumors in the head or trunk. The patient is placed on a platform that fits through the center of a circular frame. The x-ray source and the film move around in opposite directions through the frame. The platform gradually moves the patient through the frame until all the area being studied has been scanned. The CT scan provides cross-sectional, three-dimensional views of body tissue (Fig. 23–2). Images are relayed by a computer to a television screen. Details are much clearer than those obtained with plain radiographs.

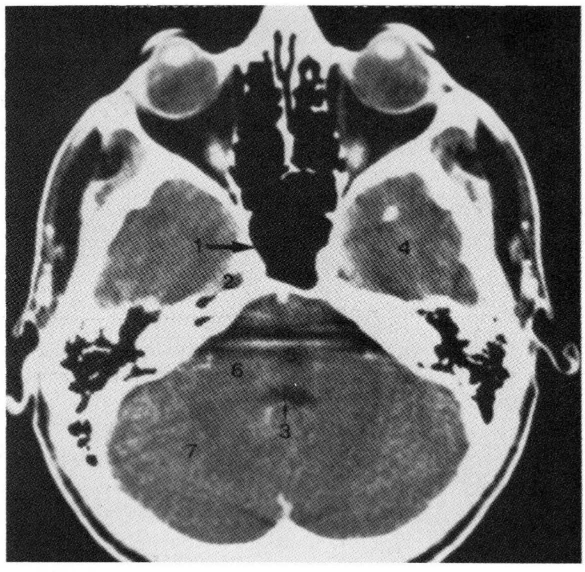

FIGURE 23–2

Computed tomography provides cross-sectional, three-dimensional views of body tissue. 1, Sphenoid sinus; 2, trigeminal ganglion; 3, fourth ventricle; 4, temporal lobe; 5, pons (partially obscured by streak artifact); 6, middle cerebellar peduncle; 7, cerebellar hemisphere. (From Seeram, E. [1994]. *Computed tomography* [p. 266]. Philadelphia: W. B. Saunders.)

A CT scan can be done with or without a contrast medium. No special preparation is usually needed, except when doing scans of the digestive tract and abdomen. Because of the use of x-rays in the CT scan, it is not appropriate for pregnant women. Also, because the patient must be able to lie quietly for 30 minutes to an hour, it may not work well for patients who are confused or restless.

Positron Emission Tomography

Positron emission tomography is a nuclear scan that reveals patterns of tissue metabolism. It can be useful in detecting tumors in the brain or breast and in measuring the effects of cancer treatment. A signed consent form may be required before doing the procedure. The patient does not need to abstain from oral intake but should avoid alcohol, caffeine, and tobacco for 24 hours in advance. The patient is seated in a reclining chair for the scan. Two intravenous lines are inserted, one to infuse an isotope and the other to draw blood samples. After the isotope is infused, the tissues of interest are scanned and a series of blood samples drawn. The patient may be asked to perform some cognitive activities like reciting something common. The patient is provided a blindfold and earplugs to reduce external stimuli. The procedure takes 1 to 1½ hours. The only postprocedure care is to force fluids to promote elimination of the isotope.

ENDOSCOPIC PROCEDURES

tissue changes

Radiographs reveal suspicious tissue changes, but usually additional studies are required to confirm the presence of cancer. Endoscopic procedures involve the insertion of lighted tubes into hollow organs or body cavities. Endoscopy is useful in diagnosing many conditions, including cancer. It permits the physician to see and to take samples of some suspicious growths for tissue examination. Examples of endoscopic procedures are bronchoscopy, colonoscopy, and cystoscopy. These and other procedures are discussed in more detail in other chapters. Every agency usually has a protocol for nursing care of the patient before and after endoscopic procedures.

MAGNETIC RESONANCE IMAGING

The technology of diagnostic procedures is changing rapidly. One of the more recent developments is magnetic resonance imaging, or simply MRI. Magnetic resonance imaging produces a type of scan that is different than from that produced by x-rays. It exposes the patient to radio frequency waves in the presence of a strong magnetic field. The process causes energy changes that can be measured and converted to computer images. Because MRI does not involve x-rays, it does not expose the patient to radiation. No known risks are associated with MRI, although its effects on the fetus are not known.

Magnetic resonance imaging is most useful in diagnosing abnormalities of the central nervous system, spinal column, neck, bones, and joints. The procedure takes little preparation. The patient takes nothing by mouth for 4 to 6 hours before the procedure only if the abdomen is being studied. Patient teaching includes the following:

1. The procedure is not painful; in fact, there are no sensations at all.
2. All metal must be removed before the procedure, including jewelry, watches, eyeglasses, hearing aids, dentures, and clothing fasteners.
3. The patient lies on a stretcher that slides into the imaging apparatus. It is like a tunnel.
4. The staff can see the patient in a mirror and can communicate over an intercom.
5. The machine makes loud metallic thumping noises.
6. The procedure can take as long as 1½ hours.
7. People who are bothered by being closed in a narrow space should let their physician know. A mild sedative may be prescribed.
8. Relaxation techniques can help reduce anxiety during the procedure.
9. Patients should empty their bladders before the procedure begins.

Because of the magnetic pull, some people cannot undergo MRI. They include people with some type of metal implant or object in their bodies, people with permanent pacemakers, those on life support systems, and those who have implanted insulin pumps. Obese patients may not fit in the narrow tunnel. Because the effects of MRI on the fetus are unknown, the procedure is not done on pregnant women.

LABORATORY TESTS

A number of laboratory tests are used during the diagnostic and treatment phases. Oncofetal antigens are found on fetal cells and on the surfaces of cancer cells. Carcinoembryonic antigen, alpha-fetoprotein, CA-125, prostate-specific antigen, CA-19-9, and pancreatic oncofetal antigen are examples of oncofetal antigens. Elevated carcinoembryonic antigen levels may occur in cancer of the digestive tract or breast cancer. They may also be elevated in heavy smokers. Alpha-fetoprotein levels can be elevated in patients with cancer of the liver and testicle, CA-125 levels in those with ovarian cancer, prostate-specific antigen levels in patients with prostate cancer, CA-19-9 levels in those with pancreatic cancer, and pancreatic oncofetal antigen levels in patients with pancreatic and lung cancers.

Oncofetal antigen tests are not used to screen the general population for cancer because the levels can also be elevated in nonmalignant conditions such as cirrhosis of the liver and ulcerative colitis. These measurements are used most often to evaluate the effects of cancer treatment. If treatment is successful in destroying the cancer, the antigen level goes down.

Other laboratory studies of body fluids cannot diagnose cancer specifically but may suggest possible malignancies. For example, an elevated serum alkaline phosphatase level may be caused by metastatic bone cancer or by hyperparathyroidism. Other potentially useful laboratory tests measure serum acid phosphatase and serum and urine calcium levels.

MEDICAL TREATMENT OF CANCER

Methods of treating cancer have traditionally included surgery, radiotherapy, and chemotherapy. A newer and less widely used treatment is immunotherapy. One treatment or a combination may be recommended, depending on the type and location of the cancer.

SURGERY

Surgery may be done to diagnose cancer, relieve symptoms, maintain function, effect a cure, or reconstruct affected structures. Surgery is the most common treatment for malignant tumors. Surgery for cancer may be extensive or simple. A thorough preoperative diagnostic evaluation enables the surgeon to plan the most appropriate procedure.

Surgery is most likely to be curative when growths are confined to one area and do not invade vital body structures. Surrounding tissues including lymph glands are often removed to eliminate malignant cells that have escaped the tumor mass. When surgery is extensive, it is often referred to as a radical procedure.

The preoperative and postoperative care of the surgical cancer patient varies with the specific surgery. General care of the surgical patient is detailed in Chapter 14. Specific surgeries are discussed in individual chapters. Following surgery, radiotherapy or chemotherapy may be recommended. The recommended treatment is based on the type of cancer, its location, and the extent of metastasis. The surgeon often consults with a radiologist and an oncologist (a physician who specializes in treating patients who have cancer) to determine the best therapy.

Adjuvant and neoadjuvant therapies are relatively recent approaches to cancer treatment. Adjuvant therapy may be used when a patient has had surgery or radiotherapy and is free of signs of disease but has a high likelihood of recurrence. Such patients may be given chemotherapy to eradicate any remaining undetected cells. Adjuvant therapy is often employed in the treatment of breast cancer. Neoadjuvant therapy employs chemotherapy to reduce the extent of the tumor before surgery or radiotherapy.

RADIOTHERAPY

Radiotherapy is the use of ionizing radiation in the treatment of disease. The units of measure for radiation doses are rads (absorbed dose of ionizing radiation) and rems (roentgen-equivalent-man). Radiation is used to treat cancer because malignant cells are more sensitive than normal cells to radiation. Radiation has immediate and delayed effects on cells. The immediate effect is cell death due to damage to the cell membrane. The delayed effect is alteration of DNA, which impairs the cell's ability to reproduce.

Radiotherapy may be given internally or externally. Internal radiation requires the introduction of the radioactive substance into the body. External radiation is given by way of a beam directed at the tumor.

Caregiver Safety

The nurse who understands radiation can work with it safely. The amount of radiation received by those who come in contact with the patient depends on the time of exposure, the distance from the radiation source, and the amount of shielding between the nurse and the source. The less time spent near the source, the less exposure the nurse incurs. Doubling the distance from the source decreases the exposure to one fourth. When the nurse triples the distance from the source, the exposure is reduced to one ninth (Fig. 23–3). Unless direct care is being given, the nurse should remain at least 6 feet away from the source. Effective shielding depends on the type of rays being emitted. In general, the denser the material composing the shield, the better protection it provides. Therefore, lead is more protective than concrete or wood. Because shielding is awkward and cannot provide complete protection during patient care, many agencies rely more on time and distance to limit exposure.

External Radiation

PROCEDURE. With external radiation therapy, the source of the radioactivity is located outside the body. A special type of x-ray machine is used to deliver a beam of radiation to the area being treated. Beams may be directed from several different angles to provide the greatest dose to the tumor and minimal exposure of other tissues. The number of treatments given is based on the radiologist's recommendation. It is not unusual for a patient to be treated five times a week for 2 to 8 weeks.

PATIENT PREPARATION. Before the first radiation treatment, the patient goes through a treatment simulation to determine the exact dosage needed and the

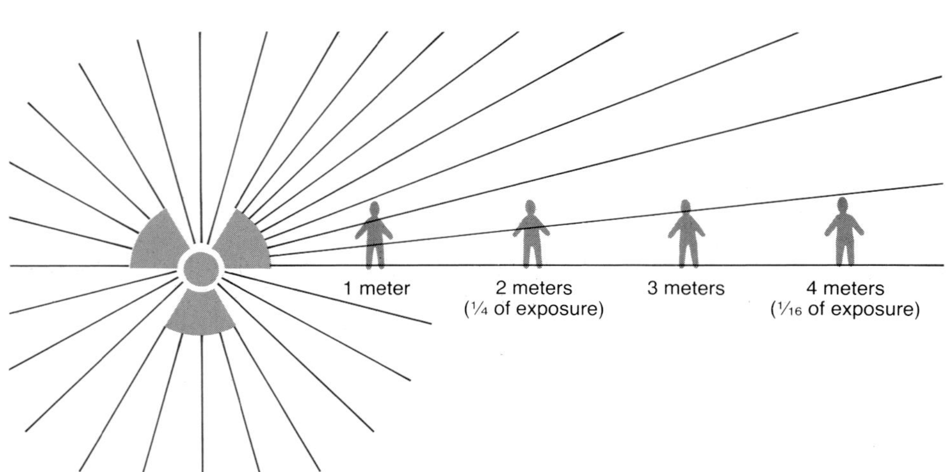

FIGURE 23-3
Radiation exposure decreases as distance from the source increases. (From Sedhorm, L. N., Yann, M. I. Y. [1985]. Radiation therapy and nurses' fears of radiation exposure. *Cancer Nursing, 8,* 129–134.)

treatment schedule. The patient is positioned in various ways while radiographs are taken. The radiologist then marks the skin over the area to be treated. The markings are made with waterproof ink and must remain visible throughout the course of radiation. The patient is instructed not to remove the markings until given permission by the radiologist.

Internal Radiation

Internal radiation involves the introduction of a radiation source into the body. Sources of radiation used for therapy include radioactive forms of iodine, phosphorus, radium, iridium, radon, and cesium. The source may be either sealed or unsealed. Sealed-source radiation is inserted into the body in a sealed container. One example of sealed-source radiation is cesium, which is contained in a sealed applicator that is inserted into body cavities to treat cancer of the mouth, tongue, vagina, or cervix. Sealed-source radiation may also be placed in threads, beads, needles, or seeds and implanted into body tissues or enclosed in a mold and applied externally. Unsealed sources are administered orally or intravenously. Iodine, taken orally, is useful in both the diagnosis and treatment of thyroid cancer. Patients being treated with internal radiation do emit radiation and do pose a threat to others until the source is removed or excreted. Therefore, the following safety measures are necessary to protect all visitors and nurses from excessive exposure to radiation.

1. The patient is placed in a private room, preferably one that is lined with lead.
2. A sign must be placed on the door to the patient's room indicating that the room is a radiation area. A standard sign is usually available for this purpose (Fig. 23–4).
3. Anyone who might enter the room for any reason needs to be informed of the proper precautions to be taken. People under the age of 18 and any pregnant female should not enter the room. This restriction applies to staff as well as others. Exposure to radiation is potentially harmful to the fetus.
4. The nurse can reduce the amount of radiation exposure by limiting time spent in the room and by working as far as possible from the radiation source. Institutional policies prescribe the time restrictions with implants. Nursing personnel who spend the most time with the patient should wear film badges to monitor their radiation exposure.
5. Work must be organized efficiently. For most patients, care can be provided in a total of 30 minutes each shift. Portable lead shields can be used to provide some protection. Lead aprons do not provide adequate protection in this situation.
6. The nurse must recognize that sealed sources can be dislodged accidentally. The placement of the source is selected to exert the direct effects of radiation on the area being treated. Specific positions may be ordered for the patient to decrease the risk of displacing the source. Bedpans and linens should be checked for any dislodged source before disposal.

   If the source moves out of position, the physician and the radiation safety personnel should be notified immediately. If the source comes out of the patient's body, it must not be touched with bare hands. Forceps and a lead container (called a *pig*) routinely placed in the room are used to retrieve and contain the source.
7. The radiologist determines how long the source is left in place.

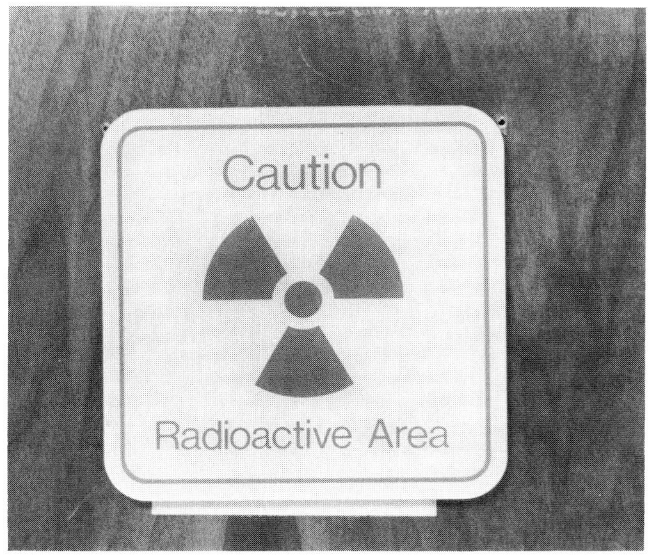

FIGURE 23-4
The radiation sign alerts others to the dangers of radiation. (Photograph by Stephen Matteson, Jr.)

When unsealed sources are used, there are some additional considerations. Gloves should be worn when working with the patient, especially when handling body fluids. Contaminated fluids, dressings, and the like may require special care as outlined in the agency policy. The radiologist can advise the staff as to how long these precautions are necessary.

SIDE EFFECTS. Side effects of radiation therapy depend on the area of the body being treated. The ideal radiation treatment destroys the tumor with the least harm to surrounding cells. Because cells that regenerate rapidly are more susceptible to radiation, both cancer and some normal cells may be harmed. Normal cells that are most sensitive to radiation include those of the hair follicle, bone marrow, lining of the digestive and urinary tracts, ovaries, testes, and lymph tissue. Radiation damage to these cells, then, explains many of the side effects of the therapy. Side effects are usually not evident until at least a week after treatments are started. Some people tolerate therapy well, whereas others become very ill.

Skin irritation and fatigue are common side effects with any type of radiation therapy. Depending on the area being radiated, the following additional side effects may occur: bone marrow suppression, alopecia (hair loss), anorexia, dry mouth, nausea and vomiting, diarrhea, and inflammation of the esophagus (esophagitis), lungs (pneumonitis), and bladder (cystitis).

Bone Marrow Suppression. In healthy persons, the bone marrow produces red blood cells, white blood cells, and platelets. Radiation suppresses the production of these cells. Anemia results from a deficiency of red blood cells. Without adequate white blood cells, the patient's ability to resist infection is reduced. Without adequate platelets, the patient is at risk for bruising and bleeding. Bone marrow suppression is most common among patients being treated for prostate or uterine cancer or for metastatic disease of the long bones.

Blood counts are usually ordered every week during radiation therapy to detect excessive bone marrow suppression. If blood counts are too low, transfusions may be required. The radiation treatments may have to be temporarily stopped until the bone marrow recovers.

Alopecia. Because the cells in the hair follicles are very sensitive to radiation, radiation of the head often produces partial or complete alopecia (loss of hair). Whether the hair grows back depends on the radiation dosage. If the hair does grow back, it may be different in color or texture than it was before treatment.

Anorexia. Anorexia is a loss of appetite. Factors that may cause the patient undergoing radiation therapy to have anorexia include inflammation of the mouth and tongue, altered taste perception, and nausea. Anorexia is an important problem because it can lead to inadequate nutrition and weight loss. It is especially problematic for patients being treated for cancer of the esophagus, neck, or head. Depression may contribute to anorexia in the patient undergoing radiation therapy.

Dry Mouth. Dry mouth, called *xerostomia*, is a special problem with radiation of the head and neck. The production of saliva decreases, putting the patient at risk for infections of the teeth and gums. Teeth are often extracted before radiation of the head or neck because the risk of radionecrosis of the teeth is so great.

Effects on Reproduction. Radiation is potentially harmful to reproductive cells as well as to the developing fetus and embryo. Therefore, radiotherapy is not recommended during pregnancy, and patients are advised to avoid becoming pregnant during the therapy.

The major side effects of radiation are summarized in Table 23–5.

CHEMOTHERAPY

Chemotherapy is the use of chemical agents in the treatment of disease. Chemical agents specifically used

TABLE 23–5
SIDE EFFECTS OF RADIATION THERAPY AND NURSING IMPLICATIONS

SITE	SIDE EFFECTS	NURSING IMPLICATIONS
Skin	Erythema (redness), desquamation (peeling) Permanent darkening	Skin is easily injured. Avoid exposure to sun, trauma, harsh chemicals, or soaps. Until therapy is completed, no lotions or topical medications should be applied. Do not remove markings.
Scalp	Partial or complete alopecia (hair loss). May be permanent. New hair may be different color and texture.	Cover scalp with wig, cap, or scarf if patient desires. Refer to American Cancer Society for free hairpieces and help with styling and care.
Digestive tract	Anorexia. Inflammation and dryness of the mouth. Decreased or altered sense of taste.	Small, frequent feedings. Respect patient preferences. Frequent oral hygiene. Suggest artificial saliva. Monitor weight to assess nutritional state.
	Dental caries	Encourage dental care. Mouth care per protocol.
	Painful swallowing	Antacids and viscous lidocaine as ordered.
	Nausea, vomiting	Antiemetics as ordered. Monitor intake.
	Diarrhea	Antidiarrheals as ordered. Perianal care.
Urinary tract	Cystitis Contracted bladder Crystalluria	Increase fluid intake. Have patient empty bladder often. Keep intake and output records.
Bone marrow	Suppressed production of red blood cells, white blood cells, and platelets.	Schedule activities to prevent overtiring. Protect from infection. Protect from injury. Watch for excessive bruising or bleeding. Check results of blood tests. Report fever. Use soft toothbrush, electric razor.
Lungs	Pneumonitis	Encourage coughing and deep breathing to prevent pneumonia. Use humidifier if ordered. Protect from respiratory infections.
Reproductive organs	Harm to embryo or fetus. Sterility, impotence	Patient advised not to become pregnant during therapy or for specified time afterward. Physician may counsel male patient about banking sperm.

to treat cancer are called antineoplastic drugs. The terms *chemotherapy* and *antineoplastic drugs* are used interchangeably in this chapter, as they are in common practice. These drugs act by destroying rapidly dividing cells and may be used alone or in combination with other forms of treatment. In some cases, chemotherapy is curative. In other circumstances, it may reduce the number of cancer cells, causing symptoms to decrease and often prolonging life.

PHARMACOLOGY CAPSULE

Adjuvant therapy is the use of chemotherapy after radiotherapy or surgery, or both, to eradicate any remaining undetected cells in patients who have a high risk for recurrence.

Types of Antineoplastic Drugs

Types of antineoplastic drugs used in chemotherapy include antitumor antibiotics, alkylating agents, antimetabolites, plant alkaloids, hormonal agents, and others. Various types of cancer are sensitive to different drugs or drug combinations. Combinations are sometimes used to attack cells at different stages of development. Table 23–6 gives examples of drugs used in chemotherapy and the cancers for which they are used.

Chemotherapy is usually administered by a nurse who has had specialized education. The drugs may be given in an inpatient or outpatient setting. The route may be oral, intramuscular, intravenous, intracavity, or intrathecal. Intracavity means the drug is instilled into a body cavity such as the bladder. Intrathecal chemotherapy is given in the subarachnoid space.

TABLE 23–6
EXAMPLES OF ANTINEOPLASTIC DRUGS USED IN CHEMOTHERAPY

Vinca alkaloids
  Vincristine
  Vinblastine
	Antimetabolites
	  Antifolates
	    Methotrexate
	  Antipyrimidines
	    Cytarabine
	    Fluorouracil

Podophyllotoxins
  VM-26
  Etoposide
	Antipurines
	  Mercaptopurine
	  Thioguanine

Nitrosureas
  Carmustine
  Lomustine
	Miscellaneous
	  Hydroxyurea
	  Procarbazine

Alkylating agents
  Mechlorethamine hydrochloride
  Melphalan
  Busulfan
  Chlorambucil
  Cyclophosphamide
	Steroids

Antracycline antibiotics
  Doxorubicin
  Dactinomycin
  Idarubicin hydrochloride
	Others
	  Bleomycin
	  Asparaginase
	  Diglycoaldehyde
	  DTIC
	  Cisplatin

Perfusion is a technique in which the drug is injected directly into an artery supplying the tumor. Perfusion is being used experimentally in the treatment of metastatic liver cancer and melanoma. The advantages of this approach, if any, are yet to be determined.

SIDE EFFECTS. Just as with radiation therapy, antineoplastic drugs act on both normal and malignant cells. The major systemic side effects of antineoplastic drugs are the same as those of radiation: bone marrow suppression, nausea and vomiting, and alopecia. Depending on the specific antineoplastic agent, the patient is also at risk for toxic effects to the heart, lungs, nerve tissue, kidneys, and bladder. These problems and related nursing interventions are discussed in the section on nursing care and are summarized in Table 23–7.

PHARMACOLOGY CAPSULE

The most dangerous adverse effect of antineoplastic drugs used in chemotherapy is bone marrow suppression.

Although bone marrow suppression is the most *dangerous* side effect, nausea and vomiting are the most distressing. Antineoplastic drugs simultaneously irritate the lining of the digestive tract and stimulate the vomiting center in the brain. Some agents, especially doxorubicin (Adriamycin), have toxic effects on the heart that may lead to heart failure. Bleomycin (Blenoxane) causes pulmonary inflammation and fibrosis that usually reverses after the therapy is completed. Vinblastine (Velban) and vincristine (Oncovin) are neurotoxic, with effects manifested most often by numbness and tingling of extremities and loss of deep tendon reflexes. Like radiation, antineoplastic drugs are hazardous to reproductive cells, and some cause impotence and sterility.

Antineoplastic agents also can cause very serious tissue injury to the vein during administration. If the agent leaks out of the vein, surrounding tissue destruction may occur. When extravasation is suspected, the infusion is stopped immediately. Various interventions may be employed by the physician or clinical nurse specialist in an effort to limit the harm caused by the agent.

BIOLOGICAL RESPONSE MODIFIERS

Surgery, radiotherapy, and chemotherapy work by destroying malignant cells and thereby reduce the size of the tumor. It is hoped that the body's natural defenses will then destroy the remaining malignant cells. The use of agents that work by promoting natural defenses have been classified as immunotherapy. Immunotherapy is now considered only one aspect of the broader classification of biological response modifiers (BRMs).

Therapy using BRMs is intended to boost the body's existing defenses. These agents act directly on malignant cells or stimulate the immune system to act against

TABLE 23-7
SIDE EFFECTS OF ANTINEOPLASTIC THERAPY AND NURSING IMPLICATIONS

SITE	SIDE EFFECTS	IMPLICATIONS
Bone marrow	Suppressed production of red blood cells, white blood cells, and platelets	Monitor blood test results. Allow rest. Prevent overtiring. Protect from infection. Report fever. Watch for excessive bruising or bleeding. Apply pressure to injection sites. Avoid rectal temperatures if white blood cell count is low. Use soft toothbrush and electric razor.
Digestive tract	Nausea and vomiting	Give antiemetics as ordered. Assess for dehydration. No fluids with meals. Pleasant environment. Respect food preferences.
	Anorexia	Small, frequent feedings. Frequent oral hygiene. Monitor weight. Give supplements as ordered.
	Xerostomia	Increase fluid intake. Recommend artificial saliva, sugarless gum or hard candy, ice chips. Moisten dry food.
	Stomatitis	Encourage dental care. Mouth care as ordered or per protocol. Assess for lesions.
	Diarrhea	Antidiarrheals as ordered. Perianal care.
	Constipation	Encourage fluids and high fiber foods, and exercise as tolerated. Give laxatives, stool softeners, enemas as ordered.
Heart	Cardiomyopathy Heart failure	Monitor for dyspnea, edema, increasing pulse pressure. Request electrocardiograms as ordered.
Lungs	Inflammation, fibrosis	Encourage turning, coughing, and deep breathing to prevent pneumonia. Use humidifier as ordered. Elevate head if dyspneic. Protect from respiratory infections. Monitor activity tolerance.
Nerve tissue	Numbness, tingling, loss of deep tendon reflexes	Protect affected areas from injury.
Scalp	Alopecia	Cover scalp with hairpiece, scarf, turban if patient wishes. Refer to American Cancer Society for free hairpieces and help with grooming.
Veins	Phlebitis at infusion site. Possible necrosis of surrounding tissue with extravasation.	Monitor infusion carefully. Protect infusion site. Report signs of extravasation immediately.
Reproductive cells	Harm to developing embryo or fetus. Sterility, impotence with some agents.	Pregnancy discouraged while on therapy and for specified period thereafter. Physician may discuss banking sperm with male patients.

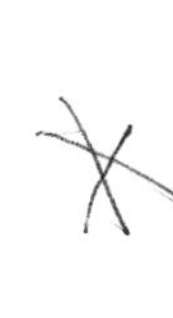

them. Such therapy is most effective if the immune system is functioning adequately. A skin test may be performed to evaluate the immune response before therapy is started. Examples of BRMs are alpha interferon, monoclonal antibodies, interleukins, tumor necrosis factor, colony-stimulating factors, and nonspecific immunomodulators.

PHARMACOLOGY CAPSULE

Biological response modifiers boost the body's natural defenses to combat malignant cells.

Because the effectiveness of BRM therapy for cancer is still being studied, it is not usually the first line of treatment. The most common side effects are extreme fatigue, headache, muscle aches, chills, and fever. Side effects are more common in older people and in people who are dehydrated, anemic, and malnourished. Previous cardiac, neurologic, gastrointestinal, hepatic, or renal disease also increases the risk of side effects. Table 23–8 outlines side effects of BRM therapy. The patient should be told to report a rash, blister, or pain at the injection site or a fever.

NURSING CARE OF THE PATIENT WHO HAS CANCER

When working with people who have cancer, it is easy for nurses to focus on the cancer and forget the person. In reality, little the nurse does has a direct effect on the cancer. Many things the nurse does affect the person who has cancer (see Care Plan: The Patient with Cancer). Assessment of the patient who has cancer is discussed along with nursing care for each phase of illness: diagnostic phase, treatment phase, rehabilitation, and recurrence or terminal illness.

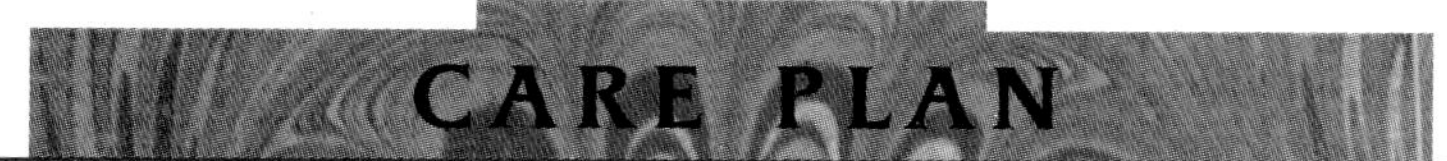

The Patient with Cancer

ASSESSMENT

Health History: Mr. Wilson is a 63-year-old African-American male who was recently diagnosed with lung cancer that is being treated with radiotherapy and chemotherapy. He reports a chronic nonproductive cough but denies dyspnea or hemoptysis. He states that he has been fatigued and weak since starting his therapy. He has had mild nausea, anorexia, and occasional diarrhea. He complains of dry mouth and is having some dysphagia. The skin over the area being radiated is tender. He is married, the father of three grown children, and is an insurance salesman. He has smoked 1 pack of cigarettes a day for 30 years, having quit smoking in 1992. At this time he continues to work part time and expresses concern about his financial situation. He states he has excellent insurance coverage.

Physical Examination: Height, 5′9″, weight, 175 lb. Vital signs: pulse, 72; respirations, 18; blood pressure, 176/92; temperature, 98°F (oral). Alert and oriented but does not initiate conversation. Dry mucous membranes and cracked lips. Skin on upper chest and neck is more darkly pigmented. Hickman catheter in place; insertion site free of swelling or drainage. Respirations are not labored, and breath sounds are clear throughout lung fields. Abdomen is soft and bowel sounds present. Extremities are warm with strong peripheral pulses. No edema. Unable to distinguish warm and cold or sharp and dull sensations in lower legs.

NURSING DIAGNOSIS	GOALS AND OUTCOME CRITERIA	INTERVENTIONS
Anxiety related to effects and uncertain outcomes of treatment.	Patient will experience reduced anxiety as evidenced by patient statements and by more relaxed behavior.	Encourage patient to talk about his illness and his feelings about it. Listen attentively and use touch to convey concern. Help patient identify sources of anxiety and strategies to deal with it such as teaching, counseling, spiritual guidance, and support groups.
Ineffective individual coping related to multiple stressors.	Patient will identify stressors and strategies to deal with them to improve coping.	Help patient set priorities during therapy. Provide information about management of therapy side effects. Encourage self-care as much as possible. Emphasize his strengths. Teach relaxation techniques. Refer to American Cancer Society for information about support services in the community.
Knowledge deficit of therapy, effects, and precautions.	Patient will correctly describe his disease, the prescribed treatment, the effects of therapy, and the precautions needed.	Determine what the patient already knows and what additional information he wants. Reinforce pretreatment teaching. Remind him not to wash skin markings off until radiologist gives permission. Do not apply lotion to irritated skin. Recommend cotton clothing over irritated skin. Provide information about specific drugs used in his chemotherapy. Refer to Cancer Information Service (1-800-4CANCER) if interested.
High risk for injury related to side effects of therapy.	Patient will have no injuries related to therapy as evidenced by absence of bleeding, dyspnea, skin lesions, or bruises.	Monitor for excessive bruising or prolonged bleeding, edema, dyspnea, impaired sensation. Report blood in stool, urine, or sputum. Handle gently. Apply pressure for 5 minutes after venipunctures or injections. Instruct to use a soft toothbrush and an electric razor. Protect feet and legs from trauma. Inspect daily for injury. Advise to wear shoes whenever out of bed.

Care Plan continued on following page

The Patient with Cancer *(Continued)*

NURSING DIAGNOSIS	GOALS AND OUTCOME CRITERIA	INTERVENTIONS
High risk for infection related to decreased white blood cells, venous access devices.	Patient will remain free of infection as evidenced by normal body temperature and absence of swelling or warmth at central line insertion site.	Advise patient to avoid crowds and people with infections. Report fever, foul wound drainage, or confusion to physician promptly. Teach patient proper care of Hickman catheter and have him return demonstration.
Altered nutrition: Less than body requirements related to anorexia and nausea.	Patient will maintain adequate nutrition as evidenced by body weight within 10 lb of usual (180 lb)	Emphasize the importance of good nutrition. Request a dietary consult. Consider small, frequent feedings. Respect preferences and aversions. Suggest soft diet eaten slowly for dysphagia. Tell the patient not to drink alcohol while receiving chemotherapy. Advise not to drink fluids with meals and to decrease intake of sweets and fatty foods. Create a pleasant environment without offensive odors. Suggest mild exercise before meals and rest afterwards. Give ordered antiemetics as necessary.
Altered oral mucous membranes related to decreased salivation, inflammation.	Patient will report successful management of dry mouth, and oral mucous membranes will be intact.	Tell patient to do frequent gentle mouth care. Recommend artificial saliva for dryness. Encourage increased fluids, sugarless gum or candies, and ice chips. Suggest moistening food before eating. When the mouth is inflammed, avoid acidic, salty, or spicy foods.
Fatigue related to anemia, effects of cancer.	Patient will report adaptations in lifestyle that reduce fatigue.	Assess patient's need for assistance and schedule activities to conserve energy.
Altered family processes related to illness and therapy.	Patient and family will discuss need to alter roles and relationships during treatment.	Include the family in patient teaching. Encourage them to plan with the patient for accomplishment of family tasks and responsibilities. Acknowledge family stress, fears, and the like. Refer to sources of help as needed. Ask the social worker to assist with financial arrangements.

TABLE 23-8

COMMON SIDE EFFECTS OF BIOLOGICAL RESPONSE MODIFIERS AND NURSING IMPLICATIONS

SITE	SIDE EFFECTS	NURSING IMPLICATIONS
Generalized	Flu-like symptoms: fever, chills, muscle aches, severe fatigue, malaise, headaches, tachycardia	Side effects may mask signs and symptoms of infection, so assess carefully. Give acetaminophen as ordered. Give meperidine as ordered for severe chills. Help patient plan for adequate rest.
Heart	Serious arrhythmias, myocardial infarction	Monitor heart rate and rhythm. Report abnormal findings.
Capillaries	Increased permeability, pulmonary and dependent edema, hypotension	Assess for edema. Monitor blood pressure. Have patient change positions slowly; avoid prolonged standing, hot baths, and showers. For hypotension, give colloids or vasopressors as ordered.
Bronchi and lungs	Anaphylaxis with bronchial constriction. Pulmonary edema.	Note signs of allergy: rash, wheezing, itching. For anaphylaxis, give epinephrine or diphenhydramine as ordered. Maintain airway. Assess lung for rales. Position for comfort (head elevated).

NOTE: Many other side effects occur with individual biological response modifiers. They include nausea, diarrhea, anorexia, weight loss, skin redness or rash, pruritus, desquamation, bone pain, renal toxicity, anemia, thrombocytopenia, leukopenia, leukocytosis, altered mental status, and liver toxicity. The nurse should identify the specific effects and implications for the specific agents the patient is receiving.

THE DIAGNOSTIC PHASE

The patient who develops one of the common signs of cancer often recognizes how serious the condition might be. Out of fear, some patients ignore the signs until the disease is advanced.

When people do seek evaluation of the symptoms, they are likely to be very worried. Patients often say that just "not knowing" is the hardest part. They go through tests and procedures, some uncomfortable, and then wait for the final word. For the patient, cancer is often what is feared most.

Assessment

When a patient is having diagnostic procedures related to an actual or a potential diagnosis of cancer, the nurse collects data needed in the planning and provision of care.

HEALTH HISTORY

Chief Complaint. The assessment begins with the chief complaint. The patient may complain of pain, lesions, lumps, or changes in some body function. The nurse elicits a complete description of the problem and the related signs and symptoms.

Past Medical History. Chronic illnesses, serious injuries, surgeries, and hospitalizations are documented.

Family History. The nurse inquires about the incidence of cancer and other serious diseases in the patient's immediate family.

Review of Systems. The review of systems records any of the following signs and symptoms, if present: pain, lumps, fatigue, activity intolerance, lesions of the skin or mucous membranes, easy bruising or bleeding, headache, vision or hearing disturbances, hoarseness, cough, dyspnea, hemoptysis, loss of appetite, difficulty swallowing, digestive disturbances, blood in the urine or stool, and change in bowel pattern.

Functional Assessment. The patient's diet, use of alcohol and tobacco, activity, and sleep routines are described. The occupation is documented and a usual day described. Health practices are assessed, including frequency of breast self-examination, testicular examination, and medical checkups. The patient's concerns are identified. The nurse asks about sources of stress and of support and usual coping strategies.

PHYSICAL EXAMINATION. The physical examination begins with measurement of vital signs, height, and weight. The nurse notes whether there has been a change in weight. The face, scalp, and oral mucosa are inspected for lesions. The neck is palpated for enlarged lymph nodes. Throughout the examination, the nurse inspects the skin for color, lesions, edema, and bruising. Breath sounds are auscultated and respiratory effort observed. The breasts are inspected for symmetry, dimpling, and abnormal skin color and are palpated for lumps or thickened areas. The abdomen is inspected for distention, auscultated for bowel sounds, and palpated for masses. The genitalia are inspected for lesions. The scrotum is palpated for descended testicles and, if present, for testicular lumps.

Nursing Diagnosis

Nursing diagnoses in the diagnostic phase may include the following:

- **Ineffective Denial** related to fear of diagnosis of cancer
- **Anxiety** related to threat of or change in health status
- **Knowledge Deficit** of diagnostic tests and procedures

Goals

Goals of nursing care for the patient who needs or is having diagnostic tests related to cancer are recognition of need for medical evaluation and treatment, reduced anxiety, and patient's knowledge of scheduled procedures.

Interventions

DENIAL. When people detect possible signs or symptoms of cancer, they may be so anxious that they cannot deal with their fears. Instead they deny the seriousness of the situation and do not seek medical care. Such delays may allow the disease to progress, making treatment more difficult and less likely to be successful. The nurse encourages people to learn the warning signs of cancer and to report them promptly. It is emphasized that these signs may be caused by conditions other than cancer, but medical evaluation is needed for a correct diagnosis. The fact that many cancers are curable, especially in the early stages, is stressed.

ANXIETY. During the diagnostic phase the patient needs encouragement, support, and honest information. The nurse must be careful to remain hopeful yet not give false reassurance ("I'm sure it will not be cancer."). Clichés are not helpful either ("Everything has a purpose."). It *is* helpful to recognize what the patient seems to be feeling ("You seem to be very worried."). Information about tests and procedures allows the patient to prepare mentally.

Nurses must remember that patients who are being evaluated for cancer are under stress. They may show this stress through anger, irritability, fear, or depression. All of these reactions are normal under the circumstances and should be accepted with understanding (Fig. 23–5).

The physician reports findings to the patient and informs the patient of the diagnosis. In the past, it was not uncommon for the diagnosis of cancer to be kept from the patient. Most patients now are told of their diagnoses. This change has come about because patients are better informed, cancer treatment has improved the odds of survival, and the patient's right to know is recognized. Nevertheless, the nurse should know what the patient has been told to avoid conflicting messages.

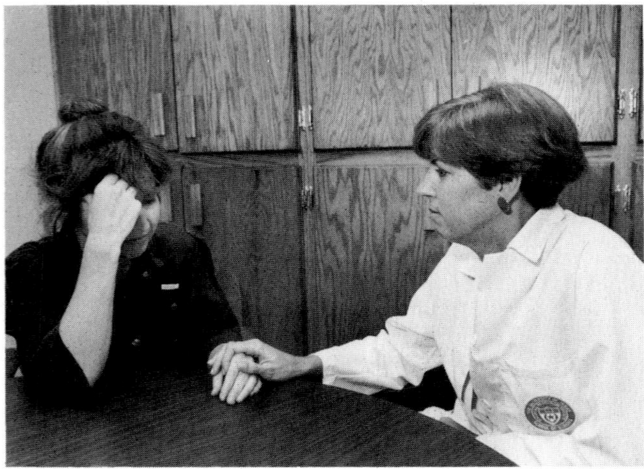

FIGURE 23-5

Listening and touching convey acceptance and caring. (Photograph by Stephen Matteson, Jr.)

Once a diagnosis of cancer has been made, the patient needs support to adapt to the situation. Even at this phase of the illness, the patient may show various responses related to grief. Responses could include denial, shock and disbelief, anger, depression, bargaining, and acceptance. It is useful for the nurse to understand and recognize how to help the grieving patient. Chapter 22 discusses nursing care of the grieving patient.

Patients struggle to adjust to the knowledge that they have cancer. For many this is the first time they have seriously considered the possibility of their own death. They are typically preoccupied with what will happen to them.

People have different ways of coping with a diagnosis of cancer. Poor coping is sometimes related to lack of information about the disease and its treatment. In that case, the oncology clinical nurse specialist may be consulted to provide patient education. Some coping styles are more effective than others. Weisman's research, cited in Dodd et al. (1993), found that patients who had the most difficulty were those who tended to try not to think about the situation, passively accepted treatment, lacked personal support, and tended to expect the worst. Patients who handled the stress of cancer better usually confronted problems directly, wanted to be well informed, had personal support, and were optimistic.

The nurse should recognize that patients employ their usual methods of dealing with stress. When coping is not effective, the nurse may want to seek a referral to a psychiatric clinical nurse specialist or a mental health counselor.

KNOWLEDGE DEFICIT. The nurse tells the patient about diagnostic procedures, including preparation, what the procedure is like, and any specific postprocedure care.

THE TREATMENT PHASE

Assessment

During the treatment phase, specific assessments depend on the type and site of cancer and the prescribed treatment. Information obtained in the initial assessment provides baseline data. The nurse frequently and systematically assesses the patient for changes related to the disease process and for effects and side effects of therapy. Areas of ongoing assessment are presented here.

HEALTH HISTORY. The nurse notes the patient's diagnosis and treatment plan. The past medical history is taken to reveal other acute and chronic conditions that require attention during cancer therapy. A complete drug profile is obtained, and allergies are recorded prominently. The systems are reviewed to detect significant symptoms related to cancer or the treatment including fatigue, weakness, headache, sore or dry mouth, dyspnea, palpitations, altered taste sensations, nausea, diarrhea, constipation, blood in stools, change in urinary frequency, hematuria or dysuria, sexual dysfunction, numbness, and tingling sensations. The functional assessment determines the effects of the illness and therapy on the daily functioning of the patient. The nurse assesses the patient's knowledge, fears, concerns, and coping strategies. Adaptations made by the patient and family are also explored during this phase.

PHYSICAL EXAMINATION. The patient's general appearance, level of consciousness, posture, and gait are noted. The nurse is alert for clues to the patient's mental and emotional state (eye contact, mannerisms, tone of voice). The patient's weight and vital signs are measured and compared with previous measurements. The skin is assessed for lesions and bruises. The scalp is inspected for hair loss. The oral mucous membranes are inspected for lesions and inflammation. The nurse observes the patient's respiratory effort and auscultates the lung fields for atelectasis or abnormal breath sounds. The abdomen is inspected for distention, and bowel sounds are auscultated. The extremities are inspected and palpated for color, edema, and peripheral pulses. Reflexes and sensation in the extremities are tested.

Assessment of the cancer patient during the treatment phase is summarized in Table 23–9.

Nursing Diagnosis

Nursing diagnoses for patients having treatment for cancer may include the following:

- **Anxiety** related to effects and outcomes of treatment
- **Ineffective Individual Coping** related to multiple stressors or overwhelming threat to self
- **Knowledge Deficit** of therapy, effects, and precautions
- **High Risk for Injury** related to side effects of therapy
- **High Risk for Infection** related to decreased white blood cells or venous access devices
- **Altered Nutrition: Less than Body Requirements** related to anorexia, nausea, and vomiting

TABLE 23-9

ASSESSMENT OF THE CANCER PATIENT IN THE TREATMENT PHASE

HEALTH HISTORY

Chief complaint: Diagnosis, prominent symptoms related to disease or treatment

Past medical history: Acute and chronic conditions, previous surgeries and hospitalizations, drug profile, allergies

Review of systems: Fatigue, weakness, headache, sore mouth, dyspnea, palpitations, altered taste sensation, nausea and vomiting, diarrhea, constipation, blood in stools or urine, urinary frequency, dysuria, numbness or tingling sensations, sexual dysfunction

Functional assessment: Effects of illness and treatment on functioning, patient knowledge and concerns, stresses and coping strategies, family adaptation

PHYSICAL EXAMINATION

General survey: Level of consciousness, posture and gait, eye contact, mannerisms, tone of voice

Height and weight: Present and previous weight

Vital signs: Present and previous readings, fever, tachypnea, tachycardia, hypotension, hypertension

Skin: Lesions, bruises, darkened or irritated areas

Scalp: Hair loss

Mouth: Condition of mucous membranes, dryness

Thorax: Respiratory effort, breath sounds

Abdomen: Distention, bowel sounds

Extremities: Color, edema, peripheral pulses, reflexes, sensation

- **Altered Oral Mucous Membranes** related to decreased salivation or inflammation (stomatitis, mucositis)
- **Colonic Constipation** related to decreased activity or drug side effects
- **Fatigue** related to anemia or effects of cancer
- **Body Image Disturbance** related to alopecia
- **Dysfunctional Grieving** related to loss of body part or altered appearance or function
- **Altered Family Processes** related to illness and therapy

Goals

Goals of nursing care for the patient having therapy for cancer are reduced anxiety, effective coping, patient's understanding of disease and treatment, absence of injury, absence of infection, adequate nutrition, decreased oral discomfort, normal bowel elimination, adaptation to decreased energy level, adaptation to hair loss, acceptance of change in body, and adjustment of family roles and relationships.

Interventions

ANXIETY. The thought of having surgery or of receiving cancer therapy may be very frightening to the patient. The nurse suspects anxiety when a patient seems tense, apprehensive, or helpless. The patient may have poor eye contact, increased pulse and respirations, perspiration, and trembling. The nurse can tactfully share his or her observations and offer the patient an opportunity to talk. The patient is encouraged to express feelings and identify the source of the anxiety. Listening and touch can be very effective in reducing anxiety. The nurse may also identify the need for patient teaching or for referrals.

INEFFECTIVE INDIVIDUAL COPING. The patient may need help in setting priorities and in coping with the side effects of therapy. Strategies to promote coping include teaching, encouraging self-care within the patient's limitations, treating physical signs and symptoms, emphasizing abilities, coaching in relaxation strategies, and encouraging the use of coping strategies that have been effective in the past.

Support groups may be most effective at this phase. People who have been through the same treatments as the patient can be especially informative and supportive. The local chapter of the American Cancer Society can provide information about services in the patient's community. Some agencies can arrange transportation for therapy and medical care. The Reach for Recovery program trains women who have had mastectomies to counsel others in adapting to their losses. Groups are also available to help patients with ostomies due to cancer of the colon, bladder, or larynx.

When a patient must be isolated physically (as when receiving internal radiotherapy), it is difficult for the nurse to provide emotional support. The nurse must remember to check on the patient frequently. Intercom conversations let the patient know he or she has not been forgotten.

KNOWLEDGE DEFICIT. A pretreatment teaching plan informs the patient what the prescribed therapy involves and what the experience will be like. The nurse should know what the physician has told the patient and reinforce that teaching. One source of information is the National Cancer Institute's Cancer Information Service. Booklets on cancer, cancer therapy, and coping can be obtained by calling CIS at 1-800-4CANCER.

External Radiation Therapy. Key points in teaching the patient about external radiation therapy are the following:

1. Having the treatment is much like having a radiograph. You are positioned on a table, and the machine is adjusted to direct the beam appropriately. During the treatment, you are alone in the room, but closed circuit television permits the staff to see you.
2. The treatment is not painful. In fact, there are no sensations at all related to the radiation. The machine that houses the radiation is controlled by a radiologist or technician. You will hear whirring or clicking sounds as the machine operates.
3. These treatments do not cause you to be radioactive. The radioactive material remains in the machine. Only the rays emitted by the material come in contact with you. When the machine is turned off, there is no radiation exposure.
4. The skin markings made by the radiologist are used to direct the radiation to the treatment site. Do not wash the marks off until the radiologist gives permission.
5. Skin over the area being treated may become irritated. Irritated skin should be kept clean and dry, but no lotions should be applied. Cotton clothing may feel

more comfortable over irritated skin. Antiperspirants should not be applied to a treatment site, but cornstarch can be used to absorb moisture.

Internal Radiation Therapy. When the patient is going to have internal radiation therapy, the teaching plan includes the following:

1. The radioactive material is given orally, injected into a vein, or implanted by a physician.
2. You are placed in a private room for a specified period of time for the treatment.
3. Visitors and staff are restricted in the amount of time they can spend in your room to limit their exposure to radiation. They also will maintain some distance from you when they are in the room.
4. If a sealed source is to be placed in a body cavity, you have to maintain a certain position to keep the source positioned correctly.

Chemotherapy. If chemotherapy is prescribed, the teaching plan includes a description of the drugs to be administered, the potential side effects, and related precautions. Written information is provided to supplement the verbal teaching. The nurse explores what the patient has heard about chemotherapy and corrects any misconceptions. Many patients have heard horror stories about drug side effects, especially nausea and vomiting. The nurse informs the patient of measures that can be taken to make the side effects more tolerable.

HIGH RISK FOR INJURY. The patient may exhibit various signs and symptoms of tissue injury associated with cancer therapy. Specific nursing measures are described for some of the injurious effects of cancer therapy.

Pneumonitis and Pulmonary Fibrosis. Patients with pneumonitis are encouraged to do coughing and deep breathing exercises to reduce the risk of pneumonia. They should be protected from exposure to people who have upper respiratory infections. If the patient has dyspnea, the nurse elevates the head and schedules care to allow adequate rest and avoid exhaustion.

Cardiac Toxicity. Patients receiving doxorubicin (Adriamycin) may show signs of heart failure, so the nurse monitors for dyspnea, increasing pulse pressure, and edema. Care of the patient with heart failure is covered in Chapter 31.

Neurotoxicity. The patient who has neurotoxic effects of chemotherapy has special needs as well. Extremities that lack normal sensation are prone to injury and must be protected.

Cystitis and Diarrhea. If the abdomen or lower back is irradiated, the patient is encouraged to increase fluid intake and empty the bladder often because of the risk of cystitis. Assessments of tissue turgor and mucous membrane moisture help the nurse detect dehydration. Diarrhea may require the administration of antidiarrheal drugs and special perianal care.

Thrombocytopenia. Both radiation and chemotherapy can suppress the production of platelets. When a patient has a low platelet count (thrombocytopenia), the blood does not clot promptly. Gentle handling is necessary to avoid trauma and bruising. Invasive procedures, including rectal temperatures, are minimized. After venipunctures or injections, pressure is applied for 5 minutes to control oozing. The patient is instructed to use a soft toothbrush and an electric razor to prevent trauma to the oral tissues or the skin.

Any blood in the stool, urine, or sputum is reported to the physician immediately. Signs and symptoms of internal bleeding include increased pulse and respirations, restlessness, pallor, decreased urine output, and falling blood pressure (a late sign).

Reproductive Cells. Because of the potential for harm to the developing embryo or fetus, females are generally advised not to become pregnant within 2 years of chemotherapy or while receiving radiotherapy. Female patients of childbearing age should discuss specific guidelines with their physicians. Because sperm production is reduced, males are counseled about the advisability of banking sperm before beginning the therapy with certain drugs.

HIGH RISK FOR INFECTION. Patients with low white blood cell counts due to radiation or chemotherapy must be protected from infection. They should avoid crowds and close contact with others who have infectious diseases. Any signs of infection (elevated temperature, foul wound drainage, confusion) are reported to the physician promptly.

If the white blood cell count is very low, compromised host precautions (or neutropenic precautions) may be needed to protect the patient. Such precautions include a private room and strict handwashing by all who enter the room. Fresh flowers, fruits, and vegetables are not allowed in the room because they harbor organisms. Additional details on compromised host precautions are in Table 30–12 in Chapter 30.

Patients who receive chemotherapy may have a venous access device implanted to permit frequent intravenous access without repeated venipunctures. Use of an access device also delivers the antineoplastic agent into a large vein with turbulent blood flow. This decreases the local tissue injury caused by the drug. The venous access device does present a potential portal for infection. Most agencies have standard procedures for care of the device. Because the device usually remains in place for the entire treatment period, the patient or a helper must know how to care for it at home. Care of venous access devices is discussed in Chapter 15.

ALTERED NUTRITION. Anorexia is common with cancer therapy, but good nutrition is essential. The patient is offered a high-protein, high-calorie diet. Small, frequent feedings are sometimes easier to take than three large meals a day. Light exercise before meals may stimulate the appetite. If patients have specific food preferences and aversions, they should be respected. Many patients find that red meat and some other foods taste bitter when on chemotherapy. Use of plastic utensils may decrease the bitter taste. Nutritional supplements (such as Ensure or Sustacal), enteral feedings, or both may be ordered if the patient has excessive weight loss.

The nurse must be familiar with the specific antineoplastic agents so that the patient can be advised of any specific food restrictions. For example, patients taking procarbazine (Matulane) may have severe hypertensive reactions if they consume foods containing tyramine while on this drug. Foods rich in tyramine include aged cheeses, bananas, beer, beverages containing caffeine, yogurt, and liver. Alcohol should not be consumed while on antineoplastic agents because the combination may produce severe nausea and vomiting, headache, and collapse.

Persistent nausea and vomiting can lead to dehydration and malnutrition. Various combinations of antiemetics and sedatives can be tried as ordered to obtain relief (Table 23–10). New drugs like ondansetron (Zofran) are often very effective when given before chemotherapy.

PHARMACOLOGY CAPSULE

Newer antiemetics and sedatives have greatly improved the management of nausea and vomiting associated with chemotherapy.

While antineoplastic drugs are being administered, sedatives are sometimes ordered so the patient can sleep. Nursing measures to manage nausea and vomiting are detailed in Chapter 34. Additional suggestions from the American Cancer Society (1987) are the following:

1. Don't drink fluids with meals.
2. Decrease intake of sweets and fatty foods.
3. Eat food at room temperature.
4. Eat slowly and chew well.
5. Drink clear, cool, unsweetened liquids.
6. Avoid offensive odors.
7. Rest after eating.

ALTERED ORAL MUCOUS MEMBRANES. A number of measures are helpful when the patient has xerostomia (dry mouth). Frequent, gentle mouth care and use of artificial saliva increase comfort. Several commercial products on the market moisten the mouth. Various protocols for mouth care can be used. For example, the patient can rinse the mouth with normal saline, a solution of 1 tablespoon of hydrogen peroxide in a glass of water, or a solution of ½ teaspoon of bicarbonate of soda in a glass of water. The patient is encouraged to increase fluid intake, chew sugarless gum or candies, suck on ice chips, and moisten dry food before eating. Lemon and glycerine swabs are no longer recommended because lemon juice dehydrates oral tissues and glycerine provides a medium for bacterial growth.

Stomatitis is a painful condition that can interfere with adequate food intake. The patient who has stomatitis should continue mouth care as prescribed, eat soft foods, and avoid foods that are acidic, salty, or spicy.

TABLE 23–10
ANTIEMETICS USED WITH CANCER THERAPY

CLASSIFICATION	SPECIFIC DRUGS	SIDE EFFECTS
Phenothiazines	Prochlorperazine maleate (Compazine) Chlorpromazine hydrochloride (Thorazine) Thiethylperazine maleate (Torecan) Promethazine hydrochloride (Phenergan) Perphenazine hydrochloride (Trilafon) Fluphenazine hydrochloride (Prolixin)	Sedation, hypotension, extrapyramidal symptoms
Antihistamines	Diphenydramine (Benadryl) Hydroxyzine hydrochloride (Vistaril) Cyclizine hydrochloride (Marezine) Meclizine hydrochloride (Bonine, Antivert) Dimenhydrinate (Dramamine)	Sedation
Butyrophenones	Droperidol (Inapsine) Haloperidol lactate (Haldol)	Extrapyramidal symptoms, sedation, hypotension
Corticosteroid	Dexamethasone (Decadron)	Fluid retention
Hypnotics or sedatives	Diazepam (Valium) Lorazepam (Ativan)	Sedation, ataxia Amnesia, sedation, dizziness
Cannabinoids	Dronabinol (Marinol)	Visual hallucinations, somnolence, ataxia, hypotension
Miscellaneous	Ondansetron hydrochloride (Zofran) Metoclopramide hydrochloride (Reglan)	Constipation, diarrhea, headache Sedation, diarrhea, dizziness, extrapyramidal symptoms

COLONIC CONSTIPATION. Some patients are constipated while on cancer therapy owing to reduced activity, narcotic analgesics, and the effects of some antineoplastic agents. The nurse monitors the patient's bowel movements to detect constipation. The physician may prescribe a high-fiber diet, stool softeners, laxatives, and phosphate or biphosphate enemas to prevent or treat constipation.

FATIGUE. Anemia and other side effects of therapy may cause the patient to tire easily. The nurse must assess the patient's need for assistance and schedule activities to conserve energy. The patient's pulse is monitored as it tends to be more rapid with anemia.

BODY IMAGE DISTURBANCE. The nurse is sensitive to the patient's concern about hair loss. At first the patient may just note extra hair in the brush or comb. Later, the hair often comes out in clumps. Hair loss may be partial or complete. Typically hair begins to grow back soon after the completion of chemotherapy and 4 to 6 months after the completion of radiotherapy. It is not unusual for the new hair to be a different color or texture. Following large doses of radiation to the head, the hair may not return. Although some patients take this in stride, others may wish to use wigs, scarves, or hats to cover the head. Some insurance companies cover the price of wigs; others do not. The American Cancer Society loans wigs to patients free of charge. The society also sponsors the "Look Good—Feel Good" program to assist patients to look their best during therapy.

DYSFUNCTIONAL GRIEVING. Treatment of cancer often results in temporary or permanent changes in body appearance or function. Changes or losses often trigger a grief response. The patient may be sad, tearful, or verbalize feelings about the loss. The nurse listens in an accepting way that lets the patient know the feelings are understood. Behaviors that suggest that the patient is beginning to accept the loss or change include talking about the loss and looking at or touching the affected part. The nurse supports the patient as needed and provides practical information about adapting to the loss.

ALTERED FAMILY PROCESSES. While undergoing treatment for cancer, the patient may be concerned with meeting responsibilities at home and at work. Some treatments extend over many months and make it difficult to maintain one's usual activities. Side effects of the treatment may make the patient feel tired and discouraged. Family and friends need to understand what the patient is going through and what they can do to help. The nurse encourages them to remain involved with the patient. Family members may need some help themselves to handle their responses to the patient's illness.

Financial concerns may be very serious for the patient and family. The nurse obtains a social work consultation if necessary to assist them with insurance and disability claims and financial assistance referrals.

Evaluation

Criteria for evaluating the effect of nursing interventions are the patient's statement of reduced anxiety and relaxed demeanor; the patient's demonstration of effective coping strategies; the patient's verbalization of content in the teaching plan; an intact skin and mucous membranes, an absence of bleeding, dyspnea, edema, diarrhea, and dysuria; a normal body temperature, an absence of purulent drainage; a stable body weight; moist mucous membranes; a bowel movement at least every 3 days; the patient's completion of essential activities without dyspnea or tachycardia; the patient's demonstration of acceptance or concealment of hair loss; the patient's discussion of feelings of loss and touching of affected parts; and the family's reassignment of roles and responsibilities.

RECOVERY AND REHABILITATION

If the outcome of treatment appears to be a cure, the patient and family are usually overjoyed. Some patients, however, become excessively concerned with their bodies, constantly monitoring for new evidence of cancer. Periodic checkups are essential but may be dreaded as the patient realizes that complete or permanent recovery cannot be guaranteed. If any signs of a possible recurrence appear, patients are understandably concerned.

As patients recover from the effects of cancer and cancer therapy, rehabilitation may be needed to restore them to the highest possible level of functioning.

TERMINAL ILLNESS

Though increasing numbers of people are surviving cancer, it is still the second leading cause of death. If treatment is unsuccessful, the patient eventually begins to decline. Patients need to know what resources are available to them and their families. The nurse can provide information about home health care, hospice, and voluntary and charitable organizations whose services might be needed. The oncology clinical nurse specialist is an excellent resource person for the patient.

Nurses must be aware of their own feelings about dying to work with these patients. Nurses can help the terminal patient in many ways. They must continue to be attentive and accepting. Nurses often fear that patients will ask them questions they cannot answer. Listening carefully is more important than talking. Patients can be guided to claim their accomplishments and find peace with their failures. Terminally ill patients should remember that although they are going to die eventually, they are living now and can still have some pleasure. Chapter 22 discusses care of the dying patient in more detail.

People with terminal cancer often express fear of having great pain as the disease progresses. Although cancer is usually painless in the early stages, advanced disease often causes pain. Cancer pain can be due to pressure on nerves, interference with circulation, obstruction of hollow structures (ureter, bowel, bronchi), and local tissue destruction.

General medical and nursing measures for the management of pain are discussed in Chapter 16. A variety of approaches should be tried to keep the patient as comfortable as possible. With severe, chronic pain it may be appropriate to medicate the patient at fixed intervals rather than on request. The nurse should not withhold ordered narcotics out of concern about causing addiction. Analgesics that may be ordered include long-acting narcotics (morphine sulfate [MS Contin, Roxanol], fentanyl patches) that may be supplemented with short-acting narcotics for breakthrough pain. Combinations of drugs, including a narcotic, a stimulant, and an antiemetic, may be effective for the cancer patient. These "cocktails," although not used as much as they once were, often control pain without excessive sedation when given regularly. The physician should be advised if pain control is not achieved.

ONCOLOGIC EMERGENCIES

The cancer patient sometimes develops conditions that require emergency intervention as a result of the disease process or the therapy. Some of the conditions requiring prompt recognition and action are hypercalcemia, syndrome of inappropriate antidiuretic hormone, disemminated intravascular clotting, superior vena cava syndrome, and spinal cord compression. Characteristics of these conditions and related interventions are outlined in Table 23–11.

UNPROVEN METHODS OF CANCER TREATMENT

A study of 5047 cancer patients in 1992 by Lerner and Kennedy found that 6% had employed some questionable method of cancer treatment. The American Cancer Society discourages the use of treatments that have not been studied and found to be safe and effective. A partial list of treatments considered unproven with regard to safety and effectiveness is presented in Table 23–12. Nurses can direct patients to the American Cancer Society for further information about questionable therapies.

TABLE 23–11
ONCOLOGIC EMERGENCIES

EMERGENCY	RISK FACTORS	SIGNS AND SYMPTOMS	TREATMENT	NURSING CARE
Hypercalcemia	Multiple myeloma, metastatic bone cancer; cancer of lung, breast, or kidney; prolonged immobility	Fatigue, confusion, weakness, constipation, polyuria, hypertension, tachycardia, poor muscle tone. If untreated, renal failure, coma, cardiac dysrhythmias, or death can occur.	IV normal saline and furosemide (Lasix). Drugs to promote excretion of calcium: plicamycin, calcitonin, etidronate disodium.	Monitor fluid status. Give IV fluids and drugs as ordered. Monitor intake and output.
Syndrome of inappropriate antidiuretic hormone	Thoracic or mediastinal tumors, thymoma, lymphomas, pancreatic cancer, cyclophosphamide (Cytoxan) or vincristine (Oncovin) therapy	Water intoxication and dilutional hyponatremia due to water retention: nausea and vomiting, anorexia, weakness, lethargy at first, followed by confusion, psychosis, loss of deep tendon reflexes, seizures, coma, and death	Fluids restricted to 500 ml/day. Demeclocycline (Declomycin). IV fluids and diuretics administered only in late stage.	Explain and enforce fluid restriction. Monitor vital signs. Keep intake and output records. Do not give demeclocycline with food or dairy products.
Disseminated intravascular coagulation	Septicemia, transfusion reaction, some drugs: vincristine, methotrexate, mercaptopurine, prednisone, asparaginase.	Normal clotting process is exaggerated, clotting factors are depleted. Early signs: petechiae, ecchymoses, prolonged bleeding from venipuncture. Late signs: signs of vascular obstruction, tachycardia, dyspnea, gastrointestinal bleeding, heart failure, and shock.	Platelets, fresh frozen plasma, other blood components. Heparin may be prescribed.	Avoid trauma. Handle gently. Give blood products and heparin as ordered. Monitor vital signs. Look for bleeding.
Superior vena cava syndrome	Breast or lung cancer, lymphoma, Kaposi's sarcoma, or metastatic testicular cancer in a position to put pressure on the superior vena cava	Redness and edema of face, conjunctiva around eyes; distended neck and thoracic veins; dyspnea, cough, tachypnea, tachycardia, cyanosis progressing to increased intracranial pressure	Radiation therapy, diuretics, steroids	Give medications as ordered. Elevate head and arms but not legs. Tell patient not to bend forward. Reassure patient that symptoms usually subside in 2–3 days.
Spinal cord compression	Lung and breast cancers, lymphomas	Tumor in epidural space presses on spinal cord, causing intense pain, weakness, altered sensation in arms or legs, impaired bowel and bladder function	High-dose radiation, corticosteroids, surgery to relieve pressure	Give analgesics as ordered. Assess for full bladder, constipation. Do neurologic checks on affected extremities.

IV, Intravenous. From Gribben, M. E. (1990). Could you detect these oncological crises? *RN, 53*(6), 36–42.

TABLE 23-12

UNPROVEN METHODS OF CANCER MANAGEMENT

Antineoplastons
Brych, Vlastimil (Milan)
Contreras methods
Dimethyl sulfoxide (DMSO)
Electronic devices
Fresh cell therapy
Gerson method
Greek cancer cure
Hoxsey method/Bio-Medical Center
Hydrogen peroxide and other "hyperoxygenation" therapies
Immunoaugmentative therapy
Iscador
Kelley malignancy index and ecology therapy
Laetrile
Livingston-Wheeler therapy
Macrobiotic diets
Metabolic therapy of Harold W. Manner, Ph.D.
"Psychic surgery"
Questionable cancer practices in Tijuana and other Mexican border clinics
Questionable "nutritional" therapies
Revici method
Simonton, O. Carl, M.D.

From American Cancer Society. (1993). *Questionable methods of cancer treatment* (p. 15). Atlanta, GA: Author.

NUTRITION CONCEPTS

- Impaired nutrition in cancer patients can result from the disease itself or from the various treatment modalities, such as chemotherapy and radiation.
- Cancer cachexia is a complex metabolic problem characterized by abnormalities in metabolism, fluid and acid-base balance, enzyme systems, and immune and endocrine functions.
- The goals of nutritional care for cancer patients are to prevent or correct nutritional deficiencies, to minimize weight loss, and to maintain or improve functional capabilities and quality of life.
- Interventions for common problems associated with cancer therapy (nausea and vomiting, food aversions, anorexia, dry mouth, diarrhea, and constipation) should be geared toward individual needs, mainly through trial and error.
- Cancer patients should have diets high in calories and protein; thus, foods high in fats (fried foods, whole milk, peanut butter) as well as snacks (nuts, ice cream, cookies) should be encouraged.
- If oral intake is inadequate, enteral tube feedings or parenteral nutrition are considered.

BIBLIOGRAPHY

American Cancer Society. (1994). *Cancer facts and figures—1994.* Atlanta, GA: Author.

Black, J. M., & Matassarin-Jacobs, E. (1993). *Luckmann and Sorensen's Medical-surgical nursing: A psychophysiologic approach* (4th ed.). Philadelphia: W. B. Saunders.

Bottomly, D. M., & Hanks, G. W. (1992). Controlling restlessness in advanced cancer patients. *American Journal of Nursing, 92*(1), 72–74.

Camp-Sorrell, D. (1991). Controlling adverse effects of chemotherapy. *Nursing 91, 21*(4), 34–41.

Cheney, C. L., & Aker, S. N. (1992). In L. K. Mahan & M. Arlin, *Krause's food, nutrition, and diet therapy* (8th ed., pp. 625–642). Philadelphia: W. B. Saunders.

DiStasio, S. A. (1993). Zofran makes chemo bearable. *RN, 56*(5), 56–59.

Doane, L. S., Fisher, L. M., & McDonald, T. W. (1990). How to give peritoneal chemotherapy. *American Journal of Nursing, 90*(4), 58–66.

Dodd, M. J., Dibble, S. L., & Thomas, M. L. (1993). Predictors of concerns and coping strategies of cancer chemotherapy outpatients. *Applied Nursing Research, 6*(1), 2–4.

Dudjak, L. A., & Fleck, A. E. (1991). BRM's: New drug therapy comes of age. *RN, 54*(10), 42–48.

Fulton, J. S. (1993). Using high-dose morphine to relieve cancer pain. *Nursing 93, 23*(2), 34–40.

Gribben, M. E. (1990). Could you detect these oncological crises? *RN, 53*(6), 36–41.

Hensley, J. R. (1991). Continuous sc morphine for cancer pain. *American Journal of Nursing, 91*(3), 98–101.

Ignatavicius, D. D., & Bayne, M. V. (1991). *Medical-surgical nursing: A nursing process approach.* Philadelphia: W. B. Saunders.

Ledermann, S. (1991). Adverse effects of chemotherapy. *Nursing 91, 21*(8), 4.

Lerner, I. J., & Kennedy, B. J. (1992). *The prevalence of questionable methods of cancer treatment in the United States.* Atlanta, GA: American Cancer Society, Inc.

Mahan, L. K., & Arlin, M. (1992). *Krause's food, nutrition, and diet therapy* (8th ed.). Philadelphia: W. B. Saunders.

McNaull, F. W. (1987). Tobaccoism in America. *American Journal of Nursing, (87)* 11, 1432.

Mettlia, C., Jones, G., Averette, H., Gusberg, S. B., & Murphy G. P. (1993). Defining and updating the American Cancer Society Guidelines for cancer-related checkup: Prostate and endometrial. *CA-Cancer Journal for Clinicians, 43*(1), 42–47.

Meyer, C. (1992). The richness of oncology nursing. *American Journal of Nursing, 92*(5), 71–78.

Mueller, R. (1992). Cancer pain: Which drugs for which patient? *RN, 55*(5), 38–45.

National Cancer Institute. (1987). *Chemotherapy and you.* (NIH Publication No. 88-1136). Bethesda, MD: National Institutes of Health.

National Cancer Institute. (1987). *Radiation therapy and you.* Bethesda, MD: Author.

National Cancer Institute. (1992). *Eating hints: Recipes and tips for better nutrition during cancer treatment.* Bethesda, MD: Author.

New drug available for nausea related to chemo. *RN, 54*(5), 121.

Pagana, K. D., & Pagana, T. J. (1992). *Mosby's diagnostic and laboratory test reference.* St. Louis: Mosby Year Book.

Patt, R., & Jubhash, J. (1990). Epidural sufentanil for cancer pain. *American Journal of Nursing, 90*(5), 122.

Plankey, E. D., & Plankey, M. W. (1990). A nuclear approach to cancer detection. *American Journal of Nursing, 90*(6), 107–108.

Radjeski, D., & Winnick, B. (1990). Oral care is part of cancer care. *RN, 53*(6), 43–46.

RH Update. (1991). Cancer society asks nurses to kick the habit. *RN, 54*(4), 18.

Spindler, J. (1991). Seeing through the mask of cancer. *Nursing 91, 21*(5), 36–40.

Unproven methods of cancer management. (1988). Atlanta, GA: American Cancer Society.

Walters, P. (1990). Chemo—A nurse's guide to action, administration, and side effects. *RN, 53*(2), 52–67.

KEY CONCEPTS

1. Cancer is the second most common cause of death in the United States.
2. Early diagnosis and treatment increase the chances of survival with many types of cancer.
3. Cells that reproduce abnormally and in an uncontrolled manner form neoplasms that can be benign or malignant.
4. Benign neoplasms do not spread to other parts of the body, whereas malignant neoplasms invade nearby tissues and can form metastases in distant parts of the body.
5. Tumors are classified by anatomic site, cell appearance and differentiation, and staging.
6. Carcinogens are factors that appear to increase the risk of developing cancer.
7. The seven warning signs of cancer are change in bowel or bladder habits, a sore that does not heal, unusual bleeding or discharge, thickening or lump, indigestion or difficulty swallowing, obvious change in a mole or wart, and a nagging cough or hoarseness.
8. A diagnosis of cancer is based on tissue studies, laboratory tests, endoscopic examinations, and radiologic and imaging procedures.
9. Surgery is the most common treatment for malignant tumors.
10. Internal or external radiotherapy is used to treat cancer because malignant cells are more sensitive than normal cells to radiation.
11. Chemotherapy is the use of chemical agents in the treatment of disease.
12. Radiotherapy and chemotherapy have serious side and adverse effects including bone marrow suppression, anorexia, alopecia, nausea and vomiting, and local inflammation.
13. Patients who receive internal radiation emit rays that can be harmful to others.

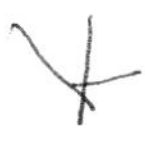

14. Biological response modifiers act directly on malignant cells and promote the body's natural defenses against cancer.

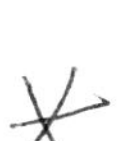

15. Patients who have suspected or confirmed cancer are very stressed and may respond with anger, irritability, fear, denial, or depression.
16. In addition to helping with specific physical problems, nursing care of the cancer patient addresses ineffective individual coping, grief response, altered nutrition, high risk for infection, and knowledge deficits.

CHAPTER 24

Adrianne Linton

The Ostomy Patient

OBJECTIVES

1. List the indications for ostomy surgery to divert urine or feces.
2. Describe nursing interventions to prepare the patient for ostomy surgery.
3. Briefly explain the types of procedures used for fecal diversion.
4. Apply the nursing process in planning care for the patient with each of the following types of fecal diversion: ileostomy, continent ileostomy, ileoanal reservoir, and colostomy.
5. Briefly explain the types of procedures done for urinary diversion.
6. Apply the nursing process in planning care for the patient with each of the following types of urinary diversion: ureterostomy, ileal conduit, continent internal reservoir.
7. Discuss major topics and content to be included in teaching patients to learn to live with ostomies.

GLOSSARY

ANASTOMOSIS Communication or connection between two organs or parts of organs

COLOSTOMY Surgically created opening in the colon

CONTINENT Capable of controlling natural impulses; in relation to an ostomy, able to retain feces or urine

ILEOSTOMY Surgically created opening in the ileum

NEPHROSTOMY Surgically created opening in the kidney to drain urine

OSTOMY Surgical procedure that creates an opening into a body structure

PROLAPSE Downward displacement

STOMA Opening created to drain contents of an organ

URETEROSTOMY Surgically created opening in the ureter

VESICOSTOMY Surgically created opening into the urinary bladder

Ostomy is the term used to describe an artificial opening into a body cavity. The site of the opening on the skin is called a stoma. An ostomy in the digestive tract may be a gastrostomy, jejunostomy, duodenostomy, ileostomy, or colostomy. The gastrostomy is used for long-term feedings and is discussed in Chapter 12. Jejunostomies, duodenostomies, ileostomies, and colostomies are created to drain fecal matter from the intestines. Examples of stomas in the urinary tract are the ureterostomy, ileal or colonic conduit, cystostomy, vesicostomy, and continent internal reservoirs. Ostomies of the urinary tract drain urine from the kidney, ureters, or bladder. Ostomies are sometimes described as means of urinary or fecal diversion. The term ostomate refers to a person who has an ostomy. Many people, however, prefer to be thought of as individuals with ostomies rather than as ostomates. This chapter describes the care of patients with ostomies created to pass urine or feces.

INDICATIONS AND PREPARATION FOR OSTOMY SURGERY

Ostomy surgery is done for a number of reasons. A temporary ostomy may be indicated following surgery or trauma or when there is severe inflammation or infection. The ostomy bypasses the diseased portion of the bowel or urinary tract, giving it time to heal. Permanent ostomies are usually necessitated by cancer of the bladder or colon or severe inflammatory bowel disease. Pouches are used with most ostomies to collect drainage. Whether ostomies are temporary or permanent, patients require considerable assistance and support to learn to manage with them.

Ideally, the patient is prepared for the ostomy before surgery. The physician informs the patient of the need for the ostomy, what it is, and whether it will be temporary or permanent. Sometimes the procedure is done in emergency situations, as when treating acute bowel obstruction or trauma. In these situations, the ostomy may come as a great shock to the patient.

An important resource for both the nurse and the patient is the enterostomal therapist (ET). The ET is a registered nurse with specialized training who has passed a certification examination. The ET is often an appropriate person to assess and teach the ostomy patient. This does not, however, relieve the staff nurse of all teaching responsibility. The staff follows up and reinforces the instructions of the ET. In settings in which specialists are not available, the responsibility for teaching may fall primarily on the nurse.

The exact placement of the stoma is very important. The ET often consults with the surgeon regarding the ideal site. Two factors must be considered: secure pouch placement and ease of self-care. The site must not be too close to the umbilicus, bony prominences, scars, folds, or creases that would prevent a good pouch seal. If the pouch does not fit smoothly around the stoma, liquid stool or urine may leak around it. The stoma is placed below the waistline if possible. If it can be placed within the margins of the rectus muscle, the muscle will help prevent peristomal hernias. The stoma must also be placed where it can be seen and touched by the patient. A patient cannot learn to care for a stoma that is located where it cannot be seen.

NURSING CARE OF THE PATIENT HAVING OSTOMY SURGERY

General preoperative nursing care is discussed in detail in Chapter 14. This section emphasizes only those aspects that are unique to the ostomy patient.

ASSESSMENT. Before ostomy surgery, the nurse is especially concerned with assessing the patient's expectations, understanding of the procedure, information desired, and fears.

NURSING DIAGNOSIS. The nursing diagnoses that require particular attention are the following:

- **Anxiety** related to perceived threat to self-image, anticipated changes in body appearance and function
- **Knowledge Deficit** of what to expect postoperatively in relation to the ostomy

GOALS. Goals of nursing care for the identified nursing diagnoses are reduced anxiety and patient's understanding of postoperative routines and procedures in relation to ostomy care.

INTERVENTIONS

Anxiety. The nurse is accepting of the patient's anxiety and tries to help the patient identify exactly what his or her concerns are. Some patients may be concerned about appearance, others about how their jobs or family lives might be disrupted. Patients are encouraged to talk and to use coping strategies that have been effective in the past. The nurse is aware that moderate or severe anxiety interferes with learning and, therefore, attempts to reduce anxiety before teaching.

Knowledge Deficit. There is some disagreement about how much teaching about the ostomy should be done preoperatively. The best guide is probably to base initial teaching on the concerns and questions raised during the assessment.

In addition to the ET, an important resource is a volunteer from an organization like the American Cancer Society or the United Ostomy Association. Volunteers are people with ostomies who have been trained to counsel other patients about adjustment to their ostomies. Their personal experiences in everyday ostomy management can make them very effective role models. Another good reason for using these volunteers is that the patient has a chance to see a well-groomed, active person who is living fully with an ostomy. When the nurse refers a patient to an ostomy group (with the patient's permission, of course), the organization will try to send a volunteer who is similar in age, sex, and occupation.

EVALUATION

Criteria for evaluating the outcomes of nursing interventions are patient's statement of reduced anxiety, relaxed manner; and patient's expression of understanding surgical routines.

FECAL DIVERSION

Intestinal ostomies divert fecal matter through a surgically created opening. Although the various types of ostomies have much in common, there are also differences that should be noted. The characteristics of the fecal material vary with the location of the ostomy and influence the type of care needed. Fecal matter in the ileum is liquid. Normally, the colon absorbs water from the fecal mass as it moves toward the rectum so that it becomes progressively more solid. When the mass is diverted from the colon, it may be liquid, semisolid, or formed.

Before fecal diversion, a low-fiber diet may be prescribed for several days. Antibiotics may be given to reduce the bacterial flora in the intestines. Cathartics and laxatives are usually ordered to empty the digestive tract.

ILEOSTOMY

An ileostomy is an opening in the ileum. The ileum is the distal portion of the small intestine that empties into the large intestine. An ileostomy is necessary when the entire colon must be bypassed or removed. Conditions that require colon bypass include congenital defects, cancer, inflammatory bowel disease, bowel trauma, and familial conditions such as multiple polyposis. Multiple polyposis is characterized by the presence of many polyps in the colon. Since these polyps often become malignant, removal of the colon may be recommended.

Procedure

A surgical incision is made in the abdomen, and a loop or the end of the ileum is brought out through a second abdominal incision (Fig. 24–1). The edges of the loop or the end of the ileal segment are everted and sutured to the abdominal skin to create a stoma. Loops may be supported with a device such as a rod or bridge instead of being sutured to the skin. Even though the patient is allowed nothing by mouth before surgery, digestive secretions quickly begin to drain from the stoma. The physician applies a temporary plastic pouch or a fluffy dressing in the operating room. The pouch collects fecal drainage to keep it from contaminating the surgical incision and to protect surrounding skin. The ileostomy frequently or intermittently drains liquid to pasty stool, so the patient will always have to wear a pouch.

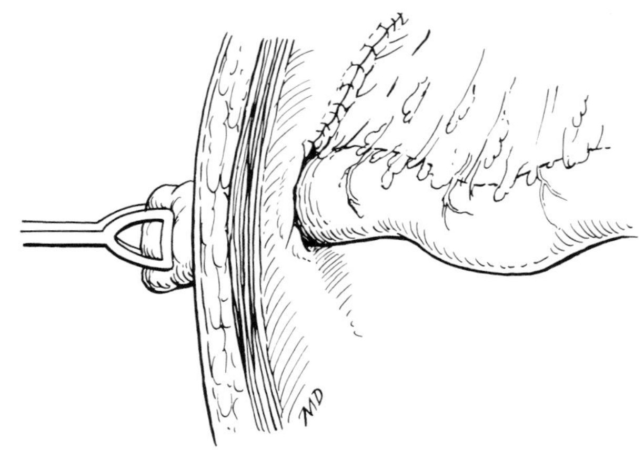

FIGURE 24–1

A surgical incision is made in the abdomen, and a loop of ileum is brought out through a second abdominal incision to create an ileostomy. (From Black, J. M., & Matassarin-Jacobs, E. [1993]. *Luckmann and Sorensen's medical-surgical nursing: A psychophysiologic approach* [4th ed., p. 1644]. Philadelphia: W. B. Saunders.)

PHARMACOLOGY CAPSULE

Ileostomy patients are usually not given timed-release capsules or enteric-coated tablets because they are likely to be eliminated before they dissolve.

Postoperative Nursing Care of the Patient with an Ileostomy

The immediate postoperative care of the patient with an ileostomy is like that of most other patients having abdominal surgery. The patient has a nasogastric tube attached to low intermittent suction. Intravenous fluids are ordered for several days, after which oral intake is gradually increased.

General care of the surgical patient is covered in Chapter 14. This section emphasizes only the special needs of the ileostomy patient.

ASSESSMENT

Health History. The health history taken preoperatively informs the nurse of the reason for the procedure. The past medical history documents other acute and chronic conditions that require management during the recovery period. Drug therapy and allergies are noted. Postoperatively, significant symptoms documented in the review of systems include pain, anorexia, nausea, vomiting, weakness, thirst, and muscle cramps. The functional assessment determines how the patient is reacting to the surgery and how he or she thinks it will affect usual functioning. The nurse also determines what stressors the patient perceives, usual coping strategies, and sources of support. The patient's understanding of ileostomy care is assessed.

Physical Examination. The physical examination begins with observation of the patient's general status: level of consciousness, orientation, posture, and expression. Vital signs and weight are taken and compared with preoperative findings. The skin is assessed for color, warmth, and turgor. The oral tissues are inspected for moisture. Respiratory effort is observed, and breath sounds are auscultated. The abdomen is assessed for distention and bowel sounds.

The stoma is inspected for color and bleeding. A new intestinal stoma should be beefy red. When healed, it should be rose red, somewhat darker than the color of the oral mucosa. A very pale, bluish, or black stoma has impaired circulation and must be reported to the physician immediately.

Swelling of the stoma is expected initially, then the stoma shrinks over a period of 6 to 8 weeks. The base of the stoma is inspected for redness, skin breakdown, and purulent drainage. A small amount of bleeding around the base of a new stoma is not unusual. In fact, it may be a positive sign indicating an adequate blood supply. If edema occurs later, it is probably due to pressure created by an improperly fitting collection device. Ileostomy drainage begins 24 to 48 hours postoperatively. The characteristics of draining fluid or fecal matter are noted. The presence of some blood and mucus in the drainage is normal at first.

Urine appearance and volume are assessed. The extremities are palpated for warmth and peripheral pulses. The nurse also observes for neuromuscular symptoms such as trembling, twitching, or cramping.

General postoperative assessment of the patient with an ostomy is summarized in Table 24–1.

TABLE 24–1

POSTOPERATIVE ASSESSMENT OF THE PATIENT WITH AN OSTOMY

HEALTH HISTORY

Chief complaint and history of present illness: Type of ostomy procedure done and reason

Past medical history: Acute and chronic conditions, prescribed drugs, allergies

Review of systems: Pain, anorexia, nausea, vomiting, abdominal cramping or pain, weakness, thirst, muscle cramps

Functional assessment: Response to surgery, anticipated effects on lifestyle, sources of stress and support, usual coping strategies

PHYSICAL EXAMINATION

General survey: Level of consciousness, orientation, posture, expression

Skin: Color, warmth, turgor

Mouth: Moisture

Thorax: Respiratory effort, breath sounds

Abdomen: Distention, bowel sounds

Stoma: Color, bleeding, edema; condition of skin at base of stoma

Characteristics of drainage: Amount, color, odor, blood, mucus

Extremities: Warmth, peripheral pulses

Neuromuscular: Trembling, twitching, cramping

NURSING DIAGNOSIS. Nursing diagnoses common to most postoperative patients (acute pain, ineffective airway clearance, high risk for infection, impaired tissue perfusion, and urinary retention) are covered in Chapter 14. Additional diagnoses specific to the ileostomy patient in the immediate postoperative phase are the following:

- **High Risk for Fluid Volume Deficit** related to nothing by mouth status, nasogastric suction, passage of liquid stool
- **Impaired Skin Integrity** related to stoma adhesive, fecal drainage
- **Body Image Disturbance** related to presence of stoma, altered body function
- **Sexual Dysfunction** related to altered body structure and function
- **Knowledge Deficit** of self-care with ostomy

GOALS. Specific goals for the identified nursing diagnoses are normal fluid balance, normal skin at stoma base, adjustment to change in body, continued sexual activities as desired by patient, and patient's knowledge of ostomy care.

INTERVENTIONS

High Risk for Fluid Volume Deficit. The loss of fluids and electrolytes through nasogastric suction and the passage of liquid stool can lead to fluid volume deficit and electrolyte imbalances. The patient is given intravenous fluids as ordered, with careful monitoring of hydration status. Accurate intake and output records must be kept. Output from all sources is measured, including urine, gastric contents, and fecal drainage. Serum electrolytes are monitored closely, but the nurse is alert for signs and symptoms of imbalances: changes in mental status (confusion, anxiety), changes in neuromuscular status (twitching, trembling, weakness), poor tissue turgor, edema, and dry mucous membranes.

Impaired Skin Integrity. The pouch is checked hourly at first to detect leakage. When the pouch is emptied or changed, the nurse tries to keep fecal matter from contaminating the primary incision. The skin around the stoma is cleaned gently but thoroughly. Maintaining skin integrity is an ongoing problem for the patient with an intestinal ostomy. The presence of fecal matter on the skin provides a medium for bacterial, fungal, and yeast infections. In addition, the materials used to hold the pouch securely can cause traumatic injuries and allergic responses.

A protective barrier must be maintained to prevent skin breakdown. A plastic pouch is used to collect fecal drainage. A good pouch is one that protects the skin, contains wastes and gas, is odor proof, permits freedom of movement, provides security for the patient, and is not noticeable. Many kinds of pouches are available, as seen in Figure 24–2, but the features are basically the same. Some type of adhesive is needed to secure the pouch around the stoma. The pouch has an opening at the bottom that allows for emptying and rinsing. Some have gas filters that allow gas to escape. There are reusable and disposable pouches, including one that is even flushable for easy disposal. The ET is a good

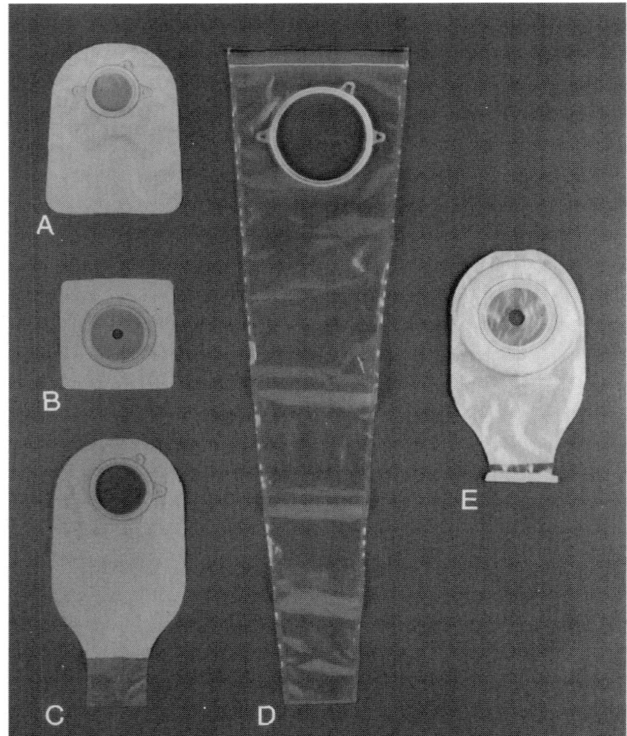

FIGURE 24-2

A variety of pouches are available to contain ostomy drainage and to protect the skin. *A,* Closed two-piece colostomy pouch. *B,* Skin barrier (second piece of two-piece pouches. *C,* Two-piece drainable colostomy and ileostomy pouch. *D,* Colostomy irrigation sleeve. *E,* One-piece drainable colostomy and ileostomy pouch with clamp. (From Black, J. M., & Matassarin-Jacobs, E. [1993]. *Luckmann and Sorensen's medical-surgical nursing: A psychophysiologic approach* [4th ed., p. 1648]. Philadelphia: W. B. Saunders.)

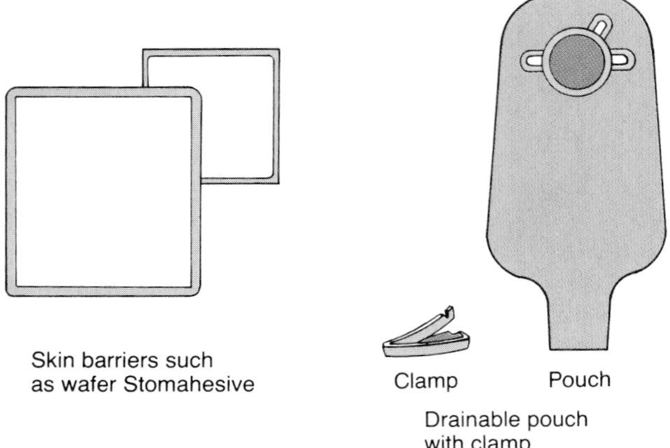

FIGURE 24-3

Protective barriers keep ostomy drainage from coming in contact with the skin and help create a seal with the pouch. (From Ignatavicius, D. D., & Bayne, M. V. [1991]. *Medical-surgical nursing: A nursing process approach* [p. 1364]. Philadelphia: W. B. Saunders.)

resource person to help the patient find the right appliance.

The appliance is removed periodically (usually every 3–5 days) for thorough cleansing of the skin surrounding the stoma. The adhesive is very gently peeled off the skin. Rough handling and frequent changes contribute to skin breakdown. Commercial adhesive removers are available if needed. The stoma and the area around it are then washed with water. If soap is used, it should be nonoily and must be rinsed off thoroughly. The skin is then patted dry. The patient may be surprised to find that the stoma itself has no sensation, but the surrounding skin may be tender.

A protective barrier must be applied before the pouch can be replaced. Skin sealants that come in the form of gels, wipes, sprays, liquids, and roll-ons may be applied to the skin. Sealants protect the skin; they do not hold the pouch in place. Next a skin barrier must be applied. Commonly used skin barriers include powders, pastes, wafers, and washers. If the skin around the stoma is irritated, powder may be applied. Excess powder is dusted away before the wafer is applied. Wafers and washers may be precut or may have to be cut to fit around the stoma. The opening should not be more than ⅛ inch larger than the stoma because a larger opening permits more fecal matter to come in contact with the skin. If a paste is used, it is applied around the stoma or on the cut edge of the wafer. The wafer is placed over the stoma and pressed down. Some pouching systems have the pouch attached to the wafer. Other systems consist of a wafer that is placed around the stoma and a pouch that then adheres to the wafer. After the pouch is securely placed, it is clamped.

Body Image Disturbance. Establishment of bowel control is an important developmental task of childhood. The patient who has an ileostomy is no longer able to control the passage of fecal matter and must learn to manage bowel elimination in a new way. This can be very distressing to the adult who fears spillage and exposure.

Inability to control odor associated with passage of gas through the stoma is another concern for the patient with an intestinal ostomy. The characteristic odor of stool is generally considered unpleasant. Since the ostomy patient may have fecal matter draining intermittently, the source of odor is almost always present.

The nurse assures the patient that odor is normal when the pouch is being changed or emptied, but that it can be controlled at other times. Causes of odor include certain foods and poor hygiene. Foods that produce gas or stimulate bowel activity are most likely to contribute to odor problems. These generally include spicy foods, onions, garlic, some vegetables like cabbage and beans, and high-fiber foods like whole grains and fresh fruits and vegetables. Reactions to specific foods depend on the individual. Therefore, the patient is advised to delete and reintroduce various foods to find those that are most troublesome. Since flatus is usually evident about 6 hours after eating gas-forming foods, the patient can eat those foods selectively at times when flatus would not be embarrassing.

Good hygiene also helps control odor. Reusable collection pouches should be washed with soap and water. Rinsing with a vinegar solution neutralizes odors that cling to the pouch. Odorproof pouches and commercial pouch deodorizers are available as well.

Sexual Dysfunction. One area that often worries patients with ostomies is sexuality. Patients are encouraged to ask questions about how the ostomy might affect sexual function or behavior. Patients may feel unattractive or fear rejection by their partners. Some males have sexual dysfunction, especially if they have had nerve damage associated with perineal surgery. The surgeon and the ET counsel these men about options, which may include penile implants. Other patients have problems because of psychological factors, which may improve with counseling.

Some practical suggestions may help the patient resume sexual activity. The pouch should be emptied and taped down before sexual intercourse. Pouch covers are available to conceal the appliance and its contents. The partner wearing the pouch should experiment with positions that are most comfortable. Female patients should know that ostomy surgery does not interfere with pregnancy or delivery.

Knowledge Deficit. After surgery, some teaching should be included every time stoma care is done. At first, the nurse may simply tell the patient what is being done and why. Then the patient is encouraged to take over more and more of the procedure. The nurse should have the patient demonstrate and practice as much as possible before discharge.

Some patients adjust more easily than others to an ostomy. A first step in accepting the stoma is looking at it. The nurse notes when the patient begins to watch stoma care. Patients are encouraged, but not forced, to participate in the care. If a patient does not begin to show some interest in learning self-care after a few days, the nurse considers supportive resources such as the ET or an ostomy club volunteer. Nurses tend to feel frustrated if patients seem unwilling to learn self-care. The nurse needs to be sensitive to the patient's feelings. An ostomy requires adjustments in body image and self-concept. Patients also have a grief response to this type of surgery. Chapter 22 explores nursing interventions to help the patient cope with feelings of loss.

The nurse or ET, or both, must help the patient plan for discharge. Topics to include in the teaching plan after ostomy surgery are skin care, pouches, diet, fluids, irrigation or drainage (if appropriate), activity, sexuality, complications, and resources. Written care instructions should be provided. The patient needs a list of supplies and places where they can be purchased. In addition, some temporary supplies should be sent home with the patient. The nurse also provides information and makes referrals as needed for resources such as home health care. The patient needs to know what activities can be done. In general, normal activities can be resumed in about 3 months. Meanwhile, heavy lifting and strenuous activities are avoided. The patient is advised to ask the physician about specific activities and contact sports.

Since the pouch and seal are waterproof, the patient can bathe or shower with the appliance in place. Regular clothing can be worn but should not apply direct pressure to the stoma.

Ostomy patients who enjoy traveling are encouraged to do so. Tips on traveling include the following:

- Take adequate supplies.
- If flying, keep the supplies in a handbag. This could avoid problems if luggage is lost or delayed.
- Include sealable plastic bags to dispose of used supplies.
- Exercise caution with new foods that may cause diarrhea or gas.
- If visiting a country where drinking the water is not advised, do not irrigate a colostomy with the water.

CONTINENT (POUCH) ILEOSTOMY

The continent ileostomy has an internal pouch created from a loop of ileum for storing fecal matter. The advantage of this type of ileostomy is that the patient does not have continuous drainage and so does not have to wear a pouch.

Not all patients are candidates for the continent ileostomy. It cannot be done for people who cannot drain the pouch or for those who do not have enough ileum for the valve to be constructed. People with ulcerative colitis are candidates for the continent ileostomy, but patients with Crohn's disease are usually not eligible.

Procedure

To create a continent ileostomy, a loop of the ileum is sutured together and then opened. A portion of the distal end of the ileum is inverted within itself to create a nipple valve. The valve prevents the leakage of fluid from the pouch. The looped section of the ileum is then closed, leaving a pouch capable of expanding and storing fecal matter. The distal end of the ileum is brought through the abdominal wall and sutured into place to create a stoma (Fig. 24–4). During surgery, a catheter is placed through the stoma into the pouch and sutured in place. The catheter is connected to low intermittent suction to keep the pouch empty. This prevents stress on the suture lines while the pouch heals.

Postoperative Nursing Care of the Patient with a Continent Ileostomy

In general, postoperative nursing care is like that described for the ileostomy patient. This section provides information on additional nursing measures that are specific to the patient with a continent ileostomy.

ASSESSMENT. Postoperative assessment of the patient who has a continent ileostomy is essentially the same as that of the ileostomy patient. When the patient has a continent ileostomy, it is especially important to assess for continuous drainage because obstruction of the catheter may occur. Absence of drainage or patient complaints of a feeling of fullness in the pouch suggest obstruction. The drainage from the catheter is bloody at first, then brownish.

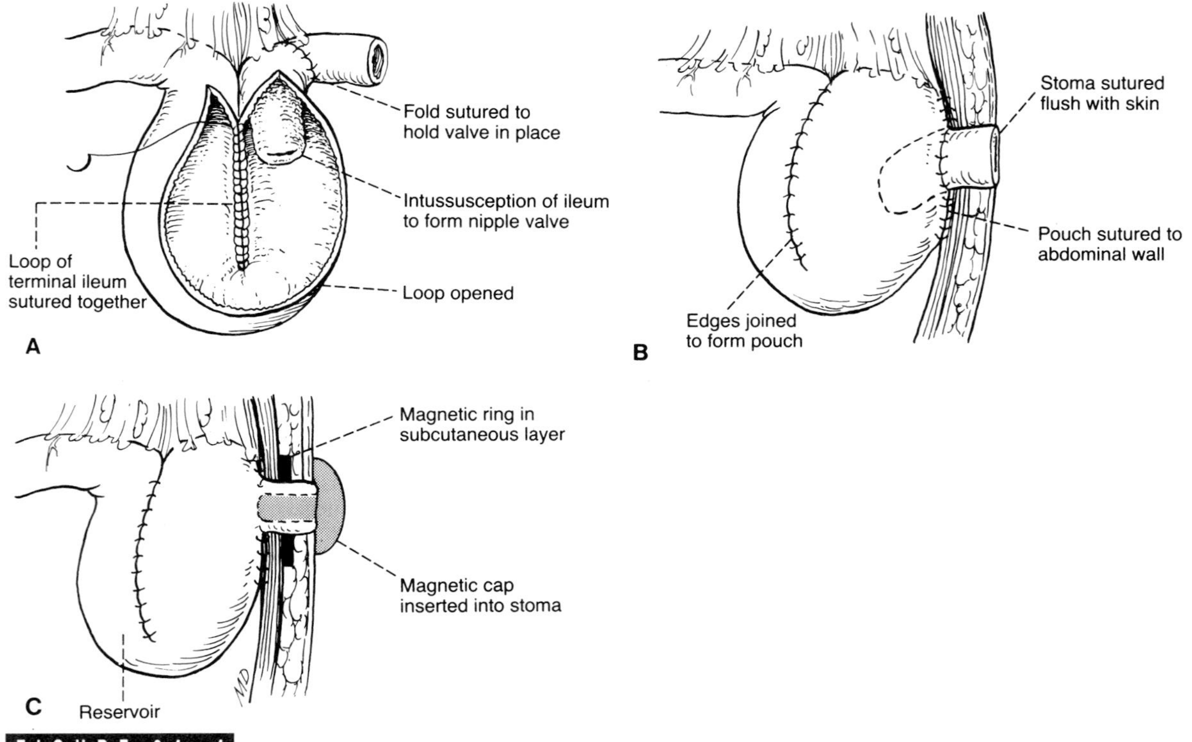

FIGURE 24-4

Continent ileostomy (Kock pouch). (From Black, J. M., & Matassarin-Jacobs, E. [1993]. *Luckmann and Sorensen's medical-surgical nursing: A psychophysiologic approach* [4th ed., p. 1645]. Philadelphia: W. B. Saunders.)

NURSING DIAGNOSIS. Nursing diagnoses in addition to those previously listed are the following:

- **High Risk for Injury** related to obstruction of the pouch drainage
- **Knowledge Deficit** of technique for draining pouch and caring for stoma

GOALS. Goals for the additional nursing diagnoses are unobstructed pouch drainage and patient's ability to drain pouch and care for stoma.

INTERVENTIONS

High Risk for Injury. In the initial postoperative period, the patient is given only intravenous fluids. The catheter is removed after several days, and the pouch is drained at intervals. At first, the pouch can hold only 70 to 100 ml of fluid. Later, it can hold as much as 600 ml. For the first 2 weeks, the pouch is drained every 3 to 4 hours. Over the next 2 weeks, the interval is lengthened to every 5 hours. Eventually, the patient will need to drain the pouch only two to four times a day. As the patient's body adapts to the ileostomy, the drainage gradually becomes thicker and the color of normal stool.

Knowledge Deficit. Key points in draining the continent ileostomy are as follows:

1. Have the patient sit or lie down for the procedure.
2. Gather supplies: lubricant, No. 28 catheter, drape, basin, irrigating syringe, irrigating solution, gauze dressing.
3. Lubricate the catheter and insert it gently into the stoma.
4. Resistance will be felt when the catheter reaches the nipple valve (about 2 inches past the stoma). Instruct the patient to bear down, then roll the catheter between your fingers and advance it into the pouch.
5. As soon as the catheter is in the pouch, gas and fecal matter will begin to drain. Drainage usually continues for about 10 minutes and produces a total volume of 50 to 200 ml.
6. If the drainage is too thick, instill 30 ml of normal saline as ordered. Gently aspirate. Do not do this unless necessary because it may cause dislocation of the nipple.
7. When drainage stops, quickly remove the catheter.
8. Place a gauze dressing over the stoma to absorb any secretions.
9. Measure, describe, and discard the drainage.
10. Instruct the patient in how to perform this procedure as soon as possible.
11. Advise the patient to wear a medical alert bracelet at all times that states he or she has a continent diversion that must be drained.

The dietitian is consulted postoperatively since the patient with a continent ileostomy will have some dietary restrictions. The diet is intended to avoid excess gas, maintain a soft stool, and avoid obstruction of the catheter. The following are foods to avoid:

- Coffee, alcohol, and gas-forming foods (initially)
- Skins, seeds, or nuts (including corn, olives, peas)
- Pineapple, berries, fresh fruit (initially)
- Milk products if they cause excessive gas.

EVALUATION. Criteria for goal achievement are the patient's pouch drains readily and the patient demonstrates proper pouch drainage procedure and stoma care.

ILEOANAL RESERVOIR

An ileoanal reservoir is somewhat like the pouch ileostomy except that fecal matter is stored and then eliminated through the rectum. It is an alternative to an ostomy and is included in this chapter because the patient has a temporary ileostomy and the nursing care is similar to that of the ostomy patient.

Procedure

The ileoanal reservoir requires a complex set of surgical procedures that are done in two stages. In the first stage, the colon is removed and an internal pouch that is created from the ileum is attached to the anorectal canal. A temporary ileostomy is made to allow the reservoir to heal. Approximately 2 months later, barium radiographs are taken to be sure that the reservoir is intact. If the reservoir does not leak, the ileostomy is closed (Fig. 24–5). The procedure is not recommended for patients with Crohn's disease or poor rectal sphincter control.

Complications

The major complications of the ileoanal reservoir are small bowel obstruction, leaking of suture lines leading to peritonitis, and inflammation of the reservoir.

OBSTRUCTION. Scar tissue or strictures may cause obstruction. Signs and symptoms of small bowel obstruction are abdominal distention, nausea and vomiting, decreased bowel sounds, and a change in bowel pattern.

PERITONITIS. If fecal matter leaks through the suture lines of the reservoir into the abdominal cavity, abscesses or peritonitis can develop. Signs and symptoms are increased pulse, respirations, and temperature; rigid abdomen and abdominal pain; and elevated white blood cell count.

INFLAMMATION. Inflammation of the reservoir may be manifested by bloody diarrhea, anorexia, and pain.

Postoperative Nursing Care of the Patient with an Ileoanal Reservoir

ASSESSMENT. The nursing assessment after surgery to create an internal reservoir is the same as for the ileostomy patient. In addition, the nurse assesses for rectal drainage and condition of the perianal skin.

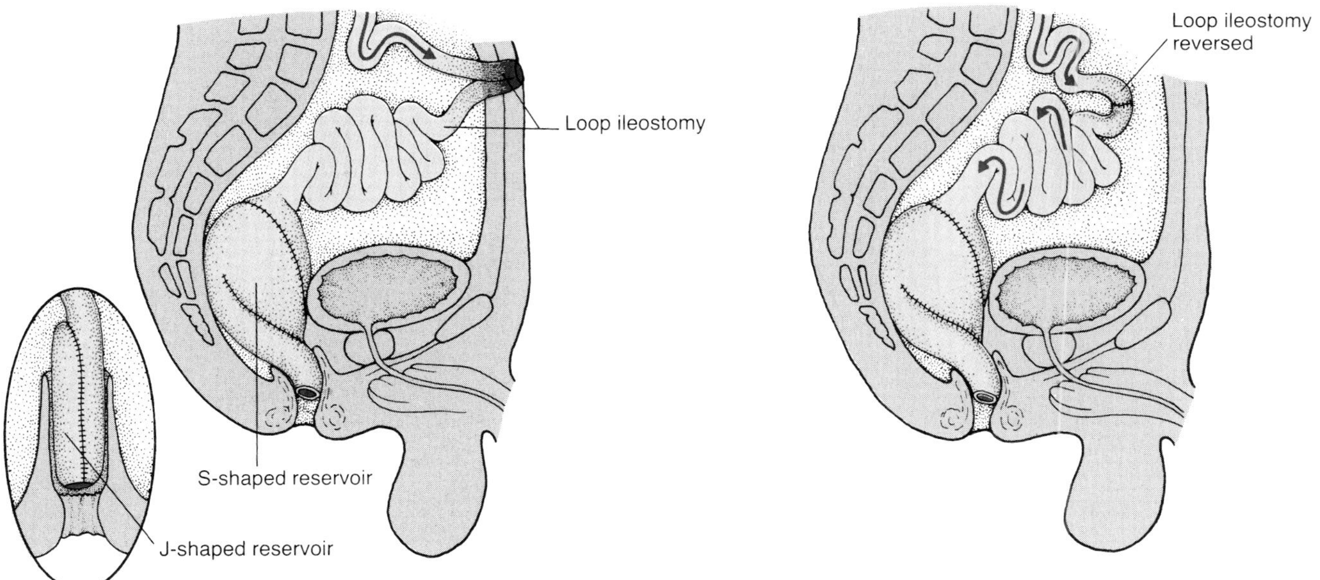

FIGURE 24-5

Creation of an ileoanal reservoir. Stage 1: The colon is removed, a temporary loop ileostomy is created, and an ileoanal reservoir is formed. The reservoir may be J or S shaped depending on the technique used. Stage 2: After the reservoir heals (usually several months), the temporary loop ileostomy is reversed and stool drains into the reservoir for storage until it is eliminated through the rectum. (From Ignatavicius, D. D., & Bayne, M. V. [1991]. *Medical-surgical nursing: A nursing process approach* [p. 1357]. Philadelphia: W. B. Saunders.)

NURSING DIAGNOSIS. In addition to the nursing diagnoses for the ileostomy patient, the following diagnoses may be appropriate for the patient with an internal reservoir:

- **High Risk for Impaired Skin Integrity** related to frequent passage of liquid stool through the rectum
- **Bowel Incontinence** related to inability to control passage of frequent liquid stools
- **High Risk for Injury** related to possible small bowel obstruction, leaking of reservoir suture line, inflammation of reservoir

Goals. Goals for nursing care for the specific nursing diagnoses identified are healthy skin; control of bowel elimination; and absence of signs and symptoms of obstruction, suture leakage, or reservoir inflammation.

INTERVENTION

High Risk for Impaired Skin Integrity. After the first surgical procedure, the patient's skin around the ileostomy stoma and in the perianal area need special care. Ileostomy care is covered earlier in this chapter. Until the reservoir is well healed, liquid discharge may be expelled without warning. Thorough, gentle cleansing and protective creams help prevent skin breakdown.

Bowel Incontinence. Initially, the patient may have as many as 20 stools a day. After a week, the number decreases to 8 to 10 daily. By 6 months, the frequency is usually only about 4 to 6 a day. Nighttime control may continue to be a problem. Perineal pads may be needed to prevent soiling of clothing.

The patient must learn to strengthen perineal muscles in order to restore control of fecal elimination. A recommended exercise is to tighten the anus, count to 10, and relax. This should be repeated five to six times, four times daily. Also, drugs can be prescribed to decrease the frequency of stools and to make them less watery.

Patients are advised to avoid fatty foods at first. There are no absolute restrictions. The patient learns through trial and error how his or her body handles specific foods. Caffeine and fresh fruits and vegetables tend to cause loose, frequent stools. Pasta, boiled rice, and low-fat cheese tend to produce thicker stools.

High Risk for Injury. The nurse is alert for signs and symptoms of bowel obstruction, peritonitis, and inflammation that should be reported to the physician. If obstruction occurs, the patient is given intravenous fluids and given nothing by mouth. A nasogastric tube is inserted to decompress the bowel. If the obstruction is caused by adhesions (scar tissue), surgery may be necessary to release the restriction.

Sometimes a stricture or narrowing develops at the site where the ileum is joined to the rectum. This is most likely to happen in the fourth week following surgery. The physician may be able to stretch the tissue manually and relieve the obstruction. If an abscess or peritonitis develops, the infection is treated with antibiotics. Intravenous fluids are ordered, and a nasogastric tube is inserted for decompression of the bowel. Surgery may be necessary to drain abscesses and repair the leaking suture line.

If the inner lining of the reservoir becomes inflamed or infected, the physician may do a proctoscopic examination to identify the cause. The condition may be treated with metronidazole (Flagyl) and steroids given orally.

EVALUATION. Goal achievement is based on intact skin without excessive redness around the rectum and the perianal area; decreasing number of incontinent stools; and absence of signs and symptoms of complications (fever, abdominal pain or distention, bloody stools, and fecal drainage).

COLOSTOMY

A colostomy is an opening in the colon through which fecal matter is eliminated. The location of the colostomy affects the characteristics of the fecal drainage: the closer to the rectum, the more formed the stool.

Procedure

A colostomy is performed by bringing a loop or an end of the intestine through the abdominal wall and creating a stoma for the passage of fecal matter. The location of the stoma depends on the portion of the intestine removed. Colostomies are classified by location in the colon. Therefore, there are ascending, transverse, descending, and sigmoid colostomies (Fig. 24–6). An ascending colostomy passes relatively liquid material. The drainage from a transverse colostomy will be liquid to semisolid. A descending or sigmoid colostomy passes softly formed stool. The colostomy begins to function on the third to fifth postoperative day.

A colostomy may be temporary or permanent. A temporary colostomy is done to allow healing of the intestine after surgery or in certain disease states. Since the intestine below the colostomy is intact, the temporary colostomy may have two stomas (Fig. 24–7). The stoma that drains fecal matter from the intestine is the proximal stoma. The distal stoma opens into the portion of the colon connected to the rectum. This is called a double-barreled colostomy. Sometimes the opening of the distal portion is brought through another location on the abdominal wall, creating a fistula through which mucus drains. An end colostomy with a Hartmann pouch for the distal segment is now more common than the double-barreled colostomy. A Hartmann pouch is created by closing the distal bowel and leaving it in place. The patient with a Hartmann pouch passes mucus through the rectum.

When it is necessary to remove a large part of the colon or the rectum, a permanent colostomy is made. Sometimes the colostomy is created in two stages. The patient returns from the first procedure with a loop of intestine protruding from an abdominal wound. The loop is held in place by a rod or a bridge. Later, the surgeon cuts the loop to create the stoma (Fig. 24–8).

The main long-term complications of colostomy are prolapse and stenosis. A prolapsed stoma protrudes farther out than usual. It is caused by increased abdominal

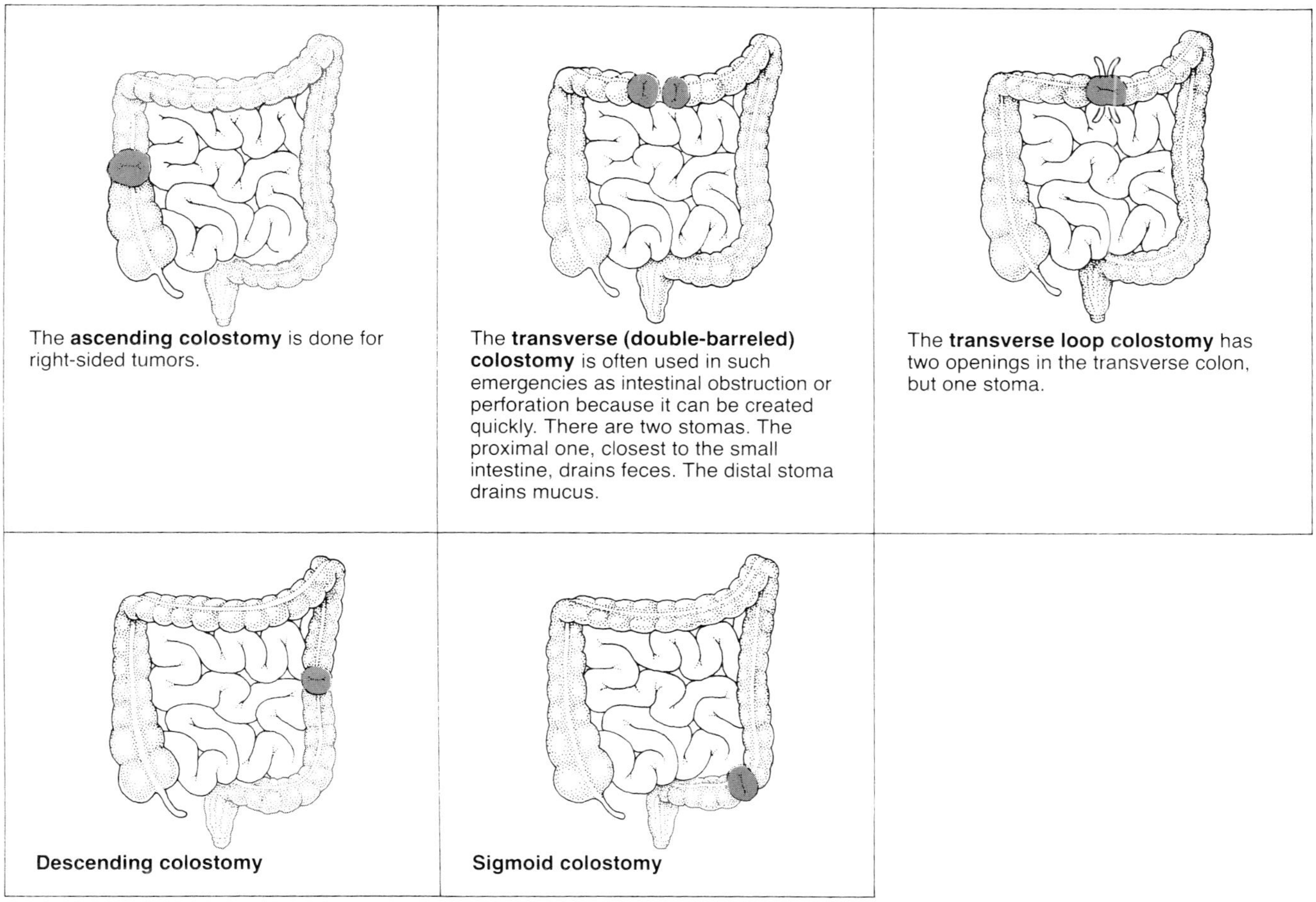

The **ascending colostomy** is done for right-sided tumors.
The **transverse (double-barreled) colostomy** is often used in such emergencies as intestinal obstruction or perforation because it can be created quickly. There are two stomas. The proximal one, closest to the small intestine, drains feces. The distal stoma drains mucus.
The **transverse loop colostomy** has two openings in the transverse colon, but one stoma.
Descending colostomy
Sigmoid colostomy

FIGURE 24-6

Types of intestinal ostomies. (From Ignatavicius, D. D., & Bayne, M. V. [1991]. *Medical-surgical nursing: A nursing process approach* [p. 1384]. Philadelphia: W. B. Saunders.)

Proximal stoma
Distal stoma

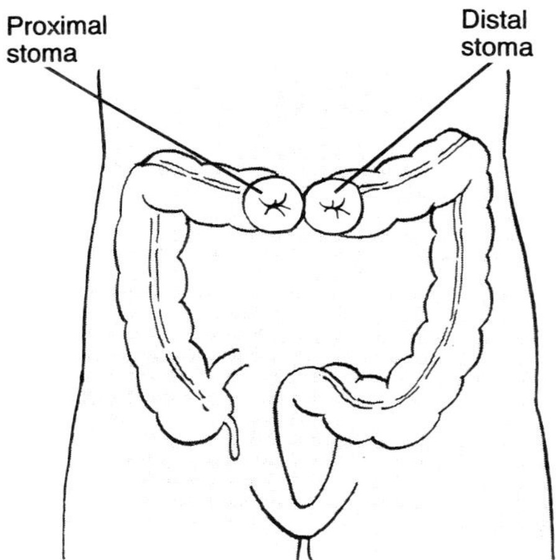

FIGURE 24-7

Double-barrel colostomy. (Adapted from Black, J. M., & Matassarin-Jacobs, E. [1993]. *Luckmann and Sorensen's medical-surgical nursing: A psychophysiologic approach* [4th ed., p. 1653]. Philadelphia: W. B. Saunders.)

MD

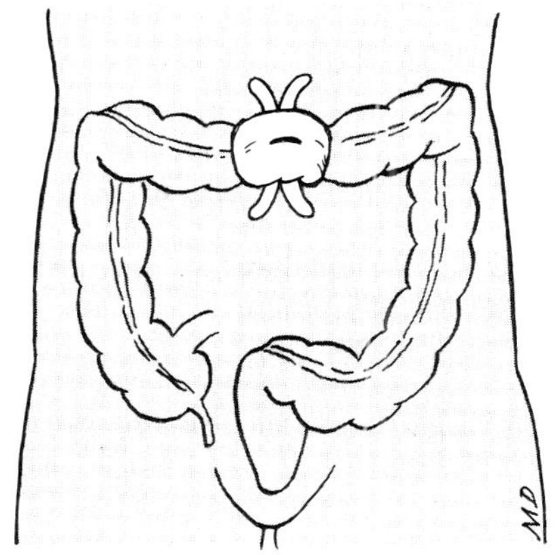

FIGURE 24-8

Loop colostomy. (Adapted from Black, J. M., & Matassarin-Jacobs, E. [1993]. *Luckmann and Sorensen's medical-surgical nursing: A psychophysiologic approach* [4th ed., p. 1653] Philadelphia: W. B. Saunders.)

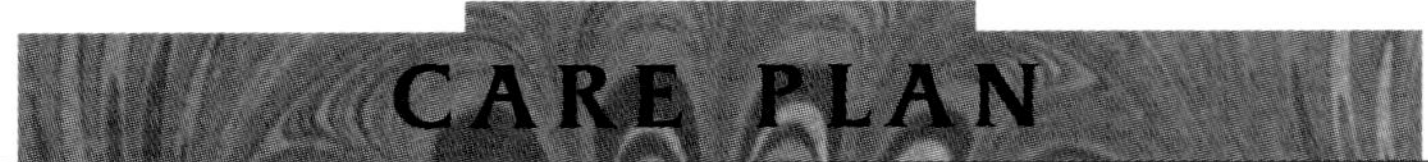

The Patient with a Colostomy

ASSESSMENT

Health History: Mr. Chin is a 47-year-old Asian American who had a bowel resection and permanent colostomy in the descending colon to remove a malignant tumor. He is 3 days post surgery. He has been receiving intravenous morphine via patient-controlled analgesia and reports adequate pain control. He has had no nausea or vomiting but has a nasogastric tube attached to low suction. He is allowed nothing by mouth (NPO) and is receiving intravenous fluids at 150 ml per hour. He participates in turning, coughing, deep breathing, and using the incentive spirometry every 2 hours. He has discussed his fear of cancer with the nurse, stating that his mother died of stomach cancer.

Physical Examination: Vital signs: temperature, 100°F orally; pulse, 92; respiration, 20; blood pressure, 118/64. The patient is alert and oriented. His skin is warm and dry with good turgor. Oral mucous membranes are moist. Breath sounds are clear to auscultation. The abdomen is soft, and bowel sounds are present in all four quadrants. The stoma is beefy red and edematous. A temporary drainage device is in place, and the collection pouch has approximately 100 ml of greenish brown liquid stool. Extremities are warm with palpable peripheral pulses. No muscle twitching or cramps are noted.

NURSING DIAGNOSIS	GOALS AND OUTCOME CRITERIA	INTERVENTIONS
High risk for fluid volume deficit related to NPO status, nasogastric suction, passage of liquid stool.	Patient will maintain normal fluid balance as evidenced by pulse and blood pressure consistent with patient's baseline, moist mucous membranes, and approximately equal fluid intake and output.	Monitor for signs of hypovolemia: tachycardia, hypotension, decreasing urine output, dry mucous membranes. Keep accurate intake and output (urine, liquid stool, gastric fluid) records. Monitor for signs of electrolyte imbalances: confusion, anxiety, twitching, trembling, muscle weakness, cardiac dysrhythmias. Give intravenous fluids as ordered, monitoring rate of flow carefully.
Impaired skin integrity related to stoma adhesive, fecal drainage.	Skin at the base of the stoma will be healed by time of discharge.	Check pouch hourly to detect leakage. When pouch is removed for emptying, prevent fecal matter from contaminating incision. When changing appliance, gently remove adhesive. Cleanse skin around stoma with soap and water, rinse, and pat dry. Apply a protective skin barrier before replacing pouch. If washers or wafers are used, make the opening not more than ⅛ inch larger than the stoma. Report rash or skin breakdown.
Body image disturbance related to presence of stoma, altered body function.	Patient will adapt to colostomy as evidenced by self-care and positive statements about self and ability to resume normal activities.	Provide an opportunity for patient to share his thoughts about colostomy. Identify specific concerns such as activity limitations, stoma care, odor control, and impact on sexuality. Provide information. Be accepting of patient's feelings. Encourage him to attend to grooming and appearance. Offer to have a volunteer from American Cancer Society or United Ostomy Association visit him. Advise of services of enterostomal therapist, mental health counselor, and spiritual counselor if patient desires.

The Patient with a Colostomy *(Continued)*

NURSING DIAGNOSIS	GOALS AND OUTCOME CRITERIA	INTERVENTIONS
Knowledge deficit of self-care with ostomy.	Patient will demonstrate proper ostomy care.	During stoma care in early postoperative period, tell patient what is being done and why. When patient begins to watch procedure, gradually encourage him to participate and then to take over care. Recognize patient's need to grieve and that patient may use denial as a coping mechanism. Develop a teaching plan that includes skin care, pouches, diet, fluids, irrigation if appropriate, activity, sexuality, complications, tips on traveling, and resources.

pressure, as can occur with coughing or sneezing. Other contributing factors might include an abdominal opening that is too large or a poorly attached stoma. Stenosis is the narrowing of the abdominal opening around the base of the stoma. If severe, stenosis blocks the passage of feces. Additional complications are associated with poor blood supply to the stoma, leading to necrosis and peristomal hernia. Peristomal hernia can limit bowel function, causing constipation, strangulation of the bowel, and poor results from colostomy irrigation.

Postoperative Nursing Care of the Patient with a Colostomy

ASSESSMENT. The postoperative care of the colostomy patient is essentially the same as that for the ileostomy patient.

NURSING DIAGNOSIS. In addition to the nursing diagnoses already identified, the following may also apply to the colostomy patient:

- **Knowledge Deficit** of irrigation procedure
- **High Risk for Injury** related to prolapse or stenosis

GOALS. Goals specific to the colostomy patient are patient's ability to perform irrigations (if ordered) and absence of signs of prolapse or stenosis.

INTERVENTIONS. Most aspects of care are the same as those discussed in relation to the ileostomy patient. A few points, specific to the colostomy patient, are presented here (see also Care Plan: The Patient with a Colostomy).

Knowledge Deficit. In the past, people with sigmoid colostomies were taught to irrigate them daily to maintain regular, controlled elimination. This procedure is no longer routinely recommended. Many patients have regular bowel movements without irrigation. Others are unlikely to establish controlled elimination and may find the procedure not worth the trouble. Patients who have liquid stools do not benefit from irrigation because they continue to drain fecal matter continuously. Irrigation is unlikely to establish control if the patient has diarrhea when under stress, has had radiotherapy, has a poor prognosis, or has a history of inflammatory bowel disease.

Irrigation can cause complications. The tube used to introduce irrigating fluid can perforate the bowel. A perforated bowel permits fecal matter to flow into the abdominal cavity, causing peritonitis, a very serious infection. The risk of perforation can be reduced greatly by using a cone-tipped catheter. Other complications are caused by the type, amount, or temperature of the solution used. Plain tap water may cause fluid and electrolyte imbalances if used repeatedly or in large amounts. If too much solution is used or if it is too cold, the patient may experience cramping, nausea, and dizziness. The physician should be advised if weakness occurs after irrigation even after the amount and temperature of the solution are adjusted.

If irrigations are indicated, the nurse or ET may perform them initially. The goal, however, is for the patient or significant other to learn to do the procedure, so an explanation of the process must be provided.

The following are key points to remember when irrigating a colostomy:

1. Have the patient select the time of day that is most convenient. The procedure should be done at approximately the same time every day. The entire process takes 45 minutes to 1 hour.
2. Have the patient sit on or in front of the toilet if possible. If the patient cannot get out of bed, the procedure can be done while the patient is in bed.
3. Remove the old pouch and apply an irrigating sleeve. This device opens at the top so that the tubing can be inserted into the stoma, and at the bottom so that fecal matter can drain into the toilet.
4. Pour 500 to 1000 ml of lukewarm irrigating solution into an enema fluid container and hold it at the

level of the patient's shoulder. Five hundred ml are used initially, but adults eventually increase the fluid to 1000 ml.

5. Clear the air from the tubing, lubricate the tubing, and insert it gently 2 to 4 inches into the stoma. The direction to insert the tubing can be assessed by first inserting a gloved, lubricated finger into the stoma. Do not use force! If a cone-tipped catheter is used, the catheter can be inserted only about 1 inch. This reduces the risk of perforation.

6. Allow the solution to flow slowly into the stoma. If the patient has cramping, slow down or stop the flow for a few minutes. Remove the catheter after the solution has been administered.

7. If the solution does not drain promptly, the bottom of the sleeve can be closed so that the patient can carry out other activities. Complete emptying may take 20 to 30 minutes.

8. When elimination is complete, the sleeve is removed, washed, and dried.

9. A clean pouch is applied if additional drainage usually occurs during the day. Some patients need only a small dressing or a stoma cap.

A few other points to remember:

- Patients with ileostomies should not be given timed-release capsules or hard-coated pills. They are likely to be eliminated before they dissolve.
- Rectal suppositories can be inserted into a colostomy stoma to stimulate evacuation. Patients who have double-barreled colostomies can be given rectal medications through the distal stoma.

High Risk for Injury. The nurse is alert for indications of colostomy complications. Although a prolapsed stoma may look frightening, it is not usually serious. There is no reason for immediate action if it continues to drain feces. It can usually be gently put back in place by the surgeon or enterostomal therapist. If the prolapse is severe or causes fecal obstruction, surgical repair is indicated.

The nurse informs the physician if the ostomy is not draining properly. The surgeon may be able to dilate the stoma and enlarge the opening. If dilation is not successful, surgery may be needed.

EVALUATION. Criteria for goal achievement are patient's demonstration of colostomy care and irrigation (if done), regular elimination of feces through the stoma, and lack of protrusion of the stoma.

URINARY DIVERSION

The most common types of urinary diversion are cutaneous ureterostomy, ileal conduit, colonic (sigmoid) conduit, cystostomy, vesicostomy, and continent internal reservoirs (Fig. 24–9). Ureterosigmoidostomy and ureteroileosigmoidostomy are not performed as commonly now as in the past.

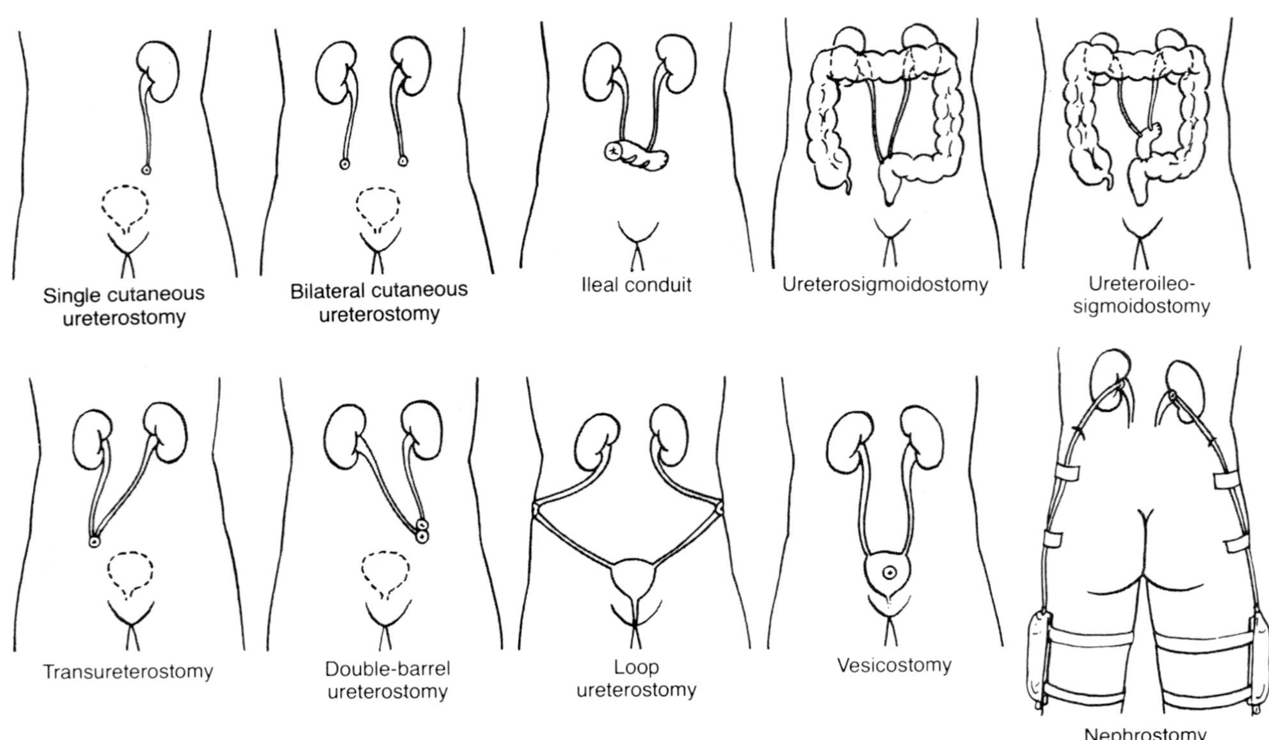

FIGURE 24–9

Types of urinary diversion. (Adapted from Black, J. M., & Matassarin-Jacobs, E. [1993]. *Luckmann and Sorensen's medical-surgical nursing: A psychophysiologic approach* [4th ed., p. 1469]. Philadelphia: W. B. Saunders.)

Urinary diversion may be temporary or permanent. Permanent urinary diversion is necessary when the bladder is congenitally absent or removed due to malignancy or trauma or when extensive pelvic malignancy obstructs urine flow. Temporary diversion may be used when there is obstruction to urine flow as might be caused by a urinary calculus or to permit healing of the ureters or bladder.

Preparation of the patient for ostomy surgery is discussed at the beginning of this chapter. Postoperative care after each type of diversion is discussed separately.

CUTANEOUS URETEROSTOMY

A cutaneous ureterostomy is created when one or both ureters are brought out through an opening in the abdomen or flank. Often the two ureters are joined surgically so that only one stoma is needed. In some situations, a stoma is created from each ureter.

A ureterostomy stoma is much smaller than an intestinal stoma. Immediately after surgery, the urinary stoma is pink, but it quickly fades to a lighter color. Since there is no reservoir to hold it, urine drains from the stoma continuously. A pouch is needed to collect the urine and protect the skin.

Complications

Complications experienced by patients with cutaneous ureterostomies include stenosis and urinary tract infections. Stenosis is a narrowing of the opening that interferes with the flow of urine. If the obstruction is not relieved, urine backs up in the kidney. The kidney may become swollen with urine, a condition called hydronephrosis, which leads to serious kidney damage. The kidneys can also be damaged by urinary tract infections.

Postoperative Nursing Care of the Patient with a Cutaneous Ureterostomy

ASSESSMENT

Health History. The preoperative health history may be used to determine the reason for ureterostomy as well as pertinent past medical history, drug profile, and allergies. In the postoperative period, the review of systems should include assessment of the presence of flank or abdominal pain, fatigue, malaise, and chills. The nurse also assesses the patient's response to the ostomy, knowledge about it, and readiness to learn.

Physical Examination. The physical examination begins with a general survey of the patient's general state. Vital signs are taken and compared with preoperative readings. Respiratory effort is observed, and breath sounds are auscultated. The abdomen is observed for distention and bowel sounds. The stoma is inspected. It is usually much smaller than an intestinal stoma and lighter in color. The amount, appearance, and odor of the urine are documented. Some blood in the urine is normal at first, but it should gradually clear. Ureterostomy drainage should not contain mucus.

NURSING DIAGNOSIS. In addition to the common diagnoses for postoperative patients (see Chapter 14), the following diagnoses may apply to the patient who has a cutaneous ureterostomy:

- **Impaired Skin Integrity** related to contact of urine with skin
- **High Risk for Infection** related to contamination of stoma
- **High Risk for Injury** related to obstruction of urine flow
- **Body Image Disturbance** related to presence of stoma, altered body function
- **Self-Care Deficit** with ostomy

GOALS. The goals of nursing care after ureterostomy are normal skin around the stoma, absence of signs of infection, unobstructed urine flow, adjustment in body image, and patient's knowledge of self-care with an ostomy.

INTERVENTIONS

Impaired Skin Integrity. Following a ureterostomy, the patient has a ureteral catheter for a week or two. The catheter is attached to a collection device. Once the catheter is removed, an appliance is needed to collect urine drainage. A variety of pouches are available (Fig. 24–2). Some have antireflux valves to prevent the flow of urine back into the stoma. A skin barrier product can be used around the stoma for protection. Karaya products are used for intestinal ostomies but not for urinary drainage because urine breaks down the product. Belts can be worn with some appliances to hold them in place. Some pouches can be connected to a leg bag for urine collection.

The pouch is generally cleaned once or twice daily. It is changed every 4 to 6 days or when it leaks because frequent changes are irritating to the surrounding skin. When it is changed, any adhesive is gently removed. A gauze pad, tampon, or tissue may be placed at the opening of the stoma to absorb urine. Pouch changes are usually done in the morning when urine production is lowest. Steps in the application of a urinary pouch are illustrated in Figure 24–10. The peristomal area is washed with water and patted dry. If soap is used, it should be nonoily and rinsed off thoroughly. If there are crystals present, a gauze pad saturated in a dilute vinegar solution can be used to dissolve them. Urinary stoma problems are summarized in Table 24–2.

High Risk for Infection. The stoma serves as a portal for pathogens to enter the urinary tract, causing infection. Urinary tract infections can have serious consequences, including kidney damage and septicemia. Pouch care is treated as a clean rather than sterile procedure because the stoma is not sterile. The nurse, however, still takes care to avoid introducing organisms to the area.

Yeast infections sometimes develop around the stoma. These are usually treated with nystatin powder applied under the skin barrier.

High Risk for Injury. If urine does not flow readily, the nurse suspects obstruction and notifies the surgeon immediately.

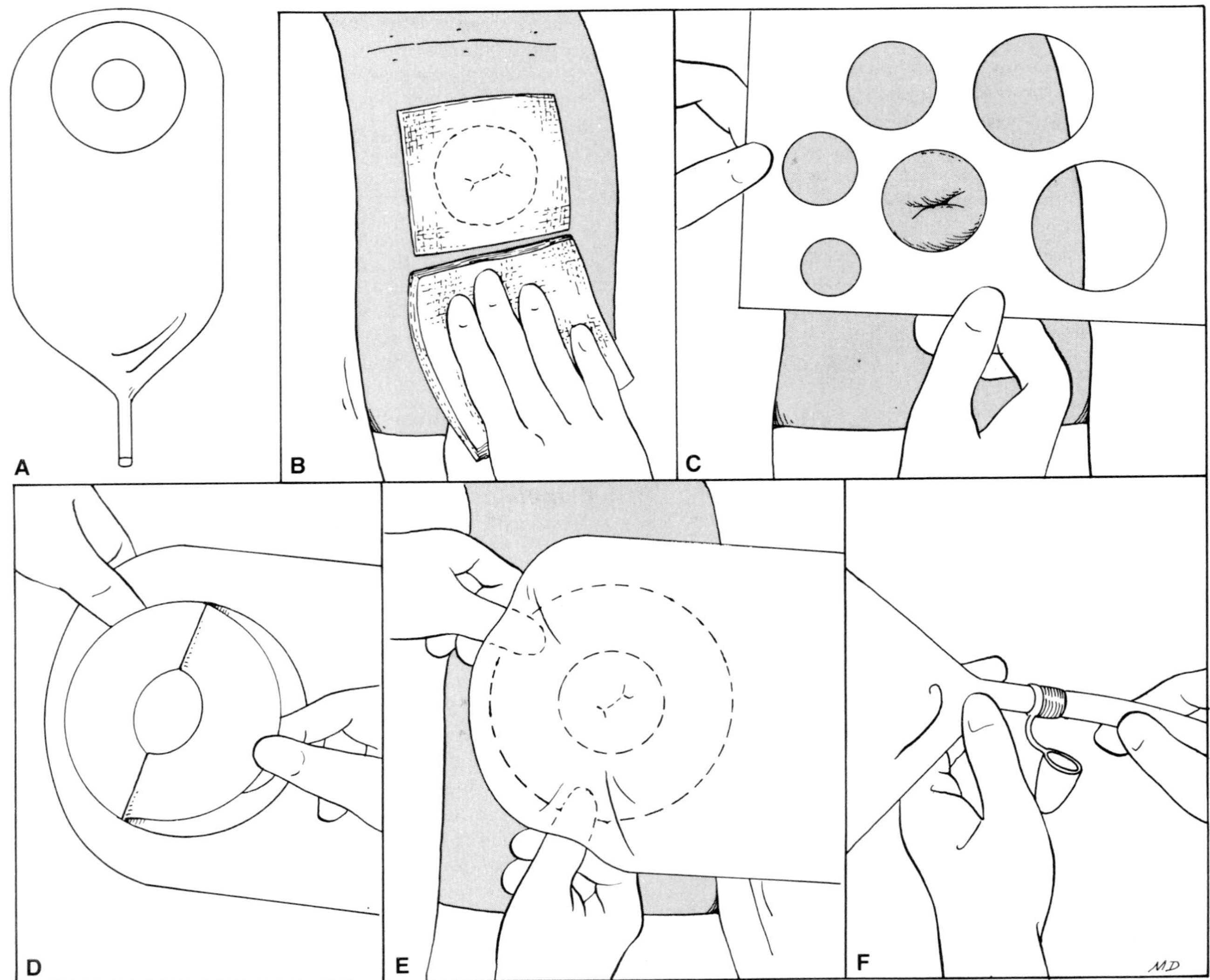

FIGURE 24-10

Procedure for applying pouch. *A,* Gather supplies: pouch, ostomy belt, skin barrier, stoma template, gauze pads, pouch clamp or rubber band, safety pin, and clean gloves. Wash hands and put on gloves. *B,* After removing the old pouch and cleaning the area around the stoma, place a gauze square over the stoma to absorb the drainage. *C,* Use a stoma template to measure the size of the stoma, and then cut an opening the same size as the stoma into the skin barrier and adhesive. *D,* Remove the backing from the adhesive of the new pouch. *E,* Place the opening in the new pouch over the stoma and gently press into place with the pouch drain pointed toward the floor. *F,* Connect the drain to the tubing or close the drain if appropriate. Secure the tubing to sheets or according to agency policy. (From Black, J. M., & Matassarin-Jacobs, E. [1993]. *Luckmann and Sorensen's medical-surgical nursing: A psychophysiologic approach* [4th ed., p. 1472]. Philadelphia: W. B. Saunders.)

Body Image Disturbance. Adjustment to a stoma can be very difficult. The patient may be afraid of leakage and odor and may feel disfigured. The nurse demonstrates acceptance of the patient and cares for the stoma in a matter-of-fact manner. The nurse also expresses understanding of the patient's feelings. The patient is encouraged to groom and dress normally. If odor is a problem, the pouch can be soaked in vinegar water for 20 to 30 minutes. Odor-proof pouches also should be recommended. Learning to care for the ureterostomy boosts the patient's self-confidence and may help to restore a more positive body image.

Patients with ostomies commonly experience grief in response to the loss of normal function and perceived disfigurement. This may be exhibited as denial, shock, anger, bargaining, or depression. Chapter 22 offers guidance for the nurse dealing with the patient who is grieving.

The change in body image may affect the patient's sexuality. The nurse provides opportunities for ostomy patients to ask questions or discuss how the ostomy might affect sexual function or behavior. Patients may feel unattractive or fear rejection by their partners. People who have had radical perineal surgeries may have

TABLE 24-2
PROBLEMS ASSOCIATED WITH URINARY STOMAS

PROBLEM	CAUSE	ASSESSMENT/INTERVENTION
Stomal laceration	Pouch opening too small Pouch not positioned correctly	Enlarge pouch opening Reposition pouch Monitor healing
Bleeding	Trauma	Apply cool cloth Cleanse gently
	Urinary tract infection	Treat infection
Stenosis	Ileal inflammation	Acidify urine Dilation by or under physician's direction
	Crystal formation	Apply vinegar compress to stoma during dressing change Put 1–2 oz of vinegar solution in pouch 20 min bid, then rinse Use vinyl or plastic pouch rather than rubber
Skin irritation	Skin barrier or wafer too small Leaking appliance	Adjust size of skin barrier or wafer to cover skin around stoma Check belt; if too tight, can break seal Replace appliance PRN
	Hair-follicle inflammation Perspiration under pouch	After skin returns to normal, shave or cut hair around stoma Dry skin well Apply protective barrier Apply powder to skin under pouch Use a soft pouch cover
	Allergy to adhesive Yeast infection	Spot test other brands to find one that does not cause irritation Dry well Apply nystatin powder as ordered Cover with sealant
Hernia/prolapse		Surgical repair
Odor	Urinary tract infection Appliance soiled or leaking	Treat infection Check seal Change appliance

bid, Twice a day; PRN, as needed.

physical barriers to sexual performance; other patients have problems because of psychological factors.

The same practical suggestions identified for the patient with an intestinal ostomy may be useful to the patient with a urinary ostomy. The pouch should be emptied before sexual intercourse. Pouch covers are available to conceal the appliance and its contents. The partner wearing the pouch should experiment with positions that are most comfortable. Female patients should know that ostomy surgery does not interfere with pregnancy or delivery.

Self-Care Deficit. Many aspects of teaching the ureterostomy patient are the same as those identified for the ileostomy patient. The topics to include in the teaching plan are ostomy care, pouches, diet, fluids, activity, sexuality, complications, and resources.

From the early postoperative period, the nurse strives to help the patient learn independent ostomy care. At first, patient teaching may take place each time stoma care is done by simply telling the patient what is being done and why. The patient is encouraged to participate and gradually assume more responsibility for the care. Practice builds confidence and provides the patient with the opportunity to identify problems while the nurse is available to help.

Some people adapt more readily to the stoma than others, but the nurse must be sensitive to their feelings and encourage them in a kind way. A volunteer from the American Cancer Society or the United Ostomy Association can be especially helpful as a role model to the new ostomy patient. With the patient's and the physician's approval, the agency can be contacted about sending a volunteer to visit the patient.

The nurse or ET, or both, must help the patient plan for discharge. Written care instructions should be provided. The patient needs a list of supplies and places where they can be purchased. In addition, some temporary supplies should be sent home with the patient. The nurse also provides information and makes referrals as needed for resources such as home health care and community organizations.

The patient needs to know what activities can be done. In general, normal activities can be resumed within 3 months, but specific directions should be obtained from the physician or ET. Since the pouch and seal are waterproof, the patient can bathe or shower with the appliance in place. Regular clothing can be worn but should not apply pressure to the stoma.

Ostomy patients who enjoy traveling are encouraged to continue to do so. When traveling, patients are advised to take adequate supplies, including sealable plastic bags to dispose of used materials. If the patient is flying, his or her supplies should be kept in a hand-carried bag to avoid problems if luggage is lost or delayed. On a long flight, a leg bag attached to the pouch may be beneficial in case the patient must remain seated owing to turbulence.

EVALUATION. Criteria for goal achievement are healed stoma base without redness or edema; absence of fever and foul urine odor; balanced fluid intake and output; patient's acknowledgment of stoma, increasing interest in self-care; patient's discussion of impact on sexuality; and patient's demonstration of proper techniques of ostomy care and description of self-care with the ostomy.

ILEAL CONDUIT

The ileal conduit is the most common type of urinary diversion. Other names for the ileal conduit are ureteroileostomy, ureteroileocutaneous anastomosis, ileal loop, and Bricker procedure.

Procedure

The ileal conduit is a urinary drainage system made out of a portion of small intestine. A 6- to 8-inch segment of ileum is first removed. The remaining ends of the ileum are then anastomosed (joined) to restore bowel function. The ureters are cut from the bladder and attached to the ileal segment at an angle to prevent reflux. One end of the ileal segment is sutured closed. The other end of the ileal segment is brought through an abdominal incision and sutured to create a stoma for urine drainage. A similar procedure that uses a segment of large intestine is called a colonic or sigmoid conduit. The stoma of an ileal or colonic conduit is bright red because it is intestinal mucosa.

Complications

During the postoperative period, the patient is at risk for a number of complications. Complications related to the surgical procedure include leakage of the anastomosed ureters and intestinal segments, ureteral obstruction, and separation of the stoma from surrounding skin.

Other problems include wound infection, necrosis of the stoma, and paralytic ileus. The stoma may become necrotic if the blood supply in the resected segment is inadequate. If the stoma turns gray or black, circulation is impaired; the physician should be notified at once.

Complications that may occur in the later postoperative period are infection, crystal formation, and calculi (stones). The patient may also have problems with the stoma: retraction, prolapse, or hernia.

Postoperative Nursing Care of the Patient with an Ileal Conduit

Nursing care of the patient who has an ileal conduit is essentially the same as that for the patient with an ileostomy. There are a few special points to make about the ileal conduit. This patient will have a nasogastric tube attached to suction to prevent abdominal distention and stress of the resected portion of the ileum while it heals. The patient is allowed nothing by mouth and is given intravenous fluids until bowel sounds return. A temporary ileus (absence of bowel activity) is expected after bowel resection. A ureteral catheter or stent may be in place to drain urine. If one is present, output is monitored because obstruction can occur. Mucus is normally present in drainage from a conduit because it is produced by the lining of the bowel segment. All patients with ileal conduits are advised to attach the pouch to a collection device during the night.

CONTINENT INTERNAL RESERVOIRS

All of the methods of urinary diversion already discussed permit urine to flow steadily through a stoma. Newer procedures have been developed that allow for the storage and controlled drainage of urine. Examples of these so-called continent internal reservoirs are the Kock pouch and the Indiana pouch (Fig. 24–11). Even more recently developed is the ileum neobladder, which eliminates the need for any stoma. The neobladder is an internal urinary reservoir that is constructed like other internal reservoirs but drains through the urethra instead of a stoma. Continence varies with the neobladder, so an artificial urinary sphincter is sometimes implanted. The neobladder is used more in males than in females.

The Kock pouch is constructed with a segment of ileum. The ureters are implanted in one side of the ileum segment. A nipple valve is constructed from the other side and attached to the skin, where a stoma is created. The valve prevents urine from flowing from the reservoir. A catheter is used to drain the reservoir at 4- to 6-hour intervals.

The Indiana pouch is similar to the Kock pouch except that it is made of a portion of the terminal ileum and the ascending colon. This reservoir is larger than that of the Kock pouch. The Indiana pouch is also drained with a catheter every 4 to 6 hours.

Complications

Complications of the continent pouches are incontinence, difficult catheterization, and urinary reflux leading to pyelonephritis, obstruction, and bacteriuria.

Postoperative Nursing Care of the Patient with a Continent Internal Reservoir

Immediately after surgery, the patient may have a Penrose drain to remove fluid from the operative site and a clear tube in place for continuous urine drainage. Irrigations may be ordered to remove clots and mucus. When the tube is removed, the pouch may be drained every 2 to 3 hours at first. Later, the patient may need to drain the pouch only every 4 to 6 hours during the day and once during the night. If the pouch functions properly, the patient does not have to wear an external appliance. A small gauze dressing may be placed over the stoma to absorb mucus drainage. The patient is advised to wear a medical alert bracelet that identifies the presence of a continent device that needs intubation to drain.

URETEROSIGMOIDOSTOMY AND URETEROILEOSIGMOIDOSTOMY

Ureterosigmoidostomy and ureteroileosigmoidostomy are not done as often now as in the past. The nurse may care for patients, however, who have had these diversions for some time and have adapted well to them. In a ureterosigmoidostomy, the ureters are implanted into the sigmoid colon. Urine drains into the colon and is eliminated through the rectum. For a ureteroileosigmoidostomy, a segment of the ileum is anastomosed to the sigmoid and the ureters implanted into that part of the ileum. Neither procedure provides continence, and both present problems with kidney infections and urinary calculi (stones). Additional complications are caused by the colon's absorption of electrolytes from the urine. Patients are at risk for deficits in potassium and bicarbonate and for excesses in sodium, chloride, and hydrogen. These imbalances may lead to metabolic acidosis.

VESICOSTOMY

Vesicostomy or cystostomy is an opening into the urinary bladder. There are several types. Some are drained continuously through a catheter, others have a nipple valve and are drained at intervals.

NEPHROSTOMY

A nephrostomy tube diverts urine directly from the kidney through a tube that exits through the skin. This device may be used as a temporary or permanent method of urinary diversion. Conditions that may be treated with these tubes are discussed in Chapter 36.

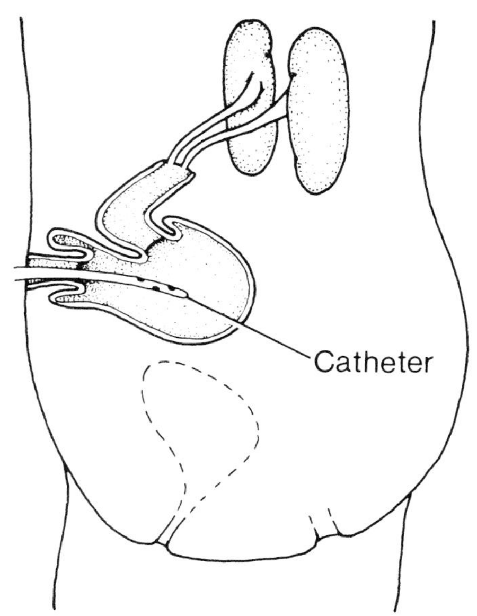

FIGURE 24-11

Continent internal urinary reservoirs: *A*, Kock pouch. (From Ignatavicius, D. D., & Bayne, M. V. [1991]. *Medical-surgical nursing: A nursing process approach* [p. 1875]. Philadelphia: W. B. Saunders.) *B*, Indiana pouch. (From Black, J. M., & Matassarin-Jacobs, E. [1993]. *Luckmann and Sorensen's medical-surgical nursing: A psychophysiologic approach* [4th ed., p. 1470]. Philadelphia: W. B. Saunders.)

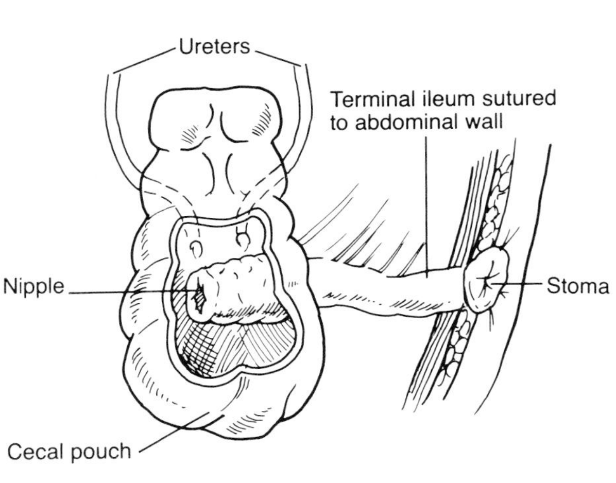

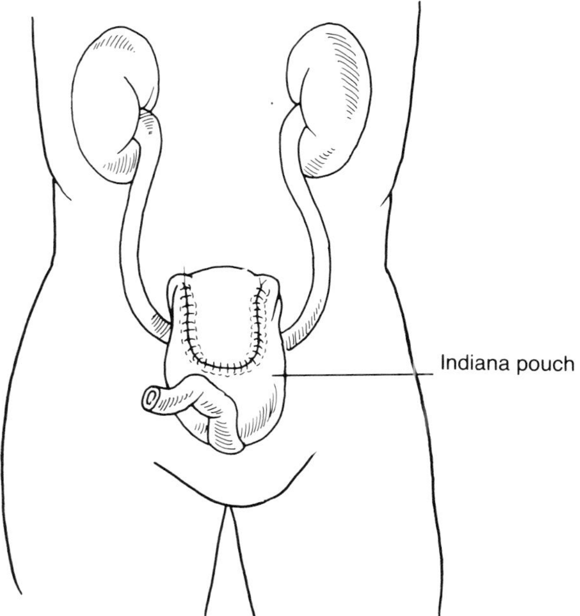

NUTRITION CONCEPTS

- Patients with an ileostomy or colostomy may eat a normal diet and simply omit foods that seem to cause problems.
- The main concern of the patient with an ileostomy or colostomy is odor, which is caused by flatulence.
- Patients should be encouraged to avoid foods tending to cause a bad odor, especially corn, dried beans, onions, cabbage, spicy foods, and fish.
- Fibrous vegetables should be avoided, and all food should be chewed well.

BIBLIOGRAPHY

Black, J. M., & Matassarin-Jacobs, E. (1993). *Luckmann and Sorensen's medical-surgical nursing: A psychophysiologic approach* (4th ed.). Philadelphia: W. B. Saunders.

Caine, R. M., & Bufalino, P. M. (1991). *Nursing care planning guides for adults* (2nd ed.). Baltimore: Williams & Wilkins.

Chernecky, C. C., Krech, R. L., & Berger, B. J. (1993). *Laboratory tests and diagnostic procedures*. Philadelphia: W. B. Saunders.

Doenges, M. E., & Moorhouse, M. F. (1993). *Nurse's pocket guide* (4th ed.). Philadelphia: F. A. Davis.

Erwin-Toth, P., & Doughty, D. B. (1992). Principles and procedures of stomal management. In B. G. Hampton & R. A. Bryant (Eds.), *Ostomies and continent diversions: Nursing management* (pp. 29–94). St. Louis: Mosby Year Book.

Henzel, B. (1992). Nursing role in management: Problems of absorption and elimination. In S. M. Lewis & I. C. Collier (Eds.), *Medical-surgical nursing* (3rd ed., pp. 1319–1355). St. Louis: Mosby Year Book.

Ignatavicius, D. D., & Bayne, M. V. (1991). *Medical-surgical nursing: A nursing process approach*. Philadelphia: W. B. Saunders.

Jarvis, C. (1992). *Physical examination and health assessment*. Philadelphia: W. B. Saunders.

Krasner, D. (1990). What's wrong with this stoma? *American Journal of Nursing, 90*(4), 46–47.

Krasner, D. (1993). Six steps to successful stoma care. *RN, 56*(7), 32–38.

Long, L. (1991). Ileostomy care. *Nursing 91, 21*(10), 73–75.

Paulford-Lecher, N. (1993). Teaching your patient stoma care. *Nursing 93, 23*(9), 47–49.

Rolstad, B. S., & Hoyman, K. (1992). Continent diversions and reservoirs. In B. G. Hampton & R. A. Bryant (Eds.), *Ostomies and continent diversions: Nursing management* (pp. 129–155). St. Louis: Mosby Year Book.

KEY CONCEPTS

1. An ostomy is an artificial opening into a body cavity; a stoma is the site of the opening on the skin.
2. Ostomy surgery may be done to bypass a section of the digestive or urinary tract either temporarily or permanently.
3. An important resource for the nurse and the ostomy patient is the enterostomal therapist—a nurse with specialized training in ostomy management.
4. Before ostomy surgery, the nurse assesses the patient's expectations, understanding of the procedure, information desired, and fears.
5. Intestinal ostomies include the ileostomy, the continent ileostomy, the ileoanal reservoir, and the colostomy.
6. The characteristics of fecal material depend on the location of the ostomy, with liquid stool draining from the ileum and softly formed stool from the descending colon.
7. The new intestinal stoma should be beefy red, and a small amount of bleeding around the base is not unusual.
8. Postoperative nursing care after intestinal ostomy surgery addresses fluid volume deficits, impaired skin integrity, body image disturbance, sexual dysfunction, and knowledge deficits.
9. Protective barriers are applied around the stoma to fill creases and create a seal, and a pouch is secured over the stoma with adhesive to collect fecal drainage.
10. Elimination of gas-forming foods and good hygiene can help control odor associated with an intestinal ostomy.
11. The continent pouch ileostomy and the ileoanal reservoir both store fecal matter, but the continent ileostomy is drained periodically with a catheter whereas the ileoanal reservoir allows fecal elimination through the rectum.
12. Routine colostomy irrigations are no longer recommended.
13. The most common types of urinary diversion are cutaneous ureterostomy, ileal conduit, colonic conduit, and continent internal reservoirs.
14. A urinary stoma is pink immediately after surgery but quickly fades to a light color.
15. Ureterostomies and ileal conduits drain urine continuously, so collection pouches are needed and meticulous skin care must be provided.
16. A continent internal reservoir allows for storage and controlled drainage of urine.
17. Complications of urinary stomas include urinary infections, obstruction of urine flow, and skin breakdown.
18. The American Cancer Society and United Ostomy Association are good resources for information about management of ostomies.

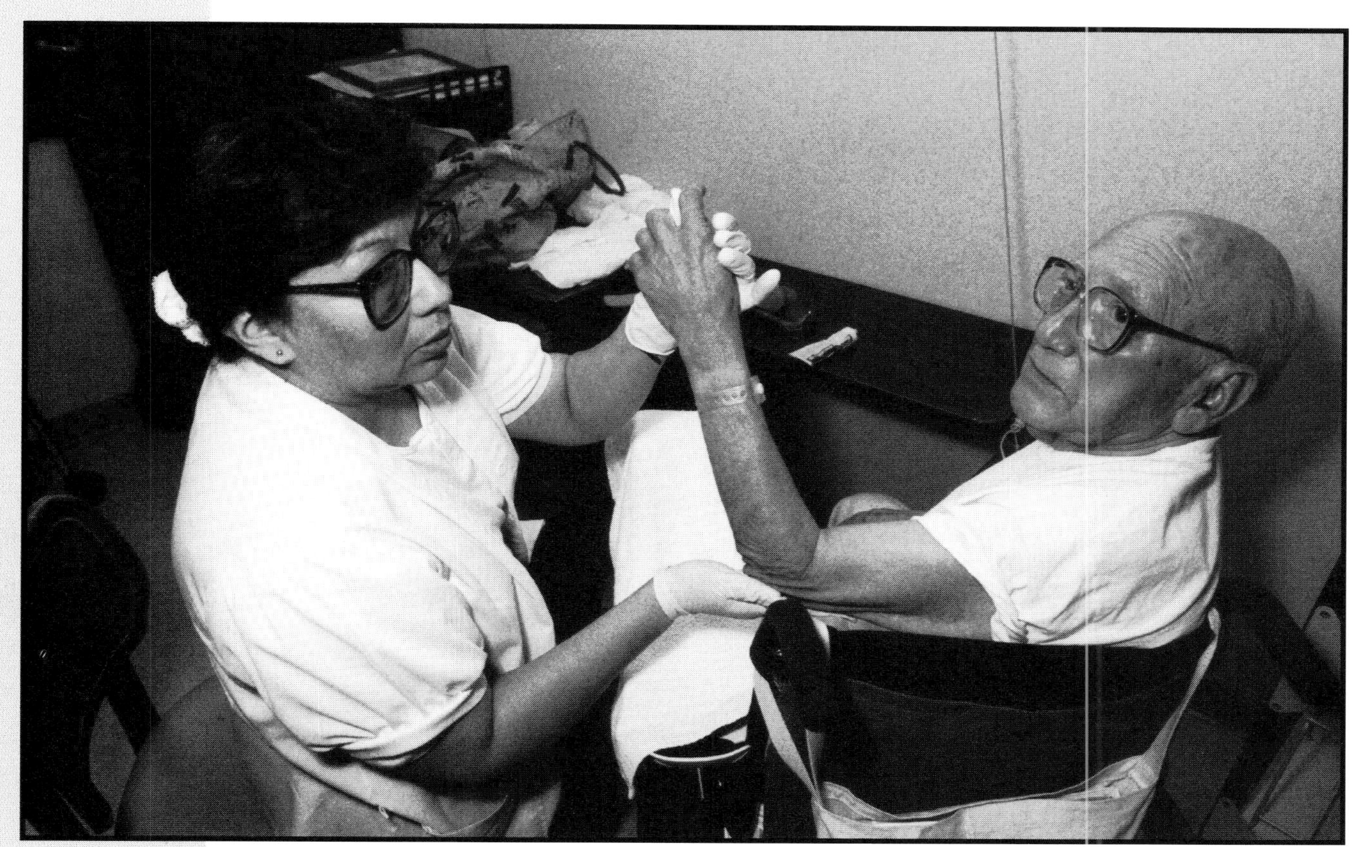

UNIT 6
Neurologic Disorders

Gayle Dasher
Adrianne Linton

CHAPTER 25

Neurologic Disorders

OBJECTIVES

1. Identify common neurologic changes in the older person and the implications of these for nursing care.
2. Describe the diagnostic tests and procedures used to evaluate neurologic dysfunction and the nursing responsibilities associated with each.
3. Identify the uses, side effects, and nursing interventions associated with common drug therapies employed in patients with neurologic disorders.
4. Describe the signs and symptoms associated with increased intracranial pressure and the medical therapies used in its treatment.
5. List the components of the nursing assessment of the patient with a neurologic disorder.
6. Describe the pathophysiology, signs and symptoms, complications, and medical or surgical treatment for patients with selected neurologic disorders.
7. Apply the nursing process to plan care for the patient with a neurologic disorder.

GLOSSARY

AURA A peculiar sensation that precedes a set of symptoms

AUTOMATISM Aimless behavior performed without conscious control or knowledge

CONTRALATERAL Affecting the opposite side

DECEREBRATE POSTURING Abnormal extension of the upper extremities with extension of the lower extremities; accompanies increased pressure on the entire cerebrum and the motor tract structures of the brain stem

DECORTICATE POSTURING Abnormal flexion of the upper extremities with extension of the lower extremities; accompanies increased pressure on the frontal lobes

ENCEPHALITIS Inflammation of brain tissue

HEMIPARESIS Weakness on one side of the body

HEMIPLEGIA Paralysis on one side of the body

INTRACRANIAL Within the skull

IPSILATERAL Affecting the same side

NEURALGIA Pain in a nerve or along the course of a nerve

Glossary continued

NEUROTRANSMITTER Biochemical messenger at nerve endings that stimulates an excitatory or inhibitory impulse

PARESTHESIA An abnormal sensation

POSTICTAL After a seizure

SEIZURE Convulsion; series of involuntary contractions of voluntary muscles

Neurologic disease and injury present some of the greatest challenges in health care today. Nurses face the challenge of caring for neurologic patients during the acute and rehabilitation phases of recovery from injuries and diseases. The long-term effects of many neurologic disorders are frequently devastating to both the patient and family. An important aspect of care is assisting the patient and family to adjust physically and emotionally to the alterations that often result from neurologic dysfunction.

ANATOMY AND PHYSIOLOGY OF THE NERVOUS SYSTEM

In this age of computers, it may be helpful to think of the nervous system as an elaborate control system. The system coordinates and regulates all bodily functions. It receives and interprets information from the external environment and initiates responses to the received information.

The functional unit of the nervous system is the neuron (nerve cell), which conducts electrical impulses from one area of the brain to another. The main cell body has branches called axons and dendrites (Fig. 25–1). Axons conduct impulses away from the cell body, and dendrites convey impulses toward the cell body. Many axons and dendrites are covered with a material called myelin, which enhances conduction along nerve fibers. Myelin gives the axons a white appearance (white matter), whereas unmyelinated cell bodies are gray (gray matter).

Neurons are classified according to their particular functions. Those that transmit information from distal parts of the body or environment toward the central nervous system are sensory neurons, also known as afferent neurons. Motor information is carried from the central nervous system to the periphery by motor neurons, also known as efferent neurons. In addition, interneurons are like relay stations between sensory and motor neurons.

Coordinated, organized function is a result of a well-integrated system of impulse transmission. When the end of a dendrite is stimulated, a series of electrochemical events is initiated. At the point of stimulation, sodium and potassium ions are exchanged, resulting in a process called depolarization. This process continues down the dendrite to the axon, until the ions return to their resting state. This return to the resting state is known as repolarization.

Impulses must be able to pass from one neuron to another across the neural synapse—the space between the axons of one neuron and the dendrites of the next neuron. When an impulse reaches the end of its axon, a biochemical messenger called a neurotransmitter is released. The known neurotransmitters are acetylcholine, norepinephrine, epinephrine, and dopamine. The neurotransmitter crosses the synapse to the neighboring dendrite, where it stimulates an electrical impulse. The process of depolarization then continues down the length of the nerve cells.

Structurally, the nervous system is divided into two main parts: (1) the brain and spinal cord compose the central nervous system, and (2) the peripheral nervous system comprises all the nerves of the peripheral parts of the body. The brain is divided into the cerebrum, cerebellum, and brain stem (Fig. 25–2). The cerebrum is composed of left and right hemispheres, which are subdivided by specific lobes. The thalamus, hypothalamus, and basal ganglia are other important structures identified in the cerebrum. Table 25–1 defines the functions of the major parts of the brain.

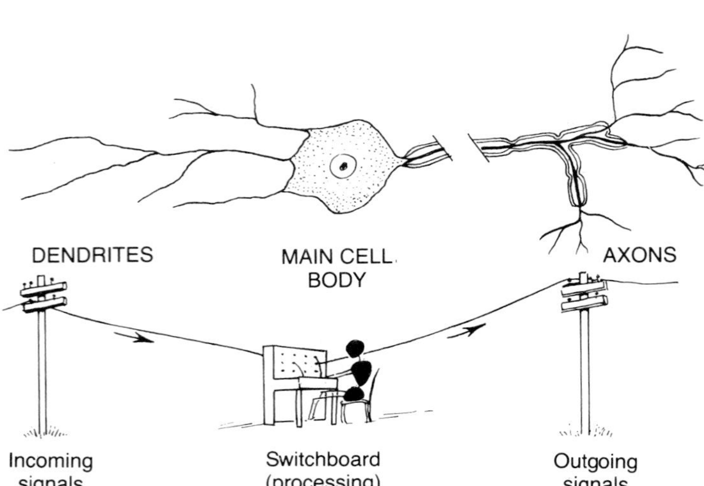

FIGURE 25-1

A neuron (nerve cell). The dendrites receive incoming messages. The axons convey outgoing signals. The process can be compared with that of a telephone communication system except that telephone signals can travel in either direction, whereas neurologic signals normally travel only from the dendrites through the neuron to the axons. (From Jacob, S. W., & Francone, C. A. [1989]. *Elements of anatomy and physiology* [2nd ed., p. 102]. Philadelphia: W. B. Saunders.)

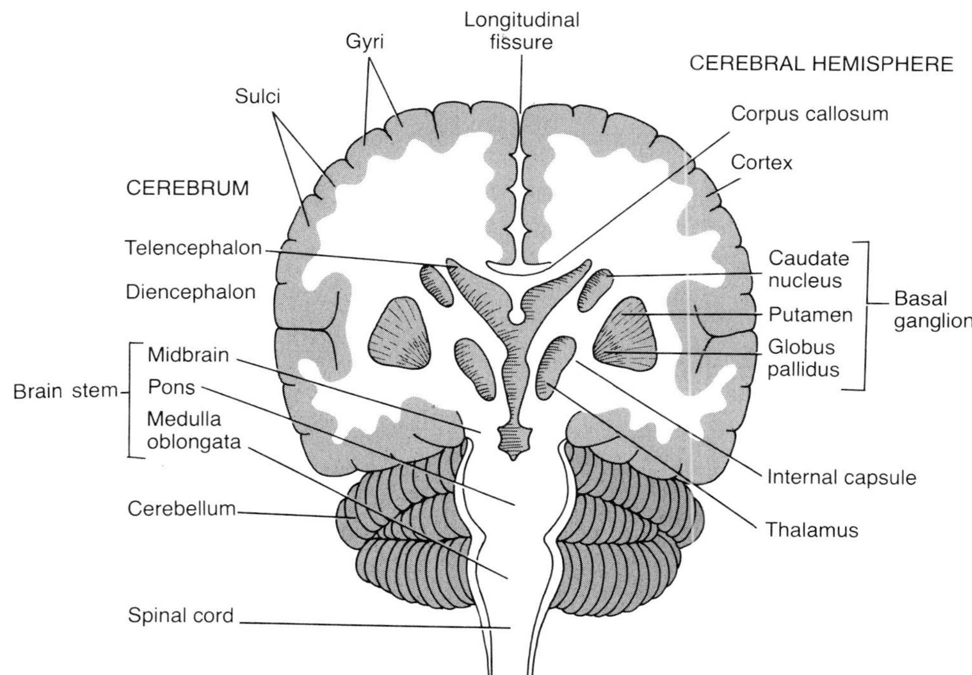

FIGURE 25-2

A cross-sectional view of the main structures of the brain. (Adapted from Black, J. M., & Matassarin-Jacobs, E. [1993]. *Luckmann and Sorensen's medical-surgical nursing: A psychophysiologic approach* [4th ed., p. 618]. Philadelphia: W. B. Saunders.)

Cerebrospinal fluid (CSF) is composed primarily of water, glucose, sodium chloride, and protein. It is produced in the ventricles of the brain and circulates within the subarachnoid space, the ventricles, and the central canal of the spinal cord (Fig. 25–3). The fluid is reabsorbed in the arachnoid villi. The CSF acts as a shock absorber for the brain and spinal cord. If excess fluid forms or fluid is not normally reabsorbed, pressure within the ventricular system increases.

The spinal cord extends from the border of the first cervical vertebra to the level of the second lumbar vertebra. Thirty-one pairs of spinal nerve roots exit from the spinal cord, each consisting of a posterior sensory (afferent) root and anterior motor (efferent) root (Fig.

TABLE 25-1

FUNCTIONS OF THE MAJOR PARTS OF THE BRAIN

Brain Stem and Diencephalon
Controls awareness or alertness through reticular activating system composed of fibers scattered throughout the midbrain, pons, and medulla.

Medulla
Links higher brain centers to other parts of the body through spinal cord. Controls muscles of respiration through respiratory reflex center. Controls heartbeat to some extent through cardiac reflex center. Constricts blood vessels to raise blood pressure through vasomotor reflex center. Is point of origin for some cranial nerves.

Pons
Relays messages from medulla to higher centers in brain. Is reflex center for some cranial nerves.

Cerebellum
Coordinates movement, balance, posture, and spatial orientation.

Midbrain
Coordinates motor function. Contains centers for visual reflexes and hearing.

Thalamus
Integrates and processes sensory stimuli.

Hypothalamus
Controls pituitary. Controls appetite, sleep, and some emotions. Controls much activity of autonomic nervous system.

Forebrain (Cerebrum)
Controls higher functions and activities: conscious mental processes, sensations, emotions, and voluntary movements.

Frontal lobe
Controls voluntary muscle movements, verbal and written speech.

Parietal lobe
Contains sensory reception areas to interpret pain, touch, temperature, distances, sizes, and shapes.

Temporal lobe
Contains auditory center for hearing and understanding of spoken language.

Occipital lobe
Contains visual center for seeing and reading. Contains olfactory center for smell.

Data from Jacob, S. W., & Francone, C. A. (1989). *Elements of anatomy and physiology* (2nd ed.). Philadelphia: W. B. Saunders.

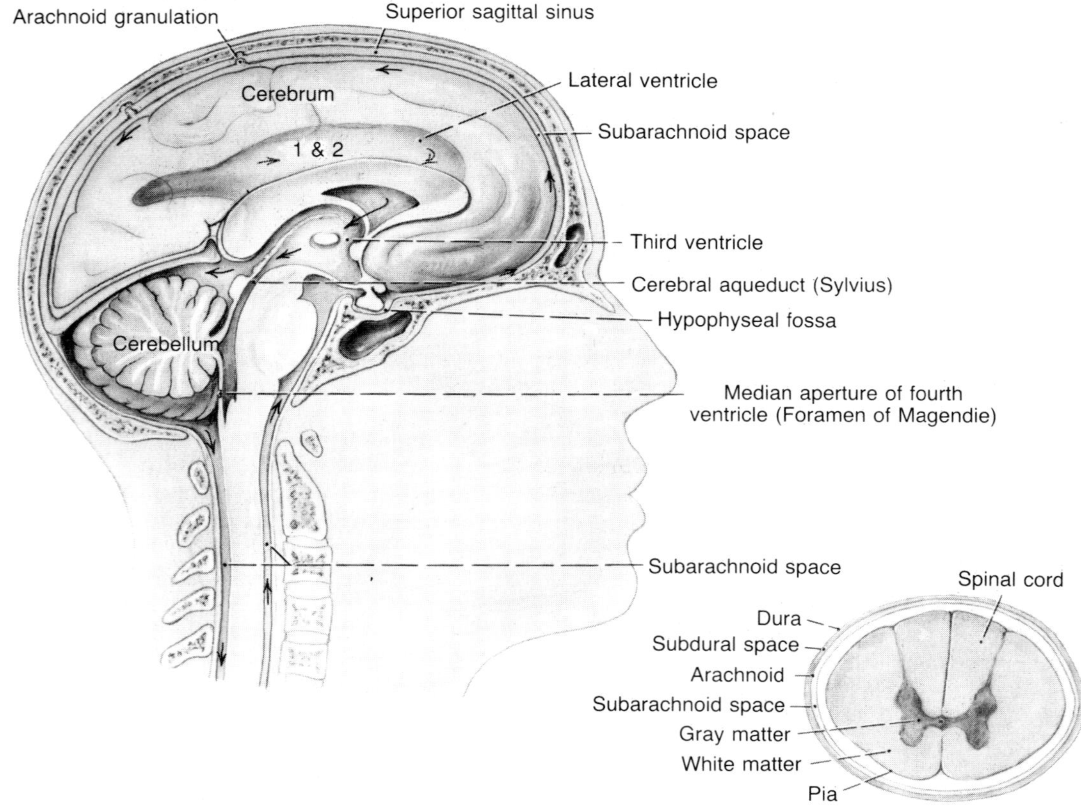

FIGURE 25-3

Cerebrospinal fluid circulates through the ventricles of the brain, the meningeal covering, and the spinal cord. (From Jacob, S. W., & Francone, C. A. [1989]. *Elements of anatomy and physiology* [2nd ed., p. 110]. Philadelphia: W. B. Saunders.)

25–4). These nerve roots, along with the twelve cranial nerves, make up the peripheral nervous system.

Part of the peripheral nervous system, known as the autonomic nervous system, helps to maintain homeostasis for the body. The autonomic nervous system controls the involuntary activities of the viscera, including smooth muscles, cardiac muscle, and glands. The two major subdivisions of the autonomic nervous system are the sympathetic nervous system and the parasympathetic nervous system.

The sympathetic nervous system is activated by stress to increase the secretion of epinephrine and norepinephrine. These neurotransmitters increase the heart rate and constrict peripheral blood vessels, causing the blood pressure to rise. This reaction to stress is called the fight or flight response. The sympathetic nervous system is also referred to as the thoracolumbar system.

Conversely, the parasympathetic nervous system mediates a rest response. Stimulation of this system results in decreased heart rate and blood pressure. The parasympathetic nervous system is also known as the craniosacral system. Specific effects of the stimulation of the sympathetic and parasympathetic nervous systems are outlined in Table 25–2.

AGE-RELATED CHANGES

With normal aging, the number of nerve cells decreases. Brain weight is reduced, and the ventricles increase in size. An aging pigment called lipofuscin is deposited in nerve cells along with amyloid, a type of protein. Increased plaques and tangled fibers are found in nerve tissue. These changes are associated with Alzheimer's disease but are also seen in the brains of people without evidence of dementia. Fortunately, there are many more nerve cells present than are needed for normal function. Therefore, most older people retain normal cognition and behavior despite the decreasing number of nerve cells.

The physical examination reveals some neurologic changes typical of aging. The pupil of the eye is often smaller and may respond to light more slowly. When asked to track (follow with the eyes) a moving object, the older person's eye movements may be jerky rather than smooth. Reflexes are usually intact except the Achilles tendon jerk, which is often absent.

Older people often demonstrate some changes in functional abilities as well. Reaction time increases with

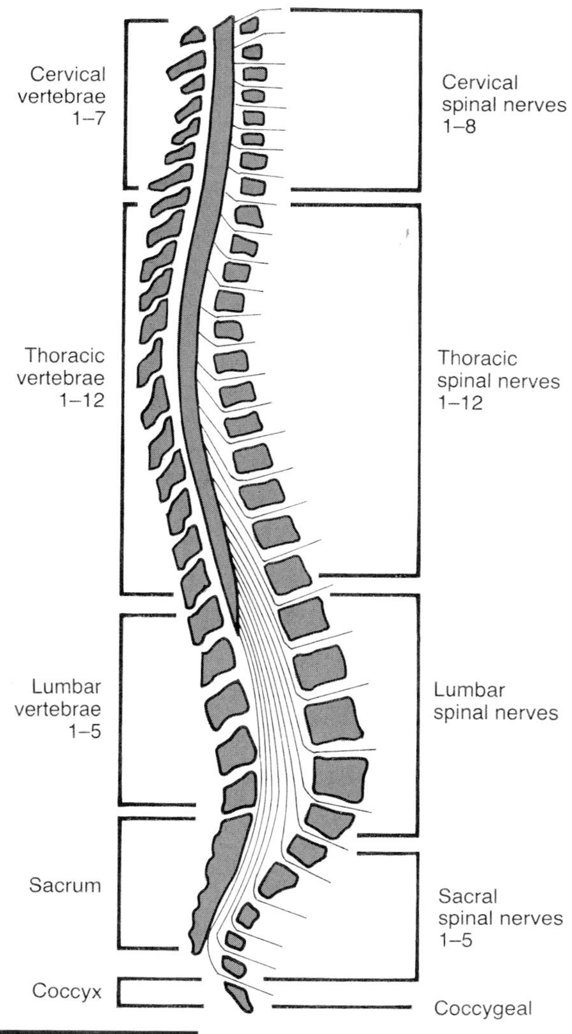

FIGURE 25-4

The spinal column depicting the vertebrae and spinal nerves. (Redrawn from Jarvis, C. [1992]. *Physical examination and health assessment* [p. 737]. Philadelphia: W. B. Saunders.)

aging, especially for complex reactions. Tremors in the head, face, and hands are common. Some older people develop dizziness and problems with balance, but these are not considered normal age-related changes.

PATHOPHYSIOLOGY OF NEUROLOGIC DISEASES

Mechanisms that can be identified as being potential causes of neurologic disorders include developmental and genetic disorders, trauma, infections and inflammation, neoplasms, degenerative processes, vascular disorders, and metabolic and endocrine disorders.

DEVELOPMENTAL AND GENETIC DISORDERS. Developmental disorders include structural problems such as hydrocephalus. An example of a genetic disorder is Huntington's disease.

TRAUMA. Central nervous system injuries arising from trauma can be life threatening or severely disabling. Trauma may be described as physical in nature, such as in accidental injury or violent crime, or chemical, such as in drug or alcohol effects on cerebral tissue.

INFECTIONS AND INFLAMMATION. Meningitis and encephalitis disease states cause inflammation of meningeal and brain tissue, respectively. Causative agents may be viral or bacterial and may be transmitted by a variety of vectors and routes.

NEOPLASMS. Central nervous system tumors may be primary or metastatic in origin. Although considerable progress has been made in treating these tumors, definitive therapy is often difficult to achieve, depending on the cell type involved in the tumor and the degree of invasion of surrounding tissue.

DEGENERATIVE PROCESSES. The primary degenerative disease of the brain is Alzheimer's disease, a progressive condition that begins with memory loss and eventually results in severe mental and physical deterioration. Alzheimer's disease is discussed in Chapter 51. Other degenerative disorders are multiple sclerosis, Parkinson's disease, amyotrophic lateral sclerosis, and Huntington's disease.

VASCULAR DISORDERS. Any factor that interferes with blood flow to nervous tissue can lead to cell death with resulting loss of function. Nerve tissue is so sensitive to hypoxia that cells begin to die after being deprived of oxygen for 5 minutes. Neurologic disorders associated with impaired blood flow include cerebrovascular accident (Chapter 26) and multi-infarct dementia. Vascular abnormalities, including aneurysms and arteriovenous malformations, can rupture or prevent delivery of adequate oxygen to affected tissue.

METABOLIC AND ENDOCRINE DISORDERS. The brain is dependent on constant supplies of glucose and other nutrients. Disturbances in glucose metabolism and electrolyte imbalances can lead to deterioration in thought processes and level of consciousness (LOC). Neurologic dysfunction can also result from accumulation of toxins as in poisoning, renal failure, and liver failure.

NURSING ASSESSMENT OF NEUROLOGIC FUNCTION

A number of diagnostic tests may be done to evaluate and diagnose neurologic problems. However, any evaluation begins with an accurate assessment, which may be initiated by the nurse. Much of the assessment may be conducted simply by observing the patient and then documenting the findings.

TABLE 25-2

EFFECTS OF SYMPATHETIC AND PARASYMPATHETIC STIMULATION

ORGAN	EFFECT OF SYMPATHETIC STIMULATION	EFFECT OF PARASYMPATHETIC STIMULATION
Eye	Pupil dilation Slight relaxation of ciliary muscle	Pupil constriction Constriction of ciliary muscle
Glands: nasal, lacrimal, salivary, gastric, pancreas	Vasoconstriction and slight secretion	Stimulation of copious secretion except pancreas
Sweat glands	Copious sweating	None
Apocrine glands	Thick, odoriferous secretion	None
Heart	Increased rate and force of contractions Coronary arteries dilate with $beta_2$ stimulation; constrict with alpha stimulation	Decreased rate and force of contractions
Lungs	Bronchial dilation Mild constriction of blood vessels	Bronchial constriction Possible dilation of blood vessels
Gut	Decreased peristalsis and tone in lumen Increased sphincter tone	Increased peristalsis and tone in lumen Decreased sphincter tone
Liver	Glucose released	Slight glycogen synthesis
Gallbladder and bile ducts	Relaxed	Contracted
Kidney	Decreased urine production and renin secretion	None
Bladder	Slight relaxation of detrusor muscle Excitation of trigone	Excitation of detrusor muscle Relaxation of trigone
Penis	Ejaculation	Erection
Systemic arterioles	Constriction of abdominal arterioles Constriction of muscle arterioles with alpha stimulation; dilation with $beta_2$ or cholinergic stimulation Constriction of skin arterioles	None
Blood	Increased coagulation and glucose	None
Basal metabolism	Increased	None
Adrenal medulla secretions	Increased	None
Mental activity	Increased	None
Piloerector muscles	Excited	None
Skeletal muscle	Increased strength and glycogenolysis	None

From Ignatavicius, D. D., & Bayne, M. (1991). *Medical-surgical nursing: A nursing process approach.* Philadelphia: W. B. Saunders. Modified from Guyton, A. C. (1991). *Textbook of medical physiology* (8th ed., p. 672). Philadelphia: W. B. Saunders.

HEALTH HISTORY

The general nursing assessment of the patient with a neurologic disorder is described here. Throughout the assessment, the nurse notes the patient's speech, behavior, coordination, alertness, and comprehension. More sophisticated assessments are discussed in the section on diagnostic tests and procedures.

CHIEF COMPLAINT AND HISTORY OF PRESENT ILLNESS. An initial portion of the neurologic assessment includes an investigation of the health history of the patient, particularly as it relates to the chief complaint. The nurse documents the event that brought the patient to seek medical attention. Any injuries are described. If the patient has pain, the onset, severity, location, and duration are noted.

PAST MEDICAL HISTORY. Past neurologic disorders and pertinent signs and symptoms are vital pieces of information. The nurse asks about a history of head injury, seizures, diabetes mellitus, hypertension, heart disease, and cancer. Dates of immunizations, including influenza, are recorded. Current medications should be listed. Allergies are recorded and highlighted per agency policy.

PHARMACOLOGY CAPSULE

Many drugs stimulate or depress the central nervous system.

FAMILY HISTORY. Inquiring about the presence of neurologic or other disease states in the immediate family may provide valuable information about risk factors, such as in stroke or neuromuscular diseases. Therefore, the nurse asks whether any immediate family members have had heart disease, stroke, diabetes mellitus, cancer, seizure disorders, muscular dystrophy, or Huntington's disease.

REVIEW OF SYSTEMS. Important signs and symptoms to be collected in reviewing the systems are fatigue or weakness, headache, dizziness, vertigo, changes in vision or hearing, tinnitus, drainage from the ears or nose, dysphagia, neck pain or stiffness, vomiting, problems with bladder or bowel function, sexual dysfunction, fainting, blackouts, tremors, paralysis, incoordination, numbness or tingling, memory problems, and mood changes.

FUNCTIONAL ASSESSMENT. The patient's usual activities and occupation are noted, as well as any interference caused by present symptoms. Sources of stress, usual coping strategies, and sources of support also are explored.

PHYSICAL EXAMINATION

A complete physical examination, including the neurologic examination, should be done when the patient is stable. A neurologic assessment provides baseline data to compare with ongoing assessments and serves as the basis for developing the nursing care plan. There are four major components of a routine neurologic examination that provide valuable information regarding the overall integrity of the central nervous system: LOC, pupillary evaluation, neuromuscular response, and vital signs. The nurse must look at the trends in neurologic status. Any assessment considered in isolation may not provide a true picture of the patient's status. For example, one elevated blood pressure reading may not be significant, but continuing increases may be associated with increased intracranial pressure (ICP).

Basic Neurologic Examination

LEVEL OF CONSCIOUSNESS. The most accurate and reliable indicator of neurologic status is LOC. Patients are evaluated for orientation to person, place, and time by asking them to state their names, where they are, and what time it is. It is important to consider the degree of stimulation required to evoke a response from the patient. If the patient responds only to vigorous physical stimulation, then LOC is more impaired than in the patient who immediately responds to a verbal greeting. Patient behavior in response to stimulation also is considered. Does the patient respond pleasantly, or is he or she combative, agitated, or lethargic? All these observations provide additional information regarding mental status.

Some of the common terms used to describe altered levels of consciousness are somnolence, lethargy, stupor, semicoma, and coma. Somnolence is unnatural drowsiness or sleepiness. Lethargy also is used to describe excessive drowsiness. Stupor suggests decreased responsiveness accompanied by lack of spontaneous motor activity. If a patient is in a stupor (stuporous) but can be aroused, the term semicomatose is used. A patient who cannot be aroused even by powerful stimuli is said to be in a coma, or comatose.

PUPILLARY EVALUATION. The second major component of the neurologic assessment is the pupillary evaluation. The size, shape, and reactivity of the pupils are assessed and compared bilaterally to evaluate equality. Pupils are generally about 3 mm in size, round, and react briskly to light. Changes in equality or reactivity from one assessment to the next may indicate neurologic deterioration.

NEUROMUSCULAR RESPONSE. Evaluation of neuromuscular response provides a means of assessing cerebral and spinal cord function. All electrical impulses responsible for eliciting motor responses are initiated in the frontal lobe of the cerebral cortex, traverse down the brain stem into the spinal cord, and stimulate muscle movement via the motor spinal nerve root. Detailed assessment techniques for specific neuromuscular responses can be found in Chapter 27.

VITAL SIGNS. Although routine monitoring of pulse, respirations, and blood pressure provides highly reliable information regarding neurologic well-being, changes are late indicators of deterioration. The significance of these values is discussed in detail in the section on increased ICP. Temperature also is monitored to detect increases that may be associated with infection or with impaired thermoregulation.

General Physical Examination

Once the neurologic assessment is done, the nurse may complete the remaining physical examination. If possible, height and weight are measured. Throughout the examination, the skin is inspected for lesions and color and is palpated for temperature. Hydration status is assessed by evaluating tissue turgor and moisture of mucous membranes. The head is inspected for lesions and palpated for masses and swelling. Respiratory effort is observed, and breath sounds are auscultated. The abdomen is inspected, auscultated for bowel sounds, and palpated for bowel and bladder distention. The extremities are inspected for injuries or abnormal positions. Assessment of motor and sensory function is detailed in Chapter 27.

Assessment of the patient with a neurologic disorder is summarized in Table 25–3.

DIAGNOSTIC TESTS AND PROCEDURES

Once an initial evaluation and history have been obtained, more detailed diagnostic tests and procedures are often indicated. Table 25–4 provides a summary of information about diagnostic tests and procedures.

Advanced Neurologic Examination

Baseline and serial examination is critical in the evaluation of the neurologic patient. Cranial nerve function,

TABLE 25-3

ASSESSMENT OF THE PATIENT WITH A NEUROLOGIC DISORDER

HEALTH HISTORY

Chief complaint and history of present illness: Event requiring medical attention.

Past medical history: Head injury, seizures, other neurologic disorders, other diseases (diabetes mellitus, hypertension, heart disease, cancer), dates of immunizations, current medications, allergies

Family history: Stroke, neuromuscular diseases, heart disease, diabetes mellitus, cancer, seizures

Review of systems: Fatigue, weakness, headache, dizziness, vertigo, changes in vision or hearing, tinnitus, drainage from nose or ears, dysphagia, neck pain or stiffness, vomiting, bladder or bowel dysfunction, fainting, blackouts, tremors, paralysis, incoordinations, numbness or tingling, memory problems, mood changes

Functional assessment: Usual occupation and activities, impact on life, sources of stress, usual coping strategies, sources of support.

PHYSICAL EXAMINATION

Level of consciousness: Response to stimulation
Pupils: Size, shape, response to light, equality
Neuromuscular status: Voluntary movement, reflexes
Vital signs: Blood pressure, pulse, respirations, temperature
When stable:
- Height and weight
- Skin: Lesions, injuries, turgor
- Head: Lesions, injuries, masses, swelling
- Oral cavity: Moisture
- Thorax: Respiratory effort, breath sounds
- Abdomen: Distention, bowel sounds
- Extremities: Injuries, abnormal positions

coordination and balance, neuromuscular function, and reflexes are those components that can assist the practitioner in localizing the area of injury or disease and in developing a plan of care relevant to the individual patient. Figure 25–5 provides an example of a flow sheet used to document periodic neurologic assessments.

CRANIAL NERVES. Various motor and sensory functions are mediated by the cranial nerves. The cranial nerves enter and exit the brain rather than the spinal cord. The primary functions of the cranial nerves are to control sensory and motor activities of the head and neck, but the vagus nerve also affects cardiac, respiratory, gastric, and gallbladder function. Each nerve may be individually assessed by the examiner with advanced assessment skills.

COORDINATION AND BALANCE. Both the cerebellum and the cerebral cortex influence coordination and balance. Cerebellar dysfunction creates loss of steady, balanced posture and gait on the ipsilateral side (same side) as the offending lesion. Lesions of the cortex, however, cause motor dysfunction on the contralateral side (opposite side) of the lesion.

Observation of routine activity, such as ambulation, feeding, or performing activities of daily living, can provide valuable information regarding coordination and balance. In the assessment of balance, the patient can be asked to walk 10 to 20 feet away from the examiner,

TABLE 25-4

DIAGNOSTIC TESTS AND PROCEDURES FOR NEUROLOGIC DISORDERS

TEST	PURPOSE/PROCEDURE	PATIENT PREPARATION	POSTPROCEDURE NURSING CARE
Lumbar puncture	A cannula is inserted into subarachnoid space of spinal column to obtain a CSF sample for analysis. Normal CSF has following characteristics: pressure, 50–175 mm H_2O; pH, 7.30–7.40; clear, colorless appearance; fasting glucose, 40–80 mg/dl; WBC, 0–10 μg/L. Analysis of CSF may also include measurement of specific gravity, bicarbonate, electrolytes, urea, and a variety of other components.	Informed consent must be obtained. Patient is told that a sample of CSF will be taken from spinal column. A local anesthetic is used to anesthetize area of puncture. No special preparation is required. During procedure, nurse assists patient to maintain a knee-chest position.	CSF specimens are placed in test tubes and labeled, with first specimen usually discarded since it may contain blood from puncture. Specimens are delivered to lab promptly. Puncture site is covered with a small bandage and assessed for CSF drainage or bleeding. Vital signs and neurologic status are monitored according to agency policy. Some agencies require patient to be kept flat for up to 8 hr to reduce risk of headache. Oral fluids are encouraged.
Electroencephalogram (EEG)	Small electrodes are placed on head to monitor electrical impulses. Used to detect seizure activity.	Test is explained to patient. Nurse emphasizes that patient will not feel any electrical shocks. Prior to test, patient's hair is shampooed. Medications such as anticonvulsants, sedatives, stimulants, and tranquilizers as well as caffeine may be withheld for up to 48 hr before EEG.	Help patient shampoo hair to remove electrode paste. Resume medications as ordered or per procedure protocol.

TABLE 25-4

DIAGNOSTIC TESTS AND PROCEDURES FOR NEUROLOGIC DISORDERS *Continued*

TEST	PURPOSE/PROCEDURE	PATIENT PREPARATION	POSTPROCEDURE NURSING CARE
		sleep-deprived EEG may be done by awakening patient and performing test shortly after onset of sleep.	
Electromyography (EMG)	Needle electrodes are placed on several points over a nerve and over muscle supplied by that nerve. Electrical activity is recorded. Useful in diagnosing neuromuscular abnormalities such as ALS, peripheral neuropathy, myasthenia gravis, and carpal tunnel syndrome.	Nurse explains procedure. Informed consent is obtained. Caffeine and smoking are restricted for 3 hr before procedure. Procedure takes 1–2 hr.	Sites of needle electrode placement are inspected. Patient may be instructed to return within 5 days to have blood drawn for enzyme tests (AST, CK, LD).
Radiologic Studies			
Brain Scan	Depicts pattern of distribution of a radioactive isotope that has been injected intravenously. Useful in diagnosing brain abscesses, tumors, contusions, vascular occlusions or hemorrhage, and hematomas. Contraindicated during pregnancy.	Nurse tells patient what to expect, that scan is painless, and that radiation exposure is minimal. Informed consent is obtained. KCl is given as ordered 2 hr before procedure.	Oral fluids are encouraged to promote elimination of isotope.
Cerebral angiography	A dye is injected into vascular system and radiography taken as dye fills cerebral blood vessels. Detects abnormalities of cerebral blood flow such as cerebral aneurysms and arteriovenous malformations.	Procedure is explained, and informed consent is obtained. All metal is removed from head area. Radiologist is informed of allergies to contrast media, shellfish, or iodine.	Pressure must be applied to puncture site, and site is monitored for bleeding. Bedrest may be ordered for up to 24 hr. If a blood vessel in arm or leg is used to inject dye, extremity is immobilized for a specified period of time and assessed for circulation and neurologic function.
Computed tomography (CT scan)	CT scans of head may be done with and without contrast media. Patient lies on a stretcher that fits into a circular machine that scans head. Used to visualize intracranial structures.	No special preparation is required except to explain procedure to patient. Assess allergies to contrast media, iodine, and shellfish.	No special aftercare is needed.
Magnetic resonance imaging (MRI)	Uses radiofrequency waves in a strong magnetic field to create images of intracranial structures without radiation. Patient lies on a stretcher that passes into a tubular structure. Drumming noises are heard while imager is in use.	Tell patient what to expect. No special preparation is required. Sedation may be ordered for confused patients or those who are claustrophobic. Patients with implanted metal cannot be exposed to MRI because magnet will affect metal. Special oxygen equipment, ventilators, and infusion pumps must be used.	No special aftercare is needed.
Pneumoencephalography	Gas is injected into the lumbar arachnoid space. It rises to the brain. Radiographs are taken that outline cerebral ventricles and cisterns. Used to diagnose masses, congenital abnormalities, cysts, and atrophy of cerebral and cerebellar cortex.	Procedure is explained to patient, and informed consent is obtained. Metal objects are removed from head area. Nurse may help support patient during lumbar puncture.	Neurologic checks are done per agency protocol. Patient is kept flat and logrolled for up to 48 hr. Inspect puncture site for CSF leakage or bleeding. Encourage oral fluids if permitted.

CSF, Cerebrospinal fluid; WBC, white blood cell count; ALS, amyotrophic lateral sclerosis; AST, aspartate aminotransferase; CK, creatine kinase; LD, lactic dehydrogenase; KCl, potassium chloride.

MISSION HOSPITAL
REGIONAL MEDICAL CENTER

ADULT NEURO FLOW SHEET

				0700	0800	0900	1000	1100	1200	1300	1400	1500	1600	1700	1800	1900	2000	2100	2200	2300	2400	0100	0200	0300	0400	0500	0600
GLASGOW COMA SCALE			Eyes Open																								
			Best Motor																								
			Best Verbal																								
			TOTAL																								
VOLUNTARY MOTOR	Right		upper extremity																								
			lower extremity																								
	Left		upper extremity																								
			lower extremity																								
CRANIAL NERVES	**PUPILS**	Right	Size																								
			Reaction																								
		Left	Size																								
			Reaction																								
	EOMS	Conjugate																									
		Dysconjugate																									
		Tracking	Right																								
			Left																								
	Blink Reflex																										
	Gag Reflex																										
	Facial Symmetry																										
			TIME	0700	0800	0900	1000	1100	1200	1300	1400	1500	1600	1700	1800	1900	2000	2100	2200	2300	2400	0100	0200	0300	0400	0500	0600

KEY

MOTOR
5+ Normal Power
4+ Weakness
3+ Anti-gravity
2+ Not anti-gravity
1+ Trace
0 No movement

Pupil Size
B = Brisk
S = Sluggish
A = Absent

2mm 3mm 4mm 5mm

6mm 7mm 8mm

✓ = Present
O = Absent
S = Symmetrical
A = Asymmetrical

Date

Speech Patterns: ______

Comments: ______

GLASGOW COMA SCALE		
Eyes Open	4	Spontaneously
	3	To verbal command
	2	To Pain
	1	No Response
Best Motor Response	6	Obeys Commands
	5	Localize Pain
	4	Flexion to pain withdraw
	3	Flexion Decorticate
	2	Extension to pain (decerebrate)
	1	No Response to pain
Best Verbal Response	5	Oriented
	4	Confused
	3	Inappropriate words
	2	Incomprehensible sounds
	1	No Response

Unit ______

R.N. Signature ______ Shift: ______

R.N. Signature ______ Shift: ______

R.N. Signature ______ Shift: ______

ADDRESSOGRAPH

Form: 408 5/92

Adult Neuro Flow Sheet

FIGURE 25-5

A neuro flow sheet is used to document assessment of neurologic function. (Courtesy of Linda R. Littlejohn, RN, BSN, CCRN, CNRN, Neuro Clinician, and Mission Hospital Regional Medical Center, Mission Viejo, CA. From Black, J. M., & Matassarin-Jacobs, E. [1993]. *Luckmann and Sorensen's medical-surgical nursing: A psychophysiologic approach* [4th ed., p. 682]. Philadelphia: W. B. Saunders.)

turn, and walk back toward the examiner. Gait and arm swing are observed. The patient is then asked to walk a straight line in a heel-to-toe fashion.

Romberg's test is done by having the patient stand, feet together and arms at sides. The patient is instructed to close the eyes and maintain that position. The examiner stays close by in case the patient starts to fall. Normally, there will be only slight swaying.

To evaluate skilled movements, the patient can be asked to perform the following activities:

1. Have the patient pat the knees with the palms of the hands and then with the backs of the hands in a rapid, alternating pattern.
2. Hold up the finger and instruct the patient to touch it with his or her index finger.
3. Have the patient touch his or her nose with his or her index finger, first with the eyes open and then with the eyes closed.

NEUROMUSCULAR FUNCTION. Individual muscle groups may be assessed by evaluating their size, tone, and strength. Upper arm strength can be evaluated by asking the patient to squeeze the examiner's fingers. The examiner puts one finger on top of another so that a firm squeeze will not painfully press the knuckles together. The patient can also be instructed to lift each hand or to raise a finger on each hand. Another means of assessing upper arm strength is to have the patient extend both arms forward with the palms up. The patient is asked to close his or her eyes and maintain the position for 10 to 20 seconds. With normal strength, the arms remain steady.

To evaluate strength of the legs, the patient is positioned supine and asked to raise one leg at a time. The patient with normal strength can lift the leg 90 degrees. Tests of strength of other muscles may be done as indicated.

SENSORY FUNCTION. There are many tests of sensory function, including evaluation of the patient's perception of pain, touch, temperature, vibration, position, and tactile discrimination. Various stimuli are applied to the skin and, without looking, the patient is asked to identify the type of stimulus perceived.

Pain. Pain can be evaluated by gently pricking the skin with a sterile needle and touching the skin with a dull object. The patient is asked to state whether sharp or dull sensations are felt. Recognition of sharp pricks indicates ability to perceive painful stimuli.

Temperature. Temperature perception can be tested by touching test tubes containing hot or cold water to the patient's skin and asking the patient to identify what temperature is perceived.

Light Touch. A wisp of cotton brushed against the skin is used to assess perception of light touch. The patient is asked to state when the sensation is felt.

Vibration. The examiner strikes a tuning fork and touches the base to a joint in the great toe or a finger. The patient is asked to report when the vibration is felt and when it stops. If the sensation is not perceived, the examiner repeats the test on more proximal areas until the patient perceives it.

Position. The examiner moves the patient's great toe or a finger up and down and asks the patient to identify the direction of the movement.

Tactile Discrimination. Tests for fine tactile discrimination include stereognosis, graphesthesia, and point location. In testing stereognosis, the examiner places a familiar object (paper clip, cotton ball) in the patient's hand and requests identification. Graphesthesia tests the patient's ability to recognize a number or letter "written" on the palm with a dull object. To test point location, the skin is touched briefly and the patient is asked to touch the place where the sensation was felt.

REFLEXES. A reflex is an unconscious, involuntary response that is entirely mediated at the level of the spinal cord, without input from higher brain centers. The knee jerk represents the simplest reflex. A stimulus is applied to the patella, with the sensory root of the spinal nerve transmitting the impulse to the spinal cord. At the cord, the impulse is relayed to the motor nerve root, which then elicits the knee jerk (Fig. 25–6). Other commonly tested reflexes are listed in Table 25–5.

Although these common reflexes are normal, others appear only with pathologic states. Babinski's reflex accompanies abnormalities in the motor pathways origi-

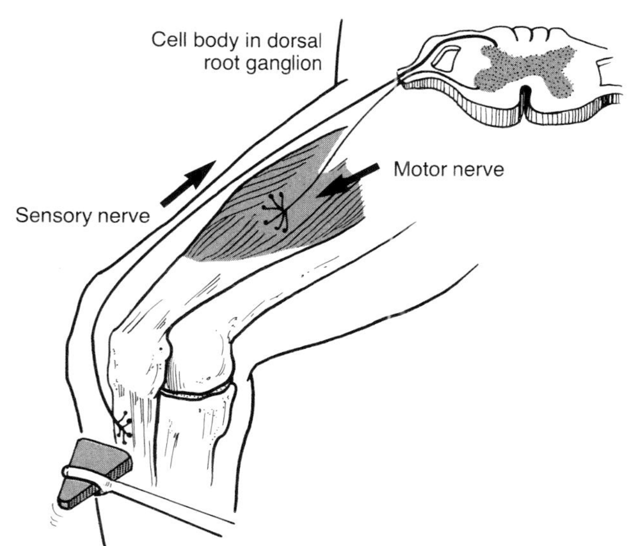

FIGURE 25-6

Reflexes are elicited by stimulating a sensory nerve, which conveys an impulse to the spinal cord. An impulse is then conveyed by a motor nerve to cause the muscle to contract. (Redrawn from Jarvis, C. [1992]. *Physical examination and health assessment* [p. 737]. Philadelphia: W. B. Saunders.)

TABLE 25–5
COMMONLY TESTED REFLEXES

REFLEX	EXPECTED RESPONSE
Biceps	Flexion of forearm
Triceps	Extension of forearm
Brachioradialis	Flexion and supination of forearm
Quadriceps	Extension of lower leg
Achilles (ankle jerk)	Plantar flexion of foot
Clonus	Absence of movement after brisk dorsiflexion of foot

nating in the cerebral cortex. It is elicited by stroking the lateral side of the bottom of the foot and observing the resulting movement of the toes. Normally, the toes curl downward. However, in the presence of cortical dysfunction, the big toe bends upward, and the other toes fan out. Figure 25–7 illustrates the response.

Lumbar Puncture

Lumbar puncture is an invasive procedure most often used to detect infections of the central nervous system, tumors, and hydrocephalus. Other indications are listed in Table 25–4. A hollow needle is inserted into the subarachnoid space at the level of the third lumbar vertebra. Entering at this level allows the physician to avoid traumatizing the spinal cord, which ends at the level of the second lumbar vertebra. Once the needle is in place, a sample of CSF is collected for laboratory analysis.

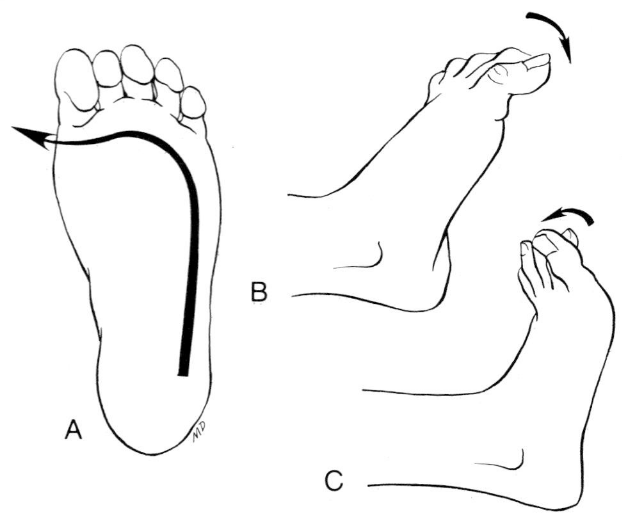

FIGURE 25–7
Babinski's reflex. *A*, The examiner scrapes the foot as shown. *B*, The normal response is plantar flexion of the toes, which may be described as an absent Babinski's reflex). *C*, An abnormal response characterized by dorsiflexion of the big toe is described as a present Babinski's reflex. The other toes may fan as part of Babinski's reflex. (From Black, J. M., & Matassarin-Jacobs, E. [1993]. *Luckmann and Sorensen's medical-surgical nursing: A psychophysiologic approach* [4th ed., p. 648]. Philadelphia: W. B. Saunders.)

Prior to the lumbar puncture, the nurse explains its purpose to the patient. Informed consent is required. The patient is instructed to void before the procedure to reduce the discomfort of a full bladder. During the procedure, the patient is required to remain on one side in a knee-to-chest position. The nurse assists the patient to maintain this position throughout the procedure (Fig. 25–8).

Because a postprocedure headache may occur, the patient is usually advised to lie flat for at least 6 hours. Increased fluid intake may help to minimize headache. Although injuries resulting from lumbar puncture are rare, postprocedure care includes assessments for numbness, tingling, or pain in the extremities; drainage from the puncture site; and changes in vital signs.

Severe headaches are sometimes treated with a blood patch created by injecting a small amount of the patient's blood into the lumbar puncture site. The blood clots, sealing the puncture site and preventing further loss of CSF.

Electroencephalogram

The electroencephalogram (EEG) is a graphic representation of electrical activity in brain cells. Small electrodes are placed at various positions on the head, which detect electrical signals generated from neurons located near the surface of the cerebral cortex. It is an excellent tool in the diagnosis of seizure activity (Fig. 25–9).

In preparation, the nurse explains the procedure in order to reduce the patient's anxiety. Many believe that some electrical stimulus will be experienced during the test, and they must be assured that this is not the case. Other misconceptions about EEG are that the examiner is able to "read the patient's mind" and that the test is done to detect mental illness. A thorough shampoo should be done to ensure that the EEG electrodes and paste will adhere to the scalp. Medications, such as anticonvulsants, sedatives, stimulants, and tranquilizers, should be withheld for 24 to 48 hours prior to the test. Caffeine-containing food and drink act as stimulants and should be restricted as well.

Fatigue stresses the brain and may evoke abnormal activity not usually seen on the EEG. Therefore, patients may be evaluated with a sleep-deprived EEG, in which they are awakened after a short sleep period in an effort to elicit such activity during the test.

No specific postprocedure activity is required. However, the nurse must ensure that all medications held prior to the EEG are resumed. In addition, the patient may need assistance with shampooing to remove the electrode paste.

Electromyography

Electromyography studies the response of peripheral motor and sensory nerves to electrical stimuli. Needle electrodes are placed on several points over a nerve and over the muscles supplied by the nerve. Stimuli are administered, and the effects are recorded on an oscilloscope.

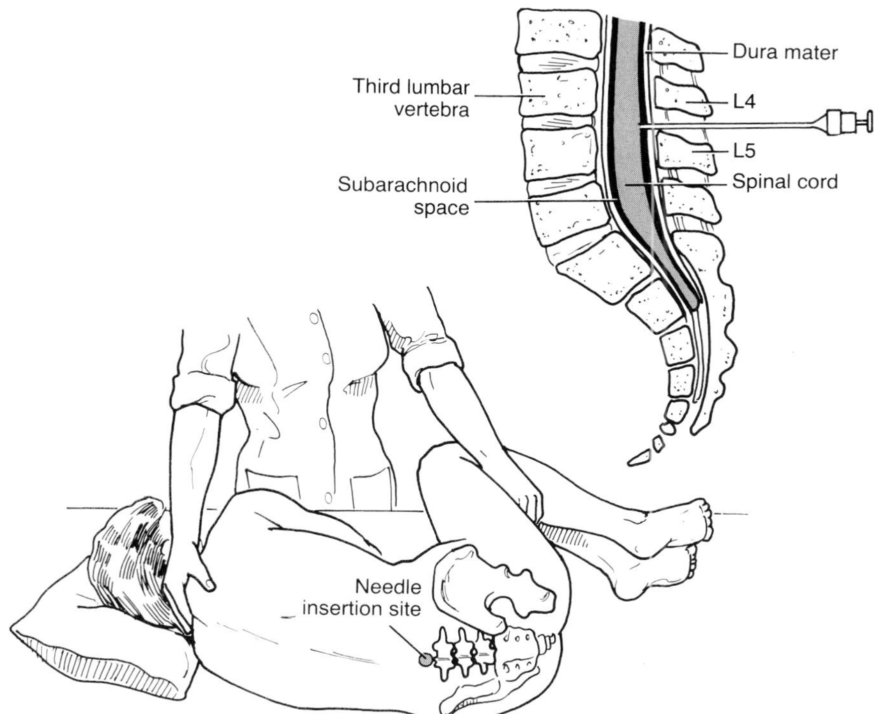

FIGURE 25-8
The nurse supports the patient in position for a lumbar puncture.

Informed consent is required for electromyography. Caffeine and smoking are restricted for 3 hours before the procedure. Some medications may be withheld according to agency procedure or physician's orders. The patient is told what to expect and that the procedure takes 1 to 2 hours.

No special postprocedure care is needed.

Radiologic Studies

BRAIN SCAN. The brain scan depicts the pattern of distribution of a radioactive isotope injected intravenously. It is useful in detecting brain abscesses, tumors, contusions, vascular occlusion or hemorrhage, and hematomas. Because radioactive material is used, the procedure is contraindicated during pregnancy.

Informed consent must be obtained for a brain scan. The patient is given potassium chloride 2 hours before the isotope is given to prevent excessive isotope uptake. The nurse tells the patient to expect an intravenous injection to be given immediately before the scan is done. The patient will lie still on a stretcher while the scanner, somewhat like an x-ray machine, moves back and forth over the head. There is no sensation associated with the scanning process. The scan is then repeated 1 hour later. The nurse assures the patient that the dose of radiation is small, quickly eliminated, and poses no threat to others.

After the test, the patient is encouraged to increase fluid intake to promote isotope elimination through the kidneys.

CEREBRAL ANGIOGRAPHY. Cerebral angiography permits visualization of the cerebral blood vessels. A cannula is usually inserted into the femoral artery, and a catheter is advanced to the carotid or vertebral arteries. A contrast dye is injected, and a series of radiographs is taken. Angiography is the most definitive diagnostic test in the diagnosis of cerebral aneurysm or congenital vascular disorders, such as arteriovenous malformation.

Informed consent is required for cerebral angiography. Any metal objects (jewelry, hairpins) must be removed from the head area. The nurse informs the radi-

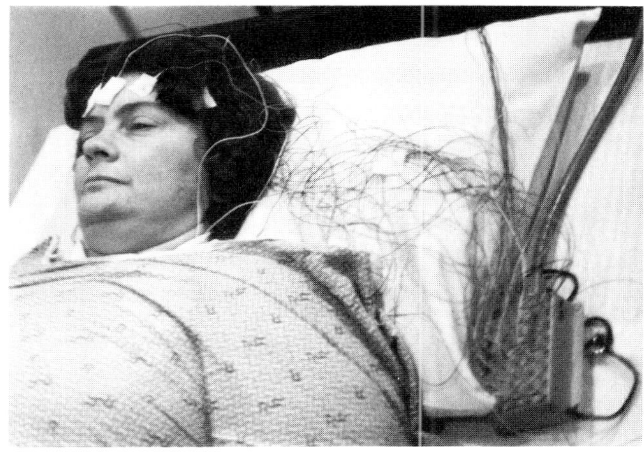

FIGURE 25-9
Electrodes are attached to the patient's scalp for an electroencephalogram. (From Black, J. M., & Matassarin-Jacobs, E. [1993]. *Luckmann and Sorensen's medical-surgical nursing: A psychophysiologic approach* [4th ed., p. 662]. Philadelphia: W. B. Saunders.)

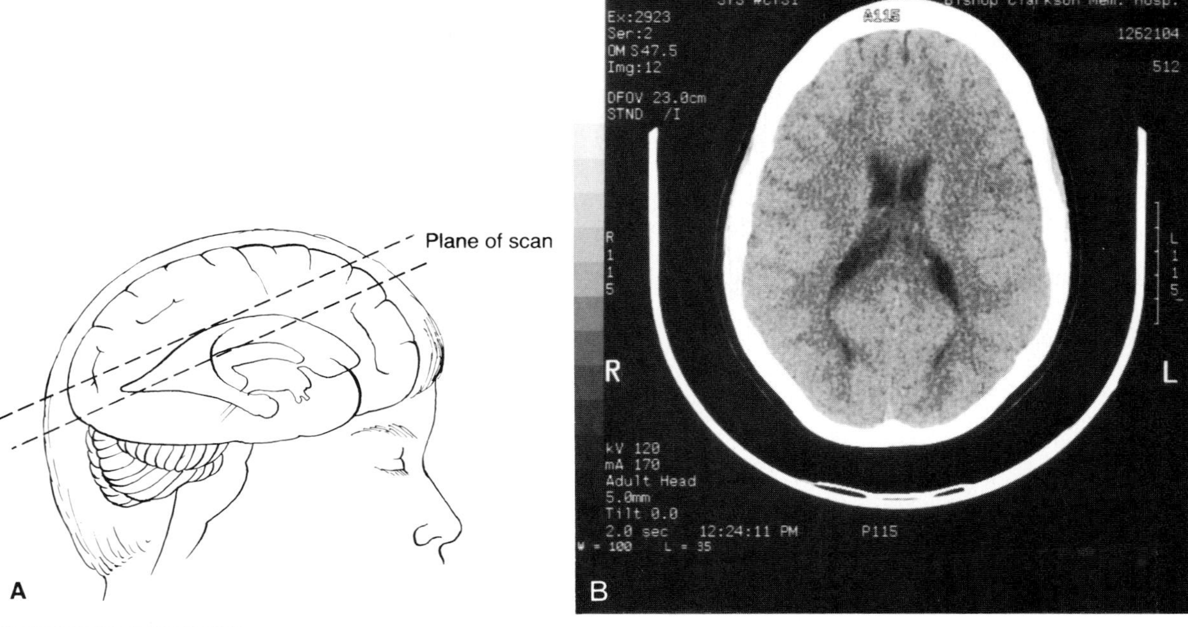

FIGURE 25-10

A computed tomography scan creates a remarkably clear image of a cross-section of the brain. (From Black, J. M., & Matassarin-Jacobs, E. [1993]. *Luckmann and Sorensen's medical-surgical nursing: A psychophysiologic approach* [4th ed., p. 659]. Philadelphia: W. B. Saunders.)

ologist about any allergies to iodine, shellfish, or contrast media. The patient is told to expect to lie still on a stretcher while the dye is injected and radiographs are taken of the head.

After the procedure, pressure is applied to the puncture site, which must be assessed for bleeding. Bedrest may be ordered for up to 24 hours. If an extremity was used for the cannula, it is usually immobilized for 12 hours and assessed for circulation and sensation. Neurologic checks are done according to agency procedure for 24 hours.

COMPUTED TOMOGRAPHY. The evolution of the computed tomographic (CT) scan represents one of the most significant developments in neurologic diagnostic procedures. It serves as an excellent tool in the evaluation of trauma, tumors, and hemorrhage (Fig. 25–10).

The patient's head is placed in the scanner, with a circular frame surrounding the head. Images of intracranial structures are created. Because air, blood, bone, tissue, and CSF have varying densities, they appear on the CT scan in various shades of gray. Enhancement of an area may be achieved by injecting contrast medium; therefore, any allergy to such media must be reported to the radiologist in advance. The entire scanning procedure lasts 15 to 30 minutes and generally requires no advance preparation.

MAGNETIC RESONANCE IMAGING. One of the latest tools in neuroradiology is magnetic resonance imaging (MRI). Unlike CT scanning, which exposes the patient to radiation, MRI does not use radiation. It is a noninvasive examination that involves placing the patient in a strong magnetic field and then applying bursts of radiofrequency waves. Sophisticated technology converts information about movement of molecules in the tissue into precise, clear images (Fig. 25–11).

This noninvasive diagnostic procedure is painless, has no known risks, and requires no preparation. The nurse tells the patient to expect to hear noises like a muffled drumbeat while in the machine. Since the patient must lie on a flat surface that rolls into a tubular structure, people who are confused or claustrophobic may require mild sedation. Because metallic objects may be adversely affected by the electromagnetic field generated by the scanner, patients with pacemakers, orthotic or prosthetic devices, aneurysm clips, or other such equipment should not be exposed to the MRI scanner. If an infusion pump is being used, the site must be converted to intermittent infusion (such as a saline or heparin lock) because the pump cannot be placed in the room where the MRI machine is located. If oxygen is required, adequate tubing is needed to allow the oxygen tank to be placed a safe distance outside the room. Special equipment is used for patients on mechanical ventilation.

PNEUMOENCEPHALOGRAPHY. For pneumoencephalography, gas injected into the lumbar subarachnoid space rises to the head. Radiographic views are then taken to outline the cerebral ventricles and cisterns. This procedure reveals masses, congenital abnor-

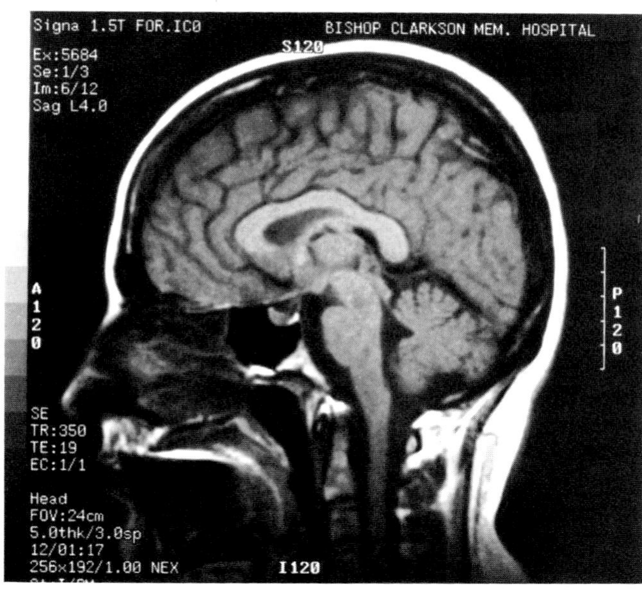

FIGURE 25-11
A magnetic resonance imaging scan uses magnetic fields to create cross-sectional views of the brain. (From Black, J. M., & Matassarin-Jacobs, E. [1993]. *Luckmann and Sorensen's medical-surgical nursing: A psychophysiologic approach* [4th ed., p. 661]. Philadelphia: W. B. Saunders.)

malities, cysts, and atrophy of the cerebral cortex. Since the advent of CT scanning, pneumoencephalography is no longer common.

COMMON THERAPEUTIC MEASURES

DRUG THERAPY

A number of drugs are used to treat neurologic disorders. They include antimicrobials, analgesics, anti-inflammatories, corticosteroids, anticonvulsants, diuretics, chemotherapeutic agents, dopaminergics, anticholinergics, cholinergics, and antihistamines. Examples of specific drugs are presented in Table 25–6.

SURGERY

A craniotomy (surgery that requires opening the skull) may be done to treat tumors, correct defects, evacuate hematomas, and relieve pressure associated with trauma. A craniectomy is the excision of a segment of the skull, and a cranioplasty is any procedure done to repair a skull defect. General care of the surgical patient is covered in Chapter 14, but interventions specific to neurologic surgery are emphasized here.

TABLE 25-6
DRUGS USED TO TREAT NEUROLOGIC DISORDERS

DRUGS	USE/ACTION	SIDE EFFECTS	NURSING INTERVENTIONS
Anticonvulsants			
Phenytoin (Dilantin)	Prevents sodium shift that causes neuron hyperexcitability; inhibits seizure activity. Reduces pain of trigeminal neuralgia.	Sluggishness, ataxia, slurred speech, nystagmus, constipation, nausea, vomiting, overgrowth of gingiva, skin rashes. Hypotension with IV route. Unusual: aplastic anemia, agranulocytosis.	Monitor pulse and report bradycardia. Monitor BP with IV dose. Safety precautions if ataxic, drowsy. Give with food to reduce GI irritation. Provide meticulous mouth care to prevent gingival overgrowth. Identify concurrent drugs to detect possible interactions that enhance or inhibit drug effect.
Barbiturates			
Phenobarbital (Luminal), primidone (Myidone)	Depress CNS and raise seizure threshold.	Drowsiness, respiratory depression, nausea, vomiting, diarrhea, constipation, rash, photosensitivity, muscle aches. With IV route: laryngospasm, bronchospasm, hypotension.	Safety precautions if drowsy. Monitor respiratory rate and BP, especially with IV route. Note other drugs for possible drug interactions. Tell patient not to stop drug without consulting physician and to avoid alcohol and excessive sunlight.
Carbamazepine (Tegretol)	Slows transmission of impulses in CNS; prevents seizures. Reduces pain of trigeminal neuralgia.	Drowsiness, ataxia, blurred vision, BP increase or decrease, heart failure, urinary retention, rash, hepatitis, aplastic anemia, agranulocytosis.	Safety precautions if drowsy. Monitor BP. Teach patient: avoid alcohol and excessive sunlight, do not change dosage or stop drug without physician's guidance, immediately report fever, sore throat, excessive bruising or bleeding, jaundice.

Table continued on following page

TABLE 25-6
DRUGS USED TO TREAT NEUROLOGIC DISORDERS *Continued*

DRUGS	USE/ACTION	SIDE EFFECTS	NURSING INTERVENTIONS
Diazepam (Valium)	Depresses CNS; inhibits impulse conduction.	Drowsiness, rash, nausea, vomiting, diarrhea, constipation, respiratory depression, psychological and physical dependence. IV route: hypotension, phlebitis.	Safety precautions if drowsy. Monitor infusion site for extravasation. Monitor BP. Give with food to decrease GI distress. Tell patient not to stop or change drug dose without physician guidance.
Clonazepam (Klonopin)	Raises seizure threshold.	Drowsiness, ataxia, agitation, rash, edema, nocturia, blurred vision, dry mouth, excitement in elderly. Toxicity causes lethargy, confusion, coma.	Avoid abrupt withdrawal; may cause restlessness, insomnia, status epilepticus. Safety measures if drowsy.
Ethosuximide (Zarontin)	Raises seizure threshold.	Nightmares, sleep and psychiatric disturbances, blood dyscrasias.	Avoid abrupt withdrawal, which can cause seizures. Monitor CBC and platelets. Assess for fatigue, bruising. Safety precautions if drowsy.
Valproic acid (Depakene)	Raises seizure threshold.	Transient nausea and vomiting, drowsiness, hepatotoxicity, blood dyscrasias.	Can give with food if GI irritation occurs. Do not crush enteric-coated tablets. Do not give liquid with carbonated drinks. Monitor CBC, platelets. Can cause seizures if withdrawn abruptly.
Antibiotics			
Penicillin G (Bicillin, Pentids, Crysticillin)	Used to treat pneumococcal, streptococcal, meningococcal, and neisserial meningitis.	Nausea, vomiting, diarrhea, epigastric distress, rash superinfections, anaphylaxis, hemolytic anemia, leukopenia.	Assess allergies before administering. Observe for anaphylaxis: rash, pruritis, wheezing. Have epinephrine, antihistamines, and resuscitation equipment on hand.
Osmotic diuretics			
Mannitol	Decreases tubular reabsorption of water so that water output rises. Used to decrease intracranial pressure related to cerebral edema and to decrease edema of spinal cord injury.	Dry mouth, blurred vision, headache, nausea and vomiting, dizziness, tachycardia, BP alterations, fluid and electrolyte imbalances, fluid volume deficit, hypokalemia, hyponatremia, circulatory overload.	Monitor BP, pulse, intake and output, tissue turgor, fluid status. If crystals form in solution, warm bottle in hot water; then cool before giving.
Corticosteroids			
Dexamethasone (Decadron)	Anti-inflammatory; used to treat cerebral edema.	Nausea and vomiting, diarrhea or constipation, hypertension, fluid volume excess, hypernatremia, hypocalcemia, hyperglycemia, increased susceptibility to infection.	Monitor intake and output, BP, electrolytes. Assess for signs of infection. Protect patients from others who have infections. Give with food or milk to reduce GI irritation. Advise patient to carry identification with information about drug therapy.

Preoperative Nursing Care

Preoperatively, the nurse assesses and documents neurologic status to provide a baseline for evaluating postoperative progress. The patient is encouraged to ask questions and to express fears. Parenteral corticosteroids may be administered as ordered to help reduce cerebral edema. Complete or partial shaving of the scalp is usually done, and the shaved hair is saved for the patient. The nurse recognizes that shaving the head can be very stressful for patients and assures them that it will grow back. Sometimes shaving is done after the patient is anesthetized to reduce the trauma. The family should be advised that a craniotomy can take as long as 12 hours and that they will get progress reports during the procedure.

Postoperative Nursing Care

Postoperative craniotomy assessment includes evaluation of LOC, vital signs, movement and strength, pupil size and response to light, and speech. Signs and symptoms that may be related to complications are headache, visual disturbances, vomiting, seizures, and respiratory

TABLE 25-6

DRUGS USED TO TREAT NEUROLOGIC DISORDERS *Continued*

DRUGS	USE/ACTION	SIDE EFFECTS	NURSING INTERVENTIONS
Antiparkinsonian agents			
Carbidopa (Sinemet)	Increases dopamine in brain; used to treat Parkinson's disease.	Nausea, dizziness, bradycardia, orthostatic hypotension, dry mouth, blurred vision, drowsiness, confusion, dystonic movements, mental status changes, urinary retention.	Monitor pulse and BP, urine output. Safety measures if dizzy or drowsy. Oral hygiene. Sustained-release tablets can be cut in half but should not be crushed.
Trihexyphenidyl (Artane)	Controls extrapyramidal symptoms caused by drug therapy.	Mental confusion and agitation in elderly. Drowsiness, weakness, urinary retention, visual and hearing disturbances, hypersensitivity, CNS depression.	Safety precautions if drowsy or weak. Assess bladder for distention. Monitor mental status, sensory status. Can give with food. Sustained-release capsules should not be crushed. Oral hygiene.
Amantadine HCl (Symmetrel)	Antiviral, antiparkinsonism.	Nausea, insomnia, dizziness, orthostatic hypotension, congestive heart failure, urinary retention.	Monitor intake and output, BP, sleep pattern. Assess for bladder distention. Safety measures if drowsy. Teach patient to manage orthostatic hypotension. Do not take within a few hours of bedtime because of tendency to cause insomnia. Tell patient not to consume alcohol while taking amantadine.
Miscellaneous Neurologic Drugs			
Interferon-β1b (Betason)	Used to reduce frequency of recurrent episodes of multiple sclerosis characterized by remissions and exacerbations.	Contraindicated with hypersensitivity to human albumin. Inflammation, pain, and necrosis at injection site. Flu-like symptoms: muscle aches, fever, chills. Menstrual problems. Depression, anxiety, confusion. Suicides and suicide attempts reported during clinical trials.	Contraindicated with hypersensitivity to human albumin. Teach patient to give injections. Monitor emotional state. Report depression. Assess injection site.
Skeletal muscle relaxant Baclofen (Lioresal)	Acts on spinal cord to decrease muscle spasms; useful with multiple sclerosis to treat spasticity.	Drowsiness, weakness, hypotension, nausea, constipation, urinary frequency. rarely causes CNS excitement, slurred speech, nocturia, impotence. Toxicity: vomiting, decreased muscle tone, seizures, respiratory depression.	Safety precautions if drowsy or weak. Monitor BP, respirations, urinary pattern, bowel elimination. Assess for signs of CNS effects. Should not be abruptly discontinued.
Acetylcholinesterase muscle stimulant Neostigmine bromide (Prostigmin) Pyridostigmine bromide (Mestinon)	Inhibits destruction of acetylcholine. Used to diagnose and treat myasthenia gravis.	Bradycardia, bronchial constriction, miosis. Toxicity: nausea and vomiting, diarrhea, flushing, hypotension, altered pulse, cholinergic crisis.	Monitor pulse and respirations. Assess for signs and symptoms of toxicity. Monitor for improved muscle strength. Oral drug best given with milk before meals.

IV, Intravenous; BP, blood pressure; GI, gastrointestinal; CNS, central nervous system; CBC, complete blood count.

depression. Vital signs and neurologic checks are usually done hourly at first. Intake and output records are maintained. The dressing is inspected for bleeding or CSF drainage. Drainage from the ears or nose is also noted. Drainage may be tested for glucose with a dipstick. Cerebrospinal fluid will be positive for glucose, whereas mucus will be negative. A dressing may be placed loosely to absorb the drainage. It should be replaced when it becomes wet because the moisture can harbor bacteria. On dressings, CSF appears as a pink stain surrounded by a lighter ring described as a "halo." The nurse reports signs of deteriorating neurologic status to the physician immediately. The patient's position is prescribed by the physician. It usually specifies that the head of the bed be elevated about 20 degrees.

If the patient has an external ventricular drainage system, the nurse uses strict aseptic technique when changing the insertion-site dressing and the drainage bag. The drip chamber of the drainage bag must be kept at the level of the external auditory canal to prevent drainage of excessive CSF. When the patient is being repositioned, the drainage tube is clamped and then restored to the correct level and unclamped.

In addition to the usual surgical complications, the patient having a craniotomy is at risk for increased ICP, CSF leak, meningitis, and seizures. Other complications depend on the area of the brain affected and could include paralysis, memory loss, confusion, and impaired speech, vision, or hearing. Since increased ICP is a concern with cranial surgery as well as with many neurologic disorders, it is described here.

INCREASED INTRACRANIAL PRESSURE. Increased ICP poses an extremely serious threat to the neurologic patient. Understanding the physiology as well as the presenting signs and symptoms can enable the nurse to recognize the problem and respond appropriately to prevent life-threatening consequences.

Pathophysiology. Anatomically, the skull is an empty cavity with three rigid sides. This cavity contains the brain, blood, and CSF, which are referred to as the components that exert pressure in the cranium. This pressure, or ICP, is normally 0 to 15 mm Hg.

In the course of a day, ICP fluctuates minimally because alterations are usually corrected rapidly. The Monro-Kellie hypothesis describes the adaptations that must occur in the three components (brain, blood, and CSF) for ICP to remain normal. If the volume of one component increases, ICP will rise unless there is a subsequent decrease in the other two components. For example, if a brain tumor increases the volume of brain tissue, ICP will rise unless the volume of both blood and CSF decrease.

As ICP increases, the perfusion (delivery of blood and oxygen) to brain tissue decreases. A minimum perfusion pressure of 60 mm Hg is necessary to ensure adequate cerebral functioning. If perfusion pressure falls to 40 mm Hg, ischemia occurs. A perfusion pressure of 30 mm Hg or less is incompatible with life. Perfusion pressure can be increased by decreasing ICP.

Signs and Symptoms. On the basis of the appearance of specific signs and symptoms, the nurse can detect increases in ICP and assess the adequacy of perfusion. The nurse assesses LOC, pupillary characteristics, motor function, sensory function, and vital signs to detect signs of increasing ICP so that treatment can be initiated promptly.

Level of consciousness is the most reliable indicator of mental status because of its extreme sensitivity to oxygen levels in the cerebral blood. As ICP increases and perfusion is reduced, oxygen delivery to cerebral tissue also is reduced. Changes in LOC are the earliest changes seen in ICP. These changes may be very subtle, with minimal agitation or drowsiness, or may be quite extreme, with profound unresponsiveness.

Classic pupillary changes are seen in increasing ICP. As pressure rises, the pupil progresses from its normal size to a dilated state described as a "blown pupil." Reaction to light is lost, and the pupil becomes dilated and fixed. These changes occur because of pressure on the oculomotor nerve (third cranial nerve).

Another major indicator of increased ICP is altered motor function. As the motor areas of the frontal lobe are compressed by rising pressure, deficits develop on the side opposite the expanding mass. When deficits are on the opposite side from brain injury, they are said to be contralateral to the injury. For example, if there is a tumor in the right side of the brain, motor deficits will appear in the left side of the body. The deficits may involve a single extremity or an entire side. Hemiparesis (weakness on one side) or hemiplegia (paralysis on one side) may be seen.

As increased pressure becomes more extensive, abnormal posturing may be evident. As increasing pressure is exerted on the cerebral tissue and frontal lobes, a pattern known as decorticate posturing can be observed. The patient exhibits abnormal flexion in the upper extremities, with extension of the lower extremities. If the total cerebrum is involved, the structures of the brain stem where the motor tracts travel toward the spinal cord are compressed, causing decerebrate posturing. The lower extremities remain extended, and the upper extremities are abnormally extended as well. These motor changes may occur spontaneously or may be seen only with painful stimuli (Fig. 25–12).

Hypothalamic impairment results in the loss of temperature control. As ICP compresses the tissue around the hypothalamus, it becomes ischemic and unable to regulate body temperature.

ICP elevations evoke an increase in systolic blood pressure with little or no associated increase in diastolic pressure. This results in a widening pulse pressure. Initially, the heart rate may be slightly accelerated. However, as ICP compresses the center for cardiac control in the brain stem, the heart rate becomes slow and irregular. Alterations in respiratory pattern are directly related to the extent of tissue compression. Figure 25–13 illustrates areas of tissue compression (types of "herniation" syndromes).

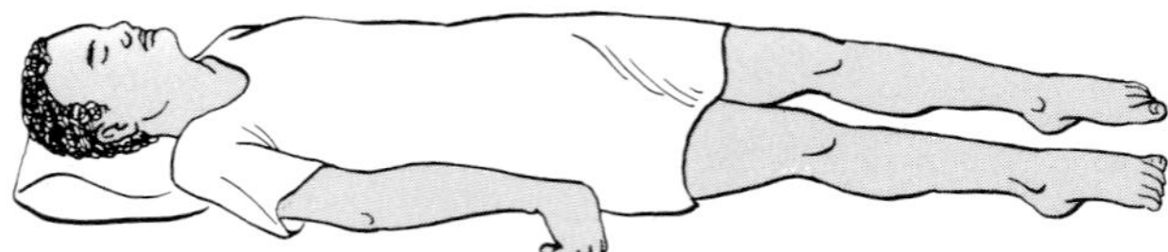

A. Extension posturing (decerebrate rigidity)

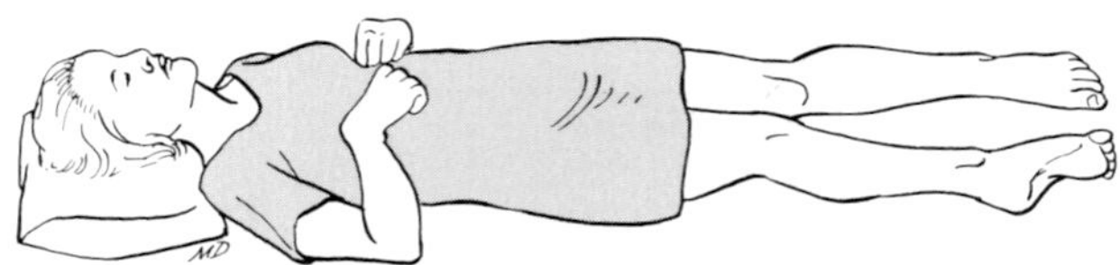

B. Abnormal flexion (decorticate rigidity)

FIGURE 25-12

Abnormal postures may be seen in the patient with neurologic impairment. *A*, Decerebrate rigidity (extension posturing); *B*, decorticate rigidity (flexion posturing). (From Black, J. M., & Matassarin-Jacobs, E. [1993]. *Luckmann and Sorensen's medical-surgical nursing: A psychophysiologic approach* [4th ed., p. 679]. Philadelphia: W. B. Saunders.)

Although it is extremely important to monitor vital signs in the neurologic patient, changes in pulse, respiratory pattern, and blood pressure are late signs of increasing ICP. The combination of hypertension, bradycardia, and a widening pulse pressure is known as Cushing's triad. Cushing's triad is generally associated with increased ICP, but it is unreliable in determining the severity of neurologic compromise.

Medical Treatment. Prompt treatment of increased ICP is vital for survival. Measures to lower ICP include positioning, hyperventilation, fluid restriction, mechanical drainage, and drug therapy.

The jugular vein is the primary route for venous outflow from the brain. It has long been thought that raising the head of the bed 30 to 45 degrees improves the flow of venous blood from the brain, thereby decreasing cerebral blood volume and ICP. However, recent research indicates that perfusion pressure may be better preserved if the head of the bed is elevated no more than 30 degrees. Further investigations may lead to some changes in current practice.

As oxygen delivery to cerebral tissue becomes more impaired, the level of carbon dioxide in the tissue increases. Increased carbon dioxide leads to dilation of cerebral blood vessels, thereby increasing the cerebral blood volume and ICP. With controlled hyperventilation, the excess carbon dioxide is eliminated, causing blood vessels to constrict and ICP to fall. Controlled hyperventilation is best achieved by mechanical ventilation. It effectively decreases ICP within 1 to 2 minutes, but its effectiveness is diminished after 36 to 48 hours.

Restriction of fluid intake reduces blood volume and can help prevent increases in ICP. All intravenous, oral, and enteral fluids should be carefully monitored to prevent fluid overload. Volumes should be sufficient, however, to maintain adequate renal function.

A specialized catheter, called a ventriculostomy catheter, can be placed in the brain to allow for the gravity drainage of excess CSF. After placement in the appropriate location, the catheter is connected to tubing and a collection bag. Drainage of CSF permits reduction of its volume, with an overall decrease in ICP. Absolute sterility must be maintained in managing this system, as it presents an open avenue for contamination.

Intravenous mannitol administration is one of the mainstays in the treatment of increased ICP. As a hyperosmolar agent, mannitol pulls edema fluid from the tissue spaces into the intravascular space. The diuretic effect of mannitol then promotes elimination of the excess fluid volume through the kidneys. Other diuretic agents, such as furosemide, also may be used in an effort to reduce edema.

PHARMACOLOGY CAPSULE

Diuretics used to treat increased intracranial pressure can cause fluid and electrolyte imbalances.

Corticosteroid administration, though controversial, may be used to help further decrease cerebral edema and ICP. Dexamethasone (Decadron) is the major agent used for neurologic patients. Additional information about drugs is presented in Table 25–6.

DISORDERS OF THE NERVOUS SYSTEM

HEADACHE

Headache is the most common type of pain. It is a symptom, rather than a disease, that has many causes.

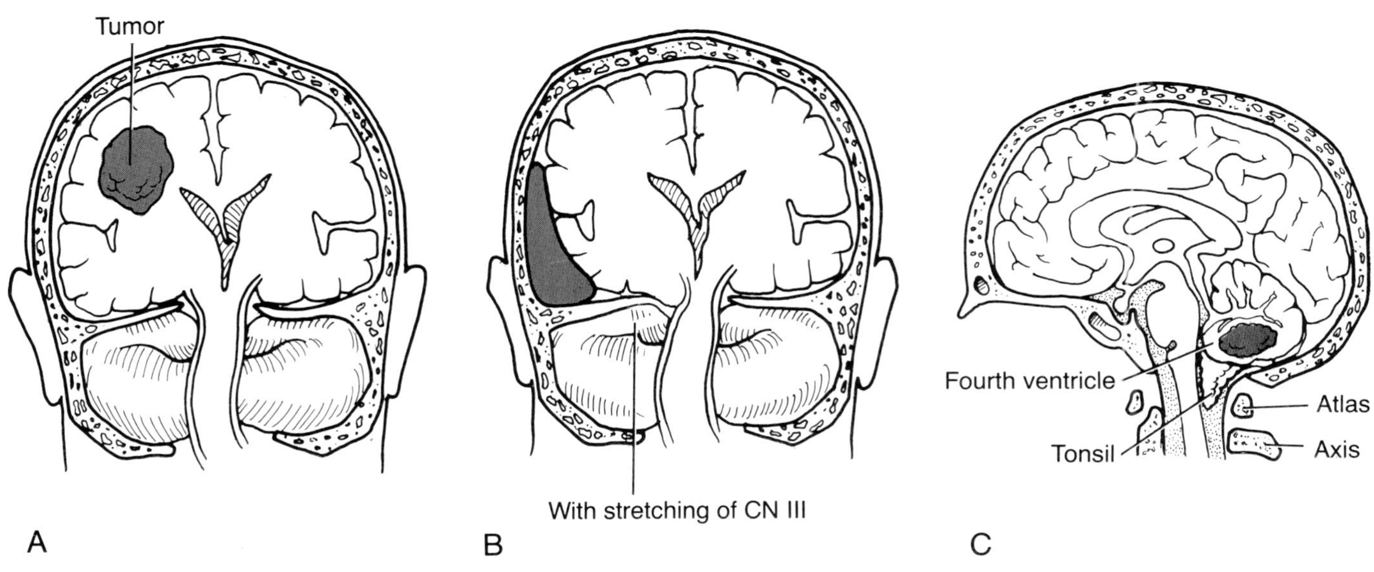

FIGURE 25-13
Types of brain herniation. *A*, Central transtentorial syndrome; *B*, lateral herniation syndrome; *C*, tonsillar herniation syndrome.

Four common types of headaches are migraine headache, cluster headache, tension headache, and headache related to disorders of the eyes, teeth, or sinuses.

MIGRAINE HEADACHE. Migraine headache is thought to be due to intracranial vasoconstriction followed by vasodilation. Although no single cause is known, it may be triggered by menstruation, ovulation, alcohol, some foods (chocolate, cheese, coffee, citrus fruits, dairy products), and stress.

Patients may experience depression, irritability, vision disturbances, nausea, and paresthesias before the onset of pain. The pain is usually unilateral, often begins in the temple or eye area, and is often very intense. Tearing and nausea and vomiting may occur. The patient is hypersensitive to light and sound and prefers a dark, quiet environment.

Prevention of migraine headaches includes avoidance of triggering factors, if known, and use of β-adrenergic blockers. Mild migraines may be treated with acetaminophen or aspirin, but more severe ones require ergot preparations or narcotic analgesics. Ergot is of value only if given in the first 30 to 60 minutes of the onset of pain.

CLUSTER HEADACHE. Cluster headaches occur in a series of episodes followed by a long period with no symptoms. They are intensely painful and seem to be related to stress or anxiety. Unlike migraines, cluster headaches usually have no warning symptoms. They are also shorter in duration than migraines. Treatment may include cold application, indomethacin (Indocin), and tricyclic antidepressants.

TENSION HEADACHES. Tension headaches result from prolonged muscle contraction associated with anxiety, stress, or stimuli from other sources such as a brain tumor or an abscessed tooth. The location of the pain may vary, and the patient may have nausea and vomiting, dizziness, tinnitus, or tearing. Tension headaches may persist for days or even years. Treatment measures include correction of known causes, psychotherapy, massage, heat application, and relaxation techniques. Analgesics, usually non-narcotic, may be prescribed along with drugs to reduce anxiety.

HEADACHES RELATED TO OTHER DISORDERS. Headaches may be associated with many conditions, including vision disturbances, glaucoma, and sinusitis. The treatment depends on the underlying cause.

SEIZURE DISORDER

The electrical impulses generated in the brain normally spread in a very organized fashion. However, in the patient with a seizure disorder, electrical impulses are conducted in a highly chaotic pattern that yields abnormal activity and behavior. Seizure activity involves a large number of hyperactive neurons that use excessive oxygen and glucose. Therefore, oxygen and glucose stores may be depleted, leading to permanent neurologic damage.

Seizure activity may be related to trauma, reduced perfusion, infection, electrolyte disturbances, poisoning, or tumors. There may also be a genetic tendency for such activity.

MEDICAL DIAGNOSIS

Diagnostic testing for seizure activity is often directed toward ruling out specific problems. Obtaining an accurate history of the seizure disorder is vital and can provide clues to possible triggering events and origin of activity. Because unexpected seizure activity is often very frightening to the family, the nurse or other health care provider may be the first reliable eyewitness. Documentation of the episode can provide valuable information in diagnosing the type of seizure disorder present. The observer should note the patient's behavior before, during, and after the seizure as well as the duration of the seizure.

As described previously, EEG records the electrical activity of the brain during rest and while subjected to some particular stimulus. The patient's EEG tracing is then compared with normally anticipated patterns to detect abnormal brain activity.

SEIZURE CLASSIFICATION

Two broad classifications of seizures may be identified based on the patterns of activity: partial seizures and generalized seizures. Abnormal electrical activity may be generated in a specific area of the brain, remain localized and stop, or the activity may spread to adjacent neurons but remain fairly localized. These patterns of activity are termed partial (or focal) seizures because they involve only a part of the brain.

If the neurons involved in the seizure recruit a sufficient number of adjacent cells, the activity can potentially spread throughout the cerebral hemispheres. Because this type of activity involves the entire brain, it produces a generalized seizure.

Some sources use the term unclassified seizures for those that are not readily classified as partial or generalized.

PARTIAL SEIZURES. Partial seizures are described as complex or simple. In a complex partial seizure (sometimes called a psychomotor seizure), the patient briefly loses consciousness. Automatism is evident, in which the patient may smack the lips, pick at clothing, or pat something. A simple partial seizure is characterized by automatism, but the person does not lose consciousness.

GENERALIZED SEIZURES. One type of generalized seizure is the tonic-clonic seizure, sometimes called a grand mal seizure. The tonic phase of the seizure is characterized by stiffening of the muscles or extremities with loss of consciousness. After the tonic phase, there is a rhythmic movement of the extremities called the clonic phase of the seizure. These phases are illustrated in Figure 25–14. The patient may be incontinent of

A

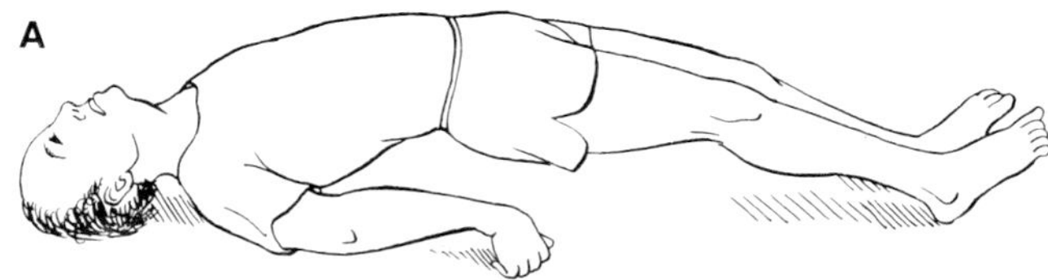

Grand mal, tonic

B

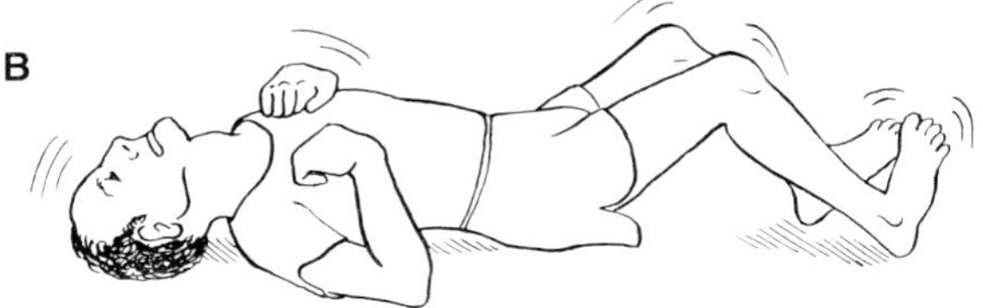

Grand mal, clonic

FIGURE 25-14

Phases of a grand mal seizure. *A*, Tonic phase; *B*, clonic phase. (From Black, J. M., & Matassarin-Jacobs, E. [1993]. *Luckmann and Sorensen's medical-surgical nursing: A psychophysiologic approach* [4th ed., p. 757]. Philadelphia: W. B. Saunders.)

urine during a grand mal seizure. Other types of generalized seizures are absence, myoclonic, and atonic seizures. Absence seizures are brief periods of loss of consciousness in which the person may appear to be daydreaming. These seizures are generally identified during childhood. During a myoclonic siezure, the person has only brief jerking or stiffening of the extremities. Atonic seizures were formerly called "drop attacks" because a sudden loss of muscle tone causes the patient to collapse.

Status Epilepticus. Status epilepticus is a medical emergency in which the patient has continuous seizures or repeated seizures in rapid succession for 30 minutes or more. The prolonged seizure activity depletes the brain of oxygen and glucose, which can lead to permanent brain damage.

Aura. Some people experience an aura preceding a seizure. The aura is a sensation such as dizziness, numbness, visual or hearing disturbance, perception of an offensive odor, or pain.

MEDICAL TREATMENT

The most desirable treatment of a seizure disorder is the resolution of the underlying condition. For example, if a tumor is causing seizure activity, surgical excision of the tumor would be the most desirable therapy. However, if a cause is not readily identifiable or correctable, medical management is implemented.

Anticonvulsant drug therapy provides satisfactory chemical control of seizure activity in about 75% of patients. A variety of drugs are available, some being more effective in particular seizure disorders than others. The selected drug is introduced and the dosage is gradually increased until a therapeutic level is achieved. If good seizure control is not accomplished with one drug, combinations of drugs may be prescribed. Table 25–6 summarizes the major drugs used in medical management of seizure disorders.

PHARMACOLOGY CAPSULE

Sudden discontinuance of anticonvulsants can trigger seizure activity.

Status epilepticus is treated with intravenous anticonvulsant drugs. If the patient does not respond to anticonvulsants, general anesthetic agents and neuromuscular blocking agents may be used.

NURSING CARE OF THE PATIENT WITH A SEIZURE DISORDER

ASSESSMENT. Assessment of the neurologic patient is summarized in Table 25–3. With a seizure disorder, it is especially important to describe the seizure episode and to document drug therapy.

NURSING DIAGNOSIS. Nursing diagnoses for the patient with a seizure disorder may include the following:

- **High Risk for Injury** related to seizure activity
- **Ineffective Individual Coping** related to social stigma of seizure disorder or chronicity
- **Knowledge Deficit** of seizure disorders, treatment, and self-care

GOALS. Nursing goals for the identified diagnoses include absence of injury, patient's ability to cope with condition in a healthy manner, and patient's knowledge of condition, treatment, and self-care.

INTERVENTIONS

High Risk for Injury. The nurse must protect the patient from injury during and after a seizure. Most agencies require that the siderails of the bed be up and padded, a suction machine be readily available, and the bed be maintained in the low position. Some experts believe that padding the siderails is unnecessary, cumbersome, and may have a negative emotional impact on the patient and visitors.

If the patient has a seizure, the nurse quickly moves objects away from the patient. If the patient falls to the floor, the head may be cradled in the nurse's lap to prevent injury. No attempt should be made to restrain the patient. In the past it was common practice to attempt to insert a tongue blade or oral airway between the teeth to prevent biting the tongue. This is no longer recommended. Attempts to force an object between clenched teeth may result in injury to the mouth and do not help if the tongue has already been bitten. The patient will not "swallow his tongue," but it may fall back and occlude the airway. Therefore, turning the patient to one side can help maintain a patent airway.

When seizure activity ceases, the patient is typically drowsy and needs to rest. Quiet and privacy should be assured. Prevention of injury can be accomplished by exercising the management described in Table 25–7. Afterward, the nurse documents the conditions and any unusual behaviors that preceded the seizure. Any lingering effects and the time before recovery are documented.

Ineffective Individual Coping and Knowledge Deficit. Ineffective individual coping can be related to lack of information or misconceptions and may be reflected in noncompliance with prescribed therapy, anxiety, or social isolation. Important aspects of nursing management include not only the care of the patient during hospitalization but also teaching the family and patient about the seizure disorder and the therapy. The teaching plan should include the following:

- Seizures: what they are, why they occur, how to control them, how to recognize an impending seizure, what to do when they occur.
- Factors that may trigger a seizure: fatigue, stress, fever, visual disturbances, alcohol, failure to take medication, large caffeine intake.
- Prescribed drugs: names, dosages, schedules, side effects, effects to be reported to the physician, importance of taking as ordered.
- Psychological factors: normal psychological response to having epilepsy, effects of stress, stress management.
- Emergency information: value of wearing a medical alert tag that identifies the patient as having a seizure disorder and the importance of carrying a card that specifies drug therapy, physician, and individuals to be contacted in an emergency.

Because a seizure disorder is frequently a lifelong problem, patient teaching must be directed toward helping the patient and family adjust to a chronic condition. Patients must adjust physically, psychologically, and vocationally to the changes brought on by the disorder itself as well as to the side effects of the medications. The nurse encourages the patient to ask questions and to express concerns. Resources in the community are identified, including the local chapter of the Epilepsy Foundation of America.

EVALUATION. Criteria for goal achievement are absence of bruises or other signs of injury; positive patient statements about life with a seizure disorder and adherence to prescribed therapy; and patient's and family's ability to explain condition, drug therapy, and interventions.

HEAD INJURY

Traumatic brain injury is a leading cause of death due to trauma in the United States. The most common causes of head injury are motor vehicle accidents, assaults, and falls, with drug and alcohol abuse being major contributing factors. Several different types of injuries can be identified.

TYPES OF HEAD INJURIES

SCALP INJURIES. Scalp injuries include lacerations, contusions, abrasions, and hematomas. They may bleed profusely and may or may not be associated with skull or brain injuries.

CONCUSSION. A concussion is head trauma in which there is no visible injury to the skull or brain. The patient has a loss of consciousness lasting less than 5 minutes and may have a headache, amnesia about the event, nausea, and vomiting.

CONTUSION. A contusion is more serious than a concussion because there is actual bruising and bleeding in the brain tissue. Contusions can be very serious, especially if the brain stem is affected.

TABLE 25–7
MANAGEMENT OF SEIZURES

"DOS"	"DON'TS"
DO remove any objects that could cause harm.	DO NOT restrain unless in grave danger of severe injury.
DO turn the person to one side if possible.	DO NOT attempt to force anything between teeth.
DO note the time the seizure began and how it progressed.	
DO assess and document postictal (postseizure) status.	
DO allow person to rest quietly.	
DO call a medical emergency if a seizure lasts more than 4 min or if seizures occur in rapid succession.	

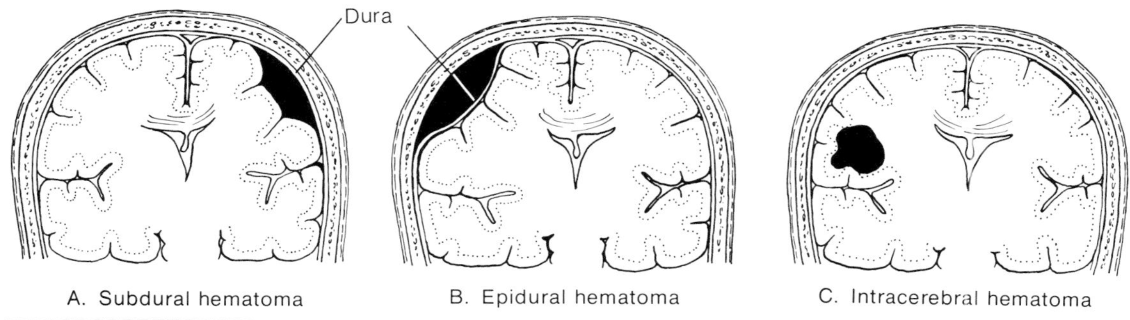

FIGURE 25-15

Hematomas. *A*, Subdural; *B*, epidural; *C*, intracerebral. (From Black, J. M., & Matassarin-Jacobs, E. [1993]. *Luckmann and Sorensen's medical-surgical nursing: A psychophysiologic approach* [4th ed., p. 763]. Philadelphia: W. B. Saunders.)

HEMATOMAS. A hematoma is a collection of blood, usually clotted, that may be classified as subdural or epidural.

Subdural Hematoma. A subdural hematoma is usually due to the tearing of the veins that drain the brain, allowing blood to accumulate in the space beneath the dura (Fig. 25–15*A*). Three types of subdural hematomas are identified: acute, subacute, and chronic. Acute subdural hematoma develops within 24 hours of the injury. Subacute subdural hematoma is seen more than 24 hours and less than 1 week after the initial injury. Chronic subdural hematoma occurs within weeks or even months of the original injury and is associated with low-impact injuries that cause very slow, diffuse bleeding. Because the bleeding associated with any hematoma can cause potentially serious consequences, astute assessment is needed to determine patient status. Surgical intervention is usually indicated for these types of injuries.

Epidural Hematoma. An epidural hematoma forms in the space between the inner surface of the skull and the outermost meningeal covering of the brain, known as dura (Fig. 25–15*B*). Generally, development of the epidural hematoma represents arterial bleeding secondary to a laceration and tearing of the middle meningeal artery. The patient typically has a momentary lapse of consciousness and then exhibits a lucid interval followed by rapid deterioration. Therefore, the nurse must be alert to any indication of increasing ICP, especially drowsiness progressing to coma. Surgical intervention may be done to relieve pressure, remove the clot, and stop the bleeding.

INTRACEREBRAL HEMORRHAGE. This bleeding represents a lesion within the tissue of the brain itself (Fig. 25–15*C*). These injuries may be small or large and may be accomplished by massive neurologic deficits.

PENETRATING INJURIES. Penetrating injuries result from sharp objects that penetrate the skull and brain tissue. In addition to the obvious brain injury, there is also external evidence of laceration of the scalp along with skull fracture. All penetrating injuries require prompt surgical intervention and present an extremely high risk of infection for the patient owing to the wound contamination that occurs.

SURGICAL TREATMENT

Surgical intervention for each of these types of trauma is directed at evacuating (removing) hematomas and débriding damaged tissue.

Nursing Care of the Patient with a Head Injury

ASSESSMENT. Nursing assessment of the patient with a neurologic disorder is outlined in Table 25–3 (see also Care Plan: The Patient with a Head Injury).

NURSING DIAGNOSIS. Nursing diagnoses for the patient with a head injury may include the following:

- **Altered Cerebral Tissue Perfusion** related to increased ICP
- **Ineffective Breathing Patterns** related to increased ICP
- **High Risk for Injury** related to seizures, decreased level of consciousness, disorientation, vision disturbances
- **High Risk for Infection** related to traumatic wounds or invasive procedures
- **Impaired Physical Mobility** related to neuromuscular impairment, decreased mental alertness
- **Body Image Disturbance** related to loss of function
- **Altered Role Performance** related to neurologic impairment

GOALS. Goals of nursing care after head injury are adequate cerebral tissue perfusion, normal oxygenation, absence of injury, absence of infection, absence of complications of immobility (contractures, decubiti, pneumonia, atelectasis, constipation, urinary retention), adaptation to altered body function, and adjustment of roles and responsibilities consistent with abilities.

INTERVENTIONS

Altered Cerebral Tissue Perfusion. The nurse monitors the patient closely for signs of increased ICP and

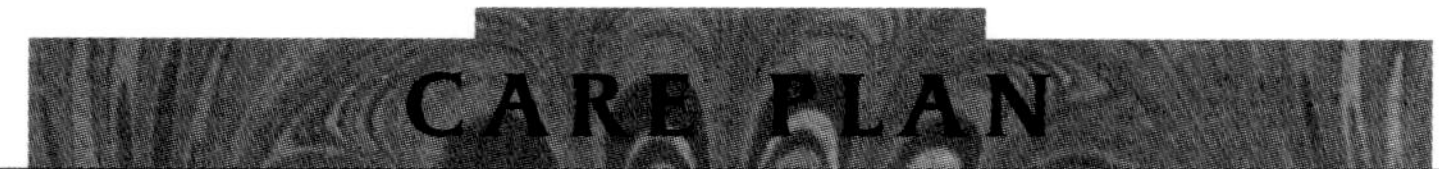

The Patient with a Head Injury

ASSESSMENT

Health History: Austin Mandrel is a 17-year-old male who was injured in a motorcycle accident 2 weeks ago. He reportedly struck his head on the pavement and was unconscious on admission. He is now alert and oriented to person and place but not to time. He is reluctant to discuss his injuries and refers to himself as a "gimp." He had a seizure the evening of admission but is being given anticonvulsants and has had none since. His mother reports that he has had no serious illnesses, hospitalization, or surgeries and that he has no known allergies. He is a high-school junior and football player. He has two close friends who visit frequently.

Physical Examination: Vital signs: temperature, 98°F orally; pulse, 62; respiration, 12; blood pressure, 150/84. The patient has a laceration on the forehead that is well healed. There are healing abrasions on the forehead and right cheek without edema or drainage. The pupils are equal and react to light. There is no drainage from the ears. There is no stiffness of the neck. Reflexes are normal in the right extremities but sluggish in the left extremities. He moves the left extremities on command, but they are weaker than the right. He is able to walk with a walker.

NURSING DIAGNOSIS	GOALS AND OUTCOME CRITERIA	INTERVENTIONS
Altered cerebral tissue perfusion related to increased intracranial pressure (ICP).	Patient will have adequate cerebral tissue perfusion as evidenced by alertness and orientation to person, place, and time.	Monitor for signs of increased ICP: decreasing level of consciousness, pupil inequality or dilation without response to light, increasing motor deficits, abnormal posture, fever, increasing blood pressure, bradycardia, respiratory depression. If increased ICP is suspected, notify physician, elevate head of bed as ordered. Monitor rate of fluid administration to prevent fluid volume excess. Administer diuretics and anti-inflammatory drugs as ordered.
Ineffective breathing pattern related to increased ICP.	Patient will have adequate oxygenation as evidenced by respiratory rate of 12 to 20 with normal arterial blood gases.	Monitor respiratory status closely for decreasing rate and depth, tachycardia. Check results of arterial blood gas studies.
High risk for injury related to lethargy, possible seizures.	Patient will remain free of injury during hospitalization.	Employ seizure precautions per agency policy. Bed in low position. Call light available and within reach of right hand. Assistance with transferring.

impaired cerebral blood flow: decreasing LOC, pupil dilation with no response to light, motor deficits, abnormal posture, fever, increased blood pressure, bradycardia, and respiratory depression. Changes are reported promptly to the physician. The head of the bed is elevated as ordered. The rate of administration of intravenous fluids is carefully regulated to prevent fluid volume excess. Urine output is monitored to ensure adequate fluid intake. If a ventriculostomy catheter is in place, the drainage is inspected and measured as ordered using strict aseptic technique. Diuretics and anti-inflammatory drugs are administered as ordered.

Ineffective Breathing Patterns. The patient's respiratory status is closely monitored by the nurse using pulse oximetry or measurement of arterial blood gases. Signs of respiratory depression are reported to the physician immediately.

High Risk for Injury. Nursing measures to prevent injuries associated with seizures and decreased LOC are discussed earlier in this chapter and are summarized in Table 25–7.

High Risk for Infection. The patient who has suffered a head injury may have serious lacerations and abrasions

The Patient with a Head Injury *(Continued)*

NURSING DIAGNOSIS	GOALS AND OUTCOME CRITERIA	INTERVENTIONS
High risk for infection related to traumatic wounds.	Patient will remain free of infection as evidenced by normal temperature and white blood cell count.	Monitor temperature for elevation. Assess wounds for increasing redness, edema, and foul drainage. Use universal precautions for wound care and when handling invasive equipment. Administer antibiotics as ordered.
Impaired physical mobility related to neuromuscular impairment, lethargy.	Patient will retain normal range of motion in all extremities and will participate in activities to restore strength to left extremities.	Explain importance of frequent position changes (at least every 2 hours) and assist patient to do so. Position affected extremities in functional alignment. Assist in active range of motion exercises at least three times a day. Apply antiembolism stockings as ordered. Assess skin, especially bony prominences, for signs of pressure or breakdown. Monitor elimination to detect urinary retention or constipation. Encourage fluids and high-fiber diet as ordered.
Body image disturbance related to loss of function.	Patient will adapt to altered body function as reflected in positive statements about self.	Encourage patient to ask questions and to express thoughts and feelings about injuries. Include him in planning sessions. Show acceptance through touch and genuine interest. Encourage friends to continue visits. Explain healing process and how rehabilitation measures can help. Emphasize abilities rather than disabilities. Promote independence as much as possible. Refer to support group.
Altered role performance related to neurologic impairment.	Patient will participate in rehabilitation efforts and explore potential new roles and activities.	Explain healing process and how rehabilitation measures can help. Help patient learn to perform activities of daily living with limitations.

that provide portals for pathogenic organisms. In addition, an intravenous fluid line and a urinary catheter may be in place. The nurse uses universal precautions for wound care as well as when handling invasive tubes. The patient's temperature is monitored for fever. Wounds are inspected for increasing redness, swelling, and foul drainage. Antibiotics are administered as ordered.

Impaired Physical Mobility. After a head injury, the patient may have temporary or permanent motor impairment. While confined to bed, the patient is turned and positioned and encouraged to deep breathe at least every 2 hours. The skin is routinely inspected for signs of pressure or breakdown. Antiembolism stockings are used if ordered. Range of motion exercises are done, and joints are positioned in functional alignment. Urine and bowel elimination is assessed frequently to detect retention or constipation. As soon as permitted, the patient should be assisted out of bed and encouraged to be as active as possible. Unfortunately, some head injury patients have permanent impairments that necessitate lifelong care. Care of the immobile patient is covered in detail in Chapter 19.

Body Image Disturbance and Altered Role Performance. The losses associated with a serious head injury can render the patient unable to resume usual activities. The injury may also leave disfiguring scars or distorted features. The nurse demonstrates acceptance of the patient through touch and genuine interest. The patient is encouraged to ask questions, express concerns, and anticipate problems and solutions. The nurse is realistic about the patient's disabilities but emphasizes abilities. Patients with serious deficits are usually treated by a team that includes rehabilitation specialists. These experts help the patient regain physical mobility, learn to carry out activities of daily living, learn new job skills, and deal with the emotional trauma of the injury and its effects.

The family is included in the rehabilitation process. In many cases, family members serve as the caregivers after head injury. Carson (1993) describes behaviors of family members of patients who had sustained head injuries. Behaviors included providing personal care, obtaining rehabilitation services, providing a safe environment, seeking remainders of the preinjury person, exploring what abilities might be regained, encouraging return to preinjury activities, encouraging active decision making, becoming active members of the rehabilitation team, and staying open to potential gains.

EVALUATION. Criteria for goal achievement are patient alert and oriented; respiratory rate of 12 to 20 with normal arterial blood gases; absence of injuries incurred during seizures or falls; normal body temperature without signs of wound or urinary infection (redness, odor) or phlebitis; intact skin, mobile joints, regular bowel movements, no bladder distention, breath sounds clear on auscultation; patient's statements of adaptation to new body image; and patient's assumption of new roles within abilities.

BRAIN TUMORS

Brain tumors account for a relatively small percentage of cancer deaths annually. Brain tumors develop in some cancer patients as a result of metastasis from other primary sites. Tumor cells can spread to the central nervous system through the blood and CSF.

Not all brain tumors are malignant. Some tumor types, such as the meningioma, a tumorous growth of the meningeal tissue, are often benign. One might assume that benign tumor cells would suggest an excellent chance of complete recovery. However, the invasion of any kind of tumor into normal brain tissue is never insignificant. This invasion can cause significant damage that may prove fatal because of increasing ICP or inaccessibility in surgery.

Etiology and Risk Factors

The causes of brain tumors are generally unknown, but some appear to be congenital in origin whereas others may be related to heredity. In addition, drug influences and environmental factors may play a role in the development of some brain tumors.

Signs and Symptoms

Signs and symptoms of brain tumors are directly related to the area of the brain that is being invaded by the tumor. Motor and sensory symptoms, visual disturbances, and headache may all be early manifestations of tumor growth. New-onset seizure activity in an adult patient often indicates the presence of a tumor. Cerebellar tumors may cause difficulties with balance and coordination. Other tumors, depending on their location, may involve cranial nerves.

Medical Treatment

Management of the patient with a brain tumor depends on the type of cells present in the tumor. Surgery can be done to remove as much of the tumor tissue as possible. If the tumor is malignant, surgery is often followed by radiation therapy with or without chemotherapeutic agents.

Nursing Care of the Patient with a Brain Tumor

Nursing care of the patient with a brain tumor depends on the specific deficits, treatment, and prognosis and may be similar to the care of the patient with a head injury. Care of the patient with cancer is discussed in Chapter 23.

ASSESSMENT. The complete neurologic assessment is summarized in Table 25–3. The assessment is especially important before brain surgery to provide a baseline for comparing postoperative findings.

NURSING DIAGNOSIS. Nursing diagnoses vary with the patient's specific symptoms and disabilities and the type of treatment employed. Common nursing diagnoses include the following:

- **Pain** related to pressure of expanding tumor mass
- **Altered Thought Processes** related to effects of tumor on brain tissue
- **Sensory Perceptual Alterations** related to impaired conduction of sensory information
- **Impaired Physical Mobility** and **Self-Care Deficits** related to motor disturbances, impaired cognition
- **Ineffective Individual** and **Family Coping** related to life-threatening disease, changes in behavior and function

GOALS. Goals for the identified nursing diagnoses are reduced pain, adaptation to altered thinking, recognition of sensory-perceptual changes, accomplishment of activities of daily living, and effective coping.

INTERVENTIONS

Pain. The nurse documents the pain and administers analgesics as ordered. Codeine or acetaminophen is often used. If pain relief is not achieved, the nurse informs the physician and assesses for signs of increased ICP.

Altered Thought Patterns. The nurse monitors for changes in cognitive function by assessing orientation and response to instructions. Evidence of delusions or hallucinations might include the patient speaking to someone who is not present or reporting something that could not be true. Sudden changes in mental status should be investigated carefully because they may be caused not only by the tumor but by correctable factors such as drugs, hypoxia, or fluid and electrolyte imbalances. The nurse listens carefully to the patient and presents reality in a straightforward manner. Devices to help the patient maintain orientation include clocks, calendars, and seasonal decorations.

Sensory Perceptual Alterations. The nurse explains that unusual sensations and perceptual alterations may be caused by the effects of the brain tumor. Safety measures are implemented as needed to prevent injury due to impaired vision or sensation.

Impaired Physical Mobility and Self-Care Deficits. The patient with a brain tumor may have varying degrees of physical impairment. The nurse assesses ability to perform activities of daily living and provides assistance as needed. The patient is encouraged to remain as active as possible. If the patient's mobility is severely impaired, there is a high risk for disuse syndrome and the associated complications. Care of the immobilized patient is described in Chapter 19.

Ineffective Individual and Family Coping. The nurse must assist the patient and family in dealing with a difficult diagnosis in addition to the obvious residual physical effects. A diagnosis of a malignant brain tumor is devastating for the family, and emotional support is vital to help them understand the nature of the disease and the anticipated problems and outcomes. Nursing care depends on the specific deficits, treatment, and prognosis and may be similar to the care of the patient with a head injury. Care of the patient with cancer is discussed in Chapter 23.

EVALUATION. Criteria for determining the outcomes of nursing interventions include patient's statement of pain relief and relaxed expression; improved mental orientation; absence of injury due to sensory or perceptual impairment; maximum possible patient mobility level and absence of complications of immobility (contractures, pneumonia, constipation, urinary retention); and patient's and family's positive statements of ability to deal with the illness.

INFECTIOUS AND INFLAMMATORY CONDITIONS

MENINGITIS

Meningitis is inflammation of the meningeal coverings of the brain and spinal cord caused by either viral or bacterial organisms. Organisms may reach the meninges through the blood, head wounds, or from other cranial structures such as the sinuses or inner ear. A number of organisms may be responsible for bacterial infection, including *Neisseria meningitidis, Streptococcus pneumonia,* and *Haemophilus influenzae.*

Complications of meningitis include seizures, septicemia, vasomotor collapse, and increased ICP. *Neisseria meningitidis* is particularly problematic because septicemia develops in approximately 10% of patients.

Signs and Symptoms

The common signs and symptoms of meningitis are generally related to meningeal irritation. These include headache, nuchal rigidity, irritability, diminished LOC, photophobia, hypersensitivity, and seizure activity. The presence of Kernig's sign and Brudzinski's sign also is indicative of meningeal irritation. To assess for Kernig's sign (Fig. 25–16*A*), the examiner flexes the patient's hip to a 90-degree angle and then extends the knee. In the presence of a meningeal infection, this movement produces pain in the hamstring area. Brudzinski's sign (Fig. 25–16*B*) is flexion of both hips when the examiner flexes the patient's neck.

Medical Diagnosis

A lumbar puncture is done to obtain a CSF sample for laboratory analysis. The sample is examined to detect the presence of microorganisms in the CSF and to identify the infecting organism. With bacterial meningitis, the CSF appears milky and purulent owing to white blood cells suspended in the fluid.

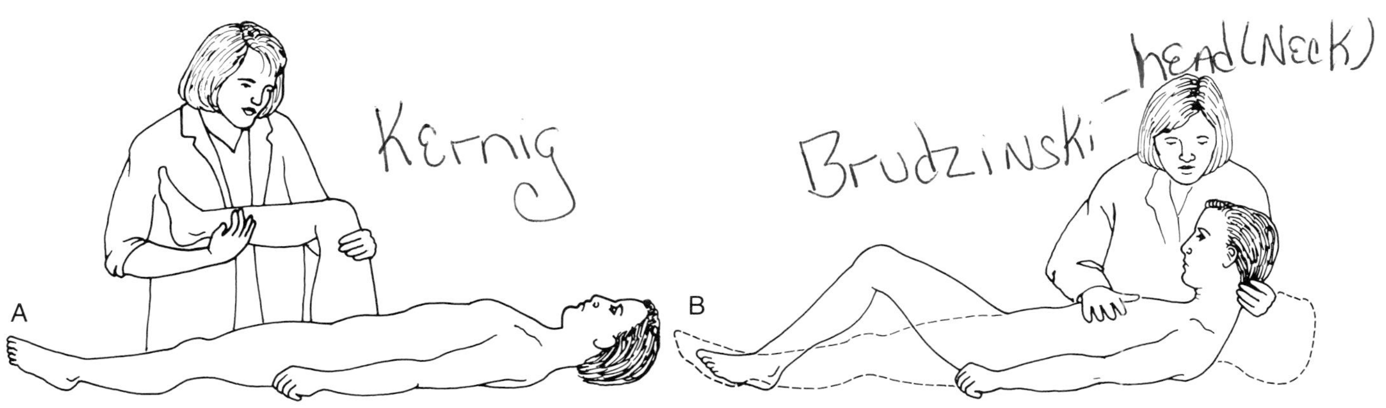

FIGURE 25–16

A, Kernig's sign: When the patient's leg is flexed as shown, the patient is unable to completely extend the leg. *B*, Brudzinski's sign: When the nurse flexes the patient's neck, hip flexion occurs. (From Black, J. M., & Matassarin-Jacobs, E. [1993]. *Luckmann and Sorensen's medical-surgical nursing: A psychophysiologic approach* [4th ed., p. 763]. Philadelphia: W. B. Saunders.)

Medical Treatment

Management of meningitis revolves around prompt recognition and treatment with antimicrobials. In severe infections, broad-spectrum antimicrobials such as penicillin G are initiated immediately. Changes in therapy may be made when the results of culture and sensitivity tests are reported. Bacterial infections usually respond to antimicrobial therapy, but there are no specific drugs effective against most viral infections of the central nervous system. Anticonvulsants are used to control seizure activity if necessary.

Nursing Care of the Patient with Meningitis

ASSESSMENT. The nurse's routine neurologic assessment is summarized in Table 25–3. When a patient has meningitis, vital signs and neurologic status are assessed frequently to determine further deterioration or the onset of complications.

NURSING DIAGNOSIS. Nursing diagnoses for the patient with meningitis may include the following:

- **Altered Cerebral Tissue Perfusion** related to increased ICP
- **Ineffective Breathing Patterns** related to depression of the respiratory center
- **Pain** related to irritation of meninges and increased ICP
- **High Risk for Injury** related to confusion, seizures, restlessness
- **Fluid Volume Deficit** related to vomiting and fever
- **High Risk for Disuse Syndrome** related to bedrest

GOALS. Nursing goals for the identified nursing diagnoses include adequate cerebral tissue perfusion, adequate oxygenation, reduced pain, absence of injury, normal fluid balance without vomiting or fever, and absence of complications of immobility.

INTERVENTIONS

Altered Cerebral Tissue Perfusion. The head of the patient's bed is elevated as ordered. The patient is instructed to avoid coughing and not to hold his or her breath during turning since these behaviors increase ICP. The use of restraints is avoided unless absolutely necessary. The nurse monitors for signs of increasing ICP: headache, nausea, vomiting, abnormal pupillary responses, and respiratory depression. If ICP does increase, treatments (e.g., diuretics, barbiturates, narcotics) are administered as ordered. Measures to lower the body temperature may be ordered to reduce the metabolic rate.

Ineffective Breathing Patterns. The respiratory status and gag and swallowing reflexes must be monitored. The patient is positioned to maintain a patent airway and suctioned if necessary. Arterial blood gas samples are drawn and analyzed as ordered. A decreasing respiratory rate is reported to the physician.

Pain. The nurse assesses the location and severity of any discomfort. Nursing measures to decrease pain include position changes and massage. Analgesics are given as ordered, and their effect is documented. Chapter 16 provides additional information about the nursing management of pain.

High Risk for Injury. Because of the prevailing risk of seizures, appropriate precautions should be taken to ensure patient safety. A subdued environment should be maintained to reduce irritability and contribute to patient comfort. The bed should be kept in low position, with the siderails padded and raised. The patient is reoriented as needed to the setting, and the call button is kept within easy reach. If the patient is dizzy, the nurse reminds the patient not to get up without assistance.

Fluid Volume Deficit. The patient's vital signs, tissue turgor and moisture, and fluid intake and output are monitored. Daily weights may be advised to assess fluid status. Oral fluids are encouraged if permitted and if the patient is alert. Intravenous fluid therapy is provided as ordered and monitored to ensure the correct flow rate. Antipyretics may be ordered for fever, and antiemetics for vomiting.

High Risk for Disuse Syndrome. The patient who is confined to the bed is at risk for all the complications of immobility, especially stasis of pulmonary secretions, pressure sores, muscle weakness, joint stiffness, and constipation. Measures to prevent these complications are discussed in detail in Chapter 19.

Isolation. If needed, isolation precautions should be initiated. Organisms responsible for meningococcal meningitis are spread by the respiratory route, and appropriate safeguards must be employed to protect other patients, family, and staff. (See Box 9–1 in Chapter 9.)

EVALUATION. Criteria for determining the outcomes of nursing care are normal vital signs and LOC, respiratory rate of 12 to 20; patient's statement of reduced pain, relaxed expression; no falls or other trauma; fluid intake equal to output, moist mucous membranes, blood pressure within patient's norms; and clear breath sounds, intact skin, normal muscle strength and joint mobility, and regular bowel movements without straining.

ENCEPHALITIS

Encephalitis is an inflammation of brain tissue that is usually caused by one of several viruses. These viruses may be prevalent during certain times of the year or in a specific geographic area. For example, certain types of mosquitoes found in the United States are carriers of a virus commonly associated with encephalitis. In addition, toxic substances or other types of viral infections, such as herpes simplex, may precipitate encephalitis.

Signs and Symptoms

The patient with encephalitis presents with symptoms directly related to the area of the brain that is involved.

Fever, nuchal rigidity, headache, confusion, delirium, agitation, and restlessness are commonly seen. However, the patient may also become comatose or exhibit aphasia, hemiparesis, facial weakness, and other alterations in motor activity.

Medical Treatment

Care for the patient with encephalitis is focused on enhancing patient comfort and increasing strength. Because seizure activity is a potential problem, appropriate precautions must be taken.

Nursing Care of the Patient with Encephalitis

The nursing plan of care parallels that of the patient with meningitis.

GUILLAIN-BARRÉ SYNDROME

Although its specific etiology is unknown, Guillain-Barré syndrome (GBS) is believed to be an autoimmune response to a viral infection. It is a rapidly progressing disease that affects the motor component of the peripheral nervous system. Although the spinal nerves are usually affected, the cranial nerves also may be involved.

Patients presenting with GBS often report some recent viral infection or vaccination. This apparently triggers an autoimmune response that destroys the myelin sheath around the peripheral nerves, slowing the conduction of impulses across the involved nerves.

Signs and Symptoms

Guillain-Barré syndrome has three phases: initial, plateau, and recovery, as described in Table 25–8. The initial phase is characterized by symmetric muscle weakness that typically begins in the lower extremities and ascends to the trunk and upper extremities. Cranial nerves may be affected by the disease process, resulting in visual and hearing disturbances, difficulty chewing, and lack of facial expression. The muscles of respiration also may be affected, resulting in the need for mechanical ventilation.

TABLE 25-8
PHASES OF GUILLAIN-BARRÉ SYNDROME

PHASE	CHARACTERISTICS	DURATION
Initial	Begins with onset of symptoms Ends when disease ceases to progress	Usually 1–3 wk
Plateau	No further changes; neither deterioration nor improvement	Several days to 2 wk
Recovery	Gradual improvement	May be as long as 2 yr; some residual effects may be permanent

Mild paresthesias or anesthesia in the feet and hands may be present in a glove or stocking distribution. In addition, some patients experience pain associated with the sensory changes. Despite all the motor and sensory changes, LOC and intellectual functioning remain unchanged.

Effects on the autonomic nervous system may include hypertension, orthostatic hypotension, cardiac dysrhythmias, profuse sweating, paralytic ileus, and urinary retention. Autonomic dysreflexia, an episode of severe hypertension and bradycardia, is a potentially life-threatening complication for the patient with GBS. Autonomic dysreflexia is triggered by overstimulation of the sympathetic nervous system, most commonly by a distended bowel or bladder.

In the plateau phase, the GBS patient remains essentially unchanged. There is no further neurologic deterioration, but there is no improvement either.

As recovery begins and progresses, remyelinization occurs and muscle strength returns in a proximal to distal pattern (head to toes). Because the underlying axon generally remains undamaged, approximately 95% of patients with GBS have a near-complete recovery. Others have residual numbness, stiffness, or paralysis.

Medical Diagnosis

The characteristic onset and pattern of ascending motor involvement provides the basis for the diagnosis of GBS. An elevated protein level in the CSF obtained by lumbar puncture provides additional evidence for the diagnosis. Nerve conduction velocity studies reveal slowed conduction speed in the involved nerves.

Medical Treatment

Management during the acute phase of the illness is directed at preserving vital function, particularly with regard to respiration. Respiratory status is closely monitored and mechanical ventilation initiated if the vital capacity falls to 15 ml per kg of body weight. Massive doses of corticosteroids may be prescribed to suppress the inflammatory process.

Because GBS is believed to be an autoimmune disease, plasmapheresis has emerged as a major treatment intervention. Plasmapheresis is a process in which blood is removed, centrifuged, and returned to the patient. In the process, antibodies that trigger the autoimmune disease are removed from the blood by a machine equipped with a special filtration system. The patient with GBS generally undergoes a series of treatments, ideally delivered within 7 to 14 days after the onset of the disease. Those patients benefiting from plasmapheresis frequently enjoy a quicker recovery.

Nursing Care of the Patient with Guillain-Barré Syndrome

ASSESSMENT. Assessment of the patient with a neurologic disorder is summarized in Table 25–3. When GBS is suspected, the health history describes the progression of symptoms. The patient's fear, coping strategies, and sources of support are noted. The nurse records information about important social data such as occupation and family roles and responsibilities. The physical examination focuses on cranial nerve, motor, respiratory, and cardiovascular function.

NURSING DIAGNOSIS. The following nursing diagnoses may apply to the patient with GBS:

- **Ineffective Breathing Patterns** related to neurologic impairment
- **Decreased Cardiac Output** related to labile blood pressure, cardiac dysrhythmias
- **High Risk for Disuse Syndrome** related to motor impairment
- **Altered Nutrition: Less than Body Requirements** related to dysphagia, endotracheal tube
- **High Risk for Injury** related to loss of sensation in hands and feet, motor impairment, inability to speak
- **Anxiety** related to paralysis, doubts about recovery, loss of verbal communication
- **Knowledge deficit** of GBS and its treatment

GOALS. Goals of nursing care for the patient with GBS are adequate oxygenation, normal cardiac output, adequate nutrition, absence of complications of immobility, absence of injury in affected body areas, decreased anxiety, and patient's knowledge of GBS and its treatment.

INTERVENTIONS

Ineffective Breathing Patterns. About 25% of patients with GBS require mechanical ventilation because of neuromuscular failure. The nurse assesses the patient's oxygenation status frequently. A respiratory rate greater than 30, abnormal chest and abdominal movements, and decreasing vital capacity signal increasingly ineffective breathing. The patient is turned at least every 2 hours and suctioned when indicated by increased pulse or adventitious breath sounds.

Decreased Cardiac Output. The nurse is alert to rapid or slow cardiac dysrhythmias and administers antidysrhythmic drugs as ordered.

Altered Nutrition: Less than Body Requirements. Impaired swallowing or the presence of an endotracheal tube requires an alternative means of feeding. Enteral feedings are usually provided by way of a gastrostomy or nasoduodenal tube. Feedings may be given continuously or intermittently. The head of the bed is elevated 30 degrees during feedings. The residual is measured at intervals to assess emptying of the stomach and prevent overfilling. In some cases, total parenteral nutrition may be employed.

High Risk for Disuse Syndrome. Immobility is a major issue to address in the patient with GBS. If mobility is severely impaired, the patient is at high risk for disuse syndrome. These patients generally benefit from the use of rotational bed therapy to help promote pulmonary hygiene, peristalsis, and urinary bladder emptying. Careful positioning is crucial, with emphasis on maintaining joint function, muscle tone, and range of motion. Active and passive exercises, splints, and continuous passive motion machines may be used to prevent contractures.

High Risk for Injury. Progressive weakness makes the patient susceptible to falls. When the patient is in bed, the nurse raises the siderails, places the call bell within reach, and puts the bed in low position. If the eyes do not close completely, ophthalmic drops or ointments are applied as ordered. Skin, especially areas without sensation, is inspected carefully to detect pressure or injury.

Anxiety. Anxiety is understandable with progressive paralysis and increasing dependence on others for basic needs. The nurse works to develop trust and establish a therapeutic relationship with the patient. If the patient is able to speak, the nurse encourages discussion of thoughts, fears, and feelings. Previously used coping strategies are explored. To promote some sense of control, the nurse gives the patient some choices about aspects of care. Equipment and procedures are explained to the patient. Other strategies to reduce anxiety include use of imagery, music, deep breathing (if possible), and controlling anxiety-producing thoughts. Boredom is a problem that must be considered for the patient with GBS. Orienting devices such as clocks, calendars, and daily schedules are helpful. The patient may enjoy television, radio, tapes, and visits from friends and family.

One source of anxiety for many patients is impaired communication. While the patient is able to speak, the nurse establishes a system of communication such as blinking (one blink means "yes," two blinks mean "no"). Then, if the condition does affect speech or if mechanical ventilation is required, the patient will have a simple means of expression.

Knowledge Deficit. From admission through rehabilitation, the GBS patient requires education about the condition and its usual course. Patients can deal with the condition better if they know what to expect, that is, how the symptoms progress and that reversal and improvement are expected.

Rehabilitation. As function is restored, emphasis is placed on both respiratory and physical rehabilitation. Total recovery of respiratory function determines how quickly physical rehabilitation can begin. Once rehabilitation is initiated, attention must be devoted to maximizing motor function through exercises and occupational therapy. Since total recovery may take several years, a prolonged rehabilitation period is sometimes necessary. Before discharge from the hospital, referrals may be made to rehabilitation or home health agencies as appropriate. The patient and family may benefit from a support group for people with long-term or chronic illnesses. The Guillain-Barré Foundation is a source of information.

EVALUATION. Criteria for evaluating the outcomes of nursing care are normal blood gases and skin color; regular pulse with rate of 60 to 100 beats per minute and blood pressure consistent with patient's norms; stable body weight; absence of skin redness or breakdown; absence of falls, bruises, corneal damage, or other injuries; patient's confirmation of reduced anxiety; and patient's confirmation of understanding or (if possible) demonstration of self-care.

PARKINSON'S DISEASE

Parkinson's disease is a progressive degenerative disorder of the basal ganglia that results in an eventual loss of coordination and control over involuntary motor movement. It is generally recognized as being a disease of the elderly, first appearing in individuals in their fifties, with males affected more frequently than females. Idiopathic Parkinson's disease has no known cause but is related to decreased levels of dopamine in the basal ganglia. A deficiency of dopamine, a neurotransmitter, contributes to the loss of motor function. Other types of parkinsonism are caused by atherosclerosis, long-term use of phenothiazines, and some toxins.

Signs and Symptoms

Several symptoms are characteristic of Parkinson's disease. The major symptoms are tremor, rigidity, and bradykinesia. Tremor is a trembling or shaking type of movement most often seen in the upper extremities of the Parkinson's patient. Tremors may occur during voluntary movements (intention tremor) or during rest. Rigidity is stiffness, and bradykinesia refers to extremely slow movements. Other signs and symptoms are loss of dexterity and power in affected limbs, aching, handwriting changes, drooling, lack of facial expression, rhythmic head nodding, reduced blinking, and slumped posture. A movement common to Parkinson's disease is "pill rolling," in which the patient moves the thumb against the fingertips as if rolling a small object. The patient with advanced disease demonstrates cogwheel rigidity (jerky movements with passive muscle stretching) and gait disturbances. The patient may seem to "freeze" and have difficulty initiating the action of walking. Depression is common, and dementia develops in some patients. Figure 25–17 illustrates the typical facial appearance, posture, and gait of individuals with Parkinson's disease.

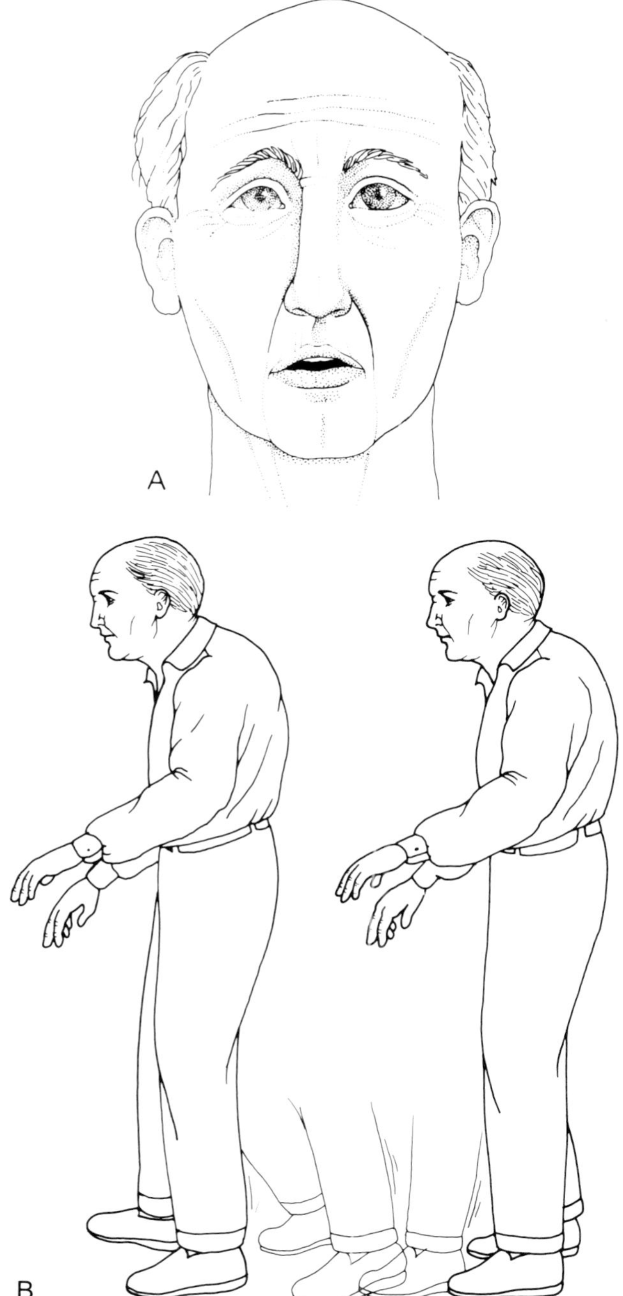

FIGURE 25-17
Parkinson's disease. *A*, Mask-like facial expression. (From Ignatavicius, D. D., & Bayne, M. V. [1991]. *Medical-surgical nursing: A nursing process approach* [p. 912]. Philadelphia: W. B. Saunders.). *B*, Posture and gait changes. (From Black, J. M., & Matassarin-Jacobs, E. [1993]. *Luckmann and Sorensen's medical-surgical nursing: A psychophysiologic approach* [4th ed., p. 784]. Philadelphia: W. B. Saunders.)

Medical Diagnosis and Medical Treatment

A diagnosis of Parkinson's disease is based on the health history and physical examination.

The management of the patient with Parkinson's disease is directed toward controlling the symptoms with physical therapy and drug therapy. The most beneficial physical therapy programs incorporate massage, heat, exercise, and gait retraining. Speech therapy has been tried, but results have generally not been encouraging.

Drug therapy relieves many of the symptoms of the disease. The cornerstone of therapy is the use of L-dopa

(L-dihydroxyphenylalanine). L-Dopa can cross the blood-brain barrier and is converted to dopamine in the basal ganglia, thereby supplementing levels of the neurotransmitter and reducing the symptoms of the disease.

The conversion of L-dopa to dopamine must occur in the basal ganglia and not in the peripheral tissue. To ensure this, inhibitors are administered to prevent the breakdown of L-dopa by decarboxylase enzymes. The decarboxylase inhibitor most commonly used is carbidopa (Sinemet). When the two drugs are used in combination, therapeutic levels may be achieved with lower dosages.

Anticholinergic drugs may be used in patients who have less severe symptoms or who are unresponsive to L-dopa. These are useful in managing tremors, rigidity, or cramping. Trihexyphenidyl (Artane) is the most commonly used anticholinergic.

Although the exact mechanism of action is unclear, amantadine (Symmetrel), an antiviral compound, is also used in the management of Parkinson's disease. Amantadine is thought to release dopamine from storage sites located in the neurons. It is often used in combination with L-dopa.

Treatment for depression may include antidepressant drug therapy, psychotherapy, and electroconvulsive therapy. Additional information about drug therapy is presented in Table 25–6.

Adrenal medullary transplant is a surgical procedure that is being studied for the treatment of Parkinson's disease. It is seen as a palliative rather than a curative procedure. Adrenal tissue is obtained from the patient and transplanted into the brain. This procedure is not widely accepted but may bring about some functional improvement in a limited number of patients with Parkinson's disease.

Nursing Care of the Patient with Parkinson's Disease

Nursing management for the patient with Parkinson's disease is primarily related to maintaining mobility and preventing injury.

ASSESSMENT. The complete neurologic assessment is summarized in Table 25–3. The health history of a patient with Parkinson's disease should specifically include assessment for weakness, fatigue, muscle cramps, sweating, dysphagia, constipation, difficulty voiding, and unusual movements. The effects of the disease on the patient's life are important to record. During the physical examination, the nurse is alert for lack of facial expression, eyes fixed in one direction, drooling, slurred speech, tearing, tremors, muscle stiffness, and poor balance and coordination.

NURSING DIAGNOSIS. The following nursing diagnoses may apply to the patient with Parkinson's disease:

- **Impaired Physical Mobility** and **Self-Care Deficit** related to neuromuscular disease
- **High Risk for Injury** related to poor balance and coordination
- **Altered Nutrition: Less than Body Requirements** related to dysphagia, difficulty with self-feeding
- **Ineffective Individual Coping** related to physical changes and effects of disease on lifestyle
- **Knowledge Deficit** of disease, management, and self-care

In addition, as the disease progresses, the patient becomes more immobilized, requiring additional nursing diagnoses as addressed in Chapter 19.

GOALS. Goals of nursing care for the patient with Parkinson's disease include patient's participation in activities to maximize mobility and self-care, absence of injury, adequate nutritional intake without aspiration, effective adaptation to disease, and patient's knowledge of disease, management, and self-care.

INTERVENTIONS

Impaired Physical Mobility. The nurse assesses the patient's mobility and ability to perform self-care. Assistance is provided as needed, but the patient is encouraged to remain as independent in self-care as possible. Assistive devices, including walkers and wheelchairs, may enable the patient to be mobile despite some deterioration in coordination and balance. The nurse stresses the value of exercise in maintaining strength and mobility. Active and passive range of motion exercises may be done. Both the physical therapist and the occupational therapist may participate in designing programs to maintain or improve function.

The following are some simple maneuvers that the patient can be taught to improve mobility:

- Scoot to the edge of a chair before trying to stand.
- Use satin sheets to make it easier to move in and out of bed.
- "March in place" before starting to walk.
- Practice lifting the foot as if to step over an object on the floor to initiate walking.

High Risk for Injury. The patient with Parkinson's disease is at special risk for injury related to falls. The nurse places the patient's call button within easy reach and instructs the patient to call for assistance when getting up. If the patient is ambulatory, the floor is kept uncluttered. Firm shoes are preferred over soft slippers because they provide better support. Assistive devices (canes, walkers, wheelchairs) are provided as needed. An unhurried atmosphere allows the patient to move at his or her own speed and decreases the risk of injury.

Altered Nutrition: Less than Body Requirements. To promote ease of swallowing, the patient is positioned comfortably for meals, with the head elevated and food conveniently arranged. Assistance is provided as needed and may involve only cutting meat and opening containers or may entail actually feeding the patient. Patients must not be rushed while eating. If the patient chokes on liquids, the nurse should consult the dietitian about the need for semisolids and thick liquids, which are often easier to swallow. Thickening agents can be added to thin fluids to facilitate swallowing. Small, frequent meals may be better tolerated than three large ones. Weight is monitored to assess adequacy of nutritional intake. Some researchers believe that Parkinson's patients benefit from a low-protein diet during the day and an evening meal high in protein, but this is still experimental.

Ineffective Individual Coping. Patients with Parkinson's disease must deal with loss of mobility that may affect their jobs, home and family responsibilities, social relationships, and leisure activities. Voice changes may severely impair verbal communication. The nurse explores how the patient is dealing with these changes. The nurse and other members of the health care team help the patient identify strategies to adapt to changing abilities. The nurse is alert to expressions of depression and informs the physician of such findings. A referral may be made to a mental health counselor, clinical nurse specialist, or support group. The nurse administers antidepressant drugs as ordered and monitors their effects.

Knowledge Deficit. The teaching plan describes the effects of Parkinson's disease and how it is treated. The nurse emphasizes the patient's role in exercising to promote mobility. Self-medication must be covered thoroughly because long-term drug therapy is usually prescribed. The nurse should supplement information about drug therapy with written material. Sources of information are the American Parkinson's Disease Association, the Parkinson's Disease Foundation, and the National Parkinson's Foundation.

EVALUATION. Criteria for evaluating the outcomes of nursing interventions are patient's participation in prescribed exercise programs and continued efforts to perform self-care; absence of bruises, lacerations, and fractures due to trauma; stable body weight; statements confirming ability to deal with the disease; and patient's adherence to prescribed therapies.

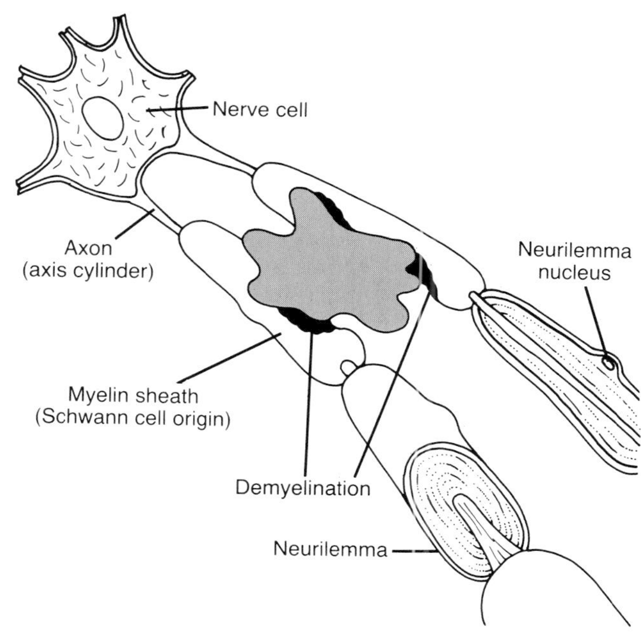

FIGURE 25-18

Changes in the nerve sheath with multiple sclerosis. The myelin coating degenerates, interfering with transmission of impulses. (From Black, J. M., & Matassarin-Jacobs, E. [1993]. *Luckmann and Sorensen's medical-surgical nursing: A psychophysiologic approach* [4th ed., p. 781]. Philadelphia: W. B. Saunders.)

MULTIPLE SCLEROSIS

A chronic, progressive degenerative disease, multiple sclerosis (MS) attacks the protective myelin sheath around axons and disrupts the motor pathways of the central nervous system (Fig. 25–18). The disease may progress steadily (chronic, progressive MS) or may be characterized by exacerbations and remissions (exacerbating-remitting MS). Young adults between 20 and 40 years of age have the highest rate of incidence, with women affected more frequently than men.

Etiology

Although the exact etiology of MS is unknown, viral infections and autoimmune processes have been implicated. Some studies have implicated a retrovirus in the disease process, but more research is needed to determine whether this is indeed the cause of MS. The myelin sheath surrounding the axons is destroyed, eventually leaving areas of sclerotic tissue (Fig. 25–18). As the sclerotic tissue develops, the patient may have a period of remission. Degeneration of the involved fibers eventually develops, yielding permanent damage. Nerve impulses, then, are no longer able to travel down the affected axon.

Signs and Symptoms

Because the exact pattern of damage varies from patient to patient, the signs and symptoms are varied as well. The most common symptoms of MS are fatigue, weakness and tingling in one or more extremities, visual disturbances, problems with coordination, bowel and bladder dysfunction, spasticity, and depression.

For patients who have exacerbating-remitting MS, the progression is variable. As the disease progresses, the periods of remission become shorter and the neurologic deficits observed during exacerbations become more severe and permanent.

Medical Diagnosis

The diagnosis of MS is based primarily on the physical examination and history of cyclic remission-exacerbation periods. A familial history of the disease is significant, as is a worsening of symptoms when the patient is exposed to warm weather. An MRI scan of the brain and spinal cord may reveal plaques characteristic of MS.

Medical Treatment

Because of its chronic, progressive nature, the treatment of MS is symptomatic and supportive. Drug therapy during periods of exacerbation may involve administration of adrenocorticotropic hormone. Prednisone also may be used to encourage remission. Other drugs that may be prescribed are cyclophosphamide and interferon-βlb (Betaseron). Interferon-βlb is used to decrease the frequency of recurrent neurologic episodes in people with exacerbating-remitting MS. The spasticity experienced by MS patients may respond to treatment with baclofen (Lioresal). Immunosuppressive agents may be used, but these carry the risk of bone marrow suppression and must be carefully monitored. Electrical neuromuscular stimulation is being used to decrease spasticity and improve active movement and function, but studies of the effectiveness have not found consistent evidence of improvement.

Nursing Care of the Patient with Multiple Sclerosis

ASSESSMENT. Complete assessment of the patient with a neurologic disorder is summarized in Table 25–3. When a patient has MS, the health history specifically includes the onset and progression of symptoms, especially those that affect mobility, vision, eating, and elimination. The nurse explores the effects of the disease on the person's lifestyle. Coping strategies are identified. Important aspects of the physical examination are evaluation of range of motion and strength and observation for gait abnormalities and tremors.

NURSING DIAGNOSIS. Nursing diagnoses for the patient with MS vary depending on the effects of the disease. Common diagnoses include the following:

- **Impaired Physical Mobility** related to weakness or spasticity
- **Sensory Perceptual Alterations** related to neurologic impairment
- **Self-Care Deficit** related to impaired voluntary movements and poor coordination
- **Functional Incontinence** related to impaired conduction of bladder nerve impulses
- **High Risk for Infection** related to inadequate resistance
- **Ineffective Individual Coping** related to chronic illness, uncertain course of disease
- **Knowledge Deficit** of disease, treatment, and self-care

GOALS. Goals of nursing care for the patient with MS are continued mobility, absence of injury associated with impaired sensation, achievement of self-care, regular bladder elimination, absence of infection, adaptation to changes in physical function, and patient's knowledge of disease, treatment, and self-care.

INTERVENTIONS

Impaired Physical Mobility. The nurse encourages the patient to be as independent as possible. Assistance with ambulation is provided as needed. A cane or walker may enable the patient to walk safely. If the patient has muscle spasms, the nurse administers muscle relaxants as ordered. Range of motion exercises are done to prevent contractures. Physical therapy may be ordered. The patient who is not able to move independently is at risk for disuse syndrome. Care of the immobile patient is covered in Chapter 19.

Sensory Perceptual Alterations. If the patient has impaired sensation, the nurse gives special attention to the skin. Extremities and pressure points are inspected for signs of pressure or trauma. The patient is encouraged to wear shoes when out of bed to prevent injury. Other measures instituted to prevent injury include caution with heat and cold.

Self-Care Deficit. The nurse encourages patients to do as much as they can for themselves. Assistance is provided as needed to carry out activities of daily living. Difficulty with feedings, especially if the patient is dysphagic, may result in inadequate food intake. Alternative means of feeding may be necessary.

Functional Incontinence. The nurse palpates the patient's lower abdomen for bladder distention. Intermittent catheterization is carried out as ordered. If urinary retention is a problem, the patient is assessed for signs and symptoms of urinary tract infection: fever, burning on urination, foul odor, sediment. If the patient has urinary incontinence, the nurse takes steps to reduce the incontinent episodes as described in Chapter 21. Incontinent briefs may be needed, and meticulous skin care is a must. Loss of bladder control is very distressing, and the nurse must be sensitive in helping the patient to deal with it.

High Risk for Infection. The MS patient who is being treated with immunosuppressive drugs has decreased resistance to infection. The nurse takes steps to reduce the risk of infection. The patient is protected from people with infections. Adequate hydration is maintained, and good hygiene practices are emphasized. The patient and family are taught the signs of infection and advised to report them promptly.

Ineffective Individual Coping. Multiple sclerosis is a chronic, progressive disease. Patients have increasing disability, requiring considerable adaptation. Since initial symptoms typically occur in young adults, patients must often learn to balance work, home, and family responsibilities. The nurse provides the patient opportunities to talk about the illness and its effects. The nurse is accepting of the patient's concerns and guides the patient to identify strengths, abilities, and usual coping strategies. A referral may be made to the clinical nurse specialist, mental health counselor, or spiritual counselor with the patient's permission. Support groups can be helpful to many patients and their families.

Knowledge Deficit. The nurse assesses what the patient knows about MS and what he or she would like to know. The teaching plan is individualized to the patient's needs and may include problems associated with immobility and measures to prevent complications.

EVALUATION. The effects of nursing interventions are determined by the following criteria: patient's demonstration of continued motor activity; absence of injury associated with impaired sensation; achievement of self-care activities; absence of bladder distention, absence of fever, lethargy, increased white blood cell count; behaviors and statements indicative of intent to maximize abilities; and patient's description of the disease, its treatment, and the importance of self-care.

AMYOTROPHIC LATERAL SCLEROSIS

Etiology

Amyotrophic lateral sclerosis (ALS), also known as Lou Gehrig's disease, is a degenerative neurologic disease. It affects males two to four times as frequently as females and strikes most often between 40 and 70 years of age. The disease generally progresses rapidly, and death ensues approximately 3 years after the onset of symptoms. Although a viral cause has been suspected, the exact etiology is unknown.

Pathophysiology

In ALS, there is degeneration of the anterior horn cells and the corticospinal tracts, so the patient demonstrates both upper and lower motor neuron symptoms. Evidence of upper motor neuron disease includes spasticity and hyperreflexia. Lower motor neuron disease is demonstrated by weakness, atrophy, cramps, and muscle twitching. Some patients have difficulty swallowing and slurred speech. Despite involvement of the motor nuclei of the brain stem, intellectual ability, sensory perception, vision, and hearing are all unaffected.

Signs and Symptoms

Initially, the patient exhibits weakness of voluntary muscles of the upper extremities, particularly the hands. In addition, some patients may experience difficulty in swallowing and speaking due to progressive weakness of the oropharyngeal muscles. Spasticity of the involved muscle groups may be seen. The disease progresses steadily until the patient is completely incapacitated. Eventually, respirations become shallow and the patient has difficulty clearing the airway of pulmonary secretions. Death results from aspiration, respiratory infection, or respiratory failure.

Medical Diagnosis and Medical Treatment

Patient history and physical examination lead to the diagnosis of ALS. Electromyography provides supporting evidence of impaired impulse conduction in the muscles. More sophisticated tests are used to rule out other degenerative motor diseases such as MS or myasthenia gravis.

Because there is no known cure or treatment for ALS, therapy is supportive.

Nursing Care of the Patient with Amyotrophic Lateral Sclerosis

ASSESSMENT. The complete neurologic assessment is outlined in Table 25–3. When a patient has ALS, the nurse's history determines the presence of dyspnea, dysphagia, muscle cramps, weakness, twitching, and joint stiffness. The effects of the disease on the patient's lifestyle are described. During the physical examination, the nurse anticipates finding weakness, muscle atrophy, abnormal reflexes and gait, and paralysis.

NURSING DIAGNOSIS. Primary nursing diagnoses addressed in caring for patients with ALS may include the following:

- **Ineffective Airway Clearance** related to paralysis of respiratory muscles
- **Impaired Physical Mobility** related to progressive weakness and atrophy
- **Altered Nutrition: Less than Body Requirements** related to dysphagia
- **Impaired Verbal Communication** related to oropharyngeal muscle weakness
- **Impaired Skin Integrity** related to immobility
- **Anticipatory Grieving** related to progressive, fatal disease
- **Situational Low Self-Esteem** related to loss of independence
- **Altered Family Processes** related to progressive illness of patient

GOALS. Nursing goals for the patient with ALS are patent airway, participation in activities to maintain mobility, adequate nutritional intake, effective communication, normal skin integrity, adaptation to losses, stable or improved self-esteem, and improved family processes.

INTERVENTIONS

Ineffective Airway Clearance. The patient's respiratory rate and effort, breath sounds, and pulse rate are monitored to detect inadequate oxygenation. The nurse instructs or assists the immobile patient in turning, coughing, and deep breathing at least every 2 hours. Chest physiotherapy may be ordered to mobilize secretions in order to prevent atelectasis and pneumonia. If the patient has difficulty removing secretions, gentle suction may be needed. Oxygen therapy is indicated if there is evidence of hypoxia (restlessness, tachycardia).

Impaired Physical Mobility. Progressive muscle wasting, spasticity, and paralysis cause increasing immobility. Active or passive range of motion exercises are performed to prevent contractures. Antispasmodic drugs are administered as ordered. Extremities are maintained in functional positions. Assistive devices (cane, walker, wheelchair) are used as needed to maintain mobility as long as possible. The nurse monitors the patient's ability to perform activities of daily living and provides assistance as needed. The patient who is immobile is at high risk for complications of immobility. Nursing care of the immobile patient is covered in Chapter 19.

Altered Nutrition: Less than Body Requirements. Muscle weakness and cranial nerve involvement eventually make it difficult for the patient to consume adequate food for good nutrition. The patient's weight is monitored to assess adequacy of the diet. Meals may be supplemented with high-protein snacks. High-fiber foods are recommended if the patient can eat them because constipation is a common problem. Adequate fluids are needed but may be difficult to swallow. The patient may be able to increase fluid intake by eating semisolids such as ice cream, milk shakes, or gelatin desserts.

The ALS patient is at risk for aspiration because of impaired swallowing. While the patient is eating, the head of the bed must be elevated or the patient must be seated in a chair. The dietitian should be consulted about providing a diet of the appropriate texture for the patient. A speech therapist can recommend techniques to facilitate swallowing. Eventually, oral intake becomes inadequate. The decision to insert a feeding tube should be based on the desires of the patient and family. The nurse administers feedings and monitors for tube placement and residual.

Impaired Verbal Communication. Speech becomes impaired by muscle weakness and dyspnea. Alternatives to verbal communication need to be established. These might include use of blinks or gestures or use of boards with pictures, words, or letters that the patient can select. The nurse should use questions that can be answered "yes" or "no" and allow the patient time to respond.

Impaired Skin Integrity. Muscle wasting, incontinence, and immobility put these patients at risk for skin breakdown. They must be repositioned at least every 2 hours, and bony prominences must be inspected for redness. Special beds that alternate or distribute pressure may be used. Wet or soiled clothing is changed promptly to avoid skin irritation. Meticulous skin care is essential.

Anticipatory Grieving. Once the implications of a diagnosis of ALS are understood, patients and their families may begin the grieving process. The nurse encourages patients to talk, listens compassionately, and helps them make realistic plans. Referrals to visiting nurse agencies and hospice services can provide needed emotional and physical support at various times in the progress of the disease.

Situational Low Self-Esteem. The nurse explores the patient's thoughts, feelings, and concerns about living with this progressive, terminal disease. Although it is difficult not to offer false reassurance, the nurse needs to let the patient ventilate, cry, or express anger. The patient's strengths, abilities, and contributions are stressed. Sources of support (family, friends, support groups, spiritual counselors, therapists) are identified and enlisted. Stress-reduction techniques include imagery, breathing exercises, and progressive relaxation. The patient's dignity is preserved by providing privacy during personal care and by attending to grooming and appearance.

Altered Family Processes. The disease is painful for both the patient and the family as it steadily takes its toll. Patients with ALS are often middle aged with family responsibilities, jobs, and places in the community. The family must plan for transfer of responsibilities and care of the patient when he or she becomes disabled. Issues that need to be discussed are patient feelings about advance directives, insurance, and wills. These topics may be difficult for them to address but are best handled while the patient's input is possible. Care of the dying patient is covered in Chapter 22.

EVALUATION. Criteria for determining the effects of nursing interventions include respiratory rate of 12 to 20 without rales or wheezes; participation in exercises to maintain mobility; stable weight; successful communication of patient's needs without excess frustration; intact skin; verbalization of losses, their importance, and acceptance; positive statements about self; and positive family communication and interactions.

HUNTINGTON'S DISEASE

Huntington's disease is an inherited degenerative neurologic disorder. It usually begins in middle adulthood with abnormal movements, emotional disturbance, and intellectual decline. Symptoms progress steadily, with increasing disability and death in 15 to 20 years. Medical and nursing care are supportive as there is no cure.

MYASTHENIA GRAVIS

Myasthenia gravis (MG) is a chronic, progressive disease in which there is a defect at the neuromuscular junction, where electrical impulses are transmitted to muscle tissue.

Etiology

There is evidence that MG may have an autoimmune basis. Some patients present with an increase in the titer of acetylcholine receptor antibody. The presence of these antibodies interferes with the normal activity at the acetylcholine receptor sites and reduces muscle strength.

Pathophysiology

Normally, as a nerve impulse travels down a peripheral nerve, the neurotransmitter acetylcholine is released

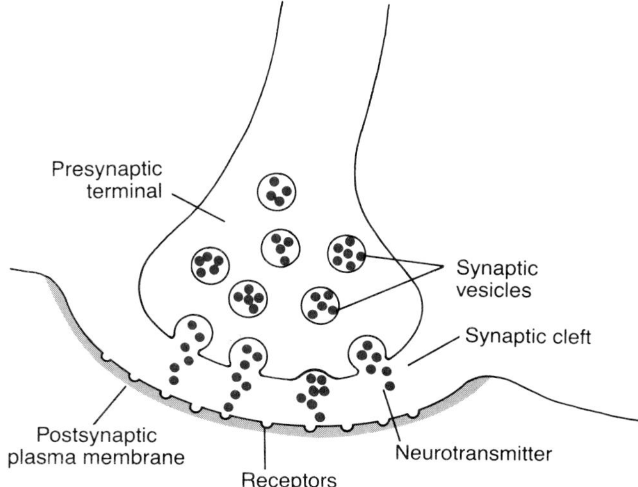

FIGURE 25-19
Neurotransmitters (norepinephrine, acetylcholine, dopamine) are released from the axon, travel across the synaptic cleft, and produce some response in the receptors of target cells. (From Black, J. M., & Matassarin-Jacobs, E. [1993]. *Luckmann and Sorensen's medical-surgical nursing: A psychophysiologic approach* [4th ed., p. 985]. Philadelphia: W. B. Saunders.)

at the presynaptic membrane (Fig. 25–19). The impulse is then transmitted across the synaptic junction to postsynaptic receptor sites on the effector muscle. This causes contraction of the involved muscle.

In MG, the amount of acetylcholine available at the neuromuscular junction is reduced. There may also be insufficient receptor sites to accommodate acetylcholine. With repeated stimulation, the muscle becomes exhausted and is eventually unable to contract at all. If respiratory muscles become involved, death from respiratory insufficiency or arrest is a possibility.

Signs and Symptoms

Myasthenia gravis is characterized by the following features: weakness of voluntary muscles, particularly those of chewing, swallowing, and speaking; partial improvements of strength with rest; and dramatic improvement with the use of anticholinesterase drugs.

Onset of symptoms is gradual, and early weakness may be so subtle that it goes unnoticed. Muscles responsible for fine movements, such as eye, facial, or hand muscles, are often affected early on in the disease process. Ptosis and diplopia are commonly seen. The patient becomes unable to perform any activity that demands sustained muscular contractions, such as brushing the hair, walking upstairs, or holding the hands over the head. The fatigue may abate with rest but rapidly returns upon repeating the activity. If the diaphragm or intercostal muscles are involved, breathing is compromised.

Medical Diagnosis

Diagnosis is made by administering edrophonium (Tensilon). This is an anticholinesterase agent that increases the relative amount of acetylcholine in the neuromuscular junction by destroying acetylcholinesterase. In the MG patient, muscle tone is markedly improved within 1 minute of injection, and this improvement persists for 4 to 5 minutes.

Medical Treatment

ANTICHOLINESTERASE DRUGS. Therapy is primarily directed toward pharmacologic management with anticholinesterase agents and corticosteroids. Neostigmine and pyridostigmine (Mestinon) are anticholinesterase drugs that increase the availability of acetylcholine at the neuromuscular junction. Both drugs inhibit the action of cholinesterase, the enzyme that destroys acetylcholine. Availability of acetylcholine is improved, thereby enhancing muscle strength. Dosages are individualized for each patient based on response and needs. Stress or sustained levels of activity can alter the need for these agents.

PHARMACOLOGY CAPSULE

Neuromuscular blocking agents must be used very cautiously in the patient with myasthenia gravis.

CORTICOSTEROIDS. Corticosteroids may be useful in those patients who do not respond well to the anticholinesterase agents. Adrenocorticotropic hormone or prednisone is administered concurrently with the anticholinesterase agent in an effort to induce remission. During the first 7 to 10 days of therapy, symptoms may worsen, requiring hospitalization to monitor for respiratory depression. With improvement, corticosteroids may be tapered and maintained at the lowest effective dose.

THYMECTOMY. Because a large number of MG patients have hyperplasia of the thymus gland, thymectomy is performed early after initial diagnosis. Close monitoring is essential postoperatively because the risk of respiratory compromise is accentuated owing to possible pneumothorax. About 40% of patients enjoy some degree of remission after thymectomy.

PLASMAPHERESIS. Plasmapheresis is an adjunctive therapy based on the autoimmune theory of myasthenia. It is a process of plasma exchange in which the acetylcholine receptor antibodies are washed from the plasma. A temporary catheter, similar to a renal dialysis access catheter, is used for venous access. Blood is then routed through a pheresis field, where the antibodies are separated from the plasma. The washed blood is then returned to the patient. The procedure takes 3 to 4 hours and is repeated over several days to ensure adequate treatment. Improvement in muscle strength may be noted within 24 to 48 hours after treatment. As progress is made with plasmapheresis, drug dosages may be decreased.

Myasthenic and Cholinergic Crises

Emergency respiratory support requiring mechanical ventilation may be necessary in the event of myasthenic or cholinergic crises. Myasthenic crisis is marked by a sudden exacerbation of myasthenic symptoms, including difficulty swallowing and breathing with possible respiratory arrest. Infection often precipitates the event, and symptoms do not decrease even with higher doses of medications.

Cholinergic crisis presents with sudden, extreme weakness and respiratory impairment. It is precipitated by overmedication with anticholinesterase drugs, which literally bombard the receptor sites with excess amounts of acetylcholine. Intubation and mechanical ventilation are required to manage the respiratory compromise.

Because the two crises present similarly, differentiation is critical. Once again, edrophonium is used to distinguish the two entities. Rapid improvement of muscle strength after administration indicates an underlying myasthenic crisis. If no improvement is observed, the patient is experiencing a cholinergic crisis.

Since MG is a chronic neurologic disease, the patient is generally managed at home. However, hospitalization is likely with initial diagnosis and during periods of crisis and respiratory compromise.

PHARMACOLOGY CAPSULE

Edrophonium rapidly reverses myasthenic crisis but has no effect on cholinergic crisis.

Nursing Care of the Patient with Myasthenia Gravis

ASSESSMENT. The complete neurologic assessment is outlined in Table 25–3. When the patient has MG, the health history describes the onset of symptoms, particularly muscle weakness, diplopia, dysphagia, slurred speech, breathing difficulties, and loss of balance. The effects of the condition on the patient's lifestyle are documented. The physical examination evaluates muscle strength, balance, respiratory effort, and oxygenation status.

NURSING DIAGNOSIS. Nursing diagnoses for the patient with MG may include the following:

- **Ineffective Breathing Patterns** related to impaired conduction of nerve impulses
- **Impaired Physical Mobility** and **Self-Care Deficit** related to muscle weakness, fatigue
- **Impaired Verbal Communication** related to weakness of the muscles involved in speech
- **Impaired Swallowing** related to muscle weakness
- **Knowledge Deficit** of disease and treatment

GOALS. Goals of nursing care for the patient with MG are adequate oxygenation, improved mobility and self-care performance, effective communication, adequate oral intake of food and fluids, and patient's knowledge of disease and treatment.

INTERVENTIONS

Ineffective Breathing Patterns. The nurse must monitor the patient for early signs and symptoms of ineffective breathing and hypoxia (tachycardia, restlessness). Progressive symptoms that do not respond to prescribed drug therapy may require mechanical ventilation. Management of the patient on a ventilator is discussed in Chapter 28.

Impaired Physical Mobility and Self-Care Deficit. Because of weakness, the patient may be relatively inactive and unable to provide self-care. The nurse monitors the patient's capabilities and assists as needed. Measures to prevent complications, discussed in Chapter 19, include turning and repositioning at least every 2 hours.

Impaired Swallowing. Patients may have difficulty chewing and swallowing. Anticholinesterase drugs may be ordered 30 minutes before meals to improve muscle strength. The patient should be seated upright for meals and allowed or assisted to eat in an unhurried manner. Small, frequent meals may be tolerated better than three large ones. A soft diet is usually ordered so that minimal chewing is required. If swallowing is severely impaired, a feeding tube may be inserted and liquid feedings given as ordered. Adequate fluid intake is important to maintain hydration and prevent constipation.

Knowledge Deficit. Patient teaching with MG is essential since this chronic condition requires lifelong treatment. The teaching plan should include an explanation of the disease, myasthenic and cholinergic crises, drug therapy, and management of symptoms. The nurse stresses the importance of taking the prescribed drugs at the proper time.

EVALUATION. Criteria for evaluating the outcomes of nursing interventions include normal respiratory rate (12–20) and effort, performance of activities of daily living without excessive fatigue, stable weight and absence of respiratory symptoms associated with aspiration, and patient's statement of essential components of the teaching plan.

TRIGEMINAL NEURALGIA (TIC DOULOUREUX)

Trigeminal neuralgia is characterized by intense pain along the distribution of one of the three branches of the trigeminal nerve (fifth cranial nerve): ophthalmic, mandibular, or maxillary (Fig. 25–20). The pain has an abrupt onset and is usually unilateral in nature, lasting from seconds to a few minutes. Despite the intense pain, there is no associated motor or sensory deficit. The pain may be crippling, restricting the patient's daily routine. Attacks may be triggered by hot or cold liquids, chewing, shaving, or washing the face. Between epi-

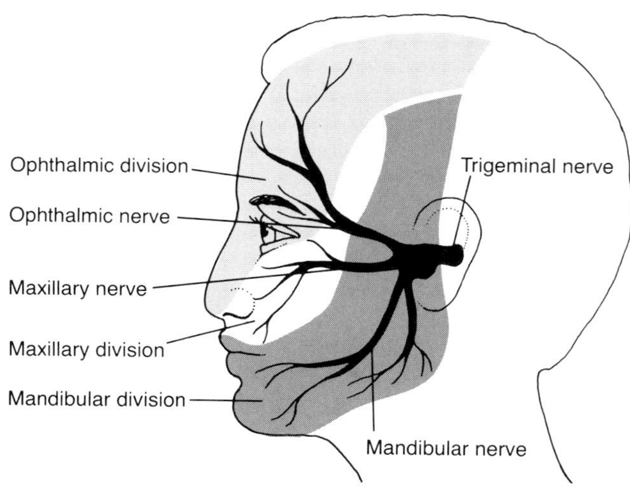

FIGURE 25-20
The area served by each of the three divisions of the trigeminal nerve is illustrated. (From Ignatavicius, D. D., & Bayne, M. V. [1991]. *Medical-surgical nursing: A nursing process approach* [p. 632]. Philadelphia: W. B. Saunders.)

sodes, the patient may experience a dull ache or be pain free.

Etiology

Although the exact etiology of trigeminal neuralgia is undetermined, various causative factors can be identified. Trauma or infection may precipitate the characteristic pain, as can compression on the nerve by an aneurysm, artery, or tumor.

Medical Diagnosis and Medical Treatment

Because there is no specific test, diagnosis is based on history. Stimulation of certain trigger points may precipitate the pain.

Pharmacologic management is the preferable course of therapy. Phenytoin (Dilantin) and carbamazepine (Tegretol) are most commonly used to suppress the pain episodes. During the acute attack, alcohol or phenol may be injected into the affected branch of the trigeminal nerve, with pain relief lasting from 8 to 16 months.

Patients with the most severe, debilitating pain may undergo surgical intervention. Electrocoagulation, a procedure in which heated electrodes are used to destroy the sensory fibers of the nerve, is effective in providing lasting pain relief without compromising motor or tactile function.

Nursing Care of the Patient with Trigeminal Neuralgia

ASSESSMENT. Assessment of the patient with trigeminal neuralgia focuses on describing the pain, factors that trigger it, and treatments found to be effective or ineffective. The effects of the condition on the patient's life are documented.

NURSING DIAGNOSIS. Nursing diagnoses for the patient with trigeminal neuralgia may include the following:

- **Pain** related to disease process
- **Self-Care Deficit** related to debilitating pain
- **Altered Nutrition: Less than Body Requirements** related to pain associated with chewing
- **Fear** related to anticipated painful episodes
- **Knowledge Deficit** of trigeminal neuralgia and its treatment

GOALS. Goals of nursing interventions for the patient with trigeminal neuralgia include reduced severity and frequency of painful attacks, performance of self-care activities, adequate nutritional intake, lessened fear, and patient's knowledge of condition and its treatment.

INTERVENTIONS. The nursing care for the patient with trigeminal neuralgia is primarily directed toward pain assessment and management. It may be beneficial to assist the patient in developing alternative strategies to pain relief, such as guided imagery or relaxation therapy. Because of the debilitating nature of the pain, the patient may require assistance in performing self-care activities. Nutrition may be affected because chewing may trigger pain. Psychological effects are also a consideration in management because the fear of engaging in some activity that may trigger pain can lead to social isolation. Chapter 16 provides additional information about care of the patient in pain. Patient teaching emphasizes the nature of the condition and avoidance of factors that trigger episodes.

EVALUATION. Criteria for evaluating the outcomes of nursing interventions are patient's statement of less frequent episodes or relief from pain; performance of activities of daily living; stable weight; statement of less fear and belief in ability to manage condition; and patient description of condition, prevention of episodes, and treatment.

NEUROFIBROMATOSIS

Neurofibromatosis, also known as von Recklinghausen's disease, is characterized by multiple tumors of peripheral, spinal, and cranial nerves. The tumors are benign but may be removed to relieve compression on the nerves or for cosmetic reasons. The patient may also have bone, muscle, and skin involvement.

BELL'S PALSY

Bell's palsy is acute paralysis of the seventh cranial nerve, which serves the face. The condition usually begins with pain behind the ear or on the face. The patient then has a "drawing" sensation followed by paralysis of the muscles on the affected side. The affected eyelids do not close, taste is impaired, and eating may be difficult. Most patients recover over a period of weeks or months, but some have residual weakness.

Bell's palsy is treated on an outpatient basis with prednisone and analgesics. Artificial tears are needed if the eyelids do not close, and the affected eye should be closed and patched at night to prevent drying of the cornea. When function begins to return, the patient can do simple exercises to improve muscle tone: grimacing, opening and closing the eyes, whistling, and puffing out the cheeks. The nurse must be sensitive to the patient's concerns about the condition and his or her appearance.

CEREBRAL PALSY

Cerebral palsy (CP) is a paralysis associated with a loss in motor coordination caused by cerebral damage. Although the etiology is uncertain, the damage is generally believed to occur at birth and to be related to hypoxia, premature birth, or birth trauma.

Individuals with CP are often frustrated by people who equate the disorder with mental retardation. Although the staggering gait and unclear speech may resemble those of some people with mental retardation, the individual with CP is fully capable of comprehending his or her situation and is willing to strive for as much independence as possible.

Types of Cerebral Palsy

Three general types of CP can be identified based on symptomatology: spastic paralysis, athetoid, and ataxic. Spastic paralysis is characterized by overall exaggerated reflexes and muscle spasms. Random, purposeless movement with extreme muscle tone is indicative of the athetoid type, whereas the ataxic variety is characterized by poor balance, an uncoordinated, staggering gait, and speech or vision defects.

Medical Treatment

Although there is no cure for CP, early muscle training and exercises can be beneficial in an effort to prevent complications and promote optimal function. Orthopedic surgery, braces, and casts may be useful in limiting deformities and disabilities.

Nursing Care of the Patient with Cerebral Palsy

Nursing care of the patient with CP is covered in depth in pediatric nursing texts because it is typically a lifelong condition diagnosed in infancy.

POSTPOLIO SYNDROME

Before the advent of the polio vaccine, many people suffered varying degrees of motor impairment caused by the polio virus. Many years after having had the initial infection, some patients once again experience progressive muscle weakness, fatigue, pain, and respiratory problems typical of polio infections. The reason for the recurrence of symptoms is not known. Medical and nursing care are primarily supportive, aimed at helping the patient adapt to the symptoms and maintain maximum possible function.

It is obvious that the management of the neurologic patient can be demanding and challenging. Astute observation and assessment are vital to any treatment plan, and other therapies are frequently driven by the nursing assessment. As is apparent in this chapter, many nursing diagnoses and modes of management are common to almost any patient with a neurologic disorder. Because of the complicated nature of many of these patients, it must be remembered that considerations for the management of other body systems also must be incorporated in a comprehensive plan.

NUTRITION CONCEPTS

- A general goal for individuals with neurologic disorders is to maintain an adequate intake of nutrients.
- Self-feeding should be promoted while maintaining feeding safety.
- Neurologically impaired people who are inactive should try to avoid obesity, which further impairs mobility.
- Inactivity may contribute to constipation, which can be somewhat relieved through diet by increasing fiber (bran, whole grains, beans, fruits, and vegetables) and encouraging a large fluid intake.
- People who have difficulty swallowing may be more likely to choke on liquids than semisolids such as gelatin, ice cream, sherbert, or puddings.

BIBLIOGRAPHY

Anderson, S. B. (1992). Guillain-Barré syndrome: Giving the patient control. *Journal of Neuroscience Nursing, 24*(3), 158–162.

Athlin, E., Norberg, A., Axelsson, K., Moller, A., & Nordstrom, G. (1989). Aberrant eating behavior in elderly Parkinsonian patients with and without dementia: Analysis of video-recorded meals. *Research in Nursing and Health, 12*(1), 41–51.

Bagley, S., Kelly, B., Tunnicliffe, N., Turnbull, N., & Walker, J. M. (1991). The effect of visual cues on the gait of independently mobile Parkinson's disease patients. *Physiotherapy, 77*(6), 415–420.

Berry, P., & Ward-Smith, P. A. (1988). Adrenal medullary transplant as a treatment for Parkinson's disease: Perioperative considerations. *Journal of Neuroscience Nursing, 20*(6), 356–361.

Black, J. M., & Matassarin-Jacobs, E. (1993). *Luckmann and Sorensen's medical-surgical nursing* (4th ed.). Philadelphia: W. B. Saunders.

Bradbury, K. M., & Bauer, M. (1990). Brain graft surgery: A new treatment for Parkinson's disease. *Critical Care Nurse, 10*(8), 15–31.

Bunting, L. K., & Fitzsimmons, B. (1991). Depression in Parkinson's disease. *Journal of Neuroscience Nursing, 23*(3), 158–164.

Caine, R. M., & Bufalino, P. M. (Eds.). (1991). *Nursing care planning guides for adults* (2nd ed.). Baltimore: Williams & Wilkins.

Carson, P. (1993). Investing in the comeback: Parent's experience following traumatic brain injury. *Journal of Neuroscience Nursing, 25*(3), 165–173.

Cummings, R. (1992). Understanding external ventricular drainage. *Journal of Neuroscience Nursing, 24*(2), 84–87.

Deglin, J. H., Vallerand, A. H., & Russin, M. M. (1991). *Davis's drug guide for nurses* (2nd ed.). Philadelphia: W. B. Saunders.

Dilorio, C., Faherty, B., & Manteuffel, B. (1992). The development of an instrument to measure self-efficacy in individuals with epilepsy. *Journal of Neuroscience Nursing, 24*(1), 9–13.

Dilorio, C., Faherty, B., & Manteuffel, B. (1993). Learning needs of persons with epilepsy: A comparison of perceptions of persons with epilepsy, nurses, and physicians. *Journal of Neuroscience Nursing, 25*(1), 22–29.

Doenges, M. E., & Moorhouse, M. F. (1993). *Nurse's pocket guide: nursing diagnoses with interventions* (4th ed.). Philadelphia: F. A. Davis.

Engli, M., & Kirsivali-Farmer, K. (1993). Needs of family members of critically ill patients with and without brain injury. *Journal of Neuroscience Nursing, 25*(2), 78–85.

Habermann-Little, B. (1991). An analysis of the prevalence and etiology of depression in Parkinson's disease. *Journal of Neuroscience Nursing, 23*(3), 165–169.

Hagen, N. A. (1991). Action STAT: Myasthenic crisis. *Nursing 91, 21*(6), 33.

Hartshorn, J. C., & Byers, V. (1992). Impact of epilepsy on quality of life. *Journal of Neuroscience Nursing, 24*(1), 24–29.

Hickey, J. V. (1991). Myasthenic crisis—your assessment counts. *RN, 54*(5), 54–59.

Hood, L. J. (1990). Myasthenia gravis: Regimens and regimen-associated problems in adults. *Journal of Neuroscience Nursing, 22*(6), 358–364.

Hubsky, E. P., & Sears, J. H. (1992). Fatigue in multiple sclerosis: Guidelines for nursing care. *Rehabilitation Nursing, 17*(4), 176–180.

Ignatavicius, D. D., & Bayne, M. V. (1991). *Medical-surgical nursing: A nursing process approach*. Philadelphia: W. B. Saunders.

Jacob, S. W., & Francone, C. A. (1989). *Elements of anatomy and physiology*. (2nd ed.). Philadelphia: W. B. Saunders.

Jarvis, C. (1992). *Physical examination and health assessment*. Philadelphia: W. B. Saunders.

Livesley, E. (1992). Effects of electrical neuromuscular stimulation on functional performance in patients with multiple sclerosis. *Physiotherapy, 78*(12), 914–917.

Marr, J. (1991). The experience of living with Parkinson's disease. *Journal of Neuroscience Nursing, 23*(5), 325–329.

Matteson, M. A., & McConnell, E. S. (1988). *Gerontological nursing*. Philadelphia: W. B. Saunders.

Michael, J. E. (1992). Vagal nerve stimulation in treatment of intractable partial seizures: Nursing implications. *Journal of Neuroscience Nursing, 24*(1), 19–23.

Miller, C. M., & Hens, M. (1993). Multiple sclerosis: A literature review. *Journal of Neuroscience Nursing, 25*(3), 174–179.

Morgante, L. A., Madonna, M. G., & Pololuk, R. (1989). Research and treatment in multiple sclerosis: Implications for nursing practice. *Journal of Neuroscience Nursing, 21*(5), 285–289.

Mulder, D. G., White, K., & Herrman, C., Jr. (1986). Thymectomy: Surgical procedure for myasthenia gravis. *AORN Journal, 43*(3), 640–646.

Murray, D. P. (1993). Impaired mobility: Guillain-Barré syndrome. *Journal of Neuroscience Nursing, 25*(2), 100–104.

O'Brien, M. T. (1993). Multiple sclerosis: Health-promoting behaviors of spousal caregivers. *Journal of Neuroscience Nursing, 25*(2), 105–112.

Rhynsburger, J. (1989). How to fight MG fatigue. *American Journal of Nursing, 89*(3), 337–340.

Shlafer, M. (1993). *The nurse, pharmacology, and drug therapy* (3rd ed.). Redwood City, CA: Addison-Wesley.

Taira, F. (1992). Facilitating self-care in clients with Parkinson's disease. *Home Health Care, 10*(4), 23–27.

Toledo, L. W. (1992). The postanesthesia patient with Parkinson's disease. *Journal of Post Anesthesia Nursing, 17*(1), 32–37.

Vernon, G. M. (1989). Parkinson's disease. *Journal of Neuroscience Nursing, 21*(5), 273–284.

Wassem, R. (1992). Self-efficacy as a predictor of adjustment to multiple sclerosis. *Journal of Neuroscience Nursing, 24*(4), 224–229.

Weeks, D. (1991). Washing the blood. *RN, 54*(5), 60–64.

Weiner, W. J., & Singer, C. (1989). Parkinson's disease and nonpharmacologic treatment programs. *Journal of the American Geriatrics Society, 37*(4), 359–363.

Yen, P. K. (1990). Does a low-protein diet help with Parkinson's? *Geriatric Nursing, 11*(1), 48.

KEY CONCEPTS

1. The functional unit of the nervous system is the neuron (nerve cell), which conducts electrical impulses from one area of the brain to another.
2. The brain and the spinal cord compose the central nervous system, whereas the nerves in the peripheral parts of the body compose the peripheral nervous system.
3. Cerebrospinal fluid circulates through the central nervous system.
4. The neurologic assessment includes evaluation of the level of consciousness, pupillary size and response, coordination and balance, sensory function, reflexes, and vital signs.
5. Increased intracranial pressure may impair cerebral tissue perfusion, resulting in ischemia and possibly respiratory arrest.
6. Signs and symptoms of increased intracranial pressure and impaired cerebral blood flow are decreasing level of consciousness, pupil dilation with no response to light, motor deficits, abnormal posture, fever, increased blood pressure, bradycardia, and respiratory depression.

7. Measures to decrease intracranial pressure include positioning, hyperventilation, fluid restriction, mechanical drainage, and drug therapy.
8. Seizures are abnormal activity and behavior caused by abnormal electrical impulses in the brain that may be treated with anticonvulsant therapy and, when possible, measures to correct the cause.
9. Nursing care of the patient with a seizure disorder addresses high risk for injury, ineffective individual coping, and knowledge deficits.
10. Nursing care of the patient with a head injury may focus on altered cerebral tissue perfusion, ineffective breathing pattern, high risk for injury, high risk for infection, impaired physical mobility, body image disturbances, and altered role performance.
11. Meningitis and encephalitis are infections of the nervous system.
12. Guillain-Barré syndrome, thought to be an autoimmune response to a viral infection, is characterized by progressive ascending neurologic deficits that eventually resolve in most people.
13. Nursing care of the patient with Guillain-Barré syndrome addresses ineffective breathing patterns, decreased cardiac output, high risk for disuse syndrome, altered nutrition, high risk for injury, anxiety, and knowledge deficit.
14. Parkinson's disease, a progressive disorder that results in loss of coordination and control over involuntary movement, is treated with physical therapy and drugs that increase dopamine in the brain.
15. The focus of nursing care for the patient with Parkinson's disease is impaired physical mobility, high risk for injury, altered nutrition, ineffective individual coping, and knowledge deficit.
16. Multiple sclerosis is a progressive degenerative disease that disrupts the motor pathways of the central nervous system and may lead to severe neurologic disabilities.
17. Amyotrophic lateral sclerosis is a rapidly progressive degenerative disease that usually results in death from respiratory complications within 3 years.
18. The patient with amyotrophic lateral sclerosis has increasing needs for nursing care, eventually becoming completely dependent for all aspects of care.
19. Myasthenia gravis is caused by a defect in impulse conduction that is manifested as weakness of voluntary muscles and is treated with anticholinesterase drugs and corticosteroids.
20. Trigeminal neuralgia is intense pain along a branch of the trigeminal nerve that may be treated with drug therapy or surgical intervention.

Marge Balzer

CHAPTER 26

Cerebrovascular Accident

OBJECTIVES

1. Explain the risk factors for cerebrovascular accident (CVA).
2. Identify the four types of CVA.
3. Describe the pathophysiology, signs and symptoms, and medical treatment for each type of CVA.
4. Describe the neurologic deficits that may result from CVA.
5. Explain tests and procedures used to diagnose a CVA.
6. Explain nursing responsibilities for patients having those tests and procedures.
7. List data to be included in the nursing assessment of the CVA patient.
8. Identify nursing diagnoses, goals, and interventions during the acute and the rehabilitation phases for the patient who has had a CVA.
9. Specify criteria used to evaluate the outcomes of nursing care for the CVA patient.
10. Identify resources for the CVA patient and family.

GLOSSARY

APHASIA The inability to understand words or the inability to respond with words, or both.

DIPLOPIA Double vision

DYSARTHRIA Inability to speak clearly due to neurologic damage that impairs normal muscle control

DYSPHAGIA Difficulty swallowing

DYSPRAXIA Partial inability to initiate coordinated voluntary motor acts

FLUENT APHASIA Ability to speak clearly but without meaning

HEMIPLEGIA Paralysis of one side of the body

HOMONYMOUS HEMIANOPSIA Loss of half the field of vision; loss is on the side opposite the brain lesion

INTRACEREBRAL Within the cerebrum

NONFLUENT APHASIA Difficulty initiating speech

PTOSIS Drooping of the upper eyelid

RECEPTIVE APHASIA Inability to comprehend words

SUBARACHNOID Between the arachnoid and pia mater layers of the membranes covering the brain

TRANSIENT ISCHEMIC ATTACK Neurologic deficits that last less than 24 hours; caused by diminished cerebral blood flow

The brain is the body's center of thinking, feeling, and physical function. In any minute, at least 800 ml of blood are circulating in the brain. Brain metabolism uses 400 calories every 24 hours. Because of the brain's circulatory demands, a block in blood supply can be damaging in a matter of minutes.

A cerebrovascular accident (CVA) is an interruption of blood flow to part of the brain. Without normal blood flow, the affected area is deprived of oxygen. The effects of oxygen deprivation vary depending on the area of the brain involved and the length of time the brain is deprived of oxygen.

A brief review of the anatomy and physiology of the brain follows. Refer to Chapter 25 for a more detailed review.

ANATOMY AND PHYSIOLOGY OF THE BRAIN

The central nervous system structures of the brain include the cerebrum, the brain stem, the reticular activating system, and the cerebellum.

CEREBRUM

The cerebrum has many complex functions including initiation of movements, recognition of sensory input, higher order thinking, emotional behavior, and regulation of endocrine and autonomic functions.

The cerebrum is divided into two halves, called hemispheres. Each hemisphere controls the opposite side of the body; that is, the right hemisphere controls the left side of the body, and the left hemisphere controls the right side of the body. For most people, the left hemisphere is dominant. This hemisphere controls the more analytic mental processes such as language ability, mathematics, and reasoning powers. The right hemisphere encompasses emotional and artistic tendencies.

A folded layer of nerve cells, the cortex, covers each hemisphere. The cortex of each hemisphere is divided into the parietal, frontal, temporal, and occipital lobes. Each lobe has a different area of function (Fig. 26–1).

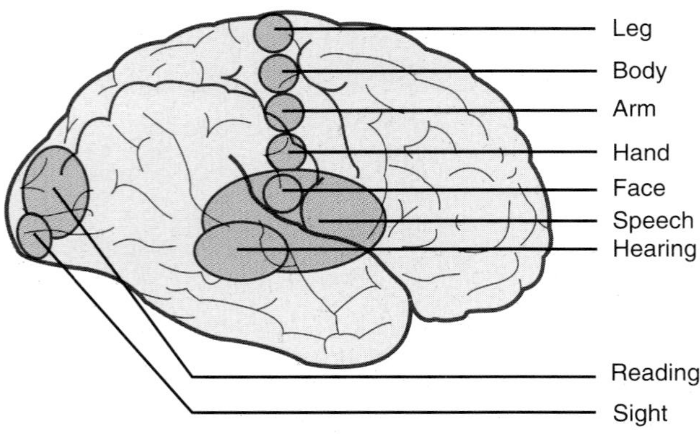

FIGURE 26–1

Control zones of the brain.

BRAIN STEM

The brain stem includes the midbrain, pons, medulla, and part of the reticular activating system. The brain stem controls vital, basic functions including respiration, heart rate, and consciousness.

CEREBELLUM

The cerebellum uses information received from the cerebrum, muscles, joints, and inner ear to coordinate movement, balance, and posture. In the cerebellum, the right side controls the right side of the body and the left side controls the left side of the body, in contrast to other parts of the brain.

CIRCULATION

The brain is rich with arterial circulation to satisfy its high need for oxygen. The circulatory system in the cerebrum is called the *cerebrovascular system.* Figure 26–2 pictures the major cerebral arteries. Individual anatomic differences in blood vessels can increase the likelihood that some people will have CVAs.

TYPES OF CEREBROVASCULAR ACCIDENTS

Cerebrovascular accidents are commonly called strokes. There are four types of CVA: transient ischemic attack (TIA), reversible ischemic neurologic deficit, completed stroke, and stroke in evolution. All types of CVAs share common signs and symptoms but differ in relation to duration and symptoms and whether the patient is stable or continues to develop new deficits.

TRANSIENT ISCHEMIC ATTACK

A TIA is a temporary neurologic deficit caused by impairment of cerebral blood flow. Blood vessels may be occluded by broken fragments of plaque or by blood clots that tend to form with certain cardiac conditions. A TIA is thought to be an important warning condition for a possible later stroke. It is believed that at least 85% of blood flow to an area must be blocked before signs and symptoms of a TIA appear.

SIGNS AND SYMPTOMS

With a TIA, neurologic signs and symptoms last from a few minutes to 24 hours. There is no remaining or residual physiologic damage. Some common signs and symptoms are dizziness, momentary confusion, loss of speech, loss of balance, tinnitus, visual disturbances, ptosis, dysarthria, dysphagia, drooping mouth, and tingling or numbness on one side of the body. The severity of the symptoms depends on the area and extent of brain involvement.

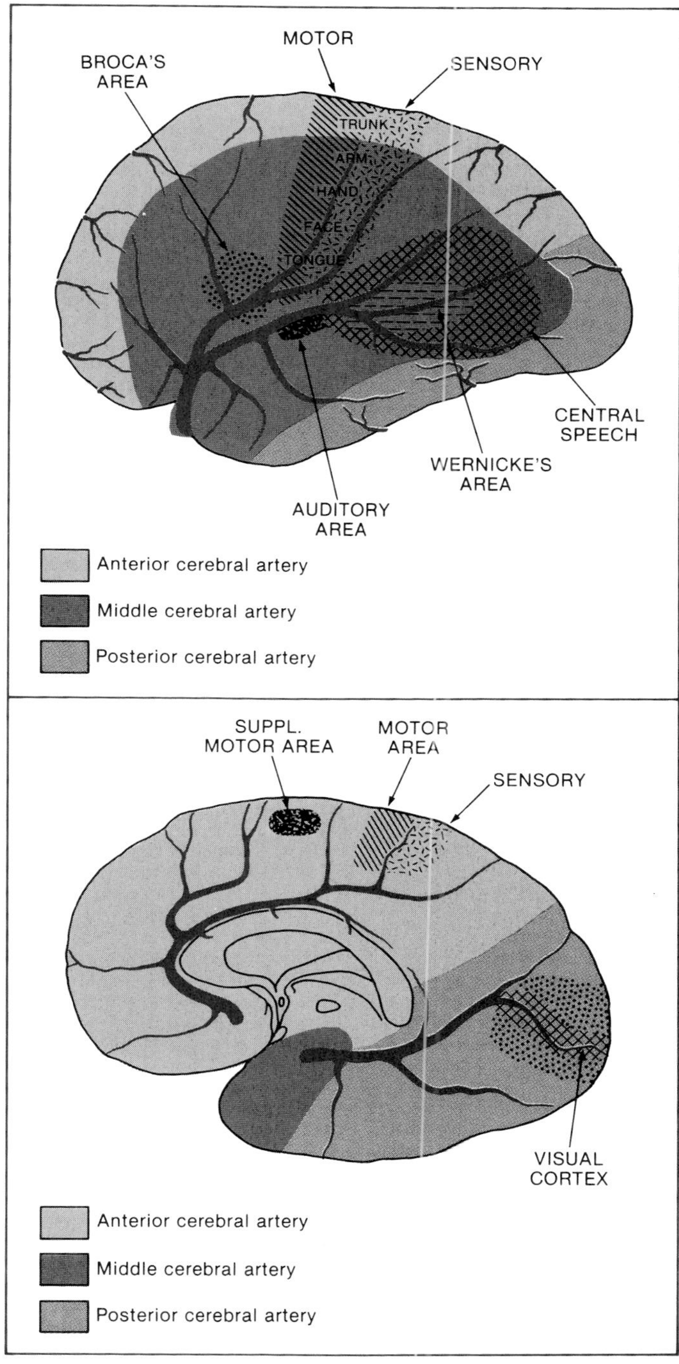

FIGURE 26-2
Cerebral circulation. (From Wyngaarden, J., & Smith, L. [1988]. *Cecil textbook of medicine* [18th ed.]. Philadelphia: W. B. Saunders.)

MEDICAL DIAGNOSIS

Diagnosis of TIA is based on the history and physical examination. The diagnosis depends on the astuteness of the physician or nurse and the ability of the patient to report the symptoms. It is difficult to say how often TIAs actually occur, because signs and symptoms may be overlooked, not reported, or attributed to old age.

In diagnosing a TIA, one can sometimes auscultate a swooshing noise in a clogged carotid artery. This sound is called a *bruit.* It is similar to a rush of water through a narrow or dammed-up area.

Angiography and radiologic studies can show a narrowing of the blood vessels. Doppler studies may also be done to assess cerebral blood flow. Ultrasonic duplex scanning is useful in detecting carotid artery disease. Computed tomography scans and electroencephalograms may be employed to rule out intracranial lesions such as tumors, aneurysms, and abscesses. Key features of diagnostic tests are presented in Table 26–1.

MEDICAL TREATMENT

Treatment of a TIA depends on the location of the narrowed vessel and the degree of narrowing. Medical treatment may include drug therapy with aspirin or dipyridamole (Persantine) to decrease platelet clumping or pentoxifylline (Trental) to improve blood flow. Warfarin (Coumadin), an anticoagulant, may be given. If warfarin is given, the patient's blood prothrombin time must be monitored regularly.

PHARMACOLOGY CAPSULE

When patients are taking anticoagulant drugs, precautions are taken to prevent injuries and bleeding.

The therapeutic range of prothrombin time during warfarin therapy should be about twice the time of a control sample or a standard designated by the lab. Additional information about drug therapy is provided in Table 26–2. Other conservative measures that may be

TABLE 26–1
CEREBROVASCULAR ACCIDENT: DIAGNOSTIC TESTS AND PROCEDURES

TEST/STUDY	PURPOSE/PROCEDURE	PATIENT PREPARATION	POSTPROCEDURE NURSING CARE
		RADIOGRAPHIC STUDIES	
Computed Tomography (CT) scan	Creates cross-sectional three-dimensional images of the brain. Is much more sensitive than traditional radiographs. Differentiates tumors from soft tissue, air from cerebrospinal fluid, and normal blood from clotted blood. Detects tumors, inflammation, edema, hematomas, and infarctions. Contrast media may be injected intravenously to outline blood vessels.	Report patient allergies to contrast media to the radiologist. Tell the patient what to expect. Advise the patient that the procedure is painless. Patients generally receive nothing by mouth (NPO) for 2–3 hr before the scan but can take prescribed medications. Diabetic diets and drugs should not be withheld. Sedatives may be ordered for patients who are unable to lie still. The patient lies on a stretcher for 20–40 min while a donut-shaped frame moves around the head. It is essential to lie perfectly still. A mechanical sound can be heard. If intravenous contrast media is given, the patient may feel flushed, warm, and nauseous and report a salty taste. Signs of allergic reaction are dyspnea, tachycardia, perspiration, and numbness.	If contrast media is used, assess for reactions to iodine: nausea, hives, swollen salivary glands. Notify physician of reaction. Administer antihistamines by mouth (PO) if ordered.
Positron emission tomography (PET) scan	Uses inhaled or injected radionuclides followed by scanning to study the brain. Provides data on brain structures, blood flow, and tissue metabolism. Can determine if speech center is still viable after a cardiovascular accident (CVA).	Explain the purpose of the test and that it is painless. The small amount of radiation is harmless. The patient should avoid alcohol, caffeine, and tobacco for 24 hr before the test. Tell the patient two intravenous (IV) lines will be started—one to inject radionuclides, the other to draw blood. Forty-five min later, the scan is done. It takes 45 min to 1 hr. The eyes and ears are covered to reduce stimuli. The patient must lie still. Relaxation techniques can be used, but the patient should not count. Sometimes the patient is asked to read, recite something from memory, or perform a mental exercise.	The patient should rise slowly after the test to avoid faintness from postural hypotension. Voiding is encouraged shortly after the test to eliminate the radionucolide from the bladder.
Brain scan	Used to visualize brain lesions including CVA. A radioactive isotope is administered intravenously and followed by scanning. Helps differentiate ischemic from hemorrhagic stroke. Ischemic changes usually not apparent until several weeks after CVA. Hemorrhage may be seen earlier. Data are used in some states to determine brain death.	Inform the patient that an IV injection that contains a small amount of radioactive material will be given. Although the dose is small and is quickly eliminated, this procedure should not be done during pregnancy. The study is painless. A blocking agent may be given PO shortly before the test to reduce concentration of the radioactive material in body tissues other than the brain. The agent contains iodine, so it is contraindicated with iodine allergy. The scan is done twice. The first is to study cerebral blood flow. It takes about 5 min. Two hr later the scan is repeated to study brain tissue. This scan takes longer. The patient must lie perfectly still during the scans. A sed-	No special care needed.

TABLE 26-1

CEREBROVASCULAR ACCIDENT: DIAGNOSTIC TESTS AND PROCEDURES *Continued*

TEST/STUDY	PURPOSE/PROCEDURE	PATIENT PREPARATION	POSTPROCEDURE NURSING CARE
		RADIOGRAPHIC STUDIES	
		ative can be ordered if the patient is unable to lie still.	
Cerebral angiography Digital subtraction angiography (DSA)	Uses computer-based images taken after injection of contrast media to visualize arteries, including carotids and vertebrals. Sometimes done just before CT scan.	The patient should be NPO for 2 hr before the test. Inform the patient that the physician will put a catheter into a vein in the arm or the groin. Fluid will be given through the catheter and images of blood vessels recorded.	Monitor vital signs. The IV catheter is removed after the procedure. A bandage is placed over the site and pressure applied. The puncture site should be inspected for hemorrhage, hematoma, or infection. Assess for signs of iodine allergy: nausea, vomiting, hives. Encourage increased fluids for 24 hr to promote elimination of the contrast media.
Angiography	Uses radiographic examinations after injection of contrast media (iodine) into an artery to visualize blood vessels. May be used to evaluate carotid and intracranial arteries.	Advise the radiologist of iodine allergy. Determine whether patient should be NPO. An intravenous infusion may be started to provide fluids and venous access if needed. Inform the patient that a catheter will be inserted in a blood vessel in the arm or the groin while in the radiology department. Contrast media will be injected and X-rays taken.	Monitor vital signs. Monitor the puncture site for bleeding and hematoma. Maintain pressure as ordered. Enforce bedrest for 6 hr or as ordered by the physician.
		IMAGING PROCEDURES	
Magnetic resonance imaging (MRI)	Creates cross-sectional images of the brain without radiation.	Advise the patient that MRI is a painless, noninvasive procedure. All metal must be removed before MRI. Tell the patient what to expect. The patient must lie still on a narrow surface. A circular device surrounds the head like a tunnel. Closing the eyes reduces claustrophobia. Mechanical noises can be heard during the procedure. Sedatives may be ordered if the patient cannot be still or is claustrophobic.	No special care is needed.
		BLOOD FLOW STUDIES	
Doppler flow	Uses an ultrasound instrument to assess carotid blood flow. A duplex scanner may be used with the doppler to detect plaques in blood vessels.	Inform the patient that the test is painless and advise what to expect. Obtain signed consent. No smoking for 30 min before test. The patient must lie on the back while an instrument is moved over the neck area.	No special care needed, unless activity limitations are prescribed.
Plethysmography	Measures blood flow volume in vessels of the eye.	Assess for contraindications: systolic pressure over 200, allergy to local anesthetics, history of lens implant or retinal detachment. Inform the patient that the test is painless but that it is necessary to relax.	Assess for conjunctival hemorrhage.
		CEREBROSPINAL FLUID EXAMINATION	
Cerebrospinal fluid (CSF) color, turbidity, pressure	Cerebrospinal fluid obtained by lumbar puncture for examination. Presence of blood is consistent with hemorrhage. The CSF pressure is also measured.	The patient should be told what to expect. The patient is positioned on the side with the head flexed and the knees drawn up. The nurse can support the patient and encourage relaxation. The physician anesthetizes the local tissue and then makes a puncture between the lumbar vertebrae. The CSF pressure is measured. If pressure is normal, 3 specimens of CSF are usually collected. The needle is then removed. Specimens must be labeled by number in order obtained and delivered promptly to the lab.	Document the procedure. A small sterile dressing is applied to the puncture site. Check for leakage and report to physician. Monitor for changes in neurologic status. Have patient lie flat if ordered for specified period of time. Encourage fluids.

TABLE 26-2
DRUG THERAPY FOR CEREBROVASCULAR ACCIDENT

DRUGS	USE/ACTION	SIDE EFFECTS	NURSING INTERVENTIONS
Corticosteroids			
Dexamethasone (Decadron)	Reduces intracranial pressure by reducing the inflammatory response in the brain after stroke; dose usually tapered over 7–10 days	Fluid retention, hypertension, hypokalemia, hyperglycemia; suppressed response to infection; abnormal fat deposits in cheeks and upper back; gastric ulcers, insomnia, easy bruising, mood swings	Monitor intake and output and blood pressure; monitor blood glucose in diabetics; protect from infection; report even minor signs of infection; protect from bumps and other minor injuries
Hyperosmotic Agents			
Mannitol (Osmitrol)	Causes diuresis to reduce intracranial pressure; mannitol is first choice	Circulatory overload. Heart failure. Hypertension. Renal failure	15–25% mannitol solutions should be filtered; monitor infusion site; stop flow and have restarted if infiltrated to avoid tissue damage; monitor for signs of fluid volume excess: hypertension, bounding pulse, edema, urine output less than fluid intake
Urea (Ureaphil) Glycerin (Osmoglyn)			
Anticoagulants			
Heparin sodium (Liquaemin Sodium)	Prevents formation of new blood clots; does not dissolve existing clots; usually given first for rapid anticoagulation; patients then gradually changed to warfarin	Bleeding or hemorrhage due to excessive anticoagulation; hyperkalemia; alopecia (hair loss); allergy; contraindicated with active bleeding	Effect is monitored by partial thromboplastin time (PTT) or by activated partial thromboplastin time (APPT); therapeutic goal is 1.5–2.0 times the control of 30–40 sec. If patient's APPT is greater, withhold drug and contact physician; assess for bruises, bleeding from gastrointestinal and urinary tract, mouth, or nose; antidote for heparin overdose: protamine sulfate; caution with venipuncture—apply pressure to site
Warfarin sodium (Coumadin, Panwarfin)	Prevents formation of new blood clots; does not dissolve existing clots	Bleeding or hemorrhage due to excessive anticoagulation; contraindicated with severe cardiac, renal, or liver disease; interacts with many other drugs	Effect is monitored by prothrombin time (PT). Therapeutic goal is 1.5–2.0 times control; check PT before each dose; physician may order dose daily based on PT;

employed to treat atherosclerosis include diet therapy and exercise.

If the blockage is severe, surgery may be advised to reduce the risk of stroke. The most common surgical procedures are endarterectomy and extracranial-intracranial bypass. Endarterectomy involves opening the obstructed blood vessel, usually a carotid artery, and removing the plaque (Fig. 26–3). Extracranial-intracranial bypass creates a detour around an obstructed blood vessel by connecting a branch of an artery outside the cranium to one inside the cranium.

REVERSIBLE ISCHEMIC NEUROLOGIC DEFICIT

If signs and symptoms persist for more than 24 hours but then disappear, the patient may be said to have had a reversible ischemic neurologic deficit. Other experts label this event a completed stroke without residual deficits.

STROKE

A stroke is a set of neurologic signs and symptoms caused by impaired blood flow to the brain. When symptoms progress over hours or days, the condition is described as stroke in evolution. When the neurologic deficits do not change for 2 to 3 days, the stroke is said to be completed.

About 500,000 people have strokes every year in the United States. Stroke is the third most common cause of death, killing almost 150,000 people each year. Unlike TIA, stroke causes lingering motor, sensory, or cognitive damage with varying disabilities. Despite these statistics, there is reason for hope. More than half of stroke victims are returned to independence in activities of daily living within 1 year after the stroke. Thirty

TABLE 26-2
DRUG THERAPY FOR CEREBROVASCULAR ACCIDENT *Continued*

DRUGS	USE/ACTION	SIDE EFFECTS	NURSING INTERVENTIONS
Anticoagulants			assess for bruising, bleeding from gastrointestinal and urinary tract, mouth, or nose; caution with venipuncture sites—apply pressure; antidote for warfarin overdose is vitamin K_1 (AquaMEPHYTON)
Thrombolytics			
Streptokinase	Dissolves fibrin clots and clot components to destroy thrombi and restore blood flow	Increased risk of minor bleeding, especially at injection sites; mild fever, mild allergic reaction; contraindicated within 2 months of intracranial bleeding	Avoid unnecessary injections; watch puncture sites closely; after arterial puncture, apply pressure at least 30 min; for major bleeding, streptokinase infusion must be stopped; whole blood, packed cells, or plasma may be ordered; antidote for excessive bleeding: aminocaproic acid (Amicar)
Tissue plasminogen activator (tPA)	Initiates dissolution of clots by breaking down fibrin	Hemorrhage, especially in the first 24 hr after administration	Minimize venipunctures; protect arterial line sites; assess for bleeding; monitor coagulation studies
Platelet Aggregation Inhibitors			
Aspirin	Reduces risk of stroke in male patients with recurrent transient ischemic attacks	Excessive bruising, bleeding; bronchoconstriction; nausea, vomiting, gastric bleeding, urticaria, confusion, drowsiness, tinnitus; contraindicated with oral anticoagulants	Monitor for side effects; tinnitus and confusion suggest overdosage; teach patients that aspirin can be harmful if not taken properly
Dipyridamole (Persantine)	Prevents thromboembolism with heart valve prostheses. Used with coumarin anticoagulants.	Hypotension, dizziness	Caution with hypotensive patients
Ticlopidine (Ticlid)	Prolongs bleeding time, decreasing the risk of stroke	Diarrhea, nausea, dyspepsia, rash; occasionally neutropenia, purpura, overdose: hypotension	Give with food or after meals; assess for bruising, signs of infection

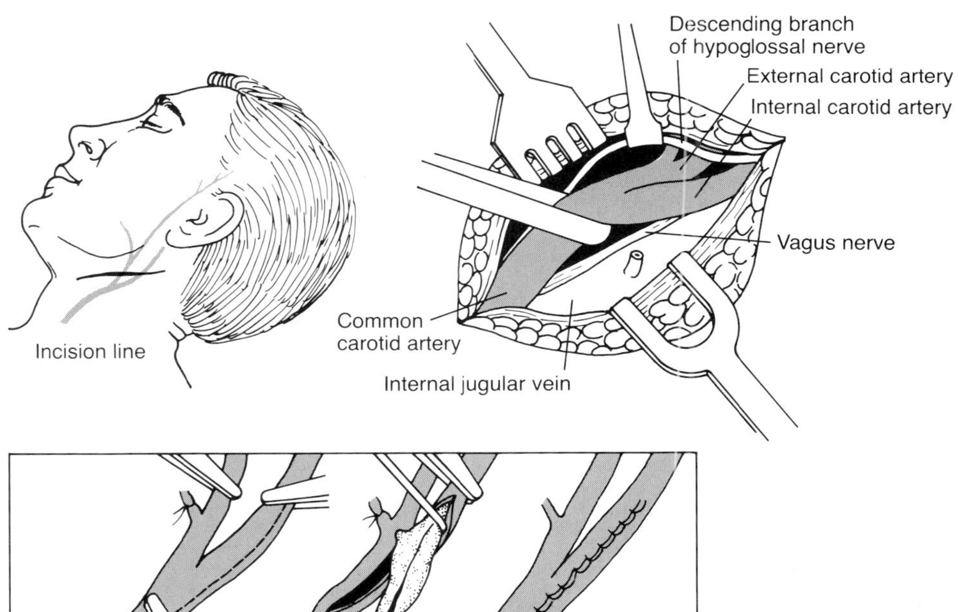

FIGURE 26-3
Carotid endarterectomy. Plaques are removed from the artery to improve blood flow. (Modified from Black, J. M., & Matassarin-Jacobs, E. [1993]. *Luckmann and Sorensen's medical-surgical nursing: A psychophysiologic approach* [4th ed.]. Philadelphia: W. B. Saunders.)

percent of stroke survivors return to work or productive lives within 1 year. These are important figures to remember when caring for the stroke patient.

PATHOPHYSIOLOGY

There are two main types of stroke: hemorrhagic and ischemic.

Hemorrhagic Stroke

Hemorrhagic stroke accounts for only about 20% of all strokes. In hemorrhagic stroke, a blood vessel in the brain ruptures and bleeding into the brain occurs. As a result, intracranial pressure may increase, disrupting normal cerebral function. Hemorrhagic strokes are further classified by location as intracerebral or subarachnoid hemorrhage.

Intracerebral (in the cerebrum) hemorrhage is frequently associated with uncontrolled hypertension. High pressure within the vessel simply breaks down the vessel structures.

A subarachnoid hemorrhage occurs between the arachnoid and pia mater layers of the brain covering. The pia mater is the thin membrane covering the brain. The arachnoid covers the pia mater. Subarachnoid hemorrhage may be due to congenital malformations of blood vessels in the brain or to rupture of an aneurysm.

Ischemic Stroke

Ischemic strokes, including embolic and thrombotic strokes, are the more common type affecting 80% of stroke patients.

An ischemic stroke is caused by the obstruction of a blood vessel, with subsequent impairment of blood flow to an area of the brain. Brain cells deprived of blood flow become ischemic and die. The effects of cell death depend on the functions of the affected cells.

The vascular obstruction is created by atherosclerotic plaques or blood clots. In an embolic stroke, the clot or plaque fragment is "traveling." It forms in some other area of the body and flows through the blood stream until it lodges in a cerebral artery. Cardiac disease is frequently a factor in the development of clots that become emboli. Patients with mitral valve stenosis, atrial fibrillation, or myocardial infarctions may develop emboli as complications of their cardiac conditions.

A thrombotic stroke develops from an obstruction that forms in a particular area in a blood vessel of the brain. Patients who have thrombotic strokes may have a history of TIAs. They may also experience stroke in evolution, or progressive stroke. In a progressive stroke, symptoms worsen over approximately 48 hours, indicating that further neurologic impairment is occurring. Figure 26–4 illustrates the development of each type of stroke.

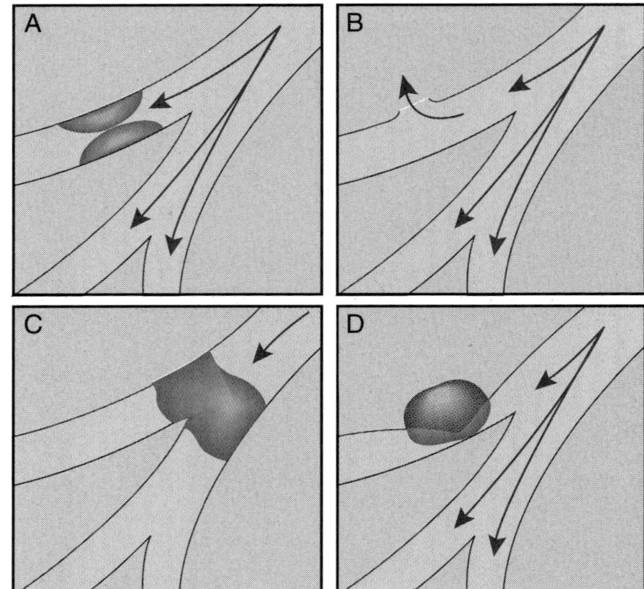

FIGURE 26–4

Causes of cerebrovascular accident *A*, Thrombus; *B*, hemorrhage; *C*, embolus; *D*, pressure.

SIGNS AND SYMPTOMS

There are some differences in signs and symptoms of stroke depending on the type, location, and extent of brain injury (Fig. 26–5). Symptoms of a hemorrhagic stroke, which generally occur suddenly, may include severe headache, stiff neck, and loss of consciousness. Vomiting and seizures may also occur.

Symptoms of an embolic stroke often appear without warning. The specific symptoms depend on the area of the brain affected by the lack of blood supply. One or more of the following signs and symptoms may be noted: one-sided weakness, numbness, visual problems, confusion and memory lapses, headache, dysphagia (difficulty swallowing), and language problems. Language problems may be in the form of difficulty understanding, speaking, or both.

The signs and symptoms of a thrombotic stroke may be the same as those seen in an embolic stroke. Because the obstruction forms in the same area in which it causes the occlusion, however, the symptoms tend to develop more gradually in a thrombotic stroke.

Regardless of the type of stroke, symptoms can be devastating. Some symptoms may improve with time and therapy, but others may be permanent. Long-term symptoms that require special attention are aphasia, dysarthria, dysphagia, dyspraxia, hemiplegia, homonymous hemianopsia, personality change, emotional lability, impaired cognition, and bladder dysfunction. Some signs and symptoms are dependent on whether the right or the left side of the brain is affected. Figure 26–5 compares right-sided and left-sided stroke.

Aphasia

The speech center is located in the dominant cerebral hemisphere so that it is in the left hemisphere for a right-handed person. When a person is left-handed, the speech center is usually located in the right hemisphere. Damage to this area may cause a stroke patient to

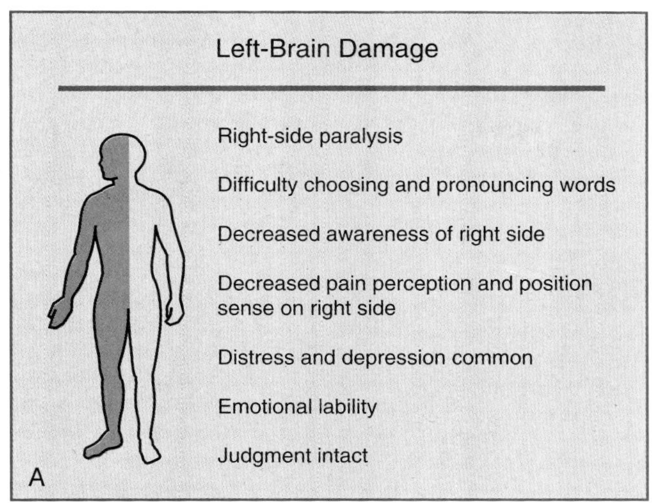

FIGURE 26–5
Comparison of right-sided and left-sided stroke.

become unable to communicate with others. Aphasia is a defect in the use of language that may impair speech, reading, writing, and comprehension of words. It is defined as receptive or expressive. The patient with receptive aphasia has difficulty understanding spoken or written words. The patient with expressive aphasia has difficulty responding appropriately. Although these types of aphasia are distinctly defined, most patients have a combination of both.

Aphasia may also be defined as fluent or nonfluent depending on the type of difficulty the patient has with speech. A patient with fluent aphasia speaks easily but makes little sense. A patient with nonfluent aphasia exerts considerable effort to initiate speech. Terms describing communication problems of the stroke patient are defined in Table 26–3.

Dysarthria

Dysarthria is defined as the inability to speak clearly. It is caused by neurologic damage that prevents normal control of muscles used in speech. Dysarthric patients may be assumed to be aphasic when they are unable to form appropriate speech with their mouths, despite comprehension and response ability. Facial weakness, usually one-sided, is a clue that the patient's speech difficulty is due to dysarthria rather than aphasia.

Dysphagia

Patients with dysarthria are also likely to have dysphagia (swallowing difficulty) that requires lengthy periods of rehabilitation. This is a very serious problem because of the risk of aspiration and because it can interfere with adequate nutrition. The problem of dysphagia can be especially discouraging for the patient when attempts to eat result in choking, frustration, and fear. Gastrostomy tubes are often inserted in these patients for long-term feeding purposes. Rehabilitation may include therapy to treat dysphagia.

Dyspraxia

Dyspraxia is the partial inability to initiate coordinated voluntary motor acts. Any part of the body with motor function may be affected. For instance, the patient may not be able to stand or walk or transfer to a chair without assistance despite the fact that the patient is not paralyzed.

TABLE 26–3
TYPES OF COMMUNICATION DISORDERS AFTER CEREBROVASCULAR ACCIDENT

TYPE	LOCATION OF BRAIN LESION	CHARACTERISTICS
Receptive aphasia	Wernicke's area	Unable to comprehend spoken or written words. Fluent: speaks easily but makes little sense.
Expressive aphasia	Broca's area	Difficulty speaking or writing. Nonfluent: much effort to initiate speech.
Dysarthria	Upper motor neurons	Speaks slowly with great effort. Words prolonged, hard to understand.

Dyspraxic patients may be able to spontaneously perform a motor act, yet be unable to initiate such an act willfully. This contradictory behavior can lead uninformed family, friends, or caretakers to assume the person is being "difficult." The difficulty initiating motor actions seen in dyspraxia is quite different from the inability to perform motor acts due to hemiplegia. The person who has apraxia can move the affected parts but cannot perform specific purposeful actions such as walking or dressing.

Hemiplegia

Hemiplegia is defined as paralysis of one side of the body. The affected side is opposite from the side of the brain in which the stroke occurred because nerve fibers in the brain cross over as they pass into the spinal cord (see Fig. 24–5). Initially, hemiplegia is characterized by flaccidity (decreased muscle tone) of the affected area. Eventually, flaccidity is replaced by spasticity (increased muscle tone). The extent of recovery from hemiplegia varies widely. Function may gradually improve to a point beyond which no further improvement occurs.

In hemiplegia, the stroke patient's sensory ability may also be impaired. Some hemiplegics with sensory involvement perceive every sensation to the affected area as painful. Patients may experience what is called *unilateral neglect,* in which they do not recognize one side as part of their bodies. Unilateral neglect is most common with right hemisphere damage and results in neglect of the left side of the body.

Homonymous Hemianopsia

Perceiving reality is especially complicated when visual disturbances accompany stroke. One of these perceptual problems is homonymous hemianopsia, which involves loss of one side of a field of vision. Homonymous hemianopsia translates to a half-blinded field of vision that occurs on the same side in both eyes, as illustrated in Figure 26–6. This problem can come to life dramatically when caring for the stroke patient who experiences it. At mealtime, the patient may leave half the plate untouched, the half on the affected side. Or the patient may shave his face completely on one side and leave whiskers untouched on his affected side.

Intellectual and Emotional Effects

Many patients experience emotional changes after a stroke, to the point of personality change from prestroke behavior. Emotional lability is a frequent problem after a stroke. The patient may be laughing and seemingly happy and suddenly burst into tears for no apparent reason. Angry outbursts, childlike behavior, and inappropriate sexual behavior may occur. Emotional changes such as these are thought to be caused by neurochemical imbalances in the brain or by loss of the brain's ability to inhibit inappropriate responses.

It has also been found that cognitive processes are slowed after a stroke even without readily apparent deficits in thinking and responses.

Elimination Disturbances

In the acute phase of stroke, and sometimes into the rehabilitation phase, the patient may experience a neurogenic bladder. A neurogenic bladder is flaccid and cannot empty completely.

Bowel incontinence is rarely a physiologic consequence of stroke. Confusion, disorientation, and immobility, however, may contribute to incontinent episodes.

RISK FACTORS

The primary risk factor for CVA is atherosclerosis—a buildup of lipid plaques in the intima of arteries. Factors that contribute to the development of atherosclerosis are hypertension, age, diabetes mellitus, and hyperlipidemia. Other factors that increase the risk of CVA are cardiac disease, atrial fibrillation, smoking (especially while taking oral contraceptives), and hypotension. Cerebrovascular accidents are more common in men than in women.

Fortunately, some risk factors can be eliminated and others controlled, thereby reducing the risk of CVA. Measures that may slow the progression of atherosclerosis include eating a healthy low-fat diet, exercising, stopping smoking, losing weight, and controlling hypertension. Good control of diabetes is advised, but the benefits in relation to preventing atherosclerosis are uncertain. Hypotension is most problematic for the elderly and can be avoided by maintaining good hydration, promptly treating blood loss, treating heart failure, and cautious monitoring of hypertensive drug therapy (Table 26–4).

MEDICAL DIAGNOSIS

When a patient is admitted to a hospital with a tentative diagnosis of a stroke, the following procedures may be ordered: blood studies, computed tomography (CT) scan, magnetic resonance imaging (MRI), positron emission tomography (PET) scan, cerebral and carotid angiography, electrocardiography, and cerebrospinal fluid examination.

Routine blood studies including complete blood count, chemistry panel, platelets, and coagulation studies may also be ordered to screen for alterations.

Brain scans (CT, MRI, PET) are useful in differentiating a hemorrhagic stroke from an ischemic stroke. Frequently, immediately following an ischemic stroke, no changes are noted on a CT scan. However, a hemor-

TABLE 26-4
MEASURES TO REDUCE THE RISK OF STROKE

1. Hypertension control.
2. Smoking cessation.
3. Treatment of atrial fibrillation.
4. Moderate alcohol consumption.
5. Detection and treatment of diabetes mellitus.
6. Dietary modification to lower serum cholesterol.

rhagic stroke produces a large dark mass on the scan. Cerebral and aortic angiography may be done to study blood vessels and to detect rupture or occlusion. Scans also are used to rule out tumors or other causes of the neurologic symptoms. A lumbar puncture may also be performed to distinguish between hemorrhage and ischemia. A lumbar puncture is *not* done if increased intracranial pressure is suspected. Grossly bloody cerebrospinal fluid indicates hemorrhage. This finding has important implications for treatment. No anticoagulants are ordered following hemorrhagic stroke. Table 26–1 summarizes diagnostic tests and procedures and nursing implications.

COMPLICATIONS

Stroke patients are at risk for many complications related to impaired neuromuscular function. The patient with severe motor impairment is at risk for constipation, dehydration, contractures, urinary tract infections, thrombophlebitis, decubitus ulcers, and pneumonia. Pneumonia is the most frequent cause of death after stroke.

Because stroke patients are typically middle-aged or elderly, they often have preexisting chronic conditions such as diabetes mellitus, heart disease, arthritis, or gastrointestinal disturbances. Management of these conditions must be taken into consideration during the acute phase of stroke.

PROGNOSIS FOR THE STROKE PATIENT

The prognosis for stroke patients is becoming increasingly hopeful. The critical variables that affect recovery are the patient's condition before the stroke, the length of time between the occurrence of stroke and the diagnosis, the support for the patient in the acute phase (usually the first 48 hours), the severity of the patient's symptoms, and the access to stimulating rehabilitative therapy. A stroke patient who is comatose for more than 36 hours has a poor chance of recovery. In addition, the recovery prospects for hemorrhagic stroke victims are significantly poorer than for ischemic stroke victims. Most recovery from stroke takes place in the first 3 months. After that time, improvement is usually slight.

The long-term recovery of the stroke patient may well depend on the care received immediately after the stroke. Therefore, the nurse's role in attending stroke patients is a vital one.

MEDICAL TREATMENT IN THE ACUTE PHASE OF STROKE

The acute phase of a stroke is defined as the time in which the patient's vital signs, particularly blood pressure, stabilize. Virtually every patient has high blood pressure during and immediately after a stroke. Blood pressure naturally decreases within 48 hours even without treatment.

A challenge for the physician is to provide for immediate care of acute problems while considering preexisting conditions as well. Chronic congestive heart failure or other cardiac problems need to be treated during the acute phase of a stroke.

Oxygen

Oxygenation is a priority immediately after a stroke, especially if the patient is unconscious. Oxygen therapy may be ordered. For patients who are comatose, tracheotomy is sometimes necessary to maintain an airway. Intubation and mechanical ventilation may be necessary to combat inadequate ventilatory effort. Respiratory exercises including incentive spirometry may be ordered for the alert patient.

Drug Therapy

Cerebral edema is sometimes treated with osmotic diuretics such as mannitol. In a newer treatment, a calcium channel blocker such as nimodipine (Nimotop) may be ordered after subarachnoid hemorrhage. Nimodipine prevents spasms in cerebral blood vessels that would impair blood flow. Corticosteroids may be prescribed to reduce intracranial pressure by reducing cerebral inflammation. Antithrombotic agents are used to prevent strokes caused by thrombi. They include acetylsalicylic acid (aspirin), dipyridamole (Persantine), sulfinpyrazone (Anturane), and ticlopidine hydrochloride (Ticlid). Tissue plasminogen activator (tPA) is being used experimentally to dissolve clots that cause acute ischemic stroke. Phenytoin (Dilantin) and phenobarbital are anticonvulsants that may be ordered if the patient has seizures. Powerful anticlotting drugs such as streptokinase are sometimes used. An experimental drug is ancrod (Arvin), a substance extracted from the venom of a pit viper that reduces blood viscosity and is given during the early signs of stroke to restore cerebral blood flow and limit the neurologic damage. Drugs used to prevent or treat CVA are included in Table 26–2.

Surgical Intervention

Surgical intervention is an option for some patients with hemorrhagic strokes. Decisions about surgery are based on the patient's age, the intracranial pressure, and the location of the hemorrhage.

Fluids and Nutrition

An order for intravenous fluids will probably be given for the stroke patient in the acute phase. This route provides fluids, electrolytes, and some calories and serves as an access for intravenous drugs. The dietary order is based on the patient's nutritional requirements and ability to eat normally. Food may be regular, soft, or pureed depending on how well the patient can chew and swallow. Vitamins and electrolyte supplementation may also be ordered.

For the malnourished patient, total parenteral nutrition may be ordered. Sometimes a nasogastric tube is inserted for feeding purposes. If long-term enteral feedings are indicated, a gastrostomy tube may be placed.

Urine Elimination

Sometimes an indwelling catheter is ordered to manage urinary incontinence. Intermittent catheterization is a method of controlling incontinence caused by the flaccid bladder that is less likely to lead to infection. This intermittent catheterization is done every 4 to 6 hours as ordered. The frequency of catheterization is based on the amount of urine obtained each time.

NURSING CARE IN THE ACUTE PHASE OF STROKE

The most important aspects of care during the acute phase of a stroke are assessment and support. Management in this phase focuses on maintenance or improvement of vital physiologic functions (see Care Plan: The Stroke Patient).

Assessment

The nursing assessment enables the nurse to recognize risk factors for CVA and to identify nursing care needs. It also provides a record of baseline data for comparison. Details of the neurologic assessment are covered in Chapter 25 and summarized in Table 25–3. Data specific to the stroke patient are presented here.

HEALTH HISTORY. The health history may be obtained from the patient or from a family member if the patient is too ill or is unable to communicate. On introduction to the stroke patient, the nurse begins to assess the patient's ability to understand language and to respond verbally and nonverbally. Responses to simple yes or no commands provide a good basis for initial assessment. Verbal responses, facial expressions, and physical reactions should be evaluated for appropriateness. If responses are not appropriate, try to identify the source of difficulty. Does the patient have trouble finding words? Do clues help the patient respond? Does the patient speak intelligibly but show little comprehension of the nurse's words? If the patient cannot provide the data needed, the nurse attempts to obtain them from a family member or friend. The informant (person who provides the history) should be noted.

Chief Complaint and History of Present Illness. In the history of the present illness, the nurse assesses the events that led the patient to seek medical care. A complete description of the illness includes the initial symptoms and how the symptoms progressed.

Past Medical History. The nurse records past serious illnesses or conditions, including hypertension, heart disease, diabetes mellitus, liver disease, gout, head trauma, and previous strokes or TIAs. Hospitalization, surgeries, and injuries are noted.

Family History. The health history documents a family history of neurologic or vascular disease as well as strokes.

Review of Systems. The patient is asked about significant problems in the review of systems. Important data to assess include weakness, impaired movement, pain (especially headache), dysphagia, bowel or bladder incontinence, visual disturbances, mental-emotional changes, and altered sensation.

Functional Assessment. The last component of the health history, the functional assessment, determines the patient's usual activities and health practices. The nurse inquires about activity level, dietary pattern, occupation, use of alcohol and tobacco, drug use, interpersonal relationships, and current stressors.

PHYSICAL EXAMINATION. During the physical examination, the nurse observes the patient's general appearance, responsiveness, and behavior. The level of consciousness is important because a decreasing level of consciousness suggests a stroke in evolution or increasing intracranial pressure. Vital signs, height, and weight are measured. The breathing pattern and effort are especially important.

The face is inspected for symmetry. The mouth is assessed for moisture and drooling. The ability to swallow is assessed in the alert patient. The pupils are inspected for size, equality, and reaction to light. By asking the patient to read something, the nurse conducts a gross vision assessment. The skin is inspected for color and palpated for moisture and turgor. Extremities are assessed for muscle tone and strength, sensation, and voluntary movement. The nurse instructs the patient to move each extremity individually and observes whether responses to commands are understood. Impaired movement may be due to aphasia or dyspraxia as well as to neuromuscular damage. The patient who has aphasia has difficulty interpreting the messages and may not perform the requested movement for that reason. The patient with dyspraxia may comprehend the instruction but be unable to direct the body part to move. Any evidence of incontinence or bladder distension should also be recorded.

Neurologic checks are repeated frequently and consist of evaluating level of consciousness, pupil appearance and response to light, response to commands, and movement and sensation of extremities. For additional neurologic assessment, see Chapter 25.

Nursing assessment of the stroke patient is summarized in Table 26–5.

Nursing Diagnosis

The nursing diagnoses following a CVA vary considerably with the location and extent of brain damage. The nursing diagnoses must be based on individual assessments. Appropriate diagnoses may include the following:

- **Ineffective Airway Clearance** related to impaired cough reflex, altered consciousness, impaired swallowing
- **Ineffective Breathing Patterns** related to impaired cerebral circulation, increased intracranial pressure
- **High Risk for Injury** related to seizure activity, confusion, motor impairment
- **Fluid Volume Deficit** related to inadequate intake or excessive diuresis

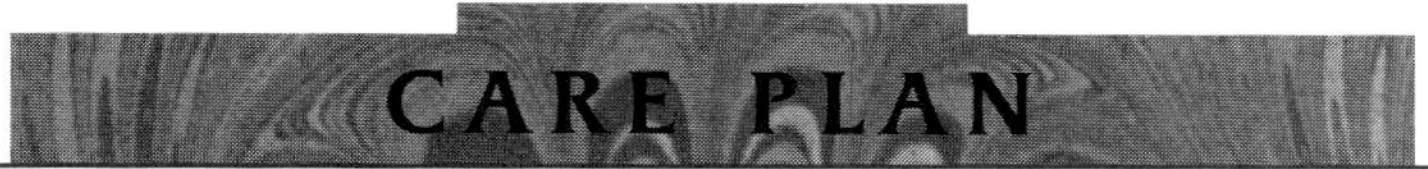

CARE PLAN

The Stroke Patient

ASSESSMENT

Health History: Mr. Gonzales is an obese 82-year-old Latino male. Admitted with weakness on right side and slurred speech. Daughter assisted with health history since patient had some difficulty responding verbally. Has had type 1 diabetes mellitus for 10 years, which he treats with oral hypoglycemic agent. Myocardial infarction at age 75. No changes in vision but does wear reading glasses; good hearing, no headaches. Is right-handed. Was unable to stand when he awoke this morning. Tried to drink some water but had difficulty swallowing. No loss of bowel or bladder control. Mr. Gonzales is divorced. An adult daughter and her two teenagers live with him. He is a retired construction worker whose hobbies are carpentry and watching television.

Physical Examination: Vital signs: Temperature, 97°F orally; pulse, 96; respirations, 22; blood pressure, 210/104. Patient is alert. Acknowledges he is in the hospital but is uncertain about day or date and time. Uses gestures to respond to some questions when he seems unable to find the right word. Pupils are equal and react to light. Ptosis of right eyelid. Hand grips, voluntary movements, and reflexes of leg, arm, and hand are normal on left side but diminished on right side. Leans toward right side.

NURSING DIAGNOSIS	GOALS AND OUTCOME CRITERIA	INTERVENTIONS
Fluid volume deficit related to inadequate intake, dysphagia.	The patient will maintain adequate hydration as evidenced by moist mucous membranes, dilute urine, pulse and blood pressure within his usual range.	Record fluid intake and output. Administer intravenous fluids as ordered. Monitor oral fluid intake and assess swallowing. Assist patient to sit up while eating and drinking. If thin fluids are difficult to swallow, try semisolids such as ice cream, puddings, popsicles. Have oral suction device available in case of choking or aspiration. Detect and report signs and symptoms of fluid volume deficit: tachycardia, concentrated urine, dry mucous membranes.
Altered nutrition: less than body requirements related to dysphagia, inability to feed self.	The patient will maintain adequate nutrition as evidenced by stable weight.	Assess food intake. Assist with meals as needed. Seat upright for meals. Do not make him feel rushed. Provide alternative means of feeding (nasogastric or gastrostomy tube, total parenteral nutrition) as ordered. Weigh weekly to assess adequacy of food intake.
Impaired verbal communication related to aphasia.	The patient will use nonverbal means to supplement verbal communication and will participate in speech therapy exercises.	Establish a code system of blinks or nods for nonverbal communication. Use pictures or cards that patient can select to express his needs. Encourage verbalization but recognize frustration and provide words if patient cannot retrieve them. Discuss referral for speech therapy with physician. Tell the patient that improvement is usually possible with therapy.
Impaired physical activity related to weakness, paralysis, poor balance.	The patient will maintain intact skin, joint mobility, regular bowel and bladder elimination, good peripheral circulation, and normal breath sounds.	While on bedrest, assist him to change positions at least every 2 hours. He should not lie on his right side for more than 30 minutes at a time. Use positioning techniques and devices to reduce pressure points. Inspect skin for redness and edema associated with pressure, and massage gently around pressure areas. Position limbs in functional alignment and perform range of motion exercises three times a day. Do not pull on the affected side. Monitor bowel and bladder function.

Care Plan Continued

The Stroke Patient *(Continued)*

NURSING DIAGNOSIS	GOALS AND OUTCOME CRITERIA	INTERVENTIONS
		Administer stool softeners and laxatives as ordered. Encourage fluids and fiber when able to take orally. Palpate lower abdomen for bladder distention and catheterize as ordered as necessary. Assess for Homans's sign. Report tenderness, pain, or swelling in calves. Exercise legs with each position change. Apply elastic stockings or alternating pressure wraps as ordered. Ambulate when able. Encourage coughing and deep breathing with each position change. Assess lung fields for atelectasis, wheezes, or rales. Report temperature elevation.
High risk for injury related to paralysis.	The patient will have no falls or injuries associated with motor impairment or altered sensory perception.	Keep the bed in low position with the siderails raised. Put the call button in reach and instruct patient to call for help to get up. Check on him frequently. Monitor position of affected extremities to prevent trauma that might not be detected because of poor sensation. Use sling or brace if ordered to support affected limbs. Assess effects of ptosis on vision. If vision is impaired, approach patient from unaffected side and arrange personal articles on that side. When patient is out of bed, be sure he is seated safely. Use pillows to prevent excessive leaning to one side. When ambulatory, use gait belt if needed and assist as appropriate.
Anxiety related to loss of function or fear of disability.	The patient will have a reduction in anxiety as evidenced by calm manner and patient statement.	Acknowledge signs of anxiety and attempt to identify sources. Provide information about what is happening, what you are doing, and what he can expect. Check on him often. Encourage family to visit.
Altered family processes related to anticipated need of patient for assistance after discharge.	The patient and family will plan for altered roles and responsibilities to support the patient during and after discharge.	Give family members an opportunity to ask questions and share their concerns. Provide information and facilitate communication with physician as needed. Refer to sources of support and resources including social worker and community agencies. Start planning for discharge. Assess family strengths and resources, willingness to help care for patient after discharge. Identify new responsibilities they might need to assume and discuss how these can be carried out.

- **Fluid Volume Excess** related to overhydration
- **Altered Nutrition: Less than Body Requirements** related to dysphagia, inability to feed self, inability to chew
- **Sensory Perceptual Alterations** related to neurologic impairment
- **Ineffective Thermoregulation** related to effects of neurologic impairment
- **Altered Thought Processes** related to impaired cerebral circulation
- **Impaired Verbal Communication** related to aphasia
- **Impaired Physical Mobility** related to weakness, paralysis, spasticity, impaired balance
- **Total or Functional Incontinence** related to impaired control, inability to manage toileting process
- **Colonic Constipation** related to immobility, dehydration, drug side effects
- **Bowel Incontinence** related to impaired conduction of impulses

TABLE 26-5

ASSESSMENT OF THE CEREBROVASCULAR ACCIDENT PATIENT

HEALTH HISTORY

Source of data: Reliability and ability of patient to provide information

Present illness: Description of onset and progression

Past medical history: Cardiovascular conditions, liver disorder, diabetes mellitus, gout, previous cerebrovascular accidents, head injury, current medications

Family history: Neurologic or vascular conditions

Review of systems: Visual disturbances, motor or sensory impairments, pain, dysphagia, incontinence, mental-emotional changes

Functional assessment: Usual activities, diet, occupation, use of alcohol and tobacco, interpersonal relationships, stressors

PHYSICAL EXAMINATION

General appearance: Level of consciousness, behavior, gait, posture

Height and weight

Vital signs: Blood pressure, temperature, pulse, respiration

Face: Symmetry

Eyes: Pupil size, equality, alignment, reaction to light; gross visual acuity, eyelid closure, ptosis

Skin: Moisture, turgor, color

Abdomen: Bowel or bladder distention

Genitalia and anus: Presence or odor of urine or stool

Extremities: Muscle tone, strength, voluntary movement, sensation

- **Ineffective Individual Coping** related to adapting to neurologic deficits
- **Altered Family Processes** related to disruption of family roles and functions

Goals

The goals of nursing care for the stroke patient include patent airway, normal respiratory rate and depth, absence of injury, adequate hydration, adequate intake of nutrients, adaptation to sensory perceptual alterations, body temperature within patient's normal range, orientation to self and environment, effective communication, absence of complications of immobility, controlled urine elimination, regular voluntary bowel elimination, use of effective coping strategies, and adaptation of the family to the patient's condition.

Interventions

INEFFECTIVE AIRWAY CLEARANCE AND INEFFECTIVE BREATHING PATTERNS. The patient's respiratory status must be monitored closely. Maintaining an open airway is essential for patients who have suffered strokes. Neurologic deficits may cause altered breathing patterns and impaired swallowing, gag, and cough reflexes. Increasing intracranial pressure may affect the respiratory center in the brain causing respiratory depression. If the patient exhibits signs of increased intracranial pressure (rising blood pressure, bradycardia, abnormal pupil response, decreasing level of consciousness), the head of the bed is elevated 30 degrees and the physician is notified.

The stroke patient is at risk for airway obstruction for a number of reasons. If the patient is unconscious, the tongue may fall back and block the airway. A side-lying position helps to prevent such obstruction. An oral or nasal airway is sometimes employed to keep the airway open.

Immobility and dehydration cause thick secretions to be retained in the respiratory tract, possibly leading to pneumonia and atelectasis. Good hydration helps to thin respiratory secretions for easier expectoration. Dysphagia may cause the patient to aspirate fluids or food, causing airway obstruction and contributing to the development of pneumonia. Pneumonia is, in fact, the most frequent cause of death after stroke. Feeding the patient with dysphagia is discussed in Chapter 12.

Suctioning and frequent position changes can help prevent aspiration and promote drainage of secretions. Respiratory treatments for the patient, with regular reminders to do deep breathing exercises, can be helpful. Forceful coughing may be discouraged in the acute phase after a hemorrhagic stroke. The nurse should ask the physician if and when coughing is permitted. Oxygen therapy is administered as ordered.

HIGH RISK FOR INJURY. Many factors place the stroke patient at risk for injury. Seizures may occur, causing the patient to lose consciousness and to have abnormal motor activity. Side rails are raised and padded according to agency protocol to reduce the trauma if the patient should strike the rails. During a seizure, the nurse turns the patient to one side and moves hard objects away from the patient. An oral airway may be placed if the patient's teeth are not clenched. Nothing should ever be forced between clenched teeth. To do so may injure the teeth and gums. Additional information about seizures is presented in Chapter 25.

Safety precautions also are essential for confused patients and patients with motor impairments. The nurse orients the patient to the surroundings and explains why the patient should not get up unassisted. The staff must respond promptly to the patient's calls for help. Although restraints are needed at times, they should be used as a last resort because they often agitate the patient and can actually cause injuries. Sufficient help should be available to assist the patient in and out of the bed.

FLUID VOLUME EXCESS OR DEFICIT. Close monitoring of fluid status is especially important in the acute phase of stroke. Accurate intake and output records are essential. Vital signs are taken and compared for trends suggesting fluid volume excess or deficit. The mouth is assessed for moisture. In a well-hydrated person the mucous membranes of the mouth are moist. Tissue turgor is evaluated, but it is not a very reliable indicator of fluid status in the older person. Age-related changes in the skin and subcutaneous structures cause a loss of tissue elasticity that may be mistaken for dehydration. Laboratory studies, including urine specific gravity, serum electrolytes, and hematocrit, are also useful indicators of fluid balance.

The patient is at risk for fluid volume excess, or overhydration, if excessive intravenous fluids are administered or the patient's kidneys are unable to eliminate excess fluid rapidly enough. Fluid volume excess may lead to edema and heart failure. Signs of fluid volume excess are fluid intake greater than output, bounding pulse, venous distention, increased blood pressure, crackles in the lungs, and edema. Evidence of excess fluid is reported to the physician. The rate of intravenous fluid may be decreased and diuretics given as ordered.

PHARMACOLOGY CAPSULE

Intake and output must be monitored while the patient is receiving intravenous fluids and drugs that reduce cerebral edema.

The patient is at risk for fluid volume deficit, or dehydration, for several reasons. The stroke patient is likely to be older, and older people are less able to conserve water through the kidneys. Also, dysphagia may occur, causing the patient's intake of oral fluids to be inadequate. If diuretics are given for fluid volume excess or increased intracranial pressure, they can precipitate excess loss of water and electrolytes. Fluid volume deficit contributes to constipation, skin dryness, and urinary tract infections and stones. Signs of fluid volume deficit are thready pulse, tachycardia, low blood pressure, low urine output, concentrated urine, dry mucous membranes, and sometimes confusion. Evidence of fluid volume deficit is reported to the physician. If intravenous fluids are being administered, the physician may order an increase in the hourly flow rate. Fluids may also be given through enteral feeding tubes. If the patient is able to take oral fluids but has difficulty swallowing, the nurse must allow time to support the patient while fluids are taken slowly. A suction machine should be on hand in case of aspiration.

ALTERED NUTRITION. The patient's nutritional status is of concern throughout stroke treatment. The patient who is malnourished is at risk for skin breakdown and infection. Obesity hampers mobility and can interfere with rehabilitation.

The patient who has dysphagia may not be able to consume adequate nutrients orally. Sometimes, a nasogastric tube is inserted for feeding purposes. The physician may order total parenteral nutrition for the malnourished patient. Aggressive treatment of dysphagia is delayed until the rehabilitative phase. Feeding the dysphagic patient is discussed in Chapter 34.

If the patient has a nasogastric or nasointestinal feeding tube, the nurse provides the correct formula and ensures that it flows at the prescribed rate. Pumps are often used to control the rate of flow, but bolus feedings may be ordered. The nurse provides the correct feeding and monitors the rate of administration. The head of the bed is elevated slightly to reduce the risk of fluid flowing back into the esophagus and being aspirated.

The tube irritates the naris and the nasal passages. The naris should be gently cleaned several times a day. Placement of the tube must be assessed according to agency policy. Concentrated formulas may cause diarrhea. If that happens, the physician is consulted about ordering dilution of the formula.

Total parenteral nutrition is given through an intravenous line inserted into a large vein (a central line). As with enteral feedings, the flow of total parenteral nutrition fluids is usually controlled with a pump. The nurse hangs new bottles of prescribed fluids. Special care is taken to prevent air entering the tubing. The insertion site also requires special care to prevent infection. Dressing changes are done according to agency protocol, using strict aseptic technique. Patients on total parenteral nutrition may develop hyperglycemia; therefore, blood glucose is monitored at regular intervals. Care of the patient receiving total parenteral nutrition is discussed in detail in Chapter 12.

SENSORY PERCEPTUAL ALTERATIONS. Sensory perceptual problems in the stroke patient may include visual disturbances, sensory deprivation or overload, and impaired tactile sensation. Among the visual disturbances are diplopia (double vision), loss of the corneal (blink) reflex, ptosis (drooping of the upper eyelid), homonymous hemianopsia, and inability to close the eyelids on the affected side. All of these pose threats to safety and to self-care. They may also contribute to confusion. The cornea is susceptible to injury when not protected and kept moist by the closed eyelid. The eyelid may be closed and patched to prevent corneal damage. Artificial tears may be used to provide moisture.

Patients who have homonymous hemianopsia see only half the field of vision. Some patients have unilateral neglect, a condition in which visual fields are intact but the patient does not attend to certain parts of the fields. Unilateral neglect is most common in patients with right brain damage. These patients may not care for one side of the body and may overlook objects on one side of the visual fields.

Encouragement to scan the affected side is helpful to these patients. Differences in the nursing approaches during the acute and rehabilitative phases are well contrasted here. In the acute phase, stroke patients with homonymous hemianopsia are positioned so that their unimpaired side is approached by the staff to reduce stress to the patient. In rehabilitation, the patient may be positioned so that deliberate scanning and use of the affected side is required. This is designed to stimulate return of function.

Balanced sensory input is essential to reduce the risk of sensory deprivation or overload. The environment should be pleasant but not overly stimulating.

Another type of sensory disturbance after stroke is diminished sensation in affected body parts. The patient who does not feel pressure or pain is susceptible to injury. A paralyzed foot can easily slip down into the side rails. Catheter tubing under the leg may create pressure that the patient cannot feel. The nurse must protect susceptible areas and remind the patient of the need for extra caution. Positioning of extremities should be checked to ensure that they are free of pressure.

INEFFECTIVE THERMOREGULATION. After a stroke, the body's temperature-regulating mechanism may be impaired, causing the temperature to rise. The nurse monitors the patient's temperature. Fever is treated aggressively with antipyretics and, if necessary, cooling blankets.

ALTERED THOUGHT PROCESSES. Stroke patients may suffer functional losses, alterations in sensation and perception, and impaired communication. In addition, they find themselves in the hospital where they are poked, monitored, and prodded by strangers and where days and nights all seem the same. All these factors combined can cause the stroke patient to become disoriented or confused.

Nurses can orient patients by introducing themselves, reminding patients where they are, why, and what is being done. Nurses should be sure that eyeglasses and hearing aids are worn if the patient normally uses them. Clocks and marked calendars are placed in view. The nurse tells the patient what time it is and what to expect next. Confused patients require frequent reassurance and reinforcement. Instructions and information need to be concise and repeated as needed. Sometimes a familiar person is helpful with a confused patient. The visitor may be disturbed by the patient's behavior, so the nurse provides guidance in how to deal with the patient.

IMPAIRED VERBAL COMMUNICATION. The alert stroke patient who has aphasia is understandably anxious about the inability to speak or to understand words, or both. Once the nurse has assessed communication deficits, adaptations in approaches are needed. The nurse uses brief, clear statements accompanied by gestures, pictures, and expressions. Questions that can be answered "yes" or "no" may allow the patient to respond more easily. The nurse should pause attentively when the patient struggles to respond. Excessive chatter can be distressing to the aphasic patient. The communication problem and approaches should be explained to the family. Speech therapy is usually not initiated until after the acute phase of the stroke. Speech rehabilitation is discussed further in Nursing Care in the Rehabilitation Phase of Stroke.

IMPAIRED PHYSICAL MOBILITY. Impaired motor function is common after stroke and places the patient at risk for complications of immobility. Care of the immobilized patient is discussed in detail in Chapter 19 and is summarized here.

Skin Integrity. The potential for skin breakdown in the stroke patient is great. Factors that contribute to this risk include motor impairment, altered consciousness or sensation, poor nutritional status, and incontinence.

Measures to maintain skin integrity include cleanliness, pressure relief, and good hydration and nutrition. When skin is dry, as it often is in older patients, bathing frequency should be reduced, soap should be used sparingly, and lotions should be applied to retain skin moisture.

One of the most important needs of the acute stroke patient is to be turned and repositioned at least every 2 hours. Breakdown can occur in vulnerable pressure points after just 30 minutes. If reddened pressure areas remain when it is time to turn the patient, the intervals between turning should be shortened. The stroke patient should not be allowed to lie on the affected side for more than 30 minutes. Because of impaired sensation, the risk of excessive pressure and trauma is much greater on that side.

Pressure must be alternated on main pressure points such as hips, knees, heels, and lower back. An air flotation mattress or fluidized bed may be used for the high-risk patient. Some of the newer therapeutic beds automatically turn patients. These beds do not stress the usual pressure points of the patient, but regular skin assessments and breathing exercises are still required. As soon as possible, the patient should be positioned comfortably in a chair for brief periods.

Good nursing care is time consuming, and the nurse can use this time to stimulate the patient with conversation and explanations of care. This is important even if the patient is unresponsive. Communicating the need for care activities to the patient is also an essential aspect of recovery.

Joint Mobility. The immobilized patient is at risk for muscle atrophy and joint contractures. In the stroke patient, the affected side is especially vulnerable when there is loss of voluntary movement. During the acute phase, the nurse is most concerned with maintaining joint mobility. This can be done by frequent gentle range of motion exercises and proper positioning. The nurse should determine whether the patient had any previous limitation of joint mobility because the older patient may have arthritic changes that reduce the range of motion. The nurse should be careful not to force resistant joints. Once the acute phase has passed, the patient is usually referred for vigorous physical therapy.

It is important never to grab or pull the extremities on the stroke patient's affected side. Dislocation or further injury can easily occur, as the patient cannot accurately perceive the pressure or pain that is normally felt.

Circulation. Another possible complication of immobility is deep vein thrombosis. Regular passive and active range of motion exercises encourage venous blood return, thereby reducing the risk of thrombus formation.

The physician may order elastic stockings or alternating pressure wraps to promote venous return. Ambulation is generally encouraged (if the patient is able) as soon as possible after the blood pressure stabilizes.

URINARY INCONTINENCE. It is not unusual for urinary incontinence to occur after stroke. This is due to a temporarily flaccid bladder. The patient is checked hourly for wetness. Wet clothing and linens are removed promptly. The skin is washed, rinsed, and patted dry. A variety of incontinence products are available to minimize the contact of urine with the skin (see Chapter 21). Sometimes an indwelling catheter is ordered to prevent incontinence. The catheter protects the skin and allows for more accurate measurement of output. The disadvantage is that an indwelling catheter is frequently the cause of urinary tract infection, which may further compromise the stroke patient. A regular toileting schedule with intermittent catheterization is a positive alternative to indwelling catheterization. External condom catheters are options for male patients. Bladder retraining, discussed in Chapter 21, is actively pursued in the rehabilitative phase.

Many older men have prostatic hypertrophy, which can cause dribbing or urine retention. Scheduled toileting may be helpful, but catheterization with a coudé or hard-tipped catheter may be required. The enlarged prostate makes catheterization more difficult. If the catheter cannot be inserted easily, it should never be forced. The physician should be notified.

COLONIC CONSTIPATION OR BOWEL INCONTINENCE. During the acute phase of stroke, it is especially important to monitor bowel elimination. It is helpful to know the patient's usual patterns, although this cannot always be determined.

Constipation may develop as a result of immobility, dehydration, and drug therapy. Incontinence, especially with loose or liquid stools, can signal a fecal impaction. Removal of an impaction usually requires repeated enemas and manual removal of hard stool. A bowel program, consisting of a mild laxative or stool softener and a high fiber diet, can assist with regular fecal elimination. It is important that the patient take in fluids sufficient to prevent dry stools.

Some older people are laxative dependent. It is unrealistic to try to reverse the effects of years of laxative use during the acute phase of stroke. The nurse informs the physician of the situation and documents bowel movements. Laxatives and enemas may be required to maintain bowel elimination.

Bowel incontinence can usually be prevented in the alert patient by regular toileting. The patient is taken to the toilet at the usual time of defecation. A raised toilet seat with arm rests is easier and safer for the patient with hemiplegia. If incontinence occurs, the nurse must take special care to clean the skin thoroughly. Caregivers must be careful not to make comments that embarrass the patient. Restoration of bowel control receives more attention in the rehabilitative phase and is detailed in Chapter 21.

INEFFECTIVE INDIVIDUAL COPING. The effects of stroke may be temporary or permanent, but it is difficult to predict how much function will be lost. Patients typically exhibit responses that reflect the grief process: shock, denial, depression, withdrawal, and bargaining. The nurse tries to understand how the patient is coping and to determine if the coping strategies are constructive. An example of unhealthy coping is the patient who denies having problems with vision or balance and refuses to call for help when getting out of bed. Or the patient who is depressed and withdrawn may resist doing therapeutic exercises that would minimize complications. The nurse can point out the patient's behavior and its consequences and encourage the patient to be actively involved in steps toward rehabilitation. Sometimes a mental health counselor or support group is needed to help the patient learn to deal with the effects of stroke more constructively.

ALTERED FAMILY PROCESSES. In the acute phase of stroke, family members are often frightened and confused. The may fear the patient's death or severe disability. They may also experience emotional and financial strain during the long rehabilitation process. Family members have to assume roles and responsibilities normally carried by the patient. Nurses must recognize that the family, as well as the patient, experiences a sense of loss when a loved one has a stroke. The nurse provides support by telling family members what is happening, what is being done, and how they can help the patient. If necessary, a referral may be made to the social worker, mental health specialist, or spiritual counselor.

Evaluation

Criteria for evaluating the effects of nursing care after stroke include normal respiratory rate and rhythm, with clear breath sounds; balanced intake and output of fluids, maintenance of body weight; successful adjustment to sensory perceptual changes as evidenced by ability to perform self-care; orientation to person, place, and time; ability to communicate needs; maintenance of joint mobility and absence of skin breakdown; voluntary control of voiding; regular voluntary bowel elimination; patient's statements of acceptance of stroke effects and intention to strive for recovery; and family's demonstration of willingness and ability to adapt to patient's condition.

NURSING CARE IN THE REHABILITATION PHASE OF STROKE

A patient's transition from the acute phase to the rehabilitation phase of stroke is an important one. Research findings have shown that early and attentive care for the stroke patient decreases the length of recovery time and increases the return of functioning. The general goal of treatment in the rehabilitation phase is restoration of self-care ability.

The stabilization of the stroke patient's vital signs, with no further observed neurologic deficits, indicates that the patient has entered the chronic phase of stroke. At this time, the patient's functional and cognitive problems can vary widely, depending on the location of the stroke in the brain and the amount of tissue damage caused by lack of blood supply. The stroke patient may regain complete independent functioning, partially recover previous abilities, or lose functional abilities completely.

The rehabilitation phase is usually managed by an interdisciplinary team. The team is composed of health care professionals such as nurses, physicians, physical therapists, occupational therapists, speech therapists, social workers, psychologists, recreational therapists, vocational rehabilitation counselors, and dietitians.

Although any improvement in functional ability may be small, vast changes can occur in the brain. Collateral blood circulation and alternative neuronal pathways may be developing at great speed. These processes determine the ultimate recovery of the patient. The goal of rehabilitation for stroke patients is to enhance this ultimate recovery of functional abilities through a program of stimulation and practice. It has been said that rehabilitation is the respectful challenging of the patient facing a chronic health problem. With this emphasis, the next section describes nursing care in the management of long-term problems that can follow a stroke.

Assessment

Nursing assessment of the stroke patient is described earlier in this chapter. In the rehabilitation phase, the nurse also assesses the patient's abilities, expectations, knowledge, motivation, and resources.

Nursing Diagnosis

Nursing diagnoses in the rehabilitation phase of stroke may include the following:

- **Self-Care Deficits** related to sensory and motor impairments
- **High Risk for Injury** related to vision and motor impairments
- **Ineffective Individual Coping** related to cognitive impairments
- **Impaired Verbal Communication** related to aphasia, dysphasia
- **Altered Nutrition: Less than Body Requirements** related to dysphagia, anorexia
- **Impaired Physical Mobility** related to residual motor impairment
- **Colonic Constipation** related to inactivity
- **Total and Functional Incontinence** related to neurologic and motor impairment

Goals

Goals of nursing care in the rehabilitation phase of stroke are increasing independence in activities of daily living, absence of injury, effective individual coping, effective communication, adequate nutrition, improved physical mobility, normal bowel elimination, and normal urine elimination.

Interventions

SELF-CARE DEFICITS. The main focus of the rehabilitation phase is to return the stroke patient to the highest level of functioning possible. Probably the most frustrating part of a stroke for many patients and caregivers is the patient's inability to complete activities of daily living. Progress requires patients to use affected parts as much as they are able.

It is important to allow time for patients to try to do things for themselves. This requires patience and a supportive attitude from the caregiver. Discouragement is a major factor in unsuccessful rehabilitation and should be addressed promptly.

Many personal devices and environmental adaptations can foster a return to independence. Prosthetic devices that assist patients with dressing, bathing, and eating are available. Simple measures such as replacing buttons with Velcro and replacing complicated trousers with elastic-waist pants can make a big difference.

Safety and accessibility of the home environment should be assessed before discharge. A home visit by the patient, nurse, and occupational therapist can be made to identify problems and make plans for adaptations. Adaptations should promote access in and out of the home and enable patients to be as independent as possible. Toileting and bathing may be facilitated by the addition of bars on bathroom walls or raised commode seats or appliances. Cooking may be assisted by adjusting the height of counters or improving access to shelves and cupboards. Patients need to practice daily tasks under conditions similar to those at home. Rehabilitation centers usually have activity centers that allow patients to practice self-care skills with their disabilities (Fig. 26–6).

HIGH RISK FOR INJURY. Alterations in sensation and vision are distressing changes that affect the patient's ability to carry out self-care and pose a threat to safety.

Sensation. As noted previously, stroke patients may have altered sensation in the affected body parts. This may appear as loss of sensation or as exaggerated response in which every sensation is perceived as painful. The stroke patient may be injured without even knowing it because of impaired sensation. When sensation is diminished, the patient must learn to assess the area frequently for signs of pressure and to protect it from injury. In addition to avoiding pressure, the patient is advised not to apply heat or cold to that area. Caregivers must also remember not to pull on the affected side or use it to move or support the patient.

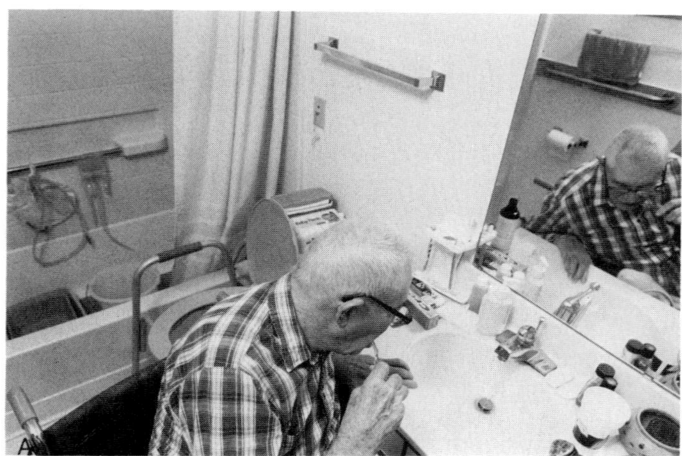

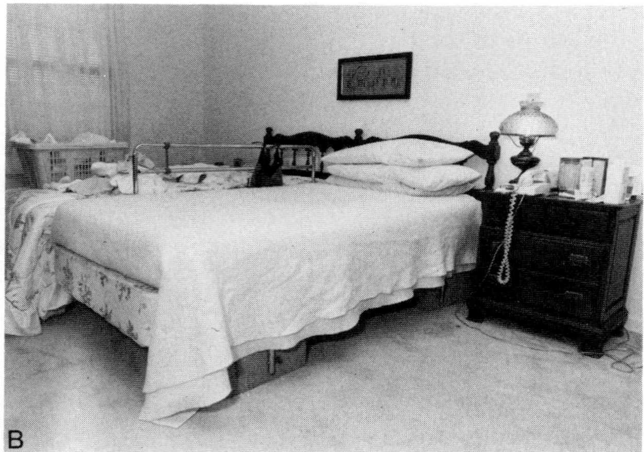

FIGURE 26-6
The home can be adapted to promote independence after a stroke.

Patients with abnormal pain perception may benefit from regular physical therapy, using a kind of desensitization. During therapy, the patient is reminded and encouraged that the pain is not real and is only misinterpreted by the brain.

Vision. Homonymous hemianopsia, in which half of the field of vision is lost, also presents problems with self-care and safety. In the acute phase, the environment is arranged so that people approach and important items are available on the unaffected side. In rehabilitation, care is shifted to a more challenging mode to promote adaptation to the disability. Things are placed in the field of visual deficit, and the patient is reminded and encouraged to scan the affected side, especially when walking, wheeling, and eating. The patient forms new habits of observation through constant practice.

INEFFECTIVE INDIVIDUAL COPING. Intellectual and emotional changes after stroke are distressing to patients and their families. The nurse needs to explain these changes and to demonstrate how to help patients adapt. Because cognitive processes may continue to be slow, the nurse is careful not to rush or frustrate the patient. Emotional lability is manifested as sudden laughing, crying, or outbursts of anger without apparent reason. Caregivers and families may attribute this emotional unpredictability to depression. It is generally believed that depression is always associated with brain trauma, so that explanation is possibly correct. However, the patient can usually be easily distracted from crying or from anger with simple redirection to the task at hand. This is an indication that the depression, if it exists, is of a different type than the usual emotional state.

IMPAIRED VERBAL COMMUNICATION. Helping the patient improve or regain effective communication is an extremely important goal of the rehabilitation phase. Communication impairments, aphasias, may take the form of inability to understand spoken words or inability to use words to express oneself. Types of aphasias were explained with signs and symptoms of stroke.

Patients with aphasia need encouragement as they struggle to communicate. The caregiver needs patience as the aphasic person requires more time to plan and deliver a response. Time must be taken to allow this to happen, but caregivers should provide verbal cues or picture boards before patients become overly frustrated in trying to respond. The physician often refers patients with severe communication impairments to speech therapists.

ALTERED NUTRITION. The patient who had dysphagia in the acute phase must be reevaluated at intervals for ability to swallow. If the patient is able to swallow saliva, the physician may allow liquids to be introduced. Initially, ¼ teaspoon of ice chips might be given with a spoon. The amount is increased and water is added until the patient is able to swallow a teaspoon of water. If problems with this simple assessment occur, a videofluoroscopic test of swallowing may be ordered. This test traces the route of swallowed fluid to detect swallowing abnormalities.

The stroke patient who has some difficulty swallowing may be placed on a supervised feeding program. Speech therapists are trained to help patients relearn swallowing, but everyday feeding falls to the nursing staff. With the head tilted forward and toward the unaffected side, the patient generally has fewer dysphagic problems. Thickeners may be added to liquids that are clear or thin for easier swallowing. Fluid intake must still be

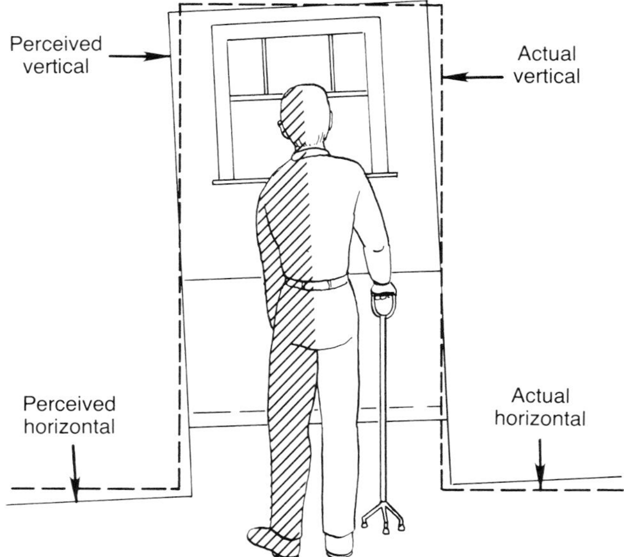

FIGURE 26-7
Perceptual disturbances in hemiplegia may affect the patient's ability to maneuver safely in the environment. (From Black, J. M., & Matassarin-Jacobs, E. [1993]. *Luckmann and Sorensen's medical-surgical nursing: A psychophysiologic approach* [4th ed.]. Philadelphia: W. B. Saunders.)

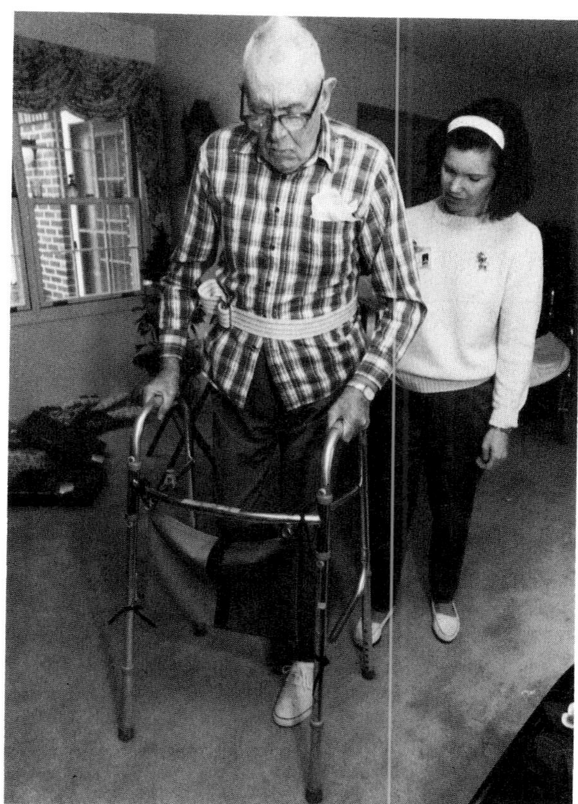

FIGURE 26-8
Nurse using a gait belt to ambulate a patient.

encouraged for the dysphagic person despite the increased work for patient and staff. Honest encouragement and pointing out small improvements are very important to the stroke patient struggling in rehabilitation.

IMPAIRED PHYSICAL MOBILITY. Mobility can continue to be a problem for stroke patients in the rehabilitation phase. Hemiplegia, dyspraxia, and visual field disturbances all create unique problems. Hemiplegia is an interesting phenomenon in that neurologic deficits cause weakness or paralysis, while musculovascular integrity remains. Hemiplegia is almost never purely a motor problem. It is usually accompanied by disturbances in balance and spatial perception (Fig. 26–7).

Regular physical therapy and occupational therapy are required for optimal return of motor function. The stimulation of regular exercise can cause dramatic return of function for the stroke patient. Therefore, affected arms and legs need to be used to maintain muscular function and vascular health if and until neurologic ability is recovered. In the meantime, assistance is needed with motor activities. When the patient is moving, the nurse assesses gait (if applicable), strength in arms and legs, and balance. Correct body mechanics and transfer techniques are essential for the nurse in working with the stroke patient. A gait belt helps the patient in transfers and in ambulation. It is a fabric belt with a toothed buckle that is applied between the nipple line and the waist that is used to support and assist the patient (Fig. 26–8).

Patients who have dyspraxia are unable to initiate voluntary motor acts. Interestingly, they sometimes exhibit those actions spontaneously. Verbal cues are provided to help them "remember" to initiate voluntary responses. Nurses need to teach other people about the nature of this dysfunction and advise them of the need for patience and cues to induce the desired motor performance.

Patients with unilateral neglect fail to recognize one side as part of their bodies. They need constant reminders to use and support their left sides.

COLONIC CONSTIPATION. Bowel elimination problems may continue into the rehabilitation phase. Incontinence is not usually a problem for the alert patient unless it is caused by inability to access toileting devices or manage clothing. The timing of episodes of bowel incontinence should be documented and a toileting schedule developed. Often simply taking the patient to the toilet at the usual time of defecation eliminates bowel incontinence. There is additional discussion of bowel incontinence in Chapter 21.

Constipation is a more common challenge in the rehabilitation phase. A regular bowel program with toileting, orientation, and reminders is an important aspect of control for this problem. Sufficient fluids are also important in promoting bowel regularity. Many stroke patients do not receive adequate fluid intake because of dysphagia or fear of incontinence. Also, caregivers may not take the extra time needed to provide fluids for the stroke patient who responds slowly. Stool softeners, laxatives, and suppositories may be used to reestablish regular bowel elimination. Dependency on laxatives should, however, be discouraged.

TOTAL INCONTINENCE. If the patient had an indwelling catheter inserted in the acute phase, it will probably be removed and efforts will be made to restore bladder control. Immediately after the catheter is removed, the patient may have poor sphincter control or may retain urine. Therefore, the nurse monitors urine output and checks for bladder distention until normal voiding is established. Pelvic muscle exercises (Chapter 21) may be prescribed to improve sphincter control.

Intermittent catheterization may continue to be necessary in the rehabilitation phase. The urine volume obtained is measured, and intermittent catheterization is done every 4 to 6 hours, depending on the volume obtained.

Urinary incontinence is more difficult to correct than bowel incontinence. A bladder program should be initiated promptly and continued to enhance the patient's sense of control. The first step is to document the patient's fluid intake and frequency of voiding. Careful observation and scheduled toileting of the stroke patient to prevent incontinence is one alternative to potential incontinence. Chapter 21 details additional measures to promote control of urination.

Evaluation

Criteria for evaluating the outcomes of nursing interventions in the rehabilitation phase are increasing patient participation in self-care; absence of falls, bruises, or pressure sores; patient's use of adaptive techniques to cope with disability; meaningful verbalizations or effective use of nonverbal communication; achievement and maintenance of ideal body weight; increasing independent physical activity; regular formed stools; and regular controlled urine elimination.

Discharge

Patients may be discharged to their homes or may go to specialized rehabilitation centers for continued therapy. Outpatient therapy is also an option for some patients. The rehabilitation phase is defined in various ways. When no improvements in function are noted in a 1- to 2-week period, some consider the rehabilitation phase to be over. Medicare defines the rehabilitation phase as 3 months after the stroke. Rehabilitation specialists say rehabilitation continues indefinitely, but progress slows down. During and after the rehabilitation phase, patients and families need to be made aware of resources to help them deal with continuing disabilities.

NUTRITION CONCEPTS

- A major nutritional concern for the stroke patient is dysphagia (difficulty swallowing), which may lead to malnutrition and dehydration because of inadequate intake.
- Swallowing thin liquids is frequently a problem. Thin liquids can be thickened with dry milk powder, cornstarch, fruit and vegetable flakes, or commercial thickening agents.
- The swallowing reflex can be stimulated better with flavorful, very warm or chilled foods than with bland, lukewarm foods.
- Foods that are better for chewing and swallowing are thickened liquids, soft bread, cooked cereal, ice cream, yogurt, cooked eggs, moist ground beef, canned fruits and vegetables, thick soups, and puddings.

Although stroke remains a major health problem, risk prevention can play a significant role in controlling it. The acute phase of stroke, from diagnosis to stabilization of blood pressure, requires support and careful evaluation of the patient's basic remaining abilities. In rehabilitation, the stroke patient is respectfully challenged to return to the highest level of function possible. Independence may not be possible, but encouraging the patient and subduing some of the major limitations of stroke can be one of the most satisfying aspects of nursing.

BIBLIOGRAPHY

Adkins, E. R. H. (1991). Nursing care of clients with impaired communication. *Rehabilitation Nursing, 16*(2), 74–76.

Baggerly, J. (1991). Sensory perceptual problems following stroke. *Nursing Clinics of North America, 26*(4), 997–1005.

Blisset, P. A. (1992). Ticlopidine hydrochloride. *Journal of Neuroscience Nursing, 24*(5), 296–300.

Boss, B. J. (1991). Managing communication disorders in stroke. *Nursing Clinics of North America, 26*(4), 985–995.

Bruckbauer, E. A. (1991). Recognizing poststroke depression. *Rehabilitation Nursing, 16*(1), 34–36.

Brust, J. C. M. (1994). Stroke. In W. R. Hazzard, E. L. Bierman, J. P. Blass, W. Ettinger, & J. Halter (Eds.), *Principles of geriatric medicine and gerontology* (3rd ed., pp. 1027–1034). New York: McGraw-Hill, Inc.

Deglin, J. H., Vallerand, A. H., & Russin, M. M. (1991). *Davis's drug guide for nurses* (2nd ed.). Philadelphia: F. A. Davis.

DeLisa, J. A. (1988). *Rehabilitation medicine: Principles and practice.* Philadelphia: J. B. Lippincott.

Granger, C. V., Hamilton, B. B., & Fielder, R. C. (1992). Discharge outcome after stroke rehabilitation. *Stroke, 23*(7), 978–982.

Gwynn, M. (1993). tPA in acute stroke—Risk or reprieve? *Journal of Neuroscience Nursing, 25*(3), 180–186.

Ignatavicius, D. D., & Bayne, M. V. (1991). *Medical-surgical nursing: A nursing process approach.* Philadelphia: W. B. Saunders.

Jahnke, H. (1991). Experimental ancrod (Arvin) for acute ischemic stroke: Nursing implications. *Journal of Neuroscience Nursing, 23*(6), 386–389.

Jarvis, C. (1992). *Physical examination and health assessment.* Philadelphia: W. B. Saunders.

Kalbach, L. R. (1991). Unilateral neglect; mechanisms and nursing care. *Journal of Neuroscience Nursing, 23*(2), 125–129.

Kelly-Hayes, M. (1991). A preventive approach to stroke. *Nursing Clinics of North America, 26*(4), 931–941.

Kottke, F. J. (1990). Krusen's *Handbook of physical medicine and rehabilitation.* Philadelphia: W. B. Saunders.

Leahy, N. M. (1991). Complications in the acute stages of stroke. *Nursing Clinics of North America, 26*(4), 971–983.

Loughrey, L. (1992). The effects of two teaching techniques on recognition and use of function words by aphasic stroke patients. *Rehabilitation Nursing, 17*(3), 137–143.

Mol, V. J., & Baker, C. A. (1991). Activity intolerance in the geriatric stroke patient. *Rehabilitation Nursing, 16*(6), 337–342.

Mulley, G. P. (1992). Stroke. In J. C. Brocklehurst, R. C. Tallis, & H. M. Fillit (Eds.), *Textbook of geriatric medicine and gerontology* (pp. 365–388). Edinburgh: Churchill Livingstone.

Olson, E. (1991). Perceptual deficits affecting the stroke patient. *Rehabilitation Nursing, 16*(4), 212–213.

Rothstein, J. M. (1991). *The rehabilitation specialist's handbook.* Philadelphia: F. A. Davis.

Shalfer, M. (1993). *The nurse, pharmacology, and drug therapy* (3rd ed.). Redwood City, CA: Addison-Wesley.

Stout, R. W. (1992). Atherosclerosis and lipid metabolism. In J. C. Brocklehurst, R. C. Tallis, & H. M. Fillit (Eds.), *Textbook of geriatric medicine and gerontology* (pp. 165–180). Edinburgh: Churchill Livingstone.

Venn, M. R., Taft, L., Carpentier, B., & Applebaugh, G. (1992). The influence of timing and suppository use on efficiency and effectiveness of bowel training after a stroke. *Rehabilitation Nursing, 17*(3), 116–120.

KEY CONCEPTS

1. A cerebrovascular accident (CVA), commonly called a stroke, is an interruption of blood flow to part of the brain.
2. The risk factors for CVA are atherosclerosis, hypertension, diabetes mellitus, cardiac disease, and, for women, smoking while taking oral contraceptives.
3. The four types of CVA are transient ischemic attack, reversible ischemic neurologic deficit, completed stroke, and stroke in evolution.
4. A transient ischemic attack is a temporary neurologic deficit caused by impaired cerebral blood flow.
5. Transient ischemic attack, sometimes considered a warning sign of impending stroke, is treated with diet, exercise, drug therapy to prevent clot formation, surgery to clear or bypass obstructed blood vessels, or a combination of these.
6. Neurologic deficits that persist for less than 24 hours and then disappear are characteristic of reversible ischemic neurologic deficit.
7. A stroke is a set of neurologic signs and symptoms persisting for more than 24 hours caused by impaired blood flow to the brain.
8. When neurologic symptoms progress over hours or days, the condition is described as stroke in evolution; with a completed stroke, the symptoms do not change for several days.
9. A hemorrhagic stroke is caused by the rupture of a blood vessel in the brain, and an ischemic stroke is caused by the obstruction of a blood vessel by an embolus or a thrombus.
10. Signs and symptoms of stroke depend on the type, location, and extent of brain injury but may include one-sided weakness, numbness, visual problems, confusion and memory lapses, headache, dysphagia, and speech problems.
11. Some symptoms of stroke improve, but patients may be left with impairments in speech, language comprehension, motor function, vision, cognition, and bladder control, as well as personality changes and emotional lability.
12. Aphasia is the inability to understand words or to respond with appropriate messages.
13. Dysarthria is the inability to speak clearly because of neurologic damage that affects the muscles of speech.
14. Dysphagia is difficulty swallowing.
15. Dyspraxia is the partial inability to initiate coordinated voluntary motor acts.
16. Paralysis of one side of the body (the side opposite the brain injury) is called hemiplegia.
17. Medical treatment of CVA may employ oxygen therapy, diuretics, corticosteroids, anticoagulants, intravenous fluids, dietary modifications, and catheterization as well as treatment of risk factors.
18. The goals of nursing care after stroke include airway maintenance, adequate hydration and nu-

trition, adaptation to sensory-perceptual and motor alterations, effective communication, prevention of injury, and control of elimination.

19. The stroke patient may regain complete independent functioning, may partially recover previous abilities, or may lose functional abilities completely.

20. The goal of rehabilitation after stroke is to enhance the recovery of functional abilities through a program of stimulation and practice.

Gayle Dasher

CHAPTER 27

Spinal Cord Injury

OBJECTIVES

1. Explain the impact of spinal cord injury.
2. Describe the diagnostic tests used to evaluate spinal cord injuries and related nursing responsibilities.
3. Explain the physical effects of spinal cord injury.
4. Describe the medical and surgical treatment during the acute phase of spinal cord injury.
5. List the data to be included in the nursing assessment of the patient with a spinal cord injury.
6. Identify nursing diagnoses, goals, and interventions for the patient with a spinal cord injury.
7. Describe the nursing care for the patient having a laminectomy.
8. State the goals of rehabilitation for the patient with spinal cord injury.

GLOSSARY

AUTONOMIC DYSREFLEXIA Abnormally exaggerated response of the autonomic nervous system to a stimulus

DERMATOME Area of skin supplied by sensory nerve fibers from a single posterior spinal root

FLACCID Soft; in relation to muscles, lacking tone

MYELINATED Surrounded with a sheath

PARAPLEGIA Loss of motor and sensory function due to damage to the spinal cord that spares the upper extremities but, depending on the level of the damage, affects the trunk, pelvis, and lower extremities

QUADRIPLEGIA Loss of motor and sensory function in all four extremities due to damage to the spinal cord

SPASTIC Increased muscle tone, characterized by sudden, involuntary muscle spasms

Few injuries prove to be as physically and emotionally devastating to a person as a permanent spinal cord injury. The latest National Head and Spinal Cord Injury survey estimates that 10,000 people sustain permanent injuries each year. One third of victims die before reaching a hospital. The remaining injured have varying degrees of disabilities, requiring care that costs more than $2 billion annually.

Young males between ages 15 and 30 are the most frequent sufferers of spinal cord injury. The leading cause of spinal cord injury is trauma sustained in vehicular accidents, falls, assaults, and sports-related mishaps. The cord can also be damaged by degenerative conditions and tumors.

Medical advances and more rapid transport of accident victims to trauma centers have made it possible for an individual with spinal cord injury to achieve a normal life expectancy. The effects of the injury, however, may lead to other health problems that require long-term care and impair quality of life. Quality nursing care during the acute and rehabilitative phases of injury can minimize the impact of lifelong problems that plague the spinal cord–injured person. Consequently, the potential for rehabilitation and full quality of life can be enhanced.

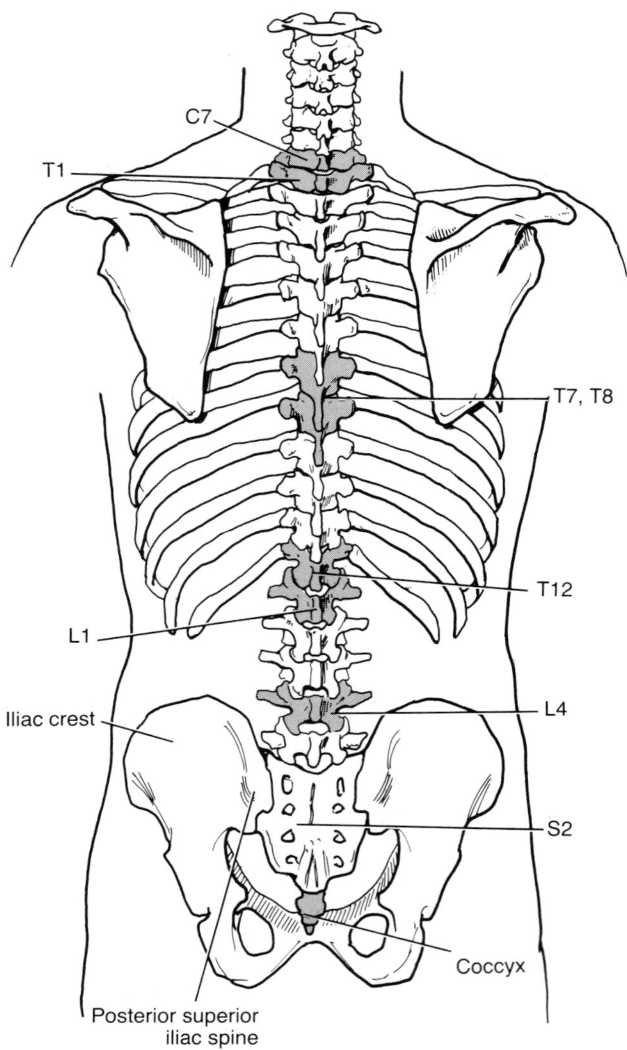

FIGURE 27–1

The bony vertebral column consists of 33 vertebrae. (Redrawn from Jarvis, C. [1992]. *Physical examination and health assessment* [p. 664]. Philadelphia: W. B. Saunders.)

ANATOMY AND PHYSIOLOGY OF THE SPINAL CORD

To understand the effects of spinal cord injury fully, it is important to know the anatomy and physiology of the spinal cord. Normal spinal cord function requires an intact cord with a good blood supply and bony support. Disruption of any one of these components can result in neurologic dysfunction.

VERTEBRAL COLUMN

The bony vertebral column consists of 33 vertebrae: 7 cervical (C1-7), 12 thoracic (T1-12), 5 lumbar (L1-5), 5 sacral (S1-5), and 4 coccygeal (fused) (Fig. 27–1). The individual vertebra consists of a body and an arch, as seen in Fig. 27–2. The body is the round structure that forms the anterior portion of the vertebra. The arch is the posterior portion of the vertebra. The spinal cord passes through an opening in the center of each arch. The structures that form the posterior section of the arch are called laminae. Each arch has many branches that attach it to the body and that provide locations for attachment of ribs and muscles. The bony column is supported by muscles and ligaments, which permit mobility and flexibility.

DISKS

Vertebrae are separated by intervertebral disks, which serve as shock absorbers for the vertebral column. Disks are composed of the anulus fibrosus and the nucleus pulposus. The anulus fibrosis is the fibrous ring of tissue that encircles the nucleus pulposus. The nucleus pulposus is the central sac-like structure with a gelatinous filling that has a high water content. As a person ages, the nucleus pulposus loses a great deal of its water, so it becomes less effective as a shock absorber. Therefore, older people are at greater risk for back injuries and herniated disks.

SPINAL CORD

The spinal cord extends from the brain stem to the level of L-2 in the pelvic cavity (Fig. 27–3). It has a central canal, which is continuous with the fourth ventricle of the brain. The cord is surrounded by three protective meningeal layers: dura mater, arachnoid, and pia mater. The dura mater is the outermost layer. The arachnoid, the middle layer, is a network of spaces containing cerebrospinal fluid (CSF). The pia mater is the innermost layer; it directly covers the spinal cord. The CSF circulates through the brain and spinal column,

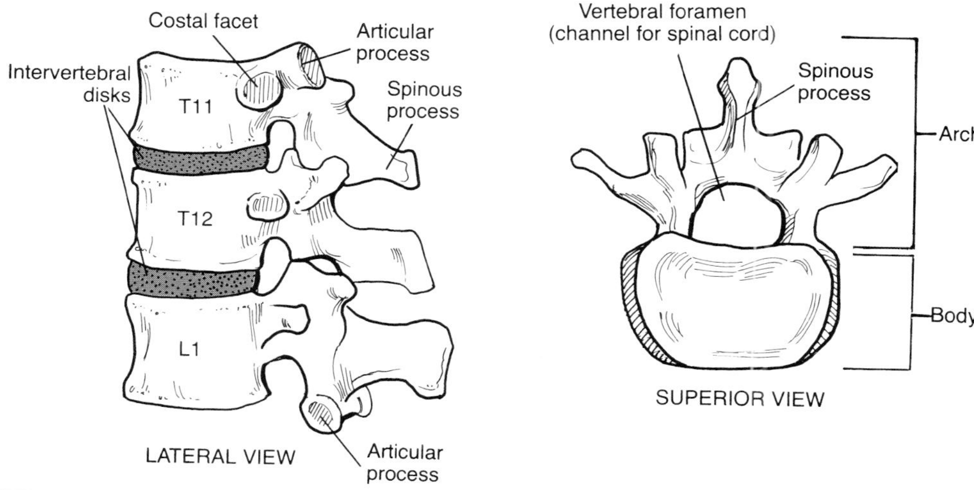

FIGURE 27-2

Intervertebral disks separate the vertebrae, each of which consists of the body and the arch. (Redrawn from Jarvis, C. [1992]. *Physical examination and health assessment* [p. 665]. Philadelphia: W. B. Saunders.)

bathing and protecting the entire central nervous system.

A cross section of the spinal cord reveals an inner area of H-shaped gray matter surrounded by white matter. The gray matter consists of the bodies of nerve cells that control motor and sensory activities. The white matter, which is myelinated (surrounded by a sheath), consists of bundles of fibers. These fibers, known as columns or tracts, convey information between the brain and the spinal cord. The tracts may be either ascending or descending. Ascending tracts carry motor and sensory information from the spinal cord to the brain. Descending tracts carry motor and sensory information from the brain to the spinal cord (Fig. 27–4).

Blood supply to the spinal cord is vital. Any disruption in blood flow can ultimately lead to neurologic damage.

Spinal cord function may be classified as either reflexive or relay in nature. With reflexive activity, the sensory stimulus is received and a response is initiated at the level of the spinal cord. The knee jerk is an example of reflexive activity. When the knee is tapped, impulses travel by sensory neurons to the spinal cord, where they are relayed to motor neurons. The impulse travels back to the muscles at the front of the thigh, causing muscle contraction and jerking of the leg. This circuit of impulse transmission is called a reflex arc.

With relay activity, the stimulus enters the spinal cord and travels up the ascending tracts to relay sensory signals from the external environment to the brain. Information is processed in the brain, and responses are initiated by impulses transmitted to the body by way of descending tracts.

The descending white matter tracts also participate in the relay function of the spinal cord. These tracts relay motor information, with messages being sent from the brain, down the cord, to muscles, which effect various kinds of responses. Four of the most important spinal cord tracts are summarized in Table 27–1.

Information is conveyed by the senses to the brain and spinal cord via the peripheral nervous system. This system comprises 31 pairs of spinal nerves, which branch from the cord and pass between the vertebrae to muscles and visceral organs. Each spinal nerve has a dorsal root, which transmits sensory information, and a ventral root, which transmits motor information. The twelve cranial nerves, arising from the brain stem, also are part of the peripheral nervous system.

DIAGNOSTIC TESTS AND PROCEDURES

Emergency care of the patient with a spinal cord injury is discussed in Chapter 13. When the victim of spinal cord injury arrives at the hospital, the extent of injury must be assessed. Specific tests are performed to determine the type of injury and to provide direction for treatment. Throughout the diagnostic process, the spine must be immobilized continuously.

NEUROLOGIC EXAMINATION. The initial neurologic evaluation of the spinal cord–injured patient provides the nurse with a baseline assessment of both function and problems. Ongoing assessment is necessary to monitor the effects of neurologic injury, detect related complications, and determine the patient's need for assistance in activities of daily living.

In the patient with spinal cord injury, neurologic evaluation focuses on the motor and sensory systems. Movement, muscle strength, and reflex activity are evaluated on an ongoing basis as described in the section on assessment. Basic neurologic assessment is covered in

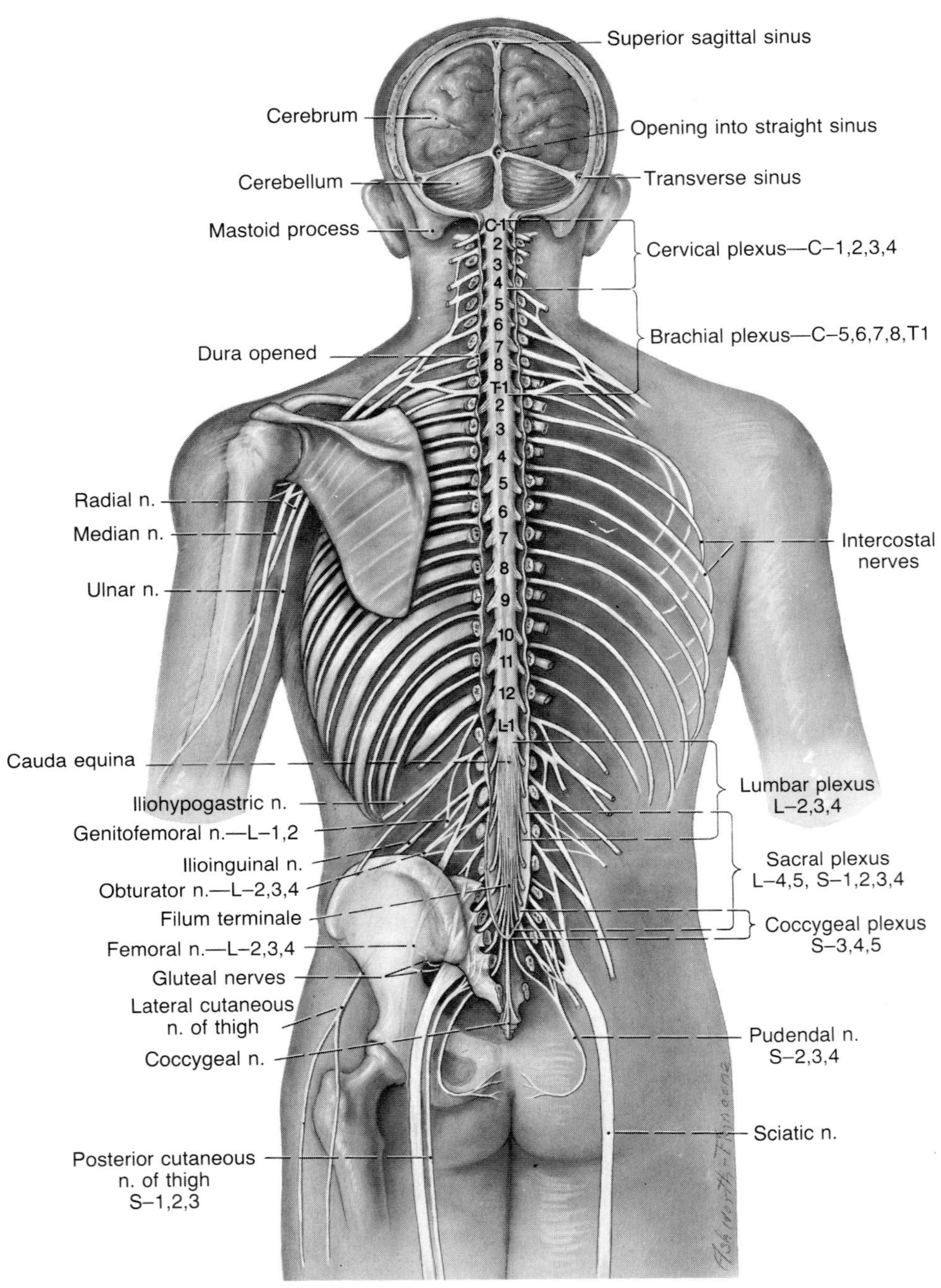

FIGURE 27-3

The spinal cord extends from the brain stem to the level of the second lumbar vertebra. (Adapted from Jacob, S. W., & Francone, C. A. [1989]. *Elements of anatomy and physiology* [2nd ed., p. 124]. Philadelphia: W. B. Saunders.)

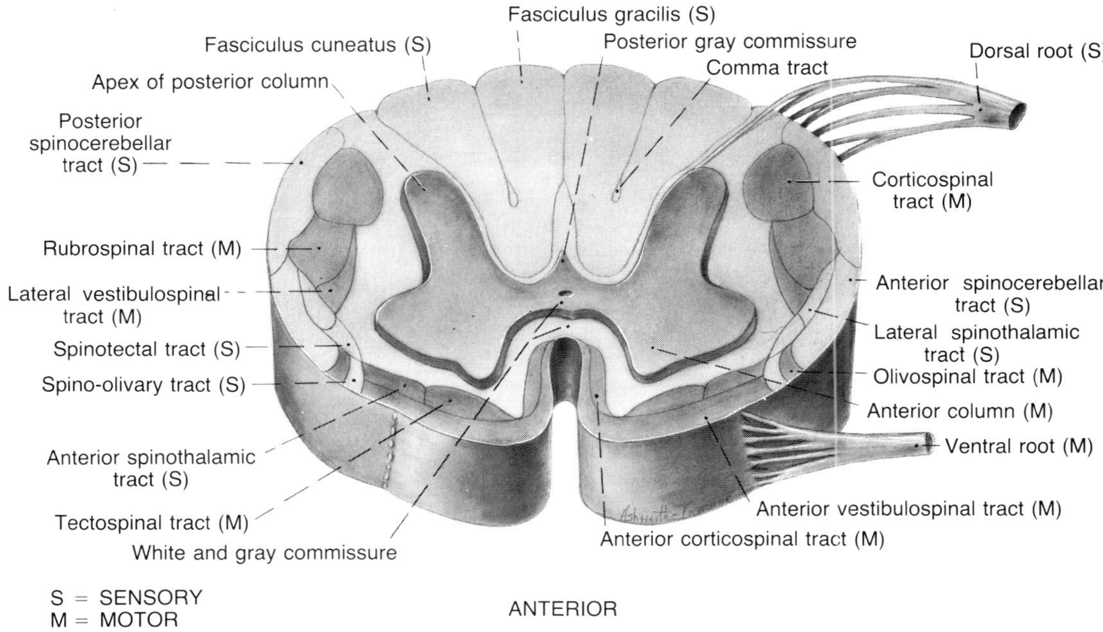

FIGURE 27-4

Cross section of spinal cord. Sensory (S) tracts convey sensory information to the brain. Motor (M) tracts convey information from the brain. (From Jacob, S. W., & Francone, C. A. [1989]. *Elements of anatomy and physiology* [2nd ed., p. 108]. Philadelphia: W. B. Saunders.)

Chapter 25. A textbook on physical assessment should be referred to for the detailed steps of the neurologic evaluation.

RADIOGRAPHY. Standard radiographs are obtained to detect vertebral compression or fractures, or both. The entire spine may be radiographed since patients sometimes have multiple fractures separated by sections of normal spine. The physician may also order special radiographs, called cone-down views, that reveal fractures more clearly. Radiography is repeated at intervals to evaluate the achievement of proper alignment with treatment.

COMPUTED TOMOGRAPHY. Computed tomography is a truly revolutionary diagnostic tool. This noninvasive procedure is used to examine small sections of tissue within any organ, allowing anatomic structures and pathologic processes to be viewed. The specific levels of the spinal cord can be visualized on the CT

TABLE 27-1

SUMMARY OF FOUR MAJOR SPINAL CORD TRACTS

TRACT	TYPE	FEATURES	FUNCTION
Spinothalamic, lateral	Ascending (sensory: pain and temperature)	Originates in spinal cord and ascends to thalamus in brain. On entering cord, impulses cross over to opposite side (contralateral).	Carries pain and temperature sensation from opposite side.
Corticospinal, lateral	Descending (motor)	Initiates in motor tract of brain, crosses over to opposite side at level of medulla, proceeds down to appropriate spinal cord level.	Controls voluntary motor action.
Spinocerebellar	Ascending (sensory)	Initiates in spinal cord and terminates in cerebellum.	Assists in coordination of muscle contraction.
Posterior columns	Ascending (sensory: touch, vibration, position sense)	Made up of several tracts that relay messages from body to brain. Initiates in sensory fibers of spinal nerves, crosses over in medulla, and terminates in sensory cortex of opposite hemisphere.	Carries touch, deep pressure, vibration, and position sense.

scan, as can the bony vertebrae and the spinal nerves. Scanning enables the physician to readily identify bony fractures, floating bone fragments, dislocations, tumors, hemorrhage, and cord and nerve compressions.

Although no special physical preparation must be made for CT, the procedure should be explained to the patient. The patient is told that he or she will be asked to lie very still for a period of time while on a small table that slowly moves through the CT scanner. Enhanced CT scanning also may be done, in which a radiopaque dye is intravenously infused into the patient. This testing is contraindicated in the patient who is allergic to this type of dye. The patient receiving the dye must be encouraged to take plenty of fluids after the procedure to promote renal excretion.

MAGNETIC RESONANCE IMAGING. Magnetic resonance imaging, unlike CT scanning, does not expose the patient to radiation. The patient is slowly moved through a strong magnetic field and then subjected to short bursts of radio waves. Sophisticated technology translates information about body tissue to produce precise, clear images of internal structures. (Fig. 27–5).

This noninvasive diagnostic procedure is painless to the patient, has no known risks, and requires no preparation. The nurse tells the patient to expect to hear a humming sound as the radio waves are turned on and off. The patient must have no metal materials or equipment on when entering the scanning suite. Because the magnetic field in the scanner is so strong, any metal object may be attracted into the field. A quartz watch would be disrupted because the magnetic field has a detrimental effect on the battery. If an intravenous pump is being used, the site must first be converted to a heparin lock because the pump cannot be placed in the scanning room. If oxygen is required, adequate tubing is needed to allow the oxygen tank to be placed a safe distance outside the suite. Patients with pacemakers cannot undergo magnetic resonance imaging because the magnetic field would inactivate the pacer.

MYELOGRAPHY. The myelogram is obtained to visualize the spinal cord and vertebrae. A puncture is made in the lumbar area between L-3 and L-4. Radiopaque dye is then injected into the subarachnoid space of the spinal cord. Any obstruction that impedes the flow of the dye can be seen on radiography. Because of the invasive nature of the procedure, informed consent must be obtained. Nursing care before and after myelography is summarized in Table 27–2.

PATHOPHYSIOLOGY OF SPINAL CORD INJURY

Traumatic injury creates abnormal forces on the neck and structural components of the spinal cord. The cervical vertebrae support the head and neck and permit movement in various directions. The thoracic vertebrae, on the other hand, permit little movement because of the restrictions of the ribs. Since the thoracic spine has limited flexibility, the neck and cervical spine are extremely vulnerable to injury.

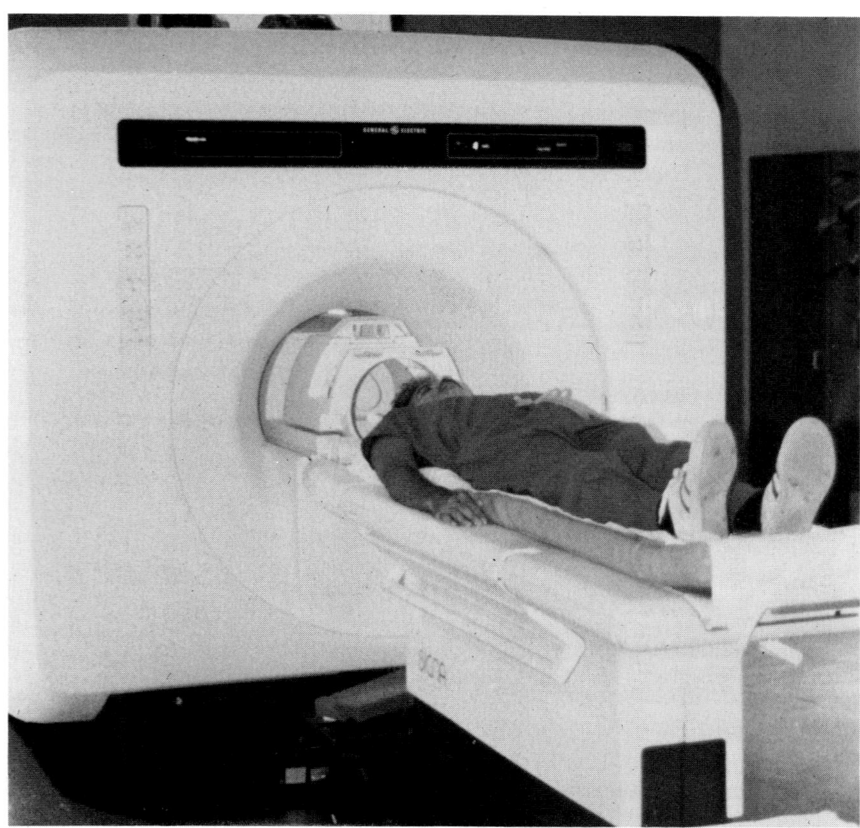

FIGURE 27-5
Patient preparing to enter magnet for magnetic resonance imaging. (From Marshall, S. B., Marshall, L. F., Vos, H. R., & Chesnut, R. M. [1990]. *Neuroscience critical care* [p. 120]. Philadelphia: W. B. Saunders.)

TABLE 27-2
NURSING CARE OF THE PATIENT HAVING MYELOGRAPHY

PREPARATION
1. Ensure that signed consent form has been obtained.
2. Inquire about allergy to dye, iodine, or shellfish; inform radiologist if allergic.
3. Allow nothing by mouth for 4–6 hr preceding procedure according to agency protocol.
4. Administer prescribed premedications.
5. Have patient empty bladder if able.
6. Determine whether any medications should be withheld.

POSTPROCEDURE CARE
1. Frequently assess vital signs and neurologic status.
2. Encourage increased fluid intake to promote elimination of dye, if not contraindicated.
3. Measure and record intake and output.
4. Position as ordered: flat or head of bed elevated 30–45 degrees depending on type of contrast medium used.
5. Administer analgesics as ordered for headache.
6. Assess for back pain, increased temperature, difficulty voiding, neck stiffness, and nausea and vomiting.

TYPES OF INJURIES

Spinal cord injuries may be classified (1) by location, (2) as open or closed, and (3) by extent of damage to the cord. Injuries classified by location are called cervical, thoracic, or lumbar depending on the level of the cord affected.

Closed injuries involve trauma in which the skin and meningeal covering outside the spinal cord remain intact. Common causes of closed injuries include compression, flexion, hyperextension, rotation, and blunt trauma (Fig. 27–6). Degeneration of the vertebrae or intervertebral disks, hematomas, or spinal cord tumors also may compress the cord or one of the spinal nerves. Fractures of the vertebral bodies may cause a subluxation (partial dislocation) of bone fragments, which may further damage the cord. Open injuries with damage to protective skin and meninges are most commonly caused by gunshot or stab wounds.

The injury may be classified as complete or incomplete depending on the extent to which the cord is transected (cut across). A complete spinal cord injury occurs when the cord has been completely severed, whereas an incomplete injury results from partial cutting of the cord. Open injuries frequently result in either complete or partial transection (cutting across) of the cord.

EFFECTS OF SPINAL CORD INJURY

Early recognition of the effects of spinal cord injury is vital to maintain maximum possible function. Factors that determine the effects of spinal cord injury include the extent of the cut and the level of the injury. A complete injury cuts all descending and ascending tracts. The result is disruption of all motor and sensory activity below the level of the injury. However, reflex activity continues below the injury because it occurs by completing the reflex arc without the transmission of impulses to and from the brain.

Trauma may also produce a variety of incomplete spinal cord injuries. These are injuries in which some function remains below the level of the injury. Specific tracts may be involved, causing particular patterns of neurologic dysfunction (Fig. 27–7). Table 27–3 describes the major types of incomplete injuries and the resulting neurologic losses.

The higher the level of the injury, the more devastating the neurologic dysfunction. High cervical spine injuries may result in the loss of motor and sensory function in all four extremities, known as quadriplegia. Injuries at or below T-2 may cause paraplegia, which is paralysis of the lower part of the body. Table 27–4 describes those activities that are possible with spinal cord injury at various levels.

RESPIRATORY IMPAIRMENT. The diaphragm is innervated by the phrenic nerve, which is formed by the nerve roots of C1-4. Therefore, injuries at or above the level of C-5 (called high cervical injuries) may result in instant death because the nerves that control respiration are interrupted. Many patients with high cervical injuries die before reaching the hospital. If these patients are fortunate enough to receive immediate attention and rapid transport to a skilled facility, mechanical ventilation may be possible. However, these patients remain dependent on ventilators and present great challenges for rehabilitation.

Modern technology affords the ventilator-dependent patient a variety of options for pulmonary rehabilitation. A small portable ventilator can be mounted on the back of a mechanized wheelchair, enabling the patient to be mobile. Phrenic nerve stimulators also may be implanted in the patient to help stimulate diaphragmatic movement and enhance respiratory function. Even with a ventilator or phrenic nerve stimulator, pulmonary hygiene is often a problem because these patients may have difficulty clearing the airway.

Cervical injuries below the level of C-4 spare the diaphragm but can involve impairment of intercostal and abdominal muscles. Patients with these injuries can usually breathe independently but often experience some degree of respiratory compromise related to weakened exhalation and cough.

SPINAL SHOCK. Spinal shock is an immediate, transient response to injury in which reflex activity below the level of the injury temporarily ceases. It may appear as early as 30 to 60 minutes after the injury and persist intermittently for days, weeks, or months. During the period of spinal shock, paralysis is described as flaccid, meaning the involved extremity or muscle group has no tone. The involved neurons in the spinal cord gradually regain their excitability. Resolution of spinal shock is marked by the appearance of spastic, involuntary movements of the extremities.

AUTONOMIC DYSREFLEXIA. One of the most serious and potentially dangerous problems for the spinal cord–injured patient is autonomic dysreflexia, an exag-

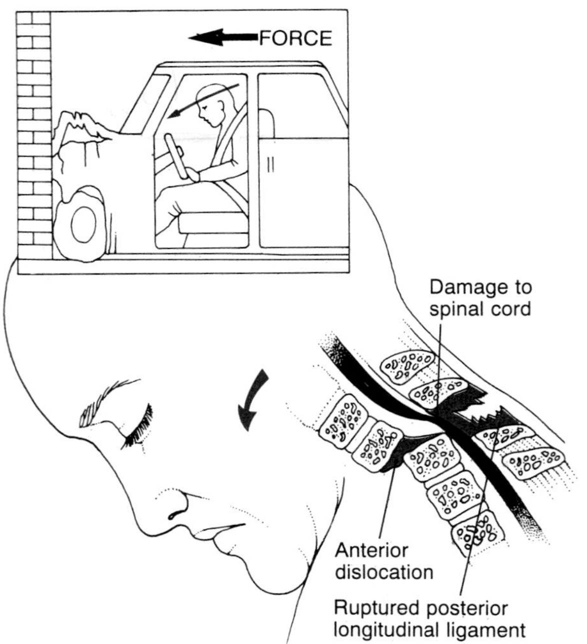

Flexion injury of the cervical spine

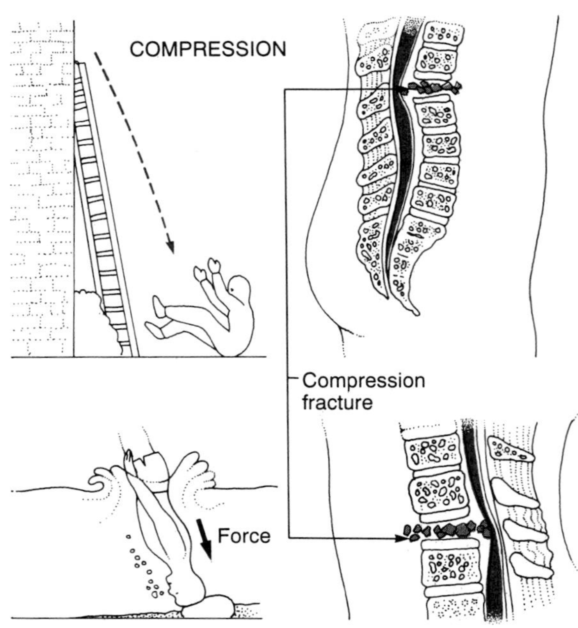

Axial loading (vertical compression) injury of the cervical spine and the lumbar spine

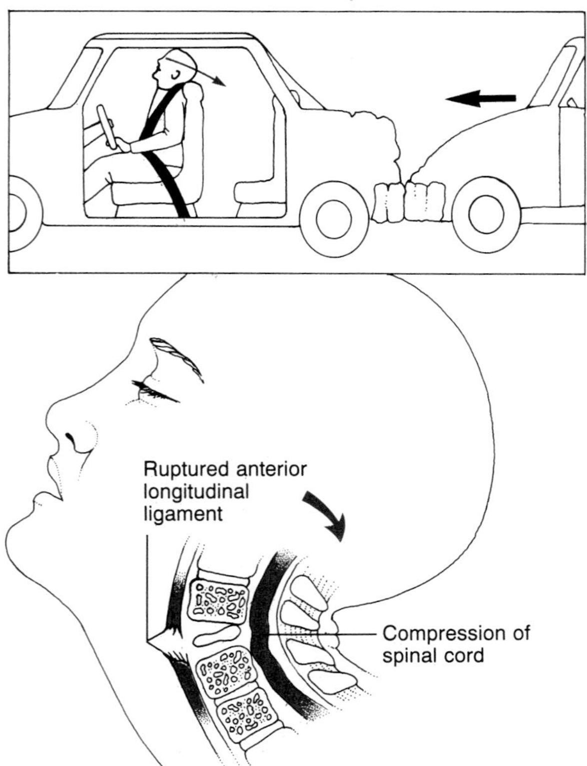

Hyperextension injury of the cervical spine

FIGURE 27-6

Mechanisms of spinal cord injury. (Adapted from Ignatavicius, D. D., & Bayne, M. V. [1991]. *Medical-surgical nursing: A nursing process approach* [pp. 939–940]. Philadelphia: W. B. Saunders.)

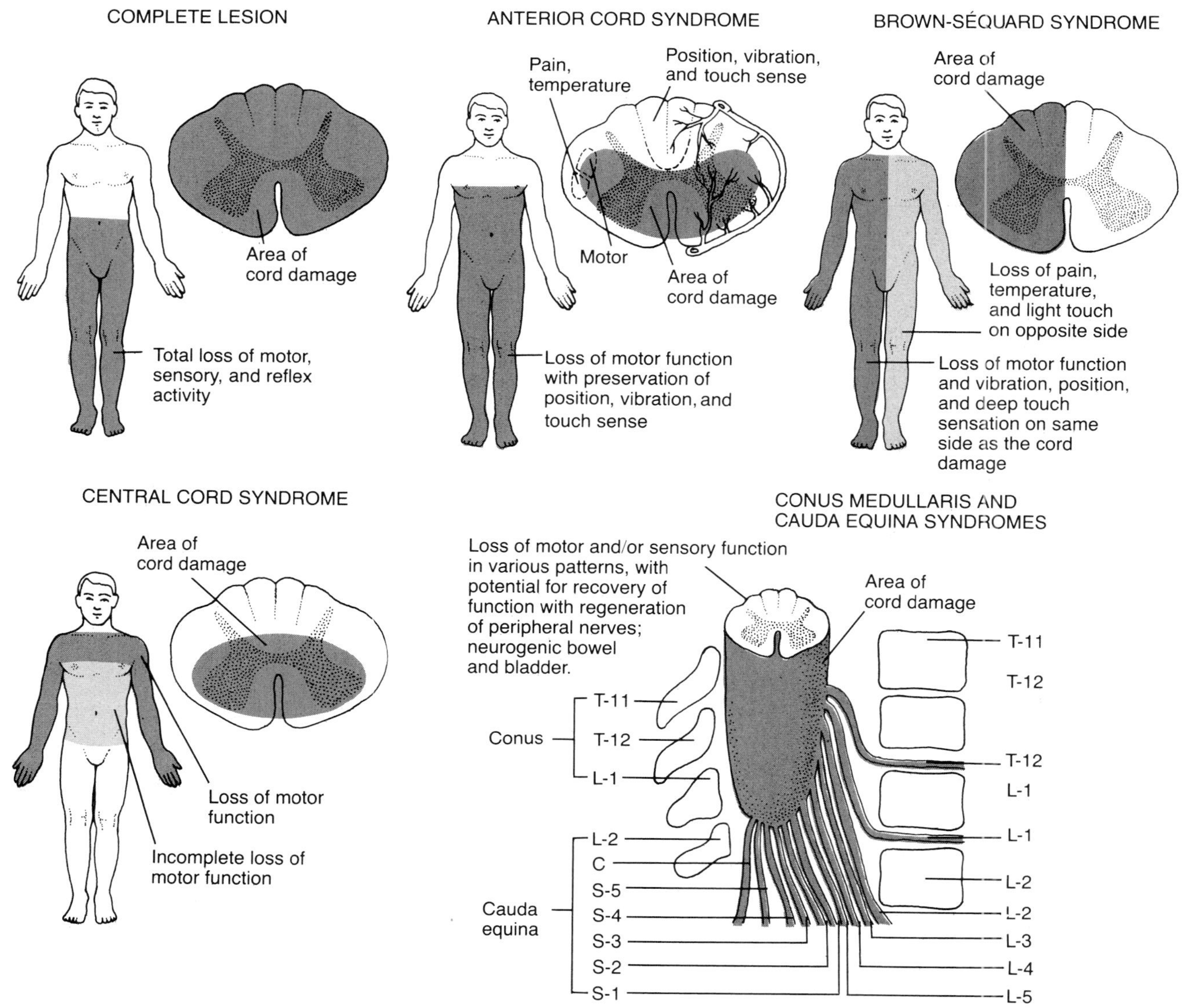

FIGURE 27-7

Patterns of injuries and neurologic dysfunction. (From Ignatavicius, D. D., & Bayne, M. V. [1991]. *Medical-surgical nursing: A nursing process approach* [p. 971]. Philadelphia: W. B. Saunders.)

TABLE 27-3

INCOMPLETE INJURIES AND RELATED NEUROLOGIC DEFICITS

INJURY	MECHANISM OF INJURY	ACCOMPANYING DEFICIT
Anterior cord syndrome	Herniation of disk occurring with flexion injury or dislocation of vertebrae	Loss of bilateral pain and temperature and motor function below level of lesion without loss of position sense.
Central cord syndrome	Hyperextension injury	Motor and sensory loss in upper extremities
Brown-Séquard syndrome	Transverse hemisection of cord	Ipsilateral loss of motor function with contralateral loss of pain and temperature

TABLE 27-4

DEGREE OF LOSS AND FUNCTIONAL CAPABILITY WITH INJURY TO EACH LEVEL OF THE SPINAL CORD

CORD LEVEL	DEGREE OF LOSS	FUNCTIONAL CAPABILITY
C1-4	Motor and sensory function from neck down Respiratory function Bowel and bladder control	Mechanical ventilation with home care
C-5	Motor and sensory function below shoulders Intercostal function in ventilation Bowel and bladder control	Has remaining head control, which facilitates use of "joystick" for writing, typing, and control of mechanical wheelchair
C-6	Motor and sensory function below shoulders but greater degree of sensation in arm and thumb Intercostal function in ventilation Bowel and bladder control	Requires some assistive devices for upper extremity use but may be able to help feed and dress self Requires mechanical wheelchair but may be capable of utilizing hand control
C-7	Motor control of portions of upper extremities Sensation below clavicle Intercostal function Bowel and bladder control	Remaining intact muscles enhance ability to carry out activities of daily living (ADL) Increased ability to manage specially equipped wheelchair and automobile
C-8	Motor control of portions of upper extremities Sensation below chest Intercostal function Bowel and bladder control	Improved upper extremity mobility enhances hand grasp, independence in ADL, and use of wheelchair Capable of self-catheterization
T1-6	Trunk muscles below midchest Sensation from midchest Some intercostal function Bowel and bladder control	Complete control of upper extremities makes independence in wheelchair and ADL possible Employment possible
T6-12	Motor control below waist Sensation below waist Bowel and bladder control	Capable of unassisted respiratory function Good upper back and abdominal strength, making increased wheelchair activities and athletics possible
L1-3	Motor and sensory function to lower extremities Sensation to lower abdomen Bowel and bladder function	Full control of upper extremities allows independence in wheelchair and appropriate athletic activity
L3-4	Motor and sensory function to distal portions of lower extremities Bowel and bladder control	Control of hip extensors remains, making ambulation possible with leg braces
L-4 to S-5	Variable motor and sensory function to knee, ankle, and foot Sensation to perineum Variable bowel and bladder control	Ambulation with braces possible Considerable independence in ADL can be expected

gerated response of the autonomic nervous system. It occurs in patients whose injury is at or above the level of T-6. As spinal shock begins to subside and reflex activity returns, the risk of autonomic dysreflexia increases. It may even occur in patients with long-standing injuries.

Excessive stimulation of sensory receptors below the level of the injury precipitates autonomic dysreflexia. The sympathetic nervous system is stimulated, but an appropriate response cannot be elicited because of the spinal cord injury. Arterioles constrict, causing severe hypertension, which may lead to seizures or a stroke if not corrected. In an attempt to reduce the excessively increased blood pressure, regulatory mechanisms cause the blood vessels to dilate. The vasodilating response is effective only above the level of the injury, where superficial vasodilation, flushing, and profuse sweating occur.

Increased blood pressure also stimulates the vagus nerve, causing bradycardia. Normally, vagal stimulation also would serve to dilate the constricted vessels. But, because the cord has been severed, these impulses never reach the affected blood vessels.

Autonomic dysreflexia is commonly triggered by a distended bladder, constipation, renal calculi, ejaculation, or uterine contractions, but it may also be caused by pressure sores, a skin rash, enemas, or even sudden position changes. In the event of autonomic dysreflexia, indwelling catheters must be inspected for possible occlusions or kinks.

SPASTICITY. Most spinal cord–injured patients display some degree of spasticity (increased muscle tone) following their injury. Muscle spasms may prove to be quite incapacitating for these patients, hampering efforts at rehabilitation. Generally, after 1 or 2 years, there is a gradual reduction in spastic episodes.

Muscle tone is evaluated by assessing the amount of resistance to passive movement. The spastic muscle displays a brief period of increased resistance, which is followed by a sudden relaxation. Reflexes also are assessed since hyperactive reflexes accompany spasticity. Spastic activity may be elicited by passive movement, positioning, or even the slight stimulation of a sheet moving over the lower extremities.

IMPAIRED SENSORY AND MOTOR FUNCTION. As stated earlier, the higher the level of the lesion, the more extensive the neurologic dysfunction. Any complete cord injury results in the loss of both motor and sensory function below the level of the lesion. The effects of incomplete lesions on sensation and motor function are variable. Impaired motor function can significantly affect the patient's mobility and self-care and thus result in complications from immobility. Loss of sensation puts the patient at risk for skin breakdown and other injuries because pressure and pain are not perceived.

IMPAIRED BLADDER FUNCTION. During the period of spinal shock, all bladder and bowel function ceases. An indwelling catheter is inserted to empty the bladder and permit close monitoring of urinary output. As soon as the patient's fluid status is stabilized, the indwelling catheter is often removed and the bladder drained by intermittent catheterization. Once spinal shock resolves, reflex activity returns. The bladder becomes spastic and may spontaneously empty. Bladder retraining protocols can be specifically designed for individual patients.

Medications may be used to aid in the prevention of urinary tract infections. Methenamine mandelate (Mandelamine) is a urinary antiseptic that may be used in the regimen. Because the action of methenamine is enhanced in an acidic environment, vitamin C (ascorbic acid) is often prescribed to lower urine pH.

IMPAIRED BOWEL FUNCTION. Loss of bowel activity in the first day or two after injury may require insertion of a nasogastric tube for decompression. Peristalsis usually returns by the third postinjury day. Most spinal cord–injured patients can maintain bowel function because the large bowel musculature has its own neural center that responds to distention by the fecal mass. To assist in evacuation of the bowel, the patient must take advantage of the abdominal muscles as well as have an appropriate diet.

IMPAIRED TEMPERATURE REGULATION. Depending on the level of the injury, the patient may have difficulty maintaining body temperature within a normal range. If a person becomes too cold, the body normally responds with vasoconstriction and shivering to increase the temperature. If a person becomes too hot, sweating helps to dissipate heat. The spinal cord–injured patient may lose these regulatory mechanisms and be unable to adapt to temperature extremes. The quadriplegic person is especially vulnerable to environmental temperature changes because such a large part of the body is affected.

IMPAIRED SEXUAL FUNCTION. Spinal levels S-2, S-3, and S-4 control sexual function, so injury at or above these levels results in sexual dysfunction. The ability of the male patient to achieve erection and ejaculation is variable, depending on the level of injury. In females, menses resume normally after injury. Women with spinal cord injuries can have sexual intercourse but lack vaginal sensation. Some women with spinal cord injuries do experience orgasm, although it is not vaginally triggered. They can also bear children regardless of the level of the lesion. In the event of pregnancy, vaginal delivery is possible if pelvic proportions are adequate. If the lesion is high, however, the woman will not be aware of labor contractions.

IMPAIRED SKIN INTEGRITY. Immobility and loss of sensation put the patient at risk for skin problems. One of the most common complications in the spinal cord–injured patient is pressure ulcers. Because the immobile patient is unable to change positions, skin in the sacral area and across the bony prominences may break down. This presents a portal for infection in the patient. In addition, the presence of a pressure sore in the sacral area impedes early rehabilitation efforts because the patient is unable to begin wheelchair training until the ulcer heals.

The complete spinal cord injury also interrupts the vasomotor tone of the vascular system. This loss of tone results in vasodilation and pooling of blood in the periphery, impeding perfusion of the skin and encouraging the development of pressure sores.

ALTERED SELF-CONCEPT AND BODY IMAGE. The impact of spinal cord injury on the patient's self-concept and body image is tremendous. Depending on the extent of the injury, every aspect of the patient's life (occupation, family roles and responsibilities, socialization, hobbies) may be affected. French and Phillips (1991) describe the effects of spinal cord injury on body image as occurring in four phases: impact, retreat, acknowledgment, and reconstruction. In the impact phase, the patient becomes aware of the devastating changes that have taken place. He or she is in emotional shock and may express a desire to die. The retreat phase is marked by depression and withdrawal as the patient considers the implications of the injury. In the acknowledgment phase, the patient begins to face the injury and deal with it realistically. The patient moves into the reconstruction phase when he or she is ready to tackle the work of rehabilitation and to begin to plan for the future. A new body image has been constructed that incorporates the injury.

MEDICAL TREATMENT IN THE ACUTE PHASE

The goals of medical treatment guide the plans for the spinal cord–injured patient through all phases of the injury. The three major medical goals for the patient with spinal injury are to save the patient's life, to prevent further injury to the cord, and to preserve as much cord function as possible. Each medical goal has specific implications for nursing care and is directed at maximizing the patient's potential for recovery and rehabilitation.

SAVING THE PATIENT'S LIFE

The patient with a spinal cord injury may have additional life-threatening injuries. As mentioned earlier, patients with high cervical cord injuries often die before arriving at the hospital owing to impaired respiratory function.

The first priority is to establish a patent airway. The conventional head-tilt–chin-lift method of opening the airway is inappropriate in spinal injury patients because of the risk of increasing cord damage. The risk of additional damage is especially high with cervical injury. Flexion of the neck, even that caused by a pillow or other support, must be avoided. The jaw-thrust method of opening the airway is preferred for these patients. Once the airway has been opened, 100% oxygen may be administered by mask and manual resuscitator (e.g., an Ambu bag).

An endotracheal or tracheostomy tube may be placed to allow direct access to the airway and to facilitate optimal oxygenation. Any injury that compromises ventilation must immediately be treated.

PREVENTING FURTHER CORD INJURY

Immobilization is essential to prevent further damage to the spinal cord after injury. Various types of devices and traction may be utilized.

TRACTION. Immobilization with skeletal traction is often used to manage cervical spinal cord injuries. A variety of skull traction devices may be used, including Gardner-Wells and Crutchfield tongs. Gardner-Wells tongs are secured just above the ears but do not actually penetrate the skull. Crutchfield tongs, which are less commonly used now than in the past, are applied directly to the skull, just behind the hairline. The tongs allow traction to be applied, which separates and aligns the vertebrae to prevent further cord damage and reduces painful muscle spasms (Fig. 27–8). After the tongs are applied, radiographs are ordered to confirm alignment of the spine. Ongoing neurologic assessment is done to monitor for further deficits.

The halo ring is used to immobilize and align the cervical vertebrae (Fig. 27–9). It is applied to the skull using four pins and then connected either to weights or to a fiberglass jacket by adjustable rods. The jacket allows the paralyzed patient to be moved out of bed and allows the patient who is not paralyzed to be ambulatory. Because such good immobilization is achieved, attention can be turned to other aspects of treatment and rehabilitation can be initiated.

SPECIAL BEDS AND CUSHIONS. A number of special beds are available to help prevent complications of immobility while maintaining spinal immobilization. A kinetic bed such as the Roto-Rest bed slowly but continually rotates the patient from side to side (Fig. 27–10). Overlay air mattresses are flotation devices that are placed on standard hospital beds. Air-fluidized and flotation beds may be used *after* the spine has been stabilized, but they are never used when a patient is in tongs because of the potential damage that could occur if the bed should unexpectedly deflate.

The Wedge-Stryker frame is a canvas and metal frame bed that may be used to help turn the patient. It is no longer used as frequently as in the past. The patient lies supine on the posterior frame for approximately 2 hours at a time. Then the anterior frame is secured on top of the patient and the device is turned over so that the patient is prone on the anterior frame. Two people are needed each time to turn the patient, and the patient must be tightly secured to the frame. Every 2 hours, the patient is turned from the supine to the prone position or vice versa. Many patients have a difficult time adjusting to such a bed because the prone position leaves the patient feeling as though suspended in midair. Because of this, most patients are managed on a conventional or specialty bed.

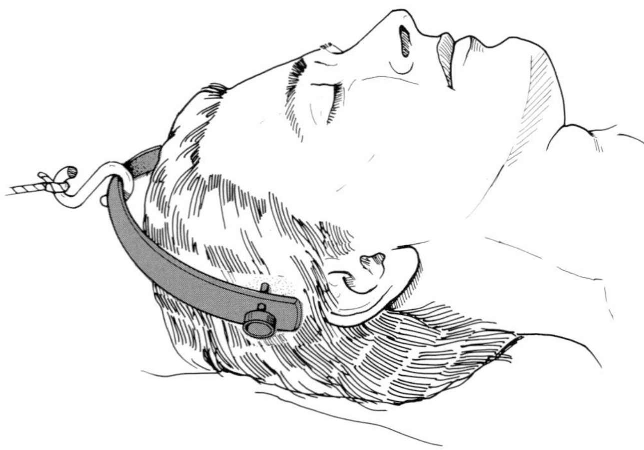

FIGURE 27-8

Gardner-Wells tongs are used to immobilize the cervical spine.

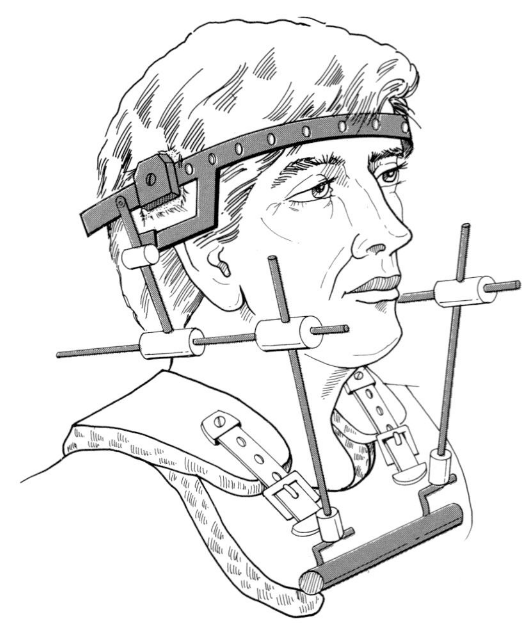

FIGURE 27-9

The halo device immobilizes and aligns the cervical vertebrae.

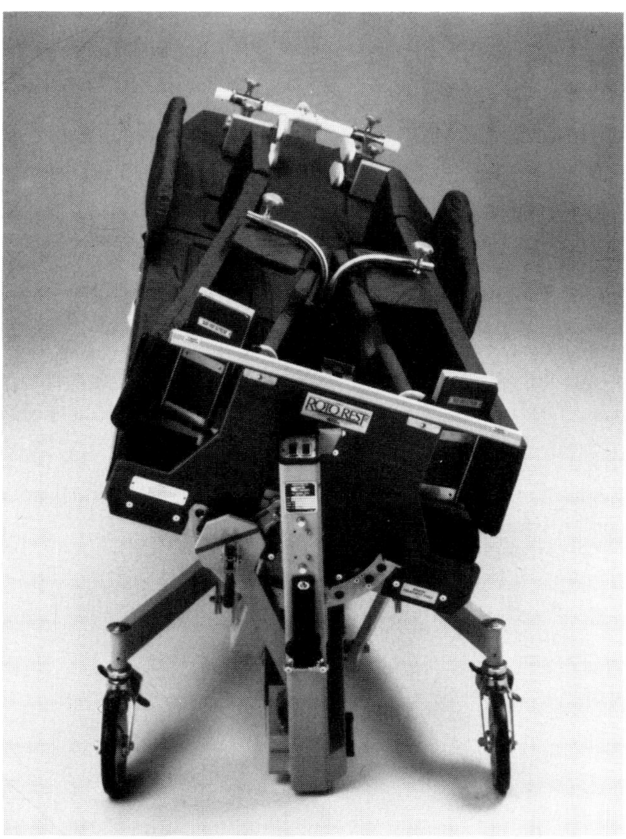

FIGURE 27-10

The Roto-Rest bed slowly turns the patient from side to side. (From Black, J. M., & Matassarin-Jacobs, E. [eds.]. [1993]. *Luckmann and Sorensen's medical surgical nursing: A psychophysiologic approach* [4th ed., p. 689]. Philadelphia: W. B. Saunders.)

Once the patient is able to be up in a chair, cushioning is needed to prevent excessive pressure and pressure ulcers. Types of cushions include those inflated with air, flotation devices, and gel pads. Examples of pressure-reducing cushions are the ROHO cushion, BBD-Bye Bye decubiti cushion, Jay cushion, Akro cushion, and Vari-Lite cushion. The cushion is selected that best meets the needs of the individual patient. The physical therapist is a good resource person for this recommendation.

DRUG THERAPY. Until recently, management of the spinal cord–injured patient has relied almost exclusively on surgical and immobilization techniques. Recent research has suggested that high doses of methylprednisolone sodium succinate (Solu-Medrol) may help decrease the deterioration of nervous tissue in the spinal cord after injury. The optimal time of administration is within the first 8 hours of injury. Although this therapy is new and still being studied, it offers hope for limiting neurologic deficits.

PHARMACOLOGY CAPSULE

The administration of high doses of methlyprednisolone sodium succinate during the first 8 hours after spinal cord injury may help to limit the neurologic effects of the injury.

PRESERVING CORD FUNCTION

Early surgical intervention may be necessary to repair cord damage. Situations in which surgery is required include cord compression by bony fragments, compound vertebral fractures, and gunshot and stab wounds. In these cases, surgery within the first 24 hours is most desirable.

A laminectomy involves removal of all or part of the posterior arch of the vertebra. This may be done to alleviate compression on the cord or spinal nerves. If multiple vertebrae are involved, a spinal fusion also may be done to stabilize the area. A spinal fusion consists of the placement of a piece of donor bone, commonly taken from the hip, into the area between the involved vertebrae. After healing, the fusion immobilizes the affected section of the spine. Postoperative immobilization of the area is necessary to allow for adequate healing, permanent fusion, and correct alignment. Neither laminectomy nor spinal fusion can be attempted until the patient has been fully stabilized during the acute phase of the injury.

NURSING CARE IN THE ACUTE PHASE

ASSESSMENT

A complete assessment as described here may be delayed until the patient is stabilized. Until then, the nurse monitors level of consciousness, vital signs, respiratory status, motor and sensory function, and intake and output.

HEALTH HISTORY

Present Illness. The nurse records the event that brought the patient to the hospital. Specific injuries incurred in the incident are noted. This may be the initial hospitalization after the injury, or the patient may be admitted at a later time for other reasons. Pain and other symptoms are described in detail.

Past Medical History. It is important not to overlook other medical problems when the patient has a spinal cord injury. The nurse inquires about other accidents or injuries and chronic illnesses such as diabetes, hypertension, heart disease, cancer, or seizure disorder. Previous hospitalizations and operations are documented. An obstetric history is obtained from the female patient.

Current medications are identified and allergies are recorded.

Family History. A routine family history is taken but is not considered specifically relevant to a diagnosis of spinal cord injury resulting from trauma.

Review of Systems. The nurse inquires about signs and symptoms that may be related to neurologic dysfunction or its consequences. Data to be collected include skin condition, headache or dizziness, vision disturbances, hearing impairment or tinnitus, nasal drainage (especially if there was a head injury), dyspnea, nausea and vomiting, constipation or diarrhea, fecal incontinence, bladder dysfunction, sexual dysfunction, and impaired motor and sensory function.

Functional Assessment. The patient's self-care abilities are assessed. The nurse explores the patient's roles and responsibilities as a family member. Occupation, hobbies, usual activity pattern, habits including use of tobacco and alcohol, and diet are recorded. It is important to know who the patient's significant others are and whether those relationships are supportive. In addition, the nurse determines the patient's emotional response to the spinal injury. Usual coping strategies are assessed. Spiritual beliefs and other sources of support are determined.

PHYSICAL EXAMINATION. The patient's reported height and weight are recorded. Actual weight may have to be delayed until the patient can tolerate the procedure. Vital signs are assessed. The nurse is alert for hypertension and bradycardia typical of autonomic dysreflexia (discussed earlier in this chapter). Temperature is taken to detect alterations that may reflect failure of regulatory mechanisms or may indicate infection. In the general survey, the nurse observes the patient's level of responsiveness, posture, and spontaneous movements.

The skin is inspected for lesions (lacerations, bruises) that may have occurred at the same time as the spinal cord injury, or for signs of pressure that may have resulted from immobility. Tissue turgor is assessed. The head is inspected for lesions and palpated for masses and swelling. The patient can be asked to read available print to assess visual acuity. The pupils of the eyes are examined for size, equality, and reaction to light.

The nurse observes the patient's respiratory effort and auscultates breath sounds. The abdomen is inspected for distention and auscultated for bowel sounds. The extremities are inspected for open fractures or abnormal positions. Range of motion, voluntary and involuntary movement, muscle strength, spasms, and sensory perception are assessed in all extremities. If conscious, the patient is asked to move the extremities through the various ranges of motion. This simply indicates whether or not the patient is capable of such movement and gives the nurse some early indication as to the involvement of particular spinal cord levels.

Muscle strength is assessed by using passive range of motion exercises and by testing strength against gravity as well as against resistance applied by the examiner. The examiner instructs the patient to try to move the extremity against the examiner's hand. Both upper and lower extremities are evaluated, and one side is compared with the other. Function is graded on a scale of 0 (complete paralysis) to 5 (normal strength) (Table 27–5). If the patient is unconscious, some noxious stimulus, such as pressure on the nailbed, must be applied to determine whether movement is possible. In the event of cranial involvement, such movement in response to noxious stimuli may be described as decorticate or decerebrate posturing. Both of these are described in Chapter 25.

Involuntary movement also may be observed in the injured patient. This type of movement is evidenced by the appearance of muscle spasms. Such spasms should be documented in terms of location and severity. Techniques for assessing the movement of the major muscle groups in both the upper and the lower extremities are described in Table 27–6.

Sensory evaluation is performed by determining the patient's ability to perceive sharp and dull sensations and touch with the eyes closed. As with the motor evaluation, one side of the body is compared with the other to assess equality. The hands, forearms, upper arms, trunk, thighs, lower legs, feet, and perineal area are included in the assessment. Sensory loss is best described by the use of a dermatome chart (Fig. 27–11). A dermatome defines an area of the skin that is innervated by a particular subcutaneous nerve root. In the initial postinjury period, sensation should be reassessed frequently because the injury may ascend and affect vital functions.

Proprioception (position sense) is tested by having the patient close his or her eyes and identify the position of a toe or finger as the nurse moves it up or down.

Nursing assessment of the patient with a spinal cord injury is summarized in Table 27–7.

NURSING DIAGNOSIS

Nursing diagnoses during the acute phase of spinal cord injury may include the following:

- **Ineffective Breathing Patterns** related to neurologic impairment
- **High Risk for Injury** related to involuntary muscle spasms, lack of motor and sensory function, orthostatic hypotension

TABLE 27-5
GRADING SCALE FOR MUSCLE STRENGTH

SCORE	FINDINGS
0	No movement. Total paralysis.
1	Weak contraction palpated or observed. No movement.
2	Muscle moves when supported against gravity.
3	Active muscle movement against gravity.
4	Active full range of motion against gravity but with some weakness when resistance is tested.
5	Full active range of motion against gravity and resistance.

TABLE 27-6

ASSESSMENT TECHNIQUES FOR MAJOR MUSCLE GROUPS

NERVE ROOT	MUSCLE ACTION	ASSESSMENT TECHNIQUE
C4-5	Abduction of shoulder	Shrug shoulder against downward pressure
C5-6	Elbow flexion (biceps)	Arm flexed toward body against resistance
C-7	Elbow extension (triceps)	Arm extended away from body against resistance
C-8	Hand grasp (finger flexors)	Hands grasped around examiner's fingers with attempts to withdraw fingers from grasp
L2-4	Hip flexion	Leg raised against resistance
L2-4	Knee extension	Knee extended away from body against resistance
L-5	Foot dorsiflexion	Foot pulled upward against resistance
L-5 to S-1	Knee flexion	Knee flexed toward body against resistance
S-1	Plantar flexion	Foot and toes pointed downward against resistance

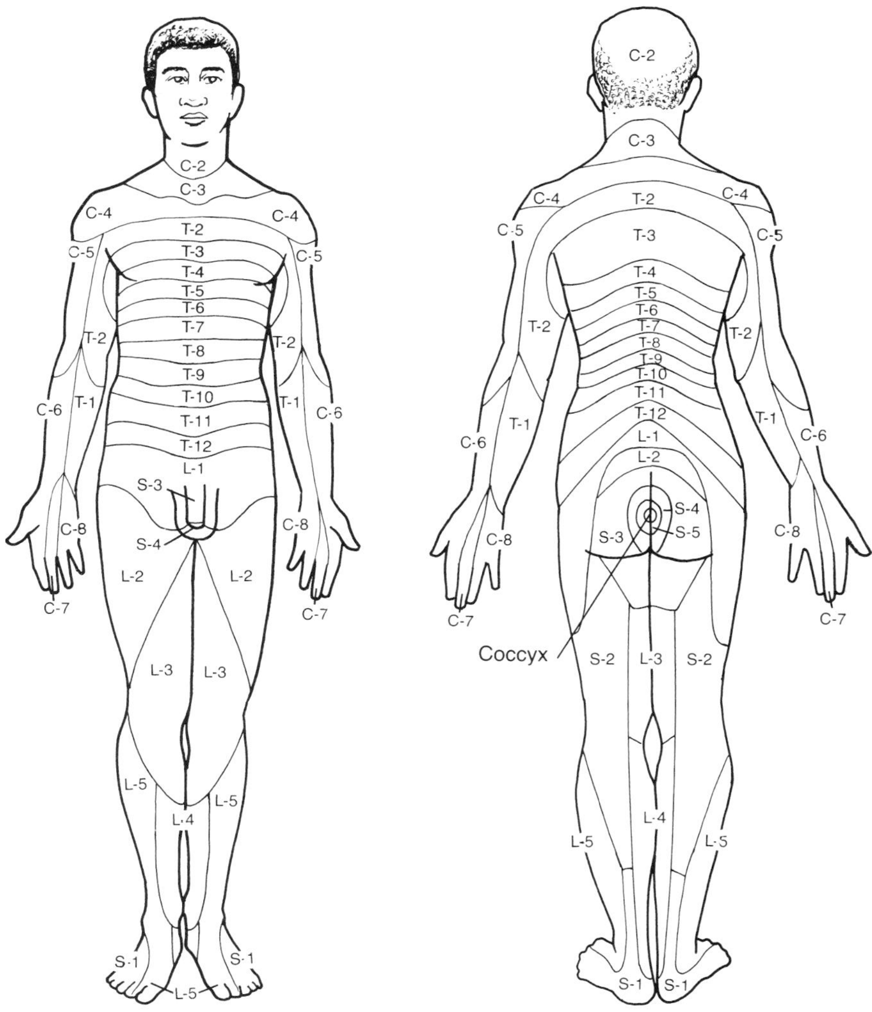

FIGURE 27-11

A dermatome chart. A dermatome defines an area of the skin that is innervated by a particular nerve root.

TABLE 27-7
ASSESSMENT OF THE PATIENT WITH A SPINAL CORD INJURY

HEALTH HISTORY

Present illness: Specific event that caused injury, other apparent injuries, pain location and severity

Past medical history: Past accidents, injuries, hospitalizations, and surgeries; history of diabetes mellitus, hypertension, heart disease, cancer, seizure disorder; obstetric history; current medications; allergies

Family history: Routine family history

Review of systems: Skin condition, headache, dizziness, vision disturbances, hearing impairment, tinnitus, nasal drainage, dyspnea, nausea, vomiting, constipation, diarrhea, fecal incontinence, bladder dysfunction, sexual dysfunction, impaired motor or sensory function

Functional assessment: Self-care abilities, roles and responsibilities, occupation, hobbies, usual activity pattern, use of tobacco and alcohol, diet, interpersonal relationships, emotional response to injury, usual coping strategies, spiritual beliefs, sources of support

PHYSICAL EXAMINATION

Height and weight

Vital signs

Level of consciousness, posture, spontaneous movements

Skin: Lesions, bruises, redness, tissue turgor

Head: Lesions, masses, swelling

Eyes: Visual acuity, pupil size, equality, reaction to light

Thorax: Respiratory effort, breath sounds

Abdomen: Distention, bowel sounds

Extremities: Range of motion, voluntary and involuntary movements, muscle strength, spasms, sensory perception, abnormal posturing, ability to recognize position of digits without looking

- **Dysreflexia** related to bladder or bowel distention, renal calculi, pressure sores
- **High Risk for Disuse Syndrome** related to pathologic or prescribed immobility, or both
- **Bowel Incontinence** related to impaired conduction of impulses
- **Altered Urinary Elimination** related to sensory motor impairment
- **High Risk for Infection** related to skeletal traction pins
- **Sensory Perceptual Alterations** (kinesthetic, tactile) related to altered sensory transmission
- **Ineffective Thermoregulation** related to spinal cord trauma
- **Self-Care Deficit** (feeding, dressing, grooming) related to neurologic impairment
- **Altered Sexuality Patterns** related to altered body function
- **Hopelessness** related to overwhelming losses and limited potential for recovered function
- **Knowledge Deficit** of condition, treatment, adaptations, expectations

GOALS

Goals of nursing care for the patient with spinal cord injury are effective breathing patterns, absence of injury, absence of signs of autonomic dysreflexia, absence of complications of immobility, controlled bowel elimination, absence of urinary retention or urinary infection, absence of pin site infection, protection of body areas with impaired sensation, effective thermoregulation, adaptation to self-care deficits, adaptation to altered sexual function, hopefulness, and patient's understanding of condition and treatment.

INTERVENTIONS

Ineffective Breathing Patterns. Respiratory problems may result from neurologic damage or may be associated with immobility. The patient with an injury at or above C-5 has complete loss of spontaneous respirations and requires mechanical ventilation. When a person has an injury to the lower thoracic cord, abdominal and intercostal muscles are affected, resulting in weakened exhalation and cough. Nursing care is individualized for these patients depending on the extent of respiratory impairment. Ventilator-dependent patients may be taught techniques to allow independent breathing for limited periods of time. The ventilator-dependent patient requires special care, as described in Chapter 28.

A variety of techniques may be used to help patients with spontaneous but impaired breathing to clear the airway more effectively. These include breathing exercises, assisted coughing, and vibration and percussion with postural drainage. For assisted coughing, the nurse applies firm pressure to the diaphragm just below the rib cage as the patient exhales or coughs. Since timing is important, the nurse establishes some form of communication with the patient (such as a blink) to identify when inspiration is completed. The nurse should be properly trained in this technique before using it.

The immobile patient is turned and repositioned as permitted to decrease pooling of secretions in the lungs. If the patient is breathing independently, the nurse coaches the patient in deep-breathing exercises and use of the incentive spirometer. Adequate hydration helps to thin secretions so that they can be more readily removed.

High Risk for Injury. Safety is of prime consideration during the period of spastic paralysis. Involuntary muscle spasms can be so violent that the patient may be thrown from the wheelchair or bedside chair. It is imperative that the patient be adequately secured with a protective strap across the chest. Even while in bed, the patient requires protection. Undue stimulation of the spastic extremity or muscle group should be avoided. When performing range of motion exercises or positioning the patient, the nurse avoids grasping the muscle itself. Rather, the joints above and below the affected muscle groups are supported with the palms of the hands.

For the patient maintained in cervical traction on a conventional bed, position changes must be done by log rolling. A minimum of three nurses is needed to correctly log roll the patient. Some prior planning must be done so that the movement is coordinated. The desired position is identified, and pillows and equipment are placed in the proper locations before turning the patient. One nurse stands at the head of the bed and stabilizes the traction by placing his or her hands firmly on the patient's head and neck without flexing the neck.

The second nurse prepares to move the shoulders while the third prepares to move the hips and legs. After explaining the procedure to the patient, the patient is turned as a unit ("log rolled") to the desired position while maintaining proper alignment. Pillows are then placed to the patient's back and shoulders and between the legs to protect any pressure spots and to promote comfort. The nurse holding the head and neck should not release the patient until all movement has been completed to ensure that traction does not slip out of place.

Ace bandages or other types of pressure stockings are applied as ordered to promote venous return, preventing a sudden drop in blood pressure and reducing the risk of thrombophlebitis.

If injections are necessary, they should be administered above the level of paralysis. There are two reasons for this. First, circulation is impaired below the level of injury, causing drug absorption to be poor. Second, the patient is at increased risk for infection when the skin integrity is broken in affected parts of the body.

Dysreflexia. The focus of nursing management for the patient at risk for AD is primarily directed toward the prevention of the triggering stimulus. The patient and family members must be taught the causes, signs and symptoms, and management of AD.

When AD occurs, it is a medical emergency. Once it is recognized, immediate action is required. Raising the patient's head to a 45-degree angle or placing the patient in a sitting position may help decrease the pressure. If the cause can be identified, every effort should be made to eliminate it. The indwelling catheter is checked for occlusion. If the bladder is distended and no indwelling catheter is present, straight catheterization may be indicated. Fecal impactions, if present, need to be digitally removed following the application of a local anesthetic as ordered. The nurse monitors the patient with severe hypertension for seizures or signs of a stroke. The physician should be immediately notified so that appropriate medications or other interventions can be initiated. Antihypertensive drugs are administered as ordered. Features of AD are summarized in Table 27–8.

High Risk for Disuse Syndrome. To avoid the development of pressure ulcers, the nurse turns the patient at least every 2 hours and massages around the bony prominences to help increase blood flow in the area. As the patient is turned, the back and sacral area are fully inspected for any breakdown or signs of pressure. Back care is performed using a gentle lotion or other agent designed specifically for the prevention of breakdown. Any reddened or broken areas noted are relieved of pressure. When the patient is resting in the lateral supine position, a pillow is placed between the legs to keep the heels free of pressure and to prevent pressure between the knees. Bed linens are kept clean, dry, and free of wrinkles. The nurse teaches the patient how to inspect the skin and to recognize signs of pressure.

Specialty beds and cushions also may be used to help alleviate pressure and enhance circulation. Patients in wheelchairs are still instructed or assisted to reposition at least every 15 minutes. Some wheelchairs designed for quadriplegic patients can be tilted backward to allow shifting of body weight.

Patients with tongs are maintained on strict bedrest. Therefore, it is imperative that meticulous skin care be provided. With the vertebral column stabilized, the patient may be turned for position changes and skin assessment.

When the patient has spasticity, nursing management is directed toward the prevention of contractures and muscle atrophy. Pharmacologic agents, such as diazepam (Valium), baclofen (Lioresal), and dantrolene sodium (Dantrium), may be effective muscle relaxants. Electrical stimulators, used with heat and physiotherapy, also may help relieve spasms. Nursing management of the patient with muscle spasms is summarized in Table 27–9.

During the time of flaccid paralysis, the nurse diligently performs passive range of motion exercises and positions and aligns the extremities to reduce the risk of subluxation or contractures.

More complete discussion of the nursing care of the immobilized person is in Chapter 19.

TABLE 27–8
AUTONOMIC DYSREFLEXIA

CAUSES
- Distended bladder or plugged catheter
- Fecal impaction
- Urinary calculi
- Pressure ulcer
- Ejaculation
- Uterine contractions

SIGNS AND SYMPTOMS
- Sudden hypertension
- Pounding headache
- Anxiety
- Flushed face
- Diaphoresis
- Nasal congestion
- Bradycardia
- Vasoconstriction below lesion with cold skin and "goose flesh"
- Vasodilation above lesion with warm, moist skin

POTENTIAL EFFECTS
- Seizures
- Stroke

MANAGEMENT
- Assessment to identify cause
- Elevation of head of bed
- Irrigation or replacement of urinary catheter
- Intermittent catheterization
- Application of topical anesthetic and digital disimpaction
- Removal of pressure from irritated skin
- Administration of antihypertensives as ordered

PHARMACOLOGY CAPSULE

Muscle relaxants may be ordered to control muscle spasticity.

TABLE 27–9

MANAGEMENT OF SPASTICITY IN THE SPINAL CORD–INJURED PATIENT

Perform passive range of motion exercises at least four times a day
Properly position and split extremities to prevent contractures
Limit tactile stimuli
Avoid incidence of noxious stimuli, such as anxiety, pain, bladder or bowel distention, and pressure ulcers
Turn and reposition at least every 2 hr
Properly administer medications to reduce spasms

Bowel Incontinence. In the early postinjury period, an ileus may develop, meaning that peristalsis ceases. The abdomen becomes distended and bowel sounds are absent. If this happens, fluids are administered intravenously and nothing is given by mouth. A nasogastric tube may be inserted and connected to suction for decompression. Peristalsis usually returns by the third day after the injury.

Once peristalsis resumes, the patient is given oral fluids and food. The nurse encourages adequate fluids and high-fiber foods to promote soft stools. Bulk laxatives, stool softeners, suppositories, and lubricants are administered as ordered. Bowel movements are documented, and measures are instituted to prevent constipation and impaction. The nurse works with the patient to determine the best schedule for bowel elimination and helps the patient to carry out the program. A bowel retraining program must be a cooperative effort between the caregiver and the patient. The program can succeed only when the patient is prepared physically and emotionally. Bowel retraining is discussed in detail in Chapter 21.

Altered Urinary Elimination. While the patient has an indwelling catheter, meticulous catheter care is essential. Since catheterization increases the risk of urinary tract infections, the nurse monitors the patient's temperature and assesses the urine for cloudiness and foul odor. Urinary acidifiers, antiseptics, and antimicrobials are administered as ordered. Oral fluids are encouraged, when permitted, to maintain dilute urine. Dairy products are discouraged because they contain calcium, which may promote formation of urinary calculi.

In the rehabilitation phase, bladder retraining is addressed. As a bladder retraining program is instituted, the nurse works with the patient to carry out the program. To help improve tone and relieve bladder spasms, the catheter may be periodically clamped and then released in an effort to increase bladder capacity. When the bladder can hold 300 to 400 ml of urine, the catheter may be removed for a trial period. Details of bladder retraining are covered in Chapter 21.

High Risk for Infection. The risks of pulmonary and urinary infections have already been discussed. If the patient has skeletal traction (Gardner-Wells tongs, halo ring), there is also a risk of infection at the pin insertion sites. Specific skin care is done as ordered or per agency policy. Pin care in some agencies involves the application of polymyxin B (Neosporin) ointment covered with sterile, dry dressings. The nurse reports increasing redness or purulent drainage at the pin sites to the physician.

PHARMACOLOGY CAPSULE

Topical antimicrobial ointments may be applied to the pin insertion sites to decrease the risk of infection.

Sensory Perceptual Alterations. Sensory loss presents definite implications for nursing care. The spinal cord–injured patient with a complete lesion is unable to detect any temperature or pain sensations below the level of the injury. The individual is not able to determine if a painful stimulus, such as a burn, is present. The nurse must ensure that meticulous skin care is provided and that all necessary measures are taken to protect the patient from harm.

Ineffective Thermoregulation. The environmental temperature should be maintained at a level that avoids chilling or overheating the patient. A room temperature of 70°F (21°C) will keep the quadriplegic's body temperature stable at 95°F. To prevent hypothermia, adequate clothing and blankets are provided. Wet clothing and linens are changed immediately.

To prevent excessive warming, the patient should avoid the outdoors during very hot, humid weather. Some patients carry a water spray bottle when outdoors in the heat or during intense activity. The water can be sprayed on the skin, where it evaporates and cools the body. Fans can also help to cool the patient. An increase in temperature is normal after exercise.

Self-Care Deficit. The nurse continually reassesses the patient's abilities and need for assistance with self-care activities. The patient may require total care initially. As soon as the patient is able, the nurse begins preparing him or her for self-care consistent with the patient's expected abilities. During rehabilitation, the patient learns to use specialized equipment and strategies in order to be as independent as possible in self-care.

Altered Sexuality Patterns. Sexuality and sexual function in the spinal cord–injured patient must be addressed when the patient first brings up the subject. Because sexual gratification is an important aspect of emotional and psychological well-being, it is an issue that requires thoughtful discussion and counseling. Patients must be apprised of their physical abilities to achieve erection or to bear children. Information is provided about the possibility of pregnancy and about birth control, if desired.

The nurse advises the patient of resources available in the agency and in the community. The expertise of a trained counselor is often needed, and the counselor is usually a member of the rehabilitation team. Honest discussion must occur between the patient and the counselor. Both parties must be willing to explore the physical and emotional aspects of the injury. Additional information on management of impaired sexual function is presented in Chapters 43 and 44.

Hopelessness. Hopelessness may be manifested by withdrawal, passive behavior, and decreased affect. A person who feels helpless sees few or no personal choices available and cannot mobilize the energy needed to move forward. The nurse offers opportunities for the patient to discuss feelings about his or her situation and future. The nurse listens actively and accepts the patient's feelings. When the patient is withdrawn, the nurse encourages, but does not force, participation in self-care. As the patient begins to acknowledge the injury and assess its impact, the nurse encourages him or her to identify strengths and coping strategies. Rehabilitation efforts are begun in earnest, with generous praise given for effort.

The health care team also works with the patient's significant others to create a supportive atmosphere that conveys hope, acceptance, and confidence. Patients and families often continue to hope for physical improvement that is unlikely. For example, they may interpret the movement associated with spastic paralysis as a return of voluntary motor function. The nurse can avoid this misconception by explaining this phenomenon in advance and emphasizing that it is expected and does not signify improved function.

Knowledge Deficit. During the acute phase of spinal cord injury, the nurse explains routines and procedures. The physician or clinical nurse specialist usually informs the patient of the extent of the injury and probable effects. The nurse reinforces that information and helps the patient and family obtain any additional information requested. An important resource is the National Spinal Cord Injury Association hotline (1-800-526-3456), which has a 24-hour service to provide information about rehabilitation, research, organizations, and local contacts. Many communities have local chapters of the Spinal Cord Society, Paralyzed Veterans of America, and National Spinal Cord Injury Association that can provide information and resources.

The following are the essential components of the teaching plan:

- Effects of spinal cord injury
- Types of treatments and their purposes
- Breathing exercises and adaptive techniques
- Range of motion exercises and positioning
- Management of orthostatic hypotension
- Skin care and assessment (Table 27–10)
- Management of bowel and bladder elimination
- Recognition of signs and symptoms of infection
- Changes in sexual function and resources for information about adaptation
- Protection of body areas that lack sensation
- Adaptive techniques and devices to maximize self-care
- Emotional responses to spinal cord injury and coping strategies
- Community resources

TABLE 27–10

SKIN CARE: KEY POINTS FOR THE PATIENT WITH A SPINAL CORD INJURY

1. Avoid excessive pressure, shearing force, and trauma.
2. Bathe in tepid water with mild soap; dry thoroughly.
3. Soak feet for 20 min once a week; keep toenails trimmed and smooth.
4. Keep skin dry and free of contact with urine or stool.
5. Avoid tight clothing with heavy seams.
6. Wear cotton undergarments and avoid clothing made of fabrics that do not absorb moisture.
7. Eat a balanced diet with adequate vitamins A and C and protein.
8. Drink 2000–3000 ml of fluid each day unless directed otherwise.
9. When in bed, turn at least every 2 hr.
10. When in a chair, shift weight at least every 15 min.
11. Inspect skin every morning and every evening for redness, bruising, blisters, and dryness and feel for swelling and hardness.
12. If redness is present, try to determine cause. Ask yourself if you are turning or shifting weight often enough, if you are transferring correctly, and if your cushions are in good condition.

EVALUATION

Criteria for evaluating the outcomes of nursing interventions are normal respiratory rate and measures of oxygenation; absence of lesions or bruises; pulse and blood pressure consistent with patient's norms; absence of pressure sores, maximal possible range of motion, clear breath sounds; regular bowel movements under controlled circumstances; no bladder distention, urine clear with normal odor; pin sites free of excessive redness or purulent drainage; intact skin without signs of pressure; normal body temperature; patient's participation in self-care to extent possible; patient's verbalization of sexual capabilities and adaptive techniques; positive patient statements; and patient's statements describing condition, effects, and treatment plan.

REHABILITATION

The saying "rehabilitation begins at admission" may sound trite, but for the spinal cord–injured patient its truth is astounding. The newly paralyzed person is faced with many sobering physical and psychological challenges. Both the acute care staff and the rehabilitation staff strive to see that the patient is fully equipped to face the challenge.

Nursing care during the acute phase of the injury focuses on preventing further disability and avoiding complications that could prolong hospitalization and hamper rehabilitation. Rehabilitation is best described as those activities that assist the individual to achieve the highest possible level of self-care and independence.

The rehabilitation process involves a well-organized interdisciplinary team that can address all aspects of function. Members of the team include the physician, nurse, physical therapist, occupational therapist, speech therapist, dietitian, social worker, psychologist, and counselor. Each plays a vital role in helping the patient achieve the highest level of independence. What was once regarded by the patient as a normal lifestyle or occupation may no longer be possible. Rather, modifications and adjustments must be made. Both the patient and the family must be emotionally and physically prepared to make those adjustments. The team not only helps the patient accomplish activities of daily living and self-care but also addresses successful adjustment to social integration and gainful employment in the workplace. Although this phase of treatment may take more than a year to accomplish, the patient, family, and rehabilitation team can take pride in the realization that a life can once again be productive and happy.

NURSING CARE OF THE LAMINECTOMY PATIENT

General care of the surgical patient is discussed in Chapter 14. This section focuses on the specific needs of the spinal cord–injured patient having a laminectomy. However, laminectomy may be done for reasons other than traumatic cord injury.

Preoperatively, the nurse assesses the patient's vital signs and neurologic status to establish baselines. The patient's understanding of surgical routines also is determined. The patient is told what to expect in the immediate postoperative period.

For the patient who has a laminectomy, postoperative care focuses on ongoing assessment of neurologic status and on promoting healing at the operative site. Specific nursing responsibilities are summarized in Table 27–11.

TABLE 27–11
NURSING CARE AFTER LAMINECTOMY

Neurologic Assessment and Vital Signs
- Frequent assessment of movement, strength, and range of motion
- Ability to localize sensory stimulus
- Frequent vital signs to determine any postoperative complications, such as hemorrhage or infection

Circulation and Respiration
- Maintain elastic stockings on lower extremities to prevent deep vein thrombosis
- Encourage range of motion exercises four times a day
- Deep breathing exercises every 2 hr
- Auscultate breath sounds every 2–4 hr
- Incentive spirometry every 2 hr while awake

Progressive Ambulation
- Progress from sitting at edge of bed to ambulating with assistance
- Encourage increasing distances and independence while ambulating
- Ensure that patient uses back brace or other apparatus as ordered

Bed or Positioning
- Bed flat or only slightly elevated to reduce strain on operative site
- Maintain soft collar for cervical laminectomy
- Encourage position changes every 2 hr

Bowel and Bladder Function
- Measure urinary output
- Assess for urinary distention and complete emptying of bladder after spontaneous void
- Encourage fluid intake
- Intermittent catheterization may be needed if patient is unable to void
- Auscultate bowel sounds
- Initiate bowel program as appropriate

Surgical Incision
- Change dressing aseptically
- Check dressing for blood or cerebrospinal fluid drainage

Pain or Discomfort
- Medicate for pain and spasms as needed
- Encourage ambulation to reduce spasms

ASSESSMENT. After a laminectomy, the nurse monitors the patient's vital signs, neurologic status, and breath sounds. Movement, strength, range of motion, and ability to localize sensory stimulus are assessed frequently. Fluid intake and output are measured. The abdomen is auscultated for bowel sounds and palpated for bladder distention. The surgical dressing is inspected for bleeding, clear CSF drainage, and foul drainage. If the patient has pain, the nurse obtains a complete description.

NURSING DIAGNOSIS. Nursing diagnoses for the postlaminectomy patient may include the following:

- **High Risk for Injury** related to immobility, neurologic trauma, spinal fluid leakage
- **Altered Tissue Perfusion** related to hypovolemia, obstruction to blood flow
- **Pain** related to tissue trauma, muscle spasms
- **Altered Urinary Elimination** related to sensory motor impairment, prescribed position restrictions
- **Colonic Constipation** related to immobility, neurologic trauma, drug therapy
- **Impaired Physical Mobility** related to neuromuscular impairment, weakness, prescribed restrictions
- **Knowledge Deficit** of course of recovery, self-care activities

GOALS. Goals of nursing care for the postoperative laminectomy patient are freedom from injury, adequate tissue perfusion, pain relief, normal urine elimination, normal bowel elimination, improved physical mobility, and patient's knowledge of routines and self-care.

INTERVENTIONS

High Risk for Injury. The nurse monitors the patient for complications of surgery. Deviations in vital signs, including increased pulse and respirations, hypotension, and fever, are reported to the physician. Neurologic findings are compared with preoperative assessments. Decreasing sensory or motor responses are reported to the physician. The patient is assisted with measures to prevent complications of immobility (breathing and leg exercises) within the limitations of postoperative restrictions. The physician is also informed if clear drainage is observed draining from the incision because this usually indicates a CSF leak. When the dressing is changed, the nurse uses aseptic technique to reduce the risk of wound contamination.

Altered Tissue Perfusion. Measures are taken to promote oxygenation and circulation. Elastic or pneumatic stockings are applied to the lower extremities as ordered to promote venous return and prevent deep vein thrombosis. Range of motion exercises are done at least four times daily or as ordered. Breath sounds are auscultated every 2 to 4 hours, and the patient is supported to deep breathe and cough to remove pulmonary secretions. The incentive spirometer may be used every 2 hours while the patient is awake. The patient is positioned in good alignment. When turning or getting out of bed, the patient is taught to keep the back straight and to avoid twisting.

A soft collar may be ordered after cervical laminectomy. Back braces may be prescribed after lumbar or thoracic spinal fusions. Typically, the braces are worn at all times at first. Use of the device is decreased as muscle strength returns. In some situations, corsets and casts are used to support and stabilize the spine. When supportive devices are worn, the nurse inspects the skin carefully to make sure they are not creating pressure that could result in skin breakdown.

Pain. The patient's level of discomfort is assessed and documented. The bed is kept flat or with the head slightly elevated to reduce strain on the operative site. Analgesics and muscle relaxants are administered as ordered. Other pain-control measures, such as relaxation techniques, cutaneous stimulation, and imagery, are described in detail in Chapter 16. If the prescribed medications and nursing interventions do not provide pain relief, the nurse discusses the problem with the physician to see if other measures can be tried.

Altered Urinary Elimination. Measures are taken to promote voiding. Intravenous fluids are usually ordered, but oral fluids also can be given as soon as the patient is able to tolerate them. Voiding is documented, urine output measured, and the bladder assessed for emptying. The nurse promotes voiding by providing privacy and positioning the patient as comfortably as allowed. Running water may stimulate voiding. If the patient is unable to void, intermittent catheterization may be ordered.

NUTRITION CONCEPTS

- Constipation and lack of bowel control are best helped by encouraging adequate fluids and high-fiber foods (whole grains, legumes, fresh fruits, and vegetables).
- Increased oral fluids help dilute urine and prevent infection when there is lack of bladder control with spinal cord injury.
- Immobility related to spinal cord injury may cause kidney and bladder calculi. A preventive measure is a calcium-restricted diet with increased fluid intake.
- Severe spinal cord injury can result in muscle wasting and weight loss, so a diet high in protein and calories is recommended, especially during the acute phase of recovery.

Colonic Constipation. Stool softeners may be ordered to prevent constipation. In addition, adequate fluids and fiber are helpful. Ambulation, when permitted, also promotes normal bowel elimination.

Impaired Physical Mobility. Patient activity progresses from sitting on the edge of the bed to ambulating with assistance. The nurse encourages the patient to gradually increase distance and independence in ambulating. If the patient is to wear a back brace or other apparatus, the nurse ensures that it is properly applied. Physical therapy may be ordered.

Knowledge Deficit. Postoperative teaching is directed toward promoting recovery from the surgery and preventing future injuries. The nurse determines activity restrictions and discusses these with the patient.

EVALUATION. Criteria for evaluating the outcomes of nursing care are stable or improving neurologic and vital signs, absence of bleeding or CSF drainage, absence of fever, and normal white blood cell count; normal pulse, blood pressure, respirations, skin color, and tissue turgor; patient's statement of pain relief and relaxed expression; spontaneous voiding without bladder distention, urine output equal to intake; regular passage of formed stool; daily increase in walking distance without fatigue; and patient's statement of appropriate self-care activities.

BIBLIOGRAPHY

Basta, S. M. (1991) Pressure sore prevention education with the spinal cord injured. *Rehabilitation Nursing, 16*(1), 6–8.

Black, J. M., & Barker, E. (1993). Assessment of clients with neurologic disorders. In J. M. Black & E. Matassarin-Jacobs (Eds.), *Luckmann and Sorensen's medical-surgical nursing: A psychophysiologic approach* (4th ed.) (pp. 637–672). Philadelphia: W. B. Saunders.

Bryant, G. A. (1992). When your patient needs back surgery. *RN, 55*(7), 46–51.

Deglin, J. H.: Vallerand, A. H.: & Russin, M. M. (1991). *Davis's drug guide for nurses* (2nd ed.). Philadelphia: F. A. Davis.

Doenges, M. E., & Moorhouse, M. F. (1991). *Nursing diagnoses with interventions* (3rd ed.). Philadelphia: F. A. Davis.

Finocchiaro, D.N., & Herzfeld, S. T. (1990). Understanding autonomic dysreflexia. *American Journal of Nursing, 90*(9), 56+.

French, J. K., & Phillips, J. A. (1991). Shattered images: Recovery for the SCI client. *Rehabilitation Nursing, 16*(3), 134–136.

Hodgson, B. B., Kizior, R. J., & Kingdon, R. T. (1993). *Nurse's drug handbook.* Philadelphia: W. B. Saunders.

Ignatavicius, D. D., & Bayne, M. V. (1991). *Medical-surgical nursing: A nursing process approach.* Philadelphia: W. B. Saunders.

Jarvis, C. (1992). *Physical examination and health assessment.* Philadelphia: W. B. Saunders.

Marshall, S. B., Marshall, L. F., Vos, H. R., & Chesnut, R. M. (1990). *Neuroscience critical care.* Philadelphia: W. B. Saunders.

Schnell, S. (1991). Nursing care of clients with disorders of the spinal cord, peripheral nerves, and cranial nerves. In J. M. Black & E. Matassarin-Jacob (Eds.), *Luckmann and Sorensen's medical-surgical nursing: A psychophysiologic approach* (4th ed.) (pp. 637–672). Philadelphia: W. B. Saunders.

Shlafer, M. (1993). *The nurse, pharmacology, and drug therapy* (2nd ed.). Redwood City, CA: Addison-Wesley.

Zejdlik, C. P. (1992). *Management of spinal cord injury* (2nd ed.). Boston: Jones and Bartlett.

KEY CONCEPTS

1. Spinal cord injury most often results from trauma but may also be caused by degenerative conditions and tumors.
2. Spinal cord injuries may be classified by location, as open or closed, and by extent of damage to the cord.
3. After spinal cord injury, motor and sensory function is monitored by assessing movement, muscle strength, sensation, and reflex activity.
4. Effects of spinal cord injury may include impairments in breathing, sensory and motor function, bladder and bowel function, temperature regulation, sexual function, skin integrity, and self-concept.
5. Injuries at or above the fifth cervical vertebra may result in instant death because of interruption of the nerves that control respirations.
6. Autonomic dysreflexia is an exaggerated sympathetic response to stimuli such as bladder distention, constipation, renal calculi, ejaculation, and uterine contractions that produces severe hypertension with the potential for seizures and stroke.
7. Muscle tone is usually flaccid immediately after injury, but spasticity develops when spinal shock resolves.
8. The goals of medical care after spinal injury are to sustain life, prevent further cord injury, and repair cord damage.
9. Immobilization is essential to prevent further damage to the cord after injury.
10. Nursing care after spinal cord injury is concerned with ineffective breathing patterns, high risk for injury, dysreflexia, high risk for disuse syndrome, bowel incontinence, altered urine elimination, high risk for infection, sensory-perceptual alterations, ineffective thermoregulation, self-care deficits, altered sexuality patterns, hopelessness, and knowledge deficits.
11. Rehabilitation assists the patient to achieve the highest possible level of self-care and independence.

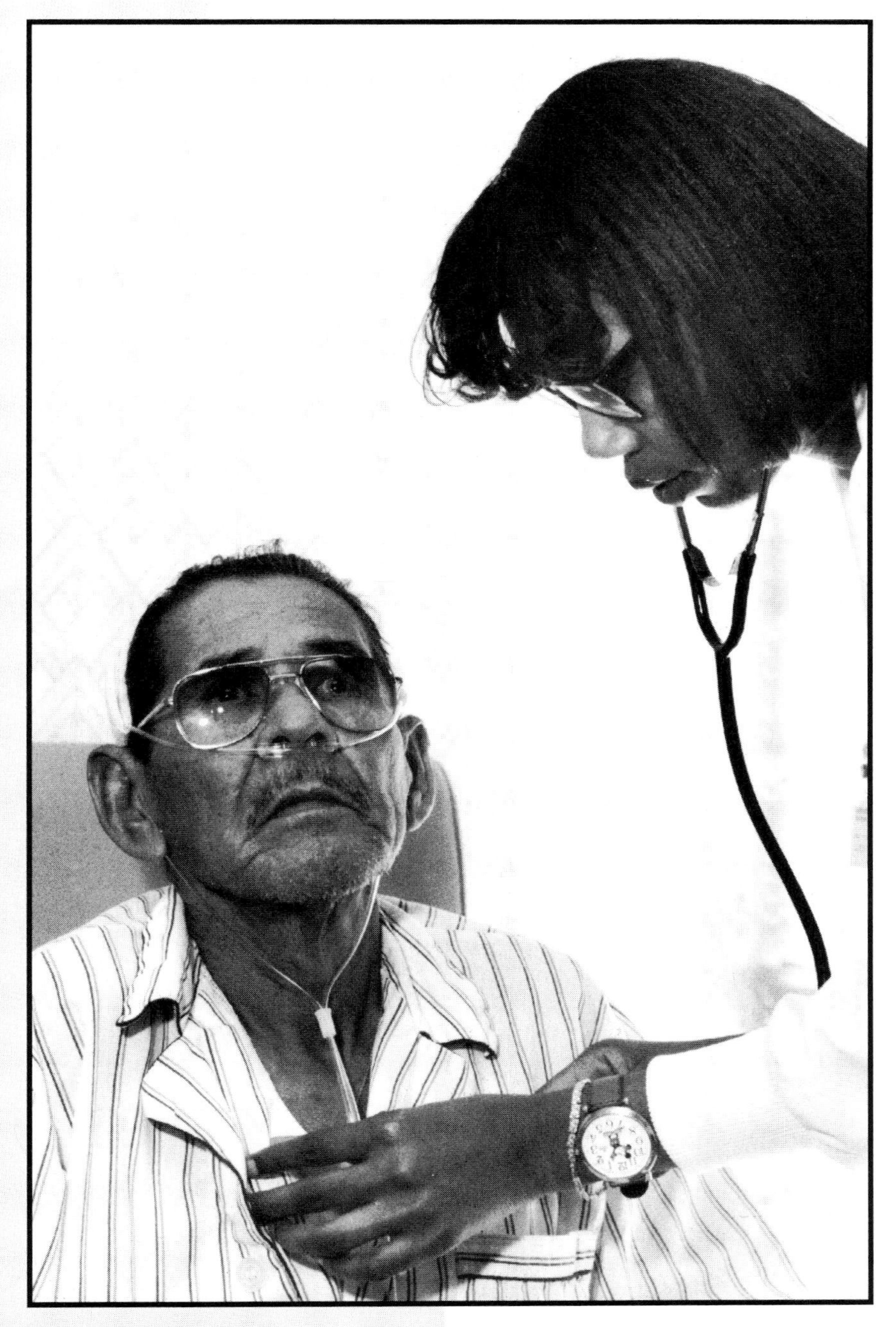

UNIT 7
Respiratory Disorders

Cheryl I. Bond
Mary Ann Matteson

CHAPTER 28

Acute Respiratory Disorders

OBJECTIVES

1. Identify data to be collected in the nursing assessment of the patient with a respiratory disorder.
2. Identify the nursing implications of age-related changes in the respiratory system.
3. Describe diagnostic tests or procedures for respiratory disorders and nursing interventions.
4. Explain nursing care of patients receiving therapeutic treatments for respiratory disorders.
5. For selected respiratory disorders, describe the pathophysiology, signs and symptoms, complications, diagnostic measures, and medical treatment.
6. Apply the nursing process to plan care for the patient who has an acute respiratory disorder.

GLOSSARY

ATELECTASIS Collapsed lung or part of a lung

CRACKLES Rales; abnormal lung sounds heard on auscultation

DYSPNEA Difficulty breathing

HEMOTHORAX Accumulation of blood in the pleural space

HYPERCAPNIA Excess carbon dioxide in the blood

HYPOXEMIA Low level of oxygen in the blood

HYPOXIA Low oxygen level

INSPISSATED Thickened and dried; often used to describe pulmonary secretions

ORTHOPNEA Difficulty breathing when lying down

PERFUSION Blood flow

PNEUMOTHORAX Accumulation of air in the pleural cavity that results in complete or partial collapse of a lung

Glossary continued

RHONCHUS Dry, rattling sound caused by partial bronchial obstruction

TACHYPNEA Rapid respiratory rate

VENTILATION Movement of air in and out of the lungs

Respiration is basic to life. The respiratory system provides "fuel" for bodily activities and energy to sustain life. Respiration is defined as the exchange of oxygen and carbon dioxide through the inspiration of air from the atmosphere and the expiration of air from the lungs. The function of the respiratory system is to supply oxygen (O_2) for the metabolic needs of the cells and to remove carbon dioxide (CO_2), one of the waste products of cell metabolism.

ANATOMY AND PHYSIOLOGY OF THE RESPIRATORY SYSTEM

ANATOMY OF THE RESPIRATORY SYSTEM

To reach the lungs, air must travel through several passages, including the nose, mouth, pharynx, larynx, trachea, and bronchi (Fig. 28–1). Each passage has an effect on the quality of the air that reaches the lungs.

Nose

The nose includes the external nose, or the part that is seen on the face, and the nasal cavity, which lies over the roof of the mouth. The external nose is made up of bones and cartilage that are covered with skin. The inside lining of the external nose consists of thick mucous membranes and small hairs. The mucous membranes also line the nasal cavity along with the cilia, which are small hair-like projections.

The mucous membranes warm and moisten the air that enters the nose. If the air is not warmed as it enters the body, the tissue lining in the respiratory tract functions poorly. If the air is not moistened, the cilia are destroyed. The mucous membranes, the hairs in the external nose, and the cilia filter out dust particles and bacteria from the air. The mucous membranes filter by trapping particles, such as dust, powder, and smoke, against the passage wall. Mucus then collects the particles and is swallowed. The cilia wave back and forth about 12 times per second to help the mucus clean the air.

Pharynx

The pharynx, or throat, is a 5-inch tube extending from the back of the mouth to the esophagus. It is divided into three parts—nasal, oral, and laryngeal. The nasopharynx lies behind the nose, the oropharynx lies behind the mouth, and the laryngopharynx lies behind the larynx.

The pharynx serves as a passage for both the respiratory and the digestive systems. It also has an important function in the formation of sounds, especially vowel sounds. The tonsils are located in the pharynx and if they become enlarged may interfere with breathing, particularly nasal breathing. In addition, speech may have a nasal sound.

Larynx

The larynx, or "voice box," is the air passage between the pharynx and the trachea. It contains vocal cords and several types of cartilage, including the thyroid cartilage and the epiglottis. The epiglottis is attached to the thyroid cartilage and has a hinged, door-like action at the entrance to the larynx. During swallowing, it acts like a lid to help prevent aspiration of food into the trachea.

The vocal cords are folds of mucous membranes that are attached to cartilage and extend from the front to the back of the larynx. The space between the folds is known as the *glottis.* Sound is produced when air from the lungs causes a rapid, repeated opening and closing of the glottis. The sounds are transformed into speech through the movements of the lips, jaws, and tongue.

Trachea

The trachea, or "windpipe," is a 4- to 5-inch tube descending from the larynx into the bronchi. It is made up of cartilage, smooth muscle, and connective tissue lined by a layer of mucous membrane. The trachea functions as a passageway for air to reach the lungs.

Bronchi

The bronchi provide a passageway for air going to and from the lungs. Two primary bronchi split to the right and left from the trachea. The right bronchus is shorter and wider and runs straighter up and down than the left bronchus. For these reasons, foreign bodies from the trachea usually enter the right bronchus.

The larger bronchi divide into smaller, or secondary, bronchi and then divide again into smaller, or tertiary, bronchi. The tertiary bronchi divide into smaller units called *bronchioles,* which eventually lead into tiny air sacs called *alveoli* located in the lungs. It is through the walls of the alveoli that the exchange of oxygen and carbon dioxide takes place (Fig. 28–2).

Lungs

The lungs are located in the right and left side of the thoracic cavity within the chest wall. The thoracic cavity is separated from the abdominal cavity by the diaphragm, a large sheet of muscle. The lungs are divided into lobes—three lobes on the right and two on the left. Each lung is covered by a membrane called the *pleura.* The pleura is a sac containing fluid that acts as a lubricant for the lungs when they expand and contract.

Louis K. Linton, RRT, CPFT, contributed to the section on Common Therapeutic Measures.

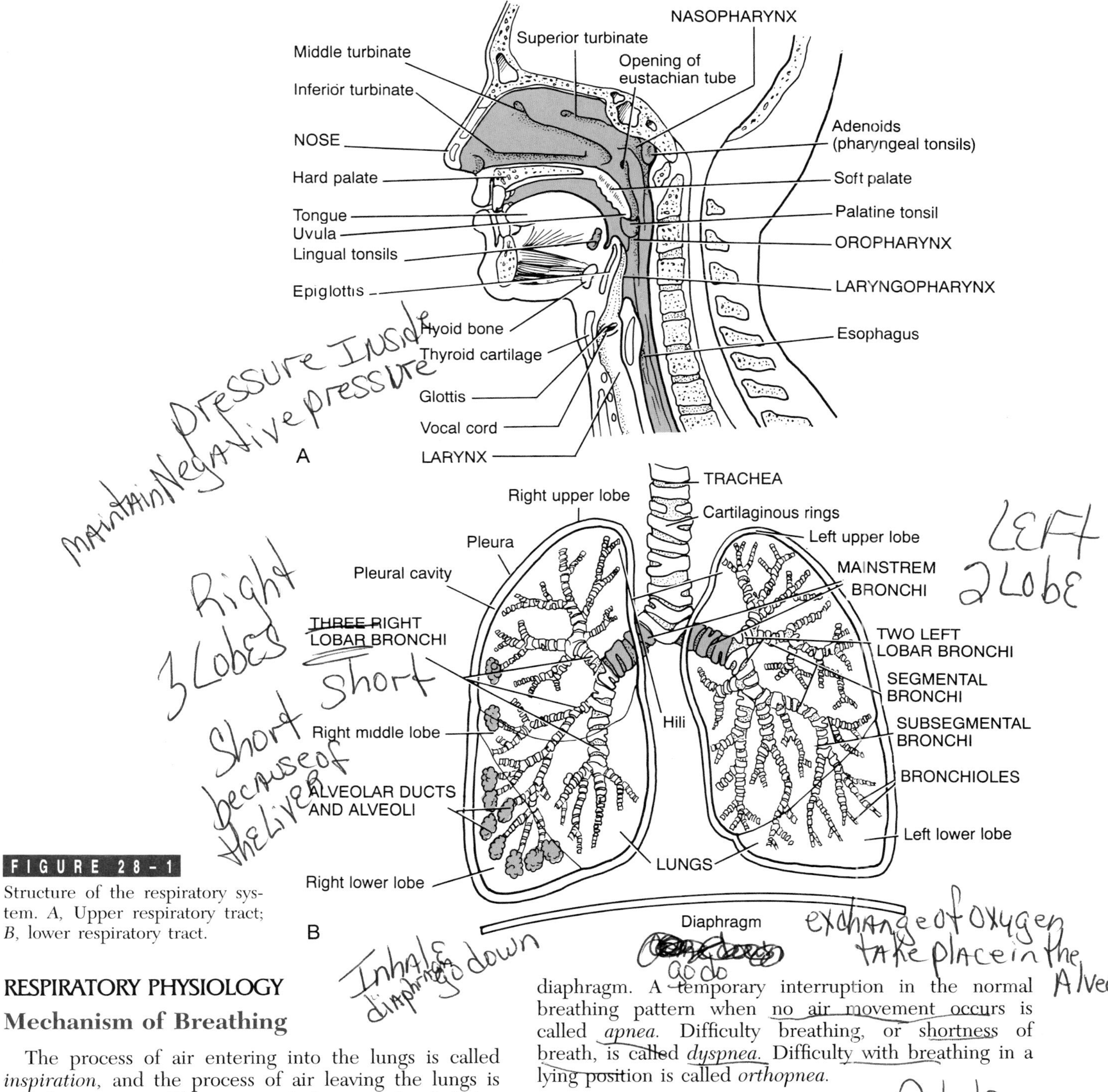

FIGURE 28–1

Structure of the respiratory system. *A*, Upper respiratory tract; *B*, lower respiratory tract.

RESPIRATORY PHYSIOLOGY

Mechanism of Breathing

The process of air entering into the lungs is called *inspiration*, and the process of air leaving the lungs is called *expiration*. The terms *inhalation* and *exhalation* are used interchangeably with inspiration and expiration. Both of these processes are accomplished by the movement of the diaphragm and the muscles in the chest. Inspiration involves an active movement of the muscles and diaphragm and can be noted by an enlargement of the chest cavity. Expiration is a passive process during which the muscles relax and the chest returns to its normal size (Fig. 28–3).

During normal, quiet breathing, about 500 ml of air are inhaled and exhaled. Most of the air movement occurs because of the contraction and relaxation of the diaphragm. A temporary interruption in the normal breathing pattern when no air movement occurs is called *apnea*. Difficulty breathing, or shortness of breath, is called *dyspnea*. Difficulty with breathing in a lying position is called *orthopnea*.

Respiratory Center

Breathing is controlled by the respiratory center, which is located in the medulla. The medulla is part of the brain stem immediately above the spinal cord. The respiratory center is stimulated by changing levels of carbon dioxide and oxygen in arterial blood. Chemoreceptors in the aorta and carotid artery monitor the pH and the amount of carbon dioxide and oxygen in the blood stream. Changes in the pH, increased levels of carbon dioxide, or decreased levels of oxygen cause sig-

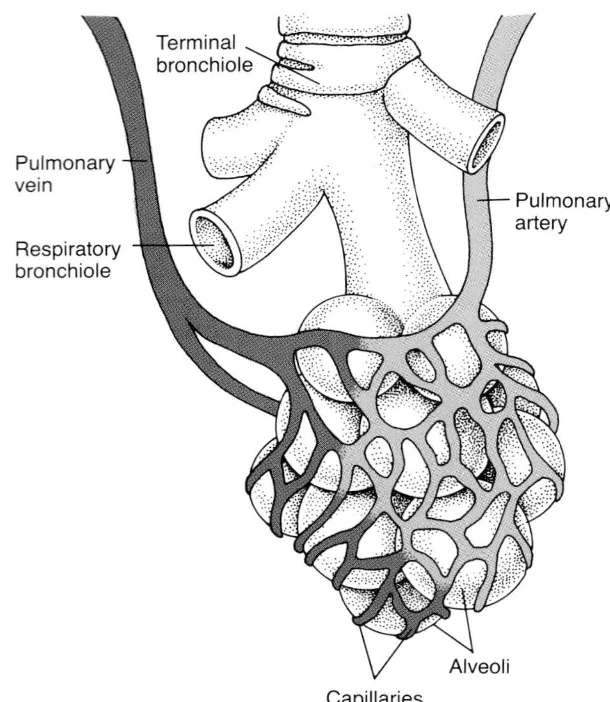

FIGURE 28-2
The terminal bronchioles, alveoli, and capillaries. (From Ignatavicius, D. D., & Bayne, M. V. [1991]. *Medical-surgical nursing: A nursing process approach* [p. 1935]. Philadelphia: W. B. Saunders.)

nals to be sent to the phrenic nerves, which in turn send signals to the respiratory muscles to carry out the major work of breathing.

AGE-RELATED CHANGES

Changes that occur with aging in the pharynx and larynx include muscle atrophy, slackening of the vocal cords, and loss of elasticity of the laryngeal muscles and cartilages. These changes may result in a gravelly, softer voice with a rise in pitch. Elders may have a difficult time communicating with one another when they already have impaired hearing and must try to understand speech that is less clear and more muted. Older adults may have a deviation of the trachea if they suffer from scoliosis of the upper spinal column.

Older persons may experience difficulty with respiration because they can have loss of lung elasticity, enlargement of the bronchioles, and decrease in the number of alveoli. In addition, the respiratory muscles atrophy, the rib cage becomes more rigid, and the diaphragm flattens. The consequences of these changes include reduced chest movement and ability to inhale and exhale, less effective cough, increased work of breathing, and less tolerance for exercise and stress.

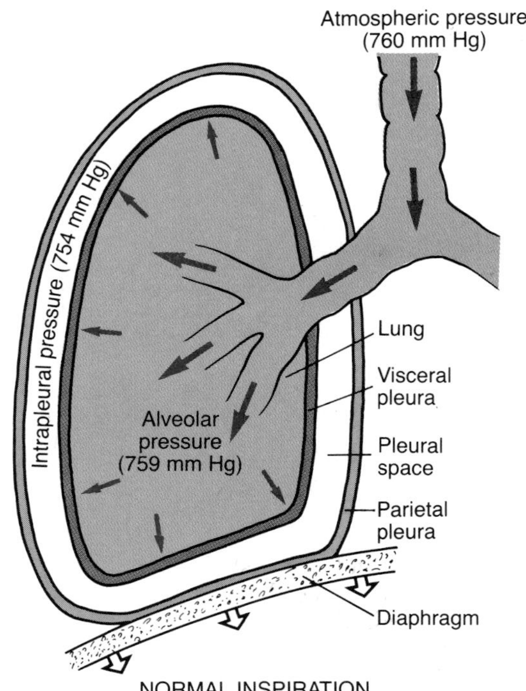

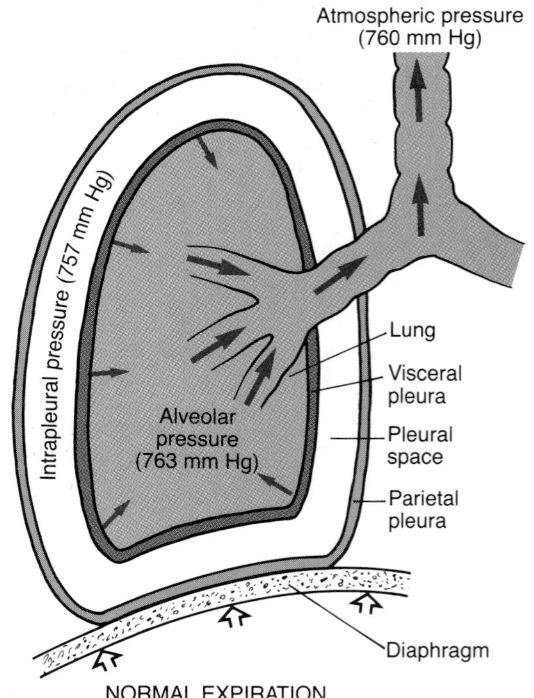

FIGURE 28-3
Normal inspiration and expiration. Note the visceral pleura, pleural space, and parietal pleura and the changes in pressure in the alveoli and pleural space on inspiration and expiration. (From Black, J. M., & Matassarin-Jacobs, E. [1993]. *Luckmann and Sorensen's medical-surgical nursing: A psychophysiologic approach* [4th ed., p. 908]. Philadelphia: W. B. Saunders.)

NURSING ASSESSMENT OF THE RESPIRATORY SYSTEM

HEALTH HISTORY

The health history encompasses the chief complaint and history of the present illness, the past medical history, the review of systems, and the functional assessment. If the patient is in respiratory distress, the nurse focuses on the immediate problem, any conditions that might affect treatment, and allergies. Detailed assessment may be deferred until the patient's respiratory status improves. The components of a complete assessment of the patient with a respiratory disorder are discussed here.

Chief Complaint and History of Present Illness

Common complaints associated with respiratory disorders are cough, pain, and dyspnea. The description of a cough must include the onset, duration, frequency, type (wet or dry), severity and related symptoms such as sputum production and pain. The frequency of expectoration and the sputum characteristics (color, consistency, odor, amount) must be documented. The patient's effort to treat the cough with measures such as medication, vaporizers, and humidifiers is recorded, as is the response to the treatments.

If the patient complains of dyspnea, the onset, duration, severity, and precipitating events are determined. The nurse notes whether the dyspnea becomes worse with activity or certain positions and whether it is more frequent during certain seasons. Associated symptoms such as fatigue or palpitations are identified. The effectiveness of methods used to manage dyspnea, which might include medications, oxygen, and positioning, is recorded.

When the patient has chest pain, the location, presence, onset, duration, and precipitating events (trauma, coughing, inspiration) are assessed. The nurse determines whether the pain causes shallow breathing and whether it radiates up to the jaw or down the arms. The presence of fever, sweating, or nausea is recorded. The nurse documents measures that bring relief such as splinting, heat, analgesics, and antitussives.

Past Medical History

The patient's past medical history determines a history of respiratory disorders, allergies, trauma, and surgery. Conditions that are important to document when a patient has a respiratory disorder include allergies, colds, pneumonia, tuberculosis, chronic bronchitis, emphysema, asthma, cancer of the respiratory tract, cystic fibrosis, sinus infections, ear infections, diabetes mellitus, and heart disease. Any other serious conditions should be noted as well. It is especially important to note conditions that suppress the immune response, making the patient more susceptible to infection. All recent and current medications are recorded, as are the dates of the most recent chest radiograph and tuberculosis test. The nurse also inquires about immunizations against pneumonia and influenza.

Family History

The nurse describes any major respiratory conditions and the smoking history of members of the household.

Review of Systems

The review of systems assesses signs and symptoms that may be directly or indirectly related to the respiratory disorder. The nurse asks about fatigue, weakness, fever, chills, and night sweats. Other data that may be significant are earaches, nasal obstructions, sinus pain, sore throat, hoarseness, edema, dyspnea, and orthopnea.

Functional Assessment

The patient's occupation is described, including any exposure to pathogens or to substances that might irritate or harm the respiratory tract. Exposure to any fumes, toxins, coal dust, silica, or sawdust is documented. The patient is asked to describe a typical day and to give particular attention to any limitations imposed by the respiratory disorder. The usual diet and fluid intake are assessed. A smoking history is important and for the cigarette smoker is usually reported in pack years. Pack years are calculated by multiplying the number of years the patient smoked cigarettes times the number of packs smoked each day. To illustrate, a person who smoked two packs a day for 30 years would have a 60 pack year smoking history. The functional assessment also includes the patient's role in the family, sources of stress, and coping strategies.

PHYSICAL EXAMINATION

The physical examination begins with observation of the patient's general appearance. The nurse notes facial expression, posture, alertness, speech pattern, and any obvious signs of distress. The vital signs are taken, and height and weight are measured. The nurse is alert to unusually rapid or slow breathing and to tachycardia, which may be a sign of hypoxia. The normal respiratory rate is 12 to 20 breaths per minute.

Head and Neck

The nurse examines the head and neck. The nose is inspected for symmetry and for deformity and gently palpated for tenderness. The patency of each naris is assessed by closing one at a time and asking the patient to breathe in through the nose. Flaring of the nares is noted because it is a common sign of air hunger. The examiner may use a nasal speculum to inspect the nasal cavity for swelling, discharge, bleeding, or foreign bodies. The nasal mucosa is normally light red in color. The patient's head is tilted back so the nurse can inspect for deviation of the nasal septum, the structure that separates the nares. A deviation may be seen as a hump in the nasal cavity. The sinuses may be palpated for tenderness by using the thumbs to apply pressure over the frontal and maxillary sinuses (see Chapter 49).

Pursed-lip breathing, a common technique for decreasing dyspnea with chronic respiratory disease, is documented. The nurse inspects the lips, the tip of the nose, the top of the auricles, the gums, and the area under the tongue for cyanosis, a bluish color related to inadequate tissue oxygenation. The pharynx is inspected for redness and tonsil exudate or enlargement, which are signs of infection.

The trachea is inspected to see if it is midline; if not midline, it is said to be deviated. A deviated trachea can be indicative of a large atelectasis, pleural effusion, aortic aneurysm, enlargement of part of the thyroid gland, and tension pneumothorax. The thumbs are placed on either side of the trachea just above the clavicles, and the trachea is gently moved from side to side. The nurse compares the spaces between the sternocleidomastoid muscles on either shoulder and the trachea. An experienced examiner palpates for enlargement and tenderness of the lymph glands. The locations of lymph glands in the neck are depicted in Figure 28–4.

Thorax

The nurse inspects the chest for deformities and lesions and observes the breathing pattern and effort. The rise and fall of the chest should be regular and symmetric. Table 28–1 illustrates the different types of breathing patterns. The thorax is palpated for tenderness and lumps. Additional, more sophisticated aspects of the examination that require special training may include palpating for symmetric chest expansion and tactile fremitus. The skilled examiner may also percuss (tap) the thorax in a systematic manner to elicit sounds that give clues about the density of underlying tissues.

Using the diaphragm of the stethoscope, the lungs are auscultated bilaterally in a systematic manner (Fig. 28–5)—usually the posterior, the sides, then the anterior chest. The nurse listens for the normal movement of air in and out of the lungs and for abnormal breath sounds: wheezes, rhonchi, and crackles. A wheeze, a high-pitched sound caused by air passing through narrowed passageways, may be present with asthma or chronic obstructive pulmonary disease. A rhonchus is a dry rattling sound caused by partial bronchial obstruction. Crackles, also called rales, are abnormal sounds associated with many cardiac and pulmonary disorders. To demonstrate the sound of fine crackles, Jarvis recommends rubbing a few strands of hair between the thumb and forefinger next to the ear. Coarse crackles are described as sounding like a Velcro fastener being separated. One other abnormal sound that may be heard on auscultation is a pleural friction rub, which is indicative of pleurisy. A pleural friction rub is a grating, scratchy noise similar to a creaking shoe.

In addition to the examination of the thorax and the auscultation of lung sounds, the nurse assesses for signs of circulatory disorders that could affect respirations.

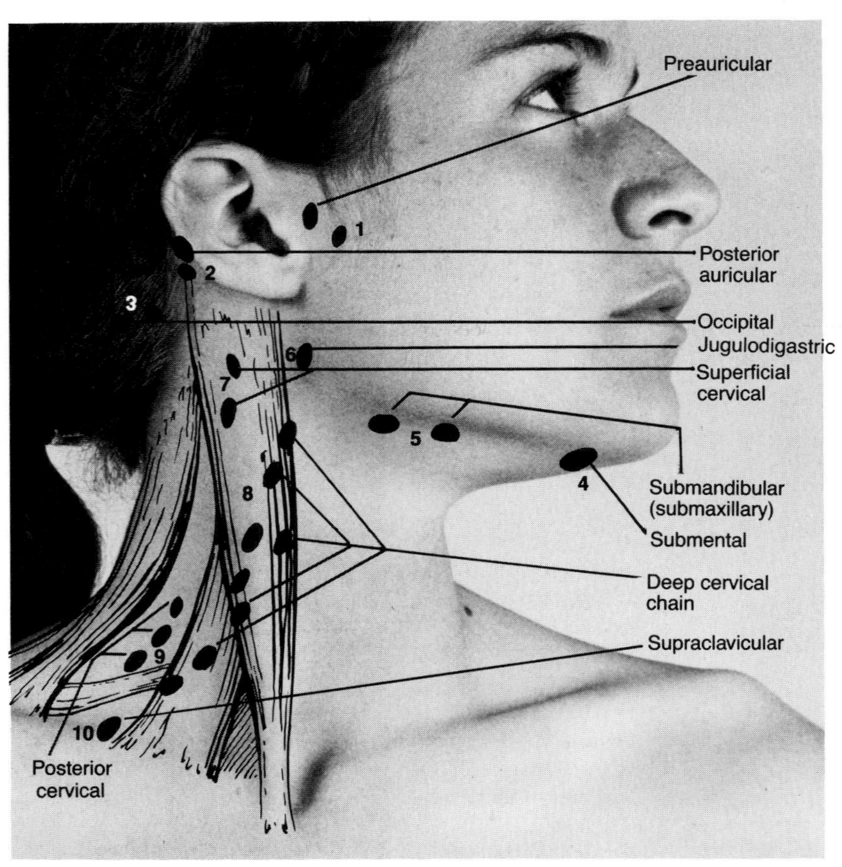

FIGURE 28–4

Lymph nodes in the neck. (From Jarvis, C. [1992]. *Physical examination and health assessment* [p. 289]. Philadelphia: W. B. Saunders.)

TABLE 28-1
TYPES OF BREATHING PATTERNS

PATTERN	CHARACTERISTICS	CAUSES
Normal	Regular pattern Even depth Rate: 12–20 breaths per minute	Normal respiratory drive
Tachypnea	Regular pattern Even depth Rate: faster than 20 breaths per minute	Fever, pain, anxiety
Bradypnea	Regular pattern Even depth Rate: slower than 12 breaths per minute	Sedatives, narcotics, alcohol; brain, metabolic, and respiratory disorders
Sighing respirations	Regular pattern Uneven depth: periodic deep breaths (more than 3 sighs per minute) Rate: 12–20 breaths per minute	Severe anxiety
Apnea Cheyne-Stokes respirations	Breaths progressively deeper, then becoming more shallow, followed by period of apnea	Severe brain pathology
Kussmaul's respirations (with hyperventilation)	Regular pattern Deep Rate: faster than 20 breaths per minute	Metabolic acidosis Diabetic ketoacidosis, renal failure
Apnea Biot's respirations	Irregular pattern Depth varies, sudden periods of apnea	Neurologic disorders
Rising end-expiratory level with forced expirations Obstructive breathing	Gradual rise in end-expiratory level during forced rapid breathing	Emphysema

Redrawn and adapted from Kersten, L. D. (1989). *Comprehensive respiratory nursing* (p. 279). Philadelphia: W. B. Saunders.

The abdomen is inspected for distention that might interfere with full expansion of the lungs. The extremities are inspected for color and palpated for edema. The fingers are examined for clubbing, which is associated with chronic respiratory problems (Fig. 28–6). Homans's sign is assessed by dorsiflexing the patient's foot. Thrombophlebitis is suspected if this maneuver elicits pain behind the knee or in the calf. This is important because the deep veins in the legs and pelvis are the source of most pulmonary emboli.

The nursing assessment of the patient with a respiratory disorder is summarized in Table 28–2.

DIAGNOSTIC TESTS AND PROCEDURES

A variety of tests and procedures may be performed to diagnose disorders of the respiratory system. These tests and procedures are described briefly here. Details of patient preparation and postprocedure care are presented in Table 28–3.

Radiologic Studies

CHEST RADIOGRAPHY. Radiographic examination of the chest is one of the most frequently used methods for respiratory screening and diagnosis. It also is used to assess progression of a disease and response to treatment. The radiograph or roentgenogram produces a picture in which the bony structures (e.g., ribs, sternum, clavicle), heart shadow, trachea, bronchi, and blood vessels are visible. Bone appears white on the film because it is very dense and does not absorb much energy. In contrast, the lungs appear black because they are filled with air and absorb the x-ray energy. Chest films usually

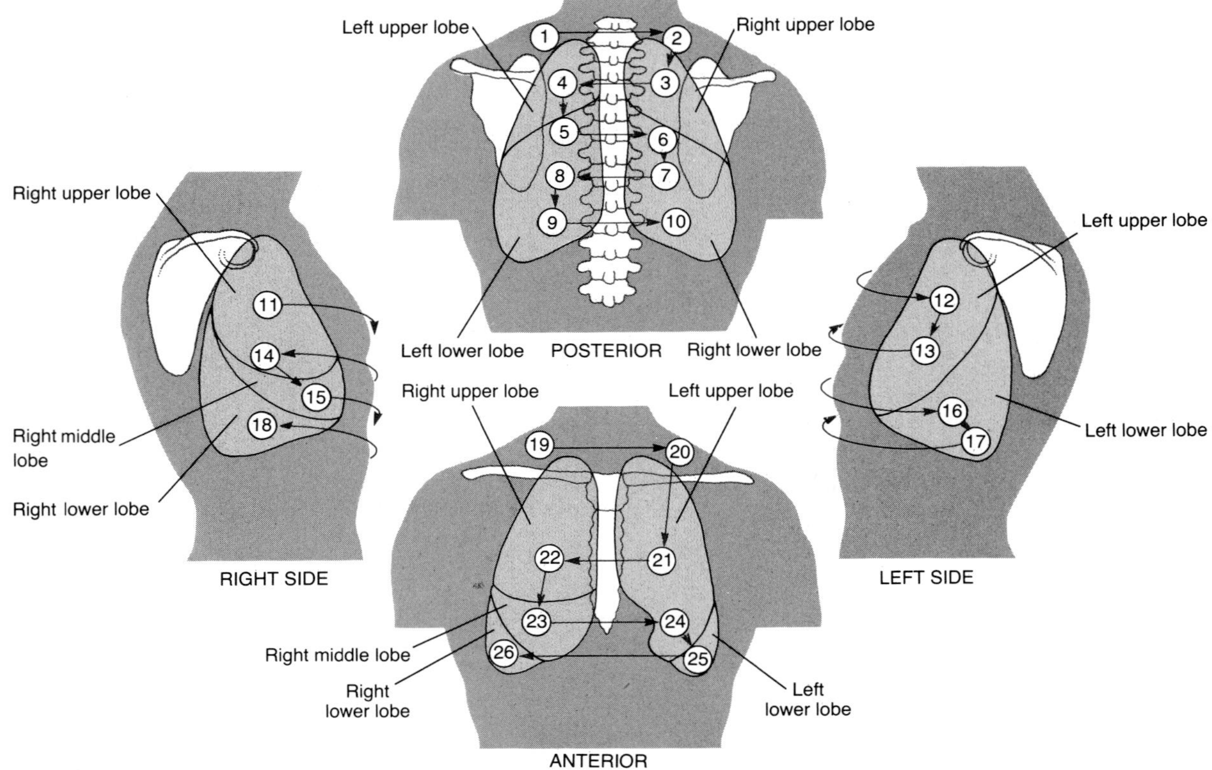

FIGURE 28-5

Sequence for percussion and auscultation of the lungs. (From Ignatavicius, D. D., & Bayne, M. V. [1991]. *Medical-surgical nursing: A nursing process approach* [p. 1942]. Philadelphia: W. B. Saunders.)

FIGURE 28-6

Clubbing is flattening of the angle between the nail and the skin. *A,* Normal angle of 160 degrees. *B,* Early clubbing—the angle is flattened to 180 degrees. *C,* Advanced clubbing—the angle is greater than 180 degrees. *D,* The Schamroth technique: The patient puts the nails of the ring fingers of each hand together and holds the other fingers straight up. The examiner looks at the space between the touching nails. If there is no clubbing, the space is diamond shaped. (Adapted from Black, J. M., & Matassarin-Jacobs, E. [1993]. *Luckmann and Sorensen's medical-surgical nursing: A psychophysiologic approach* [4th ed., p. 920]. Philadelphia: W. B. Saunders.)

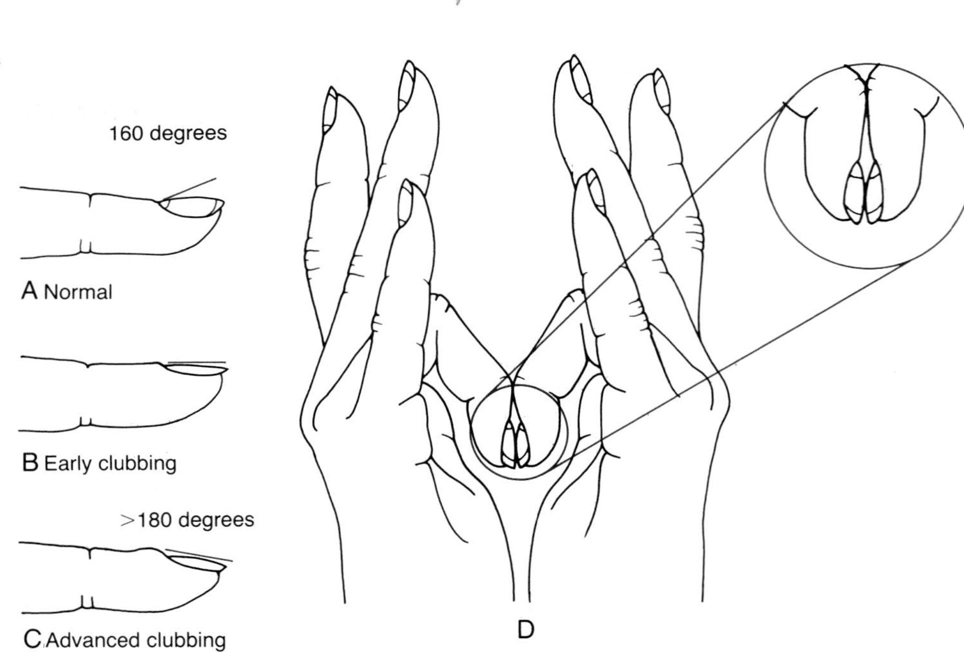

TABLE 28-2

ASSESSMENT OF THE PATIENT WITH A RESPIRATORY DISORDER

HEALTH HISTORY:

Present illness
- Cough: Onset, duration, frequency, type, severity, sputum production and characteristics, pain
- Dyspnea: Onset, duration, severity, precipitating events, associated symptoms
- Pain: Location, onset, duration, precipitating events, effects on breathing, measures that reduce or relieve, associated symptoms

Past medical history: Colds, pneumonia, tuberculosis, chronic bronchitis, emphysema, asthma, cancer of the respiratory tract, cystic fibrosis, sinus infections, ear infections, diabetes mellitus, heart disease, allergies, trauma, surgeries, hospitalizations, conditions that suppress the immune response, immunizations against pneumonia and influenza, last chest radiograph, last tuberculosis test, recent and current medications

Family history: Major respiratory conditions, smoking history

Review of symptoms: Fatigue, weakness, fever, chills, night sweats, earaches, nasal obstruction, sinus pain, sore throat, hoarseness, edema, dyspnea, orthopnea

Functional assessment: Occupation, exposure to pathogens or respiratory irritants, typical day, usual diet and fluid intake, smoking history, role in family, stressors, coping strategies

PHYSICAL EXAMINATION

General survey: Appearance, facial expression, posture, alertness, speech pattern, obvious distress

Vital signs

Height and weight

Head and neck:
- Nose: Nasal shape, tenderness, patency, flaring; swelling, discharge, bleeding, foreign bodies in nasal cavity; septal deviation
- Sinuses: Tenderness
- Lips: Pursed-lip breathing, color
- Pharynx: Redness, tonsil exudate or enlargement
- Trachea: Midline
- Lymph nodes: Enlargement, tenderness

Thorax: Breathing pattern and effort, accessory muscles, lung sounds

Abdomen: Distention

Extremities: Color, clubbing, edema, Homans's sign

TABLE 28-3

DIAGNOSTIC TESTS AND PROCEDURES FOR THE RESPIRATORY SYSTEM

TEST/STUDY	PURPOSE/ PROCEDURE	PATIENT PREPARATION	POSTPROCEDURE NURSING CARE
Arterial blood gas analysis	Measures concentrations of pH, $PaCO_2$, PaO_2, HCO_3, O_2 saturation, to detect alkalosis or acidosis, and alterations in oxygenation status that may occur with many respiratory, cardiac, and metabolic disorders. Normal values for adults are: pH: 7.35–7.45 $PaCO_2$: 35–45 mm Hg PaO_2: 75–100 mm Hg HCO_3: 22–26 mEq/L O_2 saturation: 96–100%	Tell the patient a blood sample will be drawn from an artery (usually the radial). An Allen's test *must* be done before an arterial puncture to ensure that the arteries to the hand are patent. (Arterial punctures require specialized training.)	Apply pressure to the puncture site for 5–10 min. Note the concentration of any oxygen therapy on the lab slip. Transport the blood gas syringe containing the specimen to the laboratory in an ice bath within 15 min.
Sputum analysis, culture and sensitivity, cytology	Specimens examined for volume, consistency, color, and odor. Culture reveals bacteria and fungi. Sensitivity identifies antimicrobials that are effective against the pathogens. Cytology is the study of cells to detect malignancy and inflammatory changes due to infections or irritants.	Collect the specimen early in the morning before breakfast. Provide a sterile container. Instruct the patient to: (1) Brush the teeth and rinse the mouth. (2) Cough deeply and expectorate directly into the container. (3) Immediately cap the container. (4) Inform the nurse that the specimen is ready.	Send specimen to the laboratory promptly. Refrigerate if it will be more than an hour before delivery to the lab.

Table continued on following page

TABLE 28-3

DIAGNOSTIC TESTS AND PROCEDURES FOR THE RESPIRATORY SYSTEM *Continued*

TEST/STUDY	PURPOSE/ PROCEDURE	PATIENT PREPARATION	POSTPROCEDURE NURSING CARE
		A special container and solution must be used for specimens for cytology.	
Bronchogram	Radiopaque dye is instilled in the bronchial tree through a catheter or fiberoptic bronchoscope. The dye coats the mucosal lining, and radiographs are taken to visualize the bronchial tree and detect abnormalities.	Tell the patient what to expect. Make sure consent form has been signed. The patient should have nothing by mouth 6–8 hr before procedure. Assess for iodine allergy and report to radiologist if present. Provide oral hygiene. Have patient remove dentures. Document any loose teeth. Administer sedative as ordered.	Postural drainage or aerosol therapy may be ordered to promote elimination of dye. Encourage coughing and deep breathing. Withhold food or liquids until gag reflex returns.
Chest radiograph	Creates an image of the bone structures in the thorax, the heart shadow, trachea, bronchi, blood vessels, and lungs. Used to screen and diagnose some respiratory disorders. Fluoroscopy is a radiograph that provides "motion picture" images of the lungs during inspiration and expiration.	Tell the patient what to expect. No special preparation is needed.	No special aftercare is needed.
Ventilation-perfusion scan (lung scan)	Radioactive dye is given intravenously to assess lung perfusion, followed by scanning by a special machine that detects the distribution of the dye. Then a radioactive gas is inhaled to assess lung ventilation, again followed by scanning of lungs. Demonstrates lung ventilation and perfusion. Detects pulmonary embolism and other obstructive conditions.	Explain study to patient. Assure patient that radiation dose is small and that isotope is quickly eliminated. If sedation is needed, for agitated patients or small children, the patient is usually given nothing by mouth (NPO) for 4 hr. The procedure takes about 2 hr.	Monitor patient for 1 hour for anaphylaxis. Check venipuncture site. Radioactive material is excreted in the urine. Tell patient to wash hands after voiding. If nurse handles urine, rubber gloves should be worn. Gloves and hands should be washed after urine is discarded.
Computed tomography (CT, CAT, or CAT scan)	The patient lies on a platform while a special doughnut-shaped radiographic scanner rotates around the patient and creates images of "slices" of the body. Images may be created with or without contrast media. The procedure is painless.	Explain the test to the patient. Stress the importance of remaining still during the scanning. Assess iodine allergy and report to radiologist in case contrast media is to be used. NPO may be required. Consult agency manual.	Note side effects of contrast: headache, nausea, vomiting.

are taken posteroanterior (back to front), anteroposterior (front to back), and lateral (side) to view the chest cavity from different angles.

FLUOROSCOPY. Fluoroscopy is a radiograph of the chest taken to observe deep structures in motion. It is possible to observe both lungs at the same time during inspiration and expiration. Instead of producing a single, still image, the screen registers a constant image of the chest. The fluoroscopic examination can give information about the speed and degree of lung expansion and structural defects in the bronchial tree.

TABLE 28-3

DIAGNOSTIC TESTS AND PROCEDURES FOR THE RESPIRATORY SYSTEM *Continued*

TEST/STUDY	PURPOSE/ PROCEDURE	PATIENT PREPARATION	POSTPROCEDURE NURSING CARE
Magnetic resonance imaging (MRI)	Images of multiple body planes are produced without radiation. The patient lies on a stretcher that slides into a tube-like device. Mechanical clanging noises are heard as the machine operates. Metal implants such as cardiac pacemakers and orthopedic implants may be affected by MRI, but are not absolute contraindications. Aneurysm clips, intraocular metal, heart valves made before 1964, and middle ear prostheses generally contraindicate MRI.	Explain the test to the patient. Be sure consent form has been signed. Assess for and report claustrophobia. Patients who are anxious or restless may require sedation. Special equipment must be used for oxygen therapy or mechanical ventilation. Have patient remove metal watch and jewelry.	Safety precautions if sedated; otherwise, no special aftercare is needed.
Pulmonary function tests (PFTs)	PFTs include a variety of tests used to evaluate lung function, gas exchanges, pulmonary blood flow, and acid-base balance. They are measures of total lung capacity (TLC), forced expiratory volume (FEV), functional residual capacity (FRC), inspiratory capacity (IC), vital capacity (VC), forced vital capacity (FVC), minute volume (MV), and thoracic gas volume (TGV).	Tell the patient what to expect. A clip is applied to the nose, and the patient breathes through a mouthpiece as directed while various measurements are taken. Advise not to smoke or eat a heavy meal 4–6 hr before tests. Patient should be dressed comfortably, and should void before the tests. Determine whether any medications or treatments should be withheld.	Resume medications. No special aftercare is needed.
Fiberoptic bronchoscopy	A flexible scope is inserted through the nose or mouth into the bronchial tree to visualize abnormalities, take biopsy samples of lesions, or remove foreign bodies.	Informed consent must be obtained. NPO 6–8 hr or as specified. Have patient remove dentures and provide oral hygiene. Document loose teeth. Ask the patient not to smoke. Administer sedatives and anticholinergics as ordered.	Remain NPO till gag reflex returns. Use semi-Fowler's position. Monitor vital signs. Monitor for gross hemoptysis, swelling of face and neck, stridor, decreased or asymmetric chest movement, diminished lung sounds, dyspnea. Report findings to physician.
Thoracentesis	A needle is inserted through the chest wall to obtain fluid from the pleural space. Tests on fluid specimens may measure components or reveal pathogens. Cells can be studied for malignancy.	Explain the procedure. Stress the importance of not moving or coughing during the procedure. Support the patient during the thoracentesis.	Label specimens and send to laboratory. Document amount and color of fluid. Monitor vital signs, lung sounds, chest movement. Report dyspnea, asymmetric chest movement to physician. Check dressing for bleeding.

VENTILATION-PERFUSION SCAN. When the lungs are working efficiently, there is a balance in the ventilation-perfusion ratio, so that areas receiving ventilation are well perfused with blood, and areas perfused with blood are well ventilated. When the alveolus and pulmonary blood flow are normal, ventilation and perfusion are said to "match" (Fig. 28–7).

A lung scan or ventilation-perfusion scan is used to assess lung ventilation and lung perfusion. Its chief purpose is to detect pulmonary embolism or some other obstruction. The patient is given a radioactive substance either by inhalation (to evaluate ventilation) or intravenously (to evaluate perfusion). Ventilation images are compared with the pictures taken during the perfusion

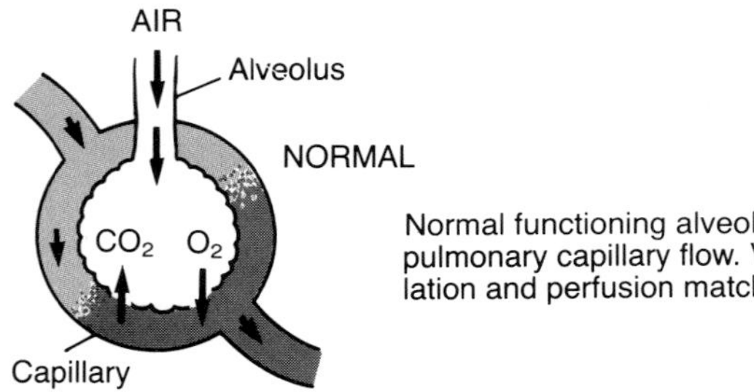

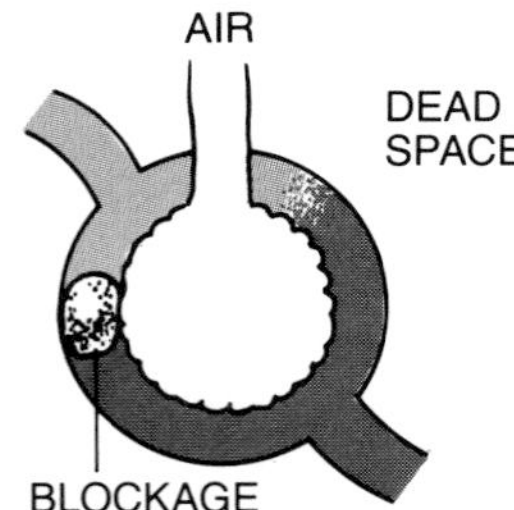

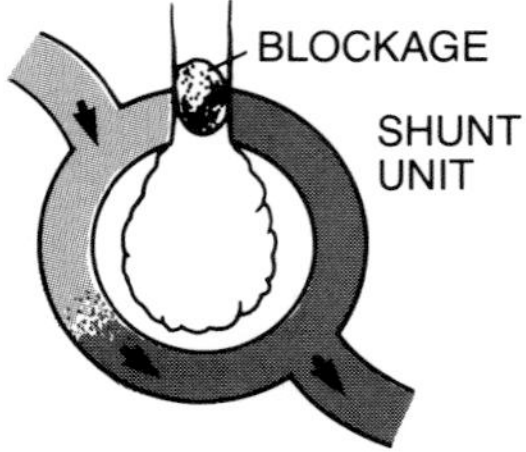

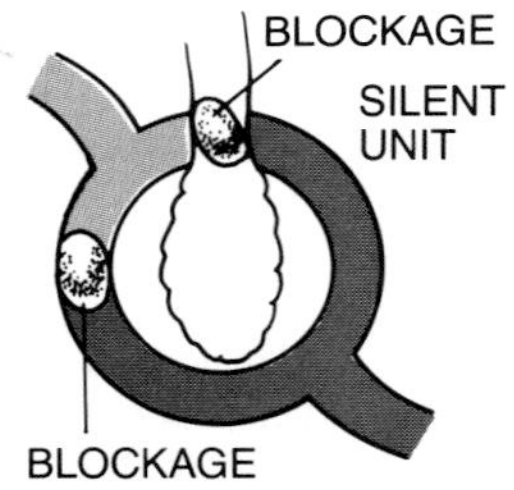

FIGURE 28–7

Normal functioning alveolus and pulmonary capillary blood flow. When both are normal, the ventilation and perfusion match. (Adapted from Black, J. M., & Matassarin-Jacobs, E. [1993]. *Luckmann and Sorensen's medical-surgical nursing: A psychophysiologic approach* [4th ed., p. 905]. Philadelphia: W. B. Saunders.)

scan to determine whether there is an equal amount of radioactivity on both the ventilation and the perfusion pictures. Any areas indicating good ventilation but poor perfusion suggest the presence of a pulmonary embolus or obstruction.

The only preparation a patient needs for a lung scan is adequate teaching about the procedure in order to allay anxiety. The only discomfort may be at the site of the injection of the radioactive dye. Very small amounts of radioactive substances are used, and they are quickly eliminated from the body without danger to the patient or to others.

Imaging Procedures

COMPUTED TOMOGRAPHY. Tomography or tomograms allow visualization of "slices" or layers of the chest. A computed tomography scan is a computerized method of tomography in which a camera rotates in a circular pattern around the body to provide a three-dimensional assessment of the thorax. The test generally is used to look for the presence of lesions or tumors.

Radioactive dye containing iodine may be injected intravenously. Each layer of the chest is photographed before and after the injection of the dye. It is extremely important to find out whether the patient is allergic to iodine before the procedure is carried out. Failure to determine sensitivity to iodine could result in an allergic reaction, anaphylaxis, and death.

MAGNETIC RESONANCE IMAGING. A magnetic resonance imaging (MRI) scan is similar to a CAT scan but without the harmful radiation. The MRI scanner encloses the patient in a doughnut-shaped magnet and picks up signals from the body to make electronic images. The patient must remain as quiet and as motionless as possible during the procedure. No preparation is necessary for the procedure, but patients should be warned that no metal may be worn inside the unit (with the exception of dental fillings).

Pulmonary Function Tests

Pulmonary function tests are used to diagnose pulmonary disease, monitor disease progression, evaluate the extent of disability, and assess the effects of medication. The tests measure lung volumes and capacities, assess the mechanics of breathing (flow rates of gas in and out of the lungs), and measure diffusion (the movement of the gas across the alveolar-capillary membrane).

SPIROMETRY. A spirometer is an instrument that measures the ventilatory function of the lung. It measures the amount of air volume that the lung can hold, the rate of flow of air in and out of the lung, and the compliance (elasticity) of lung tissue. The test enables the physician to detect impaired pulmonary function, classify the pulmonary impairment, estimate the severity of the impairment, monitor the cause of pulmonary disease and evaluate treatment, give information helpful in planning care, and provide preoperative assessment.

The test involves inserting a mouthpiece, taking as deep a breath as possible, and blowing as hard, as fast, and as long as possible. Patients should be encouraged to continue blowing out until exhalation is complete.

Spirometry measures forced vital capacity and forced expiratory volume. Interpretation of the spirometry involves first looking at the forced expiratory volume in the first second of expiration. These and other lung volumes and capacities are defined in Table 28–4.

People who are to undergo spirometry should be taught what to expect during the test and how to prepare. They may be anxious about taking a "breathing test" if they have respiratory problems because they may fear increased dyspnea or exhaustion. They should be

TABLE 28-4
LUNG VOLUMES AND CAPACITIES

VOLUME	DEFINITION	SIGNIFICANCE OF INCREASE	SIGNIFICANCE OF DECREASE
Total lung capacity (TLC)	Total lung volume when fully inflated	Overdistention of lung caused by obstructive lung disease	Restrictive lung disease
Forced expiratory volume (FEV)	Volume of air expired during specified time intervals (0.5, 1, 2, 3 sec)	Not significant	Restrictive or obstructive lung disease depending on measurements at time intervals
Functional residual capacity (FRC)	Volume of air remaining in the lungs after normal exhalation	Chronic obstructive pulmonary disease. Excessive use of positive end-expiratory pressure	Adult respiratory distress syndrome (ARDS)
Inspiratory capacity (IC)	Maximal volume of air that can be inhaled after a normal exhalation	Not significant	Restrictive lung disease
Vital capacity (VC)	Total volume of air that can be exhaled after maximum inspiration	Increased or normal VC with normal flow rates: pulmonary edema	Decreased VC with normal or increased flow rates: impaired respiratory effort
Forced vital capacity (FVC)	Total volume of air exhaled rapidly and forcefully after maximum inhalation	Not significant	Obstructive or restrictive lung disease
Minute volume (MV)	Total amount of air breathed in 1 min	Not significant	Restrictive parenchymal lung disease; fatigue
Thoracic gas volume (TGV)	Total volume of air in the lungs including ventilated and nonventilated areas	Obstructive lung disease with air trapping	Not significant

Data from Chernecky, C. C., Krech, R. L., & Berger, B. J. (1993). *Laboratory tests and diagnostic procedures.* Philadelphia: W. B. Saunders.

advised not to smoke or use bronchodilator medications for 4 to 6 hours before testing.

PHARMACOLOGY CAPSULE

Bronchodilators should not be given before pulmonary function testing because they can alter the results.

ARTERIAL BLOOD GAS ANALYSIS. Ventilation and diffusion also are measured by testing for concentrations of oxygen and carbon dioxide in the arterial blood to determine whether the exchange is adequate across the alveolar membrane. Blood gas analysis is useful in the care of patients with respiratory disorders, problems of circulation and distribution of blood, body fluid imbalances, and acid-base imbalances. Arterial blood samples are often obtained from the radial artery after first performing Allen's test to ensure adequate circulation to the hand from other arteries (Fig. 28–8).

Pulse Oximetry

Pulse oximetry permits the noninvasive measurement of arterial oxygen saturation. A sensor is clipped to an ear lobe or fingertip. A beam of light passes through the tissue, and the amount of light absorbed by oxygen-saturated hemoglobin is measured. The oxygen saturation is presented as a percentage and registered on a digital readout. Factors that interfere with accurate measurement of the oximeter are hypotension, hypothermia, vasoconstriction, and finger movement.

Sputum Analysis

Sputum is material that originates in the bronchi. Sputum analysis may be performed when respiratory disease is suspected. The mucous membrane lining of the lower respiratory tract responds to acute inflammation by increasing the production of secretions, which may contain bacterial or malignant cells. These cells may be detected by examination of sputum. Sputum specimens are also examined for volume, consistency, color, and odor. Sputum that is thick, foul smelling, and yellow, green, or rust colored usually indicates a bacterial infection. The patient is generally instructed how to

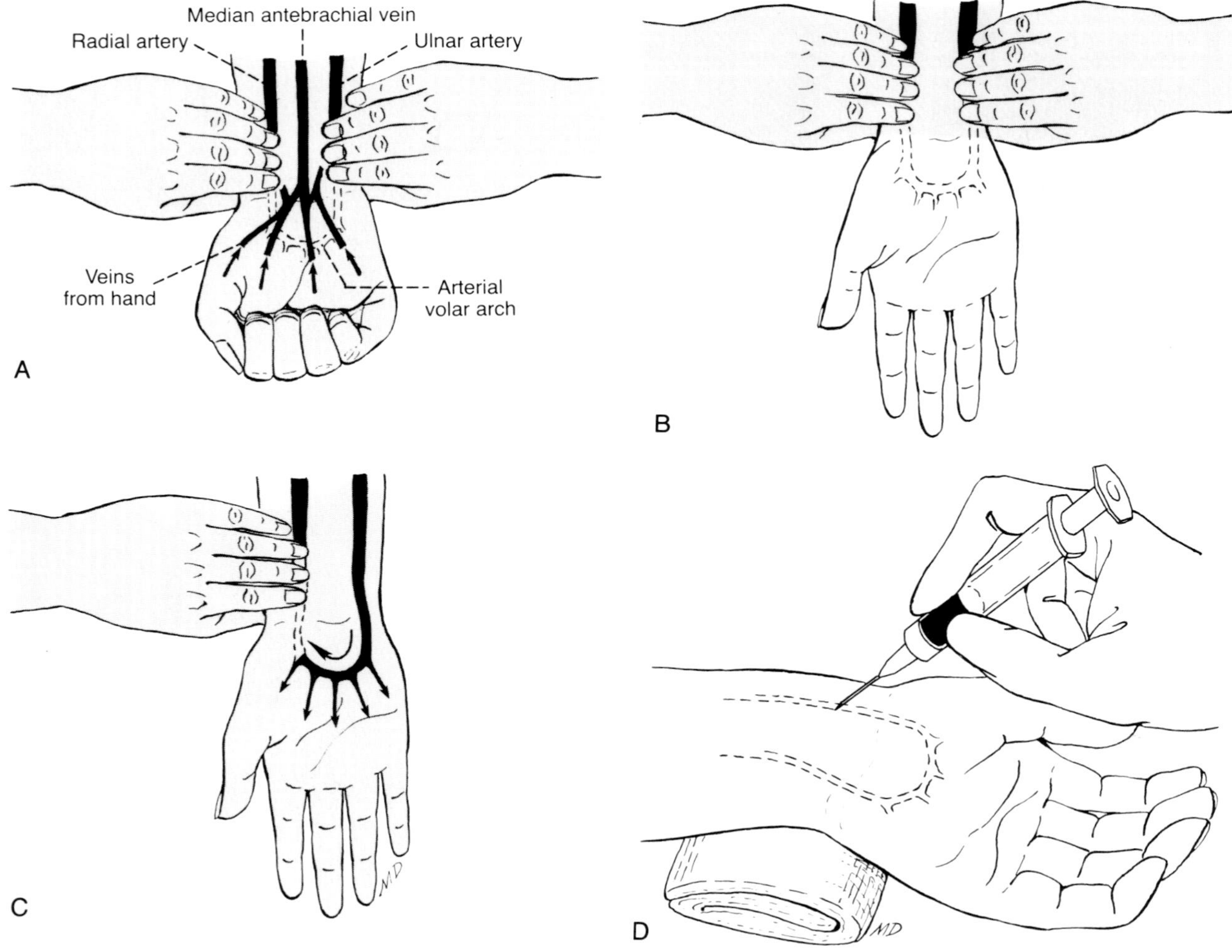

FIGURE 28-8
The Allen test should be done before each radial arterial puncture to ensure adequate collateral circulation. Because an arterial puncture may injure the radial artery, the adequacy of blood supply to the area by other arteries must be determined. A puncture is not done on an artery if other blood supply is not adequate. To perform the Allen test, occlude the radial and ulnar arteries and have the patient make a fist *(A)*. While maintaining pressure on the arteries, have the patient open the hand. The hand is pale if the arteries are occluded *(B)*. Release the pressure on the ulnar artery. If collateral circulation is adequate, color will return to the hand. This is a positive Allen test result; the puncture can proceed on the radial artery. If color does not return, the Allen test result is negative and the radial artery should not be punctured *(C)*. A blood sample is drawn from the radial artery after a positive Allen test result *(D)*. (From Black, J. M., & Matassarin-Jacobs, E. [1993]. *Luckmann and Sorensen's medical-surgical nursing: A psychophysiologic approach* [4th ed., p. 927]. Philadelphia: W. B. Saunders.)

collect the specimen. If the patient is unable to expectorate a specimen, sputum production may be induced with aerosol therapy.

CULTURE AND SENSITIVITY. Sputum culture and sensitivity tests are ordered to determine the presence of bacteria, identify the specific organisms, and identify appropriate antimicrobials. Specimens should be collected before antimicrobial therapy is begun to ensure that sufficient bacterial growth is present.

ACID-FAST TEST. An acid-fast test on a sputum specimen is performed to determine the presence of acid-fast bacilli, which include the bacteria that cause tuberculosis. Specimens are usually collected on 3 consecutive days. Each sputum specimen should be kept covered and refrigerated or delivered to the lab within 1 hour. A new sterile container is used for each collection.

CYTOLOGIC SPECIMENS. Sputum specimens are obtained for cytologic examination to determine the presence of lung carcinoma or infectious conditions. Because sputum contains cells from the tracheobronchial tree, malignant cells may be detected in the specimen. A special container with fixative solution may be used for this type of specimen collection. The agency laboratory manual must be consulted for directions.

Bronchogram

The bronchial tree can be visualized in a radiographic procedure called a bronchogram. The patient's throat and bronchi are anesthetized with a topical anesthetic. Radiopaque dye is instilled into the bronchial tree through a catheter or fiberoptic bronchoscope. The distribution of the dye is enhanced by tilting the patient in different positions. Radiographs are taken following adequate mucosal coating by the dye to reveal any pathologic condition in the bronchial tree. Complications of bronchograms include pneumonia, delayed hypersensitivity reaction, and laryngospasm.

Fiberoptic Bronchoscopy

A bronchoscopic examination is performed by inserting a flexible fiberoptic scope through the nose or mouth into the bronchial tree following local anesthesia of the patient's throat. The scope allows for direct visualization of the bronchial tree structures for assessment, diagnosis, or removal of foreign bodies or mucous plugs. Lesions suggestive of malignancy may be located and a biopsy performed as well. Complications of bronchoscopy include bronchospasm, bacteremia, bronchial perforation, pneumonia, laryngospasm, hemorrhage, and pneumothorax.

Additional details about diagnostic tests and procedures are presented in Table 28–3.

COMMON THERAPEUTIC MEASURES

THORACENTESIS

A thoracentesis is the insertion of a large-bore needle through the chest wall into the pleural space. The procedure is usually performed at the bedside by the physician. Thoracentesis is done to remove pleural fluid, blood, or air or to instill medication. Pleural fluid may be removed to reduce respiratory distress caused by fluid accumulation in the pleural space. In addition, fluid obtained in the procedure may be studied to obtain blood cell counts or to measure protein, glucose, lactic dehydrogenase, fibrinogen, or amylase levels. Study of pleural fluids may aid in the diagnosis of infectious diseases and cancer.

Preparation includes a simple explanation of the procedure. The nurse instructs the patient not to move or cough during the procedure to prevent damage to the pleural tissue. A procedural consent form is required.

The patient sits on the side of the bed and leans the upper torso over the bedside table with the head resting on folded arms or pillows (Fig. 28–9). If the patient is unable to sit up, a side-lying position with the head of the bed elevated 30 degrees may be used (Long, Phipps, & Cassmeyer, 1993). The skin is cleansed thoroughly and a local anesthetic injected. A 20-gauge or larger needle is inserted between the ribs and through the parietal membrane. Fluid or air is then aspirated. During the procedure, the nurse provides reassurance and monitors the patient's skin color, respiratory rate, and general response.

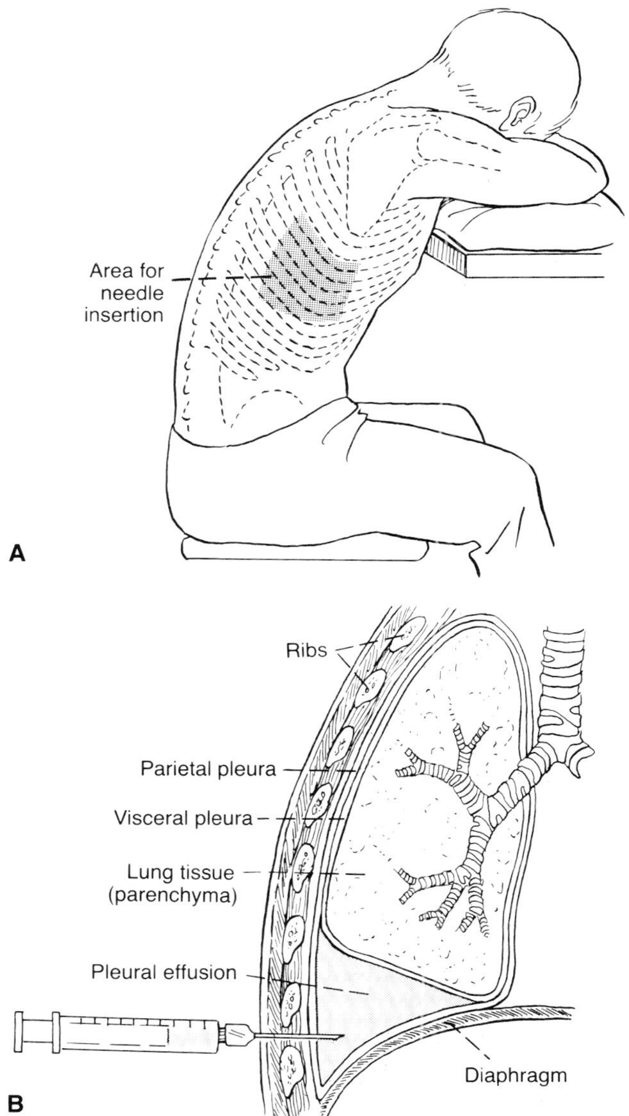

FIGURE 28-9
A, The patient is positioned for a thoracentesis. *B*, The needle is inserted into the pleural space, avoiding lung tissue and the diaphragm. The exact location of the puncture varies. (From Black, J. M., & Matassarin-Jacobs, E. [1993]. *Luckmann and Sorensen's medical-surgical nursing: A psychophysiologic approach* [4th ed., p. 938]. Philadelphia: W. B. Saunders.)

After the thoracentesis needle is removed, a sterile dressing is applied to the puncture site. The patient is positioned on the unaffected side. The amount and color of pleural fluid removed is recorded. Each specimen must be labeled according to physician's orders and sent to the laboratory promptly. Because complications of thoracentesis include air embolism, hemothorax, pneumothorax, and pulmonary edema, the nurse monitors the patient's vital signs and auscultates the lungs for diminished breath sounds. The patient is observed for uneven chest movements, respiratory distress, and hemorrhage. Any of these findings should be reported to the supervisor and the physician immediately. A chest radiograph may be ordered after the procedure to detect any pulmonary complications caused by accidental injury to the lung.

BREATHING EXERCISES

Deep Breathing and Coughing Exercises

Deep breathing and coughing exercises are performed to aid in lung expansion and expectoration of respiratory secretions. They are indicated when patients are immobilized or following general anesthesia. Instructions to the patient include the following:

1. Sit in a semi-Fowler's position for maximal lung expansion.
2. Place one hand on the abdomen to feel it rise and fall with breathing.
3. Inhale deeply through the nose, pause 1 to 3 seconds, and exhale slowly through the mouth.
4. After 4 to 6 deep breaths, cough deeply from the lungs to aid in the expectoration of sputum.
5. After thoracic or abdominal surgery, splint the incision with a pillow to minimize discomfort and support the incision.

Pursed-Lip Breathing

Another type of breathing exercise is pursed-lip breathing. It is used to inhibit airway collapse and to decrease dyspnea in patients with chronic lung disease. Patients are instructed to pucker the lips as if to whistle, blow out a candle, or blow through a straw. They should then inhale through the nose and slowly exhale through pursed lips. Exhalation should last twice as long as inhalation.

Sustained Maximal Inspiration

Sustained maximal inspiration is used to ensure deep inspiration for maximal expansion and aeration of the lungs. An incentive spirometer is an instrument that is frequently used to encourage maximal inspiration. Spirometers basically consist of a cylinder that contains balls or disks and a tube through which the patient inhales. As the patient inhales through the tube, the balls or disks rise (Fig. 28–10). The patient is instructed to inhale deeply to move the balls or disks in the cylinder upward. For maximum effect, the spirometer is kept upright because tilting the device reduces respiratory effort. Some spirometers provide a digital readout of the volume of air displaced.

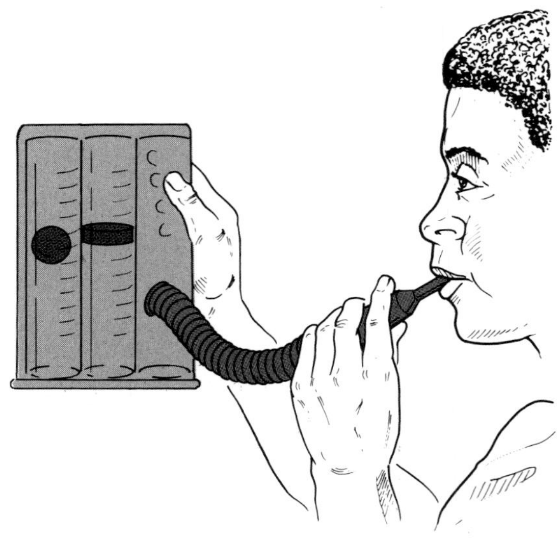

FIGURE 28-10

Incentive spirometry encourages deep breathing by providing a visual cue to the patient about the efficiency of deep breathing. (From Black, J. M., & Matassarin-Jacobs, E. [1993]. *Luckmann and Sorensen's medical-surgical nursing: A psychophysiologic approach* [4th ed., p. 957]. Philadelphia: W. B. Saunders.)

CHEST PHYSIOTHERAPY

Chest physiotherapy consists of percussion, vibration, and postural drainage. These mechanical techniques are used to facilitate the mobilization and expectoration of secretions in patients with large mucus-producing or chronic mucus-retaining respiratory disorders such as chronic bronchitis and cystic fibrosis. Although this therapy is usually performed by a respiratory therapist, the nurse should be familiar with the procedures to evaluate the patient's response. In an outpatient setting, the nurse may also monitor the caregiver's technique in administering the treatment. Chest physiotherapy should be performed before meals.

Chest Percussion and Vibration

Chest percussion and vibration are performed to facilitate the movement of respiratory secretions so sputum can be expectorated. Percussion is clapping of the cupped palms against the chest wall to dislodge and mobilize respiratory secretions (Fig. 28–11*A*). The procedure is performed with the hands cupped to create a pocket of air when striking the patient's chest, first with one hand, then with the other. Percussion is confined to areas protected by the rib cage and is never done over the sternum, kidney, liver, spleen, stomach, or spine. Generally percussion is done for 20 to 30 seconds, followed by vibration.

Vibration is performed by the therapist placing one hand on the top of the other, keeping the arms straight, and pressing the hands flat against the patient's chest (Fig. 28–11*B*). As the patient exhales, the therapist creates a shaking (vibrating) movement with the palms. The therapist pauses during inhalation. The vibration is repeated over three or four breathing cycles.

Contraindications to percussion and vibration include lung cancer, bronchospasm, pain in the area being

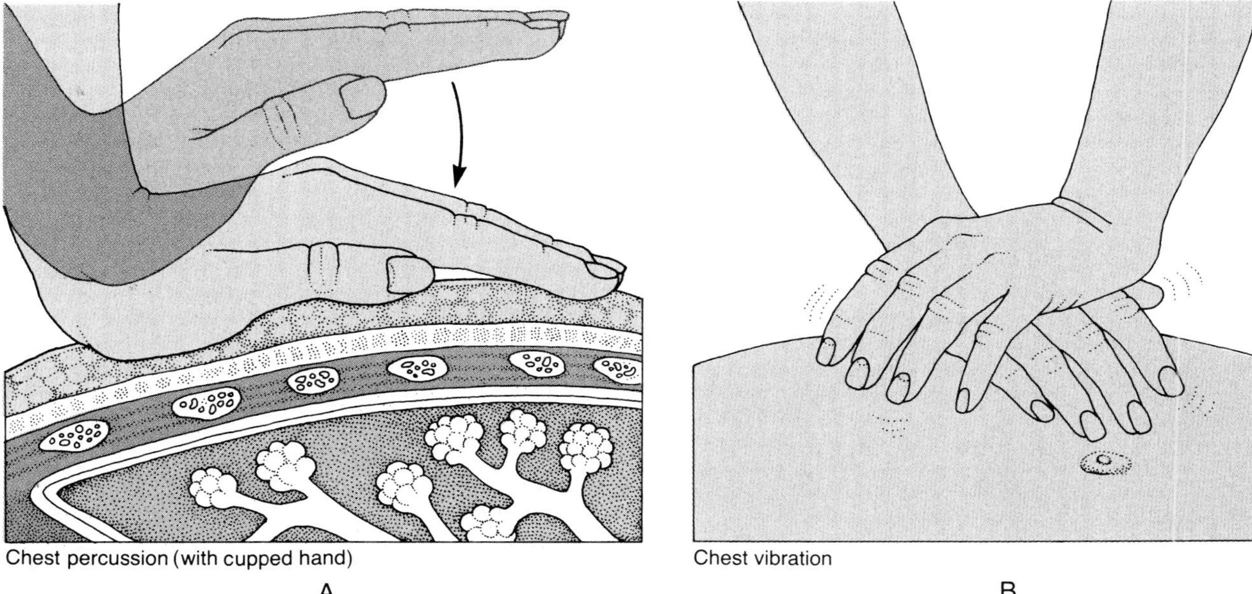

FIGURE 28-11
Chest physiotherapy. *A*, Percussion; *B*, Vibration (From Ignatavicius, D. D., & Bayne, M. V. [1991]. *Medical-surgical nursing: A nursing process approach* [p. 2035]. Philadelphia: W. B. Saunders.)

treated, hemorrhage, hemoptysis, increased intracranial pressure, chest trauma, pulmonary embolism, pulmonary edema, gastric reflux, pneumonectomy with open pericardium, extreme agitation or anxiety, and high risk for rib fractures.

Postural Drainage

Postural drainage is the technique of positioning the patient to facilitate gravitational movement of respiratory secretions toward the bronchi and trachea for expectoration. Various positions are used to drain all 18 segments of the lungs, as illustrated in Figure 28–12. If a patient cannot tolerate a specific position, it should be omitted or modified. The patient is instructed to breathe slowly and deeply throughout the procedure. The upper lobes are drained first, and the posterior basal segments of the lower lobes are drained last. The patient should not sit up between position changes. Tissues and a disposal receptacle are provided. Each position is maintained for 5 to 15 minutes. Postural drainage should be performed before meals or tube feedings. It may be ordered after respiratory treatments with bronchodilators. The frequency is ordered by the physician. If the patient experiences tachycardia over 120 beats per minute, dysrhythmias, hypertension, hypotension, dizziness, or signs of hypoxemia, the procedure should be discontinued and the physician informed.

SUCTIONING

Suctioning may be required if excessive secretions that the patient cannot expectorate accumulate in the oral or nasal airway. The goal of suctioning is to improve oxygen and carbon dioxide exchange in the lungs by removing excessive mucous secretions with a suction catheter. A procedure manual should be consulted for details, but key points when suctioning a patient include the following:

1. Use strict aseptic technique.
2. Administer oxygen before inserting the suction catheter because the procedure temporarily interferes with the patient's air flow.
3. Moisten the catheter in sterile water and insert the catheter through the nose or mouth before applying suction.
4. Apply suction intermittently as the catheter is rotated and withdrawn from the airway.
5. Maintain the pressure gauge between 80 and 100 mm Hg.
6. Limit each suction pass to 10 seconds.
7. Allow the patient to rest briefly, encourage deep breathing, and rinse the catheter with sterile solution between suction attempts.
8. Monitor the patient's response to suctioning.
9. If tachycardia or increased respiratory distress develops, stop the procedure and give the patient oxygen as ordered.
10. Document the amount, color, odor, and consistency of the patient's secretions as well as the patient's status before and after the procedure.

HUMIDIFICATION AND AEROSOL THERAPY

The upper respiratory system is designed to moisturize and warm the air that is inspired through the nose. Humidity is necessary in the respiratory tract to prevent secretions from becoming inspissated (thickened and

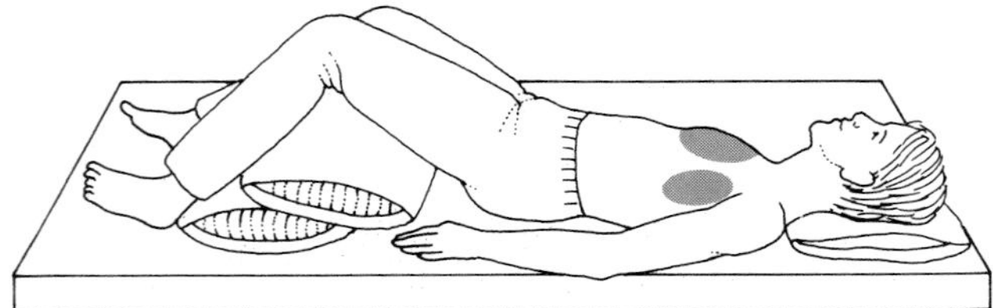

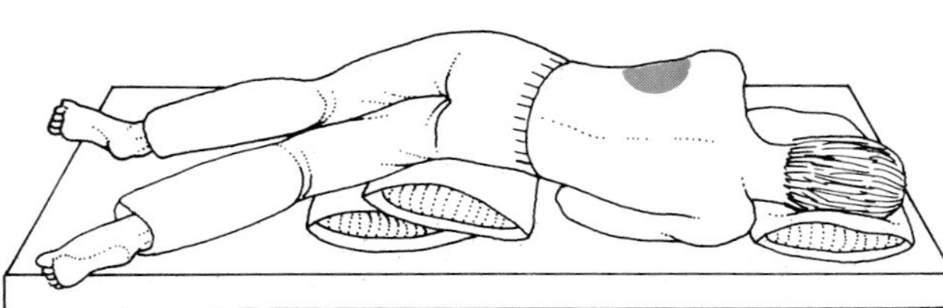

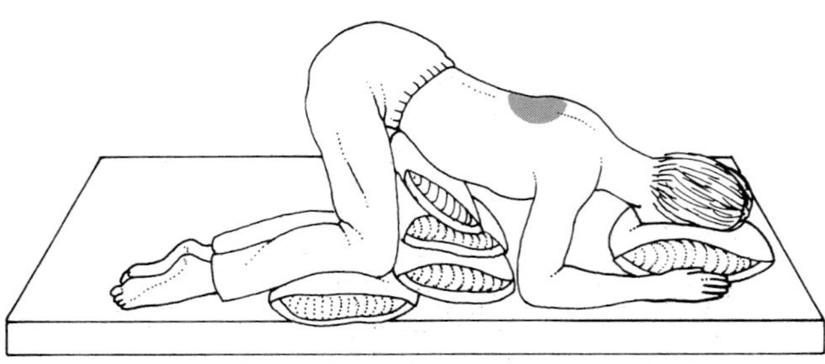

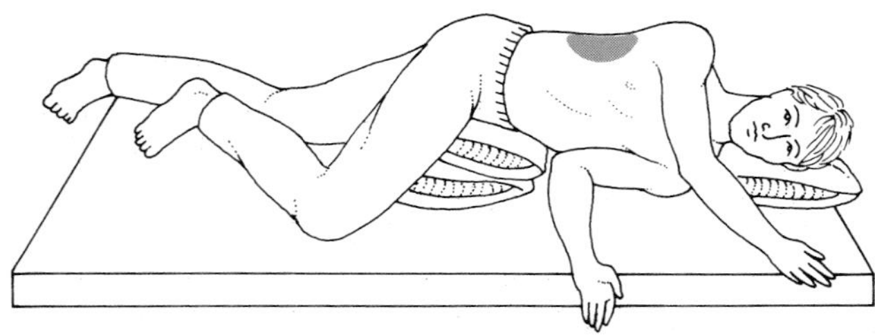

FIGURE 28-12

Positions for postural drainage of respiratory secretions. (From Ignatavicius, D. D., & Bayne, M. V. [1991]. *Medical-surgical nursing: A nursing process approach* [p. 2036]. Philadelphia: W. B. Saunders.)

dried). Inspissated secretions irritate the mucosa making it more susceptible to bacterial infection.

Humidifiers

A humidifier creates water vapor to raise the relative humidity of inspired gas to 100%. There are several types of humidifying devices available for use. Humidifiers deliver warm water vapor directly into the air. There are room humidifiers and units that are used to humidify medical oxygen. Because humidifiers require heat to create water vapor, there is a risk of heat injury when they are used. In addition, the fluid delivered to the respiratory tract can cause overhydration. The fluid reservoir can become contaminated, making it a source of airborne infection. To prevent the spread of bacteria, sterile water should be used to fill the reservoir, and the equipment must be cleaned between each use. Lastly, the equipment can present an electrical hazard.

Aerosol Therapy

Aerosol therapy is used to liquefy and mobilize respiratory secretions and to deliver medications. Aerosols are suspended liquid particles of bronchodilators or inactive fluids such as water or saline that are delivered by devices called nebulizers. Nebulizers deliver a humidified aerosol through large tubing, which may be connected to an oxygen mask or a hand-held device. When hand-held nebulizers are used, the patient should sit upright and slowly inhale the nebulizer aerosol deeply, hold the breath briefly, and exhale slowly. Once secretions are mobilized, the patient may require deep breathing and coughing techniques, postural drainage, suctioning or a combination of these, to clear the secretions. Because aerosols can cause bronchospasm, bronchodilators may be ordered before administering some types of aerosol therapy. There is also a risk of fluid retention, infection, and drug toxicity.

OXYGEN THERAPY

Air in the atmosphere contains approximately 21% oxygen. Usually this is sufficient oxygenation to meet the tissue's ability to function appropriately. In the presence of cardiopulmonary disease or injury it may be necessary to provide a patient with supplemental oxygen, that is, to enrich the atmospheric air with higher concentrations than the patient normally breathes. Oxygen should be treated as a pharmacologic agent in that there may be serious side effects as well as benefits from its use.

PHARMACOLOGY CAPSULE

Oxygen should be thought of as a pharmacologic agent with risks of adverse effects.

Oxygen therapy requires a medical order that should be carried out like any drug order. If a patient is observed becoming lethargic or bradypneic (abnormally slow breathing), a supervisor or physician should be notified immediately because these are symptoms of adverse effects of oxygen therapy.

To administer oxygen to the patient, it is necessary to alter the gas from a compressed form such as a bulk oxygen supply or cylinder to a form with a usable, safe flow rate. Nearly all modern hospitals have bulk oxygen systems with wall adapters to attach flowmeters. When patients with oxygen must be transported, a cylinder on wheels is necessary. A regulator with a flowmeter must be used. After a flowmeter has been attached to the oxygen source, it may be necessary to humidify the gas before delivering it to the patient (Fig. 28–13). Is it always necessary to humidify the oxygen? Humidification is usually unnecessary when using a low-flow cannula at a flow setting of 2 or fewer liters per minute or when using an air entrainment (Venturi) oxygen delivery system.

A tube is needed to connect the flowmeter to the specific oxygen delivery device being used. In some of the devices, the tube is incorporated as an integral component, but in others it is not. It is possible to use extension tubes for some devices, but increasing the length of the tube increases the resistance to gas flow, thus causing pressure to back up in the system, so the patient may not receive the desired oxygen flow.

Oxygen therapy is ordered in liters per minute or FI_{O_2}. FI_{O_2} means fraction of inspired oxygen. It is written, for example, as 0.30, which means 30% oxygen concentration. Various devices can deliver different amounts of oxygen (Fig. 28–14).

The most commonly used device is the nasal cannula. It fits around the face and directly into the nares by way of two prongs. It is designed to deliver a low flow of oxygen from 1 to 6 liters per minute with an approximate FI_{O_2} of 0.24 to 0.40 (24–40% oxygen). The nasal catheter is also a low-flow device that is inserted into

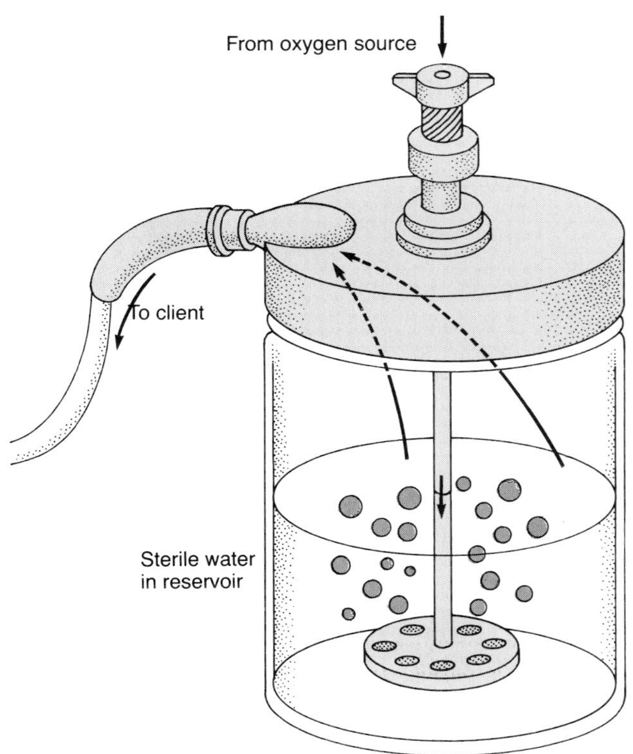

FIGURE 28–13

Bubble humidifier bottle used with oxygen therapy. (From Ignatavicius, D. D., & Bayne, M. V. [1991]. *Medical-surgical nursing: A nursing process approach* [p. 2006]. Philadelphia: W. B. Saunders.)

one naris and then into the pharyngeal space approximately at the uvula. The FI_{O_2} and flow rates are the same as those for the cannula. The catheter is colored green to avoid confusing it with a nasogastric tube. The catheter is rarely used because of the discomfort to the patient and because there is little evidence that anything is gained over the use of a cannula.

Four types of masks are available: the simple oxygen mask, the partial rebreathing mask, the nonrebreathing mask, and the air entrainment (Venturi) mask. The simple oxygen mask is designed to deliver an FI_{O_2} ranging from 0.35 to 0.55 (35–55% oxygen). Flow rates from the flowmeter may be adjusted from 6 to 10 liters per minute. The minimum flow rate of 6 liters per minute is necessary to prevent any chance of carbon dioxide buildup from occurring. The partial rebreathing mask includes a reservoir bag to elevate the potential FI_{O_2}. It is unique because the patient actually rebreathes part of the exhaled gas in the system. However, it is designed so that the rebreathed gas contains almost no carbon dioxide from the patient's lungs—only enriched oxygen. The expected FI_{O_2} range is 0.35 to 0.60 (35–60%). The flowmeter setting must be from 6 to 10 liters per minute. The nonrebreathing mask is so named because none of the patient's exhaled gas is rebreathed. Like the previous mask, it also includes a reservoir bag to enhance the FI_{O_2}, but it has a series of valves to direct the flow of oxygen in such a way that the patient receives a fresh supply of gas with each breath. The expected FI_{O_2} should be near 1.0 (100%). However, Scanlon and colleagues have shown experimentally that the highest FI_{O_2} is approximately 0.7 (70%). In addition, the air entrainment mask is designed to provide a specific FI_{O_2}. This device has been called a Venti mask or a Venturi mask in the past and still may be referred to by these names. The manufacturers of these devices list a specific flowmeter setting for the desired FI_{O_2}. It is also necessary to either adjust a setting on the device or place a specific attachment on the mask to obtain the desired results. It is recommended that the literature accompanying the mask be read, and if there is confusion a respiratory therapist should be consulted.

There may be times when an oxygen mask must be removed, as for oral care or for eating or drinking. The physician should be requested to write an order for the temporary use of a cannula during these times.

The nurse must recognize the complications of oxygen therapy, including hypoventilation, toxicity, atelectasis, and ocular damage. Patients at greatest risk for oxygen-induced hypoventilation are those with chronic respiratory disorders. They have become insensitive to high carbon dioxide levels in the blood, so that low oxygen levels in the blood serve as the stimulus for respirations. Oxygen administration raises the level of oxygen in the blood, and the patient may hypoventilate or even have apnea. Oxygen toxicity can result from exposure to a high concentration of oxygen for a prolonged period of time. Toxicity progresses from tracheobronchitis to lung fibrosis and atelectasis and may be fatal. Atelectasis can result from the replacement of nitrogen normally in the alveoli with oxygen. Oxygen is readily absorbed, predisposing the alveoli to col-

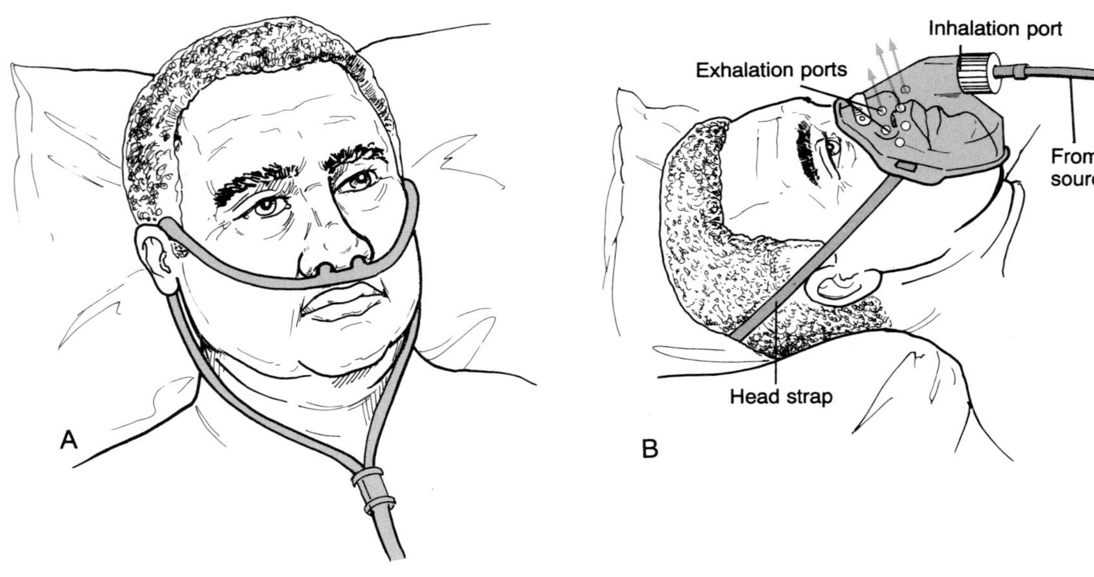

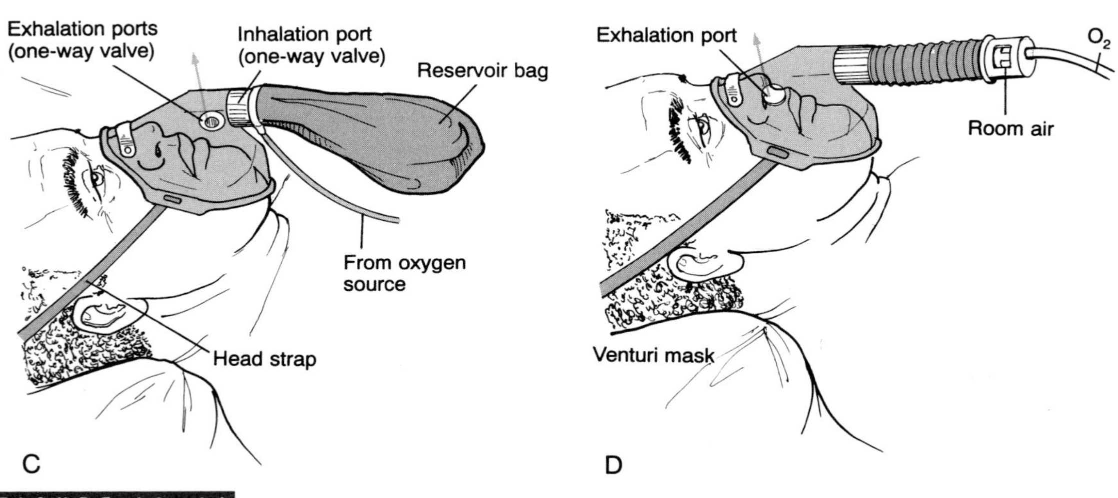

FIGURE 28-14

Oxygen delivery systems. *A,* Nasal cannula; *B,* standard oxygen mask; *C,* partial rebreathing oxygen mask; *D,* Venturi oxygen mask.

lapse. Exposure to 100% oxygen can cause retinal injury.

Key points when a patient is receiving oxygen therapy are the following:

1. Monitor the liter flow to be sure it is as prescribed.
2. Assess the patient's response to oxygen therapy; monitor reports of blood gas analyses.
3. Inspect the tubing for kinks, obstructions, loose connections; listen for a hissing sound in the oxygen mask; feel for adequate oxygen flow.
4. Maintain sterile water in the humidifier reservoir.
5. Clean and replace oxygen therapy equipment according to agency policy.
6. Advise the patient and visitors that smoking is not allowed because oxygen supports combustion.

INTERMITTENT POSITIVE-PRESSURE BREATHING TREATMENTS

Intermittent positive-pressure breathing (IPPB) treatments are used to achieve maximal lung expansion. The IPPB equipment delivers humidified gas with positive pressure, which forces air into the lungs with inhalation and allows passive exhalation. This facilitates maximal exchange of oxygen and carbon dioxide gases in the alveoli and promotes a productive cough. Aerosol medications, including mucolytics (agents that liquefy secretions) and bronchodilators, can be administered through IPPB treatments with a nebulizer device. Although most IPPB treatments are administered by respiratory therapists, they are done by nurses in some settings.

In the past, IPPB was used for a wide range of conditions. The American Association for Respiratory Care now recommends it only for specific conditions, including atelectasis, decreased lung compliance with kyphoscoliosis, and cardiogenic pulmonary edema. Intermittent positive-pressure breathing may be useful in preventing atelectasis, managing bronchospasm, and decreasing the work of breathing, but more research is needed to support these uses. In addition to its questionable usefulness, IPPB is losing favor because it may cause a tension pneumothorax in patients with chronic obstructive pulmonary disease. It may also cause respiratory alkalosis because of hyperventilation. The desired effects of IPPB can generally be achieved by other less expensive measures such as incentive spirometry and hand-held nebulizers.

To give an IPPB treatment, the patient should be seated in a Fowler's position, if not contraindicated, to maximize the ability to breathe deeply. The patient is encouraged to breathe deeply and cough so secretions may be expectorated. The lungs are auscultated before the treatment to locate secretions or areas of diminished breath sounds. After the treatment, the nurse assesses the patient's appearance, breath sounds, and vital signs to evaluate the effects of the treatment.

ARTIFICIAL AIRWAYS

Artificial airways are sometimes required to maintain a patent airway. Artificial airways include the oral airway, nasal airway, endotracheal tube, and tracheostomy tube.

Oral Airway

The oral airway is a curved tube used to maintain an airway temporarily. The oropharyngeal airway is inserted by tilting the head back, opening the mouth, and inserting the airway into the patient's mouth with the tip pointed toward the roof of the mouth. The tube is turned over while being advanced so that the end of the tube rests on the base of the patient's tongue.

Nasal Airway

A nasopharyngeal airway is a soft rubber tube that is inserted through the nose and extended to the base of the tongue. After ruling out a deviated septum, the nasal airway is coated with a water-soluble lubricant and inserted upward into the nose so that the distal end is located in the pharynx at the level of the base of the tongue. A nasal airway should be changed from one nare to the other every 8 hours.

Endotracheal Tube

An endotracheal tube is a long tube inserted through the mouth or nose into the trachea. These tubes have cuffs—inflatable balloons that seal the trachea to prevent aspiration of foreign material and to facilitate mechanical ventilation. Insertion of an endotracheal tube and care of the patient who is intubated require specialized training.

Tracheostomy

A tracheostomy is a surgically created opening through the neck into the trachea. There are a variety of tracheostomy tubes, and they may be used with or without cuffs. Care of the patient with a tracheostomy is covered in Chapter 49.

MECHANICAL VENTILATION

Mechanical ventilation is the process of providing respiratory support by means of a mechanical device called a ventilator. Ventilators are most commonly required for patients with inadequate ventilation and hypoxemia. This may be evidenced by tachypnea or bradypnea with an elevated or a stable arterial carbon dioxide tension ($Paco_2$) or a low arterial oxygen tension (Pao_2) or a low pH. To mechanically ventilate a patient, a cuffed endotracheal or tracheostomy tube must be used to deliver the air. Once the tube is in place, the cuff must be inflated to create a closed system in the patient's airway. Otherwise, air being forced into the lungs could simply flow back out of the trachea.

A volume-limited ventilator is most commonly used for patients with acute respiratory failure. It inflates the lungs with a preset volume of oxygenated air, which is delivered under pressure during the inspiratory cycle. The expiratory cycle may be conducted passively or with pressure as indicated.

There are three types of positive-pressure ventilators: volume cycled, pressure cycled, and time cycled. A volume-cycled ventilator, which delivers a constant preset amount of oxygenated air to the patient, is the most commonly used type. A pressure-cycled ventilator, which pushes air into the lungs until a preset pressure is reached, is not widely used for continuous mechanical ventilation. Time-cycled ventilators deliver oxygenated air over a preset length of time. This type is used most frequently in infants and children.

Depending on the patient's needs, ventilators may be programmed to control or assist the rate of ventilation. The most frequently used modes are intermittent mandatory ventilation and synchronized intermittent mandatory ventilation. These modes provide assistance with ventilation by allowing the patient to breathe spontaneously between a preset number of ventilator breaths. Ventilators deliver oxygen ranging in concentration from 21% oxygen (atmospheric air) to 100% oxygen. The oxygen concentration, or $F_{I_{O_2}}$, is adjusted for individual patient needs.

Tidal volume is the preset amount of oxygenated air delivered during each ventilator breath. This is usually 10 to 15 ml per kg of the patient's body weight.

The respiratory rate setting is the total number of breaths delivered per minute. The rate may be governed by the ventilator or by the ventilator and the patient's spontaneous respirations.

Positive end-expiratory pressure may be prescribed to keep the pressure in the lungs above the atmospheric pressure at the end of expiration. This reduces collapse of small airways and alveoli, thereby increasing the functional residual capacity and improving ventilation.

Other mechanical ventilation modalities include options such as pressure support, flow-by, continuous positive airway pressure, and high-frequency ventilation. These are mentioned only for completeness but not for discussion. If the nurse encounters any of these modalities, specific training is needed that is beyond the scope of this text.

Nursing care of patients on mechanical ventilation requires special training, but key aspects of care include the following:

1. Monitor settings to ensure they are set as prescribed.
2. Be sure high and low pressure alarm settings are turned on.
3. A manual resuscitator and oxygen source must be readily available.
4. Be sure water is not permitted to accumulate in the tubing.
5. Monitor the patient's vital signs and breath sounds; suction as necessary.
6. Establish an alternate method of communication because the patient cannot speak while intubated.

CHEST TUBES

Chest tubes are inserted to drain air or fluid from the pleural space of the lungs. This permits reexpansion of a collapsed lung in the patient with a hemothorax, pneumothorax, or pleural effusion. Chest tubes are inserted under sterile conditions by the physician. The procedure is usually done in the operating room but may be done at the bedside. A small incision is made to insert one chest tube in the second to fourth intercostal space to remove air. Another tube may be placed in the eighth or ninth intercostal space to remove fluids. The tubes are sutured in place, and an airtight sterile dressing is applied. The distal ends of the plastic chest tubes are connected to sterile rubber tubing that leads to a pleural drainage device composed of three compartments: the collection chamber, the waterseal chamber, and the suction chamber (Fig. 28–15). Chest fluid and air drain into the collection chamber. Air is diverted to the waterseal chamber, where it can be seen bubbling up through the water. Suction pressure is controlled in the suction control chamber. The tubing in the suction chamber is partially submerged in water; the depth of the tube in the water regulates the amount of suction. After the tubes have been inserted, a chest radiograph is obtained to confirm placement.

The nurse monitors the patient's vital signs and breath sounds frequently. The dressing is assessed to be sure a tight seal is maintained. Tubing connections are taped, and the connections are inspected frequently to detect air leaks. Extra tubing is coiled on the bed to avoid kinks and the drainage system is kept on the floor.

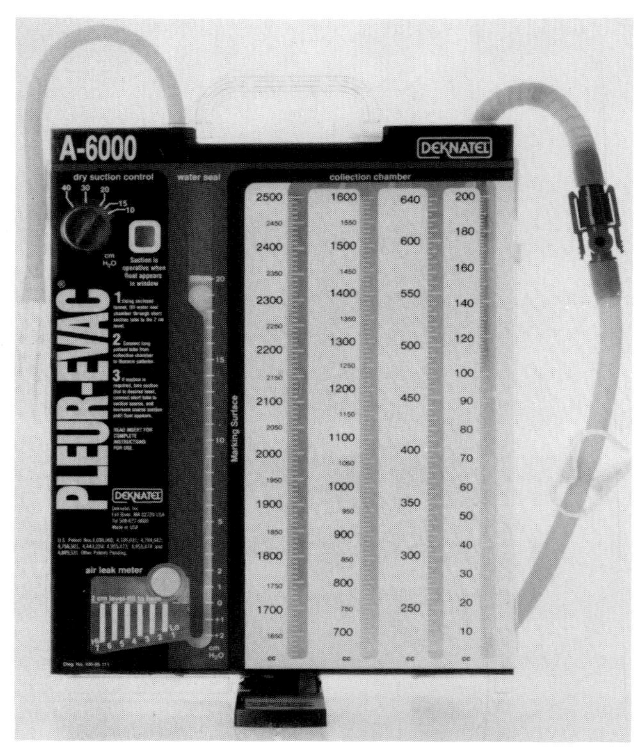

A

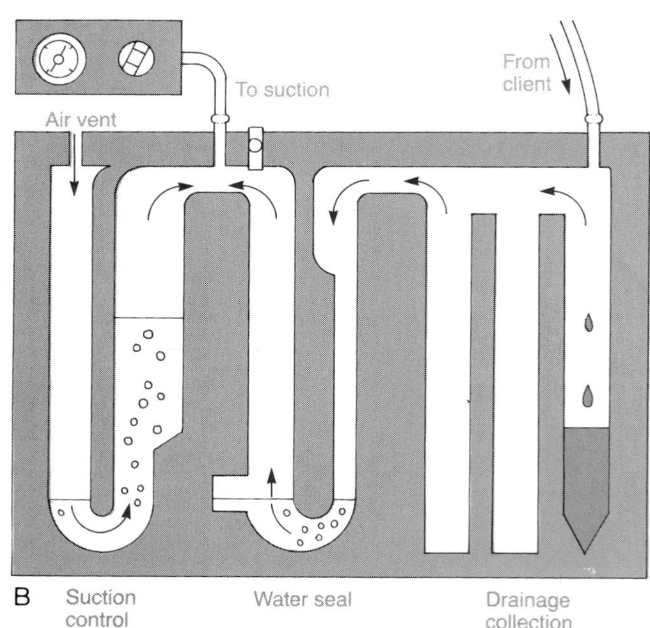

FIGURE 28–15

A, The Pleur-evac drainage system. *B,* Diagram of chambers of water seal chest drainage. (*A* courtesy of Deknatel, Inc., Fall River, MA; *B* from Ignatavicius, D. D., & Bayne, M. V. [1991]. *Medical-surgical nursing: A nursing process approach* [p. 2053]. Philadelphia: W. B. Saunders.)

The drainage is monitored for blood clots or lung tissue which may have to be gently kneaded downward to keep the tube patent. Agency and physician preferences will dictate whether chest tubes are stripped or milked (Fig. 28–16). The chambers are observed for bubbling. Bubbles are usually seen in the waterseal chamber unless the lung has reexpanded or the tubing is occluded.

The rate of drainage is monitored by marking the drainage level on the drainage receptacle. The middle waterseal chamber is observed for the expected rise in the fluid level with inspiration and the fall with expiration. Continuous bubbling in the waterseal chamber suggests an air leak. If an air leak is suspected, agency policy may permit the tubing to be clamped for a maximum of 10 seconds while locating the leak. The suction control chamber may be wet or dry. Wet chambers are regulated by maintaining the water level that is ordered by the physician. Gentle bubbling is expected in the wet suction chamber. Dry chambers are regulated by adjusting the dry suction until the float appears. The drainage receptacle is not usually changed unless the drainage chamber is full. Sterile technique must be used to change the receptacle. The nurse *must* know the agency policies and procedures for managing chest tubes.

An alternative to the large chest drainage systems is the Heimlich flutter valve (Fig. 28–17). The valve is a disposable unit that is attached to the chest tube and to a sterile drainage receptacle. Air and fluid can flow into the receptacle but cannot flow backward into the chest. The patient who has a flutter valve can assume any position and can ambulate easily. A system with a flutter valve can be attached to chest suction if necessary.

THORACIC SURGERY

A thoracotomy is the surgical opening of the chest wall. Surgical procedures on the lung include pneumonectomy, lobectomy, segmental resection, and wedge resection. Pneumonectomy is the removal of an entire lung, whereas a lobectomy is removal of one lobe of a lung. The extensive dissection and removal of a section of the lung is called a segmental resection. A wedge resection is the removal of a small, triangular section of lung tissue. Other procedures that require a thoracotomy are decortication and thoracoplasty. Decortication is stripping of the membrane that covers the visceral

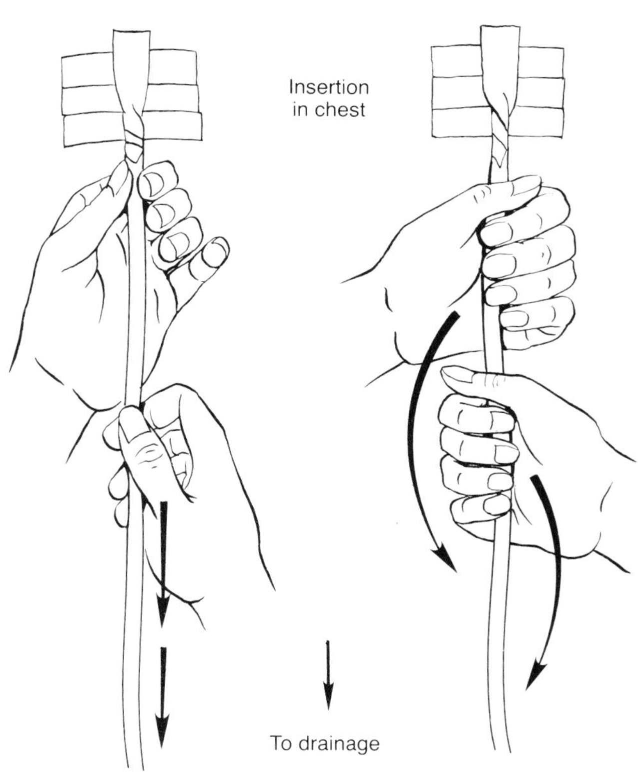

FIGURE 28-16

Two techniques for removing blood clots from chest tubes. *A*, Stripping; *B*, milking. Both can create excessive negative pressure in the pleural space, but milking is safer than stripping. The nurse follows agency policies and physician orders in relation to these procedures. (From Black, J. M., & Matassarin-Jacobs, E. [1993]. *Luckmann and Sorensen's medical-surgical nursing: A psychophysiologic approach* [4th ed., p. 1069]. Philadelphia: W. B. Saunders.)

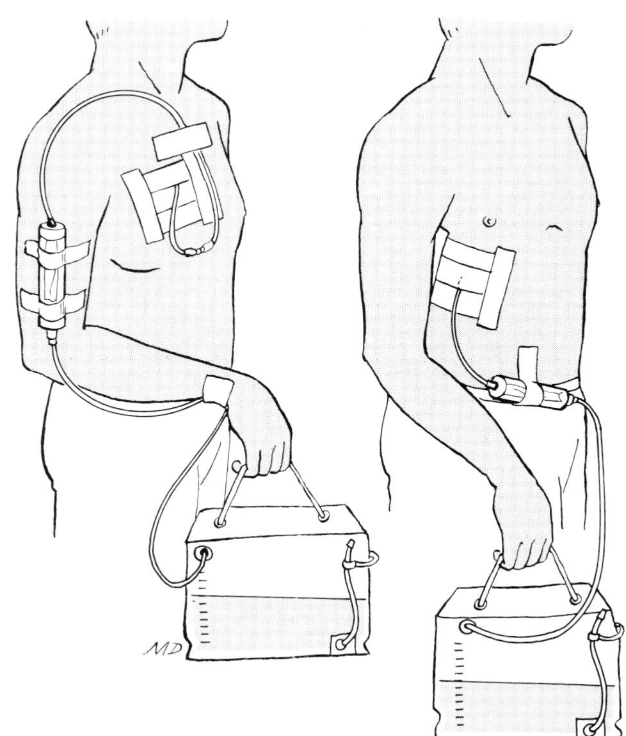

FIGURE 28-17

The Heimlich flutter valve allows chest drainage while preventing reflux of air and fluid back into the chest. It enables the patient to be more mobile than other chest drainage systems do. (From Black, J. M., & Matassarin-Jacobs, E. [1993]. *Luckmann and Sorensen's medical-surgical nursing: A psychophysiologic approach* [4th ed., p. 1071]. Philadelphia: W. B. Saunders.)

pleura, and thoracoplasty is the removal of ribs. Among the most common purposes for thoracic surgery are evaluation of chest trauma, removal of tumors and cysts, and treatment of empyema.

Preoperative Nursing Care of the Patient with a Thoracotomy

Preoperative nursing care is described in Chapter 14. Before thoracotomy, the nurse emphasizes postoperative breathing exercises. If the insertion of a chest tube is anticipated, the procedure is explained to the patient.

Postoperative Nursing Care of the Patient with a Thoracotomy

ASSESSMENT. Postoperatively, the nurse monitors vital signs, lung sounds, mental state, dressings, and chest tube function and drainage.

NURSING DIAGNOSIS. General postoperative nursing diagnoses are presented in Chapter 14. Diagnoses specific to the patient who has had a thoracotomy may also include the following:

- **Impaired Gas Exchange** related to ventilation-perfusion mismatch
- **Ineffective Breathing Patterns** related to preexisting respiratory disease or pain
- **Ineffective Airway Clearance** related to dry secretions or ineffective cough

GOALS. Goals of nursing care specific to the identified nursing diagnoses are improved gas exchange, effective breathing patterns, and improved airway clearance.

INTERVENTIONS

Impaired Gas Exchange. To improve gas exchange, the patient is usually positioned on the unaffected side. Oxygen is administered as ordered. After a thoracotomy, the patient is at risk for pneumonia and atelectasis due to the effects of anesthesia, which impairs ciliary motion, drugs that dry secretions, and immobility.

Ineffective Breathing Patterns. The patient is assisted to breathe deeply and cough. See Figure 14–13 for techniques for splinting a thoracic incision. An incentive spirometer may be used to encourage full expansion of the lungs. Adequate pain control enables the patient to breathe more effectively. Chest physiotherapy and bronchodilators are indicated for some patients. When permitted, the patient may be assisted to sit on the edge of the bed with the feet flat on the floor. An overbed table can be placed in front of the patient, who can lean on it with folded arms. This position fosters movement of the diaphragm and chest expansion.

Ineffective Airway Clearance. Good hydration thins secretions, so fluids are encouraged. If the patient cannot tolerate adequate oral fluids, intravenous fluids may be ordered. For management of chronic respiratory conditions, the reader is referred to Chapter 29.

EVALUATION. Criteria for evaluating the outcomes of nursing interventions are normal arterial blood gases and vital signs consistent with patient's norms, regular respirations without cyanosis or dyspnea, and breath sounds clear to auscultation.

VIDEO THORACOSCOPY

Many procedures that formerly required thoracic surgery can now be done with video thoracoscopy. Thoracoscopy is performed by inserting an endoscope through a small thoracic incision. Procedures that can be done with this instrument include resection of pulmonary and mediastinal lesions, biopsy, drainage of effusions, sympathectomy, vagotomy, and thymectomy. Potential complications of thoracoscopy include atelectasis, pneumonia, air leaks, and injury to thoracic organs. A chest tube is usually needed to promote full reexpansion of the lung on the operative side. Otherwise, patient care is much less complicated than it is after thoracotomy. The nurse monitors the patient's respiratory status, including lung sounds. Sudden dyspnea or other signs of respiratory distress are reported to the surgeon immediately. The amount and appearance of chest tube drainage is documented. The closed drainage system is inspected for proper functioning. Incentive spirometry may be used to encourage lung expansion. Analgesics are given as ordered, but pain is usually not as severe as it is after thoracotomy. Patients are usually permitted out of bed 4 to 6 hours postoperatively and can return to work in 1 week. Before discharge, the nurse instructs the patient to notify the physician of dyspnea or a temperature higher than 38.3°C (101°F).

DRUG THERAPY

Many types of drugs, including decongestants, antitussives, antihistamines, expectorants, antimicrobials, bronchodilators, corticosteroids, and mast cell stabilizers, may be used to treat respiratory disorders (Table 28–5).

Decongestants

Decongestants are sympathomimetic agents. They mimic the action of epinephrine and norepinephrine, causing constriction of nasal blood vessels and reducing the swelling of mucous membranes. Over-the-counter decongestants such as Sudafed are commonly used to treat the common cold. Constriction of the blood vessels is not limited to the nasal passages, so that systemic vasoconstriction and elevated blood pressure may result. Therefore, persons with hypertension, heart disease, diabetes mellitus, and hyperthyroidism are generally advised to avoid decongestant drugs except under medical supervision.

TABLE 28-5

DRUGS USED TO TREAT RESPIRATORY DISORDERS

DRUG	USE/ACTION	SIDE EFFECTS	NURSING INTERVENTIONS
Decongestants Phenylpropanolamine (PPA) Pseudoephedrine (Sudafed)	Vasoconstriction. Reduces swelling of mucous membranes. Used to treat nasal discharge, common cold.	Occasionally cause mild central nervous system stimulation, especially in the elderly. Toxicity: tachycardia, palpitations, lightheadedness, nausea, vomiting, hallucinations, seizures.	Monitor pulse and blood pressure, mental and emotional state. Contraindicated with severe hypertension, coronary artery disease, lactation. Tell patient to swallow extended release tablets whole.
Antitussives Codeine Hydrocodone bitartrate (Hycodan) Dextromethorphan	Suppression of cough reflex. Most appropriately used to control nonproductive cough or cough that interferes with rest or wound healing.	Codeine is classified as a narcotic and has abuse potential. It can also cause sedation. Dextromethorphan does not have these effects.	Encourage fluids unless contraindicated to facilitate expectoration or secretions. Safety measures with codeine.
Antihistamines Diphenhydramine (Benadryl)	Block allergic response. Dry respiratory secretions. Also act as antiemetics, local anesthetics, and sedatives.	Drowsiness, dry mouth, blurred vision, photophobia, thickening of mucous secretions, decreased sweating, constipation, urinary retention, increased heart rate.	Safety precautions if drowsy. Monitor respiratory status. Not recommended for patients with asthma. Encourage fluids if not contraindicated. Monitor elimination. Oral hygiene.
Expectorants Guaifenesin (Robitussin)	Thin respiratory secretions for easier expectoration.	Nausea and vomiting with large doses.	Assess cough productivity. Do not crush sustained-release capsules.
Antimicrobials	Kill or inhibit the growth of bacteria, viruses, or fungi.	Side and adverse effects specific to each antimicrobial classification. Common side effects are nausea, vomiting, and diarrhea. Risk of superinfections such as "yeast" infections of mouth, genitourinary tract. Risk of severe allergic response.	Assess allergies before administration. Be alert for allergic response: rash, dyspnea, loss of consciousness. Instruct patient to complete entire course of therapy. Monitor for improvement and for superinfections. Report continued symptoms.
Bronchodilators	Relax smooth muscle in the bronchial tree to relieve bronchial constriction.		
1. Methylxanthines Theophylline Aminophylline	Methylxanthines also cause increased heart rate and force of cardiac contraction, central nervous system stimulation, and increased gastric acid secretion.	Monitor for anxiety, restlessness, tachypnea, tachycardia, dysrhythmias, gastrointestinal (GI) distress. Rapid intravenous administration can cause hypotension, fatal dysrhythmias.	Monitor vital signs, mental state, drug blood levels. Measure intake and output. Give with milk or food to decrease GI distress. Do not administer before bedtime.
2. Sympathomimetics Epinephrine Isoproterenol hydrochloride (Isuprel) Ephedrine Selective $beta_2$ agonists: albuterol sulfate (Proventil), terbutaline sulfate (Brethine), isoetharine hydrochloride (Bronkosol)	Sympathomimetics also decrease mucous secretion, increase mucociliary clearance, and stabilize mast cells.	Restlessness, anxiety, tachycardia, headache, hypertension, disorientation, nausea, vomiting, diarrhea.	Do not exceed prescribed dosage. Teach patient to use inhaler. Rinse mouth after inhalation to decrease dryness. Avoid excessive caffeine. Monitor respiratory and cardiovascular status.
3. Inhaled muscarinics Ipratropium bromide (Atrovent)	Inhaled muscarinics act directly on the respiratory passages to cause bronchodilation. Not effective for acute attacks.	Increased intraocular pressure with narrow-angle glaucoma. Rarely: hypotension.	Monitor respiratory status. Evaluate for improvement. Tell patient not to use more than 2 inhalations at a time. Rinse mouth after inhaling to reduce dry mouth and throat. Avoid excessive caffeine intake.

Table continued on following page

TABLE 28-5

DRUGS USED TO TREAT RESPIRATORY DISORDERS *Continued*

DRUG	USE/ACTION	SIDE EFFECTS	NURSING INTERVENTIONS
Corticosteroids	Stabilize mast cells to reduce release of mediators that cause inflammation and edema. Restore bronchodilator response to sympathomimetics in treating acute bronchial constriction. May be given parenterally, orally, or by inhalation. Masks signs of infection.	Systemic therapy: water and sodium retention, potassium loss, abnormal fat distribution, hypertension, GI distress. Abrupt withdrawal can trigger adrenal insufficiency. Inhaled steroids: hoarseness, oral "yeast" infections, systemic effects with long-term use.	Monitor vital signs, weight, and electrolytes. Assess for subtle signs of infection.
Mast cell stabilizer Cromolyn sodium (Intal)	Reduces the production of chemicals by the mast cells that cause bronchial constriction, edema, inflammation. Helps reduce frequency and severity of asthma attacks. Does not stop asthma attack. Administered by Spinhaler, nebulization, and metered-dose inhalers.	Wheezing, sneezing, coughing. Occasional bronchoconstriction. Rare: allergies, headache, nausea, urinary frequency.	Instruct patient in self-medication. Advise that excessive use can actually cause bronchoconstriction. Rinsing mouth after use of inhaler will reduce dry mouth effects. Monitor effects.

PHARMACOLOGY CAPSULE

People with hypertension, heart disease, and hyperthyroidism should not take over-the-counter cold remedies without consulting a pharmacist or a physician. Many cold remedies stimulate the heart and raise the blood pressure.

Antitussives

Antitussives suppress the cough reflex. Antitussive action is not always desirable because coughing removes secretions from the airways. However, when a cough is nonproductive, creates pain, interferes with sleep, or impairs wound healing, temporary cough suppression may be indicated. Codeine is an effective antitussive, but it is a narcotic with many side effects and abuse potential. Therefore, dextromethorphan, which is not a narcotic, is more commonly used.

PHARMACOLOGY CAPSULE

Use antitussives cautiously. Cough is a protective mechanism that clears the airway.

Antihistamines

Antihistamines, including diphenhydramine (Benadryl), are over-the-counter medications that are frequently used because of their action in drying nasal secretions. Although they provide short-term relief, they also can cause dizziness, dry mouth, constipation, blurred vision, urinary retention, tachycardia, drowsiness, and impaired judgment. In addition, antihistamines may dry up bronchial secretions and worsen a cough. These drugs are not generally recommended for people with asthma because dry secretions contribute to difficulty clearing the airway.

Expectorants

Expectorants thin respiratory secretions so they are more readily mobilized and cleared from the airways.

Antimicrobials

Antimicrobials kill or inhibit the growth of bacteria, viruses, or fungi. Antibiotics are used to treat only bacterial infections because they are not effective against viruses or fungi. A limited number of antiviral and antifungal drugs are available. Specific antimicrobials are best selected after culture and sensitivity tests are performed on a specimen of respiratory secretions. Antimicrobials can cause allergic responses and have many side effects. The nurse instructs the patient in self-medication and stresses the importance of completing the prescribed course of therapy to prevent reinfection and the development of resistant strains of pathogens.

Bronchodilators

Bronchodilators relax smooth muscle in the bronchial airways and blood vessels. They are used to treat airway obstruction from respiratory disorders such as asthma and chronic obstructive pulmonary disease. The primary drawback to most bronchodilators is their tendency to cause cardiac and central nervous system stimulation. Some bronchodilators act primarily to prevent bronchial constriction, whereas others relieve it.

Corticosteroids

Corticosteroids are anti-inflammatory drugs that may be administered parenterally, orally, and by inhalation. The drug may be inhaled orally or nasally. They are important drugs in the treatment of asthma because they reduce inflammation and edema in the respiratory tract. These drugs are less commonly used to treat chronic obstructive pulmonary disease. Among the many systemic effects of steroids are fluid and electrolyte imbalances, hypertension, osteoporosis, and muscle wasting. Oral and parenteral steroids have more side effects than inhaled forms of the drug. Patients should know not to abruptly discontinue steroid therapy as that may lead to acute adrenal insufficiency.

PHARMACOLOGY CAPSULE

Inhaled corticosteroids can have systemic effects if used over a long time.

Mast Cell Stabilizer

Cromolyn sodium (Intal) is a drug that reduces the production of chemicals by the mast cells that cause bronchoconstriction, edema, and inflammation. This drug is used to prevent acute asthma attacks. It is not useful in stopping an attack after it starts.

DISORDERS OF THE RESPIRATORY SYSTEM

ACUTE VIRAL RHINITIS (THE COMMON COLD)

Etiology and Risk Factors

Acute viral rhinitis, also called coryza or the common cold, is the most prevalent infectious disease. It is caused by viruses that invade the upper respiratory tract through airborne droplets. The droplets are spread by an infected person through breathing, sneezing, coughing, or by direct hand contact. Touching contaminated surfaces and then carrying the virus to the nasal membranes and eyes is the most important means of spreading a cold. Therefore, careful attention to hand washing is one of the best preventive measures for avoiding a common cold.

Signs and Symptoms

Colds occur most frequently during the winter months when people tend to stay indoors and can more easily contaminate one another. A cold lasts 2 to 14 days, and people are most contagious during the first 3 days. Symptoms include a feeling of nasal dryness and stuffiness, sneezing, runny nose, headache, sore throat, lethargy, and fatigue. In severe cases, chills, fever, and marked prostration may be present.

Medical Diagnosis

The common cold is diagnosed on the basis of the patient history and physical examination.

Medical Treatment

The most common treatment for a cold is a combination of rest, fluids, proper diet, antipyretics, and analgesics. Antibiotics and currently available antiviral agents are usually not indicated because they are not effective against cold viruses. Studies have been inconclusive about the value of using large doses of vitamin C for treating and preventing a cold. Other drugs that may be used to relieve the symptoms of the common cold by drying secretions are antihistamines and decongestants.

Nursing Care of the Patient with Acute Viral Rhinitis

ASSESSMENT. The complete assessment of the patient with a respiratory disorder is summarized in Table 28–2. The health history may be limited in focus and include a complete description of symptoms, past medical history, and drug history. The physical examination focuses on the nose, throat, ears, neck, and chest.

NURSING DIAGNOSIS. The primary diagnosis for the patient with a common cold is knowledge deficit of treatment, prevention, and signs and symptoms of complications. Although most people with colds recover without incident, some patients are at high risk for infection related to viral or bacterial pneumonitis.

GOAL. The goal of nursing care is patient knowledge of treatment, self-care, prevention, and measures to avoid complications of the common cold. If the patient is at risk for secondary infection, the goal is absence of signs of worsening infection.

INTERVENTIONS. The common cold is unlikely to require inpatient care unless a patient is immunosuppressed. Therefore, the primary nursing intervention is usually patient teaching. The patient is advised to rest and to maintain a daily fluid intake of 2 to 3 liters, if not contraindicated. Good hydration is essential for keeping secretions thin for easier expectoration. A room humidifier may provide some comfort by keeping mucous membranes moist. Fever can be treated with antipyretics. The nurse identifies drugs prescribed or recommended by the physician and informs the patient of the drug names, dosages, and side effects. Many drugs used to treat symptoms of the common cold cause drowsiness, so the patient may be advised to avoid activities requiring mental alertness.

PHARMACOLOGY CAPSULE

Explain to patients that antibiotics are not usually prescribed for the common cold because it is caused by a virus, and antibiotics are only effective against bacteria.

Infection control measures are needed to prevent spread of the cold and to protect the patient who has a cold from secondary bacterial infections. During the first 3 days the patient is most contagious. The patient should avoid contact with others, especially those who are at increased risk for infection (young children, the elderly, people who are immunosuppressed), to prevent the spread of the cold. To reduce the risk of spreading the cold or of acquiring secondary bacterial infections, the nurse instructs the patient to do the following:

- Avoid close contact with other people who have bacterial infections.
- Avoid crowded places.
- Avoid sharing drinking glasses or eating utensils.
- Practice good hand washing with antibacterial soap.
- Cover the mouth when coughing or sneezing.
- Use disposable tissues for expectorated secretions; dispose of them promptly.

If the patient develops purulent sputum, chest pain, a temperature higher than 37.8°C (100°F), a red sore throat, or lung congestion, the physician must be contacted for further treatment. These signs and symptoms suggest a more severe respiratory condition that may require additional treatment.

EVALUATION. Criteria for assessing the effectiveness of patient teaching are patient's verbalization of content presented and statement of intent to follow plan of care. Absence of infection is evidenced by normal vital signs, clear breath sounds, and clear sputum.

ACUTE BRONCHITIS

Etiology and Risk Factors

Acute bronchitis is a common condition that may follow a viral infection such as a cold or influenza. Bronchitis is usually viral in origin, but bacterial causes (*Streptococcus pneumoniae* or *Haemophilus influenzae*) also are common. Irritation and inflammation may occur throughout the upper respiratory tract, resulting in an increased production of mucus. Excess production of mucus leads to coughing and sputum production.

Signs and Symptoms

Symptoms of acute bronchitis include fever, cough, yellow or green sputum, rapid breathing, and occasionally chest pain.

Medical Diagnosis

Acute bronchitis is usually diagnosed on the basis of the health history and the physical findings.

Medical Treatment

Treatment consists of a broad-spectrum antibiotic (ampicillin, tetracycline, or erythromycin) for 7 to 10 days; hospitalization is usually unnecessary.

Nursing Care of the Patient with Acute Bronchitis

Nursing care with acute bronchitis is similar to that for the common cold. In addition, patients who are taking antibiotics should be encouraged to take the full course of the medication.

INFLUENZA

The term *flu* is commonly used to describe a number of ailments involving various body systems. However, influenza is actually an acute viral respiratory infection that is accompanied by a fever. There are several strains of the influenza virus (A, B, C). A strain is further subtyped according to the place and year it was isolated. Influenza usually occurs in epidemics during the winter months. Those most susceptible to the influenza virus are very young children, elderly people, people living in institutional situations, people with chronic diseases, and health care personnel.

Complications

The most common complications of influenza are bronchitis and viral or bacterial pneumonia. Other less common complications are myocarditis, pericarditis, Reye's syndrome, confusion, seizures, Guillain-Barré syndrome, toxic shock syndrome, myositis, and renal failure.

Signs and Symptoms

Influenza is similar to the common cold in the way that it is spread, that is, through droplet infection; however, its symptoms differ from those of the common cold. Individuals with colds experience nasal symptoms, malaise, and usually are afebrile (without fever), whereas individuals with influenza typically have chills, fever, muscular pain, headache, and dry, hacking cough.

Medical Diagnosis

A diagnosis of influenza is usually based on the patient's history and physical findings. Laboratory tests for confirming infections caused by the influenza virus are improving dramatically and can provide results in less than 48 hours. However, viral tests are generally expensive and may not be available in all facilities.

Medical Treatment

Treatment of influenza is similar to the treatment of the common cold: rest, fluids, proper diet, antipyretics, and analgesics. An antiviral agent like amantadine hydrochloride (Symmetrel) or the newer rimantadine can be used to treat type A influenza, but to be effective therapy must be started within 24 to 48 hours after the onset of symptoms and continued for 10 days.

PHARMACOLOGY CAPSULE

Antiviral drugs must be administered soon after the onset of influenza symptoms to be effective.

The best treatment is prevention through immunization, especially for elderly people, people with chronic illnesses, health care personnel, and people living in crowded environments. The Immunization Practices Advisory Committee currently recommends an annual vaccination using inactivated influenza vaccine. The immunizations are usually given in the fall of the year. The protection rate for influenza vaccines is about 70% in the general population but may be lower among the elderly. Although the incidence of adverse reactions to influenza immunizations is small, some people report sore arm, headache, fever, muscle ache, nausea, and diarrhea. Acetaminophen, 325 mg taken every 4 hours for the first 12 hours, may reduce these symptoms. Other measures to reduce the risk of influenza are good nutrition and hygiene. An antiviral agent may also be prescribed for people who are at increased risk of acquiring viral infections.

Nursing Care of the Patient with Influenza

Nursing care of the patient with influenza is similar to care of the patient with the common cold. Ongoing assessment is particularly important with influenza because of the risk of serious complications, especially in the elderly. In addition, people at high risk are encouraged to be immunized against influenza: those with serious chronic cardiopulmonary disorders, residents of long-term care facilities, health care providers who have contact with high-risk patients, people older than 65, and those who have chronic metabolic disorders such as diabetes mellitus.

PNEUMONIA

Etiology and Risk Factors

The term *pneumonia* describes inflammation of certain parts of the lung such as the alveoli and bronchioles. Pneumonia may be caused by either infectious or noninfectious agents. Examples of infectious agents are bacteria, *Pseudomonas*, *Candida* and other fungi, and nonspecific viruses. Noninfectious agents may include irritating fumes, dust, or chemicals that are inhaled or foreign matter that is aspirated. Nosocomial pneumonia is a hospital-acquired infection that may be attributed to inadequate hand washing, poor sterile technique with suctioning, contaminated equipment, and exposure to others who have infectious respiratory conditions.

People who are most likely to develop pneumonia are smokers; those with altered consciousness from alcohol, seizures, anesthesia or drug overdose; those who are immunosuppressed; chronically ill people who are malnourished or debilitated; and people on bedrest with prolonged immobility.

Patients at increased risk for aspiration pneumonia are those with impaired swallowing or cough reflexes, decreased gastrointestinal motility, esophageal abnormalities, tube feedings, tracheostomies, and endotracheal tubes.

Pathophysiology

Pneumonia may be classified as lobar, bronchial, and interstitial. Lobar pneumonia involves one or more lobes of the lung, bronchopneumonia involves the bronchioles and alveoli, and interstitial pneumonia involves the lung tissue surrounding the alveoli. Pneumonia may also be classified according to the causative organism, usually bacteria or viruses. Gram-positive bacteria cause pneumococcal, staphylococcal, and streptococcal pneumonias, and gram-negative bacteria cause *Pseudomonas* and influenza pneumonias and legionnaires' disease. Viral pneumonias are caused by several different viruses, including the influenza virus. Pneumococcal pneumonia (*Streptococcus pneumoniae*) is the most common cause of bacterial and lobar pneumonia. In addition to bacteria and viruses, pneumonia may be caused by fungi, mycoplasmas, and protozoa.

The pathophysiology of pneumonia follows a predictable course. When pathogens invade the lungs, the inflammatory process causes fluid to accumulate in the affected alveoli. In a process called *hepatization*, capillaries dilate and neutrophils, red blood cells, and fibrin fill the alveoli, causing the lung to appear red and granular. Next, blood flow decreases, and leukocytes (white blood cells) and fibrin infiltrate the area and consolidate (solidify). As the infection resolves, the consolidated material dissolves and is ingested and removed by microphages.

Complications

Although most people recover from pneumonia, it remains among the most common causes of death. Relatively common pulmonary complications of pneumonia include pleurisy, pleural effusion, and atelectasis. Pleurisy is inflammation of the pleura that causes pain with breathing. Pleural effusion is the accumulation of fluid between the pleura that encases the lungs and the pleura that lines the thoracic cavity. A large amount of fluid can lead to collapse of the lung. Atelectasis refers to collapsed alveoli. Other less common pulmonary complications of pneumonia are lung abscesses, delayed resolution, and empyema. Empyema is the presence of purulent exudate in the pleural cavity. Potential systemic complications include pericarditis, arthritis, meningitis, and endocarditis.

Signs and Symptoms

Symptoms of pneumonia are fever, chills, sweats, chest pain, cough, sputum production, hemoptysis (coughing up blood), dyspnea (difficulty breathing), headache, and fatigue. Individuals with bacterial pneumonia may experience an abrupt, almost explosive onset: severe shaking chills; sharp, stabbing lateral chest pain, especially with coughing and breathing; and intermittent cough with rusty sputum. Viral pneumonia is characterized by burning or searing chest pain in the sternal area; a continuous, hacking, barking cough producing small amounts of sputum; and headache.

Medical Diagnosis

Diagnosis of pneumonia is based on the findings of the history and physical examination, sputum culture and Gram stain, chest radiograph, complete blood count, and blood culture.

Medical Treatment

Treatment usually consists of increased fluid intake (at least 3 liters every 24 hours), limited activity or bedrest, antipyretics, analgesics, and in some cases, oxygen and aerosol intermittent positive-pressure breathing therapy. Bacterial pneumonias are treated with appropriate antibiotics; however, antibiotics are not used with viral pneumonias because they do not kill viruses.

People at high risk for pneumonia may receive a pneumococcal vaccine. Vaccination is recommended for adults with chronic illnesses, particularly cardiovascular and respiratory diseases, and diabetes mellitus; people recovering from a severe illness; individuals aged 65 and older; and older adults living in nursing homes or other long-term care facilities. Vaccination is not recommended for children under 2 years of age. The vaccine is administered only once in a lifetime because there is a danger of reaction with a second dose.

Nursing Care of the Patient with Pneumonia

ASSESSMENT. Assessment of the patient with a respiratory disorder is summarized in Table 28–2 (see Care Plan: The Patient with Pneumonia).

NURSING DIAGNOSIS. Nursing diagnoses for the patient with pneumonia may include the following:

- **Ineffective Airway Clearance** related to increased sputum production, thick secretions, ineffective cough
- **Impaired Gas Exchange** related to obstruction of airways by edema and secretions or atelectasis
- **Activity Intolerance** related to fatigue, hypoxia
- **Altered Nutrition: Less than Body Requirements** related to anorexia, dyspnea, fatigue
- **High Risk for Fluid Volume Deficit** related to inadequate fluid intake, fever, mouth breathing
- **Pain** related to inflammation, cough, muscle aches
- **Knowledge Deficit** of treatment, self-care, and prevention of future pneumonia

GOALS. Goals of nursing care for the patient with pneumonia are a patent airway; adequate oxygenation; improved activity tolerance; optimal nutritional status; normal hydration; pain relief; and patient's knowledge of treatment, self-care, and preventive measures.

INTERVENTIONS

Ineffective Airway Clearance. Accumulated secretions in the respiratory tract impair gas exchange and may result in alveolar collapse. Therapeutic measures are taken to decrease the production and promote the expectoration of secretions. Antimicrobials, decongestants, and expectorants are administered as ordered. A good cough is essential for removal of secretions, but antitussives may be given as ordered if the patient becomes exhausted because of constant coughing. The patient is encouraged or assisted to change positions at least every 2 hours to help mobilize secretions. Other measures employed to mobilize secretions are deep breathing and coughing exercises, chest physiotherapy, and aerosol therapy. The patient who has a very weak cough may require suctioning. Tissues and a receptacle are provided for disposal of secretions. The nurse notes the amount, color, and consistency of secretions. Lung sounds are auscultated frequently to assess the effects of interventions to clear the airways.

Impaired Gas Exchange. The edema and secretions present with pneumonia interfere with the exchange of gases in the lungs. The patient may develop hypoxemia, meaning that the level of oxygen in the blood is low. At the same time, excess carbon dioxide may accumulate in the blood—a condition called *hypercapnia.* Because normal oxygenation is essential for all body tissues, efforts must be made to improve the patient's gas exchange.

To assess gas exchange, the nurse monitors vital signs, lung sounds, and skin color. The nurse is alert for signs of hypoxemia: restlessness, tachycardia, and tachypnea. If arterial blood gases are being measured, the nurse reports abnormal results to the physician. Hemoglobin may also be measured. A low hemoglobin is significant because it indicates the reduced oxygen-carrying capacity of red blood cells.

Measures that mobilize secretions, discussed earlier, are important in improving gas exchange. In addition,

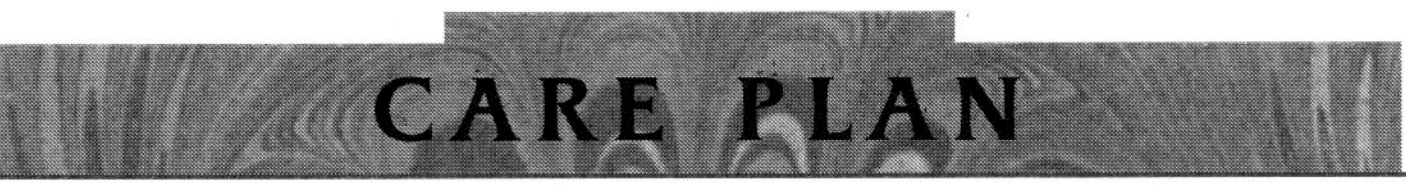

CARE PLAN

The Patient with Pneumonia

ASSESSMENT

Health History: Alice Guthrie, 77 years old, is a retired school teacher who complains of chills and fever, cough, sore throat, and chest pain. The physician diagnosed pneumonia and recommended hospitalization. Ms. Guthrie states she had a cold for about a week and seemed to get progressively worse. She states she has "a little" shortness of breath and tires very easily. Her chest pain is aggravated by coughing. She has been taking over-the-counter cold remedies. She has a history of hypertension and congestive heart failure for which she takes verapamil hydrochloride (Calan SR), 240 mg daily, and digoxin, 0.25 mg daily. Ms. Guthrie lives alone in a one-story apartment. She has a close friend next door who visits frequently.

Physical Examination: Vital signs: temperature, 100.6°F orally; pulse, 92; respiration, 24; blood pressure, 160/94. Alert, slightly dyspneic. Skin color pale. Nail beds slightly dusky. Lung sounds clear to auscultation over right lung fields. Wheezes and crackles auscultated in left lung. Frequent cough producing greenish sputum. No retractions or use of accessory muscles of respiration. Abdomen soft.

NURSING DIAGNOSIS	GOALS AND OUTCOME CRITERIA	INTERVENTIONS
Ineffective airway clearance related to increased sputum production, and thick secretions.	The patient will have a patent airway as evidenced by clear breath sounds without wheezes or crackles.	Administer antimicrobials, decongestants, and expectorants as ordered. Administer antitussives as ordered if cough interferes with rest. Suction only if necessary. Turn, deep breathe, and cough at least every 2 hours. Perform chest physiotherapy and provide aerosol therapy as ordered. Assess response. Monitor lung sounds, respiratory rate, and characteristics of secretions. Dispose of tissues in a sanitary manner.
Impaired gas exchange related to obstruction of airways by edema and secretions or atelectasis.	The patient will have adequate oxygenation as evidenced by normal arterial blood gases and vital signs.	Monitor vital signs, lung sounds, skin color, blood gas reports, and level of consciousness. Be alert for signs of hypoxemia: restlessness, tachycardia, tachypnea. Report abnormal findings to physician. Elevate head of bed. Administer oxygen therapy as ordered.
Activity intolerance related to fatigue or hypoxia.	The patient will demonstrate activities of daily living without excessive fatigue or dyspnea.	Instruct in activity restrictions as ordered. Plan care to allow periods of uninterrupted rest. Assist with activities of daily living as needed. Gradually encourage increased activity while monitoring for dyspnea and fatigue. Keep interactions short, and limit visitors.
Altered nutrition: less than body requirements related to anorexia, dyspnea, or fatigue.	The patient will maintain optimal nutritional status as evidenced by stable body weight.	Monitor food intake and weight. If intake is poor, consult with dietitian about patient preferences. Suggest small, frequent meals. Provide pleasant environment for meals. Position for comfort. Use oxygen cannula during meals if permitted. Weigh daily.
High risk for fluid volume deficit related to inadequate fluid intake, fever, or mouth breathing.	The patient's hydration will remain normal as evidenced by fluid intake equal to output, moist mucous membranes, and blood pressure consistent with patient's norms.	Monitor fluid status for signs of fluid volume deficit: decreased skin turgor, concentrated urine, decreased urine output, dry mucous membranes, elevated hemoglobin and hematocrit levels. Administer intravenous fluids as ordered. Encourage fluids by mouth up to 3 liters daily unless contraindicated. Record intake and output. Monitor temperature and treat fever as ordered. Keep dry and lightly covered. Administer tepid

Care Plan continued on following page

The Patient with Pneumonia *(Continued)*

NURSING DIAGNOSIS	GOALS AND OUTCOME CRITERIA	INTERVENTIONS
		sponge baths as ordered for fever, but do not induce shivering. Use hypothermia blanket as ordered.
Pain related to inflammation, cough, or muscle aches.	The patient will report decreased pain.	Assess pain. Administer analgesics as ordered. Reposition for comfort. Splint painful areas during coughing and deep breathing. Use massage and relaxation techniques. Document effects of interventions.

the nurse elevates the head of the bed. Some patients are more comfortable in a reclining chair that permits alterations in position. A semi-Fowler's position decreases the pressure of the abdominal organs on the diaphragm so the patient breathes more easily. Oxygen therapy is provided as ordered.

Activity Intolerance. Activity is usually restricted for the patient with pneumonia and may range from complete bedrest to limited activities. Nursing care must be scheduled to prevent overtiring and to allow for periods of uninterrupted rest. Assistance is provided as needed until the patient is able to resume self-care. Conversations should be short, and visitors should be encouraged not to tire the patient with long visits. When the patient begins to resume activities of daily living, the nurse evaluates the ability to tolerate daily activities.

Altered Nutrition: Less than Body Requirements. Good nutrition is essential to combat the infection and to promote healing. The patient's usual dietary habits are assessed to provide baseline information so that the diet may be individualized. Weight may be monitored to determine the adequacy of nutrition. The patient should be weighed before breakfast using the same scale each time. Albumin and lymphocyte blood counts are monitored to detect low levels that are common with inadequate protein.

A typical diet for the patient with pneumonia is a high protein, soft diet. Unfortunately, fatigue, dyspnea, and anorexia may interfere with adequate food intake. The nurse provides the diet as ordered, assists the patient with the meal if needed, and documents intake. To enhance the appetite, oral care is provided before meals, the head of the bed is elevated, and the tray is arranged in an attractive and convenient manner. The diet should conform to the patient's preferences as much as possible. If oxygen is needed, a nasal cannula is recommended during meals. If the patient tires quickly, more frequent meals with smaller servings may be better received.

High Risk for Fluid Volume Deficit. The patient with pneumonia may lose excess fluid because of fever and mouth breathing, and fluid intake may be inadequate because of fatigue and dyspnea. Dehydration causes respiratory secretions to be thicker and more difficult to mobilize. Signs and symptoms of fluid volume deficit include decreased skin turgor, concentrated urine, dry mucous membranes, and elevated hemoglobin and hematocrit levels. Therefore, the nurse encourages a fluid intake of 3 liters a day unless contraindicated. If the patient's oral intake is low, intravenous fluids may be ordered. Hard candy, if permitted, stimulates thirst and fluid intake. Intake and output records may be kept.

The patient's temperature is monitored every 2 to 4 hours to detect fever. Antipyretics may be administered as ordered. The patient is kept dry and lightly covered. The room is kept at a comfortable temperature that avoids chilling. Tepid sponge baths may be given for high fevers as ordered, but shivering should not be induced. A hypothermia blanket may be needed to reduce body temperature.

Pain. Pain may be treated with ordered analgesics. The nurse also uses positioning, splinting painful areas during deep breathing and coughing, and massage to promote comfort. Other measures to manage pain are detailed in Chapter 16. The effects of comfort measures are documented, and the physician is notified if pain is unrelieved or worsens.

Knowledge Deficit. The nurse explains what pneumonia is; the purpose of treatments; the need for rest, good nutrition, and good hydration; and how to reduce the risk of pneumonia in the future. The patient is encouraged to plan for discharge so that normal activities can be resumed gradually. Fatigue may persist for several weeks. If the patient will be taking drugs at home, instructions are provided. Patients with chronic respiratory or cardiovascular disorders are generally advised to be vaccinated with pneumococcal vaccine to reduce the risk of pneumococcal pneumonia. A single dose provides lifetime protection for most people. It is not repeated because there is a risk of a sensitivity reaction.

EVALUATION. Criteria for evaluating the effectiveness of nursing interventions are clear breath sounds without wheezes or crackles; normal arterial blood gases, heart rate, and respiratory rate; performance of activities of daily living with fatigue or dyspnea; stable body weight; fluid intake equal to fluid output, moist mucous membranes, and blood pressure consistent with patient norms; patient's statement of pain relief; and patient's verbalization of instructions.

Prevention of Aspiration Pneumonia

Aspiration pneumonia may be prevented by measures to avoid aspiration or to treat it promptly. If a patient is at risk for aspiration, suction equipment must be kept on hand. Patients with dysphagia (difficulty swallowing) should be positioned upright with the neck in a neutral position or slightly bent forward during meals. Because semisolids are swallowed more easily than thin liquids, thickening agents may be added to liquids.

If a patient is receiving enteral feedings, the head of the bed should be elevated while the feeding is being delivered and for 30 minutes afterward. Tube position must be checked per agency policy before each bolus feeding or at specified intervals. The aspirated fluid can be tested for acidity to ensure stomach position. Residual is measured before each bolus feeding. If it is greater than 100 ml, the feeding is withheld and the physician notified.

Continuous feedings should be stopped for 20 to 30 minutes before lowering the patient's head. If a patient must be kept flat, the best position is on the right side. Residual is checked every 4 hours. If the residual is 20% more than the hourly rate, the physician should be consulted about reducing the rate of feeding.

To reduce the risk of aspiration, the unconscious patient is positioned on alternating sides with the head of the bed elevated unless contraindicated. Fluids are not put in the patient's mouth until the presence of a gag reflex has been established.

If aspiration is suspected, suction should be used to try to remove the foreign material. A side-lying or slight Trendelenburg position, if not contraindicated, may promote drainage from the airway. Enteral feeding is stopped until it is ruled out as the source of the aspirated material. The patient is monitored closely and the physician notified. Oxygen is administered as ordered.

PLEURISY

Pleurisy is inflammation of the pleura. The most common causes are pneumonia, tuberculosis, injury to the chest wall, pulmonary infarction, and tumors. The most characteristic symptom of pleurisy is abrupt and severe pain. The pain almost always occurs on one side of the chest, and individuals can usually point to the exact spot where the pain is occurring. Breathing and coughing aggravate the pain.

Treatment of pleurisy is aimed at the underlying disease and at pain relief. Analgesics, anti-inflammatory drugs, antitussives, antimicrobials, and local heat therapy may be ordered.

Nursing Care of the Patient with Pleurisy

ASSESSMENT. Assessment of the patient with a respiratory disorder is summarized in Table 28–2.

NURSING DIAGNOSIS. The primary nursing diagnoses when a patient has pleurisy may include the following:

- **Pain** related to inflammation
- **Ineffective Breathing Patterns** related to splinting, pleural effusion
- **Knowledge Deficit** of condition, treatment, and self-care

There may be other diagnoses related to the underlying cause of pleurisy.

GOALS. The goals of nursing care for the patient with pleurisy are pain relief; effective breathing patterns; and patient's knowledge of condition, treatment, and self-care.

INTERVENTIONS

Pain. When the patient reports pain, the nurse obtains a complete description including location, severity, precipitating factors, and alleviating factors. Pain is relieved with the use of analgesics and splinting of the affected side. It also is helpful to splint the rib cage when coughing. If ordered, heat may be applied to the painful area and antitussives given to decrease painful coughing. If bedrest is prescribed, the nurse assists the patient with regular position changes. Nonsteroidal anti-inflammatory drugs (NSAIDs) are administered as ordered to reduce pain and inflammation. Patients on NSAIDs are monitored for gastrointestinal distress and bleeding.

Ineffective Breathing Patterns. The nurse monitors the patient's breathing pattern with attention to the symmetry of chest movement. The patient is encouraged to turn, take deep breaths and cough, and ambulate if permitted to mobilize secretions and maximize ventilation. The head of the bed is elevated to improve lung expansion. If pleural effusion develops, the patient experiences progressive dyspnea, decreased or absent breath sounds in the affected area, and decreased chest wall movement on the affected side. A thoracentesis may be done to remove the accumulated fluid. If the procedure is done at the bedside, the nurse assists as described in the section on Common Therapeutic Measures.

Knowledge Deficit. The nurse explains what pleurisy is and how it is treated. If a thoracentesis is necessary, the nurse reinforces the physician's explanation. If the patient is discharged on NSAIDs, the nurse cautions against taking aspirin at the same time because it increases the risk of bleeding. If the patient has gastrointestinal distress, NSAIDs may be taken with food, milk, or antacids.

EVALUATION. Criteria for evaluating the effects of nursing interventions are patient's statement of pain relief and relaxed expression, vital signs within patient's norms and normal breath sounds, and patient's verbalization of instructions.

CHEST TRAUMA

Traumatic chest injuries fall into two major categories: (1) nonpenetrating injuries and (2) penetrating injuries. Nonpenetrating or blunt injuries most commonly result from automobile accidents, falls, or blast injuries. In automobile accidents, 40% of the persons killed have sustained blunt injuries from the steering wheel. The extent of the injury depends on the force and impact of the trauma. Common nonpenetrating injuries include rib fractures, pneumothorax, pulmonary contusion, and cardiac contusion. Penetrating injuries most commonly result from gunshot or stab wounds to the chest. Common penetrating injuries include pneumothorax and life-threatening tears of the aorta, vena cava, or other major vessels.

Chest trauma can result in changes in normal pressure relationships between air inside and outside the body, interference with normal breathing patterns and protective mechanisms such as cough, disturbances in blood flow to the lungs, swelling, and pain. Individuals are therefore at risk for air entering the pleural space, infection and increased secretions in the tracheobronchial tree, hemorrhage, and abnormal fluid collection in the lung.

Signs and Symptoms

Signs and symptoms of chest injury may include obvious trauma to the chest wall (e.g., bruising); chest pain; dyspnea; cough; asymmetric movement of the chest wall; marked cyanosis of the mouth, face, nail beds, and mucous membranes; rapid, weak pulse; decreased blood pressure; deviation of the trachea; distended neck veins; and bloodshot or bulging eyes.

Medical Treatment

Immediate care of a person with a chest injury is directed at stabilization and prevention of further injury. Clothing should be removed to assess injury sites and to observe for other injuries such as bleeding. Bleeding should be treated immediately. Any open chest wound must be sealed with an airtight dressing and taped on three sides. This is called a vented dressing. It permits air to escape through the chest wound but prevents additional air from entering the chest through the wound. The danger of sealing a closed chest wound is that air may continue to leak from the lung into the pleural space, creating a tension pneumothorax (discussed in the next section). The nurse is alert for worsening respiratory status and signs of mediastinal shift, which require removal of the airtight dressing. Impaled objects should not be removed but should be stabilized with bulky dressings. Vital signs and level of consciousness should be monitored, keeping in mind the potential for shock. Oxygen may be administered via nasal cannula. To facilitate breathing, the client may be put in a semi-Fowler's position or on the injured side.

PNEUMOTHORAX

Chest injuries often cause pneumothorax, which is an accumulation of air in the pleural cavity that results in complete or partial collapse of a lung. Pneumothorax occurs in nearly half the individuals who have chest injuries. Air enters the space between the chest wall and the lung either through a hole in the chest wall or through a tear in the bronchus, bronchioles, or alveoli (Fig. 28–18).

There are two types of pneumothorax: tension and open. With a tension pneumothorax, air repeatedly enters the pleural space with inspiration, causing the pressure to rise. Because air is not escaping from the wound, the accumulating pressure causes the affected lung to collapse. The heart, trachea, esophagus, and great blood vessels shift toward the unaffected side. This is called a *mediastinal shift*, a condition that interferes with blood return to the heart. If not corrected, cardiac output falls, and the patient dies.

An open pneumothorax results from a chest wound that allows air to move in and out freely with inspiration and expiration. The lung on the affected side collapses. The heart, trachea, esophagus, and great blood vessels may shift back and forth toward the unaffected side with inspiration, then toward the affected side with expiration. This condition is called *mediastinal flutter*. Like mediastinal shift, it is potentially fatal.

Signs and Symptoms

Symptoms of pneumothorax are dyspnea, tachypnea, tachycardia, restlessness, pain, anxiety, decreased movement of the involved chest wall, asymmetric chest wall movement, diminished breath sounds on the injured side, and progressive cyanosis. In trauma cases, there may be a chest wound. If air can be heard or felt moving in and out of the wound, it is called a "sucking" chest wound.

Medical Treatment

The physician may insert an 18-gauge needle through the chest wall into the pleural space and aspirate accumulated air or fluid and then insert a chest tube. An alternative is to omit the needle aspiration and immediately insert the chest tube. If air is entering the pleural space from a tear in the lung or bronchus, surgery may be needed to repair the tear. A variety of materials are being studied for use in sealing persistent air leaks including intrapleural tetracycline, autologous "blood patches," and fibrin glue.

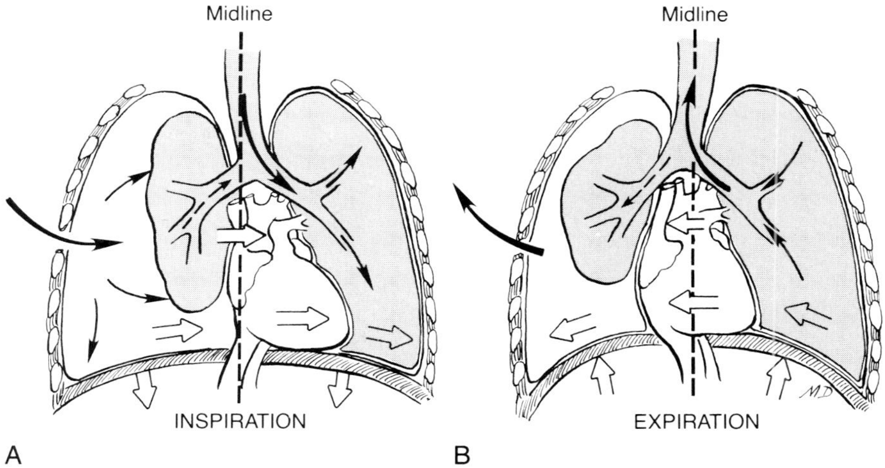

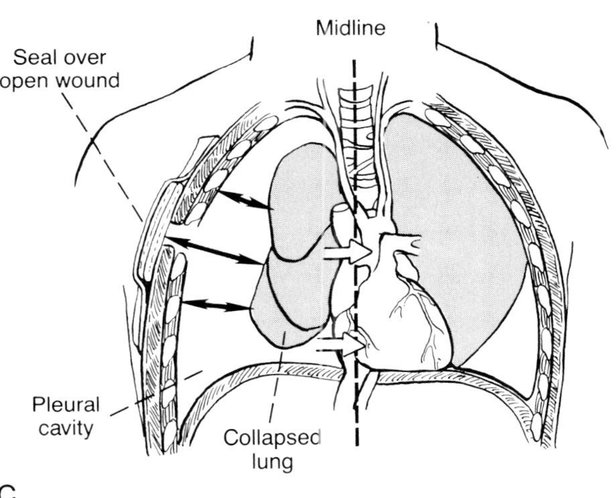

FIGURE 28–18
Pneumothorax. *A,* On inspiration, air enters the pleural space through the open chest wound. The mediastinal contents shift toward the unaffected side. *B,* On expiration, air exits through the open wound and the mediastinal contents swing back toward the affected side (mediastinal flutter). *C,* An airtight dressing can cause a tension pneumothorax. In a tension pneumothorax, air accumulates in the pleural space through a tear in the lung tissue. The air cannot exit if there is no open chest wound, and pressure builds, shifting the contents of the mediastinum toward the unaffected side and impairing circulatory and respiratory function (mediastinal shift). (Adapted from Black, J. M., & Matassarin-Jacobs, E. [1993]. *Luckmann and Sorensen's medical-surgical nursing: A psychophysiologic approach* [4th ed., pp. 2234, 2235]. Philadelphia: W. B. Saunders.)

Nursing Care of the Patient with Pneumothorax

ASSESSMENT. The complete assessment of the patient with a respiratory disorder is outlined in Table 28–2. In addition, if the patient has a chest tube, the insertion site is monitored as well as the amount and characteristics of any drainage from the tube. Care of patients with chest tubes is covered earlier in this chapter.

NURSING DIAGNOSIS. Nursing diagnoses for the patient with a pneumothorax may include the following:

- **Ineffective Breathing Patterns** related to decreased lung expansion
- **Fear** related to dyspnea
- High risk for **Decreased Cardiac Output** related to mediastinal shift
- **Pain** related to trauma, altered pressure in chest cavity, chest tube
- **High Risk for Infection** related to traumatic injury, chest tube insertion
- **Knowledge Deficit** of condition and treatment

GOALS. Goals for the care of the person with a pneumothorax are effective breathing pattern, decreased fear, adequate cardiac output, pain relief, absence of infection, and patient's understanding of condition and treatment.

INTERVENTIONS

Ineffective Breathing Patterns. The nurse monitors the patient closely for increasing respiratory distress as indicated by tachycardia, dyspnea, cyanosis, restlessness, and anxiety. The trachea is inspected for deviation that may be caused by mediastinal shift. Arterial blood gas results are checked for hypoxemia (low blood oxygen) and hypercapnia (high blood carbon dioxide). Signs and symptoms of deteriorating respiratory status are reported to the physician immediately. After the chest tube has been inserted, the nurse protects the tube and monitors its function as described earlier in this chapter.

The patient is positioned for comfort in a Fowler's or semi-Fowler's position. The side-lying position is avoided until the affected lung has reexpanded, as this position could foster mediastinal shift. The nurse supports and encourages the patient to do deep breathing and coughing exercises at least every 2 hours while awake. Oxygen is administered as ordered.

Fear. A pneumothorax is frightening. Patients feel like they are suffocating and may fear they are dying. The nurse speaks to the patient calmly and explains what is happening. The patient can be told that the chest tube will allow the lung to reexpand and relieve the dyspnea. The patient is also told how to prevent dislodging the tube. The nurse gives the patient the opportunity to ask questions and express fears.

High Risk for Decreased Cardiac Output. The patient's pulse and blood pressure are monitored. If cardiac output decreases owing to mediastinal shift, the blood pressure falls and the pulse rate increases. The physician must be notified of this potentially life-threatening change immediately.

Pain. The nurse is alert for signs of pain and documents the characteristics of the patient's pain. Analgesics are administered as ordered, and the effects are assessed. In addition to drug therapy, the nurse employs positioning, massage, distraction, and other measures described in Chapter 16. The physician is notified if pain is not relieved.

High Risk for Infection. The nurse monitors the patient for signs and symptoms of infection: fever, increased pulse and respirations, foul drainage from tube insertion site, and elevated white blood cell count. Various possible sites of infection must be considered: traumatic wounds, chest tube insertion site, intravenous infusion sites, indwelling catheter, and lungs. The nurse uses sterile technique for invasive procedures and dressing changes and administers antimicrobials as ordered. Increased activity is encouraged when permitted. The nurse monitors hydration status and promotes fluid intake of 2 to 3 liters per day unless contraindicated.

Knowledge Deficit. When the patient is acutely ill, the nurse provides brief explanations of what is being done and why. Frequent repetitions may be needed because of the patient's anxiety level and hypoxemia. Additional information is provided as the patient improves. Preparation for discharge includes care of the chest tube insertion site and signs of infection that should be reported to the physician.

EVALUATION. Criteria for evaluating the outcomes of nursing care are absence of dyspnea, normal arterial blood gases, and normal vital signs; calm demeanor, patient confirms feeling less fearful; pulse and blood pressure consistent with patient's norms; patient's statement of pain relief, more relaxed expression; absence of fever, normal white blood cell count; and patient complies with instructions and verbalizes or demonstrates content presented.

HEMOTHORAX

Hemothorax is an accumulation of blood between the chest wall and the lung that is often associated with pneumothorax. Hemothorax results from lacerated or torn blood vessels or lung tissues, lung malignancy, or pulmonary embolus. It may also be a complication of anticoagulant therapy. When air or blood collects in the pleural space, pressure around the lung increases, causing partial or complete collapse. Hemothorax is essentially treated like a pneumothorax, and the nursing care is similar. Surgical intervention may be needed to control the source of bleeding. In addition the patient is at risk for decreased cardiac output due to hemorrhage.

RIB FRACTURES

Rib fractures are the most common chest injuries. The most common cause is a blunt injury, especially the impact of the steering wheel against the chest in an automobile accident. Ribs 4 to 9 are most frequently fractured because they are least protected by chest muscles. It takes approximately 6 weeks for rib fractures to heal.

Signs and Symptoms

Signs and symptoms of fractured ribs include pain at the site of injury (especially on inspiration), occasional bruising or surface markings, swelling, visible bone fragments at the site of the injury, and shallow breathing or holding the chest protectively to minimize painful chest movements.

Medical Treatment

Treatment is aimed at relief of pain so that the patient can have good chest expansion for adequate breathing. Intercostal nerve blocks with local anesthesia are most frequently used. Analgesics, usually meperidine, along with mild sedatives also may be given for pain relief. Strapping the chest with tape or binders was once common but is now avoided because this procedure constricts the expansion of the chest and restricts deep breathing, leading to complications such as pneumonia or atelectasis.

Nursing Care of the Patient with Rib Fractures

ASSESSMENT. The nursing assessment of the patient with a respiratory disorder is outlined in Table 28–2. After rib fractures, the nurse is especially alert for signs of increasing respiratory distress that may indicate a pneumothorax caused by a bone fragment.

NURSING DIAGNOSIS. The primary nursing diagnosis for the patient who has fractured ribs is ineffective breathing patterns related to pain that occurs with ventilation.

GOAL. The goal of nursing care when a patient has fractured ribs is for the patient to have an effective breathing pattern.

INTERVENTIONS. Breathing exercises are necessary to prevent pulmonary complications after rib fractures. The nurse instructs the patient in supporting the fractured ribs while deep breathing and coughing. The patient will perform these exercises better with adequate pain control. The patient's pain is assessed every 2 hours, with the patient being asked to rank the pain from 0 (no pain) to 10 (worst pain imaginable). The nurse encourages the patient to report pain and offers reassurance that measures will be taken to provide relief. Because pain typically persists for 5 to 7 days, analgesics are administered as ordered. After medications are given, a calm environment should be provided and the patient encouraged to rest. Other nursing measures described in Chapter 16 (guided imagery, distraction, rhythmic breathing) may be employed to manage pain as well. The effects of pain management measures are evaluated, and the physician is informed if the patient's pain cannot be controlled.

EVALUATION. The criteria for evaluating goal achievement are vital signs within normal ranges, absence of dyspnea, and breath sounds clear to auscultation.

FLAIL CHEST

The term *flail chest* refers to an injury in which two adjacent ribs on the same side of the chest are each broken into two or more segments. The affected section of the rib cage is, in a sense, detached from the rest of the rib cage. This permits it to move independently, so that the segment moves in with inspiration, and moves out with expiration. The pattern of movement is exactly the opposite of the movement of an intact chest wall. Therefore, it is called *paradoxical movement.* Ventilation is impaired, and the patient becomes hypoxemic. Also, contusion (bruising) of underlying lung tissue may cause fluid to accumulate in the alveoli. Fractured ribs may tear the pleura or the lung itself, resulting in a pneumothorax or a hemothorax. The loss of chest wall stability and collapse of a lung may permit the mediastinum to "flutter"—to swing back and forth with respirations. Progressive hypoxemia and hypercapnia may be fatal.

Signs and Symptoms

Signs and symptoms of flail chest include severe dyspnea, cyanosis, tachypnea, tachycardia, and paradoxical movement of the chest.

Medical Diagnosis

Diagnosis is based on the history, physical examination, and chest radiographs. Arterial blood gases may be measured to assess the adequacy of ventilation.

Medical Treatment

The treatment of flail chest varies depending on the severity of the condition. If the patient is able to maintain adequate oxygenation, treatment may consist of deep breathing and coughing, IPPB treatment, and pain management. The patient in respiratory distress usually requires intubation and mechanical ventilation. Radiographs and arterial blood gas tests are often repeated at intervals to monitor oxygenation and detect additional pulmonary complications such as pneumonia.

Nursing Care of the Patient with Flail Chest

ASSESSMENT. The nursing assessment of the patient with a respiratory disorder is outlined in Table 28–2. When the patient has flail chest, a complete assessment is deferred until the patient's condition stabilizes. The initial assessment focuses on respiratory status, vital signs, other medical diagnoses, and a drug history.

NURSING DIAGNOSIS. For the patient with flail chest, the following nursing diagnoses may be appropriate:

- **Ineffective Breathing Patterns** related to loss of rib cage integrity
- **Pain** related to fractures
- **Anxiety** related to lack of understanding of injury and treatment

GOALS. Goals for nursing care of the patient with flail chest include effective breathing pattern, pain relief, and reduced anxiety.

INTERVENTIONS. Nursing interventions for patients with inadequate pulmonary function are similar to those for the patient with fractured ribs. Because flail chest is more serious and the patient may be acutely ill, anxiety may be very high. The nurse reduces anxiety by responding promptly to the patient's needs, providing simple explanations, and acknowledging the patient's concerns. Anxiety may be especially high if mechanical ventilation is needed. The detailed care of patients who require mechanical ventilation is beyond the scope of this book. A general discussion of mechanical ventilation is included under Common Therapeutic Measures in this chapter.

EVALUATION. Criteria for evaluating the outcomes of nursing care are normal pulse and respiratory rates, arterial blood gases within normal ranges, and absence of dyspnea; patient's statement of pain relief and relaxed manner; and patient's statement of reduced anxiety and calm demeanor.

PULMONARY EMBOLUS

An *embolus* is a foreign substance that is carried through the blood stream. Emboli are usually blood clots but may be fat, air, tumors, bone marrow, amniotic fluid, or clumps of bacteria. Risk factors for developing emboli include surgery of the pelvis or lower legs, immobility, obesity, estrogen therapy, and clotting abnormalities.

Etiology and Risk Factors

Most pulmonary emboli originate in the deep veins of the thigh or pelvis. A thrombus that develops in the veins can break away and become an embolus. The embolus flows with the blood until it reaches a vessel too narrow to pass through. The embolus lodges and obstructs blood flow so that perfusion to the area is diminished. When a portion of a pulmonary blood vessel is occluded by an embolus, the patient is said to have a *pulmonary embolism* (PE). The effects depend on the extent of the lung tissue that is deprived of blood. Small emboli generally do not cause dramatic symptoms but disrupt perfusion nevertheless. The alveoli in the affected area are ventilated but without blood flow, gas exchange cannot occur. The result is a ventilation-perfusion mismatch that results in hypoxemia. If a large pulmonary vessel is obstructed, alveoli collapse, cardiac output falls, there is constriction of the bronchi and the pulmonary artery, and sudden death may ensue.

Signs and Symptoms

Classic signs and symptoms of PE include sudden chest pain that worsens with breathing, tachypnea, and dyspnea. The patient may be apprehensive and diaphoretic with a cough and hemoptysis. Crackles may be heard on auscultation of the lungs, and the patient may have fever and tachycardia.

Medical Diagnosis

A diagnosis of PE is suggested by the history and physical findings and is confirmed by arterial blood gas analysis, electrocardiogram, lung scan, and pulmonary angiogram.

Medical and Surgical Treatment

Anticoagulation therapy is the cornerstone of treatment for PE. Intravenous heparin is usually given to establish and maintain a partial thromboplastin time of 2.0 to 2.5 times the normal rate. Heparin prevents the development of new thrombi. It prevents the extension of existing thrombi but does not dissolve them. The heparin is eventually discontinued, and the patient is maintained on an oral anticoagulant (warfarin sodium) for up to 6 months. Drugs that dissolve clots called fibrinolytics are not widely used for PE.

Hypoxemia may be managed with oxygen therapy, endotracheal intubation, and mechanical ventilation. Intravenous fluids and drugs to improve cardiac function are indicated to treat hypotension. Intravenous morphine sulfate is commonly used to relieve chest pain and apprehension.

A number of surgical interventions have been used for PE, including embolectomy, vena cava interruption, and venous thrombectomy. Embolectomy, surgical removal of the embolus from the obstructed pulmonary arteries, is a risky procedure. Vena cava interruption is most often done by placing a filter in the inferior vena cava to strain clots before they reach the pulmonary circulation (Fig. 28–19). Venous thrombectomy, removal of thrombi from veins, is not often done.

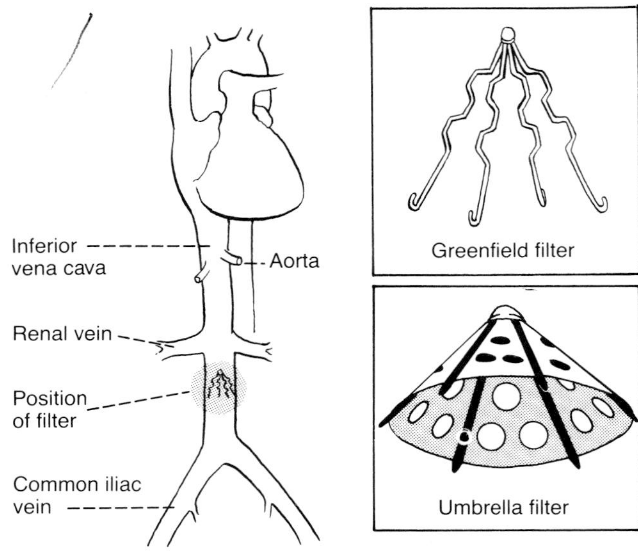

FIGURE 28-19

Greenfield and umbrella filters are examples of filters that may be placed in the inferior vena cava to prevent emboli traveling to the lung. (From Black, J. M., & Matassarin-Jacobs, E. [1993]. *Luckmann and Sorensen's medical-surgical nursing: A psychophysiologic approach* [4th ed., p. 1083]. Philadelphia: W. B. Saunders.)

Nursing Care of the Patient with a Pulmonary Embolus

ASSESSMENT. Assessment of the patient with a respiratory disorder is outlined in Table 28–2. When a patient has a PE, the nurse must monitor cardiopulmonary function but also must assess risk factors that may have led to the embolism. Homans's sign should be assessed in each leg. If this causes pain behind the knee or in the calf, the patient is said to have a positive Homans's sign, which is often associated with thrombophlebitis.

NURSING DIAGNOSIS. Nursing diagnoses vary with the extent of the area affected by the PE and the patient's symptoms. Nursing diagnoses may include the following:

- **Altered Cardiopulmonary Tissue Perfusion** related to interruption of blood flow to the alveoli
- **Anxiety** related to dyspnea, fear of death
- **High Risk for Injury** related to anticoagulant therapy
- **Knowledge Deficit** of PE, treatment, prevention, and self-care

GOALS. Goals for nursing care of the patient with a PE are normal tissue perfusion; reduced anxiety; absence of injury associated with anticoagulant therapy; and patient's understanding of PE, treatment, prevention, and self-care.

INTERVENTIONS

Altered Cardiopulmonary Tissue Perfusion. The nurse monitors the patient's respiratory rate and effort, breath sounds, skin color, pulse, and blood pressure. Arterial blood gas results are noted and reported to the physician if they are abnormal. The head of the patient's bed is elevated. Oxygen is administered as ordered, usually by nasal cannula. Strict bedrest is enforced to decrease oxygen demands. Intravenous fluids and inotropic drugs are administered as ordered. Fluid intake and output are measured and recorded.

Interventions to decrease the risk of further emboli include active and passive range of motion exercises for immobilized patients, early ambulation after surgery, and antiembolism and pneumatic compression stockings. Cushions and pillows should not be placed under the legs where circulation might be impaired.

Anxiety. The patient in respiratory distress and pain is understandably anxious. The nurse remains calm and tells the patient what is being done. Equipment and procedures are explained in terms the patient can understand. The patient is encouraged to express concerns and ask questions. A reassuring family member may be permitted to remain with the patient.

High Risk for Injury. Anticoagulant therapy poses a risk of uncontrolled bleeding. While the patient is hospitalized, the nurse assesses for excessive bruising or bleeding. Symptoms that may be caused by internal bleeding include severe headache and abdominal or back pain. The urine is inspected for hematuria. Pressure is applied to venipuncture sites to control bleeding.

To reduce the risk of bleeding, the patient's activated partial thromboplastin time is monitored every 1 to 2 days until stabilized at 1.5 to 2.5 times the normal rate. Patients with a PE are usually changed to warfarin sodium (Coumadin), an oral anticoagulant, after receiving heparin for a week or so. The effect of warfarin sodium is monitored by assessing the prothrombin time, which should be 1.5 to 2.0 times the normal rate. Prothrombin time is usually assessed and the dosage adjusted daily as needed.

PHARMACOLOGY CAPSULE

Monitor the patient's activated partial thromboplastin time when on heparin and the prothrombin time when on warfarin sodium to detect excessive anticoagulation. Watch for bleeding.

Knowledge Deficit. Patients who have had a PE must be taught how to manage their anticoagulant therapy because they usually remain on these drugs for at least several months. When patients are on anticoagulants, they are advised to use soft toothbrushes and electric razors to avoid trauma and bleeding. The nurse instructs them to report red or dark urine, which suggests urinary bleeding, hematemesis or epistaxis, and red or black stools, which suggest intestinal bleeding. Patients must also be told not to take any over-the-counter medications without consulting with the physician or pharmacist. Some drugs, especially aspirin, prolong the bleeding time, making these patients quite vulnerable to hemorrhage. To reduce the risk of a future PE, the patient is advised to avoid constricting clothing such as garters or tight girdles and to avoid prolonged pressure on the popliteal areas.

EVALUATION. Criteria for evaluating the outcomes of nursing interventions are vital signs consistent with patient's norms, absence of dyspnea, normal arterial blood gases; patient's statement of reduced anxiety and calm appearance; absence of bruising or bleeding; and patient's verbalization of instructions for self-care and prevention of future emboli.

RESPIRATORY ARREST

Respiratory arrest, the cessation of breathing, is addressed in Chapter 13.

ADULT RESPIRATORY DISTRESS SYNDROME

Etiology and Risk Factors

Adult respiratory distress syndrome (ARDS) is a progressive pulmonary disorder that follows some trauma to the lung. From 1 to 96 hours after the trauma, pulmonary infiltrates develop and lung compliance decreases. Fluid shifts into the interstitial spaces in the lungs and into the alveoli, causing pulmonary edema. Production of pulmonary surfactant decreases, leading to atelectasis. Lung compliance decreases, and the patient rapidly becomes hypoxemic.

Some patients recover and heal completely, whereas others develop lung fibrosis. The fibrosis may be mild or severe and sometimes occurs after the patient appears to be recovering. Progressive fibrosis may lead to death. Systemic complications of ARDS include cardiac dysrhythmias, renal failure, stress ulcers, thrombocytopenia, and disseminated intravascular coagulation. In addition, these patients are at risk for oxygen toxicity and sepsis.

Signs and Symptoms

The first sign of ARDS is usually increased respiratory rate. Auscultation of the lungs may reveal fine crackles. The patient may be restless, agitated, and confused. The pulse rate increases, and a cough may be present. These early signs are followed by progressively worsening dyspnea with retractions, cyanosis, and diaphoresis. Diffuse crackles and rhonchi may be heard on auscultation.

Medical Diagnosis

Adult respiratory distress syndrome is suspected on the basis of the patient's history and physical findings. Diagnostic studies include arterial blood gas analysis and chest radiographs. The blood pH rises and the $Paco_2$ falls at first because of hyperventilation. The Pao_2 falls below 70 mm Hg despite oxygen concentrations greater than 40% ($FIO_2 > 0.4$). This hypoxemia causes respiratory acidosis, as evidenced by pH below 7.35.

Medical Treatment

Early detection and treatment are critical factors in treating ARDS successfully. The patient is usually intubated and placed on a mechanical ventilator with positive end-expiratory pressure. Patient anxiety and restlessness may require sedation or even pharmacologic paralysis. Specific drug therapy depends on the underlying cause of ARDS. For example, the patient with sepsis is treated with antimicrobials. Corticosteroids are commonly used to reduce inflammation with ARDS, but there is some question about the value of this treatment.

Nursing Care of the Patient with Adult Respiratory Distress Syndrome

The patient with ARDS is critically ill and should be treated in an intensive care setting. Critical care nursing is beyond the scope of this text. However, all nurses must be aware of the risk of ARDS and respond promptly when a patient exhibits progressive respiratory distress. The rapid progression of the condition is frightening to the patient and the family. The nurse recognizes their anxiety and fear and offers emotional support and simple explanations.

NUTRITION CONCEPTS

- Adequate fluids are needed to mobilize pulmonary secretions for expectoration.
- Approximately 40% of patients admitted to intensive care units with acute respiratory failure are malnourished.
- Nutritional support for patients with respiratory failure should begin within the first 3 to 4 days of hospitalization.
- Patients who receive nutritional support are more easily weaned from ventilators than those who only receive intravenous glucose support.
- A diet for patients who have been in acute respiratory failure should be high in nutrients.
- Lung disease can substantially increase energy needs.
- The patient who is malnourished is at increased risk for respiratory infections because of impaired immunity and possible impairment of defense mechanisms.
- When a patient has a fever, each degree Celsius of elevation increases the metabolic rate 10 to 13%. For each degree Fahrenheit, the metabolic rate rises 7.2%.

BIBLIOGRAPHY

Aoki, F. Y., Yassi, A., Cheang, M., Murdzak, C., Hammond, G. W., Sekla, L. H., & Wright, B. (1993). Effects of acetaminophen on adverse effects of influenza vaccination in health care workers. *Canadian Medical Association Journal, 149*(10), 1425–1430.

Arbour, R. (1993). Weaning a patient from a ventilator. *Nursing 93, 23*(2), 52–56.

Bartlett, J. G. (1994). Pneumonia. In W. R. Hazzard, E. L. Bierman, J. P. Blass, W. H. Ettinger, & J. B. Halter (Eds.). *Principles of geriatric medicine and gerontology* (3rd ed., pp. 565–574). New York: McGraw-Hill.

Belcaster, A. (1993). Action stat! Responding to pulmonary hemorrhage. *Nursing 93, 23*(11), 33.

Berger, J. T., & Gilhooly, J. (1993). Fibrin glue treatment of persistent pneumothorax in a premature infant. *Journal of Pediatrics, 122*(6), 958–960.

Black, J. M., & Matassarin-Jacobs, E. (1993). *Luckmann and Sorensen's medical-surgical nursing: A psychophysiologic approach* (4th ed.). Philadelphia: W. B. Saunders.

Blake, G. J. (1990). Amantadine for influenza A. *Nursing 90, 20*(12), 21.

Busch, E., Barlam, B. W., Wallace, J., & Nealon, T. F. (1991). Intrapleural tetracycline for spontaneous pneumothorax in acquired immunodeficiency symdrome. *Chest, 99*(4), 1036–1037.

Campbell, J. (1993). Making sense of underwater sealed drainage. *Nursing Times, 89*(9), 34–36.

Carroll, P. (1992). Nursing the thoracotomy patient. *RN, 55*(6), 34–41.

Carruthers, D. D. (1990). Infectious pneumonia in the elderly. *American Journal of Nursing, 90*(2), 56–60.

Chernecky, C. C., Krech, R. L., & Berger, B. J. (1993). *Laboratory tests and diagnostic procedures.* Philadelphia: W. B. Saunders.

Conn, V. (1991). Self-care actions taken by older adults for influenza and colds. *Nursing Research, 40*(3), 176–181.

Connolly, A. M., Salmon, R. L., Lervy, B., & Williams, D. H. (1993). What are the complications of influenza and can they be prevented? *British Medical Journal, 306*(6890), 1452–1454.

Corbett, J. V. (1992). *Laboratory tests and diagnostic procedures with nursing diagnoses* (3rd ed.). East Norwalk, CT: Appleton & Lange.

Crimlisk, J. T., & Blansfield, J. S. (1993). Using $ETCO_2$ to confirm endotracheal tube placement. *American Journal of Nursing, 93*(3), 77–81.

Deglin, J. H., & Vallerand, A. H. (1991). *Nurse's med deck* (2nd ed.). Philadelphia: F. A. Davis Co.

deWit, S. C. (1992). *Keane's essentials of medical-surgical nursing* (3rd ed.). Philadelphia: W. B. Saunders.

Dumire, R., Crabbe, M. M., Mappin, F. G., & Fontenelle, L. J. (1992). Autologous "blood patch" pleurodesis for persistent pulmonary air leak. *Chest, 101*(1), 64–66.

Ferland, P. A. (1991). Are you ready for ventilator patients? *Nursing 91, 21*(1), 42–47.

Finesilver, C. (1992). Respiratory assessment. *RN, 55*(2), 22–30.

Fiorentini, A. (1992). Potential hazards of tracheobronchial suctioning. *Intensive and Critical Care Nursing, 8*(4), 217–226.

Fischbach, F. T. (1988). *A manual of laboratory diagnostic tests* (3rd ed.). Philadelphia: J. B. Lippincott.

Handerhan, B. (1992). Guarding against aspiration pneumonia. *Nursing 92, 22*(10), 96–97.

Hoffman, L. A., & Manzetti, J. D. (1992). Nursing assessment: Respiratory system. In S. M. Lewis & I. C. Collier. *Medi-*

cal-surgical nursing: A nursing process approach* (3rd ed.). St. Louis: Mosby Year Book.
Hunter, F., & Mitchell, S. (1993). Managing ARDS. *RN, 56*(7), 52–58.
Hurley, M. L. (1991). What's new in chest tube management. *RN, 54*(5), 34–40.
Jarvis, C. (1992). *Physical examination and health assessment.* Philadelphia: W. B. Saunders.
Johnson, E. R., McKenzie, S. W., & Sievers, A. (1993). Aspiration pneumonia in stroke. *Archives of Physical Medicine and Rehabilitation, 74*(9), 973–976.
Kersten, L. D. (1989). *Comprehensive respiratory nursing.* Philadelphia: W. B. Saunders.
Kirby, T. J., & Ginsbery, R. J. (1992). Management of the pneumothorax and barotrauma. *Clinics in Chest Medicine, 13*(1), 97–112.
Kitt, S., & Kaiser, J. (1990). *Emergency nursing.* Philadelphia: W. B. Saunders.
Long, B. C., Phipps, W. J., & Cassmeyer, V. L. (1993). *Medical-surgical nursing: A nursing process approach* (3rd ed.). St. Louis: Mosby Year Book.
Macey, B. A., & Landstrom, L. L. (1993). Replacing a chest tube drainage collection device. *American Journal of Nursing, 93*(3), 95–96.
Manzetti, J. D., & Hoffman, L. A. (1992). Nursing role in management: Upper respiratory system. In S. M. Lewis & I. C. Collier. *Medical-surgical nursing: A nursing process approach* (3rd ed.). St. Louis: Mosby Year Book.
Margolis, K. L., Nichol, K. L., Poland, G. A., & Pluhar, R. E. (1990). Frequency of adverse reactions to influenza vaccine in the elderly. *Journal of the American Medical Association, 264*(9), 1139–1141.
Margolis, K. L., Polahd, G. A., Nichol, K. L., MacPherson, D. S., Meyer, J. D., Korn, J. E. & Lofgren, R. P. (1990). Frequency of adverse reactions after influenza vaccination. *American Journal of Medicine, 88*(1), 27–30.
Mason, S. G. (1992). When a ventilator patient is going home. *RN, 55*(10), 60–64.
Mathews, P. J., Mathews, L. M., & Mitchell, R. R. (1992). *Nursing 92, 22*(2), 48–51.
Mergaert, S. (1994). STOP and assess chest tubes the easy way. *Nursing 94, 24*(2), 52–53.
Messer, R. L., & Zink, K. (1992). Nosocomial pneumonia: Combating a hospital menace. *RN, 55*(6), 48–53.
Metheny, N. (1993). Minimizing respiratory complications of nasoenteric tube feedings: State of the science. *Heart and Lung, 22*(3), 213–223.
Mitchell, J. T. (1992). Nursing role in management: Lower respiratory problems. In S. M. Lewis & I. C. Collier. *Medical-surgical nursing: A nursing process approach* (3rd ed.). St. Louis: Mosby Year Book.
Monto, A. S., & Arden, N. H. (1992). Implications of viral resistance to amantadine in control of influenza A. *Clinical Infectious Diseases, 15*(2), 362–367.
Nicholson, K. G. (1992). Clinical features of influenza. *Seminars in Respiratory Infection, 7*(1), 26–37.
Olsen, P. S. & Anderson, H. O. (1992). Long-term results after tetracycline pleurodesis in spontaneous pneumothorax. *Annals of Thoracic Surgery, 53*(6), 1015–1017.
Pachucki, C. T. (1992). The diagnosis of influenza. *Seminars in Respiratory Infection, 7*(1), 46–53.
Pagan, P. (1994). How to use a disposable end-tidal CO_2 detector. *Nursing 94, 24*(1), 50–51.
Rodman, M. J. (1993). Cough, cold, and allergy preparations. *RN, 56*(2), 38–42.
Samelson, S. L., Goldberg, E. M., & Ferguson, M. K. (1991). The thoracic vent. Clinical experience with a new device for treating simple pneumothorax. *Chest, 100*(3), 880–882.
Scanlon, C. L., Spearman, C. B., & Sheldon, R. L. (1990). *Egan's fundamentals of respiratory care* (5th ed.). St. Louis: C. V. Mosby.
Spratto, G. R., & Woods, A. L. (1994). *RN magazine's NDR-94.* Albany, NY: Delmar Publishers.
Summer, W. R., & Nelson, S. (1989). Nosocomial pneumonia: Characteristics of the patient-pathogen interaction. *Respiratory Care, 34*(2), 116–124.
Wilson, S. F., & Thompson, J. M. (1990). *Respiratory disorders.* St. Louis: Mosby Year Book.
Yeaw, E. M. J. (1992). Positioning and oxygenation: Good lung down? *American Journal of Nursing, 92*(3), 26–31.

KEY CONCEPTS

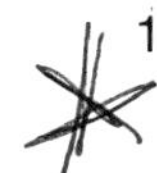

1. The function of the respiratory system is to supply oxygen for the metabolic needs of the cells and to eliminate carbon dioxide, one of the waste materials of cell metabolism.
2. Age-related changes in the respiratory system include loss of lung elasticity, enlargement of bronchioles, decreased number of alveoli, thoracic rigidity, atrophy of chest muscles, and flattening of the diaphragm.
3. A thoracentesis is the insertion of a needle through the chest wall into the pleural space to remove fluid, blood, or air or to instill medication.
4. Chest physiotherapy, which consists of percussion, vibration, and postural drainage, mobilizes respiratory secretions for expectoration.
5. Oxygen therapy is widely used and generally safe but must be used cautiously to avoid respiratory depression in chronic respiratory patients.
6. Chest tubes drain fluid and air from the pleural space, permitting a collapsed lung to reexpand.
7. Nursing diagnoses after thoracotomy may include impaired gas exchange, ineffective breathing patterns, and ineffective airway clearance.
8. Drugs commonly used for treatment of respiratory disorders include decongestants, antitussives, antihistamines, expectorants, antimicrobials, bronchodilators, corticosteroids, and mast cell stabilizers.
9. Acute viral rhinitis (the common cold), the most prevalent infectious disease, is treated symptomatically because available antimicrobials are not effective against the cold virus.

10. Influenza is an acute viral respiratory infection that can lead to pneumonia, especially in debilitated people.
11. Influenza immunizations do not protect everyone from influenza but do reduce the incidence of the infection and are recommended for people who have poor resistance to infection.
12. Pneumonia may be caused by pathogenic organisms or by noninfectious agents such as inhaled irritants, including aspirated gastric contents.
13. Nursing diagnoses for the patient with pneumonia may include ineffective airway clearance, impaired gas exchange, activity intolerance, altered nutrition, high risk for fluid volume deficit, pain, and knowledge deficit.
14. Pleurisy is inflammation of the pleura that is treated with analgesics, anti-inflammatory drugs, antitussives, antimicrobials, and local heat therapy.
15. Nursing diagnoses for the patient with pleurisy may include pain, ineffective breathing patterns, and knowledge deficit.
16. Pneumothorax is the accumulation of air in the pleural space, which may cause the lung to collapse.
17. The immediate treatment of an open chest wound is coverage with an airtight dressing followed by careful monitoring to detect signs of a tension pneumothorax.
18. With a tension pneumothorax, air accumulates in the affected side, collapsing the affected lung and causing the heart, trachea, esophagus, and great blood vessels to shift toward the unaffected side (mediastinal shift—a life-threatening condition).
19. Nursing diagnoses when a patient has chest trauma may include ineffective breathing patterns, fear, high risk for decreased cardiac output, pain, high risk for infection, and knowledge deficit.
20. Flail chest is the loss of thoracic integrity caused by fractures of two adjacent ribs into two or more segments on the same side of the chest.
21. A pulmonary embolus is a foreign substance carried through the blood stream into the lung, where it lodges and blocks blood flow.
22. Nursing diagnoses for the patient who has a pulmonary embolism may include altered cardiopulmonary tissue perfusion, anxiety, high risk for injury, and knowledge deficit.
23. Adult respiratory distress syndrome, a progressive pulmonary disorder that may lead to fibrosis of lung tissue and death, is treated with mechanical ventilation and treatment of the underlying cause.

Adrianne Linton
Louis K. Linton

CHAPTER 29

Chronic Respiratory Disorders

OBJECTIVES

1. Identify examples of chronic obstructive and restrictive pulmonary diseases.
2. Explain the relationship between cigarette smoking and chronic respiratory disorders.
3. For selected chronic respiratory disorders, describe the pathophysiology, signs and symptoms, complications, diagnostic measures, and medical treatment.
4. Apply the nursing process to plan care for the patient who has a chronic respiratory disorder.

GLOSSARY

ASBESTOSIS Interstitial fibrosis caused by inhalation of asbestos fibers

ASTHMA A condition characterized by episodes of bronchospasm that causes wheezing and dyspnea

BRACHYTHERAPY Placement of a radiation source in the body to treat a malignancy

BRONCHIECTASIS Permanent dilation of a portion of the bronchi or bronchioles

BRONCHITIS Bronchial inflammation

COR PULMONALE Right-sided heart failure associated with pulmonary disease

EMPHYSEMA Abnormal accumulation of air in body tissue; in the lung, a disorder characterized by loss of lung elasticity with trapping of air, retained carbon dioxide, and dyspnea

GRANULOMA A collection of inflammatory cells commonly surrounded by fibrotic tissue that represents a chronic inflammatory response to infectious or noninfectious agents

PNEUMOCONIOSIS One of many occupational diseases caused by inhalation of particles of industrial substances

PNEUMONITIS Inflammation of the lung

CHRONIC OBSTRUCTIVE PULMONARY DISORDERS

Chronic obstructive pulmonary disease (COPD) is the fifth leading cause of death in the United States. It is characterized as varying combinations of asthma, chronic bronchitis, and emphysema. There are individuals who have only one or two of these conditions, but the three are usually found together. Other terms used to describe COPD are chronic obstructive lung disease (COLD) and chronic airflow limitation (CAL).

A common diagnostic procedure for COPD is the pulmonary function test. Pulmonary function tests provide information about airway dynamics, lung volumes, and diffusing capacity. Airway dynamics refers to the patient's ability to inhale or to exhale by force. Some of the lung volumes measured include vital capacity, inspiratory capacity, expiratory reserve volume, residual volume, and total lung capacity. The diffusing capacity is a measurement of the ability of gases to diffuse across the alveolar capillary membrane. "Norms" are based on average measurements for healthy people who are the same age, gender, and weight as the patient. Pulmonary function tests should be performed under laboratory conditions by trained personnel to ensure a maximum degree of accuracy. It should be known that these tests are effort dependent, meaning that the patient must be mentally alert, cooperative, and able to follow directions. Additional information about pulmonary function tests is presented in Chapter 28.

BRONCHIAL ASTHMA

Asthma is a potentially reversible obstructive airway disorder that occurs from the very young to the very old. It is a highly complex condition that can be a mild nuisance or a very serious life-threatening condition.

Pathophysiology

Asthma may be generally classified into two broad categories: extrinsic and intrinsic. The population with each type of asthma is approximately equal. Extrinsic asthma, also called atopic or allergic asthma, is characterized by hypersensitivity to materials such as molds, animal dander, and pollens. These are external antigens that cause an antigen-antibody reaction in the sensitive patient. When the patient comes in contact with the allergen, immunoglobulin E (IgE) antibodies cause mast cells and basophils to release chemical mediators that constrict bronchial smooth muscle and cause edema in the airways. Allergic responses are explained in more detail in Chapter 10. People with intrinsic asthma, also called nonatopic or nonallergic asthma, respond to nonimmunologic stimuli such as infection, irritating chemical vapors, emotional distress, cold air, and even exercise. In this case, the asthmatic symptoms are caused by the release of acetylcholine in response to parasympathetic stimulation. Acetylcholine causes bronchoconstriction, which is aggravated by the effects of sympathetic stimulation of the mast cells.

The basic pathology with asthma is the narrowing of the bronchi or bronchioles as a result of contracted smooth muscle that surrounds the airways and inflammation that decreases the lumen of the airways. Constriction of the airways is called *bronchospasm* or *bronchoconstriction*. Constricted bronchi and bronchioles may be further obstructed by mucous plugs (Fig. 29–1). The obstruction causes air to be trapped in the alveoli, creating a ventilation-perfusion mismatch. That is, the alveoli are perfused with blood but not ventilated with fresh air. The effect is hypoxemia with compensatory hyperventilation.

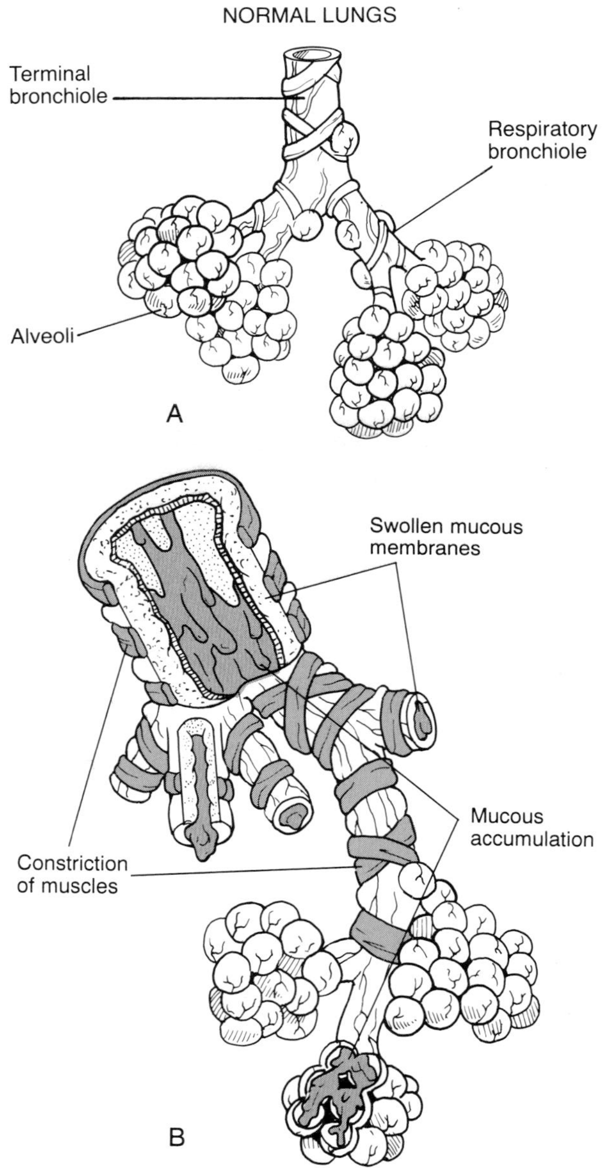

FIGURE 29–1

Comparison of terminal bronchioles, respiratory bronchioles, and alveoli in a normal lung *(A)* and in the lung of a person with bronchial asthma *(B)*. (Modified from Black, J. M., & Matassarin-Jacobs, E. [1993]. *Luckmann and Sorensen's medical-surgical nursing: A psychophysiologic approach* [4th ed., pp. 1023, 1027]. Philadelphia: W. B. Saunders.)

Complications

Severe, persistent bronchospasm is called *status asthmaticus*. If not corrected, status asthmaticus can lead to right-sided heart failure, pneumothorax, worsening hypoxemia, acidosis, and respiratory or cardiac arrest.

Signs and Symptoms

During an asthma attack, the patient may exhibit dyspnea, productive cough, use of accessory muscles of respiration (scalenes and sternocleidomastoids), audible expiratory wheezing, tachycardia, and tachypnea. The wheezing is caused by air moving through the narrowed airways.

Medical Diagnosis

A diagnosis of bronchial asthma is based on the health history, the physical examination, and the pulmonary function test results. The pulmonary function tests typically reveal that the airflow coming from the patient's lungs is significantly less than expected.

Medical Treatment

The primary goal of medical therapy is to prevent acute asthma attacks by using bronchodilators, β_2-receptor agonists, mast cell stabilizers, and, to a lesser extent, anticholinergics and corticosteroids. The exact drug therapy varies with the severity of the condition. People with mild asthma may have to use inhaled bronchodilators only when necessary, whereas those with moderate asthma may be advised to use the inhalers daily. Patients with severe asthma may require daily use of inhalers along with other agents, such as aerosol glucocorticoids.

Status asthmaticus is treated with inhaled and intravenous bronchodilators and oxygen therapy. Endotracheal intubation and mechanical ventilation are sometimes necessary. Drugs used to treat respiratory disorders are presented in Table 28–3.

Nursing Care of the Patient with Bronchial Asthma

ASSESSMENT. Complete assessment of the patient with a respiratory disorder is summarized in Table 28–2. When the patient has asthma, essential information (medications, allergies, known cardiac disease) is obtained and immediate steps are taken to relieve symptoms. Then a complete assessment is done.

Health History. It is especially important for the health history to determine the frequency and severity of attacks, the factors known to trigger attacks, the impact of the condition on the patient's life, the strategies used to manage the condition, the sources of stress and support, and the patient's knowledge about asthma and its treatment. The patient's ability to afford medical care and drug therapy should be explored.

Physical Examination. Important aspects of the physical examination include measurement of vital signs and auscultation of lung sounds. In addition, the patient's skin color and respiratory effort are assessed.

NURSING DIAGNOSIS. Nursing diagnoses for the patient with bronchial asthma may include the following:

- **Ineffective Breathing Patterns** related to air trapping
- **Impaired Gas Exchange** related to bronchospasm, air trapping, increased secretions
- **Anxiety** related to perceived threat of suffocation, hypoxemia
- **Knowledge Deficit** of asthma, its treatment, and self-care

GOALS. Goals of nursing care for the patient with asthma include normal respiratory pattern; adequate oxygenation; reduced anxiety; and patient's knowledge of asthma, its treatment, and self-care.

INTERVENTIONS

Ineffective Breathing Patterns. The nurse monitors the patient's respiratory rate, pattern, and effort. The patient is supported in a Fowler's position and given oxygen as ordered. Bronchodilators are administered as ordered, and the nurse assesses for adverse effects of drug therapy. The nurse should remain with the patient during an acute attack.

Impaired Gas Exchange. The patient is monitored for signs and symptoms of impending respiratory failure: tachypnea, shallow respirations, diaphoresis, reddening skin, tachycardia, cardiac dysrhythmias, hypertension changing to hypotension, restlessness, drowsiness, or loss of consciousness. Arterial blood gases are monitored, and the physician is contacted if the Pa_{O_2} decreases, the Pa_{CO_2} increases, and the pH falls. Oxygen is administered as ordered, usually 4 to 6 liters per minute unless the patient has chronic bronchitis and emphysema, in which case oxygen therapy is limited to 3 liters per minute. A nasal cannula is preferred over a face mask because the mask may increase the patient's feeling of suffocation.

If the patient has tenacious secretions that cannot be expectorated, chest physiotherapy and suctioning may be necessary. Because good hydration helps to thin secretions, a daily fluid intake of 2500 to 3000 ml is recommended unless contraindicated. Intravenous fluids may be ordered to improve hydration and to provide venous access for administration of emergency drugs.

Anxiety. The feeling of not being able to breathe is very frightening. In addition, with moderate to severe asthma the arterial oxygen decreases, which causes a feeling of restlessness and anxiety. Anxiety may serve to perpetuate the physical symptoms. While taking steps to improve the patient's oxygenation, the nurse also tries to reduce anxiety by remaining calm, responding to the patient's needs promptly, providing quiet reassurance, and explaining what is being done. The family may also need information and reassurance to calm their fears so they can be more supportive to the patient.

Knowledge Deficit. Because asthma is a chronic condition, the patient must learn to manage it. After the acute attack has subsided, the nurse can initiate patient teaching. The teaching plan should include the following:

- The pathophysiology of acute asthma attacks
- Factors known to trigger acute attacks: irritants in the home or workplace and stressors
- Measures to prevent attacks
- Treatment of acute attacks
- Drug therapy: correct use of inhalers (Fig. 29–2) and adverse effects (see Table 28–3)
- Resources for information and assistance in obtaining treatment and managing asthma

PHARMACOLOGY CAPSULE

To deliver drugs effectively, metered-dose inhalers must be used correctly. Teach correct use and have the patient practice, using the manufacturer's directions.

EVALUATION. Criteria for evaluating the effects of nursing interventions are a respiratory rate of 12 to 20 without dyspnea or wheezing; normal skin color, normal pulse and respiratory rates, and arterial blood gases within normal ranges; patient's statement of reduced anxiety, calm demeanor; and patient's verbalization of contents of teaching plan and statement of intent to adhere to therapeutic regimen.

CHRONIC BRONCHITIS AND EMPHYSEMA

Chronic bronchitis and emphysema can be found independently. Because they most often accompany each other, however, the two conditions are discussed together.

Pathophysiology

CHRONIC BRONCHITIS. Chronic bronchitis is bronchial inflammation characterized by increased production of mucus and chronic cough that persist for at least 3 months of the year for 2 consecutive years. Chronic bronchitis is said to be obstructive if the ratio of forced expiratory volume in 1 second to forced vital capacity falls below normal. The inflammation is caused by inhaled irritants including cigarette smoke.

Characteristic changes with chronic bronchitis are increased production of mucus, thicker mucus, and impaired ciliary action (Fig. 29–3). The patient is suscep-

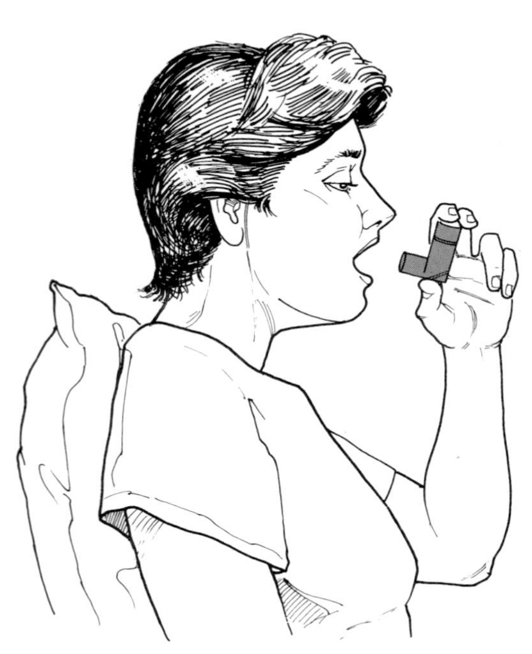

FIGURE 29–2

Use of metered-dose inhaler for administration of inhalant medication.

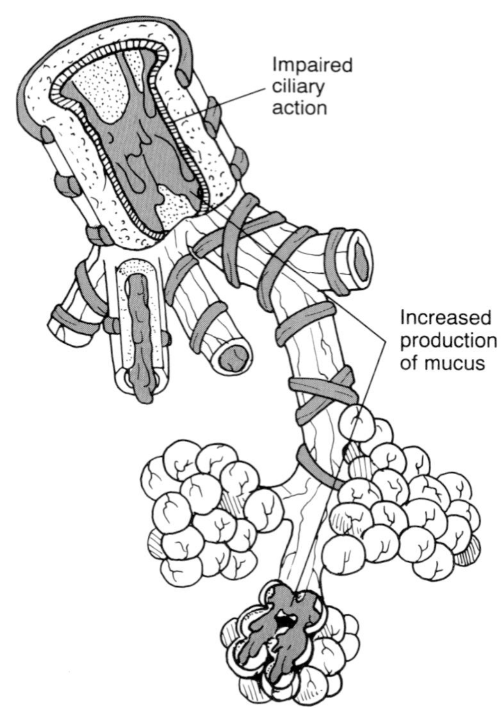

FIGURE 29–3

Chronic bronchitis. (Modified from Black, J. M., & Matassarin-Jacobs, E. [1993]. *Luckmann and Sorensen's medical-surgical nursing: A psychophysiologic approach* [4th ed., p. 1029]. Philadelphia: W. B. Saunders.)

tible to respiratory infections that aggravate the condition. At first, only large airways are affected, but smaller airways are eventually involved. Mucus obstructs the airway, causing air to be trapped in distal portions of the lungs. Alveolar ventilation is impaired, and the patient may develop hypoxemia leading to heart failure. *Cor pulmonale* is the term used to describe right-sided heart failure secondary to pulmonary disease.

EMPHYSEMA. Pulmonary emphysema is a degenerative nonreversible disease characterized by the breakdown of the alveolar septa (walls) distal to the terminal bronchioles. Two types of emphysema are centrilobular and panlobular emphysema (Fig. 29–4). Centrilobular emphysema affects mainly the respiratory bronchioles, whereas panlobular emphysema acts on the entire terminal respiratory unit. Centrilobular emphysema is associated primarily with cigarette smoking, but panlobular emphysema is more often caused by a hereditary deficiency of an enzyme inhibitor called alpha$_1$-antitrypsin. Both types may be present at the same time.

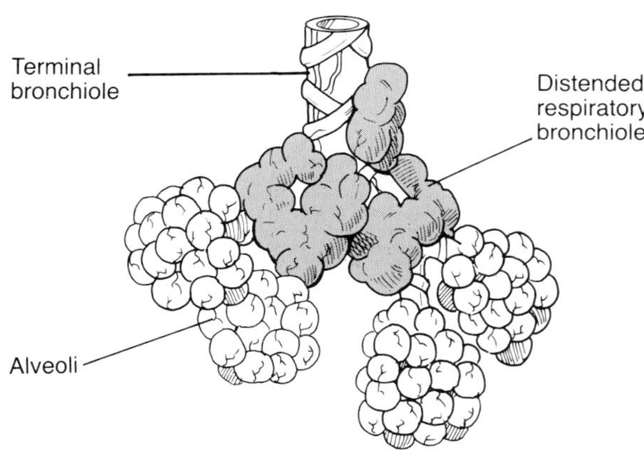

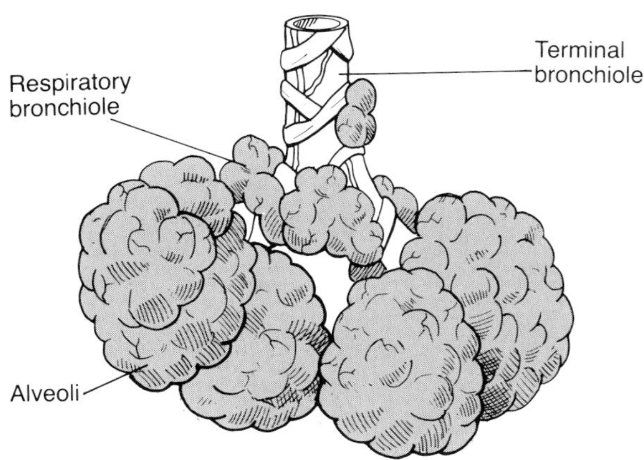

FIGURE 29-4

Types of emphysema. (Modified from Black, J. M., & Matassarin-Jacobs, E. [1993]. *Luckmann and Sorensen's medical-surgical nursing: A psychophysiologic approach* [4th ed., p. 1027]. Philadelphia: W. B. Saunders.)

Alveolar walls break down, and air spaces become permanently distended. Elastic recoil diminishes, and the airways partially collapse. Pockets of air called bullae and blebs form. Bullae are located between the alveolar spaces, whereas blebs are in the lung parenchyma. As the functional units of the lung are destroyed, the patient's ability to exchange oxygen and carbon dioxide declines. The lungs become hyperinflated, causing the diaphragm to flatten and increasing the reliance on accessory muscles for breathing. Eventually, as with chronic bronchitis, right-sided heart failure develops.

Complications

The most serious complications of chronic obstructive pulmonary disease are heart failure and respiratory failure. Respiratory failure is marked by hypoventilation and ventilation-perfusion mismatch with rising arterial carbon dioxide pressure ($Paco_2$) and declining arterial oxygen pressure (Pao_2). Factors that may lead to complications include infection, air pollution, continued smoking, left ventricular failure, myocardial infarction, pulmonary embolism, spontaneous pneumothorax, and adverse effects of drugs.

Signs and Symptoms

Chronic bronchitis and emphysema each have specific signs and symptoms owing to the differences in pathologic origin. The signs and symptoms of each are presented separately here, but the reader is reminded that the two conditions are often found together.

CHRONIC BRONCHITIS. Signs and symptoms of chronic bronchitis include productive cough, exertional dyspnea, and wheezing. With chronic hypoxemia, the red blood cell count is typically elevated to compensate for the inadequate oxygen in the blood. The patient with cor pulmonale demonstrates signs and symptoms of heart failure including increasing dyspnea, cyanosis, and peripheral edema. These signs have given rise to the term *blue bloater* to describe the patient with advanced chronic bronchitis (Fig. 29–5).

EMPHYSEMA. The main symptom of emphysema is dyspnea on exertion (Fig. 29–6). As the disease progresses, the patient may also have dyspnea when at rest. Patients are often thin and may be observed using accessory muscles of respiration. Increased anteroposterior diameter of the chest creates what is called a barrel chest. Despite dyspnea, patients who have emphysema without chronic bronchitis often have normal arterial blood gases until the disease is very advanced. Therefore, skin color may be normal. This explains the term *pink puffer* used to describe the patient with emphysema (Fig. 29–7). Depression and irritability are common in the patient with COPD.

Medical Diagnosis

Chronic obstructive pulmonary disease is suspected on the basis of patient's health history and physical examination. The most reliable diagnostic tests for

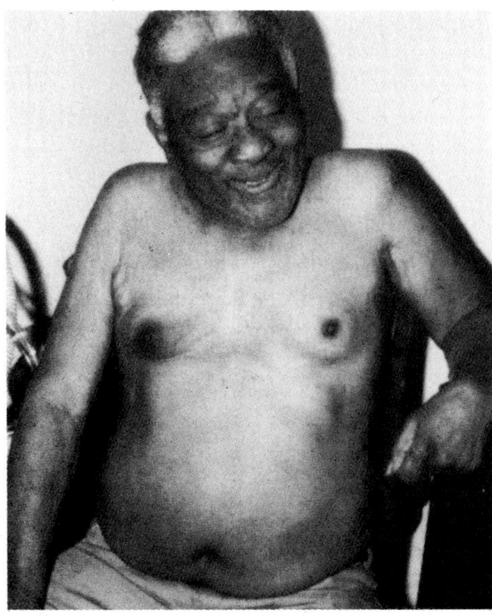

FIGURE 29-5
Patient with chronic bronchitis and all the classic findings of the "blue bloater." Note the elevation of the shoulders and the tense muscles. (From Kersten, L. D. [1989]. *Comprehensive respiratory nursing* [p. 109]. Philadelphia: W. B. Saunders.)

COPD are the pulmonary function tests, which reveal a decreased forced expiratory volume and forced vital capacity accompanied by increases in functional residual capacity, residual volume, and total lung capacity. A computed tomography scan may be done to help differentiate the type of emphysema.

Medical Treatment

DRUG THERAPY. The goals of medical treatment are improved oxygenation and decreased carbon dioxide retention. Drug therapy plays an important part in treating COPD. Bronchodilators, including beta-adrenergics and anticholinergics, are ordered to decrease airway resistance and the work of breathing. The preferred route of administration is by inhalation using a metered-dose inhaler. There is some evidence that anticholinergics such as ipratropium bromide (Atrovent) are more effective than beta-adrenergics for treating COPD. Oral theophylline is not used as commonly for bronchodilation as it once was because of the risk of drug toxicity. If theophylline is used, the sustained release form is recommended, and periodic blood levels must be determined. Corticosteroids are useful in the treatment of the inflammatory response in asthma, but there is controversy about their effectiveness with bronchitis and

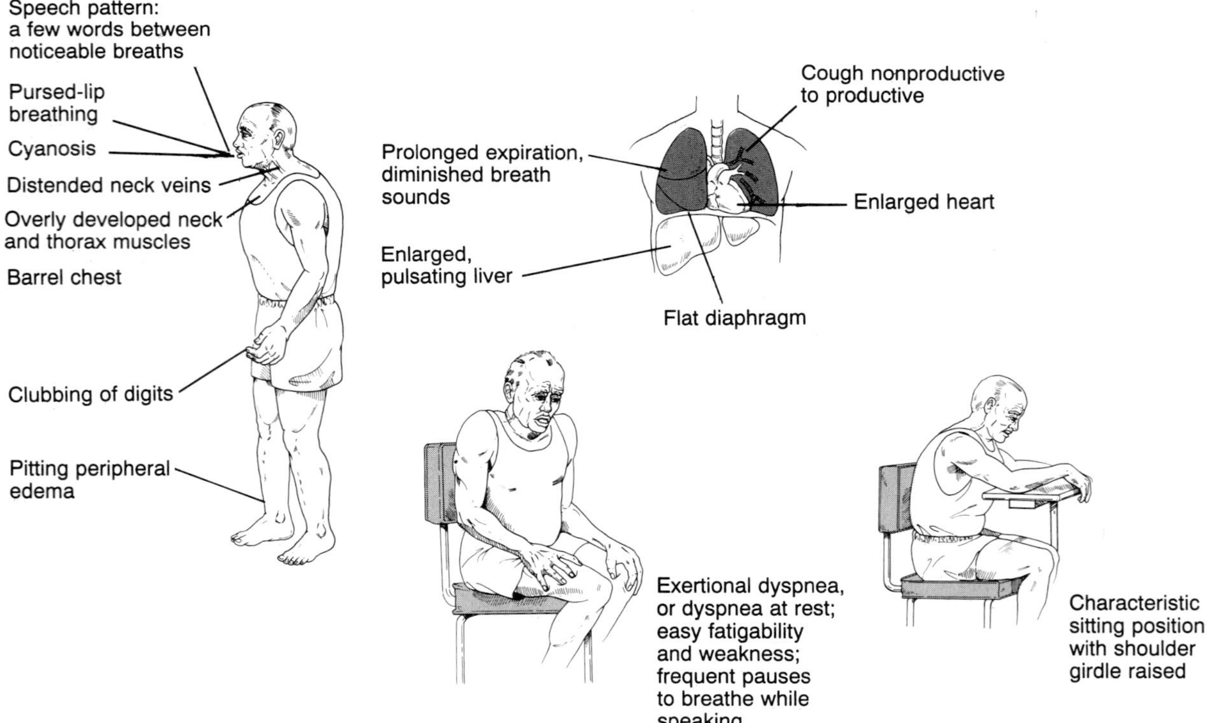

FIGURE 29-6
Signs and symptoms of chronic obstructive pulmonary disease. (Modified from Black, J. M., & Matassarin-Jacobs, E. [1993]. *Luckmann and Sorensen's medical-surgical nursing: A psychophysiologic approach* [4th ed., p. 1028]. Philadelphia: W. B. Saunders.)

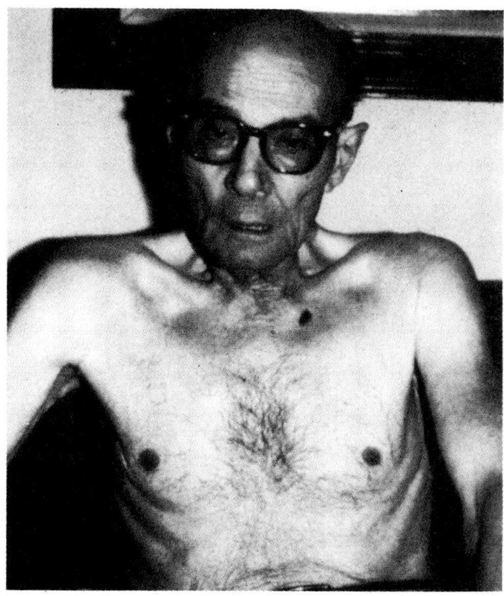

FIGURE 29-7
Patient with emphysema and all the classic findings of the "pink puffer." Note the use of accessory muscles in the neck and chest. (From Kersten, L. D. [1989]. *Comprehensive respiratory nursing.* Philadelphia: W. B. Saunders.)

emphysema. Antidepressants may be indicated and can improve the quality of life.

PHARMACOLOGY CAPSULE

Theophylline blood levels must be monitored because toxicity can be fatal. The therapeutic blood level is 10 to 20 micrograms per ml.

OXYGEN THERAPY. Oxygen therapy may be prescribed but must be used cautiously. The goal of oxygen therapy is to maintain the Pa_{O_2} between 50 and 60 mm Hg. The initial liter flow is usually 1 to 3 liters per minute. A pulse oximeter may be used while titrating the liter flow to maintain the Sa_{O_2} at 90%. Periodically, the pulse oximeter should be correlated with actual blood gas laboratory values. High levels of oxygen are not administered because COPD patients may rely on hypoxic drive to breathe. This refers to the fact that the patient has adapted to high blood carbon dioxide and relies on low blood oxygen to stimulate breathing. A high concentration of oxygen may raise the blood oxygen level so that the patient's stimulus to breathe is lost and respiratory depression may result.

CHEST PHYSIOTHERAPY. Chest physiotherapy, described in Chapter 28, may be ordered to mobilize secretions in the patient with COPD.

EXERCISE. The patient may be referred to a rehabilitation program that includes exercise reconditioning. Programs are individualized but generally employ progressive exercise—either walking or pedaling a stationary cycle. A typical program might have the patient walk 10 to 15 minutes every day or every other day. Every week or two, the exercise time is increased by 5 or 10 minutes. The goal is to enable the patient to exercise comfortably for 45 minutes to 1 hour daily or every other day. Of course, some patients may not improve this much, but improvement in walking performance and general well-being has been found in patients who consistently walked as little as 12 minutes every day for 2 months. Sometimes bronchodilators are prescribed before exercise.

NUTRITION. Nutrition is important for the COPD patient because malnutrition causes decreased energy and decreased resistance to infection and because obesity increases the work of breathing. No special diet is indicated. Supplementary feedings may be needed for some patients.

TREATMENT OF RESPIRATORY FAILURE. Respiratory failure is treated with oxygen therapy, aerosol bronchodilators, chest physiotherapy (possibly), and mechanical ventilation (if becoming exhausted).

Nursing Care of the Patient with Chronic Obstructive Pulmonary Disease

ASSESSMENT. Assessment of the patient with a respiratory disorder is summarized in Table 28–2 (see Care Plan: The Patient with COPD). When a patient has COPD, the health history should describe the presenting symptoms—often dyspnea, cough, chest pain, or a combination of these. A complete medical history should be obtained unless the patient's symptoms make it difficult to participate in a long interview. Sometimes it is necessary to break the interview into smaller sections so as not to exhaust the patient who is dyspneic. A list of current medications and drug allergies is essential. The functional assessment explores the impact of the condition on the patient's activities of daily living. Exposure to smoke or other respiratory irritants is assessed.

During the physical examination, the nurse observes the patient's posture, color, respiratory effort, and use of accessory muscles. Vital signs are measured. The patient is observed for signs of hypoxemia including restlessness, confusion, and lethargy. Pursed-lip breathing is noted. The neck is inspected for distention of veins. The shape of the thorax is inspected for the classic barrel chest. The lung fields are auscultated for diminished breath sounds. The nails are inspected for clubbing, and the nailbeds are inspected for color. The nurse inspects and palpates the feet and ankles for edema.

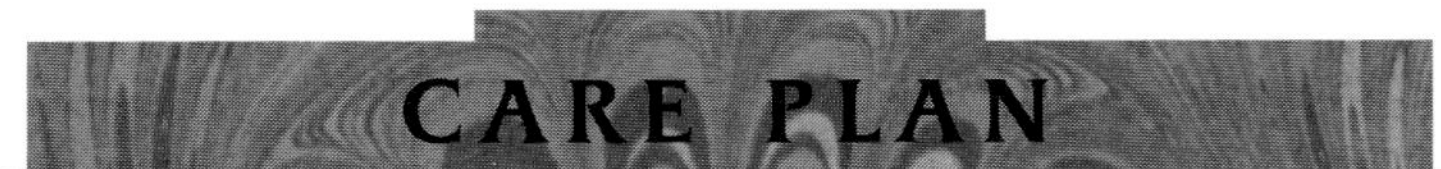

CARE PLAN
The Patient with COPD

ASSESSMENT

Health History: Susan Kellogg is a 73-year-old woman admitted for increasing dyspnea. She has had chronic bronchitis and emphysema for 3 years. Her past medical history includes frequent upper respiratory infections with two hospitalizations for pneumonia in 1993. She had a myocardial infarction in 1989 and is being treated for hypertension, for which she takes verapamil. She also uses an ipratropium (Atrovent) inhaler four times a day. She is allergic to penicillin. The review of systems notes fatigue, increasing dyspnea both with exertion and at rest, orthopnea, and productive cough with yellow sputum. Patient states she is depressed. Ms. Kellogg is a retired nurse who volunteers at a local homeless shelter 1 day a week. She lives alone and has no family in the area. She reports that her appetite is poor and that she has lost "a little" weight over the last few weeks. She has smoked one pack of cigarettes daily for 45 years. She states she knows she should quit and has tried many programs but has never lasted more than a week.

Physical Examination: Vital signs: temperature, 100.6°F orally; pulse, 100; respirations, 28; blood pressure, 140/94. Height, 5'6". Weight, 102 lb. The patient is seated with her hands on her knees to elevate her shoulders. She appears to be in mild distress. Skin color is normal. Pursed-lip breathing noted. Accessory muscles of respiration are tense. The thorax is barrel-shaped. Abdomen soft. Abdominal muscles used in respirations. No peripheral edema.

NURSING DIAGNOSIS	GOALS AND OUTCOME CRITERIA	INTERVENTIONS
Impaired gas exchange related to alveolar destruction, bronchospasm, air trapping.	The patient will have improved gas exchange as evidenced by pulse, respirations, and arterial blood gases within normal limits.	Monitor vital signs and arterial blood gases for tachycardia, tachypnea, increasing $PaCO_2$, decreasing pH. Administer oxygen at 1–3 liters/minute per nasal cannula as ordered. Assist to comfortable position: high Fowler's position in bed or supported at bedside. Reinforce pursed-lip and abdominal breathing techniques. Provide bronchodilator per inhaler as ordered. Assess technique. Assess respiratory status before and after use of bronchodilator. Monitor for adverse drug effects: dry mouth, headache, nausea, blurred vision, palpitations.
Ineffective airway clearance related to increased secretions, weak cough.	The patient will maintain a patent airway as evidenced by absence of crackles on auscultation, expectoration of secretions.	Auscultate breath sounds at least every 4 hours. Support patient during coughing and deep breathing. Document sputum amount and color. Encourage 2500–3000 ml of fluid daily. Request chest physiotherapy per order. Have suction equipment available if patient cannot expectorate secretions.
Anxiety related to hypoxemia.	The patient will verbalize decreased anxiety and will appear calm.	Respond to the patient's needs promptly. Provide comfort measures. Be accepting of irritability. Acknowledge anxiety and try to identify stressors in addition to hypoxemia. Include patient in planning care.
Altered nutrition: less than body requirements related to anorexia, dyspnea.	The patient will maintain or increase body weight during hospitalization.	Provide pleasant environment for meals. Schedule respiratory treatments at least an hour before meals. Assist with oral hygiene. Offer to arrange smaller, more frequent meals. Consult with dietitian to consider patient preferences.

The Patient with COPD *(Continued)*

NURSING DIAGNOSIS	GOALS AND OUTCOME CRITERIA	INTERVENTIONS
Activity intolerance related to inability to meet oxygen needs.	The patient will accomplish activities of daily living without dyspnea or excessive fatigue.	Allow periods of uninterrupted rest during the day. Use comfort measures such as backrub and massage to promote rest. Allow patient to do what she can for herself but assist when needed to avoid excessive tiring. Include occupational therapist and social worker to discuss plans for discharge and ways to reduce effort of activities at home. Discuss pulmonary rehabilitation program with physician. Encourage ambulation as permitted.
High risk for injury related to respiratory infection, right-sided heart failure.	The patient will have a normal body temperature, clear or white sputum, no peripheral edema.	Monitor sputum color and body temperature. Administer antimicrobials as ordered. Encourage fluid intake. Protect from people with respiratory infections. Monitor for signs of heart failure, especially peripheral edema.
Knowledge deficit of smoking cessation options.	The patient will express intent to attempt smoking cessation.	Explore smoking cessation programs that patient has tried. Be nonjudgmental and avoid scolding. Inform her of newer options such as nicotine patches, gum, and nasal spray. Tell her that drug therapy has been helpful for some people and that she may want to ask the physician about this. Provide literature from American Cancer Society and American Lung Association with suggestions to facilitate smoking cessation.

NURSING DIAGNOSIS. Nursing diagnoses for the patient with chronic bronchitis and emphysema may include the following:

- **Impaired Gas Exchange** related to alveolar destruction, bronchospasm, air trapping
- **Ineffective Airway Clearance** related to increased secretions, weak cough
- **Anxiety** related to hypoxemia
- **Altered Nutrition: Less than Body Requirements** related to anorexia, dyspnea
- **High Risk for Infection** related to decreased ciliary action, increased secretions, weak cough
- **Activity Intolerance** related to inability to meet oxygen needs
- **Decreased Cardiac Output** related to right-sided heart failure
- **Knowledge Deficit** of condition, treatment, and self-care

GOALS. Goals of nursing care for the patient with chronic bronchitis and emphysema are improved gas exchange; effective airway clearance; decreased anxiety; adequate nutrition; absence of infection; improved activity tolerance; adequate cardiac output; and patient's knowledge of condition, treatment, and self-care.

INTERVENTIONS

Impaired Gas Exchange. The nurse monitors the patient's vital signs and arterial blood gases for signs of inadequate oxygenation: tachycardia, tachypnea, increasing $Paco_2$ level, and decreasing pH level. Oxygen is administered at 1 to 3 liters per minute as ordered. The patient and family are taught not to increase the liter flow, because a sudden increase in oxygen in the blood may actually depress respirations in people with emphysema. The patient is positioned in a high Fowler's position or seated on the bedside with the arms folded on the overbed table to promote full expansion of the lungs (Fig. 29–8). The nurse teaches pursed-lip breathing by instructing the patient to breathe in through the nose and exhale slowly through the mouth with the lips almost closed. Pursed-lip breathing reduces the collapse of airways with exhalation and reduces dyspnea. Bronchodilators are administered as ordered, and the patient is assessed for therapeutic and adverse effects.

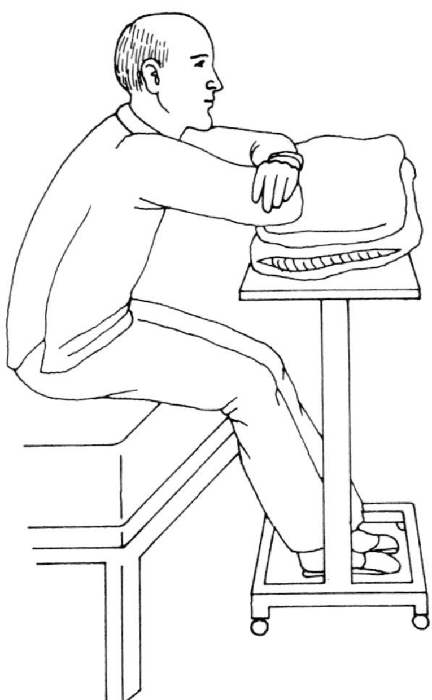

FIGURE 29-8
Sitting on the edge of the bed with the arms folded allows the accessory muscles of respiration to function more effectively. (Modified from Ignatavicius, D. D., & Bayne, M. V. [1991]. *Medical-surgical nursing: A nursing process approach* [p. 2033]. Philadelphia: W. B. Saunders.)

Ineffective Airway Clearance. The patient is monitored for signs and symptoms of airway obstruction, including tachycardia, increasing dyspnea, and abnormal breath sounds. The nurse demonstrates effective coughing techniques and assesses the patient's efforts. The patient is encouraged to drink at least 2500 to 3000 ml of fluid each day unless contraindicated to help liquefy secretions for easier expectoration. Humidification of room air can be provided to decrease the drying of secretions. Chest physiotherapy is performed as ordered, and the effects are evaluated. If the patient is unable to expectorate, suctioning may be needed to remove secretions.

Anxiety. The most important thing the nurse can do to relieve anxiety is to help the patient breathe more easily. Positioning and oxygen therapy are two simple measures that can be instituted promptly. Also, procedures and equipment are explained to the patient. The nurse must remain calm and reassuring until the patient is more comfortable and relaxed. It is important to remember that irritability and anxiety are related to hypoxemia and that the patient is not just being difficult. A family member who has a calming influence on the patient should be allowed to remain at the bedside. When leaving the patient, the nurse places the call button in reach and instructs the patient in its use. Checking on the patient often provides reassurance that help is nearby if needed.

Altered Nutrition: Less than Body Requirements. The work of breathing is increased with COPD, which in turn increases the patient's caloric requirements. Some COPD patients have difficulty maintaining adequate nutritional intake. The patient's weight may be monitored daily or weekly depending on the situation to assess the fluid or nutritional status. A patient with heart failure may gain weight owing to fluid retention. Weight loss may indicate elimination of excess fluid or loss of body weight due to inadequate nutrition. Inadequate nutrition may be associated with dyspnea, anorexia, depression, or inability to obtain and prepare food.

The patient who is dyspneic may be given a soft diet with frequent small meals rather than three large meals daily. High-calorie, high-protein supplements may be provided as well. Treatments should be scheduled so that the patient is not excessively tired or coughing during meals. To combat anorexia, the nurse consults with the dietitian to provide foods that are appealing to the patient. The patient is assisted with oral hygiene before meals. A pleasant environment is created by removing soiled tissues and emesis basins. If the agency permits, a family member might be encouraged to eat with the patient to provide a more social atmosphere. If the patient is unable to consume adequate nutrients, tube feedings or total parenteral nutrition may be instituted. If the patient is obese, weight loss should be discussed.

High Risk for Infection. Because of pooled secretions and poor nutritional status, the patient with chronic bronchitis and emphysema is at risk for respiratory infections. The nurse monitors for fever and for green or yellow sputum. Measures to promote good hydration and nutrition are employed. Prophylactic antimicrobials are administered as ordered. Patients are advised to take annual influenza immunizations and to avoid people who are ill with infectious respiratory diseases. The physician may prescribe a Pneumovax vaccine for pneumococcal pneumonia—a vaccine that is given only once.

Activity Intolerance. During hospitalization, the nurse must attempt to schedule treatments, meals, and exercise so that the patient has time to rest. If the patient becomes excessively dyspneic or develops tachycardia during activity, that activity should be stopped until the patient recovers. When preparing for discharge, the nurse helps the patient plan a daily schedule that spaces more demanding activities and allows scheduled rest periods. Portable oxygen therapy may be ordered to permit greater mobility while receiving supplemental oxygen. At home, environmental adaptations may be needed, such as rearrangement of furniture to permit easy access to bathrooms and ramps to replace steps.

If the patient is participating in a rehabilitation program to improve exercise tolerance, the nurse may monitor progress and provide encouragement and feedback.

Decreased Cardiac Output. Patients with chronic bronchitis and emphysema are at risk for right-sided heart failure that eventually affects the left side as well.

Therefore, the nurse monitors for signs of failure: increasing dyspnea, decreasing urine output, tachycardia, and dependent edema. Management of congestive heart failure is covered in Chapter 31.

Knowledge Deficit. Patients with chronic bronchitis and emphysema need to know how they can manage the condition. However, patient instruction is best done in small units to prevent overtiring and overwhelming the patient. The nurse explains the pathophysiology and treatment. Prescribed drugs are reviewed, and the patient is advised of adverse effects that should be reported to the physician. Proper instruction in the use of metered-dose inhalers is essential for maximum therapeutic benefit. If chest physiotherapy is recommended, the nurse or respiratory therapist instructs a family member in the procedure. If oxygen therapy is ordered, the equipment is demonstrated. The nurse explains safety precautions as listed in Chapter 28 and emphasizes the importance of not exceeding the prescribed liter flow. Supplementary written material should be provided. The nurse may also advise the patient of services available through the local chapter of the American Lung Association.

Smoking cessation is an important aspect of the management of chronic bronchitis and emphysema as well as of other cardiovascular and respiratory conditions. One fifth of all deaths in the United States are related to smoking. Health care providers should discourage smoking but must be careful not to be judgmental of the patient. Most patients are aware of the relationship between smoking and respiratory disease, but many find they are unable to overcome the addiction to nicotine. The nurse may ask patients if they have considered quitting smoking and if they would like information about programs that might be helpful.

The physician may order nicotine patches, gum, or nasal spray for the patient who wants to try to withdraw from smoking. Some studies have found the success rate for these products is only about 25%, but other types of smoking cessation programs typically have success rates around 10 to 20%. Success is defined as abstinence from smoking for at least 1 year. The American Cancer Society and the American Lung Association sponsor programs to support people who are trying to quit smoking.

In addition to nicotine, drugs that have been tried to discourage smoking include cimetidine hydrochloride (Tagamet), clonidine (Catapres), buspirone (BuSpar), doxepin hydrochloride (Sinequan), fluoxetin hydrochloride (Prozac), and calcium channel blockers.

EVALUATION. Criteria for evaluating the outcomes of nursing interventions are pulse, respirations, and arterial blood gases consistent with patient's norms; absence of crackles on auscultation; patient's statement of decreased anxiety, calm appearance; stable body weight; normal body temperature, white or clear sputum; completion of activities of daily living without excess fatigue; absence of dependent edema and distended neck veins; and patient's description of disease process and treatment and patient's demonstration of self-care activities.

BRONCHIECTASIS

Bronchiectasis is an abnormal dilation and distortion of the bronchi and bronchioles that is usually confined to one lung lobe or segment. It typically follows recurrent inflammatory conditions, infections, or obstructions but is sometimes congenital. The most prominent signs of bronchiectasis are coughing and the production of large amounts of purulent sputum. The patient may also have fever, hemoptysis, nasal stuffiness, sinus drainage, fatigue, and weakness.

The goals of medical treatment are to control symptoms and to prevent the spread to other areas of the lungs. Treatment consists of antibiotic therapy, bronchodilators, chest physiotherapy, and oxygen therapy. Severe bronchiectasis may be treated with surgical excision of the affected portion of the lung if the condition is confined to a limited area. The nurse administers prescribed drugs and treatments and documents the patient's response.

CYSTIC FIBROSIS

Cystic fibrosis is a hereditary disorder that is characterized by dysfunction of the exocrine glands and the production of thick, tenacious mucus. Mucus in the lungs leads to infections, emphysema, and atelectasis. At one time people with cystic fibrosis were unlikely to survive the early childhood years. Improved treatment, however, has resulted in more people with cystic fibrosis surviving to adulthood, so they may be seen in adult care settings. A pediatric textbook should be consulted for details of care of the patient with cystic fibrosis.

CHRONIC RESTRICTIVE PULMONARY DISORDERS

Generally, restrictive pulmonary disorders are those that result in reduced lung volumes with a normal to elevated ratio of forced expiratory volume in 1 second to forced vital capacity. Examples of restrictive disorders presented here are tuberculosis, sarcoidosis, pneumoconiosis, interstitial fibrosis, and lung cancer.

TUBERCULOSIS

Etiology and Risk Factors

Tuberculosis is an infection caused by *Mycobacterium tuberculosis*, an acid-fast aerobic baceterium. It is spread by droplets emitted by infected people during coughing, laughing, sneezing, and singing. Tuberculosis was a leading cause of death in the United States until effective drugs became available in the 1940s and 1950s. The incidence declined dramatically to the lowest rate in recorded history in 1984. Then in 1986 the numbers of reported cases began to rise, and that rise has continued. The rise has been variously attributed to the development of drug-resistant strains, the increasing population of immunosuppressed people with the human immunodeficiency virus infection, and the influx of immigrants from developing nations.

Anyone may become infected with tuberculosis, but most healthy people are not infected through brief contact. Those at increased risk for tuberculosis include the elderly; the economically disadvantaged and homeless; people who are substance abusers; children under the age of 5; people who are immunosuppressed; some racial and ethnic groups, including Native Americans, Eskimos, and African Americans, and immigrants from Southeast Asia, Ethiopia, Mexico, and Latin America.

Pathophysiology

A patient's initial tuberculosis infection is called the primary infection. Most people who develop primary infections do not develop active tuberculosis. When the tuberculosis bacterium invades the lung, a small area becomes inflamed. The body's immune response attempts to destroy the infecting organisms, but some may escape and be carried into the lymph nodes or throughout the body. The site of the primary infection may undergo necrotic degeneration. Cavities develop that are filled with infectious material, which eventually liquefies. This material can drain into the tracheobronchial tree and be coughed up as sputum. The infected site usually heals, creating scar tissue and sometimes sheltering inactive bacteria. In some patients, however, the infectious process progresses and the patient develops active tuberculosis. Also, it is possible for inactive bacteria to be reactivated, causing illness at a later time.

Tuberculosis is primarily an infection of the lungs, but the organisms may spread and cause infection in the kidneys, bones, meninges, genitourinary tract, lymph nodes, pleurae, pericardium, abdomen, and endocrine glands. *M. tuberculosis* infection outside the lungs is called *extrapulmonary tuberculosis.*

Signs and Symptoms

Signs and symptoms of pulmonary tuberculosis may include cough, night sweats, chest pain and tightness, fatigue, anorexia, weight loss, and low-grade fever. The cough is often persistent and productive and may produce bloody sputum (hemoptysis). Tuberculosis should be considered in patients who have pneumonia that does not respond to usual therapy.

Medical Diagnosis

The patient's history and physical examination may lead the physician to suspect tuberculosis, especially if there is known exposure to high-risk individuals. Tests to confirm the diagnosis include sputum cultures, acid-fast smears of potentially infected body fluids, tuberculin skin tests, and chest radiographs. Tuberculin skin tests are commonly used for screening. People who have been infected develop an immune response that causes a local reaction when tuberculin, a protein fraction of the tubercle bacilli, is injected intradermally. The patient is said to have a positive reaction if a hard area (induration) greater than 5 mm develops at the site within 48 to 72 hours. A positive reaction may indicate active or inactive infection. A number of factors may cause false-negative reactions, that is, an induration does not develop when the patient does have the infection.

Medical Treatment

Patients who have positive results for tuberculosis on skin tests and negative results on chest radiographs but are at increased risk for the disease are usually treated prophylactically to prevent development of active tuberculosis. The most common preventive treatment is isoniazid therapy for 9 to 12 months.

For patients with active tuberculosis, drug therapy usually consists of combinations of drugs that may include isoniazid, ethambutol, rifampin, streptomycin, pyrazinamide, and others. The course of therapy may range from 6 to 24 months. Most drugs can be given in daily doses or twice-weekly doses. The risk of adverse effects with long-term drug therapy is significant, so patient monitoring is essential. Hospitalization is sometimes indicated when drug therapy is initiated.

PHARMACOLOGY CAPSULE

Pyridoxine may be ordered with isoniazid (INH) to prevent peripheral neuritis.

Nursing Care of the Patient with Tuberculosis

ASSESSMENT. Assessment of the patient with a respiratory disorder is outlined in Table 28–2. When tuberculosis is suspected or confirmed, a complete health history and a physical examination are essential because the infection may not be confined to the lungs.

NURSING DIAGNOSIS. Specific nursing diagnoses are based on individual patient data but may include the following:

- **Impaired Gas Exchange** related to respiratory secretions, effects of the infectious process
- **Social Isolation** related to medically imposed isolation; fear of contagious disease
- **High Risk for Injury** related to the spread; reactivation of the infection secondary to lowered resistance
- **Fatigue** related to infection, weight loss, coughing
- **Altered Nutrition: Less than Body Requirements** related to anorexia, fatigue, inadequate financial resources, lack of knowledge
- **Noncompliance** related to lack of understanding of treatment and risk of reactivation, lack of financial resources
- **Knowledge Deficit** of mode of transmission, measures to present transmission and reactivation, nutrition, and drug therapy

GOALS. Goals of nursing care for the patient with tuberculosis are improved gas exchange; absence of feelings of loneliness or rejection; understanding of measures to prevent spread or reactivation; improved activity tolerance; adequate nutrition; adherence to prescribed therapy; and understanding of tuberculosis transmission, prevention, and therapy.

INTERVENTIONS

Impaired Gas Exchange. The nurse routinely monitors the patient's respiratory status. The patient is instructed in effective coughing to expectorate secretions. Ambulation as tolerated is usually encouraged, but the patient who has limited mobility may need assistance to change position at least every 2 hours. Although dyspnea is not common except with pleural effusion, the head of the bed is elevated for the patient who is dyspneic.

Social Isolation. The patient who is thought to have active tuberculosis is isolated at first. Caregivers should practice good hand washing and wear masks during contacts, but gowns are unnecessary unless there is gross contamination of clothing. The patient may feel rejected and be fearful that others will avoid contact. The nurse encourages expression of feelings about the diagnosis and the isolation. Visitors are instructed in measures to reduce the risk of infection.

High Risk for Injury. Once antibiotic therapy has been initiated and the patient's sputum cultures demonstrate low counts of acid-fast bacilli, the patient can usually be discharged. The nurse explains to the patient how the infection is transmitted and how to protect others. The patient should always cover the nose and mouth when sneezing or coughing. Disposable tissues should be used and discarded in a sanitary way. Members of the patient's household will be tested for active disease. Those who have positive skin tests but are asymptomatic are usually given prophylactic therapy to prevent development of active tuberculosis. The nurse must emphasize the importance of the patient completing the full course of therapy. Otherwise, the infection may be reactivated.

Fatigue. Fatigue is fairly common with tuberculosis. The patient's schedule should be adjusted to allow for periods of rest. The patient can be assured that fatigue diminishes as treatment progresses.

Altered Nutrition: Less than Body Requirements. Anorexia and nausea are common symptoms in the tuberculosis patient that are often adverse effects of drug therapy. The patient's weight is monitored at regular intervals. Some measures that may reduce the drug's side effects include taking the drug at bedtime and taking antinausea drugs. The nurse explains the role of nutrition in recovering from an infectious disease and encourages the patient to eat a balanced diet. Five or six small meals may be more acceptable than three large ones to the patient who has a poor appetite. Food preferences should be respected as much as possible.

Noncompliance. A major problem with treating tuberculosis is noncompliance with the lengthy prescribed drug therapy. Nurses must realize that there are many reasons that patients do not take drugs as ordered, including denial of the illness, lack of understanding, adverse drug effects, and inadequate money. Intervention should be based on the reason for the patient's noncompliance. The infectious process and its treatment are explained. The nurse reinforces the physician's instructions for the drugs and emphasizes that failure to complete the course of therapy results in reactivation of the infection. The patient is encouraged to report adverse drug effects, and solutions are sought to make them more tolerable. If the patient cannot afford the drugs, a social worker is consulted to help the patient obtain financial assistance. Sometimes patients who have difficulty taking the drugs as directed are given larger doses two to three times a week in the clinic or physician's office instead of taking daily doses at home.

Knowledge Deficit. People with tuberculosis are usually hospitalized for just a short period of time, so the nurse must implement efficient patient teaching. Verbal instructions should be supplemented with written material. Subjects to include in the teaching plan are the following:

- The effects of tuberculosis infection
- Prescribed drug therapy: name of drug, dose, directions, side effects, adverse effects that should be reported
- Importance of completing the course of therapy
- Protection of others from infection
- Importance of good hygiene, nutrition, and hydration

PHARMACOLOGY CAPSULE

Rifampin causes body fluids to become red-orange and may stain soft contact lenses.

EVALUATION. Criteria for evaluating the outcomes of nursing interventions are the absence of dyspnea, continued or restored social contacts, the patient's demonstration of measures to prevent the spread or reactivation of the infection, the patient's statement of lessened fatigue, stable body weight, the patient's statement of intention to adhere to prescribed drug therapy, and the patient's verbalization of content in teaching plan.

SARCOIDOSIS

Pathophysiology

Sarcoidosis is an inflammatory condition that may affect the skin, eyes, lungs, liver, spleen, bones, salivary glands, joints, and heart. The exact cause is unknown, but some factor triggers a series of immune processes leading to the formation of clusters of cells and debris in affected tissues called granulomas. Granulomas in the lungs may resolve or may progress to fibrosis, in which case a restrictive pulmonary condition exists. The condition more commonly affects blacks than whites and is twice as common in black females as in black males.

Signs and Symptoms

Although about one third of all patients have no symptoms, others may experience dry cough, dyspnea, chest pain, hemoptysis, fatigue, weakness, weight loss, and fever.

Medical Diagnosis

A diagnosis of sarcoidosis is based on findings on chest radiograph, pulmonary function tests, and lung biopsy.

Medical Treatment

If the patient is asymptomatic, no treatment is indicated. Symptoms usually respond well to systemic corticosteroids.

Nursing Care of the Patient with Sarcoidosis

Nursing care of the patient with sarcoidosis focuses on monitoring the patient for progressive dysfunction and teaching about corticosteroid therapy, if prescribed. Care of the patient with severe symptoms is similar to that for patients with COPD.

OCCUPATIONAL LUNG DISEASES

The inhalation of various particles in the work setting can lead to lung conditions classified as occupational lung diseases. Examples of offending substances are dust, ammonia, chlorine, plant and animal proteins, silica, asbestos, and coal dust. The Occupational Safety and Health Administration provides regulations that are intended to protect workers from exposure that could lead to occupational lung diseases.

Categories of occupational lung diseases are described here briefly. The nursing care of patients with occupational lung diseases varies with the severity of symptoms but is similar to that provided the patient with COPD.

Acute Respiratory Irritation

The inhalation of gases such as ammonia or chlorine causes acute respiratory irritation. The effects are usually temporary, but if the lower airways are affected the patient may develop pulmonary edema or alveolar damage and airway obstruction. The patient may have coughing, wheezing, and dyspnea. Symptoms resolve within a few days to several weeks, and there is usually no permanent lung damage. The treatment focuses on management of the symptoms and avoidance of future exposure.

Occupational Asthma

Inhalation of plant or animal proteins may cause an allergic reaction referred to as occupational asthma. Treatment is the same as that for bronchial asthma. Although the initial acute symptoms usually last only a few hours, the patient may continue to have a hyperreactive airway for years. This means that future exposure to irritants may trigger acute asthmatic symptoms. The patient should avoid continued exposure to the offending substance.

Hypersensitivity Pneumonitis

Hypersensitivity pneumonitis is an allergic inflammatory response of the alveoli to inhaled organic particles. The reaction may resolve within a few days, or the patient may develop pulmonary edema or interstitial fibrosis with permanent restrictive or restrictive-obstructive disease. The condition may be treated with corticosteroids and avoidance of the irritants. Respiratory support may be needed if symptoms are severe.

Pneumoconioses

Lung diseases caused by inhalation of various dusts are called pneumoconioses. Pneumoconioses develop in response to repeated exposure to silica, asbestos, or coal dust and are characterized by diffuse pulmonary fibrosis and restrictive lung disease. The effects are generally aggravated by cigarette smoking, so patients are advised to avoid both the offending dust and the cigarette smoke. Otherwise, treatment is symptomatic.

Asbestosis is a pneumoconiosis caused by occupational exposure to asbestos, an insulating material. Asbestos exposure has been linked to pleural effusions, pleural fibrosis, and malignant mesotheliomas (a specific type of lung cancer). Fear of asbestosis has led to the removal of asbestos insulation from public buildings in many cities, but there is disagreement as to whether the insulation actually poses any public health threat.

DIFFUSE INTERSTITIAL FIBROSIS

Pathophysiology

Diffuse interstitial fibrosis, also known as interstitial lung disease, is an inflammatory condition of the lower respiratory tract. It is characterized by thickening and fibrosis of the alveolar walls, rendering the alveoli nonfunctional. The condition may be caused by inhaled substances or connective tissue disorders, but sometimes no specific cause is identified.

Complications

Severe fibrosis may lead to pulmonary hypertension (increased pressure in the pulmonary artery caused by obstruction to blood flow in pulmonary vessels), cor pulmonale, and ventilatory failure, in which case the patient is said to have end-stage disease.

Signs and Symptoms

The primary symptoms are cough and progressive dyspnea. Crackles are heard in the lungs on auscultation. The patient may have clubbing of the fingertips.

Medical Treatment

The condition is treated with corticosteroids to reduce inflammation, bronchodilators, and oxygen therapy. Corticosteroid treatment may prevent additional damage but does not correct existing fibrosis. The patient should avoid additional exposure to the offending substance. Lung transplantation is relatively uncommon but may be recommended for end-stage disease.

Nursing Care of the Patient with Interstitial Fibrosis

ASSESSMENT. The complete assessment of the patient with a respiratory disorder is summarized in Table 28–2.

NURSING DIAGNOSIS. The nursing diagnoses for the patient with interstitial fibrosis may include the following:

- **Ineffective Gas Exchange** related to alveolar damage
- **Ineffective Airway Clearance** related to increased secretions.
- **Activity Intolerance** related to inadequate oxygenation
- **Anxiety** related to dyspnea or possible disabling illness

GOALS. Goals of nursing care for the patient with interstitial fibrosis are improved gas exchange, effective airway clearance, improved activity tolerance, and reduced anxiety.

INTERVENTIONS AND EVALUATION. Nursing interventions and evaluation criteria are similar to those described for the patient with COPD.

LUNG CANCER

Etiology and Risk Factors

Lung cancer is the leading cause of cancer deaths in the United States. An estimated 172,000 new cases of lung cancer are expected to be diagnosed in 1994. The incidence is decreasing among men but has been rising steadily among women. Since 1987, the death rate from lung cancer has exceeded that from breast cancer in women.

Cigarette smoking is the leading cause of lung cancer. The risk is increased even more for smokers who are exposed to other carcinogenic substances, such as arsenic, asbestos, and radioactive materials. Evidence is increasing that "secondhand" smoke poses a threat to nonsmokers as well. Air pollution may be an additional risk factor.

Pathophysiology

There are four major types of lung cancer: small cell ("oat cell") carcinoma, squamous cell carcinoma, adenocarcinoma, and large cell carcinoma. Except for small cell carcinoma, most lung cancers grow slowly. They can all metastasize to other body organs. The enlarging tumor or metastatic lesions may compress the laryngeal and phrenic nerves, the esophagus, and the major blood vessels. The small cell carcinoma, which grows rapidly, tends to metastasize early. Small cell tumors may also invade the pericardium, causing pericardial effusion (fluid accumulation in the pericardial sac) and possibly triggering dysrhythmias.

Signs and Symptoms

The warning signs of lung cancer identified by the American Cancer Society are persistent cough, hemoptysis, chest pain, and recurring pneumonia or bronchitis. Patients may also have dyspnea, weight loss, and pain in the shoulder, arm, or hand. Other signs and symptoms may be related to metastatic lesions. For example, invasion of the tumor into the ribs produces bone pain, and invasion of the pericardium may produce cardiac dysrhythmias.

Medical Diagnosis

Diagnostic tests and procedures for lung cancer include radiologic procedures (chest radiograph, computed tomography scan), fiberoptic bronchoscopy, sputum cytology studies, and biopsy of tissue obtained through bronchoscopy or thoracotomy. These procedures are explained in Chapter 28. Unfortunately, lesions are often not detectable until no longer localized. Radionuclide scans of the bones, liver, or brain may be ordered to detect metastatic lesions.

Medical Treatment

Early detection is the key to survival of lung cancer, but this is difficult because metastasis often occurs before the lesion can be seen on radiographs. Treatment decisions are made on the basis of tumor type, lymph node involvement, evidence of metastasis, and the patient's general state of health.

RADIOTHERAPY. Radiotherapy may be used alone or in combination with other treatment methods. It may be curative in some situations but may also be used to temporarily relieve symptoms by reducing the size of the lesion. Radiotherapy for lung cancer may include external beam irradiation and brachytherapy. Brachytherapy is direct irradiation by placement of the radiation source at the site of the tumor. Complications of endobronchial irradiation are pulmonary hemorrhage and radiation bronchitis and stenosis. Other general complications of radiotherapy are discussed in Chapter 23.

CHEMOTHERAPY. Chemotherapy may be used alone or with radiation and surgery in the treatment of small cell carcinoma. There is debate about the value of chemotherapy in other types of lung cancers, but research continues to explore various treatment combinations of agents such as carboplatin, vinblastine, mitomycin C, and cisplatin. These and other chemotherapeutic agents are discussed in Chapter 23.

Surgical Treatment

For early lung cancer, other than small cell carcinoma, surgical intervention is the treatment of choice. The goal of surgery is to remove the entire tumor while removing as little healthy surrounding tissue as possible. Removal of a section of tissue is called a *resection.* With lung surgery, the procedure may be a wedge resection, segmental resection, lobectomy, or pneumonectomy. These procedures are illustrated in Figure 29–9. Tumors that are accessible with a bronchoscope are sometimes treated with laser therapy. Radiotherapy, chemotherapy, or both may be used before or after surgery.

Despite advances in treatment, the 5-year survival rate for lung cancer remains 13%. Survival improves with early treatment, but American Cancer Society data indicate that only 16% of all lung cancers are detected while still localized.

NUTRITION CONCEPTS

- Malnutrition and pulmonary disease are strongly related.
- Starvation and malnutrition frequently cause impaired pulmonary function, and pulmonary disease may result in malnutrition.
- Pulmonary disease causes an increase in energy expenditure because of increased work of breathing and chronic infection.
- Reduced dietary intake in lung disease results from fluid restriction, shortness of breath, anorexia, gastrointestinal distress, and vomiting.
- Approximately 70% of patients with chronic obstructive pulmonary disease exhibit weight loss.
- Strategies for increasing intake and weight gain include eating high-calorie and high-fat foods, small frequent meals, and resting before meals.

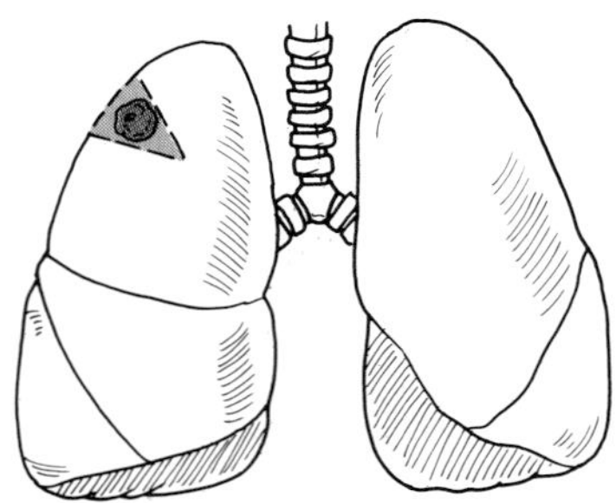

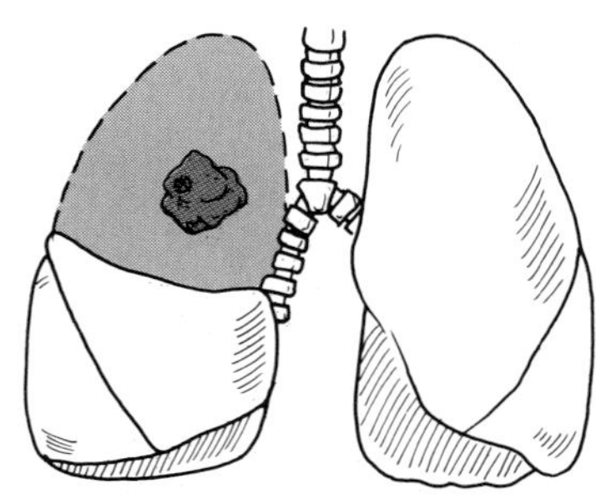

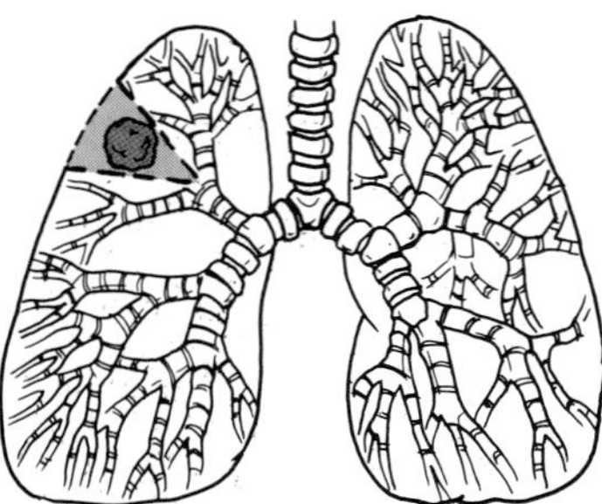

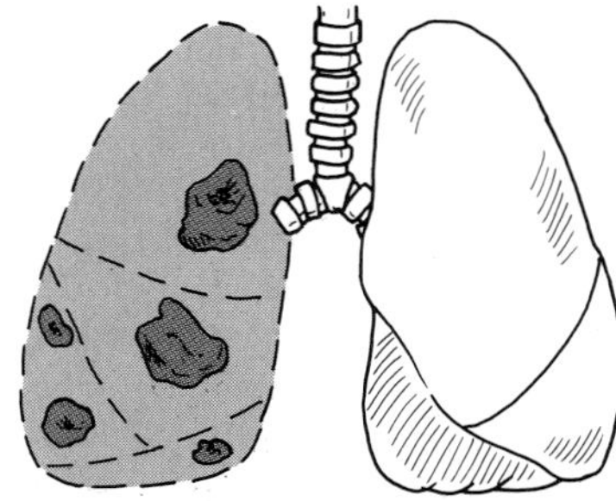

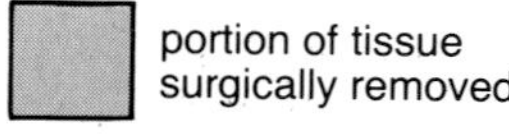

FIGURE 29–9

Pulmonary resections. (From Black, J. M., & Matassarin-Jacobs, E. [1993]. *Luckmann and Sorensen's medical-surgical nursing: A psychophysiologic approach* [4th ed., p. 1065]. Philadelphia: W. B. Saunders.)

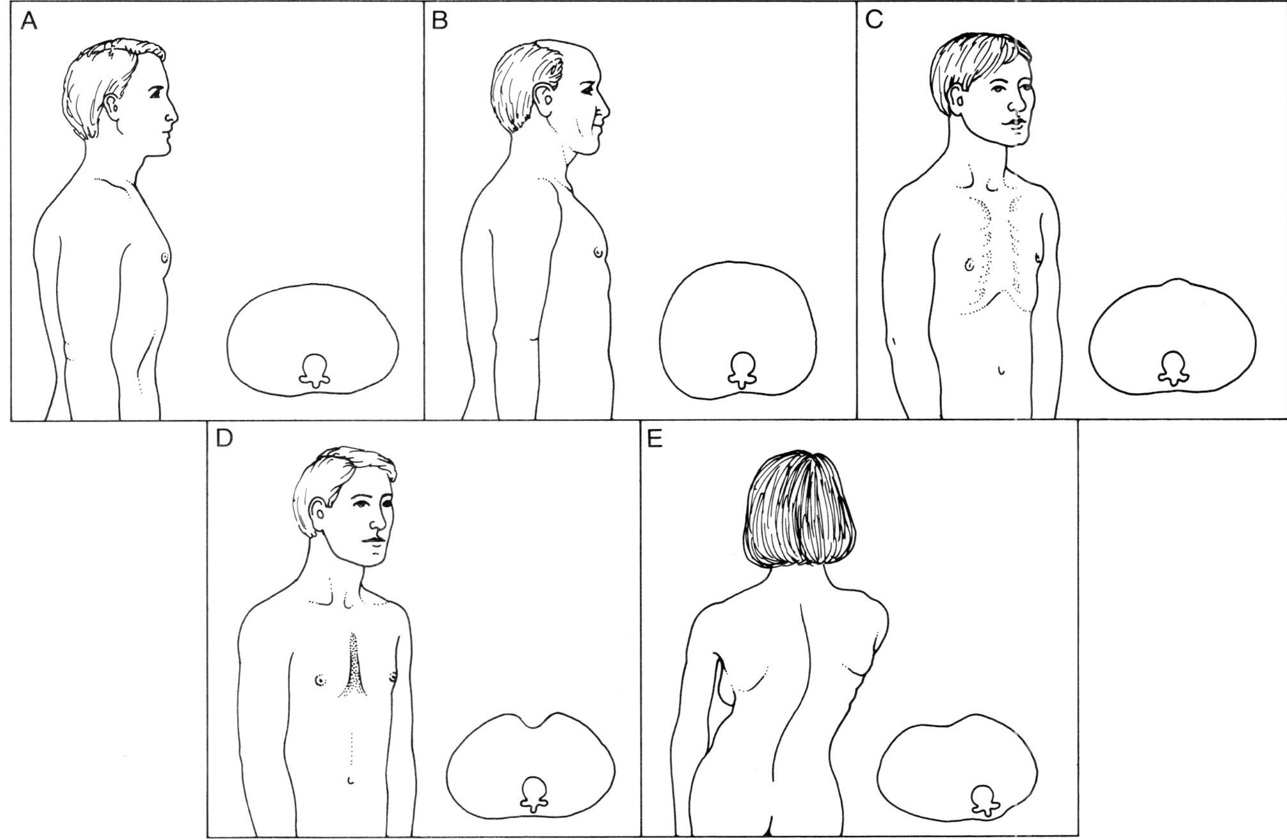

FIGURE 29–10
Normal adult chest *(A)* and chest deformities that may affect respiratory function. *B,* Increased anteroposterior diameter ("barrel chest"). *C,* Pectus excavatum ("funnel chest"). *D,* Pectus carinatum ("pigeon chest"). *E,* Thoracic kyphoscoliosis. (From Black, J. M., & Matassarin-Jacobs, E. [1993]. *Luckmann and Sorensen's medical-surgical nursing: A psychophysiologic approach* [4th ed., p. 919]. Philadelphia: W. B. Saunders.)

Nursing Care of the Patient with Lung Cancer

Nursing Care of the patient with cancer is detailed in Chapter 23. Care of the patient who has a thoracotomy is discussed in Chapter 28. In addition, nurses must continue to educate the public about the dangers of cigarette smoking to help eliminate the primary cause of lung cancer.

EXTRAPULMONARY DISORDERS

This chapter and the previous one have described disorders of the respiratory system. Many other disorders, however, can result in significant impairment of respiratory function. For example, chest deformities as seen in Figure 29–10 may interfere with lung expansion. Neuromuscular diseases such as myasthenia gravis and amyotrophic lateral sclerosis affect the muscles of respiration. Head or spinal cord injuries can disrupt the breathing center in the brain or the neural control of the diaphragm. Heart failure with pulmonary edema fills the lungs with fluid, interfering with the exchange of gases. The specific interventions are covered with these conditions in other chapters.

BIBLIOGRAPHY

Adair, N. (1994). Chronic airflow obstruction and respiratory failure. In W. R. Hazzard, E. L. Bierman, J. P. Blass, W. H. Ettinger, & J. B. Halter (Eds), *Principles of geriatric medicine and gerontology* (3rd ed., pp. 583–596). New York: McGraw-Hill.

Allen, S. C. (1992). Aging and the respiratory system. In J. C. Brocklehurst, R. C. Tallis, & H. M. Fillitt (Eds.), *Textbook of geriatric medicine and gerontology* (4th ed., pp. 739–768). Edinburgh: Churchill Livingstone.

American Cancer Society. (1993). *Cancer facts and figures—1993.* Atlanta, GA: American Cancer Society.

American Cancer Society. (1994). *Cancer facts and figures—1994.* Atlanta, GA: American Cancer Society.

Athanassiades, P., Athanassiades, H., Psychogiou, E., Kokolakis, N., & Giannioti, E. (1992). Carboplatin, vinblastine and mitomycin-C in the treatment of non–small cell bronchogenic carcinoma. *Journal of Chemotherapy, 4*(3), 196–199.

Bendayan, R., Kennedy, G., Frecker, R. C., & Sellers, E. M. (1993). Lack of effect of cimetidine on cigarette smoking. *European Journal of Clinical Pharmacology, 44*(1), 51–55.

Black, J. M., & Matassarin-Jacobs, E. (1993). *Luckmann and*

Sorensen's medical-surgical nursing: A psychophysiologic approach (4th ed.). Philadelphia: W. B. Saunders.

Boutotte, J. (1993). TB . . . the second time around . . . and how you can help to control it. *Nursing 93, 23*(5), 42–50.

Branchaud, R. M., Garant, L. J., & Kane, A. B. (1993). Pathogenesis of mesothelial reactions to asbestos fibers. *Pathobiology, 61*(3–4), 154–163.

Caine, R. M., & Bufalino, P. M. (1991). *Nursing care planning guides for adults* (2nd ed.). Baltimore: Williams & Wilkins.

Chernecky, C. C., Krech, R. L., & Berger, B. J. (1993). *Laboratory tests and diagnostic procedures.* Philadelphia: W. B. Saunders.

Corbett, J. V. (1992). *Laboratory tests and diagnostic procedures with nursing diagnoses* (3rd ed.). East Norwalk, CT: Appleton & Lange.

Deglin, J. H., & Vallerand, A. H. (1991). *Nurse's med deck* (2nd ed.). Philadelphia: F. A. Davis.

Doenges, M. E., & Moorhouse, M. F. (1993). *Nurse's pocket guide: Nursing diagnoses and interventions.* Philadelphia: F. A. Davis.

Donahoe, M., Rogers, R. M. Cottrell, J. J. (1992). Is loss of body weight in chronic obstructive pulmonary disease patients with emphysema secondary to low tissue oxygenation? *Respiration, 59 Suppl*(2), 33–39.

Finesilver, C. (1992). Respiratory assessment. *RN, 55*(2), 22–30.

Fiore, M. C. (1992). Trends in cigarette smoking in the United States. The epidemiology of tobacco use. *Medical Clinics of North America, 76*(2), 289–303.

Fischbach, F. T. (1988). *A manual of laboratory diagnostic tests* (3rd ed.). Philadelphia: J. B. Lippincott.

Foster, W. L., Gimenez, E. I., Roubidoux, M. A., Sherrier, R. H., Shannon, R. H., Roggli, V. L., & Pratt, P. C. (1993). The emphysemas: Radiologic-pathologic correlations. *Radiographics, 13*(2), 311–328.

Gaensler, E. A. (1992). Asbestos exposure in buildings. *Clinics in Chest Medicine, 13*(2), 231–242.

Gimeno, F., Postma, D. S., & van Aletena, R. (1993). Plethysmographic parameters in the assessment of reversibility of airways obstruction in patients with clinical emphysema. *Chest, 104*(2), 467–470.

Gritz, E. R. (1991). Smoking and smoking cessation in cancer patients. *British Journal of Addiction, 86*(5), 549–554.

Gross, N. J. (1991). The influence of anticholinergic agents on treatment for bronchitis and emphysema. *American Journal of Medicine, 91*(4A), 115–125.

Hoffman, L. A., & Manzetti, J. D. (1992). Nursing assessment: Respiratory system. In S. M. Lewis & I. C. Collier, *Medical-surgical nursing: A nursing process approach* (3rd ed.). St. Louis: Mosby Year Book.

Hofford, J. M. (1992). Metered dose inhaler therapy for asthma. *Journal of Family Practice, 34*(4), 485–492.

Janson-Bjerklie, S. (1990). Status asthmaticus. *American Journal of Nursing, 90*(9), 52–55.

Jarvis, C. (1992). *Physical examination and health assessment.* Philadelphia: W. B. Saunders.

Jess, L. W. (1992). Chronic bronchitis and emphysema. *Nursing 92, 22*(3), 34–41.

Jess, L. W. (1992). When your patient has asthma. *Nursing 92, 22*(4), 48–51.

Kersten, L. D. (1989). *Comprehensive respiratory nursing.* Philadelphia: W. B. Saunders.

Kim, W. D., Eidelman, D. H., Izquierdo, J. L., Ghezzo, H., Saetta, M. P., & Cosio, M. G. (1991). Centrilobular and panlobular emphysema in smokers. Two distinct morphologic and functional entities. *American Review of Respiratory Diseases, 144*(6), 1385–1390.

Lapp, N. L., Castronova, V. (1993). How silicosis and coal workers' pneumoconiosis develop—A cellular assessment. *Occupational Medicine: State of the Art Review, 8*(1), 35–56.

Leischow, S. J., & Stitzer, M. L. (1991). Smoking cessation and weight gain. *British Journal of Addiction, 86*(5), 577–581.

Lindell, K. O., & Mazzocco, M. C. (1990). Breaking bronchospasm's grip with MDI's. *American Journal of Nursing, 90*(3), 34–42.

Mark, E. J., & Shin, D. H. (1992). Asbestos and the histogenesis of lung carcinoma. *Seminars in Diagnostic Pathology, 9*(2), 110–116.

McKenna, J. P., & Cox, J. L. (1992). Transdermal nicotine replacement and smoking cessation. *American Family Physician, 45*(6), 2595–2602.

Mitchell, J. T. (1992). Nursing role in management: Lower respiratory problems. In S. M. Lewis & I. C. Collier, *Medical-surgical nursing: A nursing process approach* (3rd ed.). St. Louis: Mosby Year Book.

Nori, D., Allison, R., Kaplan, B., Samala, E., Osian, A., & Karbowitz, S. (1993). High dose rate intraluminal irradiation in bronchogenic carcinoma. *Chest, 104*(4), 1006–1011.

O'Brien, L. M., & Bartlett, K. A. (1992). TB plus HIV spells trouble. *American Journal of Nursing, 92*(5), 28–34.

Perry, M. C. (1994). Lung cancer. In W. R. Hazzard, E. L. Bierman, J. P. Blass, W. H. Ettinger, & J. B. Halter (Eds.), *Principles of geriatric medicine and gerontology* (3rd ed., pp. 607–613). New York: McGraw-Hill.

Rodman, M. J. (1993). Cough, cold, and allergy preparations. *RN, 56*(2), 38–42.

Rohatgi, P. K., & Kuzmowych, T. V. (1993). Pathogenesis and therapy of pulmonary emphysema. *Maryland Medical Journal, 42*(7), 651–661.

Sachs, D. P., & Leischow, S. J. (1991). Pharmacologic approaches to smoking cessation. *Clinical Chest Medicine, 12*(4), 769–791.

Sachs, D. P., Sawe, U., & Leischow, S. J. (1993). Effectiveness of a 16-hour transdermal nicotine patch in a medical practice setting, without intensive group counseling. *Archives of Internal Medicine, 153*(16), 1881–1890.

Scanlon, C. L., Spearman, C. B., & Sheldon, R. L. (1990). *Egan's fundamentals of respiratory care* (5th ed.). St. Louis: C. V. Mosby.

Schreur, H. J., Sterk, P. J., Venderschoot, J., van Klink, H. C., van Vollenhoven, E., & Diikman, J. H. (1992). Lung sound intensity in patients with emphysema and in normal subjects at standardized airflows. *Thorax, 47*(9), 674–679.

Speiser, B. L., & Spratling, L. (1993). Radiation bronchitis and stenosis secondary to high dose rate endobronchial irradiation. *International Journal of Radiation Oncology, Biology, Physics, 25*(4), 589–597.

Sutherland, G., Stapleton, J. A., Russell, M. A., Jarvis, M. J., Hajek, P., Belcher, M., & Feyerabend, C. (1992). Randomised controlled trial of nasal nicotine spray in smoking cessation. *Lancet, 340*(8815), 324–329.

Viskum, K., & Kok-Jenson, A. (1990). Criteria for alpha 1-antitrypsin substitution. *Lung, 168*(Suppl), 586–591.

Whyte, R. I., Schork, M. A., Sloan, H., Orringer, M. B., & Kirsh, M. M. (1992). Adjuvant treatment using transfer factor for bronchogenic carcinoma: Long term follow-up. *Annals of Thoracic Surgery, 53*(3), 391–396.

Yashar, J., Weitberg, A. B., Glicksman, A. S., Posner, M. R., Feng, W., & Wanebo, H. J. (1992). Preoperative chemotherapy and radiation therapy for stage IIIa carcinoma of the lung. *Annals of Thoracic Surgery, 53*(3), 445–448.

KEY CONCEPTS

1. Chronic obstructive pulmonary disease (COPD) includes varying combinations of asthma, chronic bronchitis, and emphysema.
2. Bronchial asthma is a potentially reversible obstructive airway disorder that is characterized by bronchospasm as a response to a variety of stimuli.
3. Status asthmaticus is severe bronchospasm that can be fatal.
4. The goal of medical therapy with asthma is to prevent acute asthma attacks using bronchodilators, β_2-receptor agonists, mast cell stabilizers, anticholinergics, and corticosteroids.
5. Nursing diagnoses for the patient with asthma may include ineffective breathing patterns, impaired gas exchange, anxiety, and knowledge deficit.
6. Chronic bronchitis is bronchial inflammation characterized by increased production of mucus and chronic cough that persists for at least 3 months of the year for 2 consecutive years.
7. Pulmonary emphysema, which often coexists with chronic bronchitis, is a degenerative nonreversible disease characterized by the breakdown of the alveolar septa distal to the terminal bronchioles.
8. Nursing diagnoses for the patient with chronic bronchitis and emphysema may include impaired gas exchange, ineffective airway clearance, anxiety, altered nutrition, high risk for infection, activity intolerance, decreased cardiac output, and knowledge deficit.
9. Smoking cessation is an important aspect of management of COPD and other cardiovascular and respiratory conditions, but success rates for stop-smoking programs are low.
10. Bronchiectasis is an abnormal dilation and distortion of the bronchi and bronchioles that causes coughing and the production of large amounts of sputum and is often associated with infection.
11. Restrictive pulmonary disorders result in reduced lung volumes with a normal to elevated ratio of forced expiratory volume in 1 second to forced vital capacity.
12. Tuberculosis is an infectious disease of the lungs and other body tissues that requires long-term drug therapy.
13. Nursing diagnoses for the patient with tuberculosis may include impaired gas exchange, social isolation, high risk for injury, fatigue, altered nutrition, noncompliance, and knowledge deficit.
14. Sarcoidosis is an inflammatory condition that may resolve with corticosteroid treatment or may lead to fibrosis.
15. Occupational lung diseases are caused by the inhalation of various substances and include acute respiratory irritation, occupational asthma, hypersensitivity pneumonitis, and pneumoconioses.
16. Diffuse interstitial fibrosis is an inflammatory condition in which there is thickening and fibrosis of the alveolar walls that renders the alveoli nonfunctional.
17. Nursing diagnoses for the patient with interstitial fibrosis may include ineffective gas exchange, ineffective airway clearance, activity intolerance, and anxiety.
18. Lung cancer, the leading cause of cancer deaths in the United States, is usually caused by cigarette smoking and is most treatable if detected while still localized.
19. Extrapulmonary causes of respiratory problems may be skeletal, neuromuscular, neurologic, or cardiac.

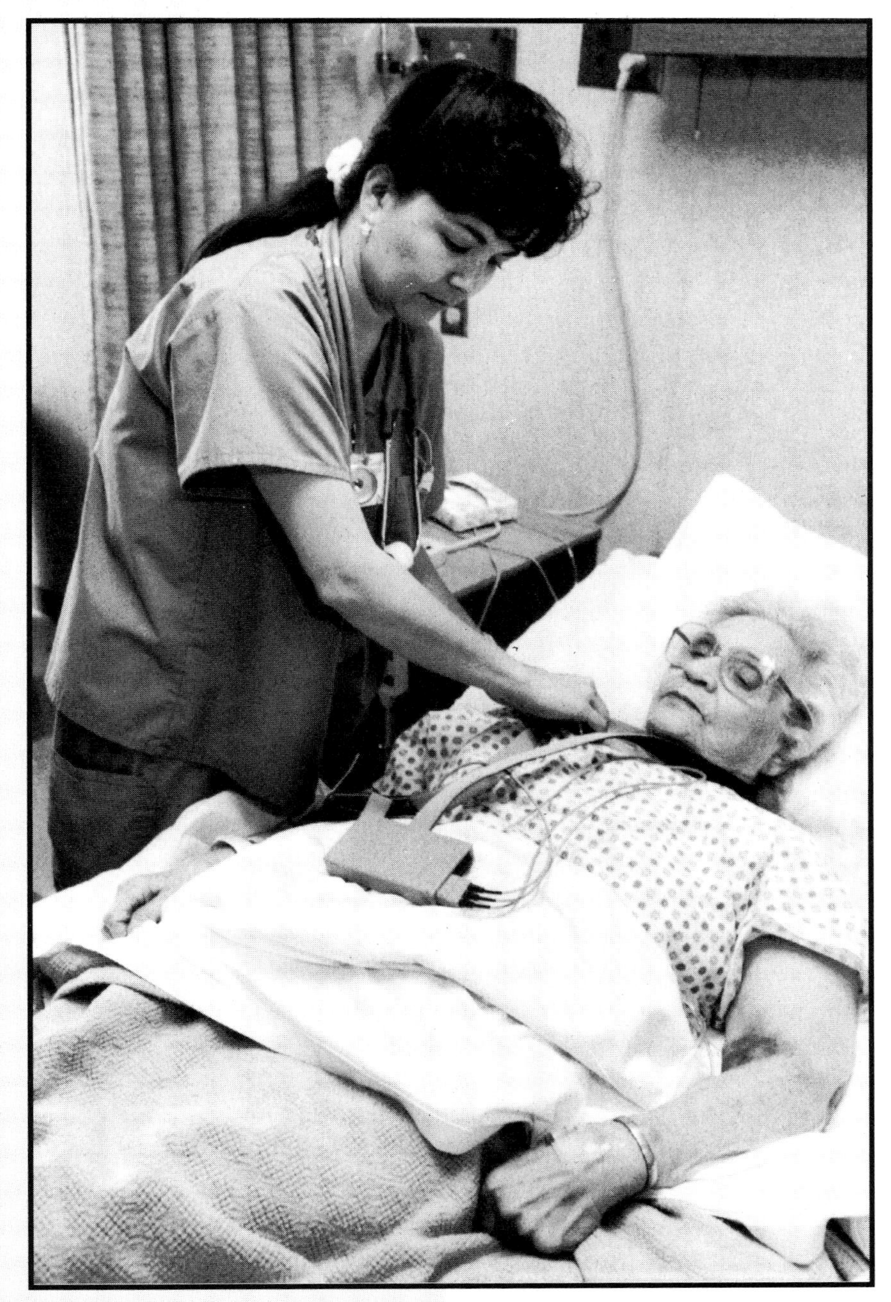

UNIT 8
Cardiovascular Disorders

Stacey Young-McCaughan

CHAPTER 30

Hematologic and Lymphatic Disorders

OBJECTIVES

1. Identify data to be collected when assessing a patient with a disorder of the hematologic or lymphatic system.
2. Describe tests and procedures used to diagnose disorders of the hematologic or lymphatic system and nursing considerations for each.
3. Describe nursing care for patients undergoing common therapeutic measures for disorders of the hematologic or lymphatic system.
4. Describe the pathophysiology, signs and symptoms, complications, and medical or surgical treatment for selected disorders of the hematologic or lymphatic system.
5. Write a nursing care plan for a patient with a disorder of the hematologic or lymphatic system.
6. Identify measures the nurse can take to reduce the risk of disorders of the hematologic or lymphatic system and to detect problems early.

GLOSSARY

ANEMIA A deficiency in the number of red blood cells, hemoglobin, or both in the blood

COMPROMISED HOST PRECAUTIONS Actions taken to help protect patients with low white blood cell counts from infection

ECCHYMOSIS A purplish skin lesion resulting from blood leaking outside the blood vessels

LEUKEMIA Cancer of the white blood cells in which the bone marrow produces too many immature white blood cells

LYMPHOMA Cancer of the lymph system

PETECHIA A small (1–3 mm) red or reddish-purple spot on the skin resulting from blood capillaries breaking and leaking small amounts of blood into the tissues

Glossary continued

The views expressed in this chapter are those of the author and do not reflect the official policy or position of the U.S. government.

PURPURA Red or reddish-purple skin lesions 3 mm or more in size that result from blood leaking outside of the blood vessels

UNIVERSAL DONOR Person with type O negative blood who can donate blood to anyone because none of the common antigens are present in the blood

UNIVERSAL RECIPIENT Person with type AB positive blood who can receive transfusions with any type of blood because all the common antigens (A, B, and Rh) are present in the blood

The hematologic system and the lymphatic system function interdependently to maintain normal physiologic functioning of the body and to protect the body from infection. Disorders of these systems can be a symptom of another disease or a primary problem of one or both of these two systems. The nurse plays an important role in helping to assess, plan, and manage the care of patients with these disorders, whatever the cause.

ANATOMY AND PHYSIOLOGY OF THE HEMATOLOGIC SYSTEM

The hematologic system includes the blood and the bone marrow. Blood is a mixture of red blood cells, white blood cells, and platelets that travel in plasma through vessels in the body performing multiple functions (Fig. 30–1). A healthy adult has approximately 6 liters of blood circulating through the body pumped by the heart. Most of the blood components are made in the bone marrow.

ERYTHROCYTES (RED BLOOD CELLS)

Red blood cells are made in the bone marrow. Once released from the marrow, they circulate in the body, transporting oxygen from the lungs to the tissues and carbon dioxide from the tissues back to the lungs. Hemoglobin in the red blood cells makes the transport of oxygen and carbon dioxide possible. Red blood cells are biconcave disks designed with a tough, flexible membrane that can fit through even the smallest capillaries. After about 120 days, the old red blood cells are filtered out of circulation by the spleen. The iron and heme in

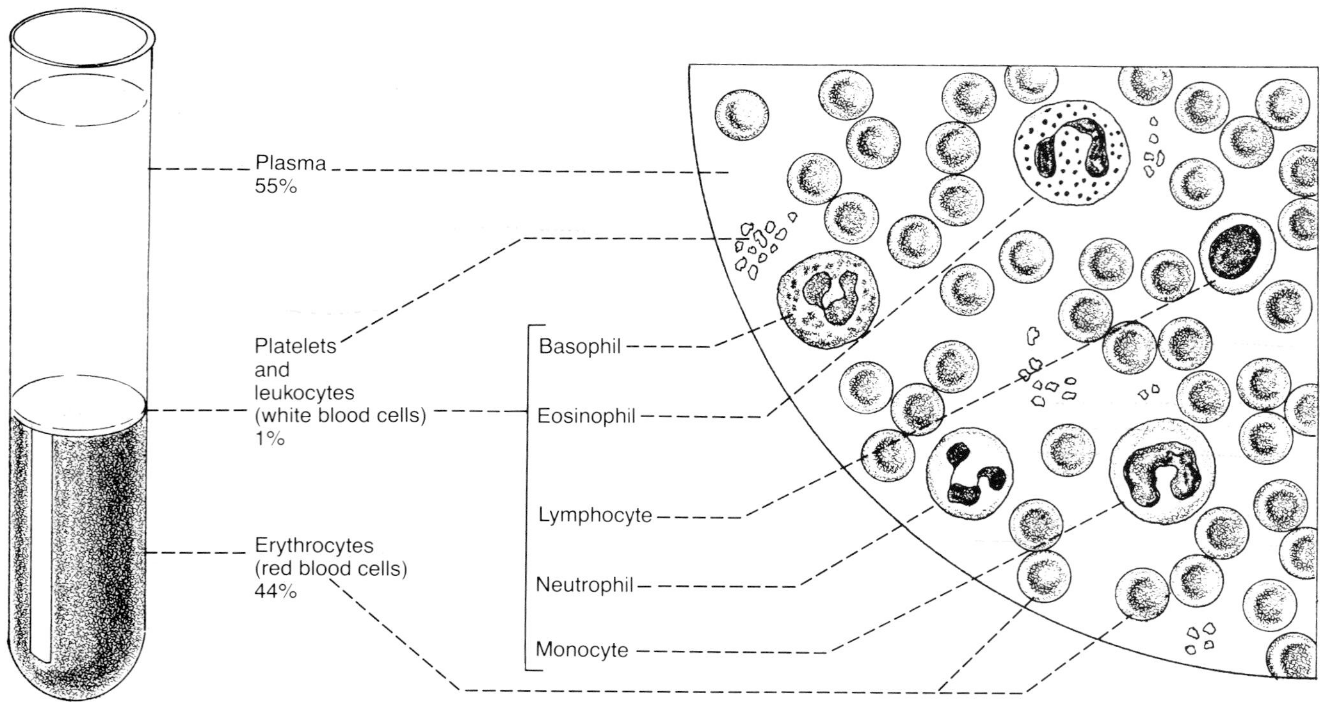

FIGURE 30–1

Blood is composed of plasma (about 55%) and cellular elements, including leukocytes, thrombocytes (platelets), and erythrocytes (about 45%). There are 600 times as many erythrocytes as leukocytes. (From Black, J. M., & Matassarin-Jacobs, E. [1993]. *Luckmann and Sorensen's medical-surgical nursing: A psychophysiologic approach* [4th ed., p. 1319]. Philadelphia: W. B. Saunders.)

the old red blood cells is reused to make new red blood cells.

The red blood cell count, the hematocrit, and the hemoglobin are the three main blood tests used to monitor the red blood cells. The red blood cell count is the total number of red blood cells found in a cubic millimeter of blood. The hematocrit is the percentage of red blood cells in whole blood. The hemoglobin tells how much hemoglobin or oxygen-carrying capacity the patient has. Table 30–1 lists normal laboratory values of the red blood cells, the hematocrit, and the hemoglobin as measured by the complete blood count (CBC). Notice that the hematocrit is roughly three times the hemoglobin.

TABLE 30–1
NORMAL LABORATORY VALUES*

Red blood cell count	
Men:	4,200,000–5,400,000/L
Women:	3,600,000–5,000,000/L
Hematocrit (Hct)	
Men:	40–54%
Women:	37–47%
Hemoglobin (Hb)	
Men:	13.5–17.5 gm/dl
Women:	12.0–16.0 gm/dl
White blood cell count (WBC):	5000–10,000
White blood cell count differential:	
Neutrophils	60–70% of total WBC
Lymphocytes	20–40% of total WBC
Eosinophils	1–4% of total WBC
Basophils	1% of total WBC
Monocytes	2–6% of total WBC
Platelets:	150,000–350,000
Prothrombin time (PT):	10–14 sec (however, normal values depend on the method used to measure the PT)
Partial thromboplastin time (PTT):	30–45 sec (however, normal values depend on the method used to measure PTT)
Bleeding time:	3–10 min (however, normal values depend on the method used to measure the bleeding time)
Serum iron	
Men:	75–175 gm/dl
Women:	65–165 gm/dl
Ferritin	
Men:	15–300 ng/ml
Women:	12–150 ng/ml
Total iron binding capcity (TIBC):	240–450 gm/dl
Direct Coombs's antiglobulin test:	negative
Hemoglobin S (Sickledex):	0
Hemoglobin electrophoresis:	
Hemoglobin A	>95.0%
Hemoglobin A_2	2.5–4.0%
Hemoglobin F	<2.0%
Hemoglobin S	0.0%
Serum protein electrophoresis (SPEP):	
Total protein	6.3–7.9 gm/dl
Albumin	3.1–4.3 gm/dl
$Alpha_1$ globulin	0.1–0.3 gm/dl
$Alpha_2$ globulin	0.6–1.0 gm/dl
Beta globulin	0.7–1.4 gm/dl
Gamma globulin	0.7–1.6 gm/dl
Urine protein electrophoresis (UPEP):	interpreted based upon SPEP results

* NOTE: Normal laboratory values may differ from hospital to hospital. Be sure to check your institution's normal values.

Adapted from Fischbach, F. T. (1992). *A manual of laboratory diagnostic tests* (4th ed.). Philadelphia: J. B. Lippincott.

LEUKOCYTES (WHITE BLOOD CELLS)

White blood cells also originate in the bone marrow. These cells protect the body from infections. Every day we are exposed to bacteria, viruses, fungi, and parasites that the white blood cells destroy before they can multiply and cause severe infections. There are five major types of white blood cells: neutrophils (known by many names including polymorphonuclear neutrophils, PMNs, polys, neuts, granulocytes, grans, or segs), lymphocytes, eosinophils, basophils, and monocytes. Each type of white blood cell combats certain types of microorganisms. Doctors and nurses follow both the total number of white blood cells in the body as well as the "differential" or percentage of each of the specific types of white blood cells in the body. Normal white blood cell counts range from 5000 to 10,000 white blood cells per cubic millimeter of blood. The majority of the white blood cells, 60%, are neutrophils. Table 30–1 lists normal laboratory values for all of the types of white blood cells. The number of neutrophils usually is of most concern to doctors and nurses because these are the cells that fight bacterial infections.

The normal life span of a white blood cell is only about 12 hours of circulation in the blood. Normally white blood cells find microorganisms, kill them by ingesting them, and in the process are themselves destroyed. Other cells called macrophages clean up the white blood cell debris. If the dead white blood cells build up faster than the macrophages can clean them up, pus is formed. This is why pus is a classic sign of infection and should be reported to a nurse or a doctor and carefully monitored.

The bone marrow is capable of producing huge numbers of white blood cells, especially neutrophils, to fight infection. It is called a *shift to the left* when the total number of white blood cells is high and the percentage of neutrophils in the differential is greater than 60%, indicating that the bone marrow is producing large numbers of neutrophils to combat a severe infection.

THROMBOCYTES (PLATELETS)

Platelets are the third major blood cell produced by the bone marrow. Platelets activate the blood clotting system by going to a break in a blood vessel and forming a platelet plug. At the same time, other clotting mechanisms are activated, and the body begins repairing itself. Normal platelet counts range from 150,000 to 350,000 platelets per cubic millimeter of blood. Many times a platelet count of 200,000 is expressed as 200 K, the K meaning "thousand." The normal life span for a platelet is 10 days once released into circulation from the bone marrow.

CLOTTING FACTORS

Once platelets initiate the blood clotting system, several clotting factors are activated. The clotting factors are numbered I through XII and include thromboplastin, prothrombin, and fibrinogen. The clotting factors act to form a fibrin matrix over the wounded area that allows the body to heal itself.

The function of the clotting factors is measured with several blood tests that include the platelet count, the prothrombin time and the partial thromboplastin time (PT/PTT), and the bleeding time. Table 30–1 lists normal laboratory values for these tests.

PLASMA

Plasma is the straw-colored fluid that carries the red blood cells, white blood cells, and platelets through the circulatory system. Plasma is primarily water. The other components of plasma are the plasma proteins (albumin, immunoglobulins, and fibrinogen) and the clotting factors.

BONE MARROW

The bone marrow is the spongy center of the bones where the red blood cells, white blood cells, and platelets are made. The marrow of all bones produces these cells; however, the majority are produced in the spinal column, pelvis, long bones of the legs, skull, ribs, and sternum.

ANATOMY AND PHYSIOLOGY OF THE LYMPHATIC SYSTEM

The lymphatic system is a completely separate vessel system in which lymph fluid flows. When blood flows through the capillary beds to deliver oxygen and pick up carbon dioxide, not all the plasma returns to the veins to be recirculated. The lymphatic system is a series of open-ended tubes in the tissues that collects plasma left behind in the tissues and returns it into the venous system. The lymphatic vessels have one-way valves, and the lymph fluid is propelled along by the normal contraction of skeletal muscles. The lymphatic vessels empty into the venous system at the right lymphatic duct of the right subclavian vein and at the thoracic duct of the left subclavian vein. Figure 30–2 shows the flow of lymph fluid and where it empties into these ducts. The lymphatic system is very important in returning plasma proteins back to the blood circulation and thereby preventing edema.

LYMPH NODES

Lymph nodes are small patches of lymphatic tissues located along the lymphatic system that filter out microorganisms from the lymph fluid before it is returned to the blood stream. Lymph nodes are located throughout the body, as depicted in Figure 30–2. The lymph nodes can become swollen with infection and with some cancers. The nodes closer to the surface of the body in the neck, under the arm, and in the groin can be palpated, or felt, when they are swollen. Many times lymph nodes deeper in the body cannot be palpated but can be visualized on computed tomography scans if they are larger than 2 cm. During surgery for cancer, the surgeon almost always takes biopsy samples from the nearby lymph nodes and has the pathologist check them to see if the cancer might have spread.

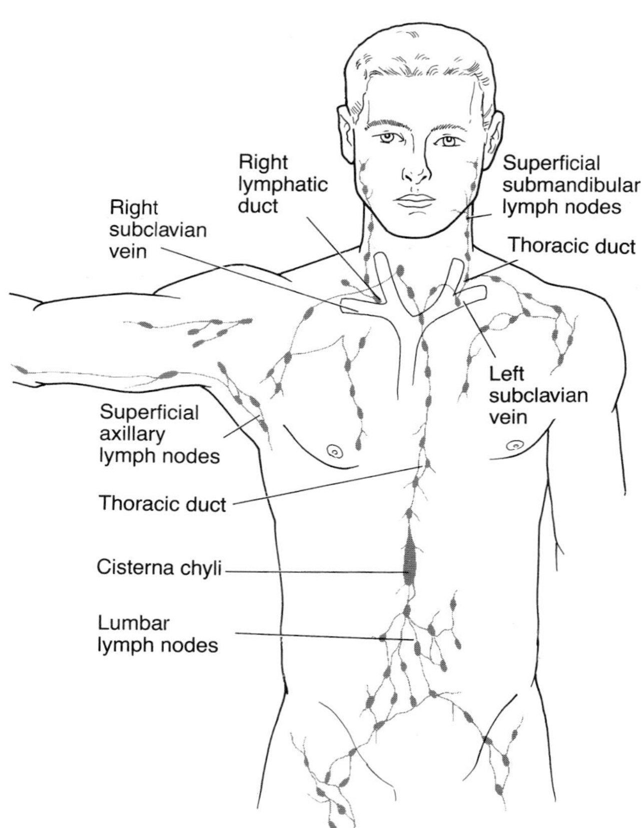

FIGURE 30–2 Diagram of the lymphatic system.

SPLEEN

The spleen is an organ that is located in the upper left quadrant of the abdomen. Like the lymph nodes, the spleen filters microorganisms from the blood. In addition to this, the spleen stores red blood cells, destroys old red blood cells, and produces antibodies. The body has many overlapping systems to protect itself from infection. Both the lymph nodes and the spleen filter microorganisms from blood and blood plasma. Once trapped, the microorganisms are destroyed by the white blood cells.

A person can live without a spleen. For example, sometimes a person who has been in a car accident has a splenectomy because the spleen was ruptured in the accident. Many times the spleen is removed during a staging work-up for Hodgkin's disease, a form of cancer of the lymph nodes. However, without a spleen, people are at greater risk for some kinds of infection, especially pneumococcal infections. If possible, patients should receive Pneumovax vaccine before the spleen is removed so that the body can form its own antibodies against pneumococcal bacteria and protect against these infections in the future. A vaccination is possible if a patient is having a planned splenectomy for Hodgkin's disease, but one is not always possible if a patient is having an emergency splenectomy after an accident.

B LYMPHOCYTES AND T LYMPHOCYTES

Another way the body protects itself from microorganisms is by utilizing specialized B and T lymphocytes. Certain lymphocytes made in the bone marrow by plasma cells undergo changes in the lymph tissue of the body to become B and T lymphocytes. B lymphocytes are responsible for the humoral immune response with the immunoglobulins IgA, IgD, IgE, IgG, and IgM. T lymphocytes are responsible for the cellular immune response.

AGE-RELATED CHANGES

With advancing age, the bone marrow becomes less productive. This is generally not hazardous to health unless a person is unusually stressed with a chronic illness, treatment for cancer, or trauma necessitating a higher production of blood cells. Even still, the bone marrow can usually respond to the increased demand given more time.

The lymphatic tissue grows very quickly between the ages of 6 and 20 years. With advancing age, lymphatic tissue shrinks, resulting in fewer lymph nodes and smaller remaining lymph nodes. But, as with the bone marrow, this change does not generally affect the overall health of an individual.

NURSING ASSESSMENT OF THE HEMATOLOGIC AND LYMPHATIC SYSTEMS

The blood is most commonly assessed through the evaluation of blood tests. However, many subtle changes in the health history and physical examination can show the nurse that changes in the patient's blood counts may be occurring and that a nurse or doctor should be notified to evaluate the patient. Table 30–2 outlines the nursing assessment of patients with disorders of the blood, bone marrow, and lymphatic system.

HEALTH HISTORY

Chief Complaint and History of Present Illness

Many times a patient with a blood problem is seen for a completely different reason and finds out that some of the symptoms are related to a blood problem. The nurse should pay special attention to patients who remark that they bruise easily or have frequent infections or are chronically fatigued, as these may be symptoms of a blood problem.

TABLE 30–2

ASSESSMENT OF PATIENTS WITH DISORDERS OF THE HEMATOLOGIC OR LYMPHATIC SYSTEM

HEALTH HISTORY

Present illness: Persistent infections, prolonged bleeding, easy bruising, chronic fatigue
Past medical history: Recent infections, recent immunizations, current medications, recent changes in medication
Family history: Blood disorders
Review of systems:
- Skin: Dryness, pruritus, lesions, bruising, change in skin color, brittle nails
- Head and neck: Headache, sore throat, enlarged lymph glands, change in vision
- Respiratory status: Dyspnea
- Cardiovascular: Palpitations, dizziness or fainting with position changes
- Gastrointestinal status: Change in eating habits, anorexia, nausea, vomiting, weight change, change in bowel habits, blood in stool
- Urinary function: Blood in urine
- Genitalia: Enlarged lymph nodes, heavy menses
- Musculoskeletal: Pain in bones or joints
- Endocrine: Fatigue, cold intolerance, night sweats

Functional assessment: Occupation and hobbies, changes in ability to do activities of daily living, roles at home and work, self-concept, activities and exercise, sleep and rest, nutrition, interpersonal relationships, stressors, coping style

PHYSICAL EXAMINATION

Vital signs: Tachycardia, tachypnea, fever
General survey: Painful or swollen areas
Skin: Color, dryness, bruising, infected lesions
Head and neck: Bleeding, infection, enlarged lymph nodes
Thorax: Respiratory rate, breath sounds, heart rate, orthostatic vital sign changes
Abdomen: Stool guaiac test, spleen or liver enlargement
Urine: Blood in urine
Genitalia: Enlarged lymph nodes, heavy menses
Musculoskeletal: Pain with movement, joint swelling or enlargement

Past Medical History

Any recent infections, recent immunizations, or recent changes in medications can affect a patient's blood counts.

Family History

Any family history of blood disorders, such as sickle cell anemia, is noted.

Review of Systems

The nurse asks about skin dryness, pruritus, brittle nails, lesions, excessive bruising, or changes in skin color. Changes in vision are noted because they may indicate bleeding in the eye. If the patient has had headaches, the nurse records the location, duration, and intensity of the pain as well as what relieves the pain. Patients with low red blood cell counts may have headaches. Also, patients with intracranial bleeding from low platelet counts may report headaches or mental status changes. Headaches or mental status changes from intracranial bleeding usually begin quickly and can be very severe. Other important signs and symptoms to document include sore throat, enlarged lymph nodes, dyspnea, palpitations, and dizziness or fainting with position changes.

The patient is asked to describe any changes in eating habits or problems with anorexia, nausea, or vomiting. Any unplanned weight loss or weight gain can be a symptom of a cancer. The patient's normal bowel function and any recent changes in frequency of bowel movements or consistency of the stool are noted. Visible blood in the patient's stool or urine should be recorded. Any musculoskeletal pain is described. Generalized bone pain can occur with a leukemia because the cancerous white blood cells are crowding the bone marrow, causing bone pain. Joint pain can occur if bleeding has occurred in the joint.

The patient is asked about fatigue or cold intolerance, which can be symptoms of low red blood cell counts. Also, night sweats, which can be a symptom of lymphoma (cancer in the lymph nodes), should be recorded. Patients with lymphoma can have such severe night sweats that they have to change nightclothes and linens several times during the night. Women are asked about unusually heavy menses that may indicate a bleeding disorder.

Functional Assessment

Patients newly diagnosed with a blood disorder may not experience dramatic changes in their functional abilities. However, many blood disorders are chronic conditions that the patient has lived with and been treated for for many years. The functional abilities of these patients may have changed because of the chronicity of their disease.

OCCUPATION AND HOBBIES. Because blood can be affected by various chemicals, any recent chemical exposure should be noted. Knowing a patient's job and hobbies can alert you to unusual chemical exposures. For example, beauticians are frequently exposed to hair dyes that may affect their blood counts. Someone who builds models for a hobby may be exposed to unusual glues or paints that may affect the blood count.

SELF-CONCEPT. The nurse assesses the patient's self-concept by exploring the patient's feelings about himself or herself. Factors that might affect self-concept include change in appearance because of the disease; whether the patient is employed; whether the patient has insurance and, if so, what kind; whether insurance is dependent upon employment; and whether the patient is on state or federal assistance.

ACTIVITY OR EXERCISE. The assessment of activity includes the patient's current activity level and the effects of treatments on the patient's usual pattern of activity and exercise. The assessment of activities should also determine the type of home the patient lives in. It may be helpful to know if the home has more than one floor and if the patient must climb stairs to enter the home. The patient's roles in the home must also be considered. The nurse asks what household chores the patient is responsible for and who does the shopping, cooking, and cleaning. If there are children to care for, note whether the patient is able to perform usual child care. The nurse also inquires what the patient does for fun and whether these activities can still be done during times of decreased energy.

SLEEP AND REST. Assessment of sleep and rest includes the number of continuous hours the patient sleeps every night, whether any sleeping aids are used, what interrupts the patient's sleep, and whether the patient naps during the day.

NUTRITION. The patient is asked to describe the usual diet and any changes in appetite, taste perception, or weight. Factors that interfere with good eating such as nausea, vomiting, financial problems, loneliness, and depression are identified.

INTERPERSONAL RELATIONSHIPS. The nurse explores the patient's view of self as a husband or wife, father or mother, son or daughter, friend, and coworker. The effect of the disease on these relationships is discussed.

COPING AND STRESS. Coping and stress are assessed by asking what the patient worries about and how the patient deals with the stress of the disease. Sources of support, which might include family, support groups, and spiritual beliefs and practices, are explored.

PERCEPTION OF HEALTH. The patient's view of his or her own health and health practices are discussed. This might include measures taken to prevent complications from the disease, and keeping regular medical appointments.

PHYSICAL EXAMINATION

The physical examination begins with measurement of vital signs and height and weight. The nurse is alert for tachycardia, tachypnea, hypotension, and fever. A temperature greater than 38.3°C (101°F) is significant because it may indicate the presence of infection.

General Survey

The patient's responsiveness, mood, expression, and posture are noted. Throughout the examination, the nurse carefully inspects and describes any swollen or painful areas the patient identifies.

Skin

The general color of the skin is noted. A patient with a low red blood cell count may appear pale. In black people this assessment may be difficult to make. The conjunctiva of the eyes, the nail beds, and the area around the mouth are inspected to detect any paleness.

Patients also may appear jaundiced, or yellow, if many red blood cells have been destroyed or if the body is having trouble clearing the blood of old red blood cells. Patients may also have dry skin and scalp or brittle nails with some vitamin deficiencies that lead to blood disorders.

The nurse describes any bruising or petechiae. Petechiae are small (1–3 mm) red or reddish-purple spots on the skin resulting from blood capillaries breaking and leaking small amounts of blood into the tissues. Petechiae almost always signal that the patient has a very low platelet count. Severe coughing can cause petechiae on the chest, neck, and face of a patient. A blood pressure cuff pumped higher than 250 mm Hg can cause petechiae on the arm of a patient with a low platelet count below the blood pressure cuff as the small capillaries break with the high cuff pressure. This is not dangerous to the patient, but it can be frightening to both the patient and the nurse when it happens.

Purpura are also red or reddish-purple spots and are the result of larger blood vessels breaking. Purpura are larger than petechiae, usually 3 mm or more. Purpura can suggest a low platelet count or a problem with clotting factors in the blood.

Ecchymoses are larger purplish areas of skin resulting from a larger amount of blood leaking outside the blood vessels. The common name for ecchymosis is a bruise. Ecchymoses do not necessarily indicate a bleeding disorder, but if the patient has a number of these areas or notes that he or she "bruises easily" it may be a symptom of a blood disorder.

Head and Neck

When evaluating the eyes, ears, nose, mouth, and throat, the nurse notes any signs of bleeding or infection. The throat is inspected for any signs of infection such as enlarged tonsils with exudate. Also, the corners of the mouth are inspected for cracking, which may be a symptom of a vitamin deficiency. The nurse palpates for any enlarged lymph nodes in the neck.

Thorax

LUNGS. The nurse assesses respiratory rate and effort. Breath sounds are auscultated for wheezing and crackles. Many times patients with low red blood cell counts are short of breath because they do not have enough red blood cells to carry oxygen to all their tissues. As a result they are tachypneic (breathing rapidly) in an attempt to oxygenate what little blood they have. Patients with respiratory infections may have abnormal breath sounds or a cough.

HEART AND VASCULAR SYSTEM. The cardiovascular assessment includes heart rate, resting blood pressure, and adaptation of blood pressure to position changes. Patients with low red blood cell counts may be tachycardic. Again, because there are not enough red blood cells to carry oxygen to all the tissues, the heart beats faster in an attempt to move what little blood there is quickly from the lungs to the body tissues to deliver oxygen.

Patients with low red blood cell counts can experience orthostatic changes in pulse and blood pressure when they stand up. The body tries to maintain a normal blood pressure when the patient changes position from lying to standing. If the patient's blood volume is inadequate, the heart rate increases and the blood pressure decreases as the patient stands. This can be why patients complain of feeling dizzy or lightheaded when they stand up quickly. To measure this, the patient's pulse and blood pressure are recorded after lying down on a bed or in a reclining chair for at least 1 minute. The patient then sits up, and the pulse and blood pressure are taken again after the patient has been sitting for 1 minute. Then the patient stands up, and the pulse and blood pressure are taken again after the patient has been standing for 1 minute. A decrease in the patient's blood pressure of 15 to 20 points from lying to standing and an increase in the patient's pulse of 15 to 20 points from lying to standing indicates that the patient is orthostatic, or "TILT positive," and needs fluids. Not all patients who are orthostatic need a blood transfusion. Most of the time people are just dehydrated and need extra fluids. However, a patient with a low red blood cell count can also be orthostatic. Some patients can experience heart palpitations or chest pain when the red blood cell count gets low as the heart tries to pump the available blood as quickly as possible.

Abdomen

If a stool specimen is available, a guaiac test may be done to detect microscopic blood. The examiner with advanced skills may palpate the abdomen for tenderness and organ enlargement. The spleen and the liver can become enlarged with blood cell disorders, causing abdominal pain.

Genitourinary Function

The patient's urine is inspected for blood. A dip stick test to detect blood may be done. The nurse palpates the groin for any enlarged lymph nodes.

DIAGNOSTIC TESTS AND PROCEDURES

Blood tests determine primarily the function of the patient's hematologic and lymphatic systems. However, other tests may be ordered by the physician to evaluate these systems more closely. Diagnostic tests and procedures with disorders of the blood and lymphatic system are described in Tables 30–3 and 30–4.

Complete Blood Count

The CBC is a common blood test done at most laboratories. It gives a count of the patient's red blood cells, white blood cells, and platelets. A differential ordered with the CBC tells how many of the different types of white blood cells the patient has. The differential is not done routinely on all CBCs, only when the total white blood cell count is higher or lower than normal.

TABLE 30–3
DIAGNOSTIC TESTS FOR EVALUATING THE HEMATOLOGIC AND LYMPHATIC SYSTEMS

TEST/STUDY	PURPOSE/PROCEDURE	PATIENT PREPARATION	POSTPROCEDURE NURSING CARE
Blood tests (CBC, PT/PTT, serum iron, TIBC, ferritin, HbS, Hb electrophoresis, direct Coombs's, serum protein electrophoresis)	Measures various blood components. Different blood tests are collected in different laboratory tubes containing specific reagents or no reagents at all. Usually the tubes have color-coded tops. Be sure and collect the blood in the blood tube specific for the blood test ordered. Usually each institution's laboratory publishes a manual identifying what colored tube to use for each blood test.	Choose the correct blood tubes to collect the blood in. Tell the patient he or she will feel a needle stick as the needle goes through the skin.	Apply bandage. Have the patient hold pressure to the site for 1 min. The bandage may be removed in 1 hr.
Bleeding time	Measures the time it takes for the platelet plug to form.	Tell the patient a blood pressure cuff is placed above the elbow and pumped up to 40 mm Hg. A puncture is made on a cleaned area of the forearm. A stop watch is started. The wound is blotted with filter paper every 30 sec until all the bleeding has stopped. The time is noted.	Apply bandage.
Urine protein electrophoresis	Performs an electrophoresis on the urine to detect abnormal amounts of protein.	Have the patient void into the toilet. Mark the time. Have the patient collect all urine for the next 24 hr. The container should be kept on ice. Exactly 24 hr after the starting time, have the patient void for the last time and submit the entire 24-hr collection to the laboratory.	No special care after this test is required.
Blood cultures	Detects and identifies microorganisms in the blood. The vein is prepared with betadine and allowed to dry. Do not touch the site. The tops of the blood culture bottles are prepared with betadine and allowed to dry.	Blood culture results are evaluated at 48 and 72 hr. Tell the patient not to expect any final results for 3 to 4 days.	Apply bandage. Have the patient hold pressure to the site for 1 min. The bandage may be removed in 1 hr.

Cultures of Blood, Sputum, Urine, and Stool

Cultures are done to detect infections in the blood, sputum, urine, or stool. When a patient has a fever without an obvious source of infection, all of these specimens are obtained to look for the source of the infection. Table 30–3 describes the procedures for collecting these specimens for culture.

Bone Marrow Biopsy

If the CBC shows abnormal changes, the physician may perform a bone marrow biopsy to see how well the blood cells are being made in the bone marrow. This procedure is also done to diagnose leukemia, a cancer of the white blood cells. Table 30–4 describes the bone marrow biopsy procedure.

Lymphangiogram

A lymphangiogram is done to evaluate the anatomy of the lymphatic vessels and the lymph nodes. Dye is injected into the lymph vessels of the feet or hand, and radiographs are taken as the dye moves up the lymph channels. A lymphangiogram is often done as part of the staging work-up for Hodgkin's disease, a cancer of the lymph nodes. However, with improved diagnostic radiology techniques, often times computed tomography scans can reveal enlarged abdominal lymph nodes and preclude the need for a lymphangiogram, which is a technically difficult procedure for the radiologist to perform. Table 30–4 describes the lymphangiogram procedure.

Spleen Sonogram or Ultrasound

The spleen sonogram is used to estimate the size of the spleen. This test is most often used if a splenectomy

TABLE 30-3
DIAGNOSTIC TESTS FOR EVALUATING THE HEMATOLOGIC AND LYMPHATIC SYSTEMS *Continued*

TEST/STUDY	PURPOSE/PROCEDURE	PATIENT PREPARATION	POSTPROCEDURE NURSING CARE
	Usually there is one anaerobic culture bottle and one aerobic culture bottle. Ten ml of blood are drawn and 5 ml are placed in each culture bottle. Send the specimen to the laboratory immediately.		
Sputum cultures	Detects and identifies microorganisms in the sputum.	Give the patient a sterile cup. Have the patient collect sputum next time he or she coughs. Caution the patient not to collect saliva. Sputum comes from the lungs with coughing. Send the specimen to the laboratory immediately.	No special care after the procedure is required.
Urine cultures	Detects and identifies microorganisms in the urine. The specimen can normally be collected by the patient as described under Patient Preparation in the next column. If the patient is unable to collect the specimen, the physician may request a straight catheterization to collect the specimen. Follow the procedures for catheterizing a patient as described in Chapter 36.	Give the patient wipes and a sterile container. Have the patient clean around the meatus of the urethra. Tell the patient to urinate a small amount into the toilet and stop. Then tell the patient to collect a urine specimen. Send the specimen to the laboratory immediately.	No special care after the procedure is required.
Stool cultures	Detects and identifies microorganisms in the stool.	Have the patient defecate into a clean bedpan or other container. Using a sterile tongue blade, collect a specimen in a sterile container. Send the specimen to the laboratory immediately. Some tests must be done while the specimen is still warm.	No special care after the procedure is required.

CBC, Complete blood count; PT, prothrombin time; PTT, partial thromboplastin time; TIBC, total iron-binding capacity; HbS, Sickle cell hemoglobin; Hb, hemoglobin.
Adapted from Fischbach, F. T. (1992). *A manual of laboratory diagnostic tests* (4th ed.). Philadelphia, J. B. Lippincott.

is planned to be sure that the surgeon knows exactly how big the spleen is. In some blood disorders, the spleen shelters platelets dramatically, reducing the number of these important blood cells that circulate. Although the bone marrow is making plenty of platelets, the spleen is holding them after they are released into circulation. Often times the spleen is several times its normal size, and so a sonogram is done to estimate the size of the spleen for the surgeon. In these cases a splenectomy can be done, which effectively increases the circulating number of platelets because there is no spleen left to hold them. Table 30–4 describes the spleen sonogram procedure.

Spleen Scan

A spleen scan is used to evaluate the size and function of the spleen. A radioactive colloid that is taken up by the spleen is injected into the patient. A single photon emission computed tomography (SPECT) machine measures how much of the radioactive colloid is taken up by the spleen. This scan is sometimes used in the staging work-up for Hodgkin's disease. Table 30–4 describes the spleen scan procedure.

COMMON THERAPEUTIC MEASURES

Treatment of disorders of the hematologic and lymphatic systems is aimed at correcting the underlying problem with medications. Many times the problem can be controlled with medications alone. Blood product transfusions are used to manage the patient's symptoms while the medications are taking effect.

TRANSFUSIONS

Table 30–5 provides an overview of blood components that can be transfused. The policy for administering blood products varies from hospital to hospital. These are some general guidelines.

Typing for Transfusions

There are four major blood groups: A, B, AB, and O. Each letter represents an antigen present on the person's red blood cells. People with type A blood have the A antigen, those with type B blood have the B antigen,

TABLE 30-4

DIAGNOSTIC PROCEDURES FOR EVALUATING THE HEMATOLOGIC AND LYMPHATIC SYSTEMS

TEST/STUDY	PURPOSE/PROCEDURE	PATIENT PREPARATION	POSTPROCEDURE NURSING CARE
Bone marrow biopsy	Used to evaluate how well the bone marrow is making red blood cells, white blood cells, and platelets. The patient is positioned on an examining table according to the location of the bone marrow biopsy. The most common site is the posterior iliac crest, although the anterior crest, sternum, and tibia are also potential sites. The selected site is prepared and draped as for a minor surgical procedure. A local anesthetic is injected. A Jamshidi needle is forced into the bone marrow. Bone marrow fluid is aspirated and a core biopsy taken through and with the Jamshidi needle. The needle is removed and a pressure dressing applied to the site. A laboratory technician must be present during the procedure to immediately fix and stain the specimens. Sometimes a short-acting anesthetic such as midazolam (Versed) is used to sedate the patient during the procedure.	Explain the purpose and procedure to the patient. A permit must be signed. No fasting is necessary. Some local discomfort may be experienced as the local anesthesia is injected before the Jamshidi needle is inserted. The patient usually feels pressure as the Jamshidi needle is inserted into the bone and a momentary sharp pain down the leg as the bone marrow fluid is aspirated. The procedure takes approximately 30 min.	If intravenous sedation is used, monitor the patient's pulse, blood pressure, respirations, and pulse oximetry every 15 min until recovery, which usually is within 30 min. The pressure dressing can be removed in 2 hr.
Lymphangiogram (LAG)	Evaluates the anatomy of the lymphatic vessels and nodes. The patient is taken to Diagnostic Radiology, where a 1–2 inch incision is made on the dorsum of each foot. The lymphatic vessels are cannulated and dye is injected. Several radiographs are taken as the dye moves up the extremity. The patient returns to Diagnostic Radiology 12–24 hr later for more radiographs of the lymph nodes and higher lymphatic channels.	Explain the purpose and procedure to the patient. A permit must be signed. No fasting is necessary. Some local discomfort may be experienced as the local anesthesia is injected to numb the top of the foot. Incisions may be blue stained from the dye. The procedure takes approximately 3 hr. The patient returns to Diagnostic Radiology 12–24 hr later for more radiographs.	Check the patient's vital signs every 4 hr for 48 hr. Monitor for an allergic reaction to the dye. Keep the incisions clean and dry after the procedure. The doctor may order the legs be elevated. Stitches may be in place that should be removed in 5 to 7 days.
Spleen sonogram or ultrasound	Used to estimate the size of the spleen. The patient lies on the back in the Ultrasound Department. A gel or lubricant that acts as a conductor is applied to the left upper quadrant of the abdomen. A technician moves a hand-held transducer over the area while watching a screen and recording the ultrasound echoes from the spleen.	Explain the purpose and procedure to the patient. The patient should fast from food 12 hr before the examination. Water is permitted. The procedure will take approximately 30–45 min.	Arrange for a meal or a snack as the patient has been fasting.
Spleen scan	Used to evaluate the size as well as the function of the spleen. In the Nuclear Medicine Department, a radioactive dye is injected into a vein. The amount of dye taken up by the spleen is measured by a machine 20–60 min after the dye is injected.	Explain the purpose and procedure to the patient. Report allergy to contrast media to radiologist. No fasting is necessary. An intravenous line must be in place to inject the dye. The procedure takes approximately 80 min.	No special care after the procedure is required.

Adapted from Fischbach, F. T. (1992). *A manual of laboratory diagnostic tests* (4th ed.). Philadelphia: J. B. Lippincott.

TABLE 30-5
BLOOD COMPONENTS THAT CAN BE TRANSFUSED

COMPONENT BLOOD	INDICATION	TYPE AND CROSS	USUAL AMOUNT IN ONE UNIT	INFUSION RATE	FILTER?
Packed red blood cells	Symptoms from a low hematocrit or hemoglobin such as shortness of breath, tachycardia, decreased blood pressure, chest pain, light-headedness, or fatigue	Yes	250–300 ml/unit	2–4 hr/unit	Yes
Platelets	Bleeding from thrombocytopenia	No, except first time	60 ml/pack; usually four to six packs are pooled together for a platelet transfusion	As quickly as the patient can tolerate	Yes
Fresh frozen plasma	Clotting deficiencies, hemophilia, for rapid reversal of warfarin (Coumadin), with massive red blood cell transfusions	No	200–280 ml/unit	10 ml/min	Yes
Cryoprecipitate	Hemophilia A	No	10 ml/bag; usually 10 bags are pooled together for a transfusion	10 ml/min	Yes

those with type AB blood have both the A and the B antigen, and people with type O blood have neither the A nor the B antigen. In addition to the ABO identification, the presence of the Rh antigen must also be determined. Persons who are Rh positive have the antigen, and those who are Rh negative do not have the antigen. People with any of these antigens cannot be given blood containing a different antigen. Therefore, patients with Type O negative blood are considered universal donors because their blood contains none of the A, B, or Rh antigens and can be given safely to anyone. Patients with AB positive blood are considered universal recipients because their blood contains the A, B, and Rh antigens. They can safely receive any type of blood. However, blood banks usually match the type of blood to be transfused with that of the patient who needs a transfusion.

Transfusions of Whole Blood

Whole blood transfusions are rarely done today because individual blood components are readily available to treat specific deficiencies.

Transfusions of Packed Red Blood Cells

Because of the risk of infection from transfusions, such as from hepatitis or human immunodeficiency virus (HIV), red blood cells are no longer given automatically when the patient's hematocrit falls below a certain number. Instead, the patient is evaluated clinically and a decision is made with the patient whether to administer a blood transfusion. Symptoms of a low hematocrit that would prompt a blood transfusion include shortness of breath, tachycardia, decreased blood pressure, chest pain, lightheadedness, and fatigue.

The patient should be counseled by the physician, and a consent form must be signed before any blood transfusion. Also before the transfusion, the patient's blood must be typed by the blood bank to determine the ABO group and whether the Rh factor is present. Then the patient's blood must be cross-matched or mixed with a small amount of the donated blood to assess compatibility. A blood tube for type and cross-match must be drawn from the patient each time the patient receives a blood transfusion.

The nurse must be familiar with and follow the institution's policies in relation to blood administration. Key points when administering blood transfusions are listed here.

1. To prepare the transfusion, select the appropriate equipment.
   A. Venipuncture equipment, including a minimum size 20-gauge cannula, preferably an 18 gauge. A large cannula is necessary to prevent lysis of cells passing through the cannula.
   B. Normal saline intravenous fluid.
   C. Blood transfusion set with built-in filter to screen for clots.
   D. Bag containing blood requested for the patient.
2. Start an intravenous infusion of normal saline using an 18-gauge needle if possible.
3. Have two licensed people check the blood when it arrives on the nursing unit.
4. Take and record the patient's vital signs.

5. Begin the transfusion within 30 minutes from the time the blood is picked up from the blood bank.
6. Piggyback the blood into the normal saline line.
7. Stay with the patient for 5 to 10 minutes after the blood is started to detect any immediate untoward reactions such as back pain, fever, chills, or decreased blood pressure that might signal a hemolytic reaction to the blood and require discontinuance of the transfusion.
8. Monitor vital signs during the transfusion according to agency policy.
9. Each unit of blood is usually 250 to 300 ml, and is administered over 2 to 4 hours.
10. When the transfusion is completed, document the procedure, the patient's vital signs, and how the procedure was tolerated.
11. Subsequent units of blood can be hung immediately, using the same blood tubing for several units if agency policy permits.

Autologous Red Blood Transfusions

One way to prevent the risks of infection and reactions with blood transfusions is to collect the patient's own blood before a planned procedure and then transfuse the patient's own blood if necessary. This method of collecting the patient's blood in advance is preferred if a lot of bleeding is expected with the procedure, especially if the patient has a rare blood type or has religious beliefs against receiving donated blood. The patient donates blood several times before the planned procedure. The blood is stored by the blood bank and is reinfused into the patient if needed intraoperatively or postoperatively.

Transfusions of White Blood Cells

White blood cell transfusions are possible but do not have any effect on a patient's white blood cell count. Also, white blood cell transfusions do not decrease the number or the severity of infections in patients. Thus, white blood cell transfusions are not performed routinely any more.

Transfusions of Platelets

Like red blood cell transfusions, platelet transfusions are not administered automatically when the patient's platelet count falls below a certain number. However, the lower a patient's platelet count, the greater the chance of bleeding. Generally, when the patient's platelet count falls below 20,000, platelets are administered. If the platelet count is higher than 20,000, platelets are usually not given unless the patient is actively bleeding. The most common sites of bleeding are the gastrointestinal tract, the lungs, and the brain.

If platelets are ordered by the physician, a one-time type and cross-match must be done by the blood bank. If the patient has been previously typed and cross-matched for a red blood cell transfusion, the blood bank can usually use this information to provide platelets. Platelets are commonly ordered in packs of four or six. Each pack contains approximately 60 ml.

The patient should be counseled by the physician, and a consent form should be signed before the platelet transfusion. Key points when administering platelets are as follows:

1. Request the platelets from the blood bank; send a sample of the patient's blood for type and cross match if this is the first platelet transfusion.
2. Start an intravenous infusion of normal saline using at least a 24-gauge cannula.
3. Have two licensed people check the platelets before administration, and prepare to administer the platelets as soon as they arrive on the nursing unit.
4. Take and record the patient's vital signs.
5. Use filtered blood transfusion tubing to deliver the platelets, which are piggybacked into the normal saline.
6. Stay with the patient 5 to 10 minutes to observe for any untoward reactions; then monitor vital signs per agency policy.
7. Platelets can be administered as fast as the patient can tolerate.
8. When the transfusion is completed, document the procedure, the patient's vital signs, and how well the procedure was tolerated.

If platelets are ordered to prevent bleeding before a procedure such as a lumbar puncture or an endoscopy, the platelets should be administered immediately before the procedure. There is no indication to "get the platelets in early" for a procedure scheduled later in the day. Instead, plan with the doctor doing the procedure to administer the platelets just before the procedure begins.

Transfusions of Plasma

Plasma is separated from whole blood by centrifugation and quickly frozen. Thus, when transfusing plasma, usually fresh frozen plasma, or FFP, is ordered. Fresh frozen plasma contains all the clotting factors as well as the plasma proteins. Cryoprecipitate, which contains only fibrinogen and factor VIII, can be further separated out from plasma and administered alone if indicated.

Reactions to Blood Transfusion

Four main types of transfusion reactions can occur with transfusions of blood or any of the blood components: hemolytic, allergic, febrile, and circulatory overload. If the patient experiences back or chest pain, fever, chills, a decreased blood pressure, urticaria, wheezing, dyspnea, or coughing during the transfusion, blood transfusion reaction procedures should be taken. The transfusion must be stopped immediately and the intravenous line kept open with the normal saline. The nurse calls for help and prepares to immediately administer oxygen, epinephrine, antipyretics, hydrocortisone sodium succinate (Solu-Cortef), furosemide (Lasix), or a combination of these as prescribed by the physician.

The unused portion of the blood is saved for the blood bank to evaluate. Blood and urine samples from the patient are taken for evaluation. Usually each institution has a blood transfusion reaction form that needs to be completed. Table 30–6 outlines the types and signs and symptoms for the different blood transfusion reactions.

COLONY STIMULATING FACTORS

Researchers have developed drugs that stimulate the bone marrow to produce more red blood cells and white blood cells. Soon drugs to raise the platelet count will also be available. Epoetin alfa (Epogen) stimulates the bone marrow to produce more red blood cells. This drug is predominantly used by hemodialysis patients who are chronically anemic as a result of dialysis. Two drugs, sargramostim (GM-CSF [granulocyte macrophage colony-stimulating factor]) and filgrastim (G-CSF [granulocyte colony-stimulating factor]), stimulate the bone marrow to produce more white blood cells. These drugs are very important to people with cancer who often experience low white blood cell counts as a side effect of chemotherapy. The colony-stimulating factors bring patients' white blood cell counts up quickly, lowering the risk of life-threatening infections. Table 30–7 describes the nursing care of patients receiving these drugs.

TABLE 30–6

SIGNS AND SYMPTOMS OF BLOOD TRANSFUSION REACTIONS

GENERAL

Fever (rise of 1°C or 2°F)

- Chills
- Muscle aches, pain
- Back pain
- Chest pain
- Headache
- Heat at site of infusion or along vein

NERVOUS SYSTEM

- Apprehension, sense of impending doom
- Tingling, numbness

RESPIRATORY SYSTEM

- Respiratory rate
  - Tachypnea
  - Apnea
- Dyspnea
- Cough
- Wheezing
- Rales

GASTROINTESTINAL SYSTEM

- Nausea
- Vomiting
- Pain, abdominal cramping
- Diarrhea (may be bloody)

CARDIOVASCULAR SYSTEM

- Heart rate
  - Bradycardia
  - Tachycardia
- Blood pressure
  - Hypotension, shock
  - Hypertension
- Peripheral circulation
  - Color cyanosis, facial flushing
  - Temperature: cool/clammy, hot/flushed/dry
  - Edema
- Bleeding
  - Generalized (DIC)
  - Oozing at surgical site

RENAL SYSTEM

- Changes in urine volume
  - Oliguria, anuria
  - Renal failure
- Changes in urine color
  - Dark, concentrated
  - Shades of red, brown, amber
  - May indicate the presence in urine of red blood cells (hematuria) or of free hemoglobin (hemoglobinuria)

INTEGUMENTARY SYSTEM

- Rashes, hives (urticaria), swelling
- Itching
- Diaphoresis

From Black, J. M., & Matassarin-Jacobs, E. (1993). *Luckmann and Sorensen's medical-surgical nursing: A psychophysiologic approach* (4th ed., p. 1397). Philadelphia: W. B. Saunders.

DISORDERS OF THE HEMATOLOGIC AND LYMPHATIC SYSTEMS

RED BLOOD CELL DISORDERS

Patients who have red blood cell disorders have either too many or too few red blood cells. Having too few red blood cells, or being anemic, is more common. Patients who are anemic can have either a lack of red blood cells or a lack of hemoglobin in the blood. Anemia can result from an acute loss of blood because too few red blood cells are being made or because too many red blood cells are being destroyed by the body. Anemia can be a primary disease or a symptom of another disease, such as gastric ulcers or cancer. The different types of the red blood disorders are described next.

Types of Red Blood Cell Disorders

POLYCYTHEMIA VERA. Polycythemia vera is a condition in which there are too many red blood cells. The increased number of red blood cells makes the blood more viscous, or thicker, so that it does not freely circulate through the body. Symptoms of polycythemia vera include headache, dizziness, ringing in the ears, and blurred vision. Patients with this disorder may have a ruddy (reddish) complexion. Treatment for polycythemia vera is to have a unit of blood phlebotomized, or taken off, to keep the patient's hematocrit normal. The procedure is usually done in the blood bank by a trained technician. A large-bore intravenous needle is inserted into the patient's antecubital vein, and one unit of blood is taken off. This is the same procedure used when a person goes to the blood bank to donate blood. However, the blood taken from the patient with polycythemia vera cannot be given to anyone else.

IRON DEFICIENCY ANEMIA. Iron deficiency anemia results from a diet that is too low in iron or from the body not absorbing enough iron from the gastrointestinal tract. As a result, the body does not have enough iron to make adequate amounts of hemoglobin. Symptoms of this anemia include fatigue and pallor. In severe cases, patients may be tachycardic, hypotensive, TILT positive, and dyspneic. Patients with iron deficiency anemia have a low serum iron level, a low ferritin level, and a high total iron binding capacity. Table 30–1 lists normal laboratory values for these tests. Doctors treat iron deficiency anemia by prescribing iron supplements and encouraging the patient to eat a diet high in iron.

TABLE 30–7

DRUGS USED TO TREAT DISORDERS OF THE HEMATOLOGIC SYSTEM

DRUGS	USE/ACTION	SIDE EFFECTS	NURSING INTERVENTIONS
Epoetin alfa, e.g., Epogen	Stimulates the bone marrow to produce red blood cells	Hypertension, headache, arthralgias	May be given by intravenous or subcutaneous injection. Patient is usually treated three times per week until the hematocrit is 30–33.
Colony-stimulating factor, e.g., G-CSF (Neupogen), GM-CSF	Stimulates the bone marrow to produce white blood cells	Bone pain	Teach the patient how to give subcutaneous injections. Generally the patient is treated until the absolute neutrophil count is >10,000. Usually the patient has a complete blood count checked three times a week to follow the white blood cell count.
Corticosteroids, e.g., dexamethasone (Decadron), methylprednisolone (Solu-Medrol), prednisone, prednisolone, hydrocortisone (Solu-Cortef)	Immunosuppressive	Stomach irritation	Give these drugs with meals. An H_2-receptor antagonist such as ranitidine (Zantac) may be prescribed to decrease gastric acid production. If the patient takes these drugs for an extended period of time, the drug should not be stopped abruptly. Instead, the drug dose should be gradually decreased over time under a physician's direction.
Ferrous sulfate, e.g., Feosol, Fer-In-Sol	Iron replacement	Constipation, black stools, mild nausea	Have the patient take the drug with food but not with milk, eggs, or caffeinated drinks because the milk and caffeine inhibit drug absorption. If the patient is taking liquid iron, dilute the drug and administer through a straw to prevent the drug from staining the teeth.
Iron dextran	Iron replacement	Hypersensitivity reactions, brown skin discoloration at the injection site	Test dose before starting treatment. Give intramuscular injections only in the upper, outer quadrant of the buttock using the Z-track technique.*
Vitamin B_{12} (cyanocobalamin)	Vitamin B_{12} replacement		Intramuscular injection. Must be given every month the rest of the person's life for pernicious anemia.

* Z-track technique—Firmly pull the skin of the upper, outer quadrant of the buttocks laterally. Insert the needle. Withdraw the plunger to check that no blood enters the syringe. Slowly inject the medication. Remove the needle and let go of the skin. Massage the area.

From Govoni, L. E., & Hayes, J. E. (1988). *Drugs and nursing implication* (6th ed.). East Norwalk, CT: Appleton & Lange.

PHARMACOLOGY CAPSULE

Iron preparations may cause diarrhea or constipation and cause the stool to darken. Antacids interfere with iron absorption.

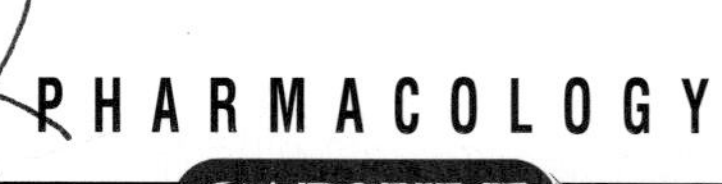

Patients who have pernicious anemia must take vitamin B_{12} injections throughout life.

Table 30–7 describes the nursing care of the patient taking iron supplements. Nurses caring for patients with iron deficiency anemia can suggest incorporating foods high in iron into the diet. Foods that are rich in iron include meats, fish, poultry, dried fruits, dark green vegetables, beans, and iron-enriched whole grain breads and cereals.

PERNICIOUS ANEMIA (VITAMIN B_{12} ANEMIA). Pernicious anemia occurs when a patient does not absorb vitamin B_{12}. The patient may lack intrinsic factor, a substance secreted by the gastric glands, which is essential for B_{12} absorption. Or the patient may have had a gastrectomy, in which part or all of the stomach was surgically removed, so the patient cannot make intrinsic factor and therefore cannot absorb vitamin B_{12}. In addition to the fatigue and pallor commonly seen with all anemias, symptoms of pernicious anemia characteristically include weakness, a sore tongue, and numbness of the hands or feet. Doctors treat pernicious anemia by prescribing a monthly intramuscular injection of vitamin B_{12} (cyanocobalamin). Patients must have these monthly injections for the rest of their lives. Table 30–7 describes the nursing care of patients receiving vitamin B_{12}.

ACQUIRED HEMOLYTIC ANEMIA. Different situations can cause a person's red blood cells to be abnormally destroyed, resulting in an acquired hemolytic anemia. This type of anemia can happen with many different diseases, such as viral infections, cancer, and autoimmune disorders such as lupus. Certain drugs, such as penicillin, can also cause an acquired hemolytic anemia. Hemolytic anemia of the newborn can occur after delivery if the mother and the baby have different blood types. Blood transfusions can cause an acquired hemolytic anemia if lymphocytes in the transfused blood make antibodies against the person receiving the blood. Sometimes people develop an acquired hemolytic anemia for no identifiable reason. Symptoms of acquired hemolytic anemia include fatigue and pallor. Patients may appear jaundiced. If the anemia is severe, tachycardia, hypotension, and dyspnea may be present. Patients with acquired hemolytic anemia have a positive result on a direct Coombs's antiglobulin blood test. Treatment of this type of anemia includes removing the cause, if possible, and administering corticosteroids to the patient. Blood transfusions may be needed. The patient usually recovers in a few days to weeks.

APLASTIC ANEMIA. Aplastic anemia results from the complete failure of the bone marrow. The name *aplastic anemia* is misleading because patients with this condition have more than an extremely low red blood cell count; they also have extremely low white blood cell counts and platelet counts because their bone marrow is not making any of these cells. Certain drugs such as streptomycin or chloramphenicol can cause bone marrow failure as can exposure to toxic chemicals or radiation. Sometimes people develop an aplastic anemia for no identifiable reason. Symptoms of aplastic anemia may include fatigue, weakness, tachycardia, dyspnea, susceptibility to infection, petechiae or purpura, gingival bleeding (from the gums), and epistaxis (nose bleeds). Patients with aplastic anemia have very low numbers on their CBCs. Their bone marrow biopsy results show decreased numbers of blood-making cells. The treatment for aplastic anemia is to eliminate the cause if possible. Transfusions are given to replace red blood cells and platelets. Antibiotics are given to prevent or treat infections. Corticosteroids may also be given. If the patient's bone marrow does not recover on its own, a bone marrow transplant may be considered if a matching donor can be found. The patient with aplastic anemia is critically ill and requires intensive nursing support similar to the care provided to a patient with acute leukemia who is undergoing chemotherapy.

SICKLE CELL ANEMIA. Sickle cell anemia is a genetic disease in which the red blood cells can become sickle shaped when oxygen levels in the red blood cells decrease (Fig. 30–3). These abnormally shaped, sickled cells become stuck in the small capillaries of the body, obstructing blood flow. The sickled blood cells are much more fragile than normal red blood cells. As a result, the sickled cells are easily ruptured when passing through small capillaries, which results in a chronic anemia. Symptoms of sickle cell anemia include persistently low red blood cell counts, fatigue, jaundice, and chronic leg ulcers. The chronically low red blood cell counts can cause the heart to enlarge (cardiomegaly) and beat faster in an attempt to oxygenate the body's tissues. Patients with sickle cell anemia periodically experience a sickle cell crisis, during which the abnormally shaped sickled cells become stuck in larger blood vessels of the body, obstructing blood flow and causing severe pain. Sickle cell disease occurs almost exclusively in blacks. Eight percent of blacks carry the genetic trait for sickle cell. Because sickle cell is carried on a recessive gene, a

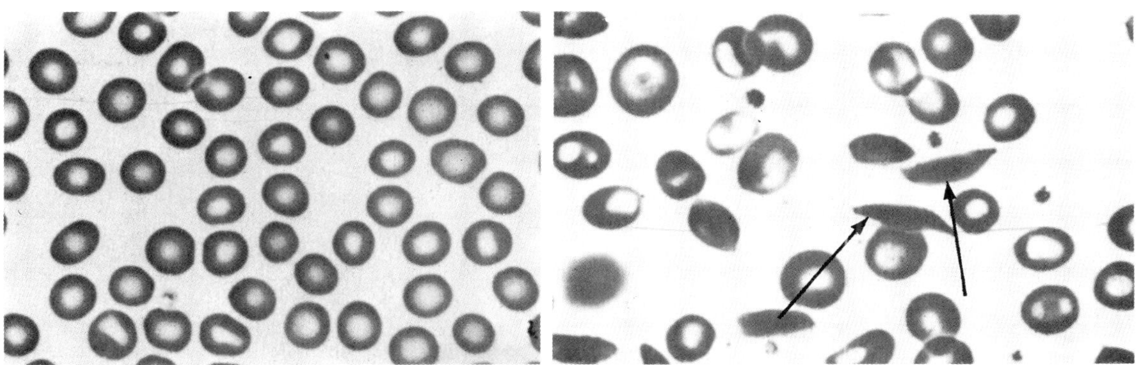

FIGURE 30-3
Comparison of normal red blood cells (*A*) and sickled cells (*B*) (magnification ×875). Sickled cells in *B* are indicated by arrows. (From Henry, J. B. [1991]. *Clinical diagnosis and management* [18th ed.]. Philadelphia: W. B. Saunders.)

person must inherit the gene from both the mother and the father to actually have the disease. Table 30–8 describes the risk of passing the sickle cell trait or disease on to children. The diagnosis of sickle cell disease is made using a hemoglobin S (Sickledex) blood test and a hemoglobin electrophoresis. Table 30–1 lists normal laboratory values for these two tests. Newborn screening for sickle cell disease can be done to identify infants with the disease and to educate parents about the disease and prevention of crises. Unfortunately, this screening is not required in every state.

Signs and Symptoms. A variety of stressors can trigger a sickle cell crisis. They include dehydration, infection, overexertion, cold weather changes, alcohol consumption, and smoking. Symptoms of a sickle cell crisis include severe pain, fever, and blocking of blood vessels by sickled cells. Symptoms vary depending on where circulation is blocked by the sickled red blood cells. Circulation is most commonly obstructed to the chest, abdomen, bones, joints, bone marrow, brain, or penis (called priapism) in a sickle cell crisis.

TABLE 30–8

RISK OF PASSING THE SICKLE CELL TRAIT OR DISEASE TO CHILDREN

		Parent with trait	
		X	X′
Healthy parent	X	X X	X′ X
	Y	X Y	X′ Y
	50% healthy child 50% chance of child with trait		
		Parent with trait	
		X	X′
Parent with disease	X′	X X′	X′ X′
	Y′	X Y′	X′ Y′
	50% chance of child with trait 50% chance of child with disease		
		Parent with trait	
		X	X′
Parent with trait	X	X X	X′ X
	Y′	X Y′	X′ Y′
	25% chance of healthy child 50% chance of child with trait 25% chance of child with disease		
		Parent with disease	
		X′	X′
Parent with disease	X′	X′ X′	X′ X′
	Y′	X′ Y′	X′ Y′
	100% chance child will have disease		

NOTE: The sickle cell trait (′) can be carried on either the X or the Y chromosome.

Medical Diagnosis. Patients with known sickle cell disease who come to the hospital in severe pain are suspected of being in crisis. There is no test to determine that a patient is in sickle cell crisis. Rather, doctors use clinical judgment to make the diagnosis. Crises can last anywhere from 1 to 10 days. Some patients experience crises every few weeks, whereas others can go months in between painful episodes. Radiographs and scans of the painful area are usually taken to look for bleeding.

Medical Treatment. There is no cure for sickle cell disease. Medical treatment for patients experiencing a sickle cell crisis is symptomatic. The physician usually prescribes intravenous fluids and pain medication. Aggressive intravenous hydration helps the kidneys clear metabolic wastes from ruptured red blood cells. Intravenous meperidine hydrochloride (Demerol) is commonly prescribed for pain relief. Patients with sickle cell disease can become addicted to narcotics, so pain needs to be carefully assessed. Usually physicians try to quickly switch the patient from intravenous narcotics to oral narcotics to nonnarcotic pain relievers as the crisis resolves so that the patient does not become addicted. However, pain can be very severe, and the patient deserves to have pain relief during these episodes even if they last for several days. Red blood cell transfusions may be prescribed to correct the anemia and help the body oxygenate tissues. Although oxygen therapy is often prescribed, it is of little benefit in reversing the crisis.

NURSING CARE OF THE PATIENT IN SICKLE CELL CRISIS

Because of the pathophysiology of the disease, patients in sickle cell crisis have specialized needs beyond treatment of simple anemia. These patients can require frequent hospitalizations, depending on the frequency and severity of their crises. A consistent nursing care plan is essential in caring for them (see Care Plan: The Patient in Sickle Cell Crisis).

Assessment. The nurse obtains a complete description of the pain that the patient in sickle cell crisis is experiencing. As discussed in Chapter 16, this includes the location, intensity, duration, and precipitating events. Vital signs are obtained every 4 hours. The nurse is especially alert for a fever, which may indicate an infection that precipitated the crisis. Any symptoms of an infection, such as abnormal breath sounds, cough, sore throat, diarrhea, skin lesions, or dysuria, are investigated as described in the Nursing Assessment section of this chapter. The patient is also assessed for signs and symptoms of dehydration, such as concentrated urine, low blood pressure, or poor skin turgor, which may have precipitated the crisis.

Nursing Diagnosis. Nursing diagnoses for the patient in a sickle cell crisis may include the following:

- Acute **Pain** related to sickle cell crisis
- **Anxiety** related to pain and hospitalization

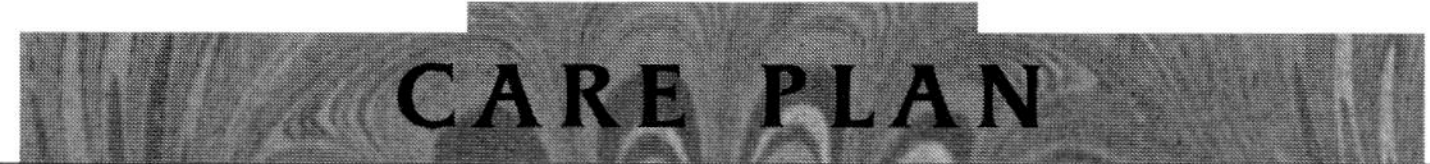

CARE PLAN

The Patient in Sickle Cell Crisis

ASSESSMENT

Health History: Miss Olivia Smith is a 22-year-old African American who was diagnosed with sickle cell anemia 7 years ago. She is small and appears younger than her stated age. She was admitted through the emergency department with chest pain and dyspnea. She reports no sensory or motor impairments. She works as an assistant in a daycare center for children. No unusual stressors are identified at this time, but she does take children outdoors to play when environmental temperature is 90°F or hotter. She does not smoke but has a few beers if socializing on weekends. Miss Smith lives with her mother, who has accompanied her to the hospital.

Physical Examination: Vital signs: temperature, 99.4°F orally; pulse, 110; respirations, 28; blood pressure, 136/92. Patient is dyspneic and anxious. Breath sounds are diminished on the left side. Oral mucous membranes are dry and sticky. Arms and legs are disproportionately long. Joints are enlarged.

NURSING DIAGNOSIS	GOALS AND OUTCOME CRITERIA	INTERVENTIONS
Acute pain related to sickle cell crisis.	The patient will state that she is comfortable and will appear more relaxed.	Give prescribed analgesics and assess effects.
Anxiety related to pain and hospitalization.	The patient will have less anxiety as evidenced by calm demeanor and verbalizations.	Be calm, offer reassurance, and respond promptly to requests. Encourage mother to stay with her until she is more comfortable.
Impaired gas exchange related to altered oxygen-carrying capacity of blood cells, possible pulmonary embolus.	The patient's respiratory status will improve as evidenced by rate of 12–20, no dyspnea, decreased restlessness.	Elevate head of bed. Administer oxygen as ordered. Allow rest until condition improves. Monitor vital signs for increasing hypoxia: increased restlessness, dyspnea, confusion. Report signs and symptoms of worsening condition to physician.
Fluid volume deficit related to inadequate fluid intake or excess loss due to activity in extreme heat.	The patient will maintain adequate hydration as evidenced by good tissue turgor, moist mucous membranes, urine specific gravity of 1.01–1.03.	Administer intravenous fluids as ordered. Monitor fluid intake and output. Weigh daily.
High risk for injury related to effects of anemia.	The patient will remain free of injury during hospitalization.	When patient is able to resume activities, assist with standing and walking in case she becomes dizzy. Have her move slowly from lying to sitting to standing positions. Allow for rest between activities. Provide extra blankets if chilly. Administer blood transfusions as prescribed.
Knowledge deficit of disease process and self-care.	The patient will acknowledge aspects of self-care, including measures to reduce the risk of complications.	Assess what patient knows, reinforce, and provide additional verbal and written information. Include: 1. Pathophysiology 2. Common stressors that can trigger crisis: infection, dehydration, hypoxia, high altitudes, strenuous activity 3. Avoidance of smoking because it constricts blood vessels 4. Need to drink 4–6 liters of nonalcoholic beverages daily to reduce risk of thrombosis

Continued on following page

The Patient in Sickle Cell Crisis *(Continued)*

NURSING DIAGNOSIS	GOALS AND OUTCOME CRITERIA	INTERVENTIONS
		5. Avoidance of travel to high altitudes where there is less oxygen 6. Importance of genetic counseling if she is interested in having children

- **Knowledge Deficit** related to the disease process
- **High Risk for Fluid Volume Deficit** related to inadequate intake or excess loss of fluids
- **High Risk for Injury** related to anemia

Goals. Goals of nursing care are pain relief, reduced anxiety, knowledge of disease process to resume self-care, adequate hydration, and absence of injury.

Interventions

Pain. Pain medications are given as prescribed. Usually intravenous meperidine hydrochloride (Demerol) is prescribed initially. Because the pain from a sickle cell crisis is so severe, patients can be medicated every hour when first admitted. Patient-controlled analgesia, or PCA, is an excellent way of administering the pain medication. The nurse closely monitors the patient's pain level. Keeping a flow sheet of patient reports of pain on a 10-point scale can be helpful, especially as different nurses care for the patient throughout the day. A 0 represents no pain, and a 10 represents the worst pain a patient ever experienced. The patient's report of pain coupled with the amount of pain medication he or she is receiving can guide the nurse and physician as to the appropriate type and amount of pain medication. A detailed discussion of pain management is presented in Chapter 16.

Anxiety. Sickle cell crises that require hospitalization can be extremely frightening to a patient especially because of the severe pain that accompanies these crises. Patients fear not obtaining adequate pain relief. The unpredictability of both the timing and the severity of the crisis can be especially frustrating to patients. The nurse provides consistent care to the patient in sickle cell crisis to establish a trusting relationship. Listening closely to the patient helps to establish this trust, thereby reducing patient anxiety. Once the patient is discharged from the hospital, he or she can contact one of the many support groups available for patients with sickle cell disease and their families. Patients should be encouraged to attend so that they can better cope with this chronic disease.

Knowledge Deficit. When patients are not in crisis, they should be taught about their disease. The nurse can help patients identify stressors that bring on a crisis and help patients take actions to avoid these stressors. Encouraging patients not to smoke or drink alcoholic beverages excessively is very important, as these are two common stressors that can bring on a crisis. Traveling to high altitudes where there is less oxygen can also bring on an attack, and patients should be warned about vacationing at high altitudes. Patients are encouraged to drink 4 to 6 liters of nonalcoholic fluids a day to maintain adequate hydration. Regular medical follow-up is of paramount importance in keeping the patient with sickle cell disease out of a crisis. Genetic counseling can be done for people with the trait and with the disease to inform them of the risk of passing the trait or disease on to their children. With this information, some people choose not to have their own children and risk passing on this painful, life-threatening disease. The National Association of Sickle Cell Disease (3345 Wilshire Boulevard, Suite 1106, Los Angeles, CA 90010, 1-213-736-5455) provides excellent free literature on sickle cell disease and can help locate groups in specific regions of the country.

Fluid Volume Deficit. The nurse administers intravenous fluids as prescribed and keeps accurate intake and output records. Daily weights are measured to assess gross fluid status. The patient is encouraged to drink 4 to 6 liters of fluids each day to maintain adequate hydration.

High Risk for Injury. The primary treatment for anemia is red blood cell transfusions. Nursing considerations in administering blood transfusions have been outlined previously in this chapter. Other precautions that should be taken when patients are anemic are outlined in Table 30–9.

Evaluation

Effective nursing interventions are determined by patient's statement of pain relief, patient's statement of reduced anxiety and calm manner, patient's verbalization of disease process and implications for self-care, consistent intake of 4 to 6 liters of fluids daily, and absence of dizziness resulting in injury.

WHITE BLOOD CELL DISORDERS

The primary white blood cell disorders are the leukemias. Leukemia is a cancer of the white blood cells in which the bone marrow produces too many immature

TABLE 30-9

SPECIFIC NURSING ACTIONS FOR THE PATIENT WHO IS ANEMIC*

1. Assist the patient with standing and moving around, as he or she can become dizzy. Move the patient slowly from lying to sitting to standing.
2. Allow for rest periods between heavy activities, as the anemic patient can tire easily.
3. Elevate the patient's head on pillows if shortness of breath occurs.
4. Provide extra blankets for these patients, as many times they feel chilly.
5. Administer oxygen as prescribed by the physician.
6. Administer blood transfusions as prescribed by the physician.

* For the patient with a hematocrit less than 30 or a hemoglobin less than 10 or both.

white blood cells. These nonfunctioning, immature white blood cells leave the patient unprotected against microorganisms and at a great risk for life-threatening infections. According to American Cancer Society statistics, an estimated 28,600 cases of leukemia will be diagnosed in 1994, accounting for 2% of all new cases of cancer diagnosed in this year. Although no cause is identified for most cases, factors that may be associated with the development of leukemia are exposure to large doses of radiation therapy or exposure to certain chemicals.

Chronic Leukemia

There are two types of chronic leukemia: chronic myelogenous leukemia (CML) and chronic lymphocytic leukemia (CLL). These forms of leukemia occur most often in adults. In both types of chronic leukemia, the patient's white blood cell count slowly goes up over months or years. The disease can usually be controlled with oral chemotherapy agents for many years. Table 30–10 describes combinations of drugs commonly used to treat the chronic leukemias. Table 30–11 describes possible side effects of the drugs. Patients being treated for chronic leukemia generally feel good. They do not lose their hair and usually do not experience nausea. Most of these patients can continue to work. The average life expectancy for a patient with CML is 4 years depending on the stage of the disease. The average life expectancy for a patient with CLL is 6 years, again depending on the stage of the disease upon diagnosis. After this time, the chronic leukemias often transform into an acute leukemia that is very difficult to treat.

TABLE 30-10

COMBINATIONS OF DRUGS USED TO TREAT LEUKEMIA AND LYMPHOMA

DISEASE	DRUG(S)
Leukemias	
Chronic myelogenous leukemia (CML)	Busulfan
Chronic lymphocytic leukemia (CLL)	Chlorambucil Prednisone
Acute myelogenous leukemia (AML)	Hydrea Ara-C and daunorubicin
Acute lymphocytic leukemia (ALL)	*Induction Chemotherapy:* Daunorubicin Vincristine Prednisone L-Asparaginase *Consolidation Chemotherapy:* Daunorubicin Vincristine Prednisone L-Asparaginase Cytarabine Methotrexate *Maintenance Chemotherapy:* Methotrexate 6-Mercaptopurine
Lymphomas	
Hodgkin's disease	MOPP (mustine, Oncovin, procarbazine, prednisone) ABVD (Adriamycin, bleomycin, vincristine, dacarbazine) Hybrid MOPP/ABD (mustine, Oncovin, procarbazine, prednisone, Adriamycin, bleomycin, dacarbazine)
Non-Hodgkin's lymphoma	CHOP (cyclophosphamide, hydroxydaunomycin or doxorubicin hydrochloride, Oncovin, prednisone) MACOP-B (methotrexate, Adriamycin, cyclophosphamide, Oncovin, prednisone, bleomycin) ProMACE CYTABOM (prednisone, methotrexate, Adriamycin, cyclophosphamide, etoposide; cytarabine, bleomycin, Oncovin, mechlorethamine)

TABLE 30-11
DRUGS COMMONLY USED TO TREAT LEUKEMIA AND LYMPHOMA

DRUG	USE/ACTION	HOW GIVEN	SIDE EFFECTS	NURSING INTERVENTIONS
L-Asparaginase (Elspar)	Miscellaneous: enzyme	Intramuscularly (IM) or intravenously (IV)	Fever, fatigue, abnormal liver function	Each time the patient receives the drug, monitor for an allergic reaction by taking vital signs every 15 min for 1 hr; the incidence of allergic reactions is higher when drug is given IV
Bleomycin sulfate (Blenoxane)	Antibiotic	IV	Fever, chills, skin changes, decreased pulmonary function test results	Test dose the patient before first dose
Busulfan (Myleran)	Alkylating	PO	Myelosuppression, pulmonary fibrosis	
Chlorambucil (Leukeran)	Alkylating	PO	Nausea, myelosuppression, secondary malignancies	
Cyclophosphamide (Cytoxan)	Alkylating	PO or IV	Myelosuppression, nausea, alopecia, nasal stuffiness, bladder inflammation	Have the patient urinate every 2–3 hr after receiving this drug
Cytarabine (Cytosaur-U, Ara-C)	Antimetabolite	IV	Myelosuppression, nausea, eye irritation with high doses	Steroid eye drops may be prescribed for patients receiving high doses of cytarabine to prevent eye irritation
Dacarbazine (DTIC)	Alkylating	IV	Myelosuppression, nausea, flu-like symptoms the day after treatment, increased sensitivity to the sun	Advise patient of side effects. Give antiemetics as ordered
Daunorubicin hydrochloride (Cerubidine)	Antibiotic	IV	Myelosuppression, nausea, alopecia, stomatitis, decreased cardiac ejection fraction	Urine may turn pink for 24 hr after the drug is given; vesicant

Patients generally die shortly after they enter this accelerated phase.

Acute Leukemia

Each of the chronic forms of leukemia—lymphocytic and myelogenous—also has an acute form. Acute lymphocytic leukemia (ALL) occurs most often in children between the ages of 2 and 6 years. Acute myelogenous leukemia (AML) occurs more often in adults. The acute leukemias appear very suddenly. The patient's white blood cell count can skyrocket in a number of days, crowding out the normal red blood cells and platelets and leaving the patient at severe risk for infection and bleeding. Treatment with chemotherapy must be started as soon as possible. Approximately 75% of patients diagnosed with ALL are alive after 5 years. Only 30% of the patients diagnosed with AML are alive after 5 years.

SIGNS AND SYMPTOMS. Patients with leukemia usually come into the hospital complaining of a persistent infection. These patients have infections because their bone marrow is producing huge numbers of immature white blood cells that cannot effectively fight infection. Usually patients with leukemia have fevers in response to the infection. Because the leukemic white blood cells crowd out the normal cells in the bone marrow, patients may have symptoms related to low platelet counts, such as petechiae or purpura, gingival bleeding (from the gums), epistaxis (nose bleeds), or melena (blood in the stool). Also, patients may have symptoms related to low red blood cell counts such as fatigue, tachycardia, and tachypnea. In addition to the symptoms related to low blood counts, patients may report weight loss, night sweats, and swollen lymph nodes. Some patients may have bone pain because of the crowding created by rapidly dividing leukemic cells in the bone marrow.

MEDICAL DIAGNOSIS. A CBC with an extremely high white blood cell count indicates that leukemia might be present. A bone marrow biopsy enables diag-

TABLE 30–11
DRUGS COMMONLY USED TO TREAT LEUKEMIA AND LYMPHOMA *Continued*

DRUG	USE/ACTION	HOW GIVEN	SIDE EFFECTS	NURSING INTERVENTIONS
Doxorubicin hydrochloride (Adriamycin)	Antibiotic	IV	Myelosuppression, nausea, alopecia, stomatitis, decreased cardiac ejection fraction	Urine may turn pink for 24 hr after the drug is given; vesicant
Etoposide (VP-16)	Plant alkaloid	IV or PO	Myelosuppression, alopecia	Patient can experience hypotension if the drug is given over less than 45 min
Hydroxyurea (Hydrea)	Miscellaneous	PO	Myelosuppression, nausea, stomatitis	Handle carefully
Mechlorethamine (nitrogen mustard, mustine)	Alkylating	IV	Myelosuppression, nausea, darkening of the veins, sterility in men	Once reconstituted, the drug must be administered within 20 min; vesicant
6-Mercaptopurine (6-MP)	Antimetabolite	PO	Nausea, stomatitis	Give mouth care and antiemetics as ordered
Methotrexate (Mexate)	Antimetabolite	IV or IM	Stomatitis, myelosuppression, diarrhea	With high doses of methotrexate, leucovorin is prescribed to start 24 hr after the methotrexate is given to "rescue" the normal cells. Give mouth care
Prednisone	Miscellaneous: steroid	PO	Stomach irritation	Give prednisone with meals. Monitor fluids and electrolytes
Procarbazine hydrochloride (Matulane)	Miscellaneous: monoamine oxidase inhibitor	PO	Nausea, myelosuppression	Patient must follow a special tyramine-free diet and avoid alcohol while taking this drug
Vinicristine (Oncovin)	Plant alkaloid	IV	Constipation, peripheral neuropathy	Vesicant. Monitor infusion site
Vinblastine (Velban)	Plant alkaloid	IV	Myelosuppression, constipation, peripheral neuropathy	Vesicant. Monitor infusion site

Data from Fischer, D. S., Knobf, M. T., & Durivage, H. J. (1993). *The cancer chemotherapy handbook* (4th ed.). St. Louis: Mosby Year Book.

nosis of the specific type of leukemia. Table 30–4 describes the procedure for a bone marrow biopsy as well as how to prepare the patient for the procedure.

MEDICAL TREATMENT

Chemotherapy. The acute leukemias are treated initially by using high doses of chemotherapy to destroy the diseased bone marrow and allow the body to regrow healthy bone marrow. Table 30–10 describes combinations of drugs commonly used to treat acute leukemias. Table 30–11 describes the possible side effects of the drugs. Patients are at great risk for infection and bleeding while their healthy bone marrow is growing back, but this is the only way the acute leukemias can be treated. Patients stay in the hospital during the chemotherapy treatments and afterward to receive antibiotics and blood transfusions until their own bone marrow grows back. Patients are generally hospitalized 4 to 6 weeks. After the initial high doses of chemotherapy called *induction therapy*, patients with ALL take lower doses of chemotherapy for the next 3 years. Patients with AML take the same high doses of chemotherapy over the next 2 to 3 months but are then finished with treatment. Subsequent doses of chemotherapy for both diseases are called *consolidation* and *maintenance therapy*.

Bone Marrow Transplantation. Bone marrow transplantation is a relatively new treatment in which even higher doses of chemotherapy and radiation therapy are given to the patient in an attempt to destroy all of the leukemia at once. This treatment also destroys all of the patient's healthy bone marrow, however, so donated bone marrow must be given to the patient after he or she is treated with the chemotherapy and the radiation therapy. The donated bone marrow is administered to the patient like a blood transfusion through an intravenous line. The transplanted bone marrow finds its way to the marrow of the bones, where it starts growing and producing healthy white blood cells, red blood cells, and platelets. Ideally, the donated bone marrow comes from a brother or a sister who has an identical human leukocyte antigen match. Human leukocyte antigen typing is similar to blood typing except that it is much more specific. If the patient does not have a sibling with an identical human leukocyte antigen match, an unrelated donor, someone who has the same match as the patient but is not related to the patient, can sometimes be found to donate bone marrow. Sometimes the patient's own bone marrow can be stored, treated with chemotherapy, and given back to the patient after the patient receives the high dose chemotherapy and radiation therapy.

Bone marrow transplantation is still a very dangerous and technically difficult treatment done only at certain hospitals. Physicians and scientists are working to find the best drugs and radiation with which to treat the patient and the best ways to support the patient while the transplanted bone marrow grows back. Even after the transplant, patients must deal with many long-term physical and psychological problems for the rest of their lives even though they may be cured of cancer.

Nursing Care of the Patient with Acute Leukemia

Patients with acute leukemia require expert nursing care. Patients are normally hospitalized for 4 to 6 weeks and are critically ill most of that time. Although the treatment trajectory for these patients can and should be anticipated, the physical and psychological nursing care of these patients is very intensive.

ASSESSMENT. Infection is the leading cause of death in patients with leukemia. Therefore, these patients are frequently assessed for any signs or symptoms of infection. The most common sites of infection are the lungs, perianal area, pharynx, genitourinary tract, and skin. Complete vital signs are taken every 4 hours. Fever is the hallmark of infection. Other vital sign changes due to sepsis, or widespread infection, include tachycardia, tachypnea, and hypotension. Breath sounds are assessed every shift and changes noted. A cough, especially a productive cough, may indicate an early pulmonary infection. If sputum is produced, the amount and color are documented. Many times the physician wants the sputum to be cultured in case of infection. The skin, including the perianal area, is carefully inspected each day for any reddened, swollen, painful, or draining areas. This is most easily done when the nurse helps the patient with the daily bath. Because patients with leukemia do not have any white blood cells during treatment, pus may not be seen even though an infection may be present. Redness, swelling, pain, or a combination of these may be the only symptom of a serious infection. The mouth and pharynx are assessed for any reddened, swollen, painful, or draining areas. The nurse asks if the patient has any pain or burning on urination, indicating a possible bladder infection.

While the nurse is assessing for infection, evidence of bleeding is also assessed. The lower the platelet count, the greater the patient's risk for bleeding. A platelet count below 50,000 is certainly cause for concern. Any petechiae, purpura, or ecchymoses are noted. Patients may have or report epistaxis, gingival bleeding, melena, and menorrhagia (heavy menstrual bleeding). A guaiac test should be performed on all stools.

PHARMACOLOGY CAPSULE

Chemotherapy can cause bone marrow suppression leading to anemia, bleeding, and inability to fight infection.

Any side effects from the chemotherapy itself, such as nausea and vomiting or stomatitis, should also be noted so the appropriate interventions can be taken. Most patients lose their hair from chemotherapy for acute leukemia beginning 1 to 2 weeks after treatment. This is to be expected.

While doing a physical assessment, the nurse also assesses how much the patient knows about the disease and treatment and how the patient is coping with this life-threatening disease.

NURSING DIAGNOSIS. Nursing diagnoses for the patient with acute leukemia may include (McNally, Somerville, Miaskowski & Rostad, 1991):

- **Knowledge Deficit** of the disease process and treatment
- **Anxiety** related to the diagnosis, treatment, change in body image, and uncertain outcome
- **High Risk for Injury** related to infection, thrombocytopenia, anemia
- **Altered Nutrition: Less than Body Requirements,** related to nausea and vomiting
- **Altered Oral Mucous Membrane** integrity related to stomatitis

GOALS. Goals of nursing care may include knowledge of disease process and treatment to manage side effects and resume self-care; reduced anxiety; absence of injury including infection, bleeding, and inadequate oxygenation; adequate intake of nutrients; and intact mucous membranes.

INTERVENTIONS

Knowledge Deficit. It is very important that the patient receive accurate, consistent information from all members of the health care team. An oncology clinical nurse specialist or other specially trained oncology nurse can usually provide comprehensive information about the disease and its treatment to the patient and family and answer questions as they arise during hospitalization. All nurses reinforce this teaching. The Leukemia Society of America (600 Third Avenue, New York, NY 10016, 1-212-573-8484) provides excellent free literature on the different types of leukemia. The National Cancer Institute (NCI), through the Cancer Information Service (1-800-4CANCER), provides excellent free literature on chemotherapy for people receiving treatment.

The American Cancer Society (1599 Clifton Road, Atlanta, GA 30320, 1-800-ACS-2345) has many support services available for people with all forms of cancer, including leukemia.

Anxiety. A diagnosis of leukemia is always a shock to patients and their families. Patients must deal not only with the disease and its treatment but also with the feeling and emotions of facing a life-threatening illness. Patients are encouraged to ask questions and to talk about their feelings. Many times a patient's fears are due to lack of knowledge about the disease and treatment. The oncology clinical nurse specialist or other specially trained oncology nurse can answer many of the patient's and family's questions. Many times information is what the patient and family need to deal with their anxiety. However, a referral to a social worker, mental health counselor, or chaplain may be indicated if the patient and family are having continued anxiety and difficulty coping. It is important for the nurse to know what the patient has been told about the disease, the treatment, and the prognosis so that correct information can be reinforced.

High Risk for Injury

Infection. Infection presents the greatest risk to patients with leukemia. Most hospitals institute "compromised host precautions" when a patient's absolute neutrophil count falls below 1000 to help protect the patient from infection. The patient is placed in a private room. Good hand washing is of paramount importance in caring for these patients. Microorganisms can be transmitted by hospital personnel who do not wash their hands thoroughly before touching the patient. Patients should be encouraged to shower every day to remove bacteria from the skin and perianal area. Because patients with low white blood cell counts often become infected with their own microorganisms through their gastrointestinal tract, patients are not allowed to eat fresh fruits or vegetables or to drink milk products. These uncooked foods naturally contain the bacteria *Escherichia coli*, *Pseudomonas aeruginosa*, and *Klebsiella* species. People with a normal immune system can easily handle ingesting small amounts of bacteria. However, patients undergoing treatment for leukemia could die from being exposed to even small amounts of these bacteria. Table 30–12 outlines typical compromised host precautions for patients with low white blood cell counts. Once the patient's absolute neutrophil count climbs above 1000, compromised host precautions can be discontinued and a regular diet eaten without restrictions.

Thrombocytopenia. Besides infection, patients with leukemia are also at great risk for bleeding related to thrombocytopenia, or low platelet count. The primary treatment for thrombocytopenia is a platelet transfusion. However, physicians try not to prescribe platelet transfusions for patients unless they are actively bleeding or their platelet count is below 20,000 because of the risks associated with blood product administration. Nursing

TABLE 30–12

SPECIFIC NURSING ACTIONS FOR THE PATIENT WHO IS NEUTROPENIC*

1. Patient should have a private room. It does not have to be an isolation room. The door may be open. A Compromised Host Precaution sign will be posted on the door.
2. All persons who enter must wash their hands before touching the patient for any reason. This is the most important way to prevent infection in these patients. Patients should be encouraged to remind all staff and visitors to wash their hands before touching them.
3. The patient should be taught to wash the hands before and after eating, using the toilet, and doing any self-care procedure. Most importantly, the patient should be encouraged to shower every day.
4. Masks are not required and are discouraged. Staff with upper respiratory or other infections should not care for the patient.
5. The patient should wear a clean mask when outside the room, especially in heavily traveled public areas such as corridors, elevators, and waiting rooms. The mask may be removed when the patient is in less public areas such as a clinic office. Patients should avoid crowded areas as much as possible. A new mask should be used during each trip out of the room.
6. Appointments should be coordinated in advance to eliminate or minimize waiting time in common waiting areas.
7. Only canned or cooked foods should be served. No raw fruits, no raw vegetables, and no milk products are served because of the risk of *Escherichia coli*, *Pseudomonas aeruginosa*, and *Klebsiella* species bacteria on or in these food items. The patient should be encouraged to choose appropriate foods from the menu. The diet roster should be annotated "Compromised Host Precautions" so that the dining room can double check that appropriate choices are being made.
8. Careful attention to aseptic technique must be observed, especially when performing phlebotomy, handling intravenous lines, or performing other invasive procedures.
9. Invasive procedures should be kept to a minimum. Invasive devices such as catheters and tubes should be removed as soon as the patient's medical condition permits.
10. Flowers and plants are allowed in the patient's room but should not be handled by the patient because of the possibility of *Escherichia coli* contamination of the water and dirt.

* Compromised host precautions for patients with an absolute neutrophil count of less than 1000 or those at significant risk of infection due to neutropenia.

Adapted from Patrick, M. A. (Ed.). (1992). *Infection control manual.* (Available from: COMMANDER, Madigan Army Medical Center, HSHJ-N (ATTN: Infection Control Nurse), Fort Lewis, WA 98431-5000).

considerations in administering platelet transfusions have been outlined previously in this chapter. Bleeding precautions that should be taken when patients are thrombocytopenic are outlined in Table 30–13.

Anemia. Anemia, or a hematocrit below 30 and a hemoglobin below 10, is a common symptom of patients with leukemia. The nurse expects anemia, just as he or she expects neutropenia and thrombocytopenia. And, just as with neutropenia and thrombocytopenia, anemia may be caused by the leukemic cells crowding out the healthy red blood cells in the bone marrow or it may be caused by the chemotherapy treatments. The primary treatment for anemia is red blood cell transfusions. Nursing considerations in administering blood transfusions have been outlined previously in this chapter. Other precautions that should be taken when patients are anemic are outlined in Table 30–9.

TABLE 30-13
SPECIFIC NURSING ACTIONS FOR THE PATIENT WHO IS THROMBOCYTOPENIC*

1. Minimize the number of invasive procedures done to the patient that might result in prolonged bleeding.
   a. Draw all laboratory samples with one daily venipuncture if possible.
   b. Avoid prolonged tourniquet use.
   c. Apply direct pressure for 3–5 min after all invasive procedures such as venipuncture or bone marrow biopsy.
   d. Avoid intramuscular injections.
2. Implement measures to avoid damage to the rectal mucosa that might cause bleeding by avoiding:
   a. rectal temperatures
   b. suppositories
   c. enemas
3. Prevent constipation by increasing fiber in the diet or administering stool softeners as ordered.
4. Pump up blood pressure cuff only until pulse is obliterated before releasing air and measuring pressure to prevent petechiae along the arm.
5. Instruct the patient to use an electric razor to shave, not a straight-edge razor that might cut the patient.
6. Instruct the patient to use a soft-bristled toothbrush, toothettes, or just mouth rinses for mouth care to prevent bleeding from the gums.
7. As much as possible and as prescribed by the physician, avoid the use of drugs that interfere with platelet function such as aspirin, ibuprofen (Motrin), and indomethacin (Indocin). Drugs that contain aspirin should also be avoided. Drugs that contain aspirin include: Excedrin, Bayer Aspirin, Vanquish, Alka-Seltzer, Percodan, and Fiorinal.
8. Administer platelet transfusions as prescribed by the physician.

* For patients with a platelet count less than 50,000 or those at significant risk for bleeding due to thrombocytopenia.

Altered Nutrition. Nausea with or without vomiting is a common side effect of chemotherapy. Persistent nausea and vomiting can adversely affect a patient's nutritional status and psychological state. Nurses play an important role in managing this most distressing side effect. A detailed discussion of the nursing management of nausea and vomiting related to chemotherapy is presented in Chapter 23.

Altered Oral Mucous Membranes. Stomatitis, an inflammation of the mucous membranes, is also a common side effect of chemotherapy. A detailed discussion of the nursing management of stomatitis is presented in Chapter 23.

EVALUATION. Effective nursing interventions are determined by patient's verbalization of disease process, treatment, and self-care; patient's report of reduced anxiety; absence of injury, platelet count greater than 100,000, hematocrit greater than 30, hemoglobin greater than 10; stable body weight; and intact mucous membranes.

LYMPHATIC SYSTEM DISORDERS

The primary lymphatic system disorders are multiple myeloma and the lymphomas. Multiple myeloma is a cancer of the plasma cells in the bone marrow. Plasma cells normally produce B lymphocytes. Lymphoma is a cancer of the lymph nodes. There are two major types of lymphoma: Hodgkin's disease and non-Hodgkin's lymphoma.

Types of Lymphatic System Disorders

MULTIPLE MYELOMA. Multiple myeloma is a cancer of the bone marrow that causes abnormal levels of blood proteins and weakened areas of the bone where the myeloma cells are growing out of control. Multiple myeloma is most commonly seen in people over the age of 60. The disease effects blacks twice as often as whites. There is no known cause for multiple myeloma; however, radiation exposure and genetic factors may play a role. Patients with multiple myeloma usually complain of bone pain. Other symptoms of the disease can be bone fractures, anemia, hypercalcemia from bone destruction, hyperuricemia if the myeloma proteins become trapped in the kidneys, and spinal cord compression in which the patient can experience lower extremity weakness or incontinence. Multiple myeloma is diagnosed with radiographs, a serum protein electrophoresis, a 24-hour urine protein electrophoresis, and a bone marrow biopsy. Table 30–1 lists the normal values for these tests. Table 30–3 describes the procedures for doing these studies. There is no cure for multiple myeloma. Treatment with radiation therapy and chemotherapy is given to control symptoms.

HODGKIN'S DISEASE. Hodgkin's disease is a type of lymphoma characterized by Reed-Sternberg cells in the lymph nodes. According to American Cancer Society statistics (1994), an estimated 7900 new cases of Hodgkin's disease will occur in 1994, accounting for less than 1% of all new cases of cancer diagnosed in that year. Incidence of the disease is highest for people in their twenties and in their fifties. Men are more likely than women to have the disease. Survival rates vary widely, depending on the stage of the disease at diagnosis. The overall 5-year survival rate for patients with Hodgkin's disease is 77%.

NON-HODGKIN'S LYMPHOMA. Non-Hodgkin's lymphoma is another cancer of the lymph system. Unlike Hodgkin's disease, non-Hodgkin's lymphoma does not have Reed-Sternberg cells. The American Cancer Society estimates 45,000 new cases of non-Hodgkin's lymphoma for 1994, which accounts for about 4% of all new cases of cancer diagnosed in that year. Patients of any age and of either gender may get non-Hodgkin's lymphoma, although the disease is more common in older people. Unlike most cancers, non-Hodgkin's lymphoma is not staged I, II, III, or IV. Instead, non-Hodgkin's lymphomas are staged as low grade, intermediate grade, and high grade. The higher the grade of lymphoma, the more aggressive the cancer. Again, survival rates vary widely, depending on the grade of the disease at diagnosis. The overall 5-year survival rate for patients with non-Hodgkin's lymphoma is 51%.

SIGNS AND SYMPTOMS. Patients with lymphoma usually notice a painless swelling of one or more of the lymph nodes. Many times this swelling is first noticed in the neck or the groin. Lymph nodes also swell when infection is present, but that swelling is usually painful and resolves quickly as the infection resolves. The swollen lymph nodes of patients with lymphoma are usually painless and remain swollen. Patients with lymphoma may also report night sweats and a recent weight loss. Patients with Hodgkin's disease may complain of itching.

MEDICAL DIAGNOSIS. The diagnosis of lymphoma is made with a lymph node biopsy. Once the diagnosis is made, various tests are done to stage the patient to determine where the cancer might have spread. Most patients have blood studies, a chest radiograph, and a computed tomography scan of the chest and abdomen. Depending on the findings from these tests, patients may also have a lymphangiogram, bone marrow biopsies, and staging laparoscopy. Table 30–4 describes these studies.

MEDICAL TREATMENT. Patients receive radiation therapy, chemotherapy, or both depending on the extent of the disease. Table 30–10 describes combinations of drugs commonly used to treat lymphoma. Table 30–11 describes the possible side effects of the drugs. Treatment for lymphoma is usually accomplished on an outpatient basis. Patients are admitted only for the staging work-up and for complications of therapy, such as infection.

NURSING CARE OF THE PATIENT WITH LYMPHOMA

Assessment. Nursing assessment of the patient with lymphoma includes an evaluation of all the lymph node chains, not just the swollen ones. Vital signs are taken every 4 to 8 hours, looking for fever. The patient is queried about night sweats, any recent weight loss, and itching.

Once treatment starts, infection and bleeding are the greatest risks to patients. Nursing assessment for infection and bleeding in the patient with lymphoma is the same as for the patient with acute leukemia. Any side effects from the chemotherapy itself such as nausea and vomiting or stomatitis should also be noted so the appropriate interventions can be taken. Many patients lose their hair from chemotherapy or from lymphoma.

While doing a physical assessment, the nurse also assesses how much the patient knows about the disease and treatment, and how the patient is coping with the life-threatening disease.

Nursing Diagnosis. Nursing diagnoses for the patient with lymphoma are similar to those for patients with leukemia and may include the following.

- **Knowledge Deficit** of the disease process and treatment
- **Anxiety** related to the diagnosis, treatment, change in body image, uncertain outcome
- **High Risk for Injury** related to infection, thrombocytopenia, anemia

Goals. Goals of nursing care may include knowledge of disease process and treatment to manage side effects and resume self-care; reduced anxiety; and absence of infection, bleeding, excessive fatigue, and inadequate oxygenation.

Interventions. Nursing interventions for the nursing diagnoses of the patient with lymphoma are the same as described previously in this chapter for the patient with acute leukemia.

Evaluation. Effective nursing interventions are determined by patient's knowledge of the disease process and treatment to manage side effects and resume self-care; reduced anxiety; and absence of fever, platelet count greater than 100,000, hematocrit greater than 30, and hemoglobin greater than 10.

COAGULATION DISORDERS

Coagulation disorders can result from a platelet abnormality or from a clotting factor deficiency.

Types of Coagulation Disorders

THROMBOCYTOPENIA. Thrombocytopenia is a condition in which a person has too few platelets circulating in the blood. This may be because not enough platelets are being made in the bone marrow or because too many platelets are being destroyed by the spleen. Certain infections, drugs, or diseases such as cancer can cause this to happen, but sometimes there is no identifiable reason.

PHARMACOLOGY CAPSULE

Thrombocytopenia can develop as an adverse effect of some drugs including penicillin and quinidine.

Symptoms of thrombocytopenia include petechiae and purpura, gingival bleeding, epistaxis, or any other unusual or prolonged bleeding. Diagnosis is made with a CBC, bleeding time, PT/PTT, and a bone marrow biopsy. Treatment for thrombocytopenia is to treat or stop the causative factor, if possible. Corticosteroids are usually given to the patient. Platelet transfusions, fresh frozen plasma, or both may be prescribed. When the spleen is thought to be destroying the platelets, a splenectomy may be done.

HEMOPHILIA. Hemophilia is a genetic disease in which the affected person lacks some of the blood clotting factors normally found in plasma. The incidence of hemophilia is 1 to 2 cases per 20,000 persons. In hemophilia A factor VIII is missing, and in hemophilia B factor IX is missing. Because the trait is carried on the X chromosome, women carry the trait and can pass it to their sons, who show the disease. Because this recessive trait is carried only on the X chromosome, it is rare for women to have the disease. Just as with sickle cell disease, genetic counseling can be done for people with the trait and with the disease to inform them of the risk of passing the trait or the disease to their children. With this information, some people choose not to have their own children and risk passing on this life-threatening disease. Table 30–14 describes the risk of passing hemophilia on to children.

SIGNS AND SYMPTOMS. Bleeding is the sign and symptom of hemophilia. Bleeding generally occurs after some sort of trauma; however, bleeding can also occur spontaneously without any clear reason. Most commonly, bleeding occurs into the joints causing swelling and severe pain. Bleeding also commonly occurs into the skin; from the mouth, gums, and lips; and from the gastrointestinal tract. Any surgical procedure puts the patient at great risk for bleeding and necessitates a complete preoperative evaluation and availability of replacement factors for transfusion.

MEDICAL DIAGNOSIS. The diagnosis of hemophilia is made by blood measurements of factors VIII and IX. Also, the PTT is prolonged in people with hemophilia.

MEDICAL TREATMENT. There is no cure for hemophilia. Medical treatment for patients experiencing a bleeding episode is symptomatic. The physician usually prescribes fresh frozen plasma, cryoprecipitate transfusions, or both. Patients with hemophilia A need factor VIII, which is found in both fresh frozen plasma and cryoprecipitate. Patients with hemophilia B need factor IX, which is found in fresh frozen plasma. Red blood cell transfusions are frequently used to replace blood lost from the profuse bleeding to which hemophiliacs are prone. Many hemophiliac patients treated with red blood cells before 1985 are now HIV positive because of transfusions with contaminated blood. Pain medication may also be prescribed to relieve pain, which is usually experienced where the bleeding occurs.

TABLE 30–14

RISK OF PASSING HEMOPHILIA ON TO CHILDREN

NOTE: The hemophilia trait X′ can be carried only on the X chromosome.

		Mother with trait	
		X	X′
Healthy father	X	X X	X′ X
	Y	X Y	X′ Y

If have daughter, 50% chance daughter carries the trait
50% chance daughter is healthy
If have son, 50% chance the son has hemophilia
50% chance the son is healthy

NURSING CARE OF THE PATIENT WITH HEMOPHILIA

Assessment. Because of the pathophysiology of the disease, patients with hemophilia have specialized needs. A consistent nursing care plan is essential in caring for these patients. The nurse assesses the patient for bleeding and pain and notes what measures have stopped the bleeding and relieved the pain in the past.

Nursing Diagnosis. Nursing diagnoses for the patient with hemophilia may include the following:

- **Knowledge Deficit** of the disease process
- **High Risk for Injury** related to bleeding
- Acute **Pain** related to bleeding into closed spaces, creating pressure on nerves

Goals. Goals of nursing care may include patient's knowledge of the disease process and self-care, absence of bleeding, and relief of pain.

Interventions

Knowledge Deficit. Hemophiliacs bleed with even the smallest bruise or abrasion. Patients and their families should be taught to prevent injury and to safeguard their environment against accidents as much as possible. Some patients and families are taught to administer the replacement concentrate at home so that if an injury does occur, prompt treatment can be initiated and blood loss minimized. The National Hemophilia Foundation (110 Green Street, Room 303, New York, NY 10012, 1-212-219-8180) provides information and support to patients with hemophilia and their families.

Bleeding. The primary treatment to control bleeding from hemophilia is to transfuse fresh frozen plasma, cryoprecipitate, or both. Nursing considerations in administering these products are outlined in Table 30–5. Bleeding precautions that should be taken when patients have hemophilia are similar to bleeding precautions taken when patients are thrombocytopenic. Refer to Table 30–13 for these bleeding precautions.

Pain. Pain medications are given as prescribed. If the patient is experiencing a great deal of pain, patient-controlled analgesia may be appropriate. The nurse closely monitors the patient's pain level using the 0 to 10 scale. Keeping a flow sheet of patient reports of pain on a 10-point scale can be helpful, especially as different nurses care for the patient throughout the day. The patient's report of pain coupled with the amount of pain medication he or she is receiving can guide the nurse and physician as to the appropriate type and amount of pain medication. A detailed discussion of pain management is presented in Chapter 16.

NUTRITION CONCEPTS

- The major treatment for iron deficiency anemia is iron replacement therapy.
- Foods rich in iron are beef, liver, dried fruits, dried peas and beans, nuts, green leafy vegetables, whole-grain breads, and cereal.
- Ascorbic acid (found in citrus fruits) promotes the absorption of iron in the body; tea taken with meals can inhibit absorption.
- The goal for a patient with leukemia, Hodgkin's disease or lymphoma is to maintain the highest level of nutrition possible. Good nutrition can promote recovery from chemotherapy and radiation therapy treatments and minimize side effects of the disease and treatments.

Evaluation. Effective nursing interventions are determined by the patient's description of hemophilia and appropriate self-care; absence of visible bleeding, pain, tachycardia, hypotension; and patient's statement of pain relief, relaxed expression.

The hematologic and lymphatic systems are vitally important in maintaining normal physiologic functioning of the body and in protecting the body from infection. Disorders of these systems can be a symptom of another disease that can be corrected easily with treatment of the underlying condition. Or the problem can be a primary disorder of the hematologic or lymphatic system. Primary disorders, such as leukemia or lymphoma, are often chronic conditions requiring intensive care in the hospital. The nurse plays an important role in helping the patient recover as quickly as possible and in helping the patient deal with the disease.

BIBLIOGRAPHY

American Cancer Society. (1994). *1994 cancer facts and figures.* New York: Author.

Bates, B. (1991). *A guide to physical examination and history taking* (5th ed.). Philadelphia: J. B. Lippincott.

Bithell, T. C. (1993). Hereditary coagulation disorders. In G. R. Lee, T. C. Bithell, J. Foerster, J. W. Athens, & J. N. Lukens (Eds.), *Wintrobe's clinical hematology* (9th ed., pp. 1422–1472). Philadelphia: Lea & Febiger.

Carlson, A. C. (1985). Infection prophylaxis in the patient with cancer. *Oncology Nursing Forum, 12*(3), 56–64.

Deisseroth, A. B., Andreeff, M., Champlin, R., Keating, M. J., Kantarjian, H., Khouri, I. F., & Talpaz, M. (1993). Chronic leukemias. In V. T. DeVita, S. Hellman, & S. A. Rosenberg (Eds.), *Cancer principles and practice of oncology* (4th ed., pp. 1965–1983). Philadelphia: J. B. Lippincott.

DeVita, V. J., Hellman, S., & Jaffe, E. S. (1993). Hodgkin's disease. In V. T. DeVita, S. Hellman, & S. A. Rosenberg (Eds.), *Cancer principles and practice of oncology* (4th ed., pp. 1819–1858). Philadelphia: J. B. Lippincott.

Fischbach, F. T. (1992). *A manual of laboratory diagnostic tests* (4th ed.). Philadelphia: J. B. Lippincott.

Fischer, D. S., Knobf, M. T., & Durivage, H. J. (1993). *The cancer chemotherapy handbook* (4th ed.). St. Louis: Mosby Year Book.

Govoni, L. E., & Hayes, J. E. (1988). *Drugs and nursing implication* (6th ed.). East Norwalk, CT: Appleton & Lange.

Guyton, A. C. (1991). *Textbook of medical physiology* (8th ed). Philadelphia: W. B. Saunders.

Jarvis, C. (1992). *Physical examination and health assessment.* Philadelphia: W. B. Saunders.

Keating, M. J., Estey, E., & Kantarjian, H. (1993). Acute leukemia. In V. T. DeVita, S. Hellman, & S. A. Rosenberg (Eds.), *Cancer principles and practice of oncology* (4th ed., pp. 1938–1964). Philadelphia: J. B. Lippincott.

Lee, G. R. (1993). Megaloblastic and non-megaloblastic macrocytic anemias. In G. R. Lee, T. C. Bithell, J. Foerster, J. W. Athens, & J. N. Lukens (Eds.), *Wintrobe's clinical hematology* (9th ed., pp. 745–790). Philadelphia: Lea & Febiger.

Long, B. C., & Wright, E. R. (1991). Management of persons with problems of the immune system. In W. J. Phipps, B. C. Long, N. F. Woods, & V. L. Cassmeyer (Eds.), *Medical-surgical nursing: Concept and clinical practice* (4th ed., pp. 775–812). St. Louis: Mosby Year Book.

Longo, D. L., DeVita, V. J., Jaffe, E. S., & Mauch, P. L. (1993). Lymphocytic lymphomas. In V. T. DeVita, S. Hellman, S. A. Rosenberg (Eds.), *Cancer principles and practice of oncology* (4th ed., pp. 1859–1927). Philadelphia: J. B. Lippincott.

Lukens, J. N. (1993). Hemoglobinopathies S, C, D, E, and O and associated diseases. In G. R. Lee, T. C. Bithell, J. Foerster, J. W. Athens, & J. N. Lukens (Eds.), *Wintrobe's clinical hematology* (9th ed., pp. 1061–1101). Philadelphia: Lea & Febiger.

Maguire-Eisen, M. (1990). Diagnosis and treatment of adult acute leukemia. *Seminars in Oncology Nursing, 6*(1), 17–24

McNally, J. C., Somerville, E. T., Miaskowski, C., & Rostad, M. (1991). *Guidelines for oncology nursing practice* (2nd ed). Philadelphia: W. B. Saunders.

Poplack, D. G., Kun, L. E., Magrath, I. T., & Pizzo, P. A. (1993). Leukemias and lymphomas of childhood. In V. T. DeVita, S. Hellman, & S. A. Rosenberg (Eds.), *Cancer principles and practice of oncology* (4th ed., pp. 1792–1818). Philadelphia: J. B. Lippincott.

Remington, J. S., & Schimpff, S. C. (1981). Please don't eat the salads. *New England Journal of Medicine, 304*(7), 433–435.

Rozzell, M. S., Hijazi, M., & Pack, B. (1983). The painful episode in sickle cell disease. *Nursing Clinics of North America, 18*(1), 185–189.

Salmon, S. E., & Cassady, J. R. (1993). Plasma cell neoplasms. In V. T. DeVita, S. Hellman, & S. A. Rosenberg (Eds.), *Cancer principles and practice of oncology* (4th ed., pp. 1984–2025). Philadelphia: J. B. Lippincott.

Wallerstein, R. Jr., & Deisseroth, A. (1993). Use of blood and blood products. In V. T. DeVita, S. Hellman, & S. A. Rosenberg (Eds.), *Cancer principles and practice of oncology* (4th ed., pp. 2262–2275). Philadelphia: J. B. Lippincott.

Walters, I., Baysinger, M., Buchanan, I., Dahl, J. A., Dorn, L., Finigan, G., Luff, J., Moore, G., Myrie, J., Noel, C., & Semper, R. (1983). Complications of sickle cell disease. *Nursing Clinics of North America, 18*(1), 139–184.

KEY CONCEPTS

1. The hematologic system includes the blood and the bone marrow.
2. A healthy adult has about 6 liters of blood circulating through the body.
3. Components of the blood are plasma, red blood cells, white blood cells, platelets, plasma proteins, and clotting factors.
4. The lymphatic system is a vessel system in which lymph fluid flows.
5. Lymph nodes are small patches of lymphatic tissue that filter out microorganisms from lymph fluid before it is returned to the blood stream.
6. The spleen filters microorganisms from the blood, stores red blood cells, destroys old red blood cells, and produces antibodies, but is not essential for life.
7. B lymphocytes are responsible for the humoral immune response, and T lymphocytes are responsible for the cellular immune response.
8. Signs of hematologic abnormalities can include petechiae, purpura, and ecchymoses.
9. The four major blood groups are A, B, AB, and O; each group may be Rh negative or Rh positive.
10. People with type O negative blood are universal blood donors, and people with type AB positive blood are universal blood recipients.
11. The four types of reaction that can occur when blood or blood components are transfused are hemolytic, allergic, febrile, and circulatory overload.
12. Anemia is a deficiency of red blood cells or hemoglobin that may be due to blood loss, iron-deficient diet, vitamin B_{12} deficiency, bone marrow failure, or genetic abnormalities.
13. Sickle cell anemia is an incurable genetic condition in which red blood cells can become abnormally sickle shaped under stress so that they rupture easily and can obstruct capillaries.
14. Sickle cell crisis, characterized by severe pain and fever, occurs when blood flow is obstructed.
15. Nursing care during sickle cell crisis focuses on the patient's acute pain, anxiety, knowledge deficit, high risk for fluid volume deficit, and high risk for injury.
16. The leukemias are cancers of the white blood cells in which immature white blood cells are produced that are unable to fight infection.
17. Leukemias are treated primarily with chemotherapy and sometimes with bone marrow transplants.
18. Multiple myeloma is cancer of the plasma cells of the bone marrow that is treated symptomatically with chemotherapy, radiation therapy, or both.
19. Hodgkin's disease and non-Hodgkin's lymphoma are cancers of the lymph system that are treated with chemotherapy, radiation therapy, or both.
20. Nursing care of patients with leukemias and lymphomas focuses on knowledge deficits, anxiety, altered oral mucous membranes, and high risk for injury related to infection, thrombocytopenia, and anemia.
21. Thrombocytopenia is a deficiency of platelets that can lead to excessive or prolonged bleeding.
22. Hemophilia, an incurable genetic disease in which some of the factors needed for blood clotting are absent, is treated with replacement clotting factors.
23. Nursing care of the patient with hemophilia addresses the patient's knowledge deficit, high risk for injury, and acute pain.

Joy M. Norton

CHAPTER 31

Cardiac Disorders

OBJECTIVES

1. Label the major parts of the heart.
2. Explain the physiology of cardiac function.
3. Explain the nursing considerations for patients having diagnostic procedures to detect or evaluate cardiac disorders.
4. Identify nursing implications for common therapeutic measures, including drug, diet, or oxygen therapy; pacemakers and cardioverters; cardiac surgery; and cardiopulmonary resuscitation.
5. For selected cardiac disorders, explain the pathophysiology, risk factors, signs and symptoms, complications, and treatment.
6. List the data to be obtained in assessing the patient with a cardiac disorder.
7. Apply the nursing process to develop a plan of care for patients with cardiac disorders.

GLOSSARY

AFTERLOAD The amount of resistance the left ventricle must generate to open the aortic valve

ARTERIOSCLEROSIS Abnormal thickening and hardening of the arterial walls

ATHEROSCLEROSIS Abnormal thickening and hardening of the arterial walls caused by fat and fibrin deposits

BRADYCARDIA Slow heart rate, usually defined as fewer than 60 beats per minute

DYSRHYTHMIA Disturbance of rhythm; arrhythmia

HEMODYNAMICS Study of the movement of blood and the forces that affect it

INFARCT An area of ischemic necrosis caused by disruption of circulation

Glossary continued

MURMUR A sound heard on auscultation; in the heart, it indicates turbulent blood flow across heart valves

PALPITATION A heartbeat that is strong, rapid, or irregular enough that the person is aware of it

PERFUSION Passage of blood through the vessels of an organ

PRELOAD The amount of blood in the left ventricle at the end of diastole; the pressure generated at the end of diastole

REGURGITATION Backward flow

SYNCOPE Fainting

TACHYCARDIA Rapid heart rate, usually defined as greater than 100 beats per minute

THROMBOEMBOLISM Obstruction of a blood vessel with a blood clot transported through the blood stream

The cardiovascular system carries oxygenated blood and nutrients to the cells and transports carbon dioxide and wastes from the cells. It requires a reservoir for blood coming from the tissues, pumping action to send blood to the lungs and the body, and an intact vasculature to transport the blood. A malfunction in any of these components may affect other body systems and may threaten the life and health of the individual.

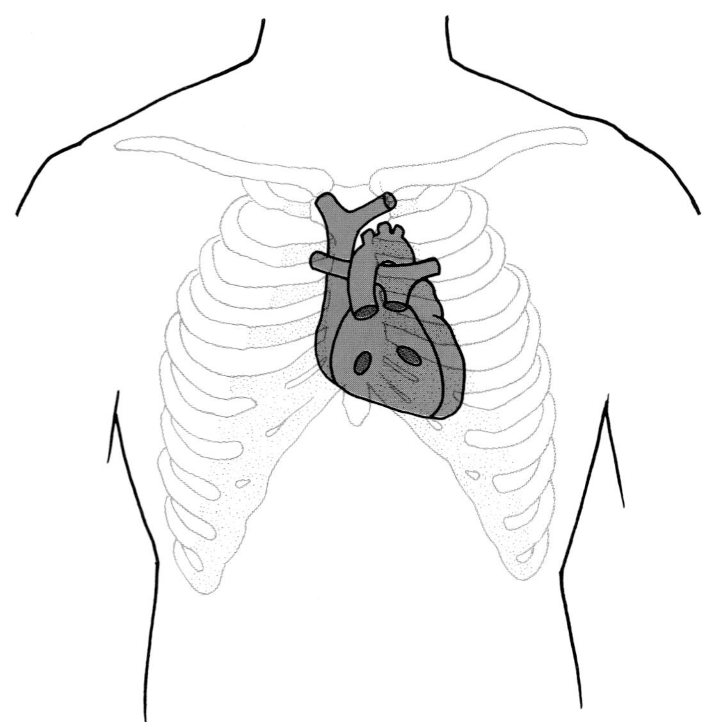

FIGURE 31-1

Anatomic location of the heart.

The heart is a hollow muscular pump located in the mediastinum (Fig. 31–1). The right and left sides of the heart receive blood from and send blood to different parts of the body. The heart is covered and protected by the sternum and the ribs anteriorly and flanked by the lungs laterally. The esophagus, the descending aorta, and the fifth through the eighth thoracic vertebrae are directly behind the heart. The heart rests on the diaphragm with two thirds of it to the left of the sternum. The right side of the heart is located under the sternum. The heart is approximately the size of the fist and weighs 10 to 14 ounces in the adult. It is covered by membranes called the visceral and parietal pericardium. The space between the pericardial membranes contains fluid that lubricates the membranes and decreases friction.

ANATOMY AND PHYSIOLOGY OF THE HEART

CHAMBERS

The heart is divided into four chambers: the right atrium, the left atrium, the right ventricle, and the left ventricle (Fig. 31–2). The four chambers are separated by septa (walls) and valves. The right atrium (RA) is a thin-walled reservoir and conduit for systemic blood. It receives blood from the inferior and the superior venae cavae and from the coronary sinuses. Normally resistance to flow in this chamber is very low, and normal pressure is 2 to 6 mm Hg. Oxygen saturation in the RA is 75%.

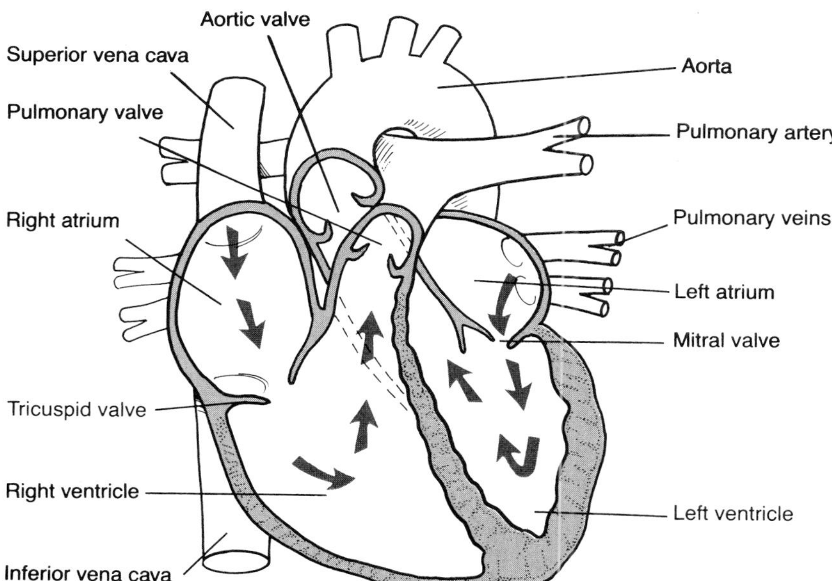

FIGURE 31-2
Normal circulation through the heart.

The right ventricle (RV) has thicker walls than the RA and receives blood from the RA through the tricuspid valve. Blood moves rather passively from the upper chamber to the lower chamber, resulting in pressure measurements of 15–30/0–5 mm Hg. Oxygen saturation in the RV is also 75%. This chamber is crescent shaped, contracts with bellows-like action, and ejects blood through the pulmonic semilunar valve into the pulmonary artery. The pulmonary artery carries the blood to the lungs where it releases carbon dioxide as waste and is resaturated with oxygen.

The left atrium (LA) receives blood saturated with oxygen from the four pulmonary veins. The wall that separates the RA from the LA is called the intra-atrial septum. This chamber has slightly higher pressure than the RA, 4 to 12 mm Hg, and an oxygen saturation of 95 to 98%.

The cone-shaped left ventricle (LV) has the thickest muscle mass of the four chambers. The LV is separated from the RV by a wall called the intraventricular septum. The LV contains the apex of the heart, which is located in the midclavicular line at the fourth or fifth intercostal space. An apical pulse is taken by auscultating the heartbeat at this location.

The LV contains the highest pressure in the heart, 120/0–10 mm Hg. The LV pressure is five times as great as the RV pressure during systole (when the chamber contracts). The oxygen saturation in the LV is 95 to 98%. Blood is received from the LA into the LV through the mitral valve. The LV contracts from apex to base, ejecting blood through the aortic semilunar valve into the aorta and systemic circulation. The systemic circulation carries oxygen and nutrients to all active cells and transports wastes to the kidneys, liver, and skin for excretion.

MUSCLE LAYERS

There are three layers of cardiac muscle tissue: the endocardium, the myocardium, and the epicardium. The endocardium is the inner layer that lines the heart chambers. The endothelial cells, connective tissue, and elastic fibers that compose the endocardium are continuous with the intima (inner lining) of the blood vessels. The middle layer, the myocardium, is made of muscle fibers. It is responsible for the pumping action of the heart. The thickness of the myocardium varies with each chamber. The outer layer, the epicardium, is also the visceral pericardium. The coronary arteries are embedded in the epicardium.

The myocardium is composed of long, narrow, branching cells that function as a coordinated unit, or syncytium. The cells are covered by a membrane, the sarcolemma. The sarcolemmas are separated from one another by intercalated disks. Inside the myocardial cells are bands of contractile proteins called myofibrils. The myocardial cells have a striped, or striated, appearance.

VALVES

There are four valves in the heart: the mitral, the tricuspid, the aortic, and the pulmonic. Their purpose is to retain blood in one chamber until the next chamber is ready to receive it. The valves keep blood flowing in one direction. They open and close passively in response to changes in pressure and volume. A valve opens when the pressure behind it is greater than the pressure ahead of it. A valve closes when the pressure ahead of it is greater than the pressure behind it.

ATRIOVENTRICULAR VALVES. The mitral and tricuspid valves are called atrioventricular (AV) valves because they separate the atria from the ventricles. The mitral valve is between the LA and the LV. The tricuspid valve separates the RA from the RV. The cusps, or leaflets, are attached by chordae tendineae to the papillary muscles that line the floor of the ventricles. These valves are closed during systole and open in diastole.

SEMILUNAR VALVES. The semilunar valves, aortic and pulmonic, separate the ventricles from the aorta and the pulmonary artery, respectively. These valves are open during systole and closed during diastole. The semilunar valves have three cusps (cup-shaped structures) each.

CORONARY BLOOD FLOW

The coronary arteries are the first branches of the systemic circulation (Fig. 31–3). These arteries supply blood to the myocardium and the conductive tissue of the heart. The two major coronary arteries, the left coronary artery (LCA) and the right coronary artery (RCA), arise from the aorta just beyond the aortic valve. Two thirds of the filling of the coronary arteries occurs during early diastole, when the aortic valve is closed and the sinuses of Valsalva are filled with blood. Myocardial fibers are relaxed at this time, thereby promoting blood flow through the coronary vessels. The LCA supplies blood to the LA, most of the LV, and most of the interventricular septum. The LCA branches into the left anterior descending and the circumflex arteries. The left anterior descending artery provides blood to the apex, and the circumflex supplies the LA and a portion of the LV. The RCA branches to supply the sinoatrial (SA) and the AV nodes, the RA and RV, part of the LA, and the inferior part of the LV. Variations in the pattern of arterial branching are common.

Collateral arteries are connections between two branches of arteries. They are more common in certain areas of the heart. It is not known whether they protect the heart or develop in response to ischemia.

The coronary arteries branch into arterioles and then into capillaries. There is approximately one capillary for each muscle fiber in the normal heart. Oxygen and nutrients are exchanged in the coronary capillaries. In the hypertrophied heart, muscle mass increases, but the capillary network appears to remain the same, resulting in reduced efficiency of oxygen and nutrient exchange.

In general the venous system parallels the arterial system: the great cardiac vein follows the left anterior descending artery, and the small cardiac vein follows the RCA. The veins meet to form the coronary sinus (the largest coronary vein), which returns blood from the myocardium to the right atrium.

CONDUCTION SYSTEM

For the heart to pump blood through the chambers, nerves must stimulate muscle contractions in an orderly fashion. The conduction pattern follows a particular route. The SA node, also called the pacemaker, initiates the impulse. The impulse is carried throughout the atria to the AV node located on the floor of the RA. The impulse is delayed in the AV node, then transmitted to the ventricles via the bundle of His. The bundle is made up of Purkinje cells and is located where the atrial and ventricular septa meet. The bundle of His divides into the left and right bundle branches. The left bundle branch divides into anterior and posterior branches called fascicles. The terminal ends of the right bundle branches are called the Purkinje fibers. When the impulse reaches the Purkinje fibers, the ventricles contract (Fig. 31–4).

CARDIAC INNERVATION. The heart is innervated by the autonomic nervous system. The cardiac plexus is a nerve network made up of both sympathetic and parasympathetic fibers that supply the SA and AV nodes as well as the atrial and ventricular tissue. Sympathetic fibers are distributed throughout the heart. Sympathetic stimulation results in increased heart rate, increased speed of conduction through the AV node, and more forceful contractions. Parasympathetic fibers, which are

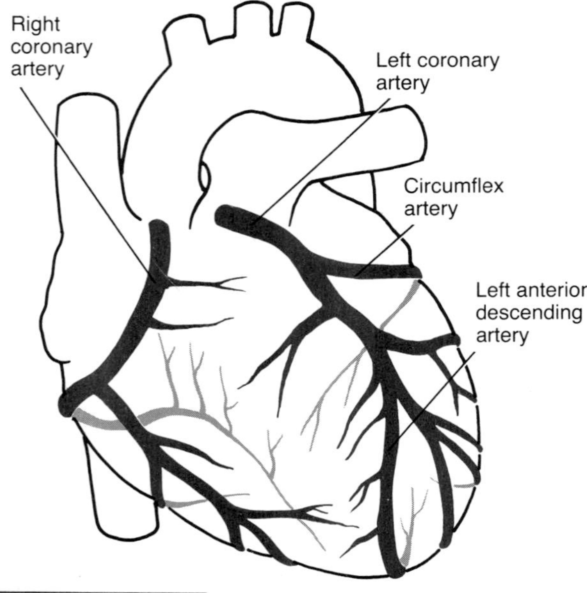

FIGURE 31–3
Coronary arteries.

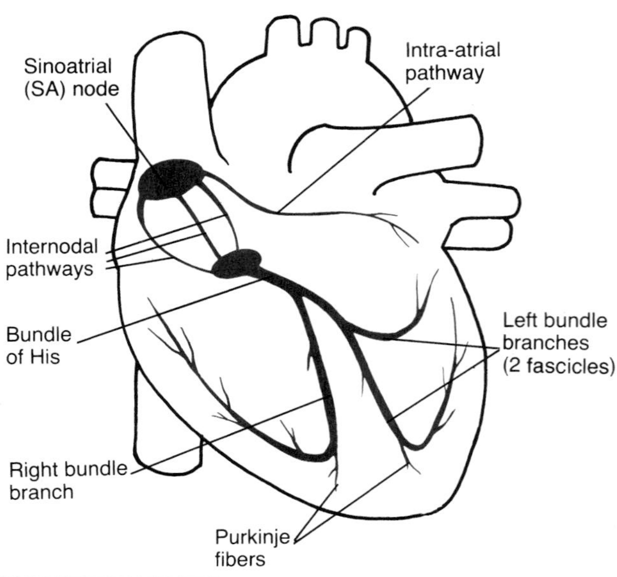

FIGURE 31–4
The conduction system of the heart.

part of the vagus nerve, are found primarily in the SA and AV nodes and the atrial tissue. Parasympathetic stimulation results in slowing of the heart rate, slowing of conduction through the AV node, and decreased strength of contraction.

CARDIAC CYCLE. Each complete heartbeat comprises the cardiac cycle. Contraction, or depolarization, is called systole. It is the first heart sound heard with a stethoscope when assessing the apical pulse. It is often referred to as "lubb" and is louder than the second sound, "dub," at the apex of the heart. The second sound is the relaxation, or repolarization, of the ventricles. It is also called diastole. In a person with a heart rate of 60 beats per minute (bpm), there would be 60 cardiac cycles per minute. Figure 31–5 illustrates the events of the cardiac cycle.

CARDIAC PHYSIOLOGY

CARDIAC MUSCLE. Essential physiologic characteristics of cardiac muscle are excitability, automaticity, conductivity, and contractility.

Excitability. Excitability is the cell's capacity to respond to an electrochemical stimulus. Cardiac cells, in their resting state, are electrically polarized. The insides of the cells are negatively charged; the outsides are positively charged. Polarity is maintained by membrane pumps that ensure the appropriate distribution of ions (sodium, potassium, and calcium) necessary to keep the insides of the cells relatively electronegative. Cardiac cells lose their internal negativity in a process called depolarization. Depolarization is the fundamental electrical event in the heart. Depolarization moves from cell to cell, producing a wave transmitted across the entire heart. Once depolarization is complete, cardiac cells restore their resting polarity through a process called repolarization.

Automaticity. Automaticity is the cell's capacity to generate an impulse without external stimulation. The SA node can spontaneously generate action potentials, allowing the heart to function independent of the autonomic nervous system. The SA node generates impulses at the rate of 60 to 100 bpm.

Conductivity. Conductivity is the cell's ability to transmit electric impulses rapidly and efficiently to distant regions of the heart. Transmission is delayed through the AV node, allowing the ventricles to fill adequately before contracting. The AV node's intrinsic rate is 40 to

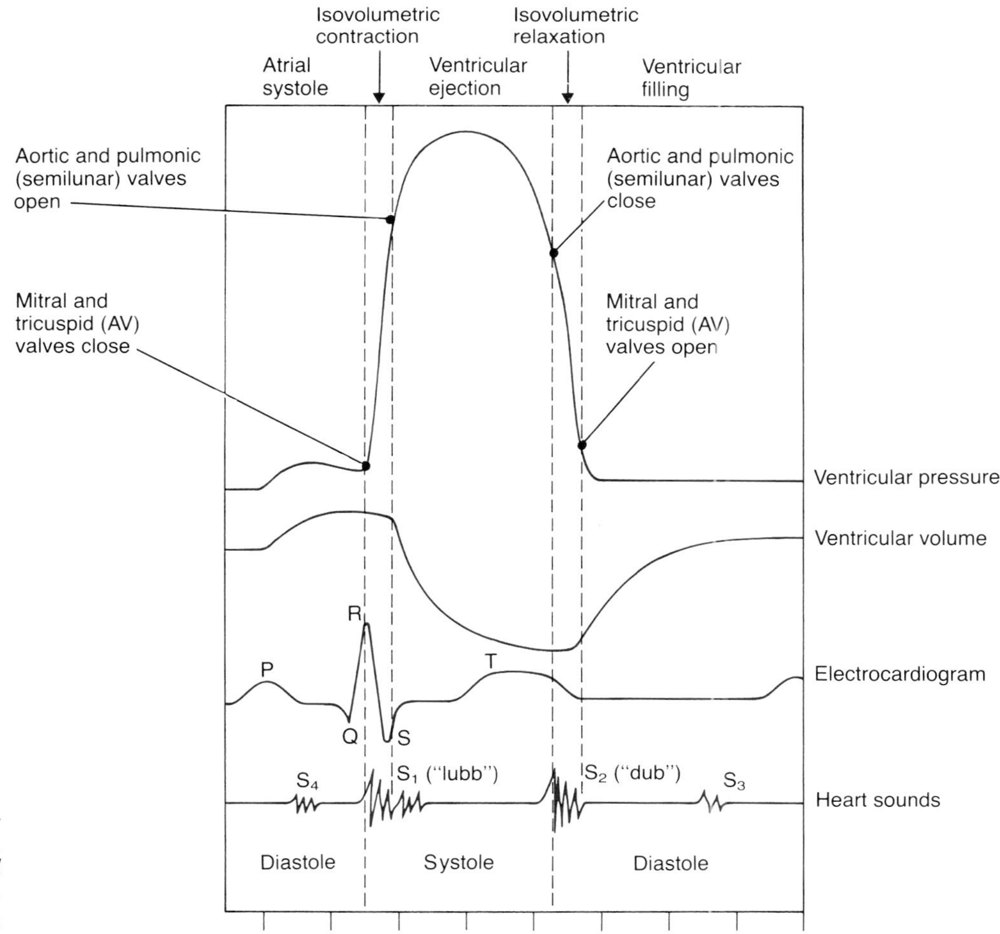

FIGURE 31–5

The cardiac cycle. (From Ignatavicius, D. D., & Bayne, M. V. [1991]. *Medical-surgical nursing: A nursing process approach* [p. 2076]. Philadelphia: W. B. Saunders.)

60 bpm. The Purkinje network's intrinsic rate is fewer than 40 bpm and for a short time can prevent cessation of heart function (Table 31–1).

Contractility. Contractility is the ability of cardiac muscle fibers to shorten when stimulated. Calcium, which is necessary for myocardial contraction, enhances contractility.

SYSTOLE AND DIASTOLE. The primary function of the heart is to pump blood through the pulmonary and systemic circulations. This is accomplished by a continually repeating pattern of contraction (systole) and relaxation (diastole).

Systole. Systole (S_1) begins with the closure of the mitral and tricuspid valves when the ventricles are full of blood. The muscle fibers tense and shorten, and intraventricular pressure increases. When the pressure in the ventricles exceeds the pressure in the aorta and the pulmonary arteries, the aortic and pulmonary valves open and blood is rapidly ejected. Two thirds of the stroke volume is ejected at this time. Rapid ejection is followed by a period of slow ejection when the pressure in the ventricles begins to decrease. Slow ejection continues until the pressure in the ventricles drops below the pressure in the aorta and pulmonary arteries; then the valves close.

Diastole. Closure of the valves produces the second heart sound, S_2, diastole. When all four valves close, the pressure in the ventricles drops rapidly as the muscle fibers relax. This continues until ventricular pressure is less than atrial pressure. Meanwhile, the atria are filling with blood from the pulmonary and systemic circulations. As the atrial pressure increases, the AV valves open, the ventricular fibers relax, and the ventricles fill.

Late diastole occurs as blood from the pulmonary system passes through the nearly empty atrium, and at this time there is optimal filling of the coronary arteries.

The final period of diastole occurs as the atria contract. Atrial contraction contributes an additional 20 to 30% to the end-diastolic volume in the ventricles. This effect is referred to as *atrial kick.* At the end of atrial contraction, the pressure in the ventricles exceeds the pressure in the atria and the AV valves close. The sound made by the closing of these valves is called systole, S_1.

CARDIAC OUTPUT. The volume of blood ejected by the heart each minute is determined by the stroke volume and the heart rate. Stroke volume is the amount of blood ejected with each ventricular contraction. The volume depends on myocardial contractility. The normal stroke volume is 60 to 100 ml. Cardiac output is the amount of blood (in liters) ejected by each ventricle per minute. It is calculated by multiplying heart rate times stroke volume ($CO = HR \times SV$). The normal cardiac output is 4 to 8 liters per minute. In the normal heart, cardiac output responds to the increased demands for oxygen and nutrients that occur with exercise, infection, or stress.

The cardiac index is a more accurate way of evaluating cardiac performance because it adjusts for body surface area. The cardiac index is obtained by dividing the cardiac output by the body surface area ($CI = CO \div BSA$). The body surface area is determined by the Dubois Body Surface Chart (Fig. 31–6). The normal cardiac index is 2.5 to 4.0 liters per minute/m^2 and indicates whether cardiac output is sufficient to meet the individual's needs.

Ejection fraction is the percentage of ventricular end-diastolic volume ejected with each stroke. The normal ejection fraction is greater than 60% and is considered a sensitive index of LV function.

Depression of ventricular function leads to decreased stroke volume, decreased ejection fraction, and increased residual ventricular volume.

Three factors affect stroke volume: preload, contractility, and afterload.

Preload. Preload is the amount of blood in the LV at the end of diastole or the pressure generated at end diastole. This is called left ventricular end-diastolic pressure. Preload is estimated at the bedside by measuring the pulmonary capillary wedge pressure or the left atrial pressure. Starling's law states that, within limits, the greater the stretch of the myocardial fiber, the more forcefully it will contract. When the preload increases, the myocardial fibers are stretched, resulting in a more forceful contraction. Increased preload results in increased stroke volume and, therefore, increased cardiac output. Factors that increase preload include increased venous return to the heart and overhydration. Factors that decrease preload include dehydration, hemorrhage, and venous vasodilation.

Contractility. Contractility is affected by biochemical changes. Inotropy is the contractile state of the cell. Factors that increase contractility (such as catecholamines) are said to have a positive inotropic effect. Factors that decrease contractility (such as acidosis and beta blockers) create a negative inotropic effect.

Afterload. Afterload is the amount of pressure the LV must generate to open the aortic valve. It is determined primarily by the diastolic pressure in the aorta. Afterload is decreased by vasodilation and increased by hypertension, vasoconstriction, and aortic stenosis. Afterload affects the rate of contraction. Decreased afterload increases heart rate and cardiac output. Increased afterload decreases heart rate and cardiac output.

Vascular resistance, the force opposing blood flow within the vessels, has a direct effect on afterload. Vascular resistance is the product of three factors: vessel

TABLE 31-1

INTRINSIC HEART RATES

INITIATION OF IMPULSE	RATE
Sinoatrial node	60–100 bpm
Atrioventricular node	40–60 bpm
Ventricle	15–40 bpm

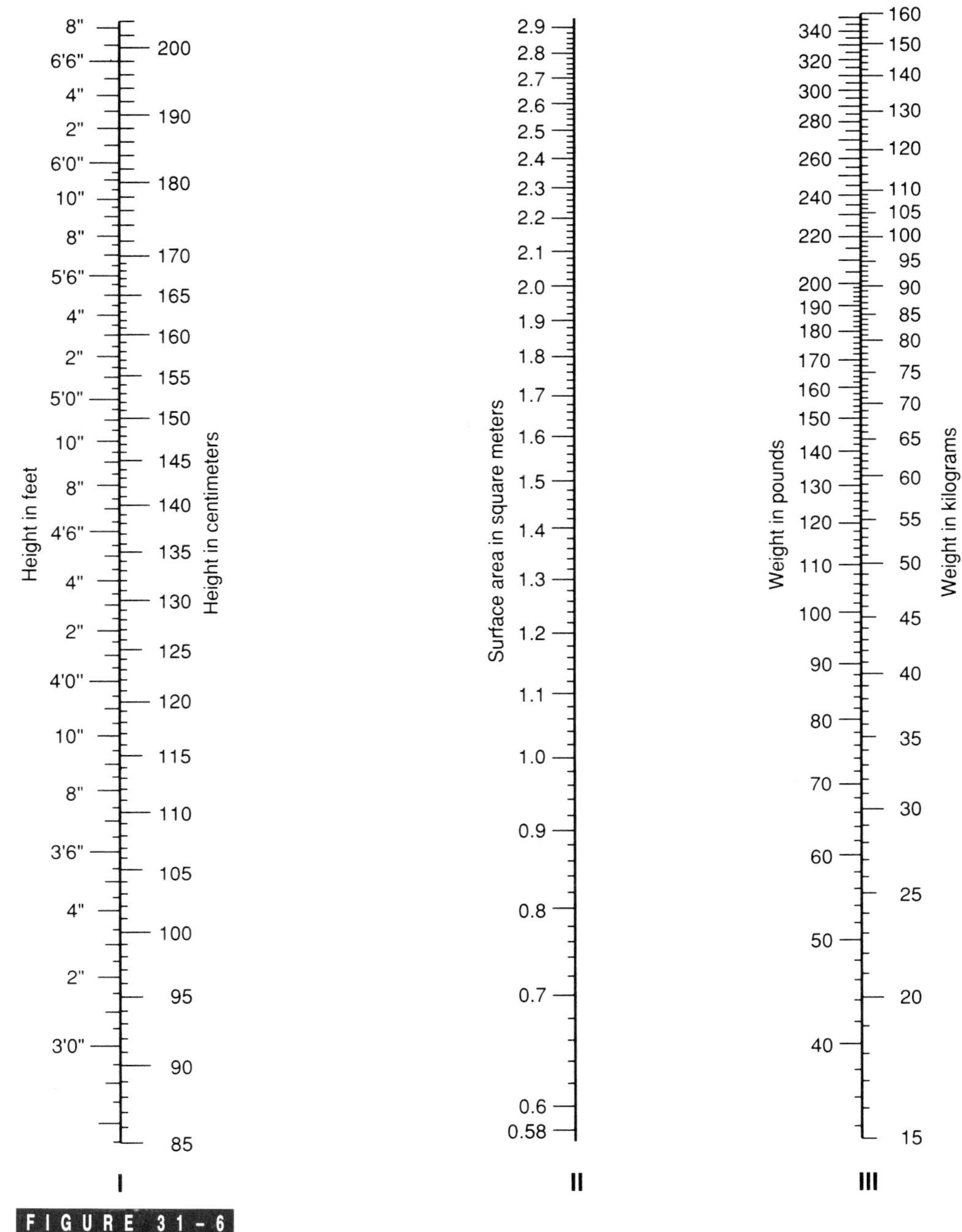

FIGURE 31–6

Dubois' body surface chart. To determine body surface area, (1) Locate the patient's height on scale I; (2) Locate the patient's weight on scale III; (3) Draw a straight line between the two points; (4) Locate the body surface area on the point where the straight line intersects scale II. (From Dubois, E. F. [1936]. *Basal metabolism in health and disease.* Malvern, PA: Lea & Febiger. Copyright 1920 by W. M. Boothby and R. B. Sandiford.)

radius, vessel length, and blood viscosity. Pulmonary vascular resistance and systemic vascular resistance are calculated to assess the patient's physiologic status. The normal pulmonary vascular resistance is 45 to 120 dynes per second per cm^2. The normal systemic vascular resistance is 900 to 1500 dynes per second per cm^2. It is derived from the mean arterial pressure, the central venous pressure, and the cardiac output. Mean arterial pressure is the sum of the systolic blood pressure plus twice the diastolic blood pressure divided by three. The normal mean arterial pressure is 80 to 100. It is a measure of peripheral tissue perfusion (Table 31–2).

MYOCARDIAL OXYGEN CONSUMPTION. Myocardial tissue routinely extracts 70 to 75% of the oxygen delivered to it via the arteries. Skeletal muscles, by

TABLE 31-2
HEMODYNAMIC MONITORING VALUES

VALUE	FORMULA	NORMAL RANGE
Cardiac output (CO)	HR × SV	4–8 L/min
Cardiac index (CI)	CO ÷ BSA	2.5–4.0 L/min/m^2
Stroke volume (SV)	CO ÷ HR	60–100 ml/beat
Ejection fraction (EF)		> 60%
Pulmonary vascular resistance (PVR)	$\frac{\text{PA mean} - \text{PCWP}}{\text{CO}} \times 80$	45–120 dynes/sec/cm^2
Systemic vascular resistance (SVR)	$\frac{\text{MAP} - \text{CVP}}{\text{CO}} \times 80$	900–1500 dynes/sec/cm^2
Mean arterial pressure	$\frac{\text{Systolic BP} + 2\text{ diastolic BP}}{3}$	80–100 mm Hg

BP, Blood pressure.

contrast, extract 35% at rest and up to 75% during exercise. The only ways to increase oxygen supply to the myocardium are to (1) increase the coronary blood flow by coronary artery vasodilation or (2) increase the oxygen tension of the blood by administering supplemental oxygen. An accelerated heart rate increases myocardial oxygen demand.

Blood pressure is the pressure exerted on blood vessels by the blood as it flows through the vessels. The pressure-regulating mechanisms include neural receptors and hormonal regulators. A detailed discussion of blood pressure regulation is presented in Chapter 33.

AGE-RELATED CHANGES

It is difficult to separate the normal age-related changes in the heart and blood vessels from the changes caused by disease. In general, age-related changes progress slowly, whereas pathogenic changes are more likely to be sudden.

HEART

Changes in the heart muscle include increased density of connective tissue and decreased elasticity. Cardiac contractility may decline, making the heart less able to adapt to changes in circulating blood volume. The valves may thicken and stiffen. If they do not close properly, the patient may have a murmur. The valves may also partially block the path of blood flow, causing incomplete emptying of the chambers.

The number of pacemaker cells in the SA node decreases, as do the number of nerve fibers in the ventricles. The aging heart takes longer to respond to stress and then responds less dramatically. It also takes longer to return to normal after exercise or stress. Cardiac dysrhythmias are more common in older people but should still be evaluated because they can be dangerous.

BLOOD VESSELS

Changes in connective tissue and elastic fibers in arteries cause them to become stiffer. Pulse pressure and systolic blood pressure generally increase. Experts disagree as to exactly what constitutes hypertension in the elderly. The American Heart Association recommends treatment of pressure exceeding 160/90, but individual physicians may use different guidelines. The veins stretch and dilate, leading to venous stasis and sometimes impaired venous return. Thrombophlebitis and varicosities are more common in older people.

The cardiovascular system adapts more slowly to changes in position, so postural hypotension may occur.

NURSING ASSESSMENT OF CARDIAC FUNCTION

HEALTH HISTORY

A complete assessment is important for the cardiac patient. If the patient is having acute symptoms, however, a detailed assessment must be deferred until the patient is stable.

THE CHIEF COMPLAINT AND HISTORY OF PRESENT ILLNESS. The nurse assesses the patient's reason for seeking medical care. Common symptoms that may be related to cardiac disorders include fatigue, edema, palpitations, dyspnea, and pain. The nurse notes when symptoms occur, what aggravates them, and what relieves them.

PAST MEDICAL HISTORY. The nurse asks if the patient has had specific conditions that may be related to cardiac disease. These include hypertension, kidney disease, pulmonary disease, stroke, rheumatic fever, streptococcal sore throat, and scarlet fever. Previous cardiac disorders and hospitalizations are documented. Recent and current medications are listed, and allergies are noted in appropriate records.

FAMILY HISTORY. Because cardiovascular problems are often familial or hereditary, the nurse assesses whether immediate relatives have had hypertension, coronary artery disease, other cardiac disorders, or diabetes mellitus.

REVIEW OF SYSTEMS. The nurse systematically assesses whether the patient has experienced the following specific symptoms: weight gain, fatigue, dyspnea (shortness of breath), cough, orthopnea (difficulty breathing in a supine position), paroxysmal nocturnal dyspnea (sudden dyspnea during sleep), palpitations, chest pain, fainting, concentrated urine, or leg edema.

If the patient has had dyspnea or orthopnea, the nurse determines when it occurred and whether the onset was gradual or sudden. Pain also requires detailed description. The pain of heart problems may radiate or be referred to other areas. The pain may radiate down either arm, to the jaw, or to just below the sternum. The severity may range from mild, intermittent discomfort to severe, crushing chest pain. The patient is asked to rate the severity of the pain on a scale of 1 (mildest) to 10 (worst possible). The nurse documents the exact description, location, severity, radiation, events causing the pain, and what relieves the pain.

FUNCTIONAL ASSESSMENT. The nurse determines how this illness has affected the patient's ability to carry out usual activities. Activity and rest patterns and usual diet are described. It is especially important to record salt and fat intake. The patient is asked about sources of stress and coping strategies.

PHYSICAL EXAMINATION

The physical examination begins with measurement of height and weight and vital signs.

Vital Signs

BLOOD PRESSURE. The correct-sized blood pressure cuff must be used. The arm is positioned at the heart level, and the blood pressure is checked in both arms. The pulse pressure (difference between the systolic and diastolic pressures) is noted because it is a noninvasive measure of cardiac output. Blood pressures and pulse rates are then measured in the lying, sitting, and standing positions. A blood pressure decrease of 20 mm Hg or more with a position change indicates decreased blood volume or an autonomic response. As blood pressure decreases the pulse should increase as a compensatory mechanism. The patient may feel dizzy or lightheaded and could faint if the blood pressure falls too much.

PULSES. The radial pulses are assessed for rate, rhythm, quality, and equality. The apical pulse is auscultated for rate and rhythm. Apical and radial pulses may be taken simultaneously to detect a pulse deficit. The normal heart rate is 60 to 100 bpm. A rate of less than 60 bpm is considered to be evidence of bradycardia; tachycardia is characterized by a heart rate in excess of 100 bpm. The rhythm is assessed as regular or irregular. The quality of the pulse is graded on a four-point scale: 0, absent pulse (not palpable); 1+, weak or thready pulse (pulse easily obliterated by slight finger pressure, returning as pressure is released); 2+, normal pulse (easily palpable); 3+, bounding pulse (forceful, not easily obliterated by finger pressure). The apical pulse is assessed at the fifth intercostal space at the midclavicular line with a stethoscope. In addition to the radial pulse, the nurse assesses the carotid, brachial, femoral, popliteal, posterior tibial, and dorsalis pedis pulses at appropriate times in the physical examination (see Fig. 32–4, Chapter 32).

RESPIRATIONS. The nurse observes the patient's respiratory effort and skin color. The respiratory rate is counted, and the stethoscope is used to auscultate the breath sounds for crackles and wheezes. The color and appearance of sputum is described.

Skin

The patient's skin is inspected for color, hair distribution, and capillary refill and is palpated for temperature. Skin color and temperature should be relatively the same over the entire body.

Heart Sounds

The heart sounds are systole (lubb) and diastole (dub). Heart sounds are auscultated with the diaphragm of the stethoscope placed firmly on the anterior chest. Figure 31–7 shows where the heart sounds, made by closing of the valves, may be heard best. With practice, the nurse can learn to distinguish these. The following pattern of auscultation is recommended:

1. Listen to the aortic area first and then the pulmonic. As the aortic and the pulmonic valves close the

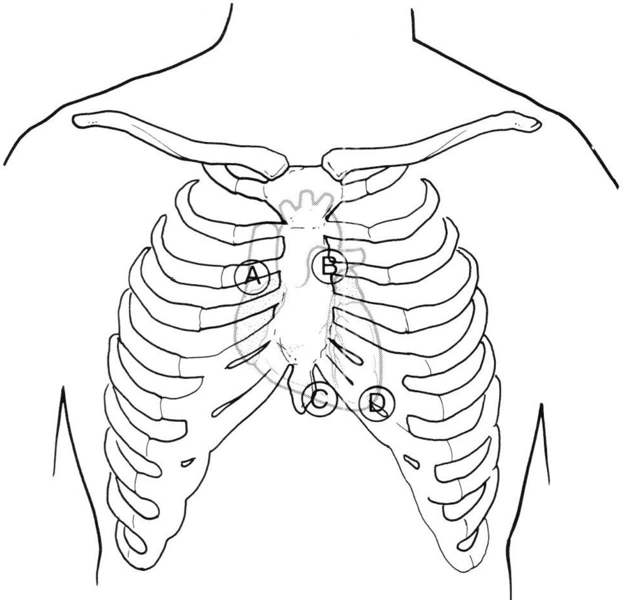

FIGURE 31–7

Auscultation of the heart. (A) *Aortic valve* at the second intercostal space to the right of the sternum; (B) *pulmonic valve* at the second intercostal space to the left of the sternum; (C) *tricuspid valve* at the fifth intercostal space to the left of the sternum; (D) *mitral valve* at the fifth intercostal space in the midclavicular line.

dub should be louder than the lubb in the aortic and pulmonic areas.

2. Listen to the tricuspid and mitral valves in the areas indicated. In these areas the lubb should be louder than the dub. In each area note the pitch, intensity, and duration of each sound.

3. After listening to each area with the diaphragm, repeat the pattern with the bell of the stethoscope. Note the additional sounds of S_3 and S_4. The S_3 and S_4 sounds are heard best with the bell of the stethoscope placed at the apex when the patient is positioned on the left side. S_3, also called a *ventricular gallop*, occurs early in diastole. S_3 is normal in children and young adults and may be pathologic after age 30. S_4, also called an

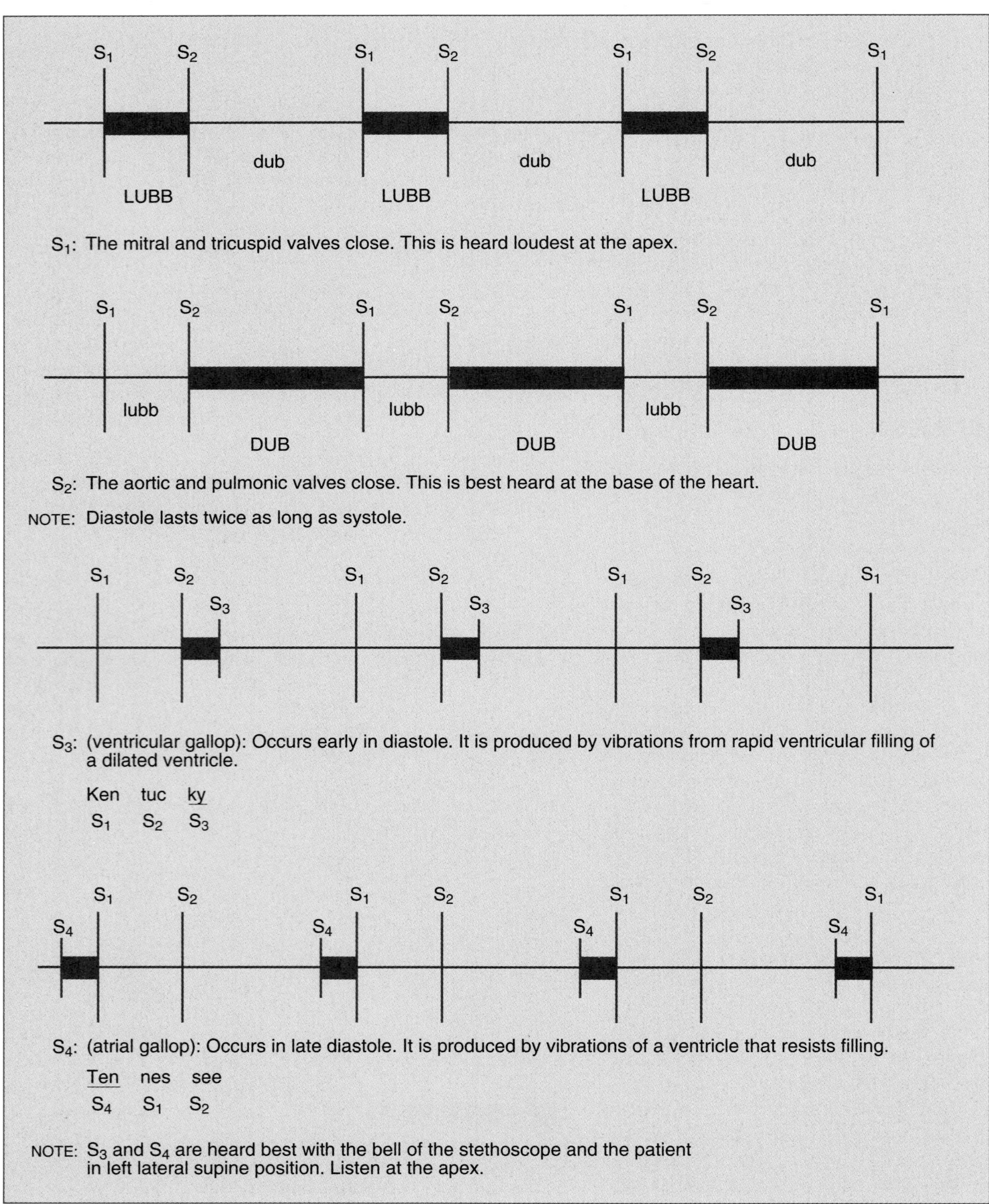

FIGURE 31-8

Listening to heart sounds.

atrial gallop, occurs late in diastole. S_4 is an abnormal heart sound. Figure 31–8 illustrates heart sounds S_1, S_2, S_3, and S_4.

HEART MURMURS. A heart murmur is the sound produced by turbulent blood flow across the valves. Murmurs are recorded as having high, low, or medium pitch, and they are located using the anatomic landmarks where they are heard best. The timing of a murmur relates to when it is heard in the cardiac cycle: early, middle, or late systole or diastole. A pansystolic murmur is heard throughout systole. A pandiastolic murmur is heard throughout diastole. A holosystolic murmur is heard throughout the entire cardiac cycle. Murmurs are graded according to intensity (Table 31–3).

A rub is heard when the pericardium is inflamed. A scratchy or muffled sound may be heard best by having the patient sit upright and lean forward. This position brings the pericardium closer to the chest wall. A pericardial friction rub is best heard along the left sternal border throughout the cardiac cycle.

Extremities

The extremities are inspected and palpated for color, edema, warmth, temperature, pulse quality, and hair distribution.

Assessment of the cardiac patient is summarized in Table 31–4.

TABLE 31-4

ASSESSMENT OF PATIENTS WITH CARDIAC DISORDERS

HEALTH HISTORY

Present illness: Fatigue, edema, palpitations, pain; aggravating and relieving factors

Past medical history: Hypertension, kidney disease, pulmonary disease, diabetes mellitus, stroke, rheumatic fever, streptococcal sore throat, scarlet fever, previous cardiac diseases or conditions, previous hospitalizations; recent and current medications; allergies

Family history: Hypertension, coronary artery disease or other cardiac conditions, diabetes mellitus

Review of systems: Weight gain, fatigue, dyspnea, cough, orthopnea, palpitations, chest pain, fainting, concentrated urine, leg edema

Functional assessment: Effects of illness on usual activities, activity and rest pattern, lifestyle, diet, sodium and fat intake, sources of stress, coping strategies

PHYSICAL EXAMINATION

General survey: Apparent distress

Height and weight

Vital signs: Blood pressure in both arms and while supine, sitting, standing; apical heart rate and rhythm; peripheral pulses: rate, rhythm, quality, equality; respiratory effort and rate

Skin: Color, hair distribution, capillary refill, temperature

Thorax: Heart sounds, heart murmurs, rubs; breath sounds, crackles, wheezes; presence and appearance of sputum

Extremities: Pulses, color, warmth, edema, hair distribution

DIAGNOSTIC TESTS AND PROCEDURES

ELECTROCARDIOGRAM

The electrocardiogram allows study of the electrical activity (conduction system) through the heart muscle. Electrical activity precedes mechanical activity in the heart. The mechanical activity is assessed by palpating the pulse. The ECG is graphed on standardized paper or viewed on an oscilloscope. Different angles allow interpretation of conduction in various planes and permit detection of conduction disturbances in specific areas of the heart.

TABLE 31-3

GRADING OF HEART MURMURS

GRADE	DESCRIPTION
I	Very faint
II	Faint, but recognizable
III	Loud, but moderate in intensity
IV	Loud and accompanied by a palpable thrill
V	Very loud, accompanied by a palpable thrill, and audible with the stethoscope partially off the client's chest
VI	Extremely loud, may be heard with the stethoscope slightly above the client's chest

From Ignatavicius, D. D., & Bayne M. V. (1991). *Medical-surgical nursing: A nursing process approach* (p. 2098). Philadelphia: W. B. Saunders.

Electrodes placed on the surface of the skin pick up the electrical impulses of the heart. The impulses are magnified and recorded on calibrated paper. Each cardiac cycle is represented by a series of P, Q, R, S, and T waves. The P wave represents atrial depolarization (as a result of the firing of the SA node) and is followed by a delay in conduction as the impulse passes through the AV node. The QRS complex represents ventricular depolarization (contraction) and is larger than the P wave because of the size of the ventricular muscle. The T wave represents ventricular repolarization (relaxation) and follows the QRS complex. A U wave, if present, may indicate a potassium imbalance.

The electrocardiogram is interpreted to detect abnormalities in rate, rhythm, or impulse conduction. The normal finding is called a *normal sinus rhythm*. It is characterized by the following:

1. A rate of 60 to 100 bpm
2. A regular rhythm
3. A P wave preceding each QRS complex
4. A PR interval that is within 0.12 to 0.20 second
5. A QRS complex that is 0.10 second or less

The common variations of normal sinus rhythm are sinus bradycardia and sinus tachycardia. In sinus bradycardia the rate is less than 60 bpm, but all other parameters fall within the normal limits. In sinus tachycardia the rate is in excess of 100 bpm, and the remaining parameters are within normal limits. Additional dysrhythmias are presented later in this chapter.

An ECG requires no special preparation, but the patient is told what to expect and that the procedure is painless.

ECHOCARDIOGRAM

The echocardiogram, or heart sonogram, is a visualization and recording of the size, shape, position, and behavior of the heart's internal structures, especially the valves. Ultrasonic waves are beamed into the heart, and their echoes are recorded. This procedure is used to evaluate some aspects of cardiac function and to diagnose a variety of cardiac disorders.

For this procedure, gel is applied to the skin and a special device called a transducer is moved over the precordium. The transducer picks up sound waves and converts them to electrical impulses. The machine converts the electrical impulses to waveforms on an oscilloscope, a videotape, or a strip chart. The patient may need to change position or to breathe in certain ways during the procedure.

The procedure requires no special preparation. The nurse explains to the patient that the procedure is noninvasive and painless and requires 30 to 60 minutes. The test may be done at the bedside or in a laboratory. Following the procedure, the conductive gel is removed from the chest wall.

PHONOCARDIOGRAM

The phonocardiogram records heart sounds graphically. The graph is compared with an ECG recorded simultaneously. The test is useful for timing events in the cardiac cycle, detecting murmurs and other abnormal heart sounds, and identifying structural valve defects. There is no patient preparation other than explanation of the test.

MAGNETIC RESONANCE IMAGING

A magnetic resonance imaging (MRI) scan provides high resolution, three-dimensional images of body structures. This procedure is superior to the computed tomography (CT) scan for differentiating diseased tissue from healthy tissue. Cardiac tissue is imaged without lung or bone interference. The patient is enclosed in a chamber for approximately 5 minutes for an MRI scan of the heart. No metallic objects are permitted in the chamber during the procedure.

MULTIPLE-GATED ACQUISITION SCANNING

In a multiple-gated acquisition scan, a camera records ventricular end-systolic and end-diastolic cardiac cycles after injection of technetium 99m–tagged red blood cells. Technetium 99m concentrates in acutely necrotic myocardial tissue. The purposes of the multiple-gated acquisition scan are to evaluate left ventricular function, detect left ventricular aneurysms, evaluate myocardial wall motion, detect intracardiac shunting, follow patients with valvular disease, locate and identify the size of a myocardial infarction, and determine left ventricular deterioration. Assessment of ventricular function can be done while resting or exercising. Sublingual nitroglycerin may be administered to assess its effect on ventricular function.

Preparation for this test includes an explanation to the patient, omission of food for 2 hours before the procedure, establishment of an intravenous infusion, placement of ECG leads, and a signed consent form.

STRESS TEST

The stress test, or exercise tolerance test, is a recording of an individual's cardiovascular response during a measured exercise challenge. The stress test is a noninvasive method of assessing the presence and severity of coronary artery disease. It is also used to measure functional capacity for work, sport, or participation in a rehabilitation program. The stress test is not a flawless procedure; false positives and false negatives abound. It is, however, the best noninvasive screening procedure available. The alternative is the much more invasive cardiac catheterization.

For the stress test the patient ambulates on a treadmill or a stationary bicycle while connected to an ECG monitor with a continuous rhythm strip (Fig. 31–9). A complete 12-lead ECG is done at frequent intervals. The blood pressure is monitored during the procedure. The speed and incline angle of the treadmill are increased until (1) the patient cannot continue for whatever reason, (2) the patient's maximum heart rate is

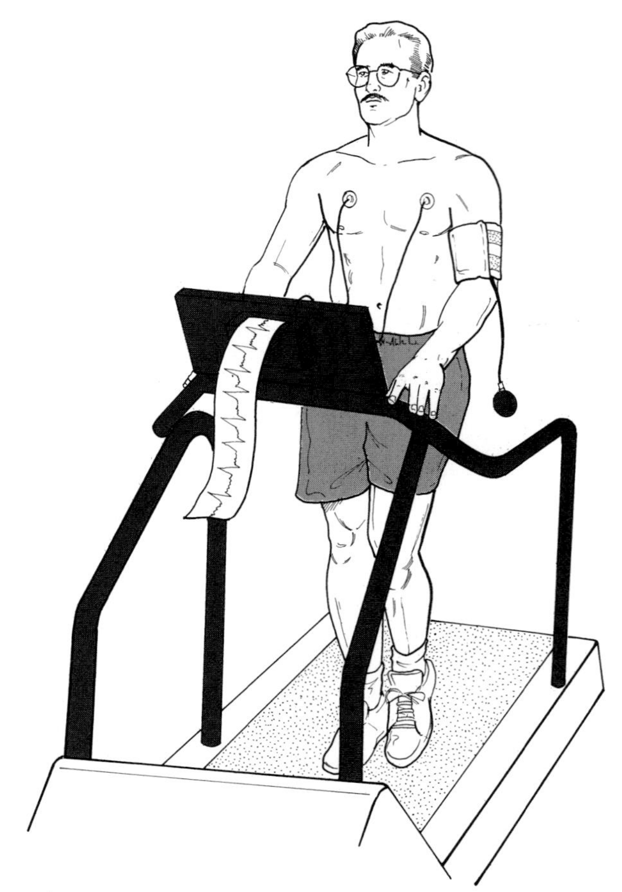

FIGURE 31–9
Stress test.

achieved, (3) symptoms intervene, or (4) significant changes are detected on the ECG. The target heart rate is 85% of the predicted maximum heart rate for the patient's age and sex. The maximum heart rate is calculated by subtracting the patient's age from 220.

Significant coronary artery disease (CAD) limits blood flow to the myocardium. The increased demands of exercise may cause symptoms of CAD to occur. The onset of such symptoms as angina, dizziness, dyspnea, or dysrhythmias or a falling blood pressure is an important sign that requires the test to be stopped immediately. A negative test result does not absolutely exclude CAD.

Contraindications for the test include acute systemic illness, severe aortic stenosis, uncontrolled congestive heart failure, severe hypertension, angina at rest, and significant dysrhythmia. Although the mortality rate for test participants is very low, cardiopulmonary resuscitation equipment must be available.

Preparation for a stress test includes a prohibition on food or fluids for 2 hours preceding the test and an explanation of how the test is performed. Informed consent must be obtained. The physician may order that beta blockers be tapered before the test. The patient should be advised to wear appropriate clothing: a loose top, a bra for women, and flat walking shoes.

Thallium Imaging

Thallium-201 may be administered for myocardial perfusion imaging during stress testing. Thallium closely parallels potassium in the normal myocardium and in particular is used to detect myocardial ischemia (old or new). The test may also be used to evaluate graft patency after coronary artery bypass graft surgery. A completely normal result on a thallium stress test may eliminate the need for the more invasive cardiac catheterization. The thallium-201 is injected, and the heart is scanned 10 to 15 minutes later to assess the areas of concentration. The scan is repeated in 4 hours to assess for redistribution.

Thallium does not enter infarcted or scarred areas and therefore shows "cold" spots in areas without blood flow. Exercise-induced ischemia resolves with rest. Scar-induced ischemia, like that caused by myocardial infarction, does not resolve with rest.

The advantages of the thallium scan include more specific detection of CAD, detection of ischemia in patients with left bundle branch block, and the ability to do the test while the patient is resting or has just completed treadmill exercise. Digoxin or left ventricular hypertrophy may hamper ECG recording during stress testing.

Preparation for thallium imaging is the same as for routine stress testing, but the patient should be told that an intravenous injection will be given. The nurse can assure the patient that the dose of radiation used is small and harmless.

HOLTER MONITOR

An ambulatory ECG, or Holter monitor, provides continuous monitoring. A portable ECG machine with a memory is worn for 24 to 48 hours. A complete record of the heart rhythm is stored and analyzed later. This type of monitoring is used to detect dysrhythmias that occur infrequently, to determine if symptoms correlate with any underlying cardiac pathology, to assess the effects of medications, and for research purposes.

While the Holter monitor is in place, the patient wears loose-fitting clothing; takes sponge baths only; avoids metal detectors, magnets, and high voltage areas; and monitors the leads and electrode placements. The nurse teaches the individual to push the event button if symptoms occur. The patient records in a diary all activity that occurs during the monitoring, such as walking, stair climbing, sleep, and sexual activity. The monitor strip is computer scanned and then interpreted by a physician.

Even more sophisticated monitoring is accomplished by transtelephonic means. An audio signal is sent over telephone lines to a station manned by personnel trained to recognize potentially dangerous dysrhythmias.

CARDIAC CATHETERIZATION (CARDIAC ANGIOGRAPHY, CORONARY ARTERIOGRAPHY)

The advent of cardiac catheterization in the 1960s greatly advanced the understanding of the heart anatomy and physiology. Cardiac catheterization is a procedure in which a catheter is inserted into a vein or artery and threaded into the heart chambers or coronary arteries, or both, under fluoroscopy, as illustrated in Figure 31–10. When the catheter tip is in place, a contrast dye is injected and films made of the visualized heart structures. In a catheterization of the right side of the heart, the catheter is inserted into a vein and threaded into the vena cava, the RA, RV, and the pulmonary artery. Pressures in the RA, RV, and pulmonary artery may be determined. The function of the pulmonic and tricuspid valves may be assessed. In a catheterization of the left side of the heart the catheter is inserted into an artery and threaded against the flow of blood into the coronary arteries or the LV. With this procedure the function of the coronary arteries and the aortic and mitral valves may be assessed. Blood samples may be taken and pressures measured in each heart chamber. The femoral vein and artery are preferred insertion sites. This procedure may be done before heart surgery for coronary artery bypass grafting or aortic or mitral valve repair. Blood samples and pressures in the various structures may be assessed with this test.

This is an invasive procedure that requires the patient's informed consent. The nurse assesses the patient for allergies, especially to iodine, seafood, and shellfish. Food and fluids are withheld for a period of time before the procedure. The physician may order intravenous heparin if the patient has been taking oral anticoagulants. The patient is informed that the room where the procedure is done has a lot of equipment, the table adjusts in several ways, and the patient will be awake and expected to cooperate with instructions to remain still, cough, or deep breathe. A hot, flushing sensation

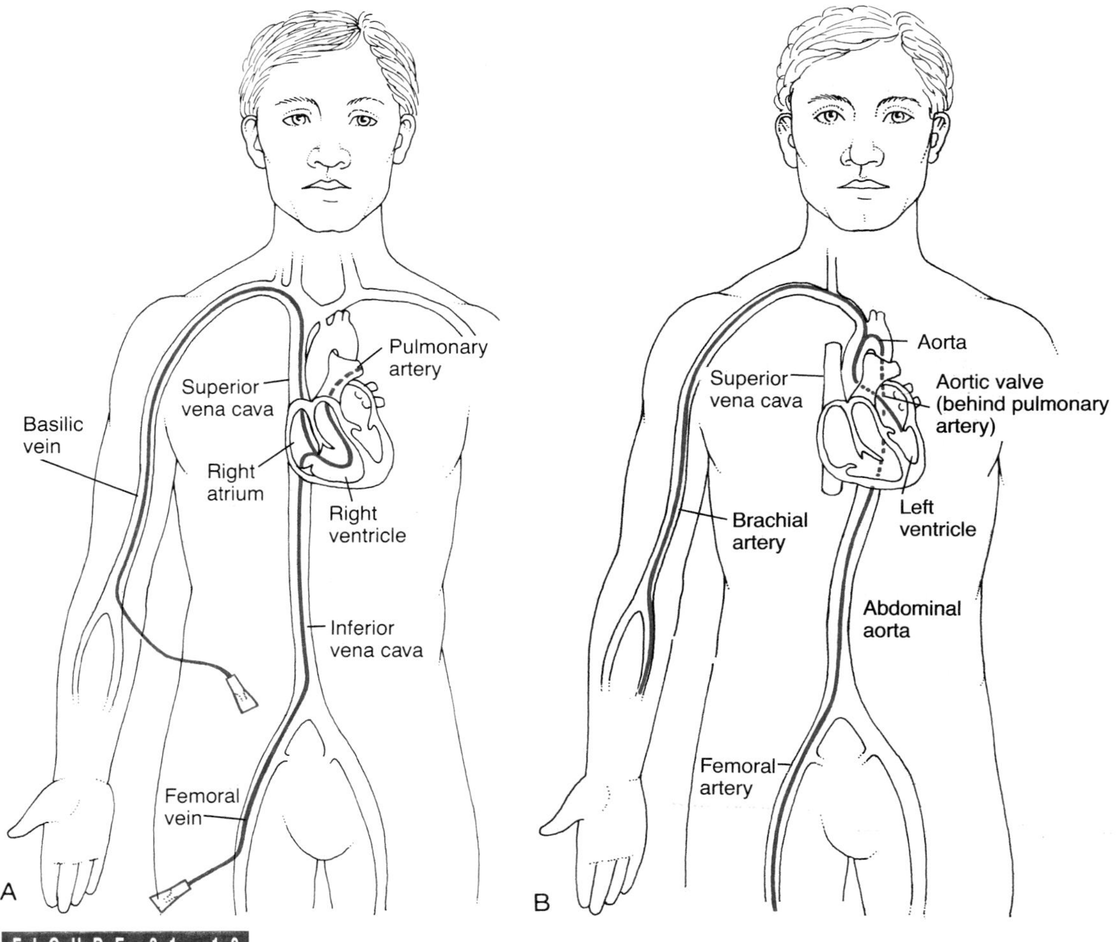

FIGURE 31-10

Right-sided *(A)* and left-sided *(B)* heart catheterization. (From Ignatavicius, D. D., & Bayne, M. V. [1991]. *Medical-surgical nursing: A nursing process approach* [p. 2108]. Philadelphia: W. B. Saunders.)

may be experienced when the dye is injected. Vital signs and ECG will be monitored during the procedure.

Following the cardiac catheterization, very firm pressure must be applied to the puncture site. Vital signs are assessed every 15 minutes for 1 hour and every 30 minutes until stable. The cannula insertion site is inspected for bleeding or hematoma formation with each assessment of vital signs. A dressing or pressure treatment (sandbag) may be applied to the site. Peripheral pulses are assessed as frequently as vital signs. The patient is instructed not to move the cannulated leg for 8 to 12 hours and not to ambulate for 24 hours. The patient is encouraged to drink large amounts of fluids to help remove the dye from the body. Generally the patient is allowed to eat as soon as the procedure is completed. Patients are often anxious to know the results of the test if these were not discussed during the procedure. The physician should explain the findings as soon as possible after the procedure. Complications of cardiac catheterization include bleeding, hematoma formation, infection, and embolus or thrombus formation.

HEMODYNAMIC MONITORING

In addition to noninvasive cardiac assessment such as blood pressure measurement and ECG monitoring, more sophisticated measures may be needed to determine what is going on within the heart itself. Two invasive catheters have been developed to assess the pressures within the heart and the lungs: the central catheter and the pulmonary artery catheter. Nurses who work in intensive care areas frequently work with patients who have these catheters.

Central Catheter

The central catheter is placed through the skin, into a blood vessel (brachial, femoral, subclavian, or jugular sites), and threaded into the RA. The catheter may have one to three lumens. With this catheter the pressure in the RA (called right atrial pressure [RAP] or central venous pressure [CVP]) can be measured (Fig. 31–11). This measurement is used as an indication of fluid volume. The normal CVP or RAP is 2 to 6 mm Hg. Meas-

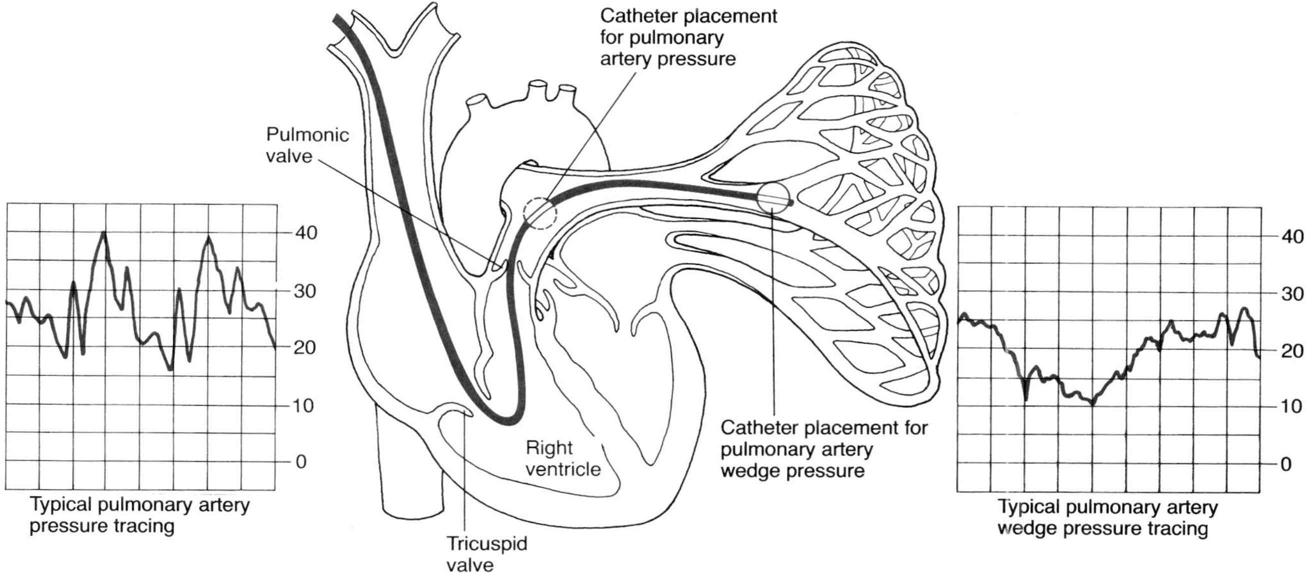

FIGURE 31-11

Central venous catheter and pressure waveform. (From Ignatavicius, D. D., & Bayne, M. V. [1991]. *Medical-surgical nursing: A nursing process approach* [p. 2111]. Philadelphia: W. B. Saunders.)

urements below normal indicate hypovolemia, and measurements above normal indicate hypervolemia. This catheter may also be used to infuse fluids, blood and blood products, and medications as well as to withdraw blood for analysis.

Pulmonary Artery Catheter

The pulmonary artery catheter, frequently called a Swan-Ganz catheter, is longer than the central venous catheter. It is inserted like the central venous catheter and is threaded through the RA, the tricuspid valve, the RV, the pulmonic valve, and into the pulmonary artery. The catheter is balloon-tipped and flows with the blood. Different waveforms are seen on an oscilloscope as the catheter moves through the different areas of the heart (Fig. 31–12). Pulmonary artery catheters may have 2 to 5 lumens and are approximately 110 cm (44 inches) long. Various lumens are used to measure the pulmonary capillary wedge pressure, inflate the balloon, measure RAP, determine cardiac output, and administer fluids and drugs. Newer catheters incorporate fiberoptics for continuous monitoring of saturated venous oxygenation (Svo_2), a measure of tissue perfusion.

The purpose of pulmonary artery catheters is to assess left-sided heart function based on measurements in the right side of the heart. The proximal port is used to measure the RAP or CVP (normal value 2–6 mm Hg). The distal port measures the pulmonary artery pressure (normal value 20–30/0–10). The lungs are low pressure organs unless the patient has chronic obstructive pulmonary disease (COPD).

PULMONARY CAPILLARY WEDGE PRESSURE. To determine the pulmonary capillary wedge pressure, the balloon is inflated with 1.5 ml of air. This allows the tip of the catheter to float into a pulmonary capillary until it occludes the capillary. This measures the pressure ahead of the catheter, therefore, the left ventricular heart function. The normal pulmonary capillary wedge pressure is 4 to 12 mm Hg. Once the pressure is recorded, the balloon is deflated.

The pulmonary capillary wedge pressure is used to assess preload. The pressure is low when fluid is restricted, when diuretics are being administered, and when patients are receiving vasodilators such as nitroglycerin or morphine. The pressure is elevated with excess fluid or when fluid volume expanders such as albumin, dextran, or hetastarch are being administered.

CARDIAC OUTPUT. Cardiac output is most frequently measured by the thermodilution method. In this procedure, 5 or 10 ml of solution is injected through the proximal port at end expiration. A special tip called a thermistor measures the changes in temperature when the solution is injected. The cardiac output is calculated based on the time it takes to detect the change in temperature. In the past, iced solution was used. Current research, however, indicates that room temperature solution (5% dextrose in water or normal saline) is usually reliable for most patients. The procedure is repeated three times. The average of the three measurements is calculated by the cardiac monitor. The normal cardiac output is 4 to 8 liters per minute. Stress increases the cardiac output. Cardiac output may decrease with myocardial infarction, congestive heart failure, bradycardia, tachycardia, and some drugs. It is important for the nurse to use consistent technique in measuring cardiac output. Hemodynamic monitoring values are summarized in Table 31–2.

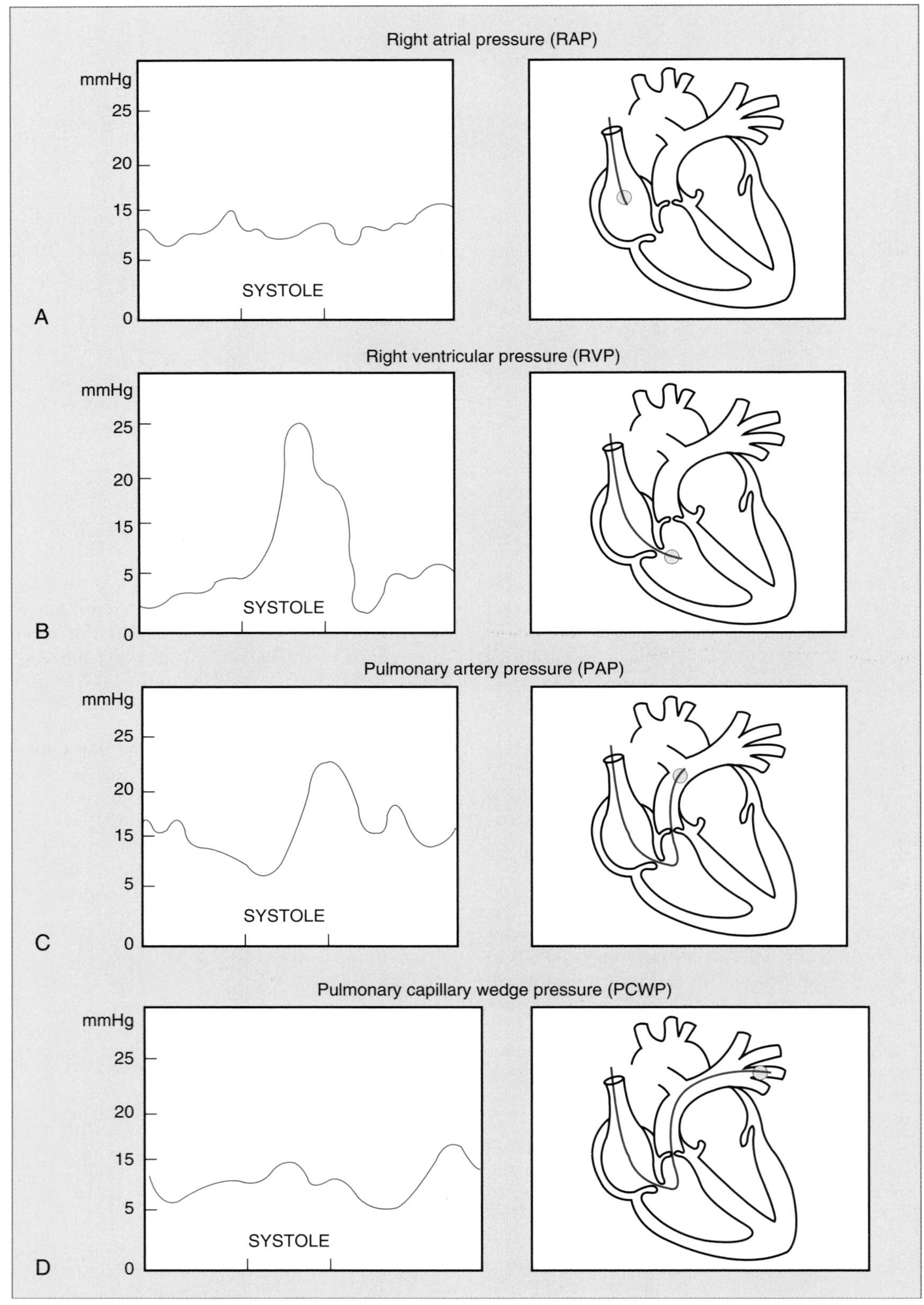

FIGURE 31-12
Pressure waveforms.

ARTERIAL LINES. An arterial line may be inserted (most often in the radial artery) to provide a direct measurement of systolic and diastolic blood pressures. Once the line is inserted, it is connected to a pressurized solution to keep the catheter patent and to a transducer to assess pressure. The mean arterial pressure is an indication of tissue perfusion. This pressure is elevated with sympathetic stimulation and increased heart rate.

LABORATORY TESTS

Complete Blood Count

The complete blood count is a basic screening test. Included in this test are the white blood cell count (WBC), the red blood cell count (RBC), the hemoglobin (Hgb) and hematocrit (Hct) measurements, the RBC indices, and in some laboratories the platelet count. The patient is advised that a blood specimen will be drawn. No special preparation is usually required, although the nurse should follow agency procedures. Components of the complete blood count are presented in Table 31–5.

WHITE BLOOD CELL COUNT. The WBC count indicates the body's ability to defend itself against infection and inflammation. The WBC level is generally elevated with inflammatory processes such as myocardial infarction and bacterial infections but may be below normal with viral infections and bone marrow depression.

RED BLOOD CELL COUNT. The RBC count is assessed to determine the ability of the blood to carry oxygen from the lungs to the tissues and carbon dioxide from the tissues to the lungs. The RBC level may be below normal with anemias and malignancies and may be elevated in dehydration.

TABLE 31–5
COMPLETE BLOOD COUNT

TEST		NORMAL VALUES
White blood cells		5000–10,000/ml
Differential:	Neutrophils	60–70%
	Eosinophils	1–4%
	Basophils	0.5–1.0%
	Lymphocytes	20–40%
	Monocytes	2–6%
Red blood cells		
Males		4,200,000–5,400,000/mm^3
Females		3,600,000–5,000,000/mm^3
Hematocrit		
Males		40–54%
Females		37–47%
Hemoglobin		
Males		13.5–17.5 gm/dl
Females		12–16 gm/dl
Platelets		150,000–350,000/mm^3

HEMATOCRIT. The Hct is the percentage of packed RBCs in the total sample of whole blood. With severe dehydration, the plasma portion of the blood decreases and the Hct is elevated. In anemias and hemorrhage, the Hct is below normal. In general, the Hct is three times the Hgb measurement.

HEMOGLOBIN. Hemoglobin is the main component of the RBCs. Its function is to transport oxygen to the cells. The Hgb measurement may be below normal in anemias and hemorrhage. It is elevated in dehydration, COPD, and congestive heart failure. A Hgb of less than 5 gm% leads to heart failure and death if not corrected.

PLATELET (THROMBOCYTE) COUNT. The platelets are the smallest of the formed elements in the blood. They are necessary for coagulation. The platelet count is below normal with anemias, bone marrow depression, and bleeding. The count may be increased in acute infections and some heart diseases. A count of less than 20,000 may result in spontaneous bleeding.

Erythrocyte Sedimentation Rate

The erythrocyte sedimentation rate measures the rate of settlement of RBCs in unclotted blood. It is a nonspecific test that detects inflammation or tissue necrosis. It is elevated with a variety of conditions, including acute myocardial infarction. It may also be elevated with malignancies, bacterial infections, and following surgery. The erythrocyte sedimentation rate may be below normal with congestive heart failure, mononucleosis, and angina.

Cardiac Enzymes

Cardiac enzymes are released when heart cells die as a result of damage. These enzymes are measured in the serum, and their values rise as indicators of damage to the heart cells. The tests usually require no preparation, although the nurse should consult the agency laboratory guidelines for any special instructions. The patient is advised that a blood sample will be drawn. Table 31–6 lists normal cardiac enzyme levels.

CREATINE PHOSPHOKINASE. This enzyme is found in three tissues in high concentration: brain, heart, and skeletal muscle. The type of creatine phosphokinase (CPK) specific to heart tissue is CPK-MB. Elevation of the CPK-MB level indicates damage to the myocardial cells. The CPK-MB can be expected to rise 4 to 6 hours after an acute myocardial infarction, peak in 12 to 24 hours at more than six times the normal value, and return to normal within 2 to 3 days if no new damage occurs. Serial trends should be observed. The nurse can plot these trends. An important point to remember is to draw the first CPK before any other invasion of the skin such as intramuscular injections and insertion of intravenous lines. Musculoskeletal injuries

TABLE 31–6
CARDIAC ENZYMES

TEST	NORMAL VALUES*
Creatine phosphokinase (CPK)	
Males	38–174 u/L
Females	96–140 u/L
CPK Isoenzymes	
MM	100%
MB	0%
BB	0%
Lactate dehydrogenase (LDH)	70–180 mg/dl 95–200 u/L
LDH isoenzymes	
LDH_1	17.5–28.3%
LDH_2	30.4–36.4%
Serum glutamic oxaloacetic transaminase (SGOT) or aspartate aminotransferase (AST)	
Males	7–21 u/L
Females	6–18 u/L

* Values may vary according to the laboratory equipment used.

(especially fractures and surgery) and recent excessive athletic activity can also elevate the CPK level.

LACTIC DEHYDROGENASE. Lactic dehydrogenase (LDH) is an intracellular enzyme with highest concentration in the heart, skeletal muscle, RBCs, liver, kidney, lung, and brain. There are five forms (isoenzymes) of LDH; LDH_1 and LDH_2 are primarily cardiac. Generally LDH_1 is lower than LDH_2. Causes of elevated LDH isoenzymes 1 and 2 are myocardial infarction, infections, liver disease, cancer, and blood transfusions.

ASPARTATE AMINOTRANSFERASE. Aspartate aminotransferase (AST) is also called serum glutamic oxaloacetic transaminase. This enzyme is found primarily in heart muscle and the liver. It is elevated with an acute myocardial infarction and in liver damage.

Arterial Blood Gases

Arterial blood gases are analyzed to determine the body's ability to maintain the acid-base balance. Acidity or alkalinity is determined by pH. If the serum pH is less than 7.35, the blood is acidic; greater than 7.45 indicates alkalinity. Carbonic acid dissociates into carbon diozide and water. The lungs regulate carbon dioxide. The partial pressure of carbon dioxide in the blood is abbreviated Pco_2. A Pco_2 greater than 45 with an acidic pH is a respiratory acidosis and indicates that the body is unable to excrete the excess carbon dioxide through the lungs. With a pH in excess of 7.45 and a Pco_2 of less than 35, a respiratory alkalosis is present.

The kidneys regulate bicarbonate (HCO_3) through excretion and retention. The HCO_3 (and or base excess, a combination of all serum bases) is assessed to determine metabolic causes of imbalance. If the pH is less than 7.35 and the HCO_3 is less than 22, the body is in metabolic acidosis. With a pH greater than 7.45 and a HCO_3 greater than 26, the interpretation is metabolic alkalosis (Table 31–7).

TABLE 31–7
INTERPRETING ARTERIAL BLOOD GASES

NORMAL RANGE	pH (7.35–7.45)	Pco_2 (35–45)	HCO_3 (22–26)
Respiratory acidosis	↓	↑	Normal
Respiratory alkalosis	↑	↓	Normal
Metabolic acidosis	↓	Normal	↓
Metabolic alkalosis	↑	Normal	↑

↑, Elevated; ↓, decreased.
NOTE: If the arrows are in the same direction a metabolic problem exists. If the arrows are in opposite directions a respiratory problem exists.

Patients with acute myocardial infarction often exhibit metabolic acidosis. Nursing responsibilities include preparing the patient for the procedure, preparing a heparinized syringe, performing the arterial stick or drawing blood from the arterial line, excluding air bubbles from the sample, inserting an airtight cap, icing the sample, and sending the sample to the laboratory. Following a direct arterial stick, pressure must be applied to the site for at least 5 minutes. The nurse interprets the results of the arterial blood gases test and communicates them to the physician.

Lipid Profile

A lipid profile is a battery of tests that measure the most common serum lipids: cholesterol, triglycerides, and phospholipids.

CHOLESTEROL. Cholesterol is a blood lipid produced by the liver. It is used to form bile salts for the digestion of fat and for the production of adrenal, ovarian, and testicular hormones. The normal adult serum cholesterol level is less than 200 mg per dl. Elevated cholesterol levels (hypercholesterolemia) are associated with increased risk of coronary artery disease, hypertension, and myocardial infarction. The cholesterol accumulates in the arterial lumen and in time results in decreased blood flow and occlusion.

Three forms of cholesterol are identified: high-density lipids (HDLs), low-density lipids (LDLs), and very low density lipids (VLDLs). The HDLs are desirable as they promote the excretion of LDLs and VLDLs. The normal LDL level is 60 to 160 mg per dl. The risk for coronary artery disease is increased if LDL levels are elevated. The risk for coronary artery disease is decreased if HDL levels are elevated. Normal HDL levels are 30 to 70 mg per dl. A good way to remember the difference is that HDLs are "healthy" and LDLs are "lethal."

TRIGLYCERIDES. Triglycerides are a major contributor to coronary artery disease. They are produced in the liver. Triglyceride levels increase when LDL levels increase. The normal triglyceride level is 40 to 150 mg per dl.

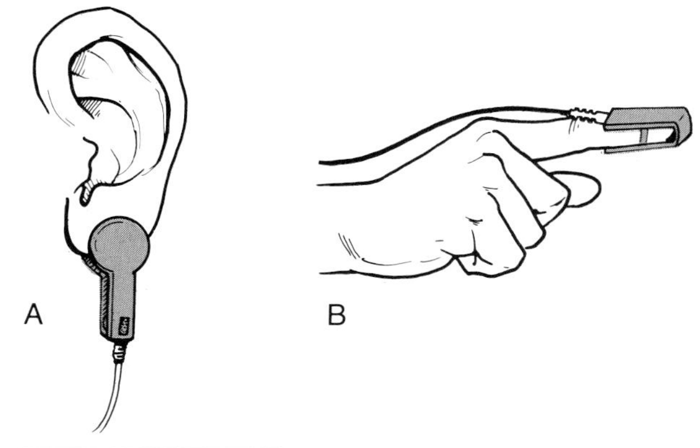

FIGURE 31–13

Pulse oximeter. *A*, Ear probe; *B*, clip on finger.

PULSE OXIMETRY

A pulse oximeter is a noninvasive measurement of arterial oxygen saturation. Light is passed through a pulsating artery and interpreted mechanically to determine the oxygen saturation. The transdermal clip or patch may be applied to a digit (finger or toe), the ear, or the nose (Fig. 31–13).

MIXED VENOUS OXYGEN SATURATION

The Svo_2 is monitored to assess the balance between oxygen delivery and oxygen utilization by the tissues. A fiberoptic flow-directed pulmonary artery catheter can be used to continuously monitor Svo_2. Normal Svo_2 for adults is 60 to 80%. This indicates adequate tissue perfusion. A slowly decreasing Svo_2 may indicate bleeding as the tissues have less oxygen delivered to them. Readings of less than 60% indicate cardiopulmonary failure or increased peripheral oxygen consumption. A reading of less than 20% indicates permanent cellular damage. Readings greater than 80% may occur with increased oxygen delivery, decreased oxygen demand, increased cardiac output, or an inability of the tissues to extract oxygen.

Table 31–8 summarizes diagnostic tests and procedures and nursing implications.

COMMON THERAPEUTIC MEASURES

DRUG THERAPY

Commonly used cardiac drugs are cardiac glycosides, antianginals, antidysrhythmics, and miscellaneous and emergency drugs. Examples of these drugs, their actions, their adverse effects, and nursing considerations are summarized in Table 31–9.

TABLE 31–8

THE HEART: DIAGNOSTIC TESTS AND PROCEDURES

TEST	PURPOSE/PROCEDURE	PATIENT PREPARATION	POSTPROCEDURE NURSING CARE
Electrocardiogram (ECG)	Electrodes are placed on the skin to detect electrical activity of the heart. Detects abnormalities in conduction of impulses including changes caused by heart damage.	Tell the patient what to expect and that the procedure is painless. No special preparation is required.	Remove gel from skin. No special care needed.
Echocardiogram	Uses ultrasound to create images of the heart. Gel is placed on the patient's skin and a transducer moved over the area. Detects valve abnormalities, left ventricular hypertrophy, hypertrophic cardiomyopathy.	Tell the patient what to expect and that the procedure is painless. There is no special preparation.	Remove gel from skin. No special care needed.
Phonocardiogram (PCG)	Electrodes are placed on the chest and microphones over the heart apex and base. PCG and ECG are done simultaneously. The patient may be asked to assume several positions and to change breathing patterns. Takes about 30 min.	Tell the patient what to expect and that the procedure is painless. No special preparation is required.	Remove gel from skin. No special care needed.
Magnetic resonance imaging (MRI)	Creates images of body structures without radiation. The patient lies on a firm pad that rolls into a circular device. Clanging sounds are heard as the machine works.	All metal must be removed. Sedation may be ordered if patient is very anxious or unable to be still.	No special care needed. Safety precautions if sedative has been given.
Multiple-gated acquisition scanning (MUGA)	Radioactive material is injected intravenously and the heart scanned to evaluate function. May be done at rest or during exercise.	Tell patient what to expect. NPO for 2 hr before procedure. Intravenous infusion started as ordered. Signed consent required.	No special care needed.

Table continued on following page

TABLE 31-8
THE HEART: DIAGNOSTIC TESTS AND PROCEDURES *Continued*

TEST	PURPOSE/PROCEDURE	PATIENT PREPARATION	POSTPROCEDURE NURSING CARE
Stress test (exercise tolerance test or ETT)	Assesses presence and severity of coronary artery disease by having the patient exercise during ECG monitoring. Blood pressure is monitored and the test stopped if symptoms of coronary artery disease occur.	Tell the patient what to expect. Nothing by mouth (NPO) for 2 hr before test. Give beta blocker if ordered. Have patient wear loose clothing and comfortable shoes. Signed consent required.	No special care needed.
Thallium imaging	Thallium-20 is given intravenously and the heart scanned to assess blood flow. Scanning may be done at rest or after exercise.	Same as stress test. Tell patient intravenous injection will be given and that radiation dose is small and quickly eliminated.	No special care needed.
Holter monitor	Provides continuous ECG monitoring for a 24- to 48-hr period. Detects occasional dysrhythmias that may be correlated with specific activities noted in patient's diary.	Tell patient to wear loose clothing, take only sponge bath, avoid magnets and metal detectors, and monitor placement of electrodes. Emphasize keeping accurate diary of activities and to push "event button" if symptoms occur.	Return at scheduled time. ECG recording will be retrieved for interpretation.
Cardiac catheterization	A catheter is passed through a vein or artery and dye injected. Radiographs are taken to visualize heart structures and blood vessels. The procedure is done in a special room. Blood pressure, pulse, and ECG are monitored throughout test.	Tell patient what to expect. Assess allergies to seafood or iodine and inform radiologist. NPO for specified time before procedure. Tell patient to expect flushing sensation when dye injected. Give sedative if ordered. Signed consent required.	Check puncture site. Maintain pressure per protocol. Monitor vital signs and peripheral pulses on affected extremity. Enforce bedrest as ordered.
Complete blood count (CBC)	Counts white and red blood cells, hemoglobin and hematocrit, red blood cell indices, and sometimes platelets. Normal values in Table 31–7.	Tell patient a blood sample will be drawn. No special preparation.	Check venipuncture site. Apply pressure if oozing.
Erythrocyte sedimentation rate (ESR)	Measures rate at which red blood cells settle in unclotted blood. Elevated with infections and inflammation. Decreased with CHF.	Same as CBC.	Same as CBC.
Cardiac enzymes	Measures CPK, LDH, and AST to detect elevation associated with heart damage.	Same as CBC. To detect acute myocardial infarction, draw specimen before other invasive procedures.	Same as CBC.
Arterial blood gases (ABGs)	Assesses acid-base balance by measuring pH, CO_2, PCO_2, HCO_3, and base excess.	Tell patient about arterial puncture. Prepare heparinized syringe and obtain blood sample.	Remove air bubbles from sample. Place tube on ice and send for immediate analysis. Apply pressure to puncture site for 5 min. Report results.
Lipid profile	Measures common serum blood lipids (cholesterol, triglycerides, phospholipids). Used to evaluate risk of coronary artery disease.	Tell patient to expect venipuncture. NPO for 12 hr before sample drawn. Usual diet for 2 weeks before test.	Same as CBC.

Cardiac Glycosides

The cardiac glycosides are also called cardiotonics or digitalis glycosides. Examples are digoxin (Lanoxin) and digitoxin. These drugs have several important pharmacologic actions on the heart. They slow the heart rate (negative chronotropic effect) and increase the force of myocardial contraction (positive inotropic effect), causing increased stroke volume and cardiac output. Cardiac glycosides are the most widely used drugs in the treatment of congestive heart failure. They are also used to treat some cardiac dysrhythmias.

When rapid effects are needed, a patient can be given a loading dose (called a digitalizing dose) of cardiac glycosides. Once therapeutic blood levels are obtained, a maintenance dose is prescribed to maintain the therapeutic effects. These drugs have high potential for toxicity and require close monitoring. Common practice is to count the apical pulse before giving each dose. If the rate is below 60 bpm in adults, the dose is withheld and the physician contacted. Because patients are often on cardiac glycosides for long-term therapy, they must be taught to monitor their own pulse and to report symptoms of toxicity (anorexia, nausea, visual disturbances).

TABLE 31-9
CARDIOVASCULAR DRUGS

DRUG, DOSE, ROUTE	USE/ACTION	NURSING INTERVENTIONS
Cardiac Glycosides		
Digoxin (Lanoxin) *Loading dose:* 0.5–1.0 mg intravenously (IV) over 5–10 min or orally (po) in divided doses over 24 hr *Maintenance dose:* 0.125–0.5 mg IV or po daily	Delays impulse conduction through atrioventricular (AV) node (slows heart rate (HR); negative chronotropic effect). Increases strength or force of myocardial contraction (positive inotropic effect). Increases stroke volume and cardiac output (CO). Used for congestive heart failure (CHF), atrial fibrillation and flutter, and paroxysmal atrial tachycardia.	Obtain baseline vital signs, electrocardiogram (ECG), and electrolytes before administering first dose. Assess apical pulse for 1 min; notify physician if <60. Cannot be administered intramuscularly (IM). Monitor K^+ levels; administer K^+ supplements as ordered if K^+ <3. Decreased renal function may delay excretion and lead to toxicity. Toxic effects may be indicated by dysrhythmias, pulse <60, anorexia, nausea, syncope, and yellow halos around lights. Therapeutic level: 0.8–2.0 ng/ml Toxic level: >2 ng/ml Teach the patient: Take radial pulse for 1 min Take at the same time daily
Antianginals		
Diltiazem hydrochloride (Cardizem)	Calcium channel blocker. Dilates coronary arteries; increases availability of oxygen to the myocardium. Decreases total peripheral vascular resistance (PVR), afterload, and systolic blood pressure. Slightly decreases myocardial contractility. Prolongs AV node refractory period. Used in chronic stable angina, coronary artery spasm, and hypertension.	Dosage may need to be reduced in elderly patients. Teach the patient: Take radial pulse for 1 min Limit caffeine intake Change positions with caution to prevent postural hypotension Take before meals and at bedtime
Isosorbide dinitrate (Isordil)	Vasodilator through relaxation of smooth muscles. Decreases preload, afterload, left ventricular end-diastolic pressure (LVEDP), and myocardial oxygen consumption. Used for acute angina and maintenance of chronic angina.	Assess vital signs before administration. Teach the patient: Take 1–2 hr before meals and at bedtime Sit when taking the sublingual or chewable medications Change positions slowly to avoid orthostatic hypotension Avoid hot showers, tubs, saunas Headache decreases over time Alcohol potentiates hypotension If 3 sublingual or chewable doses do not relieve angina, go to the emergency department
Nadolol (Corgard). Dosage increased gradually until optimal response is achieved.	Beta-adrenergic blocker. Decreases HR and CO at rest and with exercise. Decreases conduction velocity through the AV node. Used in hypertension and prophylactically for chronic stable angina.	Assess blood pressure (BP) and apical pulse before administration. Monitor weight. Teach the patient: Take radial pulse for 1 min Hold medication and notify physician if HR <60 or irregular Weigh daily; report a gain of 3–4 lb Do not discontinue this drug abruptly; taper off over 1–2 weeks
Nifedipine (Procardia)	Calcium channel blocker. Decreases myocardial oxygen consumption. Dilates coronary arteries. Decreases PVR. Increases CO. Used for angina, mild to moderate hypertension, vascular headaches, coronary artery spasms.	Monitor BP during titration. Teach the patient: Smoking is contraindicated (nicotine constricts coronary arteries) Do not discontinue this drug abruptly Limit caffeine intake

Table continued on following page

TABLE 31-9
CARDIOVASCULAR DRUGS *Continued*

DRUG, DOSE, ROUTE	USE/ACTION	NURSING INTERVENTIONS
Antianginals		
Nitroglycerin (NTG)	Vasodilator (arteries and veins). Relaxes all smooth muscles, especially vascular smooth muscle. Decreases preload, afterload, BP, CO, and systemic vascular resistance (SVR). Used to prevent and treat angina. Available as sublingual tablets, ointment, transdermal patch, buccal tablets, mist, and sustained release oral tablets.	Assess BP and pulse before administration. Apply ointment in uniform layer on paper provided; apply to nonhairy skin (chest, back, upper arm); do not touch (causes headache); rotate sites. IV drug is delivered in glass containers with special tubing; use an infusion pump; monitor closely. Teach the patient: Sit or lie down at onset of chest pains Place tablet under tongue; tablet should tingle if effective (elderly may not detect this) Repeat q5 min for total of 3 doses; if chest pains not relieved have someone else drive to emergency department Keep tablets in containers in which supplied; drug decomposes on exposure to light and air Headache decreases with tolerance Drug may be taken before activities likely to cause angina (exercise, sex)
Propranolol (Inderal)	Nonselective beta-adrenergic blocker. Decreases HR, myocardial irritability and contractility. Decreases BP in hypertension. Decreases CO. Used in dysrhythmias, myocardial infarction, hypertension, migraines, and chronic stable angina.	Monitor vital signs. May be administered with diuretic to decrease Na^+ and water retention. May cause bronchial constriction. Use with caution in all patients with obstructive lung disease. Auscultate lungs for crackles and heart for S_3 and S_4 sounds. Monitor weight daily; check for peripheral edema. Monitor blood glucose with diabetes. Teach the patient: Do not discontinue this drug abruptly; taper over 2 weeks Take at the same time(s) each day Moderate alcohol No smoking Decrease Na^+ intake with this drug There is not the normal increase in HR with exercise and stress; increase activity slowly Weigh daily, check for edema
Verapamil hydrochloride (Calan, Isoptin)	Calcium channel blocker. Slows AV conduction. Vasodilates peripheral and coronary arteries. Increases oxygen to myocardium. Used to treat supraventricular tachycardias, atrial fibrillation and flutter, angina, hypertension, and vascular headaches.	Assess baseline vital signs, hepatic and renal function. Assess for signs of CHF (pulmonary and/or peripheral edema). Monitor pulse and BP before each dose. Administer IV bolus more slowly to the elderly. Teach the patient: Take radial pulse for 1 min; report irregular or slow pulse No caffeine (opposes calcium channel blocking effect) Change position slowly until tolerance develops Exercise with caution: drug's effects may give false impression of tolerance
Antidysrhythmics		
Amiodarone hydrochloride (Cordarone)	Antidysrhythmic. Increases action potential duration and effective refractory period. Increases CO. Decreases PVR, coronary artery resistance, and HR. Used for severe tachycardia and supraventricular tachycardias.	Continuously monitor ECG for a decrease in dysrhythmia. Observe for thyroid dysfunction (each 200-mg tablet contains 75 mg of iodine) and neurologic effects (tremors, ataxia, headache, insomnia). Teach the patient: Take radial pulse daily Photosensitivity and photophobia may occur Pharmacologic action may have a delayed onset of 5 days to 3 mo Skin discolorations fade with time

TABLE 31-9
CARDIOVASCULAR DRUGS *Continued*

DRUG, DOSE, ROUTE	USE/ACTION	NURSING INTERVENTIONS
Antidysrhythmics		
Bretylium tosylate (Bretylol)	Adrenergic blocker. Suppresses ventricular fibrillation and ventricular tachycardia. Used for short-term treatment of life-threatening ventricular tachycardias in patients who do not respond to conventional therapy, ventricular fibrillation, and cardioversion.	Monitor vital signs, ECG. Have resuscitation equipment available. If nausea and vomiting occur, decrease the rate of infusion.
Disopyramide phosphate (Norpace)	Reduces the rate of spontaneous diastolic depolarization in pacemaker cells. Increases SVR. Decreases myocardial conductivity. Suppresses ectopic focal activity. Used to suppress and prevent recurrent PVCs and ventricular tachycardia.	Assess apical pulse before administration; hold if <60 or >120 and notify physician. Monitor BP. Monitor intake and output; urinary retention and constipation may occur. Teach the patient: Take radial pulse daily Daily weight; observe for edema Change position slowly No alcohol (severely decreases BP) Relieve dry mouth with sugarless gum or hard candy Avoid sunlight (photosensitivity)
Flecainide acetate (Tambocor)	Antidysrhythmic. Decreases conduction velocity. Increases ventricular refractory period. Used to treat PVCs, atrial tachycardia, and other dysrhythmias not responsive to other antidysrhythmics.	Monitor ECG.
Lidocaine (Xylocaine)	Increases the electrical stimulation threshold of the ventricular conduction system. Used for rapid control of ventricular dysrhythmias during myocardial infarction, cardiac surgery, cardiac catheterization, and digitalis intoxication.	Administer with an infusion pump. Monitor BP and ECG. May precipitate malignant hyperthermia (tachycardia, tachypnea, elevated temperature). Assess breath sounds for crackles.
Mexiletine hydrochloride (Mexitil)	Antidysrhythmic structurally similar to lidocaine. Used to suppress symptomatic ventricular dysrhythmias.	Administer with food or antacids. Monitor ECG.
Phenytoin sodium (Dilantin)	Used to treat paroxysmal atrial tachycardia and ventricular dysrhythmias.	Mix IV solution immediately before administration. Administer only in normal saline (drug crystallizes in dextrose). Do not exceed 50 mg/min IV. Decreased dosage in the elderly may be needed. Teach the patient: Alcohol potentiates the action and therefore may precipitate toxicity
Procainamide hydrochloride (Pronestyl, Procan SR)	Depresses myocardial excitability. Peripheral vasodilator. Used to treat life-threatening ventricular dysrhythmias and prophylactically to maintain a normal sinus rhythm after conversion of atrial or ventricular dysrhythmias.	Administer with an infusion pump. Monitor BP and ECG continuously. Watch for prolonged PR and QT intervals and widened QRS interval, heart block, and dysrhythmias. Monitor complete blood count (CBC) during long-term therapy for leukopenia and agranulocytosis. Hypotensive effects may be treated with dopamine or norepinephrine. Assess apical pulse before administration of oral doses. May precipitate malignant hyperthermia. Teach the patient: Record fibrillation episodes (lightheadedness, weakness, syncope)

Table continued on following page

TABLE 31–9
CARDIOVASCULAR DRUGS *Continued*

DRUG, DOSE, ROUTE	USE/ACTION	NURSING INTERVENTIONS
Antidysrhythmics		
Propranolol (Inderal). See description under Antianginals		
Quinidine	Antidysrhythmic. Depresses myocardial excitability, contractility, automaticity, and conduction velocity. Anticholinergic effects increase the ventricular rate. Relaxes muscles. Used for atrial and ventricular dysrhythmias.	If administered with digoxin may produce toxicity or unpredictable dysrhythmias. Administer with meals to decrease gastric distress. Severe hypotension may occur with large doses. Monitor electrolytes; continuing diarrhea may indicate electrolyte imbalance.
Tocainide hydrochloride (Tonocard)	Antidysrhythmic. Primary analogue of lidocaine. Used for life-threatening ventricular dysrhythmias associated with prolonged QT interval.	Monitor ECG. Administer with food or antacids to decrease gastrointestinal side effects. Monitor CBC for blood dyscrasias (agranulocytosis, leukocytosis, neutropenia).
Verapamil (Calan, Isoptin). See description under Antianginals		
Miscellaneous and Emergency Drugs		
Amrinone lactate (Inocor)	Cardiac inotrope. Vasodilator. Increases myocardial contractions without increasing HR. Increases blood flow through collateral coronary vessels. Increases stroke volume and CO. Decreases preload and afterload. Used to treat CHF refractory to other medications.	Administer with an infusion pump. Titrate to target BP. Monitor intake and output. Avoid extravasation. Discard solution 24 hr after preparation.
Atropine sulfate	Vagal blocker. Increases HR and CO in heart blocks and severe bradycardia. Used in symptomatic bradycardia and bradydysrhythmias.	Assess HR and rhythm and BP.
Calcium chloride	Necessary for cardiac rhythm, tone, and contraction. Increases muscle tone and force of contraction. Used in cardiac resuscitation and in cardiac irregularities associated with hyperkalemia.	Monitor ECG, BP, and arterial blood gases. Avoid extravasation; causes necrosis. Alkalosis decreases the absorption of calcium. Acidosis increases the absorption of calcium.
Dobutamine (Dobutrex)	Synthetic catecholamine. Beta-adrenergic agonist. Increases CO with less increase in HR and BP than other catecholamines. Used in CHF and after cardiac surgery to increase myocardial contractility, stroke volume, and CO.	Continuous monitoring of ECG, cardiac parameters, and urinary output; titrate to HR and BP. Urinary output should increase with improved CO and renal function. Often used with nitroprusside or dopamine for additive effects. Causes less increase in HR, PVR, and dysrhythmias than dopamine. At a rate <7 μg/kg/min expect increased myocardial contraction, CO, and renal blood flow. At a rate >7 μg/kg/min expect peripheral vasoconstriction and increased mean arterial pressure (MAP).

Other specific nursing considerations are presented in Table 31–9.

Antianginals

Drugs used to treat angina (chest pain related to myocardial ischemia) include calcium channel blockers, vasodilators, and beta-adrenergic blockers. Examples of each classification and nursing considerations are presented in Table 31–9.

Antidysrhythmics

Drugs used to treat abnormal cardiac rhythms are called antidysrhythmics or antiarrhythmics. There are four main classes of antidysrhythmics with various actions. In general, they work by slowing conduction rates, depressing automaticity, or increasing resistance to premature stimulation. All antidysrhythmics have the potential to cause additional dysrhythmias. Specific drugs and nursing considerations are presented in Table 31–9.

TABLE 31-9
CARDIOVASCULAR DRUGS *Continued*

DRUG, DOSE, ROUTE	USE/ACTION	NURSING INTERVENTIONS
Miscellaneous and Emergency Drugs		
Dopamine hydrochloride (Intropin)	Neurotransmitter; precursor to norepinephrine. Increases CO and BP. Improves renal blood flow and therefore urine output with lower doses. Used for hemodynamic support in shock.	Avoid extravasation; causes necrosis. Monitor vital signs, ECG, urine output, and extremity color. Titrate to target BP; use an infusion pump. Peripheral vasoconstriction is noted with cold upper and lower extremities.
Epinephrine hydrochloride (Adrenalin Chloride)	Catecholamine. Strengthens myocardial contraction; increases BP, HR, and CO. Dilates bronchial tree. Used in anaphylactic shock and to restore cardiac rhythm in cardiac arrest.	Monitor vital signs and ECG continuously. Avoid extravasation; causes sloughing. Titrate to cardiac response. Caution: available in several concentrations (1 : 100, 1 : 1000, 1 : 10,000); be sure to check for prescribed solution. May be administered via endotracheal tube as drug is rapidly absorbed from the lungs.
Isoproterenol hydrochloride (Isuprel)	Cardiac stimulant (positive inotropic and chronotropic effects). Bronchodilator. Peripheral vasodilator. Increases HR and contractility. Decreases PVR and diastolic BP resulting in increased CO and systolic BP, decreased MAP, and increased myocardial oxygen consumption. Used as a cardiac stimulant in cardiac arrest, cardiogenic shock, ventricular dysrhythmias, and heart block.	Continuous monitoring of ECG. Monitor vital signs, urine output, and peripheral blood flow. Titrate to desired HR, BP, and urine output. Avoid extravasation.
Sodium nitroprusside (Nipride)	Vasodilator. Decreases preload and afterload. Used in hypertensive crises.	Light-sensitive preparation; wrap in aluminum foil. Administer with an infusion pump. Titrate to maintain CO. Continuously monitor BP. Discard solution 4 hr after preparation. Assess thiocyanate levels daily for patients on long-term therapy.
Norepinephrine (Levophed)	Catecholamine. Vasoconstriction. Cardiac stimulant: increased BP, myocardial oxygen, and coronary artery blood flow. Used in acute hypotensive states, myocardial infarction, and cardiac arrest.	Mix only with dextrose in water or dextrose in saline. Administer with an infusion pump. Report decreased urine output immediately. Continuously monitor and titrate to BP. Monitor peripheral blood flow.
Sodium bicarbonate	Systemic alkalinizer. Used to correct metabolic acidosis in cardiac arrest.	Do not infuse with calcium. Monitor arterial blood gases. Avoid extravasation; causes severe tissue damage.

Diuretics

Diuretics are often prescribed for cardiac conditions. Many patients with heart problems have fluid retention that is treated with diuretics. The most frequently used diuretics are furosemide (Lasix) and hydrochlorothiazide (Esidrix, HCTZ, and Oretic). Information about these and other diuretics is presented in Table 36–4 in the chapter on urologic disorders.

Anticoagulants

Anticoagulants are used to treat or prevent clot formation. Heparin and warfarin are the most commonly used preventive anticoagulants.

HEPARIN. Heparin interferes with factor III in the clotting process. It is administered by continuous intravenous drip or subcutaneously. When a patient has a clotting episode, a heparin bolus is administered and a continuous infusion is started. The infusion rate is set to deliver a prescribed number of heparin units per hour. The physician adjusts the heparin dosage based on the partial thromboplastin time (PTT). When the PTT has stabilized (generally at 1.5 to 2.0 times the control level), the drug is changed to the subcutaneous route. Because heparin cannot be administered orally, the patient must remain hospitalized during its administration.

WARFARIN. The anticoagulant that may be administered orally, warfarin (Coumadin), is started as soon as possible. The warfarin dosage is regulated by the prothrombin time (PT). The PT is also kept in a therapeutic range of 1.5 to 2.0 times the normal level. Patients who have had artificial valve replacements must remain on anticoagulant therapy for life.

PHARMACOLOGY CAPSULE

Heparin dosage is adjusted based on the patient's partial thromboplastin time. Warfarin dosage is adjusted based on the patient's prothrombin time.

Antiplatelet Agents

Antiplatelet therapy is often used after a myocardial infarction to prevent strokes. The dosage of aspirin as an antiplatelet agent in stroke prevention is under investigation. Some studies have shown that one baby aspirin (60 mg) a day is sufficient, and other studies indicate that an even smaller dosage may produce a therapeutic effect. Dipyridamole (Persantine) also exhibits an antiplatelet effect and may be prescribed for patients who are unable to tolerate aspirin.

Thrombolytic Agents

Whereas anticoagulants and antiplatelet agents prevent the continued formation of clots, the thrombolytic agents act to destroy clots that have already formed. Streptokinase, urokinase, and tissue plasminogen activator are examples of thrombolytics. They are best used as soon as there is evidence of clot formation. They are administered intravenously when certain criteria have been met. Administration is continued until there is evidence of reperfusion or until the maximum dosage has been given.

PHARMACOLOGY CAPSULE

Anticoagulants and antiplatelet agents prevent formation of new clots, but thrombolytic agents destroy clots that have already formed.

Analgesics

The patient who has a myocardial infarction experiences severe chest pain. The first medication administered to a patient with chest pain is nitroglycerin, a vasodilator. When this drug does not relieve the pain, morphine is the preferred analgesic. Morphine relieves pain, reduces anxiety, and reduces the workload of the heart by trapping some of the venous blood in the periphery of the body. An alternative to morphine is meperidine hydrochloride (Demerol). Meperidine is less effective in relieving anxiety and cardiac workload than morphine. Morphine and meperidine are most effective when administered intravenously.

DIET THERAPY

Reduction of body weight reduces the workload on the heart. A low-fat high-fiber diet is generally recommended for cardiac patients. The recommended diet contains less than 30% of the daily calories from fat. Of the 30%, 10% should be from saturated fats and 20% from unsaturated fats. High-fiber foods include whole grains, fruits, and vegetables. An exercise program may help the patient achieve optimal weight.

Sodium

If fluid retention accompanies the cardiac problem, the physician may order sodium restriction. A diet containing 2 grams of sodium per day is most often prescribed. Restrictions greater than this are difficult to achieve, and studies have shown that patients quickly become noncompliant with the dietary regimen.

Potassium

Patients taking potassium-wasting diuretics (e.g., furosemide and hydrochlorothiazide) need to include adequate potassium in the diet to counteract the depletion. Patients taking large doses of potassium-wasting diuretics need to have potassium supplements prescribed.

PHARMACOLOGY CAPSULE

Potassium-wasting diuretics such as furosemide and hydrochlorothiazide may cause hypokalemia, which can lead to dangerous dysrhythmias.

OXYGEN THERAPY

The myocardium needs an adequate blood supply to function properly. Any patient complaining of chest pain unrelieved by nitroglycerin should have supplemental oxygen administered. A nasal cannula or face mask should be applied, set to deliver the prescribed liter flow, and the patient's response to this therapy monitored.

PACEMAKERS

Pacemakers were first introduced in 1958. Their purpose is to restore regular rhythm and to improve cardiac output and tissue perfusion. Pacemakers may be temporary or permanent and transcutaneous, transvenous, or implantable. A transcutaneous pacemaker has an electrode that delivers an impulse through the skin. A transvenous pacemaker has an electrode that is threaded through a vein to the heart. An implantable pacemaker is surgically placed in the chest. Impulses are conducted from the power source, the pacemaker, to the heart through a lead that stimulates the contraction of the myocardium.

Modes

The pacemaker generator can be set in three modes: chambers paced, chambers sensed, and mode of response. The international code developed for pacemakers is shown in Table 31–10.

TABLE 31-10
INTERNATIONAL CODE FOR PACEMAKERS

CHAMBERS PACED	CHAMBERS SENSED	MODE OF RESPONSE	PROGRAMMABILITY	TACHYARRHYTHMIA FUNCTIONS
V = ventricle	V = ventricle	I = inhibited	P = programmable rate	B = burst
A = atrium	A = atrium	T = triggered	M = multiprogrammability	N = normal rate competition
D = dual	D = dual	D = dual: atrium triggered and ventricle inhibited	C = programmable with telemetry	S = scanning
	O = none	O = none	O = none	E = external

The most common setting is DDD, as it simulates normal cardiac physiology most closely. This means that both the ventricles and the atria are monitored. If no impulse is generated to initiate a contraction, the pacemaker provides one. Dual mode of response means that the atria are triggered if they do not spontaneously initiate an impulse and the ventricles are inhibited from responding on their own.

Modes are described as fixed rate, demand rate, or AV sequential. The fixed-rate mode delivers a set number, generally 72 or 80, of impulses per minute regardless of the intrinsic cardiac activity. The demand pacemaker delivers impulses when spontaneous beats are less than the minimum number set. This is the most common mode. The AV sequential mode detects activity in both chambers and delivers impulses as needed.

Temporary Pacemakers

A temporary pacemaker is inserted for bradycardia with syncope, tachycardia, myocardial infarction, and heart block. The leads are threaded into the RV through the venous system (transvenous), through a closed chest puncture, or during open chest surgery. Pulmonary artery catheters are available with pacemaker capability. Leads may also be applied directly to the chest wall (transcutaneous) for emergency temporary pacing.

Permanent Pacemakers

A permanent implantable pacemaker is inserted under local anesthesia. The batteries, generally lithium, have an 8- to 10-year expected life. Permanent pacemakers are inserted in the operating room, catheterization laboratory, or special procedures area. The electrodes are sutured to the epicardium in the atrial and the ventricular areas or both. The generator is placed in a subcutaneous pocket, generally under the clavicle.

NURSING CARE OF THE PATIENT WITH A PACEMAKER. Patients having pacemakers inserted recover in the postanesthesia care unit and then go to a unit with telemetry capability. The patient is monitored for proper pacemaker functioning. The ECG is examined for rhythm, pacemaker spike, and dysrhythmias (premature ventricular contractions and ventricular tachycardia are seen most often). The pacemaker spike is a mark observed on the ECG tracing that represents the impulse generated by the pacemaker. The nurse assesses vital signs and cardiac output and inspects the incision frequently. Patients rest for 24 hours after the insertion of a permanent pacemaker. They are ambulated as soon as possible and encouraged to resume normal activities.

Following insertion of a temporary pacemaker, no electrical devices (bed, razor, call light) should be in contact with the patient. The ECG is monitored, and the patient is transported with a portable cardiac monitor and a nurse in attendance. The pacemaker is assessed for misfiring. A gradual increase of activities is planned.

The nurse teaches the patient how to count the pulse for 1 full minute daily. Wound care and the healing process are discussed. The patient is advised to notify the physician of symptoms of decreased cardiac output. These symptoms may be dyspnea, dizziness, syncope, weakness, fatigue, and chest pain. The patient is also instructed to carry an identification card describing the type of pacemaker implanted.

CARDIOVERSION

Cardioversion is the delivery of a synchronized shock to terminate atrial or ventricular tachydysrhythmias (rapid abnormal heart rhythms). It may be done as an emergency or elective procedure. The shock is synchronized with the R wave to avoid shocking during the vulnerable period of the T wave. A shock delivered during ventricular relaxation can initiate ventricular fibrillation.

If the patient is receiving digoxin, the drug is withheld for 24 hours before the procedure. Emergency drugs are made available and the patient has a patent intravenous infusion in place before the procedure. The procedure is explained, and informed consent is obtained. The patient is then given a short-acting sedative as ordered. The cardioverter is set to the synchronized mode, and two electrodes are placed on the chest. One electrode is placed to the right of the sternum just below the clavicle and the other at the apex of the heart. The initial impulse varies from 25 to 100 joules depending on the type of dysrhythmia. If the initial impulse does not convert the dysrhythmia to normal sinus rhythm, the joules are increased and the procedure repeated.

Following cardioversion the patient usually responds very quickly from the sedation and does not remember the event. The skin under the electrodes is inspected for irritation. The patient's heart rate and rhythm, vital signs, and neurologic status are assessed. Transient dysrhythmias and a drop in blood pressure are common.

The nurse is especially alert for atrial fibrillation, which can lead to atrial wall thrombus and emboli formation.

CARDIAC SURGERY

The most common surgical procedures involving the heart are pacemaker insertion, open-heart surgery to repair or replace valves or septa or remove tumors, and arterial bypass surgery. Pacemaker insertion is described earlier in this section. Arterial bypass surgery is described later as a surgical treatment for acute myocardial infarction.

With open-heart surgery, the heart muscle must be at rest during the repair. This involves placing the patient on a machine to reroute the blood away from the heart and lungs and to maintain appropriate oxygen and carbon dioxide levels. The heart's rhythm is interrupted by a cold electrolyte solution and may be restarted after the surgery by electrical stimulation. During this type of surgery, the patient's core temperature is reduced to decrease the oxygen needs of the entire body, especially the brain. Rewarming begins when the heart is restarted and continues until a normal core temperature is reached.

Preoperative Nursing Care of the Cardiac Surgery Patient

ASSESSMENT. Nursing assessment of the patient with cardiac disorders is summarized in Table 31–4. When a patient is facing cardiac surgery, the nurse must also assess the patient's fears and anxiety. Patients are usually upset and very concerned when heart surgery is recommended. The nurse also determines what the patient knows about the surgery and what more he or she would like to know.

NURSING DIAGNOSIS. Preoperative nursing diagnoses for the patient may include the following:

- **Fear** related to perceived threat of death or unfamiliarity with setting and procedures
- **Anxiety** related to threat to health status or uncertain outcome
- **Knowledge Deficit** of surgical routines and expectations of the patient

GOALS. Goals of preoperative nursing care are reduced fear and anxiety and patient's knowledge of surgical routines and expectations.

INTERVENTIONS

Fear and Anxiety. The nurse encourages the patient to identify feelings and then explores the basis of those feelings. It is important that nurses not assume they know how patients feel. The nurse accepts the patient's feelings and does not give trite reassurance ("Don't worry; everything will be fine"). Accurate information about what to expect helps reduce fear of the unknown. Physical comfort measures such as a massage or back rub may also be soothing. If the patient's anxiety level remains high, the physician should be notified.

Knowledge Deficit. The physician reviews the diagnostic tests that led to the recommendation for surgery, the surgical procedure itself, and what to expect after surgery. Nevertheless, the nurse must be able to clarify and further explain what the patient will experience. If the surgery is to be done as an emergency, little time is available to do preoperative teaching. Planned cardiac surgery allows time for the patient to accept the need for surgery and to explore why the procedure is necessary. Patients having pacemakers inserted can usually expect to return to their same units postoperatively. Patients having more extensive surgery will go to an intensive care unit. It is desirable to show the patient the room and the equipment before surgery. The patient must be taught how to turn, cough, deep breathe, and exercise the leg muscles following surgery. Most patients are intubated for approximately 24 hours after surgery. A means of communication should be established before surgery. Inclusion of the family in the preoperative teaching makes them feel more informed and helpful postoperatively.

EVALUATION. Criteria for evaluating the outcome of nursing interventions are patient's statement of reduced fear or anxiety and more relaxed manner and patient's description of usual routine and activities that promote recovery and reduce complications.

Postoperative Nursing Care of the Cardiac Surgery Patient

Nursing care needs vary considerably depending on the type of surgical procedure. Care specific to certain conditions is discussed with those conditions. In addition, the reader is referred to Chapter 14 for thorough coverage of care of the surgical patient. This section addresses needs common to many patients having cardiac surgery.

ASSESSMENT. Assessment of the cardiac patient is summarized in Table 31–4. Postoperatively, the nurse is especially alert to changes in vital signs, breath sounds, urine output, mental alertness, and color. Cardiac rhythms, arterial blood gases, and hemodynamic pressures are monitored. Chest tube function is evaluated. All dressings are inspected frequently for type and amount of drainage. The surgical wound and insertion sites of tubes and cannulas are examined for redness, swelling, and purulent drainage. Urine is assessed for amount, appearance, and odor.

NURSING DIAGNOSIS. Nursing diagnoses for the patient having cardiac surgery may include the following:

- **Ineffective Breathing Patterns** related to mechanical ventilation, general anesthesia, pain, or restrictive surgical dressings
- **Pain** related to tissue trauma
- **Ineffective Thermoregulation** related to cooling during surgery
- **Decreased Cardiac Output** related to fluid loss or decreased fluid intake

- **High Risk for Infection** related to altered skin integrity
- **Anxiety** related to unfamiliar routines and stressful experience
- **Knowledge Deficit** of postoperative self-care and rehabilitation

GOALS. Common goals for the patient having cardiac surgery are normal oxygenation, reduced pain, normal body temperature, normal cardiac output, absence of infection, reduced anxiety, and knowledge of postoperative care.

INTERVENTIONS. Nursing care is individualized on the basis of the assessment data.

Ineffective Breathing Patterns. Patients with open-heart or bypass surgery are unresponsive on arrival in the intensive care unit. Ventilatory assistance is of prime importance. Breath sounds and arterial blood gases are reassessed frequently. Chest tubes are in place and are connected to underwater seal drainage. (See Chapter 28 for the care of chest tubes.) The patient is repositioned often to promote removal of pulmonary secretions and improve respiratory excursion.

When the patient is extubated, an oxygen mask or nasal cannula is ordered to provide supplemental oxygen. The patient is assisted to cough and deep breathe frequently. A pillow or a blanket in a pillow case can be used as an incisional splint during coughing. An incentive spirometer is usually ordered, and the nurse monitors its use and reminds the patient to use it. Early ambulation, as ordered, also reduces the risk of pulmonary complications.

Pain. Effective pain relief makes it easier for the patient to turn, cough, and deep breathe. The nurse assesses the patient's pain: location, severity, aggravating factors, and relieving factors. Analgesics are administered as ordered. Intravenous morphine in small doses is most frequently prescribed for analgesia. The nurse also employs independent measures, including position changes, back rubs, relaxation techniques, and imagery. The nurse assesses the effectiveness of the interventions in managing pain.

Ineffective Thermoregulation. Warmed blankets, heating blankets, and warming lights may be used to assist rewarming. Body temperature is monitored continuously until stable.

Decreased Cardiac Output. Cardiac pressures continue to be monitored every 5 to 15 minutes until stable. Medications are titrated based on vital signs, hemodynamic pressures, and cardiac rhythms. Pacing wires are connected to a temporary pacemaker. Fluid and blood administration and assessment of urinary and other drainage outputs are monitored by the nurse. Volume expanders (albumin, dextran, hetastarch) and vasoactive drugs may be necessary to maintain blood pressure. Oral fluids are ordered shortly after extubation.

High Risk for Infection. The patient is at risk for incisional, respiratory tract, and urinary tract infections. In addition, the presence of multiple tubes and cannulas provides additional sites for potential infection. To reduce the risk of infection, the nurse practices good hand-washing technique and uses aseptic technique when handling dressings and invasive equipment. Wound care is provided as ordered or per agency policy. Antibiotics are administered as ordered.

Anxiety. The nurse informs the patient and the family what is being done and how the patient is responding. The nurse must remember to talk to the patient and offer reassurance. When the patient is on a ventilator, a nonverbal means of communication needs to be established. It is often necessary to repeat instructions because of the effects of pain, medications, and anxiety.

Knowledge Deficit. Before discharge, the nurse begins teaching the patient self-care, including wound care and recognition of signs of infection. The importance of follow-up care and rehabilitation is stressed. Specific discharge instructions are discussed with specific disorders.

EVALUATION. Criteria for evaluating the effectiveness of nursing interventions are normal arterial blood gas results, patient's statement of pain relief, body temperature of at least 36.7°C (98°F) orally, fluid intake equal to output, patient's statement of reduced anxiety, and patient's verbalization of postoperative self-care and rehabilitation methods.

CARDIOPULMONARY RESUSCITATION

Cardiopulmonary resuscitation is the restoration of heart and lung function after cardiac arrest. The procedure is employed in basic life support, basic cardiac life support, and advanced cardiac life support. Basic life support is addressed in Chapter 13. The reader is referred to materials prepared by the American Heart Association for current, in-depth coverage of the procedure.

CARDIAC DISORDERS

CORONARY ARTERY DISEASE

Coronary artery disease occurs when the major coronary arteries supplying the myocardium are partially or completely blocked. It is the leading cause of death in the United States. Blockage of the arteries is caused by coronary artery spasm, arteriosclerosis, or atherosclerosis. Blockage of the coronary arteries results in ischemia and infarction of myocardial tissue.

ARTERIOSCLEROSIS

Arteriosclerosis is an abnormal thickening and hardening of arterial walls. Smooth muscle cells and collagen migrate into the tunica intima (innermost layer of the artery) and cause the arterial wall to stiffen and thicken and the lumen to decrease in diameter. Lipids, cholesterol, calcium, and thrombi adhere to the damaged arterial wall. This process limits the elasticity of the wall and decreases the flow of oxygen-carrying blood to tissues. Some effects of arteriosclerosis are hypertension, impaired tissue perfusion, and aneurysms.

ATHEROSCLEROSIS

Atherosclerosis is a form of arteriosclerosis in which thickening and hardening of the vessel wall are caused by soft deposits of intra-arterial fat and fibrin that harden over time. The disease process may take several forms depending on the anatomic location (e.g., coronary or cerebral), age, genetic and physiologic status, and other individual risk factors. Low-density lipid deposits occur early when cholesterol accumulates in the arterial wall. Lesions occur primarily within the tunica intima and are of three types: fatty streaks, fibrous plaque, and advanced lesions.

TYPES OF LESIONS

Fatty Streak. The fatty streak is a flat, yellow, lipid-filled smooth muscle cell that causes no obstruction of the affected vessel. It is commonly found in the aorta by age 10 and in coronary arteries by age 15 regardless of race, sex, or environmental factors. The fatty streak is thought to be reversible. There are no symptoms associated with these lesions.

Fibrous Plaque. The fibrous plaque is the characteristic lesion of advanced atherosclerosis. It is rarely found in people younger than 25 years. The lipid-laden smooth muscle cells become surrounded by collagen, elastic fibers, and a mucoprotein matrix. The white, raised lesion protrudes into the lumen. The mass fixes itself to the inner wall of the tunica intima and may invade the muscular tunica media. If the lesion enlarges sufficiently, it may occlude the lumen. This lesion occurs most frequently at bifurcations (the points at which blood vessels divide into two smaller vessels), curves, and where arteries taper.

Advanced Lesions. Advanced lesions develop as hemorrhage, calcification, cellular necrosis, and thrombi of the intima alter the fibrous plaques and contribute to the loss of elasticity and resulting occlusion of the vessels.

COLLATERAL CIRCULATION. If plaque formation occurs slowly, collateral circulation may develop. Collateral blood vessels are new branches that grow from existing arteries to provide increased blood flow.

Risk Factors

Factors that increase the risk of atherosclerosis include diabetes mellitus with increased glucose, decreased protein, and decreased high-density lipoproteins. Other factors that increase the risk of CAD are nicotine, hypertension, and obesity. The nicotine in cigarette smoke is a potent vasoconstrictor. With hypertension, vasoconstriction increases the work of the heart. Obesity increases the workload of the heart, and increased fat around vessels decreases the vessel elasticity.

Signs and Symptoms

Generally CAD is asymptomatic until the tissue's blood supply is reduced by at least 60%. Then clinical manifestations depend on the vessels involved and the sites of the lesions. In CAD, the left anterior descending artery is most often affected.

Pain is the most frequent symptom. Pain represents lack of oxygen to tissues. The pain resulting from lack of oxygen to the myocardium is called *angina pectoris.* It occurs most often with exercise or activity and generally subsides with rest. Other precipitating factors are smoking, physical exertion, emotional stress, and heavy meals. It may be caused by spasms of the coronary arteries, thrombosis, or occlusion of the lumen. The pain is usually substernal and described by the patient as vise-like, burning, squeezing, or smothering. The pain may radiate to either arm, the shoulder, the jaw, the neck, or the epigastrium. Accompanying symptoms are diaphoresis, dyspnea, nausea, and vomiting. Angina that is not relieved by drug therapy suggests progressive ischemia that can result in infarction of tissue.

Two less common types of angina are unstable angina and Prinzmetal's angina. Unstable (crescendo) angina indicates acute coronary insufficiency. It may occur at rest or with minimal exertion and is often unrelieved by nitroglycerin. Patients with unstable angina are at increased risk for myocardial infarction and sudden cardiac death. Prinzmetal's, or variant, angina occurs at rest and may occur without evidence of atherosclerosis. It is caused by coronary artery spasm.

Medical Treatment

Treatment of CAD includes diet therapy, drug therapy, and reduction of risk factors (smoking, obesity, hypertension). Calcium channel blockers (verapamil, diltiazem, and nifedipine) are used to decrease coronary artery spasm and myocardial oxygen demand.

DIET THERAPY. Treatment begins with dietary adjustment. The aim of the dietary regimen is to decrease the serum cholesterol to 200 mg for those older than 30 years of age and to 180 for those younger than 30 years. Fat intake should be decreased to 30% or less of the daily calories; saturated fat should constitute less than 10%. Daily cholesterol intake is restricted to 250 to 300 mg.

DRUG THERAPY. Drug therapy may be initiated if dietary control does not reduce cholesterol sufficiently. Antilipemics (agents that reduce serum lipids) include cholestyramine resin (Questran), clofibrate (Atromid-S), colestipol hydrochloride (Colestid), gemfibrozil (Lopid), lovastatin (Mevacor), and niacin.

The goals of drug therapy for the CAD patient may also include reduction of angina and reduction of cholesterol. Various forms of nitroglycerin are prescribed for treatment of acute angina. These are administered sublingually or buccally at the onset of pain. They are quickly absorbed and usually effective. Oral, topical, and transdermal nitrates may be ordered to prevent angina attacks. Other drugs used for prophylaxis (prevention) of angina are calcium channel blockers and beta-adrenergic blockers.

Additional information about selected antianginal and antilipemic drugs is presented in Table 31–9.

SURGICAL INTERVENTION. Surgical procedures to treat CAD are discussed under treatment of myocardial infarction.

ACUTE MYOCARDIAL INFARCTION

An acute myocardial infarction (AMI) is the destruction of myocardial tissue as a result of lack of blood and oxygen supply. Approximately 1.5 million AMIs with 500,000 deaths from AMI per year occur in the United States. Men predominate in patients younger than 65 years; after age 65 the incidence is approximately equal in men and women.

Risk Factors

Risk factors for AMI include obesity, smoking, high-fat diet, hypertension, family history, male gender, diabetes mellitus, sedentary lifestyle, and excessive stress. Smoking, high-fat diet, and hypertension are considered modifiable risk factors. This means that risk can be reduced by cessation of smoking, diet modification, and management of hypertension.

Pathophysiology

An AMI begins with the occlusion of a coronary artery. Over a period of 4 to 6 hours a process of ischemia, injury, and infarction develop. Ischemia results from a lack of blood and oxygen to a portion of the heart muscle. If ischemia is not reversed, then injury occurs. Deprived of blood and oxygen, the affected tissue becomes soft and loses its normal color. With continued ischemia an infarction, death of myocardial tissue, occurs. Ischemia lasting 20 minutes or more is sufficient to produce irreversible tissue damage.

Within 24 hours after an infarction, the healing process begins. By the third day, necrotic tissue has been broken down by enzymes and removed by macrophages. Collateral circulation develops to supply the injured area, and scar tissue begins to form. Ten to 14 days after the AMI, the myocardium is especially vulnerable to stress because of the weakness of the healing tissue. Complete healing takes about 6 weeks.

Complications

Up to 90% of patients with AMI suffer complications. The major complications are dysrhythmias, cardiac failure, cardiogenic shock, thromboembolism, and ventricular rupture.

DYSRHYTHMIAS. Dysrhythmias are disturbances in heart rhythm, including excessively rapid, slow, or irregular heartbeats. They occur in approximately 80% of all AMI patients. Because some dysrhythmias are life threatening, continuous cardiac monitoring is usually ordered for AMI patients. This permits early detection and prompt treatment of dysrhythmias. Recognition and treatment of specific dysrhythmias are addressed later in this chapter.

CARDIAC FAILURE. The AMI may cause the heart to fail as a pump. The injured left ventricle is unable to meet the body's circulatory demands. The ventricle fails to empty efficiently. Increased preload leads to systemic and pulmonary edema. Cardiac output and blood pressure fall. Untreated cardiac failure progresses to cardiogenic shock and death. Early symptoms of congestive failure are dyspnea, restlessness, and increasing heart rate.

CARDIOGENIC SHOCK. Cardiogenic shock is the most frequent cause of death after an AMI. It is generally related to extensive injury to the left ventricle and is more common when the patient has had a previous infarction. Cardiogenic shock is marked by hypotension; cool, moist skin; oliguria; and decreasing alertness.

THROMBOEMBOLISM. Following an AMI, thrombi may form in the injured heart chambers or in the veins of the legs. The thrombi may break loose, travel through the circulation, and lodge in the lung. Pallor, cyanosis, and heart failure may be caused by pulmonary emboli. Massive pulmonary embolism is characterized by sudden, severe dyspnea. It is usually fatal. Pulmonary emboli are discussed in detail in Chapter 28.

VENTRICULAR RUPTURE. Weakened areas of the ventricular wall may bulge during contractions. If scar tissue is inadequate to strengthen the wall, an aneurysm may develop and rupture. Ventricular rupture is fatal.

Signs and Symptoms

Pain is the classic symptom of AMI. It is typically a heavy or constrictive pain located below or behind the sternum as described with CAD. It may radiate to arms, back, neck, or jaw. The pain may begin with or without exertion. It progresses if not relieved by rest and nitroglycerin. The patient becomes diaphoretic, lightheaded, and may experience nausea, vomiting, and dyspnea. The skin is frequently cold and clammy. The patient experiences great anxiety and often a feeling of impending doom. Dyspnea is sometimes the only symptom experienced by elderly people with AMIs. Anyone with chest pain unrelieved for 30 minutes should go to an emergency department for treatment.

Medical Diagnosis

The diagnosis of an AMI is based primarily on the patient's history and the physical signs and symptoms. The AMI can be confirmed by laboratory evidence and ECG changes.

CARDIAC ENZYMES. A blood sample is drawn from anyone with prolonged chest pain to measure cardiac enzymes. With sustained ischemia the cell membrane is impaired, and enzymes are released from their intracellular location into the interstitial fluid. These enzymes can be measured in the serum and are assessed at regular intervals to confirm an AMI. Creatine phosphokinase and its isoenzyme CPK-MB (myocardial) elevate most rapidly with infarction. Beginning 4 to 6 hours after infarction, the CPK rises to five or more times the normal level within 12 to 24 hours and returns to normal in 2 to 3 days. Lactate dehydrogenase elevates 8 to 12 hours after infarction, peaks in 3 to 4 days, and returns to normal in 10 to 14 days. Five isoenzymes have been isolated from LDH. Altered LDH_1 and LDH_2 are associated with myocardial infarction. Normally LDH_2 has a higher value than LDH_1. When this is reversed (called a *flipped LDH*), it confirms an AMI. Serum glutamic-oxaloacetic transaminase begins to rise in 6 to 8 hours, peaks in 1 to 2 days, and returns to normal in 4 to 8 days (Fig. 31–14). Serum glutamic-oxaloacetic transaminase, today called aspartate aminotransferase, is the least reliable of the three enzymes measured.

Changes in the normal waveform and dysrhythmias can be seen on ECG. With ischemia, the T wave is inverted. With injury, there is ST segment elevation. With infarction, there is a significant Q wave (Fig. 31–15). A significant Q wave is one that is greater than one third the height of the R wave. The most frequently observed dysrhythmias are premature ventricular contractions, ventricular tachycardia, and ventricular fibrillation.

Medical Treatment

The overall goal of medical therapy is to preserve myocardial tissue. This can best be accomplished by early treatment and risk modification.

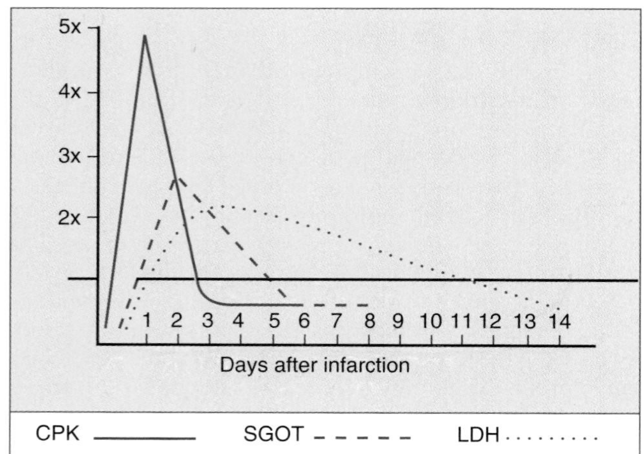

FIGURE 31–14
Cardiac enzyme levels. CPK, Creatine phosphokinase; SGOT, serum glutamic-oxaloacetic transaminase; LDH, lactate dehydrogenase.

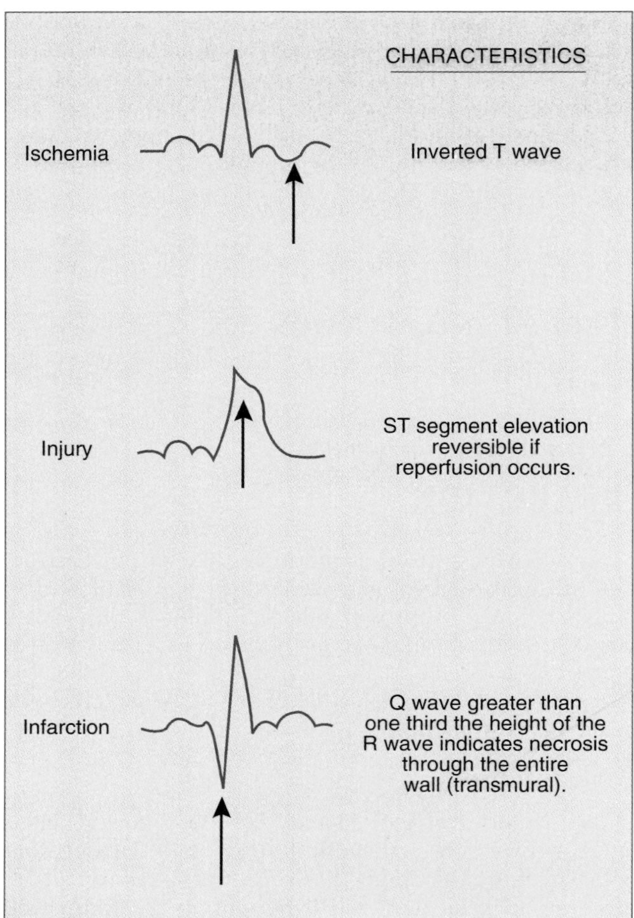

FIGURE 31–15
The process of infarction.

DRUG THERAPY. Nitroglycerin, sublingual or intravenous, is administered to dilate coronary arteries and increase blood flow to the damaged area. If the nitroglycerin produces relief of pain, the infarction may not extend. Morphine sulfate is also used for chest pain. It has many effects in addition to analgesia. Morphine causes peripheral pooling of blood, which decreases the blood returning to the heart and lungs, diminishes anxiety, decreases tachypnea, and relaxes bronchial smooth muscles, thereby improving gas exchange. If the patient cannot tolerate morphine, meperidine (Demerol) may be used, but it does not have all the nonanalgesic properties of morphine and may increase the heart rate.

Thrombolytic therapy is useful for patients whose infarctions are diagnosed early. Streptokinase and tissue plasminogen activator are administered intravenously or into the coronary arteries (during cardiac catheterization) to dissolve thrombi. This treatment is most effective when initiated within 6 hours of the onset of chest pain. The patient must meet strict criteria (no recent surgery or active bleeding, no history of a stroke, no bleeding disorders) and provide informed consent before the administration of thrombolytics. Following the administration of the thrombolytics, heparin is administered to prevent further clot formation. Once the patient is stable, oral aspirin may be ordered as the anticoagulant of choice.

Lidocaine may be administered for ventricular tachycardia. Digitalis may be ordered to increase myocardial contractility and decrease the heart rate. Calcium channel blockers decrease conduction through the AV node, thereby slowing the heart rate; decrease myocardial oxygen demand; dilate arteries; and decrease systemic vascular resistance. Unstable patients may require dopamine or dobutamine or both as inotropic agents. As the myocardium receives blood and oxygen, reperfusion dysrhythmias that require treatment may be noted.

ANGIOPLASTY. A percutaneous transluminal angioplasty may be performed if one vessel is occluded. In some cardiac centers, percutaneous transluminal angioplasty is being done on multiple vessels as technology improves. The procedure involves passage of a catheter through a peripheral artery into the occluded coronary artery. The tip of the catheter contains a balloon that is inflated to compress the atherosclerotic plaque and dilate the artery.

At this time, there are many requirements that candidates for percutaneous transluminal angioplasty must meet. When appropriate, this procedure is preferred over coronary artery bypass surgery because it can be done under local anesthetic, is less invasive, and has a faster recovery time. The procedure is safer than bypass surgery but is not without risks. Complications of percutaneous transluminal angioplasty include coronary artery rupture, occlusion of distal vessels, dysrhythmias, coronary spasm, and death. In approximately 30% of patients, the vessel narrows again within 6 months.

A newer procedure is laser angioplasty. It employs a catheter with a laser on the tip. The laser is used to widen the lumen of the artery by destroying atherosclerotic plaques.

CORONARY ARTERY BYPASS GRAFT SURGERY. Coronary artery bypass graft surgery may be performed to improve the blood supply to the myocardium. Arterial bypass surgery uses the patient's own vasculature as replacement for occluded coronary arteries. From one to six vessels may be bypassed. The saphenous veins and the internal mammary artery are most commonly used. The saphenous veins are removed from one or both legs, inspected for patency, and reversed so that the valves do not inhibit blood flow. The replacement vessels are attached above and below the occlusions in the coronary arteries and serve as new conduits for oxygenated blood to the myocardium (Fig. 31–16). This is major surgery. The survival rate is higher in patients who are in stable condition.

Nursing Care of the Patient with Coronary Artery Disease

ASSESSMENT. General assessment of the cardiac patient is summarized in Table 31–4. When a patient has CAD, the nurse is especially concerned with assessment of pain. When chest pain is present, early evaluation and treatment are paramount. The patient is asked to describe the pain, including type, location, duration, and severity. The nurse records what the patient was doing

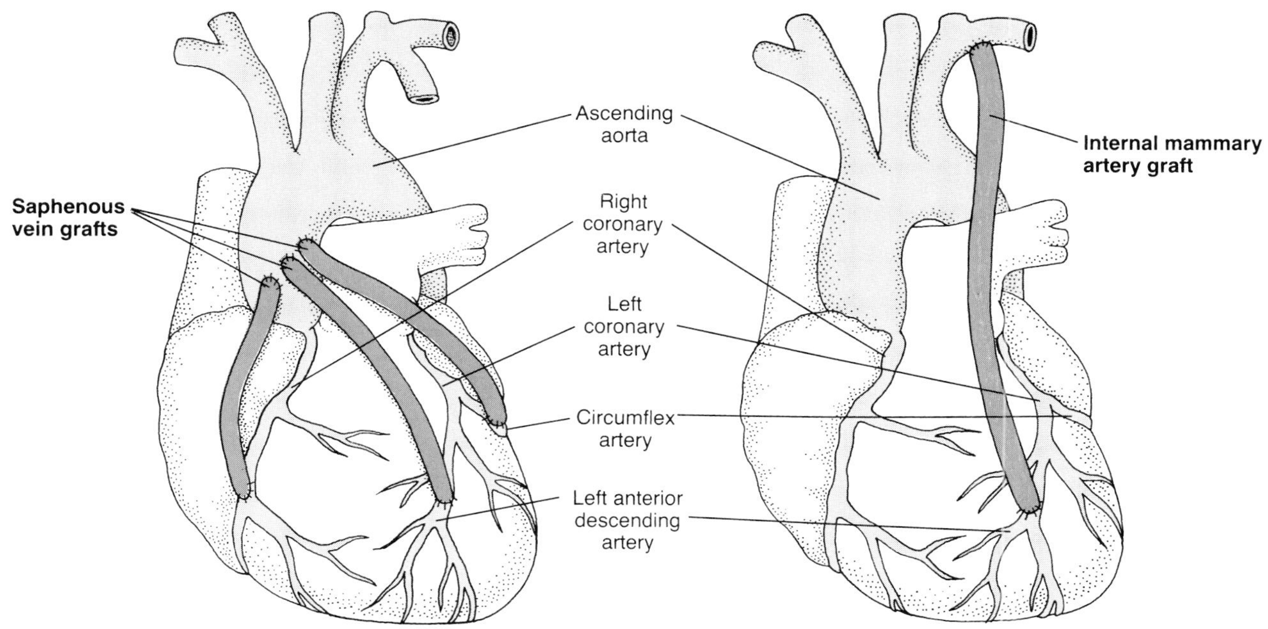

FIGURE 31–16

Coronary artery bypass grafting surgery. (From Ignatavicius, D. D., & Bayne, M. V. [1991]. *Medical-surgical nursing: A nursing process approach* [p. 2158]. Philadelphia: W. B. Saunders.)

when the pain started, what action was taken, and the effects of any actions or treatments. The patient's skin is inspected for color and palpated for temperature and moisture. Vital signs are assessed frequently. The mental status and level of anxiety are documented. When cardiac monitoring is initiated, the nurse evaluates the rate and rhythm.

NURSING DIAGNOSIS. Nursing diagnoses for the patient with a suspected or confirmed AMI may include the following:

- **Anxiety** related to feeling of impending doom
- **Pain** related to lack of oxygen to the myocardium
- **Decreased Cardiac Output** related to dysrhythmia and heart rate
- **Knowledge Deficit** of cardiac care or patient role in recovery

GOALS. Goals for the patient include reduced anxiety, pain relief, normal cardiac output, and patient's knowledge of routine and self-care.

INTERVENTIONS

Anxiety. The nurse provides as calm an environment as possible. Procedures and equipment are explained simply to the patient and family. Family members are also kept informed of the patient's progress. They can be helpful in calming the patient during the acute episode.

Pain. The nurse administers analgesics as ordered and monitors for relief of pain. Morphine is usually administered in small amounts (2–4 mg) intravenously every few minutes until pain relief is evident. Supplemental oxygen is provided generally through nasal cannula at 2 to 4 liters per minute to provide adequate oxygen to the heart muscle. The head of the bed is usually elevated at least 30 degrees. The nurse informs the physician if the patient has an increasing respiratory rate or dyspnea.

Decreased Cardiac Output. The nurse monitors vital signs hourly or more frequently until stable. The ECG is monitored for changes in normal waveform (inverted T wave, ST elevation, and Q wave) and for dysrhythmias. The physician is notified of changes in the rhythm. In an intensive care unit, standing orders prescribe drug therapy for specific dysrhythmias. An intravenous line is usually established so that emergency drugs can be administered quickly and directly. Prompt treatment of dysrhythmias may prevent fatal alterations in rhythm. The nurse monitors the patient for fluid volume excess (rales, cough, jugular vein distention) and reports any such evidence to the physician.

Interventions to decrease demands on the heart include assisting the patient to rest, spacing activities and providing rest periods, adequate ventilation and oxygenation, relief of pain, and maintenance of a calm, quiet environment.

Knowledge Deficit. During the acute phase of AMI, the nurse provides simple explanations of the procedures and routines. The nurse may also reinforce information given by the physician about the diagnosis and treatment. Patient teaching is especially important in the rehabilitation phase.

CARDIAC REHABILITATION. As soon as the patient is stable the nurse can begin rehabilitation by teaching the patient and family about exercise, medications, and diet. If surgical intervention has been proposed, the nurse may also teach the patient about that procedure.

The purpose of rehabilitation is to minimize the risk of repetition of adverse cardiac events. The goal of rehabilitation is to enable patients to attain the highest level of wellness and work ability.

The program is individualized to the patient for maximal success. The four phases of cardiac rehabilitation are I, inpatient management; II, immediately after discharge; III, later cardiac rehabilitation; and IV, maintenance. A team of medical professionals (e.g., nurse, physician, physical therapist, nutritionist, social worker) plans the individual program.

Phase I. Phase I occurs from the onset of the cardiac incident to discharge from the hospital. Activities are gradually increased and the patient's response to them evaluated and documented. Minimal physical deconditioning is desired. Breathing exercises can be initiated early, while the patient is still on bedrest. The patient is instructed to take five slow deep breaths inhaled through the nose and exhaled through pursed lips each hour. Also included in phase I are arm and leg exercises, pulse assessment, assessment of the effects of medications on pulse and blood pressure, dietary instructions, and walking exercises.

Phase II. Phase II begins at discharge and extends 3 months after discharge. During this time delayed emotional responses (anger, anxiety, depression) may occur. The support provided by the rehabilitation team is most important to help the patient with continued physical training and lifestyle changes. During this phase many patients are able to return to work while being monitored for response to activities.

Phase III. Phase III begins at 3 months after discharge and extends to 1 year. Stress management and modification of risk factors are emphasized. Risk factor modification includes diet, exercise, and medications. Fat in the diet should be less than 30% of the total calories; saturated fats are limited to 10%. Total calories are determined by height and weight. Cholesterol intake is limited to less than 300 mg per day. Salt may be restricted to 2 grams per day. Exercise begins gradually and is monitored with periodic stress tests. During this phase the patient is reassessed for the need for further treatment.

The patient is taught about the prescribed medications, including desired effect on the heart and blood pressure, dose, potential side effects, and signs and symptoms that should be reported to the physician. Commonly used medications are vasodilators (nitroglycerin), antihypertensives, antidysrhythmics, beta-adrenergic blocking agents (propranolol, nadolol, timolol, and atenolol), calcium channel blockers (nifedipine, verapamil, and diltiazem), antilipemics (cholestyramine resin, clofibrate, gemfibrozil, lovastatin, and niacin), antiplatelet agents (aspirin and dipyridamole), and stool softeners. These and other related drugs are summarized in Table 31–9.

Phase IV. Phase IV begins at 1 year and lasts throughout life. It is a continuation of phase III and provides progressive evaluation of exercise tolerance and lifestyle changes.

EVALUATION. Criteria for achievement of nursing goals are patient's statement of reduced anxiety, calm demeanor; patient's statement of pain relief, relaxed appearance; normal pulse, blood pressure, and cardiac rhythm; and patient's demonstration of knowledge of routines and rehabilitation measures. The nurse evaluates the patient's knowledge of the disease process; compliance with medication, diet, and exercise regimens; and lifestyle changes. The patient's weight control is often a good estimate of compliance.

CONGESTIVE HEART FAILURE

Congestive heart failure (CHF) is the inability of the heart to meet the metabolic demands of the body.

Etiology and Risk Factors

Causes of CHF are primarily of two types: disorders that increase the workload of the heart and disorders that interfere with the pumping ability of the heart. Therefore, patients at risk for CHF include those with CAD, myocardial infarction, cardiomyopathy, hypertension, COPD, pulmonary hypertension, anemia, disease of the heart valves, and fluid volume overload. Other conditions that increase metabolic needs such as fever and pregnancy may also precipitate heart failure.

Pathophysiology

The left ventricle, right ventricle, or both fail as pumps. Usually the left side of the heart fails first. In time, the right side fails as a result of the left-sided failure. There is a 50% mortality over a 4-year time frame.

COMPENSATION. Compensation is a term used to describe the cardiac and circulatory adjustments that maintain or restore cardiac output to normal or near normal. Compensation occurs through three mechanisms: sympathetic nervous system stimulation, regulation of blood volume by the kidneys, and enlargement of the ventricular myocardium.

Sympathetic Compensation. The sympathetic nervous system responds to decreased cardiac output and blood pressure. Catecholamines are released that increase heart rate, stroke volume, cardiac output, and venous tone. Increased venous tone increases systemic vascular resistance, venous return, and ventricular filling.

Renal Compensation. The second mechanism that responds to decreased cardiac output is renal compensation. When cardiac output falls, so does renal perfusion. This initiates the renin-angiotensin mechanism. Renin, secreted by the kidneys, activates angiotensinogen to angiotensin I. Angiotensin I is converted to angiotensin II, which causes vasoconstriction and triggers release of aldosterone. Vasoconstriction raises the blood pressure by increasing peripheral resistance to blood flow. Aldosterone causes the kidneys to retain sodium and water, which increases blood volume.

Ventricular Hypertrophy. The third mechanism is enlargement of the ventricular myocardium, called *ventricular hypertrophy,* which results from strain. The increased blood volume raises the pressure in the ventricles, which can also cause the ventricles to dilate.

After a period of time, the compensatory mechanisms may no longer be able to meet the increased demands. Contractility decreases; the heart muscle can stretch just so far before becoming inefficient. The force of contraction of the LV decreases. Stroke volume and cardiac output decrease as pumping action fails. Afterload increases with left-sided heart failure. Blood backs up in the LA and then the pulmonary veins. Because of the high pressure in the pulmonary veins (pulmonary hypertension), fluid leaks from the capillaries, causing pulmonary edema. Pulmonary hypertension eventually causes the right side of the heart to fail as well. Then blood returning to the heart from the body meets resistance, which causes systemic pressure to rise. This results in peripheral edema and enlargement of the liver and spleen. If heart failure is not corrected, death eventually ensues.

With left-sided heart failure there is increased left ventricular end-diastolic pressure, increased left atrial pressure, increased pulmonary pressure, and resulting pulmonary edema as the excess fluid leaks into the lung tissues. In right-sided CHF right ventricular pressure increases, right atrial pressure increases, and fluid accumulates in the systemic vasculature.

Signs and Symptoms

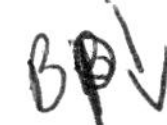

The patient with left-sided heart failure is typically very anxious, pale, and tachycardic. Consecutive blood pressure readings may show a downward trend. Auscultation of the lung fields may reveal crackles, wheezes, dyspnea, and cough. When assessing heart sounds, S_3 and S_4 may be heard as a result of the backup of fluid and the heart's inability to handle the excess fluids.

With right-sided heart failure there is increased central venous pressure, jugular venous distention, abdominal engorgement, and dependent edema. Anorexia, nausea, and vomiting may result from the abdominal engorgement. Fatigue, weight gain, and decreased urinary output are common complaints.

Medical Diagnosis

The diagnosis of CHF is made on the basis of the history, physical examination, radiographs, and laboratory test results. A chest radiograph may reveal hazy lung fields, distended vasculature, and cardiomegaly. An echocardiogram may reveal heart enlargement and ineffective ventricular contraction. Laboratory tests indicative of CHF are decreased serum sodium and hematocrit from hemodilution and decreased saturated arterial oxygenation from poor pulmonary perfusion. The blood urea nitrogen (BUN) and creatinine are elevated with decreased renal function. Liver function tests are elevated with hepatomegaly (liver enlargement). The patient who is critically ill with CHF may require more intensive monitoring of hemodynamics.

Medical Treatment

Medical treatment includes management of the underlying cause, drug therapy to improve cardiac output and eliminate excess fluid, and conservative measures to decrease demands on the heart.

Treatment of the underlying problem may involve such interventions as correction of dysrhythmias, management of hypertension, and valve replacement or repair.

DRUG THERAPY. Drugs used to treat CHF and their actions are cardiac glycosides or inotropic agents, diuretics, and vasodilators. Digoxin, an inotropic agent, is prescribed to improve pump function by increasing contractility and decreasing heart rate. Dopamine, dobutamine, and amrinone are other inotropic agents that may be prescribed to improve cardiac contractility, improve renal perfusion, and decrease fluid retention. Diuretics are prescribed to decrease circulating fluid volume and decrease preload. Morphine may be used to decrease anxiety, dilate the vasculature, and reduce myocardial oxygen consumption in the acute stage. Table 31–9 provides additional information about drugs used to treat CHF.

Decreasing cardiac workload and increasing oxygenation to the myocardium are accomplished by using vasodilators, the intra-aortic balloon pump, the semi-

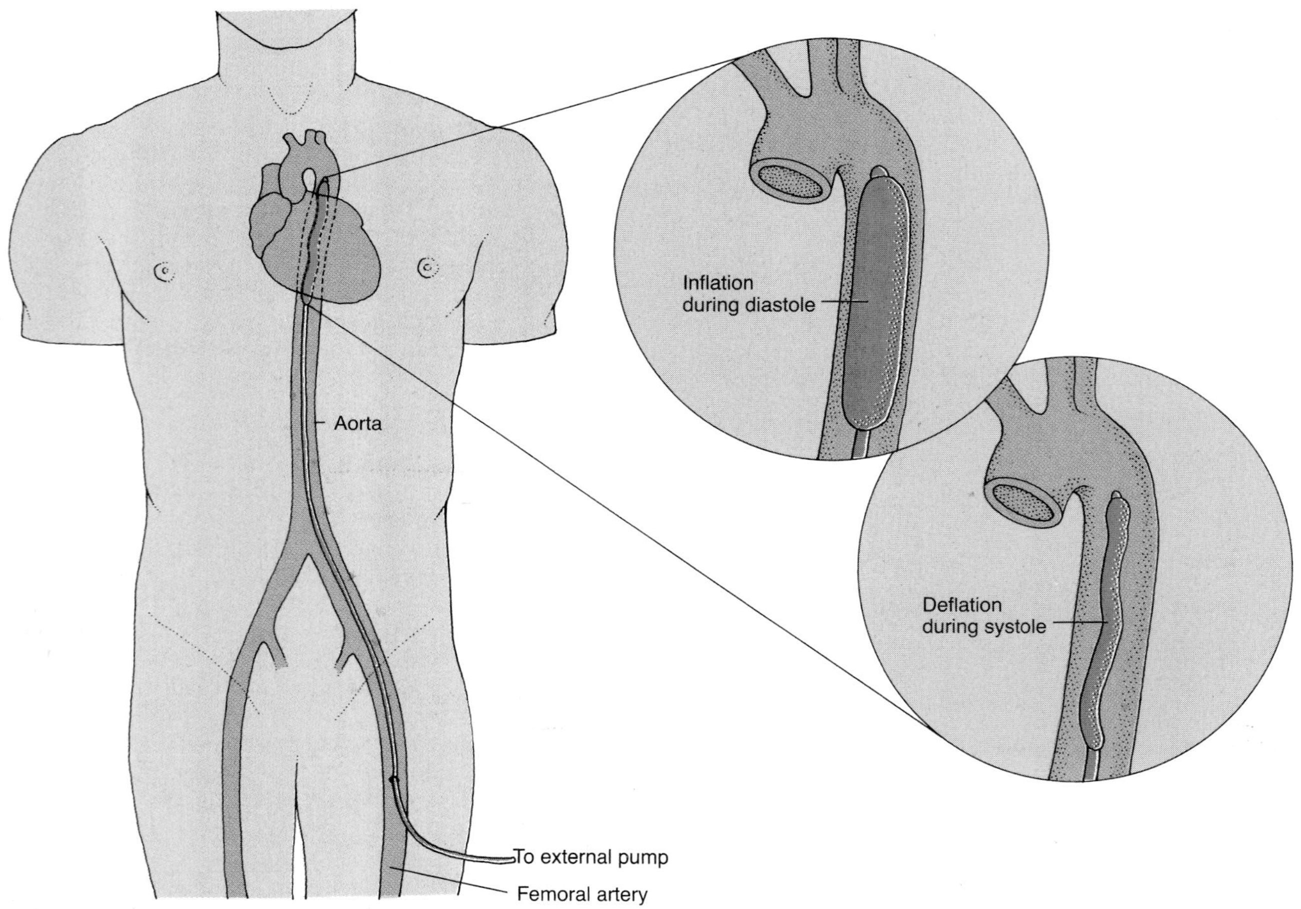

FIGURE 31-17

Intra-aortic balloon catheter is inserted into the femoral artery and advanced into the descending aorta. The balloon lies just distal to the left subclavian artery. Immediately after it is inserted, the catheter is connected to the external pump. (From Ignatavicius, D. D., & Bayne, M. V. [1991]. *Medical-surgical nursing: A nursing process approach* [p. 2157]. Philadelphia: W. B. Saunders.)

Fowler's position, and mechanical ventilation. The intra-aortic balloon pump is a temporary device used to increase cardiac output and coronary artery perfusion. The balloon inflates in diastole to perfuse the coronary arteries and deflates in systole to decrease systemic vascular resistance (Fig. 31–17).

ROTATING TOURNIQUETS. Rotating tourniquets may be used for rapid reduction of circulating volume. Tourniquets (usually blood pressure cuffs) are placed proximally on each extremity. Three tourniquets are inflated one at a time to trap volume in the extremities and relieve the heart of a substantial workload. A flow sheet must be organized so that the inflation of tourniquets is rotated at the prescribed time.

Complications

Dysrhythmias, cardiac failure, and ventricular aneurysm with potential rupture of the aneurysm are possible complications of CHF.

Nursing Care of the Patient in Congestive Heart Failure

ASSESSMENT. Complete assessment of the cardiac patient is outlined in Table 31–4 (see also Care Plan: The Patient in Congestive Heart Failure). It is especially important to assess heart sounds, rate, and rhythm. The point of maximum impulse is noted. The apical and radial pulses are assessed frequently. The nurse inspects for jugular vein distention. A baseline respiratory assessment of rate, rhythm, and breath sounds is vital. The nurse also assesses for preload and afterload by measuring weight and blood pressure accurately. The skin is inspected and palpated for turgor and edema. Intake and output records and daily weights may be done to evaluate fluid retention or loss. If ordered, central venous pressure and hemodynamic readings may be taken as well. If cardiac monitoring is done, the nurse observes for dysrhythmias. Nurses who work in intensive care units routinely interpret ECGs. Interpretation is discussed later in this chapter.

PHARMACOLOGY CAPSULE

Before each dose of digitalis, the apical pulse is counted for 1 full minute. If the heart rate is less than 60 bpm, the drug is withheld and the physician notified.

NURSING DIAGNOSIS. The most common nursing diagnoses with CHF are the following:

- **Fluid Volume Excess** related to ineffective cardiac pumping
- **Impaired Gas Exchange** related to decreased pulmonary perfusion
- **Anxiety** related to edema and inability to breathe
- **Decreased Cardiac Output** related to mechanical failure
- **Fatigue** related to inability to perform usual activities
- **Knowledge Deficit** of CHF, its treatment, and self-care

GOALS. The overall goals for the treatment of the CHF patient are to reverse the decompensatory process and to maximize cardiac function. The specific goals of nursing care include normal fluid volume, adequate oxygenation, reduced anxiety, improved cardiac output, increased activity tolerance, and patient's knowledge of self-care.

INTERVENTIONS

Fluid Volume Excess. Fluid retention is a response to CHF, an attempt to maintain normal cardiac output. Unfortunately, it compounds the problem by increasing the workload on the heart. Therefore, measures are taken to reduce the fluid volume to normal while improving the function of the heart. The nurse administers diuretics as ordered and monitors the patient for adverse effects. The most common adverse effects of diuretic therapy are fluid and electrolyte disturbances. Signs and symptoms that may indicate fluid or electrolyte disturbances include cardiac dysrhythmias, muscle weakness or twitching, cramps, changes in mental status, and abdominal distention. Frequent serum electrolyte measurements are usually ordered. The nurse notes the results and notifies the physician of abnormal findings. If hourly urine output is being measured, the nurse reports an output of less than 30 ml per hour to the physician as well.

PHARMACOLOGY CAPSULE

The most common adverse effects of diuretic therapy are fluid and electrolyte imbalances.

Intravenous fluids are usually administered to provide a line for drug administration. The nurse monitors the rate of fluid administration carefully and adjusts the rate as needed. If fluid retention is not relieved by other means, fluid restriction may be instituted. All staff should know the exact amount of fluid allowed and must record all intake. Fluid restriction can be very uncomfortable for the patient. Even with fluid volume excess, the patient may feel thirsty because of electrolyte imbalances. Oral fluids are presented in small containers and offered at reasonable intervals. Mouth care is provided frequently. The patient and family must understand why fluids are restricted so that the patient does not exceed the prescribed intake.

Impaired Gas Exchange. Hypoxia is a common finding with left-sided heart failure due to pulmonary edema and with right-sided heart failure due to decreased blood flow to the lungs. The patient with CHF generally breathes more easily in a semi- or high

CARE PLAN

The Patient in Congestive Heart Failure

ASSESSMENT

Health History: Mrs. Ling is a 73-year-old Chinese-American woman. She is a retired business owner who lives alone and has no immediate family in the area. She began having dyspnea and orthopnea that has become progressively worse over the last 3 days. Her past medical history includes a myocardial infarction 1 year ago, and a 10-year history of hypertension controlled with diet and verapamil, 240 mg daily. In addition to the verapamil, she takes only an occasional laxative. She complains of fatigue, restlessness, insomnia, and anorexia and a productive cough with pink sputum.

Physical Examination: Vital signs: temperature, 98°F orally; pulse, 104 slightly irregular; respiration, 24; blood pressure, 168/96. Height, 5′2″; weight, 152 (a 7-lb increase in 1 week). Patient is alert but appears anxious. Skin is pale and diaphoretic. An S_3 murmur is present. Jugular vein distention is noted. Auscultation of the lungs reveals crackles in the lower lobes of both lungs. The abdomen is distended. Bowel sounds are present in all four quadrants. 3+ pitting edema is present in both feet and ankles.

Mrs. Ling is being admitted to the coronary care unit for treatment, where she will have continuous electrocardiogram (ECG) and hemodynamic monitoring.

NURSING DIAGNOSIS	GOALS AND OUTCOME CRITERIA	INTERVENTIONS
Decreased cardiac output related to decreased myocardial contractility.	The patient's cardiac output will improve as evidenced by normal heart rate and rhythm, normal blood pressure, normal hemodynamic measures, and breath sounds clear to auscultation.	Monitor vital signs, heart and lung sounds, level of consciousness, ECG. Monitor hemodynamics: blood pressure, pulmonary artery pressure, pulmonary capillary wedge pressure, cardiac output, cardiac index, and systemic vascular resistance. Enforce bedrest with head of bed elevated. Schedule activities to allow rest. Request small, frequent meals. Administer cardiotonics, vasodilators, and angiotensin inhibitors as ordered.
Fluid volume excess related to decreased glomerular filtration rate, increased aldosterone, sodium and water retention, and increased antidiuretic hormone release.	The patient will have normal fluid balance as evidenced by weight of 145, absence of edema, absence of crackles and wheezes in the lungs, and ability to participate in activities of daily living (ADLs) without dyspnea.	Monitor for jugular venous distention and peripheral edema. Auscultate heart and lung sounds every 4 hr. Measure weight daily and intake and output accurately. Maintain intravenous lines and correct fluid infusion rate. Administer diuretics as ordered. Teach about sodium restriction and rationale. Protect edematous extremities from pressure or injury.
Impaired gas exchange related to pulmonary congestion.	The patient's gas exchange will be normal as evidenced by normal arterial blood gases, normal skin color, absence of dyspnea, and clear lung sounds.	Assess lung sounds and respiratory status every 4 hr. Monitor arterial blood gases, pulmonary artery mean pressure, and pulmonary capillary wedge pressure. Elevate head of bed. Administer oxygen as ordered. Assist to cough and deep breathe every 2 hr. Administer diuretics and morphine sulfate as ordered.
Activity intolerance related to imbalance between oxygen supply and demand.	The patient's activity tolerance will improve as evidenced by performance of ADLs without excessive fatigue or dyspnea.	Assess response to activity when permitted. Monitor for dyspnea, changes in vital signs. Limit fatiguing activities. Gradually increase activity as tolerance improves.

The Patient in Congestive Heart Failure *(Continued)*

NURSING DIAGNOSIS	GOALS AND OUTCOME CRITERIA	INTERVENTIONS
Anxiety related to hypoxia, life-threatening situation.	The patient's anxiety will be reduced as evidenced by calm demeanor and statement that she feels less anxious.	Explain procedures and equipment. Tell patient about congestive heart failure (CHF) and how it is being treated. Point out signs of improvement. Visit often and respond to call light promptly. Offer spiritual counselor if desired.
Knowledge deficit of condition, treatment, self-care, and resources.	The patient will verbalize information about her condition, treatment, self-care measures, and resources.	Provide simple explanation of CHF, its effects, and its treatment. As discharge nears, discuss diet, exercise, and drug therapy. Explain signs and symptoms that should be reported to physician. Advise of services of American Heart Association for information. Explore sources of support and need for visiting nurse or home health services.

Fowler's position. Elevation of the upper body facilitates breathing by reducing pressure of the abdominal organs on the diaphragm. Supplemental oxygen is usually prescribed at 4 to 6 liters per minute per nasal cannula. The flow rate is reduced to 2 liters per minute for patients with chronic hypoxia. Respiratory status and blood gases are assessed frequently.

Prescribed bedrest can lead to other pulmonary complications related to immobility: hypostatic pneumonia and pulmonary emboli. The patient is taught to cough and deep breathe at least every 2 hours to promote respiratory excursion and to mobilize secretions. Other interventions to prevent complications of immobility are detailed in Chapter 19.

Anxiety. Factors that may cause the patient to become anxious are dyspnea, unfamiliar setting and routines, and uncertainty about what is happening. The nurse acknowledges the patient's anxiety and attempts to identify the basis. While taking immediate measures to relieve dyspnea, the nurse calmly explains what is being done. It may be helpful to tell the patient how specific measures help relieve symptoms. The presence of a family member may have a calming effect if the nurse takes time to explain that the relative must remain calm too.

Decreased Cardiac Output. Inotropic drugs, vasodilators, and diuretics are given as ordered, and the patient is monitored for therapeutic and adverse effects. Bedrest and stress reduction reduce the cardiac workload. When the patient is acutely ill, the nurse eliminates unnecessary activity. Partial baths are given rather than complete bed baths. The patient is assisted to change positions at least every 2 hours so the skin can be inspected for signs of pressure. Gentle massage of pressure points stimulates local circulation. Visitors may be permitted but should be advised to sit quietly with the patient for short periods of time.

Fatigue. Frequent rest periods, pacing of activities, and relaxation techniques help the patient conserve energy. As the fluid volume is decreased and the cardiac output is increased, the patient can expect to be less fatigued.

Knowledge Deficit. Patients with chronic CHF require instruction on diet, medications, exercise routines, and recognition of significant changes in signs and symptoms.

The most common therapeutic dietary measure for CHF is sodium restriction. The patient may be limited to 2 grams of sodium per day. In severe cases, a limitation of 500 to 1000 mg per day may be prescribed. Reduced sodium intake decreases fluid retention, thereby reducing the cardiac workload. For a 2-gram sodium diet, the patient is advised to avoid foods high in sodium (a list should be provided), not to add salt before or after cooking, and to use no more than 2 cups of milk products daily. Patients often have difficulty changing their use of seasonings. The nurse acknowledges the difficulty and explains how sodium limitation contributes to improvement of cardiac function. It is best to identify the type of diet to be prescribed on discharge as early as possible. This allows time for a dietary consultation to be arranged, which should be followed by reinforcement by the nurse. The person who prepares the patient's meals at home must be included in the teaching sessions.

The patient may be discharged on medications, often inotropic drugs and diuretics. The nurse tells the patient what type of medication is being prescribed and explains dosage, schedule, side and adverse effects, and any special aspects of administration. Elderly patients are more susceptible to adverse drug effects because they may metabolize and excrete drugs more slowly. This is especially true when the older patient is taking digitalis. The patient is advised to report early signs of digitalis toxicity: anorexia, nausea, visual disturbances.

PHARMACOLOGY CAPSULE

Elderly people are more susceptible to adverse drug effects because they metabolize and excrete drugs more slowly.

The patient may be referred to a rehabilitation facility for exercise training. In general, the patient is advised to plan rest periods before and after tiring activities. Activity should be increased gradually, with rest periods taken when fatigue or dyspnea occurs. The physician may prescribe vasodilators for patients who experience chest pain with some activities. If monitoring is indicated after discharge, a referral to a home nursing agency should be requested.

The nurse instructs the patient to notify the physician if the following problems develop: increasing dyspnea or edema, excessive fatigue, or pain that is not relieved by rest or prescribed medications. In addition, the patient is advised to avoid smoking and smoky environments and to refrain from wearing constricting clothing on the lower extremities.

Sources of information and assistance in the community are identified. For example, the American Heart Association has information on diet and exercise. The Visiting Nurses Association or a home health agency can provide assessments and assistance in the home. The physician may order portable oxygen for use at home. The nurse or a respiratory therapist instructs the patient in the use of the equipment and the safety precautions to take when using oxygen (see Chapter 28).

EVALUATION. Criteria for evaluating goal achievement include normal fluid volume as evidenced by normal blood pressure and absence of edema or dyspnea; clear breath sounds and normal respiratory rate; patient's statement of reduced anxiety and calm demeanor; regular heart rate and rhythm; performance of normal activities without fatigue; and patient's demonstration of knowledge of medical therapy and self-care.

INFLAMMATORY DISORDERS

Inflammation of the heart most often results from systemic infections. The endocardium, myocardium, and pericardium may be affected.

INFECTIVE ENDOCARDITIS

Etiology and Risk Factors

Microbial infections of the endocardium primarily affect the valves. Organisms present in the blood easily colonize on valves damaged by rheumatic heart disease, congenital defects, or a mitral valve that is prolapsed.

Although the incidence of infective endocarditis (IE) has decreased with the use of antibiotics, there has been a resurgence of the problem in intravenous drug abusers. The more frequent use of invasive intravascular catheters for severely compromised patients has also contributed to the frequency with which IE occurs.

Patients with known valvular disease are also at risk for IE. They should be treated with prophylactic antibiotics before dental or invasive procedures. Immunosuppression or any source of bacterial contamination (lacerations, pneumonia, invasive procedures, intravenous drug use with contaminated needles) places patients at risk.

Pathophysiology

Bacteria enter the blood stream via any of the previously mentioned means. The most common organisms are *Staphylococcus aureus*, β-hemolytic streptococcus, *Streptococcus viridans*, and *Escherichia coli*. The bacteria accumulate on the heart valves and form vegetations. The mitral valve is the most common site for these vegetations. The turbulence of the blood flow through the heart weakens the vegetations and causes pieces to break off. These emboli can then obstruct circulation and impair tissue perfusion in the lungs, brain, kidneys, and heart.

Complications

Complications of IE include ventricular septal defect, CHF, and embolization. Congestive heart failure is the most frequent cause of death with IE.

Signs and Symptoms

Patients generally present with fever, malaise, and weight loss. The temperature may be low grade (37.2–38.9°C [99–102°F]) or higher (38.9–40.6°C [102–105°F]). The fever is accompanied by chills and night sweats. Chest or abdominal pain may be reported, possibly indicating embolization.

Medical Diagnosis

The diagnosis of IE is based on the history, physical examination, and results of laboratory studies. A history of recent dental or surgical procedures may precede IE. Auscultation may reveal a heart murmur. Echocardiogram helps to visualize lesions and valvular regurgitation. Right-sided or left-sided heart failure may be evident. Serial blood cultures may give clues to the causative organism or organisms. The WBC count may be elevated.

Medical Treatment

Antimicrobials, rest, and limitation of activities are the primary therapeutic measures for IE. Antimicrobials are given intravenously for 2 to 6 weeks depending on the organism. The patient is usually hospitalized for at least 1 week and then receives home intravenous therapy if that is available. Prophylactic anticoagulants may be necessary. Surgery may be necessary to replace an infected prosthetic valve.

Nursing Care of the Patient with Infective Endocarditis

ASSESSMENT. The patient's history should be reviewed for risk factors, recent invasive procedures, known pathologic cardiac conditions, and onset of symptoms. The nurse assesses for temperature elevation, heart murmur, evidence of CHF (cough, peripheral edema) and embolization. Complete assessment of the cardiac patient is summarized in Table 31–4.

NURSING DIAGNOSIS. Potential nursing diagnoses for IE include the following:

- **Decreased Cardiac Output** related to impaired valve function
- **Knowledge Deficit** of disease process and treatment
- **Impaired Physical Mobility** related to fatigue and prolonged intravenous therapy
- **Alteration in Tissue Perfusion** related to embolization

GOALS. The goals for IE include normal cardiac output, patient's knowledge of disease process and treatment, resumption of usual physical activities without symptoms, and normal tissue perfusion.

INTERVENTIONS. The nurse administers the prescribed antibiotics. Throughout the course of the illness, the nurse continues to assess cardiac output and monitor for complications. The patient is taught about the medications prescribed and any restrictions imposed. Adequate rest is necessary during the healing process. Range of motion exercises may be necessary during the acute stage and until the patient is ambulatory.

EVALUATION. Achievement of goals is determined by normal pulse and blood pressure; patient's demonstration of knowledge of IE and treatment; patient's performance of activities of daily living without fatigue; and absence of dyspnea or signs of circulatory obstruction.

MYOCARDITIS

Myocarditis is a local or diffuse inflammation of the myocardium. It may be caused by a viral or bacterial organism, an autoimmune process, or a toxicity to a drug or to lead. It may result in cardiomyopathy.

The incidence is not well known. Myocarditis often affects those 20 to 40 years of age. Those who are immunocompromised are at risk.

Pathophysiology

Myocarditis is characterized by degeneration and necrosis of myocardial tissue that is different from the ischemia associated with myocardial infarction. Tissue next to the necrotic area hypertrophies. The extent of the damage is directly related to the number of areas of myocardial destruction. The hypertrophied areas may lose elasticity, which can result in CHF or dysrhythmias. It is possible that myocarditis is a phase of dilated cardiomyopathy.

Complications

The complications of myocarditis are CHF, dysrhythmias, embolization, and cardiomyopathy.

Signs and Symptoms

Myocarditis is asymptomatic in some patients. Others have fever, fatigue, sore throat, dyspnea, and muscle aches. Lymph nodes may be enlarged. Cardiac symptoms, mainly chest pain, typically develop 7 to 10 days after a viral infection. Patients often present in CHF or with dysrhythmias.

Medical Diagnosis

Diagnosis is based on history, symptoms, and testing. The physical examination may detect a friction rub, rales in the lungs, and jugular vein distention. A chest radiograph and an echocardiogram may reveal cardiac hypertrophy. Dysrhythmias may be evident on ECG. A myocardial biopsy shows lymphocytic infiltration and cell necrosis.

Medical Treatment

Treatment of myocarditis is aimed at stabilizing the patient hemodynamically. Bedrest, activity restriction, and supplemental oxygen assist with decreasing the workload of the heart. Drug therapy may include inotropic agents, anticoagulants, antidysrhythmics, and antibiotics. Immunosuppressant drugs may be ordered after the infectious stage of this disease has passed, although this treatment is controversial.

Nursing Care of the Patient with Myocarditis

ASSESSMENT. While taking the health history, the nurse asks about recent illnesses, medications, and exposure to toxins. In the review of systems, the nurse assesses the patient's activity tolerance. Signs of CHF (edema, dyspnea) are recorded. Vital signs are assessed to detect fever and tachycardia. The breath sounds are assessed for crackles. The skin is inspected and palpated for color and edema. The complete assessment of the cardiac patient is outlined in Table 31–4.

NURSING DIAGNOSIS. Potential nursing diagnoses for the patient with myocarditis may include the following:

- **Decreased Cardiac Output** related to complications of inflammation
- **Anxiety** related to prolonged incapacity
- **Activity Intolerance** related to fatigue
- **Knowledge Deficit** of disease process

GOALS. The major goals of nursing care for the patient with myocarditis are normal cardiac output, reduced anxiety, improved activity tolerance, and patient's knowledge of myocarditis and treatment.

INTERVENTIONS. Medications to control inflammation and to decrease the workload of the heart are administered as ordered. The nurse provides for adequate rest and assesses tolerance of activity. The patient is taught about the disease and lifestyle modification.

EVALUATION. Criteria for goal achievement are vital signs within patient's usual range, patient's statement of reduced anxiety and calm manner, increasing activity without fatigue, and patient's description of disease process, treatment, and self-care.

PERICARDITIS

Etiology and Risk Factors

Pericarditis is an inflammation of the pericardium. It may be a primary disease or associated with another inflammatory process. The disease may be acute or chronic. Acute pericarditis is caused by viruses, bacteria, fungi, chemotherapy, or myocardial infarction (Dressler's syndrome). Chronic pericarditis is caused by tuberculosis, radiation, or metastases.

Pathophysiology

In acute pericarditis, the inflammatory process causes an increase in the amount of pericardial fluid and inflammation of the surrounding tissues. With effusion, clear or turbid fluid accumulates in the pericardial space. In effusive-constrictive pericarditis adhesions occur. In constrictive pericarditis scarring of the pericardium fuses the visceral and parietal pericardia together. Loss of elasticity occurs from the scarring. This constrictive process prevents adequate ventricular filling.

Complications

The major complication with pericarditis is pericardial effusion or accumulation of fluid in the pericardial space. This may lead to cardiac tamponade when sufficient fluid accumulation decreases ventricular filling. The resulting drop in cardiac output is an emergency. It is treated with pericardiocentesis to remove the fluid accumulation.

Signs and Symptoms

Chest pain is the hallmark symptom of pericarditis. The pain is most severe on inspiration. It is most often sharp and stabbing but may be described as dull or burning. It is relieved by sitting up and leaning forward. Dyspnea, chills, and fever accompany pericarditis. Slowly progressing pericardial effusion does not result in hemodynamic compromise until 400 to 500 ml of fluid have accumulated. Rapidly accumulating fluid may precipitate very sudden symptoms with accumulation of fluid up to 250 ml.

Medical Diagnosis

The diagnostic challenge is to differentiate pericarditis from AMI. The WBC count is elevated with pericarditis. Serial ECGs show that the ST segment elevation resolves in several weeks. QRS voltage may decrease from the accumulated fluid in the pericardial space. An echocardiogram may show pericardial thickening and effusion. Atrial fibrillation often occurs from the irritation. The CPK-MB may be elevated. Blood cultures may identify the causative organism or organisms.

Medical Treatment

The patient is treated with analgesics, antipyretics, anti-inflammatory agents, and antibiotics. With constrictive pericarditis, the patient would be treated as for CHF. Surgical creation of a pericardial window (removal of a segment of parietal pericardium to allow continuous drainage of pericardial fluid) may be necessary for treating chronic pericarditis with effusion.

Nursing Care of the Patient with Pericarditis

ASSESSMENT. General nursing assessment of the cardiac patient is summarized in Table 31–4. With pericarditis, assessment of heart sounds is especially important.

NURSING DIAGNOSIS. Potential nursing diagnoses for the patient with pericarditis include the following:

- **Pain** related to pericardial inflammation
- **Decreased Cardiac Output** related to pericardial constriction
- **Anxiety** related to illness
- **Knowledge Deficit** related to the disease process

GOALS. The goals of nursing care for the patient with pericarditis include pain relief, improved cardiac output, decreased anxiety, and patient's knowledge of condition and self-care.

INTERVENTIONS. Rest and reduction of activity decrease the workload of the heart. The nurse administers medications and teaches the patient about the medications. Emotional support from the nursing staff and significant others is vital. The patient can be instructed in relaxation techniques. The nurse monitors vital signs and auscultates for a pericardial friction rub. The rub is heard during inspiration with the diaphragm of the stethoscope placed between the second and the fourth intercostal spaces at the left sternal border. It is heard when there is no fluid accumulation. Distant heart sounds may be heard when there is fluid accumulation. Pain characteristics and response to analgesics and anti-inflammatory agents are noted. The ECG is monitored for dysrhythmias.

EVALUATION. Criteria for evaluating the effectiveness of nursing care are patient's statement of pain relief, pulse and blood pressure consistent with patient's norms, patient's statement of decreased anxiety and calm manner, and patient's descriptions of condition and self-care.

CARDIOMYOPATHY

Etiology and Risk Factors

Cardiomyopathy is disease of the heart muscle. Its cause is unknown. The disease generally leads to heart failure. Three types of cardiomyopathy are recognized: dilated, hypertrophic, and restrictive (Fig. 31–18). Dilated cardiomyopathy (DC) is the most common type and is found primarily in men 40 to 60 years of age. There is an increased incidence in black men. A relatively poor prognosis exists for DC, with a 50% mortality in 5 years. Hypertrophic cardiomyopathy (HC) is generally of genetic origin. Persons with HC generally die by age 40, and the incidence of sudden cardiac death with this diagnosis is high. Restrictive cardiomyopathy (RC) is the least common type and occurs in young men and women.

Three risk factors are associated with DC: excessive use of alcohol, pregnancy, and infections. The genetic predisposition with HC is known to skip generations. Amyloidosis, sarcoidosis, and other immunosuppressive disorders may predispose young people to RC.

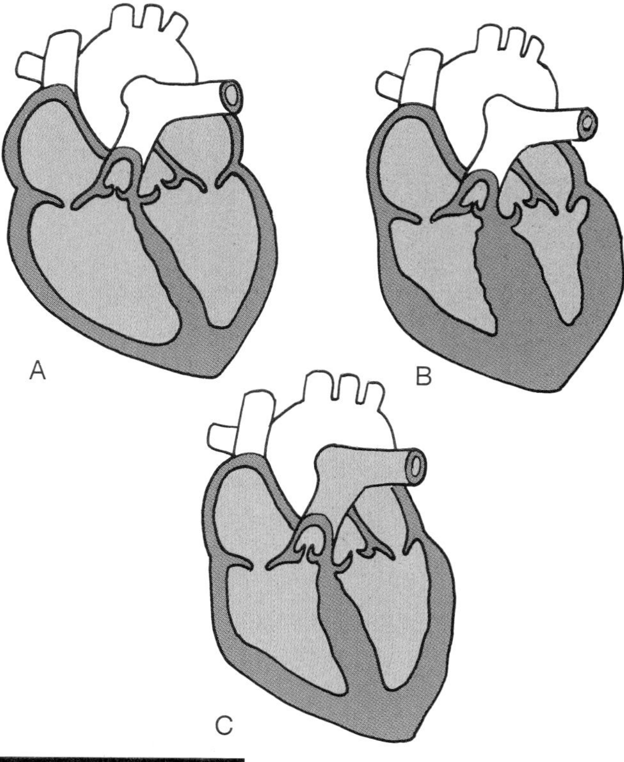

FIGURE 31–18

Cardiomyopathy. *A*, Dilated cardiomyopathy; *B*, hypertrophic cardiomyopathy; *C*, restrictive cardiomyopathy.

Pathophysiology

With DC there is an interference with calcium uptake. This causes decreased cellular contractility, decreased ejection fraction and stroke volume, and increased left ventricular end-diastolic pressure. Pressure backup results in dilation of all four chambers and is most pronounced in the ventricles. Left ventricular failure and resulting CHF are seen as the result of excessive back pressure (see Fig. 31–18*A*).

In HC the left ventricle hypertrophies and there is thickening of the ventricular septum and of the mitral valve. The left ventricular capacity decreases and narrows the left ventricular outflow. The size of the LA increases as a result of the back pressure. Ventricular dysrhythmias are common (see Fig. 31–18*B*).

In RC the myocardium becomes rigid and less distensible in systole. This reduces ventricular filling and cardiac output. Pulmonary and systemic congestion result. The exterior heart size remains normal, but all four chambers decrease in size (see Fig. 31–18*C*).

Signs and Symptoms

Dilated cardiomyopathy is a progressive, chronic disease. The onset is gradual, with dyspnea, fatigue, left-sided heart failure, and moderate to severe cardiomyopathy. Mitral valve regurgitation and S_3 and S_4 sounds are evident.

With HC the progression of symptoms is slow. Dyspnea, orthopnea, angina, fatigue, syncope, palpitations, ankle edema, and S_4 sounds are found.

With RC the primary symptom is exercise intolerance. Dyspnea, fatigue, right-sided CHF, S_3 and S_4 sounds, and mitral valve regurgitation are also noted.

Medical Diagnosis

Diagnosis of DC is made primarily on the basis of echocardiogram results. Cardiac enlargement may be noted on chest radiograph. The echocardiogram and chest radiograph are also used to diagnose HC. Other findings include an aortic murmur and atrial and ventricular dysrhythmias. An enlarged LV may be accompanied by left atrial enlargement. The diagnosis of RC is demonstrated by decreased cardiac output and CHF. It must be differentiated from pericarditis.

Medical Treatment

Supportive measures are used for DC. Positive inotropic drugs to improve cardiac output, diuretics and nitrates to decrease preload, and vasodilators to decrease afterload provide this type of therapy. Anticoagulants may be used to prevent thrombi. If all other measures fail, the patient needs a heart transplant. Surgery, in the form of a myomectomy, ventriculomyomectomy, or mitral valve replacement are considered for HC. Medical treatment for HC includes antidysrhythmics, antibiotics, anticoagulants, verapamil, and beta blockers. Positive inotropic drugs, diuretics, and nitrates are contraindicated with HC. With DC the tachycardia helps to maintain cardiac output. When this compensatory mechanism fails, supportive measures, as indicated with DC, are used. Complications observed with all types of cardiomyopathy are dysrhythmias, CHF, and death. There is a poor prognosis with cardiomyopathy.

Nursing Care of the Patient with Cardiomyopathy

ASSESSMENT. These patients are primarily assessed for heart failure. The nurse is alert for dyspnea, cough, edema, dysrhythmias, and decreased cardiac output.

NURSING DIAGNOSIS. Nursing diagnoses for patients with cardiomyopathy include the following:

- **Decreased Cardiac Output** related to ventricular failure
- **Activity Intolerance** related to poor tissue perfusion
- **Hopelessness** related to poor prognosis
- **Knowledge Deficit** of disease process and self-care

GOALS. The goals of care are improved cardiac output, increased activity tolerance, a more positive outlook, and patient's knowledge of disease process and self-care.

INTERVENTIONS. The care of these patients is similar to that of patients with CHF. In addition, a hopeful atmosphere and a careful explanation of care requirements are necessary. The family is encouraged to support the patient. The teaching plan guides the patient to make lifestyle changes. The nurse encourages the patient to make decisions and choices.

EVALUATION. Criteria for evaluating the success of nursing interventions are normal pulse and blood pressure; patient's performance of activities of daily living without excessive fatigue; patient's expression of feelings about condition and hopeful statements; and patient's description of condition, treatment, and self-care.

CARDIAC TRANSPLANTATION

The first heart transplant was performed in 1967 in South Africa by Dr. Christiaan Barnard. Today heart transplants in the United States, approximately 1800 per year, are done for end-stage heart disease. Most of the cases of end-stage heart disease that require transplantation are caused by cardiomyopathy or valvular heart disease. Most recipients are younger than 50 years and without evidence of other major diseases (e.g., diabetes mellitus, malignancy, peptic ulcer disease). Psychological makeup is carefully assessed before transplantation. Individuals with a history of depression, noncompliance, and inability to cope with stress are poor candidates. In the United States there are federal regulations that prohibit the sale of human organs.

The donor must meet the criteria for brain death, have no malignancies outside the central nervous system, be free of infection, and not have experienced severe chest trauma. Prolonged advanced life support measures are avoided. The donor and recipient organs must be carefully matched. The donor heart size must be sufficient to meet the needs of the recipient. The donor heart may be preserved for 4 to 6 hours before transplantation.

The recipient must be free of infection at the time of transplantation. The patient is prepared for surgery as with any open heart procedure. Cardiopulmonary bypass is initiated and the recipient's heart is removed except for the posterior portions of the atria (Fig. 31–19). The donor heart is trimmed and anastomosed to the remaining native heart. The patient is removed from bypass, the heart restarted, and the chest is closed.

Aftercare of the heart transplant patient is similar to that of the patient after coronary artery bypass surgery. Hemodynamic monitoring, ventilation, cardiac assessment, care of chest tubes, and accurate intake and output measurements are vital. Immediately after surgery the patient is placed in a private room in the intensive care unit. Modified protective isolation is employed. The use of gowns, masks, and careful hand washing have been found to be superior to strict isolation techniques. The removal of invasive lines (endotracheal tube, pulmonary artery catheter, Foley catheter, and chest tubes) is accomplished as rapidly as possible to decrease the chance of infection. Postoperatively the prevention of infection is a major goal. Pulmonary infections are most frequently found after heart transplants. Moving the patient from the intensive care unit to a private room and to home as soon as possible decreases the incidence of nosocomial infections. Patients and families are taught the signs and symptoms of infection and to avoid crowds and others with infections.

In addition, the patient with a transplant receives immunosuppressive medications. Lifelong immunosuppression is administered to prevent the body from rejecting the donated heart, which it recognizes as foreign tissue. Initially large doses of corticosteroids are administered, and the dose is decreased over time. At the first indication of rejection (increased temperature, infection, dyspnea, malaise, fatigue, dysrhythmia) the steroid dose is generally increased. Other drugs being used to prevent and treat rejection are azathioprine (Imuran), cyclosporine (Sandimmune), the monoclonal antibody OKT-3, antithymocytic globulin (ATG), antilymphocytic globulin (ALG), FK-506, and rapamycin. Protocols using several immunosuppressive agents are considered most effective. Reduced dosages of each drug provides for a lower incidence of toxicity.

Rejection is monitored through endomyocardial biopsies. These are performed frequently in the immediate period after transplantation and less frequently over time. Patients are taught to monitor their own progress and to report problems promptly. Patients are followed closely by the transplant team and are observed for infection, rejection, quality of life, and complications. Common complications noted after heart transplant are hypertension, elevated cholesterol, obesity, and malignancies.

SUDDEN CARDIAC DEATH

Sudden cardiac death (SCD) occurs when heart activity and respirations cease abruptly. It is the leading

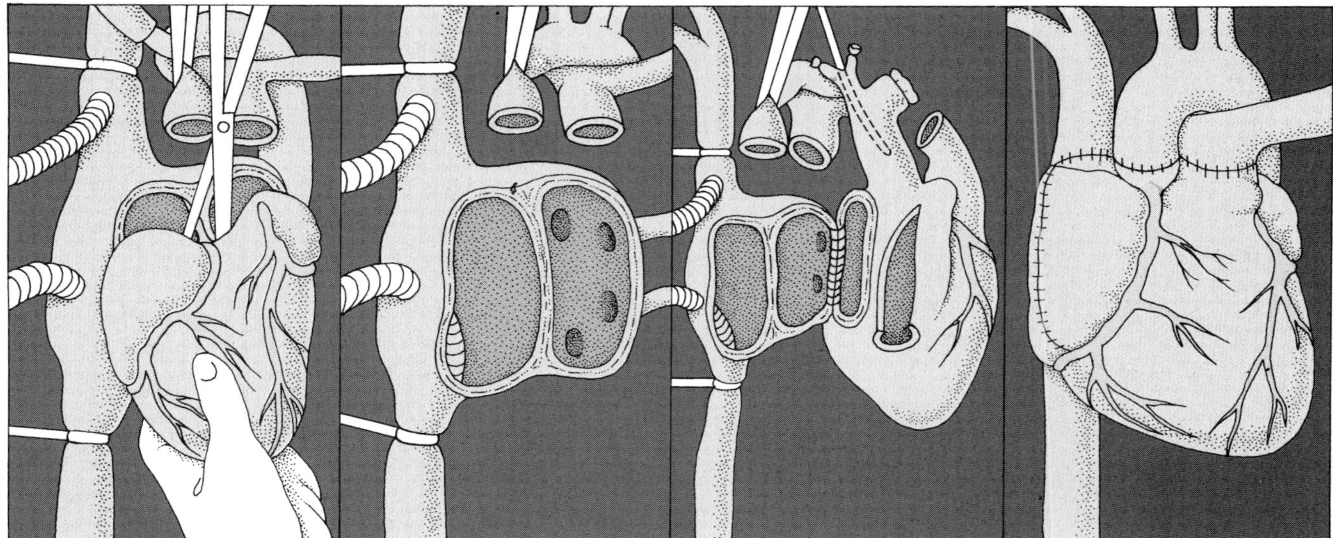

FIGURE 31-19

Heart transplantation. (From Ignatavicius, D. D., & Bayne, M. V. [1991]. *Medical-surgical nursing: A nursing process approach* [p. 2170]. Philadelphia: W. B. Saunders.)

PHARMACOLOGY CAPSULE

Patients taking immunosuppressive drugs to prevent rejection of transplanted tissue have reduced resistance to infection.

cause of death in the United States and occurs in over half a million people per year. Eighty percent of the victims are males between the ages of 20 and 65. Approximately 80% do not live to or through resuscitation. There is a high incidence of recurrence among survivors.

The SCD event generally occurs during ordinary activity. It is often preceded by ventricular tachycardia or ventricular fibrillation and occasionally by severe bradydysrhythmias (slow abnormal cardiac rhythms). An episode of SCD may be the first indication of coronary artery disease. Other causes include complex and multifocal PVCs, ventricular tachycardia, left ventricular dysfunction, cardiomyopathy, hypokalemia, antidysrhythmics, liquid protein diets, and high alcohol consumption.

Those who survive an episode of SCD need to have extensive testing done to determine the nature and cause of the dysrhythmia. Antidysrhythmics are the treatment of choice. If they are ineffective, the patient may be considered a candidate for an automatic implantable cardioverter-defibrillator. Surgery to destroy the irritable focus is an option in a limited number of patients.

AUTOMATIC IMPLANTABLE CARDIOVERTER-DEFIBRILLATOR

The automatic implantable cardioverter-defibrillator (AICD), a relatively new device, is used to treat patients with life-threatening recurrent ventricular fibrillation who are unresponsive to medications or pacemakers. Its use has greatly decreased the mortality from sudden cardiac death. The device senses heart rate and interprets waveform shape. The AICD generator is implanted in the subcutaneous tissue of the abdomen, weighs about 10 ounces, and is larger than a package of cigarettes. The electrodes are implanted in the pericardium (Fig. 31–20). The cardioverter recognizes ventricular fibrillation and uses the shocks to convert the dysrhythmia to normal sinus rhythm. When the AICD senses ventricular fibrillation, it delivers a shock of 25 to 30 joules to defibrillate. If the heart rhythm does not return to normal, the device can deliver up to four or five shocks, pause, and repeat the cycle. The generator can deliver up to 300 shocks over a 5- to 6-year time frame. The patient is instructed to sit or lie down when experiencing a shock and to keep a record of the number of shocks delivered. Patients report the shocks feel like a blow to the chest.

The AICD is inserted in an open chest procedure under general anesthesia. One or more chest tubes are present postoperatively. Patients require analgesia to turn, cough, and deep breathe. The device may not be

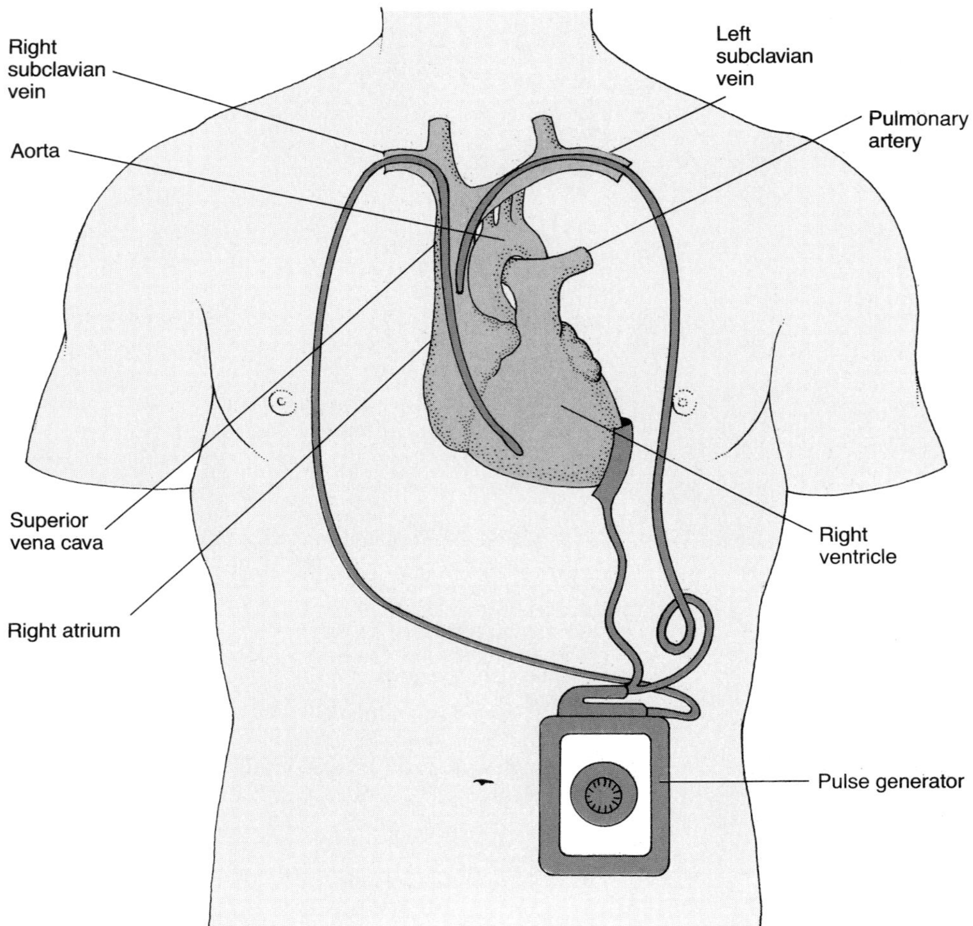

FIGURE 31-20 Automatic implantable cardioverter-defibrillator. (From Ignatavicius, D. D., & Bayne, M. V. [1991]. *Medical-surgical nursing: A nursing process approach* [p. 2148]. Philadelphia: W. B. Saunders.)

activated for several days after surgery until there is less pericardial and ventricular irritability. These patients may need a cardiac rehabilitation program for optimal well-being. An exercise tolerance test may be performed before discharge to determine whether adjustments in the device are necessary.

Complications

Complications associated with the AICD are inappropriate shocks, broken or displaced leads, and failure to deliver shocks as a result of battery failure or failure to recognize a dysrhythmia.

Nursing Care of the Patient with an Automatic Implantable Cardioverter-Defibrillator

The nurse can promote psychosocial adaptation. The patient may be concerned with body image change and a fear of shocks. It is important to decrease anxiety about being shocked. Some patients become very dependent on the machine. These patients and families need much teaching and support. Individuals who touch the patient during a shock will feel a tingling sensation, which is not harmful. An established support group for the patient and family is very helpful. The family is instructed in cardiopulmonary resuscitation. An identification bracelet and a card with instructions about the AICD setting are carried at all times. Patients are told to avoid strong magnetic fields (metal detectors, power plants, and magnetic resonance imaging). Beeps from the generator indicate the need to move away from a magnetic field. Regular follow-up care is important.

VALVULAR DISEASE

The purpose of the heart valves is to maintain blood flow in one direction. If the valves are damaged through a congenital defect or acquired disease, their function is compromised. Stenosis and insufficiency are the two major valve problems. Stenosis is narrowing of the valvular opening. A stenotic valve limits the amount of blood ejected from one chamber to the next and results in increased afterload. Insufficiency is the inability of the valve to close completely. Insufficiency, also called regurgitation, allows the blood to flow backward when a valve does not close efficiently. This increases the pressure behind the valve and therefore increases preload. In stenosis and insufficiency, affected are not only the valve leaflets or cusps but also the chordae tendineae and the papillary muscles. The left side of the heart is most often affected, and the mitral valve is the most frequently affected of all the valves. The pulmonic valve is infrequently affected. Only left-sided valvular disease is discussed here.

Antibiotics have decreased the incidence of valvular disease from rheumatic fever, but nonrheumatic valvular disease has increased. Longer life span and intravenous drug abuse are the primary causes of the increasing incidence of nonrheumatic valvular disease.

MITRAL STENOSIS

Mitral stenosis is the narrowing of the opening in the mitral valve that impedes blood flow from the LA into the LV. The mitral valve leaflets become thickened and fibrotic. Young women, 20 to 40 years of age, are most often affected by mitral stenosis.

Rheumatic heart disease is the leading cause of mitral stenosis. Congenital malformations of the mitral valve occur but are not common. Other causes are calcium accumulation on valve leaflets and atrial myxomas (tumors).

Pathophysiology

The thickening of the valve structures reduces the outflow of blood from the LA to the LV. The LA dilates to accommodate the amount of blood not ejected, left atrial pressure increases, pulmonary artery pressure increases, and the RV hypertrophies. Eventually, the RV fails, and cardiac output decreases because less blood is delivered to the LV.

Signs and Symptoms

Symptoms may begin soon after the disease process or may be delayed for many years. Dyspnea, fatigue, cough, chest pain, and activity intolerance are the most frequent symptoms. Exertional dyspnea and pulmonary edema occur as blood backs up in the pulmonary system and serous fluid leaks into the pulmonary tissues.

Medical Diagnosis

Diagnosis is made on the basis of the patient history, physical examination, and results of diagnostic procedures. The chest radiograph shows left atrial, right ventricular, and pulmonary vascular enlargement. Echocardiogram is used to visualize the mitral valve. Cardiac catheterization is used to confirm the diagnosis and determine the extent of the disease process.

Medical Treatment

When symptomatic, the patient with mitral stenosis is treated as for CHF with drug therapy, sodium and fluid restrictions, and activity restriction. Digoxin, diuretics, beta blockers, and antidysrhythmics may be prescribed. If the patient has atrial fibrillation, anticoagulants may be prescribed also. Prophylactic antibiotics are prescribed before any invasive procedure for patients with mitral stenosis because bacteria tend to cluster on the damaged valves.

Surgical Treatment

Surgical treatment includes commissurotomy, mitral valve replacement, and balloon valvuloplasty. Commissurotomy is excision of parts of the leaflets to enlarge the opening. The mitral valve is replaced with a biologic or synthetic valve (Fig. 31–21). Both commissurotomy and mitral valve replacement require major surgery with cardiopulmonary bypass.

Balloon valvuloplasty is a procedure done in the cardiac catheterization laboratory that has been very successful in dilating stenosed heart valves. It is less invasive than valve replacement or commissurotomy. To dilate the mitral valve, one catheter is threaded through the venous circulation to the RA. The atrial septum is perforated, and a balloon catheter is passed into the LA and through the mitral valve. The balloon is inflated until the valve opens sufficiently. After the procedure, the patient is observed closely in an intensive care unit for dysrhythmias and complications. The perforated atrial septum closes in most cases. Complications include cardiac tamponade, valve regurgitation or restenosis, and hemorrhage. The expected complication, embolization of valve pieces, occurs infrequently.

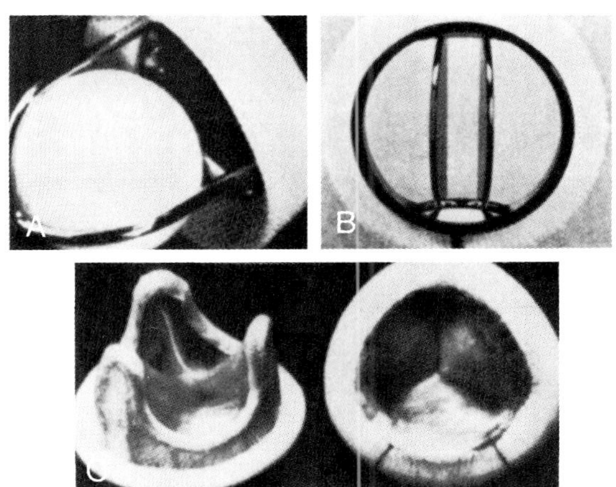

FIGURE 31-21

Examples of biologic and synthetic heart valves. *A,* Starr-Edwards caged-ball valve with cloth sewing ring and bare struts; *B,* St. Jude medical bileaflet valve; *C,* Carpentier-Edwards porcine prosthetic valve. (*A* from Starek, P. J. K. [1987]. In Technical aspects of uncomplicated valve replacement. In P. J. Starek [Ed.], *Heart valve replacement and reconstruction.* Chicago: Year Book Medical Publishers. Reproduced with permission from Mosby–Year Book, Inc.; *B* from Crawford, F. A., Jr. [1987]. In F. A. Crawford [Ed.], *Cardiac surgery: Current heart valve prostheses [Vol. 1].* Philadelphia: Hanley and Belfus; and *C* from Magilligan, D. J., Jr. [1987]. In F. A. Crawford [Ed.], *Cardiac surgery: Current heart valve prostheses [Vol. 1].* Philadelphia: Hanley and Belfus.)

Nursing Care of the Patient with Mitral Stenosis

ASSESSMENT. It is most important to obtain a complete history as summarized in Table 31–4 and record of signs and symptoms being experienced. The nurse takes the vital signs and auscultates for heart murmurs. The murmur of mitral stenosis is a rumbling, low-pitched, diastolic type. It is heard best with the bell of the stethoscope at the apex of the heart with the patient in left lateral position. The ECG may show a notched P wave, indicating left atrial enlargement. Atrial fibrillation is frequently seen. Tachycardia and tachypnea are common signs. The pulse pressure may be decreasing, indicating low cardiac output. Jugular venous distention and crackles are found with pulmonary congestion.

NURSING DIAGNOSIS. The nursing diagnoses for mitral stenosis are the same as those for CHF and for all valvular diseases:

- **Decreased Cardiac Output** related to narrowing or insufficiency of valvular competence
- **Impaired Gas Exchange** related to pulmonary congestion
- **Activity Intolerance** related to imbalance between oxygen supply and demand
- **Fluid Volume Excess** related to decreased glomerular filtration rate, increased aldosterone, sodium and water retention, and increased antidiuretic hormone release

See the nursing care for CHF for the rest of the nursing process.

MITRAL INSUFFICIENCY

Mitral insufficiency often accompanies mitral stenosis as a result of rheumatic fever. One or both of the valve leaflets become rigid and shorten preventing complete closure of the valve. Mitral insufficiency occurs more in males when the cause is other than rheumatic disease.

The LA and LV hypertrophy as a result of the backflow of blood against the incompetent valve. Left ventricular hypertrophy is compensatory in an attempt to maintain cardiac output. Eventually the left side of the heart fails, and symptoms are then the same as described under mitral stenosis.

The murmur of mitral insufficiency is high pitched, blowing, and occurs during systole. It is best heard at the apex and may radiate to the axilla. With severe disease S_3 and S_4 sounds may be auscultated. Atrial fibrillation occurs as the LA enlarges.

Mitral insufficiency is treated with vasodilators to decrease the afterload and therefore the regurgitation. Other medical treatment includes activity restriction, dietary sodium limitation, diuretics, and digitalis. Surgical treatment includes annuloplasty and mitral valve replacement. Annuloplasty is reconstruction of the leaflets and the annulus.

MITRAL VALVE PROLAPSE

The mitral valve prolapses when one or both leaflets enlarge and protrude into the LA during systole. It has a tendency to run in families and may be caused by heart infections, rheumatic fever, or a wide variety of congenital anomalies. The disease is usually benign but may progress to mitral insufficiency. Mitral valve prolapse occurs in 5 to 10% of the population. Most victims are women 20 to 55 years of age.

In most patients symptoms do not occur or may occur with stress. Symptoms include chest pain, palpitations, dizziness, and syncope. Some patients exhibit dysrhythmias. The ECG usually shows normal findings. Evidence of prolapse of the valve may be found with echocardiogram.

The problem is treated with stress reduction techniques.

AORTIC STENOSIS

Etiology and Risk Factors

Stenosis of the aortic valve occurs when the valve cusps become fibrotic and calcify. It may be caused by a congenital malformation or result from rheumatic fever, syphilis, or the aging process (atherosclerosis and calcification). When seen in younger patients, it is most often caused by a congenital malformation. The aortic valve is most commonly diseased in the aging population. The disease occurs predominantly in men.

Pathophysiology

The valve opening decreases to one third normal size before symptoms occur. As flow is impeded through the narrowed valve, the LV hypertrophies to compensate for the extra pressure needed to eject blood. The LA also compensates by delivering a strong atrial kick. These compensatory mechanisms allow normal function until atrial fibrillation disrupts the atrial kick or until the LV hypertrophies to the point of dysfunction with decreased cardiac output and myocardial ischemia. With left ventricular dysfunction the blood will back up into the left atrium and the pulmonary system. If uncorrected, eventually the right side of the heart will fail.

Signs and Symptoms

The patient complains of dyspnea on exertion, angina, and syncope. Fatigue, orthopnea, and paroxysmal nocturnal dyspnea are late symptoms and indicate heart failure.

Medical Diagnosis

The chest radiograph shows atrial and ventricular enlargement, and these are late signs. The murmur of aortic stenosis is harsh and systolic. It is heard best in the aortic area, second intercostal space to the right of the sternum. The echocardiogram shows left ventricular wall thickening. An exercise tolerance test may be ordered to evaluate heart function.

Medical Treatment

Prophylactic antibiotics are prescribed to prevent infective endocarditis with dental and invasive procedures.

Heart failure is treated with digoxin, diuretics, low-sodium diet, and activity restriction. Surgical treatment includes balloon valvuloplasty and aortic valve replacement.

Nursing Care of the Patient with Aortic Stenosis

The nurse monitors for a bounding arterial pulse and widened pulse pressure. The nursing process is the same as for CHF (see Care Plan: The Patient in Congestive Heart Failure).

AORTIC INSUFFICIENCY

Fibrosis and thickening of the aortic cusps progress until the valves no longer maintain unidirectional blood flow. Aortic insufficiency is caused primarily by rheumatic fever. Other causes include IE, blunt chest trauma, calcification of the valve, and chronic hypertension. Seventy-five percent of the patients with aortic insufficiency are men. However, when both the aortic and the mitral valves are diseased, women predominate.

Regurgitation of blood into the LV during diastole increases the amount of blood in the LV. The LV dilates and hypertrophies. Myocardial ischemia and left ventricular failure occur. Blood backs up into the pulmonary system and eventually right ventricular failure occurs.

The murmur of aortic insufficiency is high pitched, blowing, and occurs in diastole. It is auscultated best at the aortic area. The point of maximal impulse may be shifted to the left and down. Tachycardia and palpitations are compensatory mechanisms. Later signs of CHF such as fatigue, dyspnea, and ascites develop. A widened pulse pressure results from a low diastolic pressure. S_3 and S_4 sounds are often auscultated.

Left atrial and ventricular dilation are noted on chest radiograph. The echocardiogram shows left ventricular dilation. Cardiac catheterization is used to determine the extent of incompetence.

As with other patients with valve disease, these patients have prophylactic antibiotics prescribed before invasive procedures. Digoxin and diuretics are prescribed for left ventricular hypertrophy. Aortic valve replacement provides long-term correction.

ELECTROCARDIOGRAM MONITORING

Nurses working in critical care areas are responsible for monitoring and interpreting ECGs. Patients are generally monitored continuously at the bedside and have intermittent monitoring through a 12-lead ECG.

12-LEAD ELECTROCARDIOGRAM

A 12-lead ECG looks at the heart from 12 directions or perspectives. This permits more precise evaluation of the heart's electrical activity. Three leads are placed on the limbs, three leads are augmented, and there are six chest, or precordial, leads. Electricity flows from the negative to the positive lead. If the depolarization wave flows toward the positive pole (electrode), the deflection will be upright. If the wave flows away from the positive pole, the deflection will be negative.

There are three standard limb leads: I, II, and III. Lead I records electrical activity between the RA and the LA. Lead II records activity between the RA and the left leg. Lead III records activity between the LA and the left leg. Leads I and II follow the conduction pathway most closely and provide the clearest, most upright complexes (Fig. 31–22).

The augmented leads increase the amplitude of the deflections. The augmented leads are AVR, AVL, and AVF (Fig. 31–23).

The six precordial leads (V_1 to V_6) are placed on the chest. The V leads give definitive descriptions of ventricular function. Leads V_1 and V_2 depict right ventricular activity. Leads V_3 through V_6 show left ventricular function (Fig. 31–24).

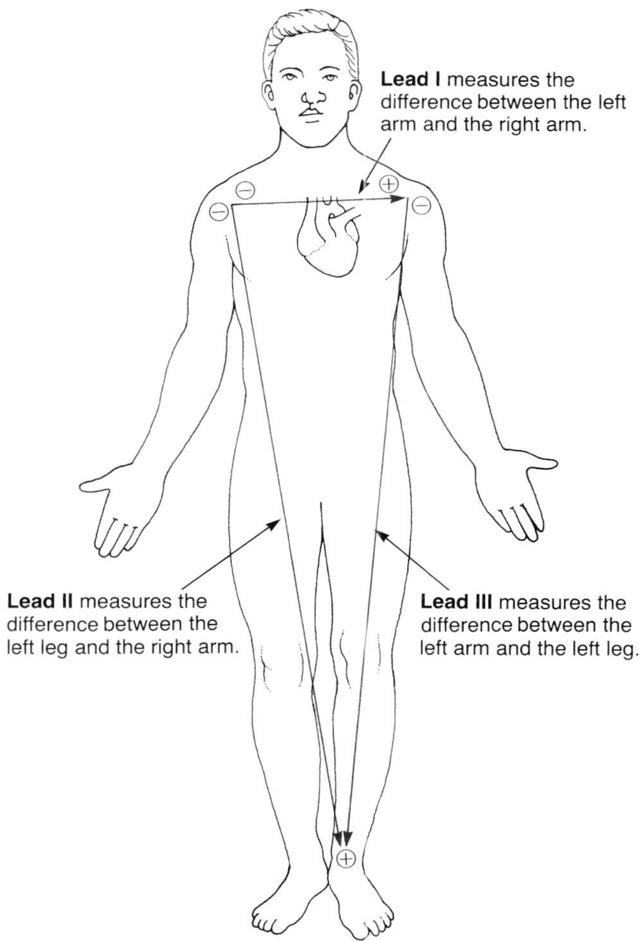

FIGURE 31–22
Electrode placement for leads I, II, and III. (From Ignatavicius, D. D., & Bayne, M. V. [1991]. *Medical-surgical nursing: A nursing process approach* [p. 2103]. Philadelphia: W. B. Saunders.)

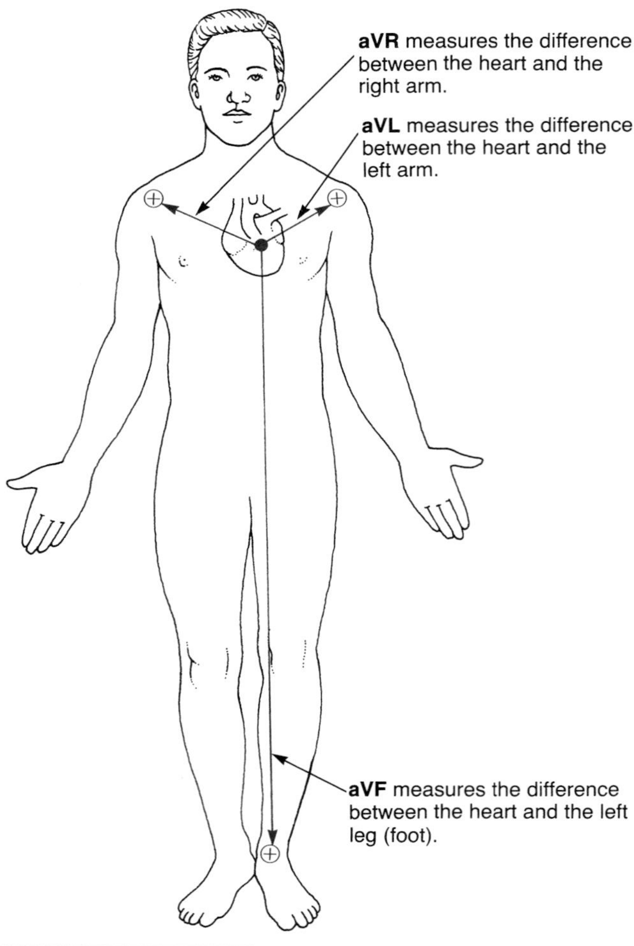

FIGURE 31-23

Augmented leads. (From Ignatavicius, D. D., & Bayne, M. V. [1991]. *Medical-surgical nursing: A nursing process approach* [p. 2104]. Philadelphia: W. B. Saunders.)

CONTINUOUS MONITORING

For continuous monitoring only one or two single leads are used. Three electrodes are applied to the chest. Conductive gel is applied to the skin under the electrode. The electrodes are held in place by adhesive pads. The electrode sites are cleaned thoroughly before the pads are applied. The pads are changed according to agency policy. The skin is monitored for irritation or breakdown.

Lead II is the most commonly monitored lead. In that lead the P, QRS, and T waves are upright. Two other commonly used leads are the modified chest leads 1 and 6 (MCL_1, MCL_6) (Fig. 31–25). They are often used in telemetry units, where patients are ambulatory and many patients are monitored at a remote station.

INTERPRETATION OF ELECTROCARDIOGRAMS

To interpret an ECG strip, the reader is referred to the following diagram (Fig. 31–26). The graph paper consists of horizontal and vertical small and large squares. The horizontal axis measures time; the vertical axis measures voltage. Each small square represents 0.04 second on the horizontal axis and 1 mm on the vertical axis. Each large square, bounded by heavy lines, is made up of 5 small squares and represents 0.20 second and 5 mm. The electrical activity of the heart is represented by deflections, positive and negative, from the baseline. A deflection is an upward or downward movement from the baseline. The baseline is called the *isoelectric line*. The first positive deflection (upward movement) is the small, rounded P wave that represents atrial depolarization. The second positive deflection is the peaked QRS complex that represents ventricular depolarization. The

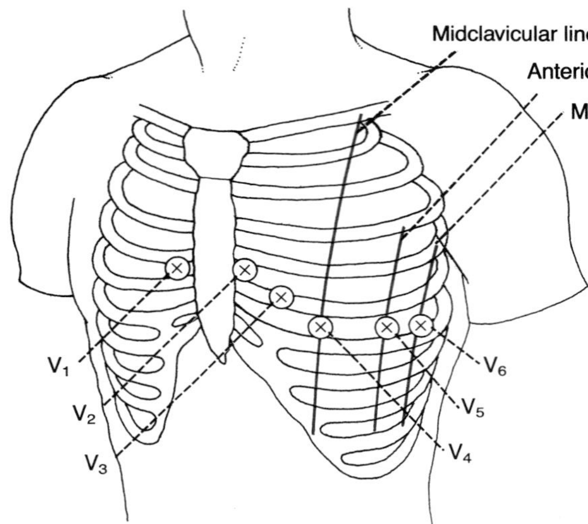

FIGURE 31-24

Precordial leads. (From Ignatavicius, D. D., & Bayne, M. V. [1991]. *Medical-surgical nursing: A nursing process approach* [p. 2104]. Philadelphia: W. B. Saunders.)

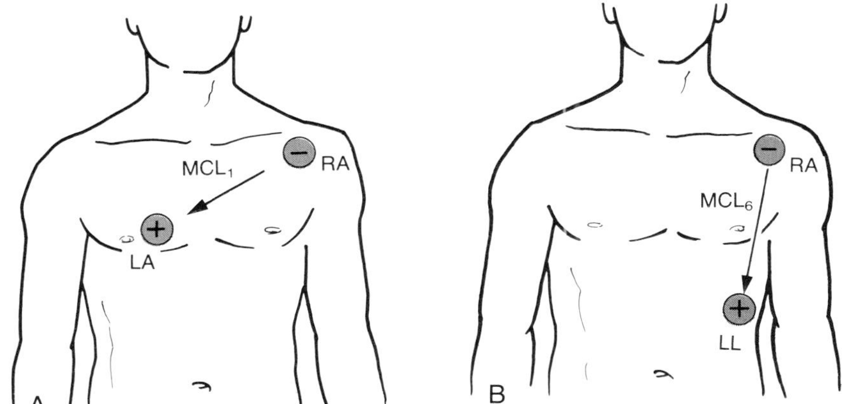

FIGURE 31-25
Modified chest leads. *A,* MCL$_1$; *B,* MCL$_6$.

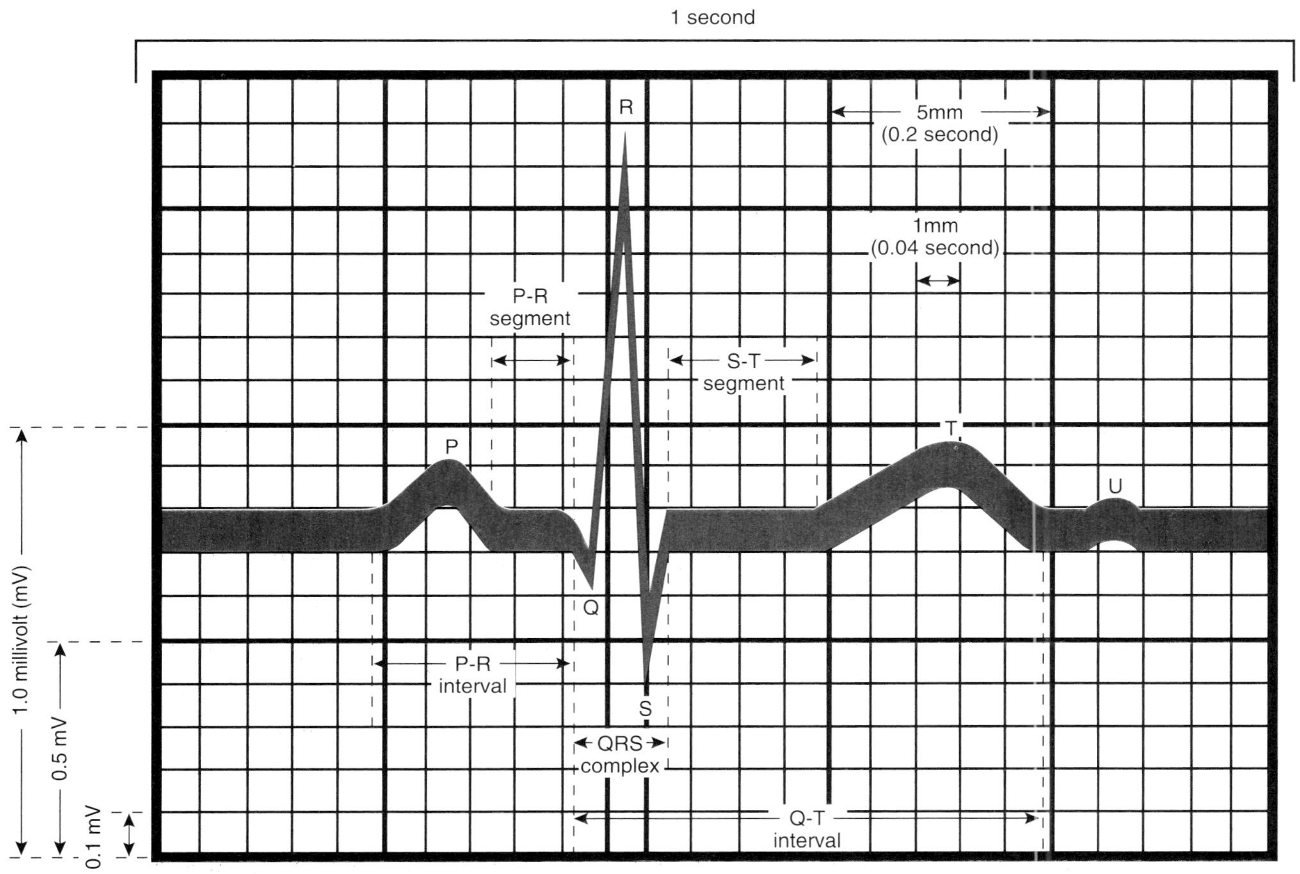

FIGURE 31-26
Interpreting the electrocardiogram. (From Black, J. M., & Matassarin-Jacobs, E. [1993]. *Luckmann and Sorensen's medical-surgical nursing: A psychophysiologic approach* [4th ed., p. 1122]. Philadelphia: W. B. Saunders.)

TABLE 31-11

CRITERIA FOR ELECTROCARDIOGRAM INTERPRETATION

Rate	Are the atrial and ventricular rates the same as measured by the P-P and R-R intervals?
Rhythm	Is the rate regular or irregular? If irregular, is there a pattern? Are there ectopic beats? Where do they occur?
P waves	Is there a P wave before every QRS complex? Does each of the P waves have the same size and shape?
PR interval (PRI)	Are all the PRIs the same length? If not, is there a pattern to the irregularity? Are the PRIs within the normal range?
QRS complexes	Do all the QRS complexes look alike? Are all the QRS complexes within the normal range (0.06–0.10 sec)?
T waves	Do all the T waves look alike? Are the T waves upright or inverted?

Q is the first negative deflection, meaning the line moves below the isoelectric line. The R wave corresponds to the patient's pulse. Atrial repolarization occurs during ventricular depolarization and is obscured by the QRS complex. The third deflection is the rounded T wave, which represents ventricular repolarization. The fourth deflection, if present, is the U wave. It is small, rounded, and generally indicates electrolyte imbalance (hypokalemia).

The PR interval represents the time it takes the impulse to travel from the atria through the AV node to the ventricles. The PR interval is measured from the beginning of the P wave to the Q wave. The normal PR interval is from 0.12 to 0.20 second. The QRS complex is measured from the point at which the Q leaves the isoelectric line to the point at which the S returns to the isoelectric line. The normal QRS complex is 0.06 to 0.10 second. The ST segment represents the time from ventricular depolarization to ventricular repolarization. The ST segment should be along the isoelectric line. The QT segment represents ventricular refractory time. It is measured from the beginning of the QRS complex to the end of the T wave. The normal QT segment time range is 0.36 to 0.44 second. The QT segment is affected by age, sex, and heart rate.

Criteria have been established for interpreting an ECG strip. The ECG is evaluated for rate, regularity, P waves, PRI, and QRS complexes (Table 31–11).

RATE CALCULATION. Most ECG strips have tic marks indicating 3-second time periods. There are several ways to calculate heart rate from the ECG strip. The quickest but least accurate method is to count the number of R waves in a 6-second strip (between three tic marks or 30 large squares) and multiply by 10 for the estimate of the number of beats per minute. For example, if there are six R waves in a 6-second strip, the heart rate is 60 bpm.

Another method is to find an R wave on a heavy line. Count the number of heavy lines until the next R as 300, 150, 100, 75, 60, 50, 43, and 37. For example, if there are three heavy lines between two consecutive R waves, the heart rate would be 100 bpm. A third method, the most accurate, uses the number of small squares between two R waves. Divide 1500 by the number of small squares. For example, if there are 25 small squares between two R waves the rate is 60 bpm (1500 divided by 25). The atrial rate is determined by

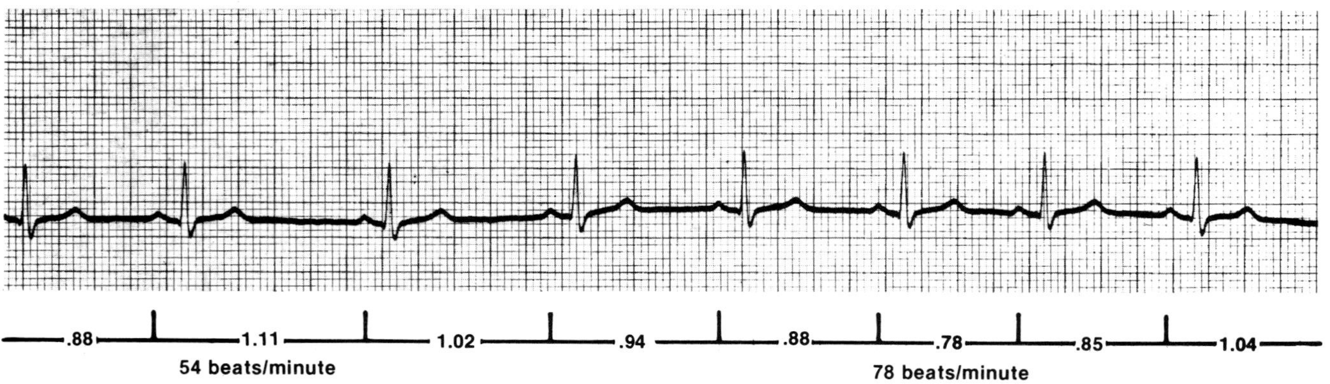

FIGURE 31-27

Normal sinus rhythm. Each segment between the dark lines (above the monitor strip) represents 3 sec, when the monitor is set at a speed of 25 mm/sec.

Characteristics: **Rate**—60–100 bpm; **regularity**—regular (P to P and R to R intervals are regular); **P wave,** PR interval—there is a P before every QRS; each P wave is the same size and shape; PR interval is between 0.12 and 0.20 sec; **QRS**—falls between 0.06 and 0.10 sec; **T wave**—rounded, all the same shape.

Interpretation: Normal sinus rhythm.

(From Phillips, R. E., & Feeney, M. K. [1990]. *The cardiac rhythms* [3rd. ed., p. 85]. Philadelphia: W. B. Saunders.)

the number of P waves and the ventricular rate by the number of QRS complexes. The normal rate is from 60 to 100 bpm.

REGULARITY. The consecutive R to R intervals are measured for consistency. Using calipers or a blank piece of paper, note the distance between R waves. If the distances do not vary more than 1 small square the rhythm is considered regular. If the distances are greater than 1 small square the rhythm is irregular.

P WAVES. The next evaluation is of P waves. Is there a P wave before each QRS complex? If so, the rhythm originates in the SA node. Do all the P waves appear the same size and shape? If so, the impulse originates in the SA node.

PR INTERVAL. Does the PR interval fall within the normal range of 0.12 to 0.20 second? If so, there is no interference in conduction from the SA to the AV node.

QRS COMPLEX. Does the QRS complex fall within the 0.06 to 0.10 second range? If the QRS is prolonged (0.12 second or greater), there is a delay in conduction through the ventricles.

T WAVES. Are the T waves rounded and the same size and shape? Do the T waves follow the QRS complexes?

NORMAL SINUS RHYTHM

The most common cardiac rhythm is sinus in origin because the impulse originates in the SA node, is conducted normally, and meets all of the criteria established earlier. Normal sinus rhythm is displayed in Figure 31–27.

COMMON DYSRHYTHMIAS

A dysrhythmia is a disturbance of the rhythm of the heart caused by a problem in the conduction system. Dysrhythmias are categorized according to the site of the origin of the impulse formation. Dysrhythmias originating in the SA node are atrial. Dysrhythmias originating in the AV node are called junctional or escape rhythms. Dysrhythmias originating below the AV node are called ventricular. Blocks are interruptions in impulse conduction. Dysrhythmias and blocks have characteristics that are noted on the ECG. See Figures 31–28 though 31–41 for examples.

PHARMACOLOGY CAPSULE

Antidysrhythmic drugs are used to treat dysrhythmias and restore normal sinus rhythm.

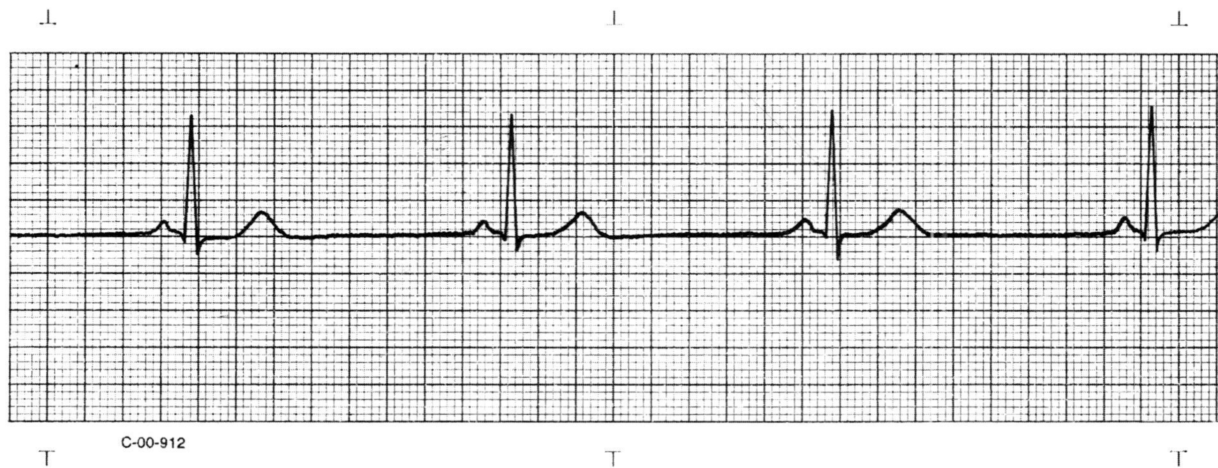

FIGURE 31-28

Sinus bradycardia.

Characteristics: **Rate**—less than 60 bpm; **regularity**—normal; **P wave,** PR interval—normal; **QRS**—normal; **T wave**—normal.

Interpretation: All characteristics are within normal ranges except for the rate, which is slow.

Causes: Drugs including digitalis and beta blockers, vagal stimulation (Valsalva maneuver), severe pain, hyperkalemia, infection, and myocardial infarction. Frequently seen in athletes as a result of conditioning.

Symptoms: Dizziness and syncope, if any.

Treatment: Not treated unless the patient is symptomatic. The underlying cause is treated. Atropine or isoproterenol may be given to increase the heart rate. A pacemaker may be necessary.

(From Ignatavicius, D. D., & Bayne, M. V. [1991]. *Medical-surgical nursing: A nursing process approach* [p. 2120]. Philadelphia: W. B. Saunders.)

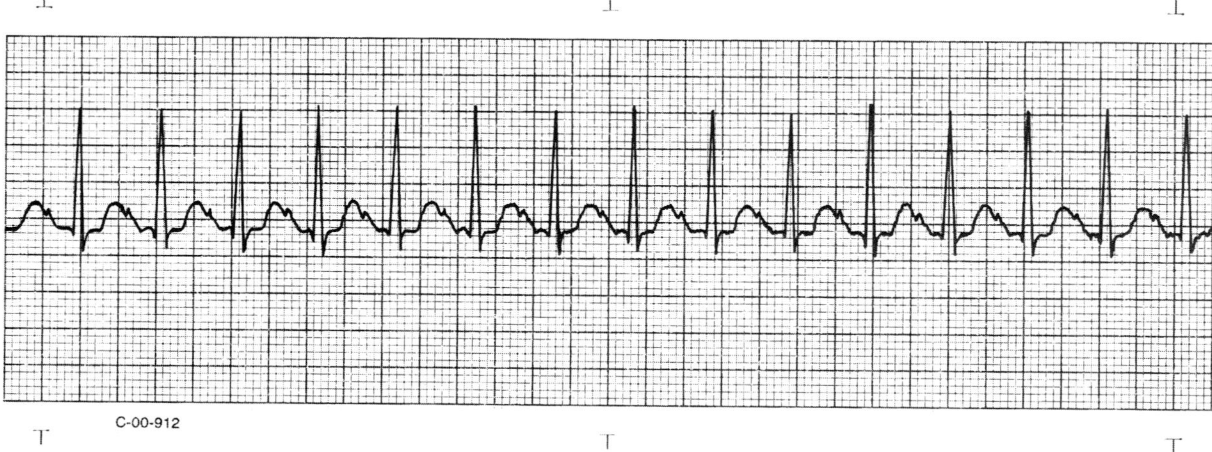

FIGURE 31-29

Sinus tachycardia.

Characteristics: **Rate**—greater than 100; usually less than 160 bpm; **regularity**—regular; **P wave,** PR interval—P waves may be buried in T wave of preceding beat with very rapid rates, more than 140 bpm; **QRS**—normal; **T wave**—normal.

Interpretation: All characteristics are within normal range except for the rate, which is excessive.

Causes: Fever, dehydration, hypovolemia, increased sympathetic nervous system stimulation, stress, exercise, and acute myocardial infarction.

Symptoms: Palpitations most common. Angina and decreased cardiac output from the decreased ventricular filling time may also occur.

Treatment: Correction of underlying cause. Elimination of caffeine, nicotine, and alcohol. Vagal stimulation may decrease the rate but does not treat the cause.

(From Ignatavicius, D. D., & Bayne, M. V. [1991]. *Medical-surgical nursing: A nursing process approach* [p. 2119]. Philadelphia: W. B. Saunders.)

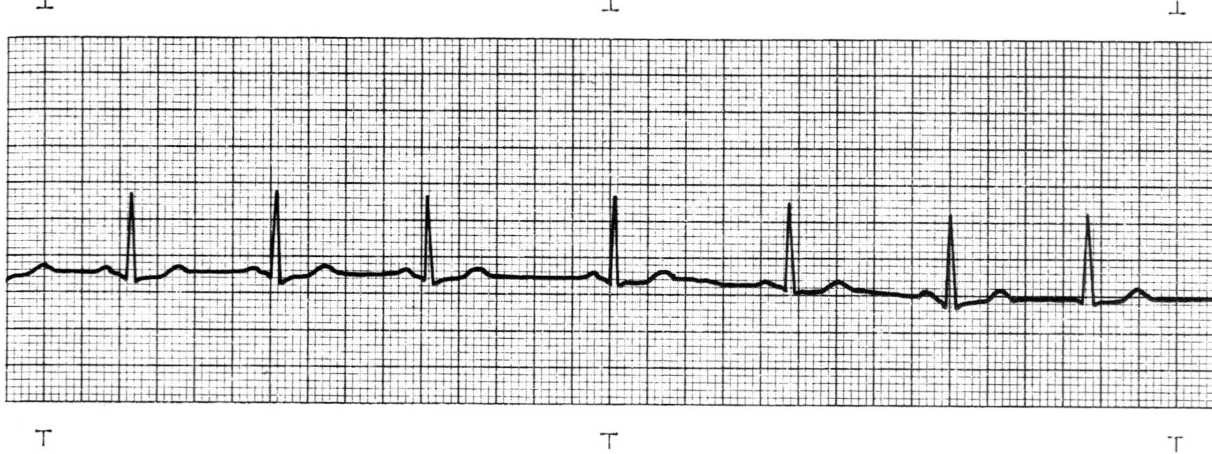

FIGURE 31-30

Sinus dysrhythmia.

Characteristics: **Rate**—normal; **regularity**—slightly irregular, varies with respirations; **P wave,** PR interval—P to P intervals vary, the difference between the shortest and longest P to P interval is greater than 0.12 sec; the PR interval is normal; **QRS**—normal; **T wave**—normal.

Interpretation: The rate varies with respirations. Considered normal when the rhythm varies in relation to the respiratory cycle: The R to R interval is shorter during inspiration; therefore, the rate is increased; the R to R interval is longer during expiration; therefore, the rate is decreased.

Causes: When unrelated to respirations, is often the result of digoxin toxicity, increased intracranial pressure, or inferior wall myocardial infarction. In the elderly, marked variation may indicate a condition known as *sick sinus syndrome.*

Symptoms: Generally none.

Treatment: If treatment is necessary, atropine is used and the underlying problem is treated.

(From Ignatavicius D. D., & Bayne, M. V. [1991]. *Medical-surgical nursing: A nursing process approach* [p. 2119]. Philadelphia: W. B. Saunders.)

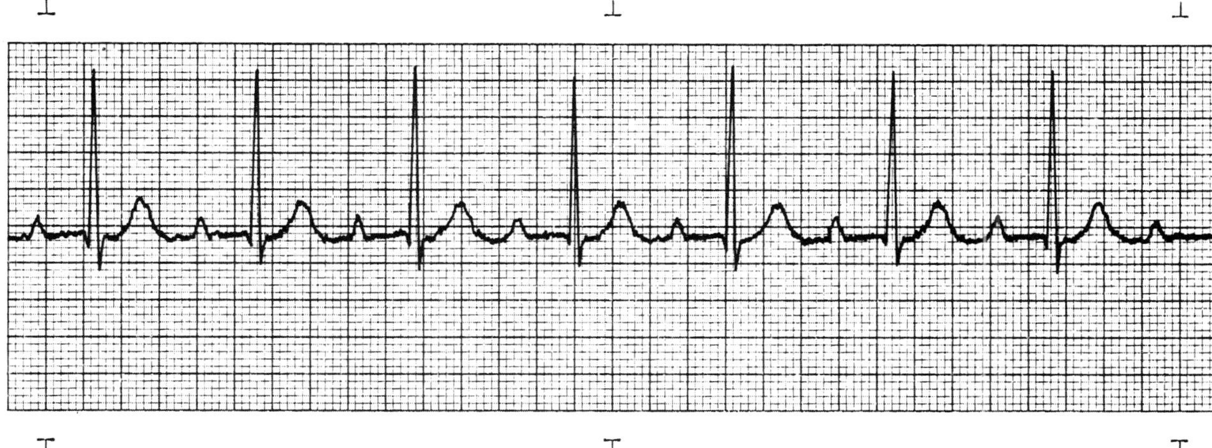

FIGURE 31-31

First degree atrioventricular (AV) block.
Characteristics: **Rate**—normal; **regularity**—regular; **P wave,** PR interval—all P waves are conducted to the ventricles, but AV conduction is prolonged through the AV node; PR interval is greater than 0.20 sec and constant; **QRS**—normal; **T wave**—normal.
Interpretation: The PR interval is prolonged.
Causes: Increased vagal tone, coronary artery disease, digoxin toxicity, heart infections, and quinidine.
Symptoms: May be bradycardic.
Treatment: Correction of underlying cause.
(From Ignatavicius, D. D., & Bayne, M. V. [1991]. *Medical-surgical nursing: A nursing process approach* [p. 2126]. Philadelphia: W. B. Saunders.)

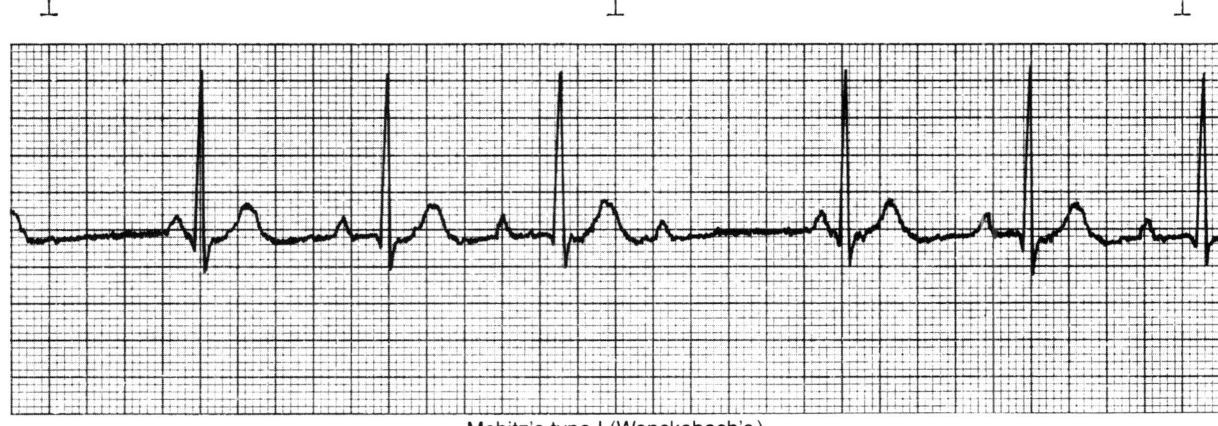

FIGURE 31-32

Second-degree atrioventricular block: Type I (Mobitz I) (Wenckebach).
Characteristics: **Rate**—atrial rate is greater than ventricular rate; **regularity**—atrial rate is regular; ventricular rate is irregular; **P wave,** PR interval—there are more P waves than QRS complexes; the PR interval increases until a P is not followed by a QRS; **QRS**—some are absent; **T wave**—absent when the QRS is dropped.
Interpretation: Progressively lengthening PR interval and a dropped beat.
Causes: Myocardial ischemia with progressive increase in conduction time through the sinoatrial node, inferior wall myocardial infarction, digoxin toxicity, and electrolyte imbalance.
Symptoms: Decreased blood pressure and syncope, if any.
Treatment: Atropine, pacemaker.
(From Ignatavicius, D. D., & Bayne, M. V. [1991]. *Medical-surgical nursing: A nursing process approach* [p. 2126]. Philadelphia: W. B. Saunders.)

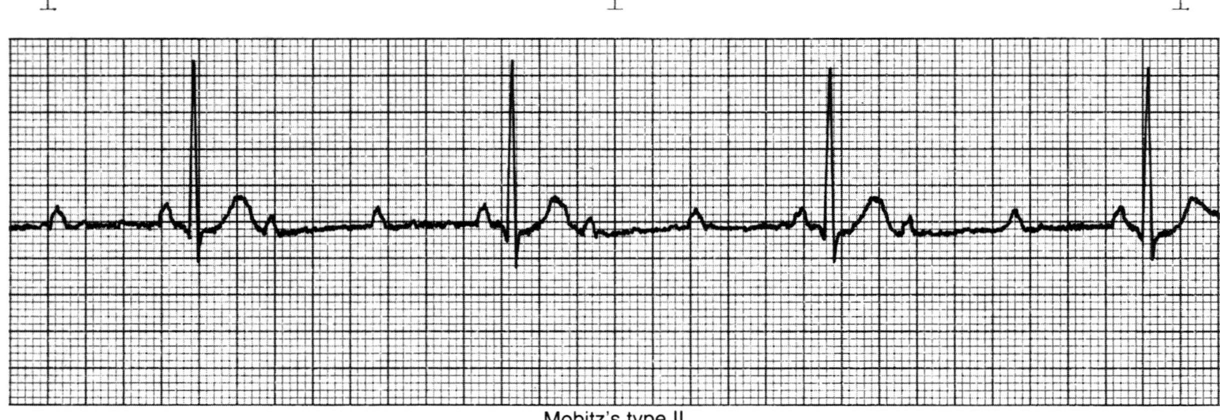

FIGURE 31-33

Second degree atrioventricular (AV) block: Type II (Mobitz II).
Characteristics: **Rate**—atrial rate regular; ventricular rate may be less than atrial; **regularity**—irregular; **P wave,** PR interval—P to P intervals are regular; PR interval is fixed at normal or greater than 0.20 sec; **QRS**—QRS complexes do not always follow P waves; the QRS may be normal or widened; **T wave**—normal after completed conduction.
Interpretation: Sudden blocking of a QRS.
Causes: Conduction abnormalities in the ventricles, acute myocardial infarction.
Symptoms: Hypotension, bradycardia; decreased cardiac output with frequent blocks.
Treatment: Pacemaker may be necessary to prevent third-degree AV block or asystole; isoproterenol helps to increase cardiac output.
(From Ignatavicius, D. D., & Bayne, M. V. [1991]. *Medical-surgical nursing: A nursing process approach* [p. 2126]. Philadelphia: W. B. Saunders.)

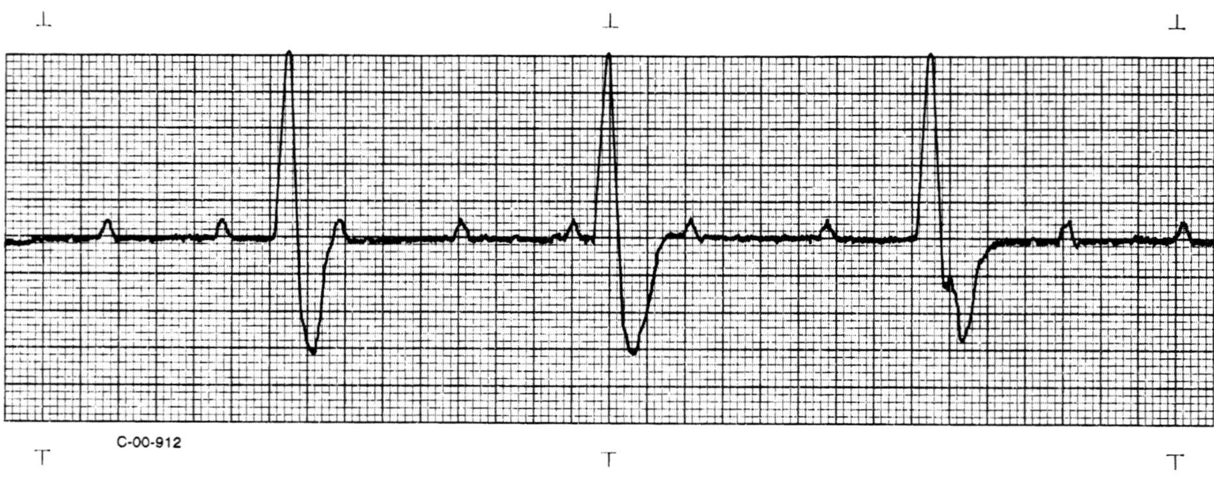

FIGURE 31-34

Third-degree atrioventricular (AV) block.
Characteristics: **Rate**—atrial rate is faster than ventricular rate; ventricular rate is generally less than 45 bpm; **regularity**—irregular; **P wave,** PR interval—no relationship exists between the P waves and the QRS complexes; **QRS**—atria and ventricles are beating independently; the QRS is ventricular in origin; **T wave**—normal.
Interpretation: Impulses originating in the sinoatrial node are blocked at the AV node. The ventricles respond to a secondary pacemaker.
Causes: Digoxin toxicity, conduction damage during mitral valve replacement, hypoxia, and rheumatic fever.
Symptoms: Hypotension, syncope, decreased cardiac output. The underlying cause is treated.
Treatment: Atropine or isoproterenol; pacemaker.
(From Ignatavicius, D. D., & Bayne, M. V. [1991]. *Medical-surgical nursing: A nursing process approach* [p. 2127]. Philadelphia: W. B. Saunders.)

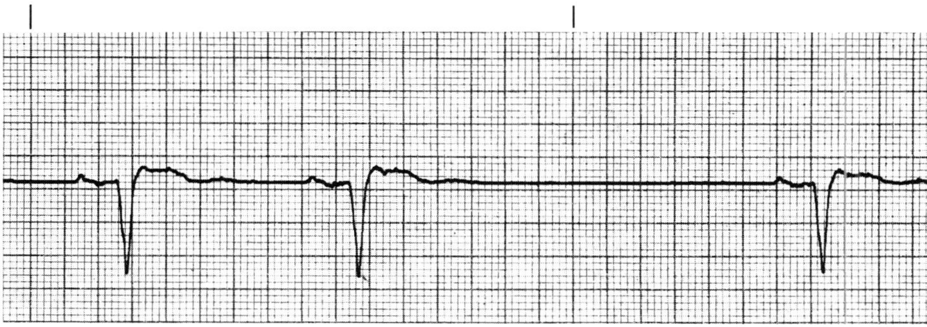

FIGURE 31-35

Sinus arrest.

Characteristics: **Rate**—normal or slow before arrest; **regularity**—regular except when interrupted by a dropped beat; **P wave,** PR interval—normal when present; absent during pause; **QRS**—normal to absent during pause; **T wave**—normal to absent during pause.

Interpretation: A pause in the cardiac cycle as the sinoatrial node fails to generate an impulse.

Causes: Degenerative heart disease, myocardial infarction, digoxin toxicity.

Symptoms: Bradycardia, decreased cardiac output.

Treatment: Pacemaker if the patient experiences repeated episodes.

(From Black, J. M., & Matassarin-Jacobs, E. [1993]. *Luckmann and Sorensen's medical-surgical nursing: A psychophysiologic approach* [4th ed., p. 1123]. Philadelphia: W. B. Saunders.)

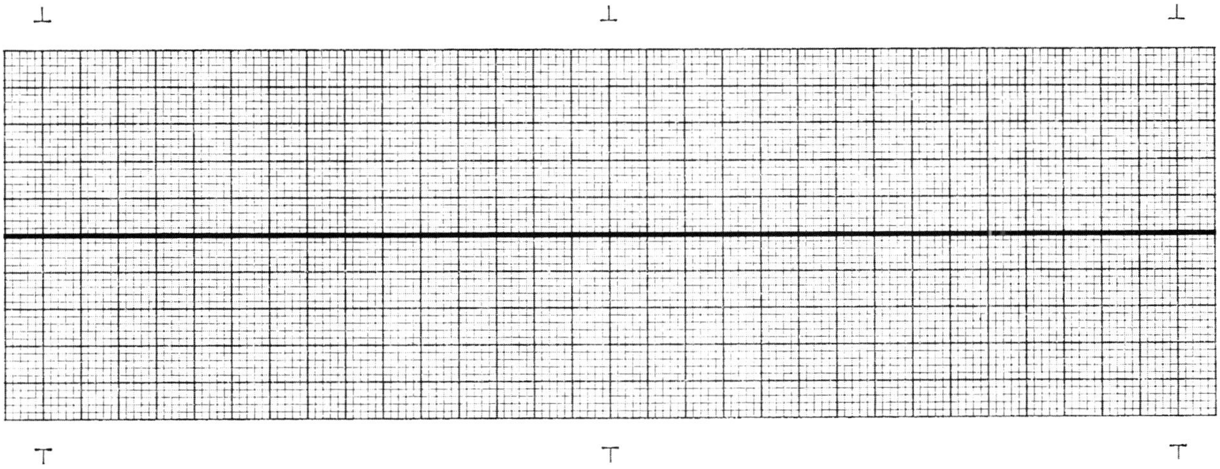

FIGURE 31-36

Asystole.

Characteristics: **Rate**—none; **regularity**—none; **P wave,** PR interval—there may be P waves but none is conducted; the PR interval is not measurable; **QRS**—absent; **T wave**—absent.

Interpretation: Straight or only slightly wavy baseline.

Causes: Severe metabolic deficit, acute respiratory failure, and myocardial damage.

Symptoms: Loss of consciousness, no pulse.

Treatment: Immediate response with cardiopulmonary resuscitation and advanced cardiac life support; may require permanent pacemaker.

(From Ignatavicius, D. D., & Bayne, M. V. [1991]. *Medical-surgical nursing: A nursing process approach* [p. 2130]. Philadelphia: W. B. Saunders.)

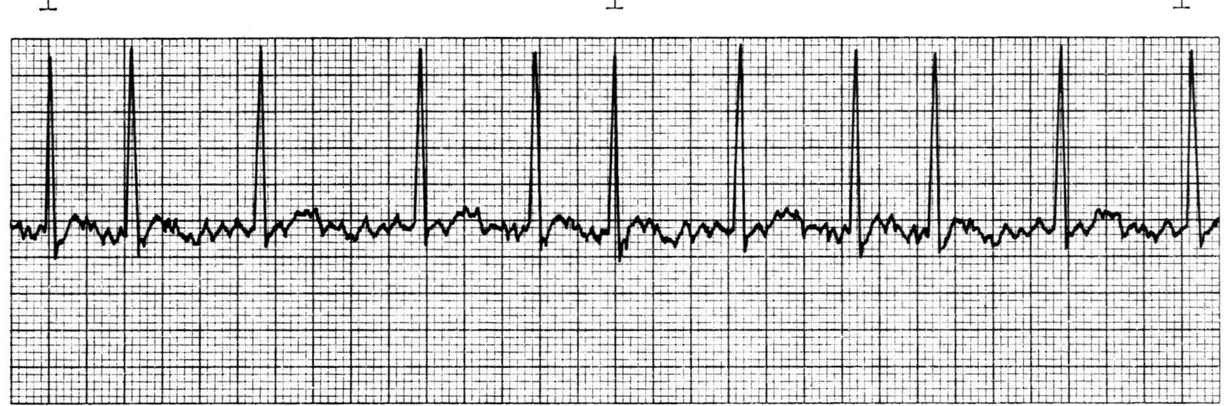

FIGURE 31-37

Atrial fibrillation.
Characteristics: **Rate**—atrial rate is greater than 400 bpm if it can be determined at all; the ventricular rate is 100–150 bpm; **regularity**—very irregular; **P wave,** PR interval—no P waves; cannot measure the PR interval; **QRS**—normal; **T wave**—cannot determine.
Interpretation: The baseline between QRS complexes is wavy.
Causes: Rheumatic fever, mitral valve stenosis, coronary artery disease, hypertension, cardiomyopathy, myocardial infarction, hyperthyroidism, chronic obstructive pulmonary disease, and congestive heart failure. It is frequently seen in the elderly after the administration of anesthesia.
Symptoms: May have palpitations, angina, and decreased cardiac output. The concerns with atrial fibrillation are development of an atrial thrombus and loss of atrial kick from ineffective atrial function.
Treatment: Digoxin, verapamil, propranolol, and quinidine to increase cardiac output; a Valsalva maneuver may temporarily reduce a rapid ventricular response; anticoagulants to prevent embolization; synchronized cardioversion to restore a normal rhythm.
(From Ignatavicius, D. D., & Bayne, M. V. [1991]. *Medical-surgical nursing: A nursing process approach* [p. 2124]. Philadelphia: W. B. Saunders.)

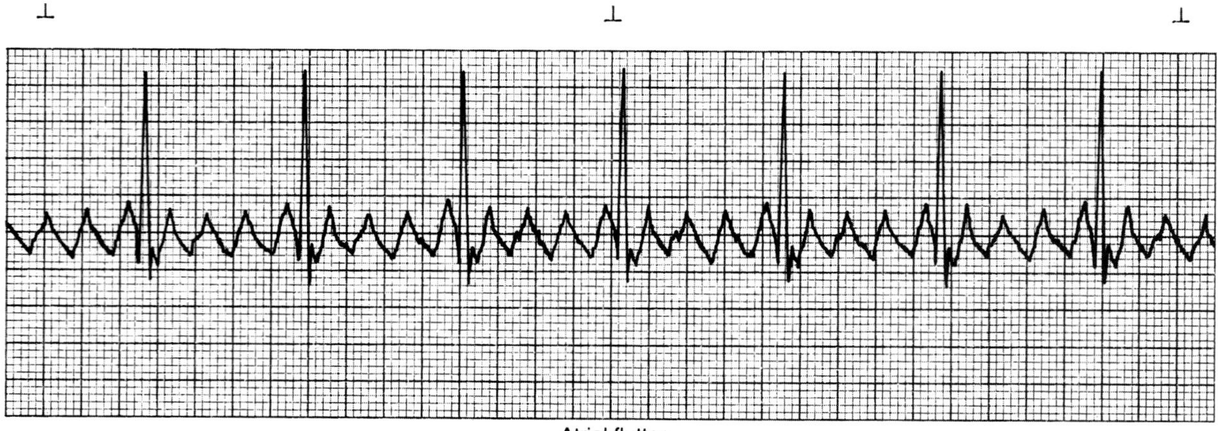

FIGURE 31-38

Atrial flutter.
Characteristics: **Rate**—atrial rate 250–350 bpm; ventricular rate 60–100 bpm; **regularity**—atrial rate regular; ventricular regular or irregular; **P wave,** PR interval—P waves are rounded "F" or flutter waves; PR interval is not measurable; **QRS**—generally normal; **T wave**—cannot determine.
Interpretation: The sawtooth P waves are characteristic; there may be a pattern to the number of flutter waves and ventricular response: 4 to 1, 3 to 1, or 2 to 1.
Causes: Coronary artery disease, myocardial damage, valvular disease, heart infections, and digoxin toxicity.
Symptoms: Palpitations, decreased cardiac output.
Treatment: Harder to treat than atrial fibrillation. Verapamil, digoxin (if not the cause), propranolol, quinidine, and beta blockers. Synchronized cardioversion.
(From Ignatavicius, D. D., & Bayne, M. V. [1991]. *Medical-surgical nursing: A nursing process approach* [p. 2124]. Philadelphia: W. B. Saunders.)

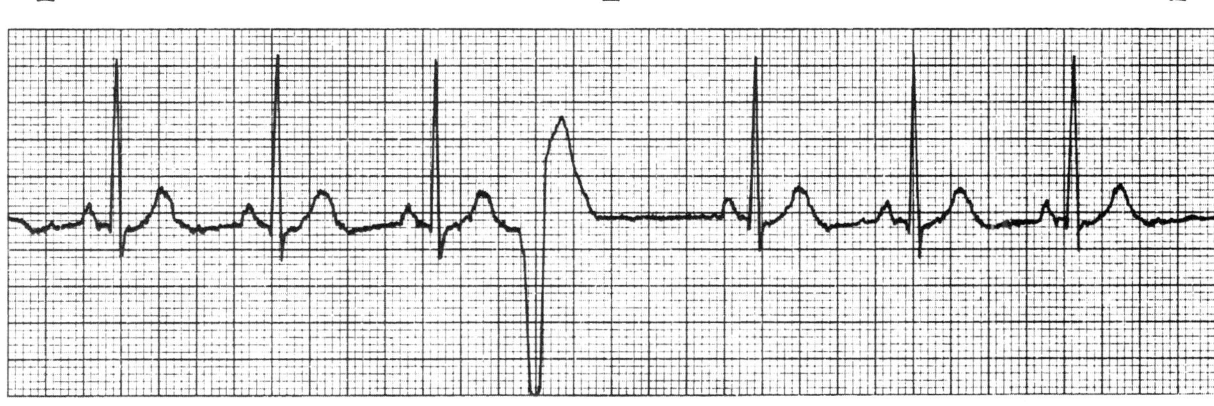

FIGURE 31-39

Premature ventricular contractions (PVCs).
Characteristics: **Rate**—normal; **regularity**—irregular because of PVCs; **P wave,** PR interval—no P wave with the PVC; inverted P wave may follow a PVC; there is no PR interval with the PVC; **QRS**—wide and bizarre in the PVC; **T wave**—opposite deflection to the PVC.
Interpretations: Wide QRS. Unifocal PVCs originate from one site. Multifocal PVCs arise from different ventricular sites and have a poorer prognosis.
Causes: Digoxin toxicity, hypokalemia, hypercalcemia, sympathetic nervous system stimulation (stress, caffeine, nicotine), and excess catecholamine release.
Symptoms: The patient may or may not note a "skipped" beat. The PVCs are not palpable at peripheral pulse sites, but a pause may be observed. Cardiac output diminishes with frequent PVCs.
Treatment: No treatment necessary for infrequent PVCs, which probably occur undetected in most people; antidysrhythmics for symptomatic or frequent PVCs.
(From Ignatavicius, D. D., & Bayne, M. V. [1991]. *Medical-surgical nursing: A nursing process approach* [p. 2121]. Philadelphia: W. B. Saunders.)

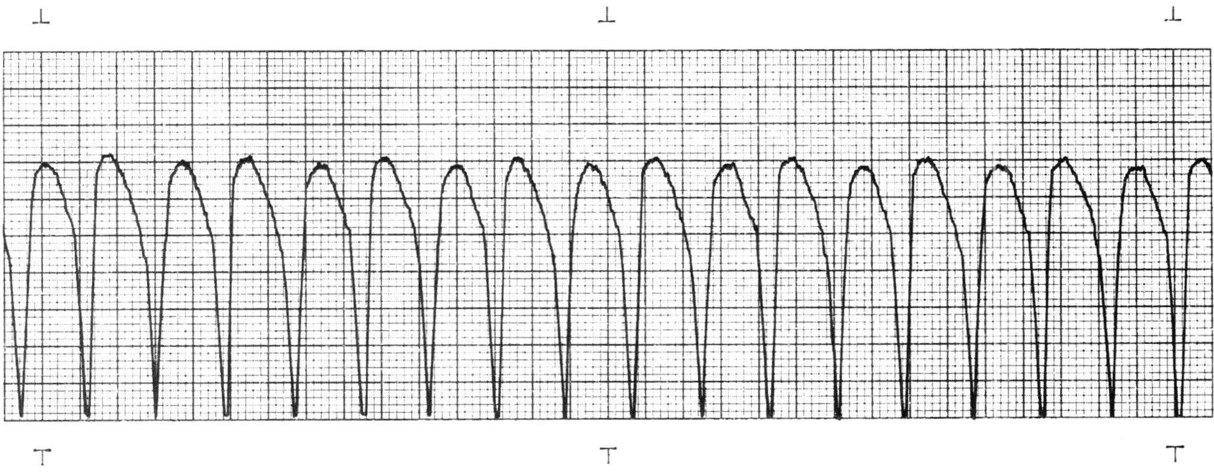

FIGURE 31-40

Ventricular tachycardia.
Characteristics: **Rate**—100–250 bpm; there is no relationship between the atrial and the ventricular contractions; **regularity**—irregular; **P wave,** PR interval—absent; **QRS**—wide, bizarre; greater than 0.12 sec; may look like PVCs; **T wave**—opposite deflection to QRS.
Interpretation: This is a life-threatening dysrhythmia that often precedes ventricular fibrillation.
Causes: Myocardial irritation, myocardial infarction, coronary artery disease, rheumatic heart disease, hypokalemia, and digoxin toxicity.
Symptoms: Initially palpitations, dizziness, and chest pain progressing to decreased cardiac output and loss of consciousness.
Treatment: If there is hemodynamic compromise antidysrhythmics (lidocaine, procainamide, or bretylium) are administered. Cardiopulmonary resuscitation and advanced cardiac life support are used to provide tissue perfusion. An automatic implantable cardioverter-defibrillator may be necessary to stabilize the patient.
(From Ignatavicius, D. D., & Bayne, M. V. [1991]. *Medical-surgical nursing: A nursing process approach* [p. 2129]. Philadelphia: W. B. Saunders.)

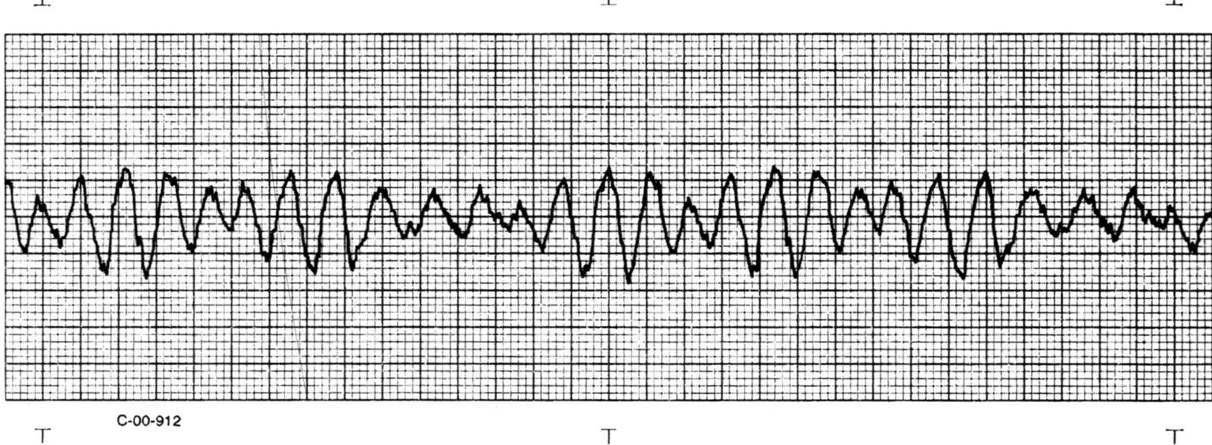

FIGURE 31-41

Ventricular fibrillation.

Characteristics: **Rate**—undeterminable; **regularity**—chaotic, wavy baseline; **P wave,** PR interval—undeterminable; **QRS**—undeterminable; **T wave**—undeterminable.

Interpretation: This life-threatening dysrhythmia must be terminated quickly if the patient is to resume useful function.

Causes: Coronary artery disease, acute myocardial infarction, untreated ventricular tachycardia, electrolyte and acid-base imbalances, electric shock, and hypothermia.

Symptoms: Loss of consciousness, cessation of heart beat and respirations, dilation of pupils.

Treatment: Cardiopulmonary resuscitation, defibrillation, and advanced cardiac life support measures are used to treat ventricular fibrillation.

(From Ignatavicius, D. D., & Bayne, M. V. [1991]. *Medical-surgical nursing: A nursing process approach* [p. 2130]. Philadelphia: W. B. Saunders.)

NUTRITION CONCEPTS

- A major part of treatment for persons with heart disease is reduction of fat and cholesterol in the diet.
- When fats are used in cooking or eating, unsaturated fats (vegetable oil such as corn oil, canola oil, or olive oil) should be substituted for saturated fats (animal fat such as butter or lard).
- Fats and oils used in cooking or eating should be limited to 5 to 8 servings daily in normal adults.
- Saturated fat can be limited by eating only 5 to 7 ounces of meat daily.
- Foods that contain omega-3 fatty acids (certain fish, walnuts, and soybeans) lower serum triglycerides and decrease the number of deaths due to heart disease.

BIBLIOGRAPHY

Abou-awdi, N. (1991). High-tech help for failing hearts. *RN, 54*(5), 42–44.

Abou-awdi, N., Rountree, W. D., Kelly, A. M., & Rutan, P. M. (1991). New support for the failing heart. *American Journal of Nursing, 91*(1), 38–41.

Appel-Hardin, S., & Dente-Cassidy, A. M. (1991). *Nursing 91, 21*(5), 58–65.

Bavin, T. K., & Self, M. A. (1991). Weaning from intra-aortic balloon pump support. *American Journal of Nursing, 91*(10), 54–59.

Berry, S. L., & Schleicher, C. A. (1992). Adjusting the beat: What to teach about antiarrhythmias. *American Journal of Nursing, 92*(6), 28–33.

Bucher, N. (1992). A safer way to get hemodynamic data. *RN, 55*(11), 56–61.

Campbell, C. D., & Newsome, J. A. (1992). Action stat: Treating a lethal arrhythmia. *Nursing 92, 22*(2), 33.

Chernecky, C. C., Krech, R. L., & Berger, B. J. (1993). *Laboratory tests and diagnostic procedures.* Philadelphia: W. B. Saunders.

Collings, S. (1991). Coronary atherectomy takes a new direction. *American Journal of Nursing, 91*(10), 16.

Drew, B. J. (1992). Using cardiac leads: The right way. *Nursing 92, 22*(5), 50–54.

Finesilver, C., & Metzler, D. J. (1991). Right ventricular infarction: The critically different MI. *American Journal of Nursing, 91*(4), 32–36.

Gawlinski, A., & Jensen, G. A. (1991). The complications of cardiovascular aging. *American Journal of Nursing, 91*(11), 26–32.

Gegaris, C. N. (1991). Everyone was pulling for Edna. *Nursing 91, 21*(10), 44–48.

Gortner, S. R., Kirks, J., & Wolfe, M. M. (1992). The road for recovery for elders after CABG. *American Journal of Nursing, 92*(8), 44–49.

Grab, C. (1992). The cutting alternative to PTCA. *RN, 55*(7), 22–27.

Green, E. (1992). Solving the puzzle of chest pain. *American Journal of Nursing, 92*(1), 32–40.

Hochrein, M., & Sohl, L. (1992). Heart smart: A guide to cardiac tests. *American Journal of Nursing, 92*(12), 22–25.

Hodgson, B. B., Kizior, R. J., & Kingdon, R. T. (1993). *Nurse's drug handbook.* Philadelphia: W. B. Saunders.

Holcomb, S. S. (1993). Atherectomy. *Nursing 93, 23*(2), 44–47.

House, M. A., & Griego, L. (1992). Nursing role in management: Congestive heart failure and cardiac surgery. In S. M. Lewis, & I. C. Collier (Eds.), *Medical-surgical nursing.* St. Louis: Mosby Year Book.

House, M. A., & Griego, L. (1992). Nursing role in management: Coronary artery disease. In S. M. Lewis & I. C. Collier (Eds.), *Medical-surgical nursing.* St. Louis: Mosby Year Book.

Howard, P. (1990). Ischemic risks for patients on IABP. *American Journal of Nursing, 90*(3), 29.

Howard, P. (1991). Elevated cholesterol: A nurse's guide to drug therapy. *RN, 54*(8), 26–30.

Ignatavicius, D. D., & Bayne, M. V. (1991). *Medical-surgical nursing: A nursing process approach.* Philadelphia: W. B. Saunders.

Jarvis, C. (1992). *Physical examination and health assessment.* Philadelphia: W. B. Saunders.

Johns, C. I. (1992). Nursing role in management: Dysrhythmias. In S. M. Lewis & I. C. Collier (Eds.), *Medical-surgical nursing.* St. Louis: Mosby Year Book.

Kater, K. M., Kuhrik, N. S., & Kuhrik, M. (1992). Corralling atrial fibrillation with "maze" surgery. *American Journal of Nursing, 92*(7), 34–38.

Kuhrik, N., Kuhrik, M., Williams, J., & Orlando, A. (1992). Defibrillation over the phone. *American Journal of Nursing, 92*(11), 28–31.

Kupper, N. S., & Duke, E. S. (1992). Nursing role in management: Inflammatory and valvular heart disease. In S. M. Lewis & I. C. Collier (Eds.), *Medical-surgical nursing.* St. Louis: Mosby Year Book.

Letterer, R. A., Carew, B., Reid, M., & Woods, P. (1992). Learning to live with congestive heart failure. *Nursing 92, 22*(5), 34–41.

Luquire, R., & Houston, S. (1993). Cardiomyopathy: How to buy time. *RN, 56*(5), 28–33.

Matteson, M. A., & McConnell, E. S. (1989). *Gerontological nursing.* Philadelphia: W. B. Saunders.

Mercer, M. E. (1992). Rate-responsive pacers. *RN, 55*(5), 34–36.

Merva, J. A. (1992). Temporary pacemakers. *RN, 55*(5), 28–33.

Merva, J. (1993). A closer look at the heart SAECG. *RN, 56*(5), 50–54.

Moore, K. (1992). Do you konw these new emergency protocols? *RN, 55*(11), 34–35.

Olbrych, D. D. (1993). Interpreting CPK and LDH results. *Nursing 93, 23*(1), 48–49.

Owen, A. (1991). Keeping pace with temporary pacemakers. *Nursing 91, 21*(4), 58–64.

Palarski, V., & Washburn, S. (1992). Overcoming LVD in cardiac rehab. *American Journal of Nursing, 92*(9), 52–57.

Reyes-Vargas, A. V., & Gillett, P. (1991). Pulmonary artery catheters do more than ever. *RN, 54*(5), 46–51.

Ruth-Sahd, L., & Martin, D. (1991). Myths and facts about implantable cardioverter defibrillators. *Nursing 91, 21*(11), 86.

Saul, L. (1991). Arrhythmia mimics. *American Journal of Nursing, 91*(3), 40–43.

Scalzo, T. (1992). Managing a patient on remote telemetry. *Nursing 92, 22*(3), 57–59.

Schaefer, Y. G., Chicca, C., & Fisher, C. (1992). Caring for a patient with an AICD. *Nursing 92, 22*(12), 48–50.

Schultz, S. J., Foley, C. R., & Gordon, D. G. (1991). Preparing your patient for a cardiac P.E.T. scan. *Nursing 91, 21*(9), 63–64.

Shaffer, R. B., & Lynn-McHale, D. (1991). Action stat: Responding quickly to asystole. *Nursing 91, 21*(9), 33.

Shlafer, M., & Marieb, E. N. (1989). *The nurse, pharmacology, and drug therapy.* Redwood City, CA: Addison-Wesley.

Smith, A. (1991). Case example: Myocardial rupture. *American Journal of Nursing, 91*(10), 25–26.

Smith, C. E. (1991). Assessment under pressure: When your patient says, "my chest hurts." *Nursing 91, 21*(11), 66–70.

Snowberger, P. (1991). Wandering atrial pacemaker. *RN, 54*(9), 36–37.

Snowberger, P. (1992). Atrial fibrillation. *RN, 55*(9), 42–44.

Snowberger, P. (1992). Sinus arrhythmia. *RN, 55*(1), 50–51.

Snowberger, P. (1993). Second-degree AV block. *RN, 56*(2), 43–45.

Snowberger, P. (1993). Third-degree heart block. *RN, 55*(6), 52–54.

Solomon, J. (1991). Managing a failing heart. *RN, 54*(8), 46–51.

Starks-Bledsoe, D., & Vespe, M. (1992). Heading off sudden cardiac death. *Nursing 92, 22*(11), 52–56.

Wilson, D. D., & Smith, C. E. (1992). Nursing assessment: Cardiovascular system. In S. M. Lewis & I. C. Collier (Eds.), *Medical-surgical nursing.* St. Louis: Mosby Year Book.

Witherell, C. L. (1990). Questions nurses ask about pacemakers. *American Journal of Nursing, 90*(12), 20–28.

Yacone-Morton, L. A. (1991). Cardiac assessment. *RN, 54*(12), 28–35.

KEY CONCEPTS

1. The primary function of the heart is to pump blood through the pulmonary and systemic circulation.
2. The heartbeat has two phases: systole (contraction) and diastole (relaxation).
3. Cardiac output is the amount of blood ejected by each ventricle per minute; stroke volume is the amount of blood ejected by a ventricle in a single contraction.
4. The factors that affect stroke volume are preload, contractility, and afterload.
5. The heart sounds are "lubb" heard during systole and "dub" heard during diastole.
6. The most common cardiac surgical procedures are pacemaker insertion, valve repair or replacement, septal repair, and arterial bypass surgery.
7. Nursing concerns after cardiac surgery include ineffective breathing patterns, pain, ineffective

thermoregulation, decreased cardiac output, high risk for infection, anxiety, and knowledge deficit.

8. Pacemakers are electronic devices that deliver impulses to stimulate contraction of the myocardium.
9. Coronary artery disease, the leading cause of death in the United States, is treated with drug therapy, diet modifications, lifestyle modifications, surgical intervention, or a combination of these.
10. Risk factors for atherosclerosis are diabetes mellitus with elevated blood glucose, decreased serum high-density lipoproteins, nicotine, hypertension, and obesity.
11. Angina pectoris is the pain that results from myocardial ischemia. It is treated with vasodilators and rest.
12. Procedures used to improve myocardial blood flow include percutaneous coronary balloon angioplasty, laser angioplasty, and coronary artery bypass grafts.
13. Acute myocardial infarction, caused by occlusion of a coronary artery, can lead to dysrhythmias, cardiac failure, cardiogenic shock, thromboembolism, and ventricular rupture.
14. Nursing care of the myocardial infarction patient addresses anxiety, pain, decreased cardiac output, altered gas exchange, and knowledge deficits.
15. Patients with acute cardiac conditions often have continuous cardiac monitoring to detect potentially fatal dysrhythmias for prompt treatment.
16. Cardiac rehabilitation begins with a cardiac incident, lasts throughout life, and includes the patient and family in teaching about exercise, diet, and medications.
17. Congestive heart failure, the inability of the heart to meet the metabolic demands of the body, may be caused by disorders that increase the workload of the heart or interfere with the pumping action of the heart.
18. The cornerstone of treatment of congestive heart failure is cardiotonic glycosides, also called inotropic agents, that increase the pumping effectiveness of the heart.
19. Treatment of congestive heart failure may include correction of underlying causes, drug therapy to improve cardiac function and eliminate excess fluid, and measures to decrease demands on the heart.
20. Complications of congestive heart failure are dysrhythmias, cardiac failure, and ventricular aneurysms and rupture.
21. Nursing care of the patient with congestive heart failure focuses on fluid volume excess, impaired gas exchange, anxiety, decreased cardiac output, fatigue, and knowledge deficits.
22. Cardiac inflammatory conditions (endocarditis, myocarditis, and pericarditis) are treated with drug therapy and rest.
23. Cardiomyopathy is a disease of the heart muscle that is treated with supportive measures but may lead to cardiac failure that eventually requires cardiac transplantation.
24. Patients who have had heart transplants require immunosuppressive drugs for the remainder of their lives to prevent rejection of the foreign tissue.
25. Signs and symptoms of cardiac transplant rejection are fever, dyspnea, fatigue, and dysrhythmias.
26. Sudden cardiac death, the abrupt cessation of heart activity and respirations, is fatal in 80% of all cases.
27. An automatic implantable cardioverter-defibrillator is an implanted device that monitors cardiac activity, detects life-threatening dysrhythmias, and delivers a shock to convert the rhythm to a normal one.
28. The primary disorders of the heart valves are stenosis, which interferes with blood movement from one chamber to the next, and insufficiency, which allows blood to flow backward.
29. Valve disease may be treated with drug therapy to improve cardiac function, with balloon valvuloplasty to dilate stenosed valves, with commissurotomy to enlarge the opening, and with mitral valve replacement using a biologic or synthetic valve.
30. A dysrhythmia is a disturbance of the heart rhythm caused by a problem in the conduction system.

Carol Boswell

CHAPTER 32

Peripheral Vascular Disorders

OBJECTIVES

1. Identify specific anatomic and physiologic factors that affect the peripheral blood supply and tissue oxygenation.
2. Indicate appropriate parameters for assessing a patient with peripheral vascular involvement.
3. Discuss tests and procedures used to diagnose peripheral vascular disorders and the nursing considerations for each.
4. State the pathophysiology, signs and symptoms, complications, and medical or surgical treatments for selected peripheral vascular disorders.
5. Use the nursing process to plan care for patients with peripheral vascular disorders.

GLOSSARY

BRUIT A murmur detected by auscultation

EMBOLISM Sudden obstruction of an artery by a floating clot or foreign material

HEMOCONCENTRATION Concentration of the blood

ISCHEMIA Deficient blood flow due to obstruction or constriction of blood vessels

PARESTHESIA An abnormal sensation

PHLEBITIS Inflammation of a vein

PHLEBOTHROMBOSIS Development of venous thrombi without venous inflammation

POIKILOTHERMIA Coolness in an area of the body due to decreased blood flow

THROMBOPHLEBITIS Development of venous thrombi in the presence of venous inflammation

THROMBOSIS Development or presence of a thrombus

VASOCONSTRICTION Decrease in blood vessel diameter

VASODILATION Increase in blood vessel diameter

VISCOSITY Resistance to flow related to the friction between two components; thickness

Adequate perfusion (blood flow), which delivers oxygen and nutrients to the tissues, is dependent on a functionally intact cardiovascular system. When this system is compromised by peripheral vascular disease, the homeostasis of the body is affected. Advanced age, heredity, smoking, obesity, physical inactivity, hypertension, and diabetes mellitus are risk factors that contribute to the growing prevalence of peripheral vascular disease. This disease process affects both the arterial and the venous components within the vascular systems. Close to 1 million individuals in the United States are affected each year by atherosclerotic peripheral vascular disease. People over the age of 70 have an increased chance of being affected by this disease process with resulting functional impairment. Approximately 500,000 individuals each year are diagnosed with deep vein thrombosis; nearly 140,000 die each year as a result of complications.

Atherosclerosis is covered in Chapter 31. Other peripheral vascular disorders are presented here.

ANATOMY AND PHYSIOLOGY OF THE PERIPHERAL VASCULAR SYSTEM

The peripheral vascular system comprises arteries, capillaries, veins, and the lymph vessels (Fig. 32–1). The function of this system is to maintain blood flow to supply adequate oxygenation and nourishment of the tissues. Any interruption of the blood flow to the body tissues results in hypoxia, which can lead to tissue death (necrosis) if untreated.

ARTERIES

Arteries are the vessels that carry the blood away from the heart toward the tissues. These vessels are normally elastic and have greater tensile strength than the veins. Arteries branch into smaller vessels called arterioles as they travel away from the heart. When the arteries and arterioles work effectively, oxygen and nutrients are transferred to the tissues for utilization.

Arteries and arterioles are thick-walled structures formed by three layers: the intima, the media, and the adventitia (Fig. 32–2). The *intima* is composed of endothelial cells that form the smooth inner surface of the arteries, allowing the blood to flow with little resistance. The middle layer is the *media.* This layer is the primary structure of the artery. The media is composed of smooth muscle, elastic fibers, and connective tissue fibers. It functions to control the dilation and constriction of the vessels to ensure the even, constant flow of blood to the peripheral areas of the body.

Smooth muscles, which encircle the vessels, control the diameter of each vessel. The autonomic nervous system acts on the smooth muscles, resulting in arterial dilation and constriction. These changes in the diameter of the arteries result in increased resistance to the blood flow. In addition to the autonomic nervous system's effect on the vessels, other chemical and hormonal factors influence the size and activities of the smooth muscles. The outer layer of the arteries and arterioles is the *adventitia.* Connective tissue is the primary component of this layer. The adventitia works to secure the artery or arteriole to the surrounding structure.

CAPILLARIES

Transfer of oxygen and nutrients between the blood and the tissue cells occurs at the level of the capillaries in the vascular system. As the arteries and arterioles branch into progressively smaller and smaller vessels, the capillaries are formed. The capillaries are formed by a single layer of endothelial cells, which allow the efficient movement of nutrients and oxygen into the tissues and the extraction of metabolic wastes from the tissues. Red blood cells have to conform to the size of these vessels by changing their shape owing to the small diameter of the capillaries. The distribution of capillaries is determined by the metabolic activity occurring in the tissue. Tissues such as skeletal muscles and digestive tract lining have a rich capillary network, but tissues such as bones and cartilage have a scanty capillary network.

Because capillaries lack the smooth muscles that are present in the arteries, the amount of blood in the capillary is controlled by precapillary sphincters. Other factors such as chemical stimulation and hormonal

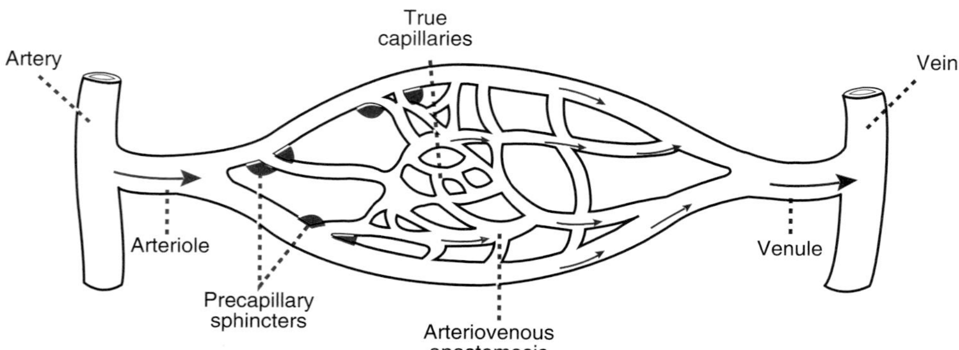

FIGURE 32–1
Capillary bed. Food, fluids, and oxygen are delivered to tissues through the capillaries, and wastes are collected from the capillaries for recycling or excretion. Precapillary sphincters help regulate the flow.

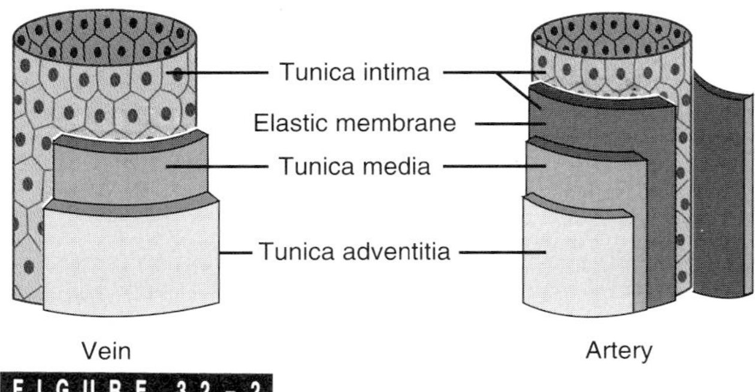

FIGURE 32–2
Tissue layers of veins and arteries.

changes influence blood flow and fluid shifts in the capillaries.

VEINS

The blood is returned to the heart by way of the veins and venules. These vessels are formed as the capillaries organize into larger and larger vessels. The venous system is less sturdy and more passive than the arterial system. The walls of veins and venules are composed of the same three layers as the walls of the arteries and arterioles, but the layers are less defined (see Fig. 32–2). Because the walls of the veins and venules are thinner and less muscular, these vessels have a greater capacity for distensibility than those of the arterial system. Therefore, the venous system permits the storage of a large volume of blood under relatively low pressure. As much as 75% of the total blood volume within the body is housed in the venous system.

Valves

The venous system is equipped with valves that are composed of endothelial leaflets (Fig. 32–3). These valves aid in the transportation of blood toward the heart against gravity. Each valve allows the blood to move in one direction only and prevents distal reflux of the blood in the dependent extremities.

Innervation

The innervation of the venous system is accomplished by the sympathetic nervous system. The sympathetic nervous system acts on the musculature of the veins to stimulate venoconstriction. As the valves and skeletal muscles knead the veins, the blood is forced back toward the heart. This process of massaging the venous system reduces venous pooling and increases the circulating blood volume. As the blood is moved toward the heart, the unoxygenated blood and metabolic waste materials are carried out of the tissues.

LYMPH VESSELS

The lymph system is an organization of small, thin-walled vessels that resemble the capillaries. These vessels accommodate the collection of lymph fluid from the peripheral tissues and the transportation of the fluid to the venous circulatory system. Because the lymph system interacts with the venous system, it is classified as part of the cardiovascular system. The lymph system comprises two main trunks: the thoracic duct and the right lymphatic duct. Each of these trunks is responsible for the collection and drainage of specific areas of the body.

Lymph fluid is composed of plasma-like fluid, large protein molecules, and foreign substances. Because these protein molecules are too large to enter the capillaries or the venules, the lymph fluid carries them to the lymphatic ducts, where they are emptied into the subclavian and the internal jugular veins. The movement of lymph fluid is accomplished by the contraction of muscles, which encircle the lymphatic walls and surrounding tissues.

FACTORS THAT AFFECT BLOOD FLOW

The body has multiple homeostatic mechanisms to increase and decrease the circulating blood flow either systemically or locally. The mechanisms basically work by changing resistance within the vessels or by changing the blood viscosity.

Resistance

The resistance within the vascular system is controlled by nervous and hormonal factors that regulate the diameter of the vessels. When vascular diameter increases, peripheral resistance falls and blood flow increases.

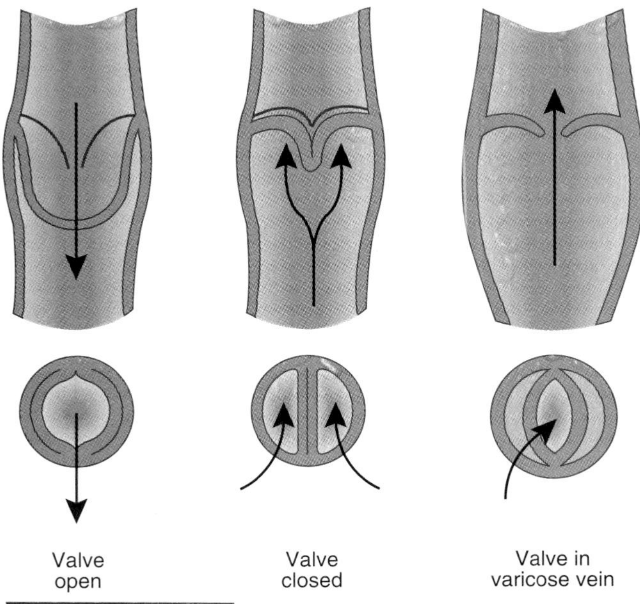

FIGURE 32–3
Veins contain bicuspid valves that open in the direction of blood flow but prevent regurgitation of flow when pockets become filled and distended.

When vascular diameter decreases, however, peripheral resistance increases, thereby reducing blood flow. The diameter of blood vessels is controlled by the central nervous system, hormones, some ions, and blood pH.

The sympathetic nervous system plays a major role in adjusting vascular resistance. The sympathetic nervous system regulates the size of peripheral blood vessels through the vasomotor center located in the medulla and the pons. The stimulation of the sympathetic nervous system by either physiologic or psychological stressors also triggers the release of norepinephrine and epinephrine, which cause vasoconstriction. The primary action of epinephrine, which is secreted by the adrenal medulla, is vasoconstriction.

Other factors that cause changes in vascular resistance are angiotensin, serotonin, histamine, the kinins, and the prostaglandins. Angiotensin is a potent chemical released by the kidneys that causes intense vasoconstriction and retention of salt and water by the kidneys. The kinins, histamine, and prostaglandins cause vasodilation, which decreases peripheral resistance. Serotonin, a chemical that is liberated from platelets when vessel walls are damaged, can cause vasoconstriction or vasodilation depending on tissue conditions.

Blood Viscosity

In addition to changes in peripheral resistance, modification of blood viscosity also helps regulate blood flow to peripheral tissues. Viscosity describes the thickness of the blood. The blood viscosity is usually constant but can be affected by changes in the proportions of the solid or liquid components. An increase in red blood cells or a decrease in body water produces hemoconcentration, which increases blood viscosity. When blood is concentrated, the kidneys generally begin to retain water and the movement of fluid out of the capillaries is restricted.

An important factor that affects blood viscosity is capillary permeability. Hydrostatic and osmotic pressures normally maintain balanced movement of fluids in and out of the capillaries. Any mechanism that alters capillary permeability changes the amount and direction of fluid movement, resulting in a change in blood viscosity. Factors that increase capillary permeability include histamine, bradykinin, and prostaglandins. Certain muscle metabolites, hypoxemia, malnutrition, and pH imbalances can also increase capillary permeability. When the proportion of serum in the blood is higher than normal, the kidneys excrete excess fluid.

AGE-RELATED CHANGES

Aging compromises the systems of the body in multiple ways. The vascular system is no exception to this process. The primary age-related change in the peripheral vessels is the stiffening of the vessel walls, called arteriosclerosis. As arteriosclerosis develops, the delivery of oxygen and nutrients to the tissue is compromised and a buildup of waste products in the tissue is experienced.

The stiffening of the peripheral vessels associated with aging occurs in both the intima and the media of the vessel wall. The intima is thickened and hardened by the proliferation of cells. It becomes roughened, which increases the risk of emboli. The connective and elastic tissue fibers in the media become calcified. This process produces a thinner and fragmented layer within the peripheral vessels. This loss of elasticity in the peripheral vessels increases the peripheral resistance, impairs the flow of blood, and results in an increase in the workload of the left ventricle. As a result of these changes in the peripheral vascular system, the transportation of oxygen and nutrients to the tissues and the removal of wastes from the tissues is affected adversely.

The transportation of oxygen may also be compromised by the decrease of hemoglobin seen in some aging patients. A reduction of hemoglobin in the blood produces a decline in the oxygen-carrying capacity of the blood. Because the stiffening blood vessels cause a decrease in the blood flow and a decrease in hemoglobin causes a compromise in the oxygen-carrying capacity, homeostasis of the peripheral tissues is substantially affected.

Overall, aging in the vascular system may cause a slowing of the heart rate and a decrease in the stroke volume, which may result in a decrease in cardiac output of approximately 30 to 40%. If the cardiac output is altered, the older person may adapt more slowly to changes in the peripheral vascular system.

NURSING ASSESSMENT OF THE PERIPHERAL VASCULAR SYSTEM

HEALTH HISTORY

Chief Complaint and History of Present Illness

The nursing assessment of a patient who may have a peripheral vascular disorder requires a thorough cardiovascular assessment as described in Chapter 31. Assessment of the peripheral circulation focuses on the six classical P's characteristic of peripheral vascular disease: pain, pulselessness, poikilothermia, pallor, paresthesia, and paralysis. Each of these characteristics needs to be evaluated to some extent.

PAIN. A thorough pain history provides invaluable information for diagnosing peripheral vascular disease. Acute pain is indicative of acute embolic occlusion of an artery. Chronic pain directs the investigation toward intermittent claudication or rest pain. The nurse addresses the nature of any pain or discomfort in the calf, thigh, hip, or buttock areas. The assessment should identify the nature of the pain (e.g., sharp, throbbing, continuous, intermittent), the location of the pain, and the precipitating factors (e.g., exercise, lying down in bed). The length of the pain episodes and the measures that relieve the pain are documented.

When pain is caused by a venous disorder, it is described as tenderness, heaviness, or fullness in the extremity. The history should note whether the pain was alleviated by elevating the extremity or wearing support stockings.

Intermittent Claudication. Intermittent claudication is pain that is associated with a decrease in perfusion that is aggravated by exercise and relieved by rest. An occlusion of the artery restricts the blood flow to the distal extremity. Intermittent claudication can affect any major muscle group distal to the point of arterial occlusion. The pain is described as a feeling of tightness, burning, fatigue, aching, or cramping. Exercise causes the muscle group to become ischemic, resulting in the development of pain. When the exercise is stopped, the pain is relieved.

Rest Pain. Rest pain reflects the presence of a severe arterial occlusion. As a result of the occlusion, tissue ischemia develops in the extremity, with the consequence of burning pain in the foot area. Patients who have rest pain experience severe foot pain after lying flat for a period of time. The pain is relieved when the extremity is dangled in a dependent position. Frequently, the history reveals the patient's habit of sleeping in a chair or with the feet maintained in a dependent position.

PULSELESSNESS. The peripheral pulses are assessed for rate, rhythm, and quality. The pulses are assessed and compared bilaterally to detect any differences.

POIKILOTHERMY AND PALLOR. The presence or absence of poikilothermy and pallor should be assessed in the health history. Poikilothermy is decreased temperature at an ischemic site. The rest of the extremity is warmer than the poikilothermic area. Pallor is paleness over an area of reduced blood supply.

PARESTHESIA AND PARALYSIS. Paresthesia and paralysis are important symptoms that need to be identified during the history part of the assessment. Paresthesia is defined as an abnormal sensation such as numbness, tingling, pins and needles sensation, or a crawling sensation. These abnormal sensations as well as paralysis may be associated with impaired conduction of nerve impulses caused by the reduction of oxygen and nutrients to the nerve tissues and the accumulation of waste materials.

Past Medical History

The past medical history includes the cardiovascular assessment as described in Chapter 31. A history of hypertension, coronary artery disease, myocardial infarctions, or atherosclerosis is documented. Because atherosclerosis affects the cerebral, renal, and respiratory blood vessels, each of these areas is included in the discussion of past medical problems. The presence of diabetes is also recorded because peripheral vascular disease is a common complication of diabetes.

Family History

The family history centers around the existence of any cardiovascular disorders in the immediate family members. Relevant cardiovascular disease processes include hypertension, coronary artery disease, myocardial infarction, and atherosclerosis. A family history of diabetes is documented.

Review of Systems

Careful attention is given to the integumentary system because changes in the integument provide important clues to the presence and severity of peripheral vascular disease. Changes that may be associated with peripheral vascular disease are thick and brittle nails; shiny, taut, scaly, and dry skin; skin temperature variations; skin ulcerations; muscle atrophy; localized redness and hardness; and hair loss on the extremities.

Another component of the review of systems is the assessment for chest pain and dyspnea. These symptoms are important because 10% of people with deep vein thrombosis develop a pulmonary embolus.

Functional Assessment

The functional assessment determines the impact of the disease process on the patient's life. The pain associated with the disease can interfere with work time and recreational activities. Because of the reduction of activities, the patient's stamina can be negatively affected. If limb amputation is necessary because of tissue necrosis, it is especially important to consider the effect of the limb loss on all aspects of the patient's functioning.

PHYSICAL EXAMINATION

The physical examination findings help determine whether the disease process is arterial or venous in nature. Generally, arterial complications involve multiple areas, whereas venous complications remain more localized, usually in the lower extremities. The skin is inspected for color and lesions. Paleness suggests peripheral vasoconstriction or inadequate arterial blood flow. A reddish-brown discoloration called rubor in a dependent lower extremity suggests the presence of damaged, dilated vessels as a result of arterial occlusive disease. In venous disorders, the affected areas of the skin may have a brownish discoloration and be cyanotic when the extremity is dependent. The nurse is alert for open ulcers and for scars around the ankles that may be associated with either arterial or venous disease. The existence of stasis dermatitis must also be noted. Stasis dermatitis appears as brown pigmentation with flaky skin over the edematous areas of the ankles. It may take on a bluish cast when the ankle is in a dependent position. Arterial stasis dermatitis begins as ulcerations in the toes. They are painful, pale, crusty, and located over bony prominences. Venous stasis dermatitis starts as ulcers in the ankle area. They develop very slowly, are generally painless, and are difficult to heal.

Capillary refill time in the nail beds is assessed to determine the adequacy of the peripheral perfusion. The nail bed is pressed until it blanches (turns pale). The pressure is then released, and the nurse notes the length of time in seconds required for the color to return. Usually a finding exceeding 3 seconds denotes a reduction in peripheral perfusion.

The nurse palpates the affected areas to evaluate the temperature, the presence and extent of edema, and the peripheral pulses. Skin temperature is palpated bilaterally and proximally to distally to determine the existence of any ischemic areas. A cool limb suggests an arterial problem, and a warm limb suggests a venous problem.

Swelling or edema develops in a dependent site as a result of systemic disorders, lymphatic dysfunction, deep vein thrombosis, or chronic venous insufficiency. To assess edema, the nurse should determine the severity, location, and indentation of the affected area. A comparison between the same area on each of the extremities is made. The severity is determined by pressing the thumb into the edematous area for approximately 5 seconds. The severity is graded from 1+ to 4+ depending on the depth of depression: $<\frac{1}{4}$ inch = 1+; $\frac{1}{4}$ to $\frac{1}{2}$ inch = 2+; $\frac{1}{2}$ to 1 inch = 3+; and >1 inch = 4+. If the depression of the thumb remains in the edematous area, the edema is said to be pitting.

Another aspect of the assessment is the evaluation of the peripheral pulses (Fig. 32–4). Each pulse is assessed for presence, symmetry, volume, and rhythm. The peripheral pulses assessed in the upper extremities include the brachial, ulnar, and radial arteries. The peripheral pulses appraised in the lower extremities are the femoral, popliteal, dorsalis pedis, and posterior tibial arteries. A comparison among bilateral pulses is evaluated and recorded. Absent or asymmetric pulses should be documented. The palpation of the arteries provides valuable information concerning the condition of the vessels. A sclerotic vessel feels stiff and cord-like, whereas a normal vessel can be palpated as soft and springy.

When peripheral vascular disease is suspected, Homans's sign should be evaluated. With the knee slightly flexed, the patient's foot is dorsiflexed sharply. If dorsiflexion causes pain in the calf area or behind the knee, Homans's test is positive for venous thrombosis. Approximately 50% of patients with venous thrombosis experience deep calf pain during the testing process. However, many patients with a positive Homans's sign prove not to have venous thrombosis.

Another test that can be beneficial in the assessment of the peripheral vascular system is Allen's test. Allen's test is used to determine the adequacy of arterial circulation to the hand. The patient is asked to clench the fist tightly while the examiner occludes the radial and ulnar arteries. The patient is instructed to open the fist, and pressure on the ulnar artery is released. If the ulnar artery is patent, the palm should promptly return to a normal color. A persistence of pallor in the palm area indicates an occlusion of the ulnar artery. The test can be repeated with the ulnar artery being occluded instead of the radial artery to detect occlusion within the radial artery (see Fig. 28–8).

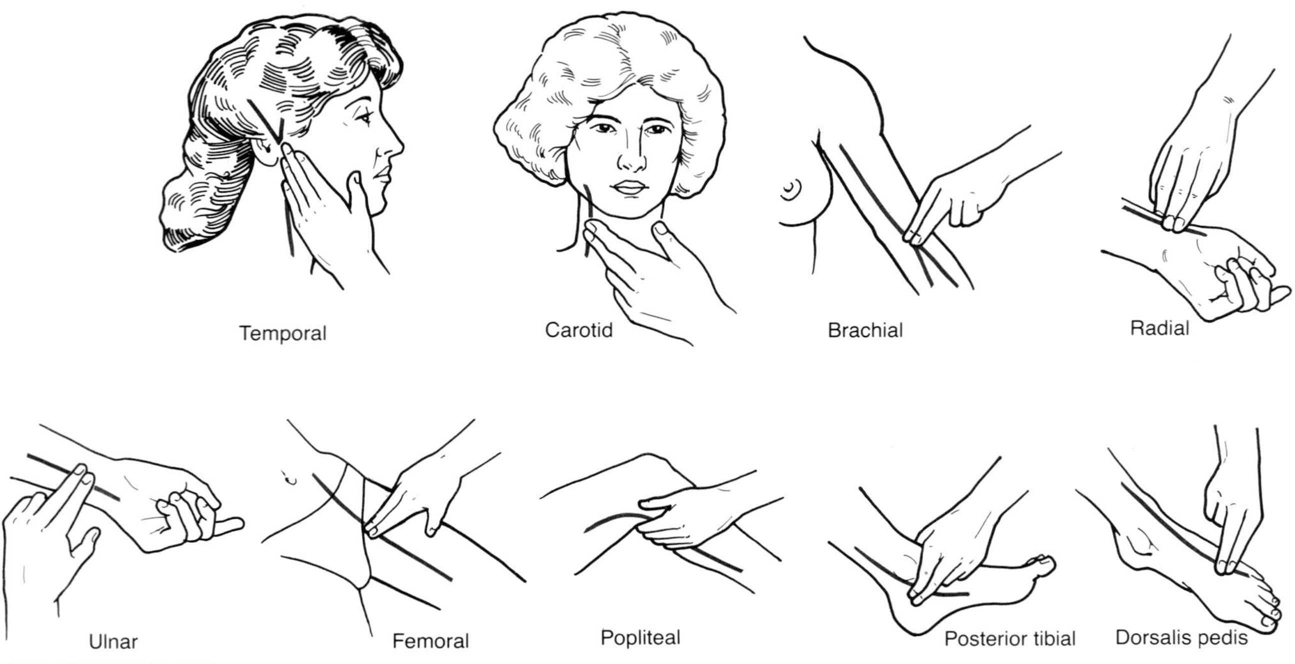

FIGURE 32-4

Peripheral pulses are assessed bilaterally from head to toe and rated for volume, rhythm, and symmetry.

TABLE 32-1

ASSESSMENT OF PATIENTS WITH PERIPHERAL VASCULAR DISEASE

HEALTH HISTORY	
Present illness:	Complaints of pain, pulselessness, poikilothermia, pallor, paresthesia, and paralysis
Past medical history:	Hypertension, coronary artery disease, myocardial infarction, amputations, atherosclerosis, diabetes mellitus
Family history:	Hypertension, coronary artery disease, myocardial infarction, atherosclerosis, diabetes mellitus
Review of systems:	Hairlessness on lower extremities; peripheral edema, discoloration of dependent areas, temperature changes in compromised areas, ulcerations on lower extremities, limb pain; thick, brittle toenails; temperature variation over involved area; muscle atrophy; localized redness and induration in affected extremity; chest pain; dyspnea
Functional assessment:	Mobility restricted by pain, decreased stamina
PHYSICAL EXAMINATION	
General survey:	Posture, gait, presence of pain in affected extremities
Cardiovascular:	Symmetric peripheral pulses, capillary refill time, Homans's sign
Integumentary:	Temperature of affected area, edema in dependent area, color of affected extremity, development of rubor in lower extremities, presence of stasis dermatitis or ulcers

The nurse with advanced education can further evaluate the peripheral vascular function by auscultating the sounds of the blood flow through the arteries. Bruits sound like turbulent, fast-moving fluid. The presence of bruits can signal the development of chronic arterial occlusive disease long before other signs appear.

Nursing assessment of the patient with peripheral vascular disease is summarized in Table 32–1.

DIAGNOSTIC TESTS AND PROCEDURES

Based on the findings of the physical examination, selected diagnostic studies will be ordered by the physician to confirm the disease process and determine the severity of the compromised vessels. The procedures and tests commonly used to diagnose peripheral vascular disease are Doppler ultrasound, plethysmography, pressure measurement, stress testing, and angiography, which includes both arteriography and venography (Table 32–2). Imaging procedures include magnetic resonance imaging (MRI), computed tomography (CT) scanning, and venous duplex scanning, which aid in the determination of the severity of the disease process.

Doppler Ultrasound

Doppler ultrasound is a noninvasive, inexpensive, highly reliable diagnostic tool. Low-intensity, high-frequency sound waves are directed toward the artery or vein being tested. These sound waves strike the moving blood cells and transmit a sound back to the receiver. The purposes of this test are to facilitate the diagnosis of peripheral vascular disease and to monitor the changes in the blood flow associated with vascular diseases. The frequency of the rebounded sound changes proportionally with the blood flow velocity. Arteries reflect a high-pitched sound, whereas veins produce sounds that vary with respirations and reflect a blowing tone. In the presence of an occlusion or narrowed vessel, the sounds are diminished. The entire test can be performed in approximately 10 to 20 minutes. The primary vessels examined are the posterior tibial, popliteal, and common femoral veins.

In preparation for the test, the patient is instructed that the test is risk-free and painless. During the examination, the patient might be asked to change the position of the extremity being evaluated and to perform breathing exercises.

Plethysmography

Plethysmography is a noninvasive examination that measures the blood volume and graphs changes in the flow of blood. These tests are used to detect deep vein thrombosis in the proximal areas of the lower extremities, to screen patients who are at risk for developing peripheral vascular disease, and to investigate the possibility of pulmonary emboli. Five different types of plethysmography are utilized to gain the information needed concerning blood volume changes. The primary type used to assess peripheral vascular disease is impedance plethysmography.

With the patient in a supine position, the leg being tested is raised to a 30- to 35-degree angle. The elevation of the extremity aids in the venous drainage of the area. A pressure cuff is placed on the thigh and inflated to allow for full venous distention. Electrodes measure electrical resistance and provide information about blood flow changes. The cuff pressure is deflated rapidly after the pressure readings have indicated complete venous filling. A strip chart tracing of the venous volume readings and venous volume changes is made following the deflation of the cuff. When a thrombus is present, the tracings reflect a reduction in the venous volume and venous volume changes.

To prepare the patient for the test, the procedure should be described. The test is painless and safe. Both

TABLE 32-2
DIAGNOSTIC TESTS AND PROCEDURES FOR PERIPHERAL VASCULAR DISEASE (PVD)

TEST/STUDY	PURPOSE/ PROCEDURE	PATIENT PREPARATION	POSTPROCEDURE NURSING CARE
Doppler ultrasound	To facilitate the diagnosis of PVD; to monitor the changes in blood flow associated with vascular disease Test is risk free and painless; low-intensity, high-frequency sound waves reflected off moving blood produce sound tracings; primary vessels evaluated are posterior tibial, calf, popliteal, and common femoral veins	Tell patient what to expect; patient may be asked to change position of extremity being evaluated and perform breathing exercises	No special care after procedure
Plethysmography	Primary type used is impedance plethysmography; to detect deep vein thrombosis in the proximal areas of the lower extremity; to screen patient who is at risk for developing PVD; to investigate the possibility of pulmonary emboli Noninvasive; measures the blood volume and graphs changes in the flow of blood; painless; safe; extremity is elevated and pressure cuff placed; following full venous distention, cuff is released and venous volume tracing done; three to four tracings per leg done to provide comparison	Tell patient what to expect and that test takes approximately 30 to 45 min	No special care after procedure
Pressure measurement	Types—segmental limb pressures or pulse volume measurements; pressures taken in systolic blood pressure, ankles, and multiple sites over the extremities. Noninvasive; safe; measurements are taken while at rest and during activities; painless	Tell patient what to expect	No special care after procedure
Exercise (treadmill) test	Evaluates the functional disabilities experienced by the patient Noninvasive; pulse volume measurements taken at rest, with exercise, and after exercise; patient is asked to walk for about 5 min at a rate of 1½ miles per hr on a treadmill; if dyspnea or pain begins, the test is stopped	Tell patient what to expect and that the test will be stopped if it exceeds the patient's tolerance	Careful monitoring of any complications that may develop as a result of the test
Angiography	Types—venography and arteriography; injection of dye into the vessels to make them visible on radiographs; to confirm the diagnosis of PVD; to distinguish clot formation from venous obstruction; to locate a suitable vessel for grafting Invasive; patient exposed to somewhat high doses of radiation	Operative permit must be signed; explain procedure; nothing by mouth for about 4 hr before testing; warn about possible transient burning sensation at injection site. Assess allergy to dye or iodine and report to radiologist	Risks are hemorrhage at insertion site, dye-induced allergic reaction, thrombosis at the insertion site; order bedrest after arteriography; monitor vital signs; assess injection site for hematoma; if deep vein thrombosis is diagnosed, bedrest may be ordered

legs are tested to allow for comparison of the readings. Because the test may require the completion of three to five tracings per leg, the test usually takes approximately 30 to 45 minutes.

Pressure Measurement

Pressure measurements can be completed as segmental limb pressures and pulse volume measurements. The pulse volumes are recorded as waveforms. These waveforms provide information concerning the progression of arterial occlusion. All pressure measurements are noninvasive and safe. Blood pressure is measured at multiple sites over the extremities to be examined. Measurements are taken while the patient is at rest. When a vessel has a stenotic or occluded area, the pressure readings are reduced at that level.

The patient is informed concerning the specific test to be completed. The segmental limb pressure test and pulse volume measurement test are painless.

Exercise (Treadmill) Test

The exercise test is sometimes referred to as a stress test. This test is noninvasive. The treadmill helps to evaluate the functional disabilities experienced by the patient. Pulse volume measurements are taken with the patient at rest and throughout the exercise period. The final measurements are taken after a period of rest.

The preparation of the patient must include education regarding the expected procedure. The patient is asked to walk for approximately 5 minutes at a 1.5 miles per hour rate on a treadmill. The pulse measurements are taken at designated times throughout the test. During this test, the patient is observed for any signs of distress such as claudication or dyspnea. If distress begins, the test is stopped immediately. Following the test, the nurse is responsible for carefully monitoring the patient for the development of any distress.

Angiography

Angiography is an invasive procedure that requires the injection of dye into the vascular system. The vessels become visible on radiographs. The two types of angiography are classified by the vessels examined during the procedure: arteriography, which examines arteries, and venography, which examines veins. Abnormalities can be visualized directly during the process to establish the location and severity of the problem. Because this procedure is invasive, the patient is exposed to relatively high doses of radiation and to the risks from the dyes utilized during the procedure. The purposes of these tests are to confirm the diagnosis of peripheral vascular disease, to distinguish clot formation from venous obstruction, or to locate a suitable vessel for grafting. The risks that are associated with these tests are hemorrhage at the insertion site, dye-induced allergic reactions, thrombosis at the insertion site, and emboli as a result of the procedure.

In preparation for the test, the patient must complete a consent form that lists the risks of the procedure. The procedures require that the patient take nothing by mouth for approximately 4 hours before the testing is done. A warning should be given to the patient that the injection of the dye causes a transient burning sensation at the site and some feelings of uneasiness during the procedure.

The postprocedure evaluation directs the nurse to assess the patient approximately every hour for a 6-hour period. The patient should be checked for any signs of an allergic reaction, hemorrhage at the site, diminished pulses, and infection.

COMMON THERAPEUTIC MEASURES

The primary goals with peripheral vascular disease are to increase the arterial blood supply to the extremities; reduce venous congestion; dilate blood vessels to increase arterial blood flow; prevent vascular compression; provide relief of pain; attain or maintain tissue integrity; and encourage adherence to the treatment plan.

Exercise programs, stress management, pain management, smoking cessation, elastic stockings, intermittent pneumatic compression units, body positioning, drug therapy, surgical interventions, and patient education are employed in the management of the disease process.

EXERCISE

The simple act of walking stimulates the movement of the blood from the dependent areas of the extremities toward the heart. The process of walking contracts the muscles of the lower extremities, pushing venous blood upward toward the heart and promoting the development of improved collateral circulation.

A specific type of exercise program that is effective in the management of peripheral vascular disease is the use of Buerger-Allen exercises or active postural exercises (Fig. 32–5). To perform the Buerger-Allen exercises, the individual is assisted to a supine position on a bed or flat surface. The legs are raised above the level of the heart for approximately 2 minutes or until blanching occurs. Then the legs are lowered to a dependent position. While the patient is in this position, the feet are flexed and extended for approximately 3 minutes or until the legs return to a pink coloration. Then the legs are positioned in a horizontal position for about 5 minutes. This entire process is repeated approximately six times in each session, with three to four sessions a day providing the best results. These exercises allow gravity to fill and empty the blood vessels. The exercises are stopped immediately if the patient has pain or severe skin color changes during the performance of the exercises.

With a disease process that can result in necrosis and gangrene, any exercise program must be prescribed by the physician. Patients who display leg ulcers, gangrene, or acute thrombotic occlusion may be restricted to bedrest until the disease process improves.

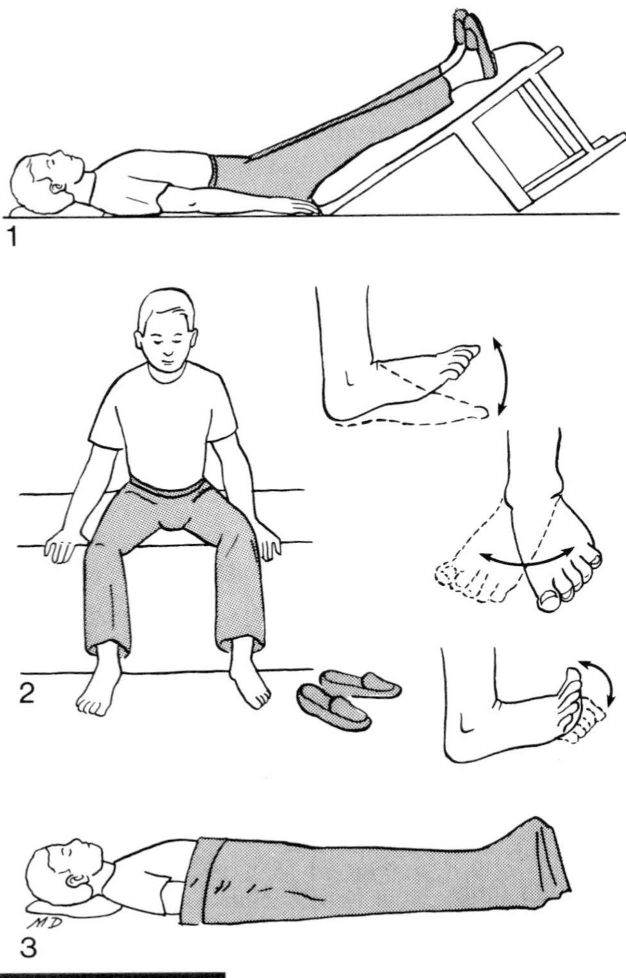

FIGURE 32-5

Buerger-Allen exercises. *1,* Elevate feet on padded chair or board for ½ to 3 minutes. *2,* Sit in relaxed position while each foot is flexed and extended, then pronated and supinated for 3 minutes. The feet should become entirely pink. If the feet are blue or painful, elevate them and relax as necessary. *3,* Lie quietly for 5 minutes, keeping legs warm with a blanket. (From Black, J. M., & Matassarin-Jacobs, E. [1993]. *Luckmann and Sorensen's medical-surgical nursing: A psychophysiologic approach* [4th ed., p. 1289]. Philadelphia: W. B. Saunders.)

STRESS MANAGEMENT

Emotional stress affects the entire body, including the peripheral vascular system. Stress results in peripheral vasoconstriction, which is detrimental to a compromised peripheral vascular system. The resistance to blood flow is increased, which results in a decrease in the blood available to the tissues. Emotional stress cannot be avoided entirely but can be reduced with a stress management plan.

PAIN MANAGEMENT

The presence of pain causes the patient with peripheral vascular disease to restrict the amount of mobility attempted. As mobility decreases with peripheral vascular disease, the disease process escalates. Therefore, pain management is an important aspect of care. Pain management can be accomplished by promoting improved circulation to the affected area, administering the prescribed analgesics, or both. With intermittent claudication, simply stopping the exercise decreases circulatory demands and alleviates the pain. Pain can result from the wearing of constrictive garments such as girdles, garters, belts, and tight pantyhose. The patient should be advised to avoid all constrictive clothing.

SMOKING CESSATION

A simple therapeutic measure to aid in the management of peripheral vascular disease is smoking cessation. This is very important because smoking causes vasoconstriction (constriction of the blood vessels). The nicotine in the tobacco causes vasospasms, which drastically restrict the peripheral circulation. The vasoconstriction can be documented for up to 1 hour after a cigarette has been smoked.

ELASTIC STOCKINGS

Another therapy that is effective in the management of peripheral vascular disease is the employment of elastic stockings or antiembolism hose. These stockings provide sustained and consistently distributed pressure over the entire surface of the calves and thighs. The correct placement of elastic stockings reduces the diameter of the superficial veins, resulting in improved blood flow to the deeper veins. Care must be taken when applying these stockings because they can become tourniquets if applied incorrectly. The proper size of elastic stockings must be determined for each patient by utilizing the instruction sheet provided by the manufacturer. Elastic stockings are best applied in the morning before rising from bed because swelling is usually at its lowest level at this time of the day. With the stockings inside out, start the placement by pulling the stocking onto the foot with firm, even support (Fig. 32–6). Once the elastic stocking is positioned over the heel, pull from the sides so it distributes evenly over the entire length of the leg. The stockings should be smooth when the application process is completed. If the top is allowed to roll or turn down, circulatory stasis occurs. The stockings are removed for 10 to 20 minutes twice a day. During the time the stockings are off, it is best for the patient to be resting in bed or with the extremities in a nondependent position. When the elastic stockings are removed, the skin is inspected for any signs of irritation, pressure, or tenderness, which could reflect developing complications.

INTERMITTENT PNEUMATIC COMPRESSION

Intermittent pneumatic compression or a pulsatile antiembolism system may be utilized for patients who are confined to bed following surgery or a traumatic episode. The primary function of these devices is to pre-

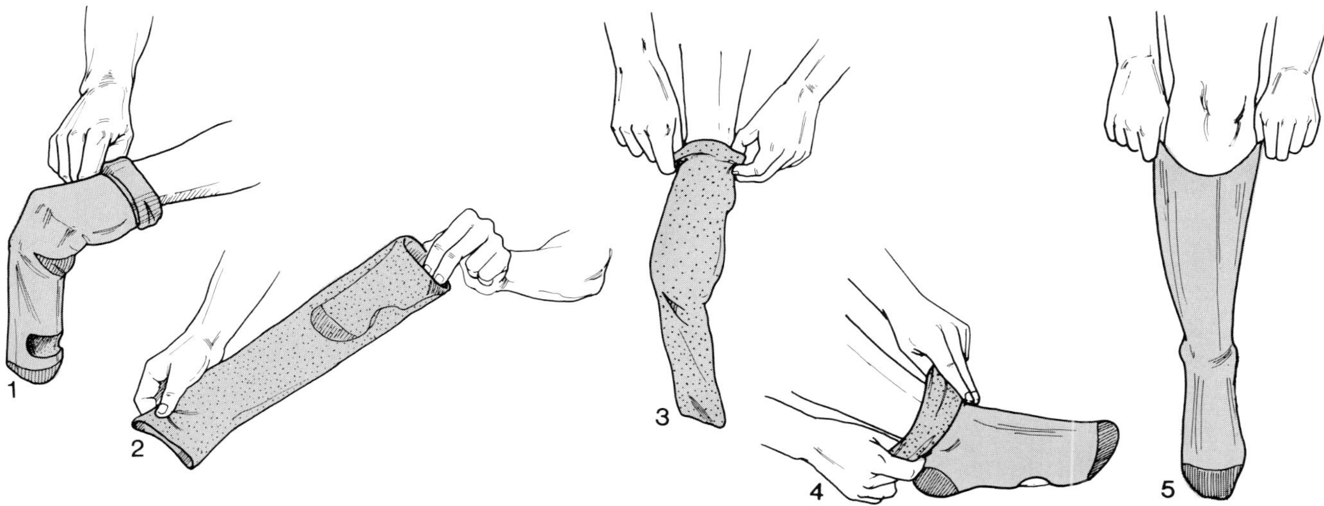

FIGURE 32-6
Elastic stockings provide sustained, consistently distributed pressure over the entire surface of the calves and thighs to promote venous return.

vent deep vein thrombosis. With intermittent pneumatic compression, elastic stockings are applied that are sequentially inflated from the ankles, calves, and thighs and then deflated. This expansion and contraction simulates the muscle pump of the lower extremities, prevents venous pooling, and stimulates the circulation.

POSITIONING

Body positions play an important part in the management of peripheral vascular disease. Frequently, patients are restricted to bed during the acute phases of the disease process. It becomes important to utilize different positions to mobilize the blood volume that has become stagnant in the dependent areas. Lowering the extremities below the level of the heart enhances the arterial blood supply. Elevating the lower extremities above the level of the heart promotes the venous return and reduces venous stasis. For patients who are not restricted to bed, prolonged standing enhances the strain on the venous system. On every possible occasion, the patient is instructed to sit down and elevate the extremity to a nondependent position.

THERMOTHERAPY

Thermotherapy with either warm or cold can be employed for its effects on the circulatory system. Heat, whether dry or moist, works as a vasodilator that promotes arterial flow to the peripheral tissues. Care must be employed when using heat because patients with peripheral vascular disease may have impaired sensation as a result of tissue ischemia. (Blood vessels constrict in response to cold.) Clothing can be used effectively to promote warmth and to prevent vasoconstriction from chilling.

PROTECTION

Affected extremities must be protected from trauma because the healing process is usually compromised with peripheral vascular disease. To prevent injury to blood-deprived tissues, the patient must avoid scratching and vigorous rubbing. The patient is cautioned not to walk about barefoot, to wear properly fitting shoes and clean socks or hose, and to keep fingernails and toenails trimmed and smooth. Ingrown toenails, blisters, or skin injuries should be reported to the physician for prompt treatment.

PATIENT TEACHING

Patient education is important in the management of peripheral vascular disease. The patient must understand the disease process and the prescribed therapies. The teaching plan should include cleanliness, warmth, safety, comfort measures, prevention of constricting blood flow, exercise, signs and symptoms that should be reported to the health care provider, and the importance of smoking cessation.

SURGICAL PROCEDURES

As peripheral vascular disease progresses, surgical intervention may become necessary. Embolectomy, percutaneous transluminal angioplasty (PTA), endarterectomy, sympathectomy, ligation and vein stripping, and sclerotherapy are procedures that may be employed.

Embolectomy

Embolectomy is the removal of a blood clot located in a large vessel. The process involves an incision into the vessel and the removal of the clot under direct visualization of the site or via a catheter. This procedure is employed when an arterial embolism is present and the patient has complicating factors that restrict the use of thrombolytic agents. Another method for completing an embolectomy is the use of a Fogarty embolectomy catheter. The catheter, which has a soft inflatable balloon near the tip, is positioned in the artery with the use of an arteriotomy. The tip of the catheter is passed through the embolus and inflated. Once the balloon is inflated, a steady tension is placed on the catheter to withdraw the entire embolus and apparatus from the vessel.

Percutaneous Transluminal Angioplasty

Percutaneous transluminal angioplasty does not require the actual incision of the vessel. The procedure is employed to gain access to the arteries in the lower extremities in people who are poor surgical risks. The primary purpose of this technique is to relieve arterial stenosis in such areas as the superficial femoral and iliac arteries. Under local anesthesia a balloon catheter is passed into the vessel to the stenotic area. Once the catheter is maneuvered into the optimal position, the balloon is inflated. This inflation of the balloon compresses the stenotic area or lesion against the vessel walls, which dilates the lumen of the artery and improves blood flow. Heparin is injected through the catheter at the time of removal to prevent clot formation. Pressure must be applied to the catheter insertion site for approximately 10 to 20 minutes to prevent hemorrhage from the site. Complications of percutaneous transluminal angioplasty are hematoma formation, embolus, arterial dissection, and allergic reactions.

Endarterectomy

An endarterectomy requires an incision into the obstructed vessel. Once the vessel is entered, the emboli and atherosclerotic plaque are stripped away from the intima of the vessel. After the removal of the obstructive material, the vessel is surgically closed.

Sympathectomy

A sympathectomy is an alternate method that may be used to improve vascular circulation. It is used when the patient has intermittent claudication. The process involves the excision of the sympathetic ganglia, which results in arteriolar dilation and increased blood flow. When a lumbar sympathetic block shows that poor circulation is related to atherosclerotic vessels, a sympathectomy is not the treatment of choice because the causative factor is not managed by the surgical procedure.

Vein Ligation and Stripping

Vein ligation and stripping is used primarily in the treatment of varicose veins. The patency of the deep veins must be established before the surgical procedure. The greater or lesser saphenous systems, or both, are the vessels removed through this process. The vessels are ligated at the proximal area near the femoral vein and the distal area in the ankle. A vein stripper is inserted from the ankle to the groin area. The stripping action progresses in a downward fashion. Pressure and elevation are employed during the procedure to reduce the bleeding.

Sclerotherapy

Sclerotherapy is another method for managing varicose veins. Because the complications of thrombosis, injection site necrosis, vasospasm, hemolysis, and allergic reaction are common, this process is not employed frequently at this time. Sclerotherapy requires the injection of a chemical that irritates the venous endothelium. This irritation results in the development of localized phlebitis and fibrosis, which closes the vein lumen. Sclerotherapy is a palliative therapy used for small varicosities and in conjunction with vein ligation and stripping. Following the procedure, an elastic stocking is positioned and left in place for approximately 5 days. Support stockings are required for an additional 5 weeks following the therapy. An exercise program of walking is emphasized to encourage and facilitate the blood flow to the extremity.

NURSING CARE RELATED TO SURGERY

PREOPERATIVE NURSING CARE. General preoperative care is covered in Chapter 14. With the major surgical procedures utilized in the cardiovascular system, the patient may have severe activity limitations until the surgical procedure is done to reduce the demands on the circulatory system. The affected extremity is placed in a level or slightly dependent position as ordered. To optimize peripheral circulation, the warmth of the extremity is maintained. The limb is protected from further injury.

POSTOPERATIVE NURSING CARE. Tissue perfusion must be monitored closely in the postoperative period. This tissue perfusion can be evaluated by assessing color of the extremity, temperature of the area, complaints of pain or tenderness in the area, capillary refill time, presence of edema or swelling in the area, peripheral pulses, and exercise tolerance. Disappearance of a peripheral pulse alerts the nurse to the possible development of a thrombotic occlusion at the site.

The primary goal of the postoperative period is the stimulation of circulation by encouraging movement and the prevention of stasis within the extremity. Anticoagulants are usually continued postoperatively to prevent the formation of a thrombus at the operative site. During the recovery period, the nurse emphasizes that the patient should not cross the lower extremities or place the affected extremity in a dependent position for excessive time periods. The elevation of the extremity aids in the prevention of edema formation.

DRUGS

Drugs used to treat peripheral vascular disease include anticoagulants, thrombolytics, vasodilators, hypoglycemic agents, antihypertensives, antiplatelet agents, nonsteroidal anti-inflammatory drugs, adrenergic blocking agents, and analgesics (Table 32–3). Each of these classifications of medication acts to improve peripheral circulation or treats a condition that affects blood flow.

Anticoagulants

Anticoagulant therapy is employed to prolong the clotting time, to hinder the extension of a thrombus,

TABLE 32–3

DRUGS USED TO TREAT PERIPHERAL VASCULAR DISEASES

DRUGS	USE/ACTION	SIDE EFFECTS	NURSING INTERVENTIONS
Anticoagulants			
Heparin sodium (Liquaemin Sodium)	Interferes with blood clotting; prevents formation of new clots; does not affect existing clots	Thrombocytopenia, bleeding, hemorrhage, nausea and vomiting, local irritation at injection site	Frequent laboratory work drawn to monitor effects on clotting. Check activated partial thromboplastin time (APTT) before each dose. Goal is APTT 1.5 to 2.5 times normal. Monitor for bleeding. Avoid trauma. Heparin given intravenously or subcutaneously. After subcutaneous injection, apply pressure but do not massage. Rotate injection sites.
Warfarin sodium (Coumadin)	Interferes with blood clotting; may prevent extension of existing clots and formation of new clots	Bruising, hemorrhage, nausea, anorexia	Check prothrombin time before each dose. May be required to notify physician before each dose. Monitor for bleeding. Teach patient not to take aspirin with warfarin.
Thrombolytics			
Streptokinase (Kabikinase) Urokinase (Abbokinase) Alteplase (Activase)	Dissolves existing clots	Minor to major bleeding; transient thrombocytopenia and alopecia; hypersensitivity rare; cardiac arrhythmias	Monitor lab tests of clotting activity. Monitor electrocardiogram and vital signs. Assess for bleeding. Protect from trauma.
Antiplatelet Agent			
Aspirin	Inhibits platelet aggregation; decreases inflammation and fever; reduces pain	Gastrointestinal (GI) irritation, tinnitus, pruritus, headache, bleeding	Assess for bruising, bleeding. Give with milk or food if GI irritation occurs.
Vasodilators			
Papaverine (Pavabid)	Works directly on smooth muscle in vascular walls to relax blood vessels	Sweating, vertigo, headache, flushing, GI distress, tachycardia, tachypnea. Large doses: sedation, cardiac arrhythmias, tremors, postural hypotension, nausea, and vomiting	Assess vital signs. Notify physician of flushing, rash, abdominal pain. Administer with food or antacid. Safety precautions if drowsy. Avoid sudden position changes. Report nausea and vomiting.
Nylidrin hydrochloride (Arlidin)	Dilates peripheral blood vessels by acting on beta-adrenergic receptors		
Hemorrheologic Agent			
Pentoxifylline (Trental)	Reduces fibrinogen concentration; increases flexibility of red blood cells to allow passage through small vessels; used to treat intermittent claudication	Dyspepsia, epistaxis, dizziness, nausea, vomiting, angina, tachycardia, cardiac arrhythmias	Assess vital signs. Administer with meals. Take safety precautions if dizzy.

and to inhibit the formation of a thrombus during the postoperative period. The two primary anticoagulant medications used are warfarin sodium (Coumadin) derivatives, which are given orally, and heparin, administered parenterally. When administering heparin parenterally, it is given intravenously for immediate response and subcutaneously for maintenance or prophylaxis. The clinical indications for anticoagulant treatment are venous thrombosis, pulmonary embolism, and patient susceptibility to embolism. When anticoagulant therapy is employed, regular coagulation tests are done to assess the effectiveness of the treatment regimen. The effective range for the partial thromboplastin time during heparin treatment is 1½ times the control. Because anticoagulants interfere with blood clotting, careful attention must be given to signs of bleeding. The fundamental complication of anticoagulant therapy is spontaneous bleeding that can occur anywhere in the body and be evident in the urine, stool, emesis, or integument. Because this complication can occur, the antidotes for each type of anticoagulant should be accessible. The antidote for heparin is protamine sulfate and for warfarin sodium is vitamin K. Medications such as antibiotics, mineral oil, salicylates, and tolbutamide can intensify the anticoagulant effects of warfarin sodium. The effectiveness of warfarin sodium may be decreased by antacids, barbiturates, oral contraceptives, and adrenal corticosteroids. Knowledge of the interactions of all prescribed medications with the anticoagulants is important to avoid excessive or inadequate anticoagulation.

Patient teaching with anticoagulant therapy should include a discussion of (1) the current medication regimen and interactions, (2) adverse effects that should be reported, (3) the avoidance of adding medications without first talking to the health care provider, (4) the importance of scheduling and completing regular blood testing to ensure maintenance drug levels, (5) the importance of checking for signs of bleeding, and (6) the need to wear a MedicAlert bracelet.

PHARMACOLOGY CAPSULE

Anticoagulants prevent the formation of blood clots; thrombolytics dissolve existing blood clots.

PHARMACOLOGY CAPSULE

Patients taking anticoagulant drugs must be monitored for bleeding.

Thrombolytics

Thrombolytic therapy is given intravenously to dissolve an existing clot. The commonly employed thrombolytic medications are streptokinase, urokinase, and tissue plasminogen activator. Uncontrolled bleeding can result from the medication; therefore, the patient must be assessed continuously during the treatment regimen. The disorders that necessitate the use of thrombolytic therapy are pulmonary embolus and occlusion of the peripheral and coronary arteries.

Other Medications

Multiple other types of medications are used during the treatment phase for peripheral vascular diseases. Vasodilators are employed to relax the vascular smooth muscle, which reduces resistance in the vessels, resulting in increased blood flow. Analgesics are used to relieve the pain response from ischemia. Nonsteroidal anti-inflammatory medications are also employed to allow the patient greater mobility without the effects of discomfort. A patient with reduced pain can participate more in exercises. Hypoglycemic and antihypertensive medications are used to control diabetes mellitus and hypertension, respectively, which complicate the peripheral vascular circulation. Antiplatelets such as aspirin are commonly prescribed in doses of 300 to 325 mg every day or every other day to make the platelets less likely to adhere to other platelets. Adrenergic blocking agents are utilized in some cases to block the sympathetic effects resulting in the dilation of the vessels and improved blood flow. Pentoxifylline is used to treat peripheral vascular disease by improving the passage of red blood cells through small vessels.

PHARMACOLOGY CAPSULE

Monitor patients taking vasodilators for hypotension.

Each of these medications may be utilized during the treatment of peripheral vascular disease. The use of specific pharmacologic agents depends on the individual's symptoms.

DIETARY INTERVENTIONS

The dietary interventions employed with peripheral vascular disease follow the plan for cardiovascular management. Diets low in fats lower cholesterol levels in the blood and restrict the development of atherosclerotic plaque. Dietary measures which aid in the reduction of atherosclerotic plaque lessen the roughness of the vessel walls and decrease the development of peripheral vascular complications. A weight reduction diet may be prescribed if the patient is obese. Obesity causes a strain on the heart, increases venous congestion, and reduces circulation to the peripheral areas. A diet low in fats, coupled with exercise, expedites weight loss, which helps control peripheral vascular disease.

Other nutritional considerations for managing peripheral vascular disease are the utilization of a balanced diet plan with the inclusion of vitamin B, vitamin C, and adequate protein. These elements advance the healing processes of the tissue and prevent tissue breakdown.

DISORDERS OF THE PERIPHERAL VASCULAR SYSTEM

VENOUS THROMBOSIS

Pathophysiology

The terms *phlebitis, thrombophlebitis, phlebothrombosis,* and *deep vein thrombosis* are often used interchangeably. Each term in reality describes a slightly different process. Phlebitis is an inflammatory process of the vein wall. Thrombophlebitis denotes the formation of a clot at the site of inflammation within a vein. Phlebothrombosis describes the development of a thrombus in a vein as a result of stasis, deviation of the intima, or hypercoagulability. Deep vein thrombosis refers to the development of a clot in one of the deep veins rather than the superficial vessels. A grave risk with deep vein thrombosis is the development of a pulmonary embolus. The superficial vein that is frequently affected by thrombus formation is the saphenous vein. The deep veins commonly involved with thrombi are the diofemoral, popliteal, and small calf veins.

Risk Factors

Some of the risk factors that may predispose a person to the development of thrombi are the following:

1. Bedrest prescribed as treatment for myocardial infarction, congestive heart failure, fractures, or other conditions treated with bedrest.
2. General surgery for individuals over the age of 40
3. Leg trauma resulting in immobilization from casts or traction
4. Previous venous insufficiency
5. Obesity
6. Use of oral contraceptives
7. Malignancy

Research has identified three factors (called *Virchow's triad*) that contribute to the formation of clots in the venous system: (1) stasis of the blood, (2) damage to the vessel walls, and (3) hypercoagulability. Research findings indicate that at least two of the three antecedent factors must be present for a thrombus to form.

Signs and Symptoms

The signs and symptoms of each of the disease processes are slightly different. Phlebothrombosis frequently has no clinical signs because no inflammation develops at the site of thrombosis. As many as 50% of patients with venous thrombosis display no visible signs or symptoms. When the obstruction occurs in a deep vein, the patient may demonstrate edema or swelling of the affected extremity, warmth and tenderness at the area of compromise, positive Homans's sign, and prominent superficial veins. In comparison, if the obstruction is located in the superficial vessels, the symptoms may be limited to pain, redness, warmth or tenderness in the affected area. The signs and symptoms depend on the size of the thrombus, the amount of obstruction, the location of the thrombus, the adequacy of the established collateral circulation, and the existence of other medical problems.

Medical Diagnosis

The primary diagnostic examinations used in the detection of thrombus formation are venography, plethysmography, and Doppler ultrasound. These tests are instrumental in the confirmation of the disease process and the determination of the treatment plan.

Medical and Surgical Treatment

The treatment plan is directed toward the prevention of thrombus extension, the prevention of pulmonary emboli, the reduction of the risk of further thromboembolus formation, and the reduction of pain and discomfort. Anticoagulant or thrombolytic therapy, or both, is begun as soon as possible following the diagnosis. The treatment plan typically includes patient teaching concerning the disease process; the ongoing assessment for pulmonary emboli; bedrest; elevation of the extremity; warm moist soaks to the affected area; antiembolism hose; and the initiation of ambulation following the acute phase of the disease. Surgery may be considered when the patient cannot receive anticoagulants or thrombolytic therapy or when the possibility for the development of pulmonary emboli is grave.

Nursing Care of the Patient with Thrombosis

ASSESSMENT. Assessment of the patient with peripheral vascular disease is summarized in Table 32–1.

NURSING DIAGNOSIS. The nursing diagnoses for the patient with phlebitis, thrombophlebitis, phlebothrombosis, and deep vein thrombosis may include the following:

- **Impaired Skin Integrity** related to venous stasis
- **Pain** related to impaired circulation and tissue ischemia
- **Anxiety** related to hospitalization and uncertainty of disease process
- **Knowledge Deficit** related to the developing disease process, treatment, self-care
- **Activity Intolerance** related to leg pain or swelling
- **Altered Tissue Perfusion** related to impaired peripheral circulation
- **Impaired Gas Exchange** related to pulmonary emboli

GOALS. The goals of nursing care for the identified nursing diagnosis are skin integrity, pain relief, reduced anxiety, improved patient understanding of disease process, improved activity tolerance, adequate tissue perfusion, and improved gas exchange.

INTERVENTIONS

Impaired Skin Integrity. Careful attention to ensure the intactness of the skin is of utmost importance. The skin must be inspected carefully to identify early signs of breakdown or compromise. The extremities are monitored for symmetry in color, warmth, pulses, and circumference. The elevation of the extremity promotes venous return and aids in the improvement of circulation to the area. Adequate circulation provides the tissues with the oxygen and nutrients that are necessary to ensure the intactness of the site. Edematous tissue is easily injured and heals with difficulty, so it must be protected from trauma, including pressure.

Pain. The patient's pain must be reduced before the activity intolerance can be managed. The discomfort that develops as a result of the disease process can be managed by prescribed analgesics at times. Other comfort measures may be ordered, such as warm, moist soaks and elevation of the extremity. The area should not be massaged or rubbed because this action can enhance the development of emboli, particularly pulmonary emboli by causing thrombi to break free from the wall of the vein.

Anxiety and Knowledge Deficit. Anxiety may be caused, in part, by lack of knowledge about the disease and its treatment. Also, the patient may have concerns about the effects of the condition on employment, activities of daily living, and quality of life. The patient may even restrict activities out of fear of pain. The relief of anxiety can help the patient move toward an acceptable level of activity. Anxiety and the knowledge deficit can be managed in much the same manner. With the development of any teaching plan, the current understanding level of the patient must be assessed and addressed to promote adherence to the treatment plan. The nurse provides factual and timely information concerning the disease process, treatment regimen, progress reports, and home maintenance plans to help reduce fears and concerns. This information allows patients to participate actively in their own health care. Control reduces patients' feelings of anxiety and possible fear. Patient teaching should include information regarding proper positioning, avoidance of crossing the legs, initiation of active exercise, medication regimen, application and use of antiembolism hose, and avoidance of periods of prolonged standing.

Activity Intolerance. Because activity intolerance aggravates the disease process, attention must be directed toward getting the inactive patient mobile again. It is important to establish a realistic exercise or activity plan. The plan should begin at the patient's current level and slowly add activities over a period of several weeks. The patient is instructed to stop the activity temporarily if pain, such as intermittent claudication, develops. Once the pain subsides, the activity may be continued.

Altered Tissue Perfusion. Improvement of tissue perfusion accomplishes several goals. Improved peripheral circulation aids in tissue perfusion, which results in decreased of pain or discomfort, the improvement of skin integrity, the reduction of anxiety, and increased physical activity. Anticoagulants, thrombolytics, or both are administered as ordered to dissolve the clot or to prevent new clots and reestablish blood flow to the affected area. The affected extremity is elevated as ordered during the acute phase. Once the acute phase is over, the patient is aided in the development of the exercise plan. Warm, moist packs are employed as ordered to improve circulation to the affected area. The nurse instructs the patient in the placement of antiembolism hose used to prevent stasis and improve circulation. The reduction of stress and cessation of smoking also improve tissue perfusion.

Impaired Gas Exchange. The possibility of developing a pulmonary embolus during the treatment of venous thrombosis is an ever-present concern. The nurse monitors for signs and symptoms of pulmonary embolism, which include dyspnea, chest pain, and anxiety. Interventions that the nurse can implement to improve the gas exchange of the patient who has a pulmonary embolism include elevating the head of the bed to a 45-degree angle, using oxygen when ordered, monitoring and documenting any changes in the patient's respiratory pattern, addressing anxiety, teaching the patient deep breathing and coughing techniques, and assisting with position changes every 2 hours. Each of these interventions helps the patient maintain open airways.

EVALUATION. Criteria for evaluating the outcomes of nursing interventions are absence of skin redness, rash, pallor, or lesions; patient's verbalization of pain relief and relaxed manner; patient's verbalization of reduced anxiety, calm manner; patient's description of condition, treatment, and self-care; increasing activity without pain; pulses present and symmetric, normal skin color and warmth; and respiratory rate of 12 to 20, absence of dyspnea and chest pain.

ARTERIAL EMBOLISM

Pathophysiology

The development of an arterial embolism is a potentially life-threatening event that requires immediate attention. The arterial embolus forms within the heart approximately 85% of the time. A roughened atheromatous plaque in any artery can also lead to the formation of a thrombus. If the thrombus breaks loose, it becomes an embolus traveling through the circulatory system until it lodges in a vessel, resulting in the immediate cessation of blood flow distal to the occlusion. The severity of the effects of occlusion depends on the size of the embolus formed, the organs involved in the compromised area, and the extent to which collateral circulation can maintain sufficient blood flow to affected tissues.

Signs and Symptoms

The clinical manifestations of an obstructed artery may vary from none to the presence of severe pain and other symptoms of tissue ischemia. When the collateral circulation is unable to compensate for the compromised blood flow, the patient develops distinct symptoms of reduced blood flow to the tissues. Tissues that do not have adequate blood supply develop the following signs and symptoms:

1. Severe and acute pain
2. Gradual loss of sensory and motor function to the areas
3. Pain aggravated by movement or pressure
4. Absent distal pulses
5. Pallor and mottling
6. A sharp line of color and temperature demarcation.

Medical and Surgical Treatment

Arterial embolism is managed with the administration of intravenous anticoagulants to prohibit the development of further thrombosis and reduce the extent of tissue necrosis that develops. Thrombolytic agents are used to dissolve the thrombus. When these medications cannot be used, as in cases of active internal bleeding, cardiovascular accident, recent major surgery, uncontrolled hypertension, and pregnancy, the patient may be prepared for an embolectomy. The thrombus is removed surgically to prevent the further development of tissue necrosis as a result of impaired circulation.

Nursing Care of the Patient with Arterial Embolism

ASSESSMENT. The assessment of the patient with arterial embolism is displayed on Table 32–1.

NURSING DIAGNOSIS. The nursing diagnoses that can be utilized in the management of arterial emboli are the following:

- **Altered Tissue Perfusion** related to the compromised circulation
- **Fear** related to the treatments, environment, and risk of death
- **Knowledge Deficit** of surgical procedure
- **Impaired Skin Integrity** related to ischemic changes from the reduction of peripheral circulation
- **Impaired Physical Mobility** related to the surgical procedure and compromised circulation

GOALS. The nursing goals are improved circulation, reduced fear, patient's knowledge of self-care, healthy skin integrity in the affected area, and improved physical mobility.

INTERVENTIONS. The interventions utilized by the nurse are focused on the improvement of circulation and the prevention of further damage to the affected tissue.

Altered Tissue Perfusion. Circulation can be facilitated by maintaining the affected extremities at a horizontal level or a level slightly below the horizontal, administering prescribed medications such as anticoagulants and analgesics, and performing range of motion exercises as ordered.

Fear. Fear can be decreased by orienting the patient to the environment and the expected therapies, using simple direct statements to explain the disease process and procedures, encouraging the expression of feelings of helplessness and anxiety, and helping the patient identify coping mechanisms that have worked in other situations.

Knowledge Deficit. To correct the patient's knowledge deficit, the nurse provides up-to-date, factual information in a professional, nonthreatening manner. Content of the teaching plan includes the disease process, treatment, and self-care measures.

Impaired Skin Integrity. With arterial embolism, the affected tissue is highly susceptible to injury and must be protected from pressure, trauma, and temperature extremes.

Impaired Physical Mobility. Improved physical mobility requires instruction regarding the correct way to perform range of motion exercises and development of a progressive exercise plan. This exercise plan usually is limited to 15 minutes, three times a day, for the initial days following surgery or treatment. A slow, regular progression of exercise intensity is determined that meets the patient's individualized plan of care.

EVALUATION. The criteria for the achievement of patient goals are normal skin color and palpable pulses, capillary refill time less than 3 seconds; calm manner; patient's statement of disease process and treatment, demonstration of self-care; absence of skin lesions; and increasing patient activity without increasing discomfort.

PERIPHERAL ARTERIAL OCCLUSIVE DISEASE

Pathophysiology

Peripheral arterial occlusive disease is identified by the terms *atherosclerosis obliterans, arterial insufficiency,* and *peripheral vascular disease.* It is characterized by pathologic changes in the arteries, typically plaque formations that arise where the arteries branch, veer, arch, narrow, or taper (Fig. 32–7). The most common sites for arterial occlusion are the distal superficial femoral and the popliteal arteries. Occlusions interfere with blood flow and therefore impair the delivery of oxygen and nutrients to the tissues. Hypoxia affects all tissues distal to the areas of occlusion. Peripheral nerves and muscles are more susceptible to harm from hypoxia than the skin and subcutaneous tissues. Severe oxygen deprivation may lead to ischemia and then to necrosis (tissue death) or gangrene.

Because peripheral arterial occlusive disease develops gradually, several compensatory mechanisms attempt to maintain circulation and tissue function. These compensatory mechanisms include the development of collateral blood vessels, vasodilation, and anaerobic metabolism. The severity of symptoms depends on the extent of collateral circulation that develops.

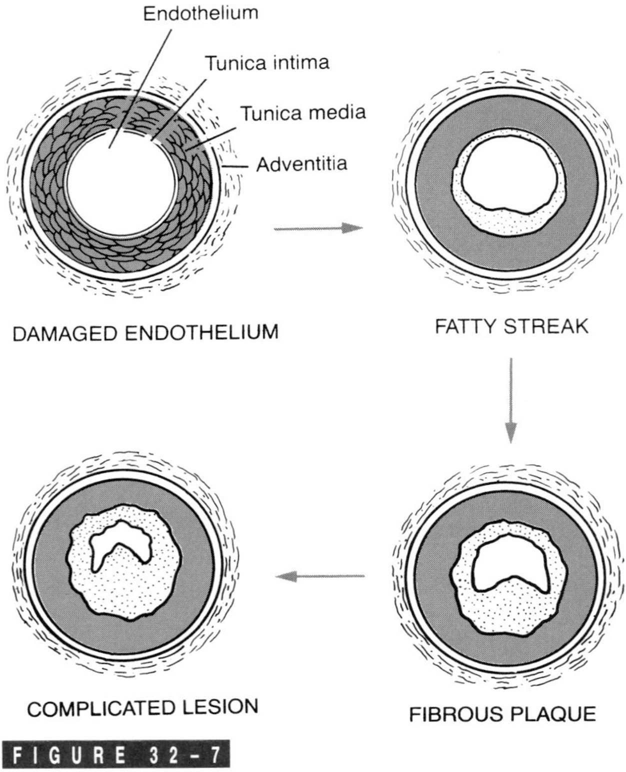

FIGURE 32-7
Development of atherosclerosis.

Peripheral arterial occlusive disease is most common in men older than 50. Factors that contribute to the development of this disease include atherosclerosis, embolism, thrombosis, trauma, vasospasm, inflammation, and autoimmune responses. Other risk factors that are more controllable are hyperlipidemia, diabetes mellitus, hypertension, cigarette smoking, and stress.

Signs and Symptoms

The clinical manifestations of peripheral arterial occlusive disease develop gradually. Intermittent claudication is the hallmark sign, with its insidious development of aching, cramping, tiredness, and weakness in the legs that is relieved by rest. Rest pain is another common occurrence with the disease process. The pain that develops during rest is described as persistent and aching. Complaints of tingling or numbness or both in the toes are frequently voiced. The affected extremity is cold and numb owing to the reduction in the flow of blood to the area. The skin color of the affected area changes to a pallor owing to reduced blood flow. When the extremity is in a dependent position, the color becomes red. This reduction of blood supply to the skin and toenails causes changes to occur such as ulcerations, gangrene, muscle atrophy, and thickening of the nails. Another clinical manifestation of peripheral arterial occlusive disease is the absence of peripheral pulses below the occlusive area. A comparative assessment of the two extremities must be made to determine changes in size and diameter. Other signs of arterial occlusion are shiny, scaly skin; subcutaneous tissue loss; hairlessness on the affected extremity; and ulcers with a pale gray or yellowish hue especially at the ankles.

Medical Diagnosis

The diagnostic tests used to confirm a diagnosis of peripheral arterial occlusive disease are Doppler ultrasonography, plethysmography, angiography, segmental limb pressures, pulse volume measurements, and exercise testing. A lumbar sympathetic block is used at times to evaluate the peripheral circulation. A local anesthetic is injected into the lumbar epidural space to block the sympathetic nervous system to the lower extremities. This process of blocking the nerves should produce vasodilation and an increase in temperature to the lower extremities. If the vessels are compromised by atherosclerotic changes, the vessels are ill adapted for vasodilation. This failure of the vessels to dilate following the lumbar epidural block alerts the physician to possible occlusive vascular disease.

Medical and Surgical Treatment

Drug therapy may include vasodilators and the hemorrheologic agent pentoxifylline. Surgical interventions that are utilized in the treatment of peripheral arterial occlusive disease are sympathectomy, endarterectomy, and percutaneous transluminal angioplasty. A sympathectomy is employed to increase the collateral circulation. An endarterectomy with a graft is the surgical removal of the diseased segment and the replacement of the segment with a graft of some type—either synthetic or from another blood vessel. Percutaneous transluminal angioplasty is the placement of a balloon catheter into the diseased area. The inflation of the balloon compresses the obstruction with resulting improvement in the blood flow through the area. Complications that are possible with percutaneous transluminal angioplasty are hematoma formation, embolus, arterial dissection, and allergic reaction. These procedures are discussed earlier in this chapter.

Nursing Care of the Patient with Peripheral Arterial Occlusive Disease

ASSESSMENT. Complete assessment of the patient with peripheral vascular disease is summarized in Table 32–1. When the patient has had surgical intervention, it is especially important to assess the pulses distal to the surgical site and compare them with the same pulses in the unaffected extremity. Cessation of a pulse alerts the nurse to possible arterial occlusion, and the surgeon must be notified immediately. Other important aspects of the postoperative assessment are vital signs, color and temperature of the affected extremity, fluid intake and output, central venous pressure, and mental status. If the patient has pain, the nurse documents the location, severity, and nature of the pain.

NURSING DIAGNOSIS. The nursing diagnoses for the patient with peripheral arterial occlusive disease may include the following:

Activity Intolerance related to impaired blood flow to extremities

- **Chronic Pain** related to ischemia
- **Knowledge Deficit** of disease process, treatment, self-care
- **Impaired Skin Integrity** related to inadequate circulation
- **Body Image Disturbance** related to muscle atrophy, stasis ulcers, and skin discoloration
- **Altered Peripheral Tissue Perfusion** related to vascular occlusion

If surgical intervention is performed, additional diagnoses may include the following:

- **High Risk for Infection** related to surgical incision, graft placement
- **Decreased Cardiac Output** related to hemorrhage, diuresis, fluid shifts
- **Altered Peripheral Tissue Perfusion** related to graft thrombosis
- **Acute Pain** related to surgical incision
- **Impaired Physical Mobility** related to weakness, fear, surgical procedure

GOALS. The goals of nursing care with peripheral arterial occlusive disease are improved activity tolerance, reduced pain, patient's knowledge of self-care, intact skin, positive body image, and adequate tissue perfusion. Additional goals for the postoperative patient are absence of infection, normal cardiac output, patent graft, relief of acute pain, and increased physical mobility.

INTERVENTIONS

Activity Intolerance. To monitor the patient's activity tolerance, the nurse assesses the patient before, during, and after planned activities. Progress is then monitored as treatment progresses. When planning an exercise regimen, the following guidelines may be used:

1. Allow the patient to participate in planning the activity schedule and goals.
2. Gradually increase the exercise time as tolerance increases.
3. Discontinue activity if the patient reports chest pain, bradycardia, dyspnea, or intermittent claudication. After rest relieves the pain of intermittent claudication, the patient may resume activity.
4. Reduce the intensity of the activity if the pulse takes longer than 3 to 4 minutes to return to the baseline rate, or if the patient has severe dyspnea.
5. For bedfast patients, start exercises with range of motion exercises twice daily.
6. Patients should *not* exercise when they have leg ulcers, cellulitis, deep vein thrombosis, or gangrene.

Chronic Pain. The chronic pain associated with ischemia is exhausting and greatly reduces the patient's quality of life. Therefore, measures must be taken to help the patient learn to manage the pain. The most direct measure is to increase circulation or decrease metabolic demands of ischemic tissues. Resting the extremities in a dependent position may help relieve the pain of arterial occlusive disease. Analgesics may be administered as prescribed, but there are also many comfort measures the nurse can employ or teach the patient that reduce the pain. Nonpharmacologic pain relief measures include relaxation techniques, warm baths, breathing exercises, and backrubs. See Chapter 16 for a detailed discussion of pain management.

Impaired Skin Integrity. The nursing interventions for maintaining skin integrity are the same as those for patients with arterial embolism. To maintain skin integrity, measures are taken to improve circulation and to avoid tissue trauma. If ulcers develop, bedrest is usually prescribed. The ulcerated area must be kept clean and free of pressure. Treatment protocols vary but may include wet to damp dressings, whirlpool therapy, and surgical débridement followed by the application of occlusive dressings. The feet are especially susceptible to injury and require special care. The patient is advised not to go barefoot, to wear only shoes that fit properly, to inspect the feet daily for signs of pressure or lesions, and to keep the toenails neatly trimmed. Nails should not be trimmed too short because of the risk of ingrown nails. Toenails should always be cut straight across rather than in a curved shape. The patient should see a peripheral vascular specialist promptly if any foot problems develop.

Knowledge Deficit. The patient must have reliable information regarding the disease process and treatment. Any misconceptions must be clarified for the patient and the family. The nurse should include the family in patient teaching because their fears and concerns can have an enormous impact on the patient's perception of the situation.

Body Image Disturbance. The patient is encouraged to express feelings that result from problems associated with peripheral arterial occlusive disease such as activity intolerance, stasis ulcers, discoloration of the extremities, and, for some, amputations. The nurse is supportive and helps the patient identify coping strategies to deal with the feelings.

Altered Tissue Perfusion. Vasodilators and other drugs that improve blood flow are administered as ordered. Exercise is encouraged according to the individualized exercise plan. Adequate warmth is maintained, and smoking is discouraged. Elevation of the extremities is generally not recommended with arterial disease.

Additional interventions are indicated for the postoperative patient.

High Risk for Infection. Postoperatively, patients are at risk for infection in the surgical incision and in the grafts (especially synthetic grafts) that are used to replace the diseased blood vessel. An infected synthetic graft is very serious because it necessitates removal of the graft and often amputation. The nurse monitors the patient's temperature and reports elevations to the surgeon. The incision is inspected for increasing redness, edema, and drainage that suggest infection. Antimicrobials are usually ordered preoperatively and may be continued postoperatively.

Decreased Cardiac Output. The nurse monitors for signs and symptoms of fluid volume deficit: tachycardia, restlessness, decreased urine output, pallor, and hypotension. Intravenous and oral fluids are provided as ordered, and intake and output records are kept. Daily weights may be measured as well. The surgical dressing is inspected for bleeding, which must be reported immediately to the surgeon.

Altered Tissue Perfusion. Thrombus formation can occur in the graft causing occlusion and impaired blood flow. The nurse monitors the pulses, warmth, and color of the operative extremity and promptly informs the surgeon of diminishing pulses, coolness, and pallor or cyanosis. Some patients are given anticoagulants or thrombolytics to decrease the risk of graft occlusion. Edema for 4 to 8 weeks is common after bypass surgery. The leg is usually wrapped in a light dressing or vascular boot and kept flat initially. Elastic stockings are not used immediately after a vein graft.

Pain. Acute postoperative pain is treated with analgesics, positioning, and relaxation techniques as described in Chapters 14 and 16.

Impaired Physical Mobility. Postoperatively, the patient's activities are increased gradually. A specific program of exercises may be prescribed. The nurse assists the patient and assesses muscle strength and tolerance of activity.

EVALUATION. Criteria for evaluating the outcomes of nursing interventions are patient's statement of improved tolerance of activity; patient's statement of reduced pain and relaxed expression; patient's description and demonstration of self-care measures; absence of skin lesions; positive patient statements about self, efforts to maintain good physical appearance; and palpable pulses. Postoperatively, additional outcome criteria include normal body temperature and absence of increasing wound redness or drainage; pulse and blood pressure consistent with patient's norms; warmth, improved color, and palpable pulses in operative extremity; patient's statement of pain relief and relaxed manner; and increasing activity without pain.

RAYNAUD'S DISEASE

Pathophysiology

Raynaud's disease and phenomenon are forms of an intermittent constriction of arterioles that affects the hands primarily although it can affect the toes and tip of the nose. The temporary vasoconstriction of the peripheral vessels in the hands is demonstrated by an increased or unusual sensation of coldness, pain, and pallor in the area. Gangrene is not common, but can develop in the skin on the tips of the digits. The cause of this condition is unknown, but it may be related to hypersensitivity to cold or release of serotonin. Stress and cold climates seem to aggravate the disease process. Women from the ages of 16 to 40 years are primarily affected, especially during the winter months or in northern areas where cold weather is more common. Raynaud's phenomenon follows the same general pattern but is typically secondary to connective tissue or collagen vascular disease, and is unilateral rather than bilateral.

Signs and Symptoms

The cardinal signs and symptoms of Raynaud's disease are chronically cold hands, numbness, tingling, and pallor. Involvement in the fingers is not symmetric in nature. The thumb is usually unaffected by the arterial spasms. The classical sequence of color changes seen during the arterial spasm episode progresses from pallor to cyanosis to redness. Pallor is the result of sudden vasoconstriction. The pallor of the skin turns to cyanosis as the oxygen supply to the tissue is compromised by the vasoconstriction. As the spasm resolves, vasodilation begins in the area, resulting in the development of a reactive hyperemia on rewarming of the area that produces a red color.

Medical Diagnosis

The diagnosis of Raynaud's disease is based on the signs and symptoms and the absence of evidence of occlusive vascular disease.

Medical and Surgical Treatment

The goals of the medical treatment plan for Raynaud's disease are to prevent pain and to promote vasodilation in the extremities. The medical treatment incorporates the use of vasodilators, calcium antagonists, alpha-adrenergic blockers, and sympatholytic agents to restrict the development of vasoconstriction in the area. Postural hypotension is a frequent complication noted with the use of these medications. At times the physician may resort to the use of a sympathectomy to interrupt the sympathetic nerves. This surgical procedure aids some selected patients but is not used routinely.

Nursing Care of the Patient with Raynaud's Disease

ASSESSMENT. Assessment of the patient with Raynaud's disease includes the data described at the beginning of this chapter and summarized in Table 32–1.

NURSING DIAGNOSIS. The nursing diagnoses that are considered with this disease process may include the following:

- **Pain** related to the ischemia that develops from vasoconstriction
- **Altered Peripheral Tissue Perfusion** related to vasoconstriction
- **Fear** related to the potential loss of work, difficulty performing activities of daily living

GOALS. Goals of nursing care with Raynaud's phenomenon include reduced pain, improved oxygenation of the peripheral tissues, and relief from fear.

INTERVENTIONS

Pain and Altered Tissue Perfusion. Nursing interventions to reduce pain and improve tissue perfusion are directed toward teaching the patient to avoid the stimuli that cause the vasoconstriction: exposure to cold, smoking, and uncontrollable stress. Because cold and smoking result in vasoconstriction, the patient is encouraged to take part in a smoking cessation program and is advised to dress warmly when going out in cold weather. Pain can be managed by careful warming of the area when the vasoconstriction occurs. The affected areas must also be protected from trauma. Care should be taken not to use hot water to warm the extremity because this practice can result in burns due to lack of sensation during the period of vasoconstriction.

Fear. Fear can be addressed in much the same manner as anxiety. The nurse attempts to determine the actual cause of fear—loss of work, loss of limb, or pain. Once the reason for the fear is identified, the steps used to reduce or manage anxiety can be incorporated into the management of fear. The nurse explores and accepts the patient's feelings, provides factual information, encourages problem solving, and helps the patient learn to live with the condition and to manage the prescribed therapy.

EVALUATION. Goal achievement is based on patient's verbalization of decreased pain, decreased episodes of vasoconstriction, and patient's statement of reduced fear.

ANEURYSMS

Pathophysiology

An aneurysm is a dilated segment of an artery caused by weakness and stretching of the arterial wall. Aneurysms can be congenital or acquired. Conditions associated with congenital aneurysms are Marfan's syndrome and Ehlers-Danlos syndrome. Acquired aneurysms can be caused by arteriosclerosis, trauma, or infection. The most common cause of aneurysms is atherosclerosis. Hypertension is apparently a contributing factor. With atherosclerosis, plaques form on the intima—the innermost layer of the arterial wall. The media—middle layer of the arterial wall—that contains elastic fibers weakens, allowing the vessel to balloon out. Infections including syphilis can also damage the media and result in the formation of aneurysms. The abdominal aorta is the most common site of aneurysm formation.

Signs and Symptoms

Signs and symptoms, if any, vary with the location of the aneurysm. People with thoracic aneurysms usually have no symptoms, but some report deep, diffuse chest pain. If the aneurysm puts pressure on the recurrent laryngeal nerve, the patient may complain of hoarseness. Pressure on the esophagus may cause dysphagia (difficulty swallowing). If the superior vena cava is compressed, the patient may have edema of the head and arms. Signs of airway obstruction may be present if the aneurysm presses against pulmonary structures.

Abdominal aneurysms are usually detected during routine physical examinations or radiologic studies. The aneurysm may be palpated as a pulsating mass in the area slightly left of the umbilicus. Although most abdominal aneurysms are asymptomatic, pressure on abdominal organs and nerves may cause back pain, epigastric pain, or constipation.

Complications

Complications of aneurysms include rupture, thrombus formation that obstructs blood flow, emboli, and pressure on surrounding structures.

Medical Diagnosis

Diagnosis is made on the basis of physical findings and radiologic studies. Studies performed to obtain better visualization of the aneurysm include echocardiography, ultrasonography, computed tomography, and aortography.

Medical Treatment

Repair of aneurysms may be done by replacing the dilated segment of the artery with a synthetic graft or, in some cases, suturing or patching the defective area. Repair is usually done as soon as possible but may be delayed until the patient is evaluated for other problems that create additional surgical risks.

Decisions to attempt repair of aneurysms are based on the size of the defect and the patient's general status. For example, an abdominal aortic aneurysm smaller than 5 cm is usually monitored with periodic ultrasound studies. If it begins to enlarge, surgical repair may then be recommended.

Complications of aneurysm surgery vary with the location of the defect. Complications of aortic abdominal aneurysm surgery include myocardial infarction, sexual dysfunction, renal failure, emboli, spinal cord ischemia with paralysis, bowel and bladder incontinence, and impaired sensation.

Preoperative Nursing Care

When surgical repair of an aneurysm is planned, the nurse prepares the patient physically and emotionally as described in Chapter 14. It is important to document chronic conditions such as emphysema or heart disease that increase the risk of postoperative complications.

Postoperative Nursing Care

Following aortic aneurysm repair, the patient is usually kept in a critical care area for 24 to 48 hours. Mechanical ventilation may be employed initially to maintain good oxygenation status.

ASSESSMENT. General postoperative assessment is outlined in Table 14–4. Assessment after repair of an aortic aneurysm focuses on vital signs, hemodynamic monitoring, renal function, and fluid balance. The extremities are assessed for color, warmth, and peripheral pulses.

NURSING DIAGNOSIS. In addition to the routine problems of the postoperative patient (see Chapter 14), nursing diagnoses for the patient who has had an aortic aneurysm repair may include the following:

- **Altered Renal Perfusion** related to interrupted blood flow
- **High Risk for Injury** related to ileus and distention
- **Ineffective Breathing Patterns** related to abdominal incision or splinting
- **Decreased Cardiac Output** related to myocardial infarction, occlusion of blood vessels, graft leakage
- **Altered Peripheral Perfusion** related to vascular occlusion

GOALS. Goals of nursing care for the postoperative patient after aneurysm repair are normal fluid and electrolyte balance, absence of injury related to ileus, effective breathing patterns, adequate cardiac output, and normal peripheral circulation.

INTERVENTIONS

Altered Renal Perfusion. During repair of an abdominal aneurysm, the aorta is clamped for a period of time. This poses a risk of renal damage and subsequent renal failure. Therefore, fluid intake is recorded and urine output measured hourly. Blood urea nitrogen, creatinine, and electrolyte levels are usually assessed daily to detect increases associated with renal failure. The nurse reports declining urine output to the physician. The nurse also assesses for edema, which may be caused by fluid retention or by circulatory obstruction. Intravenous fluids are administered as ordered.

High Risk for Injury. Following abdominal surgery, peristalsis ceases temporarily. A nasogastric tube is usually inserted and attached to suction to prevent gaseous distention of the bowel, which is uncomfortable and places stress on the abdominal incision. The nurse ensures that the suction is working properly and monitors for distention and the return of bowel sounds.

Ineffective Breathing Patterns. Whether the patient has an abdominal or a thoracic incision, there is a risk of poor lung expansion. After thoracic surgery, patients are at especially high risk for atelectasis and pneumonia. Mechanical ventilation for the first 24 hours maintains adequate ventilation until the patient is able to breathe effectively. Thereafter, the patient is assisted to turn, deep breathe, and cough frequently. An incentive spirometer may be used to encourage lung expansion. The patient's incision should be supported during the breathing exercises. Analgesics are administered and other pain relief measures employed. The patient can breathe more effectively if good pain relief is achieved. Lung sounds are monitored frequently to assess for abnormalities.

Decreased Cardiac Output. Cardiac output may fall as a result of myocardial infarction, cardiac dysrhythmias, heart failure, or hemorrhage. Hemorrhage may occur in the incision or by separation of the graft. The patient's vital signs and hemodynamics are monitored closely. The nurse assesses the wound dressing and drains for increasing bleeding. Early signs of circulatory failure are restlessness and tachycardia. Later signs are hypotension, cyanosis, and decreased alertness. The physician is notified immediately if there is evidence of decreasing cardiac output.

Altered Peripheral Perfusion. There is a risk of impaired blood flow below the level of the aneurysm. The nurse monitors peripheral pulses and the color and warmth of the extremities. This assessment is especially important when a patient has had a femoral or popliteal aneurysm repair. Signs and symptoms of occlusion include pain, pallor or cyanosis, and coldness. These must be reported to the physician at once.

EVALUATION. Criteria for evaluating the outcomes of nursing interventions are urine output equal to fluid intake, normal blood urea nitrogen and creatinine; intact wound margins, no abdominal distention, bowel sounds present; regular respirations, 12 to 20 per minute, clear breath sounds; pulse and blood pressure consistent with patient's norms, absence of increasing bleeding; and warm extremities with palpable pulses.

AORTIC DISSECTION

Aortic dissection is different from an aneurysm. A small tear in the intima permits blood to escape into the space between the intima and the media. Blood accumulates between the layers possibly causing the media to split lengthwise. The split may extend up and down the aorta where it can occlude major arteries. If no complications occur, the patient may be managed with antihypertensives and drugs to decrease the strength of cardiac contractions. Otherwise, the affected area is replaced with a synthetic graft. A key aspect of postoperative care is keeping the blood pressure at the lowest possible level. In other respects, the care is similar to that of a patient who has had an aneurysm repair.

VARICOSE VEIN DISEASE

Pathophysiology

Varicose veins are referred to as varicosities. Varicosities are dilated, tortuous, superficial veins, often the saphenous veins in the lower extremities (Fig. 32–8). The dilation of the vessels results from the incompetence of the valves within the veins as a result of hereditary weakness, occupations requiring prolonged standing, aging, pregnancy, obesity, or a combination of these. Typically the onset is gradual and progressive. The wearing of restrictive clothing aggravates the process. The two types of varicose veins are primary, which does not involve the deep veins, and secondary, which has deep vein obstructive involvement. Varicosities can occur in areas other than the peripheral veins, such as the esophageal and hemorrhoidal veins. Incompetent valves are irreversible.

Signs and Symptoms

When only the superficial veins are involved, the signs and symptoms are minimal except for the cosmetic

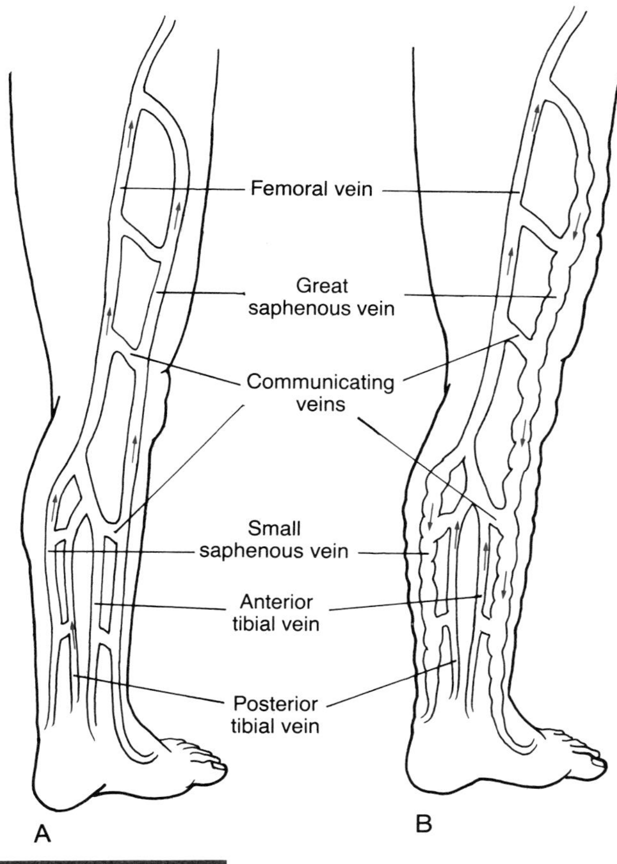

FIGURE 32-8
Venous return from the legs. *A*, Normal flow. *B*, Varicosities and retrograde venous flow.

changes that occur. The dilated veins are seen as oversized, discolored (purplish), and tortuous. Symptoms typically include dull aching sensations when standing or walking, feeling of heaviness in the affected legs, muscle cramps especially at night, increased fatigue of the muscles in the affected area, and ankle edema. Nodes can be palpated along the veins by the experienced practitioner.

Medical Diagnosis

The diagnosis of varicose veins utilizes plethysmography, lower limb venography, Doppler ultrasonography, and the Brodie-Trendelenburg test. The Brodie-Trendelenburg test demonstrates the backward flow of blood in the venous system. The patient is asked to lie down with the affected leg elevated to accommodate the emptying of the blood from the vessels. A soft tourniquet is positioned around the upper thigh to restrict the veins. The patient is asked to stand and walk around. The response of the vessels before and after the release of the tourniquet demonstrates to the health care provider the extent of incompetent valves located in the deep veins and the superficial vessels. Information about other diagnostic tests and procedures is presented in Table 32–2.

Medical and Surgical Treatment

Conservative medical treatments of varicosities are used whenever possible. The avoidance of activities that aggravate the symptoms and the reduction of any excess weight are recommended. The patient is encouraged to avoid restrictive garments, prolonged standing or sitting, crossing the legs or knees, and injury to the compromised areas. Use of support stockings may be recommended.

When surgery is necessary, sclerotherapy, ligation and stripping, or both are done. Surgery may be recommended for cosmetic reasons or if stasis ulcers develop.

Nursing Care of the Patient with Varicose Vein Disease

ASSESSMENT. When a patient has varicose veins, the health history determines the presence of pain, edema, cramps, and muscle fatigue. A family history of varicose veins is noted. The patient's occupation and usual activities are recorded. During the development of a pain and discomfort history, the nurse needs to take time to learn what has worked for the patient in the past in regard to pain control for the chronic pain. When the nurse takes time to listen carefully, additional information concerning pain, fears, and lack of knowledge can be obtained and addressed. The physical examination focuses on inspection of the legs for color, edema, turgor, and capillary refill. The nurse palpates for the presence of tenderness. Postoperative assessment is especially concerned with monitoring peripheral circulation and tissue perfusion.

NURSING DIAGNOSIS. The nursing diagnosis for use with the patient who has varicose veins are the following:

- **Pain** related to engorgement of the veins
- **Activity Intolerance** related to feelings of heaviness and fatigue
- **Knowledge Deficit** related to the management of the varicosities

GOALS. Specific goals for the identified nursing diagnoses are reduced pain, increased activity, and patient's understanding of the disease process and treatment plan.

INTERVENTIONS

Pain and Activity Intolerance. Many nursing interventions reduce pain and improve activity tolerance, so they are discussed together. The nursing interventions to manage pain and activity intolerance are the use of antiembolism hose or support hose; the performance of exercises to promote circulation; the avoidance of prolonged standing or sitting; the avoidance of restrictive clothing; the elevation of extremities when possible to aid in emptying the veins, and the use of analgesics as needed. The nurse also teaches nonpharmacologic methods for pain relief. Frequent position changes reduce discomfort by promoting venous return.

Knowledge Deficit. The patient needs to understand varicose veins and management techniques. For the surgical patient, patient teaching is of paramount importance because the procedure is often done as a same-day surgical procedure. The teaching plan should emphasize the points discussed under pain and activity tolerance.

Pressure bandages are placed on the extremities while in the surgical suite. These bandages are replaced with elastic stockings. The elastic stockings are required for approximately 3 to 4 weeks following surgery. Bedrest is necessary for the first 24 hours after surgery with the extremities elevated at a 30-degree angle. The regimen allows the patient to walk approximately every 2 hours for 5 to 10 minutes.

EVALUATION. The evaluation criteria are the patient's statement of decreased pain with activity; a regular, gradual increase in activity with less discomfort; and the patient's verbalization and demonstration of self-care as outlined in a teaching plan.

CHRONIC VENOUS INSUFFICIENCY

Pathophysiology

Another name used for chronic venous insufficiency is postphlebitic syndrome. Postphlebitic syndrome is the culmination of long-standing venous stasis and primary varicose veins. Primary varicosities and thrombophlebitis impair the valves of the deep veins, causing chronic venous stasis and ineffective peripheral tissue perfusion. The principal vessels affected are the iliac and femoral veins. The disorder is long standing, challenging to manage, and often disabling.

Signs and Symptoms

The individual with postphlebitic syndrome has edema in the dependent areas, altered pigmentation, pain, stasis dermatitis, and stasis ulcerations. The leg edema results from the venous stasis in the superficial veins around the ankles and calf areas. The altered pigmentation is seen as brownish areas in the same ankle and calf areas. Pain is described as heaviness and burning in the early stages of chronic venous insufficiency. Prolonged venous insufficiency eventually results in the reduction of innervation of the area. Stasis dermatitis is the initial sign of the development of ulcerations. The primary site for pigmentation changes and ulcerations is the medial malleolus of the ankle. Dermatitis develops as the veins become congested and unable to meet the oxygen requirement of the peripheral tissue. Cellular ischemia may progress to tissue necrosis, which is seen as stasis ulcerations. Stasis ulcerations are evident as open sores with inflammation. These areas can begin to drain or become covered with a thick black eschar. The risk of infection is high in the poorly perfused ulcers.

Medical Diagnosis

Noninvasive screening is done via the Doppler ultrasound and plethysmography to confirm the diagnosis of postphlebitic syndrome or chronic venous insufficiency. The symmetry of peripheral pulses is assessed. A culture may be ordered to determine the infectious agent if the stasis ulcer is draining.

Medical and Surgical Treatment

The medical treatment plan employs medications such as antibiotics for the infections and Unna boots for the ulcerations. Unna boots are medicated dressings used in conjunction with the antibiotics to promote healing of the ulcerations. The medical management of stasis ulcerations is constantly changing. The wound is débrided of necrotic tissue. Once the wound is débrided, the treatment regimens are individualized. Some examples of the regimens are the following:

1. Flushing the wound with saline
2. Application of topical agents and soaps to débride the area
3. Application of an enzymatic débridement agent
4. Use of wet to dry soaks
5. Hyperbaric oxygen therapy
6. Excision of large ulcers with skin grafting to cover the area

The overall goal for medical management of ulcerations is the preservation of the extremity by the stimulation of granulation tissue in the ulcer.

Nursing Care of the Patient with Chronic Venous Insufficiency

ASSESSMENT. The overall assessment is summarized in Table 32–1. When the patient has chronic venous insufficiency, the assessment emphasizes skin temperature, presence of a Homans's sign, presence of pain in the affected extremity, development of rubor in the lower extremities, and presence of stasis dermatitis (see Care Plan: The Patient with a Venous Stasis Ulcer).

NURSING DIAGNOSIS. The nursing diagnoses are much the same as those for other peripheral vascular disease processes.

- **Altered Peripheral Tissue Perfusion** related to reduced vascular circulation
- **Body Image Disturbance** related to chronic, open stasis ulcerations
- **High Risk for Infection** related to compromised circulation and impaired skin integrity
- **Impaired Skin Integrity** related to stasis dermatitis and ulcerations

NURSING GOALS. The nursing goals for the patient with chronic venous insufficiency are improved circulation to the peripheral areas and decreased venous pooling, patient's adaptation to body image changes, absence of infections; and improved tissue perfusion, and restored skin integrity.

INTERVENTIONS

Altered Tissue Perfusion. Measures that benefit the circulation in areas of compromised vascular function

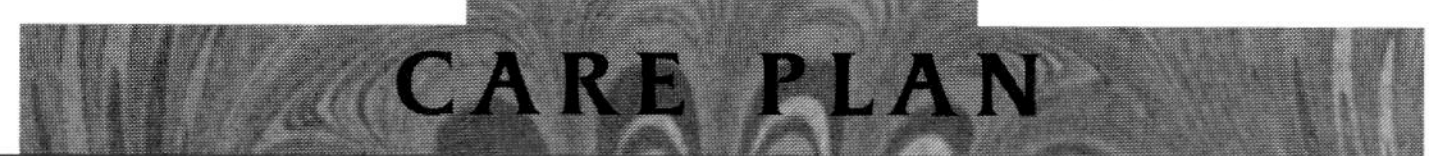

CARE PLAN
The Patient with a Venous Stasis Ulcer

ASSESSMENT

Health History: Wayne Barry is a 75-year-old man who is being seen in the community clinic for an ulcer on the medial malleolus of the right ankle. The ulcer is shallow and measures 1.5 cm × 2.5 cm. He describes a "heavy," burning sensation in the lower legs. He worked for many years as a toll booth attendant and has had chronic venous insufficiency for 5 years. He reports having had hypertension in the past but is taking no medication for it. Otherwise, he has been in good health and remains active. He is the caregiver for his wife who has been disabled for 3 years owing to a stroke. He has a daughter who helps with her care and who has been dressing the leg ulcer.

Physical Examination: Vital signs: Temperature, 97° F orally; pulse, 64; respiration, 16; blood pressure, 194/102. Alert and oriented. Walks with slight limp. 1+ edema both ankles. Varicosities noted in both legs. Stasis dermatitis in ankles and calves. Ulcer is 1.5 cm × 2.5 cm and shallow. The ulcer is slightly moist, pink, with no drainage or odor. Ankles and feet are cooler than calves. Pedal pulses faint but palpable, slightly stronger in left foot.

NURSING DIAGNOSIS	GOALS AND OUTCOME CRITERIA	INTERVENTIONS
Altered peripheral tissue perfusion related to compromised circulation.	The patient will carry out prescribed measures to improve tissue perfusion. Tissue perfusion will improve as evidenced by reduced pain, redness, and edema; skin warm to touch.	Instruct the patient in measures to improve circulation: exercise moderately each day, elevate the legs above the level of the heart when resting, avoid smoking, use support stockings as ordered, avoid prolonged periods of walking or standing still. Teach wound care as ordered. At each visit, assess condition of ulcer, peripheral pulses, skin color and warmth, pain, and edema.
High risk for infection related to open wound.	The patient will remain free of signs and symptoms of infection: fever, increasing redness, foul drainage.	Teach hygienic techniques of handwashing and wound care. Encourage diet with adequate protein and vitamins. Teach signs and symptoms of infection that should be reported to physician. Instruct in antimicrobial therapy if prescribed.
Chronic pain related to circulatory impairment.	The patient will report pain relief.	Encourage the patient to increase movement and maintain warmth to improve circulation. Teach pain relief measures including relaxation, deep breathing techniques, cutaneous stimulation, and behavior modification. Explain the use of prescribed analgesics. Assess effectiveness of measures.
Impaired skin integrity related to circulatory impairment.	The patient's wound will heal completely.	Assess and document the condition of the ulcer during each clinic visit. Advise the patient to use gentle soaps for bathing, to avoid trauma, and not to rub the ulcer. Encourage good nutrition and adequate fluid intake. Discuss wound care with physician or clinical nurse specialist in wound care.
Knowledge deficit of chronic venous insufficiency and treatment of stasis ulcer.	The patient will correctly explain chronic venous insufficiency and demonstrate correct care of ulcer.	Assess the patient's understanding of condition and self-care. Advise to avoid restrictive clothing, smoking, and weight gain. Explore sources of stress and coping strategies.

Care Plan continued on following page

The Patient with a Venous Stasis Ulcer *(Continued)*

NURSING DIAGNOSIS	GOALS AND OUTCOME CRITERIA	INTERVENTIONS
Knowledge deficit of importance of treating hypertension.	The patient will verbalize understanding of need to have blood pressure evaluated and will make an appointment for evaluation.	Explain importance of detecting and treating hypertension. Refer to physician or blood pressure clinic for evaluation.

are the elevation of the affected areas, the avoidance of restrictive clothing, protection from injuries or trauma to the area, the maintenance of adequate nutrition, and the use of antiembolism stockings.

Body Image Disturbance. The patient is encouraged to share feelings about body image changes. The nurse is accepting and supportive. The patient is encouraged to pay attention to grooming. Strategies for concealing ulcers are discussed.

High Risk for Infection. The patient is carefully assessed for signs of a developing infection such as elevated temperature, chills, general malaise, localized redness, and pain. The patient is taught to take an active part in the prevention of infections by thorough handwashing techniques, general hygiene, and appropriate wound care.

Impaired Skin Integrity. The nurse assesses for dermatitis and ulcerations. Thorough attention is given to patient education because the patient is the primary manager of the care. These ulcerations are frequently treated on an outpatient basis. The patient and family must be carefully instructed in the management of the ulcerations while in the home setting.

EVALUATION. Criteria for evaluating the outcomes of nursing interventions are absence of edema and lesions; verbalization of concerns about body image, efforts to maintain appearance; absence of fever, local redness, or drainage; and intact skin in affected areas.

LYMPHANGITIS

Pathophysiology

An acute inflammation of the lymphatic channels is identified as lymphangitis. The inflammation is the result of an infectious process in the lower extremities. Hemolytic streptococcus is the common infectious agent involved with lymphangitis.

Signs and Symptoms

The primary characteristic of lymphangitis is the enlargement of the lymph nodes along the lymphatic channel. Each node can be palpated along the course of the channel. The patient complains of tenderness as these nodes are assessed. A red streak from the infected wound extends up the extremity along the path of the lymphatics, as each node drains into the lymphatic system and the cardiovascular system. These nodes are located in the groin, the axilla, and the cervical regions. The symptoms of a generalized infection—elevated temperature and chills—are present. The infectious material can localize into an abscess with the symptoms of necrotic, suppurative discharge from the area.

Medical Diagnosis

The lymphatic system is assessed by lymphangiography. This technique can detect metastatic carcinoma, lymphoma, or infections. Lymphangiography allows for the radiologic visualization of the lymphatic system with a contrast medium.

Medical and Surgical Treatment

The medical management of lymphangitis necessitates the administration of antimicrobial agents to combat the infection. When an abscess develops, the area is incised to drain the suppurative material.

Nursing Care of the Patient with Lymphangitis

ASSESSMENT. The assessment of the patient diagnosed with lymphangitis is palpation of the lymph nodes in the groin and underarm areas for any enlargements. The skin is inspected for red streaks along the paths of lymphatic channels.

NURSING DIAGNOSIS. The nursing diagnoses for the patient with lymphangitis may include the following:

- **Pain** related to the inflammatory process in the lymphatic system
- **Activity Intolerance** related to the discomfort identified with movement
- **High Risk for Infection** related to the inflammatory process

GOALS. The goals for the patient are relief of the pain and discomfort, increased activity tolerance, and absence of infection.

NUTRITION CONCEPTS

- Edema frequently is treated with a low-sodium diet, and sodium-restricted diets vary from 4 grams (least restrictive) to 250 mg (severe sodium restriction) daily.
- Foods high in sodium that should be *avoided* are salt, monosodium glutamate (MSG), smoked or processed meats (ham, bacon, frankfurters, cold cuts), salted foods (potato chips, pretzels, salted nuts, popcorn), prepackaged frozen foods, and canned foods.
- Older adults taking diuretics are not encouraged to restrict sodium intake because they are at risk for low sodium syndrome.
- Salt substitutes are a source of potassium, which is desirable in patients receiving diuretics; however, salt substitutes should always be approved by a physician before using.

INTERVENTIONS

Pain. Nursing interventions to relieve pain include the administration of the prescribed analgesics and antimicrobials and elevation of the extremity to reduce the development of lymphedema. Nonpharmacologic measures should be used as well as analgesics. The application of warm, moist soaks to the infected areas as prescribed improves the circulation to the area. As the circulation is improved, white blood cells, nutrients, and oxygen are delivered, which aid in the recovery of the healthy tissue. Elastic support hose are utilized for several months following an acute attack of lymphangitis to prevent the formation of lymphedema.

Activity Intolerance and High Risk for Infection. Nursing care of the patient with lymphangitis is essentially the same as that for chronic venous insufficiency.

EVALUATION. Criteria for evaluating the outcomes of nursing interventions are patient's verbalization of pain relief, patient's verbalization of improved activity tolerance without increased pain; and absence of fever, lymph node enlargement, or redness along lymph channels.

BIBLIOGRAPHY

Bright, L. D., & Georgi, S. (1992). Peripheral vascular disease: Is it arterial or venous? *American Journal of Nursing, 92*(9), 34–48.

Carpenito, L. J. (1991). *Handbook of nursing diagnosis* (4th ed.). Philadelphia: J. B. Lippincott.

Carroll, P. (1992). Using cuffs to prevent clots. *RN, 55*(4), 57–59.

Chernecky, C. C., Krech, R. L., & Berger, B. J. (1993). *Laboratory tests and diagnostic procedures.* Philadelphia: W. B. Saunders.

Corbett, J. V. (1992). *Laboratory tests and diagnostic procedures with nursing diagnoses.* (3rd ed.). East Norwalk, CT: Appleton & Lange.

Dennison, P. D., & Black, J. M. (1993). Nursing care of clients with peripheral vascular disorders. In J. M. Black & E. Matassarin-Jacobs (Eds.), *Luckmann and Sorenson's medical-surgical nursing: A psychophysiologic approach.* (4th ed., pp. 1253–1314). Philadelphia: W. B. Saunders.

Diagnosis and management of peripheral vascular disease. (1992). *American Family Physician, 1*(45), 2750–2752.

Fahey, V. A. (1989). An in-depth look at deep vein thrombosis. *Nursing 89, 19*(1), 86–93.

Fellows, E., & Jocz, A. (1991). Getting the upper hand on lower extremity arterial disease. *Nursing 91, 21*(8), 34–43.

Gehring, P. E. (1992). Perfecting the art: Vascular assessment. *RN, 55*(1), 40–50.

Hamilton, H. K. (Ed.). (1989). *Diagnostics* (2nd ed.). Springhouse, PA: Springhouse Corporation.

Hodgson, B. B., Kizior, R. J., & Kingdon, R. T. (1993). *Nurse's drug handbook.* Philadelphia: W. B. Saunders.

Kee, J. L. (1991). *Laboratory and diagnostic tests with nursing implications* (3rd ed.). East Norwalk, CT: Appleton & Lange.

Loeb, S. E. (Ed.). (1991). Vascular problems. *Nurse Review.* Springhouse, PA: Springhouse Corporation.

Lueckenotte, A. G. (1990). *Pocket guide to gerontologic assessment.* St. Louis: C. V. Mosby.

Mathewson Kuhn, M. (1989). *Pharmacotherapeutics: A nursing process approach* (2nd ed.). Philadelphia: F. A. Davis.

Ruby, E. B., & Gray, V. R. (1986). *Handbook of health assessment* (2nd ed.). East Norwalk, CT: Appleton-Century-Crofts.

Smeltzer, S. C., & Bare, B. G. (Eds.). (1992). *Brunner and Saddarth's textbook of medical-surgical nursing* (7th ed.). Philadelphia: J. B. Lippincott.

Smith Suddarth, D. (Ed.). (1991). *The Lippincott manual of nursing practice* (5th ed.). Philadelphia: J. B. Lippincott Company.

KEY CONCEPTS

1. The peripheral vascular system comprises arteries, capillaries, veins, and lymph vessels, each of which plays a critical role in the oxygenation and nourishment of body tissues.
2. Risk factors for peripheral vascular disease include older age, heredity, smoking, hypertension, and diabetes mellitus.
3. Stiffening of blood vessel walls occurs with aging.
4. The six P's characteristic of peripheral vascular disease are pain, pulselessness, poikilothermia, pallor, paresthesia, and paralysis.
5. Intermittent claudication is pain in any major

KEY CONCEPTS (continued)

muscle group that is precipitated by exercise and relieved by rest.

6. Poikilothermia describes an area of the body that is cooler than the rest of the body owing to local ischemia.
7. Tests and procedures used to diagnose peripheral vascular disease include Doppler ultrasound, plethysmography, pressure measurement, stress testing, angiography, and venography.
8. Common therapeutic measures used in the management of peripheral vascular disease are exercise programs, stress management training, pain management, smoking cessation, prescribed body positions, and the use of elastic stockings or intermittent pneumatic compression devices.
9. Blood flow may be improved with drug therapy using anticoagulants, thrombolytics, and vasodilators.
10. Surgical interventions for peripheral vascular disease include embolectomy, angioplasty, endarterectomy, sympathectomy, ligation and vein stripping, and sclerotherapy.
11. A low-fat diet is usually prescribed and a weight reduction program may be advised if appropriate.
12. Phlebitis is inflammation of a vein wall, whereas thrombophlebitis describes clot formation in an inflamed vein.
13. Thrombosis is clot formation, and deep vein thrombosis indicates the clot is located in deep veins—a condition that poses a high risk for pulmonary emboli.
14. Risk factors for thrombus formation are bedrest, surgery in people older than age 40, leg trauma and immobilization, previous venous insufficiency, obesity, oral contraceptives, and malignancy.
15. Nursing care of the patient with peripheral vascular disease addresses impaired skin integrity, pain, anxiety, knowledge deficit, activity intolerance, altered tissue perfusion, and impaired gas exchange.
16. An arterial embolus, an unattached clot or other material in an artery, can lodge in an artery and obstruct blood flow; it may be dissolved with thrombolytic therapy or may be removed surgically.
17. Nursing care of the patient with an arterial embolus focuses on altered tissue perfusion, fear, knowledge deficit, impaired skin integrity, and impaired physical mobility.
18. Peripheral arterial occlusive diseases impair blood flow and may be treated surgically.
19. Nursing care of the patient with peripheral arterial occlusive disease focuses on activity intolerance, chronic pain, knowledge deficit, impaired skin integrity, body image disturbance, and altered tissue perfusion.
20. Raynaud's disease and phenomenon are characterized by intermittent arteriolar vasoconstriction that is usually treated with vasodilators and sympatholytic agents.
21. Varicose veins are dilated, tortuous, superficial veins that result from incompetent venous valves; they may lead to chronic venous insufficiency and are treated with conservative measures to improve venous return and sometimes with surgical intervention.
22. Lymphangitis is an inflammation of the lymphatic channels that is treated with antimicrobials, analgesics, heat therapy, and rest.

Joy M. Norton

CHAPTER 33

Hypertension

OBJECTIVES

1. Define hypertension.
2. Explain the physiology of blood pressure regulation.
3. Discuss the risk factors, signs and symptoms, diagnosis, treatment, and complications of hypertension.
4. Identify the nursing considerations when administering selected antihypertensive drugs.
5. List the data to be obtained in the nursing assessment of a person with known or suspected hypertension.
6. Identify the nursing diagnoses for the patient with hypertension.
7. Describe the nursing interventions for the patient with hypertension.

GLOSSARY

EPISTAXIS Nosebleed

HYPERLIPIDEMIA Excess insoluble fats in the blood

HYPERTENSION Persistent elevation of arterial blood pressure greater than 140/90 mm Hg

HYPERTROPHY Enlargement

ORTHOSTATIC HYPOTENSION Sudden drop in systolic blood pressure when changing from a lying or sitting position to a standing position

SYNCOPE Fainting

THROMBUS (*pl.* THROMBI) Stationary blood clot

Hypertension is considered the most common cardiovascular problem in the United States today. Approximately 60 million people, or about 20% of the U.S. population, have hypertension that requires monitoring or treatment, or both.

The condition is usually detected in people aged 30 to 50; however, it is being found with increasing frequency in children. Hypertension occurs twice as often in blacks as in whites and is more common in females than in males.

Hypertension is called the silent killer because it often has no symptoms and is not discovered until a serious complication develops. It is estimated that 50% of those with hypertension do not know they have it.

Complications of hypertension, including damage to the heart, kidneys, brain, and eyes, increase after age 50. Males, especially black males, suffer serious complications more often than females. Cardiac disease is the leading cause of death in hypertensives.

DEFINITIONS

Hypertension has been defined as a persistent elevation of arterial blood pressure greater than 140/90 mm Hg. Severity of hypertension is defined according to the diastolic blood pressure (DBP). In mild hypertension, the DBP ranges from 90 to 104. Moderate hypertension is diagnosed when the DBP ranges from 105 to 114. A DBP of 115 or greater is considered severe hypertension. Complications and death increase directly with the degree of hypertension. Even though these criteria are widely used, some sources recommend more conservative criteria that classify readings by stages (Table 33–1).

Some people have only occasional elevations in blood pressure and normal readings at other times. These findings are called isolated pressure elevations. Isolated systolic blood pressure (SBP) elevations of 160 mm Hg or more frequently occur in the elderly. The elevations are most often due to atherosclerosis.

TABLE 33-1

CLASSIFICATION OF STAGES OF HYPERTENSION FROM THE JOINT NATIONAL COMMITTEE ON DETECTION, EVALUATION, AND TREATMENT OF HIGH BLOOD PRESSURE

Stage I	Systolic: 140–159 mm Hg Diastolic: 90–99 mm Hg
Stage II	Systolic: 160–179 mm Hg Diastolic: 100–109 mm Hg
Stage III	Systolic: 180–209 mm Hg Diastolic: 110–119 mm Hg
Stage IV	Systolic: ≥210 mm Hg Diastolic: ≥120 mm Hg

From Johannsen, J. M. (1993). Update: Guidelines for treating hypertension. *American Journal of Nursing, 93*(3), 42–49.

TYPES OF HYPERTENSION

Hypertension is classified as essential (primary) or secondary. Essential hypertension accounts for 90 to 95% of all cases of hypertension. Its cause is unknown. Secondary hypertension is caused by underlying factors such as kidney disease, certain arterial conditions, some drugs, and occasionally pregnancy.

ANATOMY AND PHYSIOLOGY OF BLOOD PRESSURE REGULATION

Two factors determine blood pressure: cardiac output and peripheral vascular resistance. Blood pressure (BP) equals cardiac output (CO) times peripheral vascular resistance (PVR); that is, BP = CO × PVR.

CARDIAC OUTPUT

Cardiac output is the volume of blood pumped by the heart in a specific period of time (usually 1 minute). It is determined by the strength, rate, and rhythm of the contraction of the left ventricle and by the blood volume.

PERIPHERAL VASCULAR RESISTANCE

Peripheral vascular resistance is the force in the blood vessels that the left ventricle must overcome to eject blood from the heart. Resistance to blood flow is primarily determined by the diameter of the blood vessels and blood viscosity (thickness). Increased peripheral vascular resistance results from a narrowing of the arteries and arterioles and an increased fluid volume in the blood vessels that occurs as a result of sodium and water retention. Increased peripheral vascular resistance is the most prominent characteristic of hypertension.

The diameter of blood vessels is regulated largely by the vasomotor center. The vasomotor center is located in the medulla of the brain. Sympathetic nervous system tracts from the medulla extend down the spinal cord to the thoracic and abdominal regions. Stimulation of the sympathetic nervous system causes release of the hormones norepinephrine and epinephrine. These hormones, called catecholamines, are potent vasoconstrictors, meaning that they cause the blood vessels to constrict, making the diameter smaller. By constricting blood vessels, norepinephrine increases peripheral vascular resistance and raises blood pressure. Epinephrine constricts blood vessels and increases the force of cardiac contraction, causing blood pressure to rise.

Vasoconstriction decreases blood flow to the kidneys, which then release renin. Renin leads to the formation of angiotensin, another potent vasoconstrictor. Angiotensin stimulates the adrenal cortex to secrete aldosterone, a hormone that promotes sodium and water retention. This results in an increased blood volume. Vasoconstriction, cardiac stimulation, and retention of fluid all con-

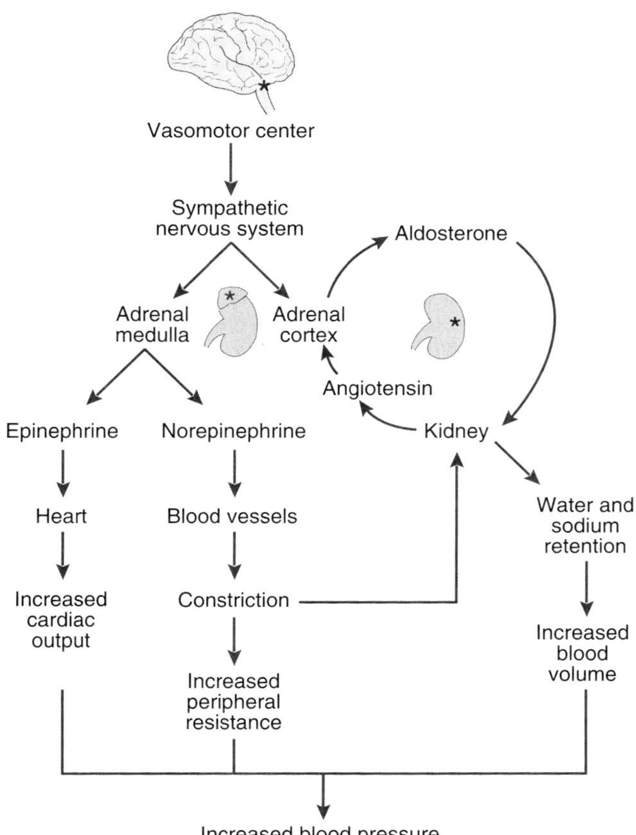

FIGURE 33-1
Factors that increase blood pressure.

tribute to hypertension. Figure 33–1 illustrates how various factors raise blood pressure.

ESSENTIAL HYPERTENSION

RISK FACTORS

The primary risk factors for essential hypertension are obesity, atherosclerosis, cigarette smoking, and sedentary lifestyle.

A person whose weight is 20% over ideal body weight is considered obese. The additional weight and fat cause increases in the number of blood vessels, circulating blood volume, and cardiac workload.

Atherosclerosis decreases the elasticity of the arteries and arterioles, causing increased systemic and peripheral vascular resistance.

Nicotine in cigarettes constricts blood vessels and causes the release of epinephrine and norepinephrine. These hormones, as already mentioned, also constrict blood vessels and raise heart rate and blood pressure.

Lack of physical activity leads to pooling of blood in the extremities and increases the workload of the cardiovascular system.

Other risk factors include stress, overstimulation, and a family history of obesity, hypertension, or hyperlipidemia. Hyperlipidemia is excess insoluble fats in the blood, a factor that contributes to atherosclerosis. Stress caused by such factors as a high-pressure job, financial worries, or family problems increases secretion of catecholamines.

Stimulants that may contribute to or aggravate hypertension include caffeine, nicotine, and amphetamines. Caffeine is found in tea, coffee, and chocolate. Nicotine is obtained by smoking or chewing tobacco products.

AGE-RELATED CHANGES AFFECTING BLOOD PRESSURE

Some age-related changes affect blood pressure. With aging, atherosclerotic changes reduce the elasticity of the arteries, causing a decrease in cardiac output and an increase in peripheral vascular resistance. After age 60, peripheral vascular resistance increases about 1% per year. Systolic pressure increases in response to increased peripheral vascular resistance. In addition, pulse pressure (the difference between the SBP and the DBP) widens in response to decreased ability of the aorta to distend (stretch).

In the past, elevated blood pressure was considered normal in the older person and was often untreated. Since research has shown that older people do benefit from controlling hypertension, age is no longer considered a barrier to aggressive treatment.

SIGNS AND SYMPTOMS

Many people who are hypertensive have no symptoms. Symptoms that may accompany hypertension include occipital headaches that are more severe on arising, lightheadedness, and epistaxis (nosebleed). If hypertension has damaged blood vessels in the heart, kidneys, eyes, or brain, the patient may have symptoms of impaired function of those organs.

COMPLICATIONS

The long-term effect of prolonged hypertension is replacement of elastic arteriolar tissue with stiffer fibrous collagen tissue. Thickening of the arteriolar wall decreases its ability to distend, resulting in increased peripheral vascular resistance and decreased blood flow to various organs. The effects are most significant in the eyes, heart, kidneys, and brain. Patients with hypertension must be assessed frequently for damage to these sensitive organs (Fig. 33–2).

Eyes

Damage to the eyes may include narrowing of the retinal arterioles, retinal hemorrhages, and papilledema (edema of the optic nerve). These changes may lead to blindness.

Heart

Coronary artery disease develops in patients with hypertension two to three times more frequently than in people with normal blood pressures. Coronary artery

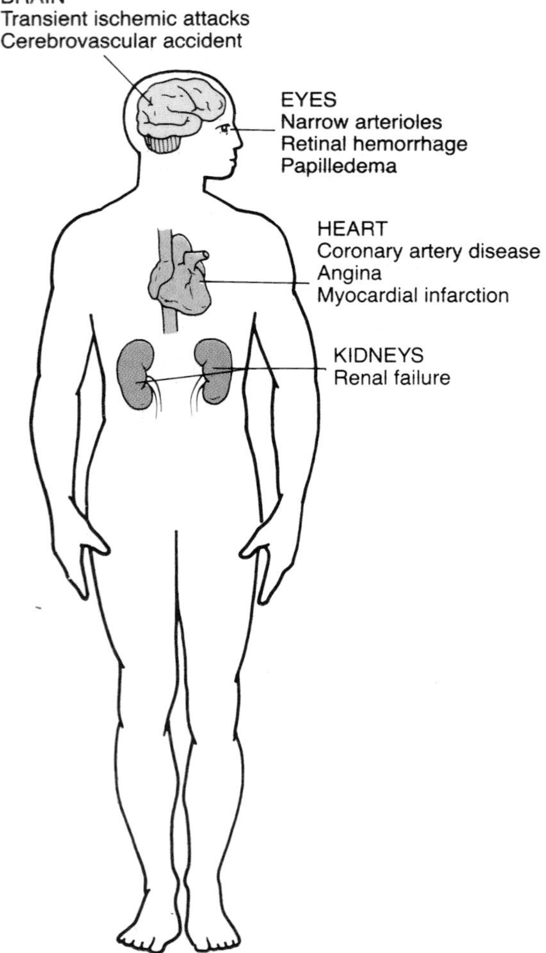

FIGURE 33-2
Long-term effects of hypertension on body organs.

disease causes an inadequate blood supply to the myocardium, resulting in angina, myocardial infarction, and congestive heart failure. Myocardial infarction, commonly called a heart attack, results when the blood supply to the heart muscle is inadequate and the myocardium is deprived of oxygen.

Sustained hypertension requires the left ventricle to work harder to overcome increased peripheral resistance. The increased workload may cause the left ventricle to become hypertrophied (enlarged), and it may eventually fail.

Kidneys

Narrowing of the renal arteries may decrease renal function and lead to chronic renal failure. Initial indicators of renal failure are nocturia (need to urinate during the night) and azotemia (accumulation of nitrogen waste products in the blood). In addition, urinalysis may reveal protein (proteinuria) or blood (hematuria), or both, in the urine.

Brain

Prolonged hypertension constricts and damages cerebral arteries, putting the patient at risk for transient ischemic attacks and cerebrovascular accidents. A transient ischemic attack, sometimes called a TIA or "little stroke," is a temporary neurologic dysfunction caused by cerebral ischemia.

A cerebrovascular accident (called a CVA or stroke) results from interrupted blood flow in the brain caused by a rupture of a blood vessel or a thrombus (clot) occluding the vessel. People with hypertension have a seven times greater incidence of cerebrovascular accidents than those with normal blood pressures.

DIAGNOSTIC TESTS

Diagnosis of hypertension is based on direct and indirect data. Hypertension is confirmed by averaging two or more blood pressure measurements on two or more occasions and finding the averages above 140/90.

On finding an elevated blood pressure, the physician examines the patient for effects of hypertension on other parts of the body. An eye examination with an ophthalmoscope may reveal retinal hemorrhages or narrowed retinal arteries. An electrocardiogram may reveal left ventricular hypertrophy or myocardial ischemia.

Blood samples are usually drawn for a complete blood count and assessment of liver and kidney function. If there is kidney damage, the blood urea nitrogen and serum creatinine levels are elevated. Elevated serum cholesterol may indicate atherosclerosis. A chest radiograph may show enlargement of the heart or pulmonary blood vessels.

Physicians disagree about the need for trying to determine the cause of hypertension. If there is no evidence to suggest an underlying disease process, the general consensus is to limit diagnostic tests to those that are most significant. This reduces patient care costs.

MEDICAL TREATMENT

The goal of therapy for hypertension is to gradually reduce peripheral vascular resistance and blood pressure. Optimal blood pressure is generally defined as a DBP of 90 mm Hg or less. Some experts accept a DBP of 95 in the older person.

A conservative, nonpharmacologic method (without drugs) is generally tried first. Drug treatment may be added if needed.

Lifestyle Modifications

A nonpharmacologic approach includes weight reduction, smoking cessation, sodium restriction, exercise, relaxation techniques, and modified alcohol intake. Reduction of weight to an optimal level can reduce blood pressure by reducing the workload of the heart. Stopping smoking can eliminate the vasoconstriction caused by nicotine. Reduction of sodium in the body reduces water retention, thereby decreasing the circulating blood volume.

A planned program of exercise improves cardiac efficiency by increasing cardiac output and decreasing peripheral vascular resistance. Exercise also decreases the patient's blood glucose and cholesterol levels and promotes a sense of well-being. Isotonic exercises such as walking, bicycling, and swimming help to reduce weight and promote relaxation.

Relaxation therapy, biofeedback, and behavior modification techniques also may be employed to reduce stress and lower blood pressure. Alcohol intake should not exceed 2 ounces per day because alcohol can increase blood pressure as well as alter the effects of some antihypertensive drugs.

Pharmacologic Therapy

Drug therapy is indicated if conservative therapies are not effective or if the blood pressure is very high initially. Drug therapy must be individualized for each patient. The goal of drug therapy is to normalize blood pressure using the smallest number of the safest drugs at the lowest effective dosages. Antihypertensive drugs are listed in Table 33–2.

STEPPED-CARE APPROACH. The stepped-care approach (Table 33–3) is a plan for selecting drugs to treat hypertension. It begins with administration of a single, relatively safe drug. The physician progresses to the next step until good control is achieved.

TABLE 33–2
DRUGS USED TO TREAT HYPERTENSION

SITE OF ACTION	GENERIC NAME	TRADE NAME
Central nervous system	Clonidine	Catapres
	Methyldopa	Aldomet
Sympathetic ganglia	Trimethaphan	Arfonad
Adrenergic nerve endings	Phentolamine	Regitine
	Prazosin	Minipress
	Propranolol	Inderal
	Atenolol	Tenormin
	Metoprolol	Lopressor
	Nadolol	Corgard
	Labetalol	Normodyne
Vascular smooth muscle	Hydralazine	Apresoline
	Diazoxide	Hyperstat IV
	Minoxidil	Loniten
	Nitroprusside	Nipride
	Hydrochlorothiazide	HCTZ
	Verapamil	Calan
	Nifedipine	Procardia
	Diltiazem	Cardizem
Kidney and afferent arterioles	Hydrochlorothiazide	HCTZ
	Furosemide	Lasix
	Spironolactone	Aldactone
Renin-angiotensin system	Captopril	Capoten
	Enalapril	Vasotec

TABLE 33–3
STEPPED-CARE APPROACH

Step One
Low dose of one of the following:
Thiazide diuretic
Beta-adrenergic receptor blocker
Angiotensin-converting enzyme inhibitor
Calcium antagonist

Step Two
Increased dosage of the first drug or addition of another Step One drug

Step Three
Increased dosage of Step Two drug
OR
Addition of a third drug
OR
Prescription of a different drug from Step One

Step One. The first step recommends starting the patient on a low dose of one of the following: thiazide diuretic, beta-adrenergic receptor blocker (beta blocker), calcium antagonist (calcium channel blocker), or angiotensin-converting enzyme inhibitor (ACE inhibitor).

Step Two. If the first drug is not effective, step two is an increase in the dosage of the first drug or the addition of a second drug from step one. An alternative drug also might be selected.

Step Three. The third step is implemented if the patient does not respond to the step one or two drugs. In step three, there are three options: increase the dosage of those drugs prescribed in step two, add a third drug, or try a different drug from step one.

SPECIFIC ANTIHYPERTENSIVE DRUGS

Diuretics. Diuretics lower blood pressure by reducing blood volume through promotion of renal excretion of sodium and water. They also seem to decrease the sensitivity of blood vessels to catecholamines. There are several types of diuretics: thiazide, loop (high ceiling), and potassium sparing. Among the diuretics that may be used to treat hypertension are hydrochlorothiazide (HCTZ) and spironolactone (Aldactone).

Patients taking diuretics must be monitored for fluid and electrolyte imbalances, especially hypovolemia and potassium imbalances. Intake and output records may be kept on hospitalized patients who are taking diuretics.

Hypokalemia is a potentially serious problem except with potassium-sparing diuretics. The nurse should monitor for signs of hypokalemia: confusion, irritability, muscle weakness, and anorexia. To prevent hypokalemia, the patient should consume additional dietary potassium. Sources of potassium include bananas and orange juice. Some patients require supplementary potassium.

PHARMACOLOGY CAPSULE

When patients are taking diuretics, monitor for signs and symptoms of hypokalemia: cardiac dysrhythmias, muscle weakness, and diminished bowel sounds.

Beta-Adrenergic Receptor Blockers. These agents, commonly called beta blockers, reduce blood pressure by blocking the beta effects of catecholamines. A commonly used beta blocker is propranolol (Inderal). When beta receptors are stimulated, they stimulate the heart and relax bronchial smooth muscle. Beta blockers prevent this stimulation, resulting in decreased heart rate, decreased strength of cardiac contraction, and bronchial constriction. There are a number of beta blockers that have slightly different effects. Some affect cardiac function more, others have a greater effect on the bronchi.

Common side effects of beta blockers include bradycardia and hypotension, hypoglycemia, and increased low-density lipoprotein in the blood. Beta blockers are used cautiously in patients with asthma, diabetes, and chronic obstructive pulmonary disease. When a patient is taking a beta blocker, the nurse should monitor for bradycardia and hypotension. People with diabetes should be watched carefully for hypoglycemia since beta blockers lower blood glucose and mask the usual signs of hypoglycemia. Diaphoresis (excessive perspiration) may be the only sign of hypoglycemia when people with diabetes are taking beta blockers.

PHARMACOLOGY CAPSULE

Monitor people with diabetes for low blood glucose if they are taking beta blockers.

Calcium Antagonists. Calcium antagonists are called calcium channel blockers because they block the movement of calcium into cardiac and vascular smooth muscle cells. This action reduces the heart rate, decreases the force of cardiac contraction, and dilates peripheral blood vessels. Since dilated vessels present less resistance to blood flow, blood pressure is reduced. Verapamil (Calan) is an example of a calcium channel blocker used for hypertension.

Common side effects of calcium channel blockers are flushing, dizziness, and headache. The nurse should also monitor for hypotension and bradycardia.

Angiotensin-Converting Enzyme Inhibitors. These inhibitors prevent the conversion of angiotensin I to angiotensin II, a potent vasoconstrictor. Blocking the production of angiotensin II decreases peripheral resistance. ACE inhibitors also decrease fluid retention by decreasing the production of aldosterone. Examples of ACE inhibitors are captopril (Capoten) and enalapril (Vasotec).

Adverse effects can include a skin rash, neutropenia, and proteinuria. Acute renal failure occurs in some patients.

OTHER ANTIHYPERTENSIVE DRUGS. Other drugs used to treat hypertension include central adrenergic blockers, alpha-adrenergic blockers, and direct vasodilators.

Central Adrenergic Blockers. Central adrenergic blockers inhibit impulses from the vasomotor center in the brain that maintain the muscle tone in blood vessels. The effect of this type of drug is to reduce peripheral resistance and lower blood pressure. Examples of centrally acting adrenergic blockers are clonidine (Catapres) and methyldopa (Aldomet).

Alpha-Adrenergic Receptor Blockers. Stimulation of alpha receptors produces constriction of arterioles. Drugs such as prazosin (Minipress) block alpha receptor effects and lower blood pressure by reducing peripheral resistance. The most important adverse effect is orthostatic hypotension, which is most severe with initial or increased dosages. Patients should lie down for 2 hours after taking a first or increased dose of this drug. Alpha blockers can also cause dizziness, headache, and drowsiness.

Direct Vasodilators. Direct vasodilators lower blood pressure by relaxing arteriolar smooth muscle. Examples of direct vasodilators are hydralazine (Apresoline), diazoxide (Hyperstat IV), and sodium nitroprusside (Nipride). Diazoxide and sodium nitroprusside are used to treat hypertensive crisis. Diazoxide is given by direct intravenous injection. Sodium nitroprusside is diluted in intravenous fluids and administered at the rate needed for the desired results.

NURSING IMPLICATIONS. The nurse needs to be familiar with the drugs commonly prescribed for hypertension. Nursing responsibilities include administering the drugs to inpatients, monitoring for therapeutic and adverse effects, and teaching patients about their drugs. Additional information about antihypertensive drugs and nursing interventions is presented in Table 33–4.

The elderly respond differently to drug therapy. Older patients are at risk for adverse effects of medications because of reduced liver and kidney function. They are especially susceptible to orthostatic hypotension because their blood vessels respond more slowly to position changes. This creates increased risk for falls.

Older people may respond differently to beta blockers and to diuretics. The effectiveness of beta blockers may be reduced because beta receptor activity is lessened in the elderly. In addition, diuretics may produce a more profound decrease in blood volume in these patients.

Often elderly patients are also taking medications for other diseases. Drug interactions can alter therapeutic effects or enhance side effects. Dosages for antihyper-

TABLE 33-4

ANTIHYPERTENSIVE DRUGS AND NURSING INTERVENTIONS

DRUG	USE/ACTION	SIDE EFFECTS	NURSING INTERVENTIONS
General Considerations 1. Monitor blood pressure (BP) regularly with patient in supine, sitting, and standing positions. 2. Encourage patients to take medications and keep follow-up appointments even when feeling well. 3. Teach patients with orthostatic hypotension to rise slowly, avoid prolonged standing, and avoid hot baths and showers. 4. Advise patients to consult physician or pharmacist about safety of over-the-counter drugs. 5. Do not stop drugs abruptly because rebound hypertension may occur.			
Centrally acting drugs	Act on central nervous system to block vasoconstriction, which lowers BP. Also reduces anxiety.	Drowsiness, dry mouth, weakness, depression, retention of sodium and water. Orthostatic hypotension with some drugs.	Monitor BP. Safety precautions. Oral hygiene. Assess for edema. Teach patient to manage orthostatic hypotension.
Ganglionic blockers	Block transmission of nerve impulses that constrict blood vessels. Vessels dilate, reducing BP.	Sodium and water retention, bradycardia, impaired ejaculation, nasal stuffiness, gastrointestinal disturbances. Some drugs cause orthostatic hypotension.	Monitor pulse and BP. Assess for edema, sexual dysfunction. Give with meals to reduce gastrointestinal distress. Teach patient to manage orthostatic hypotension.
Alpha-adrenergic blockers	Block effects of norepinephrine, causing vasodilation.	Reflex tachycardia, palpitations, headache, dizziness, drowsiness, nausea. Potentially severe orthostatic hypotension with first or increased dose of prazosin.	Monitor pulse and BP. Advise patient that most side effects diminish over time. Give first or increased dose of prazosin at bedtime. Advise of possible orthostatic hypotension.
Beta-adrenergic blockers	Decrease cardiac stimulation.	Bradycardia, fatigue, drowsiness, depression, hypoglycemia, bronchial constriction.	Monitor pulse, BP, and respiration. Assess emotional status. Monitor asthmatics for dyspnea, diabetics for low blood glucose.
Direct vasodilators	Relax vascular smooth muscle, causing vasodilation.	Reflex tachycardia, headache, dizziness, nausea and vomiting, anorexia, hypotension.	Monitor pulse and BP.
Calcium channel blockers	Decrease force of cardiac contraction and dilate peripheral blood vessels.	Bradycardia, flushing, dizziness, headache.	Monitor pulse.
Angiotensin-converting enzyme inhibitors	Reduce aldosterone secretion and prevent formation of angiotensin II, which decreases peripheral resistance and fluid volume.	Skin rash, neutropenia. Renal failure in patients with renal artery stenosis.	Monitor blood cell counts. Report changes in urine output.
Diuretics	Reduce fluid volume. May cause vasodilation. Sodium loss may reduce vasoconstriction.	Fluid volume deficit, hyponatremia, hypokalemia (except with potassium-sparing diuretics).	Monitor fluid balance: hydration, urine output, mental status, muscle tone. Recommend foods high in potassium (bananas, orange juice) unless on potassium-sparing diuretics.

tensive medications may need to be reduced or adjusted depending on what diseases the patient has.

NURSING CARE OF THE PATIENT WITH HYPERTENSION

ASSESSMENT

Early detection, education, and promotion of adherence are the keys to blood pressure control. Periodic blood pressure checks detect new or unknown hypertensives and provide data to evaluate the effect of therapy in known hypertensives.

The nursing assessment of the known or suspected hypertensive begins with a complete history and physical examination.

Health History

The patient's reason for seeking health care is noted. Since hypertension often has no symptoms, the visit may be related to some other problem. The past medical history is explored to determine whether the patient has ever had renal, cardiac, or endocrine disorders or hypertension. The date and readings of the last blood pressure measurement are noted. If the patient is female, the nurse asks about pregnancy. Current medications, including over-the-counter drugs, are listed. A family health history includes the presence of hypertension, myocardial infarction, or cerebrovascular accidents among the patient's relatives.

The nurse then reviews the body systems for significant signs and symptoms, particularly headaches, epistaxis, dizziness, visual disturbances, dyspnea, angina, or nocturia. The functional assessment may detect some potential risk factors for hypertension. It includes occupation, exercise and activity, sleep and rest, nutrition, interpersonal relationships, and stressors.

Physical Examination

While taking the health history and beginning the physical examination, the nurse observes the patient's general appearance, noting any obvious distress. Height and weight and vital signs are measured. The nurse may be the first to detect elevated pressure, so accurate measurement of blood pressure is very important. The proper cuff size is essential. Too small a cuff may give a false high reading, whereas a cuff that is too large may give a false low reading.

The blood pressure should be assessed in both arms in the supine, sitting, and standing positions. Blood pressure assessment begins with the patient resting supine for at least 10 minutes. Following supine blood pressure assessment, the sitting and then the standing readings are taken after 1 to 3 minutes in each position. When body position is altered from supine to standing, the SBP normally falls approximately 10 mm Hg and the DBP rises approximately 5 mm Hg. The apical and peripheral pulses are assessed for rate, rhythm, and quality or character in each position.

TABLE 33-5

ASSESSMENT OF THE PATIENT WITH KNOWN OR SUSPECTED HYPERTENSION

HEALTH HISTORY

Present illness: Description of reason for seeking care
Past medical history: Renal, cardiac, or endocrine disorders; hypertension; last blood pressure reading; pregnancy; current medications
Family history: Hypertension, myocardial infarction, cerebrovascular accident
Review of systems: Headache, dizziness, epistaxis, visual disturbances, dyspnea, angina, nocturia
Functional assessment: Occupation, activity and exercise, sleep and rest, nutrition, interpersonal relationships, current stressors

PHYSICAL EXAMINATION

General appearance: Distress
Height and weight
Vital signs
  Blood pressure: supine, sitting, standing
  Pulse
  Respiration
  Temperature
Extremities: Edema
Neuromuscular: Abnormalities

If blood pressure is elevated initially, it should be reassessed after 1 to 5 minutes. If the pressure remains elevated, the patient should be referred for medical evaluation. The nurse should remember that a single elevated reading does not mean that the patient has hypertension. If the blood pressure is severely elevated (DBP of 115 or more), the patient is in imminent danger of a stroke and immediate medical care is needed.

In addition to blood pressure and pulses, the nurse assesses respiratory rate and effort. Extremities are inspected for edema and color. Any abnormalities in neurologic or muscular function are also noted.

Nursing assessment of the patient with known or suspected hypertension is summarized in Table 33–5.

NURSING DIAGNOSIS

Nursing diagnoses for the patient with hypertension may include the following:

- **Knowledge Deficit** of hypertension and measures to control it
- **Noncompliance** related to negative side effects of prescribed drug therapy
- **High Risk for Injury** related to orthostatic hypotension secondary to antihypertensive drug therapy, sedation
- **Ineffective Individual Coping** related to depression secondary to antihypertensive drug therapy
- **Sexual Dysfunction** related to medication side effects

GOALS

The goals of nursing care are patient's understanding of hypertension and its treatment, patient's adherence to prescribed treatment, absence of injury, effective coping with depression, and satisfactory sexual function.

INTERVENTIONS

Knowledge Deficit

Frequent communication with a health care provider and active participation in a wellness program are encouraged for each person with hypertension. Members of the patient's household, especially a spouse, should be included in the teaching. Their understanding and cooperation can be very supportive to the patient.

Education begins as soon as the condition is diagnosed and continues throughout life. The patient should be able to understand the disease process and adhere to the treatment regimen with minimal adverse effects. Patient teaching focuses on understanding hypertension and managing it with diet, exercise, smoking cessation, stress management, and drug therapy. Complications are discussed, but the nurse emphasizes that controlling hypertension reduces the risk of complications.

As with any patient teaching, the nurse begins by finding out what the person already knows and is most interested in learning. By addressing the patient's immediate concerns first, the nurse builds trust that should facilitate further teaching. Measures to manage hypertension should not be presented as a long list of "don'ts" but, rather, as health practices that are beneficial to everyone.

Patients are taught to take their own blood pressures on a regular basis and report the findings to a health care provider. Generally, blood pressure readings obtained in the home are more valid measures because patients are more relaxed there than in a clinic or office.

DIET. The goals of diet therapy for the person with hypertension are to maintain ideal body weight and to prevent fluid retention. Total calorie intake may need to be adjusted to achieve that goal. A diet low in saturated fats with no more than 2 grams of sodium is often prescribed. Sodium restriction is more effective for some patients than for others.

Potassium intake may need to be increased if the patient is taking diuretics that result in excretion of potassium. Potassium supplements may be necessary for patients taking potassium-wasting diuretics.

The nurse and the dietitian should cooperate in teaching patients about their prescribed dietary alterations. If someone other than the patient prepares the food at home, that person should be included during the dietary teaching.

EXERCISE. Nutrition and exercise go hand in hand. It is very difficult to maintain or lose weight without engaging in some form of exercise. Walking is highly recommended as an exercise that increases cardiovascular functioning, burns calories, relieves stress, and promotes well-being. An exercise program can benefit people of all ages, even the elderly. The nurse advises patients to ask their physicians before beginning new exercise programs. They are told to gradually increase their activities over a period of time.

When people engage in a program of good nutrition and exercise, it is often possible to decrease or eliminate medications used to control hypertension.

STRESS MANAGEMENT. Patients need to understand how stress affects blood pressure. The nurse can help them to identify stressors in their lives and explore ways to reduce them. Referrals to professional counselors may be in order for patients with complicated or multiple stressors. Some agencies or community centers offer classes in stress management or relaxation techniques.

DRUG THERAPY. Patients need to be well informed about their medications. The name, dosage, purpose, and side effects of any prescribed medication are reviewed with the patient. The nurse advises the patient not to discontinue the drug or change the dosage without consulting with the physician. Suddenly stopping antihypertensive drugs may produce adverse effects, including rebound hypertension (sudden return of elevated blood pressure), myocardial infarction, and cerebrovascular accident.

Noncompliance

Adherence to therapy requires commitment and active participation on the part of the patient. Lifestyle changes may be required, and pharmacologic side effects may be unpleasant. Failure to follow the prescribed regimen is referred to as noncompliance. Some people prefer the term nonadherence. In counseling the patient, it must be stressed that hypertension is a chronic disease requiring long-term management. Lack of symptoms or reduction of blood pressure often prompts patients to discontinue drug therapy inappropriately.

Teaching patients about their medications will hopefully promote adherence. Information in writing and a chart with times for medication administration may be helpful.

Patients who do not take their medications as prescribed often cite the adverse side effects as reasons for noncompliance. It is important to teach patients to report unpleasant drug side effects to the physician promptly. A change in dosage or in the medication itself may reduce undesirable effects, but the patient should not make changes unless advised to do so by the physician. Common side effects of antihypertensive drugs that may affect adherence are orthostatic hypotension, sedation, sexual dysfunction, and depression.

PHARMACOLOGY CAPSULE

Advise patients not to discontinue antihypertensive therapy simply because they feel well. Blood pressure can be very high with no symptoms.

Injury

The patient taking antihypertensive medications may be at risk for injury owing to drug side effects. The effects that pose the greatest potential for injury are orthostatic hypotension and sedation.

ORTHOSTATIC HYPOTENSION. Orthostatic or postural hypotension is a sudden drop in SBP, usually 20 mm Hg, when going from a lying or sitting position to a standing position. Patients at risk for orthostatic hypotension are monitored for lightheadness, dizziness, and syncope (fainting). This is an especially dangerous side effect for the elderly person, who may be seriously injured in a fall.

Patients who are prone to orthostatic hypotension are instructed to rise slowly from a lying or sitting position. Contraindicated are activities that cause blood pressure to fall, such as prolonged standing in one place and taking very hot baths or showers.

PHARMACOLOGY CAPSULE

Tell patients how to manage orthostatic hypotension associated with antihypertensive therapy.

SEDATION. Sedation may be dealt with by taking medications at bedtime to promote sleep. Advise patients if drowsiness is likely so that dangerous activities or those requiring alertness can be avoided during times of peak drug effect.

Coping

If depression occurs as a side effect of an antihypertensive drug, the physician should be consulted so that another drug may be substituted. This side effect should be taken very seriously. Patients with severe depression are referred to a mental health professional.

Sexual Dysfunction

A common side effect of many antihypertensive medications is sexual dysfunction. Dysfunctions may take the form of decreased libido, inability to achieve an erection, or delayed ejaculation.

Many patients consider sexual function to be a very personal subject, so it must be handled in a sensitive manner. Some patients volunteer information about sexual changes. Others may fail to relate the problem to their medications and not report it to the nurse or the physician. The nurse can introduce the subject by saying, "Some people taking this medication have changes in sexual function. Has this been a problem for you?" If it is a problem for the patient, the physician should be advised so that an alternative medication can be considered.

EVALUATION

The following criteria are used for evaluating the outcomes of nursing interventions: patient's correct explanation of hypertension and its treatment, evidence of adherence to prescribed treatment (weight loss, cessation of smoking, lowered blood pressure), absence of injury related to orthostatic hypotension or sedation, positive emotional state, and patient's statement of ability to manage effects of drug therapy on sexual function.

OLDER PATIENTS

Planning nursing care for older hypertensive patients requires some additional considerations. Response to drug therapy is more difficult to predict, and side effects are more common. Orthostatic hypotension and sedation are especially problematic for the older person, who is prone to fall and suffer serious injuries. Depression also must be taken very seriously because it lowers motivation, impairs quality of life, and can lead to suicide.

Health care providers tend to assume that the elderly are not sexually active. Therefore, they often fail to assess sexual function or dysfunction in older people. This is a real disservice to the older person whose sexual functioning is impaired as a result of antihypertensive drugs. The older patient should be treated just like a younger patient in the assessment and management of distressing drug effects.

HYPERTENSIVE EMERGENCIES

Hypertensive crisis is a life-threatening medical emergency. The patient presents with severe headache, blurred vision, nausea, restlessness, and confusion. Along with a very elevated DBP (130 mm Hg or more), the heart and respiratory rates are increased. This episode may result from having stopped taking antihypertensive drugs or may be caused by malignant hypertension, hypertensive encephalopathy, eclampsia, pheochromocytoma (adrenal tumor), or a cerebrovascular accident.

Without appropriate treatment, the patient may develop cardiac and renal damage. Death may ensue as a result of a cerebrovascular accident, renal failure, or cardiac failure.

Malignant hypertension is a specific type of hypertensive emergency in which the DBP exceeds 140 mm Hg. It has a sudden onset and is seen most often in black males aged 30 to 40.

MEDICAL DIAGNOSIS

Assessment in the emergency room reveals elevated blood pressure, pulse, and respiratory rate. Retinal hemorrhage or papilledema, or both, can be observed in the fundus (back, interior portion) of the eye.

The physician orders blood drawn for arterial blood gases, complete blood count, electrolytes, blood urea nitrogen, creatinine, and cardiac enzymes. A chest ra-

TABLE 33-6
EMERGENCY ANTIHYPERTENSIVE DRUGS

Hydralazine (Apresoline)
Sodium nitroprusside (Nipride)
Diazoxide (Hyperstat)
Labetalol (Normodyne)
Methyldopa (Aldomet)
Nitroglycerin (Nitro-Bid)
Trimethaphan (Arfonad)
Mecamylamine (Inversine)

Data from Shlafer, M. (1993). *The nurse, pharmacology, and drug therapy* (2nd ed., p. 673). New York: Addison-Wesley.

diograph may be requested. Direct blood pressure monitoring through an arterial catheter is preferred.

MEDICAL TREATMENT

The goal of drug therapy is to rapidly reduce the pressure to a non–life-threatening level and then to slowly bring it within normal range. This is done with diuretics and potent vasodilators. Examples of drugs that may be ordered include diazoxide, hydralazine, phentolamine, labetalol, and nitroprusside. An intravenous line is usually established because many drugs are given by that route. Drugs used to treat hypertensive crisis are listed in Table 33–6.

NURSING CARE OF THE PATIENT IN HYPERTENSIVE CRISIS

ASSESSMENT

The patient in hypertensive crisis must be closely monitored. The nurse assesses the patient's blood pressure, pulse, respiration, and level of consciousness frequently. Some drugs are given in intravenous fluids, requiring continuous monitoring and adjustment. A careful record of fluid intake and output should be kept.

Nausea and vomiting should alert the nurse to observe the patient closely since these symptoms may indicate an impending seizure or coma.

NURSING INTERVENTIONS

The nurse's role in caring for the patient in hypertensive crisis includes administering prescribed drugs, monitoring vital signs before and after each drug dose, assessing cardiac and renal function, starting and maintaining intravenous therapy and oxygen as ordered, and comforting the patient.

Appropriate safety measures should be taken if the patient shows signs of seizure activity or a decreasing level of consciousness. Bed siderails should be raised and padded if necessary. Elevation of the head of the bed facilitates breathing. An oral airway and suction equipment should be at the bedside. Brief explanations or words of encouragement may help to allay some of the patient's anxiety.

As the patient's condition improves, it is important for the nurse to explain how to manage hypertension and to prevent future crises from developing. Adherence to the prescribed regimen and regular follow-up care are necessary for all patients with hypertension.

NUTRITION CONCEPTS

- Diet and lifestyle changes, including weight reduction, exercise, and stress management, are important in the treatment of hypertension.
- Weight loss in obese individuals lowers blood pressure at a rate of 1 mm Hg per kg (2.2 pounds) of body weight.
- Sodium-restricted diets help lower blood pressure in many individuals with hypertension.
- A high potassium intake may help lower blood pressure as well as replace potassium lost with potassium-wasting diuretics. Foods particularly high in potassium are fresh fruits and vegetables.
- An adequate calcium intake may help in preventing and treating hypertension. Two to three cups of milk or yogurt per day, 4 ounces of low-sodium cheese, or calcium supplements (calcium carbonate, 1–2 grams/day) can provide adequate calcium intake.

Hypertension is a common and serious chronic condition. The nurse is often the first person to detect it in symptom-free patients. Nurses can promote adherence to treatment plans by teaching and counseling patients about hypertension. Effective management significantly reduces the risk of complications in many patients.

BIBLIOGRAPHY

Barrows, J. J. (1992). Nursing role in management: Blood pressure disturbances. In S. M. Lewis & I. C. Collier (Eds.), *Medical-surgical nursing*. St. Louis: Mosby Year Book.

Cerrato, P. L. (1990). Hypertension: The role of diet and lifestyle. *RN*, *53*(12), 46–51.

Hill, M. N., & Grim, C. M. (1991). How to take a precise blood pressure. *American Journal of Nursing*, *91*(2), 38–42.

Ignatavicius, D. D., & Bayne, M. V. (1991). *Medical-surgical nursing: A nursing process approach*. Philadelphia: W. B. Saunders.

Jarvis, C. (1992). *Physical examination and health assessment*. Philadelphia: W. B. Saunders.

Johannsen, J. M. (1993). Update: Guidelines for treating hypertension. *American Journal of Nursing*. *93*(3), 42–52.

Matteson, M. A., & McConnell, E. S. (1989). *Gerontological nursing*. Philadelphia: W. B. Saunders.

Nash, C. (1990). New once daily antihypertensive is added to beta-blocker group. *American Journal of Nursing, 90*(3), 65–66.

Nash, C. (1992). How do you test a digital sphygmomanometer? *American Journal of Nursing, 92*(1), 66–70.

Newborn, V. B. (1991). Cautionary tales on using beta-blockers. *Geriatric Nursing, 12*(3), 119–122.

Shlafer, M. (1991). Solid grounds for treating elders' systolic hypertension. *American Journal of Nursing, 91*(10), 18.

Shlafer, M. (1993). *The nurse, pharmacology, and drug therapy* (2nd ed.). Redwood City, CA: Addison-Wesley.

Trottier, D. J., & Kochar, M. S. (1992). Hypertension and high cholesterol: A dangerous synergy. *American Journal of Nursing. 92*(11), 40–43.

KEY CONCEPTS

1. Hypertension is called the silent killer because it often has no symptoms and is not discovered until a serious complication develops such as damage to the blood vessels in the kidneys, eyes, heart, or brain.
2. Hypertension is defined as a persistent elevation of arterial blood pressure greater than 140/90 mm Hg.
3. Essential hypertension has no known cause, whereas secondary hypertension is caused by an underlying factor such as kidney disease.
4. The two factors that determine blood pressure are cardiac output and peripheral vascular resistance.
5. The primary risk factors for essential hypertension are obesity, atherosclerosis, cigarette smoking, and sedentary lifestyle.
6. Blood pressure tends to rise as people age, but age is not a barrier to aggressive treatment of hypertension.
7. Hypertension often has no symptoms, but some people experience occipital headaches, lightheadedness, and epistaxis.
8. A diagnosis of hypertension is usually based on multiple readings and is accompanied by tests to rule out possible correctable causes.
9. Conservative measures to treat hypertension include weight reduction, smoking cessation, sodium restriction, exercise, relaxation techniques, and modified alcohol intake.
10. Pharmacologic treatment is based on the stepped-care approach, which begins with the prescription of a single, relatively safe drug and advances through specific steps until good control is achieved.
11. Types of drugs used to treat hypertension include diuretics, beta-adrenergic receptor blockers, calcium channel blockers, angiotensin-converting enzyme inhibitors, central adrenergic blockers, alpha-adrenergic blockers, and direct vasodilators.
12. Nursing care of the hypertensive person addresses knowledge deficits, noncompliance or nonadherence, high risk for injury, ineffective individual coping, and sexual dysfunction.
13. Hypertensive crisis, defined as a diastolic blood pressure of 130 mm Hg or more, is a life-threatening medical emergency that is usually treated with diuretics and potent vasodilators.
14. Complications of hypertensive crisis include stroke, heart failure, and kidney failure.

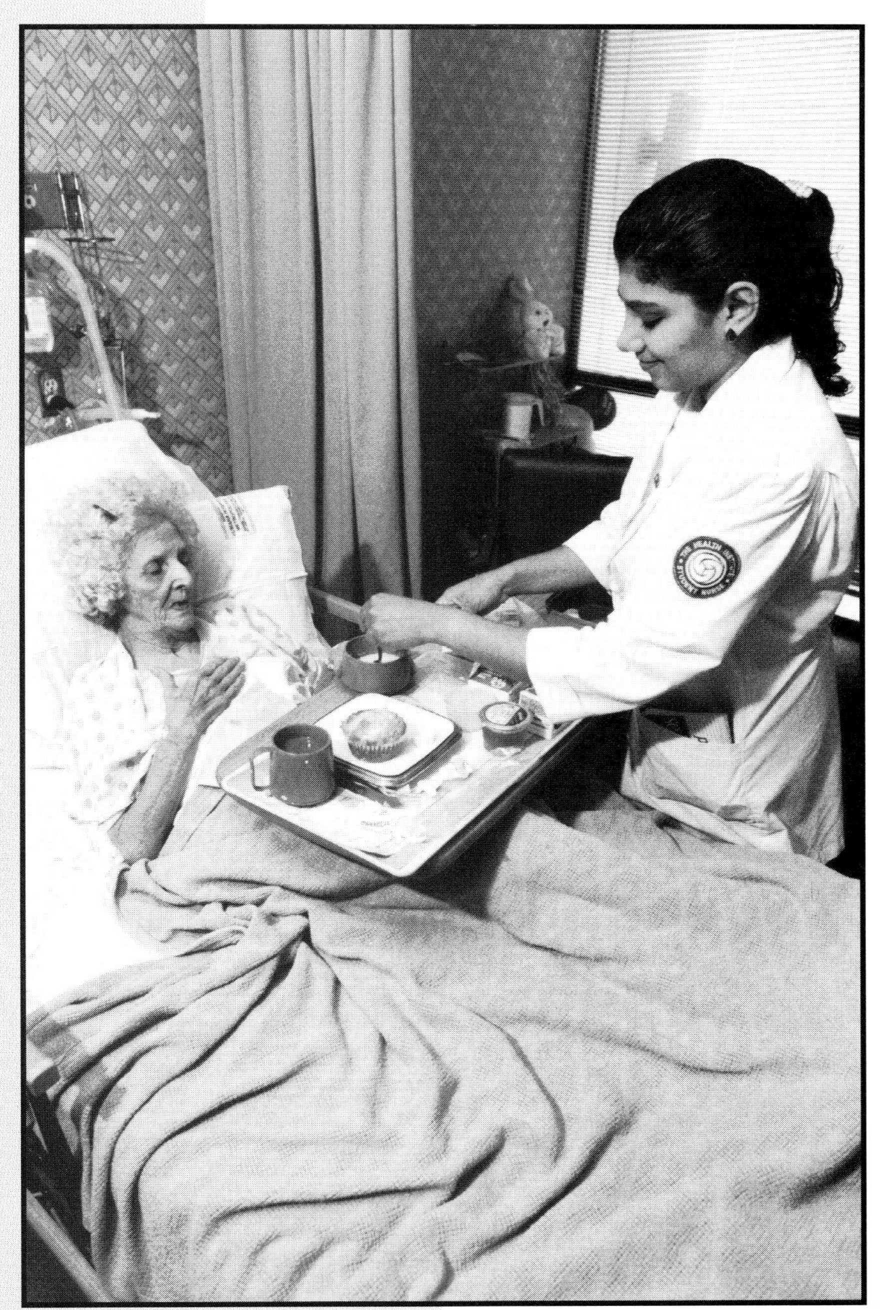

UNIT 9 Digestive Disorders

Adrianne Linton

CHAPTER 34

Digestive Tract Disorders

OBJECTIVES

1. List the nursing responsibilities in the care of patients undergoing diagnostic tests and procedures for disorders of the digestive tract.
2. List the data to be included in the nursing assessment of the patient with a digestive disorder.
3. Describe the nursing care of patients with gastrointestinal intubation and decompression, tube feedings, total parenteral nutrition, digestive tract surgery, and drug therapy for digestive disorders.
4. Describe the pathophysiology, signs and symptoms, complications, and medical treatment of selected digestive disorders.
5. Apply the nursing process to develop nursing care plans for patients receiving treatment for digestive disorders.

GLOSSARY

ANOREXIA Lack of appetite for food

CARIES Destructive process of tooth decay

CATHARTIC Agent that stimulates bowel evacuation; usually rapid in effect and producing a watery stool

DYSPEPSIA Epigastric discomfort after meals, caused by impaired digestion

DYSPHAGIA Difficulty swallowing

EMESIS Vomiting

ERUCTATION Expulsion of gas from the stomach through the mouth; belching

FLATULENCE Formation of excessive gas in the stomach or intestines

FLATUS Gas in the digestive tract that is expelled through the rectum

Glossary continued

GINGIVITIS Inflammation of the gums

LAXATIVE Agent that softens stool and promotes bowel evacuation

PERITONEUM Membrane that lines the walls of the abdominal and pelvic cavities

PERITONITIS Inflammation of the peritoneum

REGURGITATION Gentle ejection of stomach contents into the mouth without nausea or retching

STOMATITIS Inflammation of the oral mucosa

To remain healthy, the human body must have a steady supply of nutrients and fluids. The primary role of the digestive tract is to extract the essential molecules from food and fluids to maintain cellular function. Disorders of the digestive tract can threaten the patient's nutritional status, leading to disorders in the structure and functioning of other body systems.

ANATOMY AND PHYSIOLOGY OF THE DIGESTIVE TRACT

The functions of the digestive tract are digestion, absorption, and elimination. Digestion is the breakdown of food into simple nutrient molecules that can be used by the cells. The process of digestion requires (1) the adequate intake of food and fluids, (2) the mechanical and chemical breakdown of food, and (3) the movement of food through the digestive tract. Absorption is the transfer of digested food molecules from the digestive tract into the blood stream. Elimination is the removal of solid food wastes from the body.

The digestive tract is also called the gastrointestinal tract (or GI tract) and the alimentary tract (Fig. 34–1). It is a muscular tube about 30 feet long. The main parts of the digestive tract are the mouth, pharynx, esophagus, stomach, small intestine, large intestine, and anus.

Other organs that are outside the digestive tract but considered part of the digestive system are called accessory organs. Accessory organs include the salivary glands, liver, gallbladder, and pancreas. Each of these secretes fluid containing specialized enzymes into the digestive tract. These enzymes play a part in the breakdown or metabolism of foodstuffs (Table 34–1).

A two-layer membrane, the peritoneum, lines the abdominal cavity and covers the surfaces of the abdominal organs. Lubricating fluid between the two layers permits the organs to move without friction during breathing and digestive movements.

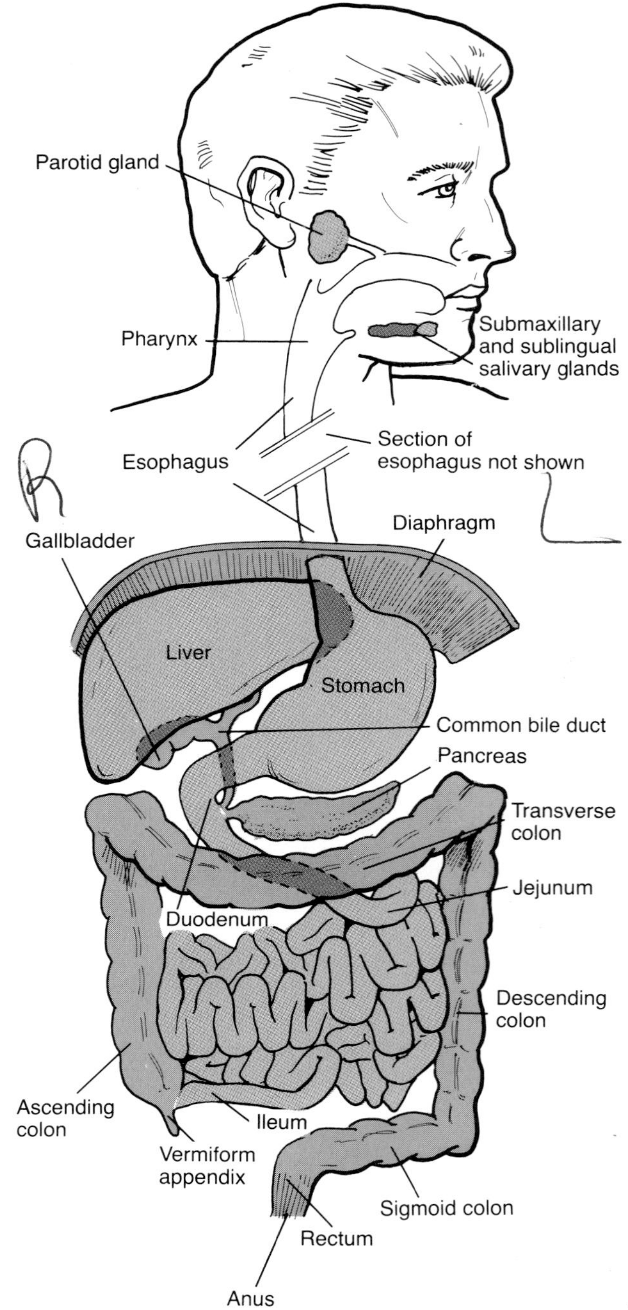

FIGURE 34–1

The digestive tract and associated structures.

MOUTH

Food is taken into the mouth, where the teeth, tongue, and salivary glands begin the process of food digestion. As the teeth cut and grind the food, the salivary glands secrete saliva, a watery solution that contains ptyalin. Ptyalin is an enzyme that initiates the breakdown of carbohydrates. The tongue helps by mixing saliva with the food and pressing it against the teeth. When the bolus is to be swallowed, the tongue forces the food into the pharynx.

PHARYNX

The pharynx is a muscular structure that is shared by the digestive and respiratory tracts. It joins the mouth and nasal passages to the esophagus. During swallowing,

TABLE 34-1
DIGESTIVE ENZYMES AND SUBSTRATES

SITE	ENZYME	SUBSTRATE		
		Carbohydrates	Protein	Fats
Mouth	Ptyalin	X		
Stomach	Rennin		X	
	Pepsin		X	
	Lipase			X
Small intestine	Pancreatic enzymes:			
	Trypsin		X	
	Chymotrypsin		X	
	Carboxypolypeptidase		X	
	Ribonuclease		X	
	Deoxyribonuclease		X	
	Elastase		X	
	Lipase			X
	Cholesterase ester			X
	α-Amylase	X		
	Small intestine enzymes:			
	Carboxypeptidase		X	
	Aminopeptidase		X	
	Dipeptidase		X	
	Nucleosidase		X	
	Enterokinase		X	
	Lipase			X
	Sucrase	X		
	α-Dextrinase	X		
	Maltase	X		
	Lactase	X		

the epiglottis covers the airway like a trapdoor to prevent food from entering the respiratory tract.

ESOPHAGUS

Food moves from the pharynx into the esophagus, a long muscular tube that passes through the diaphragm into the stomach. Gravity helps, but is not essential for, the movement of food through the esophagus. Circular, wave-like contractions of the muscles of the digestive tract propel food down the tract. This movement is called peristalsis.

STOMACH

The stomach is the widest section of the digestive tract. It is separated from the esophagus by the cardiac sphincter. The stomach is not very large when empty, but it expands considerably when food is present. It consists of three sections: the fundus, the body, and the pylorus. A unique arrangement of muscle layers allows the stomach to churn the food, mixing it with gastric secretions until it becomes a semiliquid mass called chyme. Gastric secretions include rennin, pepsin, hydrochloric acid, and lipase. Rennin starts to break down milk proteins, lipase breaks down fats, and pepsin and hydrochloric acid partially digest proteins. The pyloric sphincter between the stomach and the small intestine keeps food in the stomach until it is properly mixed.

SMALL INTESTINE

Chyme leaves the stomach and enters the small intestine, where chemical digestion and absorption of nutrients take place. The small intestine is approximately 20 feet long and consists of three sections: the duodenum, the jejunum, and the ileum.

Liver and pancreatic secretions enter the digestive tract in the duodenum. Bile, produced in the liver and stored in the gallbladder, breaks down large fat globules. Pancreatic enzymes further reduce the fat to glycerol and fatty acids, which can easily be absorbed. The functions of the liver, gallbladder, and pancreas are discussed in greater detail in Chapter 35.

Three layers of tissue make up the walls of the small intestine. The inner layer is lined with thousands of microscopic projections called villi. Digested food molecules are absorbed through the villi into the blood stream.

The mucous membrane layer secretes the digestive enzymes sucrase, lactase, maltase, carboxypeptidase, aminopeptidase, dipeptidase, nucleosidase, lipase, and enterokinase. Functions of these enzymes are listed in Table 34–1. Muscle layers contract to continue mixing the chyme, moving it toward the large intestine.

LARGE INTESTINE AND ANUS

Chyme enters the large intestine through the ileocecal valve. The first section of the large intestine is the cecum, where the appendix is located. The large intestine goes up the right side of the abdomen (the ascending colon), across the abdomen just below the waist (the transverse colon), and down the left side of the abdomen (the descending colon). The part of the descending colon between the iliac crest and the rectum is called the sigmoid colon. The last 6 to 8 inches of the large intestine is the rectum, which ends at the anus, where wastes leave the body. The presence of sphincters in the anus allows wastes to be stored until voluntary elimination occurs.

Unlike the small intestine, the large intestine has no villi and secretes no digestive enzymes. Its function is to absorb water from the chyme and eliminate the remaining solid wastes in the form of feces.

AGE-RELATED CHANGES

Normal aging generally does not significantly impair ingestion, digestion, absorption, or elimination. When acute or chronic illnesses occur, however, the older person is at increased risk for problems with digestion and elimination.

The teeth are mechanically worn down with age. They appear darker and somewhat transparent. Gingiva (gums) tend to recede. Although tooth loss is not a normal effect of aging, about half of all Americans 65 and older are edentulous. The main reasons for tooth loss are caries and periodontal disease. Many older people have complete or partial dentures. There is a significant loss of tastebuds with age. Xerostoma (dry mouth) is common but may be caused by poor hydration and drug side effects rather than aging.

The walls of the esophagus and stomach become thinner with aging, and secretions lessen. The production of hydrochloric acid and digestive enzymes decreases. Gastric motor activity slows; thus, gastric emptying is delayed and hunger contractions diminish. There are no significant changes in the small intestine with age. In the large intestine, the muscle layer and mucosa atrophy. Smooth muscle tone and blood flow decrease, and connective tissue increases.

Constipation is a frequent complaint among the elderly, and they use laxatives more often than young people. Many experts believe that constipation is not a normal age-related change but, rather, is caused by such factors as low fluid intake, lack of dietary fiber, inactivity, drugs, depression, and hypothyroidism.

NURSING ASSESSMENT OF THE DIGESTIVE TRACT

A thorough assessment of digestive function provides data about the intake, digestion, and absorption of nutrients and the elimination of solid wastes. The essential data are obtained by interview, objective measurements, inspection, palpation, and auscultation.

HEALTH HISTORY

Chief Complaint and History of Present Illness

The health history begins with a detailed description of the present illness. Complaints may include weight changes, problems with food ingestion, symptoms of digestive disturbances, or alterations in bowel elimination.

Past Medical History

The past medical history documents recent surgery, trauma, burns, or infections. Serious illnesses such as diabetes, hepatitis, anemia, peptic ulcers, gallbladder disease, and cancer are noted. The nurse should also identify any alternative methods of feeding or fecal diversion (ileostomy, colostomy). If feedings are given via nasogastric, gastrostomy, enterostomy, or esophagogastrostomy tubes, the type and amount of feedings should be noted as well as the feeding schedule. The past history also includes a list of recent and current medications, both prescription and over the counter. Use of antacids and laxatives is especially important to elicit. Food allergy or intolerance should be documented, preferably with a description of the reaction that occurs when the offending food is eaten.

Family History

The nurse inquires whether the patient has a family history of diabetes, cancer of the digestive tract, peptic ulcers, gallbladder disease, hepatitis, alcoholism, intestinal polyps, or obesity.

Review of Systems

The review of systems begins with an assessment of general health state. The patient is asked about changes in the skin, including jaundice (yellow color) and pruritus (itching). The nurse assesses the presence of mouth problems, specifically dental caries, lesions, bleeding, increased or decreased salivation, abnormal tastes or odors, and pain. Any difficulties with chewing or swallowing are important to note. The nurse also inquires about changes in appetite, food intake, and weight. If nausea, vomiting, dyspepsia (indigestion), heartburn, or pain is present, the nurse identifies factors that seem to be related to the symptoms. Pain location should be described, along with precipitating factors, relationship to meals, and measures that relieve the pain. Assessment of elimination includes usual bowel habits and recent changes, flatulence (gas), change in stool characteristics (frequency, amount, color, consistency), bleeding, and painful defecation.

PHARMACOLOGY CAPSULE

Many drugs affect gastrointestinal function, causing anorexia, nausea, vomiting, and diarrhea or constipation.

Functional Assessment

The functional assessment focuses on nutrition, activity, and stressors. Information about general dietary habits should include daily pattern of food intake (mealtimes, food eaten in a typical day, food likes and dislikes, and use of food supplements), attitudes and beliefs about food, and changes in dietary habits related to health problems. The effects of the chief complaint on usual functioning are described.

PHYSICAL EXAMINATION

The physical examination begins with the measurement of height, weight, and vital signs. The nurse observes the patient's general appearance and then begins the head and neck examination.

Head and Neck

The mouth should be inspected to determine the condition of the lips, teeth, gums, tongue, and mucous membranes. Moisture, color, and lesions are described. Any unpleasant or unusual odors of the mouth are noted. If the patient has dentures, the mouth should be examined with and without the dentures in place. A tongue blade is needed to depress the tongue and examine the pharynx. The patient is instructed to say "ah" while the nurse observes the movement of the uvula and soft palate. Normally, the uvula and soft palate move upward, with the uvula remaining midline.

Abdomen

For the abdominal examination, the patient should be supine, with the head raised slightly and the knees slightly flexed. The areas of the abdomen are commonly described as quadrants. An imaginary line is drawn horizontally across the abdomen at the level of the umbilicus. A second imaginary line extends from the sternum to the pubic bone. This creates the four quadrants: the right upper quadrant, the left upper quadrant, the right lower quadrant, and the left lower quadrant. Findings can then be documented as to anatomic location (Fig. 34–2).

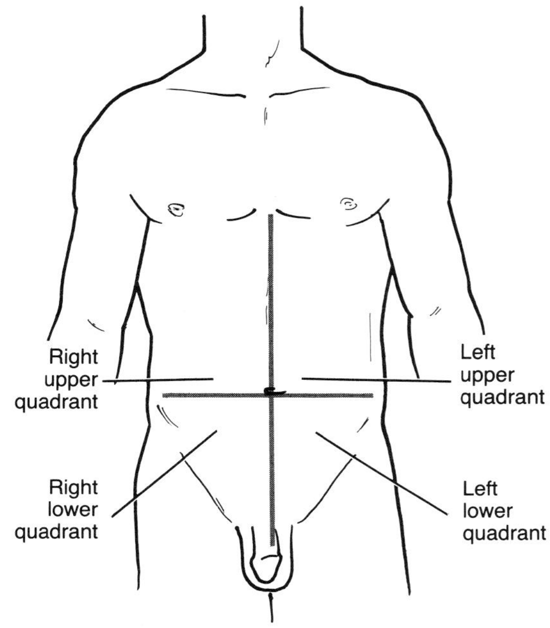

FIGURE 34-2
The abdomen is divided into four quadrants.

INSPECTION. The skin of the abdomen is inspected for color, texture, scars, striae, rashes, lesions, and dilated blood vessels. The general contour of the abdomen is assessed and described as flat, convex (rounded), concave (sunken), protuberant, or distended. The location and contour of the umbilicus are noted. Aortic pulsations and peristalsis are sometimes observed, especially in thin people.

AUSCULTATION. After inspecting the abdomen, the nurse auscultates the abdomen to assess bowel sounds. Auscultation is done before palpation since palpation can alter normal bowel sounds. The diaphragm of the stethoscope should be warmed and used to listen to each quadrant. Normal bowel sounds include clicks and gurgles that occur 5 to 30 times per minute. The nurse should listen for at least 2 minutes in each quadrant. If no sounds are heard, the nurse listens for a full 5 minutes before documenting absence of bowel sounds. Bowel sounds may be described as present, absent, increased, decreased, high pitched, gurgling, tinkling, or gushing. Loud gurgling sounds are called borborygmi.

PERCUSSION. Nurses with advanced training in physical examination use percussion and palpation to collect additional data. Percussion is tapping on the skin to detect the presence of air, fluid, or masses in the underlying tissues. It can also be used to locate the margins of internal organs. Percussion over an air-filled organ produces a high-pitched, hollow sound called tympany. Tympany is similar to the sound made by a kettle drum. Percussion over a solid or fluid-filled structure sounds dull and flat. All four quadrants of the abdomen should be percussed. Normally, tympany is heard more than dullness.

PALPATION. Palpation is done to detect tenderness, sensitivity, masses, swelling, and muscular resistance. The fingers are held together and used to depress the abdomen gently in all four quadrants. Light palpation depresses the abdominal wall only about 1 cm. Deep palpation uses more pressure. To assess for rebound tenderness, the abdomen is depressed and then quickly released. Deep palpation and tests for rebound tenderness should be done only by people who are trained in these techniques.

Rectum and Anus

Gloves should be worn to examine the anal and perianal areas. The perianal skin is inspected for color, rashes, and lesions. External hemorrhoids are noted if present. The rectal examination is performed by a trained examiner. A gloved, lubricated finger is inserted into the rectum pointed toward the umbilicus. The patient is instructed to "bear down" as if to have a bowel movement. This relaxes the anal sphincter. The examiner palpates for lumps and tenderness in the rectum.

Assessment of the patient with a digestive tract disorder is summarized in Table 34–2.

TABLE 34-2

ASSESSMENT OF THE PATIENT WITH A DISORDER OF THE DIGESTIVE TRACT

HEALTH HISTORY

Present illness: Weight changes, problems with food ingestion, symptoms of digestive disturbances, alterations in bowel elimination

Past medical history: Recent surgery, trauma, infections; history of diabetes mellitus, hepatitis, anemia, peptic ulcers, gallbladder disease, cancer; alternative methods of feeding: type, amount, schedule; fecal diversion: type; allergies: food, drugs

Family history: Diabetes mellitus, cancer of the digestive tract, peptic ulcers, gallbladder disease, hepatitis, alcoholism, intestinal polyps, obesity

Review of systems: Skin color, pruritus.

- Oral cavity: Presence and condition of teeth, condition of gums, moisture, pain, abnormal tastes or odors, difficulty chewing
- Appetite
- Dysphagia
- Digestive disturbances: Nausea, vomiting, dyspepsia, heartburn, pain
- Bowel elimination: Changes, pain, flatulence, bleeding, stool characteristics

Functional assessment: Dietary pattern, attitudes and beliefs about food, activity, stressors

PHYSICAL EXAMINATION

Height and weight

Vital signs

General appearance

Head and neck: Condition of teeth, gums, tongue, mucous membranes, odors, uvula position

Abdomen: Skin color, texture, scars, striae, rashes, lesions, dilated blood vessels; abdominal contour, distention; umbilicus location and contour; bowel sounds; abdominal tenderness, masses, swelling, muscular resistance, rebound tenderness

Perianal skin: Color, rash, lesions; hemorrhoids

DIAGNOSTIC TESTS AND PROCEDURES

Diagnostic tests for digestive disorders include radiographic studies, endoscopic examinations, ultrasound studies, magnetic resonance imaging, laboratory studies, and biopsies of gastrointestinal contents.

RADIOGRAPHIC STUDIES

Radiographic studies include the upper gastrointestinal (UGI or GI) series (barium swallow), small bowel series, and barium enema. Radiographs of the gallbladder are obtained as well and are discussed in Chapter 35. These studies allow the radiologist to study the structure and function of the digestive tract. A contrast medium is used in some studies. This is a substance, such as barium sulfate, that can be given orally or by enema. Sometimes air is introduced into the bowel for radiographic studies. This is called an air contrast procedure. When radiographs are taken, the contrast medium outlines the hollow organs of the digestive tract (Fig. 34–3).

PATIENT PREPARATION. When radiographs are ordered, very precise preparation is usually required. Patient instructions include information about the preparation, what to expect during the procedure, and any care needed after the procedure. Details of specific diagnostic tests and procedures are given in Table 34–3. Most hospitals and clinics have a specific protocol to be followed prior to the examination. If the patient is not properly prepared for the procedure, it may have to be repeated.

In general, the preparation is designed to cleanse the upper or lower digestive tract, whichever is being examined. This is done by limiting the intake of food and fluids and by promoting the elimination of wastes. The patient may be limited to clear liquids for a specific period of time, then allowed nothing by mouth for 8 to 12 hours. Bowel cleansing can be accomplished with oral cathartics, rectal suppositories, and enemas. Fluid restriction and bowel cleansing can be difficult for elderly or debilitated patients. If they become exhausted or have changes in their vital signs, the preparation should be stopped and the physician notified.

POSTPROCEDURE CARE. After a patient has taken barium, it is very important to monitor the patient's stools to be sure the barium is eliminated from the body. If it stays in the digestive tract, it can harden and cause an obstruction. Laxatives may be ordered to hasten passage of the barium. Oral fluids also should be encouraged to promote elimination. Stools should be examined until normal color returns. As long as barium remains in the digestive tract, stools are light in color. Figure 34–4 illustrates the time required for food or other substances to move through the digestive tract.

ENDOSCOPIC EXAMINATIONS

Endoscopic examinations permit direct inspection of hollow, interior organs through a lighted tube called an endoscope. Endoscopes may be rigid tubes or flexible fiberscopes.

Endoscopic examinations of the upper gastrointestinal tract include esophagoscopy, gastroscopy, gastroduodenoscopy, esophagogastroduodenoscopy, and endoscopic retrograde cholangiography. The latter is discussed in Chapter 35. Endoscopic examinations of the lower digestive tract include colonoscopy, proctoscopy, and sigmoidoscopy. The names of these examinations sound complicated but can easily be broken down to determine what structures are being studied. Table 34–4 lists prefixes for parts of the digestive system that can be combined with the suffix *-scopy,* meaning "to examine."

PATIENT PREPARATION. Prior to endoscopic examinations, a signed consent may be required. Patients are usually not permitted food or fluids for 6 to 8 hours prior to the examination. Bowel cleansing may be very thorough or may just require enemas. A sedative may be ordered before the procedure to reduce anxiety.

POSTPROCEDURE CARE. Following endoscopic examination of the upper digestive tract, the patient is allowed nothing by mouth (no oral fluids or food) until

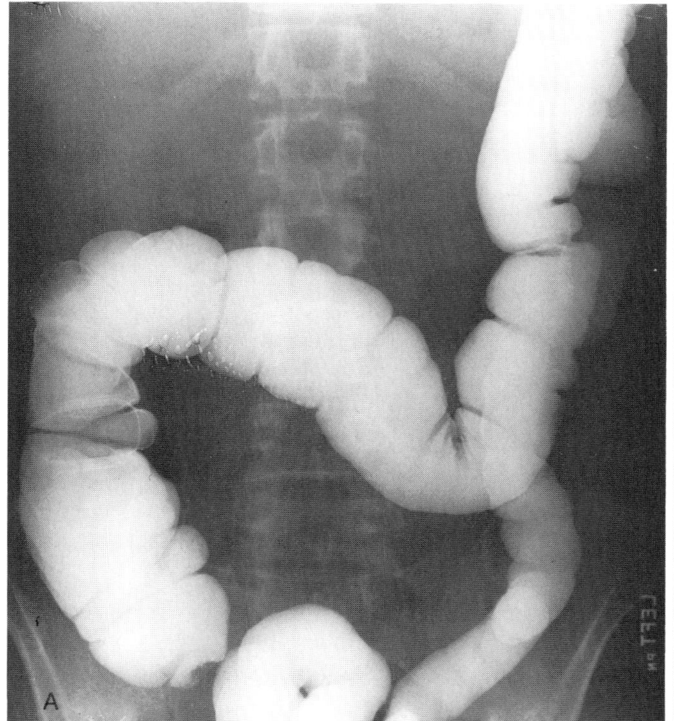

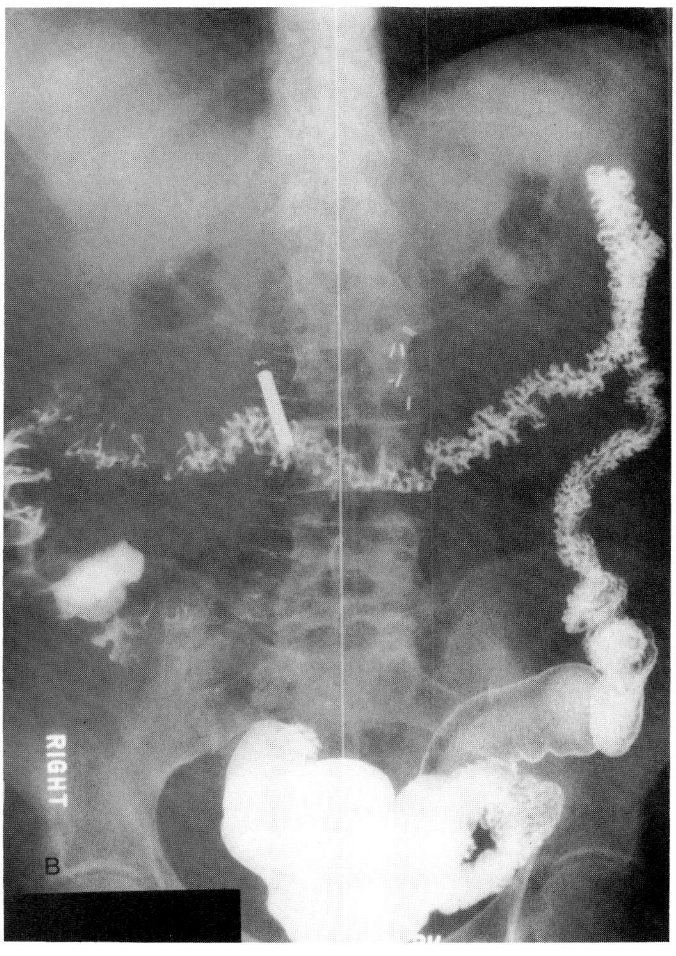

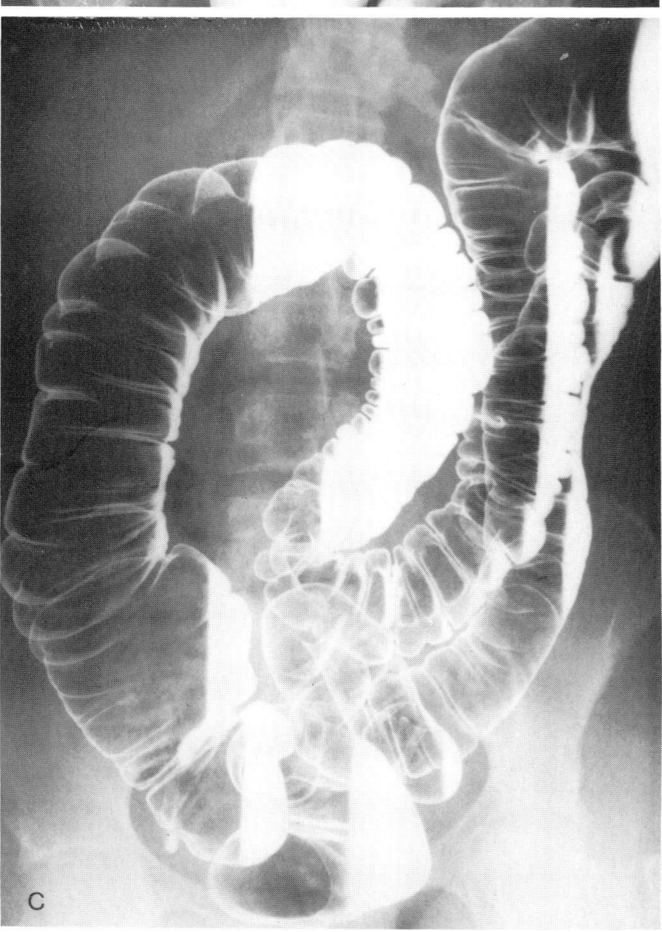

FIGURE 34-3

Contrast media outlines the hollow organs of the digestive tract. (From Laufer, I., & Levine, M. C. [1992]. *Double contrast gastrointestinal radiology* [2nd ed., p. 3]. Philadelphia: W. B. Saunders.)

TABLE 34-3
DIAGNOSTIC TESTS AND PROCEDURES FOR THE DIGESTIVE TRACT

TEST	PURPOSE/PROCEDURE	PATIENT PREPARATION	POSTPROCEDURE NURSING CARE
Radiographic Tests			
Upper gastrointestinal (UGI or GI) series Barium swallow	Detects abnormalities of esophagus and stomach. Patient drinks a contrast solution while radiologist observes filling and emptying of esophagus, stomach, and duodenum via fluoroscope. Films taken 6 hr later show how much barium has passed through the stomach.	NPO 8–12 hr before procedure.	Monitor stools at least 2 days for passage of white stools that show that barium is being eliminated (normal stool color returns in ~3 days). Laxatives may be ordered to promote elimination. Provide food, fluids, and rest.
Small bowel series	Detects abnormalities of small intestine. Patient drinks a contrast solution. Films are taken at 20–30-min intervals as solution passes through small intestine. Patient will be asked to assume various positions for x-rays. Procedure may take several hours.	Same as for UGI series.	Same as for UGI series.
Barium enema	Detects abnormalities of large intestine. Contrast solution is administered by enema. X-rays are taken with patient in a variety of positions. Procedure may take as long as 1¼ hr.	Patient may be restricted to clear liquids day or evening before procedure. Usually NPO after midnight. Laxatives and enemas given on previous day. Enemas till clear on morning of procedure.	Same as for UGI series.
Gallbladder (GB) series (oral cholecystogram)	Evaluates functioning of gallbladder and bile ducts. Visualizes stones if present. Patient is given an oral contrast substance day before. X-rays are taken in a variety of positions. A high-fat drink or a medication may be given to cause gallbladder to contract. Study takes an hour or more.	Ask about sensitivity to iodine before giving contrast substance. Hold substance and notify physician if patient reports allergy. Give contrast substance as ordered and tell patient to drink large amounts of clear liquids. No food is permitted until exam is completed. A low-fat meal is ordered evening prior to study. A laxative or stool softener may be ordered after meal.	Provide food, fluids, and rest. Monitor for allergic reaction to contrast substance.
Intravenous cholangiography	Permits visualization of bile ducts, usually done when gallbladder does not visualize on cholecystogram. X-rays are taken before and at intervals after an intravenous contrast agent is injected. Takes 4 to 6 hr.	Withhold food and fluids as ordered. Usually NPO after midnight before study. A laxative also may be ordered night before. Ask about iodine sensitivity.	Same as for oral cholecystogram. If solution is given through liver (percutaneous transhepatic cholangiography), watch for signs of bleeding and respiratory distress.
T-tube cholangiogram	Evaluates whether bile ducts are open after gallbladder surgery. Contrast agent is injected into T-tube prior to taking x-rays. Takes about 15 min.	Same as for intravenous cholangiography.	Same as for oral cholecystogram.
Endoscopic Tests			
Upper Digestive Tract			
Esophagoscopy	Visualizes esophagus.	Upper digestive exams: NPO for 6–8 hr. Sedative shortly before exam if ordered.	NPO till gag reflex returns. Monitor for signs of perforation: fever, abdominal distention, cramping pain.
Gastroscopy	Visualizes stomach.		
Gastroduodenoscopy	Visualizes stomach and duodenum.		
Esophagogastroduodenoscopy	Visualizes esophagus, stomach, and duodenum.		
Endoscopic retrograde cholangiography	Visualizes bile ducts and gallbladder.		

TABLE 34-3

DIAGNOSTIC TESTS AND PROCEDURES FOR THE DIGESTIVE TRACT *Continued*

TEST	PURPOSE/PROCEDURE	PATIENT PREPARATION	POSTPROCEDURE NURSING CARE
Endoscopic Tests			
Lower Digestive Tract			
Colonoscopy Proctoscopy	Visualizes colon. Visualizes rectum.	NPO for 6–8 hr before exam. May be restricted to liquids previous day or evening. Bowel cleansing procedures include cathartics, suppositories, and enemas.	Monitor for signs of perforation: fever, abdominal distention, cramping pain. Assess for rectal bleeding.
Sigmoidoscopy	Visualizes rectum and sigmoid colon.	Cathartics and suppositories are usually given evening before test. Enemas till clear may be ordered on morning of test.	

NPO, Nothing by mouth.

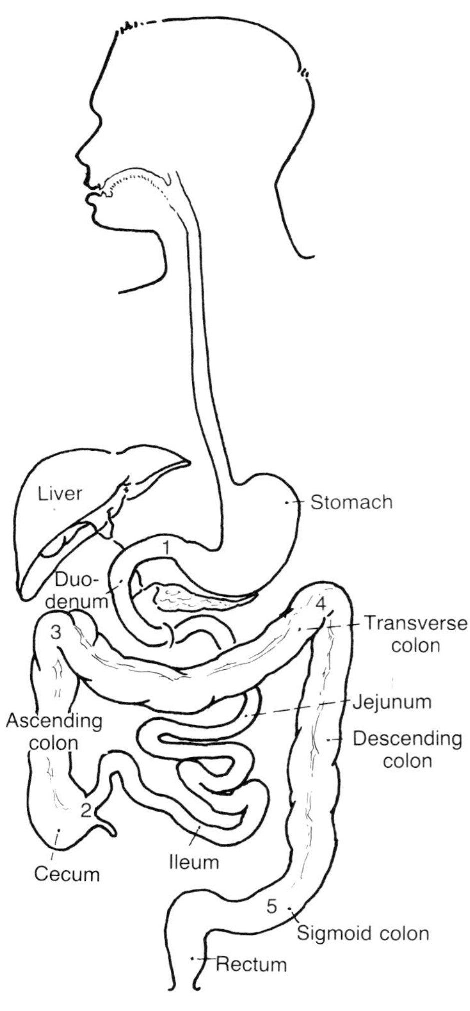

FIGURE 34-4

Time required for the passage of substances through the digestive tract. (From Jacob, S. W., & Francone, C. A. [1989]. *Elements of anatomy and physiology* [2nd ed., p. 254]. Philadelphia: W. B. Saunders.)

the gag reflex returns. The most serious complication of endoscopy is perforation, or puncture, of the digestive tract. The nurse should be alert for bleeding from the throat or rectum that could indicate trauma or perforation. Elevated temperature, abdominal distention, cramping pain, and vague discomfort also are signs and symptoms of perforation.

LABORATORY STUDIES

The most common laboratory studies are performed on gastric secretions and stool specimens.

GASTRIC ANALYSIS. Gastric analysis is performed to determine the hydrochloric acid content of the gastric fluid. A nasogastric tube is inserted, and gastric secretions are withdrawn every 15 minutes for 1 hour. The nurse may be responsible for withdrawing the specimens, labeling them in order, and sending them for analysis. This enables measurement of basal gastric secretions. If a gastric acid stimulation test is ordered as well, a drug that stimulates acid secretion (e.g., pentagastrin [Peptavlon]) is administered to the patient. Once again, specimens are collected at 15-minute intervals, labeled, and sent for analysis.

TABLE 34-4

TERMINOLOGY FOR DIAGNOSTIC STUDIES OF THE DIGESTIVE TRACT

PREFIX	REFERS TO
Esophag-	Esophagus
Gastr-	Stomach
Duoden-	Duodenum
Sigmoid-	Sigmoid colon
Proct-	Rectum
Cholangi-	Gallbladder
Pancreat-	Pancreas

How to interpret new terms:
Scopy = "to examine"
Proctoscopy = *Proct* + *scopy*
Proctoscopy = to examine the rectum
Esophagogastroduodenoscopy = *esophag* + *gastr* + *duoden* + *scopy*
Esophagogastroduodenoscopy = to examine the esophagus, stomach, and duodenum

Tubeless gastric analysis detects the presence of gastric hydrochloric acid. A gastric stimulant is given, followed an hour later by a resin dye (azuresin [Diagnex Blue]). The dye is given orally. It reacts with gastric hydrochloric acid to release the dye, which is excreted in the urine. If hydrochloric acid is present in the stomach, the dye appears in the urine 2 hours later.

OCCULT BLOOD TEST. One test that is frequently done on the nursing unit detects occult blood in body fluids. Occult blood is blood that cannot be seen with the naked eye. Specimens most often tested for occult blood are vomitus, gastric secretions, and stool.

STOOL EXAMINATION. Stool specimens are most often examined for blood, bile, pathogenic organisms, and parasite ova (eggs). Several important points must be remembered when stool examinations are ordered:

1. The specimen should be collected in a clean, dry container. Urine should not be in the container because it destroys parasites. Bathroom tissue should not be discarded in the container since the paper contains bismuth. Bismuth interferes with some tests.
2. It is best to deliver stool specimens to the laboratory immediately. If temporary storage is necessary, specimens for ova and parasites must be kept warm. Specimens for pathogens should be refrigerated.
3. When a stool specimen is being tested for occult blood, the patient should not eat red meat for 2 to 3 days before the specimen is collected. Red meat interferes with the test results.
4. If visible blood or mucus is present in the stool, it should be included in the specimen sent to the laboratory.

COMMON THERAPEUTIC MEASURES

GASTROINTESTINAL INTUBATION

Tubes are most often inserted into the stomach or intestines to deliver feedings or to keep the digestive tract empty (decompression). Tubes that are passed through the nose are called nasogastric, nasoduodenal, or nasoenteric tubes, depending on whether the end is located in the stomach or the small intestine.

There are a variety of tubes for special purposes (Fig. 34–5). Levin and gastric sump tubes are nasogastric tubes and may be used for feedings or decompression (Fig. 34–6). Gastrostomy tubes, used for feedings, are placed in the stomach through an opening (stoma) in the abdominal wall. Smaller nasoduodenal tubes, such as the Dobbhoff feeding tube, are weighted so that they pass through the stomach into the duodenum.

Nasoenteric tubes used for decompression of the small intestine include the Miller-Abbott, Cantor, and Harris tubes. Care of the patient with tubes for feeding or decompression is discussed separately.

The Sengstaken-Blakemore esophageal-gastric balloon tube is a special tube used to control bleeding in the esophagus. It is generally used in patients with severe complications of liver disease and is therefore discussed in Chapter 35.

Tube Feedings

Patients who are unable to eat or swallow normally may have feeding tubes inserted. Once the tube is in place, exact feeding orders are written. Feedings may be delivered by gravity flow or by infusion pump. Without a pump, the nurse uses a syringe barrel or a packaged

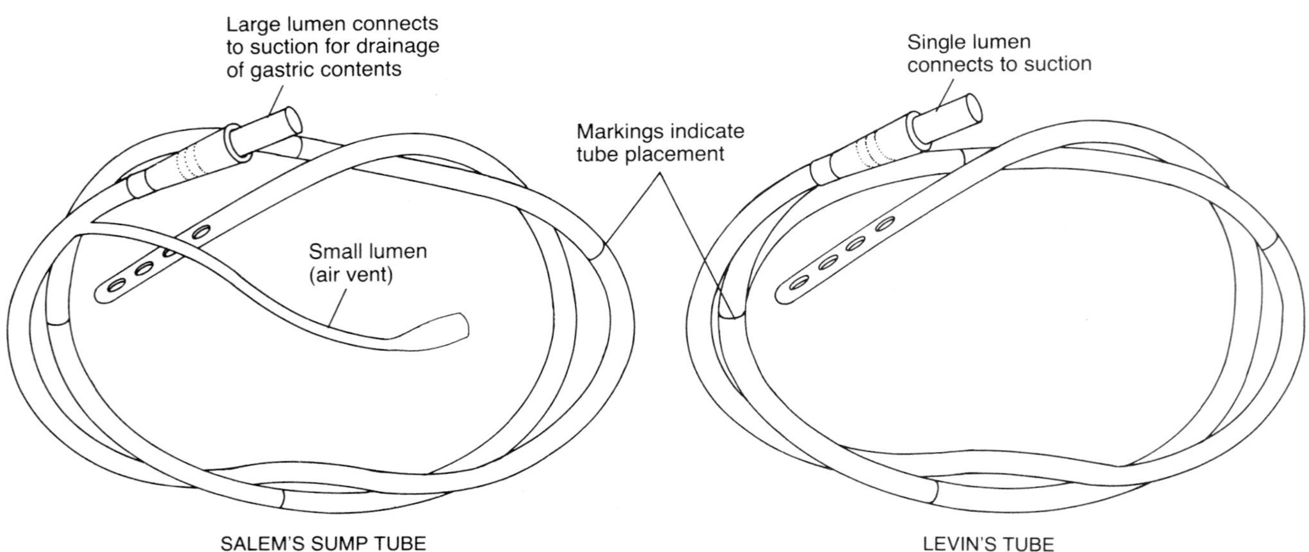

FIGURE 34–5
A variety of tubes are used in the digestive tract. (From Ignatavicius, D. D., & Bayne, M. V. [1991]. *Medical-surgical nursing: A nursing process approach* [p. 1317]. Philadelphia: W. B. Saunders.)

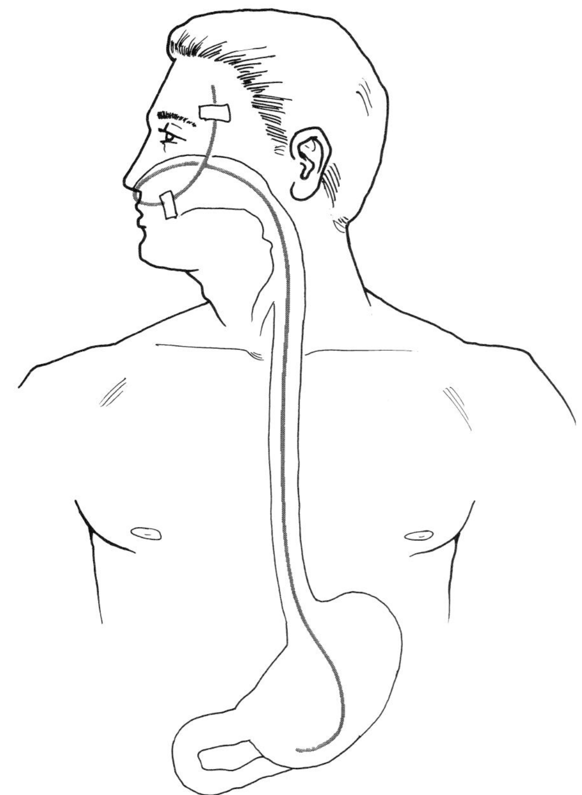

FIGURE 34-6
A Levin tube in place.

delivery set to put the feeding into the tube. Regardless of the method used, several key points must be remembered about this procedure:

1. Assist the patient into Fowler's or an elevated side-lying position to reduce the chance of aspiration (regurgitation and passage of fluids into the respiratory tract). Keep the head and chest elevated for about 30 minutes after the feeding is completed.
2. Check to be sure that the end of the tube is in the stomach or the duodenum before starting the feeding. This can be done by injecting 5 ml of air through the tube while listening over the stomach area with a stethoscope. A popping or gurgling sound confirms the location of the tube. A second method is to use a syringe to apply suction to the tube. Obtaining digestive tract contents ensures that the tube is in place. The pH of the fluid can be assessed for acidity, which is characteristic of stomach fluids. When a nasoduodenal tube is used, a radiograph is usually ordered to check the tube location. Feedings are not started until placement is certain.
3. Residual is monitored to help prevent overfilling the stomach. Check for residual (formula remaining in the stomach from the previous feeding) before each feeding or according to agency procedure. Use a syringe to withdraw and measure the formula. Agency policies dictate what action should be taken based on the amount of residual formula. The physician may need to be notified. The amount of the residual may be subtracted from the next feeding, or feedings may be discontinued for a specified period of time. The residual formula should be returned through the tube to prevent loss of electrolytes.
4. Obtain the correct formula. In the hospital setting, feedings are commercially prepared. There are many varieties of formulas. Be sure to give the right formula, in the right amount, at the right dilution, on the right schedule, to the right patient.
5. When tube feedings are first started, they are often diluted to one-half or one-fourth strength. If the patient tolerates the formula well, the concentration is gradually increased.
6. Stop the feeding and notify the physician if the patient has nausea or pain.
7. Rinse the tube by flushing it with at least 30 ml of water after each bolus feeding. Extra water may be ordered.
8. If diarrhea occurs, contact the physician regarding decreasing the concentration or the rate of delivery, or both, of the formula.
9. Dumping syndrome may occur with rapid feedings of concentrated formula. Signs and symptoms are cold sweat, abdominal distention, dizziness, weakness, rapid pulse rate, nausea, and diarrhea.
10. If using a syringe to give the feeding, do the following:
    a. Remove the plunger from the barrel of the syringe.
    b. Attach the barrel to the feeding tube.
    c. Pinch or kink the tube while the syringe barrel is filled with formula to prevent air from being forced into the stomach.
    d. Hold the barrel about 12 inches above the level of the stomach, and allow the fluid to flow by gravity.
11. If an infusion pump is used to deliver the feeding, remember the following:
    a. The tubing should be filled with formula before connecting it to the feeding tube. Otherwise, air will be forced into the digestive tract.
    b. Bolus feedings are given at specified intervals. They usually consist of 200 to 300 ml over 30 to 45 minutes for each feeding.
    c. Continuous feedings are usually given at a rate of 80 to 150 ml per hour. No more than 6 hours' worth of formula should be hung because it can become contaminated.

PHARMACOLOGY CAPSULE

Oral drugs can usually be given through a nasogastric tube, but some drugs should not be crushed. Consult a drug reference.

Gastrointestinal Decompression

Gastrointestinal decompression is used for the relief or prevention of distention. A tube is passed through a nostril, into the stomach or intestines or both, and attached to suction. The suction removes fluid and gases that accumulate when gastrointestinal motility is impaired. Conditions that slow motility include peritonitis, obstruction, and any type of surgery under general anesthesia. Handling of the bowel in abdominal surgery often causes a temporary loss of peristalsis. Decompression may be ordered until bowel activity returns, usually in 3 to 5 days.

Several types of tubes are used for gastrointestinal decompression. As mentioned earlier, the Levin and gastric sump tubes can be used for gastric decompression (often called GI suction). Miller-Abbott, Cantor, and Harris tubes are weighted and are used for intestinal decompression (Fig. 34–7). The patient may return from surgery with the tube in place, or it can be inserted on the nursing unit. The following are key points to remember when caring for the patient with gastrointestinal suction:

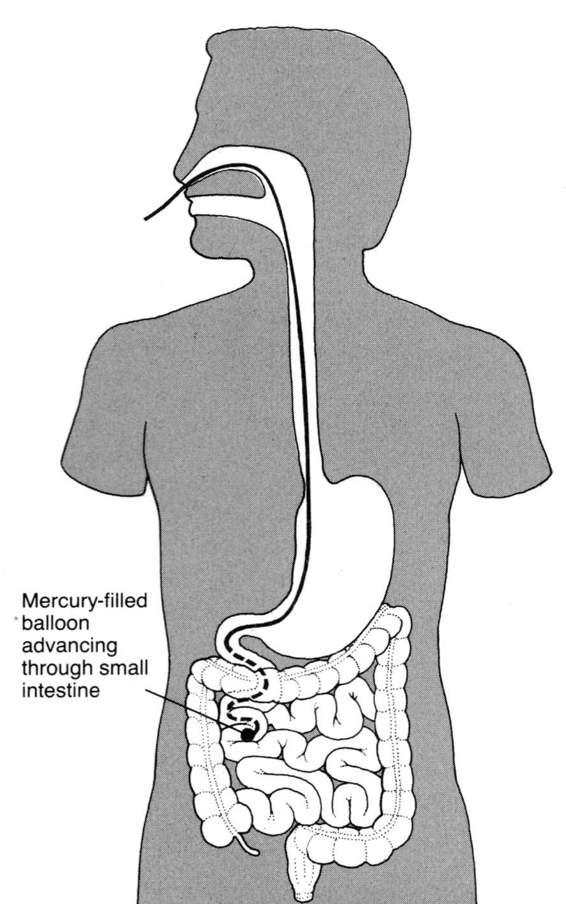

FIGURE 34-7
A nasointestinal tube has a mercury-filled balloon that stimulates peristalsis and advances the tube through the intestines. (From Ignatavicius, D. D., & Bayne, M. V. [1991]. *Medical-surgical nursing: A nursing process approach* [p. 1397]. Philadelphia: W. B. Saunders.)

1. Attach the tube to a suction apparatus as ordered. The suction pressure should be set on "low" and "intermittent." These settings should prevent trauma to the mucosa, which can occur if tissue is drawn into the suction tubing.
2. Monitor the patency of the tube. Observe for the movement of fluids through the tubing into the suction container. If the tube does not seem to be draining, change the patient's position. Gently rotate the tube or pull it out very slightly. (*Exception:* Do not reposition tubes after gastric surgery.) Notify the physician if drainage does not resume.
3. Irrigations should not be done routinely, but they may be ordered occasionally as needed. Frequent irrigations cause acid-base disturbances. For adults, irrigations are usually done with 20 to 30 ml of normal saline. Check the physician's order or the agency procedure manual.
4. Monitor the suction output. Record the amount, color, and characteristics every shift. When blood is present, the drainage may be bright red, dark red, brown, or black. Dark brown or green fluid suggests that there is an obstruction below the point where bile enters the digestive tract.
5. Monitor the patient for successful decompression. If distention is not being effectively relieved, the patient may have nausea and vomiting, shortness of breath, a feeling of fullness, and enlargement of the abdomen.
6. Assess for the return of peristalsis, indicated by the presence of bowel sounds and passing of flatus (gas) through the rectum.
7. Provide comfort measures. The nasopharynx and throat are often very tender. Since the patient is allowed nothing by mouth, mouth dryness is another source of discomfort. Handle the tubing gently. Cleanse the nostrils and apply a water-soluble lubricant to reduce drying and irritation. Provide mouth care frequently. Moisturize the lips. Offer oral spray or lozenges as ordered to provide temporary relief of sore throat.
8. Once the tube is in place, it will be taped to keep it from being pulled out unless it is the type of tube intended to move through the digestive tract. Tape should secure the tube to the upper lip and cheek or nose (Fig. 34–8). The tubing should not be taped to the forehead because this puts excessive pressure on the nasal tissues. The tube should be moved carefully during activity to avoid trauma to the nasopharynx. The tube may be wrapped with a piece of tape and then pinned to the patient's gown to prevent accidental traction on the tube.

TOTAL PARENTERAL NUTRITION

Sometimes the digestive tract cannot be used for feedings. Total parenteral nutrition (TPN) bypasses the digestive tract by delivering nutrients directly to the blood stream. A catheter inserted into a large vein such as the subclavian is used for the feedings (Fig. 34–9). The feeding passes directly into the superior vena cava

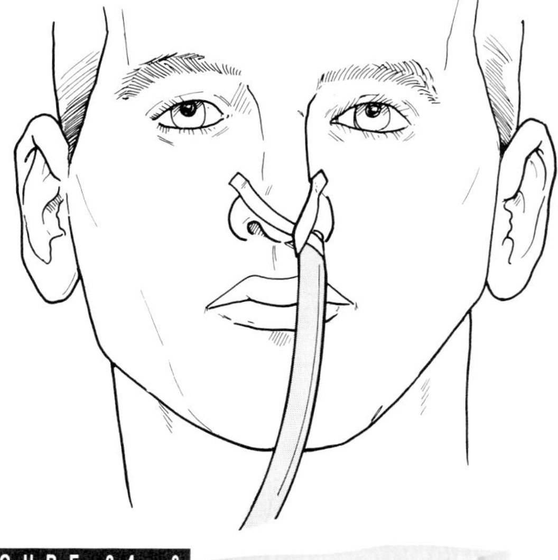

FIGURE 34-8
Tape secures the nasogastric tube to the nose.

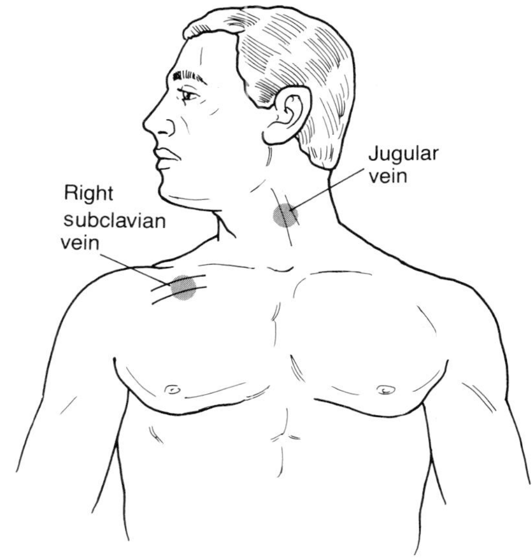

FIGURE 34-9
Preferred sites for intravenous lines to deliver total parenteral nutrition.

or the right atrium. This placement allows for rapid dilution of the concentrated feeding. If the solution were given in a smaller vein, it would cause thrombophlebitis (inflammation of the vein).

When the catheter is inserted, it is sutured to the skin and the insertion site is covered with a sterile dressing. A radiograph is ordered to check placement before the catheter is used for feedings.

Regular intravenous feedings can provide only water, glucose, electrolytes, minerals, and vitamins. This is adequate for short-term problems but does not provide all the nutrients necessary to maintain health or promote healing.

Two types of solutions are used for TPN therapy. The first is a concentrated solution of glucose, amino acids, vitamins, and minerals. It is administered using a special filter. A lipid solution also can be given through a peripheral vein. The lipids are not mixed with the TPN solution.

Important points when caring for the patient receiving TPN include the following:

1. Take great care to prevent infection at the insertion site. Sterile technique should always be used for site care. The exact procedure should be ordered or written in the agency procedure manual. Each time the dressing is changed, inspect the site for signs of infection (redness, swelling, foul odor, or purulent drainage). Monitor the patient's temperature for an elevation.
2. Monitor the flow rate. If given too rapidly, the patient may have circulatory overload, changes in blood sugar, or excessive diuresis (urine output). If the feeding falls behind schedule, do not speed up the rate to "catch up."
3. Monitor the patient for signs and symptoms of blood glucose changes. The concentrated glucose solution can raise the blood glucose excessively (hyperglycemia). Elevated glucose stimulates the pancreas to produce more insulin, which may then cause a drop in blood glucose (hypoglycemia). Urine or blood should be monitored to detect abnormal glucose levels.
4. Do not use the TPN catheter to administer drugs.
5. Be sure that all staff who give medications differentiate TPN lines from small-bore enteral feeding tubes. Patient deaths have occurred as a result of oral medications being administered through a TPN line.
6. Be alert for depression that often occurs with illnesses requiring TPN. Talk to the patient about his or her feelings. Report sadness and discouragement to the nursing team and the physician.

PHARMACOLOGY CAPSULE

A total parenteral nutrition (TPN) line should *not* be used to administer any drugs.

GASTROINTESTINAL SURGERY

Many conditions of the digestive tract require surgical treatment. Surgery on the mouth and esophagus may be needed to correct defects or in the treatment of cancer. Surgical conditions of the stomach include bleeding ulcers, hiatal hernia, and cancer. Less commonly, surgery is done to decrease the capacity of the stomach for the treatment of extreme obesity. Conditions of the large intestine that may require surgery include cancer, diverticulosis, appendicitis, polyps, obstruction, and ulcerative colitis. General care of the surgical patient is covered in Chapter 14.

Preoperative Care

Radiographic examinations of the digestive tract are often done prior to surgery. These may be done on an outpatient basis or after admission to the hospital.

The digestive tract is usually cleansed prior to gastrointestinal surgery. The extent of the cleansing depends on the exact site of the surgery. Oral preparations such as magnesium citrate or large-volume cathartic (laxative) solutions may be prescribed. Use of enemas until the returning fluid is clear also may be ordered. This process is tiring and may exhaust the very ill or elderly patient. The nurse should offer assistance with toileting and hygiene. Changes in vital signs or mental state during the bowel cleansing process should be reported to the physician.

Diet is usually limited to liquids for 24 hours before the surgery. Of course, the patient should have nothing to eat or drink from midnight until the morning of surgery. Intravenous fluids may be ordered, especially if gastrointestinal suction is being used.

General anesthesia and abdominal surgery cause a temporary loss of peristalsis. Therefore, before or during surgery, a nasogastric tube may be inserted and attached to suction. This prevents the accumulation of fluid and gas in the digestive tract until peristalsis returns.

Postoperative Care

Usual postoperative care, discussed in Chapter 14, includes measures to relieve pain, detect complications (hemorrhage, infection), and prevent adverse effects of immobility, anesthesia, and drug therapy. Immediately after surgery on the digestive tract, the nurse is especially concerned with preventing gastric or abdominal distention, replacing lost fluids, and maintaining urine elimination. The patient usually has a nasogastric tube in place for decompression. The continuous removal of fluids and gas decreases the stimulation of the digestive tract and reduces pressure on the internal incisions. The nurse monitors gastrointestinal suction to be sure it is draining. The drainage is inspected, described, and measured. The abdomen is assessed for distention and bowel sounds. The nurse must check the physician's orders regarding irrigation. After gastric surgery, the nurse does *not* irrigate or reposition the tube because of the possibility of traumatizing healing tissue. If the tube is not draining properly or distention is noted, the nurse notifies the physician.

Intravenous fluids are given until gastrointestinal suction is discontinued and oral intake is adequate. Careful intake and output records are kept. The patient is at risk for fluid and electrolyte imbalances when gastrointestinal suction is used. Since the patient often has difficulty voiding after abdominal surgery, an indwelling catheter is usually inserted during the procedure. If there is no catheter, the patient may require nursing measures to promote voiding. These measures are discussed in Chapter 36.

DRUG THERAPY

Drugs that are used because of their effects on the digestive tract include emetics, antiemetics, laxatives, cathartics, antidiarrheals, antacids, anticholinergics, mucosal barriers, histamine$_2$ (H_2) receptor blockers, and antibiotics. These drugs are discussed with the conditions for which they are prescribed. In addition, Table 34–5 summarizes these drugs, their actions, and nursing interventions.

DISORDERS OF THE DIGESTIVE TRACT

DISORDERS AFFECTING INGESTION

Anything that interferes with the ability to eat a balanced diet can cause nutritional deficiencies. Problems can be as basic as anorexia, inability to feed oneself, or dysphagia, or they may occur secondary to other problems, such as oral infection and inflammation, dental problems, oral cancer, and parotitis.

ANOREXIA

The intake of food is largely dependent on having an appetite. Lack of appetite is called anorexia.

Causes

Anorexia can occur with many physical and emotional disturbances. The presence of nausea, decreased sense of taste or smell, mouth disorders, and medications are some physical factors that may decrease one's appetite. Emotional problems such as anxiety, depression, or unpleasant thoughts also may cause anorexia. The environment can influence appetite as well. Unpleasant odors or sights can quickly dampen a patient's enthusiasm for a meal. Therapeutic diets such as pureed, low-salt, and low-fat diets are unappetizing to some people. Older people often report decreased appetite. This may be attributed to diminished senses of taste and smell, drug effects, decreased activity, and social isolation.

Medical Diagnosis

The physician assesses the patient for evidence of malnutrition. Weight may be monitored over several weeks. A complete history and physical are done to detect underlying problems and effects of inadequate intake. Initial diagnostic tests that are likely to be ordered include serum hemoglobin, iron, total iron-binding capacity, transferrin, calcium, folate, B_{12}, and zinc. Tests of thyroid function may be ordered to detect metabolic disorders, as well as skin tests to evaluate allergic responses. A stool specimen may be tested for occult blood. If indicated, the physician may perform additional procedures to detect possible cancers of the digestive system, lungs, and breasts.

Medical Treatment

Correctable causes of anorexia are treated, but sometimes no physical cause is found. Nutritional supple-

TABLE 34-5
DRUGS USED TO TREAT DISORDERS OF THE DIGESTIVE TRACT

DRUG	USE/ACTION	NURSING INTERVENTIONS
Antacids Magnesium hydroxide Aluminum hydroxide Calcium carbonate Sodium bicarbonate	Reduce pain of peptic ulcers by neutralizing acid in stomach, decreasing irritation of stomach lining, and inhibiting action of pepsin on stomach lining.	Antacids are nonprescription drugs, but they still have side effects and can be abused. Calcium and aluminum salts tend to cause constipation. Magnesium salts tend to cause diarrhea. Combinations may be used to neutralize these effects. Shake liquids before pouring. Follow dose with water or milk to deliver antacid to stomach. Antacids interfere with absorption of oral drugs if given within 1–2 hr of each other. Tablets should be chewed before swallowing.
H_2 Receptor Antagonists Cimetidine (Tagamet) Ranitidine (Zantac) Famotidine (Pepcid) Nizatidine (Axid)	Reduce secretion of gastric acid and promote healing of ulcers.	Give with or after meals. Do not give ranitidine at same time as antacids. Side effects: diarrhea, muscle pain, rash, confusion, drowsiness. Cimetidine can cause impotence and gynecomastia and impairs metabolism of many common drugs.
Sucralfate (Carafate)	Coats ulcer surface to allow healing.	Give on empty stomach: 1 hr before meals and at bedtime. Do not give within 30 min of antacids. Interferes with absorption of some other drugs.
Synthetic Prostaglandins Misoprostol (Cytotec)	Decrease gastric acid secretion and protect gastric mucosa.	Often used to prevent gastric ulcers due to nonsteroidal anti-inflammatory drugs. Contraindicated during pregnancy. Side effects: diarrhea, abdominal pain. Usually given with meals and at bedtime.
Antispasmodics Atropine Belladonna **Anticholinergics** Dicyclomine (Bentyl) Glycopyrrolate (Robinul) Propantheline bromide (Pro-Banthine)	Reduce pain by reducing tone of smooth muscle in GI tract.	Contraindicated with narrow-angle glaucoma, renal disease, prostatic hypertrophy, or intestinal obstruction. Best given ½ to 1 hr before meals and at bedtime. Side effects: dry mouth, constipation, visual disturbance, urinary retention. Elderly may become confused, agitated, or drowsy. Provide oral hygiene. Monitor stools and urine output. Report changes in behavior. Tincture of belladonna can be mixed with applesauce to disguise taste.
Laxatives	Facilitate bowel elimination.	Monitor stools. Encourage adequate fluids and fiber to reduce need for laxatives. Laxatives are intended for temporary, occasional relief of constipation and are contraindicated with undiagnosed abdominal pain and inflammatory conditions of GI tract.
Stimulants Bisacodyl (Dulcolax) Phenolphthalein (Ex-Lax) Senna (Senokot)	Stimulate GI tract by irritating mucosa.	Tend to produce diarrhea-like stool.
Bulk-forming laxatives Psyllium (Metamucil) Methylcellulose (Citrucel)	Increase bulk and fluid in stool to stimulate peristalsis with passage of formed, soft stool.	One of safest laxatives for long-term therapy and during pregnancy. Patient must take adequate fluids, or mass can harden. May take up to 3 days before effect evident, so used primarily for prevention of constipation.

Table continued on following page

TABLE 34-5
DRUGS USED TO TREAT DISORDERS OF THE DIGESTIVE TRACT *Continued*

DRUG	USE/ACTION	NURSING INTERVENTIONS
Laxatives		
Saline laxatives		
Magnesium citrate Magnesium hydroxide (milk of magnesia) Sodium phosphate (Fleet Phospho-Soda)	Draw water into bowel to distend and stimulate evacuation.	Risk of dehydration with prolonged use. Short-term use only.
Lubricants		
Mineral oil	Lubricate feces for easier passage.	Impair absorption of fat-soluble drugs and nutrients, so should be given on an empty stomach. Risk of lipid pneumonia if aspirated.
Fecal wetting agents Docusate calcium (Surfak) Docusate sodium (Colace)	Soften fecal mass.	May take up to 3 days before effects evident, so used primarily for prevention of constipation. Liquid forms can be given in milk or juice to mask taste.
Suppositories Glycerin Bisacodyl (Dulcolax)	Stimulate evacuation by irritating or distending bowel.	Usually act within an hour.
Lactulose (Cephulac)	Increases fecal water content to stimulate evacuation. Promotes passage of ammonia through rectum.	Can be mixed with full glass of water, milk, or juice to disguise taste. More effective on empty stomach. Used in hepatic encephalopathy. Side effects: cramps, flatulence, diarrhea, hyperglycemia with diabetes.
Polyethylene Glycol-electrolyte solution (GoLYTELY)	Rapidly causes diarrhea by allowing a large volume of water to be retained in colon.	Four liters given over approximately 3 hr cleanses bowel in about 4 hr. Rapid, dramatic effect, so be sure toilet is convenient. Most often used to prepare GI tract for diagnostic procedures or surgery.
Antidiarrheal Agents		
Opiates Morphine Diphenoxylate HCl (Lomotil) Loperamide HCl (Imodium)	Decrease intestinal motility so that liquid portion of feces is reabsorbed.	Sometimes given after each stool for acute diarrhea, but do not exceed maximum dosage. Side effects: CNS depression, drowsiness, dizziness, constipation, nausea, dry mouth. Take safety precautions. Oral hygiene.
Adsorbents Kaolin Aluminum hydroxide	Bind to substances that may cause diarrhea.	Shake suspension before pouring. Do not administer with other oral drugs since adsorbents will interfere with absorption.
Lactobacillus products	Replace normal bacterial flora of bowel.	May require refrigeration.

ments may be ordered. The oral route is preferred, but, in extreme cases, enteral feedings or TPN may be indicated.

Nursing Care of the Patient with Anorexia

ASSESSMENT. The general assessment of the patient with digestive disturbances is summarized in Table 34–2. In assessing the patient with anorexia, the nurse explores factors that may be affecting appetite. Chronic and recent illnesses, hospitalizations, medications, and allergies are recorded. The patient's obstetric history should be obtained as well. The review of systems may provide clues to anorexia. Significant symptoms include pain, nausea, dyspnea, or extreme fatigue. The functional assessment reveals patterns of activity and rest, usual dietary patterns, current stressors, and coping strategies—all factors that can affect appetite. In the physical examination, the nurse is especially alert for signs of malnutrition: glossitis (inflammation of the tongue), cheilosis (cracked lips), edema, jaundice, and muscle wasting. The examination should also assess for inflammation or lesions of the mouth and dental problems. If the patient has dentures, the fit should be evaluated. It is very important to have the patient remove the dentures before the gums are assessed.

NURSING DIAGNOSIS. The primary nursing diagnosis for the patient with anorexia is altered nutrition: less than body requirements related to anorexia. It is helpful

TABLE 34-5
DRUGS USED TO TREAT DISORDERS OF THE DIGESTIVE TRACT *Continued*

DRUG	USE/ACTION	NURSING INTERVENTIONS
Emetics		
Ipecac syrup	Cause vomiting. Used to treat some types of poisoning and oral drug overdose.	Follow ipecac with water according to age: <1 yr: ½–1 glass; Older children: 1–2 glasses; Adults: 3–4 glasses. Emetic action inactivated by charcoal. Milk interferes with action of ipecac. Side effects: CNS depression (use cautiously with other CNS depressants).
Antiemetics	Prevent and treat nausea.	
Antihistamines: Promethazine HCl (Phenergan); Dimenhydrinate HCl (Dramamine)	Decrease sensitivity of vestibular apparatus of inner ear. Suppress vomiting center.	Side effects: drowsiness and confusion, especially if given with other CNS depressants. Cautious use with asthma, glaucoma, prostatic hypertrophy.
Sedatives: Hydroxyzine; Anticholinergics: Scopolamine (Transderm Scop)	Decrease sensitivity of vestibular apparatus and suppress vomiting center.	Transderm Scop is a medicated adhesive disk that is placed behind ear. Often used to prevent motion sickness.
Metoclopramide (Reglan)	Speeds up gastric emptying into small intestine.	Contraindications: GI perforation, obstruction, or hemorrhage, epilepsy. Side effects: CNS depression, GI upset, Parkinson-like symptoms.
Anti-infectives		
Sulfasalazine (Azulfidine)	Treatment of ulcerative colitis.	Contraindications: allergy to aspirin. Adequate fluid intake needed to prevent crystalluria and urinary stone formation. Side effects: orange-yellow color to urine and skin, photosensitivity. Avoid direct sunlight.
Olsalazine (Dipentum)	Treatment of ulcerative colitis	Adverse effects: abdominal pain, diarrhea, headache, nausea. Discontinue if hives, rash, wheezing occur. Encourage fluids.
Antifungals		
Nystatin (Mycostatin); Clotrimazole (Mycelex)	Effective against *Candida albicans* ("yeast") infections.	Instruct patient to dissolve lozenges in mouth. Shake suspensions well. Swish nystatin in mouth before swallowing. Side effects: nausea, vomiting, diarrhea with nystatin. Nausea, vomiting, itching with clotrimazole.

GI, Gastrointestinal; CNS, central nervous system.

if the nurse can identify factors that contribute to the patient's anorexia.

GOALS. The goals of nursing care for the patient with anorexia are patient's statement of improved appetite and adequate food intake.

INTERVENTIONS. Depending on the reason for the anorexia, a number of interventions may be successful in improving the patient's appetite. If the patient has a dry mouth or bad taste in the mouth, frequent oral hygiene is indicated. If the teeth or gums are in poor condition, the nurse can teach proper oral hygiene and refer the patient for dental care. Poorly fitting dentures need to be relined for a tighter fit or replaced.

When a patient is nauseated, measures should be taken to relieve the nausea before presenting a meal tray. Nausea and anorexia can both be related to unpleasant stimuli in the environment. Before serving a meal tray, the nurse should remove bedpans and emesis basins from sight, conceal drains and drainage collection devices, and deodorize the room if necessary.

Many people enjoy meals more when they are in the company of others. Socialization during mealtime can greatly improve a person's appetite. A family member might be encouraged to visit during meals or accompany the patient to a dining facility so that they can eat together. Some facilities provide guest trays for patients' family members. In long-term care facilities, a central dining room is usually available for those who enjoy company during meals. On nursing units, small groups of patients often enjoy having their meals together in a sunroom or lounge.

Even people with good appetites eat some foods more willingly than others. For the patient with anorexia, it is especially important to respect food likes and dislikes. If the food being served is unappealing, the nurse can ask the dietitian to discuss the diet with the patient. Sometimes food from home is a special treat. Before food is brought in by family or friends, they should be advised of any dietary restrictions. Small servings are more acceptable than large ones to the anorexic person. Additional nutrients can be provided by between-meals snacks. In the inpatient setting, the nurse has little control over the specific food served, but, in the home, the meal preparer can be encouraged to provide foods that vary in color, texture, and taste.

Sometimes nurses overlook the obvious when trying to get patients to eat. The patient should be positioned comfortably and have easy access to the food. If the patient cannot cut food or open packages, someone should be sure to do this. Tiring activities should not be scheduled immediately before mealtime.

Fortunately, anorexia is a temporary problem for most people. For others, however, it is a chronic problem. The patient needs to be taught the importance of adequate nutritional intake. When they understand how nutrition is related to their health goals, most patients will make an effort to eat. If the patient seems to be anxious or depressed, the nurse can ask about concerns that he or she may have. The physician should be consulted about possible counseling if emotional distress persists.

EVALUATION. The criteria for evaluating the effects of nursing interventions are patient's statement of improved appetite, increased food intake, and stable or increased weight.

FEEDING PROBLEMS

Patients may require assistance with meals because of temporary impairments or long-term disabilities. Those likely to need assistance include patients with paralysis, arthritis, neuromuscular disorders, confusion, weakness, or visual impairment. Thorough assessments and individualized interventions are needed to ensure adequate nutrition despite disability.

Medical Diagnosis and Treatment

Medical diagnosis is directed at identifying the basic problems and prescribing treatment as appropriate. Patients are often referred to physical therapy and occupational therapy to help them regain basic self-care skills.

Nursing Care of the Patient with Feeding Problems

ASSESSMENT. Nurses must assess each patient's ability to feed himself or herself independently. The nursing assessment focuses on determining the nature of the patient's difficulty and identifying remaining abilities. Some patients are temporarily impaired because they are immobilized or confined to restricted positions as part of their medical treatment. Important aspects of the physical examination are visual acuity, range of motion and muscle strength in both arms, and range of motion and grip strength in both hands. The patient's ability to follow instructions is evaluated as well.

NURSING DIAGNOSIS. The primary nursing diagnoses for patients who are unable to feed themselves are the following:

- **Self-Care Deficit** (feeding) related to paralysis, weakness, poor coordination, confusion, visual impairment
- **Altered Nutrition: Less than Body Requirements** related to inability to feed self

GOALS. Goals of nursing care for patients who cannot feed themselves are improved self-feeding and adequate food intake.

INTERVENTIONS. In general, patients should be encouraged to be as independent in feeding as possible. For some, proper positioning and arrangement of the meal tray are all that is needed. Assistive devices designed for paralyzed and arthritic patients are available. These can be obtained through the physical therapy or occupational therapy department. Simple adaptations such as padding the handles of utensils may enable the patient with limited grasping ability to feed himself or herself.

When patients need only partial assistance, the nurse may open milk cartons, cut meat, butter bread, and season food. Before seasoning food or sweetening drinks, the nurse should ask about patient preferences. Most people feel very strongly about these preferences. Confused patients can often feed themselves if the task is made simple. They may require occasional reminders to continue eating. Sometimes a group dining situation works well for these patients because they may imitate the behavior of others who are eating.

The term *feeder* is sometimes used to refer to patients who must be fed. This label is demeaning and threatens the patient's self-esteem. The patient should be addressed as an adult. Pleasant conversation should be directed to the patient while he or she is being fed. The nurse should remember the following points when feeding a patient:

1. The patient should be seated upright, and the head should be tilted slightly forward.
2. A napkin or towel should be tucked at the patient's chin to catch spills.
3. The patient who is able to communicate should be asked in what order the food should be offered. The practice of mixing all food together "to make sure the patient gets a little of everything" is unappetizing and not recommended.
4. Some patients do not open their mouths voluntarily. Touching the lips with the spoon or gently pressing just below the lower lip with a finger may encourage them to do so.

5. Pacing is important, so the nurse should observe that the patient has swallowed before offering more food.

6. In stroke patients, food may accumulate in the affected side of the mouth. The mouth should be checked at intervals for accumulated food.

At the completion of the meal, the nurse should provide mouth care and record the amount of food taken.

EVALUATION. Criteria for evaluating the success of nursing interventions when a patient requires help with feeding are patient participation of feeding within his or her capabilities and patient consumption of adequate food to maintain or achieve ideal body weight.

ORAL INFLAMMATION AND INFECTIONS

Stomatitis

Stomatitis is a general term for inflammation of the oral mucosa. It may result from the mechanical trauma of poorly fitting dentures, the irritation of excessive tobacco or alcohol use, poor oral hygiene, inadequate nutrition, pathogenic organisms, radiation therapy, or drug therapy. Disorders of the kidney, liver, or blood also can cause stomatitis. Emotional tension and excessive fatigue seem to make people more susceptible to some types of stomatitis. Medical treatment is directed at determining the cause and eliminating it. If specific pathogenic organisms are identified, appropriate antibiotics (usually topical) or antiviral agents may be prescribed. A soft, bland diet may be ordered.

Vincent's Infection

Vincent's infection is caused by bacteria. It has been called trench mouth because it frequently developed among soldiers in the field in World War I. It is a bacterial infection that causes bleeding ulcers and a metallic taste in the mouth, foul breath, and increased salivation. The patient may also have signs of a general infection, such as fever, enlarged lymph nodes, and anorexia. Topical antibiotics and mouthwashes are used to treat the infection. Rest, a nutritious diet, and good oral hygiene are helpful.

Herpes Simplex

Herpes simplex is caused by the herpes simplex virus, type I. Ulcers and vesicles develop in the mouth and on the lips. People commonly refer to these lesions as cold sores or fever blisters. They tend to occur in people who have upper respiratory infections, have had excessive sun exposure, or are under stress. Spirits of camphor, topical steroids, and antiviral agents may be prescribed as treatment.

Aphthous Stomatitis

Aphthous stomatitis ("canker sore") may be caused by a virus. It is characterized by ulcers of the lips and mouth that recur at intervals. Topical or systemic steroids may be used to treat this chronic condition.

Candida Albicans

Candida albicans, a yeast-like fungus, causes the oral condition known as thrush or candidiasis. Bluish white lesions can be seen on the mucous membranes of the mouth. Patients at high risk for candidiasis include those on steroid or long-term antibiotic therapy. Oral medications are usually prescribed to treat candidiasis.

Nursing Care of the Patient with Oral Inflammation or Infection

Patients with only oral inflammation or infections are usually treated as outpatients, so the nurse's role is limited to reinforcing medical instructions. These conditions, however, may develop in patients who are hospitalized for other reasons. The nurse then has a more active role in treating and teaching them.

ASSESSMENT. The nursing history includes a thorough description of the patient's symptoms. Pain location, onset, and precipitating factors are described. Measures that have helped relieve the pain are noted as well. The nurse documents any known illnesses and treatments, including drugs and radiation therapy. Habits, including diet, oral care practices, alcohol intake, and use of tobacco, are described. The patient's stress level also is assessed. The oral cavity is inspected for redness, swelling, and lesions.

NURSING DIAGNOSIS. Nursing diagnoses for the patient with an infectious or inflammatory oral condition may include the following:

- **Pain** related to tissue trauma, irritation, infection
- **Altered Oral Mucous Membrane** related to trauma, ineffective oral hygiene, infection, drug adverse effects
- **Altered Nutrition: Less than Body Requirements** related to inflamed or infected oral tissue

GOALS. The goals of nursing care for the patient with inflammation or infection of the oral cavity are pain relief, healthy oral mucous membranes, and adequate nutritional intake.

INTERVENTIONS. When acute inflammation is present, gentle oral hygiene and the use of prescribed mouthwashes are soothing. The teeth and tongue can be cleansed with a soft-bristle toothbrush, sponge, or cotton-tipped applicator. Medications must be given as ordered. It is important to read the directions carefully for these medications. Instead of just swallowing the medication, the patient may need to be told to swish liquid medication in the mouth or to permit tablets to dissolve in the cheek. If the patient is discharged while taking a medication, the nurse should emphasize the importance of completing the entire prescription. The patient should also be taught proper techniques for brushing and flossing the teeth. The nurse emphasizes the importance of daily oral hygiene and good nutrition in preventing recurrences.

EVALUATION. Criteria for evaluating the outcomes of nursing interventions are patient's verbalization of pain relief, intact mucous membranes without redness or lesions, and stable body weight.

PHARMACOLOGY CAPSULE

When drugs are given for stomatitis, for example, the directions may be to "swish and swallow" the medication. Be sure to instruct patients appropriately.

DISORDERS OF THE TEETH AND GUMS

Dental Caries

The term dental caries refers to a destructive process of tooth decay. Dental decay starts with the presence of plaque on the teeth. Plaque is a substance made up of bacteria, saliva, and cells that sticks to the surface of the teeth. Bacteria produce acids that destroy the protective tooth enamel, permitting decay. Untreated decay erodes into the canal of the tooth, causing intense pain and death of the pulp. The only treatment for dental caries is removal of the decayed part of the tooth followed by filling the cavity with a restorative material.

Tooth decay can largely be prevented by good oral hygiene and nutrition. Fluoride is so effective in strengthening tooth enamel that many cities add it to the public water supply. In addition, a dentist may apply fluoride directly to tooth surfaces. Toothpastes containing fluoride are recommended by the American Dental Association to reduce the risk of tooth decay. Patients are encouraged to limit sugar intake as well.

Periodontal Disease

Periodontal disease begins with gingivitis (inflammation of the gums) and progresses to involve the other structures that support the teeth. In gingivitis, the gums are typically red, swollen, painful, and bleed easily. Gingivitis results primarily from inadequate oral hygiene. Food particles accumulate between the teeth and the gums, causing irritation. Gingivitis is more common in people who are missing some teeth or whose bite does not close properly. Other contributing factors are poor general health, anemia, vitamin deficiencies, and some blood dyscrasias.

Early detection and treatment of gingivitis can stop the progression. Treatment in the early stage consists of professional dental care for teeth cleaning and correction of contributing problems. If the condition is not treated, abscesses develop around the roots, the teeth loosen, and extraction becomes necessary. In more advanced cases, treatment may include not only removing calculus (hardened plaque) but also smoothing root surfaces and surgical removal of the soft, diseased gum tissue (Fig. 34–10). Abnormalities of the teeth and gums are illustrated in Color Plate I.

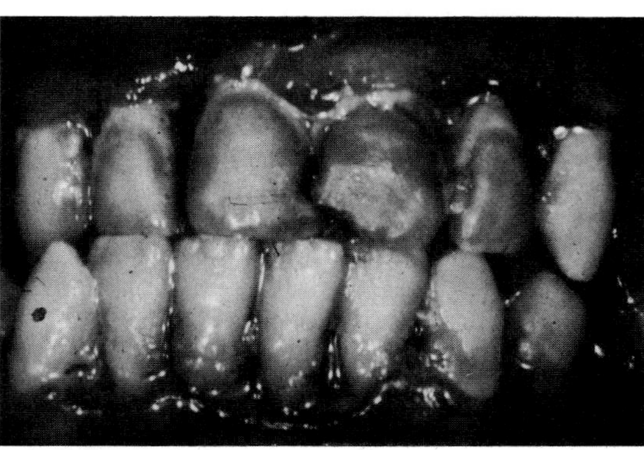

FIGURE 34-10

Acute gingivitis. (From Shafer, W. G., Hine, M. K., & Levy, B. M. [1983]. *A textbook of oral pathology* [4th ed., p. 779]. Philadelphia: W. B. Saunders.)

Nursing Care of the Patient with a Tooth or Gum Disorder

ASSESSMENT. In the health history, the nurse determines the presence of oral pain or soreness. The patient's usual diet, frequency of dental examinations, and mouth care practices are noted. When examining the mouth, the nurse observes the condition of the teeth and gums. Missing or broken teeth, caries, redness or lesions of the gums, and gum recession are documented. It is especially important for nurses in long-term care to assess patients' mouths at frequent intervals. Oral problems are often overlooked until they are quite advanced.

NURSING DIAGNOSIS. Nursing diagnoses for the patient with problems of the teeth or gums may include the following:

- **Pain** related to dental caries, tissue inflammation
- **Altered Nutrition: Less than Body Requirements** related to oral pain
- **Knowledge Deficit** of recommended mouth care practices

GOALS. Goals for the patient with dental or gum problems are pain relief, adequate nutritional intake, and improved mouth care practices by the patient.

INTERVENTIONS. Most patients are treated for dental and gum conditions in dentists' offices. Sometimes, however, dental problems develop when the patient is receiving nursing care for some other reason. In that case, interventions may be directed at minimizing pain until the problem is corrected by a dentist. The physician or dentist may order analgesics for acute pain. Gentle mouth care should be performed several times daily.

The nurse is in a position to teach patients how to prevent dental caries and gingivitis. Periodic dental examinations are advised so that expert instruction in mouth care may be obtained. Patients are encouraged to brush the teeth at least twice daily, to floss every day, to limit sugar intake, and to eat a balanced diet.

Nurses must provide oral care for patients who cannot do it themselves. Nurse aides and attendants need to understand the importance of regular mouth care and know how to provide it. The nurse should clearly include this care in the aide's daily instructions.

EVALUATION. Criteria for evaluating the effectiveness of nursing interventions are patient's statement of pain relief, adequate nutritional intake to maintain body weight, patient's demonstration of correct mouth care techniques, and evidence of good mouth care (absence of odor and food debris).

ORAL CANCER

The most life-threatening disorder affecting the mouth is cancer. Two types of malignant tumors develop in the mouth: squamous cell carcinoma and basal cell carcinoma. Squamous cell carcinomas occur on the lips, buccal mucosa, gums, floor of the mouth, tonsils, and tongue. The most common site for basal cell carcinoma is the lip.

Risk Factors

Cancer of the lip is related to prolonged exposure to irritants, including sun, wind, and pipe smoking. Factors that increase the risk of cancers inside the mouth include tobacco and alcohol use (especially in combination), poor nutritional status, and chronic irritation.

Signs and Symptoms

Symptoms of oral cancer include tongue irritation, loose teeth, and pain in the tongue or ear. Malignant lesions may appear as ulcerations, thickened or rough areas, or sore spots. The presence of hard, white patches in the mouth is called leukoplakia. Leukoplakia is considered a premalignant condition.

Medical Diagnosis and Treatment

A biopsy of suspicious lesions is done to make a medical diagnosis. When a malignancy is confirmed, the physician often orders endoscopic examinations and radiographs of the upper digestive and respiratory tracts to see if there is evidence of metastases. Depending on the extent of the cancer, treatment may include surgery, radiation, or chemotherapy, or a combination. Small lesions may simply be excised and sutured. Larger lesions that are more invasive usually require more extensive surgery. An incision can be made along the jawbone for access to the oral cavity. Grafts are sometimes needed to close large defects caused by the surgical procedures. The donor site is usually the patient's anterior thigh. Surgical procedures are illustrated in Figure 34–11.

Nursing Care of the Patient with Oral Cancer

ASSESSMENT. Assessment of the patient with a disorder of the digestive tract is summarized in Table 34–2. When a patient is being evaluated for possible oral cancer, it is especially important to note a history of prolonged sun exposure, tobacco use, or alcohol consumption. The nurse asks whether the patient or immediate family members have a history of cancer. Significant signs and symptoms to be documented include difficulty swallowing or chewing, decreased appetite, weight loss, change in fit of dentures, and hemoptysis. The physical examination should focus on examination of the mouth for lesions. In addition, the nurse assesses the neck for limitation of movement and enlarged lymph nodes.

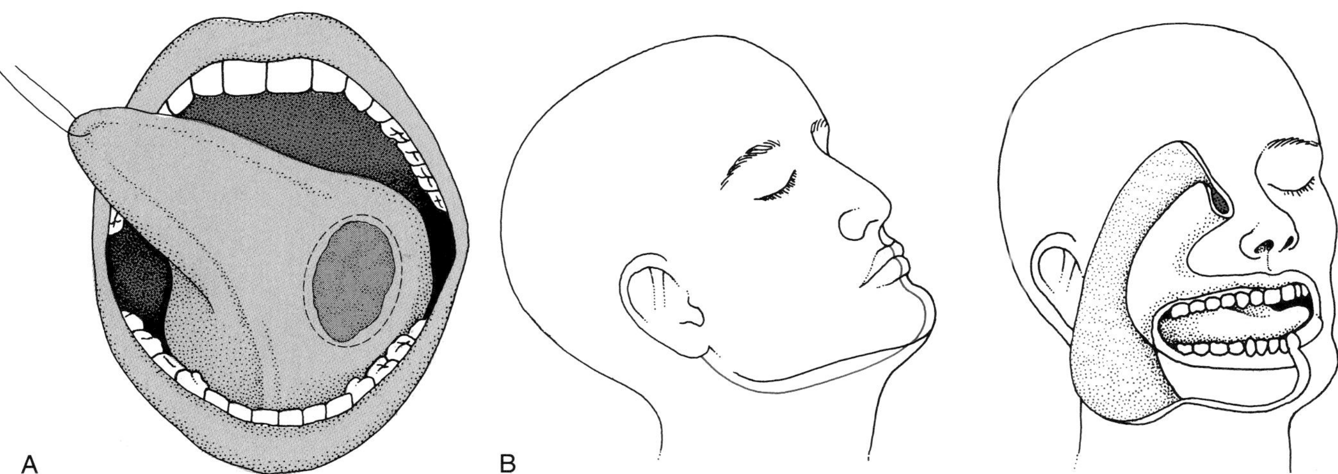

FIGURE 34-11

Approaches to surgery of the oral cavity for cancer. *A*, Peroral (through the mouth) (Adapted from Ignatavicius, D. D., & Bayne, M. V. [1991]. *Medical-surgical nursing: A nursing process approach* [p. 1259]. Philadelphia: W. B. Saunders.) *B*, External approach. (Adapted from Thawley, S. E., & Panje, W. R. [1987]. *Comprehensive management of head and neck tumors.* Philadelphia: W. B. Saunders.)

NURSING DIAGNOSIS. Nursing diagnoses for the patient with oral cancer may include the following:

- **Altered Oral Mucous Membrane** related to tumor, edema, secretions
- **Ineffective Breathing Patterns** related to tumor, tissue trauma
- **Knowledge Deficit** of treatment and prevention of oral cancer

When surgery is performed, additional nursing diagnoses may include the following:

- **Pain** related to tissue trauma
- **Altered Nutrition: Less than Body Requirements** related to pain, edema, medical restrictions on oral intake
- **Impaired Verbal Communication** related to edema, tissue trauma
- **Body Image Disturbance** related to surgical or radiation treatment
- **High Risk for Infection** related to broken skin, traumatized tissue
- **Altered Tissue Perfusion** of graft related to inadequate blood flow

GOALS. Goals for nursing care of the patient with oral cancer may include intact oral mucosa, effective breathing pattern, patient's understanding of treatment and prevention, pain relief, adequate caloric intake, effective communication, adjustment to altered appearance, absence of infection, and survival of grafted tissue.

INTERVENTIONS

Altered Oral Mucous Membrane. Mouth care varies with the type of lesion and the treatment performed. Surgical incisions can be extensive with considerable tissue trauma. Radiation therapy causes edema and increased secretions. Dry mouth is often a problem after radiation of the mouth. The physician should be consulted before doing any mouth care for the patient who has had oral surgery or radiation. Temperatures are usually taken by the rectal route after oral surgery. The physician may order specific solutions for rinsing the mouth. One solution that soothes and cleans is half hydrogen peroxide and half normal saline. Another is made by mixing ½ teaspoon of baking soda in 8 ounces of water. Good hydration keeps the oral mucosa moist and thins secretions.

Ineffective Breathing Patterns. Edema, secretions, and an enlarging tumor can cause obstruction of the airway. The nurse monitors respiratory status frequently and reports signs of inadequate oxygenation (dyspnea, restlessness, tachycardia). If edema is present, the head of the bed should be elevated. Steroids may be ordered to decrease inflammation and production of secretions. Oral suction may be ordered to remove secretions that might be aspirated. A tracheotomy may be performed to prevent or treat airway obstruction. Care of the patient with a tracheostomy is covered in Chapter 49.

Pain. Patients with oral cancer may have pain as a result of the lesion, surgical trauma, or the effects of radiation. Patients who have had grafts often report more pain in the donor site than in the grafted site. Analgesics should be administered as ordered to manage pain. The physician should be informed if the medication is not controlling the patient's pain. In addition to drug therapy, the nurse can use relaxation, imagery, and other strategies, as described in Chapter 16.

Altered Nutrition. If the patient is able to swallow, a soft or liquid diet may be prescribed. Mouth care before and after meals may improve appetite and keeps the mouth free of food particles. If the patient cannot or should not take oral nutrition, a feeding tube (nasogastric or gastrostomy) will probably be needed. Another option is TPN. Intake and output records and daily weights are monitored to assess adequate intake. With large tumors that cannot be completely removed or following extensive oral surgery, the feeding tube may be needed indefinitely. See the section on common therapeutic measures earlier in this chapter for care of the patient with a feeding tube. When the patient is able to take oral fluids, the nurse assesses swallowing and monitors the amount of food taken. Therapy may be needed to help the patient learn to swallow again. Speech therapists are experts in evaluating and managing swallowing disorders.

Impaired Verbal Communication. A large tumor or one that interferes with movement of the tongue is likely to affect speech. In addition, surgical procedures can damage structures involved in normal speech. The nurse assesses the patient's ability to read and write. A system is devised to enable the patient to communicate with others. A "magic slate" or pen and pad can be provided and kept within the patient's reach. The call button also must be within reach at all times. The intercom system at the nurse's station should be marked so that staff know to go to the patient's room rather than asking what is needed over the intercom. If the speech organs are intact, the patient may need speech therapy to regain clear oral communication. The nurse and others need to realize how traumatic it is for the patient who is unable to express thoughts verbally. Caregivers should be patient and not rush the patient. Successful communication should be complimented.

Body Image Disturbance. Patients with oral cancer may have body image disturbances as a result of impaired speech, inability to eat, and altered physical appearance. Sometimes external incisions are extensive and disfiguring. Patients need to feel accepted by caregivers and family. Acceptance is demonstrated by attentive care, patience, touching, and listening. Patients can be assured that edema related to surgery will resolve. Some disfigurement, however, may be permanent. The nurse encourages the patient to resume grooming and explores ways to improve appearance. Professional counseling may be needed to help the patient learn to cope with body image changes.

High Risk for Infection. Patients with open lesions or surgical incisions are at risk for infection. If a graft has been done, the patient's donor site is also a potential site for infection. The nurse is alert for signs and symptoms of infection (fever, redness, swelling, purulent drainage), and the physician is advised of their presence. Prophylactic antibiotics may be ordered. Care of external incisions is done according to physician's orders and agency policy.

Altered Tissue Perfusion. When living tissue is grafted, the primary concern is maintaining adequate blood supply so that the tissue remains alive. The nurse monitors graft color and warmth and protects the graft from pressure. Coolness or darkness is reported to the physician.

Knowledge Deficit. Nurses promote prevention of oral cancer by teaching patients to avoid known risk factors (tobacco and alcohol use, excessive sun exposure). Any dental problem or pain in the mouth should be reported to a dentist or physician for early evaluation.

Following surgery for oral cancers, the nurse teaches the patient the importance of good nutrition and mouth care for wound healing. If the patient is discharged with a feeding tube or tracheostomy, the nurse teaches the patient how to manage it. Teaching for self-care should begin as soon as the patient is well enough to participate, not a few hours before discharge. If the patient and family appear to need assistance, the nurse contacts the physician about a referral to a home health agency.

EVALUATION. Criteria for evaluating nursing interventions are healed surgical incision; normal respiratory rate and effort; accurate patient statement of treatments and ways to reduce risk of recurrence; patient statement of pain relief; stable or increased weight; patient ability to communicate needs; patient statement of acceptance of physical alterations; absence of fever, elevated white blood cell count, increased redness of incision or purulent drainage; and warm grafted tissue with normal color.

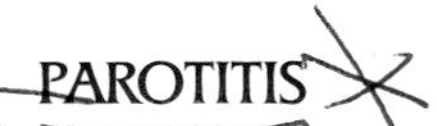

PAROTITIS

Parotitis refers to inflammation of the parotid glands. This condition causes painful swelling of the salivary glands below the ear next to the lower jaw. Pain increases during eating. Parotitis may develop in patients who are unable to take oral liquids for a long time, especially if their oral hygiene is poor. Patients who are very weak and have little resistance to infection also are at risk for parotitis.

The condition is treated with antibiotics, mouthwashes, and warm compresses. If chronic inflammation develops, surgical drainage or removal may be necessary. Otherwise, the infected gland can rupture, spreading infection into surrounding tissues. Parotitis might be prevented in susceptible patients by providing chewing gum or citrus-flavored hard candy (if allowed) to stimulate saliva production. The nurse assesses the patients temperature and comfort level and monitors swelling of the infected gland. Antibiotics and mouth care are provided as ordered.

ESOPHAGEAL CANCER

Pathophysiology

Cancer of the esophagus is not common, but it has a very poor prognosis. Most esophageal cancers are located in the middle or lower portion of the esophagus. There is no known cause, but predisposing factors are cigarette smoking, excessive alcohol intake, chronic trauma, poor oral hygiene, and eating spicy foods.

Cancer of the esophagus has often begun to metastasize by the time it is diagnosed. The liver and lung are common sites of metastasis. The lesion can also extend to the aorta, causing erosion and hemorrhage. Other complications are esophageal obstruction and perforation.

Signs and Symptoms

Progressive dysphagia (difficulty swallowing) is the primary symptom of esophageal cancer. The patient has difficulty with meat first, then with soft foods, and eventually with liquids. Pain associated with swallowing may be substernal, epigastric, or located in the back with radiation to the neck, jaws, ear, or shoulder. Some patients report sore throats and choking. Obstruction is a late sign of esophageal cancer. Weight loss may be dramatic.

Medical Diagnosis

Radiographic studies used to diagnose cancer of the esophagus include barium swallow and computed tomographic scan. Esophagoscopy may be done to permit the physician to visualize and biopsy the lesion. Endoscopic ultrasonography also may be used to assess the lesion and surrounding tissue. Additional information about common diagnostic tests and procedures is summarized in Table 34–3.

Medical Treatment

Esophageal cancer may be treated with surgery, radiation, chemotherapy, or various combinations of these. Three surgical procedures can be done to treat this type of cancer (Fig. 34–12):

- Esophagectomy—removal of all or part of the esophagus and replacement of the resected part with a Dacron graft
- Esophagogastrostomy—resection of the diseased part of the esophagus and attachment of the remaining esophagus to the stomach
- Esophagoenterostomy—replacement of the diseased part of the esophagus with a segment of colon

The use of a segment of bowel to create a new esophagus is being attempted in some settings. Radiation therapy may be done before or after surgery.

Patients who are considered poor surgical risks may receive palliative treatment, which may include the following:

- Dilation of the esophagus to decrease dysphagia

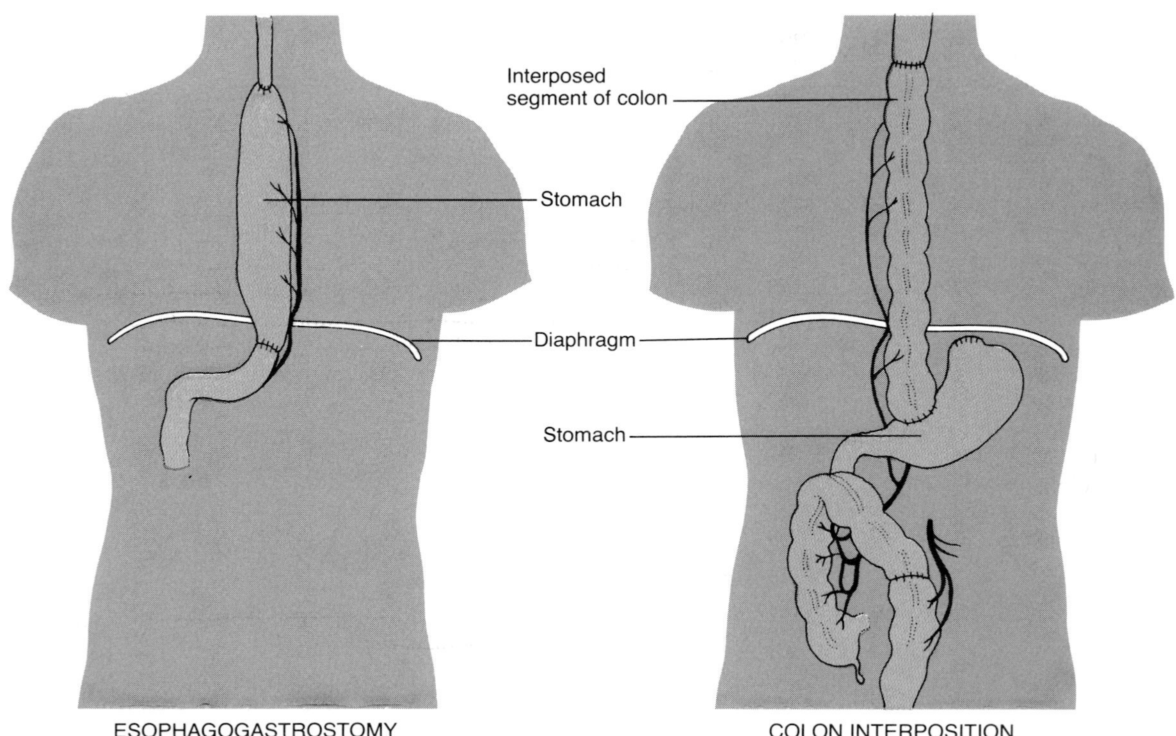

FIGURE 34–12
Surgical approaches to the treatment of esophageal cancer. (From Ignatavicius, D. D., & Bayne, M. V. [1991]. *Medical-surgical nursing: A nursing process approach* [p. 1292]. Philadelphia: W. B. Saunders.)

- Placement of a stent (a rigid tube) in the esophagus to keep it open
- Laser treatment through an endoscope
- Radiation therapy, usually a 6- to 8-week course of therapy
- Chemotherapy

The physician may insert a feeding tube, often a gastrostomy tube, to provide adequate nourishment.

Nursing Care of the Patient with Esophageal Cancer

ASSESSMENT. Assessment of the patient with a digestive tract disorder is summarized in Table 34–2. When caring for the patient with cancer of the esophagus, key data in the health history are dysphagia, pain, and choking. The nurse obtains a thorough description of the patient's pain, including location, severity, precipitating factors, and measures that bring relief. Nursing assessment of dysphagia includes the patient's description of the problem and observations of the patient while eating. The conditions under which the patient has dysphagia should be noted, as should the temperature and texture of foods that cause problems. The nurse also assesses the presence of hoarseness, cough, anorexia, weight loss, and regurgitation. The functional assessment documents the use of alcohol and tobacco and dietary practices.

Important aspects of the physical examination are general physical appearance and height and weight. It is helpful to observe the patient eating. The nurse notes body position, size of bites, chewing efforts, and speed of eating.

NURSING DIAGNOSIS. Nursing diagnoses for the patient with esophageal cancer may include the following:

- **Pain** related to esophageal lesion, effects of radiation therapy
- **Altered Nutrition: Less than Body Requirements** related to dysphagia
- **Anxiety** related to diagnosis, therapy, uncertain outcome

If the patient undergoes surgery, additional nursing diagnoses may include the following:

- **High Risk for Injury** related to leakage at anastomosis sites
- **Impaired Gas Exchange** related to incisional pain, splinting
- **Knowledge Deficit** of treatment and self-care

GOALS. Goals of nursing care may include pain relief, adequate intake of nutrients, reduced anxiety, healed incision and anastomoses, normal respirations, and patient's ability to resume self-care.

INTERVENTIONS

Pain. The nurse monitors the patient's comfort level. Analgesics are given as ordered. Independent measures to reduce or relieve pain are discussed in Chapter 16.

Altered Nutrition. Nutrition is a major problem for the patient with esophageal cancer. Daily weights, intake and output measurements, and calorie counts may all be kept to monitor adequacy of intake. A high-calorie, high-protein diet is recommended. The texture is adjusted as needed (e.g., soft, semisolid), depending on the patient's ability to swallow.

Some general interventions may be helpful in managing dysphagia. A quiet, relaxed environment helps the patient concentrate on effective swallowing. An erect position is preferred. The head should be tilted slightly forward. Some patients think that they can swallow better with the head thrown back. In reality, that position actually makes swallowing more difficult and increases the risk of aspiration. If dysphagia prevents adequate nutritional intake, an alternative feeding method must be used. Options include nasogastric and gastrostomy feedings and TPN.

Postoperatively, patients usually have nasogastric tubes inserted and attached to suction. The nurse does not irrigate or reposition nasogastric tubes in patients who have had esophageal surgery. The physician should be notified if the tube is not draining properly. Drainage is typically bloody for the first 8 to 12 hours and then gradually turns yellowish. After bowel sounds return, the physician orders oral fluids introduced in small amounts. At first, only water is given. The nurse assesses the patient's ability to swallow. Intake and output and daily weights are recorded to evaluate nutrition.

PHARMACOLOGY CAPSULE

The patient with dysphagia may be able to take liquid medications more easily than capsules or tablets.

Anxiety. A diagnosis of cancer evokes many questions and fears. It is important for the nurse to know what the patient has been told about the treatment and the prognosis so that correct information can be reinforced. Unfortunately, esophageal cancer is often fatal. Patients are encouraged to ask questions and to talk about fears. The nurse is accepting of the patient's feelings and avoids using trite phrases and false reassurance. A referral to a spiritual or mental health counselor may be indicated.

During the diagnostic period, the nurse assesses the patient's understanding of tests and procedures and offers explanations as needed. The patient is helped to select foods that are comfortably swallowed.

Preoperative teaching emphasizes the importance of turning, coughing, and deep breathing after surgery. The patient is told to expect a nasogastric tube, chest tube, and intravenous fluids.

High Risk for Injury. Depending on the surgical procedure, the patient may have multiple incisions and wound drains. The nurse assists the patient to support the wounds during coughing and position changes. Like any surgical patient, the patient who has surgery for esophageal cancer must be monitored for signs and symptoms of hemorrhage (restlessness, tachycardia, hypotension) and infection (fever, increased white blood cell count, erythema, and purulent wound drainage). In addition to the risk of infection, the patient is at risk for leakage of anastomosis sites. If the anastomosis is not secure, digestive fluids leak into the thoracic or abdominal cavity. The risk of leakage is greatest 5 to 7 days after surgery. Signs and symptoms of leakage are fever, tachycardia, tachypnea, and fluid accumulation. The physician should be notified immediately if leakage is suspected.

Impaired Gas Exchange. Immediately after surgery, the patient may be artificially ventilated to maintain adequate oxygenation. Chest tubes are needed to remove fluid from the thoracic cavity. When the ventilator is discontinued, the nurse encourages and supports the patient to turn, cough, and deep breath. Chest physiotherapy or incentive spirometry may be ordered. The patient's head is elevated to ease chest expansion and to reduce the risk of reflux of gastric contents into the esophagus.

Patients who have stents placed in the esophagus should be told how to reduce the risk of regurgitation of stomach contents. They are instructed to eat only small meals, to remain upright for several hours after meals, and to avoid lying flat at any time. The head of the bed should be elevated at least 30 degrees at all times.

Knowledge Deficit. Postoperatively, the nurse prepares the patient for discharge. The patient is encouraged to continue breathing exercises and to gradually increase activity. Bedrest is discouraged. The nurse points out the characteristics of the healing incisions and teaches the patient signs of wound complications that should be reported. The importance of small, high-calorie, high-protein meals is stressed. If nasogastric feedings are continued, the nurse instructs the patient and family in management of the feedings. Since esophageal cancer often recurs, the patient should know to report increased pain or dysphagia. A referral may be made to a home health agency for assistance after discharge.

EVALUATION. Effective nursing interventions are determined by patient's statement of pain reduction or relief; stable or increased body weight; patient's statement of lessened anxiety; absence of signs and symptoms and of wound complications; normal respiratory rate, effort, and clear breath sounds; and patient's demonstration of self-care.

DISORDERS AFFECTING DIGESTION AND ABSORPTION

NAUSEA AND VOMITING

Nausea is a feeling of discomfort sometimes referred to as queasiness. It may or may not be accompanied by abdominal pain, pallor, perspiration, and cold, clammy skin. Causes of nausea include irritating foods, infectious diseases, radiation, drugs and other chemicals, hormonal changes and imbalances, and distention of the digestive tract. It is common after surgery and in patients with motion sickness and inner ear disorders.

Nausea and vomiting often occur together. Vomiting is the forceful expulsion of stomach contents through the mouth. It occurs when the vomiting reflex in the brain is stimulated. Very forceful ejection of stomach contents is called projectile vomiting. Regurgitation is the gentle ejection of food or fluid without nausea or retching. Just before vomiting occurs, a person usually senses what is about to happen. Tachycardia and increased salivation are common just before vomiting.

Complications

Prolonged or severe vomiting can lead to significant losses of fluids and electrolytes. In addition to dehydration, metabolic alkalosis may develop due to loss of stomach acids. Patients who are very weak or unable to move are at risk for aspirating the vomited stomach contents. Therefore, nausea and vomiting must be treated to relieve patient discomfort and to prevent complications.

Medical Treatment

Drugs that prevent or treat nausea and vomiting are classified as antiemetics. Most antiemetic drugs have multiple uses. They may have local effects (adsorbents), or they may act on the central nervous system. Centrally acting antiemetics include anticholinergics, antihistamines, phenothiazines, and marijuana derivatives. Examples of these drugs are listed in Table 34–5. A common side effect of most centrally acting antiemetics is drowsiness. They may also cause tachycardia, hypotension, constipation, urinary retention, and dry mouth. Antiemetics are generally contraindicated in glaucoma, myocardial infarction, bowel or urinary obstruction, and pregnancy.

Intravenous fluids may be ordered to prevent dehydration. Oral fluids may be limited to clear liquids or withheld completely until the vomiting stops. At times, a nasogastric tube is inserted and attached to suction to keep the stomach empty. Severe or prolonged vomiting may necessitate TPN to meet the patient's metabolic needs.

PHARMACOLOGY CAPSULE

A common side effect of most antiemetics is drowsiness, so safety precautions may be necessary.

Nursing Care of the Patient with Nausea and Vomiting

ASSESSMENT. The nurse's assessment plays an important part in the management of nausea and vomiting. The health history should elicit a description of the onset, frequency, and duration of the present illness. The conditions under which nausea and vomiting occur are noted. For example, is it before or after meals, at a certain time of day, or after taking a certain medication? If vomiting occurs, the amount, color, odor, and contents of the vomitus should be recorded. Contents might include undigested food or medications. Vomitus containing bile has a characteristic green color. A bright red color suggests recent bleeding in the esophagus or stomach, although it could be due to recently ingested red food or liquid. When blood has been in the stomach long enough to be acted on by stomach secretions, it turns dark brown and resembles wet coffee grounds.

A complete health history should be obtained when the patient is able to participate. Surgeries, chronic illnesses, allergies, and medications are recorded. The nurse inquires about pregnancy since many drugs are contraindicated in the pregnant woman.

In the physical examination, the patient's general appearance, vital signs, and height and weight are recorded. Hydration status is evaluated on the basis of pulse and blood pressure, tissue turgor, mental status, and muscle tone. Respiratory rate, effort, and breath sounds are evaluated. The abdomen is assessed for distention, the presence or absence of bowel sounds, and tenderness.

NURSING DIAGNOSIS. Nursing diagnoses for the patient with nausea and vomiting include the following:

- **Altered Nutrition: Less than Body Requirements** related to nausea and vomiting
- **High Risk for Fluid Volume Deficit** related to loss of fluids through vomiting
- **High Risk for Aspiration** related to decreased level of consciousness, impaired swallowing, wired jaws, depressed gag reflex, vomiting

GOALS. Goals of nursing care for the patient with nausea and vomiting include adequate food intake, normal fluid balance, and normal respirations.

INTERVENTIONS

Altered Nutrition and Fluid Volume Deficit. When a patient complains of nausea, he or she is assisted to assume a still, comfortable position. The room temperature should be cool, and any unpleasant stimuli should be removed. An emesis basin is provided. A cool, damp cloth applied to the face and neck is comforting. Taking deep breaths and swallowing may be effective in suppressing the vomiting reflex. Unless the episode passes promptly, an antiemetic drug should be given as ordered. In situations in which nausea can be anticipated, antiemetics are best given before nausea occurs. It is easier to prevent nausea than to treat it.

If the patient does vomit, the nurse remains close by and offers reassurance. The emesis basin is emptied as promptly as possible and returned in case it is needed again. Soiled clothing and linen are replaced. Mouth care to remove unpleasant tastes can be done when the urge to vomit subsides.

Severe or prolonged vomiting puts the patient at risk for fluid volume deficit. Infants and the elderly are especially susceptible to fluid volume deficit because their kidneys are less efficient in conserving body fluids. The nurse monitors intake and output, vital signs, and other measures of hydration. Signs of fluid volume deficit include tachycardia, hypotension, oliguria, confusion, and poor tissue turgor.

When the patient is ready to resume oral intake, he or she is usually started on clear liquids. Tea, broth, flat carbonated liquids, and gelatin are generally best tolerated. Other liquids may be added if nausea and vomiting do not recur. If permitted, dry toast or crackers may be given to help relieve nausea. The patient should be advised to eat slowly.

When regular meals are resumed, fluids should be taken between meals rather than with meals. As mentioned earlier, alternative methods of feeding will be necessary if nausea and vomiting threaten the patient's fluid or nutritional status.

High Risk for Aspiration. The patient who is unconscious or has impaired swallowing or a depressed gag reflex is at risk for aspiration. This risk is much greater when the patient is vomiting. The patient must be positioned on the side so that vomitus can drain from the mouth. Suction apparatus should be kept on hand and used as needed to clear the mouth and upper airway. The nurse monitors the patient's respiratory rate and effort and breath sounds. Increasing respiratory rate, dyspnea, and abnormal breath sounds are reported to the physician.

EVALUATION. Evidence of achievement of nursing goals includes stable body weight, patient's report of decreased nausea, no vomiting; pulse and blood pressure consistent with patient's normal level, moist mucous membranes; and respiratory rate of 12 to 20 with clear breath sounds.

HIATAL HERNIA

Pathophysiology

The esophageal hiatus is the opening in the diaphragm through which the esophagus passes (Fig. 34–13). A hiatal hernia is the protrusion of the lower esophagus and stomach upward through the diaphragm, into the chest. Figure 34–14 illustrates the two types of hiatal hernias: sliding hernia and paraesophageal (rolling) hernia. In a sliding hernia, the gastroesophageal junction is above the hiatus. The stomach slides into the thoracic cavity when the patient reclines. It slides back into place when the patient stands or sits up.

In a rolling hernia, the gastroesophageal junction remains in place but a portion of the stomach herniates up through the diaphragm. Weakness of the esophageal sphincter permits gastric fluids to flow backward into the esophagus. Acidic gastric fluids can cause inflammation of the esophagus, called esophagitis.

Complications of hiatal hernia include ulcerations, bleeding, and aspiration of regurgitated stomach contents.

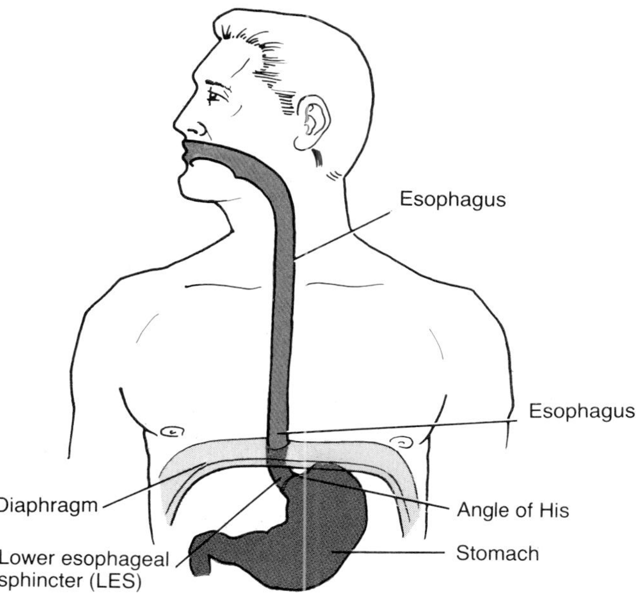

FIGURE 34–13
The esophagus and related structures.

Causes

Hiatal hernia is thought to be caused by weakness in the lower esophageal sphincter (LES) of the diaphragm. The LES is located where the esophagus and the stomach join. Factors that contribute to development of hiatal hernia include excessive intra-abdominal pressure, trauma, and long-term bedrest in a reclining position. Intra-abdominal pressure is increased by obesity, pregnancy, abdominal tumors, ascites, and repeated heavy lifting or strain. Hiatal hernia develops in about half of all people over 60 years of age.

Signs and Symptoms

Many patients with hiatal hernias have no symptoms at all. Others report feelings of fullness, dysphagia, eructation (belching), regurgitation, and heartburn. Heartburn is a feeling of burning and tightness rising from the lower sternum to the throat. It is triggered by foods and drugs that decrease LES pressure and by lying down or bending over.

Medical Diagnosis

When hiatal hernia is suspected, several tests and procedures may be ordered. A barium swallow with fluoroscopy outlines the esophagus and demonstrates esophageal peristalsis. In the patient with hiatal hernia, the reflux of gastric contents is evident. Esophagoscopy is direct examination of the esophagus with an endoscope. Structural abnormalities and tissue inflammation may be detected. Tissue specimens can be taken for biopsy during endoscopy.

Esophageal manometry measures the pressures in the stomach and the esophagus. With the patient sitting up,

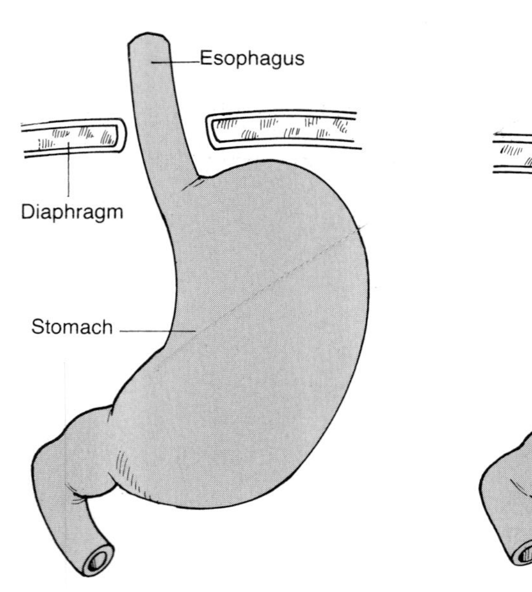

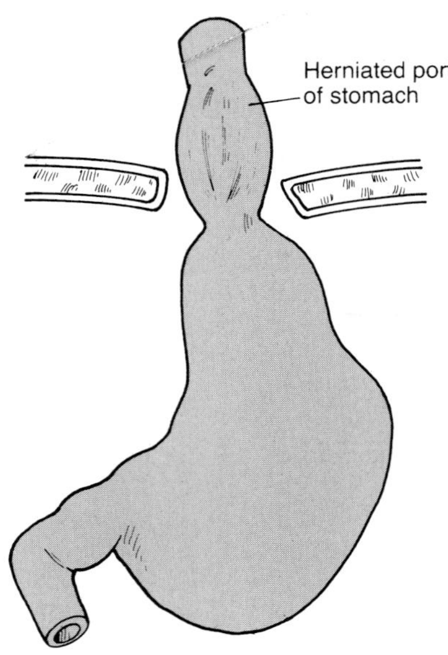

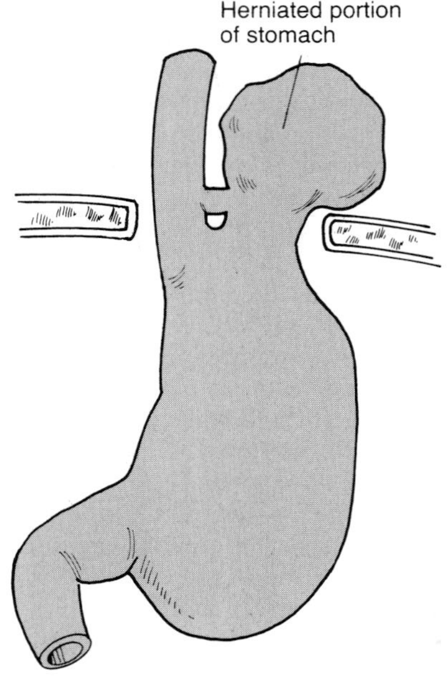

FIGURE 34–14
Hiatal hernia.

a small tube is inserted through the nose into the stomach. The patient is then placed in a supine position. Small amounts of water or gelatin are given to the patient to swallow. Pressure measurements are taken in the stomach and esophagus. For acid reflux testing, a second probe that is sensitive to acid is inserted through the nose into the esophagus. The detection of acid in the esophagus is consistent with esophageal reflux.

Medical Treatment

In many cases, hiatal hernia can be managed with drug therapy, diet, and measures to avoid increased intra-abdominal pressure. Drug therapy includes antacids and, sometimes, drugs such as cimetidine (Tagamet) to reduce gastric acid secretion. Bethanechol chloride (Urecholine) may be ordered to increase the tone of the LES.

Surgery may be necessary if severe bleeding or narrowing of the esophagus occurs. Surgical options to treat hiatal hernia include fundoplication and placement of the synthetic Angelchik prosthesis. Fundoplication (Fig. 34–15) strengthens the LES by suturing the fundus of the stomach around the esophagus and anchoring it below the diaphragm. The Angelchik prosthesis, illustrated in Figure 34–16, is a C-shaped silicone device. It is tied around the distal esophagus, anchoring it below the diaphragm. For these procedures, incisions may be made in either the abdomen or the chest. Either way, there is a risk of postoperative respiratory complications.

Nursing Care of the Patient with Hiatal Hernia

ASSESSMENT. Assessment of the patient with a digestive tract disorder is summarized in Table 34–2. When a patient has hiatal hernia, the nurse assesses the patient's symptoms (pain, dysphagia, eructation). Factors that trigger the symptoms are recorded as well as measures that aggravate or relieve them. The past medical history should include any abdominal trauma. The patient's dietary habits, use of alcohol and tobacco, and medication history are recorded. The nurse inquires about activities requiring lifting or intense physical exertion. In the physical examination, the nurse measures the patient's height and weight.

NURSING DIAGNOSIS. Nursing diagnoses for the patient with hiatal hernia may include the following:

- **Chronic Pain** related to esophageal inflammation
- **High Risk for Aspiration** related to regurgitation of gastric contents
- **Altered Nutrition: Less than Body Requirements** related to dysphagia
- **Knowledge Deficit** of measures to manage hiatal hernia

GOALS. Goals of nursing care for the hiatal hernia patient may include pain relief, absence of aspiration, adequate nutrient intake, and knowledge of self-care to manage hiatal hernia.

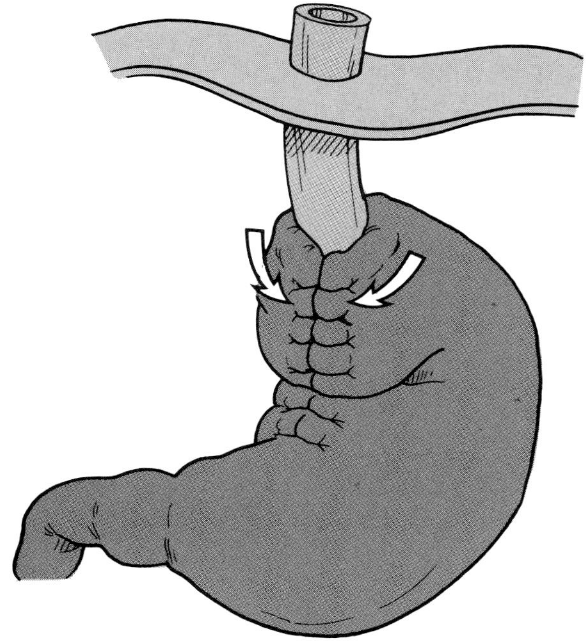

FIGURE 34-15
Nissen fundoplication for hiatal hernia repair.

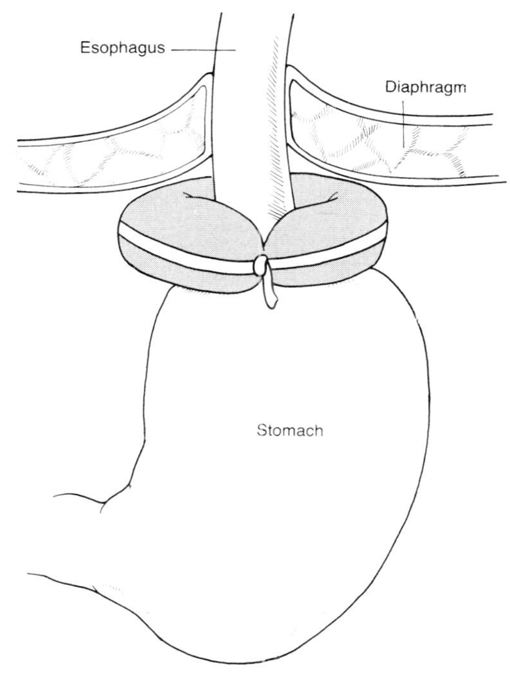

FIGURE 34-16
Placement of the Angelchik prosthesis.

INTERVENTIONS

Chronic Pain. Pain is caused by the reflux of acid into the inflamed esophagus. Therefore, pain can be reduced by increasing LES pressure, which keeps gastric contents from passing into the esophagus. Drugs that increase LES pressure, neutralize acid, and reduce acid secretion are administered as ordered. The nurse evaluates the effects of drug therapy. Dietary alterations, discussed later, are helpful in reducing the symptoms of hiatal hernia.

High Risk for Aspiration. Gastric contents that are regurgitated into the esophagus may be aspirated into the respiratory tract, causing aspiration pneumonia. To reduce the risk of aspiration, food and fluids should not be taken for 2 to 3 hours before bedtime. This reduces reflux of stomach contents during sleep. Patients with hiatal hernia should sleep with their heads elevated 6 to 12 inches. Wooden blocks can be placed under the legs of the head of the bed if a mechanical or electrical bed is not available. This sleeping position requires a period of adjustment but is very important to prevent nighttime reflux.

Altered Nutrition. The nurse assesses weight changes and notes excessive weight loss. Measures to control pain, as discussed earlier, help the patient eat more comfortably. Small, frequent meals are advised because large meals increase pressure in the stomach and delay gastric emptying. The nurse encourages the patient to avoid foods that are known to decrease LES pressure: fatty foods, coffee, tea, cola, chocolate, and alcohol. Also, acidic and spicy foods may be irritating when the esophagus is inflamed. The patient who is obese needs to be counseled about the relationship between obesity and increased intra-abdominal pressure.

Knowledge Deficit. The nurse teaches the patient the importance of drug therapy, diet, weight control, and positioning in the management of hiatal hernia. Patients are encouraged to avoid smoking and to learn stress management since smoking and stress aggravate the condition. Patients are also taught how to prevent increased intra-abdominal pressure. The nurse cautions the patient to avoid bending forward, lifting, or straining and to avoid clothing that is tight around the waist or abdomen.

EVALUATION. Criteria for evaluating the outcomes of nursing interventions are patient's statement of decreased pain; normal pulse, respirations, and temperature, clear breath sounds; stable body weight; and patient's description and demonstration of self-care measures.

POSTOPERATIVE CARE. Postoperative care after hiatal hernia repair is similar to that after any major abdominal surgery. Turning, coughing, and deep breathing are particularly important for these patients. The patient will probably have a nasogastric tube in place and connected to suction for a day or two after surgery.

Until bowel function returns, the patient is given only intravenous fluids. The patient can be advised to expect mild dysphagia for several weeks.

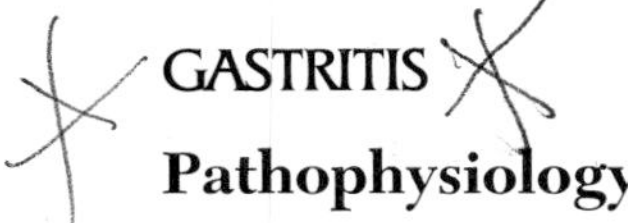

GASTRITIS

Pathophysiology

Gastritis is an inflammation of the lining of the stomach. It may be acute or chronic and may range from mild to severe. Acute gastritis can be caused by excessive intake of food or alcohol, food poisoning, or chemical irritation. It usually lasts several hours to several days, until the irritant has been eliminated. The most serious complication of acute gastritis is hemorrhage.

The patient usually has a full recovery, but repeated bouts of acute gastritis can lead to chronic gastritis. Sometimes chronic gastritis has no apparent cause. Chronic irritation and inflammation can lead to atrophic gastritis and gastric atrophy. These changes in the stomach lining result in decreased production of acid and intrinsic factor. Intrinsic factor is needed for the absorption of vitamin B_{12}, which is essential for the maturation of red blood cells. Without intrinsic factor, a serious condition called pernicious anemia develops. The management of pernicious anemia is discussed in Chapter 30.

PHARMACOLOGY CAPSULE

Oral vitamin B_{12} is ineffective in pernicious anemia; only the parenteral form is appropriate.

Signs and Symptoms

Symptoms of acute gastritis usually include nausea, vomiting, a feeling of fullness, and pain in the stomach area. Chronic gastritis may have the same symptoms as acute gastritis. Some patients, however, have only mild indigestion with chronic gastritis.

Medical Diagnosis

The best means of diagnosing gastritis is gastroscopy. The physician is able to visualize the interior of the stomach and biopsy any suspicious areas. A barium swallow may be done as well. Laboratory studies may be performed to detect occult blood in the feces, low blood hemoglobin and hematocrit, and low serum gastrin.

Medical Treatment

The medical management of acute gastritis is concerned with treatment of the symptoms and fluid replacement. If hospitalization is considered necessary, oral fluids and foods are usually withheld until the acute symptoms subside. Intravenous fluids can be ordered to prevent or treat dehydration. Medications to reduce gastric acidity (antacids and H_2 receptor blockers) and to relieve nausea may be given. Topical anesthetics (oxethazaine) and analgesics may be ordered for pain relief. When nausea and vomiting stop, oral fluids are gradually increased. Typically, the patient progresses from clear liquids to full liquids and then to a soft, bland diet.

The medical management of chronic gastritis focuses on elimination of the cause (e.g., alcohol, drugs) and treatment of pernicious anemia. A bland diet given in six small feedings is usually prescribed, with antacids ordered after meals. Corticosteroids also may be used. Vitamin B_{12} injections must be given regularly to prevent long-term complications.

Surgical intervention may be needed if conservative measures fail to correct or control gastritis. Specific procedures and nursing implications are the same as for peptic ulcer disease, which is discussed later.

Nursing Care of the Patient with Gastritis

ASSESSMENT. In taking the health history, the nurse first describes the patient's present illness. Patients often complain of pain, indigestion, nausea, and vomiting. The nurse determines the onset, duration, and location of pain. Factors that trigger or relieve the symptoms are noted. Chronic illnesses are recorded, as are current and recent medications. The nurse asks whether the patient has had any unexplained weight loss. The functional assessment provides information about dietary practices, use of alcohol and tobacco, and activity and rest patterns. The patient is asked if there are significant sources of stress at present.

In the physical examination, the nurse observes the patient's general appearance for signs of distress. Vital signs and height and weight are measured for comparison to previous readings. Skin color and turgor are assessed. The abdomen is inspected for distention and palpated for tenderness and guarding. The nurse auscultates the abdomen for increased bowel sounds.

NURSING DIAGNOSIS. Nursing diagnoses for the patient with gastritis may include the following:

- **Pain** related to inflammation of gastric mucosa
- **Altered Nutrition: Less than Body Requirements** related to anorexia, pain, nausea and vomiting
- **High Risk for Fluid Volume Deficit** related to vomiting, bleeding
- **Ineffective Individual Coping** related to chronic illness
- **Knowledge Deficit** of self-care measures

GOALS. Goals of nursing care for the patient with gastritis are pain relief, adequate nutritional intake, normal hydration, absence of signs of bleeding, effective coping strategies, and patient's knowledge of gastritis and self-care measures.

INTERVENTIONS

Pain. Medications including antacids, H_2 receptor blockers, analgesics, and topical anesthetics are given as ordered. The nurse assesses drug effectiveness and informs the physician if pain is not relieved. Nonpharmacologic methods of pain control as described in Chapter 16 may be employed as well.

Altered Nutrition. The nurse encourages the patient to identify foods that seem to aggravate the symptoms and to eliminate them from the diet. The patient should be taught that a soft, bland diet taken in small meals may decrease symptoms. Caffeine is usually eliminated from the diet. The patient's dietary intake is noted. Daily weights may be appropriate to determine whether the patient is receiving adequate nourishment.

Fluid Volume Deficit. Fluid volume deficit may result from dehydration or from hemorrhage. The patient may become dehydrated owing to poor oral intake or severe vomiting. The nurse is alert for signs of fluid volume deficit (oliguria, tachycardia, dry skin and mucous membranes, poor tissue turgor, and hypotension). Intake and output are recorded. Vomited fluids are inspected for bright red blood or dark brown particles that indicate bleeding in the stomach. The stool is inspected for the maroon or tarry black appearance characteristic of bleeding from the stomach. Intravenous fluids are given as ordered, with the nurse monitoring the rate of infusion.

Ineffective Individual Coping. Chronic illness drains the patient physically and emotionally. The nurse explores how the patient is dealing with gastritis and what additional supports are needed. Professional counseling may be needed to help the patient learn relaxation and stress management techniques. When alcohol abuse contributes to gastritis, the nurse can provide information about community resources such as Alcoholics Anonymous.

Knowledge Deficit. The nurse prepares the patient for discharge by teaching how gastritis can be treated with diet, medications, and stress management. The patient should know that bloody vomitus or dark, tarry stools should be reported to the physician.

EVALUATION. Criteria for effective nursing care are patient's statement of pain relief; stable weight; fluid output equal to intake and absence of signs of dehydration; patient's knowledge of stress management techniques and resources; and patient's statement of self-care measures.

PEPTIC ULCER

Pathophysiology

A peptic ulcer is a loss of tissue from the lining of the digestive tract. Normally, a mucus barrier protects the lining from the digestive fluids. When that barrier fails, pepsin and hydrochloric acid cause injury to the unprotected tissue.

Peptic ulcers may be acute or chronic, depending on the layers of tissue affected. Acute ulcers affect only the superficial layers of the digestive lining, whereas chronic ulcers extend into the muscle layer. Acute ulcers are sometimes called acute gastric lesions.

Peptic ulcers are classified as gastric or duodenal, depending on their location. Gastric and duodenal ulcers differ in depth of injury, amount of gastric secretions, incidence, and signs and symptoms. These differences are presented in Table 34–6.

Gastric ulcers occur most often in men and in the elderly. Women who have ulcers are more likely to have gastric ulcers than duodenal ulcers. The incidence rate of gastric ulcers is higher among people with type A blood than among people with other blood types. Although people think of ulcers as a condition of the rich and powerful, gastric ulcers are actually more common among unskilled laborers.

Eighty percent of peptic ulcers occur in the duodenum. Duodenal ulcers are more common in younger men and in people with type O blood. There is an increase in the secretion of gastric acid. Duodenal ulcers are found among people in all occupations and income levels.

Causes

Causes of acute gastric lesions include drugs and stress. Extremely stressful events such as shock, burns, and trauma are thought to cause a temporary decrease in blood flow to the gastric mucosa. Inadequate blood flow interferes with the mucosal barrier, permitting breakdown of the stomach lining. Spicy foods are often blamed for ulcers, but this link has not been proved. With gastric ulcers, gastric acid production is usually normal or decreased.

Conditions that cause a high gastric acid concentration seem to contribute to the development of duodenal ulcers. Examples of such conditions are chronic obstructive pulmonary disease, cirrhosis of the liver, chronic

TABLE 34-6
COMPARISON OF GASTRIC AND DUODENAL ULCERS

CHARACTERISTIC	GASTRIC ULCER	DUODENAL ULCER
Incidence	More common in older men, working class, blood type A, substance abusers, people under severe stress.	More common in younger men, all social classes, blood type O, people with chronic illnesses.
Ulcer depth	Shallow	Deep
Gastric secretions	Unchanged or decreased	Increased
Signs and symptoms	Burning and pressure in upper left abdomen below rib cage and in back. Pain 1–2 hr after meals. Relieved by food or fluids.	Burning and pressure in upper middle abdomen and back. Pain 2–4 hr after meals. Relieved by antacids or foods.
Complications	Hemorrhage, perforation, obstruction	Hemorrhage, perforation, obstruction

pancreatitis, and hyperparathyroidism. Heavy alcohol and tobacco use also is associated with duodenal ulcers, as well as with gastric ulcers.

Signs and Symptoms

Gastric ulcers typically produce burning pain in the epigastric area 1 to 2 hours after meals. Nausea, anorexia, and weight loss are sometimes present. Some patients have no pain at all until serious complications develop.

Although some patients with duodenal ulcers have no pain, others experience a burning or cramping pain 2 to 4 hours after meals. The pain is located in the area just beneath the xyphoid process. It is often relieved by antacids or food. The patient commonly reports pain that lasts for several weeks or months, disappears, and returns.

Complications

Peptic ulcers can lead to serious, even life-threatening complications. Intractability is the term used to describe symptomatic peptic ulcer disease that does not respond to treatment. Hemorrhage is more common in the elderly and in people with gastric ulcers. If not brought under control, the patient can bleed to death.

Perforation is a break in the wall of the stomach or the duodenum that permits digestive fluids to leak into the peritoneal cavity, causing inflammation of the peritoneum (peritonitis).

The pylorus is the opening between the stomach and the duodenum. With peptic ulcer disease, pyloric obstruction may develop as a result of edema and scarring. Pyloric obstruction causes persistent vomiting that can lead to severe fluid and electrolyte imbalances.

Medical Diagnosis

Tests and procedures used to detect peptic ulcers include barium swallow, gastroscopy, and esophagogastroduodenoscopy. These studies, including patient preparation and aftercare, are described in Table 34–3.

Gastric analysis may be done to determine the acidity of stomach secretions. Although some patients with ulcers have high acid levels, others do not. Variations in the process of collecting the specimens can produce unreliable results. Therefore, the value of this test is in doubt. Gastric analysis is thought to be more accurate if pentagastrin is given to stimulate gastric secretions prior to collection of the specimens.

Medical Treatment

The goals of medical treatment of peptic ulcer are to relieve symptoms, promote healing, prevent or detect complications, and prevent recurrence. Interventions include drug therapy, diet, and stress management.

DRUG THERAPY. Drug therapy is intended to relieve pain, protect the ulcer from further damage, reduce gastric acid secretion, and alleviate anxiety. Drugs used to treat peptic ulcer disease include antacids, sucralfate, H_2 receptor blockers, and anticholinergics. Antacids relieve pain by neutralizing gastric acid. They also prevent the formation of pepsin. Antacids are available as liquids and as chewable tablets. They are usually ordered 1 and 3 hours after meals and at bedtime. Antacid therapy may be prescribed after the ulcer has healed to prevent recurrence. Since antacids are available without a prescription, patients may think they can do no harm. In fact, they can have serious side effects. They also impair the absorption of many other drugs if taken at the same time. The patient should be cautioned to take the exact amount prescribed and not to adjust it on his or her own.

Sucralfate (Carafate) clings to the surface of the ulcer and protects it so that healing can take place. Histamine$_2$ receptor antagonists are used to decrease hydrochloric acid production and to promote healing of the ulcer. Examples of H_2 receptor antagonists include cimetidine (Tagamet) and ranitidine (Zantac). Anticholinergic drugs such as propantheline bromide (Pro-Banthine) may be used to improve the action of both cimetidine and antacids. Metoclopramide (Reglan) causes the stomach to empty more quickly, removing food and drugs that stimulate acid production.

PHARMACOLOGY CAPSULE

Antacids are drugs and can have adverse effects if taken excessively!

DIET THERAPY. The recommended diet therapy for ulcer patients has changed over the years. The current approach is to permit the patient most any foods that do not produce discomfort. The patient is usually discouraged from taking in foods that stimulate acid secretion but do not neutralize acids. These foods include coffee, tea, meat broth, and alcohol. The effect of spicy foods is debated, but they should be excluded if they cause pain. Symptoms occur more often when the stomach is empty. Therefore, frequent, small feedings throughout the day are recommended. The ulcer patient should be advised not to skip meals.

MANAGING COMPLICATIONS. Complications may be treated medically or surgically. If hemorrhage is suspected, a nasogastric tube is inserted and attached to suction to remove and measure blood in the stomach. After the stomach has been suctioned, the physician may use saline lavage to control bleeding. The patient is placed on the left side, and 50 to 200 ml of saline (usually iced to cause vasoconstriction) is instilled in the stomach through the nasogastric tube. The saline is then suctioned out, and the procedure is repeated until the returning fluid is clear and free of clots. Iced saline has traditionally been used for saline lavage. Some experts, however, recommend that room-temperature saline be used to decrease the risk of damage to the gastric mucosa and to avoid stimulation of the vagal nerve. Vasopressin may be given intravenously to control hemorrhage. Arterial embolization is a procedure that uses the patient's own blood and other substances to seal bleeding arteries. Once bleeding is controlled, antacids and H_2 receptor blockers are usually ordered at frequent intervals.

Perforation is treated initially with gastric decompression and intravenous fluids and antibiotics. A small perforation may close spontaneously, otherwise surgical repair is needed.

Obstruction may be due to edema and spasm, which often respond to medical treatment. A nasogastric tube is inserted to decompress the stomach, and intravenous fluids are provided. The nasogastric tube is clamped after 72 hours. If there is no evidence of continued obstruction, oral fluids are introduced. Continued obstruction requires surgical intervention.

Complications of peptic ulcer disease, signs and symptoms, related treatments, and nursing care are summarized in Table 34–7.

SURGERY. Surgical intervention is indicated for treatment of complications that do not respond to conservative treatment or to decrease acid secretion. Procedures that decrease acid secretion include vagotomy, pyloroplasty, gastroenterostomy, antrectomy, and subtotal gastrectomy. In extreme cases, total gastrectomy is necessary. These procedures are described in Table 34–8 and illustrated in Figure 34–17.

Nursing Care of the Patient with Peptic Ulcer Managed Medically

Nursing care of the patient with peptic ulcer disease can be quite complicated, depending on the severity of the condition and the medical or surgical treatment. Therefore, nursing care of the medical patient and the surgical patient is discussed separately (see also Care Plan: The Patient with a Peptic Ulcer).

ASSESSMENT. Complete assessment of the patient with a disorder of the digestive tract is summarized in Table 34–2. When a patient has peptic ulcer disease, the nurse describes the symptoms that caused the patient to seek medical care. The presence of pain is documented, including location, aggravating factors, and measures that bring relief. The relationship between pain and food intake also is noted.

Important aspects of the past medical history include recent serious illnesses, previous peptic ulcer disease, and a medication history. A family history of ulcers is assessed as well. Significant symptoms include nausea, vomiting, and indigestion. The nurse asks if blood has been noted in vomitus and if stools have changed color or consistency. The functional assessment records the patient's usual diet, use of alcohol and tobacco, activities, sleep patterns, and stressors.

The physical examination begins with general observations of the patient. Vital signs are taken to detect tachycardia and hypotension, which may indicate complications in the acutely ill patient. Height and weight are measured. The skin and mucous membranes are assessed for turgor and moisture. The abdomen is inspected for distention and palpated for tenderness. Bowel sounds are auscultated.

NURSING DIAGNOSIS. Nursing diagnoses for the patient with peptic ulcer disease may include the following:

- **Pain** related to ulceration of stomach or duodenum
- **Altered Nutrition: Less than Body Requirements** related to nausea, vomiting, anorexia, dietary restrictions, nothing by mouth status
- **High Risk for Injury** related to hemorrhage, perforation, obstruction
- **Ineffective Individual Coping** related to prescribed alterations in lifestyle
- **Knowledge Deficit** of self-care to manage peptic ulcer disease

GOALS. The goals of nursing care for the patient with peptic ulcer disease are pain relief, adequate nutrition, absence of complications, adjustment to prescribed changes in lifestyle, and patient's knowledge of self-care measures.

INTERVENTIONS

Pain. The most important means of reducing pain associated with peptic ulcer disease are drug therapy, rest,

TABLE 34–7

COMPLICATIONS OF PEPTIC ULCER DISEASE

COMPLICATION	SIGNS AND SYMPTOMS	TREATMENT	NURSING CARE
Hemorrhage	Thready pulse, restlessness, diaphoresis, chills, oliguria, hematemesis, tarry stools, hypotension.	Saline lavage Vasopressin Arterial embolization	Assist with procedure. Monitor effects of treatment. Monitor for water intoxication: headache, coma, tremor, sweating, anxiety. Monitor vital signs, intake and output. Maintain patent NG tube. IV fluids as ordered.
Perforation	Sudden, sharp midepigastric pain that spreads over entire abdomen. Rigid abdomen. Absence of bowel sounds. Shock.	NG suction Antibiotics IV fluids	Monitor vital signs, intake and output. Enforce NPO order. Give fluids and blood as ordered. Keep NG tube patent.
Obstruction	Feeling of fullness, nausea after eating, persistent vomiting.	NG suction	Monitor vital signs, intake and output. Keep NG tube patent.

NG, Nasogastric; IV, intravenous; NPO, nothing by mouth.

TABLE 34-8

SURGICAL TREATMENT OF PEPTIC ULCER DISEASE

SURGERY	PROCEDURE	PURPOSE	ADVERSE EFFECTS
Vagotomy			
Truncal	Vagus nerve that supplies stomach is severed.	Decreases stimulation of gastric acid secretion.	May have delayed gastric emptying. Feeling of fullness, dumping syndrome, diarrhea.
Selective or superselective	Severs that part of vagus nerve that stimulates acid production. Spares nerve supply to pyloric sphincter.	Decreases stimulation of gastric acid secretion.	Delayed gastric emptying.
Pyloroplasty	Widens pylorus.	Improves passage of stomach contents into duodenum. Usually done with vagotomy to prevent gastric stasis.	Dumping syndrome due to rapid emptying of stomach into duodenum.
Simple gastroenterostomy	Creates passage between body of stomach and jejunum.	Permits passage of alkaline intestinal secretions into stomach to neutralize gastric acid.	May actually increase gastric acid secretion.
Antrectomy	Removal of antrum of stomach.	Reduces gastric acid by removing source of acid secretion.	Diarrhea, feeling of fullness after eating, dumping syndrome, malabsorption, anemia.
Subtotal gastrectomy			
Gastroduodenoscopy (Billroth I)	Part of distal portion of stomach, including antrum, is removed. Remaining stomach is anastomosed to duodenum.	Reduces acid by removing source of gastric acid secretion.	Dumping syndrome (less often than with other procedures), anemia, malabsorption, weight loss, bile reflux.
Gastrojejunostomy (Billroth II)	Part of distal portion of stomach, including antrum, is removed. Remaining stomach is anastomosed to jejunum.	Removes source of acid secretion.	Dumping syndrome, weight loss, malabsorption, duodenal infection, pernicious anemia, afferent loop syndrome (obstruction of duodenal loop).
Total gastrectomy	Removal of entire stomach. Esophagus anastomosed to duodenum.	Removes source of gastric acid secretion.	Can only consume small, frequent meals of semi-solid foods. Pernicious anemia; dumping syndrome.

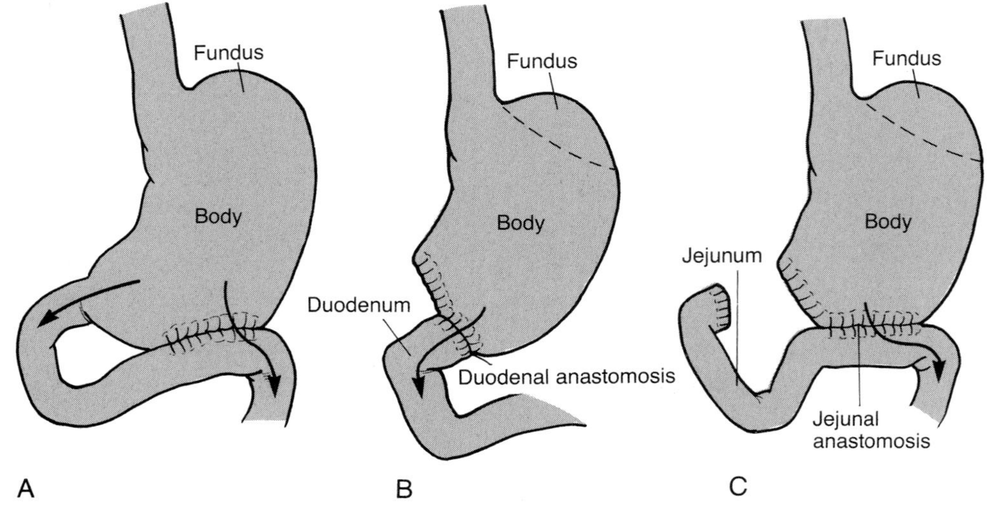

FIGURE 34-17

Gastric surgical procedures: *A*, Gastroenterostomy: passage created between stomach and jejunum. *B*, Billroth I (gastroduodenoscopy): distal portion of stomach removed and remainder anastomosed to duodenum. *C*, Billroth II (gastrojejunostomy): lower portion of stomach removed and remainder anastomosed to jejumun. Shaded area represents portion removed.

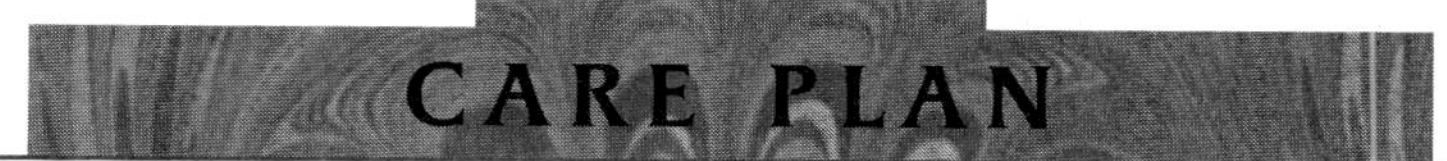

CARE PLAN
The Patient with a Peptic Ulcer

ASSESSMENT

Health History: Mr. Louis Kennon is a 47-year-old male who has recently been diagnosed as having duodenal ulcers. He has a history of burning pain 2 to 3 hours after meals. The pain is located just beneath the xyphoid process and is relieved by antacids. Symptoms are sometimes accompanied by nausea but not vomiting. He noticed that his stools have been darker than usual this week. Mr. Kennon describes his health as good but is being treated for hypertension. He states that he rarely drinks alcoholic beverages but smokes 1½ packs of cigarettes daily. He is a truck driver who usually eats only two meals each day at irregular hours.

Physical Examination: Vital signs: temperature, 97.6°F; pulse, 76; respiration, 16; blood pressure, 136/82. His height is 5 feet 10 inches, and his weight is 210 pounds. He is alert and oriented. The abdomen is soft. Bowel sounds are present in all four quadrants.

NURSING DIAGNOSIS	GOALS AND OUTCOME CRITERIA	INTERVENTIONS
Acute pain related to ulceration of duodenum.	Patient will verbalize pain relief and appear relaxed.	Administer drugs that decrease acid secretion, neutralize acid, or coat ulcer surfaces as ordered. Promote a restful environment and explain importance of rest to patient. Teach relaxation techniques.
Altered nutrition: less than body requirements related to nausea, vomiting, anorexia, dietary restrictions.	Patient will maintain adequate nutrition as evidenced by stable body weight.	Provide diet as ordered: often bland, low-fat diet given in six small feedings. Administer antiemetics for nausea and vomiting. Monitor weight. Consult dietitian if patient is losing weight.
High risk for injury related to hemorrhage, perforation, and obstruction.	Patient will remain free of complications as evidenced by normal vital signs, no vomiting, hematemesis, or tarry stools.	Monitor for signs and symptoms of bleeding: hematemesis, tarry stools, weakness, tachycardia, pallor, and hypotension. If hemorrhage occurs, notify physician and monitor vital signs. Perform lavage via nasogastric tube as ordered. Keep patient quiet and enforce nothing by mouth order. Maintain intravenous lines to ensure venous access in emergency. Monitor for signs and symptoms of perforation: sudden, sharp pain in midepigastric region that spreads across abdomen, patient drawing knees up toward chest. If perforation occurs, notify physician and monitor vital signs. Withhold oral fluids. Anticipate need for nasogastric suction and intravenous fluids. Monitor for signs and symptoms of pyloric obstruction: persistent vomiting. Carry out orders, including nasogastric suction, intravenous fluids, and antibiotics.
Ineffective individual coping related to prescribed alterations in lifestyle.	Patient will express intent to implement lifestyle alterations.	Identify behaviors such as use of alcohol and tobacco that aggravate peptic ulcer disease. Explain effects of behaviors on disease. Offer information about resources (American Cancer Society, American Lung Association) that provide services to help patients give up tobacco.

Care Plan continued on following page

The Patient with a Peptic Ulcer *(Continued)*

NURSING DIAGNOSIS	GOALS AND OUTCOME CRITERIA	INTERVENTIONS
Knowledge deficit of self-care to manage peptic ulcer disease.	Patient will correctly describe self-care measures to promote healing of duodenal ulcers and prevent recurrence.	Tell patient to avoid foods that stimulate release of gastrin: alcohol, tobacco, caffeine. Stress importance of taking drugs as prescribed. Explain side and adverse effects and their management. List drugs that are contraindicated: aspirin, nonsteroidal anti-inflammatory drugs, and corticosteroids. Supplement verbal instruction with written information. Encourage follow-up care.

and diet. Drugs reduce pain by neutralizing acid, decreasing acid secretion, or coating the ulcer surface. For maximum effect, the nurse should give the medications at the recommended times. For example, antacids are most effective when given 1 hour after meals and at bedtime. The nurse should know the side effects of these drugs and monitor for them. The physician should be notified if pain persists or worsens despite drug therapy.

Rest reduces symptoms of peptic ulcer disease because physical activity stimulates gastric secretions. The environment should be as restful as possible. The nurse can encourage relaxation techniques and stress management strategies as described in Chapter 16.

Altered Nutrition. Dietary restrictions have long been part of the treatment of peptic ulcer disease. Many experts now question the impact of special diets on ulcers. When the patient has acute symptoms, a bland low-fiber diet is often given in six small feedings. The patient is advised to avoid any foods that have caused gastric distress in the past. In general, alcohol, tobacco, and beverages that contain caffeine are discouraged because they stimulate release of gastrin. The physician may advise the patient to adhere to a low-fiber diet with limited protein and calcium. Some patients tolerate decaffeinated coffee, but it contains peptides that can also stimulate gastrin release.

When nausea and vomiting are present, oral fluids may be restricted to clear liquids, or the patient may be allowed nothing by mouth. The nurse administers antiemetics as ordered. Emesis basins are promptly removed, and vomited fluid is measured. The patient is helped to wash, and soiled clothing is replaced.

High Risk for Injury. The nurse monitors the patient for signs and symptoms of complications. Signs of bleeding are hematemesis (vomiting blood) and the presence of blood in the feces. Blood that has passed through the digestive tract is maroon to black and causes the stool to have a sticky or tarry quality. Vomited fluid and stools may be tested for occult blood. When blood loss is significant, the patient may go into shock. Early signs of shock are weakness, tachycardia, and pallor. Hypotension is a relatively late sign.

If hemorrhage occurs, the nurse notifies the physician and continues to monitor the patient's vital signs. Insertion of a nasogastric tube and saline lavage should be anticipated. The nurse assists with the procedures and reassures the patient. The patient is kept quiet and is given nothing by mouth. Intravenous lines should be maintained, and fluid intake and output recorded. The patient may have to be prepared for transfer to intensive care or to surgery.

Perforation is characterized by sudden, sharp pain starting in the midepigastric region and spreading across the entire abdomen. Digestive fluids in the abdomen cause peritonitis (inflammation of the peritoneum). With peritonitis, the abdomen is rigid and tender. The patient tends to draw the knees up toward the chest.

When perforation is suspected, the nursing care is much like that provided for hemorrhage. The physician is notified, and the patient's vital signs are monitored. Nothing is given by mouth. The nurse anticipates the need for nasogastric intubation and decompression and for intravenous fluids. The patient may be prepared for surgery.

The most prominent symptom of pyloric obstruction is persistent vomiting. The patient may also have signs and symptoms of fluid deficit and electrolyte imbalances. The nurse inserts a nasogastric tube for decompression as ordered. Intravenous fluids and antibiotics are administered. When the nasogastric tube is removed, the nurse monitors the patient's tolerance of fluids.

Ineffective Individual Coping. During periods of acute discomfort, patients are often receptive to measures that bring relief. Once acute symptoms resolve, however, many patients return to behaviors such as use of alcohol and tobacco that aggravate peptic ulcer disease. The nurse needs to explore what the patient thinks about prescribed treatments and how they will affect lifestyle. Resources to help patients who may have difficulty giving up alcohol or tobacco are available.

Knowledge Deficit. Patients with peptic ulcer disease are often discharged on drug therapy and with some dietary prescription. The nurse needs to assess and reinforce the patient's understanding of the instructions.

Patients should be advised of the importance of taking medications as they are prescribed. If they have problems related to the medications, the physician should be contacted. The nurse should also emphasize the need to avoid aspirin, nonsteroidal anti-inflammatory drugs such as ibuprofen, and corticosteroids. Written instructions are preferred because patients forget much of what they are told verbally. The nurse also reinforces the importance of follow-up care even if symptoms are under control.

EVALUATION. Criteria for evaluating the outcomes of nursing care are patient's statement of pain relief; stable weight; absence of complications as evidenced by normal vital signs and absence of vomiting, hematemesis, or tarry stools; patient's planning to incorporate therapy into lifestyle; and patient's description of self-medication and dietary restrictions, if any.

Nursing Care of the Patient with Peptic Ulcer Managed Surgically

Preoperative nursing care is like that outlined in Chapter 14 for any patient having major surgery. This section emphasizes the special postoperative needs of the patient who has gastric surgery for peptic ulcer disease.

ASSESSMENT. Postoperatively, the nurse assesses the patient for pain, nausea, and vomiting. If the patient has pain, the nurse describes the severity (using a scale of 1 to 10), location, and related factors. Vital signs are taken at frequent intervals until stable. The amount and type of intravenous fluids are noted, and the infusion site is checked for swelling or redness. If a nasogastric tube is present, the nurse assesses patency of the tube as well as the color and amount of drainage. The skin around the nostril where the tube is located is checked for irritation. The patient's breath sounds are auscultated. The wound dressing is inspected for bleeding. Once the dressing is removed, the wound is examined for increased redness, swelling, drainage, and incomplete closure. Any drainage from the wound or from drains is described. The abdomen is inspected for distention and auscultated for bowel sounds. The nurse monitors urine output and assesses for bladder distention.

NURSING DIAGNOSIS. General postoperative diagnoses are discussed in Chapter 14. Nursing diagnoses specific to the patient who has had gastric surgery for peptic ulcer disease may also include the following:

- **High Risk for Injury** related to gastric dilation, obstruction, perforation
- **Altered Nutrition: Less than Body Requirements** related to decreased capacity for absorption of nutrients
- **Decreased Cardiac Output** related to hypovolemia secondary to dumping syndrome
- **Knowledge Deficit** of self-care and prevention of recurrence

GOALS. Nursing goals for the patient after gastric surgery are absence of signs of complications; adequate nutrition; normal cardiac output; and patient's knowledge of treatment and prevention of peptic ulcer disease.

INTERVENTIONS

High Risk for Injury. Potential complications of gastric surgery include gastric dilation, obstruction, and perforation. Gastric dilation results from accumulation of fluid in the stomach. The patient complains of feeling full and having epigastric pain. Tachycardia, hypotension, and hiccups may develop. Obstruction can result from edema at the surgical site, causing pain and vomiting.

A nasogastric tube is usually inserted preoperatively and remains in place after surgery. Specific orders for suction will be written. It is very important to maintain suction and drainage as ordered. Excessive fluid and gas in the stomach put pressure on the incision that could cause perforation. Perforation could result in hemorrhage and peritonitis.

Following gastric surgery, the nurse should *not* irrigate or reposition the tube. To do so may cause the suture line in the stomach to tear. Nasogastric drainage is usually bright red immediately after surgery. The color darkens over the first 24 hours and then turns yellow or green. The tube is removed when peristalsis returns, usually the third to fifth postoperative day. The nurse documents the presence of bowel sounds and the passage of flatus through the rectum.

Altered Nutrition. After the tube is removed, the diet is gradually advanced from clear liquids to full liquids and then to solid foods. As the diet is progressed, the nurse should assess the patient for nausea, vomiting, or abdominal distention. Special dietary needs depend on the type of surgery. After subtotal gastrectomy, small, frequent meals are given until the stomach stretches enough to tolerate three regular meals a day. After total gastrectomy, small, frequent meals of semisolid foods are usually necessary for the rest of the patient's life.

Gastric surgery can have serious effects on the patient's nutritional status. The absorption of vitamin B_{12}, folic acid, iron, calcium, and vitamin D may be impaired, so supplements will be needed. Without vitamin B_{12}, the patient develops pernicious anemia. Pernicious anemia is more common after a total gastrectomy but can follow a subtotal gastrectomy. As discussed earlier, the parietal cells in the stomach produce intrinsic factor, a substance that is needed to absorb vitamin B_{12}. Vitamin B_{12} is essential for the production of red blood cells. When all or part of the stomach is removed, the patient develops a vitamin B_{12} deficiency and, eventually, severe anemia. The condition is easily treated with regular injections of vitamin B_{12}.

Decreased Cardiac Output. Some patients experience dumping syndrome after gastric surgery. This occurs because the absence or decreased size of the stomach prevents normal pacing of chyme moving into the intestine. Within 15 to 30 minutes after the patient eats, the concentrated liquid chyme moving into the intestine draws fluid out of the blood. The patient's blood volume falls, causing weakness, dizziness, diaphoresis, and palpitations. The increased fluid in the intestines causes cramps, loud bowel sounds, and the urge to defecate. Symptoms may last as long as an hour after meals.

Dumping syndrome usually disappears within a few months. Meanwhile, the following directions for the patient will help:

1. Take a diet low in carbohydrates and refined sugar, moderate in fat, and moderate to high in protein. It should be divided into six meals daily.
2. Drink fluids between meals, not with them.
3. Lie down for about 30 minutes after meals.

Knowledge Deficit. The nurse teaches the patient about medications that will be needed after discharge. Alterations in eating habits and diet are reinforced. The patient is taught to report signs of complications (nausea, vomiting, abdominal pain, and dark, tarry stools).

To reduce the risk of recurrence, the patient is advised of risk factors that should be avoided. Caffeine and alcohol should be eliminated from the diet. Smoking cessation is strongly recommended. The patient must know not to take aspirin or nonsteroidal anti-inflammatory drugs. Although the relationship between ulcers and emotional stress is not clear, stress seems to aggravate peptic ulcer disease. Therefore, the patient is encouraged to recognize stressors and learn techniques of stress management. Personal counseling or therapy may be appropriate.

EVALUATION. Criteria for evaluating the outcomes of nursing care after gastric surgery are normal vital signs and minimal vomiting; absence of signs of nutritional deficiencies, normal red blood cell count, and hemoglobin; no decrease in blood pressure after meals; and patient description of prescribed self-care.

STOMACH CANCER

Pathophysiology

Cancer of the stomach is diagnosed in more than 25,000 people in the United States each year. The incidence is highest among males, African Americans, people over age 70, and people of lower socioeconomic status.

Stomach carcinoma begins in the mucous membranes, invades the gastric wall, and spreads to the regional lymphatics, liver, pancreas, and colon. Distant metastases are found in the lungs and bones. Unfortunately, there are no signs or symptoms in the early stages. Late signs and symptoms are vomiting, ascites, liver enlargement, and an abdominal mass. By the time late signs appear, the cancer is advanced and the patient's chance of 5-year survival is only about 10%.

Risk Factors

No specific cause of gastric cancer is known. Risk factors include pernicious anemia, chronic atrophic gastritis, and achlorhydria. Other factors that seem to be related to stomach cancer are cigarette smoking and a diet high in starch, salt, pickled foods, salted meats, and nitrates. Patients who have had the Billroth II procedure (gastrojejunostomy) also have increased incidence of stomach cancer.

Medical Diagnosis

Gastroscopy is used to examine the interior of the stomach and to take specimens for microscopic study. The physician may also order an upper GI series to detect masses and obstructions. Laboratory studies include hemoglobin and hematocrit, serum albumin, liver function tests, and carcinoembryonic antigen. Stool specimens may be tested for occult blood.

Medical Treatment

Treatment of stomach cancer may employ surgery, chemotherapy, radiation, or a combination of these. Surgery and chemotherapy are most commonly recommended. If the cancer is detected early, surgical options include subtotal gastrectomy with lymph node dissection and total gastrectomy (Fig. 34–18). Sometimes part of the esophagus or duodenum is resected. In more advanced cancer, the surgeon may remove as much of the tumor as possible to relieve or prevent obstruction without removing the entire stomach.

Preoperative Nursing Care of the Patient with Stomach Cancer

In the preoperative period, the nurse assesses the patient's understanding of the condition and what to expect after surgery. It is important to know what the physician has told the patient so that conflicting messages are not sent.

Nursing diagnoses focus on knowledge deficit and ineffective coping.

Nursing goals are for the patient to know what to expect and to be emotionally prepared for the surgery.

The nurse informs the patient about the nasogastric tube, intravenous fluids, and so on and teaches cough-

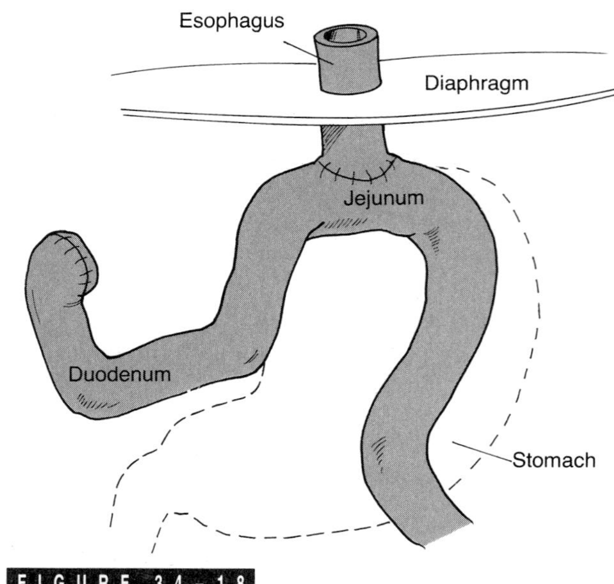

FIGURE 34-18
Total gastrectomy.

ing, deep breathing, and leg exercises. The patient's usual coping methods are identified and supported. Sources of support such as family members or a spiritual counselor are included in the preoperative care.

Effective preoperative care is evaluated by the patient's demonstration of exercises and statement of being ready for the surgery.

Postoperative Nursing Care for the Patient with Stomach Cancer

General nursing care for the postoperative patient is covered in Chapter 14. Special needs of patients having surgery for gastric cancer are discussed here. Chapter 24 presents general care of the patient who has cancer.

ASSESSMENT. Data that are especially important after surgery for stomach cancer are comfort, appetite, and nausea and vomiting. Weight changes are monitored, and dietary preferences are determined. The patient's support system and coping strategies are identified.

NURSING DIAGNOSIS. Nursing diagnoses that are especially important after surgery for stomach cancer include the following:

- **Pain** related to tumor or surgical trauma, or both
- **Altered Nutrition: Less than Body Requirements** related to anorexia, pain, nausea and vomiting
- **Ineffective Individual Coping** related to diagnosis of cancer, poor prognosis
- **Knowledge Deficit** of therapy and self-care

GOALS. Goals of nursing care are pain reduction and relief, adequate nutrition, patient's acceptance of cancer treatment, and patient's knowledge of therapy and self-care.

INTERVENTIONS

Pain. Analgesics should be given as ordered, but other nursing measures also should be tried to manage pain. Massage, relaxation techniques, and mental imagery are examples of measures to treat pain.

Altered Nutrition. Nutritional needs are much like those of the patient who has surgery for peptic ulcer disease. When nasogastric suction is discontinued, oral fluids are introduced. If the patient tolerates clear liquids, the diet is gradually advanced. Small servings of bland foods are tolerated best. If dumping syndrome is a problem, it is managed with a diet that is low in carbohydrates and refined sugar, moderate in fat, and moderate to high in protein. Food is served in six small meals, and fluids are taken between meals, not with them. The patient is advised to lie down for 30 minutes after eating. The patient's weight is monitored carefully. If weight is not maintained with oral intake, TPN may be instituted.

Ineffective Individual Coping. The patient and family may need help in coping with this life-threatening illness. The nurse encourages the patient to talk and is accepting of the thoughts and feelings expressed. The nurse also guides the patient to think about changes that may be necessary in daily routines after discharge. If chemotherapy or radiation therapy is planned, the patient needs to know what to expect. The nurse can share information about community resources such as home health agencies or the American Cancer Society.

Knowledge Deficit. Details of patient teaching are dictated by the individual assessment. Areas that may require teaching are nutrition, drug therapy, self-care during chemotherapy or radiation therapy, and wound care.

EVALUATION. Criteria for evaluating the outcomes of nursing care include patient's statement of pain relief, stable body weight, patient's use of healthy coping strategies, and patient's verbalization of therapy and self-care.

OBESITY

Obesity is defined as increased body weight caused by excessive body fat. The term is used to describe body weight that is greater than 20% higher than ideal. The term morbid obesity is used when a person weighs twice as much as his or her ideal weight.

Causes

Factors related to obesity include heredity, body build and metabolism, and psychosocial factors. Although many factors may contribute to obesity, the basic problem is that caloric intake exceeds metabolic demands. Excess food energy is converted to fat cells, which are capable of great expansion. When fat cells reach a certain size, they divide to form new fat cells. Fat cells decrease in size, but not in number, when a person loses weight.

Many attempts have been made to explain why some people become obese. There may be a mechanism in the hypothalamus that regulates weight within a certain range. When a person's nutrient intake falls below the level required to maintain the set weight, the body conserves energy to maintain that weight. This may explain why some people always seem to return to a certain weight despite strict dieting and temporary weight loss.

Complications

Complications of obesity include cardiovascular and respiratory problems, polycythemia, diabetes mellitus, cholelithiasis (gallstones), infertility, endometrial cancer, and fatty liver infiltration. Obesity also aggravates degenerative joint disease. In addition, obesity can take its toll on the patient's emotional well-being. Very obese people may be ostracized and experience discrimination. Even health care providers sometimes treat obese patients as uncooperative and unmotivated.

Medical Diagnosis

Obesity may be defined on the basis of comparison to standard weight tables. The amount of body fat can be estimated by measuring skin-fold thickness at selected body sites. The physician may order tests of endocrine function to rule out correctable causes of obesity. Additional diagnostic tests and procedures may be done to detect complications associated with obesity.

Medical Treatment

The primary treatment of obesity is a weight reduction diet accompanied by a planned exercise program. The ideal diet consists of foods from the basic four food groups and takes individual preferences into account. The calorie allowance may be as little as 800 calories a day. Amphetamines are effective in suppressing appetite but are not widely prescribed because their effects are temporary and they aggravate cardiac disease and hypertension.

When extreme obesity persists over a period of years despite conservative treatment, surgical intervention may be recommended. Surgical procedures include the following:

- Liposuction—the removal of adipose tissue from selected sites through a suction cannula. This procedure is used mainly for cosmetic surgery.
- Lipectomy—the surgical excision of folds of adipose tissue. Effects are seen immediately but may not last.
- Jaw wiring—the wiring of the jaws so that the patient cannot open the mouth; only liquids can be taken orally. This procedure is sometimes done when immediate weight loss is needed in preparation for surgical procedures. Weight loss is often significant but temporary.
- Intragastric balloon—the placement of a plastic balloon in the stomach, which is inflated and left in place to decrease the stomach's capacity for food. The patient feels full with little food. The balloon has been effective for some, but complications include stomach ulcers, intestinal obstruction, and stomach perforation.
- Gastric bypass—the stapling of the stomach to create an upper pouch that is anastomosed to the jejunum. Food intake is limited by the reduced stomach capacity. Dumping syndrome and malabsorption are common.
- Gastroplasty—the stapling of the stomach to create two chambers with a small path for food to move through the stomach. Food intake is limited by the small upper chamber, and emptying is delayed.
- Jejunoileal bypass—the anastomosis of the stomach to the ileum. Many complications can occur, including prolonged diarrhea, malnutrition, renal failure, cholelithiasis, and liver dysfunction.

Nursing Care of the Obese Patient

ASSESSMENT. Assessment of the obese patient identifies factors that may contribute to obesity and explores the physical and psychosocial effects. The patient's reason for seeking care is recorded. The past medical history documents pertinent chronic illnesses such as cardiac, respiratory, and orthopedic problems and diabetes mellitus. The nurse assesses usual dietary practices. Factors that trigger overeating and reactions to overeating are identified. The nurse inquires about interpersonal relationships, stresses, and coping strategies. In addition, the nurse collects data about previous efforts to lose weight and current interest in losing weight.

During the assessment, it is essential for the nurse to convey an attitude of respect and concern. Nurses need to be aware of their personal feelings about obese people and to consider how these feelings affect the nurse-patient relationship.

NURSING DIAGNOSIS. Nursing diagnoses for the patient who is obese may include the following:

- **Altered Nutrition: More than Body Requirements** related to excessive calorie intake for metabolic needs
- **Altered Tissue Perfusion:** cardiac, respiratory, renal, peripheral related to increased workload on heart
- **Ineffective Breathing Patterns** related to restricted lung expansion
- **Body Image Disturbance** related to excessive weight, perceived unattractiveness
- **Knowledge Deficit** of measures to achieve and maintain ideal body weight

GOALS. Goals of nursing care for the obese patient are appropriate nutrient intake, adequate tissue perfusion, absence of respiratory complications, improved body image, and patient's knowledge of weight loss measures.

INTERVENTIONS

Altered Nutrition. Before nutrition teaching begins, the nurse must know what the patient already knows and what he or she is motivated to learn. The following points in relation to nutrition should be emphasized:

- A balanced, low-calorie diet is more effective over time than a faddish, quick weight loss program.
- Eating habits must be changed, or weight loss will be temporary.
- Goal weight should be determined with the physician and the dietitian. Realistic goals for weight loss should be set at 1 or 2 pounds per week.
- Weighing food portions at the beginning of the diet makes the patient aware of portion sizes.
- Written materials should list foods to include and those to avoid.

While the patient learns about improved eating patterns, the need for increased physical activity also should be stressed. A person who has been sedentary must gradually increase activity as tolerance increases.

Altered Tissue Perfusion. The nurse monitors the patient's tolerance of physical activity. Tachycardia and dyspnea suggest that the patient's tolerance has been exceeded. When an obese patient is hospitalized for a medical or surgical condition, extra precautions must be taken to maintain circulation and respirations. Position changes, deep breathing, and leg exercises reduce the risk of cardiopulmonary complications.

Ineffective Breathing Patterns. The nurse monitors the patient's respiratory rate, effort, and breath sounds. During hospitalization, position changes and breathing exercises are especially important. The patient often breathes easier with the head of the bed elevated.

Body Image Disturbance. The nurse demonstrates acceptance of obese patients by spending time with them, avoiding judgmental comments, and touching. The patient is encouraged to problem solve how to overcome perceived limitations imposed by weight. Good grooming and attention to appearance are noted and complimented.

Knowledge Deficit. Topics to include in teaching plans include basic nutrition, diet planning for weight loss, goal setting, exercise, motivation, and self-esteem. It is important for the nurse to know and use resources to assist the patient in weight loss efforts.

EVALUATION. Criteria for evaluating the outcomes of nursing interventions are decreasing body weight; pulse and blood pressure within normal ranges; respiratory rate of 12 to 20 without dyspnea; positive patient statements about self, good grooming; and patient's demonstration of healthy food selections.

DISORDERS AFFECTING ABSORPTION AND ELIMINATION

MALABSORPTION

Malabsorption is a term used to describe a condition in which one or more nutrients are not digested or absorbed. Among the many causes of malabsorption are bacteria, deficiencies of bile salts or digestive enzymes, alterations in the intestinal mucosa, and absence of all or part of the stomach or intestines. The specific effects of malabsorption depend on the type of deficiencies that are present. Likewise, treatment is directed at replacing deficient enzymes or avoiding substances that cannot be absorbed. Two examples of malabsorption are sprue and lactase deficiency.

There are two types of sprue: celiac (nontropical) and tropical. Celiac sprue is caused by a genetic abnormality. It is characterized by severe changes in the intestinal mucosa and impaired absorption of most nutrients. Tropical sprue is caused by an infectious agent and results in malabsorption of fats, folic acid, and vitamin B_{12}.

People with lactase deficiency do not have adequate lactase to reduce lactose to glucose and galactose. These people are said to have lactose intolerance. Lactase deficiency may be inherited or acquired. Inherited lactase deficiency is most prevalent among blacks, Asians, and South Americans. Causes of acquired lactase deficiency include inflammatory bowel disease, gastroenteritis, and sprue syndrome.

Signs and Symptoms

A common sign of malabsorption is steatorrhea, the presence of excessive fat in the stool. Stools are large, bulky, foamy, and foul smelling. Patients may also have weight loss, fatigue, decreased libido, easy bruising, edema, anemia, and bone pain.

Bloating, cramping, abdominal cramps, and diarrhea are symptoms of lactase deficiency that commonly occur within several hours of consuming milk products.

Medical Diagnosis

Diagnosis of sprue is based on laboratory studies, endoscopy with biopsy, radiographic procedures, and ultrasound studies. Lactase deficiency is diagnosed on the basis of the health history, the lactose tolerance test, a breath test for abnormal hydrogen levels, and if necessary biopsy of the intestinal mucosa.

Medical Treatment

Diet and drug therapy constitute the cornerstone of treatment for sprue. Foods that aggravate the patient's symptoms are eliminated from the diet. Celiac disease is treated by avoiding products that contain gluten (wheat, barley, oats, and rye). Severe symptoms may be treated with corticosteroids. Tropical sprue is treated with antibiotics and folic acid supplements.

Lactase deficiency can be treated by eliminating milk and milk products from the diet, although many adults can tolerate small amounts of lactose without symptoms. Lactase enzyme can be mixed with milk or taken before drinking milk to avoid symptoms. Some milk and milk products that have been treated with lactase are also available. If milk products are limited, the diet must be assessed for adequacy of calcium, vitamin D, and riboflavin. Supplements may be advised.

Nursing Care of the Patient with Malabsorption

The nurse assesses the patient's symptoms. Stool characteristics are noted. In the case of celiac sprue, emphasis is on teaching the patient how to eliminate gluten from the diet. Antibiotics are given as ordered for tropical sprue. If folic acid therapy is to be continued, the patient should be instructed in self-medication. The effect of therapy is evaluated by the return of normal stool consistency. The patient with lactase deficiency is advised of dietary restrictions and alternative products.

DIARRHEA

Diarrhea is defined as the passage of loose, liquid stools with increased frequency. The patient may also have cramps, abdominal pain, and a feeling of urgency before bowel movements.

Causes

Many factors can cause diarrhea. They include spoiled foods, allergies, infections, diverticulosis, malabsorption, cancer, stress, fecal impactions, and tube feedings. Some medications cause diarrhea, but it is usually mild and painless.

Complications

Diarrhea is usually temporary and causes no serious problems. It does pose a greater threat, however, to the very old, the very young, and those in poor health. These individuals are more likely to become dehydrated and experience electrolyte imbalances and metabolic acidosis. Chronic diarrhea interferes with absorption of nutrients and can lead to malnutrition and anemia.

Medical Treatment

Acute diarrhea is usually treated by resting the digestive tract and giving antidiarrheal drugs. In the outpatient setting, the patient is advised to consume only clear liquids. A variety of liquids, such as broth, gelatin, and clear fruit juices, provide water, electrolytes, and some calories. Hospitalized patients may be allowed nothing by mouth and be given intravenous fluids. Severe, persistent diarrhea may require TPN. When diarrhea begins to improve, the diet is gradually expanded to include full liquids, bland solids, and then all other foods.

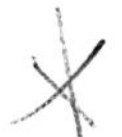

Nursing Care of the Patient with Diarrhea

ASSESSMENT. Nursing assessment of the patient with diarrhea can help determine possible causes, the severity and progress of the condition, complications, and the effect of treatment. The history should record the presence of diarrhea and detail the onset, severity, precipitating factors, and measures that bring relief. Pain accompanying diarrhea is documented. The patient is asked about stool characteristics, including amount, color, odor, and unusual contents such as blood, mucus, or undigested food. The functional assessment focuses on usual diet, dietary changes, recent and current medications, and recent travel to a foreign country. It is also important to assess the patient's ability to get to the toilet independently or to call for assistance with toileting.

Important aspects of the physical examination include vital signs, weight, and tissue turgor. Tissue turgor is often assessed by gently pinching the tissue on the forearm. If the pinched tissue flattens as soon as it is released, tissue turgor is generally considered good. This test is not a good indicator of hydration in the elderly because their tissue is less elastic, regardless of hydration. The abdomen is palpated for distention or tenderness, and the perianal area is inspected for irritation. A rectal examination should be performed if the nurse suspects fecal impaction.

NURSING DIAGNOSIS. Diarrhea is a nursing diagnosis, but other related diagnoses, including the following, may be appropriate for the patient with diarrhea:

- **Fluid Volume Deficit** related to fluid loss from diarrhea
- **Impaired Skin Integrity** related to irritation of diarrhea stool
- **Pain** related to abdominal cramping and rectal irritation
- **Altered Nutrition: Less than Body Requirements** related to failure to absorb nutrients
- **Self-Care Deficit:** toileting difficulties related to weakness or decreased level of consciousness

GOALS. Goals of nursing care for the patient with diarrhea include adequate hydration, patient comfort, intact skin, adequate nutrition, and self-care toileting ability.

INTERVENTIONS

Fluid Volume Deficit. Prevention of serious fluid and electrolyte imbalances requires careful monitoring and replacement of fluid losses. When patients have severe diarrhea, intake and output records should be kept. Whenever possible, liquid stools are measured. The characteristics of the stools also are important and should be recorded. Signs and symptoms that alert the nurse to possible fluid imbalances may include fluid output greater than intake; decrease in blood pressure; changes in pulse rate or rhythm; changes in respiratory rate or depth; confusion; muscle weakness, tingling, or twitching; and poor tissue turgor. These changes may indicate serious imbalances in water and electrolyte balance. They should be recorded and reported promptly.

If oral fluids are permitted, the patient should take 2000 to 3000 ml of various fluids each day. Flow rates of intravenous fluids should be monitored carefully. Excessive or rapid fluid replacement can cause heart failure, especially in the elderly.

Impaired Skin Integrity. Liquid stool is very irritating to the anal and perianal areas. With frequent bowel movements, skin breakdown may occur. The nurse assists the patient, if necessary, with perianal care after each stool. The area is washed thoroughly and gently with warm water and mild soap, then patted dry with a soft towel. Protective creams, sprays, or lotions can be applied.

Pain. Abdominal cramping associated with diarrhea is often relieved by antidiarrheal drugs that reduce intestinal activity. The nurse records the severity, duration, and location of the pain as well as the effects of drug therapy.

Self-Care Deficit. Frail elderly or those who are acutely ill may have difficulty with toileting during diarrhea episodes. If possible, they are placed in rooms close to the nurse's station. Staff should be aware of the need to respond to call lights promptly. A bedside commode is recommended if the toilet is too far from the bed. Patients who are unable to call for help must be checked frequently for the presence of diarrhea stools.

EVALUATION. Criteria for evaluating nursing interventions include passage of formed stools, normal pulse, blood pressure, and tissue turgor; intact perianal skin; patient's statement of pain relief; stable body weight; and patient's management of own toileting within capabilities.

CONSTIPATION

The frequency of defecation varies among healthy people. Bowel movements may occur as often as two or three times daily or as seldom as twice a week. If the stool is soft and is passed without difficulty, the patient is not constipated. Constipation is a condition in which a person has hard, dry, infrequent stools that are passed with difficulty.

Causes

Many factors can contribute to constipation. When stool is present in the rectum, the urge to defecate occurs. If the urge is ignored, stool remains in the rectum longer than usual and becomes dry. It is then more difficult, and sometimes painful, to have a bowel movement. People who frequently ignore the urge to defecate may become chronically constipated. Frequent use of laxatives or enemas also contributes to chronic constipation. These agents keep the lower digestive tract empty and eventually interfere with the normal pattern of elimination.

Since physical activity promotes normal bowel elimination, people who are inactive are at risk for constipation. Inadequate water intake can lead to constipation because more water will be reabsorbed from the stool in the large intestine. Diet significantly affects the stool. A diet that is low in fiber and high in foods such as cheese, lean meat, and pasta promotes constipation.

Drugs that slow intestinal motility or increase urine output also contribute to constipation. Examples of these drugs are those used for anesthesia, pain relief, and cold symptoms. Medical conditions that may be related to constipation include diseases of the colon or rectum, as well as brain or spinal cord injury. Abdominal surgery causes a loss of intestinal activity, but it should be temporary.

Many people believe that constipation is normal for older people. Normal age-related changes in the large intestine do not explain the frequent complaints of constipation by the elderly. More likely, when constipation does occur, it is related to inactivity, drug therapy, long-term laxative or enema abuse, or some medical condition.

Many elderly people grew up believing that a daily bowel movement was necessary for health. If a day passed without a bowel movement, they used laxatives or enemas to produce one. Over time, this practice fosters laxative or enema dependence. Eventually, the person is unable to have a bowel movement without the laxative or enema. This dependence, established over many years, is very difficult to correct.

Complications

When people are constipated, they have to strain to have bowel movements. Straining occurs when a person attempts to exhale with the glottis closed, causing increased pressure in the chest and abdominal cavities. This is called the Valsalva maneuver. The pressure slows the flow of circulating blood back into the chest, causing a brief drop in pulse and blood pressure. Relaxation allows a rush of blood back into the chest with a resulting rise in pulse and blood pressure. The rapid changes in blood flow can be fatal to a patient with heart disease. Therefore, prevention of constipation and straining is very important in the care of cardiac patients. Chronic constipation contributes to the development of hemorrhoids. Another complication of constipation is fecal impaction, which is discussed later.

Medical Treatment

Treatment of constipation is directed toward immediate relief of the problem and prevention of future episodes. Laxatives, suppositories, enemas, or a combination are ordered to get prompt results. The physician may prescribe stool softeners as well. Stool softeners, as the name suggests, promote normal elimination by allowing more water to be held in the stool so that it is softer and more easily passed. It takes several days for the effects to be seen, so stool softeners are not used for acute constipation. They are relatively safe drugs that are often prescribed over a long period of time. The trade names of some stool softeners are Colace, Surfak, and Metamucil.

Metamucil is an example of a bulk-forming stool softener. In the intestinal tract, it absorbs water to produce a gel-like mass to aid in the passage of a soft stool. If the patient does not take adequate fluids, the mass can harden and cause obstruction in the intestine. Table 34–5 provides additional information about drugs.

PHARMACOLOGY CAPSULE

Laxatives, cathartics, enemas, and suppositories usually relieve constipation promptly, but the effects of stool softeners are not seen for several days.

Nursing Care of the Patient with Constipation

ASSESSMENT. The nurse should assess bowel elimination to detect constipation or risk factors that may cause it. The patient's usual pattern of bowel elimination should be described, including frequency, amount, color, unusual contents (blood, mucus, undigested food), and pain associated with defecation. Recent changes in any of these factors should be noted. Information about diet, exercise, and drug therapy is helpful in revealing potential risk factors for constipation. If any aids to elimination (laxatives, enemas, suppositories) are used, the type and frequency should be recorded.

The abdomen is examined for distention or visible peristalsis. The nurse auscultates for bowel sounds in all four quadrants of the abdomen. When severe constipation is accompanied by mild diarrhea, a rectal examination should be done to detect a fecal impaction if agency policy permits.

NURSING DIAGNOSIS. Constipation is a nursing diagnosis. It may be related to drug therapy, diet, inadequate fluid intake, inactivity, neuromuscular disorders, or laxative abuse. Another nursing diagnosis that may apply to the patient with constipation is knowledge deficit of measures to promote normal bowel elimination.

GOALS. Goals of nursing care for the patient who is constipated include establishment of normal bowel elimination and patient's knowledge of measures to promote normal bowel elimination.

INTERVENTIONS

Constipation. The nurse's first action is directed at relieving the patient's constipation. Sometimes the physician will write an order for "laxative of choice or enema as needed." An enema or suppository is preferred if the patient is very uncomfortable because it usually acts within an hour. A laxative may take as long as 8 to 10 hours.

When a laxative is truly needed, it should be given. It is, however, often abused. As mentioned earlier, frequent use can lead to physical and psychological dependence. Laxatives can also produce diarrhea, which may lead to excessive loss of fluids and electrolytes.

Nurses are often responsible for managing bowel elimination of severely disabled people. This is especially true in long-term care facilities. It is critical for the staff to record and describe all stools so that problems can be found and treated early. Nurse's aides need to be taught the importance of keeping accurate records. If detected early, constipation may be easily treated with a mild laxative or suppository. Severe constipation may require repeated enemas and laxatives for relief.

In most cases, bowel elimination can be maintained with diet, fluids, exercise, and regular toilet habits. Occasional use of elimination aids is not harmful. Some patients, however, require nursing interventions to promote elimination for a long time.

Megacolon is a condition in which the large intestine loses the ability to contract effectively enough to propel the fecal mass toward the rectum. These patients usually require regular enemas for bowel cleansing. Other measures are not generally adequate. Patients who have special problems with constipation are those with neurologic conditions such as spinal cord injuries and cerebrovascular accident (stroke). The management of bowel elimination for these patients and the process of bowel retraining is discussed in Chapter 21.

Fecal Impaction. All nursing staff should understand the possibility of fecal impaction in the physically or mentally impaired person. Fecal impaction refers to the retention of a large mass of stool in the rectum that the patient is unable to pass. Some liquid stool trickles around the impaction and may be mistaken for diarrhea.

The nurse should suspect impaction when a patient who has not had a bowel movement for several days has repeated episodes of mild diarrhea. If agency policy permits, the nurse can assess for impaction by inserting a gloved, lubricated finger into the rectum. The fecal mass is usually easily felt. It may be very hard or soft.

The impaction is removed using the agency protocol or specific physician's orders. This process usually requires administration of a mineral oil enema to soften hard stool, followed by a soapsuds enema. It may be necessary to break up and remove the mass manually. This procedure is painful and embarrassing for the patient. Rectal procedures stimulate the vagus nerve, possibly causing a drop in heart rate. With good nursing care, manual extraction should rarely be necessary.

Knowledge Deficit. The following are key points to emphasize in patient teaching to maintain normal bowel elimination:

- Include high-fiber foods in the diet. Examples are fruits, raw vegetables, greens, and whole grains.
- Drink six to eight 8-ounce glasses of water each day unless the physician has restricted fluid intake for some reason.
- Do some type of exercise each day. It does not have to be strenuous; walking is excellent exercise.
- Try to keep a regular pattern of bowel elimination. Go to the bathroom promptly in response to the urge to have a bowel movement.
- Use a toilet that is comfortable. Feet should touch the floor, causing the hips to bend slightly. Use a footstool if necessary. This helps use of the abdominal muscles.
- Contrary to popular opinion, it is not necessary to have a bowel movement every day. A bowel movement every 2 or 3 days without pain or straining is normal for some people.
- Laxatives can be used safely for occasional constipation. If they are used frequently, however, they can interfere with normal elimination. Consult the physician for a recommended laxative.

EVALUATION. Criteria for evaluating the outcomes of nursing interventions are passage of regular formed stools without straining and patient's verbalization of measures to prevent constipation.

PATIENT EDUCATION TO PROMOTE NORMAL BOWEL FUNCTION. The nurse often has the opportunity to teach patients how to promote normal bowel function and detect problems early. Acute gastrointestinal disorders can be caused by irritants or infectious agents. Patients should be encouraged to identify and avoid foods that create distress.

The ingestion of infectious agents can be reduced by practicing good hand washing and food handling. Food poisoning can be acquired from food that has been improperly stored, poorly cooked, or exposed to contaminated containers or utensils. The nurse can provide guidance in proper food handling.

Food poisoning is often a problem for frail elderly who live at home. Poor vision and smell can make food management difficult. It is a good idea for the home health nurse to check the patient's refrigerator and food cabinets to identify potential problems.

Many people recognize that they have changes in their gastrointestinal function when they are under a lot of stress. These people may benefit from relaxation and stress management training.

In addition, nurses can promote health by teaching patients how to detect possible serious digestive problems in the early stages. Gastrointestinal symptoms that could indicate gastric cancer include persistent gastric distress, anorexia, and weight loss. Rectal bleeding or a change in bowel habits, or both, often occurs with intestinal cancer. As part of the annual physical examination for people over age 40, many physicians do a rectal examination and test the stool for occult blood.

Teaching patients what is normal, how to promote normal function, and how to detect problems can all help to avoid serious gastrointestinal dysfunction.

INTESTINAL OBSTRUCTION

Causes

Intestinal obstruction can be caused by many factors, including strangulated hernia, tumor, paralytic ileus, stricture, volvulus (twisting of the bowel), intussusception (telescoping of the bowel into itself), and postoperative adhesions. When the bowel is obstructed, digestive contents cannot progress. Volvulus and intussusception are illustrated in Fig. 34–19.

Signs and Symptoms

Symptoms are most acute when an obstruction is located in the proximal portion of the small intestine. Early symptoms of obstruction are vomiting (possibly projectile), abdominal pain, and constipation. Gastric contents are vomited first, followed by bile, then fecal matter. Blood or purulent drainage may be passed rectally. Abdominal distention may develop, especially with colon obstruction.

Complications

Vomiting can lead to fluid and electrolyte imbalances and metabolic alkalosis. If blood supply to the intestine is impaired, gangrene and perforation of the bowel may occur. Untreated obstruction can result in shock and death.

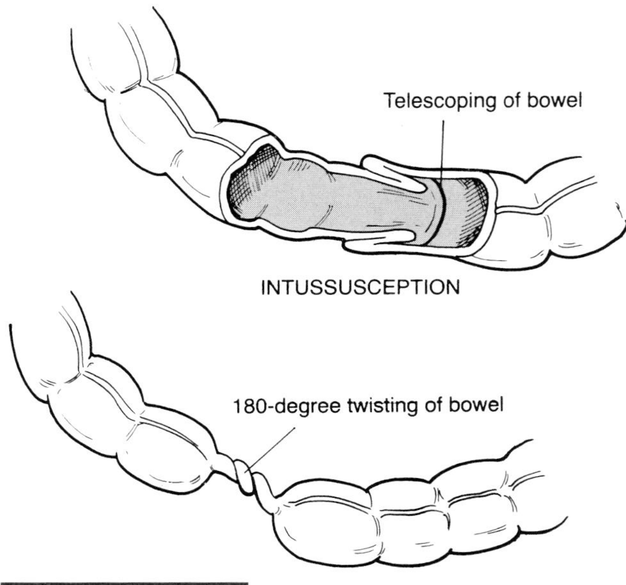

FIGURE 34–19
Mechanical bowel obstruction. *A*, Intussusception; *B*, volvulus.

Medical Diagnosis

Intestinal obstruction is suspected on the basis of the history, physical examination, and laboratory studies. It is confirmed by radiologic studies.

Medical Treatment

The initial treatment of obstruction is gastrointestinal decompression. A nasoenteral tube is passed and connected to suction. Intravenous fluids are provided. Depending on the cause of the obstruction, surgical intervention may be necessary.

Nursing Care of the Patient with Intestinal Obstruction

ASSESSMENT. The nurse assesses the patient's symptoms, including pain and nausea. The onset and progression of symptoms are documented. The past medical history should include potentially related conditions, such as hernia, cancer of the digestive tract, and abdominal surgeries. The nurse asks when the patient's last bowel movement was and if the characteristics were normal.

Vital signs are measured to detect signs of infection (fever, tachycardia) and impending shock (tachycardia, hypotension). Skin moisture and tissue turgor are assessed, along with moisture of the mucous membranes. The abdomen is inspected for distention and visible peristalsis, ausculatated for rapid, high-pitched tinkling bowel sounds, and gently palpated for tenderness and guarding. Rectal bleeding or drainage is noted.

NURSING DIAGNOSIS. In the preoperative period, the nursing diagnoses generally include the following:

- **Pain** related to distention
- **Fluid Volume Deficit** related to vomiting, intestinal suction
- **High Risk for Infection** related to complications of obstruction
- **Ineffective Breathing Patterns** related to abdominal distention
- **Anxiety** related to pain, anticipated surgery

GOALS. Goals of nursing care are pain relief, balanced fluid intake and output, absence of infection, return of bowel sounds, adequate ventilation, and reduction of anxiety.

INTERVENTIONS

Pain. Analgesics are given as ordered. If the physician is withholding analgesics while making a diagnosis, the nurse informs the patient of this and uses other strategies, such as massage and relaxation.

Fluid Volume Deficit. The nurse promotes fluid balance by providing intravenous fluids as ordered. Vital signs and intake and output are monitored. If nasoenteral suction is ordered, the nurse monitors output and ensures free drainage at all times.

High Risk for Infection. The patient's temperature is monitored. Signs of intestinal rupture (increasing tenderness, sudden sharp pain, and abdominal rigidity) are reported to the physician immediately.

Ineffective Breathing Patterns. The patient's head is elevated to relieve pressure on the diaphragm. Deep breathing and coughing are encouraged. Oxygen is administered as ordered. When surgery is planned, the nurse carries out preoperative orders, which often include an enema and intravenous fluids.

Anxiety. The patient is given simple explanations of what is being done and what to expect postoperatively if surgery is scheduled. The importance of deep breathing, turning, coughing, and leg exercises is stressed.

Postoperative Care. Postoperative care depends on the surgical procedure performed.

EVALUATION. The nurse evaluates the outcomes of care by the patient's statement of pain relief, absence of signs of infection (fever, tachycardia, increased white blood cell count) or dehydration (dry mucous membranes, oliguria), clear breath sounds, cessation of vomiting, return of active bowel sounds, and patient's statement of reduced anxiety.

APPENDICITIS

Pathophysiology

The appendix is a blind pouch in the cecum. Appendicitis is an inflammation of the appendix. Inflammation occurs when feces block the opening of the appendix to the large intestine. The tissue becomes infected by bacteria in the digestive tract. Pus accumulates, blood supply is impaired, and the appendix may rupture. A ruptured appendix allows digestive contents to enter the abdominal cavity, causing peritonitis. Early detection of appendicitis may permit treatment before the appendix ruptures.

Signs and Symptoms

The initial symptom of appendicitis is usually pain in the epigastric region or around the umbilicus, which then shifts to the right lower quadrant. The classic symptom of appendicitis is pain at McBurney's point, which is located midway between the umbilicus and the iliac crest (Fig. 34–20). The patient may have a temperature elevation and nausea and vomiting. Because of the pain, the patient may assume a position of hip flexion. The right leg cannot be straightened without pain. An elevated white blood cell count shows the presence of infection.

Signs and symptoms of peritonitis are absence of bowel sounds, severe abdominal distention, increased pulse and temperature, nausea, and vomiting. The abdomen may be rigid and board-like, although this sign is often absent with peritonitis in older patients. Shock should be suspected if the patient begins to lose consciousness and is cool and pale.

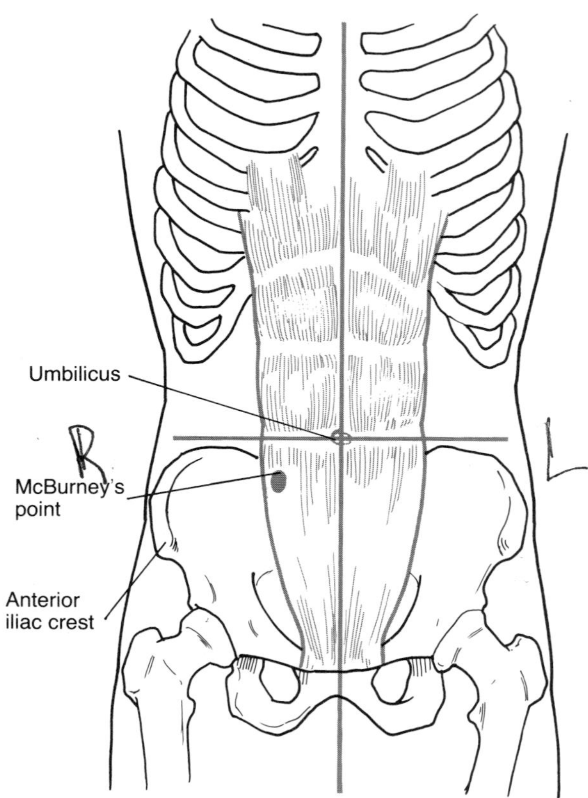

FIGURE 34–20
McBurney's point is located midway between the anterior iliac crest and the umbilicus in the right lower quadrant. Localized tenderness here is typical of appendicitis.

Medical Diagnosis

A diagnosis of appendicitis is based on classic signs and symptoms and a white blood cell count of 10,000 to 15,000.

Medical Treatment

When appendicitis is suspected, the patient is allowed nothing by mouth. A cold pack to the abdomen may be ordered. Laxatives and heat applications should *never* be given for undiagnosed abdominal pain. If the appendix is inflamed, heat or laxatives may cause it to rupture.

If rupture has not occurred, immediate surgical treatment is indicated. With a ruptured appendix, surgery may be delayed 6 to 8 hours while antibiotics and intravenous fluids are given.

Nursing Care of the Patient with Appendicitis

ASSESSMENT. The patient's chief complaint is usually pain. The nurse assesses the location, severity, onset, duration, precipitating factors, and alleviating measures in relation to the pain. In the past medical history, the nurse notes previous abdominal distress, chronic illnesses, and surgeries. Allergies and medications are recorded as well. The presence of nausea and vomiting is determined in the review of systems. Significant data in the physical examination are temperature; abdominal pain, distention, and tenderness; and the presence and characteristics of bowel sounds.

NURSING DIAGNOSIS. Nursing diagnoses for the patient with appendicitis may include the following:

- **High Risk for Infection** (peritonitis) related to appendix rupture
- **Fluid Volume Deficit** related to nausea, vomiting, medical restriction of fluid intake
- **Pain** related to inflammation of appendix or surgical tissue trauma
- **Ineffective Breathing Patterns** related to incisional pain or anesthesia
- **Fear** related to sudden emergency status, minimal preoperative teaching
- **Knowledge Deficit** of surgical routines and of self-care after discharge

GOALS. Goals of nursing care for the patient with appendicitis may include absence of infection, normal fluid balance, pain relief, effective breathing, decreased fear, and patient's knowledge of self-care after discharge.

INTERVENTIONS

Preoperative Care. Before surgery, the patient will probably be most comfortable in a semi-Fowler or side-lying position with the hips flexed. While the physician determines the diagnosis, analgesics may be withheld. The location and pattern of the pain are needed to make a diagnosis. The nurse can explain this to the patient. If the appendix has not ruptured, surgery is usually done promptly upon diagnosis. With a ruptured appendix, surgery may be delayed while antibiotics and intravenous fluids are given. If rupture is suspected, the patient's head is elevated to localize the infection.

Postoperative Care. Postoperatively, the patient receives antibiotics, intravenous fluids, and possibly gastrointestinal decompression. The patient is assisted to turn, cough, and deep breathe to promote expansion of the lungs. Incentive spirometry also can be useful. The nurse should show the patient how to splint the incision during deep breathing. Early ambulation is usually ordered to reduce the risk of postoperative complications. The abdominal wound is assessed for redness, swelling, and foul drainage. Wound care is carried out as ordered or according to agency policy.

If there are no complications, the patient is usually discharged in a few days. Normal activities can be resumed in 2 to 3 weeks.

EVALUATION. Criteria for evaluating the effects of nursing interventions include normal temperature and white blood cell count; normal pulse and blood pressure, moist mucous membranes; patient's statement of reduced pain; respiratory rate of 12 to 20 with clear breath sounds; patient's statement of reduced fear, calm manner; and patient's description of surgical routines and postoperative self-care.

PERITONITIS

Pathophysiology

Peritonitis is inflammation of the peritoneum caused by chemical or bacterial contamination of the peritoneal cavity. Chemical contamination may follow rupture of a digestive tract structure, including the appendix. Bacterial contamination may be caused by rupture of a digestive tract structure or fallopian tube or from nonsterile, traumatic wounds.

When a chemical or bacterial contaminant is present, the body's defenses attempt to "wall off" the area to contain the injury. Fluid shifts out of the blood stream into the peritoneal cavity. Peristalsis slows or stops. If defenses are adequate, the offending fluid remains localized and is eventually eliminated. Complications of peritonitis include abscesses, adhesions, septicemia, hypovolemic shock, paralytic ileus, and organ failure.

Signs and Symptoms

Signs and symptoms of peritonitis include pain over the affected area, rebound tenderness, abdominal rigidity and distention, fever, tachycardia, tachypnea, nausea, and vomiting. The elderly patient may have more subtle symptoms with less pain and the absence of abdominal rigidity.

Medical Diagnosis

A diagnosis of peritonitis is suspected on the basis of the patient's history and physical examination. Diagnostic tests and procedures done to confirm the inflammation include complete blood cell count, serum electrolytes, abdominal radiograph, computed tomographic scan, and ultrasound. Paracentesis may be done to obtain a specimen of fluid for culture.

Medical Treatment

A nasogastric tube is inserted for gastrointestinal decompression. Intravenous fluids, antibiotics, and analgesics are ordered. Surgery may be done to close a ruptured structure and to remove foreign material and fluid from the peritoneal cavity.

Nursing Care of the Patient with Peritonitis

ASSESSMENT. The nurse begins with assessment of the patient's present illness. Pain is the prominent symptom, and the nurse documents the onset, location, severity, and related symptoms. When peritonitis is suspected, the nurse records a history of abdominal trauma, including surgery. Vital signs are recorded. The abdomen is inspected for distention and auscultated for the presence of bowel sounds. Measures of fluid status are noted, including tissue turgor, moisture of mucous membranes, and intake and output.

NURSING DIAGNOSIS. Nursing diagnoses for the patient with peritonitis may include the following:

- **Pain** related to inflammation
- **Decreased Cardiac Output** related to decreased blood volume
- **Altered Nutrition: Less than Body Requirements** related to nausea, vomiting, nothing by mouth status
- **Anxiety** related to threat of serious illness and invasive treatment

GOALS. Goals of nursing care for the patient with peritonitis may include pain relief, normal cardiac output, adequate nutrition, and reduction of anxiety.

INTERVENTIONS

Pain. Narcotic analgesics are administered as ordered for pain. The nurse positions the patient with the head elevated and provides comfort measures such as massage and relaxation techniques. The physician is notified if pain relief is not obtained.

Decreased Cardiac Output. The shift of fluid from the blood into the peritoneal cavity may be so great that the patient develops fluid volume deficit. Cardiac output falls, and perfusion of vital organs is reduced. The nurse administers intravenous fluids as ordered and monitors fluid intake and output. The nurse monitors vital signs and reports increasing pulse, restlessness, pallor, and decreasing blood pressure. In addition to fluid volume deficit, the patient may go into shock because of septicemia (presence of bacteria in the blood).

Altered Nutrition. Gastrointestinal decompression usually eliminates nausea and vomiting, but antiemetics may be ordered as needed. The nurse must check to be sure that the nasogastric tube is draining at all times.

Anxiety. The patient is likely to be anxious owing to pain and uncertainty about what is happening. Even when there is a sense of urgency in caring for the patient, the nurse gives simple explanations for procedures and tells the patient what to expect. The patient is encouraged to ask questions. If surgery is planned, essential preoperative teaching may have to be done quickly. The patient is told the importance of breathing and leg exercises after abdominal surgery. The physician may order sedatives to calm the patient.

Postoperative care is like that for any major surgery as described in Chapter 14.

EVALUATION. Evidence of effective nursing care includes patient's statement of pain relief, normal pulse and blood pressure, stable body weight, and calm manner.

ABDOMINAL HERNIA

Pathophysiology

Muscles play an important role in keeping the abdominal organs in place. Weakness in those muscles may allow a portion of the large intestine to push through the abdominal wall. The bulging portion of intestine is called a hernia. Hernias most often occur in areas where the abdominal wall is already weak. Weak locations include the umbilicus and the lower inguinal areas of the abdomen (Fig. 34–21).

Hernias are classified as reducible or irreducible. A reducible hernia slips back into the abdominal cavity with gentle pressure or when the patient lies on his or her back. An irreducible hernia, sometimes called incarcerated, is trapped. If a hernia cannot be reduced, blood flow to the trapped loop of intestine is impaired and may become gangrenous. The intestine is also obstructed. At that point, the hernia is considered to be strangulated.

Signs and Symptoms

Hernias are usually diagnosed when a patient reports a smooth lump on the abdomen. The lump may disappear when the patient is lying down or at rest but returns when he or she stands or strains. Heavy lifting or coughing usually causes the hernia to appear.

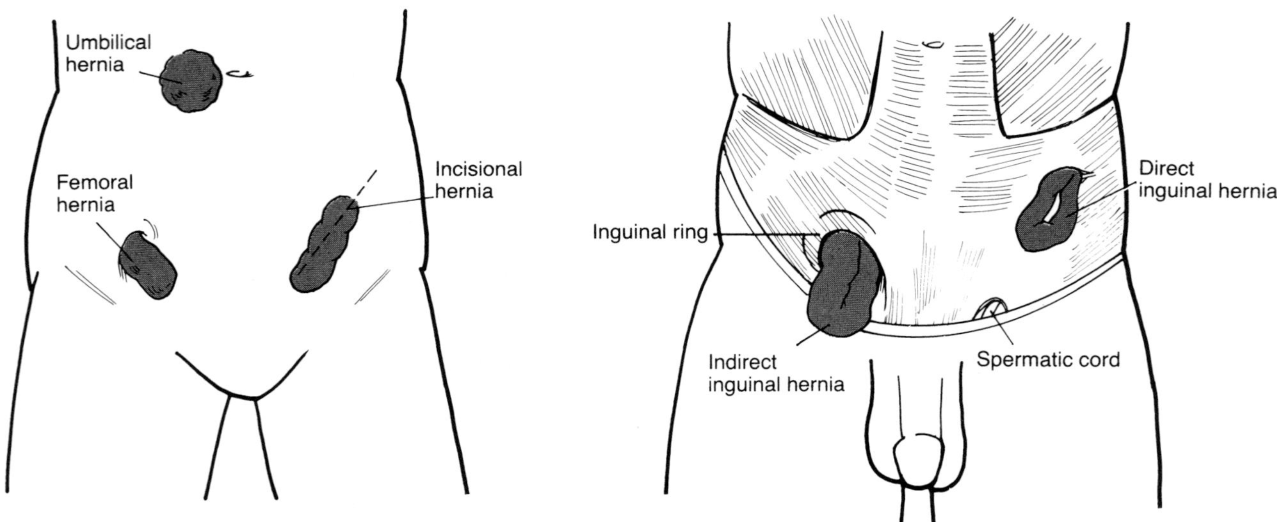

FIGURE 34–21
Abdominal hernias.

Hernias are usually not painful unless they become incarcerated. With incarceration, the patient has severe abdominal pain and distention, vomiting, and cramps.

Medical Diagnosis

Hernias are diagnosed on the basis of the health history and physical examination.

Medical Treatment

Surgical repair of hernias is usually recommended even if they are reducible. Repair prevents the possibility of incarceration. Two surgical procedures are used to repair hernias. Herniorrhaphy is the repair of the muscle defect by suturing. If additional measures are needed to strengthen the abdominal wall, a hernioplasty is done. Strong materials are used to cover and reinforce the defect.

Some patients cannot tolerate the stress of surgical hernia repair. For them, a truss may be advised, although they are not as widely used as in the past. A truss consists of a pad that is placed over the hernia and a belt that holds it in place. It provides support for the weak muscles.

Nursing Care of the Patient with Abdominal Hernia

ASSESSMENT. The nurse begins the assessment with the patient's chief complaint, usually a smooth lump in the abdomen that appears and disappears with various activities and positions. The nurse asks about pain and vomiting, which may be present if the hernia is strangulated. The patient's work and home responsibilities are explored to identify the type of physical exertion required. The most relevant aspect of the physical examination is the assessment of the abdomen. The nurse inspects for abnormalities and listens for bowel sounds in all four quadrants. If the patient wears a truss, the nurse inspects the skin underneath it for signs of irritation.

If the patient has surgery, the general postoperative care is discussed in Chapter 14. In addition to the routine postoperative assessments, after hernia repair the nurse is especially concerned with assessing bowel and bladder elimination, wound healing, and patient's knowledge about postoperative care to avoid stress on the healing surgical wound.

NURSING DIAGNOSIS. Preoperative nursing diagnoses may include the following:

- **High Risk for Injury** related to hernia strangulation
- **Impaired Skin Integrity** related to pressure created by the truss
- **Knowledge Deficit** related to self-care

If the patient has surgical correction of the hernia, additional nursing diagnoses may be the following:

- **Altered Urinary Elimination** related to abdominal surgery, anesthesia
- **Colonic Constipation** related to immobility, effects of anesthesia, and abdominal surgery
- **High Risk for Injury** related to wound dehiscence
- **Knowledge Deficit** related to activity restrictions, postoperative self-care

GOALS. Goals of nursing care for the patient with an abdominal hernia are absence of complications (strangulation), healthy skin while wearing truss, and patient's knowledge of self-care. Additional goals for the postoperative patient are normal bladder function, normal bowel function, absence of wound dehiscence, and patient's knowledge of postoperative limitations and self-care.

INTERVENTIONS. The nurse monitors the patient for signs and symptoms of strangulation (nausea, vomiting, pain, abdominal distention, fever, and tachycardia). If these symptoms develop, the physician should be notified immediately. It is important for the nonsurgical patient to know that these symptoms should be reported.

Instructions to the patient who uses a truss should include the following:

- Put the truss on before rising each morning.
- Check under the pad and the belt several times daily for skin irritation.
- The truss does not cure a hernia, so measures to prevent straining should still be taken.

The nurse should determine what restrictions the patient has in relation to physical exertion. The patient needs clear written instructions. If surgery is planned, the nurse informs the patient of surgical routines and demonstrates how to do deep breathing exercises and to support the incision.

Many patients have temporary problems urinating after hernia repair surgery. The nurse keeps intake and output records, documents voiding, and assesses for bladder distention. Bowel activity may also cease temporarily in response to the anesthesia and manipulation of the bowel during surgery. Therefore, the nurse monitors bowel sounds and notes the passage of flatus. Like any other patients having major surgery, these patients need to keep their lungs clear to prevent complications. They are encouraged to turn and deep breathe, but they should not cough or sneeze. Coughing and sneezing put tension on the surgical incision and repaired tissues. Scrotal swelling is common after inguinal hernia repair. A scrotal support and an ice pack can greatly reduce the painful swelling. Activities are usually restricted for 2 to 6 weeks. The nurse reinforces the physician's instructions about refraining from exertion and lifting. The patient is also advised to report fever or wound drainage to the physician.

EVALUATION. Criteria for evaluating the outcomes of nursing interventions are normal pulse and temperature without abdominal pain or distention, intact skin without redness under truss, and patient's verbalization of self-care with the hernia. Postoperatively, outcome criteria include urine output equal to fluid intake without bladder distention, active bowel sounds, intact wound margins, and patient's verbalization of postoperative routines and measures to reduce strain on surgical incision.

INFLAMMATORY BOWEL DISEASE

Pathophysiology

Inflammatory bowel disease (IBD) is a term used to refer to both ulcerative colitis and Crohn's disease. Crohn's disease is also known as regional enteritis. In both conditions, there is inflammation and ulceration of the lining of the intestinal tract. The two conditions have similar symptoms and are treated much the same way medically.

A patient with IBD may have a few isolated attacks or may have a chronic condition. With chronic IBD, attacks may last days or even months, followed by remissions of several weeks to several years.

Causes

The exact cause of IBD is unknown. Possible causes that are being studied include infectious agents, autoimmune reactions, allergies, and heredity. In the past, it was thought that IBD might be caused by stress. Current thinking, however, suggests that stress results from the condition rather than causing it.

Signs and Symptoms

Bloody diarrhea and abdominal pain are the most common symptoms of IBD. In severe cases, the patient may also have fever and weight loss.

Complications

The local complications of IBD include hemorrhage, obstruction, perforation (rupture), abscesses in the anus or rectum, fistulas, and megacolon. Patients who have had ulcerative colitis for 10 years have a greatly increased risk of cancer of the large intestine. Patients with Crohn's disease do not have such a high risk.

Systemic complications also may be found with ulcerative colitis. These are conditions outside the intestine but related to the colitis. They include inflammation of the joints and eyes, skin lesions, urinary stones, and liver disease. Of course, severe or prolonged diarrhea can result in malnutrition, anemia, and fluid and electrolyte imbalances.

Medical Diagnosis

Inflammatory bowel disease is suspected on the basis of the history and physical examination. It is confirmed by barium enema with air contrast and colonoscopy with biopsy and cell studies.

Medical Treatment

Treatment of IBD addresses both the local and the systemic effects of the disorders. Intestinal inflammation is treated with drug therapy, diet, and rest. Medical treatment of IBD includes the following drugs:

- Anti-inflammatory and immunosuppressants to decrease inflammation
- Antidiarrheals to control diarrhea
- Anticholinergics to reduce gastrointestinal motility and secretions
- Antibiotics to prevent or treat infections (usually sulfasalazine or olsalazine)
- Iron supplements and vitamin B_{12} to treat anemia

Steroids may be given orally, rectally, or intravenously for their anti-inflammatory action. Drugs that suppress the immune response may be ordered if steroids are not effective. Because they reduce the patient's ability to resist infection, however, immunosuppressants are used with caution.

A low-roughage diet without milk products is prescribed for mild to moderate IBD. Intravenous fluids or TPN may be needed to provide fluid, electrolytes, and nutrients when symptoms are severe.

Although most patients respond to medical treatment, some require surgery. Removal of the colon (colectomy) is curative for ulcerative colitis. When the colon is removed, an artificial opening from the small intestine through the abdominal wall is needed to allow elimination of digestive wastes. The opening is called an ileostomy. Although good health is usually restored after this surgery, an ileostomy is permanent and requires special care. Therefore, surgery is not usually done unless all other measures have failed. Care of the patient with an ostomy is covered in Chapter 24.

Surgical treatment of Crohn's disease is more likely to be removal of the diseased portion of the intestine. In more than half of these patients, the disease appears in another section of the intestine after surgery.

PHARMACOLOGY CAPSULE

Corticosteroids suppress the inflammatory response, so the patient is more susceptible to infection.

Nursing Care of the Patient with Inflammatory Bowel Disease

The nursing care of a patient during an acute attack of IBD is concerned with ongoing assessment, comfort measures, skin care, emotional support, and the administration and monitoring of drug therapy. The nursing needs of the IBD patient who undergoes surgery are like those of other patients who have gastrointestinal surgery, as discussed earlier in this chapter.

ASSESSMENT. Assessment of the patient with IBD should identify the symptoms that caused the patient to seek care, usually pain and diarrhea. The onset, location, severity, and duration of pain are documented. Factors that contribute to the onset of pain, such as specific foods or stressors, are noted. The onset and duration of diarrhea are noted, as well as the presence of blood. The nurse assesses the impact of the illness on the patient's life and explores how the patient copes.

Important aspects of the physical examination are vital signs, height and weight, and measures of hydration (tissue turgor, moisture of mucous membranes). The perianal area should be inspected for irritation or ulceration. Accurate intake and output records should be kept. Diarrhea stools are measured if possible and counted as output.

NURSING DIAGNOSIS. Nursing diagnoses for the patient with IBD may include the following:

- **Pain** related to abdominal cramping, perianal irritation
- **Diarrhea** related to intestinal inflammation
- **Fluid Volume Deficit** related to diarrhea
- **Altered Nutrition: Less than Body Requirements** related to malabsorption
- **Ineffective Individual Coping** related to chronic illness
- **High Risk for Injury** related to adverse drug effects
- **Knowledge Deficit** of IBD and self-care

GOALS. Goals of nursing care for the patient with IBD are pain relief, cessation of diarrhea, adequate hydration, adequate nutrition, patient's adaptation to management of IBD, absence of adverse drug effects, and patient's knowledge of IBD and self-care.

INTERVENTIONS

Pain. Perianal pain is treated with gentle cleansing, sitz baths, and skin protectants. Measures to relieve abdominal pain include administration of analgesics and antispasmodics and application of heat to the abdomen as ordered. The nurse also uses positioning, massage, relaxation, imagery, and other strategies described in Chapter 16.

Diarrhea. Easy access to a toilet and prompt response to calls for help reduce the chance of episodes of bowel incontinence. Following each stool, gentle cleansing should be done and the perianal area assessed. Bedpans or bedside commodes, if used, are removed and cleaned immediately. Room deodorizers are used to eliminate odors.

Prescribed drugs for diarrhea usually include antidiarrheals, antispasmodics, anticholinergics, antibiotics, and corticosteroids. The patient may be allowed nothing by mouth or may be given only clear liquids when diarrhea is severe. Bedrest may be prescribed, or the patient may just be encouraged to rest.

Fluid Volume Deficit. Severe diarrhea can quickly deplete the patient's fluid volume. Fluid status must be assessed on an ongoing basis. Signs of fluid volume deficit are dry mucous membranes, hypotension, tachycardia, and decreased urine output. The nurse administers intravenous fluids and TPN as ordered.

Altered Nutrition. When the patient is allowed nothing by mouth, TPN is used for nourishment. When symptoms are less severe, elemental feedings such as Ensure may be ordered. The patient who is able to take solid food is usually placed on a low-residue diet without caffeine, pepper, or alcohol. Foods that are not allowed include whole grains, nuts, and raw fruits and vegetables. A dietitian should be consulted to teach the patient about the prescribed diet. Weight is monitored on a routine basis.

High Risk for Injury. Nursing responsibilities in relation to drug therapy for IBD include administering the drugs, monitoring their effects, and teaching the patient about long-term drug therapy. Sulfasalazine is the antibiotic most often prescribed for patients with ulcerative colitis. It is useful in treating acute attacks and preventing future attacks. After an acute attack has subsided, the drug dosage is gradually reduced. A low-maintenance dose may be given for as long as a year. The patient should be taught that discontinuing the drug early may result in another acute attack.

Sulfasalazine can cause crystals to form in the urine (crystalluria), which can damage the kidneys. Therefore, patients taking this drug should take enough fluids to maintain a urine output of 1500 ml daily. A high urine output reduces the risk of crystalluria.

Corticosteroids are used in IBD for their ability to reduce inflammation. Unfortunately, this action also decreases the ability of the body to resist infection. Patients on steroids must be monitored for any signs and symptoms of infections. They should be told to avoid unnecessary exposure to others with infectious conditions.

Steroid therapy can have many other serious side effects as well. These effects include fluid and electrolyte imbalances, ulcers, increased blood sugar, weight gain, elevated blood pressure, acne, capillary fragility, and hirsutism (abnormal growth of hair).

Ineffective Individual Coping. Inflammatory bowel disease is painful, stressful, and can interfere with the patient's everyday life. The nurse tries to establish a trusting relationship with the patient. The nurse encourages independence, participation in care and decision making, and realistic goal setting. People who have IBD may benefit from courses or therapy that assist them with stress management. With the patient's approval, referrals may be made to mental health professionals or spiritual counselors. Sadness and discouragement should be recognized and reported to the physician.

Knowledge Deficit. Topics for patient teaching include information about IBD, diet therapy, drug therapy, resources, and signs and symptoms requiring medical attention. The patient is encouraged to explore individual factors that precipitate acute attacks and measures that bring relief.

EVALUATION. Criteria for evaluating the outcomes of nursing care are patient's statement of pain relief; passage of formed stools; moist mucous membranes, normal pulse rate and blood pressure; stable body weight; patient's reporting of adaptation to IBD; absence of signs of crystalluria, electrolyte imbalances, hyperglycemia, hypertension, and bruising.

DIVERTICULOSIS

Pathophysiology

Diverticulosis is a condition characterized by small sac-like pouches in the intestinal wall called diverticula. Diverticula occur when weak areas of the intestinal wall

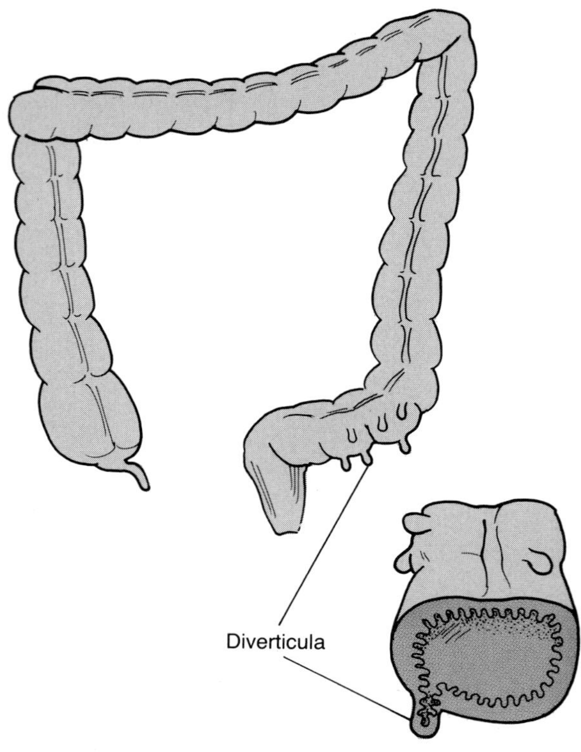

FIGURE 34-22
Diverticula in the sigmoid colon.

allow segments of the mucous membrane to herniate outward (Fig. 34–22). Most diverticula are found in the sigmoid colon, and there is usually more than one.

Risk Factors

Since diverticulosis is most common in developed countries, it is thought that lack of dietary residue is a contributing factor. Other related factors are age, constipation, obesity, and emotional tension.

Signs and Symptoms

Diverticulosis is often asymptomatic, but many people report changes in bowel habits. The change may be constipation, diarrhea, or periodic bouts of both. Other symptoms might include rectal bleeding, pain in the left lower abdomen, nausea and vomiting, and urinary problems.

Complications

Intestinal contents can lodge in diverticula, causing inflammation or infection. The patient is then said to have diverticulitis. Diverticulitis may be related to irritating foods, alcohol, chronic constipation, and persistent coughing. Symptoms of pain and bleeding are more severe with diverticulitis. The patient may also have a fever.

Possible complications of diverticulitis are severe bleeding, obstruction, perforation (rupture), peritonitis, and fistula formation. A fistula is an abnormal opening. In this case, it is most likely to develop between the colon and the bladder or vagina. The fistula permits bowel contents to pass into these other structures.

Medical Diagnosis

Diverticulosis may be suspected on the basis of the patient's symptoms. The stool is tested for occult blood. Colonoscopy and barium enema allow the physician to confirm the presence of diverticula. Since these procedures are invasive, they are delayed if there are signs and symptoms of acute inflammation.

Medical Treatment

Diverticulosis is currently being treated with a high-residue diet without spicy foods. Stool softeners or bulk-forming laxatives are used to treat constipation, and antidiarrheals are prescribed for those who have diarrhea. If pain is severe, it may be treated with meperidine (Demerol). Anticholinergics may be given to decrease spasms in the colon. Opiates (e.g., morphine) should not be given because they cause constipation and increased pressure in the sigmoid colon. Broad-spectrum antibiotics are often prescribed.

During periods of acute inflammation, the patient is placed on bedrest and given nothing by mouth. Intravenous fluids are ordered. Gastrointestinal decompression also may be instituted.

If symptoms persist and complications occur, surgical intervention may be necessary. The affected portion of the colon is removed. A temporary colostomy may be created to "rest" the colon while the surgical incisions heal. Sometimes elective surgery is recommended because the risk of surgical complications is much lower than it is with emergency surgery.

Nursing Care of the Patient with Diverticulosis

The nurse assesses the patient's comfort and stool characteristics. Nausea and vomiting are noted. The patient's temperature is monitored. The abdomen is assessed for distention and tenderness.

NURSING DIAGNOSIS. Nursing diagnoses for the patient with diverticulitis may include the following:

- **Fluid Volume Deficit** related to diarrhea and vomiting
- **Pain** related to inflammation
- **High Risk for Infection** related to perforation
- **Knowledge Deficit** of self-care

GOALS. Goals of nursing care are adequate hydration, pain relief, absence of infection, and patient's knowledge of self-care measures.

INTERVENTIONS. The nurse provides fluids as permitted and monitors the patient's intake and output. Antiemetics are given for nausea. Analgesics and anticholinergics may be given as ordered for pain. The nurse is alert for signs of perforation (fever, abdominal distention, and rigidity). The patient is given information about diverticulosis, including the pathophysiology, treatment, and symptoms of inflammation.

If surgery is performed, the nursing care is similar to that described for any major abdominal surgery. General surgical care is included in Chapter 14, and care of the patient with an ostomy is discussed in Chapter 24.

EVALUATION. Criteria for evaluating the outcomes of nursing interventions are moist mucous membranes and normal pulse and blood pressure; patient's statement of reduced pain; absence of fever and abdominal distention; and patient's verbalization of self-care measures.

COLORECTAL CANCER

Pathophysiology

Colorectal cancer, or cancer of the large intestine, occurs equally in men and women over the age of 40. People at greater risk for colorectal cancer are those with histories of ulcerative colitis or family histories of multiple intestinal polyps. There is some evidence that a high-fat, low-fiber diet also may contribute to the development of this type of cancer.

Colorectal cancer can develop anywhere in the large intestine. Three fourths of all colorectal cancers are located in the rectum or lower sigmoid colon (Fig. 34–23). These portions of the intestine are easy to examine with a sigmoidoscope. Therefore, sigmoidoscopy is often included in routine physical examinations of older adults.

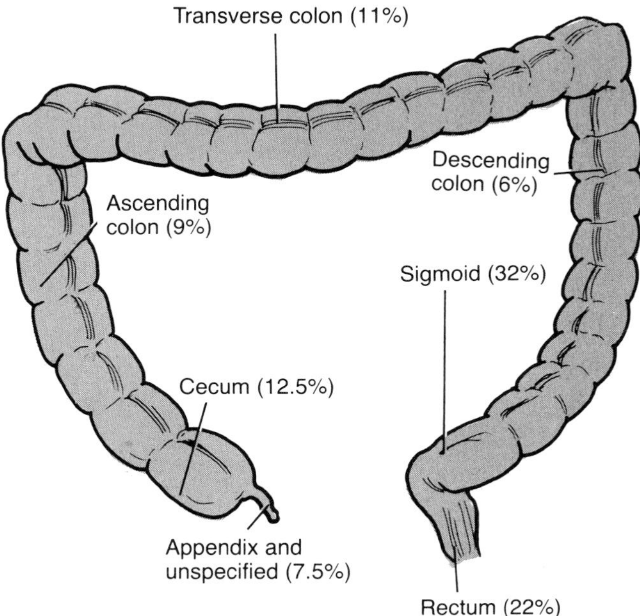

FIGURE 34–23
Sites of colorectal cancer.

Signs and Symptoms

Signs and symptoms of colorectal cancer depend on the location of the disease. In the early stages, symptoms are usually mild. If the cancer is located on the right side of the abdomen, the patient may have only vague cramping until the disease is advanced. Unexplained anemia, weakness, and fatigue related to blood loss may be the only early symptoms of right-sided colon cancer.

Cancers on the left side or in the rectum cause more obvious changes in bowel function. Patients may develop diarrhea or constipation and may notice blood in the stool. Stools may become very narrow, causing them to be described as "pencil-like." This is due to pressure on the bowel from the growing tumor, which causes a narrowed lumen. The patient may report a feeling of fullness or pressure in the abdomen or rectum. If untreated, obstruction of the bowel eventually occurs regardless of the tumor site.

Medical Treatment

Colorectal cancers are usually treated surgically. The exact surgical procedure depends on the location and extent of the cancer. For cancers above the rectum, the diseased portion of the intestine can often be removed. The healthy ends of the remaining intestine are then anastomosed (connected).

Rectal cancers often require more extensive surgery, with incisions in both the abdomen and the perineum (abdominoperineal resection). With removal of the rectum, a permanent colostomy must be created for fecal elimination.

A relatively new stapling procedure can be used to attach the rectal stump to the anus in patients with certain rectal cancers. When this is possible, normal bowel elimination can be maintained and a colostomy can be avoided.

Nursing Care of the Patient with Colorectal Cancer

Since the primary treatment for colon cancer is surgery, nursing care focuses on the surgical patient. Preoperative care includes bowel preparation, hydration, emotional support, and teaching of postoperative routines to prevent surgical complications. Care of the patient with an ostomy is covered in Chapter 24.

ASSESSMENT. In the postoperative period, the nurse assesses vital signs, intake and output, breath sounds, bowel sounds, and pain. The appearance of wounds and wound drainage is noted. If there is a colostomy, the fecal drainage is measured and described. The patient's reactions to the surgical procedure and any other anticipated therapies are assessed.

NURSING DIAGNOSIS. Nursing diagnoses for the patient who has had surgery for colon cancer may include the following:

- **High Risk for Injury** related to extensive surgical trauma, open wounds

- **Altered Tissue Perfusion** (cardiopulmonary) related to effects of anesthesia, immobility
- **Pain** related to tissue trauma
- **Knowledge Deficit** of self-care and therapy
- **Sexual Dysfunction** related to perineal surgery
- **Ineffective Individual Coping** related to life-threatening illness

GOALS. Goals for the patient who has had surgery for colon cancer are wound healing without infection, adequate tissue perfusion, pain relief, patient's knowledge of self-care and therapy; patient's understanding of potential sexual dysfunction, and identification of patient's strengths and resources.

INTERVENTIONS

High Risk for Injury. The nursing care of a patient following an abdominoperineal resection is very demanding. The patient has three incisions: one on the abdomen, a second for the colostomy, and a third on the perineum. All three should be checked for bleeding or drainage. The perineal wound normally drains a large amount of serosanguineous fluid. Serosanguineous fluid is made up of serum and blood. It is a pinkish color and thin in consistency. The wound may be open and packed, partly closed with Penrose drains, or closed and drained with a suction device. An example of a suction drainage system is the Jackson-Pratt drain and fluid collection device. Dressings should initially be reinforced when saturated. Disposable waterproof pads under the patient's hips protect bedding and can easily be changed. A T-binder holds the perineal dressing securely in place.

With so many wounds, especially open ones, these patients are at great risk for infection. Any handling of wound dressings should be done wearing sterile gloves. The wound should always be assessed for signs of infection (unusual odor, excessive redness or swelling around the wound, and purulent drainage).

If there is packing in a wound, it will gradually be removed. Once the packing has been completely removed, the physician may order the wound to be irrigated on a regular schedule. Gentle irrigations promote healing by keeping the wound clean. Strict sterile technique must be used during wound irrigations.

Altered Tissue Perfusion (Cardiopulmonary). Since the abdominoperineal resection requires several incisions and is a lengthy procedure, the patient is at risk for respiratory and circulatory complications. Coughing, deep breathing, and incentive spirometry help prevent fluid accumulation in the lungs. The patient should also be encouraged and assisted to change positions at least every 2 hours. Leg exercises are important because the pressure on abdominal blood vessels during the long surgery may contribute to the formation of blood clots in the legs.

Pain. Pain is severe for several postoperative days. Narcotic analgesics should be given as ordered. If they do not provide relief, the physician should be told. In addition to drug therapy, the nurse should try comfort measures such as position changes and back rubs. At first, the patient will probably be most comfortable in a side-lying position. Later, he or she will be able to tolerate being supine as well.

When the patient is allowed to be up, sitz baths may be ordered several times a day. The warm water cleans, soothes, and increases circulation to the perineum. The patient should be supervised in the sitz bath the first few times in case of dizziness or faintness.

Knowledge Deficit. As the patient improves, the nurse needs to consider long-term needs. The patient must learn to cope with a colostomy, possible changes in sexual functioning, and possibly a partially healed perineal wound. The enterostomal therapist, an expert in the care of patients with ostomies, is an excellent resource person for colostomy management. Before discharge, either the patient or a caregiver must know how to care for the colostomy. Ostomy care is explained in Chapter 24.

Sexual Dysfunction. Extensive perineal surgery can cause various types of sexual dysfunction. The nurse should be open and sensitive to questions that the patient may bring up about sexual function. Questions about the specific effects of particular surgical procedures on sexual function should be referred to the physician. This is not to say that the nurse should dismiss or ignore patient concerns about sexuality but, rather, to stress that the information given must be accurate. Once the correct answers are known, the nurse can reinforce them.

Ineffective Individual Coping. Patients with colorectal cancer and their families often face a difficult period of adjustment. For many people, the thought of having cancer brings up fears of pain, suffering, and a lingering death. These fears may not surface until after the patient recovers from the acute postoperative period. The nurse can help by encouraging the patient to express fears and ask questions and by being a kind listener. Referrals to mental health or spiritual counselors or to support groups can be helpful.

While learning to deal with changes in body image and the threat of a potentially deadly disease, the patient may be faced with receiving chemotherapy as well. Most patients have heard about the side effects of the powerful drugs used in chemotherapy, and they may be genuinely fearful of the treatments. The nursing care of patients receiving chemotherapy is discussed in detail in Chapter 23.

EVALUATION. Criteria for evaluating the outcomes of nursing interventions are intact wounds free of excessive redness, normal body temperature; vital signs consistent with patient's baseline norms; patient's statement of pain relief; patient's verbalization of therapy and self-care; patient's acknowledgement of potential sexual dysfunction; and use of healthy coping strategies.

POLYPS

Polyps are small growths in the intestine. Most are benign, but they can become malignant. Two inherited syndromes, familial polyposis and Gardner's syndrome, are characterized by multiple colorectal polyps and almost always lead to cancer. Polyps are usually asymptomatic and are found on routine testing. Potential complications are bleeding and obstruction. Polyps are diagnosed by a barium enema or an endoscopic examination. Some of the growths can be removed during the endoscopic examination. Colectomy may be advised for patients with familial polyposis or Gardner's syndrome because of the high risk of malignancy.

The nurse encourages patients who are at risk for cancer to seek medical attention. If the patient has surgery, the postoperative care is similar to that of the patient with cancer of the colon. If a colostomy is created, the patient needs special support and teaching, as described in Chapter 24.

HEMORRHOIDS

Hemorrhoids are dilated veins in the rectum. They may be above the sphincter muscles of the anus (internal hemorrhoids) or below these muscles (external hemorrhoids) (Fig. 34–24). If blood clots form in external hemorrhoids, they become inflamed and very painful. Hemorrhoids containing clotted blood are said to be thrombosed.

Risk Factors

A key factor in the development of hemorrhoids is increased pressure in the rectal blood vessels. Pressure is increased by constipation, pregnancy, and prolonged sitting or standing.

Signs and Symptoms

The most common symptoms of hemorrhoids are rectal pain and itching. Bleeding may occur with defecation, especially if the hemorrhoids are internal. External hemorrhoids are easy to see and appear red or bluish.

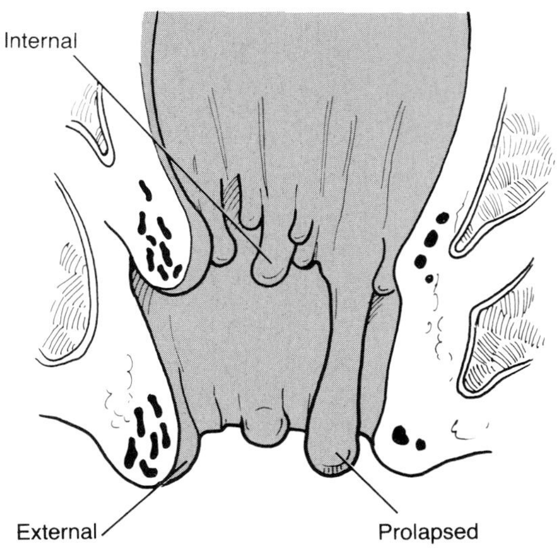

FIGURE 34-24
Internal, external, and prolapsed hemorrhoids.

Medical Diagnosis and Treatment

Hemorrhoids are diagnosed upon visual inspection. Nonsurgical treatment of hemorrhoids attempts to relieve pain, swelling, and pressure. Topical medications such as creams, lotions, or suppositories may be ordered to soothe and shrink inflamed tissue. Sitz baths are often comforting. The physician may order heat or cold applications. Sometimes, especially with thrombosed hemorrhoids, ice packs may be applied for a few hours, followed by warm packs.

In severe cases, removal of hemorrhoids is necessary. Methods of removing hemorrhoids include ligation, sclerotherapy, cryotherapy, and hemorrhoidectomy.

Ligation means "tying off." Sometimes internal hemorrhoids can be ligated with rubber bands. The bands cut off the blood supply so that the vessels shrink and die. Dead tissue eventually breaks off and is eliminated.

Sclerotherapy is the injection of an agent into the tissue around the hemorrhoids that causes them to shrink. It is a relatively simple procedure but often provides only temporary results.

Cryotherapy uses a cold probe to freeze the hemorrhoid. The procedure has many disadvantages, so it is not commonly used now.

A hemorrhoidectomy is the surgical excision (removal) of hemorrhoids. It is necessary when symptoms are very severe. After the hemorrhoids are removed, the wound may be closed with sutures or packed and left open to heal.

Nursing Care of the Patient with Hemorrhoids

Medical management of hemorrhoids does not usually require hospitalization. Therefore, this section emphasizes the care of the surgical patient. Preoperative care includes bowel preparation and patient teaching of postoperative measures to prevent complications of immobility and anesthesia.

ASSESSMENT. After hemorrhoidectomy, the nurse monitors vital signs, intake and output, and breath sounds. The perianal area is assessed for bleeding and drainage.

NURSING DIAGNOSIS. Nursing diagnoses after hemorrhoidectomy may include the following:

- **Pain** related to tissue trauma
- **Impaired Skin Integrity** related to surgical procedure
- **Constipation** related to delay of defecation
- **Knowledge Deficit** of postoperative self-care and prevention of recurrence

GOALS. Following hemorrhoid surgery, the goals of nursing care are pain relief, wound healing, normal bowel elimination, and patient's knowledge of self-care and preventive measures.

INTERVENTIONS

Pain. Hemorrhoidectomy patients have severe postoperative pain that requires narcotic analgesics for relief.

Cold packs over the rectal dressing may be ordered initially. Imagery and relaxation techniques may also help control pain.

Impaired Skin Integrity. The physician removes the wound packing a day or two after surgery. After the packing is removed, the nurse should assess for rectal bleeding. Sitz baths may then be ordered to soothe and cleanse the area and to promote circulation. A soft pad or cushion can be provided for more comfortable sitting.

Constipation. It is especially important to assess and record any stools passed after rectal surgery. The patient will probably dread the first bowel movement, expecting severe pain. Stool softeners will probably be ordered to reduce the trauma of defecation. The nurse can give pain medication before the patient tries to defecate. The nurse should stay close by in case the patient feels weak or faint.

Knowledge Deficit. Before discharge, the patient should be advised of any prescribed activity limitations and signs and symptoms that should be reported to the physician (fever, bleeding). Whether surgical treatment or conservative treatment is needed for hemorrhoids, the patient should be taught how to avoid recurrence. Once the acute symptoms are relieved, the nurse should teach the patient how to reduce the risk of hemorrhoids in the future.

Patients should be advised to avoid constipation, prolonged sitting or standing, or straining to have a bowel movement. A high-fiber diet with plenty of fluids is recommended to promote regular, soft stools. Routine use of stool softeners may be prescribed. The patient should be reminded to follow a regular pattern of bowel elimination and not to delay defecation when the urge occurs.

EVALUATION. The desired outcomes of nursing interventions are measured by the patient's statement of pain relief, well-healed surgical incisions, passage of soft stool, and patient's verbalization of self-care to promote healing and to prevent recurrence.

ANORECTAL ABSCESS

An anorectal abscess is an infection in the tissue around the rectum. Signs and symptoms are rectal pain, swelling, redness, and tenderness. The patient often reports a history of diarrhea. If the abscess becomes chronic, it causes bleeding, itching, and discharge.

Anorectal abscess is treated with antibiotics followed by incision and drainage. The procedure may be done under local or general anesthesia, depending on how extensive the abscess is. Preoperatively, pain is treated with ice packs, sitz baths, and topical agents as ordered. Postoperatively, nursing care is similar to that after hemorrhoidectomy. Pain is treated with narcotic analgesics. Patient teaching emphasizes the importance of thorough cleansing after each bowel movement. The nurse advises the patient to consume adequate fluids and a high-fiber diet to promote soft stools.

ANAL FISSURE

An anal fissure is a laceration between the anal canal and the perianal skin. Fissures may be related to constipation, diarrhea, Crohn's disease, tuberculosis, leukemia, trauma, or childbirth. Sometimes there is no apparent cause. Signs and symptoms include pain before and after defecation and bleeding on the stool or tissue. If the fissure becomes chronic, the patient may experience pruritus, urinary frequency or retention, and dysuria. Fissures usually heal spontaneously, but they can become chronic. Conservative treatment of anal fissures employs sitz baths, stool softeners, and analgesics. Surgical excision may be necessary. Postoperatively, the patient is instructed to cleanse the perianal area after defecation. Pain-relief measures and stool softeners are continued.

ANAL FISTULA

An anal fistula is an abnormal opening between the anal canal and the perianal skin. Fistulas can develop from anorectal abscesses or be related to IBD or tuberculosis. The patient typically complains of pruritus and discharge. Sitz baths provide some comfort. The surgical treatment is excision of the fistula and surrounding tissue. Sometimes a temporary colostomy is done to allow the surgical site to heal. Postoperative care includes analgesics and sitz baths for pain.

NUTRITION CONCEPTS

- People with gastric ulcers experience more pain after eating.
- People with duodenal ulcers experience less pain after eating.
- A peptic ulcer diet is individualized and usually consists of small to moderate-sized meals, avoiding foods that cause an increase in gastric acid secretions or consistently cause distress.
- Diarrhea is caused by pathogenic organisms, diet, intestinal lesions, or irritations associated with various diseases or conditions.
- The major nutritional goal of therapy for diarrhea is to replace lost fluids.
- Constipation is caused by insufficient fiber intake, insufficient fluid intake, lack of exercise, and habitual use of laxatives.
- Dietary treatment of constipation consists of increasing fluid (8–10 glasses of water per day) and fiber intake.
- A hot drink such as coffee or tea enhances peristalsis and promotes defecation.

Normal functioning of the digestive tract is essential for health. The nurse plays an important role in promoting normal function by teaching patients about healthy dietary and elimination practices. The nurse also applies the nursing process to the care of patients with disorders of the digestive tract.

BIBLIOGRAPHY

Beachley, M., & Farrar, J. (1993). Abdominal trauma: Putting the pieces together. *American Journal of Nursing, 93*(11), 26–35.

Black, J. M., & Matassarin-Jacobs, E. (1993). *Luckmann and Sorensen's medical-surgical nursing: A psychophysiologic approach* (4th ed.). Philadelphia: W. B. Saunders.

Brenton, L., & Sich, A. (1991). Caring for the morbidly obese. *American Journal of Nursing, 91*(8), 40–43.

Bryant, G. A. (1992). When the bowel is blocked. *RN, 55*(1), 58–67.

Caine, R. M., & Bufalino, P. M. (1991). *Nursing care planning guides for adults* (2nd ed.). Baltimore: Williams & Wilkins.

Chernecky, C. C., Krech, R. L., & Berger, B. J. (1993). *Laboratory tests and diagnostic procedures.* Philadelphia: W. B. Saunders.

Deters, G. E. (1992). Nursing role in management: Problems of digestion. In S. M. Lewis & I. C. Collier (Eds.), *Medical-surgical nursing* (3rd ed.) (pp. 1037–1073). St. Louis: Mosby Year Book.

Deters, G. E. (1992). Nursing role in management: Problems of nutrition. In S. M. Lewis & I. C. Collier (Eds.), *Medical-surgical nursing* (3rd ed.) (pp. 1003–1036). St. Louis: Mosby Year Book.

Dilorio, C., & Price, M. E. (1990). Swallowing: An assessment and practice guide. *American Journal of Nursing, 90*(7), 38–46.

Doenges, M. E., & Moorhouse, M. F. (1993). *Nurse's pocket guide* (4th ed.). Philadelphia: F. A. Davis.

Elrod, R. (1992). Nursing assessment: Gastrointestinal system. In S. M. Lewis & I. C. Collier (Eds.), *Medical-surgical nursing,* (3rd ed.) (pp. 952–977). St. Louis: Mosby Year Book.

Elrod, R. (1992). Nursing role in management: Problems of ingestion. In S. M. Lewis & I. C. Collier (Eds.), *Medical-surgical nursing* (3rd ed.) (pp. 978–1002). St. Louis: Mosby Year Book.

Gardner, S. S., & Messner, R. L. (1992). Upper GI bleeds. *RN, 55*(12), 42–47.

Haas, L. B. (1992). Nursing role in management: Endocrine problems. In S. M. Lewis & I. C. Collier (Eds.), *Medical-surgical nursing* (3rd ed.) (pp. 1319–1355). St. Louis: Mosby Year Book.

Henzel, B. (1992). Nursing role in management: Problems of absorption and elimination. In S. M. Lewis & I. C. Collier (Eds.), *Medical-surgical nursing* (3rd ed.) (pp. 1074–1120). St. Louis: Mosby Year Book.

Hodgson, B. B., Kizior, R. J., & Kingdon, R. T. (1993). *Nurse's drug handbook.* Philadelphia: W. B. Saunders.

Holmgren, C. (1992). Abdominal assessment. *RN, 55*(3), 28–34.

Ignatavicius, D. D., & Bayne, M. V. (1991). *Medical-surgical nursing: A nursing process approach.* Philadelphia: W. B. Saunders.

Jarvis, C. (1992). *Physical examination and health assessment.* Philadelphia: W. B. Saunders.

Johns, J. L. (1991). When the patient has an ulcer. *RN, 54*(11), 44–51.

Lehmann, S., & Barber, J. R. (1991). Giving medications by feeding tube. *Nursing 91, 21*(11), 58–61.

Matteson, M. A., & McConnell, E. S. (1989). *Gerontological Nursing.* Philadelphia: W. B. Saunders.

McVey, L. (1992). A direct assault on abdominal cancers. *RN, 55*(2), 46–53.

Norris, M. K. (1992). Action stat! Emergency treatment for tooth avulsion. *Nursing 92, 22*(3), 33.

Nursing grand rounds: Tom was a big challenge. (1992). *Nursing 92, 22*(10), 60–64.

Rich, J. (1993). Acute abdominal pain: Revealing the source. *Nursing 93, 23*(9), 34–42.

Roberts, M. K. (1992). Assessing and treating volvulus. *Nursing 92, 22*(2), 56–58.

Schmelzer, M., & Wright, K. (1993). Say nope to soap. *American Journal of Nursing, 93*(3), 21.

Shlafer, M., & Marieb, E. N. (1989). *The nurse, pharmacology, and drug therapy.* Redwood City, CA: Addison-Wesley.

Surratt, S., Ryan, A. B., Hallenbeck, P., Blandon, M. M., & Sugarbaker, P. (1993). Troubleshooting a sump pump. *American Journal of Nursing, 93*(1), 42–44.

Treating ulcerative colitis. (1991). *Nursing 91, 21*(8), 75–76.

Understanding peptic ulcers. (1992). *Nursing 92, 22*(3), 32C–32D.

Webber-Jones, K. M. (1992). How to declog a feeding tube. *Nursing 92, 22*(4), 62–64.

Young, C., & White, S. (1992). Preparing patients for tube feeding at home. *American Journal of Nursing, 92*(4), 46–53.

KEY CONCEPTS

1. Any disorder of the digestive tract can cause nutritional deficiencies by disrupting one or more of its three functions: digestion, absorption, and elimination.
2. Anorexia, lack of an appetite, may be caused by illness, drugs, or emotional factors.
3. Oral inflammations and infections can be caused by irritants, bacteria, viruses, and fungi and can interfere with food intake and enjoyment.
4. Disorders of the teeth and gums require meticulous oral hygiene and professional dental care to prevent tooth loss.
5. Cancers inside the oral cavity are usually squamous cell carcinomas related to poor nutrition, chronic irritation, or combined tobacco and alcohol use.
6. Cancers of the lip are usually basal cell carcinomas attributed to prolonged exposure to irritants, including sun, wind, and pipe smoking.
7. Nursing care of patients being treated for oral

cancers focuses on pain, impaired communication, altered nutrition, body image disturbance, and impaired skin integrity.

8. Cancer of the esophagus may be treated with surgery, radiotherapy, chemotherapy, or a combination of these, or by palliative measures to maintain a patent esophagus.
9. Vomiting, which can result in fluid and electrolyte imbalances, aspiration, and nutritional deficiencies, is treated with antiemetics, fluid and electrolyte replacement, and sometimes gastrointestinal decompression.
10. Treatment of hiatal hernia, the protrusion of the lower esophagus and stomach upward through the diaphragm, may include drug therapy, diet, measures to avoid increased intra-abdominal pressure, or surgery.
11. Gastritis is inflammation of the stomach lining caused by excessive intake of food or alcohol, food poisoning, or chemical ingestion.
12. Peptic ulcer is loss of tissue from the lining of the stomach or duodenum that can lead to hemorrhage, perforation, and obstruction.
13. Nursing care of peptic ulcer patients focuses on pain, altered nutrition, high risk for injury, ineffective individual coping, and knowledge deficit.
14. Dumping syndrome may occur after gastric surgery, causing weakness, dizziness, diaphoresis, and palpitations.
15. Nursing care of the patient with stomach cancer, which is often advanced when diagnosed, focuses on pain, altered nutrition, ineffective individual coping, and knowledge deficit.
16. The term obesity is used to describe body weight greater than 20% more than the person's ideal body weight and is treated with diet, planned exercise, and, in some cases, surgical intervention.
17. There are a variety of types of malabsorption, conditions in which one or more nutrients are not digested or absorbed.
18. Diarrhea is the frequent passage of loose or liquid stools that can lead to fluid and electrolyte imbalances, metabolic acidosis, and malnutrition.
19. Constipation is the difficult passage of hard, dry stools that may be related to inactivity, dehydration, laxative dependence, low-fiber diet, some drugs, and a variety of medical conditions.
20. Fecal impaction is the retention of a large mass of stool in the rectum that the patient cannot pass and that may require removal with enemas and manual extraction.
21. Factors that can cause intestinal obstruction include strangulated hernia, tumor, paralytic ileus, stricture, volvulus, intussusception, and postoperative adhesions.
22. Appendicitis is inflammation of the appendix that requires surgical treatment to prevent rupture and peritonitis.
23. A hernia is a portion of intestine that bulges through a weak area in the muscles of the abdominal wall and can become incarcerated (trapped) and obstructed.
24. Inflammatory bowel disease (IBD), characterized by inflammation and ulceration of the lining of the intestines, includes ulcerative colitis and Crohn's disease.
25. Nursing care of the patient with IBD focuses on pain, diarrhea, fluid volume deficit, altered nutrition, ineffective individual coping, high risk for injury, and knowledge deficit.
26. Diverticulosis is characterized by small, sac-like pouches in the intestinal wall that can become inflamed, causing obstruction, perforation, peritonitis, and fistula formation.
27. Nursing care of the patient with colorectal cancer, which is usually treated surgically, focuses on high risk for injury, altered tissue perfusion, acute pain, knowledge deficit, sexual dysfunction, and ineffective individual coping.
28. Polyps are small growths in the intestine that are usually benign but may be removed because they may bleed, cause obstructions, or become malignant.
29. Hemorrhoids are dilated rectal veins that can become inflamed and thrombosed; they are treated with topical medications, sitz baths, heat or cold, sclerotherapy, or surgical excision.
30. Anal disorders include abscesses, fissures, and fistulas, all of which may be treated surgically.

Adrianne Linton

CHAPTER 35

Disorders of the Liver, Gallbladder, and Pancreas

OBJECTIVES

1. Identify nursing assessment data related to the functions of the liver, gallbladder, and pancreas.
2. Identify the nurse's role in tests and procedures performed to diagnose disorders of the liver, gallbladder, and pancreas.
3. Describe the care of the patient who has an esophageal balloon tube in place.
4. Explain the pathology, signs and symptoms, diagnosis, complications, and medical treatment of selected disorders of the liver, gallbladder, and pancreas.
5. Apply the nursing process to develop a nursing care plan for the patient with liver, gallbladder, or pancreatic dysfunction.

GLOSSARY

ASCITES Accumulation of excess fluid in the peritoneal cavity

CHOLECYSTECTOMY Removal of the gallbladder

CHOLECYSTITIS Inflammation of the gallbladder

CHOLEDOCHOLITHIASIS Obstruction of the common bile duct by a gallstone

CHOLELITHIASIS Presence of gallstones in the gallbladder

CIRRHOSIS Chronic, progressive liver disease

ENDOCRINE GLAND Gland that secretes a substance directly into the blood

ERUCTATION Ejection of gas from the stomach through the mouth; belching

GLUCONEOGENESIS Synthesis of glucose from sources other than carbohydrates

GLYCOGENESIS Conversion of glucose from glycogen

Glossary continued

GLYCOGENOLYSIS Splitting of glycogen into glucose

HEPATIC Pertaining to the liver

HEPATITIS Inflammation of the liver

HEPATOMEGALY Enlargement of the liver

ICTERUS Jaundice; golden yellow skin color caused by deposition of bile

JAUNDICE Golden yellow color of the skin, sclerae, and mucous membranes caused by deposition of bile pigments; associated with liver dysfunction or bile obstruction

THE LIVER

The liver is the largest internal organ in the body. It is located under the diaphragm in the upper right abdomen, as illustrated in Figure 35–1. The term hepatic refers to the liver.

ANATOMY AND PHYSIOLOGY OF THE LIVER

The liver is made up of four lobes that divide into many lobules (Fig. 35–2). The hepatic artery delivers blood from the aorta to the liver. The portal vein delivers blood from the intestines to the liver. Portal blood circulates through the liver and is transported to the inferior vena cava by the hepatic veins. Figure 35–3 illustrates hepatic circulation.

Specialized hepatic cells allow the liver to carry out many critical functions. Reticuloendothelial cells, called Kupffer's cells, ingest old red blood cells and bacteria. Parenchymal cells carry out various metabolic functions, including metabolism of carbohydrates, fats, proteins, and steroids and detoxification of potentially harmful substances.

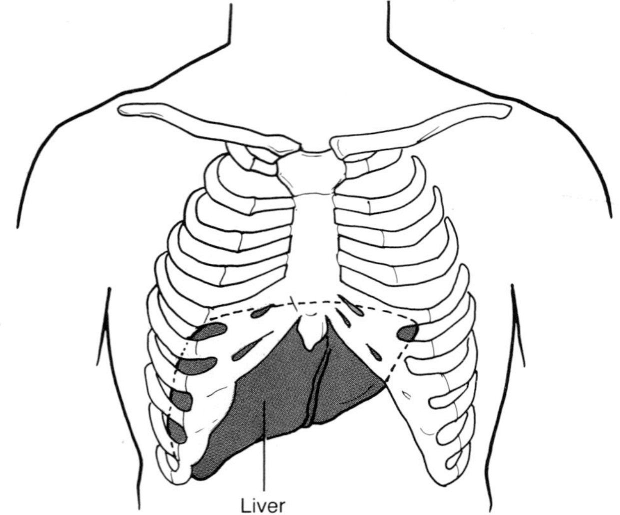

FIGURE 35–1
The liver is located under the diaphragm in the right upper abdomen.

BILE PRODUCTION AND EXCRETION

Bilirubin is a product of the normal breakdown of old red blood cells in the liver. The initial breakdown product is unconjugated or indirect bilirubin. The liver then converts unconjugated bilirubin into conjugated bilirubin and secretes it into the bile. Bile produced in the liver passes through the cystic duct into the gallbladder for storage.

When fats pass into the duodenum, the gallbladder and the liver respond by delivering bile through the common bile duct into the small intestine. Bile emulsifies fat, meaning that it breaks it into small particles that can easily be absorbed. It also neutralizes the acidic chyme as it leaves the stomach. Bile plays a role in the absorption of fat-soluble vitamins and the removal of some toxins.

Bile travels through the intestines with the chyme. In the large intestine, it is converted to urobilinogen and then to stercobilin. This final breakdown product of bilirubin gives stool its characteristic brown color.

METABOLISM

Glucose Metabolism

The liver helps maintain the blood glucose within a certain range. After a meal, excess glucose molecules are taken up by the liver, combined, and then stored as glycogen. This process is called glycogenesis. When the glucose level in the blood falls, the process is reversed by glycogenolysis, and the glucose molecules are returned to the blood. Gluconeogenesis is the third process by which the liver maintains blood glucose. Fats and protein are broken down in response to low blood glucose, and the molecules are used to make new glucose.

Protein Metabolism

Some nonessential amino acids, plasma proteins (albumin and globulin), and clotting factors are synthesized in the liver. Another important liver function in relation to protein metabolism is the conversion of ammonia to urea. Ammonia is a byproduct of the metabolism of amino acids. If ammonia accumulates in the blood, it produces toxic effects on brain tissue.

Lipid Metabolism

The liver synthesizes lipids from glucose, pyruvic acid, acetic acid, and amino acids. It also synthesizes fatty acids, breaks down triglycerides, and synthesizes and breaks down cholesterol.

Blood Coagulation

Normal blood coagulation (clotting) is a complex process. Two essential elements for coagulation, prothrombin and fibrinogen, are synthesized by the liver.

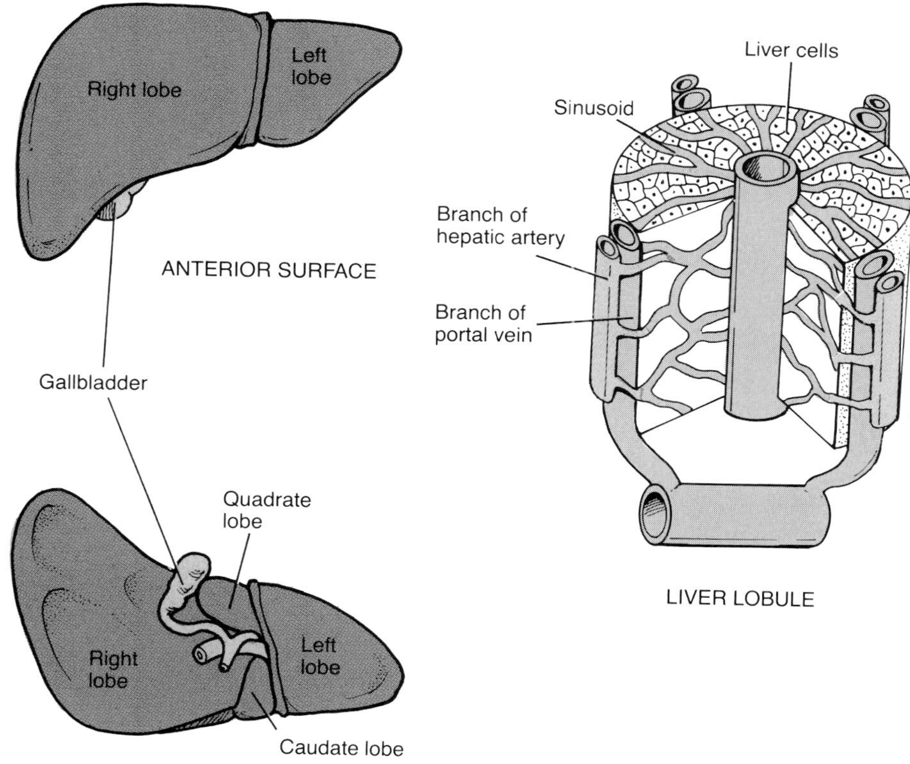

FIGURE 35-2

The liver has four lobes, each made up of many lobules.

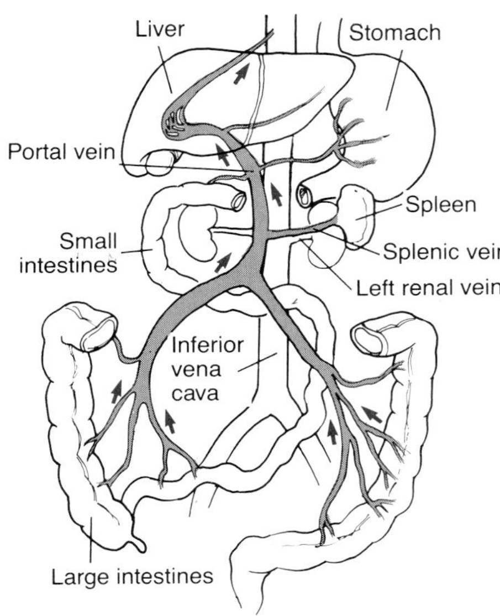

FIGURE 35-3

Hepatic circulation. Venous blood from the spleen, stomach, pancreas, and intestines passes through the liver via the portal vein and is delivered through the hepatic veins to the inferior vena cava.

Detoxification

The liver filters the blood and inactivates many chemicals, including most medications. Therefore, medications are prescribed very cautiously for patients with poor liver function. Patients with liver disease are at increased risk for drug toxicities. With age, there is some decrease in liver function, so lower drug dosages may be adequate. Especially with long-term therapy, the older person should be assessed frequently for signs of toxicity.

PHARMACOLOGY CAPSULE

Since many drugs are metabolized in the liver, patients with liver disease are at increased risk for drug toxicities.

Immunity

An important protective mechanism is the development of antibodies to resist pathogens. Antibodies and other substances that aid resistance to infection are produced in the liver.

Hormone Metabolism

The liver plays an important role in the metabolism of adrenocortical hormones, estrogen, testosterone, and aldosterone. If these hormones are not metabolized, they accumulate, causing an exaggerated effect on target organs.

NURSING ASSESSMENT OF THE LIVER

The liver has so many important functions that alterations may cause a number of systemic signs and symptoms. The health history and physical examination may detect liver dysfunction or may be used to assess responses to treatment of liver disorders.

HEALTH HISTORY

The nurse begins by asking about the patient's chief complaint. The present illness is explored and described.

Past Medical History

The past medical history documents any previous or chronic liver disorders. Recent surgeries, injuries, or blood transfusions are documented since they sometimes expose the patient to the hepatitis virus. A complete list of medications is compiled.

Family History

The nurse assesses whether any of the patient's family members have had cancer of the liver or colon, hepatitis, or alcoholism.

Review of Systems

The nurse inquires about the patient's general health status and systematically assesses for signs and symptoms related to liver dysfunction. People who have impaired liver function often complain of general fatigue. They may have had personality or behavior changes, but the patients are not always aware of these. The nurse inquires about any changes in weight, skin color, itching, easy bruising, headaches, enlarged lymph nodes, breast enlargement in men, or dyspnea.

Gastrointestinal symptoms are common with liver disease. Therefore, the patient is asked about the presence of anorexia, abdominal pain, nausea and vomiting, diarrhea, or gastrointestinal bleeding. The color of stool is noted because clay-colored stools are characteristic of bile obstruction. Changes in urine color also may be significant since patients with liver disease often have dark urine.

The nurse asks whether the patient has had any numbness, tingling, or edema in the extremities.

Functional Assessment

The patient's daily routines are explored, including dietary intake and patterns of activity and rest. Since liver disease may be associated with exposure to toxins, the nurse assesses the patient's exposure to potentially toxic chemicals and pattern of alcohol use. Some people are reluctant to discuss alcohol use, so the subject must be handled tactfully. People tend to understate the amount of alcohol they typically consume. Use of street drugs, especially those taken intravenously, must be noted.

The last part of the functional assessment is the identification of stressors, usual coping strategies, and sources of support.

PHYSICAL EXAMINATION

The physical assessment begins with the measurement of vital signs and weight and observation of the patient's general appearance. Skin color is especially important in relation to the liver. Jaundice is a golden yellow skin color associated with liver dysfunction or bile obstruction. It is relatively easy to recognize in fair-skinned people.

The color of the sclera of the eyes is inspected. Like the skin, the sclera may turn yellow, a condition called scleral icterus. This sign is especially useful when jaundice cannot be seen elsewhere in dark-skinned people.

The nurse assesses for enlargement of breast tissue in males. Such enlargement is called gynecomastia. When inspecting the chest, the nurse also looks for spider angiomas. Spider angiomas are small, visible vessels shaped like spiders.

The examination of the abdomen is especially important in detecting liver disease. The nurse inspects the shape of the abdomen. The presence of prominent veins is noted. If significant ascites (fluid accumulation in the peritoneal cavity) is present, the abdomen appears distended. The abdomen can be measured at the largest circumference in order to permit comparative measurements later (Fig. 35–4).

The abdomen is palpated for distention and tenderness. Experienced examiners may be able to palpate the liver, but, unless it is enlarged, it is difficult to locate under the right rib cage. An enlarged, diseased liver may be felt well below the rib margin. Liver enlargement is called hepatomegaly.

The extremities are examined for bruising, edema, muscle wasting, and impaired sensation. The hands are inspected for palmar erythema (redness of the palms).

The assessment of a patient with a liver disorder is summarized in Table 35–1. Findings associated with liver disease are illustrated in Figure 35–5.

DIAGNOSTIC TESTS AND PROCEDURES

The physician uses a number of tools to assess liver function, including laboratory and radiographic studies, scans, ultrasonography, imaging, and biopsies. Details

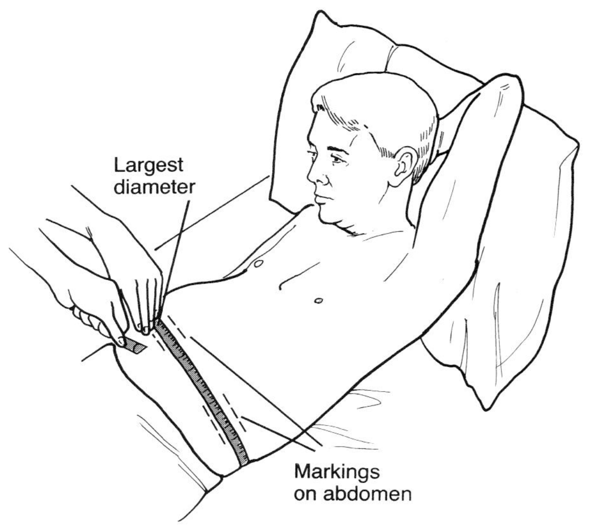

FIGURE 35-4

How to measure abdominal girth. Marks are made on the abdominal midline and both sides so that subsequent measurements can always be made at the same place.

of specific tests and procedures are provided in Table 35–2.

Laboratory Studies

Laboratory studies of blood specimens are done to measure serum and urine bilirubin, serum proteins, ammonia, prothrombin time, vitamin K production, and serum enzymes. Examples of serum enzymes include alkaline phosphatase (ALP), alanine aminotransferase (ALT), serum glutamic-pyruvic transaminase (SGPT), aldolase (ALS), aspartate aminotransferase (AST), serum glutamic-oxaloacetic transaminase (SGOT), and lactic dehydrogenase (LDH).

TABLE 35-1

ASSESSMENT OF THE PATIENT WITH LIVER DISEASE

HEALTH HISTORY

Present illness: Fatigue, weight changes, digestive disturbances, skin changes
Past medical history: Previous liver disease, hepatitis B immunization, recent and current medications taken
Review of systems: Weakness, fatigue, pruritus, dyspnea, anorexia, abdominal pain, nausea and vomiting, diarrhea, bloody stools, changes in urine or stool color, numbness or tingling of extremities
Functional assessment: Diet, alcohol intake, occupation, exposure to toxins, stress, coping strategies, interpersonal relationships

PHYSICAL EXAMINATION

Vital signs: Hypertension, tachypnea
Height and weight
Skin: Dryness, scratches, jaundice, bruises
Eyes: Scleral icterus
Thorax: Spider angiomas
Breasts: Gynecomastia
Abdomen: Distention, prominent veins, girth, liver enlargement

The nurse should check the agency procedure manual for patient preparation. Many liver function tests require a fasting blood sample. The blood sample may also require special treatment such as refrigeration or protection from light.

Since gastrointestinal bleeding is sometimes a problem with liver disease, gastric fluids and stools may be tested for the presence of occult blood. Urine specimens may also be tested for bilirubin and urobilinogen, and stool specimens for urobilinogen.

A dye excretion test also may be ordered in which indocyanine green is administered intravenously to determine the liver's ability to extract the chemical. Blood samples are then taken at 5-minute intervals for up to 30 minutes to assess the amount of dye remaining in the blood.

Radiographic Studies

Radiographic studies are used primarily to visualize the circulatory and biliary systems in the liver. The liver scan employs a radioactive substance that is injected into a vein. The substance accumulates in the liver. Radiographs are then taken to reveal tumors and abscesses.

Ultrasonography

Ultrasonography uses sound waves to create an image of the liver, spleen, pancreas, gallbladder, and biliary system. It is a noninvasive and painless procedure.

Computed Tomography and Magnetic Resonance Imaging

Computed tomography (CT) and magnetic resonance imaging are used to obtain scans of internal organs, including the liver. They are noninvasive, painless procedures.

Liver Biopsy

A liver biopsy is a procedure that involves removal of a small specimen of liver tissue for examination. The specimen can be obtained through an incision under general anesthesia (open biopsy). Another method (needle biopsy) involves the use of a special type of needle inserted through the abdominal wall to obtain the specimen.

Prior to either procedure, baseline vital signs and blood coagulation studies should be done. Signed consent is required. If having a needle biopsy, the patient should be told what to expect during the procedure. For a needle biopsy, the patient is positioned supine with the right arm behind the head. A pad is placed under the right chest. The physician instructs the patient to take a deep breath and hold it during the actual puncture.

A pressure dressing is placed over the puncture and should be checked for bleeding. The physician may order the patient kept on the right side for a period of time to maintain pressure to the area. Following the procedure, the nurse monitors vital signs for signs of blood loss (tachycardia, restlessness, hypotension) or pneumothorax (restlessness, tachypnea).

NEUROLOGIC FINDINGS
Asterixis
Portal-systemic encephalopathy
Paresthesias of feet
Peripheral nerve degeneration
Reversal of sleep-wake pattern
Sensory disturbances

GASTROINTESTINAL (GI) FINDINGS
Abdominal pain
Anorexia
Ascites
Clay-colored stools
Diarrhea
Esophageal varices
Fetor hepaticus
Gallstones
Gastritis
GI bleeding
Hemorrhoidal varices
Hepatomegaly
Hiatal hernia
Hypersplenism
Malnutrition
Nausea
Small nodular liver
Vomiting

RENAL FINDINGS
Hepatorenal syndrome
Increased urine bilirubin

ENDOCRINE FINDINGS
Increased aldosterone
Increased antidiuretic hormone
Increased circulating estrogens
Increased glucocorticoids
Gynecomastia

IMMUNE SYSTEM DISTURBANCES
Leukopenia
Increased susceptibility to infection

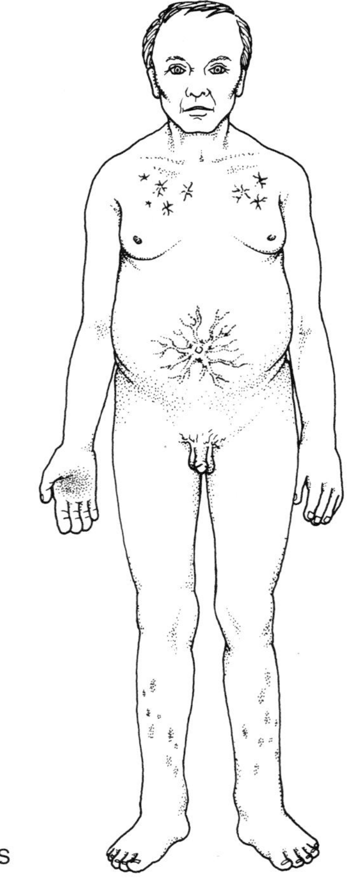

CARDIOVASCULAR FINDINGS
Cardiac arrhythmias
Development of collateral circulation
Hyperkinetic circulation
Peripheral edema
Spider angiomas
Fatigue
Portal hypertension

PULMONARY FINDINGS
Dyspnea
Hydrothorax
Hyperventilation
Hypoxemia

HEMATOLOGIC FINDINGS
Anemia
Disseminated intravascular coagulation
Impaired coagulation
Splenomegaly
Thrombocytopenia

DERMATOLOGIC FINDINGS
Axillary and pubic hair changes
Increased skin pigmentation
Jaundice
Pruritus
Spider angiomas
Caput medusae
Palmar erythema
Ecchymosis

FLUID AND ELECTROLYTE DISTURBANCES
Ascites
Decreased effective blood volume
Dilutional hyponatremia or hypernatremia
Hypocalcemia
Hypokalemia
Peripheral edema
Water retention

FIGURE 35-5

Findings associated with liver disease. Early signs and symptoms are in red. (From Ignatavicius, D. D., & Bayne, M. V. [1991]. *Medical-surgical nursing: A nursing process approach* [p. 1481]. Philadelphia: W. B. Saunders.)

The primary complications of liver biopsy are hemorrhage and pneumothorax. Bleeding is a possibility because of the liver's rich blood supply and the potential for impaired coagulation in the patient with liver disease. Pneumothorax occurs if the lung is accidentally punctured during the biopsy. Air escapes into the pleural cavity, and the lung on the affected side collapses.

DISORDERS OF THE LIVER

HEPATITIS

Hepatitis is inflammation of the liver caused by a viral infection or exposure to toxic chemicals. It is estimated that 100,000 cases of viral hepatitis occur in the United States each year.

Pathophysiology

Hepatitis has both local and systemic effects. Locally, the inflammatory process causes the liver to swell. If swelling is severe, there are two important effects. First, the bile channels are compressed, damaging the cells that produce bile. This results in an elevation in serum bilirubin and jaundice. Second, blood flow through the liver is impaired, causing pressure to rise in the portal circulation.

Systemic effects are related to altered metabolic functions normally performed by the liver and to the infectious response in viral hepatitis. Systemic signs and symptoms of hepatitis include rash, angioedema, arthritis, fever, and malaise.

Types of Hepatitis

Hepatitis may be caused by one of several viruses or by toxic agents. Viral hepatitis is classified as hepatitis A,

TABLE 35-2
DIAGNOSTIC TESTS AND PROCEDURES FOR THE LIVER AND GALLBLADDER

TEST/STUDY	PURPOSE/PROCEDURE	PATIENT PREPARATION	POSTPROCEDURE NURSING CARE
Laboratory Tests			
Blood Studies			
Serum bilirubin	Assesses liver function by measuring bilirubin in the blood. Normal values include: Total bilirubin: 0.2–1.0 mg/dl *or* 3.4–17.1 μmol/L Conjugated bilirubin: 0.0–0.2 mg/dl *or* 0.0–3.4 μmol/L Unconjugated bilirubin: 0.2–0.8 mg/dl	Tell the patient a blood sample will be drawn before breakfast. Bilirubin tests should not be done for 24 hr after contrast media has been given.	Monitor venipuncture site for bleeding. Apply pressure for 5 min if evidence of impaired clotting.
Alkaline phosphatase	Detects increases associated with liver or bone disease. Normal value: 25–92 U/L		Same as serum bilirubin
Prothrombin time	Detects increased clotting time possibly caused by liver disease or vitamin K deficiency. Normal Value: 11.0–12.6 sec		Same as serum bilirubin
Serum enzymes AST (SGOT) ALT (SGPT) LDH	Detects elevations in enzymes related to diseases of the liver. Normal values: AST: Men 7–21 μ/L Women 6–18 μ/L ALT: Men 6–24 U/L Women 4–17 U/L LDH: Varies with type of test	Consult agency guidelines to see if fasting is necessary. Tell patient a blood sample will be drawn.	Same as serum bilirubin
Serum protein electrophoresis	Detects decreased levels of proteins consistent with liver disease.		Same as serum bilirubin
Dye excretion	Measures the ability of the liver to filter a dye (indocyanine green) from the blood.	Tell the patient a dye will be injected into a vein and blood samples will then be drawn at 5-min intervals for up to 30 min to see how much dye remains.	Same as serum bilirubin
Radiographic Studies			
Computed tomography (CT scan)	Creates cross-sectional images of liver and other organs. Is much more sensitive than traditional radiographs.	Patient allergies to contrast medicine should be reported to the radiologist. Advise the patient that the procedure is painless and noninvasive. NPO status may be ordered before a CT scan, but routine drugs can usually be taken. The patient will lie still on a stretcher while a donut-shaped machine moves around him or her. Contrast dye is sometimes injected intravenously. It can create a feeling of warmth, a salty taste, and nausea. Sedation can be ordered if patient has difficulty lying still.	No special care usually needed. Inform the physician of any signs of allergic response to contrast dye. Give antihistamines as ordered for allergy.

Table continued on following page

TABLE 35-2

DIAGNOSTIC TESTS AND PROCEDURES FOR THE LIVER AND GALLBLADDER *Continued*

TEST/STUDY	PURPOSE/PROCEDURE	PATIENT PREPARATION	POSTPROCEDURE NURSING CARE
Radiographic Studies			
Angiography			
Percutaneous transhepatic cholangiography	Iodine is given and radiographs are used to visualize the biliary duct system.	Report patient allergies to iodine or seafood before the test. During procedure, the patient must lie still while a needle is inserted into liver and dye is injected. Radiographs are used to place the needles and observe the outline of the bile ducts or blood vessels.	Bedrest for 8 hr. Check the puncture site for bleeding. Monitor vital signs to detect signs of bleeding.
Portal venography and hepatic arteriography	Use intravenous contrast dye followed by radiographs to study blood vessels in liver.		
Liver scan	A radioactive substance is given that collects in liver. A scanner maps uptake of radiation, revealing tumors and abscesses.	During procedure, the radioactive substance is given intravenously. The patient should be assured that small dose of radiation is harmless. The patient is then helped to assume various positions while radiographs are taken.	
Imaging Procedures			
Ultrasonography	Uses high-frequency sound waves to create an image of the liver, spleen, pancreas, gallbladder, and biliary system.	The patient may be NPO for 8–12 hr before procedure. Patient teaching: During the procedure, the patient will lie on a table. A technician applies gel to the abdomen and moves an instrument called a transducer over the abdomen. Images are projected onto a screen. The procedure is not painful.	No special care needed after the procedure.
Magnetic resonance imaging (MRI)	Creates cross-sectional images of the liver and other organs without radiation.	Advise the patient that MRI is a painless, noninvasive procedure. All metal must be removed before MRI. The patient must be still on a narrow surface. A circular device surrounds the body like a tunnel. Closing eyes reduces claustrophobia. Machine is noisy.	No special care needed.
Tissue Examination			
Liver biopsy	Removes a small specimen of liver tissue for examination.	Baseline vital signs and blood coagulation studies should be obtained.	Monitor vital signs for indications of bleeding (tachycardia, tachypnea, restlessness, hypotension) and pneumothorax (dyspnea, tachycardia).
Needle biopsy	The specimen is obtained by inserting a special needle into the liver through the abdominal wall.	The patient is positioned supine with the right arm behind the head.	Check pressure dressing for bleeding. Position the patient on the right side as ordered.
Open biopsy	An incision is made under general anesthesia.	Done in the operating room and requires standard preoperative procedures. Informed consent must be obtained from the patient.	

AST, Aspartate aminotransferase; SGOT, serum glutamic-oxaloacetic transaminase; ALT, alanine aminotransferase; SGPT, serum glutamic-pyruvic transaminase; LDH, lactate dehydrogenase; NPO, nothing by mouth.

B, C, D, or E. Key features of each type of hepatitis are summarized in Table 35–3.

HEPATITIS A. Hepatitis A has been called infectious hepatitis and epidemic hepatitis. It is caused by the hepatitis A virus, which is transmitted from one person to another by way of water, food, or medical equipment that has been contaminated with infected fecal matter.

HEPATITIS B. Hepatitis B, caused by the hepatitis B virus, is often called serum hepatitis. Since the hepatitis B virus is found in all body fluids of infected persons, modes of transmission include intimate contact with carriers as well as contaminated blood or medical equipment.

HEPATITIS C. Hepatitis C is also called non-A, non-B hepatitis. There are two types of hepatitis C: one is parenterally transmitted, and the other is enterically transmitted. Several viruses are thought to be responsible for hepatitis C. It too is transmitted by contaminated blood or medical equipment.

HEPATITIS D. Hepatitis D is transmitted with hepatitis B. It is caused by a virus known as the delta agent.

HEPATITIS E. Hepatitis E has only recently been described. It is similar to hepatitis A and is transmitted in the same way.

NONINFECTIOUS HEPATITIS. Noninfectious hepatitis is caused by exposure to toxins such as carbon tetrachloride, alcohol, benzene, halothane, aspirin, and methyldopa.

Signs and Symptoms

Regardless of the cause, the signs and symptoms of hepatitis are similar. Differences occur in the number and severity of the symptoms from one person to the next. Many patients have no symptoms at all. For those who are symptomatic, the course of the disease is marked by three phases: preicteric, icteric, and posticteric.

PREICTERIC PHASE. Common findings in the preicteric phase include malaise, severe headache, right upper quadrant abdominal pain, anorexia, nausea, vomiting, fever, arthralgia, rash, enlarged lymph nodes, urticaria, and enlargement and tenderness of the liver. The preicteric phase lasts 1 to 21 days and is the period when the patient is most infectious.

ICTERIC PHASE. The icteric phase is characterized by jaundice, light or clay-colored stools, and dark urine typical of impaired bile production and secretion. Pruritus may be present, caused by the accumulation of bile salts under the skin. Gastrointestinal symptoms from the preicteric phase often persist. The icteric phase lasts 2

TABLE 35–3

KEY FEATURES OF EACH TYPE OF VIRAL HEPATITIS

TYPE	CAUSE	TRANSMISSION ROUTE	INCUBATION PERIOD	PREVENTION
Hepatitis A	Hepatitis A virus (HAV)	Fecal-oral route. Often via contaminated water or food.	3–5 wk	Hand washing after toileting. Clean water and food supplies. Gloves to handle stool specimens, soiled articles. Immune globulin before or within 48 hr after exposure.
Hepatitis B	Hepatitis B virus (HBV)	Introduction of contaminated blood through skin or mucous membranes. Often via contaminated needles or other medical or dental equipment. Also by sexual contact. Newborns may be infected before, during, or after birth.	2–5 mo	Vaccine given to people at risk for exposure. Use disposable needles. Avoid contaminated articles. Screen blood donors. Caution with body fluids. Hepatitis B immune globulin given after exposure.
Hepatitis C (non-A, non-B)	Hepatitis C virus (HCV)	Introduction of contaminated blood through skin or mucous membranes, usually by needles or other medical or dental equipment.	7 wk	Use disposable needles. Avoid contaminated articles. Screen blood donors. Caution with body fluids. No vaccine.
Hepatitis D	"Delta agent" hepatitis D virus (HDV)	Transmitted only with HBV via contaminated blood or equipment, sexual contact.	1–6 mo	Hepatitis B vaccine.
Hepatitis E		Fecal-oral route often via contaminated water or food.	3–6 wk	Hand washing after toileting. Clean water and food supplies. Gloves to handle stool specimens, soiled articles. Immune globulin before or within 48 hr after exposure.

to 4 weeks. Hepatitis patients in whom jaundice does not develop are said to have anicteric hepatitis.

POSTICTERIC PHASE. In the posticteric phase, fatigue, malaise, and liver enlargement persist for several months.

Complications

Most people recover fully from hepatitis, but there can be residual damage and complications. Some patients become carriers. About one fourth of those who become carriers will have chronic active hepatitis, which can lead to cirrhosis. Carriers are also at increased risk for liver cancer. People who have had hepatitis cannot donate blood because of the risk of transmission of the disease to the recipient.

Complications of hepatitis include chronic persistent hepatitis, chronic active hepatitis, and fulminant hepatitis. Chronic persistent hepatitis is characterized by a prolonged recovery with continuing fatigue and liver enlargement that eventually resolves. With chronic active hepatitis, signs and symptoms persist for more than 6 months. Liver damage continues and may lead to cirrhosis. If necrosis of damaged cells occurs without regeneration, fulminant hepatitis results. It is marked by severe liver failure and is often fatal. Hepatitis D virus, which coexists with the hepatitis B virus, can contribute to the development of fulminant hepatitis.

Medical Diagnosis

A diagnosis of hepatitis is supported by abnormal liver function tests. Typical findings consistent with hepatitis include elevated serum enzymes, serum and urinary bilirubin, and urinary urobilinogen. The prothrombin time is prolonged. Albumin may be normal or low, and globulin may be normal or high. The types of viral hepatitis can be identified by the presence of specific viral antigens and antibodies.

Medical Treatment

There is no specific cure for hepatitis. Treatment is designed to promote healing and to manage symptoms. Physician's orders usually include antipyretics for fever and antiemetics for nausea. Corticosteroids may be ordered if the patient is very ill or fulminant hepatitis is suspected. The selection of drugs is important since hepatotoxic drugs should not be given. Suggested antiemetics are dimenhydrinate (Dramamine) and trimethobenzamide (Tigan). Phenothiazines are contraindicated. If sedatives are needed, chloral hydrate or diphenhydramine (Benadryl) is recommended.

The prescribed diet is usually high in carbohydrates with a moderate to high protein allowance, moderate to low fat content, and supplementary vitamins. The amount of activity allowed is based on the patient's signs and symptoms and liver function tests. Bedrest may be ordered during the icteric phase, but practices vary.

PHARMACOLOGY CAPSULE

Hepatotoxic drugs are contraindicated for the hepatitis patient.

NURSING CARE OF THE PATIENT WITH HEPATITIS

Assessment

Nursing assessment of the patient with liver disease is outlined in Table 35–1. When assessing the patient with hepatitis, the health history includes information about general health state, drug and alcohol use, chemical exposure, dietary habits, blood transfusions, recent travel, gastrointestinal disturbances, and changes in skin, urine, or stools.

Ongoing physical assessment includes vital signs, inspection of skin, weight changes, and mental status.

Nursing Diagnosis

Common nursing diagnoses for the patient with hepatitis include the following:

- **Activity Intolerance** and **Impaired Physical Mobility** related to fatigue, impaired metabolism, prescribed bedrest
- **Altered Nutrition: Less than Body Requirements** related to anorexia, nausea and vomiting
- **Fluid Volume Deficit** related to inadequate intake, vomiting
- **Impaired Skin Integrity** related to pruritus and scratching
- **Body Image Disturbance** related to jaundice
- **Anxiety** related to hospitalization, unfamiliar procedures, serious illness
- **Knowledge Deficit** related to mode of transmission of hepatitis, self-care

Goals

The goals of nursing care for the patient with hepatitis are improved activity tolerance and absence of complications of immobility, adequate dietary intake, normal fluid status, decreased pruritus, patient's understanding that jaundice is temporary, reduced anxiety, and knowledge of self-care and practices to prevent transmission of hepatitis to others.

Interventions

ACTIVITY INTOLERANCE AND IMPAIRED PHYSICAL MOBILITY. When the patient is on bedrest or some other activity limitation, the nurse explains that rest allows the liver to heal by regenerating new cells to replace those damaged by hepatitis. The nurse promotes rest by planning activities to permit times when the patient is not disturbed. Diversions such as reading or television can be offered.

Complete bedrest is usually not necessary; however, if it is ordered, the patient is at risk for complications of immobility. The skin should be inspected for early signs of pressure (redness, especially over bony prominences). Gentle massage with moisturizing lotions stimulates circulation and protects the skin. If the patient is unable to turn independently, the nurse should assist with turning at least every 2 hours.

The patient should also be taught and reminded to cough and deep breathe every 2 hours to reduce the risk of pneumonia. Gentle exercise of the legs promotes circulation and discourages the formation of thrombi.

Inactivity tends to lead to constipation and may cause urinary stasis. Bowel movements and urine output are therefore recorded. The nurse also describes any abnormal characteristics of stool and urine. Care of the immobilized patient is discussed in detail in Chapter 19.

ALTERED NUTRITION. Good nutrition is essential to decrease demands on the liver and provide protein for healing. Unfortunately, anorexia is a common symptom of hepatitis. Measures to manage anorexia include small, frequent meals; a pleasant eating environment; frequent oral hygiene; and explanations of the need for a balanced diet. Occasionally, a feeding tube is inserted to increase nutritional intake.

Nausea and vomiting also can contribute to nutritional deficits and fluid and electrolyte imbalances. Best results are usually obtained by administering antiemetics as soon as nausea is reported. A cool, damp cloth to the face and neck is sometimes helpful. When the patient vomits, the nurse should note the amount and contents of vomited material (emesis) as well as any visible or occult blood. Emesis is measured and recorded as output. Soiled clothing, linens, and basins should be removed from sight promptly and handled according to agency infection-control guidelines. Nursing management of nausea and vomiting is discussed in greater detail in Chapter 34.

FLUID VOLUME DEFICIT. The patient with hepatitis needs to maintain fluid intake of 3000 ml per day unless contraindicated. Intake and output records are maintained. The nurse should be alert for signs of fluid retention, such as edema, increasing abdominal girth, and rising blood pressure. If the patient's fluid intake is low or vomiting is present, the nurse should also monitor for dehydration. Signs of dehydration include dry mucous membranes, tachycardia, concentrated urine, and confusion. Patients who are at risk for dehydration may receive intravenous fluids as prescribed.

IMPAIRED SKIN INTEGRITY. Pruritus, or itching, is an annoying symptom. Patients naturally respond by scratching and may cause breaks in the skin. Nursing measures are designed to reduce dryess and irritation. The skin is bathed in cool water and then patted dry. Mild soap may be used unless it seems to increase symptoms. Lubricating lotions or topical antipruritics may be applied. Older, soft sheets should be selected. If a patient is confused, the fingernails should be trimmed. Mittens may be needed to prevent excessive scratching. If conservative measures are not effective, the physician should be consulted about ordering an antihistamine.

BODY IMAGE DISTURBANCE. The patient may be self-conscious about his or her appearance because of jaundice. The nurse can help by demonstrating acceptance of the patient and explaining that the skin color usually returns to normal in 2 to 4 weeks.

ANXIETY. Hospitalization and diagnostic tests and procedures can provoke anxiety in the hepatitis patient. The patient may also be fearful about the expected course of the disease and the risk of complications. The nurse encourages questions and finds out what the patient wants to know. Explanations about what to expect reduce the fear of the unknown. The nurse can also explore how patients usually deal with stress and help them to identify coping strategies.

KNOWLEDGE DEFICIT. The patient with hepatitis needs to know how to avoid exposing others to the virus. Precautions vary with the type of hepatitis. People who have had close contact with the patient should be vaccinated with immune globulin to boost temporarily the body's natural resistance to infection. People who live with the hepatitis patient should not share personal items or utensils. Patients should exercise good hand washing after toileting. When the patient has hepatitis B, others should avoid sexual contact with the patient or exposure to the patient's blood. Table 35–3 summarizes precautions to be used to prevent the transmission of hepatitis.

STAFF PROTECTION. When patients are hospitalized, universal precautions are implemented. Nurses are at risk for exposure to hepatitis because they often handle body fluids. The Centers for Disease Control and Prevention estimate that 15 to 25% of all health care providers contract hepatitis B. For that reason, vaccination for hepatitis B is required by the Occupational Safety and Health Administration for nurses and other health care providers. The vaccine is given in a series of three injections and confers long-term immunity on most people.

Evaluation

Criteria for evaluating goal achievement are patient's statement of less fatigue and absence of signs of complications of immobility (skin intact, breath sounds clear, no calf tenderness), stable body weight, fluid output equal to intake with normal vital signs and tissue turgor, patient's acknowledgment that jaundice is temporary, patient's statement of decreased anxiety and calm demeanor, and patient's description of correct preventive practices and self-care.

CIRRHOSIS

Pathophysiology

Cirrhosis is a chronic, progressive disease of the liver. It is characterized by degeneration and destruction of liver cells. Fibrotic bands of connective tissue impair the flow of blood and lymph and distort the normal liver structure.

As cirrhosis progresses, there is significant disruption of many physiologic processes. The effects of liver disease include metabolic disturbances, blood abnormalities, fluid and electrolyte imbalances, decreased resistance to infection, accumulation of drugs and toxins, and obstruction of blood vessels and bile ducts in the liver.

Incidence

The highest incidence of cirrhosis is in people between the ages of 40 and 60. It is the fifth leading cause of death in people in that age range in the United States. It is more common in men than in women and is often, but not always, related to excessive alcohol intake.

Types of Cirrhosis

There are four types of cirrhosis, classified on the basis of cause: Laënnec's, postnecrotic, biliary, and cardiac cirrhosis.

LAËNNEC'S CIRRHOSIS. Laënnec's cirrhosis is caused by nutritional deficiencies or exposure to alcohol or other toxins. The liver enlarges, becomes "knobby," and then shrinks. The process can be reversed if the underlying problem is corrected early enough.

POSTNECROTIC CIRRHOSIS. Postnecrotic cirrhosis can be a complication of hepatitis in which there is massive liver cell necrosis.

BILIARY CIRRHOSIS. Biliary cirrhosis is also called obstructive or idiopathic cirrhosis. As the name suggests, it develops as a result of obstruction to bile flow.

CARDIAC CIRRHOSIS. Cardiac cirrhosis follows severe right-sided heart failure. Venous congestion and hypoxia lead to necrosis of liver cells.

Signs and Symptoms

In the early stage, signs and symptoms of cirrhosis are usually subtle. The patient may report slight weight loss, unexplained fever, fatigue, and dull heaviness in the right upper abdomen. These symptoms are probably due to inflammation and enlargement of the liver. The liver may be palpable below the right rib margin.

As the disease progresses, impaired metabolism of carbohydrates, fats, and protein causes gastrointestinal disturbances such as anorexia, nausea, vomiting, diarrhea or constipation, flatulence, and dyspepsia (heartburn). Resistance to blood flow from the intestines to the liver causes circulation to become congested in the intestines, stomach, and esophagus. Elevated pressure in veins in the gastrointestinal tract causes them to dilate and bulge. Dilated veins in the esophagus are called esophageal varices, and those in the rectum are hemorrhoids. Prominent veins may be visible on the abdomen.

Hematologic disorders seen with cirrhosis include anemia, leukocytopenia, thrombocytopenia, and prothrombin deficiency. As a result, patients tend to be easily tired and are more susceptible to infections. They bruise easily and may bleed excessively from minor trauma. Epistaxis (nosebleed) is common.

Later signs and symptoms of cirrhosis reflect the liver's inability to perform normal functions. Jaundice develops owing to elevated serum bilirubin. Two factors contribute to jaundice in the patient with cirrhosis. First, diseased liver cells may be unable to conjugate and excrete bilirubin. Second, structural changes in the liver prevent the normal flow of bile out of the liver. Another effect of impaired bilirubin excretion is the deposition of bile salts under the skin that can cause intense pruritus.

The diseased liver is unable to metabolize estrogen, testosterone, aldosterone, and adrenocortical hormones. The patient, therefore, exhibits signs and symptoms of hormone excesses. Testicular atrophy, impotence, and gynecomastia (breast enlargement) may be noted in males, and amenorrhea in females. Redness of the palms of the hands, called palmar erythema, and spider angiomas also are attributed to hormone excess. Excess aldosterone contributes to sodium and water retention. The failing liver is also unable to metabolize ammonia, a product of protein metabolism. Excess ammonia affects the central nervous system, leading to confusion and decreasing consciousness.

Cirrhosis impairs the liver's ability to manufacture albumin. Albumin plays a critical role in creating the colloid osmotic pressure that retains water in the vascular compartment. With low serum albumin, water leaks from the capillaries, causing decreased blood volume and edema. Ascites is the accumulation of fluid in the peritoneal cavity.

Peripheral neuropathy, characterized by tingling or numbness in the extremities, is common with cirrhosis. This is thought to be caused by dietary deficiencies of vitamin B_{12}, thiamine, and folic acid.

Figure 35–5 illustrates the clinical picture of the cirrhosis patient.

Complications

The patient with cirrhosis is at risk for many complications, including portal hypertension, esophageal varices, ascites, hepatic encephalopathy, and hepatorenal syndrome.

PORTAL HYPERTENSION. The portal vein delivers blood from the intestines to the liver. Changes in the liver with cirrhosis obstruct the flow of incoming blood, causing blood to back up in the portal system. High portal pressure, portal hypertension, causes collateral vessels to develop. Collateral vessels commonly form in the esophagus, the anterior abdominal wall, and the rectum.

ESOPHAGEAL VARICES. Distended, engorged vessels in the esophagus are called esophageal varices. They are fragile and bleed easily, with the potential for fatal hemorrhage. Circumstances that may trigger bleeding include irritation and increased intra-abdominal pressure. Sources of irritation are alcohol, coarse foods, and stomach acid. Intra-abdominal pressure is increased by vomiting, coughing, heavy lifting, and straining at stool.

ASCITES. Ascites is an accumulation of fluid in the peritoneal cavity. Factors that contribute to the development of ascites with cirrhosis include portal hypertension, leaking of lymph fluid and albumin-rich fluid from the diseased liver, low serum albumin, increased aldosterone, and water retention.

HEPATIC ENCEPHALOPATHY. The failing liver is unable to detoxify ammonia, a breakdown product of protein metabolism. Excessive ammonia in the blood causes neurologic symptoms, including cognitive disturbances, declining level of consciousness, and changes in neuromuscular function. If the condition is not reversed, the patient lapses into unconsciousness, referred to as hepatic coma.

Factors that may precipitate hepatic encephalopathy are infection, fluid and potassium depletion, gastrointestinal bleeding, constipation, and some drugs.

HEPATORENAL SYNDROME. Hepatorenal syndrome is renal failure in the cirrhosis patient that often follows diuretic therapy, paracentesis, or gastrointestinal hemorrhage. The kidney structure appears unchanged, so the reason for failure is not known.

Medical Diagnosis

When the patient's history and physical examination suggest cirrhosis, tests and procedures may be ordered to confirm or rule out the disease. These include blood tests, liver biopsy, liver scan, ultrasonography, CT scan, and magnetic resonance imaging. Results of blood tests that are consistent with cirrhosis include elevated serum and urine bilirubin, elevated serum enzymes, decreased total serum protein, decreased cholesterol, and prolonged prothrombin time. The complete blood count may reveal deficiencies of red and white blood cells and platelets.

The liver biopsy is performed to obtain a tissue specimen for microscopic study. Typical cellular changes occur with cirrhosis. Scans and imaging procedures outline the liver features. The liver is enlarged in the early stage of cirrhosis, but later it becomes smaller and knobby.

Table 35–2 summarizes tests and procedures used to diagnose liver disorders.

Medical Treatment

The goals of medical treatment for cirrhosis are to limit deterioration of liver function and to prevent complications, but there is no specific medical treatment. The approach is to promote rest so that the liver can regenerate. The earlier the condition is diagnosed and measures are taken to promote healing, the better the chance of recovery.

Bedrest is usually ordered if the patient is in liver failure. A diet high in carbohydrates and vitamins with moderate to high protein is typically ordered unless the patient's blood ammonia level is elevated. In that case, protein is restricted until the ammonia level falls. Supplementary iron and vitamins (B complex, K, and C) also may be ordered. The amount of fat allowed in the diet varies with the patient's condition. Anorexia is frequently a problem with cirrhosis, so small semisolid or liquid meals may be better received.

Other medical treatments may be ordered to correct complications of cirrhosis. Intravenous fluids may be needed to correct fluid and electrolyte imbalances. Anemia may require blood transfusions. Water and sodium are likely to be restricted in patients with severe fluid retention.

ASCITES. The medical management of ascites aims to promote reabsorption and elimination of the fluid by means of salt restriction and diuretics. Salt-poor albumin may be given intravenously to help maintain blood volume and to increase urinary output. Albumin raises the serum colloid osmotic pressure, causing water to be drawn into the blood stream. (See Table 35–4 for drugs used to treat the patient with ascites.)

If ascites does not respond to conservative treatment, fluid can be removed with a needle, a procedure called paracentesis. An alternative is the placement of a peritoneal-venous shunt.

Paracentesis. Paracentesis is the removal of ascitic fluid from the peritoneal cavity. A special instrument called a trocar is inserted through the abdominal wall, and a catheter is placed to allow the fluid to drain. This procedure is indicated only when ascites interferes with the patient's breathing. It is not used frequently because it removes essential protein and electrolytes. In addition, it provides a potential portal for pathogens.

If paracentesis is done to remove ascitic fluids, the nurse needs to prepare the patient, assist and support the patient during the procedure, and provide aftercare. The physician should explain what will be done and obtain patient consent. The nurse reinforces explanations and may obtain the written consent form, depending on agency policy. The nurse obtains baseline vital signs, weight, and abdominal girth. The patient is instructed to void. The procedure is often done at the bedside with the patient in a sitting position.

During paracentesis, the nurse supports and encourages the patient, as illustrated in Figure 35–6. The physician may request vital signs during the process. Two to 3 liters of fluid is usually removed slowly. Rapid removal of ascitic fluid could result in circulatory collapse. After paracentesis, a sterile dressing is applied to the puncture site. Vital signs are taken every 15 minutes until stable, and the dressing is checked for bleeding. The fluid obtained should be measured and a specimen sent for laboratory analysis. The procedure should be documented, including the amount and color of the fluid.

Peritoneal-Venous Shunts. Peritoneal-venous shunts are implanted permanently to allow ascitic fluid to drain from the abdomen and return to the blood stream.

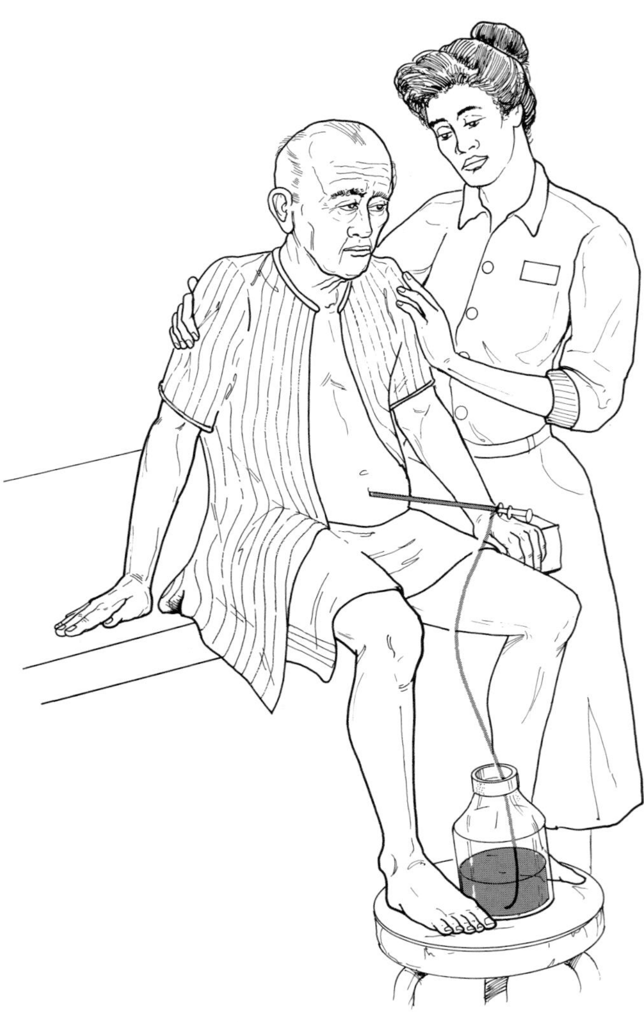

FIGURE 35-6
The nurse supports and encourages the patient during paracentesis.

The LeVeen peritoneal-venous shunt (Fig. 35–7) is a tube that is placed in the abdomen, running from the peritoneal cavity to the jugular vein or superior vena cava. The tube has a one-way valve that permits excess fluid to drain into the venous circulation when pressure rises in the abdomen. When the patient inspires, intra-abdominal pressure rises, causing the valve to open.

A second type of peritoneal-venous shunt involves a manual pump placed under the skin. It can be compressed to cause fluid to flow from the peritoneum to the venous system. The advantage to shunting ascitic fluid is that protein-rich serum is retained and returned to the vascular compartment.

Potential complications of peritoneal-venous shunts are peritonitis and tubing obstruction.

BLEEDING ESOPHAGEAL VARICES. Several techniques can be used to control bleeding esophageal varices. These include placement of an esophageal-gastric balloon tube, surgical ligation, and sclerotherapy.

Esophageal-Gastric Balloon Tube. Esophageal-gastric balloon tubes may be used to apply direct pressure to bleeding veins in the esophagus and stomach. Examples of tubes used for this purpose are the Sengstaken-Blakemore esophageal-gastric balloon tube and the Minnesota tube. The Sengstaken-Blakemore tube has three ports. One is used to inflate the esophageal balloon, another to inflate the gastric balloon, and the third to suction the stomach. The Minnesota tube is like the Sengstaken-Blakemore tube, but it has one additional port that allows suction of esophageal secretions (Fig. 35–8).

The tube is inserted by a physician. The gastric balloon is inflated first and gently pulled upward to apply pressure to veins in the upper part of the stomach. The esophageal balloon is then inflated. The gastric suction tube is connected to continuous suction. It may also be irrigated to remove clots and maintain patency of the tube. It is important to remove old blood from the stomach so that it will not be digested. Digested blood produces ammonia, which increases the likelihood of hepatic encephalopathy. Gastric suction also reduces the risk of vomiting, which would force the balloons out of place. The tube is usually left inflated for 24 to 48 hours. It is then deflated but left in place so that it can be reinflated if needed.

Surgical Treatment of Bleeding Varices. In an emergency situation, the surgeon may ligate (tie off) bleeding varices directly. The patient can then be stabilized prior to a more extensive corrective procedure. Corrective procedures surgically shunt blood from engorged varices to other veins. A portacaval shunt diverts blood to the vena cava, whereas a splenorenal shunt routes the blood to the splenic vein.

Sclerotherapy. Sclerotherapy is a procedure in which a solution is injected into the varices or into the veins that supply them, causing the varices to harden and close (Fig. 35–9). The procedure can be done through an endoscope or through a small surgical incision. Sclerotherapy can be done to prevent or to treat bleeding.

After sclerotherapy, patients often report chest discomfort for several days. The physician usually orders a mild analgesic. If it does not relieve the pain, the physician should be notified because this may indicate perforation of the esophagus. Once a patient has had sclerotherapy, extra care must be taken in the insertion of nasogastric tubes.

HEPATIC ENCEPHALOPATHY. Medical treatment of hepatic encephalopathy consists of elimination of protein intake, intravenous fluids and vitamins, and avoidance of drugs. Antibiotics that disinfect the bowel may be given to decrease ammonia production by intestinal bacteria. If the patient has been bleeding into the gastrointestinal tract, laxatives and enemas may be ordered to remove old blood and protein.

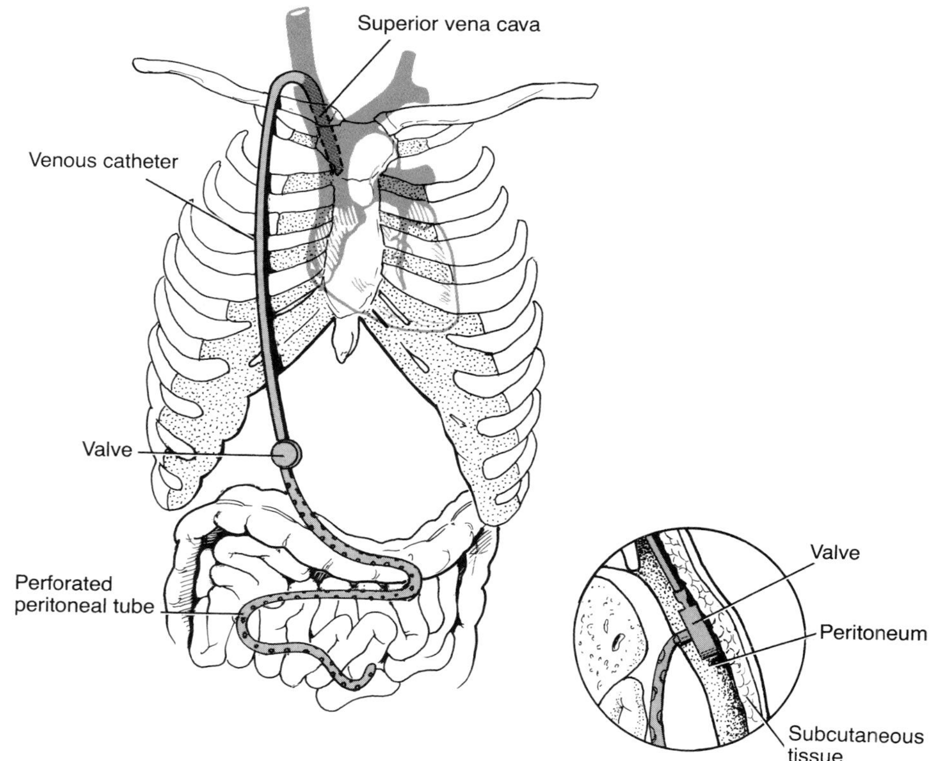

FIGURE 35-7
A peritoneal venous shunt drains ascitic fluid from the abdominal cavity into the superior vena cava.

HEPATORENAL SYNDROME. Hepatorenal syndrome is treated with salt-poor albumin, diuretics, and sodium and water restriction.

DRUG THERAPY. A variety of drugs may be used to treat the effects of cirrhosis. These drugs and nursing implications are summarized in Table 35–4.

NURSING CARE OF THE PATIENT WITH CIRRHOSIS

Assessment

Ongoing assessments of the cirrhosis patient should include daily weights, measurements of intake and out-

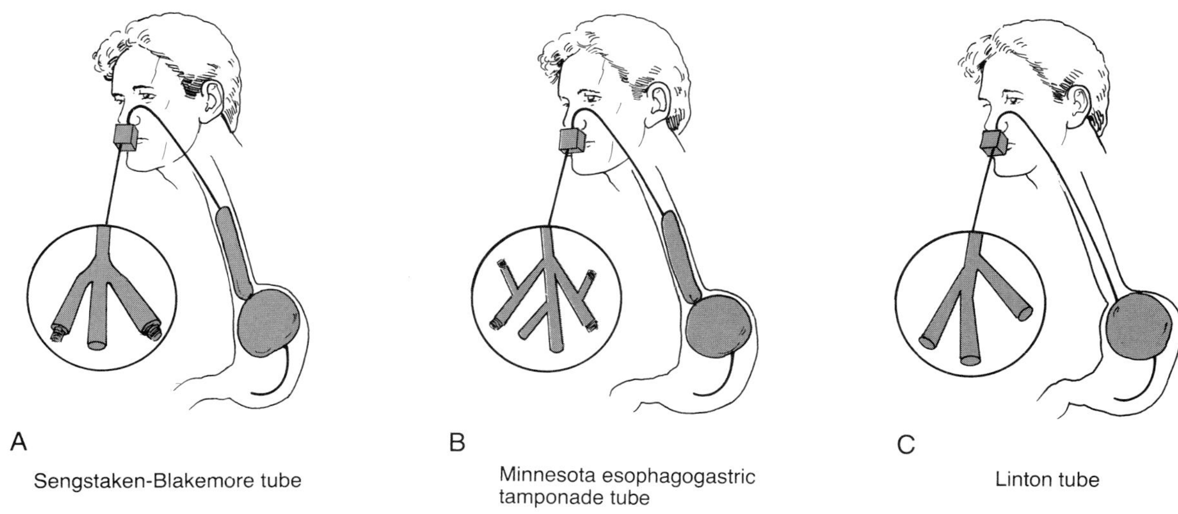

FIGURE 35-8
Esophageal tubes.

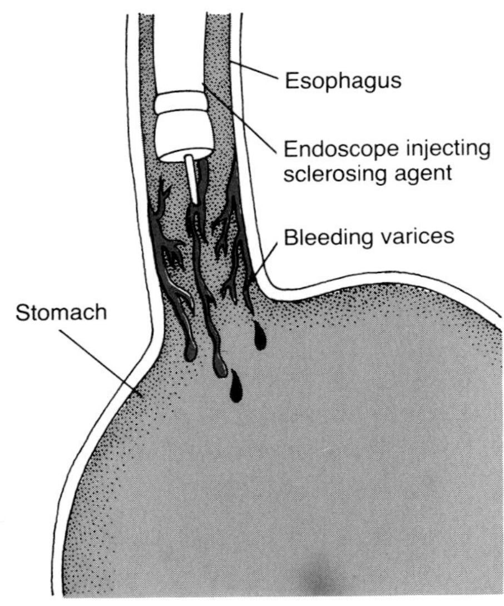

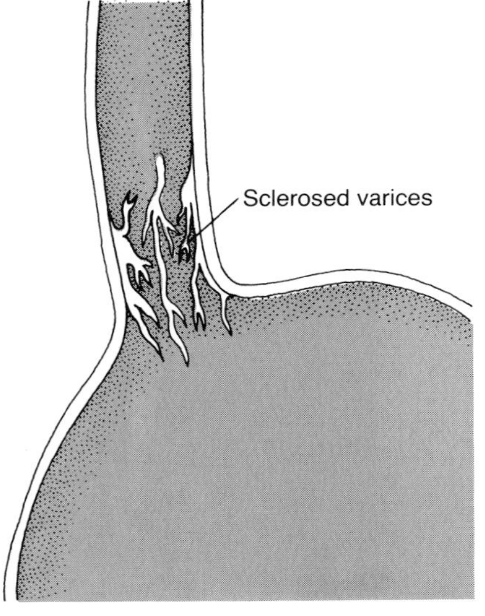

FIGURE 35-9
Injection sclerotherapy. (From Ignatavicius, D. D., & Bayne, M. V. [1991]. *Medical-surgical nursing: A nursing process approach* [p. 1493]. Philadelphia: W. B. Saunders.)

put, and abdominal girth. Special attention is given to monitoring for signs and symptoms of complications: bleeding, ascites, encephalopathy, and renal failure.

Nursing Diagnosis

Although nursing diagnoses must be based on individual assessments, the following are common with cirrhosis:

- **Altered Nutrition: Less than Body Requirements** related to anorexia, metabolic imbalances
- **Activity Intolerance** related to fatigue
- **High Risk for Impaired Skin Integrity** related to edema, immobility, pruritus, hypoproteinemia
- **Ineffective Breathing Patterns** related to ascites
- **High Risk for Injury** related to impaired coagulation
- **Altered Thought Processes** related to elevated blood ammonia
- **Fluid Volume Deficit** (hypovolemia) and **Fluid Volume Excess** (in third space) related to hypoproteinemia, increased aldosterone
- **High Risk for Infection** related to liver dysfunction, impaired response to infection, malnutrition
- **Fear** related to dyspnea, life-threatening illness
- **Knowledge Deficit** of disease, treatment, and self-care

Goals

Goals of nursing care for the cirrhosis patient are adequate nutrition, improved activity tolerance, intact skin, normal breathing, absence of bleeding, normal cognitive function, normal fluid distribution in body fluid compartments, absence of infection, reduced fear, and patient's knowledge of cirrhosis, treatment, and self-care.

Interventions

ALTERED NUTRITION. Good nutrition is essential for regeneration of liver tissue. However, it is a challenge for the cirrhosis patient, who often has anorexia, indigestion, nausea, and vomiting. Furthermore, the diet may be made less palatable by protein or salt restriction.

The nurse explains the need for adequate food intake to the patient and encourages eating even when not hungry. Small, frequent meals may be more acceptable to the anorexic patient. A dietary consult can be arranged for the patient to report likes and dislikes.

Mealtimes are made as pleasant as possible. Bedpans, emesis basins, and drainage collection devices are put out of sight. The room is ventilated to reduce odors. Tiring activities are not scheduled immediately before meals. Daily weights are usually ordered to assess both nutritional and fluid status.

ACTIVITY INTOLERANCE. Some activity limitations are usually imposed, depending on the patient's overall status. Nursing care should be scheduled to allow some periods of undisturbed rest. The patient can generally assume any position that is comfortable. The head of the bed is elevated if ascites is present to facilitate breathing. Some patients are more comfortable sitting in a chair with the feet elevated.

If the patient spends all or most of the day in bed, there is a risk of complications related to immobility. The nurse assists the patient to change positions, deep breathe, and exercise extremities regularly.

HIGH RISK FOR IMPAIRED SKIN INTEGRITY. The patient with cirrhosis is at risk for skin breakdown for the following reasons:

1. Bile salts deposited under the skin may cause intense pruritus.
2. Patients with advanced disease usually have a loss of muscle and fat tissue. This reduces the padding that normally protects the skin from pressure.

TABLE 35-4

DRUG THERAPY FOR CIRRHOSIS

GENERAL NURSING IMPLICATIONS

1. No drug can cure cirrhosis.
2. Drug therapy treats symptoms: fluid retention, portal hypertension, encephalopathy, and bleeding.
3. Patients with liver dysfunction may not metabolize drugs normally, so be alert for adverse effects.

DRUG	USE/ACTION	SIDE EFFECTS	NURSING INTERVENTIONS
Diuretics Spironolactone (Aldactone) Amiloride (Midamor) Furosemide (Lasix) Chlorothiazide (Diuril)	Promote excretion of excess fluid in edema and ascites.	Fluid and electrolyte imbalances including fluid volume deficit and hyponatremia. Hypokalemia can occur except with potassium-sparing diuretics like spironolactone.	Monitor intake and output, abdominal girth. Check laboratory values for electrolyte imbalances.
Pituitary hormone Vasopressin (Pitressin)	Reduces pressure in portal veins to treat bleeding esophageal varices.	Tissue necrosis with extravasation. Water intoxication, hyponatremia, intestinal and uterine cramping.	Inspect infusion site hourly for blanching; if present, stop infusion and notify charge nurse or physician.
Vasodilators	Given with vasopressin to decrease side effects.		Follow directions for administration carefully.
Nitroglycerin		Tachycardia, hypotension, flushing, and headache.	
Nitroprusside (Nipride)	Lowers blood pressure.	Tachycardia, hypotension, acidosis, and fluid retention.	Nitroprusside must be diluted. Monitor vital signs continuously.
Beta-adrenergic blocker Propranolol (Inderal)	Reduces pressure in portal veins to reduce risk of bleeding.	Bradycardia, bronchoconstriction. Masks signs of hypoglycemia.	Monitor pulse; if below 60, withhold and notify physician. Monitor blood sugar in diabetics.
Antibiotic Neomycin sulfate	Reduces gastrointestinal bacterial flora, decreasing ammonia production. Used to prevent or treat hepatic encephalopathy.	Toxic to kidney and eighth cranial nerve (hearing and balance). Increases action of neuromuscular blocking agents like anesthetics.	Monitor intake and output. Assess for hearing impairment, tinnitus (ringing in ears), nausea, loss of balance.
Laxative Lactulose (Cephulac)	Promotes elimination of ammonia in feces. Used to prevent or treat hepatic encephalopathy.	Cramps, distention, flatulence, eructation. Hyperglycemia with diabetes.	May be ordered every hour at first. Can be mixed with fruit juice, water, or milk. Monitor diabetics.
Dopaminergic agent Levodopa	Replaces dopamine lost in process of protein breakdown. Used to prevent or treat hepatic encephalopathy.	Nausea, vomiting, orthostatic hypotension.	Teach patient to manage orthostatic hypotension. Comfort measures for nausea. Report vomiting. Give antiemetics as ordered.
Vitamins B Complex	Needed for production of red blood cells and for normal growth and development.	Allergic reaction to thiamine (anaphylaxis). Adverse effects rare.	Intradermal test dose may be ordered to detect sensitivity to thiamine. Check site for reaction: redness, swelling. Check reference for incompatibility with other intravenous drugs.
K Menadiol (vitamin K_3) Phytonadione (Aqua-MEPHYTON)	Treats serious bleeding disorders caused by deficiency of prothrombin. Used cautiously with severe liver disease.	Gastric upset (oral route only), rash, urticaria, flushing, hemolytic anemia. Pain and swelling at injection site.	Check lab results for prothrombin time. Report abnormalities. Monitor complete blood count. Assess for bleeding. Apply pressure to needle puncture sites for 5 min.

3. Many patients have edema, which makes tissue more fragile and impairs healing.

Nursing measures to relieve the itching of pruritus include gentle bathing with mild soap and warm water, thorough rinsing, and application of moisturizing lotions. The patient's nails should be kept short. If scratching persists, soft cotton mittens or gloves can be applied to reduce trauma. If itching is severe, the physician may be consulted about ordering a medication to relieve the discomfort.

INEFFECTIVE BREATHING PATTERNS. Ascitic fluid can cause the abdomen to become greatly distended. While in bed, the patient breathes easier with the head of the bed elevated. Sitting in a chair with the feet elevated, if allowed, may be even more comfortable.

HIGH RISK FOR INJURY. The patient with cirrhosis is at great risk for injury or hemorrhage due to impaired coagulation and fragile varices. The nurse should handle the patient gently to avoid trauma. A soft toothbrush or swab should be used for mouth care. Firm pressure should be applied to injection sites to minimize oozing. Siderails can be padded if the patient is restless.

If the patient has bleeding esophageal varices, an esophageal-gastric balloon tube may be inserted. The patient with this type of tube is usually in an intensive care unit since close monitoring is necessary. The tube is uncomfortable, and the patient is likely to be frightened about both the bleeding and the treatment. When the tube is in place, the patient must be monitored for signs of continued or renewed bleeding, including restlessness, increasing pulse and respirations, and falling blood pressure. Stool characteristics are noted. Bleeding from the esophagus or stomach usually produces a sticky (tarry) maroon to black stool. The aspirated stomach and esophageal contents also should be examined for evidence of fresh bleeding. Old blood in the stomach is usually brownish and may be described as resembling coffee grounds. Fresh blood is bright to dark red.

Since the esophagus and the trachea are adjacent to each other, upward movement of the esophageal balloon can cause airway obstruction. Therefore, when the balloon tube is in place, the patient must be monitored for sudden respiratory distress. Should this occur, both balloon ports must be promptly cut and the tubes removed by a properly trained person.

ALTERED THOUGHT PROCESSES. Cognitive changes in the cirrhosis patient are usually due to hepatic encephalopathy. Nursing care of the patient with hepatic encephalopathy includes monitoring of mental and neurologic status. The physician should be informed of changes in status. The patient who is confused or unconscious requires close attention to prevent injury or complications of immobility. The nurse talks to the patient to provide basic information and reassurance. The family may also need an explanation of the patient's behavior. Dietary protein restrictions are enforced, and drugs that decrease bacteria in the intestines such as neomycin and lactulose are given as ordered. The nurse is alert for adverse effects of drug therapy, which may include diarrhea, vitamin K deficiency, and ototoxicity.

FLUID VOLUME DEFICIT AND EXCESS. Fluid needs vary with the patient's condition. Sodium and water are likely to be restricted if there is marked edema or ascites. Despite the excess in total body water, the patient's blood volume may be dangerously low. Without adequate albumin in the serum, colloid osmotic pressure falls and water shifts out of the capillaries into the tissues. Intravenous fluids and salt-poor albumin are administered as ordered. In addition to monitoring vital signs, the nurse needs to evaluate fluid intake and output.

HIGH RISK FOR INFECTION. The cirrhosis patient is at risk for infection for several reasons. The liver is no longer able to filter bacteria from the blood as it comes from the intestines. The function of the spleen also is impaired, which lowers resistance to infection. In addition, these patients tend to be malnourished, so they lack the building materials for tissue repair. The nurse monitors for fever and malaise that suggest infection. The patient is protected from others with infections. Caregivers practice good hand washing and use aseptic technique for invasive procedures.

FEAR. Patients with cirrhosis can experience frightening complications, including confusion, dyspnea, and hemorrhage. With advanced cirrhosis, the prognosis is poor and patients often have repeated emergency admissions. Treatments and diagnostic procedures may be painful and anxiety producing. The nurse can help by recognizing the patient's fear and acknowledging it.

To provide emotional support to cirrhosis patients, nurses need to be aware of their personal reactions to these patients. There is a stigma attached to cirrhosis because of its association with alcohol abuse. Nurses must treat patients in a nonjudgmental manner.

KNOWLEDGE DEFICIT. When the patient is acutely ill, simple explanations are given and questions answered. When the patient improves, the nurse explores what he or she knows about cirrhosis and determines what additional information is needed. Aspects of the disease to be covered include pathology (simple explanations), purposes of medical treatment, diet and drug therapy, signs and symptoms that should be reported to the physician, and management of symptoms. If the patient's history includes alcohol abuse, the nurse may need to explain the effects of alcohol on the disease. Information about community resources for assistance with alcoholism should be provided. Nurses must realize that alcoholism is a complex chronic disease that is not easily controlled. For the severely debilitated person, home nursing services may be recommended.

PHARMACOLOGY CAPSULE

Many drugs, including acetaminophen, can be toxic to the liver.

Evaluation

Criteria for successful nursing interventions include stable weight; ability to perform activities without excessive fatigue; intact skin, no scratching; respiratory rate of 12 to 20 without dyspnea; absence of blood in emesis or stool, vital signs consistent with patient's normal values; absence of injury when confused, mentally alert and oriented; balanced fluid intake and output without edema or ascites; temperature less than 100°F; expressed lessening of fear; and verbalization of correct self-care measures and support resources.

CANCER OF THE LIVER

Cancer rarely begins in the liver, but it is a frequent site of metastasis. Cirrhosis is a predisposing factor for liver cancer. Signs and symptoms of liver cancer include liver enlargement, weight loss, anorexia, nausea, vomiting, and dull pain in the upper right quadrant of the abdomen. As the disease progresses, the signs and symptoms are essentially the same as those of cirrhosis. Since early signs and symptoms of liver cancer are vague, the condition is often not diagnosed until it is advanced.

Tests and procedures used to diagnose liver cancer are liver scan and biopsy, hepatic arteriography, endoscopy, and measurement of alpha-fetoprotein. If cancer is confined to one area, a lobectomy may be done. Otherwise, chemotherapy is the primary treatment. It is generally considered to be palliative, meaning that it may slow the progress of the cancer and increase patient comfort but is unlikely to be curative.

During the course of the illness, the patient's needs are much like those of the cirrhosis patient, which are covered earlier in this chapter. Additional aspects of nursing care of the patient with cancer are discussed in Chapter 23.

LIVER TRANSPLANTATION

The only possible cure for end-stage liver disease is liver transplantation. It is also appropriate in cancer that is confined to the liver and for certain congenital disorders.

Patients who are recommended for transplantation are ranked by acuity and need and entered into a national computer network. When a liver becomes available by donation, the best recipient can be identified. Patients awaiting transplant must be on standby status in case a donor is located. This is a time of alternating hope and fear for patients and families, marked by the recognition that they are waiting for someone else to die.

Following liver transplantation, the patient is cared for in a specialized unit. A transplant patient often has a T tube, wound drainage devices, a nasogastric tube, and a central line for total parenteral nutrition (TPN). Mechanical ventilation also is used initially.

Nursing assessments focus on neurologic status, vital signs, central venous pressure, respiratory status, and indicators of bleeding. If stable, the patient is moved out of the unit after 3 or 4 days. The nurse continues to monitor vital signs, intake and output, and neurologic status. Usual postoperative care, including turning, coughing and deep breathing, and progressive activity, are instituted.

Drugs must be given to prevent rejection of the donor liver. Cyclosporine is the most commonly used antirejection drug. Since it is toxic to the kidneys, the patient may be given diuretics and dopamine to support kidney function.

The transplant patient must be monitored for signs of rejection. These include fever, anorexia, depression, vague abdominal pain, muscle aches, and joint pain. Rejection may be treated with corticosteroids or other immunosuppressants. If this treatment is unsuccessful, retransplantation may be needed.

Prior to discharge, the patient should be taught signs and symptoms of rejection and infection, wound care, dietary restrictions (usually sodium restriction), and self-medication.

THE BILIARY TRACT

ANATOMY AND PHYSIOLOGY OF THE BILIARY TRACT

Bile is a yellow-green liquid that has several impor tant functions. It contains bile salts that are essential for the emulsification and digestion of fats. It also provides a medium for the excretion of bilirubin from the liver.

The biliary tract is made up of the gallbladder and the bile ducts. The function of the biliary tract is to deliver bile from the liver to the duodenum. Bile is produced in the liver and channeled into the common hepatic duct. The common hepatic duct joins the cystic duct to form the common bile duct. The cystic duct leads to the gallbladder, a sac-like organ located beneath the liver. Bile flows from the liver to the gallbladder, where it is stored and concentrated (Fig. 35–10).

When fats enter the duodenum, the gallbladder contracts and delivers bile to the intestine through the common bile duct.

NURSING ASSESSMENT OF THE BILIARY TRACT

The nursing assessment of the gastrointestinal system is outlined in Table 34–2 in the previous chapter. When

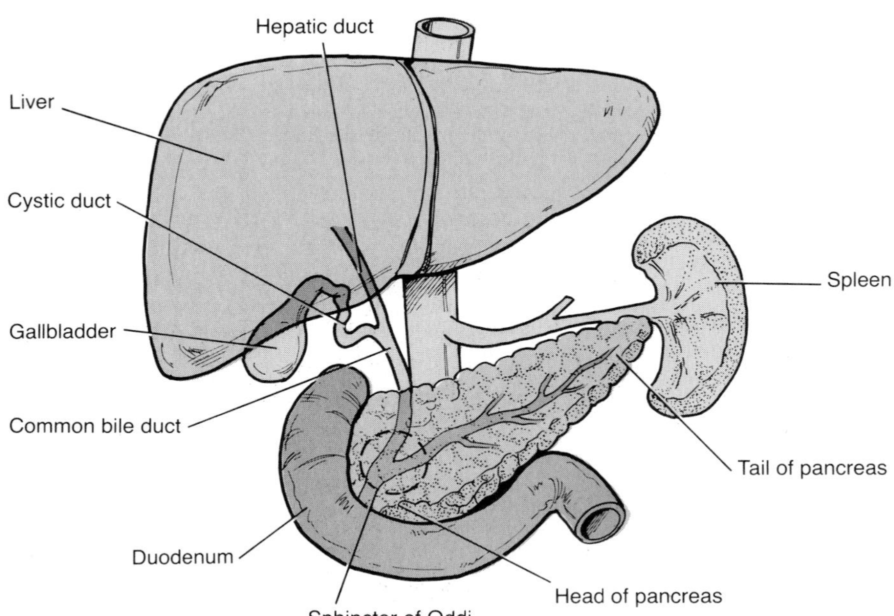

FIGURE 35-10
Anatomy of the liver, gallbladder, and pancreas.

a patient has known or suspected gallbladder dysfunction, specific data that are especially important are identified here.

HEALTH HISTORY

Common reasons for seeking medical care for biliary problems are digestive disturbances and pain. The nurse elicits a complete description of these symptoms. Factors that seem to bring on or relieve the symptoms are noted. The relationship between symptoms and meals may be significant. The use of estrogen or oral contraceptives is recorded. The nurse also inquires about factors known to be associated with gallbladder disease: family history, obesity, Native American ancestry, and inactivity. In the review of systems, the nurse asks whether the patient has had dry skin, indigestion, fat intolerance, dyspepsia, nausea, vomiting, light-colored stools, or dark urine.

PHYSICAL EXAMINATION

When a patient has gallbladder disease, significant findings in the physical examination include dry skin, fever, jaundice, tachycardia, tachypnea, and abdominal guarding and distention. Assessment of the patient with a biliary tract disorder is summarized in Table 35–5.

DIAGNOSTIC TESTS AND PROCEDURES

Tests and procedures used to diagnose gallbladder disorders are ultrasonography, oral cholecystography, intravenous cholangiography, endoscopic retrograde cholangiopancreatography (ERCP), and percutaneous transhepatic cholangiography. Laboratory studies include liver function tests, serum and urine bilirubin, and a complete blood count. Table 35–2 describes common diagnostic tests and nursing implications.

DISORDERS OF THE GALLBLADDER

Gallbladder disease is one of the most common health problems in the United States. Risk factors for gallbladder disease include obesity, familial tendency, sedentary lifestyle, and use of estrogen or oral contraceptives. Women are at greater risk than men, especially women who have had multiple pregnancies. Whites and Native Americans also are at increased risk.

The two most common gallbladder disorders are cholecystitis and cholelithiasis. Carcinoma of the gallbladder occurs but is unusual.

TABLE 35-5
ASSESSMENT OF THE PATIENT WITH GALLBLADDER DISEASE

HEALTH HISTORY

Present illness: Digestive disturbances, pain: location, onset, intensity, duration, relationship to meals, aggravating and relieving factors
Past medical history: Gallbladder disease, pregnancy, surgery, recent and current medications
Family history: Gallbladder disease
Review of systems: Pruritus, indigestion, fat intolerance, dyspepsia, nausea, vomiting, light-colored stools, dark urine

PHYSICAL EXAMINATION

Vital signs: Tachycardia, tachypnea, fever
Skin: Dryness, jaundice
Abdomen: Guarding, distention

CHOLECYSTITIS AND CHOLELITHIASIS

Cholecystitis is inflammation of the gallbladder. It is most often caused by the presence of gallstones but can be due to bacteria, toxic chemicals, tumors, anesthesia, starvation, and narcotics. The inflamed gallbladder and cystic duct become swollen and congested with blood. The cystic duct may actually become occluded.

When gallstones are present, the patient is said to have cholelithiasis. Most gallstones are composed of cholesterol mixed with bile salts, bilirubin, calcium, and protein. It is not known exactly why gallstones form, but the process is associated with high concentrations of cholesterol. The concentration of cholesterol rises when there is stasis of bile (as occurs with pregnancy, immobility, and inflammation of the biliary tract).

Gallstones may be found anywhere in the biliary tract: the gallbladder, the cystic duct, or the common bile duct (Fig. 35–11). The stones may move through the biliary tract with bile flow. If a stone cannot pass through the tract, it lodges and causes an obstruction. Ducts respond to obstruction with spasms in an effort to move the stone. This is responsible for an intense spasmodic pain, called biliary colic.

If the cystic duct is obstructed, bile cannot leave the gallbladder and inflammation develops. Cystic duct obstruction does not prevent the flow of bile into the duodenum from the liver. If the common bile duct is obstructed (choledocholithiasis), bile is unable to flow into the duodenum.

Signs and Symptoms

Signs and symptoms of cholecystitis vary from one patient to the next. Some have only mild indigestion, whereas others have severe pain, fever, and jaundice. Other symptoms are nausea, eructation, fever, chills, and right upper quadrant pain that radiates to the shoulder. Symptoms typically occur about 3 hours after a meal, especially if the food had high fat content.

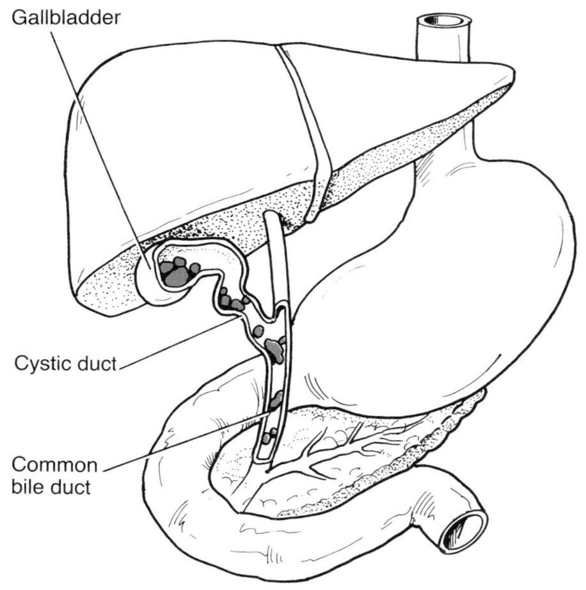

FIGURE 35–11
Gallstones within the gallbladder that are obstructing the common bile duct and the cystic duct.

With obstruction to bile flow, bile production in the liver decreases and the serum bilirubin rises, leading to obstructive jaundice. Some excess bilirubin is excreted in the urine, creating a dark, amber color. Digestion of fats is impaired, causing intolerance of fatty foods and steatorrhea (excess fat in feces). The absence of urobilinogen in the stool causes it to be a characteristic clay color. The patient is unable to absorb fat-soluble vitamins and may show signs of vitamin deficiencies. Vitamin K deficiency interferes with normal blood clotting, and thus the patient bleeds and bruises easily.

Complications

The most serious complications of cholecystitis and cholelithiasis are pancreatitis, abscesses, cholangitis (inflammation of the biliary ducts), and rupture of the gallbladder.

Medical Diagnosis

A tentative diagnosis of cholelithiasis based on the history and physical is usually easily confirmed with ultrasonography. This noninvasive study uses sound waves to create an image of the gallbladder and to reveal the presence of stones. Intravenous cholangiography or percutaneous transhepatic cholangiography uses dye to outline the biliary tract and locate stones.

Blood and urine studies provide additional information. With inflammation or infection, the white blood cell count is elevated. If bile flow is obstructed, serum and urinary bilirubin and serum enzymes may be elevated. Nursing considerations with specific diagnostic tests and procedures are summarized in Table 35–2.

Medical Treatment

Acute cholecystitis is managed symptomatically. Analgesics and anticholinergics are ordered to relieve pain and smooth muscle spasm. Antibiotics are given to treat infection. Intravenous fluids are selected to maintain fluid balance, especially if the patient has been vomiting. A nasogastric tube may be inserted and attached to suction. This relieves nausea and vomiting and reduces the stimulation of the gallbladder by intestinal contents.

Among the options available for the treatment of cholelithiasis are drug therapy, shock-wave lithotripsy, endoscopic sphincterotomy, and cholecystectomy.

DRUG THERAPY. Two types of drugs are used to dissolve gallstones: oral bile salts and dissolution agents. Oral bile salts include chenodeoxycholic acid (Chenix) and ursodeoxycholic acid (UDCA; Actigall). They may be prescribed when the patient has small cholesterol stones. The main side effects of these drugs are diarrhea, cramps, and elevated serum enzymes. Side effects are milder with UDCA, but it is very expensive. Dissolution of stones with these agents can take from 6 months to 2 years, and the treatment is successful in only about one third of those treated.

Methyl-tert butyl ether (MTBE) and monooctanoin (Moctanin) are dissolution agents. The agent MTBE is instilled in the gallbladder through a transhepatic catheter. The physician instills and aspirates the drug repeatedly until fluoroscopy shows that the stones either have dissolved or are not responding to the treatment.

Monooctanoin is used to treat larger stones in the common bile duct. It is given through a nasal-biliary catheter per continuous infusion for 1 to 3 weeks. The patient is allowed to have a bland diet, and the infusion is stopped during meals. Side effects include anorexia, nausea, vomiting, diarrhea, and abdominal pain. Slowing the infusion rate may decrease side effects. Antiemetics and antidiarrheals can be given as ordered. Cholangiograms are obtained periodically to assess the effects of the drug. It is effective about half the time.

Drugs used to treat conditions of the biliary tract are described in Table 35–6.

EXTRACORPOREAL SHOCK-WAVE LITHOTRIPSY. This procedure, ESWL, is appropriate for patients with few stones and mild to moderate symptoms. Prior to ESWL, the physician uses ultrasonography or contrast dye to locate the stones. Contrast dye can be given through a nasal-biliary catheter or through a percutaneous transhepatic catheter.

For ESWL, the patient sits in a tank of water or lies on a table with a water-filled cushion positioned next to the treatment area. The lithotriptor delivers a series of shock waves through the water or through the cushion, causing the stones to break up. The shocks are coordinated with the patient's heartbeat to prevent triggering arrhythmias. A typical treatment consists of 1500 shocks. The sensation feels like a fluttering or light slap. It should not be painful, but analgesics or sedatives may be given if the patient reports pain or is excessively anxious. At the completion of the treatment, the physician may give a dissolution agent if the patient has a biliary catheter.

After the treatment, the patient is observed for hematuria, fever (suggestive of pancreatitis), and cardiac dysrhythmias. A low-fat diet is advised initially. Biliary colic may occur as stone fragments move through the biliary system. This moderate to severe right upper quadrant pain is treated with narcotics or antispasmodics as needed. The physician may prescribe oral bile acids for several months. Follow-up ultrasonography is done at specific intervals to evaluate the effects of the treatment. Remaining fragments can sometimes be removed through endoscopy. Lithotripsy can be repeated if necessary.

ENDOSCOPIC SPHINCTEROTOMY. Endoscopic sphincterotomy involves the use of endoscopic instruments to incise the sphincter of Oddi and extract stones from the common bile duct, as illustrated in Figure 35–12. The patient is given a sedative but remains conscious during the procedure. Lidocaine spray is used to deaden the gag reflex so that the endoscope can be passed through the mouth. A choledochoscope also can

TABLE 35–6
DRUG THERAPY FOR CHOLELITHIASIS

GENERAL NURSING IMPLICATIONS

1. Drugs are effective only against small cholesterol stones.
2. Drug therapy is successful in only about one third to one half of patients treated.

DRUG	SIDE EFFECTS	NURSING INTERVENTIONS
Oral bile salts		
Chenodeoxycholic acid (Chenix) Ursodeoxycholic acid (UDCA; Actigall)	Diarrhea, cramps, nausea, vomiting, elevated serum enzymes, low-density lipoproteins, and cholesterol. UDCA has milder side effects but is very expensive. Contraindications: biliary tract infection, pancreatitis, pregnancy.	Advise patients not to become pregnant while on this drug. Stress importance of periodic blood tests of liver enzymes and serum cholesterol.
Dissolution agents		
Methyl-tert butyl ether (MTBE)	Abdominal pain and nausea during treatment.	Oral contrast dye given previous evening. Position patient on right side afterward to reduce bleeding. Monitor for hemorrhage, shock, and pneumothorax. Vital signs every 15 min until stable then every 4 hr times 3. Bedrest for 24 hr.
Monooctanoin (Moctanin)	Anorexia, nausea, vomiting, diarrhea, abdominal pain. Rarely, acute pancreatitis.	Give antiemetics and antidiarrheals PRN, as ordered. With physician's approval, stop infusion for meals. Keep nasal biliary tube securely anchored. Slowing the rate of infusion may control gastrointestinal distress.

PRN, As needed.

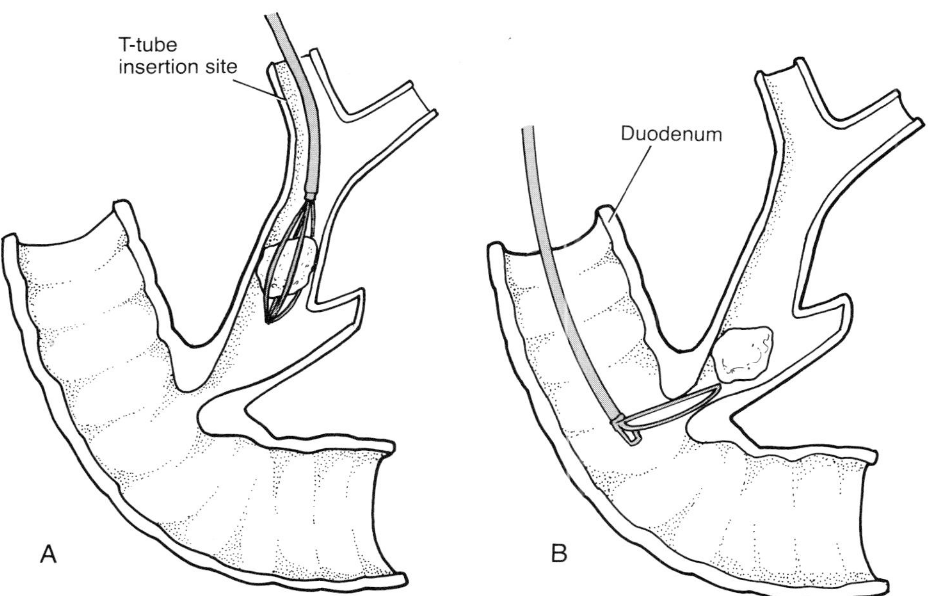

FIGURE 35-12
Choledoscopic removal of gallstones.

be inserted through a T tube into the common bile duct. A special basket is used to extract the stones.

After endoscopic sphincterotomy, the patient is usually kept on bedrest for 6 to 8 hours. Nothing is given by mouth until the gag reflex returns. The patient is monitored for signs of complications. Bloody stools and tachycardia may indicate hemorrhage secondary to trauma. Fever and abdominal pain may indicate pancreatitis or perforation of the duodenum.

CHOLECYSTECTOMY. Cholecystectomy is the most frequently used treatment for cholelithiasis. In the classic procedure, an incision is made below the right rib margin. The gallbladder is removed, and the common bile duct is explored for stones. Exploration of the bile duct may cause it to swell and obstruct bile flow from the liver. A T tube may be placed in the common bile duct to maintain bile flow until swelling in the duct subsides (Fig. 35–13). One part of the tubing is brought through the patient's skin and connected to a closed gravity drainage receptacle.

When the patient first returns from surgery, the drainage from the T tube may be bloody, but it should soon become greenish brown. Drainage should gradually decrease as edema subsides in the common bile duct. The amount of drainage is measured, and the physician is notified if it exceeds 1000 ml in 24 hours.

The patient is placed in low Fowler's position with the tube arranged to drain freely. The nurse protects the tube during movement to prevent dislodging it. The physician specifies the level of the drainage bag and when it should be clamped. Orders may call for the tube to be clamped for 1 to 2 hours before meals so that bile is available for digestion. The tube is clamped for increasingly longer periods of time. If the patient experiences pain, fever, chills, nausea, or distention, the tube should be unclamped. The physician removes the T tube when the patient tolerates clamping for a prolonged period of time.

If the patient is discharged with the T tube in place, the patient must be taught how to care for the tube, including emptying it, caring for the insertion site, and recognizing when to clamp and unclamp it.

A newer surgical procedure is a laparoscopic cholecystectomy. The surgeon inserts a laparoscope with a camera through a small abdominal incision. Using the camera, the surgeon guides forceps and a laser toward the gallbladder through other small abdominal incisions. The gallbladder is grasped with the forceps, cut free with the laser, and pulled out through one of the small incisions. Complications are rare, and patients usually resume regular activities in 2 or 3 days.

NURSING CARE OF THE PATIENT WITH A GALLBLADDER DISORDER

Assessment

General assessment of patients with problems of the biliary tract is outlined in Table 35–5.

Nursing Diagnosis

Nursing diagnoses for the patient with cholecystitis and cholelithiasis may include the following:

- **Pain** related to biliary colic
- **Fluid Volume Deficit** related to vomiting, inadequate intake
- **Impaired Skin Integrity** related to pruritus
- **Anxiety** related to disease, anticipation of invasive procedures
- **High Risk for Injury** (bleeding) related to vitamin K deficiency
- **Knowledge Deficit** of disease, diet, and drug therapy

Goals

The nursing goals for the patient with cholecystitis and cholelithiasis include reduced pain, adequate hydra-

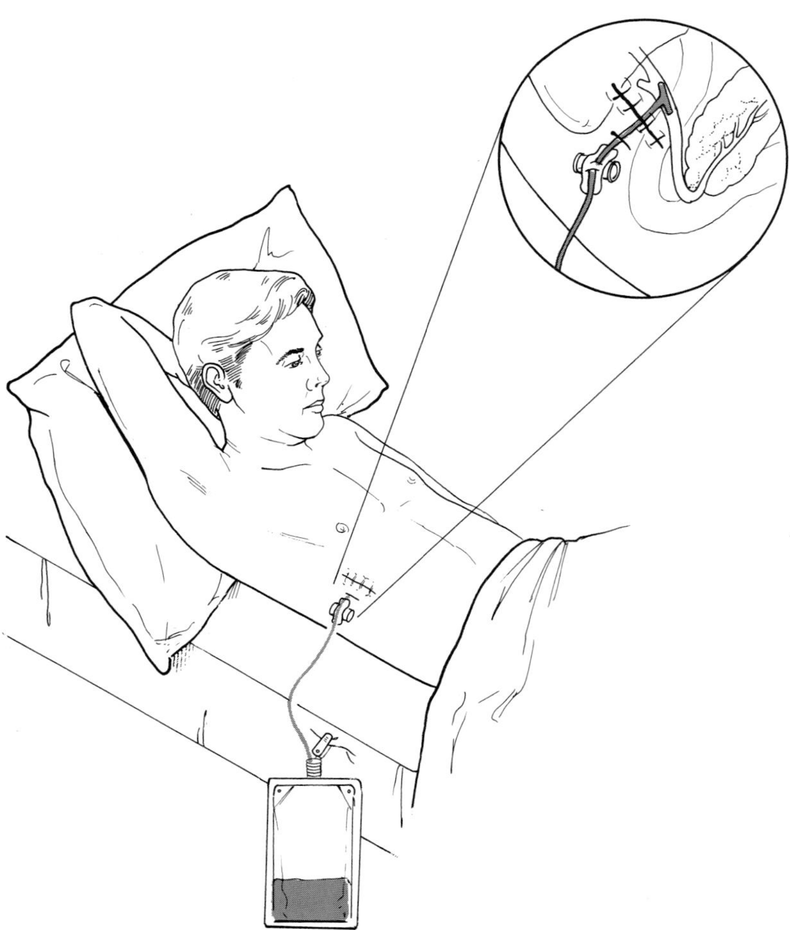

FIGURE 35-13
A T-tube in the common bile duct.

tion, intact skin, reduced anxiety, absence of bleeding, and patient's knowledge of the disease, diet, and treatment.

Interventions for Cholecystitis

PAIN. The degree of pain with cholecystitis varies, but many patients experience severe pain. Narcotic analgesics and anticholinergics are usually ordered. The nurse assesses comfort often and medicates the patient as soon as pain is reported instead of waiting for it to become severe. When narcotic analgesics are given, safety precautions must be taken because of the sedative effects of the drugs. The nurse employs other comfort measures in addition to medications. Position changes, smooth linens, back rubs, and mouth care also may promote comfort.

Attacks of biliary colic are caused by stimulation of the gallbladder, most often by fats in the duodenum. A low-fat diet is recommended to decrease the incidence of acute symptoms.

FLUID VOLUME DEFICIT. If nausea and vomiting are present, the patient is at risk for fluid and electrolyte imbalances. Antiemetics are given as ordered. Intake and output records should be kept. The nurse monitors for signs of fluid volume deficit (hypovolemia): tachycardia, hypotension, dry skin, concentrated urine, decreased urine output.

If vomiting is severe, a nasogastric tube may be inserted and attached to suction. Fluids are provided intravenously. The nurse notes the amount and characteristics of aspirated fluid. A problem associated with nasogastric decompression is the continuous removal of gastric secretions. When the fluid is continually drained, the patient loses significant water, electrolytes, and acid. This puts the patient at risk for fluid volume deficit, potassium deficit, sodium excess, and metabolic alkalosis. Serum electrolytes are monitored, and specific intravenous fluids are ordered to maintain or restore balance.

IMPAIRED SKIN INTEGRITY. Patients who have obstructive jaundice due to blockage of the bile ducts often have pruritus caused by accumulated bile salts under the skin. Measures to promote comfort include tepid baths with baking soda or oily lotions, use of soft linens, and maintaining a comfortable room temperature. Patients should be advised not to scratch, but that can be difficult. Short fingernails or even cotton gloves may be proposed to avoid skin injury from scratching. The physician may order a drug such as cholestyramine (Questran) to reduce the discomfort.

ANXIETY. Acute pain and unexpected hospitalization can be anxiety-provoking for patients and their families. They need clear explanations about what is being done and what they can expect. The nurse acknowledges their anxiety and takes time to offer reassurance.

HIGH RISK FOR INJURY. A patient who has obstructed bile flow may have a deficiency of vitamin K since absorption of this vitamin in the digestive tract requires bile salts. Vitamin K is needed for the production of prothrombin, an essential element for clotting. Indications of vitamin K deficiency include bleeding gums and oozing of blood at injection sites. Trauma can be minimized by using a soft toothbrush or swab for mouth care and by applying gentle pressure to injection sites.

KNOWLEDGE DEFICIT. Whether cholelithiasis is treated conservatively or surgically, the patient needs to be well prepared for discharge.

Conservative treatment consists of a low-fat diet usually supplemented with fat-soluble vitamins. The dietitian can explain the details of the diet to the patient, but the nurse needs to be able to reinforce them. The nurse should also advise the patient to report signs of bile duct obstruction: light stools, dark urine, jaundice, and pruritus.

Patients who are taking oral bile salts to dissolve gallstones need to know about their medications. The physician needs to be informed if gastric upset occurs because it can lead to gastric ulcers. Diarrhea is another side effect that can usually be managed with antidiarrheals. Some bile acids are hepatotoxic, so serum enzymes are monitored. One last important teaching point is that bile salts interfere with oral contraceptives, so patients should use alternative methods of contraception while on these drugs.

PHARMACOLOGY CAPSULE

Caution patients that supplementary bile salts interfere with oral contraceptives.

Evaluation

Criteria for evaluating goal achievement for the patient with cholecystitis are patient's statement of absent or reduced pain, balanced intake and output and vital signs consistent with patient's norms, intact skin without itching or redness, patient's statement of reduced anxiety and relaxed manner, absence of bleeding, and patient's verbalization of diet and drug therapy.

NURSING CARE OF THE PATIENT FOLLOWING SURGERY FOR CHOLELITHIASIS

Common nursing interventions for the patient who has abdominal surgery for cholelithiasis are presented here. Detailed assessment and care of the surgical patient is presented in Chapter 14. Nursing care after laparoscopic cholecystectomy is much simpler as patients usually recover quickly and are hospitalized less than 24 hours. They usually do not require postoperative nasogastric intubation or T tubes.

Assessment

Postoperatively, the nurse takes the patient's vital signs until stable. Chest expansion is observed, and breath sounds are auscultated. The dressing is inspected for bleeding. If there is a T tube present, the color and amount of drainage are noted. Passive drains are examined to be sure that they are functioning properly. The skin around the incision or the drain is inspected for redness or breakdown. If a nasogastric tube is in place, the nurse observes the characteristics and amount of the drainage and ensures that the suction is operational. The patient's nares are inspected for irritation or pressure from the tube.

Nursing Diagnosis

If the patient undergoes a surgical procedure, nursing diagnoses may include the following:

- **Pain** related to surgical incision, nasogastric tube
- **Ineffective Breathing Patterns** related to splinting of surgical incision
- **Impaired Skin Integrity** related to wound drainage, surgical incision
- **Fluid Volume Deficit** related to gastrointestinal suction
- **High Risk for Infection** related to surgical incision, invasive procedure
- **Knowledge Deficit** of surgical routines and postoperative self-care

Goals

Goals of postoperative nursing care are reduced pain, effective breathing patterns, wound healing without skin breakdown, normal fluid status, absence of infection, and patient's knowledge of surgical routines and postoperative self-care.

Interventions

PAIN. When the patient undergoes a procedure that requires a surgical incision, pain is expected. In addition to administering ordered analgesics, the nurse repositions the patient for comfort and checks to see that any drainage tubes are functioning. The patient is taught how to support the incision with hands or a pillow during coughing and deep breathing. Other pain relief measures are described in Chapter 16. If pain continues despite these measures, the physician should be notified.

The patient who has a nasogastric tube has an additional source of discomfort. The nose and throat may become very sore. The nurse secures the tube to the patient's upper lip or nose so that it is not easily moved or tugged. The nares are cleansed gently, and water-soluble lubricant is applied to keep the area moist. Frequent mouth care is provided.

INEFFECTIVE BREATHING PATTERNS. Potentially ineffective breathing patterns are most likely to be a problem when the patient has a subcostal incision. The incision is located close to the diaphragm, so full lung expansion is painful. The patient tends to guard the surgical area by not breathing deeply. The nurse explains the importance of deep breathing to prevent atelectasis and pneumonia. The patient is also shown how splinting the area makes breathing and coughing more comfortable. Adequate pain management also enables the patient to breathe more effectively. Respiratory rate and breath sounds are monitored.

IMPAIRED SKIN INTEGRITY. Patients who have subcostal incisions often have wound drains in place. These drains allow for removal of fluids that collect at the surgical site. A Penrose drain diverts fluids directly onto the wound dressings. This requires frequent dressing changes to prevent skin irritation. It is especially important if bile is present in the drainage because bile contains digestive enzymes that are even more irritating. A pouch collection device like those used for stomas can be applied if needed to protect the skin. A passive drain such as the Jackson-Pratt has a fluid collection device that keeps fluid away from the skin.

FLUID VOLUME DEFICIT. Postoperatively the nurse measures fluid intake and output. Until oral fluids are permitted, fluids are administered intravenously as ordered. Blood studies may be ordered to assess serum electrolytes. If nasogastric suction is ordered, the nurse checks frequently to be sure it is working properly. Otherwise, the patient may have distention that causes vomiting and further loss of fluids and electrolytes.

HIGH RISK FOR INFECTION. The patient who has gallbladder surgery is at risk for infection of the surgical wound. Draining wounds provide a moist environment for bacterial growth. Meticulous wound care can reduce that risk.

A complication of endoscopic sphincterotomy is pancreatitis caused by accidental entry of the endoscope into the pancreatic duct. Early signs of pancreatitis are pain and fever.

KNOWLEDGE DEFICIT. Cholecystectomy patients are sometimes discharged with T tubes in place. The nurse instructs the patient in care of the tube several days before discharge so that the patient can practice under supervision. A low-fat diet may be advised for 4 to 6 weeks. Postoperative limitations also are discussed. The nurse should inquire about the physician's postoperative instructions. In general, the patient is advised not to do any heavy lifting for 4 to 6 weeks. Other activities, including sexual intercourse, can usually be resumed when the patient feels well enough.

After laparoscopic cholecystectomy, the patient is usually instructed to avoid fatty foods for several weeks, remove the dressings and bathe or shower normally the next day, and notify the physician if there is redness, drainage, or pus from the incision. The patient should also report any signs of peritonitis: severe abdominal pain, chills and fever, and vomiting.

Evaluation

Evaluation of nursing care of the cholecystectomy patient is based on patient's statement of absent or reduced pain, breath sounds clear on auscultation, intact skin and clean wound margins without excessive redness, balanced intake and output, normal temperature and white blood cell count, and demonstrated patient self-care ability.

CANCER OF THE GALLBLADDER

Cancer of the gallbladder is rare and is thought to be related to chronic cholecystitis and cholelithiasis. Diagnosis is often delayed because early signs and symptoms are essentially the same as those of cholecystitis and cholelithiasis.

Treatment options include surgery, chemotherapy, and radiation therapy, but the prognosis is generally poor. Often only supportive, symptomatic care is given. Nursing care is similar to that of other patients with gallbladder disease. The nurse also needs to focus on the needs of the cancer patient, as discussed in Chapter 23.

THE PANCREAS

The pancreas is a gland that has both endocrine and exocrine functions. As an endocrine gland, it secretes hormones into the blood that regulate the blood glucose level. The exocrine function is the production of digestive enzymes that are secreted into the duodenum through a duct. This section focuses on disorders of the pancreas, with the exception of diabetes mellitus, which is covered in Chapter 41.

ANATOMY AND PHYSIOLOGY OF THE PANCREAS

The pancreas is a fish-shaped organ located in the upper left quadrant of the abdomen behind the stomach. The head of the pancreas lies against the duodenum, and the tail lies next to the spleen. The pancreatic ducts connect the pancreas to the duodenum. One duct goes directly to the duodenum, the other merges with the common bile duct, as seen in Figure 35–10.

EXOCRINE FUNCTION

The exocrine function of the pancreas is carried out by acinar tissue. Acinar tissue is composed of tiny grape-like clusters of cells that produce pancreatic juice. Pancreatic fluid contains enzymes needed for digestion of proteins, fats, and carbohydrates. It is secreted into the duodenum through the pancreatic duct.

Pancreatic enzymes trypsin, amylase, and lipase act on partially digested foods in the small intestine. Trypsin plays a role in the digestion of protein by breaking proteases and peptones into small polypeptides. Normally, trypsin is not activated until it enters the duodenum. Otherwise, it would digest the protein tissue of the pancreas itself. Amylase acts with intestinal enzymes to reduce starch, sucrose, and fructose to glucose, fructose, and galactose. Lipase acts on emulsified fats to yield fatty acids, glycerides, and glycerol.

ENDOCRINE FUNCTION

The endocrine function of the pancreas is carried out by clusters of specialized cells scattered throughout the pancreas. These cells are called islets of Langerhans. The islets contain alpha, beta, delta, and PP cells. Alpha cells produce and secrete glucagon. Beta cells produce and secrete insulin. Delta cells produce somatostatin, which inhibits the release of glucagon and insulin. PP cells secrete pancreatic polypeptide—a hormone of uncertain function.

Glucagon is secreted when the blood glucose level falls. It stimulates the liver to convert glycogen into glucose. Insulin is secreted when the blood glucose rises, as after a meal. It stimulates the use of glucose by the cells so that a normal glucose blood level is maintained. The function of insulin is reviewed more thoroughly in Chapter 41.

NURSING ASSESSMENT OF THE PANCREAS

Assessment of the patient with a pancreatic disorder is outlined in Table 35–7. The assessment focuses on digestive and metabolic functions.

TABLE 35-7
ASSESSMENT OF THE PATIENT WITH A PANCREATIC DISORDER

HEALTH HISTORY

Present illness: General well-being, digestive disturbances, pain
Past medical history: Disorders of the biliary tract or duodenum, abdominal trauma or surgery, metabolic disorders; medication history, especially thiazides, furosemide, estrogens, corticosteroids, sulfonamides, and opiates
Family history: Pancreatic disorders
Review of systems: Pruritus, respiratory distress, nausea and vomiting, abdominal pain
Functional assessment: Dietary habits, alcohol intake

PHYSICAL EXAMINATION

General survey: Restlessness, flushing, diaphoresis
Vital signs: Low-grade fever, tachycardia, tachypnea, hypotension
Skin: Jaundice, dryness, scratches
Abdomen: Distention, tenderness, diminished bowel sounds, discoloration

HEALTH HISTORY

The nurse inquires about the patient's general health status because pancreatic disorders are often accompanied by weakness and fatigue. The past medical history documents previous disorders of the biliary tract or duodenum, abdominal trauma or surgery, and metabolic disorders such as diabetes mellitus. The medication history should be detailed and specifically include the use of thiazides, furosemide, estrogens, corticosteroids, sulfonamides, and opiates. A family history of pancreatic disorders is noted. In the review of systems, the nurse obtains a complete description of any pain in the upper abdomen or epigastric area. Symptoms that may be important in relation to pancreatic disorders are dyspnea, nausea, and vomiting. The functional assessment includes data about the patient's dietary habits and use of alcohol.

PHYSICAL EXAMINATION

The nurse notes any restlessness, flushing, or diaphoresis during the examination. Vital signs are taken and may detect low-grade fever, tachypnea, tachycardia, and hypotension. The skin is inspected for jaundice. The abdomen is assessed for distention, tenderness, discoloration, and diminished bowel sounds.

DIAGNOSTIC TESTS AND PROCEDURES

Tests and procedures used to diagnose pancreatic disorders include laboratory analyses of blood, urine, stool, and pancreatic fluid; ultrasonography; CT; and ERCP.

Specific blood studies used to assess pancreatic function include serum amylase, lipase, glucose, calcium, and triglycerides. Urine amylase and renal amylase clearance tests also may be ordered. Stool specimens may be analyzed for fat content.

The secretin stimulation test measures the bicarbonate concentration of pancreatic fluid after secretin is given intravenously to stimulate the production of pancreatic fluid.

If cancer is suspected, blood levels of carcinoembryonic antigen or pancreatic oncofetal antigen may be measured. Unfortunately, these antigens are elevated with many types of cancer, so their presence does not specifically indicate pancreatic cancer.

Additional information about diagnostic tests and procedures for the pancreas is provided in Table 35–8.

DISORDERS OF THE PANCREAS

PANCREATITIS

Pancreatitis is inflammation of the pancreas. It may be acute or chronic. Chronic pancreatitis may follow the acute condition but often develops independently.

Pancreatitis is most often caused by biliary tract disorders or alcoholism. Other causes include viral infections, peptic ulcer disease, cysts, metabolic disorders (renal failure, hyperparathyroidism), and trauma from

TABLE 35-8
DIAGNOSTIC TESTS AND PROCEDURES FOR THE PANCREAS

TEST/STUDY	PURPOSE/PROCEDURE	PATIENT PREPARATION	POSTPROCEDURE NURSING CARE
Laboratory Tests			
Serum enzymes			
Amylase	Detects increases associated with pancreatitis, parotitis, cholecystitis. Detects decreases associated with liver disease, burns, thyrotoxicosis. Normal value: 50–150/L.	Advise patient that a blood sample will be drawn.	No special aftercare is needed except to check venipuncture site for bleeding or swelling.
Lipase	Detects increases associated with pancreatic inflammation, carcinoma. Normal values vary with type of test used.		
Serum glucose	Detects disorders of glucose metabolism and is used to monitor management of diabetes mellitus. Normal value: 70–110 mg/dl.	If patient to do self-testing, teach correct technique and how to interpret findings.	Record reading. Check to see if insulin should be given. Administer insulin as ordered.
Serum calcium	Detects decreases associated with many conditions, including pancreatic disorders.	Advise patient to expect venipuncture.	Check venipuncture site for bleeding or swelling.
Serum triglycerides	Detects increases associated with pancreatitis and many other conditions.	Same as serum calcium.	Same as serum calcium.
Tumor markers: carcinoembryonic antigen (CEA); pancreatic oncofetal antigen (POA)	Detects increases associated with many types of cancer, including pancreatic. Also increases with pancreatitis, cirrhosis, hepatitis, and chronic cigarette smoking.	Same as serum calcium.	Same as serum calcium.
Secretin stimulation test	Secretin is given intravenously. Gastric and duodenal fluids are aspirated through a double-lumen tube. Fluid is analyzed. Decreased volume of secretions and bicarbonate is consistent with pancreatitis.	Tell patient that a medication will be given in a vein and that a tube will be passed through nose into stomach so that fluid can be removed from stomach for study.	Remove tube unless instructed otherwise. Provide comfort measures.
Urine amylase	Detects increases of amylase in urine associated with acute pancreatitis, peptic ulcer, and choledocholithiasis. Test may be ordered for a 1-hr, 2-hr, or 24-hr specimen.	Advise patient of time for collection of specimens. Encourage fluids during test if not contraindicated.	
Ultrasonography			
Abdominal ultrasound	Uses sound waves to visualize pancreas directly. Is noninvasive.	Some labs require NPO before procedure. Study cannot be done if barium or excessive gas is in digestive tract. Tell patient that he or she will lie on back on an examination table. A gel or oil is applied to skin, and an instrument is moved over upper abdomen. Images are seen on a screen and recorded.	No special aftercare is needed.
Radiographic Studies			
Computed tomography (CT) scan	Uses x-rays with a special scanner to provide detailed information about internal organ position and structure. Contrast medium may be given orally or intravenously.	NPO is needed prior to some CT scans. Tell patient to expect to lie on a narrow stretcher. Scanner is a donut-shaped machine that moves back and forth and around stretcher. It makes clicking noises. Contraindicated during pregnancy. Assess allergies to dye and inform radiologist.	No special aftercare is needed.
Endoscopic retrograde cholangiopancreatography (ERCP)	Uses an endoscope to examine gallbladder and pancreas to evaluate bile obstruction and to confirm pancreatic disease. Contrast medium is injected into bile duct.	A consent form must be signed. Patient will be NPO as long as 12 hr. Physician may order patient to gargle with a topical anesthetic. An intravenous line may be started to administer sedatives.	Monitor vital signs for 4 hr. Check gag reflex before giving fluids or food. Monitor for urinary retention. Report temperature elevation that may indicate inflammation.

NPO, Nothing by mouth.

external injury, surgery, or endoscopic procedures. In addition, chronic pancreatitis is sometimes associated with cancer of the duodenum or pancreas.

Normally, pancreatic enzymes are activated in the small intestine. With pancreatitis, digestive enzymes (trypsin, elastase, and phospholipase A) are activated by some unknown mechanism and begin to digest pancreatic tissue (a process called autodigestion), fat, and elastic tissue in blood vessels. Pancreatic fluid may leak into the surrounding tissues. The effect of this escaped fluid has been compared to an internal chemical burn, and the effects can be devastating.

Chronic pancreatitis is often related to alcohol abuse. It is usually characterized by obstruction of the pancreatic duct, leading to progressive destruction of the pancreas.

Signs and Symptoms

Abdominal pain is the most prominent symptom of pancreatitis. The pain is typically severe, with a sudden onset, and is centered in the upper left quadrant or the epigastric region and radiates to the back. Severe vomiting, flushing, cyanosis, and dyspnea often accompany the pain. Other signs and symptoms are low-grade fever, tachypnea, tachycardia, and hypotension.

The abdomen may be tender and distended. Bowel sounds may be absent, suggesting an ileus. Trypsin may damage blood vessels, causing pancreatic hemorrhage and discoloration of the abdomen. Findings might include cyanosis or greenish discoloration of the abdominal wall, the flanks, and the area around the umbilicus. Enzymes released into the abdominal cavity increase capillary permeability, permitting protein-rich serum to leak from blood vessels. Bleeding and shifting of fluid reduce blood volume and may lead to shock. Early signs and symptoms of shock are restlessness and tachycardia. Hypotension is a late sign.

Symptoms of chronic pancreatitis are similar to those of the acute disease but usually appear as periodic attacks that become more and more frequent. In addition, patients with chronic pancreatitis may develop diabetes mellitus and malabsorption with steatorrhea.

Complications

Complications of pancreatitis include pseudocyst; abscess; hypocalcemia; and pulmonary, cardiac, and renal complications.

A pseudocyst is a fluid-filled pouch attached to the pancreas. It contains products of tissue destruction and pancreatic enzymes. The fluid can leak into the digestive tract or the abdominal cavity. Symptoms of pseudocyst include abdominal pain, nausea, vomiting, and anorexia. Sometimes a mass can be palpated in the epigastric area. Necrosis within the pancreas can lead to pancreatic abscess, a fluid-filled cavity in the pancreas. Symptoms are similar to those of pseudocyst. Patients usually run a high fever.

Hypocalcemia (low serum calcium) is caused by the action of fatty acids on calcium and increased loss of calcium in the urine. Pulmonary complications of pancreatitis are pneumonia and atelectasis. Pancreatitis can be fatal. In the early stage of acute pancreatitis, causes of death are usually cardiovascular, renal, or pulmonary failure. Later, sepsis and abscesses are the leading causes of death.

A person may recover completely from an attack of acute pancreatitis, have repeated acute episodes, or experience chronic pancreatitis.

Medical Diagnosis

The most important diagnostic findings in acute pancreatitis are elevated serum amylase, serum lipase, and urinary amylase. When the kidneys clear amylase more rapidly than they clear creatinine, acute pancreatitis is strongly suspected. Other findings with acute pancreatitis are elevated serum lipids and glucose, and decreased serum calcium. Ultrasonography and ERCP may reveal the presence of gallstones, cysts, or abscesses.

Tests for chronic pancreatitis include the secretin stimulation test and fecal studies in addition to the tests used for acute pancreatitis. Findings consistent with chronic pancreatitis are decreased volume and bicarbonate concentration of pancreatic fluid and high fecal fat content.

Medical Treatment

The patient is usually allowed nothing by mouth, and a nasogastric tube is inserted and connected to suction. This removes the stimulus for secretion of pancreatic fluid.

Intravenous fluids are ordered to restore and maintain fluid balance. Total parenteral nutrition may be needed to provide adequate nutrients. Blood or plasma expanders are given if the blood volume is low. Since the inflamed pancreas is susceptible to infection, some physicians order prophylactic antibiotics.

DRUG THERAPY. Pain control is a major problem with pancreatitis. Meperidine (Demerol) is the analgesic of choice because opiates (like morphine) cause more spasm in the pancreatic ducts. With chronic pancreatitis, there is concern about addiction to narcotic analgesics. Drugs such as nitroglycerin that relax smooth muscle also may be ordered.

The patient with chronic pancreatitis needs to take pancreatic enzymes in order to digest food. The enzymes can be taken with meals or snacks. The effect of the enzymes can be determined by examining the stools. Steatorrhea results from inadequate enzymes. If diabetes mellitus develops, insulin or oral hypoglycemic drugs are needed. The patient requires diabetes education. Other drugs that may be needed are antacids, anticholinergics, and histamine blockers to decrease hydrochloric acid secretion in the stomach. Bile salts also may be needed to enhance absorption of fat-soluble vitamins. Drugs used to treat pancreatitis are described in Table 35–9.

TABLE 35-9
DRUGS USED TO TREAT PANCREATITIS

DRUG	USE/ACTION	SIDE EFFECTS	NURSING INTERVENTIONS
Acute Pancreatitis			
Narcotic analgesics Meperidine (Demerol)	Relieve pain.	Sedation, confusion, hypotension, nausea, vomiting, constipation.	Monitor BP, P, R. Assess bowel elimination. Safety precautions. Give antiemetics as ordered.
Smooth muscle relaxants Nitroglycerin	Relieve spasm, reduce pain.	Headache, dizziness, flushing, tachycardia, hypotension.	Monitor BP and P. Use special containers and tubing for IV administration.
Antispasmodics Propantheline bromide (Pro-Banthine)	Decrease bicarbonate and pancreatic enzyme secretion.	Tachycardia, dry mouth, constipation, urinary retention and hesitancy, drowsiness.	Administer 30 min before meals. Don't give within 1 hr of antacids or antidiarrheals. Safety precautions if drowsy. Mouth care. Monitor stools.
Antacids	Neutralize gastric acid; indirectly decrease production of pancreatic secretions.	Constipation with aluminum; diarrhea with magnesium.	Monitor electrolytes. Give 1 hr apart from other oral drugs. Give on empty stomach. Chew tablets and follow with full glass of water. Shake liquids well.
Carbonic anhydrase inhibitors Acetazolamide (Diamox)	Reduce bicarbonate concentration in pancreatic secretions.	Rash, drowsiness, nausea, vomiting, renal calculi, hypercalcemia, aplastic anemia, leukopenia, seizures, hypokalemia.	Encourage 2000–3000 ml fluid/day unless contraindicated. Give with food to decrease GI distress. Safety precautions. Monitor electrolytes and blood cell counts.
Somatostatin	Inhibits secretion of pancreatic enzymes.		
Histamine$_2$ receptor blockers Cimetidine (Tagamet) Ranitidine (Zantac)	Decrease production of HCl so that pancreatic enzymes cannot be activated.	Confusion, nausea, diarrhea, constipation, drowsiness, headache, rash, agranulocytosis.	Administer with or immediately after meals. Discourage smoking, which counteracts these drugs. Safety precautions. Report sore throat or fever.
Vitamin and mineral supplements	Supplement poor dietary intake or impaired absorption. Calcium treats hypocalcemia.	Potential for overdose of fat-soluble vitamins and calcium. Calcium potentiates cardiac glycosides.	
Adrenocortical steroids	Decrease inflammation.	Fluid retention, hypokalemia, hyperglycemia, hypocalcemia, decreased resistance to infection, mood swings.	Monitor BP, P, and blood glucose. Assess for edema. Protect from infection. Explain that emotional/personality changes are temporary.
Chronic Pancreatitis			
Pancreatic enzymes Pancreatin Pancrelipase (Cotazym, Viokase, Pancrease)	Supplement normal pancreatic enzyme secretion; aid in digestion of fats, carbohydrates, and proteins. Goal is less frequent stools with lower fat content.	Diarrhea, nausea, stomach cramps, abdominal pain.	Give with meals or snacks. Capsule contents can be sprinkled on food but should not be chewed. Mix powders with fruit juice or applesauce to mask taste. Do not mix with protein foods. Have patient wipe lips with wet cloth to prevent skin irritation. Evaluate drug effect by noting number and consistency of stools.
Hypoglycemia agents Insulin Oral hypoglycemics	Needed when pancreas is unable to produce insulin.	Hypoglycemia.	See Chapter 41 for details on hypoglycemic drug therapy.

BP, Blood pressure; P, pulse; R, respiration; IV, intravenous; GI, gastrointestinal; HCl, hydrochloric acid.

PHARMACOLOGY CAPSULE

Morphine is not recommended to treat the pain of pancreatitis because morphine tends to increase spasms in the pancreatic ducts.

SURGICAL INTERVENTION. If an abscess, pseudocyst, or severe peritonitis develops, surgical intervention is indicated. Surgical débridement involves resection of necrotic tissue and irrigation of the cavity to remove harmful fluid. The procedure may have to be repeated more than once. Following surgical débridement, multiple sumps are placed in the abdomen for continuous postoperative irrigation. Each sump tube is connected to a separate suction apparatus. Irrigations may be alternated as ordered.

NURSING CARE OF THE PATIENT WITH A PANCREATIC DISORDER

Assessment

General nursing assessment of the patient with possible pancreatic disorders is outlined in Table 35–7 (see also Care Plan: The Patient with Pancreatitis). When a patient has acute pancreatitis, it is especially important to assess for signs of hypovolemic shock: restlessness, tachycardia, tachypnea, hypotension, decreased urinary output, and discoloration of the abdomen and flanks. In addition, the patient's mental status should be assessed. Alterations may be due to metabolic imbalances. The alcoholic patient may develop confusion and agitation due to alcohol withdrawal.

If the patient has surgery, general postoperative assessment should include data covered in Chapter 14.

Nursing Diagnosis

Common nursing diagnoses for the patient with pancreatitis include the following:

- **Pain** related to inflammation, infection, biliary obstruction, autodigestion
- **Fluid Volume Deficit** related to vomiting, bleeding, fluid shift from the blood to the abdominal cavity
- **High Risk for Infection** related to tissue necrosis
- **Impaired Gas Exchange** related to pain, pulmonary complications
- **Altered Nutrition: Less than Body Requirements** related to anorexia, vomiting, digestive disturbance
- **Anxiety** related to unfamiliar setting and procedures; acute illness
- **Knowledge Deficit** about condition and treatment

Goals

Nursing goals for the patient with pancreatitis include pain reduction, fluid balance, absence of infection, normal gas exchange, adequate nutritional intake, reduced anxiety, and knowledge of pancreatitis and self-care.

Interventions

PAIN. The nurse should assess the patient's pain and provide ordered analgesics and antispasmodics promptly. The patient should be repositioned for comfort. Other nursing measures for pain are described in Chapter 16 and include distraction, imagery, and cutaneous stimulation. The effectiveness of pain-control measures should be evaluated and documented. The physician should be consulted if pain is not relieved.

FLUID VOLUME DEFICIT. The nurse inserts a nasogastric tube and connects it to suction as ordered. Intravenous fluids also are administered as ordered. The nurse monitors the patient's fluid status by monitoring vital signs, intake and output, and weight. Signs of fluid volume deficit include tachycardia, hypotension, dry skin, concentrated urine, and intake that exceeds output. Depletion of blood volume causes hypovolemic shock and leads to death if not corrected. Other potential fluid imbalances are metabolic alkalosis from severe vomiting, hypokalemia, hyponatremia, hypocalcemia, and hypochloremia. Hypocalcemia is manifested by muscle twitching or cramping. If symptoms of hypocalcemia appear, serum electrolytes are usually measured and calcium gluconate given if needed.

HIGH RISK FOR INFECTION. Necrosis of the pancreas and surrounding tissue provides a site for infection. If a surgical procedure is done, there is also risk of wound infection. The nurse should report fever, purulent drainage, or separation of wound margins—all signs of infection. Special care should be taken to maintain asepsis during wound care.

IMPAIRED GAS EXCHANGE. Fluid accumulation in the peritoneal cavity puts upward pressure on the diaphragm, thereby limiting lung expansion. Because the acutely ill patient is inactive, secretions may pool in the lungs. Poor lung expansion and inactivity combine to invite pneumonia and atelectasis. The nurse should monitor for tachypnea, dyspnea, and abnormal breath sounds.

Measures to prevent pulmonary complications in the patient with pancreatitis include frequent turning, coughing, and deep breathing. Semi-Fowler's position promotes lung expansion.

ALTERED NUTRITION. Oral intake is restricted with acute pancreatitis because it stimulates pancreatic fluid secretion. Nutrients are usually ordered as TPN. When a patient is on TPN, the nurse must monitor for hyperglycemia. Insulin may be added to the TPN fluid or given by continuous intravenous infusion. Daily weights are used to evaluate the adequacy of the nutrition plan.

Once oral intake is resumed, a high-protein, moderate- to high-carbohydrate, low-fat diet is usually prescribed. Spicy foods, caffeine, and alcohol should be avoided. At first, small, frequent meals may be tolerated better than large meals.

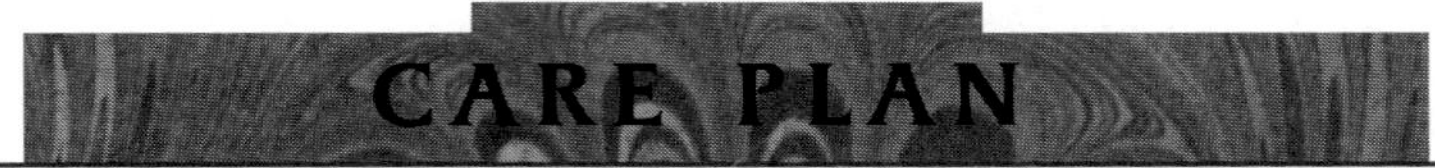

CARE PLAN

The Patient with Pancreatitis

ASSESSMENT

Health History: Mrs. Sanchez is a 57-year-old Latina admitted with repeated attacks of severe pain in the upper left quadrant that radiates to her back. She reports having vomited repeatedly over the past 24 hours. When the pain is severe, she reports feeling flushed, faint, and short of breath. She has no other related symptoms. Mrs. Sanchez reports having had a gallbladder attack several months ago that resolved without surgery. She is a high school teacher who lives with her husband.

Physical Examination: The patient appears to be in acute distress, but she is alert and oriented. Vital signs: temperature, 100.2°F orally; pulse, 92; respiration, 24; blood pressure, 144/84. Her abdomen is tender and distended with hypoactive bowel sounds in all four quadrants.

NURSING DIAGNOSIS	GOALS AND OUTCOME CRITERIA	INTERVENTIONS
Acute pain related to inflammation, biliary obstruction, autodigestion.	The patient will report decreased pain and will appear more relaxed.	Document painful episodes and treat promptly with analgesics and antispasmodics as ordered. Use distraction, imagery, and relaxation techniques to enhance drug therapy. Advise physician if pain is unrelieved.
Fluid volume deficit related to vomiting, bleeding, fluid shift from blood to abdominal cavity.	The patient's fluid status will stabilize as evidenced by stable blood pressure and pulse, normal skin color, urine output equal to fluid intake.	Insert nasogastric tube and connect to low suction as ordered. Initiate intravenous fluid therapy and administer as ordered. Monitor vital signs, intake and output, weight, and electrolyte studies. Report signs of fluid volume deficit: tachycardia, hypotension, dry skin, concentrated urine.
High risk for infection related to tissue necrosis.	The patient will be free of signs and symptoms of infection: fever, tachycardia, increased white blood cell count.	Monitor vital signs and blood cell counts. Report signs of infection. Administer antimicrobials as ordered. Use universal precautions for invasive procedures.
Impaired gas exchange related to pain, pulmonary complications.	The patient will remain free of pulmonary complications as evidenced by absence of dyspnea, tachypnea, and abnormal breath sounds.	Assess respirations and breath sounds. Assist to change positions, cough, and deep breathe at least every 2 hours. Use semi-Fowler's position to promote lung expansion.
Altered nutrition: less than body requirements related to anorexia, vomiting, digestive disturbances.	The patient's body weight will decrease by no more than 5 pounds during hospitalization.	Administer TPN if ordered. Monitor for hyperglycemia and administer insulin as ordered. Take daily weights. When oral intake is permitted, monitor patient tolerance. Discourage spicy foods, caffeine, and alcohol.
Anxiety related to acute symptoms.	The patient will report decreased anxiety and will be calm.	Check on patient often. Respond to her needs promptly. Ask what questions she has and provide explanations of the condition and the treatment she is receiving.
Knowledge deficit of condition and treatment.	The patient will acknowledge understanding of pancreatitis and its treatment.	Explain condition, treatments, and equipment. Assess understanding. Reinforce as needed.

ANXIETY. The nurse attempts to determine the reasons for the patient's anxiety. Some concerns can be alleviated by telling the patient what is happening and what to expect. The nurse responds quickly to the patient's needs and offers comforting reassurance by checking on the patient frequently. Anxiety can be related to pain or hypoxia as well as to emotional distress, so the nurse assesses comfort and oxygenation status and takes appropriate corrective actions.

KNOWLEDGE DEFICIT. During acute attacks, the nurse should answer questions and give simple explanations. As the patient improves, instruction should include information about nutrition, wound care, drug therapy, and prevention of future acute attacks of pancreatitis. If alcoholism is a factor, the nurse should emphasize the relationship between it and pancreatitis. The nurse should know community resources that assist with alcohol abuse, such as Alcoholics Anonymous. It is very important to present information about alcohol use in a nonjudgmental manner.

Evaluation

Criteria for evaluating the effectiveness of nursing interventions are expressed pain reduction, stable weight and vital signs consistent with patient norms, intact skin and wound margins free of excessive redness, normal breath sounds, patient's statement of reduced anxiety and calm demeanor, and patient's description of self-care.

CANCER OF THE PANCREAS

Cancer of the pancreas is extremely serious. About 28,000 new cases are diagnosed each year in the United States. Most of these people die within a year. Factors that seem to be related to the development of pancreatic cancer are smoking, high-fat diet, and cirrhosis of the liver. Diabetes mellitus and chronic pancreatitis also seem related to pancreatic cancer, but the relationship is unclear. Tumors may develop in the head, body, or tail of the pancreas. Pancreatic cancer quickly spreads to the duodenum, stomach, spleen, and left adrenal gland.

Signs and Symptoms

When located in the head of the pancreas, tumors typically obstruct the common bile duct, causing jaundice. In the early stage of the disease, jaundice may be the only sign present. If the patient seeks medical care early, the chance of survival is somewhat better. Other signs and symptoms may be weight loss, upper abdominal pain, anorexia, vomiting, weakness, and diarrhea.

When the tumor is in the body or the tail of the pancreas, the patient may not have any symptoms until the disease is advanced. Then the liver, gallbladder, and spleen may be enlarged. Pressure on the portal veins may cause esophageal and gastric varices (dilated veins) that bleed easily into the gastrointestinal tract. Pressure on nerves may cause back pain.

Medical Diagnosis

Diagnostic tests and procedures used when pancreatic cancer is suspected include blood studies, CT, ultrasonography, ERCP, and percutaneous transhepatic cholangiography.

Blood values associated with pancreatic cancer include elevated serum amylase, lipase, bilirubin, and enzymes. Carcinoembryonic antigen and CA 19-9 are usually elevated, although CA 19-9 is more specific for pancreatic cancer than is carcinoembryonic antigen.

Percutaneous transhepatic cholangiography and ERCP allow the physician to detect obstructed pancreatic ducts and to take samples of pancreatic fluid and tissue. The patient is allowed nothing by mouth for at least 4 hours before either of these procedures. A sedative is given. Afterward, the nurse monitors vital signs for indications of bleeding. After percutaneous transhepatic cholangiography, the patient should lie on the right side for 4 hours to prevent bleeding. During ERCP, medication is used to suppress the gag reflex. Therefore, the patient who has undergone ERCP is not given fluids or food until the gag reflex returns.

Medical Treatment

Treatment depends on the location and extent of the malignant tissue. If the tumor is confined to the head of the pancreas, surgery may be an option. Procedures include total pancreatectomy or the Whipple procedure. The Whipple procedure involves the removal of the diseased portion of the pancreas, the duodenum, and part of the stomach. The stomach, pancreatic duct, and common bile duct are then anastomosed to the jejunum as illustrated in Figure 35–14. Potential complications of the Whipple procedure are listed in Table 35–10.

Sometimes surgical procedures are done primarily to relieve obstruction and improve patient comfort. Narcotic analgesics are ordered for pain management. At times, a jejunostomy tube is placed below the obstruction so that the patient can be given tube feedings.

Radiation or chemotherapy, or both, may be ordered. These therapies are discussed in detail in Chapter 23.

NURSING CARE OF THE PATIENT WITH PANCREATIC CANCER

Assessment

General assessment of the patient with a pancreatic disorder is outlined in Table 35–7. With pancreatic cancer, the nurse should pay particular attention to assessment of gastrointestinal function, pain, and emotional state. If surgery is planned, the patient's knowledge about pre- and postoperative care should be assessed.

Nursing Diagnosis

Nursing diagnoses for the patient with pancreatic cancer may include the following:

- **Pain** related to obstruction, extensive malignancy
- **Fear** related to diagnosis or poor prognosis

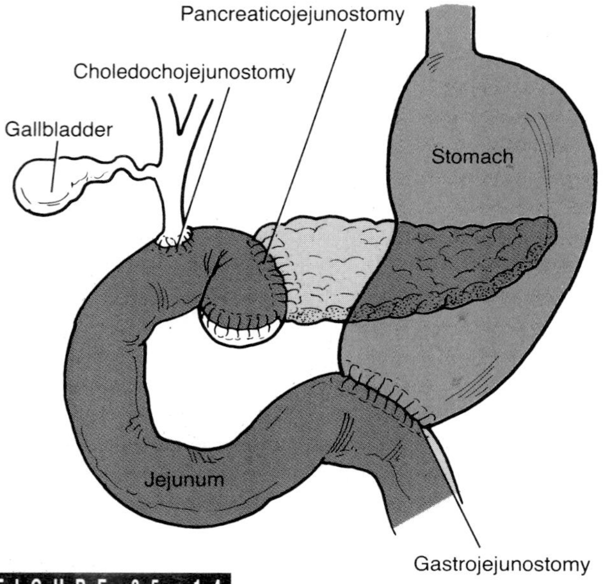

FIGURE 35-14
The Whipple procedure.

- **Knowledge Deficit** of diagnostic and therapeutic procedures
- **Altered Nutrition: Less than Body Requirements** related to anorexia, nausea, vomiting
- **Impaired Skin Integrity** related to pruritus, inactivity, nutritional deficiencies
- **Body Image Disturbance** related to jaundice, weight loss

Goals

The goals of nursing care for the patient with pancreatic cancer are pain reduction, lessened fear, demonstrated understanding of medical and nursing interventions, adequate intake to maintain body weight, skin integrity, and effective coping with body image changes.

Interventions

In many ways, the care of the patient with pancreatic cancer is like that of the patient with pancreatitis, as discussed earlier. Chapter 23 also provides details of caring for the patient with cancer. Areas requiring special attention with pancreatic cancer are discussed here.

PAIN. Narcotic analgesics are usually needed for pain management. The physician may order meperidine (Demerol), morphine, or hydromorphone (Dilaudid). Radiation and chemotherapy can reduce pain by shrinking the tumor. The nurse can also employ distraction, imagery, and cutaneous stimulation, as discussed in Chapter 16.

FEAR. The nurse can help the patient by assessing and acknowledging fear, showing compassion, teaching, and providing attentive care. A referral to a mental health professional or spiritual counselor can be made with the patient's consent.

TABLE 35-10
POTENTIAL COMPLICATIONS OF THE WHIPPLE PROCEDURE

COMPLICATION	NURSING INTERVENTIONS
Hemorrhage	Monitor vital signs for tachycardia, falling blood pressure. Assess for restlessness. Check dressings and drains for excess or bright bleeding.
Fluid and electrolyte imbalances	Assess for cardiac dysrhythmias, muscle weakness or twitching, changes in mental status. Monitor intake and output, tissue turgor. Check laboratory reports and notify physician of abnormalities.
Respiratory failure	Monitor respiratory rate and effort, skin color, breath sounds.
Circulatory failure	Monitor for dysrhythmias, tachycardia, falling blood pressure.
Renal failure	Measure intake and urine output. Report output of less than 30 ml/hr. Assess for edema. Maintain prescribed fluid intake.
Hepatic failure	Assess for jaundice, fatigue, confusion, digestive disturbances.
Wound infection, dehiscence, and fistulas	Assess dressing and drains for excess bleeding, foul odor, purulent drainage. Check temperature for fever. Note elevation in white blood cell count.
Hyperglycemia	Monitor blood glucose as ordered. Note drowsiness, thirst, polyphagia, polyuria.

KNOWLEDGE DEFICIT. The nurse determines what the patient knows and wants to know about diagnostic and therapeutic measures. People under stress retain only part of what they hear, so the nurse must repeat and reinforce teaching. The patient's family also may need information and support. The nurse refers questions about medical decisions and prognosis to the physician. Referrals to community resources including the American Cancer Society and home health services may be appropriate to provide information, support, and assistance.

ALTERED NUTRITION. The nurse monitors the patient's dietary intake and weight. If intake is poor, the dietitian should be consulted. Small, frequent meals may be ordered. Sometimes a jejunostomy is placed, and feeding is delivered by pump. Feedings are usually started with dilute formula given at a slow rate. Both the concentration and the rate are gradually increased. The physician should be informed if the patient develops diarrhea. Some patients require TPN to get adequate nutrition.

IMPAIRED SKIN INTEGRITY. If pruritus is a problem, special skin care and protection are needed. Bath soaps should be eliminated and emollient lotions ap-

NUTRITION CONCEPTS

- People with gallbladder disease should follow a low-fat diet because fat intake usually causes pain.
- For a person with hepatitis, the diet should be high in calories and vitamins with moderate to high protein and moderate to low fat.
- When the liver is damaged, such as with cirrhosis, protein may be restricted to lower blood ammonia.
- In both hepatitis and cirrhosis, carbohydrates should provide most of the calories.
- A clear liquid diet with a gradual progression to low-fat, high-carbohydrate foods is recommended following an attack of acute pancreatitis.
- For chronic pancreatitis patients, a diet high in carbohydrates and protein is used, with restriction of fats as needed to prevent or reduce pain.

plied. The nails are kept short. Mittens can be supplied if the patient is unable to avoid scratching. The physician may order diphenhydramine (Benadryl) to reduce pruritus. If a patient has drains or fistulas, irritating digestive fluids may come in contact with the skin. The exposed skin must be carefully cleaned. Skin barriers and pouches may be effective in protecting the skin. An enterostomal therapist may be consulted for advice on skin care.

BODY IMAGE DISTURBANCE. Weight loss and jaundice alter the patient's appearance and may be distressing. The nurse assists patients with grooming and encourages them to look their best.

Surgical Complications and Postoperative Nursing Care

In general, the postoperative care of the patient with pancreatic cancer is like that of any patient undergoing major abdominal surgery. If the Whipple procedure is performed, the patient is at risk for many complications. These include hemorrhage; fluid and electrolyte imbalances; respiratory, circulatory, renal, and hepatic failure; wound infection and dehiscence; fistulas; and hyperglycemia. Therefore, ongoing nursing assessments are critical. Vital signs, intake and output, and blood glucose are monitored closely. The wound is assessed for bleeding, infection, and separation of margins. Mental status is evaluated to detect changes associated with electrolyte imbalances, poor circulation, and hepatic or renal failure.

Evaluation

Criteria for measuring the effects of nursing care for the patient with pancreatic cancer are patient's statement of pain reduction, patient's statement of lessened fear and improved ability to cope, patient's description of diagnostic and therapeutic measures, stable or increased weight, intact skin, and patient's efforts to improve appearance.

BIBLIOGRAPHY

Black, J. M., & Matassarin-Jacobs, E. (1993). *Luckmann and Sorensen's medical-surgical nursing* (4th ed.). Philadelphia: W. B. Saunders.

Butler, L. (1992). Hepatitis: A nurse's story. *RN, 55*(4), 66–68.

Butler, R. W. (1994). Managing the complications of cirrhosis. *American Journal of Nursing, 94*(3), 46–49.

Cerrato, P. L. (1989). Would a new diet help your gallstone patient? *RN, 52*(7), 59–61.

Cerrato, P. L. (1992). When your patient has liver disease. *RN, 55*(3), 77–80.

Chernecky, C. C., Krech, R. L., & Berger, B. J. (1993). *Laboratory tests and diagnostic procedures.* Philadelphia: W. B. Saunders.

Doherty, M. M., & Carver, D. K. (1993). New relief for esophageal varices. *American Journal of Nursing, 93*(4), 58–63.

Driscoll, D. W. (1992). Perinatal transmission of hepatitis B. *RN, 55*(4), 65.

Fischbach, F. T. (1988). *A manual of laboratory diagnostic tests* (3rd ed.). Philadelphia: W. B. Saunders.

Grau, P. A. (1991). Are you at risk for hepatitis B? *Nursing 91, 21*(3), 44–46.

Greifzu, S., & Dest, V. (1991). When the diagnosis is pancreatic cancer. *RN, 54*(9), 38–42.

Guyton, A. C. (1991). *Textbook of medical physiology* (8th ed.). Philadelphia: W. B. Saunders.

Heeg, J. M., & Coleman, D. A. (1992). Hepatitis kills. *RN, 55*(4), 60–66.

Holmgren, C. (1992). Abdominal assessment. *RN, 55*(3), 28–34.

Ignatavicius, D. D., & Bayne, M. V. (1991). *Medical-surgical nursing: A nursing process approach.* Philadelphia: W. B. Saunders.

Jackson, M. M., & Rymer, T. E. (1994). Viral hepatitis: Anatomy of a diagnosis. *American Journal of Nursing, 94*(1), 43–48.

Jarvis, C. (1992). *Physical examination and health assessment.* Philadelphia: W. B. Saunders.

Jurf, J. B., Clements, L., & Llorente, J. (1990). Chloecystectomy made easier. *American Journal of Nursing, 90*(12), 38–39.

Lancaster, S. (1992). PV shunts relieve ascites. *RN, 55*(8), 58–61.

Lisanti, P., & Talotta, D. (1990). Hepatitis D: Another reason to get your HBV vaccine. *American Journal of Nursing, 90*(4), 29–30.

Martin, F. (1992). When the liver breaks down. *RN, 55*(8), 52–57.

Marx, J. F. (1993). Viral hepatitis: Unscrambling the alphabet. *Nursing 93, 23*(1), 34–42.

McConnell, E. A. (1991). Diagnosing rectal bleeding. *Nursing 91, 21*(8), 102–103.

McConnell, E. A. (1993). Caring for a biliary drainage tube. *Nursing 93, 23*(6), 26.

Norris, M. K. G. (1991). Assessing serum bilirubin levels. *Nursing 91, 21*(5), 18.

Norris, M. K. G. (1991). RN master care plan: The patient with pancreatic cancer. *RN, 54*(9), 43–44.

Ondrusek, R. (1993). Cholecystectomy: an update. *RN, 56*(1), 28–33.

Shlafer, M. (1993). *The nurse, pharmacology, and drug therapy*. Philadelphia: W. B. Saunders.

Smith, A. (1991). When the pancreas self-destructs. *American Journal of Nursing, 91*(9), 38–52.

Thompson, C. (1992). Managing acute pancreatitis. *RN, 55*(3), 52–57.

Whiteman, K., Nachtmann, L., Biondo, M., & Formella, L. (1990). Liver transplantation. *American Journal of Nursing, 90*(6), 68–72.

KEY CONCEPTS

1. The liver plays an important role in bile production and excretion; glucose, protein, and lipid metabolism; blood coagulation; detoxification; immunity; and hormone metabolism.
2. Signs of liver dysfunction include jaundice (a golden yellow skin color) and scleral icterus (yellowing of the sclera of the eyes).
3. Hepatitis is liver inflammation caused by a viral infection or exposure to toxic substances that can lead to hepatic failure.
4. Nursing care of the hepatitis patient addresses activity intolerance and impaired physical mobility, altered nutrition, altered comfort, impaired skin integrity, fluid volume deficit, body image disturbances, anxiety, and knowledge deficit.
5. Health care providers should be vaccinated against hepatitis B since it can be spread through contact with body fluids.
6. Cirrhosis is chronic, progressive liver failure that disrupts metabolism and causes blood abnormalities, fluid and electrolyte imbalances, decreased resistance to infection, accumulation of drugs and toxins, and obstruction of blood vessels and bile ducts in the liver.
7. Cirrhosis may be caused by nutritional deficiencies, toxins (including alcohol), hepatitis, biliary obstruction, and heart failure.
8. Complications of cirrhosis include portal hypertension, esophageal varices, ascites, hepatic encephalopathy, and hepatorenal syndrome.
9. Nursing care of the patient with cirrhosis addresses altered nutrition, activity intolerance, high risk for impaired skin integrity, altered comfort, ineffective breathing patterns, high risk for injury, altered tissue perfusion, altered thought processes, fluid volume deficit, high risk for infection, and fear.
10. The only cure for end-stage liver disease is liver transplantation, which requires lifelong treatment with antirejection drugs that suppress the immune system and put the patient at risk for infection.
11. Signs and symptoms of transplanted organ rejection are fever, anorexia, depression, vague abdominal pain, muscle aches, and joint pain.
12. Bile is produced in the liver, stored in the gallbladder, and delivered to the intestine, where it is essential for emulsification and digestion of fats.
13. Cholecystitis is inflammation of the gallbladder usually caused by gallstones that may obstruct bile flow, causing symptoms from mild indigestion to nausea, chills and fever, and right upper quadrant pain that radiates to the shoulder.
14. Cholelithiasis (stones in the bile) may be treated with oral bile salts, dissolution agents, lithotripsy, endoscopic sphincterotomy, or cholecystectomy.
15. Nursing care of the patient with cholecystitis and cholelithiasis focuses on pain, fluid volume deficit, pruritus, anxiety, high risk for injury, and, for surgical patients, ineffective breathing patterns, impaired skin integrity, high risk for infection, and knowledge deficit.
16. The pancreas has both an endocrine function (insulin secretion) and an exocrine function (secretion of digestive enzymes).
17. Pancreatitis is inflammation of the pancreas, which can lead to pseudocyst, abscess, hypocalcemia, and pulmonary, cardiac, and renal complications.
18. Nursing care of the patient with pancreatitis addresses pain, fluid volume deficit, high risk for infection, impaired gas exchange, altered nutrition, anxiety, and knowledge deficit.
19. Most patients with pancreatic cancer die within a year, especially if the cancer is in the body or the tail of the pancreas.
20. Nursing care of the patient with pancreatic cancer usually focuses on pain, fear, knowledge deficit, altered nutrition, impaired skin integrity, and body image disturbance.

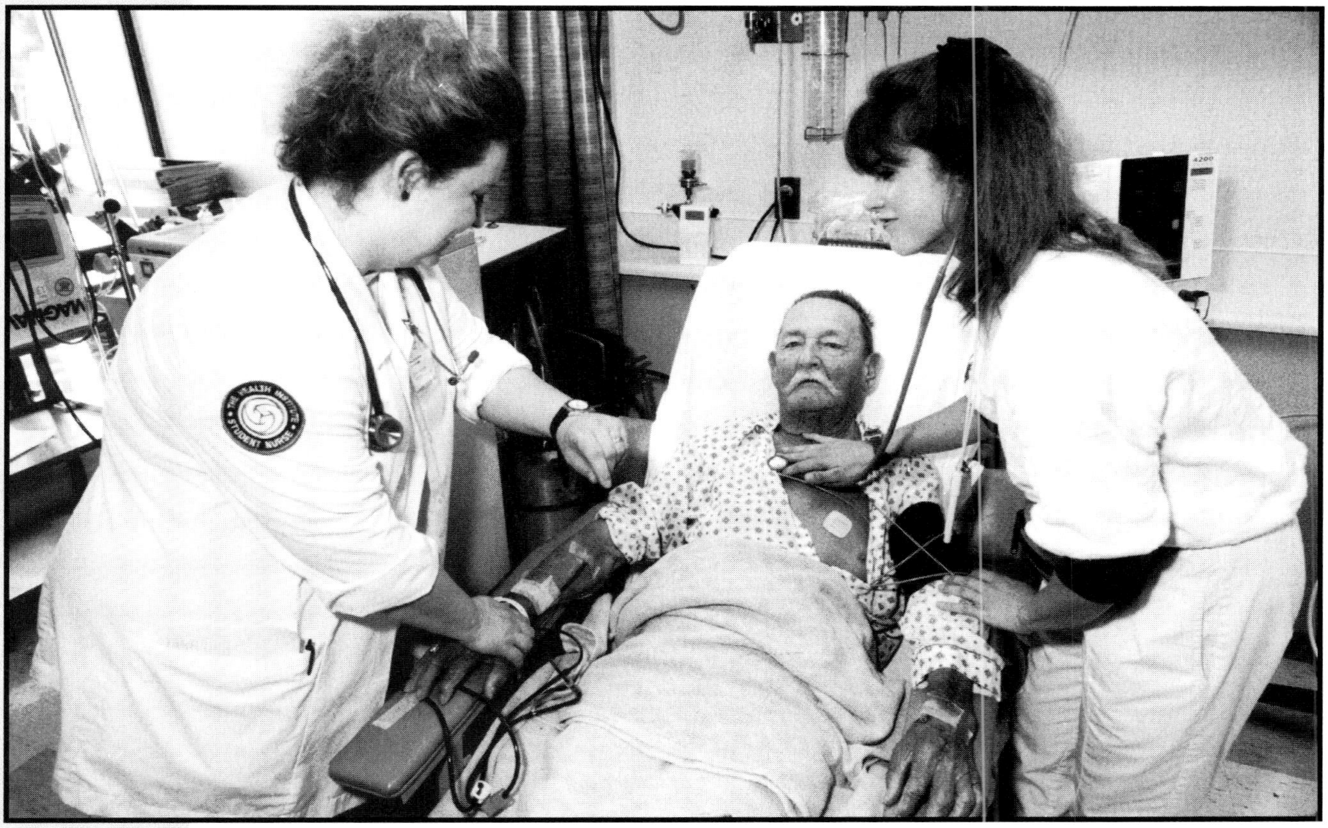

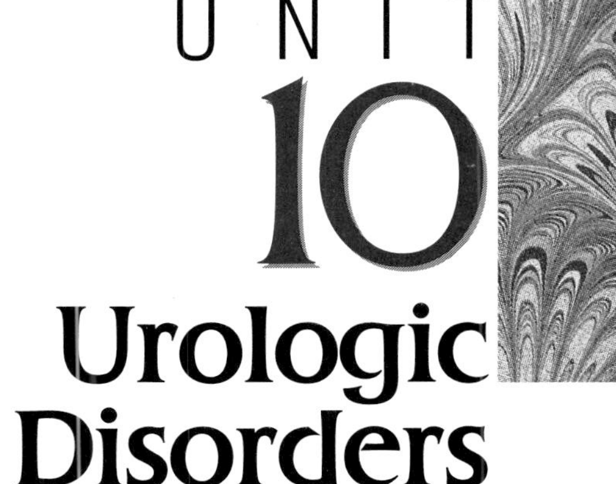

UNIT 10
Urologic Disorders

Joy M. Norton

CHAPTER 36

Urologic Disorders

OBJECTIVES

1. List the data to be collected when assessing a patient who has a urologic disorder.
2. Describe the diagnostic tests and procedures for patients with urologic disorders.
3. Explain the nursing responsibilities for patients having tests and procedures to diagnose urologic disorders.
4. Describe the nursing responsibilities for common therapeutic measures employed to treat urologic disorders.
5. Explain the pathophysiology, signs and symptoms, complications, and treatment of disorders of the kidney, ureters, bladder, and urethra.
6. Apply the nursing process to plan care for patients with urologic disorders.

GLOSSARY

ANURIA Absence of urine production

AZOTEMIA Accumulation of nitrogenous compounds in the blood

CALCULUS Concentration, commonly called a stone, formed of mineral salts in hollow organs or their passages (plural *calculi*)

CYSTECTOMY Removal or resection of the urinary bladder or of a cyst

DIURESIS Increased production of urine

DYSURIA Difficult or painful urination

HEMATURIA Blood in the urine

LITHOTOMY Removal of calculi through an incision in a duct or organ

LITHOTRIPSY Crushing or disintegration of calculi

NEPHROTOXIC Having a harmful effect on kidney tissue

NOCTURIA Excessive urination during the night

OLIGURIA Decreased urine output

POLYURIA Excessive urine volume

UREMIA Azotemia; the signs and symptoms typical of chronic renal failure

The urinary tract plays a vital role in maintaining homeostasis and removing metabolic wastes. Because body systems are interdependent, disease processes in other body systems may have a direct and harmful effect on the urinary system. Similarly, urinary system diseases may significantly affect the respiratory and circulatory systems. Serious alterations in urinary function eventually affect all other systems. A person can live with one functioning kidney, but the body cannot support life with the loss of both kidneys.

ANATOMY AND PHYSIOLOGY OF THE URINARY SYSTEM

ANATOMY

The urinary system consists of the kidneys, ureters, bladder, and urethra (Fig. 36–1).

Kidney and Ureters

The two kidneys are located on each side of the lower thoracic vertebrae, at about the level of the waist. Each kidney is surrounded and protected by a fibrous capsule, fat, and muscle layer. The kidneys lie behind the peritoneum, a membrane that separates them from the abdominal contents.

The layers of the kidney are the cortex and the medulla. The cortex (outer layer) receives a large blood supply and is very sensitive to changes in blood flow. The cortex contains the glomeruli and most of the tubules. The medulla (inner portion) contains 8 to 18 pyramids, triangular-shaped structures that collect urine and drain it into the calices. The calices join to form the pelvis of the kidney. The renal pelvis is the cavity located at the hilus of the kidney. The pelvis serves to collect urine produced by the kidney. From each kidney pelvis, a ureter arises and transports urine to the bladder. The ureters are approximately 25 to 30 cm long and 2 to 8 mm in diameter.

The renal artery, along with a vein, nerves, and lymphatic vessels, enters and exits the kidney through the hilus. The right and left renal arteries that branch off the abdominal aorta deliver blood to the kidneys. One fourth of the body's blood supply is filtered per minute, or the entire blood supply every 4 to 5 minutes. Each renal vein returns blood directly to the inferior vena cava. These structures are illustrated in Figures 36–1 and 36–2.

The nephron is the functional unit of the kidney. Each kidney has 1 to 1.25 million nephrons. A nephron

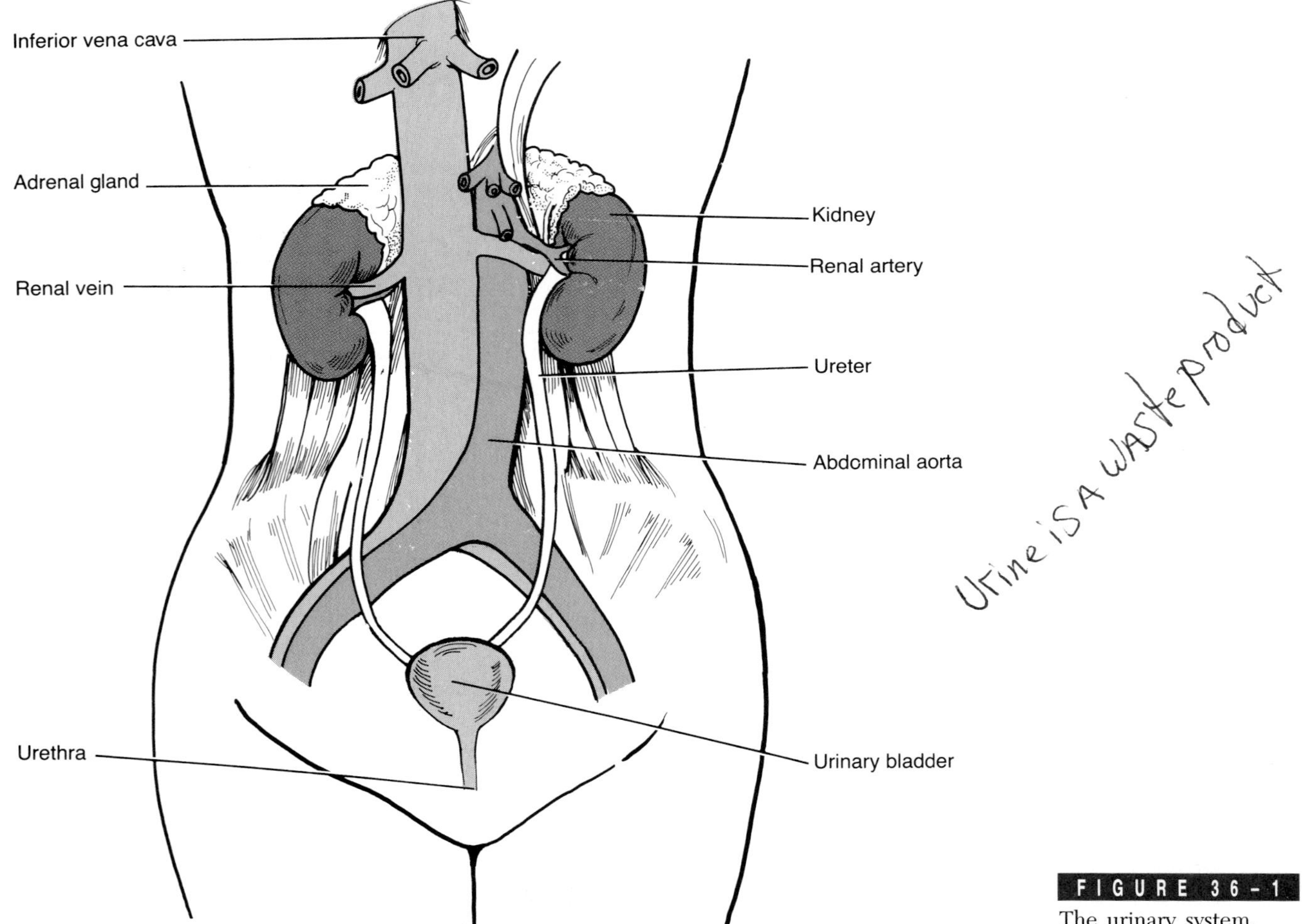

FIGURE 36–1
The urinary system.

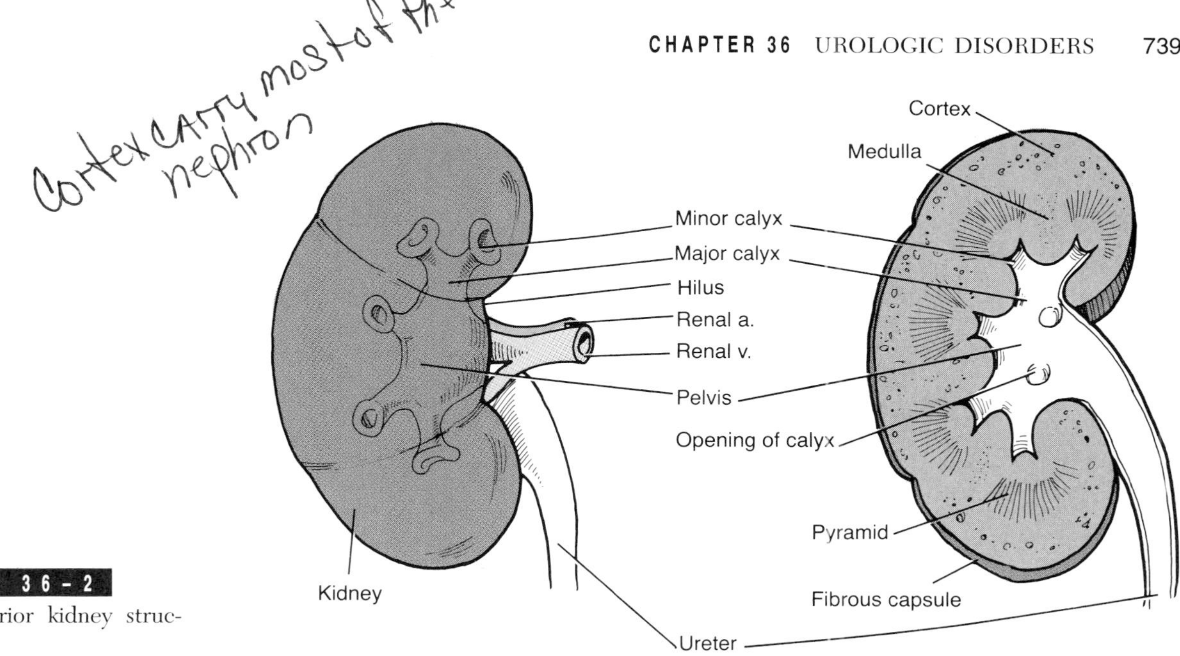

FIGURE 36-2
View of interior kidney structures.

is a vascular tubular system consisting of a glomerulus, a Bowman's capsule, and a tubule. A glomerulus is a mass of blood vessels tucked into the cup-like Bowman's capsule. Each tubule consists of a proximal tubule, Henle's loop, distal tubule, and collecting duct (Fig. 36–3).

Bladder and Urethra

The bladder is a muscular sac that readily stretches to store urine. The bladder rests on the floor of the pelvic cavity behind the peritoneum. It is located in front of the rectum in males and in front of the vagina and uterus in females. The upper portion of the bladder is called the fundus, and the apex is close to the pelvic floor. The bladder neck, containing the internal sphincter, is the most inferior portion. The trigone is a triangular-shaped area on the posterior wall bounded by the two ureters and the urethra. The trigone closes the opening of the ureters into the bladder during micturition (urination). This mechanism keeps urine from being forced back into the ureters.

Sensory and motor nerves supply the bladder. Sympathetic fibers from T-9 through L-2 and parasympathetic and somatic nerves from S-2 through S-4 provide bladder control. Parasympathetic stimulation to the detrusor muscle causes it to contract to empty the bladder. Sympathetic stimulation causes the trigone to close the ureteral openings. The pudendal nerve, which supplies the external sphincter and the pelvic floor muscles, is under voluntary control. When 300 to 400 ml of urine collects in the bladder, bladder distention causes the urge to micturate. The bladder muscle that contracts to empty the bladder is the detrusor muscle (Fig. 36–4).

The urethra is a muscular tube lined with mucous membranes that carries urine from the bladder out of the body. The urethra functions as a sphincter, meaning that it contracts to hold urine in the bladder and relaxes to allow urine to flow from the bladder. In the male, the urethra is encircled by the prostate gland. The urethra is 20 cm long in males and 3 to 5 cm long in females. The short length and close proximity of the urethra to the female anus are two reasons for the increased incidence of bladder infections in women.

PHYSIOLOGY

The functions of the urinary system are regulatory, excretory, and hormonal. Regulatory functions are per-

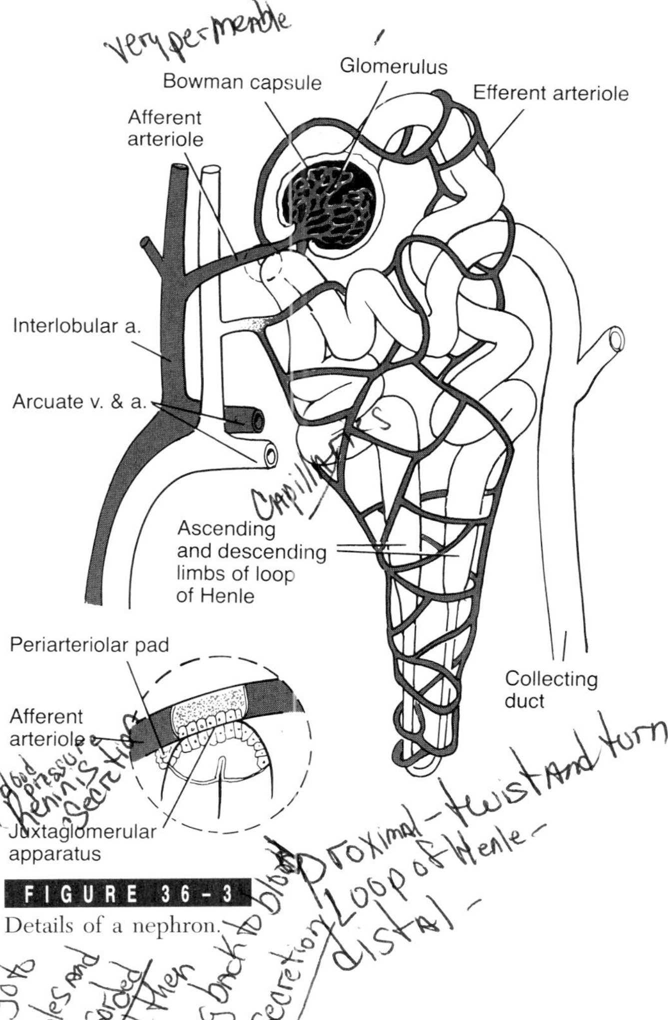

FIGURE 36-3
Details of a nephron.

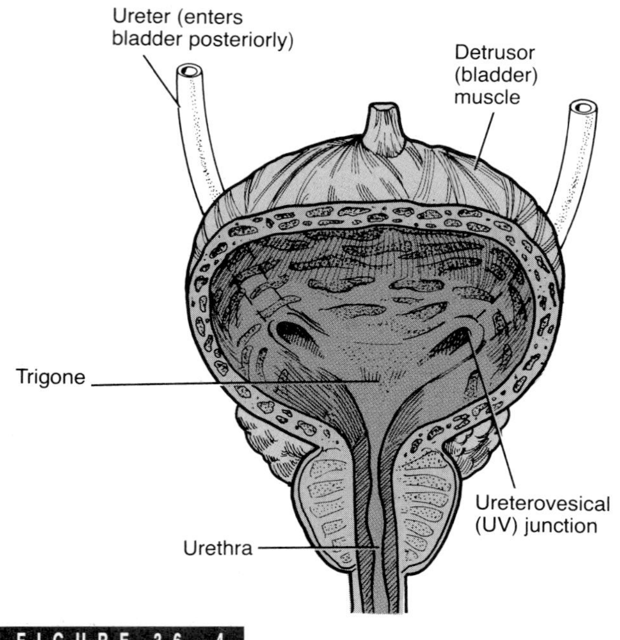

FIGURE 36-4
The urinary bladder cut to reveal the interior.

formed by the formation of urine and by the secretion of renin, which affects blood pressure. Regulatory processes maintain fluid balance, keep electrolytes in normal range, and maintain acid-base balance. The excretory function of the kidney is the elimination of urine. The hormonal function is to stimulate red blood cell production.

Regulation and Excretion

URINE PRODUCTION. Three processes occur in urine production: glomerular filtration, tubular reabsorption, and tubular secretion.

Glomerular Filtration. Glomerular filtration is an ultrafiltration process across the semipermeable membrane, the glomerular capsule. Fluids, electrolytes, and certain nonelectrolytes are filtered out of the blood as it passes through the glomerulus. Plasma proteins are too large to pass through the membrane and, therefore, remain in the blood. The ultrafiltration process requires adequate blood volume and hydrostatic pressure from the pumping of the heart and the resistance of the blood vessels. The product of glomerular filtration is called the glomerular filtrate. It contains water, electrolytes (sodium, potassium, calcium, magnesium, chloride, bicarbonate, phosphate, and other anions), glucose, urea, creatinine, uric acid, and amino acids. Glomerular filtrate and blood plasma are essentially the same except that the filtrate does not have proteins. Most of the filtrate is returned to the blood through tubular reabsorption.

Tubular Reabsorption. Tubules reabsorb water, some electrolytes, and nonelectrolytes as needed to maintain normal fluid balance. Reabsorption occurs through diffusion, active transport, and osmosis. Some nonelectrolytes (urea, creatinine, and uric acid) are not readily reabsorbed and are excreted in the urine. The reabsorption of water reflects the ability of the kidney to concentrate or dilute urine as necessary. The amount of water reabsorbed is influenced by antidiuretic hormone and aldosterone. Antidiuretic hormone, stored in the posterior pituitary, alters permeability of the distal tubules and collecting ducts to control the amount of water reabsorbed. The more hormone released, the more water the tubules reabsorb. Aldosterone is secreted by the adrenals in response to concentrated urine. It causes the reabsorption of sodium and water.

Tubular Secretion. The tubules secrete ions into the lumen to be excreted in the urine. The tubular secretion of potassium and hydrogen ions regulates serum potassium level. This is the kidney's acid-base regulating mechanism. The kidneys regulate acids and bases in conjunction with the buffers in the blood and with the lungs. The kidneys secrete fixed acids produced by normal (primarily protein) metabolism. The lungs excrete the volatile acids. The kidneys regulate fixed acid secretion by conserving bicarbonate, by excreting sodium in exchange for hydrogen ions, and by excreting ammonia. The normal pH of urine is 5 to 7.

The end product of glomerular filtration and tubular reabsorption is urine. Urine is composed mostly of water, sodium, potassium, chloride, urea, creatinine, and uric acid. The body normally excretes 1 to 2 liters of urine each day, which is about 1% of the water filtered by the glomeruli in the same period of time. Glucose and proteins are substances present in blood but not normally present in the urine. Glucose is normally completely reabsorbed in the tubules. The presence of proteins in urine indicates glomerular damage. Urine is delivered to the renal pelvis, where it flows into the ureter. The production of urine is illustrated in Figure 36–5.

URINE ELIMINATION. Peristaltic waves move urine from the kidney through the ureter to the bladder. The presence of 200 to 400 ml of urine in the bladder causes the urge to micturate. However, the bladder can distend to hold several times that amount. Micturition is a complex process that is under a variety of neural controls. The control is voluntary for the toilet-trained person with intact motor and sensory nerve pathways. Micturition generally occurs five to six times a day and may occur once at night. The amount of urine produced is affected by fluid intake, temperature, diaphoresis, vomiting, diarrhea, and medications such as diuretics.

A series of events allows the release of urine. The pelvic floor muscles and the urethral sphincter relax. The trigone contracts, closing the ureters to prevent backflow of urine into the ureters. The detrusor muscle contracts, and urine is forced through the urethra. After the bladder empties, the detrusor muscle relaxes, the bladder neck closes, the trigone relaxes, and the perineal muscles resume normal tone. Voiding is primarily an involuntary reflex act. Voluntary control of voiding is exhibited in the initiation, restraint, and interruption of micturition.

REGULATION OF SERUM CALCIUM AND PHOSPHATE. Parathormone is a hormone secreted by the parathyroid glands to maintain serum calcium levels. When serum calcium is low, parathormone is secreted and acts on the tubules to promote reabsorption of calcium ions. At the same time, tubular reabsorption of phosphate is decreased. This mechanism maintains normal serum calcium and phosphate levels.

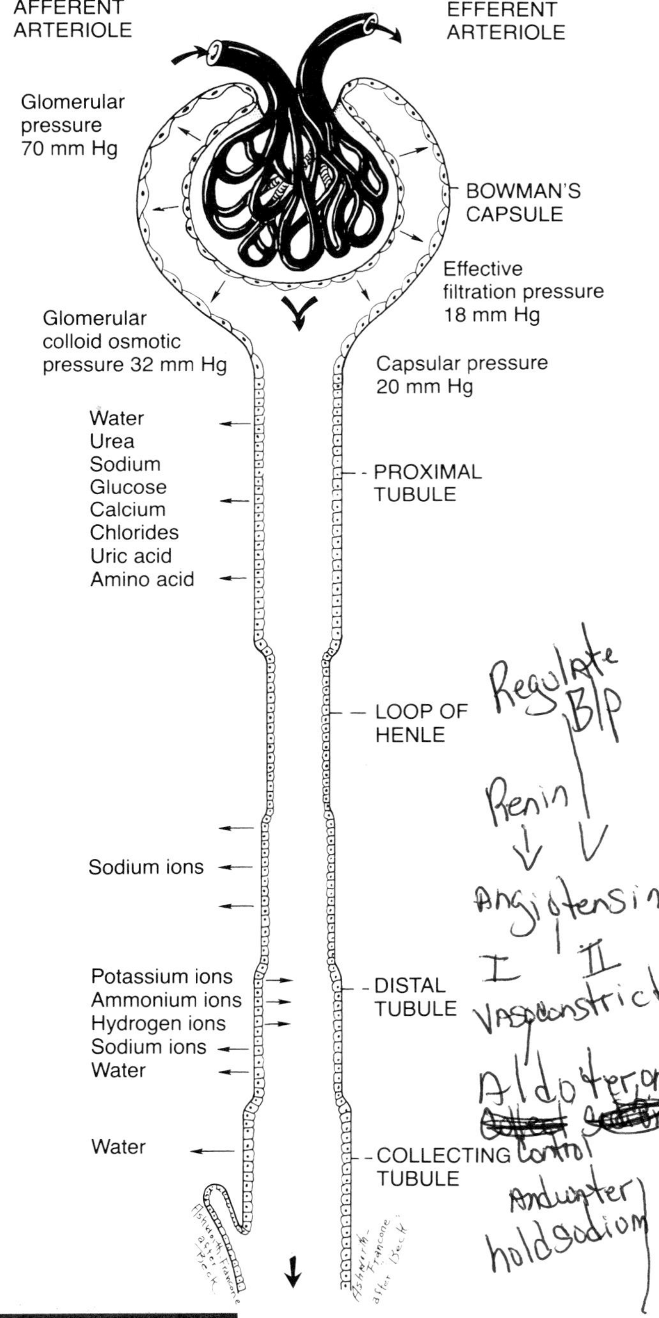

FIGURE 36-5

Urine production. (From Jacob, S. W., & Francone, C. A. [1989]. *Elements of anatomy and physiology* [2nd ed., p. 271]. Philadelphia: W. B. Saunders.)

REGULATION OF BLOOD PRESSURE. Blood pressure is regulated through fluid volume maintenance and release of the hormone renin from the kidneys. One way to raise or lower blood pressure is to change blood volume. This can be done by retaining additional fluid or by eliminating excess fluid. When plasma is very concentrated, it is said to be hypertonic. Dehydration is a common condition that leads to hypertonic plasma. Hypertonic plasma stimulates the release of antidiuretic hormone from the posterior pituitary. Antidiuretic hormone causes reabsorption of water in the renal tubules, decreasing urine volume. The retained fluid expands blood volume, with a subsequent rise in blood pressure.

A second mechanism by which the kidneys affect blood pressure is the secretion of renin. Renin is released in response to inadequate renal blood flow or low arterial pressure. Renin acts on angiotensinogen, a hormone produced by the liver, and converts it to angiotensin I. A lung enzyme converts angiotensin I to angiotensin II. Angiotensin II is a powerful peripheral vasoconstrictor. Also, angiotensin II triggers the release of aldosterone from the adrenal cortex. Aldosterone stimulates tubular reabsorption of sodium and water, and plasma volume is expanded.

With severely decreased cardiac output, as seen in hemorrhage and shock, the renal arteries constrict to prevent fluid loss and to shunt blood to more vital organs (heart, lungs, brain). This vasoconstriction limits renal blood flow. If blood flow is not restored, death of renal tissue may occur.

Hormonal Stimulation of Red Blood Cell Production

Erythropoietin is secreted in the kidneys and stimulates the bone marrow to produce red blood cells. This process is triggered by decreased oxygen in renal blood. Patients in renal failure have a deficiency of erythropoietin, which causes them to become anemic.

AGE-RELATED CHANGES IN THE URINARY SYSTEM

As people age, significant changes occur in the urinary system. Fortunately, the kidneys have enough reserve that normal function is usually maintained. When older people are stressed, however, the kidneys do not adapt as well as they do in younger people.

Structural changes in the kidney include loss of nephrons, thickening of membranes in nephrons, and sclerosis of renal blood vessels. As a result of these changes, renal blood flow and glomerular filtration decline. In addition, plasma renin and aldosterone levels fall and tubules are less responsive to antidiuretic hormone. As a result of all these changes, the older person's kidneys are less able to concentrate and dilute urine in response to serum osmolality.

Creatinine clearance decreases with age. This means that the rate at which the kidneys are able to remove creatinine from the blood is diminished. Creatinine clearance is a better indicator of kidney function than serum creatinine. There is also some decline in erythropoietin, a factor that may contribute to anemia. Aging also affects the renal threshold for glucose. Serum glucose can be considerably elevated before it is detected in the urine.

In younger people, urine production peaks during waking hours. This pattern is lost with age such that urine production does not decrease at night. Therefore, older persons often have nocturia, meaning that they awaken from sleep to void.

The bladder also undergoes changes with age. Bladder muscles weaken, and connective tissue increases. The effect is decreased capacity and incomplete emptying. The mechanism that prevents the reflux of urine from the bladder into the ureters is less effective. Urine reflux can be an important source of kidney infection.

Incontinence is not a normal consequence of age, but it is common. Female urinary incontinence is often caused by relaxed pelvic musculature related to childbirth trauma and lack of estrogen after menopause. For detailed information on incontinence, see Chapter 21. In males, urethral obstruction is more often a problem. It is often caused by the enlarged prostate closing in on the urethra. Prostate enlargement is discussed in Chapter 44.

NURSING ASSESSMENT OF THE URINARY SYSTEM

Elimination is considered to be a very personal activity, and people are not accustomed to discussing it with others. Assessment of urinary function and problems, therefore, may be embarrassing to the patient. Privacy and a calm, accepting manner help put the patient at ease.

HEALTH HISTORY

Chief Complaint

The nurse begins the assessment by exploring what caused the patient to seek health care. Patients with urinary problems most often report changes in urine quality or quantity, pain, or changes in urination.

History of Present Illness

The nurse assesses the patient's normal or usual pattern of urination. Important data include volume of urine, frequency of voiding, and appearance of urine. The patient may have difficulty estimating the amount of urine voided but can usually recognize an increase or decrease from normal. If intake and output records are available, the recent pattern is noted. Terms used to describe urine volume are *polyuria, oliguria,* and *anuria.* Polyuria refers to a large urine output, oliguria to a low output, and anuria to the absence of output. Urine characteristics to record include color, clarity (clear or cloudy), presence of particles, and odor. *Hematuria* is the presence of blood in the urine.

Pain may or may not occur, but it is more common with acute conditions. The nurse assesses the presence of pain or discomfort. The characteristics of the pain are described: intensity, location, distribution, onset, duration, frequency, relationship to urination, precipitating factors, and measures that provide relief. Painful urination is called *dysuria.* Urologic conditions may also cause pain in the flank, abdomen, symphysis pubis, and genitalia. The pain may be so severe that it causes nausea and vomiting.

The nurse also assesses any problem the patient has had initiating or controlling urination. Circumstances under which these problems occur is documented. For example, incontinence (involuntary loss of urine) may occur with laughing or sneezing. This is called stress incontinence.

Past Medical History

After the present illness has been fully described, the patient's past medical history is explored. Significant findings include a history of streptococcal infections, recurrent urinary tract infections, renal calculi, gout, or hypercalcemia. The nurse asks if the patient has had urologic surgery, catheterization, examination (such as cystoscopy or radiography), or trauma and if the patient has used any type of urinary diversion or collection device. Recent and current medications, including both prescription and over-the-counter drugs, are documented because some medications are nephrotoxic (harmful to the kidneys). Exposure to toxic chemicals in the home or the workplace is assessed.

PHARMACOLOGY CAPSULE

Nephrotoxic drugs are harmful to the kidneys.

Family History

The patient's family medical history is assessed as well. Conditions of importance are congenital kidney problems such as polycystic kidneys or urinary tract malformations, diabetes mellitus, and hypertension.

Review of Systems

The body systems are reviewed to detect other problems that may be related to the urinary complaints. The patient is asked about the occurrence of changes in skin color, respiratory distress, edema, fatigue, nausea, vomiting, chills, and fever.

Functional Assessment

The functional assessment includes information about habits and practices that might affect or contribute to urinary tract disorders. The nurse assesses daily fluid intake because urine production varies with fluid intake. It is also helpful to determine the patient's usual exercise pattern because excessive exercise or prolonged immobility affects the urinary system. The effects of the chief complaint on daily life are assessed as well.

PHYSICAL EXAMINATION

The physical examination begins with inspection of the skin for color (ashen, yellow) and the presence of crystals on the skin (uremic frost). Tissue turgor is evaluated to detect dehydration or edema. The area around the eyes is examined for periorbital edema, which suggests fluid retention. The mouth is inspected for moisture and odor. Patients in renal failure may have an odor of urine on their breath.

Respiratory rate, pattern, and effort are observed. Respirations may be rapid with metabolic acidosis, infection, and fluid overload. Kussmaul respirations, seen with metabolic acidosis, are rapid and deep. Dyspnea may be evident with fluid overload. The lungs are auscultated for crackles or rhonchi that may indicate fluid overload. Heart irregularities may be noted with potassium imbalances.

The abdomen is inspected for scars and contours and is palpated for tenderness and bladder distention. Auscultation of the kidney area over the costovertebral angle (Fig. 36–6) is done to detect renal bruits. Bruits are swishing sounds caused by the turbulence of blood. Renal bruits indicate renal artery stenosis (narrowing). The abdomen is then percussed. A dull sound may be heard over a distended bladder. Pain may be elicited over one or both kidneys.

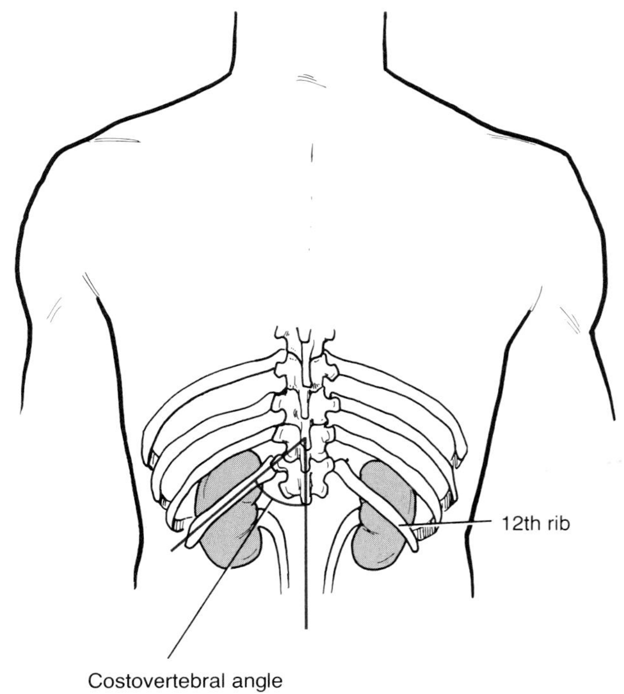

FIGURE 36-6
The costovertebral angle.

The nurse observes for edema throughout the examination. With renal failure, edema is generalized, not dependent. The skin may be dry and flushed over the edematous area.

The last part of the physical examination is inspection of the genitalia. Universal precautions should be observed. The penis is examined for lesions, scars, or discharge. If there are penile lesions or urethral discharge, smears are obtained for culture. A nurse with advanced skills or the physician may also perform rectal and pelvic examinations, especially if symptoms suggest problems of the reproductive system. The pelvic examination may reveal gynecologic rather than urologic problems. The male rectal examination helps detect prostate enlargement, which often creates problems with voiding. Nursing assessment of urologic function is outlined in Table 36–1.

DIAGNOSTIC TESTS AND PROCEDURES

Urine Tests

URINALYSIS. A voided or catheterized urine specimen is examined for color, pH, specific gravity, glucose, protein, blood, ketones, and bilirubin. Urine appearance is very important. Normal urine is the color of straw. Gross hematuria appears bright red in acid urine and tea colored in alkaline urine. Smaller amounts of blood may give the urine a cloudy or smoky appearance. A bacterial infection may also make the urine cloudy. Colorless urine may indicate excessive fluid intake, chronic renal failure, diabetes mellitus, or diabetes insipidus.

TABLE 36-1
ASSESSMENT OF UROLOGIC FUNCTION

HEALTH HISTORY

Present illness: Changes in urine quality or quantity, voiding pattern, pain
Past medical history: Streptococcal infections, urinary tract infections or calculi, gout, hypercalcemia, urologic surgery or instrumentation, urinary diversion, recent and current medications.
Family history: Urinary disorders, diabetes mellitus, hypertension
Review of systems: Fatigue, pruritus, dyspnea; urine quantity: polyuria, oliguria, anuria; urine quality: color, odor, components; frequency of voiding; pain: onset, intensity, frequency, location, duration, precipitating and relieving factors
Functional assessment: Fluid intake, diet, activity

PHYSICAL EXAMINATION

General appearance: Level of consciousness, orientation
Vital signs
Weight
Skin: Color, moisture, turgor, crystals
Respirations: Rate, pattern, effort, breath sounds
Circulation: Dysrhythmias, blood pressure alterations
Abdomen: Scars, contour, tenderness, bruits
Genitalia: Lesions, scars, discharge

Dark yellow to orange urine may be related to dehydration, some medications, and some foods.

Normally, urine is sterile and slightly acidic. Microscopic examination of the urine is used to assess for cells, casts, bacteria, and crystals. Urine electrolytes and osmolality indicate the kidneys' ability to excrete or conserve electrolytes. Urine osmolality is compared with serum osmolality. If serum osmolality is elevated, the kidneys should conserve water and excrete concentrated urine (i.e., urine with high osmolality). If serum osmolality is low, the kidneys should excrete water and produce dilute urine (i.e., urine with low osmolality). The ratio of urine to serum osmolality should be greater than 1:1. Data reported from a routine urinalysis are summarized in Table 36–2.

URINE CULTURE AND SENSITIVITY. A urine culture permits identification of microorganisms present in the urine. Sensitivity testing determines which antibiotics will be effective against the specific organisms. The first voided urine of the day is preferred for this test. A clean-catch or midstream specimen is obtained. The patient is instructed to cleanse the penis or vulva thoroughly, void a small amount, stop the urine stream, and then void into a sterile container. If catheterization must be done to obtain the urine, the specimen is collected after allowing a small amount of urine to be discarded. The container is capped and immediately sent to the laboratory. If delivery to the laboratory is delayed, the specimen is refrigerated. Culture and identification of the organism or organisms require 24 to 36 hours.

CREATININE CLEARANCE. Creatinine clearance is the best test of overall kidney function. It is an estimate of glomerular filtration rate. This test requires collection of all urine for 12 or 24 hours, as ordered. Normal levels vary for males and females, depending on muscle mass. Values are usually lower in females. A creatinine clearance rate of 100 ml per minute or greater is considered 100% normal. A rate of 50 ml per minute is 50% of normal function.

Urine and serum creatinine levels are compared to determine kidney function. They should be opposite from one another. As one rises, the other falls.

Blood Tests

BLOOD UREA NITROGEN. This test is a general indicator of the kidneys' ability to excrete urea, an end product of protein metabolism. In addition to renal failure, factors that increase blood urea nitrogen (BUN) are a high-protein diet (especially with renal disease), gastrointestinal bleeding, dehydration, and some drugs (aspirin, chemotherapeutic agents, diuretics, gentamicin, lithium carbonate, morphine, steroids, sulfonamides, and tobramycin).

SERUM CREATININE. Creatinine is a waste product of skeletal muscle breakdown. The level of creatinine in the blood is an indication of the kidneys' ability to excrete wastes. Serum creatinine is elevated only in renal disorders and is a better measurement of kidney function than BUN. Unlike BUN, creatinine is not influenced by diet, hydration, nutritional status, or liver function. With normally functioning kidneys, the serum creatinine level is very low and the urine level is high. The normal ratio of BUN to creatinine is 10:1.

SERUM ELECTROLYTES. Serum electrolytes must be monitored in the renal patient because imbalances can have very serious consequences. In renal failure, sodium and potassium levels are elevated and calcium levels are decreased.

Ultrasonography

Ultrasonography (ultrasound) uses sound waves to detect urinary tract malformations as well as cysts, tumors,

TABLE 36-2
URINALYSIS DATA

COMPONENTS	NORMAL VALUES	IMPLICATION OF ABNORMAL VALUES
Color	Light yellow to amber	Dilute, colorless: overhydration, diabetes insipidus, chronic kidney disease Concentrated dark amber: dehydration Red, brown: blood in urine
Appearance	Clear	Cloudy, hazy: bacteria, pus, RBCs
pH	5–7	<5: acidosis, starvation, diarrhea >7: alkalosis, bacteriuria, UTI
Specific gravity	1.005–1.030	<1.005: diabetes insipidus, overhydration, renal disease, severe hypokalemia >1.030: dehydration, diabetes mellitus
Protein	Up to 8 mg/dl; reagent strip negative	>8: exercise, severe stress, fever, renal disease, malignancy
Glucose	Negative	Positive: diabetes mellitus, stroke, Cushing's syndrome, anesthesia, severe stress
Ketones	Negative	Positive: diabetes mellitus, starvation, excessive protein ingestion
Bilirubin	Negative	Positive: liver disease (jaundice)
Microscopic		
RBCs	0–2	>2 (hematuria): kidney trauma, renal disease, anticoagulants
WBCs	0–4	>4: UTI, strenuous exercise
Casts	Negative to occasional hyaline casts	Positive: fever, renal disease, heart failure
Crystals	Negative	Positive: renal stone formation
Bacteria	Negative	Positive: UTI

RBCs, Red blood cells; UTI, urinary tract infection; WBCs, white blood cells.

and renal calculi. Ultrasound may also be used to guide a needle inserted to aspirate specimens from cysts or tumors. Before ultrasound, the patient is usually instructed to drink a certain amount of water and not to empty the bladder. The full bladder enhances visualization of organs and tissues. The procedure is painless and takes only about 15 minutes. The patient lies still while the technician applies lubricant to the abdomen and flank. An instrument called a transducer is then moved over the lubricated skin surface. Images are recorded for study by the radiologist. When the procedure is over, the lubricant is wiped off and the patient is permitted to go to the bathroom to void.

Radiographic Tests and Procedures

FLAT PLATE. A flat plate of the abdomen is also called a KUB (for kidneys, ureters, and bladder) or a plain film. Tumors, malformations, and calculi may be found with this type of radiograph. It provides a general outline of the kidneys, revealing their approximate size and contour. This procedure requires no special preparation or aftercare. It is not done on pregnant patients. It should be scheduled before any other studies that require contrast media.

INTRAVENOUS PYELOGRAM. Also called an excretory urogram, intravenous pyelogram (IVP) permits visualization of the kidneys, ureters, and bladder. It allows assessment of kidney function and structures, ureter size and patency, bladder size and shape, and presence of calculi. The procedure involves the use of a contrast medium, fluoroscopy, and radiography. A contrast medium (an iodine dye) is injected intravenously. Several radiographs are then taken at 5-minute intervals while the dye is concentrated by the kidneys and excreted via the ureters and bladder. The procedure is contraindicated in elderly patients with known renal insufficiency and in patients with diabetes mellitus or multiple myeloma.

Before the procedure, the nurse explains the test to the patient and administers a laxative and enemas as ordered, and the patient has nothing by mouth (NPO) for 8 to 10 hours. The nurse asks about iodine allergy and informs the radiologist if the patient is allergic to iodine. The patient can be told to expect a flushed, warm feeling and a salty taste in the mouth when the dye is injected. The procedures takes about 45 minutes. The only aftercare is to encourage fluids to promote excretion of the dye and to assess for any signs of allergic response to the iodine. Symptoms of an allergic reaction to iodine dye include itching, hives, wheezing, and respiratory distress. The allergic reaction is treated by discontinuing the iodine dye administration, giving antihistamines, and administering cardiopulmonary resuscitation if necessary.

ANGIOGRAM. A renal angiogram permits study of the renal blood vessels. It is used to diagnose renal artery stenosis, aneurysms, vascular tumors, renal cysts, and renal infarctions. In angiography, a catheter is inserted through the femoral artery and threaded into the aorta. A contrast medium is injected into each renal artery, and radiographs are taken as the dye passes through the kidneys.

Patient preparation includes explanation of the procedure and assessment of iodine allergy. If the patient is allergic to iodine, the radiologist must be advised before the procedure. The nurse informs the patient what the procedure involves and to expect a warm sensation when the dye is injected. A consent form must be signed. Preparatory measures usually include a laxative and enemas to cleanse the bowel and nothing by mouth for 8 to 12 hours. Anticoagulants are withheld for 12 to 24 hours before the procedure to reduce the risk of excessive bleeding. Premedications may be ordered to reduce anxiety. The patient is encouraged to void before the premedications are given.

When a patient returns from undergoing angiography, assessments are frequently done to detect signs of blood loss (restlessness, tachycardia, hypotension, decreasing urine output). The catheter insertion site is assessed for bleeding or hematoma. A sandbag or ice bag may be ordered for the insertion site for the first several hours. Peripheral pulses, color of the extremity, and temperature on the side of the arterial puncture are monitored frequently. Complaints of abdominal or flank pain are promptly reported to the physician as they may indicate significant bleeding. The patient may be kept on bedrest for 12 to 24 hours. Intravenous fluids are often ordered, but oral fluids should be encouraged as well.

RENAL SCAN. A renal scan indicates the size, shape, and location of the kidneys; detects renal infarction, atherosclerosis, trauma, or rejection of a transplant; and identifies primary renal disease. An intravenous radioisotope is injected, and radiographs are taken to demonstrate blood flow to each kidney. The test is not done on pregnant women but can be used for patients who are allergic to the iodine dye used for the IVP.

In preparing the patient for the scan, the nurse explains that it takes about an hour and is painless except for venipuncture. The patient can be assured that the dose of radiation is very small and that it is quickly excreted in the urine. After the scan, patients who are able may use the toilet. For incontinent patients, the nurse wears gloves and discards soiled articles in containers for special handling. Pregnant caregivers should not be exposed to these patients for at least 24 hours after the scan.

Invasive Procedures

RENAL BIOPSY. A renal biopsy is performed to obtain a specimen of renal tissue for direct examination. It is usually done to evaluate conditions leading to renal failure. The procedure may be done through open or closed methods. The open method is a surgical procedure. An incision is made in the flank, and a specimen of kidney tissue is excised. The closed procedure involves insertion of a needle under fluoroscopy or ultrasonography to aspirate the tissue specimen. The closed procedure requires patient cooperation. The patient must be able to lie in the prone position with a blanket roll under the lower abdomen for up to 45 minutes. Patients with breathing problems may not be able to tolerate this position or alter their breathing patterns as needed during the procedure.

Before a renal biopsy, clotting studies (prothrombin time, partial thromboplastin time and platelet count) need to be within normal limits and hypertension should be under control. Elevated blood pressure may increase postoperative bleeding. Informed consent is obtained before the procedure. The nurse answers any questions the patient may have and explains the need to have nothing by mouth for 6 hours before the biopsy.

After the biopsy, the patient must be assessed frequently for bleeding. Serious bleeding is not common, but it can occur. A pressure dressing will be in place. It should be inspected each time vital signs are taken. Tachycardia, restlessness, hypotension, and flank pain radiating to the front of the abdomen suggest significant bleeding and should be reported to the physician immediately. The patient is kept on bedrest for 24 hours in a supine position, with a sandbag or blanket roll under the flank area. Hemoglobin and hematocrit are checked 6 and 24 hours after the biopsy. Pink-tinged urine or small amounts of frank blood in the urine are to be expected during the first 24 hours. If bleeding is suspected, the patient is given intravenous fluids to restore fluid volume. Surgery is necessary if bleeding persists. The patient is advised to avoid heavy exercise, lifting, and sports activities for 1 to 2 weeks after a renal biopsy.

CYSTOSCOPY. Cystoscopy is the direct visualization of the interior of the urethra, bladder, and ureteral orifices. The procedure may be done for diagnostic or treatment purposes. As a diagnostic procedure, the cystoscopy allows the physician to observe lesions, locate sources of bleeding, and take biopsy samples. Treatments that can be done with this procedure include cauterization of lesions; removal of calculi, tumors, or foreign materials; implantation of radium seeds; insertion of ureteral catheters; and control of bleeding. A lighted tube called a cystoscope is inserted through the urethra into the bladder under sterile conditions. Local or general anesthesia may be used for the procedure. Retrograde pyelography, which involves injecting dye into the ureters, also can be done during cystoscopy.

Before cystoscopy, the nurse explains the purpose of the procedure and tells the patient that mild to moderate discomfort may be experienced. Informed consent is obtained. Enemas are given, if ordered, before the procedure. The patient may have a liquid breakfast if the test is to be done under local anesthesia but will have nothing by mouth if general anesthesia is planned. Preprocedure medications are usually ordered to reduce anxiety and bladder spasms.

Postprocedure assessment includes intake and output, vital signs (especially temperature), and urine color. The urine will be pink tinged to wine colored after the procedure and should lighten to its usual color within 24 to 48 hours. Back pain, bladder spasms, urinary frequency, and burning on urination are common and may be relieved by warm sitz baths and mild analgesics. Belladonna and opium (B & O) suppositories may be ordered to reduce bladder spasms. Bladder perforation is rare but may be indicated by severe abdominal pain. The patient is encouraged to drink 2 to 3 liters of liquids a day, unless contraindicated. Antibiotics may be ordered for a day before and 2 to 3 days after a cystoscopy.

Urodynamic Studies

Urodynamic studies are performed to determine the physiology of micturition. They are done to assess innervation of the bladder, incontinence, and other variations in urinary patterns. Urodynamic studies measure the rate of urine flow during voiding. The rate of flow is decreased with obstruction or decreased innervation.

CYSTOGRAM AND VOIDING CYSTOURETHROGRAM. The cystogram outlines the contour of the bladder and shows reflux of urine. Reflux is the backward movement of urine from the bladder into the ureters. Cystograms can also help diagnose neurogenic bladders, fistulas, tumors, and ruptured bladders. For a cystogram, a catheter is inserted into the bladder, dye is injected, and radiographs are taken.

A voiding cystourethrogram gives the physician additional information on strictures and uretheral disorders during voiding. The bladder is filled with dye, and radiographs are taken during urination and repeated after urination. This procedure may be embarrassing for the patient. The nurse explains the need for the test and provides as much privacy as possible during the procedure.

CYSTOMETROGRAM. The cystometrogram is used to evaluate bladder tone in the patient with incontinence or with a neurogenic bladder. A catheter is inserted into the bladder, and fluid is instilled until the patient reports the urge to void. When the patient feels urgency, the catheter is removed, the patient voids, and residual urine is measured. Drugs may be given to see if they effectively enhance or relax bladder tone in the individual patient.

Summary

Diagnostic tests and procedures for urinary disorders are summarized in Table 36–3.

COMMON THERAPEUTIC MEASURES

CATHETERIZATION

Catheterization is the introduction of a catheter through the urethra into the bladder for the purpose of removing urine. Catheters are inserted when patients are unable to void as a result of the effects of anesthesia, paralysis, trauma, unconsciousness, or certain surgical procedures. The major concern with catheterization is the potential for introduction of bacteria into the normally sterile bladder. Catheterization is the primary

TABLE 36-3

DIAGNOSTIC TESTS AND PROCEDURES FOR URINARY DISORDERS

TEST/STUDY	PURPOSE/PROCEDURE	PATIENT PREPARATION	POSTPROCEDURE NURSING CARE
Laboratory Studies			
Urine culture and sensitivity	Culture identifies microorganisms in urine. Sensitivity determines which antibiotic will be effective. Normal: no growth.	Have patient collect specimen of first voided urine of day. Instruct in midstream, clean-catch technique. Provide sterile container. Send specimen to lab promptly.	Cap specimen and refrigerate or send to lab promptly.
Creatinine clearance	Estimates glomerular filtration rate. Decreases with renal disease. Normal value: 100 ml/min.	Provide specimen container. Document first void and save all urine for next 24 hr.	
Blood urea nitrogen (BUN)	Indicates kidneys' ability to excrete urea, an end product of protein metabolism. Normal values: 7–18 mg/dl or 2.5–6.3 mmol/L. Increased with impaired renal function, infection, diabetes. Decreased with liver failure, malnutrition, overhydration.	Advise patient that blood specimen will be drawn. Consult agency lab manual to see if patient should be NPO.	Check venipuncture site for bleeding, hematoma.
Serum creatinine	Measures kidneys' ability to excrete waste based on amount of creatinine in blood. Normal values: varies with method used; should be small. Increased with impaired renal function, urinary obstruction, muscle disease. Decreased with muscular dystrophy.	Advise patient that blood specimen will be drawn. Consult agency lab manual to see if patient should be NPO.	Check venipuncture site for bleeding, hematoma.
Serum electrolytes	Detects alterations reflecting inability of kidney to retain or excrete electrolytes. Sodium and potassium elevated and calcium decreased in renal failure. Normal values: see Chapter 11.	Advise patient that blood specimen will be drawn. Consult agency lab manual to see if patient should be NPO.	Check venipuncture site for bleeding, hematoma. Electrolyte imbalances can be life threatening. Check lab reports and notify physician of abnormalities. See Chapter 11 for details on specific electrolytes.
Ultrasound			
Abdominal and renal ultrasound	Uses sound waves to detect cysts, tumors, urinary calculi, urinary tract malformations. Can be used to guide needle insertion for closed biopsy.	Patient may have to drink a specified amount of water so that bladder will be full during ultrasound. Tell patient that procedure is painless. Gel is applied to skin, and an instrument is moved over skin surface.	Wash gel off skin. No special aftercare.
Radiographic Studies			
Flat plate (KUB)	Provides radiographic view of kidneys, ureters, and bladder.	No special preparation. Schedule before studies that use contrast media.	No special care.
Intravenous pyelogram (IVP)	Uses x-rays and fluoroscope to outline kidneys, ureters, and bladder. Uses contrast medium to show urine flow. Detects urinary abnormalities, calculi, and obstructions.	Assess and report iodine allergy. Tell patient that "dye" will be injected and radiographs taken to study urinary tract. A feeling of warmth and a salty taste are expected after injection. Give laxatives and enemas as ordered prior to test. NPO 8–10 hr.	Encourage fluids to flush contrast medium from body. Monitor for signs of iodine allergy: urticaria, rash, nausea, swollen parotid glands. Check injection site for inflammation.
Angiogram	Uses x-rays and contrast medium to examine blood vessels of kidney.	Tell patient that physician will insert catheter into blood vessel (usually in groin) and inject "dye." Radiographs are then taken as dye circulates through kidneys. A warm feeling is expected when dye is injected. Assess and report any iodine allergy. Usual preparation: NPO for 8–12 hr, laxatives and enemas. Anticoagulant drugs usually withheld before test.	Assess for signs of bleeding: tachycardia, dyspnea, restlessness. Check injection site for bleeding. Keep sandbag or ice pack over site as ordered (usually several hours). Monitor pulse, color, and warmth of extremity in which catheter was inserted. Report abdominal or flank pain. Maintain bedrest for 12–24 hr as ordered. Encourage fluids. Measure intake and output.

Table continued on following page

TABLE 36-3

DIAGNOSTIC TESTS AND PROCEDURES FOR URINARY DISORDERS *Continued*

TEST/STUDY	PURPOSE/PROCEDURE	PATIENT PREPARATION	POSTPROCEDURE NURSING CARE
Renal scan	Uses radioisotopes and x-rays to study renal blood flow. Detects infarctions, trauma, atherosclerosis, transplant rejection, some renal diseases.	Contraindicated in pregnancy. Tell patient that isotope will be injected and radiographs taken. Radiation dose is small and quickly eliminated.	No special care unless patient is incontinent. Then, wear gloves to handle urine and change linens. Discard per agency protocol. Continent patients can use toilet. Pregnant caregivers should avoid these patients for 24 hr.
Urodynamic Studies			
Cystogram and cystourethrogram	Uses dye injected into bladder through catheter followed by x-rays to outline bladder and demonstrate reflux of urine from bladder to ureters. For voiding cystourethrogram, bladder and urethra are radiographed during urination. Rate of urine flow is measured.	Tell patient that catheter will be inserted and dye instilled into bladder.	Monitor urine output and vital signs. Encourage increased fluids unless contraindicated. Observe for allergic reaction to dye. Assess for urinary retention.
Cystometrogram	Evaluates bladder tone. Fluid is instilled into bladder through urethral catheter. When patient feels urge to void, catheter is removed. Patient voids, and residual urine is measured. Drugs may be given to test bladder response.	Explain procedure to patient.	Encourage increased fluids unless contraindicated. Monitor intake and output. Administer drugs as ordered for bladder spasms.
Invasive Procedures			
Renal biopsy	Excision of small amount of kidney tissue for examination. May be obtained through incision (open biopsy) or with special needle (closed biopsy).	Physician explains procedure selected. For closed biopsy, patient is positioned prone with rolled blanket under abdomen about 45 min. Be sure reports of clotting studies (PT, PTT, platelets) are on chart. Report elevated blood pressure. NPO as ordered.	Monitor vital signs and dressing for bleeding (tachycardia, restlessness, flank pain radiating to abdomen). Position supine with roll or sandbag under flank area. Bedrest for 24 hr. Assure patient that pink-tinged urine or small amount of blood in urine is expected first 24 hr. Advise patient of no heavy lifting or exercise for 1–2 wk.
Cystoscopy	Uses lighted scope inserted through the urethra to see urethra, bladder, and ureteral openings. Allows diagnosis of problems, removal of bladder calculi, biopsy, some treatments. Local or general anesthesia may be used. Dye may be injected into kidneys through ureters (retrograde pyelography).	Tell patient that procedure is done in operating room or special room under sterile conditions. For local anesthesia, liquids may be allowed. NPO before general anesthesia. Laxatives or enemas as ordered. Give medications as ordered to reduce anxiety and bladder spasms.	Safety precautions first time up, as orthostatic hypotension common. Monitor intake and output, vital signs, urine color. Report severe pain. Give medications or assist with sitz baths as ordered for pain or urinary frequency. Encourage 2–3 L of fluids daily. Tell patient that pink-tinged urine is expected for 1 or 2 days.

NPO, Nothing by mouth; PT, prothrombin time; PTT, partial thromboplastin time.

cause of nosocomial (hospital acquired) infections. Therefore, it is essential that strict aseptic techniques be followed when catheterization is necessary.

Urinary catheters are available in a variety of sizes for adults (generally from the small 12 French to the larger 20 French) and may be of a retaining or nonretaining design. Examples of retaining catheters are the coudé, Foley, Malecot, and Pezzer. Robinson and whistle-tip catheters are nonretaining or straight catheters. Nurses are most familiar with Foley catheters that have either double or triple lumens. Malecot and Pezzer catheters are used most frequently as suprapubic catheters.

Occasionally, patients are catheterized to measure residual urine. This procedure is often part of a bladder training program for patients who have lost control over bladder function. To measure residual volume, the patient must be catheterized immediately after voiding. Less than 50 ml of residual urine is considered normal.

The reader should refer to a fundamentals of nursing textbook for detailed information on the insertion and care of urethral catheters. The following are key points to remember when catheterization is necessary:

1. Catheterize only after other noninvasive measures have failed or when absolutely necessary for diagnostic purposes.
2. Use sterile technique and equipment to insert the catheter.
3. With an indwelling catheter, do the following:
   a. Secure the tubing to the patient's inner thigh (females) or abdomen (males).

b. Handle the catheter gently to avoid trauma to the urethra.
c. Keep the urine collection bag below the level of the patient's bladder.
d. Keep the drainage system closed as much as possible.
e. Provide perineal care twice daily (*Note:* antibiotic ointments are not recommended).
f. Practice good hand washing before and after handling the catheter.

URETERAL CATHETER

A ureteral catheter is threaded through a ureter into the renal pelvis. It can be inserted through the bladder during cystoscopy or through an abdominal incision. A ureteral catheter permits urine to flow through the swollen ureter after traumatic surgery. The catheter is connected to a drainage system, and output is measured frequently. Output from this catheter is recorded separately from other urine output. The nurse makes certain that the catheter is not kinked or clamped, as pressure would build up in the kidney, causing tissue damage. If irrigation is ordered, a maximum of 5 ml of lukewarm, sterile normal saline is instilled slowly because the capacity of the renal pelvis is only 3 to 5 ml. Unless both ureters are completely obstructed, urine continues to drain into the bladder. This urine output must be recorded as well.

NEPHROSTOMY TUBE

When a ureter is completely obstructed, the physician may insert a nephrostomy tube through a flank incision directly into the kidney pelvis. The tube is connected to a drainage system and assessed frequently. Drainage must be continuous, so the nurse must ensure that the tube is not kinked or clamped at any time. Some urine usually leaks around the tube and flows through the flank incision. Sterile dressing changes and skin care are performed as needed. Irrigation with a small amount of sterile normal saline may be ordered. Because of the small capacity of the renal pelvis, only about 5 ml of irrigating fluid is used.

URINARY STENT

A stent is a hollow tube that is placed in a structure to give it support and allow fluid to flow through. A urinary stent may be placed in the ureter to maintain alignment or to provide a route for urine drainage. The stent is inserted by the physician. It may be completely internal or it may extend through the urethra or skin. Several types of stents are available. The double-J stent has one end in the bladder and the other end in the pelvis of the kidney.

UROLOGIC SURGERY

Urologic surgery may be done on any part of the urinary tract. *Nephrectomy* is removal of the kidney because of cancer, massive trauma or bleeding, severe chronic failure with infection, or polycystic kidney disease or for donation. Many types of surgery are used to remove calculi, depending on their location. A surgical opening may be made in the renal parenchyma, renal pelvis, ureter, or bladder. *Lithotripsy* is a noninvasive procedure to break up calculi, but patient care is similar to that of the surgical patient. Bladder surgery may be necessitated by bleeding, functional problems, or cancer. Removal of the bladder is a *cystectomy;* opening of the bladder is a *cystotomy*. Some surgical procedures can be done through a cystoscope, so there is no external incision. Surgical procedures that reroute the flow of urine are called *urinary diversions*.

Preoperative Care

Preparation for urologic surgery includes a complete diagnostic work-up to rule out other medical problems. Fluid status is evaluated, and any imbalances are corrected. Usual preoperative care measures are taken as described in Chapter 14. Bowel cleansing may be ordered before some procedures. If the patient will have a stoma for urine drainage, an enterostomal therapist is usually consulted for patient counseling and teaching.

Postoperative Care

Postoperatively, particular attention is given to urine output, respirations, and bowel function. Output is closely monitored, with drainage from various tubes recorded separately. Output less than 30 ml per hour should be reported to the physician. Flank or abdominal incisions cause pain on deep breathing. The nurse explains the risk of atelectasis and supports the patient to cough and deep breathe. Breath sounds are routinely auscultated to assess lung aeration. Urologic surgery often involves manipulation of the bowel, which can lead to paralytic ileus. Therefore, the return of bowel sounds is monitored, and fluids are withheld until they are present.

DRUG THERAPY

A number of drugs are available to treat urinary tract disorders. Major classifications of commonly used drugs are diuretics, antihypertensives, antibiotics, antacids, stool softeners and laxatives, vitamin and mineral supplements, and synthetic hormones. These classifications, specific drugs, their actions and adverse effects, and nursing interventions are summarized in Table 36–4. Immunosuppressant drugs are addressed separately in Table 36–5.

DISORDERS OF THE URINARY TRACT

URINARY TRACT INFECTIONS

Urinary tract infections (UTIs) are common, especially among women. They can involve any part of the

TABLE 36–4
DRUGS USED TO TREAT URINARY DISORDERS

GENERAL CONSIDERATIONS
1. Drugs are selected carefully because many drugs are nephrotoxic.
2. Drug dosages need to be reduced if renal function is impaired and the drug is excreted in the urine.

DRUGS	USE/ACTION	SIDE EFFECTS	NURSING INTERVENTIONS
Diuretics and Antihypertensives			
Diuretics	Cause kidneys to excrete water and sodium. Lower blood pressure.		Monitor intake and output, blood pressure, weight. Administer in morning to avoid nocturia. (Assess for electrolyte imbalances.) Monitor serum potassium level. Potassium supplements may be ordered except with potassium-sparing drugs.
Osmotic diuretics (mannitol, urea)		Dehydration, electrolyte imbalances.	Monitor injection site for extravasation. Administer only freshly prepared solutions.
Thiazide diuretics (hydrochlorothiazide [HydroDIURIL] metolazone [Zaroxolyn])		Hypokalemia, hypercalcemia.	Monitor diabetics for hyperglycemia. Encourage potassium-rich foods.
Loop diuretics (furosemide [Lasix])		Orthostatic hypotension, hypokalemia, hyponatremia.	Monitor diabetics for hyperglycemia. Encourage potassium-rich foods. Teach patient to cope with orthostatic hypotension.
Potassium-sparing diuretics (spironolactone [Aldactone])		Hyperkalemia. Drowsiness. Gynecomastia in males on long-term therapy.	Safety measures. Assess for hyperkalemia: diarrhea, muscle twitching, dysrhythmias.
Antihypertensives	Lower blood pressure.		Monitor blood pressure. Do not discontinue suddenly. For orthostatic hypotension, teach patients to change position slowly and avoid prolonged standing.
Centrally acting antiadrenergics (methyldopa [Aldomet], clonidine [Catapres])		Drowsiness, hemolytic anemia, liver damage. Rebound hypertension if stopped suddenly.	Administer at bedtime. Safety precautions. Advise patient to discontinue drug only under medical direction.
Peripherally acting antiadrenergics (prazosin [Minipress])		Hypotension (especially with initial dose).	Give first dose or increased dose at bedtime. Teach patient to manage orthostatic hypotension.
Beta-adrenergic blockers (propranolol [Inderal])		Bronchoconstriction, bradycardia, hypoglycemia.	Monitor respirations in asthmatics and COPD patients. Masks symptoms of low blood glucose.
Vasodilators (hydralazine [Apresoline])		Tachycardia, palpitations, headache, lupus-like syndrome.	Report lupus-like signs: fever, sore throat, skin rash.
Phosphate Binders			
Aluminum hydroxide gel (Amphojel)	Binds with phosphate in intestines to prevent absorption. Given to prevent renal osteodystrophy. Raises serum calcium.	Hypophosphatemia: muscle weakness, anorexia, bone pain. Constipation.	Monitor for hypophosphatemia. Record bowel movements. Give laxatives and stool softeners as ordered.

urinary tract and can be acquired through the blood or lymph or may enter through the urethra. Infections are called "ascending" when pathogens move from the urethra to the bladder and "descending" when pathogens travel from the kidney to the bladder. Nosocomial infections are those acquired during hospitalization. Urinary tract infections are the most common nosocomial infections. Most UTIs are bacterial, but they can be caused by viruses, yeasts, and fungi. It is important to treat UTIs in order to prevent renal scarring that can lead to failure. Risk factors for UTI are listed in Table 36–6.

URETHRITIS

Urethritis is inflammation of the urethra. Inflammation may be caused by microorganisms, trauma, or hypersensitivity to chemicals in products such as vaginal deodorants, spermicidal jellies, or bubble bath detergents. The most frequently identified causative microor-

TABLE 36-4
DRUGS USED TO TREAT URINARY DISORDERS *Continued*

DRUGS	USE/ACTION	SIDE EFFECTS	NURSING INTERVENTIONS
Vitamin and Mineral Supplements			
Ferrous sulfate	Treats iron deficiency anemia.	Constipation or diarrhea, dark stools.	Administer on empty stomach with water. Can give liquid with water or fruit juice to disguise taste.
Folic acid	Supplements dietary intake.	Few adverse effects. Occasional hypersensitivity.	
Calcium gluconate	Treats hypocalcemia.	Hypercalcemia.	Monitor blood studies. Administer in divided doses 1 hr after meals.
Hormones			
Recombinant human erythropoietin (epoetin alfa)	Improves red blood cell formation. Reverses anemia. Requires adequate serum iron and ferritin to be effective.	Headache, tachycardia, hypertension, dyspnea, diarrhea, hyperkalemia, nausea, vomiting, clotted vascular access, seizures.	Monitor blood pressure. Contraindicated in uncontrolled hypertension. Dosage is adjusted to maintain hematocrit between 30 and 33%.
Antibiotics			
Sulfonamides			
Sulfisoxazole (Gantrisin)	Treats UTIs.	Drowsiness, dizziness. Agranulocytosis, anemia, thrombocytopenia. Nausea, vomiting, diarrhea. Liver dysfunction. Crystalluria leading to renal tubular damage. Photosensitivity. Allergy. Infertility.	Tell patient urine will be orange. Monitor blood cell counts. Give with full glass of water. Maintain urine output of 1500 ml/day to prevent crystalluria. Have patient avoid excessive sun exposure. Do not give if patient has history of sulfonamide allergy.
Methenamine (Mandelamine)	Antibacterial. Effective only in acid urine. Used to prevent or suppress recurrent UTIs.	Nausea, vomiting, diarrhea.	Give with meals to reduce gastrointestinal effects. Encourage adequate fluids. Discourage large intake of milk products.
Nalidixic acid (NegGram)	Antibacterial. Used for chronic UTIs.	Headache, malaise, vertigo, syncope, confusion, peripheral neuritis, vision disturbances. Nausea and vomiting. Photosensitivity.	Advise patient to avoid prolonged sun exposure. Administer 1 hr before meals unless gastrointestinal upset occurs. Encourage adequate fluids.
Nitrofurantoin (Furadantin, Macrodantin)	Used to treat acute and chronic UTIs.	Dyspnea. Nausea and vomiting. Numbness and tingling of legs.	Administer with food or milk to reduce gastric distress.
Trimethoprim (Trimpex)	Used to treat acute or chronic UTIs. Especially effective against recurrent UTIs in males.	Nausea, vomiting, glossitis. Skin rash.	Tell patient to report skin rash—may be allergic response.

COPD, Chronic obstructive pulmonary disease; UTIs, urinary tract infections.

ganisms are *Escherichia coli, Chlamydia, Trichomonas, Neisseria gonorrhoeae,* and herpes simplex virus type 2.

Signs and Symptoms

Signs and symptoms of urethritis include dysuria, frequency, urgency, and bladder spasms. A urethral discharge may be noted.

Medical Diagnosis

Urethritis is diagnosed based on patient signs and symptoms, urinalysis, and urethral smear.

Medical Treatment

Antimicrobials are used to treat the condition when it is caused by microorganisms. If the patient is sexually active, both the patient and the sexual partner may be treated with antimicrobials to prevent reinfection.

Nursing Care of the Patient with Urethritis

ASSESSMENT. Assessment of the patient with a urologic disorder is outlined in Table 36–1. Important aspects of assessment when a patient has urethritis are comfort, possible causative factors, and understanding of treatment and prevention.

NURSING DIAGNOSIS. The primary nursing diagnoses for the patient with urethritis are the following:

- Acute **Pain** related to tissue inflammation
- **Knowledge Deficit** of cause, treatment, and prevention of urethritis

TABLE 36-5
IMMUNOSUPPRESSANT DRUGS

GENERAL CONSIDERATIONS
1. Patients on immunosuppressants have reduced resistance to infection, so they must be monitored for subtle signs of infection.
2. Protect patients from infections.
3. Teach patients the importance of taking drugs as prescribed and keeping follow-up appointments.

DRUG	USE/ACTION	SIDE EFFECTS	NURSING INTERVENTIONS
Corticosteroids Prednisone (Deltasone) Methylprednisolone (Medrol) Methylprednisolone sodium succinate (Solu-Medrol)	Anti-inflammatory: prevent movement of leukocytes into transplanted tissue	Retention of water and sodium; loss of potassium. Elevated blood glucose. Hypertension. Gastrointestinal bleeding. Mood swings. Psychosis. Infections. Impaired healing.	Monitor intake and output. Assess for fluid and electrolyte imbalances: edema, increased blood pressure, cardiac dysrhythmias, muscle weakness, confusion. Antacids are often ordered to protect stomach.
Antilymphocyte preparations	Coat antigens of transplanted organ so immune system does not recognize them as foreign.	Fever, chills, joint pain, phlebitis, anaphylaxis.	Monitor closely for anaphylaxis, especially with first dose. Check infusion site. Have site changed if evidence of extravasation.
Monoclonal antibodies Muromonab-CD3 (Orthoclone OKT3)	React with T cell antigens and destroy them. Used to treat acute rejection in renal transplant patients.	Fever, chills, headache, tremor, dyspnea. Flushing, anaphylaxis. Nausea, vomiting, diarrhea. Chest pain.	Monitor closely for anaphylaxis, especially with first dose. Monitor for fluid overload. Check infusion site. Have site changed if evidence of extravasation.
T Cell suppressors Cyclosporine (Sandimmune)	Interferes with T lymphocyte activity. Enhances transplant survival with less risk of infection.	Nephrotoxicity (elevated serum creatinine). Fluid retention. Hypertension. Hyperkalemia. Hirsutism. Venous thrombosis. Gingival hyperplasia. Tremors. Seizures. Viral infections. Anemia. Leukopenia. Thrombocytopenia. Anaphylaxis with intravenous administration.	Monitor serum creatinine and electrolytes. Check for edema. Monitor blood pressure. Have epinephrine 1:1000 available during intravenous administration. Report adverse effects to physician. Mix oral form with food or chocolate to disguise unpleasant oiliness.

GOALS. Goals of nursing care are reduced pain and patient's ability to describe treatment and prevention measures.

INTERVENTIONS. Sitz baths are soothing and may reduce the pain of urethritis. The nurse instructs the patient in self-care measures. Females are told to wipe from front to back after toileting and to void before and after sexual intercourse as a means of preventing urethritis. Bubble baths and vaginal deodorant sprays are discouraged. Uncircumcised males are instructed to clean the penis under the foreskin regularly.

EVALUATION. Criteria for evaluating nursing interventions include patient's statement of pain relief and correct patient's description of prevention and treatment.

TABLE 36-6
RISK FACTORS FOR URINARY TRACT INFECTIONS

Female gender
Vaginal infections
Bubble baths and vaginal deodorant sprays
Dehydration
Tight-fitting, synthetic undergarments
Infrequent voiding
First trimester of pregnancy
Trauma during delivery

CYSTITIS

Cystitis is inflammation of the urinary bladder. The most common cause is bacterial contamination. Other factors that increase the incidence of cystitis are prolonged immobility, renal calculi, urinary diversion, and indwelling catheters. Females are more susceptible than males to cystitis because the female urethra is shorter and closer to the vagina and rectum. The longer urethra and antibacterial substances in prostatic fluid are thought to decrease the incidence of UTIs in males.

Signs and Symptoms

Symptoms of cystitis include urgency, frequency, dysuria, nocturia, bladder spasms, incontinence, and low-grade fever. Urine may be dark, tea colored, or cloudy. Fever, fatigue, and pelvic or abdominal discomfort are common. Bladder spasms may be manifested by pain behind the symphysis pubis. Spasms may occur during or after urination.

Medical Diagnosis

A urine specimen is usually obtained for urinalysis, culture, and sensitivity.

Medical Treatment

Cystitis is treated with antibiotics that concentrate in the urine. The physician may order an antibiotic while awaiting the results of the culture and sensitivity. The order will be changed if the results show that another antibiotic would be more effective. A mild analgesic such as acetaminophen is useful for relieving discomfort. Phenazopyridine (Pyridium) may be ordered for 2 to 3 days to decrease discomfort and bladder spasms. Belladonna and opium suppositories may be ordered to relax urinary sphincters and allow more complete bladder emptying. The use of suppositories is preferred to catheterization.

Nursing Care of the Patient with Cystitis

ASSESSMENT. The general assessment of the patient with a urinary tract disorder is outlined in Table 36–1. The nursing assessment of the patient with cystitis focuses on patient symptoms, possible causative factors, and understanding of treatment and prevention.

NURSING DIAGNOSIS. Priority nursing diagnoses are the following:

- **Pain** related to tissue inflammation
- **Knowledge Deficit** of cause, treatment, and prevention of cystitis

GOALS. Goals of nursing care are reduced pain and patient's ability to explain and carry out self-care measures.

INTERVENTIONS. The nurse administers analgesics as ordered for pain. Warm sitz baths are also comforting. Patient teaching emphasizes the need for a high fluid intake, instructions about prescribed drugs, and measures to avoid future infections. The patient needs to consume at least 3 liters of fluid per day and void frequently. Fluids should be consumed during the day and at night so that the urinary tract is continually flushed. The patient is instructed to complete the entire course of prescribed antibiotics. The nurse also advises the patient that phenazopyridine turns urine an orange-red color that may stain clothing.

PHARMACOLOGY CAPSULE

Instruct patients to complete the entire course of antimicrobial therapy to ensure that the infection is eradicated.

PREVENTION. It is especially important to teach the patient measures to reduce the risk of future infections. Hygiene practices described in the nursing care of the patient with urethritis are also appropriate for patients with cystitis. Women are taught that a moist environment encourages bacterial growth. Cotton undergarments keep the perineum drier than synthetic materials. Tight-fitting clothing in the perineal area should be avoided. Showers are preferred over tub baths. Cranberry juice is sometimes recommended to make the urine more acidic and discourage bacterial growth. There is some disagreement about the value of the juice and the amount needed to be effective, but it is a safe, simple measure to try. Patients are taught to avoid coffee, tea, carbonated beverages with caffeine, and apple, grapefruit, orange, and tomato juices as these irritate the bladder. Many physicians instruct cystitis patients to return for follow-up urinalyses to evaluate the effects of treatment. The nurse reinforces this instruction.

EVALUATION. Criteria for evaluating the effectiveness of nursing interventions include patient's statement of pain relief and patient's description of correct self-care measures.

PYELONEPHRITIS

Pyelonephritis is inflammation of the renal pelvis. It may affect one or both kidneys. Acute pyelonephritis is most frequently caused by an ascending bacterial infection, but it may be blood borne. Chronic pyelonephritis may be persistent or recurrent and results in renal parenchymal damage. It is most often the result of reflux of urine from inadequate closure of the ureterovesical junction during voiding. Progressive scarring results in atrophy of the affected kidneys. Hypertension and renal ischemia develop. Chronic pyelonephritis is usually caused by recurrent acute pyelonephritis. Chronic pyelonephritis may lead to renal insufficiency. If the patient progresses to renal atrophy and end-stage renal disease, dialysis or transplantation are the only means of keeping the patient alive.

Signs and Symptoms

Signs and symptoms of acute pyelonephritis include high fever, chills, nausea, vomiting, and dysuria. Severe pain or a constant dull ache occurs in the flank area. The patient with chronic pyelonephritis often complains of bladder irritation, chronic fatigue, and a slight aching over one or both kidneys.

Medical Treatment

The goal of treatment for pyelonephritis is to prevent further damage. Antibiotics, urinary tract antiseptics, analgesics, and antispasmodics may be ordered. Long-term antibiotic therapy may be prescribed for repeated acute infections or chronic infection. Additional medications may be needed to treat hypertension. Dietary salt and protein restriction may be imposed on the patient with chronic disease. If an obstruction or congenital anomaly is present, it may be surgically removed. Urine samples must be obtained for follow-up cultures to determine whether the infection has been resolved.

Nursing Care of the Patient with Pyelonephritis

ASSESSMENT. The general assessment of the patient with a urinary tract disorder is outlined in Table 36–1.

When assessing the patient with pyelonephritis, the nurse records the presence of related signs and symptoms, a history of previous urinary tract disorders, any predisposing factors, and the effects of the infection on daily activities.

NURSING DIAGNOSIS. Nursing diagnoses typically include the following:

- **Pain** related to inflammation
- **Activity Intolerance** related to fatigue
- **Fluid Volume Deficit** related to vomiting, anorexia
- **Altered Nutrition: Less than Body Requirements** related to anorexia, nausea, vomiting
- **Knowledge Deficit** related to treatment and future prevention of pyelonephritis

GOALS. Goals of nursing care for the patient with pyelonephritis include pain relief, completion of activities of daily living without excessive fatigue, adequate fluid and food intake, and understanding of the treatment and prevention of pyelonephritis.

INTERVENTIONS

Pain and Activity Intolerance. Analgesics are given as ordered when the patient reports pain. Antibiotics and antiseptics do not provide direct pain relief but eventually help by eliminating the cause of the inflammation. The pain and systemic symptoms of infection contribute to fatigue and activity intolerance. The nurse helps by assisting with activities of daily living and by scheduling activities to allow for periods of uninterrupted rest.

Fluid Volume Deficit and Altered Nutrition. Adequate food and fluids are very important for the patient with pyelonephritis. If nausea and vomiting occur, the nurse informs the physician and administers antiemetics as ordered. Food intake and fluid intake and output are recorded. If the patient is unable to take the recommended 2 to 3 liters of fluid daily, intravenous fluids may be prescribed. The nurse must be careful when "forcing fluids" to prevent circulatory overload. The older patient, unable to handle a suddenly increased fluid volume, may develop congestive heart failure. Possible signs of this complication are bounding pulse, rising blood pressure, dyspnea, and edema.

Knowledge Deficit. If the patient is discharged with medications, the nurse reviews the drugs and stresses the importance of taking them as prescribed. The patient is encouraged to seek follow-up evaluation and to report suspected recurrence to the physician immediately. Patients with chronic pyelonephritis must be adequately prepared for self-care after discharge. The teaching plan emphasizes how and why to take prescribed medications, limitations on physical activity and exercise, the importance of adequate fluid intake, and any prescribed dietary alterations.

EVALUATION. Criteria for evaluating the effectiveness of nursing care are patient's statement of pain reduction or relief, improved activity tolerance, balanced fluid intake and output, maintenance of body weight, and patient's ability to describe prescribed treatment correctly.

POLYCYSTIC KIDNEY DISEASE

Polycystic kidney disease is a hereditary disorder. Grape-like cysts replace normal kidney tissue (Fig. 36–7). The disease usually appears by age 40.

Signs and Symptoms

The bilateral cysts enlarge, compress functional renal tissue, and eventually result in renal failure. This slowly progressive disorder begins with dull, aching lower back or flank pain. Chronic infection contributes to the progressive loss of function. The kidneys lose the ability to concentrate urine. Hypertension and congestive heart failure develop. Often, cystic lesions are found on other organs. As the cysts enlarge, they create pressure on other organs.

Medical Treatment

Supportive treatment is recommended to preserve kidney function, treat UTI, and control hypertension. As the disease progresses, kidney function decreases and end-stage renal disease develops. Dialysis and transplantation are treatment options at that point. Genetic counseling is advised for these patients.

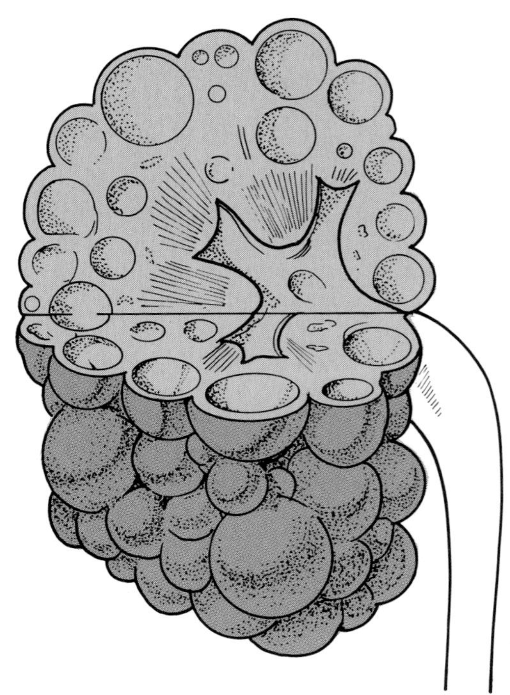

FIGURE 36-7
Polycystic kidney.

Nursing Care of the Patient with Polycystic Kidney Disease

See nursing care of patients having renal surgery, dialysis, and transplantation.

ACUTE GLOMERULONEPHRITIS

Glomerulonephritis is inflammation of the capillary loops in the glomeruli. Although there are many types of acute glomerulonephritis, the most common type follows a streptococcal infection of the respiratory tract. The group A *β-hemolytic streptococcus* is most often implicated. An antigen-antibody reaction results in inflammation of the glomeruli. Scar tissue forms in the glomeruli. Glomerular permeability increases, and proteins are found in the urine. The glomerular filtration rate decreases and nitrogenous wastes accumulate in the blood. Both BUN and serum creatinine rise. Tea-colored urine is noted, and urine output decreases. Peripheral and periorbital (around the eyes) edema is evident. Mild to severe hypertension occurs as glomerular filtration decreases and hypervolemia (increased blood volume) results. Anemia may result from the loss of red blood cells. Acute glomerulonephritis may resolve or progress to a chronic form of the disease.

Medical Diagnosis

Diagnosis is based on patient assessment and laboratory tests. A urinalysis is done to detect proteinuria and red blood cell casts. Blood studies measure BUN, creatinine, and albumin. Streptococcal antibody tests indicate whether the patient has had a streptococcal infection. Renal ultrasound, renal biopsy, or both also may be ordered.

Medical Treatment

Acute glomerulonephritis is treated with diuretics and antihypertensive medications. Antibiotics are indicated if there is evidence of streptococcal infection. In the acute phase, bedrest is ordered to prevent or treat heart failure and severe hypertension from fluid overload. Activity restriction is usually continued as long as urine tests show blood or protein, or blood pressure is elevated. Fluids, sodium, potassium, and protein may be restricted until there is sufficient recovery of kidney function. When fluid overload has been corrected, moderate activity is permitted, but the patient still needs sufficient rest to allow the kidneys to heal. Since approximately one half of patients with acute glomerulonephritis experience progressive renal insufficiency, consistent follow-up is needed. If renal failure develops, dialysis is necessary. Patients who progress to chronic glomerulonephritis develop end-stage renal disease in 1 to 30 years. (See section on chronic renal failure.)

Nursing Care of the Patient with Acute Glomerulonephritis

ASSESSMENT. Assessment of patients with urinary tract disorders is outlined in Table 36–1. This section identifies the data that are especially relevant when the patient has acute glomerulonephritis. Assessment includes the documentation of signs and symptoms, recording of recent infections (especially sore throat or skin lesion), and changes in urine characteristics.

During the physical examination, the nurse inspects the area around the eyes, the extremities, and the abdomen for fluid accumulation. Tissue turgor is assessed. Respiratory and cardiac function is evaluated for evidence of fluid volume excess: dyspnea, tachycardia, hypertension. Accurate intake and output records and daily weights help to assess the kidney's ability to excrete excess fluid.

NURSING DIAGNOSIS. Nursing diagnoses for the patient with acute glomerulonephritis include the following:

- **Fluid Volume Excess** related to renal dysfunction
- **Activity Intolerance** related to retention of chemical wastes, fatigue, prescribed bedrest
- **Self-Care Deficit** related to prescribed bedrest, lack of knowledge of treatment measures
- **Anxiety** related to possibility of chronic illness

GOALS. Goals for nursing care are restoration of fluid balance, improved activity tolerance, performance of self-care measures, and reduced anxiety.

INTERVENTIONS

Fluid Volume Excess. The nurse maintains careful records of fluid intake and output. Patients and family members are instructed in the importance of accurate records. If fluids are restricted, the nurse explains the need for the restriction and helps the patient plan the timing and amounts of allowed fluids. Fluid restriction can be very distressing. It is better to present fluids in small containers than to serve an ounce or two in a large glass. If the patient has edema, special skin care is needed. Taut, swollen tissue is easily damaged and heals slowly. The patient must be handled carefully and encouraged to change positions often to prevent pressure.

Activity Intolerance. Activity intolerance may be due to infection, accumulated toxins, or anemia. During the acute illness, activity is discouraged to allow the kidneys to heal. The nurse explains the importance of rest for recovery. Activities must be scheduled to allow for periods of uninterrupted rest. Of course, the patient on bedrest is at risk for complications of immobility: skin breakdown, pneumonia, muscle weakness, joint stiffness, and thrombus formation. Therefore, the nurse has the patient change position, cough and deep breathe, and gently exercise joints periodically. Nursing measures to prevent the complications of immobility are described in Chapter 19.

Self-Care Deficit. The nurse provides assistance with activities of daily living. The patient needs to understand how rest, dietary restrictions, and medications promote recovery. The need for follow-up care is emphasized. When the patient is discharged, the nurse reinforces the importance of reporting any signs of recurrence such as changes in urine characteristics or edema. The patient is instructed to increase activities gradually as the edema and fatigue resolve.

Anxiety. The patient with acute glomerulonephritis may be very concerned about the possibility of developing a chronic, life-threatening condition. The nurse can explore the patient's thoughts and feelings about the condition. Helpful interventions may be in the form of empathetic listening, factual information, or referrals to other professionals.

EVALUATION. Criteria for evaluating the success of nursing interventions include balanced intake and output, patient's statement of improved activity tolerance, patient's adherence to treatment regimen, and patient's statement of lessened anxiety.

URINARY TRACT OBSTRUCTIONS

RENAL CALCULI

The condition characterized by formation of calculi in the urinary tract is called *lithiasis*. It is common, especially in men. There is a familial tendency toward calculi and a high incidence of recurrence.

Pathophysiology

Most calculi are precipitations of calcium salts (calcium phosphate or calcium oxalate), uric acid, magnesium ammonium phosphate (struvite), or cystine. All these substances are normally found in the urine. Factors that influence the development of calculi are hydration, diet, urine components, and activity. A consistent fluid intake of less than 1500 ml per day may contribute to the formation of calculi. When a person is dehydrated, the kidneys conserve water, causing urine to be concentrated. Calculi are more likely to form in concentrated urine. A diet that is high in calcium or purines or one that affects urine pH also can contribute to calculus formation. The fact that most people who consume a high-calcium diet do not develop calculi suggests that some people are predisposed to the condition and others are not. Other factors that contribute to calculi are hyperparathyroidism, immobility, and excessive intake of vitamins C or D or antacids. Most calculi originate in the kidney (nephrolithiasis) and travel through the ureters into the bladder (urolithiasis).

Urine is normally acidic, with a pH ranging from 5 to 7. Some substances tend to precipitate, causing calculus formation in acid urine; others precipitate in alkaline urine. The kidneys excrete substances that are believed to inhibit formation of calculi. A decrease in these substances may contribute to calculus formation. Calculus formation is also enhanced by urinary stasis, UTI, the presence of crystals, and scar tissue formed by previous injury to the urinary tract.

Signs and Symptoms

The patient's chief complaint is pain. The location and characteristics of the pain may provide clues to the site of the calculus. Dull flank pain suggests a calculus in the renal pelvis or stretching of the renal capsule from urine retention (hydronephrosis). If a calculus lodges in a ureter, the patient usually has excruciating pain in the abdomen that radiates to the groin or the perineum. The ureter goes into spasm (colic) in an attempt to move the calculus along and relieve the obstruction. Nausea, vomiting, and hematuria may accompany the pain. The patient may also show signs and symptoms of UTI.

Medical Diagnosis

The presence and location of calculi in the urinary tract may be confirmed by KUB, IVP, or ultrasound. A routine urinalysis will probably be ordered as well. If a calculus can be obtained, its composition can be determined by laboratory analysis.

Medical Treatment

The majority of calculi are passed spontaneously. Ambulation and adequate hydration facilitate the passage of many calculi. Narcotic analgesics and antispasmodics are ordered to relieve the intense, colicky pain. Antibiotics are ordered if infection is present or if internal manipulation of the calculus is necessary. If the calculus does not pass and symptoms continue, several procedures may be used to destroy or remove it.

LITHOTRIPSY. Lithotripsy (shattering of the calculus) may be accomplished by a variety of means. Extracorporeal shock wave lithotripsy uses a device called a lithotriptor to deliver a series of shock waves to disintegrate the calculi. The patient is placed in a tank of water, or a water-filled cushion is placed on the abdomen or flank. General or epidural anesthesia is given because the series of 1000 to 1500 shocks is painful. A fluoroscope is used to monitor the procedure. The lithotriptor bombards the area where the calculi are located. The shock waves break the calculi into small pieces. The procedure takes 30 to 45 minutes. The pulverized calculi are excreted in the urine in 1 to 4 weeks. Bruising and hemorrhage are possible complications of lithotripsy (Fig. 36–8).

Newer methods are being sought that will deliver lower doses of shock waves, eliminate the need for general anesthesia, and localize the shock waves to the calculi. The use of laser beams also is being explored. If calculi are not passed spontaneously or with a lithotriptor, surgery may be necessary.

LITHOTOMY. The incision of an organ or a duct to remove a calculus is a lithotomy. A nephrolithotomy is the surgical procedure used if the calculus is in the kidney. The removal of a calculus from the renal pelvis is a pyelolithotomy. A ureterolithotomy is removal of a calculus from a ureter (Fig. 36–9).

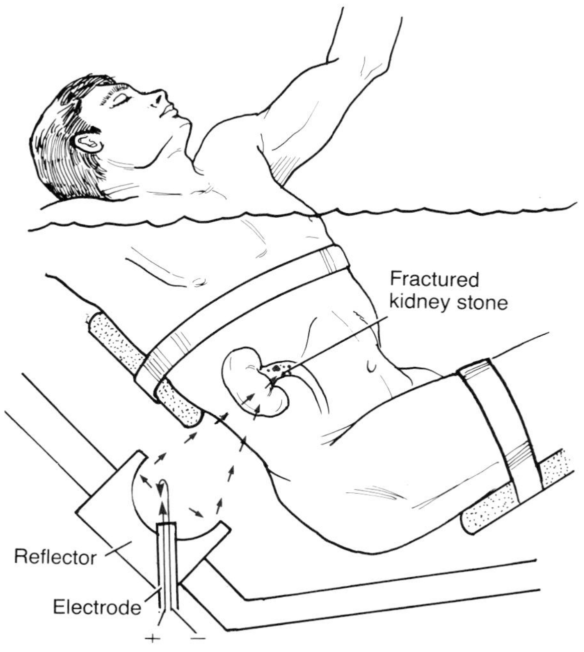

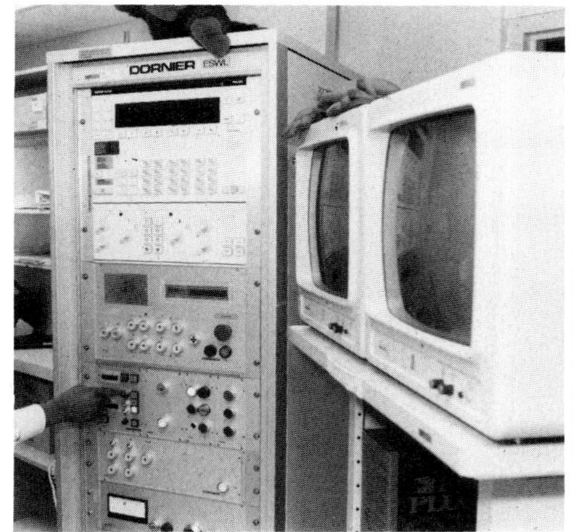

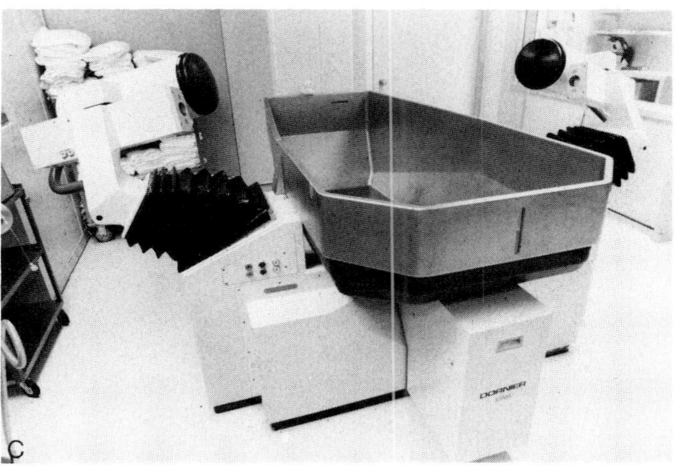

FIGURE 36-8

A, Extracorporeal lithotripsy. *B* and *C*, A lithotriptor. (*B* and *C*, Photographs by Stephen Matteson, Jr.)

Prevention

An important medical goal is to prevent recurrence of renal calculi. Long-term medical management of these patients includes a high fluid intake to keep urine dilute, dietary restrictions for specific elements (i.e., calcium and purines), regular exercise, and occasionally medications to alter the urine pH. Medications are less effective than dietary management.

Nursing Care of the Patient with Renal Calculi

ASSESSMENT. Assessment of the patient with a urinary tract disorder is discussed earlier in this chapter (also see Care Plan: The Patient With Renal Calculi). When the patient has known or suspected urinary calculi, the nurse pays particular attention to a personal or family history of calculi. The patient's usual fluid intake and diet, including vitamin and mineral supplements, are described. If pain is present, the nurse describes the location, severity, and nature of the pain. Any changes in urine amount or characteristics also are recorded. The temperature is taken to detect the presence of fever. A nurse who is trained in physical examination palpates and percusses the flanks and the abdomen, noting the presence of pain, tenderness, or a distended bladder.

NURSING DIAGNOSIS. Nursing diagnoses for the patient with urinary calculi may include the following:

- **Pain** related to obstruction, trauma, and renal colic
- **Altered Urinary Elimination** related to obstruction
- **High Risk for Fluid Volume Deficit** related to anorexia, nausea, and vomiting
- **Knowledge Deficit** of prevention and treatment of calculi

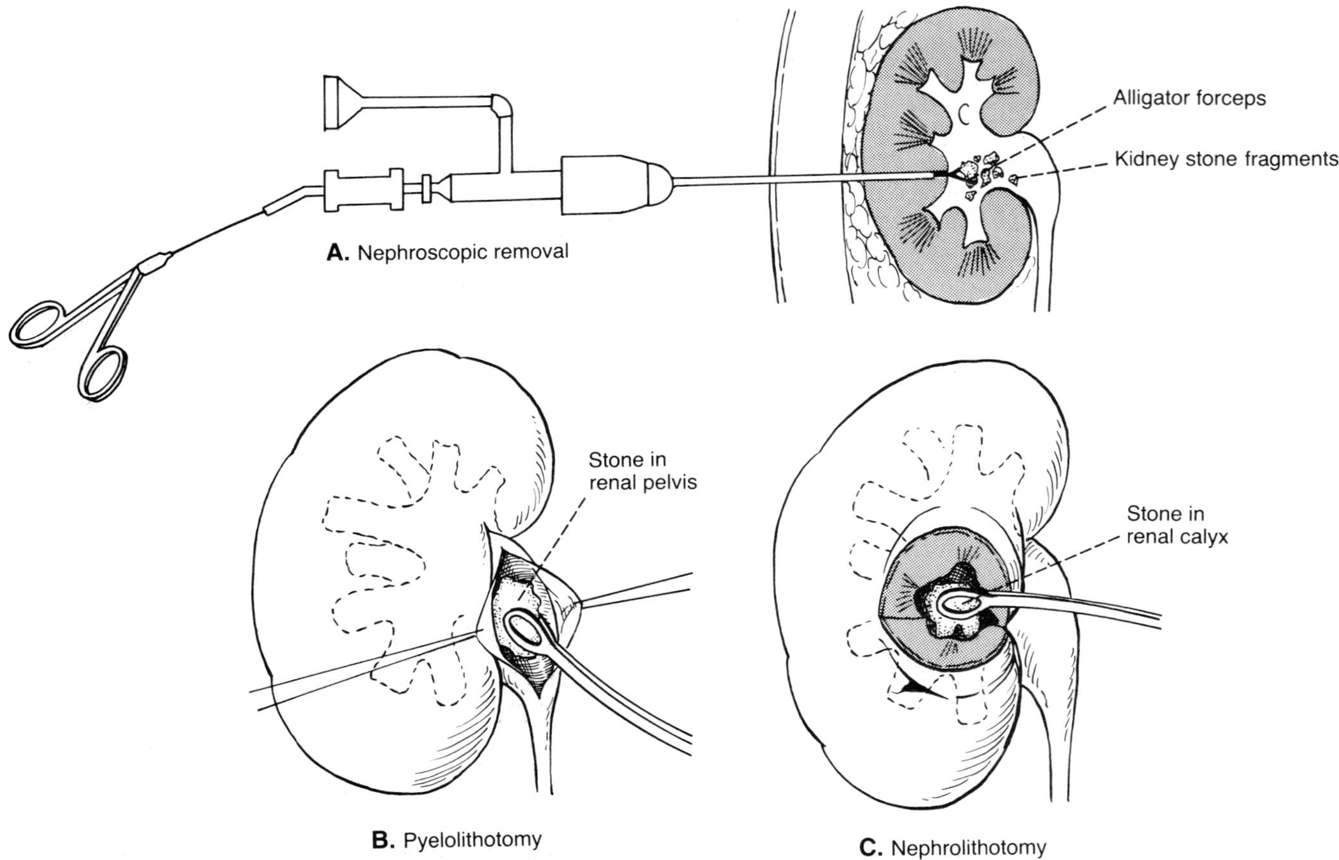

FIGURE 36-9

Surgical procedures for renal calculi. *A*, Nephroscopy; *B*, pyelolithotomy; *C*, nephrolithotomy. (Adapted from Black, J. M., & Matassarin-Jacobs, E. [1993]. *Medical-surgical nursing: A psychophysiologic approach* [4th ed., p. 1528]. Philadelphia: W. B. Saunders.)

If surgery is performed, additional nursing diagnoses are the following:

- **High Risk for Infection** related to invasive procedures
- **Decreased Cardiac Output** related to blood loss
- **Ineffective Breathing Patterns** related to painful incision

GOALS. Goals of nursing care are pain relief, normal urine output, normal fluid balance, and patient's understanding of treatment and prevention of calculi. Additional goals for the surgical patient are absence of infection, normal pulse and blood pressure, and effective breathing patterns.

INTERVENTIONS

Pain. Because calculi in the urinary tract can be excruciating, pain relief is a major nursing concern. Initially, it may be necessary to administer morphine intravenously to relieve the pain. Antispasmodics also are usually ordered to reduce the smooth muscle spasms in the ureters. If pain is intermittent, the patient may be permitted to ambulate when comfortable. Ambulation may actually help the calculus move through the urinary tract. Of course, safety precautions are needed if narcotics have been given. The pain may resolve suddenly if the calculus moves into the bladder or is passed through the urethra.

Altered Urine Elimination. Depending on its size and location, a calculus may obstruct urine flow. If urine backs up into the kidney, hydronephrosis may develop. Hydronephrosis is distention of the kidney with urine, a condition that can cause permanent damage (Fig. 36–10). The nurse maintains accurate records of fluid intake and output and reports low output to the physician. In addition, urine is usually strained and examined for calculi. If any calculi are recovered, they should be sent to the laboratory for analysis.

High Risk for Fluid Volume Deficit. Renal colic is often accompanied by nausea and sometimes vomiting. Antiemetics should be given promptly as ordered. The physician will probably order intravenous fluids to maintain dilute urine and to flush the urinary tract. A fluid intake of 4 liters per day is usually recommended. Large volumes of fluids like this must be given carefully to the older patient, who can easily develop fluid volume excess. Vital signs must be monitored for signs of circulatory overload (tachycardia, bounding pulse, dyspnea, edema, hypertension).

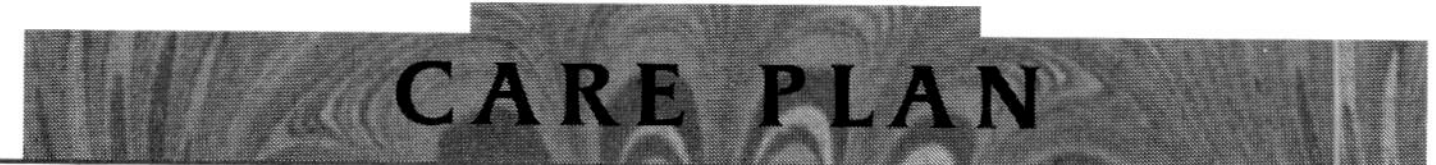

The Patient with Renal Calculi

ASSESSMENT

Health History: Mr. Frank Scarpino, age 43, was admitted with excruciating abdominal pain radiating to the groin. He experienced nausea and vomiting with the pain. The review of systems revealed a history of hypertension controlled with verapamil, 200 mg per day. He has also had repeated urinary tract infections, most recently 1 month ago. At that time, he was treated with antibiotics and the symptoms subsided. Radiologic studies detected a calculus lodged in the right ureter. Lithotripsy was done under general anesthesia to shatter the calculus. Mr. Scarpino returned to his hospital room 3 hours ago. He is complaining of soreness in the right lower abdomen.

Physical Examination: Mr. Scarpino is fully oriented but drowsy. Vital signs: temperature, 100°F orally; pulse, 88; respiration, 20; blood pressure, 138/74. His abdomen is soft but tender. There is no bladder distention. He voided 350 ml pink-tinged urine. Intravenous fluids are infusing at 150 ml per hour.

NURSING DIAGNOSIS	GOALS AND OUTCOME CRITERIA	INTERVENTIONS
Acute pain related to obstruction, trauma, renal colic.	Patient will report pain relief and will appear more relaxed.	Assess pain characteristics. For severe pain, administer morphine as ordered. Administer antispasmodics as ordered. Assist with ambulation when permitted to promote passage of calculus fragments. Milder pain may be treated with nonnarcotic analgesics. Position changes, backrubs, relaxation, and imagery may be used to enhance analgesia. Document effects of pain relief interventions.
Altered urine elimination related to obstruction.	Patient's urine output will be approximately equal to fluid intake.	Measure all fluid intake and output. Report low output to physician. Strain all urine to collect calculi fragments. Send fragments to laboratory for analysis. Maintain intravenous fluids.
High risk for fluid volume deficit related to NPO status, nausea, and vomiting.	The patient will be adequately hydrated as evidenced by moist mucous membranes, dilute urine, and vital signs consistent with patient's norms.	Administer intravenous fluids as ordered. Assess for fluid volume deficit: hypotension, tachycardia, sticky mucous membranes, concentrated urine. Encourage oral fluids when permitted. Administer antiemetics as ordered for nausea and vomiting.
Ineffective breathing pattern related to abdominal pain, splinting.	Patient's breath sounds will be normal throughout the lung fields.	Assess respiratory status: rate, effort, breath sounds. Encourage deep breathing and coughing every 2 hours until fully ambulatory.
Decreased cardiac output related to blood loss.	Patient's cardiac output will remain normal as evidenced by vital signs consistent with patient's norms and by absence of tachycardia, hypotension, or restlessness.	Assess the abdomen and groin area for bruising—some is expected. Note red color and increased viscosity of urine associated with bleeding. Report increased redness. Monitor vital signs to detect decreasing cardiac output: tachycardia, restlessness, hypotension.
Knowledge deficit of prevention and treatment of calculi, self-care after lithotripsy.	Patient will describe self-care after lithotripsy and measures to prevent recurrence of calculi.	Tell the patient that the fragments are usually passed in the urine over a period of several weeks and may cause some pain. Administer antibiotics as ordered and emphasize importance of treating

Care Plan continued on following page

The Patient with Renal Calculi *(Continued)*

NURSING DIAGNOSIS	GOALS AND OUTCOME CRITERIA	INTERVENTIONS
		any new UTIs to reduce the risk of calculi formation. Advise patient to consume 3 to 4 liters of fluid daily unless the physician prescribes less. Fluids should be taken around the clock to prevent concentration during the night. If any dietary restrictions are imposed, request a dietary consult to explain them to the patient.

Postoperative Care. Preoperatively, the patient needs to have the expected procedure explained and any questions answered. Goals of postoperative care are maintenance of urine drainage, prevention of UTI, and prevention of pulmonary and circulatory complications.

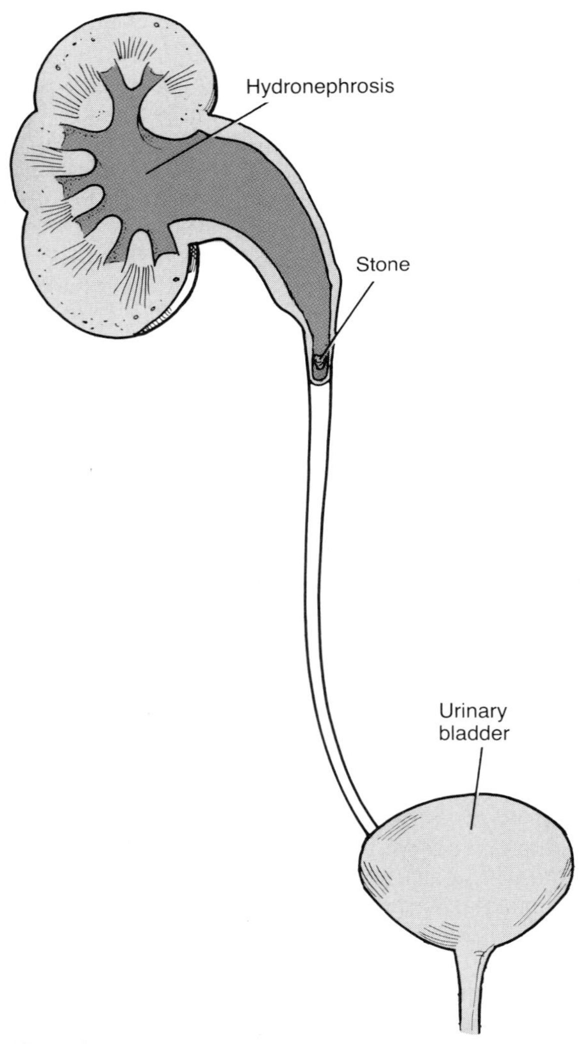

FIGURE 36-10
Hydronephrosis caused by ureteral obstruction.

High Risk for Infection. The patient is apt to have drains, catheters, a ureteral stent (to splint the ureter until it heals), or a combination of these. Each tube is connected to its own closed drainage system. Tubes must be positioned for free flow of urine at all times. Accurate account must be kept of drainage from each tube. If the patient has a flank incision, the area around the dressing must be checked frequently for drainage, as urine tends to leak from the incision. A large amount of serosanguineous drainage is normal immediately after surgery. In about 2 days, the drainage changes to serous. Frequent dressing changes using sterile technique may be required. In some cases, an ostomy appliance is used to accumulate drainage and to permit accurate measurement of the drainage.

Some patients have nephrostomy tubes placed directly in the kidney. The tube is placed for drainage or for instillation of irrigating fluid. It also diverts urine flow from the ureter until adequate healing has occurred. If irrigations are ordered, strict aseptic technique should be followed and not more than 5 ml of warm sterile normal saline used at a time.

Decreased Cardiac Output. The patient is at risk for the same postoperative complications as any surgical patient. The nurse should be especially alert for any signs of excessive bleeding, infection, or pulmonary complications. To detect bleeding, the nurse inspects the dressing and drainage hourly for the first 24 hours. Bright bleeding, excessive serosanguineous drainage, increasing pulse, restlessness, or decreasing blood pressure are reported to the physician immediately. Indications of infection such as odor, cloudy drainage, or temperature above 100°F also should be reported. Measures to reduce the risk of infection include maintaining closed drainage systems, changing wet dressings promptly, and use of strict aseptic technique when handling tubes or dressings.

Ineffective Breathing Patterns. The nurse must monitor the patient's pulmonary status carefully. A flank incision makes taking a deep breath very painful. The patient is assisted to turn, cough, and deep breathe at least every 2 hours. An incentive spirometer helps determine how much the patient is able to inflate the lungs. When the patient coughs, the incision needs to be splinted with pillows or folded blankets. For the first 1 or 2 postoperative days, analgesics administered before turning, coughing, and deep breathing make these activities more comfortable. Adequate fluid intake thins respiratory secretions and makes them easier to expectorate. Early and frequent ambulation promotes improved respiratory function. All of these efforts help prevent atelectasis and pneumonia, a primary treatment goal.

Prevention. When the patient is discharged, the nurse reinforces the need to continue to consume 4 liters of fluid daily unless contraindicated. The fluid needs to be consumed over the 24-hour period so that urine does not become concentrated at night. The patient is advised to drink 2 glasses of water before bed and another 2 glasses when awakening at night to void. This pattern should be followed for life to reduce the risk of calculus formation in the future. If the physician has prescribed a special diet or dietary restriction, the nurse provides instructions or has the dietitian do so.

EVALUATION. Criteria for evaluating the effects of nursing interventions include patient's statement of pain relief, balanced intake and output, and accurate patient's description of prevention and treatment of calculi. The outcomes for the surgical patient should also include absence of signs and symptoms of infection (fever, cloudy urine, elevated white blood cells), pulse and blood pressure consistent with the patient's norms and clear breath sounds throughout the lung fields.

UROLOGIC TRAUMA

The kidneys sustain 50% of all urologic injuries. Trauma may be penetrating or blunt. Penetrating injuries most often result from knives or guns. Blunt trauma occurs when a force is applied to the abdominal wall and the energy is diffused into the abdominal cavity. Examples of blunt force are motor vehicle accidents, contact sports injuries, falls, and intentional injuries. Blunt injuries to the kidneys produce lacerations or contusions. The ureters are rarely injured with blunt trauma. They are most often disrupted by penetration and require surgical anastomosis. The bladder is rarely injured by blunt trauma if empty. If the bladder is full, it may rupture with blunt trauma. The urethra is most apt to be injured in males because of its unprotected anatomic location.

When blunt trauma is suspected, the patient is observed for bruising on the abdomen or in the flank area. The nurse assesses for signs of shock (tachycardia, restlessness, hypotension, pallor), pain, and a palpable abdominal or flank mass. The presence of bruises over the flank and lower back that occur with retroperitoneal bleeding is called Grey Turner's sign.

The physician may order a KUB, urography, computed tomography, or ultrasound to further determine the extent of injury. Diagnostic peritoneal lavage may be performed to determine whether there is bleeding in the peritoneal cavity. A positive finding necessitates surgery to find and eliminate the source of bleeding.

The most frequent indication of urologic trauma is hematuria. It is best if the patient can void, but this may not be possible with other injuries. Before catheterizing a patient with suspected trauma, the nurse carefully inspects the urethral meatus. If there is blood in or around the meatus, a urologist should perform the catheterization or insert a suprapubic catheter.

If the injury is not severe, there is little bleeding, and there are no signs of shock, the patient is observed and closely monitored. More severe injuries most likely require surgery to repair damage. Postsurgical care of these patients is similar to the care of the patient with a nephrectomy, urinary calculi, or cystectomy.

CANCERS OF THE URINARY SYSTEM

Care of the patient with cancer is covered in Chapter 23. This section focuses on the specific needs of the patient with cancer of the urinary tract.

RENAL CANCER

Malignancies of the kidney account for 3% of all reported cancers. Eighty percent of renal malignancies are adenocarcinomas, which primarily affect males 55 to 60 years of age. Less common squamous cell carcinomas of the renal pelvis affect males and females equally.

A renal tumor may reach considerable size before it is detected. Renal malignancies metastasize to the liver, lungs, long bones, and other kidney. Direct extension of the tumor may be found in the ureter. Early symptoms are anemia, weakness, and weight loss. Painless, gross hematuria is the classic symptom, but it generally occurs in the advanced stage. A dull ache in the flank area also is a late symptom.

Medical Diagnosis

The physician may be able to palpate a mass in the flank area. Diagnostic tests and procedures to study the mass may include excretory urography, retrograde pyelography, ultrasound, arteriography, computed tomography, magnetic resonance imaging, and renal biopsy. Care of the patient undergoing these procedures is detailed in Table 36–3.

Medical Treatment

Radical nephrectomy is the treatment of choice for renal cancer. Removal of a kidney is a nephrectomy. Radical nephrectomy involves removal of the kidney and its adjacent tissue, adrenal gland, renal artery and vein, and local lymph glands. Prior to nephrectomy, the renal artery may be occluded to reduce the blood supply to the tumor. In general, renal tumors are not responsive to radiation or chemotherapy, but radiation is sometimes used as a palliative measure for inoperable cancer. Currently, researchers are studying the use of biologic response modifiers in the treatment of bladder cancer. Interferon-α has produced encouraging results in some studies.

Nursing Care of the Patient with Renal Cancer

ASSESSMENT. Nursing assessment of the patient with a urologic disorder is outlined in Table 36–1. When a patient has a suspected or confirmed renal malignancy, there may be very few signs and symptoms. The nurse inquires about weakness, fatigue, and any changes observed in the urine. The patient's emotional state, usual coping strategies, and support systems are explored.

Preoperative Care. General preoperative nursing care is discussed in detail in Chapter 14. Before nephrectomy, the patient's primary nursing diagnoses are ineffective individual coping related to potentially fatal disease and knowledge deficit of tests, procedures, and effects of nephrectomy. The goals of nursing care are for the patient to feel emotionally prepared for the surgery and to understand what is being done and what to expect.

Thorough explanations of diagnostic tests and preoperative teaching provide needed information. The patient can be assured that one functioning kidney can sustain adequate kidney function. Tests are done to confirm that the unaffected kidney functions adequately before a nephrectomy. It should be noted that older patients are more likely to have renal insufficiency. They may eventually need renal dialysis after nephrectomy. The teaching plan includes what to expect in the postoperative period and how to turn, cough, and deep breathe. Serum and urine laboratory tests are usually ordered to serve as baseline data for postoperative comparison. Other preoperative care is the same as that for any other major surgery.

Postoperative Care. Common aspects of postoperative care are covered in Chapter 14. After nephrectomy, the nurse monitors vital signs to detect fluid volume alterations related to blood loss or fluid retention. Intake and output are recorded as another measure of fluid balance and renal function. Drains and tubes are checked routinely to ensure proper function. Dressings are monitored for drainage. Once the dressings have been removed, the wound is assessed for intactness and signs of infection (excessive redness or swelling, purulent drainage). The patient's comfort level is assessed. Breath sounds and bowel sounds are auscultated. The nurse anticipates some emotional distress and encourages the patient to express thoughts and feelings about cancer.

NURSING DIAGNOSIS. In the postoperative period, the nursing diagnoses are the following:

- **Pain** related to incisional tissue trauma
- **High Risk for Fluid Volume Deficit** related to dehydration, blood loss
- **Ineffective Breathing Patterns** related to proximity of incision to diaphragm
- **High Risk for Injury** related to decreased peristalsis caused by bowel manipulation during surgery
- **High Risk for Infection** related to break in skin
- **Ineffective Individual Coping** related to diagnosis of cancer
- **Knowledge Deficit** of postoperative self-care and future treatment regimen

GOALS. The goals of nursing care after surgery for urologic cancer are pain reduction or relief, adequate fluid volume, effective breathing, absence of abdominal distention, absence of signs and symptoms of infection, effective coping, and patient's statement of postoperative restrictions.

INTERVENTIONS

Pain. The nurse obtains a complete description of the patient's pain. Incisional pain is intense at first and deserves prompt administration of prescribed analgesics. Because of the patient's position in surgery, there may be muscle aches in the opposite side and flank area. Medication can be supplemented with position changes and back rubs. Other comfort measures are described in Chapter 16.

High Risk for Fluid Volume Deficit. Intravenous fluids are given initially. The physician normally orders about 3 liters of fluid daily. Accurate intake and output records must be kept. At first, the urine may be measured every 1 to 2 hours. If less than 30 ml is produced in an hour, the physician is notified. When the patient is able, daily weights are an even better measure of fluid balance. Blood urea nitrogen, serum creatinine, serum electrolytes, and urine specific gravity are assessed and compared with preoperative values.

The nephrectomy patient must also be monitored for bleeding. The dressing is checked frequently for drainage. The nurse is careful to check *under* the patient since blood flows to the most dependent area. Sometimes, the dressing is "dry and intact" but the patient is lying in a pool of blood.

Ineffective Breathing Patterns. The location of the flank incision causes pain with expansion of the thorax. Patients tend to protect the area by not breathing deeply. This may lead to pneumonia and atelectasis. It is especially important to have the patient turn, cough, and deep breathe every 1 to 2 hours. The nurse helps by supporting the incision during respiratory exercises. An incentive spirometer is used to encourage deeper inspiration. As soon as ambulation is permitted, the patient is assisted out of bed. The time and distance walked are gradually increased.

High Risk for Injury. Anesthesia and manipulation of abdominal organs cause temporary cessation of peristalsis in the intestines. Until peristalsis returns, the patient is not permitted to take anything by mouth. If peristalsis does not return within 3 to 4 days, the patient is said to have paralytic ileus. Because paralytic ileus is fairly common after nephrectomy, a nasogastric tube may be inserted and attached to suction during surgery. Suction keeps the stomach empty, reducing the risk of nausea and abdominal distention. The return of peristalsis is detected by active bowel sounds and the passage of flatus (gas). The nurse auscultates the abdomen for bowel sounds and observes for abdominal distention. Ambulation promotes the return of peristalsis.

High Risk for Infection. During dressing changes, strict aseptic technique is used. Montgomery straps may decrease irritation from the adhesive tape if frequent dressing changes are required.

Ineffective Individual Coping. The patient facing cancer fears the possibility of death, mourns the loss of an organ, and may dread additional cancer therapy. The nurse can help by encouraging the patient to talk and clarify concerns, listening empathetically, providing requested information, and referring the patient to expert counselors. Usual coping strategies and sources of support are explored. Chapter 23 provides additional detail on nursing care of the cancer patient.

Knowledge Deficit. Before discharge, the patient is cautioned not to lift or participate in other strenuous activities for 8 weeks. Contact sports are prohibited for life because trauma to the remaining kidney could eliminate all kidney function.

EVALUATION. Evaluation of the effectiveness of nursing interventions is based on the patient's statement of pain relief, normal blood pressure and tissue turgor, clear breath sounds, active bowel sounds, absence of fever, statement of lessened anxiety, and correct description of treatment and self-care.

BLADDER CANCER

Cancer of the bladder is the most common malignancy of the urinary tract. It occurs most often in men 50 to 70 years of age. The ureteral orifices and the bladder neck are the most frequent sites of bladder cancer. Over the years, chemical agents have been suspected as carcinogens. The tars found in smoking tobacco, aniline dyes found in industrial compounds, and tryptophan have all been implicated in the development of bladder cancer.

Signs and Symptoms

The most frequent symptom of bladder cancer is painless, intermittent hematuria. Other symptoms include bladder irritability; infection, with dysuria, frequency, and urgency; and decreased stream of urine.

Medical Diagnosis

When the patient's signs and symptoms suggest bladder cancer, the physician may order a urinalysis, IVP, and computed tomography scan. Cystoscopy may also be done to visualize the bladder and permit biopsy of any observable lesions. Details of these tests and procedures and nursing implications are provided in Table 36–3.

Medical Treatment

Bladder malignancies respond more favorably to chemotherapy than do kidney tumors, but surgery is the treatment of choice. The type of surgery depends on whether the cancer is superficial, invasive, or metastatic. Superficial cancers involve only the bladder mucosa or submucosa, or both. Superficial lesions with low recurrence rates may be treated with cystoscopic resection and fulguration or with laser photocoagulation. Cystoscopic resection is the removal of tissue through a cystoscope with a special cutting instrument. Fulguration is the use of electric current to burn and destroy tissue. Laser photocoagulation is the use of an intense beam of light (argon laser) to destroy tissue.

Two other surgical procedures for bladder cancer are segmental bladder resection and radical cystectomy. A segmental bladder resection is done for a single, primary tumor too large to remove by cystoscopic resection. It involves removal of the tumor and adjacent bladder muscle, a procedure that decreases the size of the bladder. A radical cystectomy is removal of the entire bladder and adjacent structures with diversion of the ureters. This procedure is reserved for malignancies that are untreatable with less conservative measures. This is very extensive surgery, and an optimal state of health before surgery is desirable. Radiation or chemotherapy may be done before surgery.

URINARY DIVERSION. When the bladder must be removed completely, urine must be allowed to drain through another route, called urinary diversion. There are several types of urinary diversions: ileal and sigmoid conduits, ureterosigmoidostomy, ureteroileosigmoidostomy, ureterostomy, and nephrostomy. These diversions are illustrated in Figure 36–11.

To form an ileal conduit, a portion of the ileum is resected from the small bowel. The ureters are implanted in the ileum, one end of the ileum is closed, and the open end is implanted on the abdominal surface as a stoma. Urine is excreted through the ileal conduit rather than through the urethra. A urinary drainage pouch is attached to the skin to collect the urine. A sigmoid conduit is formed by the same procedure except that a section of sigmoid colon instead of ileum is used. Ureterosigmoidostomy and ureteroileosigmoidostomy are anastomoses of one or both ureters to the intestine so that urine is eliminated with the feces. A ureterostomy brings the ureter to the abdominal surface, where urine is eliminated through a stoma. A nephrostomy is the placement of a tube in the kidney so that urine may drain through the tube into an external collection device. Detailed information about urinary diversion is presented in Chapter 36.

Nursing Care of the Patient with Bladder Cancer

ASSESSMENT. Assessment of the patient with possible or confirmed bladder cancer includes a complete description of urinary signs and symptoms. Fatigue and weight loss are significant and should be noted. The health history may reveal use of tobacco or exposure to carcinogenic chemicals. The patient's emotional state, coping strategies, and sources of support are assessed.

Preoperative Care. In addition to the common nursing care described in Chapter 14, important preoperative nursing diagnoses for the patient facing segmental resection for cancer may be fear related to life-threatening diagnosis and ineffective individual coping related to

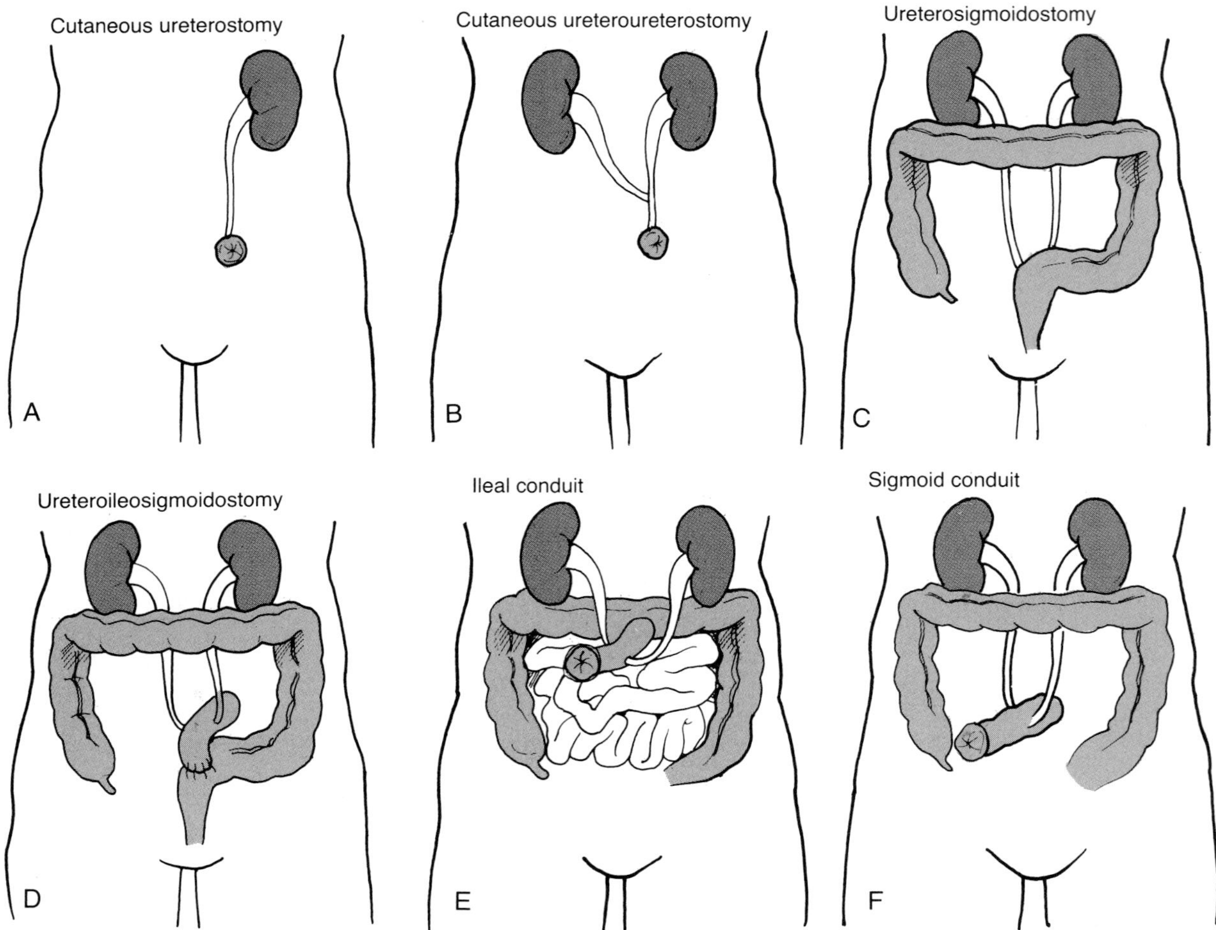

FIGURE 36-11

Urinary diversion. *A,* Cutaneous ureterostomy; *B,* cutaneous ureteroureterostomy; *C,* ureterosigmoidostomy; *D,* ureteroileosigmoidostomy; *E,* ileal conduit; *F,* sigmoid conduit. (Modified from Ignatavicius, D. D., & Bayne, M. V. [1991]. *Medical-surgical nursing: A nursing process approach* [pp. 1872–1875]. Philadelphia: W. B. Saunders.)

lifestyle change. The nurse's goals are reduced fear and effective coping strategies. To accomplish these goals, the nurse explores the patient's fear and provides information and encouragement. The thought of having cancer is frightening, and nurses must educate the public that it is often curable. Coping strategies are assessed and resources provided as needed. The patient needs support to accept the diagnosis and follow through with the treatment.

The patient having radical cystectomy faces a more difficult adjustment—that of permanent urinary diversion. The patient needs to be prepared psychologically as well as physically to deal with a change in body image. The enterostomal therapist is a valuable resource to both the nurse and the patient in preparing for this surgery. The therapist selects the stoma site with the patient. The patient may be advised to wear a water-filled pouch for several days before surgery to help ensure proper stoma placement. If the patient would like to talk to someone who has had a cystectomy, this can often be arranged through a local chapter of the American Cancer Society.

Preoperative care for an ileal or sigmoid conduit includes thorough preparation of the intestinal tract. Bowel preparation requires several days. The patient begins with a low-residue diet and then a clear-fluid diet. Oral neomycin, an antibiotic that is not absorbed from the intestinal tract, is administered to reduce bacteria in the bowel. Enemas also are administered as ordered before surgery.

Evidence of effective preoperative nursing interventions is patient's expression of reduced fear and patient's use of realistic problem solving.

Postoperative Care. Postoperative assessment includes vital signs, intake and output, patency of tubes, bowel sounds, comfort, and appearance of the drainage, stoma, and wound.

NURSING DIAGNOSIS. Priority nursing diagnoses after bladder surgery may include the following:

- **Pain** related to tissue trauma
- **Altered Urinary Elimination** related to urinary diversion

- **Impaired Skin Integrity** related to surgical incision
- **High Risk for Infection** related to tissue trauma
- **High Risk for Injury** related to absence of peristalsis secondary to bowel manipulation during surgery
- **Knowledge Deficit** of postoperative self-care

Additional nursing diagnoses such as body image disturbance and knowledge deficit of stoma care are appropriate if the patient has ostomy surgery. These are discussed in Chapter 24.

GOALS. Nursing goals are reduced pain, unobstructed urine flow, well-healed surgical incision, absence of infection, absence of abdominal distention, and knowledge of self-care.

INTERVENTIONS. Routine postoperative nursing care aimed at the prevention of complications includes turning, coughing, and deep breathing. Leg exercises and early ambulation are especially important because lymph nodes are excised and this contributes to edema of the legs.

Pain. Prescribed analgesics and other comfort measures are employed to control pain.

Altered Urine Elimination. Urethral and suprapubic catheters are inspected and care provided as detailed earlier in this chapter. Urine should be free of sediment, blood, or casts. Once the catheters are removed, the patient who has had a segmental resection is encouraged to void frequently. Bladder capacity will increase up to 250 to 300 ml over several months.

If a patient has had a radical cystectomy, the nurse inspects the stoma for inflammation and irritation. Details of stoma care are provided in Chapter 24.

Impaired Skin Integrity. The surgical incision is monitored to ensure that it is healing without increasing redness or swelling or purulent drainage. Wound care is provided as ordered or per agency protocol. Sites of urine drains and the stoma also must receive care to prevent skin irritation and breakdown.

High Risk for Infection. These patients are at risk for infections in the surgical incisions, drain sites, and urinary tract. The nurse monitors the patient's vital signs, blood work, and wounds for evidence of infection (fever, elevated white blood cell count, and foul odor). Strict aseptic technique is used when providing wound care.

High Risk for Injury. Oral fluids are withheld until bowel sounds provide evidence that peristalsis has returned. Intravenous fluids are administered as ordered. When oral intake is permitted, an adequate fluid intake (2500–3000 ml daily) is encouraged.

Knowledge Deficit. Patient teaching must begin in the early postoperative period because the patient needs to learn self-care before discharge. It includes wound care, signs of infection, care of any type of urinary diversion, and activity restrictions as prescribed by the physician. The enterostomal therapist is an invaluable resource for the person who has a stoma.

EVALUATION. Measures of successful nursing interventions are patient's statement of reduced pain and relaxed expression; urine output equal to intake; intact wound without signs of infection; absence of temperature elevation; active bowel sounds; and patient's verbalization of correct self-care measures. For the patient with urinary diversion, the nurse also evaluates adaptation to altered body image and ability to care for the stoma. The patient should demonstrate the ability to care for the stoma and be able to identify significant signs and symptoms that should be reported to the physician.

RENAL FAILURE

Any condition that decreases blood flow to the kidneys may impair renal function and result in renal failure. Renal failure is classified as acute or chronic based on onset and reversibility. Acute renal failure has a rapid onset (1–7 days) and is usually reversible. Chronic renal failure has a slow onset (months to years) and is characterized by progressive, irreversible damage.

ACUTE RENAL FAILURE

Causes

Causes of renal failure can be prerenal, intrarenal, or postrenal. Prerenal failure results from decreased blood flow to the glomeruli. A systolic blood pressure of 70 or greater is necessary to sustain glomerular filtration. If the systolic pressure drops below 70 and is not corrected, renal failure may develop.

Intrarenal failure may be caused by nephrotoxic agents, kidney infections, occlusion of intrarenal arteries, or direct trauma to the kidney parenchyma. Antibiotics (particularly the mycins), heavy metals (lead and mercury), cleaning compounds, pesticides, and poisonous mushrooms may be toxic to the kidneys. Pyelonephritis, glomerulonephritis, renal tuberculosis, and polycystic kidney disease are examples of kidney conditions that may lead to kidney failure. The arteries in the renal parenchyma may become narrowed as a result of atherosclerosis, hypertension, nephrosclerosis, or blood components (sickled red cells, hemoglobin, or myoglobin). Trauma from motor vehicle accidents, contact sports injuries, and other direct blows also may be intrarenal causes of failure.

Postrenal causes of renal failure are obstructions beyond the kidneys that cause urine to back up. Ureteral calculi and benign prostatic hypertrophy are examples of postrenal causes of failure.

Patients at risk for acute renal failure include those having major surgery, experiencing major trauma, or receiving large doses of nephrotoxic drugs. These patients should have their blood pressures and fluid balances assessed more frequently than usual. Older people are also at risk for acute renal failure because they are less able to adapt to alterations in fluid balance or cardiac output. Renal function should always be assessed with any acute condition in the older patient. Early detection and treatment may significantly decrease the death rate from acute renal failure.

Stages of Acute Renal Failure

The four stages of acute renal failure are onset, oliguria, diuresis, and recovery.

ONSET STAGE. The onset stage is short (1–3 days) and characterized by increasing BUN and serum creatinine with normal to decreased urine output. The primary treatment goal during this stage is reversal of failing renal function to prevent further damage.

OLIGURIC STAGE. During the oliguric stage, the urine output decreases to 400 ml per day or less. The serum values for BUN, creatinine, potassium, and phosphorus increase. Serum calcium and bicarbonate decrease. The oliguric stage follows the onset stage and continues for up to 14 days. Urine specific gravity becomes fixed at 1.010 (normal range, 1.005–1.030), indicating the inability of the tubules to concentrate urine. The patient becomes hypervolemic, meaning that the blood volume is greater than normal. Urine osmolality decreases and serum osmolality increases as waste products are retained.

DIURETIC STAGE. The diuretic stage begins when urine output exceeds 400 ml per day and may rise above 4 liters per day. Despite the production of large quantities of urine, few waste products are excreted, and wastes accumulate in the blood. Toward the end of the diuretic stage, the kidneys begin to excrete BUN, creatinine, potassium, and phosphorus and retain calcium and bicarbonate. This is an indication of return of kidney function.

RECOVERY STAGE. As renal tissue recovers, serum electrolytes, BUN, and creatinine return to normal. This recovery stage lasts 1 to 12 months. If complete recovery does not occur, the patient may develop renal insufficiency or chronic renal failure. Renal insufficiency is indicated by loss of approximately 80% of function. It is possible to lead a relatively normal life with renal insufficiency unless there are other illnesses that place an additional burden on kidney function.

Medical Treatment

The primary goal of treatment for acute renal failure is to prevent further damage. Supportive measures aim to control symptoms and to prevent complications. Support measures include fluid and dietary restrictions, restoration of electrolyte balance, and dialysis if needed. Additional treatment depends on the cause of the failure.

DRUG THERAPY. Oliguria is treated with diuretics, most often an osmotic diuretic like mannitol or a high-ceiling diuretic like furosemide (Lasix) or ethacrynic acid (Edecrin). Hyperkalemia, which typically accompanies oliguria, is treated aggressively since it can be life threatening. Drugs given intravenously to lower serum potassium include hypertonic glucose and insulin, sodium bicarbonate, and calcium gluconate. Sodium polystyrene sulfonate (Kayexalate), given orally or rectally, also lowers serum potassium.

PHARMACOLOGY CAPSULE

Oliguria may be treated with diuretics such as mannitol or furosemide.

DIET. Dietary modifications for acute renal failure are based on consideration of serum electrolytes and urea. Sodium and potassium allowances are individually determined. Adequate carbohydrates are provided to prevent the breakdown of fat and protein. Essential amino acid supplements may be ordered. If the patient's nutritional needs are not being met by oral intake, total parenteral nutrition may be instituted.

FLUIDS. Daily fluid needs are generally calculated by adding 500 ml to the previous day's fluid output. The extra 500 ml represents the daily insensible loss. Since the oliguric patient may have an output of only 400 ml in a day, the next day's fluid allowance would be 400 ml plus 500 ml, for a total of 900 ml.

DIALYSIS. If conservative measures fail to maintain adequate urine output, dialysis is indicated. A cannula placed in the femoral vein can be used for temporary dialysis. If the cannula is left in place between dialysis treatments, the patient must be immobile. If the cannula is removed and replaced repeatedly, however, there is a risk of hematoma formation. An alternative is to use a subclavian cannula that can be left in place between treatments. The disadvantage of leaving the cannula in place is that the risk of infection increases.

HEMOFILTRATION. Hemofiltration is another option for treating the patient in acute renal failure. This procedure is also called continuous arteriovenous hemofiltration. A femoral or subclavian cannula is connected to tubing that contains a blood filter and a collection device. The patient's blood flows through the tubing. Excess fluids, electrolytes, and wastes are filtered into the collection device. The blood is then returned to the patient. The procedure is typically carried out continuously over 2 to 5 days.

Nursing Care of the Patient in Acute Renal Failure

ASSESSMENT. Complete assessment of the patient with a urinary disorder is summarized in Table 36–1. For the patient in acute renal failure, monitoring fluid status is critical. Intake and output records must be carefully kept. Daily weights are an effective means of assessing changes in fluid status (500 ml of fluid weigh ~1 pound). To be useful, daily weights must be done at the same time each day, using the same scale, and with the patient wearing the same amount of clothing. Because hypervolemia (fluid volume excess) is a major problem during the oliguric stage, the nurse must assess for signs and symptoms of impending heart failure: hypertension, bounding pulse, edema, cough, dysrhythmias.

Electrolyte imbalances can include alterations in serum potassium, sodium, calcium, phosphate, and magnesium. Signs and symptoms of each of these imbalances are discussed in Chapter 11. General assessment of electrolyte balance includes cardiac rate and rhythm, neuromuscular status, edema, and mental status. The acutely ill patient must also be monitored for signs and symptoms related to immobility: pressure sores, impaired circulation, constipation, and atelectasis.

One final area of assessment is the patient's understanding of the condition and its treatment. Fears, anxiety, coping strategies, and sources of support are identified.

NURSING DIAGNOSIS. Specific nursing diagnoses vary with the stage of acute renal failure but may include the following:

- **Fluid Volume Excess** related to impaired kidney function (oliguric stage) or **Fluid Volume Deficit** related to high-output renal failure (diuretic stage)
- **Decreased Cardiac Output** related to fluid and electrolyte imbalances
- **Anxiety** related to life-threatening illness
- **Disuse Syndrome** related to immobility
- **Knowledge Deficit** of condition, treatment, and self-care

GOALS. The nursing goals for the patient in acute renal failure include normal fluid and electrolyte balance, normal cardiac output, reduced anxiety, patient's ability to care for self, and absence of complications of immobility.

INTERVENTIONS

Fluid Volume Excess. The nurse assesses and documents fluid status on an ongoing basis. In the oliguric stage, fluid is likely to be restricted. Fluid restrictions are explained and reinforced. The fluid allowance during the oliguric stage can be very limited. Measures to help the patient cope with fluid limitations include considering patient preferences in fluid selection and carefully planning fluid intake throughout waking hours. Nurses must remember to plan for fluids needed to take medications. When only a few ounces of fluids are allowed at a time, a small juice cup should be used rather than a large glass that is only one quarter full. This creates an illusion of volume that may make the patient feel less deprived. To obtain patient cooperation, it is essential for the patient and family to understand the importance of adhering to the fluid restriction.

Diuretics are given as ordered, and the patient is monitored for adverse effects. A fluid challenge of normal saline may be rapidly infused while diuretics are given to promote improved renal perfusion.

Decreased Cardiac Output. In the diuretic stage, patients produce large volumes of dilute urine. Fluid volume deficit becomes a possibility. The nurse is concerned about cardiac status because the heart rate must increase to make up for the diminished blood volume. Eventually the heart may fail. Oral and intravenous fluids are given as ordered with careful monitoring of output at the same time.

Anxiety. Anxiety is understandable when a vital organ fails. The patient may fear death or chronic illness, with the potential for financial ruin, loss of vitality, and dependence on medical care. The nurse provides honest information to questions about renal failure and its treatment. Details about the prognosis should be referred to the physician.

The patient in acute renal failure may have a complete recovery. This may take up to 1 year. Unfortunately, some do not recover but develop chronic renal failure. Those patients who do not improve need special support in learning to accept and deal with this major health deviation.

Disuse Syndrome. The patient with acute renal failure is very ill and may be immobilized. Therefore, the nurse must attend to prevention of complications of immobility as well as to the acute renal problem. This includes skin care, turning, coughing, deep breathing, leg exercises, and measures to promote bowel elimination. Care of the immobilized patient is described in Chapter 19.

Knowledge Deficit. The acutely ill patient is given basic information about the disease, diagnostic tests and procedures, and treatments. The nurse explains the reasons for interventions such as fluid restrictions, turning, deep breathing, and leg exercises. As the patient improves, patient teaching includes fluids, diet, drug therapy, activity, and signs and symptoms that should be reported to the physician (dyspnea, edema, fever).

EVALUATION. Criteria for evaluating the outcomes of nursing interventions for the patient in renal failure are absence of edema and dyspnea, normal serum electrolyte values; pulse and blood pressure consistent with patient's norms; patient's statement of decreased anxiety; absence of skin breakdown and constipation, breath sounds clear to auscultation; and patient verbalization of condition, treatment, and self-care.

CHRONIC RENAL FAILURE

When 90 to 95% of kidney function is lost, the patient is considered to be in chronic renal failure. Chronic renal failure is characterized by azotemia (increased nitrogen waste products, BUN and creatinine, in the blood). Uremia is the term used when the condition advances to the point that the kidneys are unable to maintain fluid and electrolyte or acid-base balance. Uremia is also called end-stage renal disease. All of the causes of acute renal failure listed earlier may lead to chronic renal failure. In addition, chronic renal infections may predispose the patient to progressive renal failure. The most frequent causes, however, are hypertension, diabetes mellitus, and atherosclerosis.

Signs and Symptoms

AZOTEMIA. The first function lost in chronic renal failure is the ability to concentrate urine. This results in an increase of waste products in the blood, despite producing large amounts of dilute urine. As the disease progresses, urine output typically declines until very little to no urine is produced.

Blood urea nitrogen is an approximate estimate of the glomerular filtration rate. It is affected by protein breakdown. Normal BUN ranges from 10 to 20 mg per dl. When BUN reaches or exceeds 70 mg per dl, dialysis is needed to reduce it.

Serum creatinine is a waste product of skeletal muscle breakdown. It is a more reliable measure of kidney function than BUN. It is not affected by diet, hydration, hepatic function, or metabolism. Normal serum creatinine is 0.5 to 1.5 mg per dl. A serum creatinine level that is twice normal reflects a 50% loss of function. When the value reaches or exceeds 10 times normal or greater, 90% of function has been lost. The kidneys are able to adapt to a loss of up to 80% of function. The kidney hypertrophies (increases in size) in an attempt to maintain function.

Creatinine clearance (a urine test) is the best indicator of renal function. It is ordered less frequently than serum creatinine, however, because it requires collection of all urine in a 12- or 24-hour period. Normal creatinine clearance exceeds 100 ml per minute.

HYPERKALEMIA. The primary means of potassium excretion is through the kidneys. As kidney function fails, potassium is retained. Hyperkalemia is the most life-threatening effect of renal failure. The normal range for serum potassium is 3.5 to 5 mEq per liter. Elevated serum potassium interferes with normal cardiac function, causing cardiac dysrhythmias. The patient becomes apathetic and confused and may have nausea, abdominal cramps, muscle weakness, and numbness of the extremities. Serum potassium greater than 6 mg per dl requires cardiac monitoring. Peaked and elevated T waves, widened QRS complexes, and flat to absent P waves may be noted. If the serum potassium is not reduced, the patient may develop bradycardia (pulse <50/min) or asystole (no heartbeat).

Hyperkalemia is treated with intravenous glucose and insulin or with sodium bicarbonate. These drugs drive potassium back into the cells, reducing the serum potassium level. They are used as temporary emergency measures. Kayexalate, administered orally or rectally, exchanges sodium for potassium and eliminates potassium in the feces. The most frequently used method of reducing elevated serum potassium is dialysis.

HYPOCALCEMIA. Diseased kidney tissue lacks the enzyme that activates vitamin D. Without active vitamin D, calcium absorption from the bowel decreases. The body tries to compensate by shifting calcium from the bones into the blood. Serum phosphate binds with calcium, further depleting calcium levels. The normal serum calcium level is 9 to 11 mg per dl or 4.5 to 5.5 mEq per liter. Abnormally low serum calcium is called hypocalcemia. Patients with hypocalcemia experience tingling sensations, muscle twitches, irritability, and tetany. Tetany is sustained, painful muscle contraction. Hypocalcemia is treated with calcium supplements, active vitamin D, and phosphate binders. Phosphate binders such as aluminum hydroxide gel should be administered with meals but not with other medications. Side effects of phosphate binders include hypophosphatemia and constipation. Antacids with magnesium, such as milk of magnesia, magnesium carbonate, magnesium oxide, and magnesium trisilicate, should be avoided.

METABOLIC ACIDOSIS. Failure of the renal tubules to excrete acid ions and acid waste products causes the body's acid level to rise. Decreased bicarbonate reabsorption renders the body unable to neutralize the excess acid. Excess acid leads to metabolic acidosis. The lungs attempt to compensate by eliminating more carbon dioxide through hyperventilation. Indications of metabolic acidosis are headache, lethargy, and delirium.

FLUID BALANCE. Most patients with chronic renal failure retain sodium and water, causing hypernatremia and hypervolemia. Elevated blood pressure and edema are signs of hypervolemia. Without correction, the hypervolemic patient may develop congestive heart failure. Prevention and treatment of hypervolemia include fluid restriction, diuretics, and dialysis if necessary. A few patients are sodium wasters. These patients lose excess sodium and water in the urine and develop hyponatremia and hypovolemia.

INSULIN RESISTANCE. With renal failure, cells become resistant to the action of insulin. As a result, blood insulin and glucose levels rise. Hyperinsulinemia stimulates the liver to produce triglycerides. Patients in chronic renal failure have high serum levels of very low density lipoproteins. Elevated lipids in the blood (hyperlipidemia) contribute to accelerated atherosclerosis.

ANEMIA. Patients in chronic renal failure produce less erythropoietin, a hormone necessary for red blood cell production. Even the red blood cells that are produced have a shorter life span than usual because of the toxic environment in which they live. Therefore, patients in chronic renal failure have anemia. Iron supplements and folic acid may be ordered. Transfusions may be required if the hematocrit drops below 20% (normal value, 35–45% for females and 45–55% for males). A genetically engineered erythropoietin (epoetin alfa) has been approved for human use. It is administered intravenously following hemodialysis or subcutaneously for patients on peritoneal dialysis. This product improves red blood cell formation and has reversed anemia and the need for transfusions in some patients in chronic renal failure.

IMMUNOLOGIC FUNCTION. Because the inflammatory response diminishes with chronic renal failure, fewer white blood cells gather at the site of an infection or injury. The general immune response is suppressed, and antibody production declines.

CARDIOVASCULAR SYSTEM. The cardiovascular system is affected by hypervolemia, hyperkalemia, and hypocalcemia. Hypervolemia increases the workload of the heart, possibly leading to congestive heart failure. Signs of congestive heart failure are moist breath sounds, bounding pulse, dependent edema, and dyspnea. Dysrhythmias may be caused by hyperkalemia or hypocalcemia. Thirty to 50% of patients with chronic renal failure develop a transient pericardial friction rub that is a chemical response to accumulated waste products.

NEUROLOGIC SYSTEM. Neurologic effects of chronic renal failure are mental status changes (lethargy, irritability, confusion) and peripheral neuropathy. Peripheral neuropathy may be evident initially as a "restless" feeling and later as footdrop or paralysis of the legs. Many physicians treat the development of peripheral neuropathy as a signal to begin dialysis.

Disequilibrium syndrome may occur with hemodialysis. The rapid removal of urea from the blood does not allow time for the spinal fluid to adjust. Confusion, lethargy, headache, nausea, and vomiting may progress to coma or seizures if not treated. Disequilibrium is corrected with the administration of hypertonic glucose.

INTEGUMENTARY SYSTEM. The integumentary system is also affected by the waste product accumulation. Calcium phosphate crystals and urea accumulate in the skin, causing itching. Dryness results from decreased oil gland production and decreased perspiration. A pale gray to yellow color may result from anemia and from unexcreted bilirubin and uremic pigments. Hair and nails become dry and brittle. Uremic frost is the term used when whitish crystals composed of urea and other salts precipitate on the skin. Uremic frost is most often noted around the mouth. It is a very late sign in chronic renal failure.

GASTROINTESTINAL SYSTEM. Ammonia is a breakdown product of urea. When ammonia accumulates in the gastrointestinal tract, it causes irritation, nausea, vomiting, a metallic taste in the mouth, and bleeding. Antacids administered every 2 hours help to relieve the irritation. A diet high in carbohydrates and low in protein is prescribed to reduce the accumulation of urea. Other common gastrointestinal disturbances with chronic renal failure are stomatitis (inflammation of the mouth), anorexia, nausea, vomiting, constipation, and diarrhea.

MUSCULOSKELETAL SYSTEM. Renal osteodystrophy refers to the skeletal changes characteristic of chronic renal failure. The three major changes are metastatic calcification, bone demineralization, and osteitis fibrosa. Metastatic calcification is deposition of calcium phosphate complexes in blood vessels and in joints, lungs, muscles, and eyes. Deposits in blood vessels can impair blood flow so severely that fingers and toes may become gangrenous. Bone demineralization is directly related to hypocalcemia. Low serum calcium triggers increased production of parathormone. Parathormone mobilizes calcium from the bone and shifts it into the blood. Over time, there can be significant loss of bone mass. When calcium is lost from bones, it is replaced with fibrous tissue. This condition is called osteitis fibrosa.

REPRODUCTIVE SYSTEM. Chronic renal failure affects the reproductive systems of both males and females. The production of sex hormones declines and libido is diminished. Ovulation and menstruation usually cease in females. Males typically have low sperm counts and impotence. One must consider that the general effects of a chronic illness undoubtedly affect sexual desire and function.

ENDOCRINE FUNCTION. Patients with chronic renal failure are usually hypothyroid for unknown reasons.

EMOTIONAL AND PSYCHOLOGICAL EFFECTS. Emotional and psychological effects of chronic renal failure include emotional lability, depression, anxiety, and slowed intellectual functioning.

Medical Treatment

Treatment of chronic renal failure aims to promote elimination of wastes, maintain fluid balance, and manage the systemic effects of the disease. Conservative treatment of systemic effects of chronic renal failure are provided in the preceding section. To summarize, these treatments include

- Intravenous glucose and insulin, sodium bicarbonate, or sodium polystyrene sulfonate to treat hyperkalemia
- Calcium, active vitamin D, and phosphate binders to treat hypocalcemia
- Fluid restriction and diuretics to treat hypervolemia
- Iron supplements, folic acid, blood transfusions, and synthetic erythropoietin to treat anemia
- Hypertonic glucose to treat disequilibrium syndrome
- High-carbohydrate, low-protein diet to prevent excess urea

DIALYSIS. When kidney failure can no longer be managed conservatively, dialysis is required to sustain life. Dialysis is the passage of molecules through a semipermeable membrane into a special solution called dialysate solution. Dialysis operates like the kidney on the principles of osmosis, diffusion, and ultrafiltration. Small molecules like urea, creatinine, and electrolytes pass out of the blood, across the membrane, and into the solution by diffusion. Glucose increases the osmotic pressure in the dialysate solution, causing excess water to be drawn across the membrane and into the solution. Ultrafiltration is the movement of fluid caused by pressure. In hemodialysis, pressure in the blood is higher than that in the dialysate solution, so fluid is forced into the solution.

Pores in the semipermeable membrane do not allow passage of larger molecules such as proteins and blood cells. Dialysis does not affect production of erythropoietin and renin or the activation of vitamin D.

The goals of dialysis are to

- Remove the end products of protein metabolism from the blood
- Maintain safe concentrations of serum electrolytes
- Correct acidosis and replenish the body's bicarbonate buffer system
- Remove excess fluid from the blood

Dialysis enables many patients to maintain or regain self-esteem and to be productive members of society. Two primary means of dialysis are available: hemodialysis and peritoneal dialysis.

Hemodialysis. Hemodialysis is a process by which blood is removed from the body and circulated through an artificial kidney (hemodialyzer; synthetic semipermeable membrane) for removal of excess fluid, electrolytes, and wastes. The dialyzed blood is then returned to the patient (Fig. 36–12).

Hemodialysis requires vascular access (access to the patient's blood stream). This may be accomplished by temporary catheter, cannula, graft, or fistula. Subclavian or femoral catheters can be used for temporary access for dialysis during acute renal failure while a graft or fistula matures or for patients on peritoneal dialysis who need immediate access for hemodialysis. The catheters may be used for up to 1 week.

A cannula, also called an arteriovenous (or AV) shunt, provides an external connection between an artery and a vein (Fig. 36–13). The synthetic tubings are connected and provide temporary (6–12 months) access for hemodialysis. An advantage to the cannula is that venipuncture is not needed to initiate dialysis. Because the cannula is external, however, the danger of hemorrhage is ever present if the tubing should be disrupted. Therefore, arteriovenous shunts are no longer the preferred type of access. A dressing is required over the cannula. Clamps should be attached to the dressing at all times. In the event the cannula should break or become disconnected, the clamps are used to close it and prevent exsanguination (bleeding to death). A second possible complication is skin breakdown around the cannula insertion site. The dressing is changed daily using sterile technique. The external shunt is inspected for any signs of infection (redness, excess warmth, and swelling). Showering, swimming, and contact sports are prohibited. The arm with the shunt should never be used to take blood pressures.

An alternative to the external shunt is an internal connection between an artery and a vein using a bovine or synthetic (Gore-Tex, PFTE) graft. This requires a surgical procedure. One to 2 weeks should be allowed for healing before the internal graft is used. These grafts may last as long as 7 to 9 years.

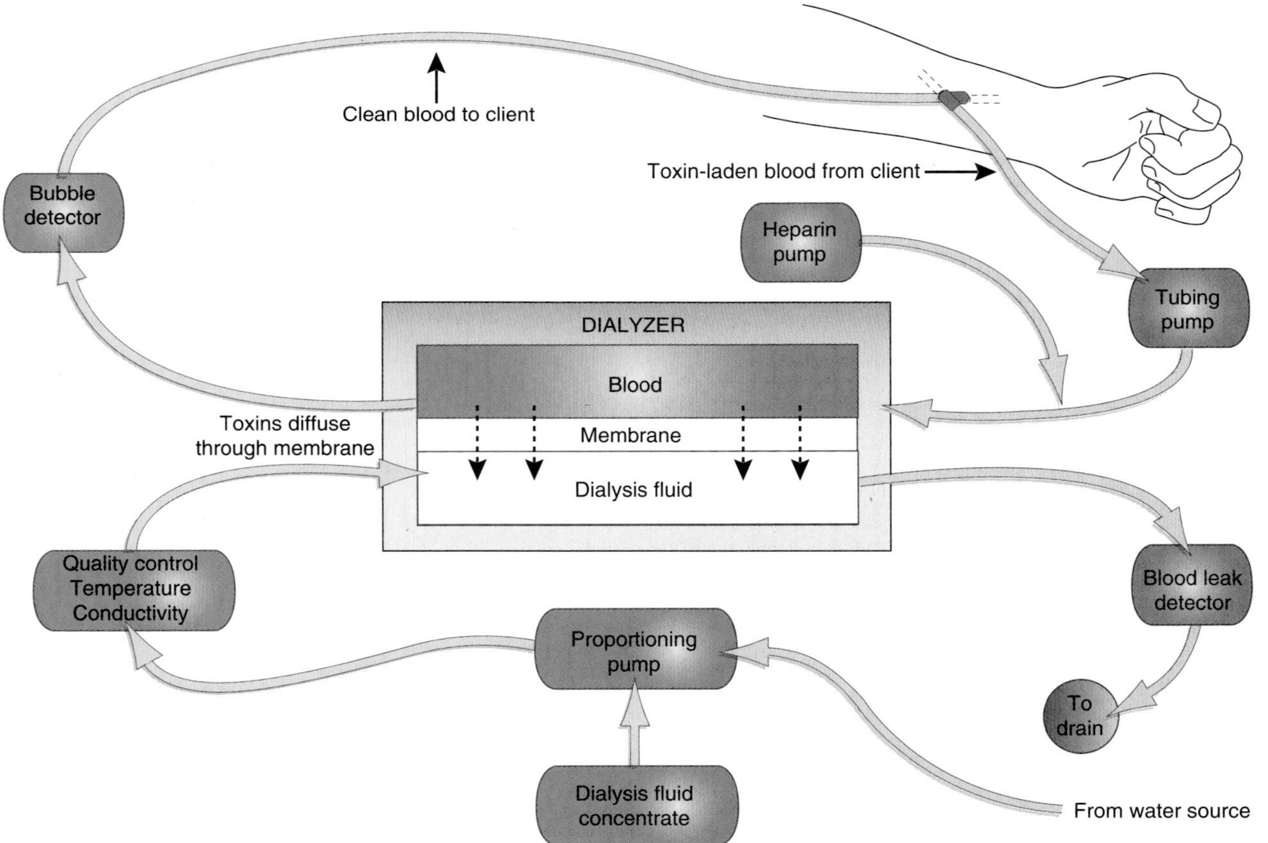

FIGURE 36–12
Schematic diagram of hemodialysis.

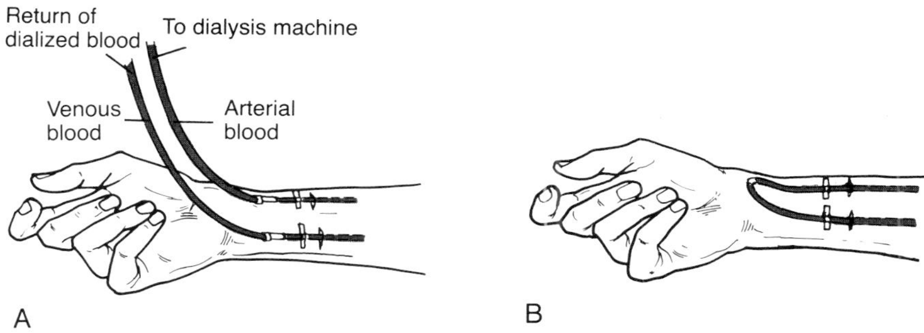

FIGURE 36–13
An arteriovenous shunt in use for dialysis *(A)* and not in use *(B)*.

Another option is a fistula, which is an internal connection of an artery and a vein. Following the surgical anastomosis of the two vessels, the vein wall thickens and becomes more muscular. It requires 6 to 12 weeks to mature before use and may last 3 to 5 years. The nondominant arm is preferred for a fistula.

Internal shunts do not require dressing changes. The nurse monitors the site for bleeding after venipunctures. Pulses below the shunt should be checked to ensure adequate circulation. Circulatory impairment distal to the shunt is called steal syndrome. To prevent damage to the shunt, blood pressures are not taken in the arm where the shunt is located.

Vascular access sites must be assessed for patency. A "thrill" is a rippling sensation palpable on the venous side of the cannula or fistula. A bruit is a rushing or roaring noise or a "swoosh" heard through a stethoscope with each heartbeat. Absence of these signs may indicate occlusion of the vessel and makes it unsuitable for hemodialysis.

Once vascular access is established, the patient may be hemodialyzed. Blood is withdrawn from the artery, circulated through the dialyzer, and returned through the venous line. Heparin is used as an anticoagulant to prevent blood from clotting. Hemodialysis requires specially trained personnel and expensive equipment. Although dialysis is usually performed in a dialysis center, home dialysis is available. The hemodialysis process takes approximately 4 hours and is generally done three times weekly.

Advantages of hemodialysis include its use in emergencies and the rapid removal of wastes, electrolytes, and fluid. Disadvantages include the need for vascular access, the use of an anticoagulant and the potential for hemorrhage, anemia, rapid fluid and electrolyte shifts (dialysis disequilibrium syndrome), muscle cramps, nausea and vomiting, and air emboli.

Complications. Complications of hemodialysis include atherosclerotic cardiovascular disease, anemia, gastric ulcers, disturbed calcium metabolism, and hepatitis. Atherosclerotic cardiovascular disease is the leading cause of death for hemodialysis patients.

Peritoneal Dialysis. Peritoneal dialysis uses the patient's own peritoneum as a semipermeable dialyzing membrane. Fluid is instilled into the peritoneal cavity. Waste products are drawn into the fluid, which is then drained from the peritoneal cavity (Fig. 36–14).

Peritoneal dialysis may be done on a temporary or permanent basis. For temporary use, a trocar is used to insert a catheter into the peritoneal cavity through the abdominal wall. For long-term use, a catheter is implanted into the peritoneal cavity. Over time, a bacterial barrier forms at the insertion site and provides some protection against infection.

Advantages of peritoneal dialysis over hemodialysis include less anemia, reduced cost of equipment, few dietary and fluid restrictions, independence, and closer resemblance to normal kidney function. Disadvantages include peritonitis (the major complication), hernias, low back pain, respiratory distress, and decreased serum albumin. Peritoneal dialysis cannot be used for patients with recent abdominal surgery, extensive abdominal trauma, or open abdominal wounds.

Continuous ambulatory peritoneal dialysis allows the patient freedom from a machine and the independence to perform dialysis alone. Fluid is allowed to flow into the peritoneal cavity (generally 2 liters over 10 minutes).

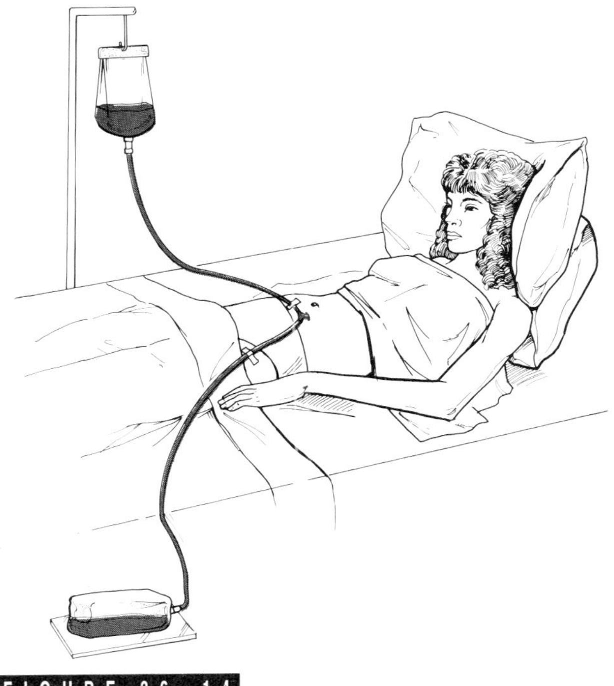

FIGURE 36–14
Peritoneal dialysis.

The fluid remains in the cavity for 4 to 8 hours while osmosis and diffusion occur. The fluid is then drained from the cavity over about 20 minutes. The patient exchanges the outflow container for a new inflow container. This procedure is repeated four to five times. Strict aseptic technique must be used with the initiation of the process and with each exchange. The patient or a reliable caregiver must be taught the process by someone who understands it well.

Continuous cyclic peritoneal dialysis is a newer method that allows the patient to have dialysis performed at night by a machine. Three cycles are usually performed, and the last dialysate remains in the peritoneal cavity during the day. This allows the patient freedom during the day. It also reduces the risk of infection because the system is interrupted less often.

Complications. A complication of peritoneal dialysis is peritonitis, an infection of the peritoneum. The fluid in the outflow container must be inspected for evidence of infection (cloudiness, particles). Any signs of infection should be reported to the physician immediately. Peritonitis is usually treated with antibiotics administered through the peritoneal catheter.

Nursing Care of the Patient in Chronic Renal Failure

ASSESSMENT. The general nursing assessment of the patient with a urologic disorder is outlined in Table 36–1. For the patient in chronic renal failure, frequent monitoring for changes in status is especially important. Fluid balance is closely evaluated. During hospitalization, accurate intake and output records must be kept. The nurse is alert for signs and symptoms of fluid volume excess that can lead to cardiac failure. Warning signs are increasing edema, dyspnea, tachycardia, bounding pulse, and rising blood pressure.

Serum electrolytes are measured frequently, but the nurse is always alert for signs and symptoms of electrolyte imbalances. With chronic renal failure, the nurse is most concerned with detecting hyperkalemia, hypocalcemia, and metabolic acidosis. Hyponatremia and hypovolemia are less common. Assessment of fluid and electrolyte imbalances includes characteristics of pulse and respirations, blood pressure, mental status, and neuromuscular activity.

Assessment of nutrition includes appetite, usual daily intake, weight gain or loss pattern, and prescribed diet. The nurse also needs to determine how well the patient understands and follows the prescribed diet.

Mental and emotional status must not be overlooked when assessing the patient with renal failure. Increasing confusion or loss of consciousness can be due to accumulated toxins or electrolyte imbalances. Emotional responses to a diagnosis of chronic renal failure vary. The nurse determines the patient's perceptions of the situation and identifies usual coping strategies. Anxiety, fear, altered body image, and lowered self-esteem are common.

The long-term effects of chronic renal failure and its treatment put the patient at risk for many complications. The nurse assesses bowel elimination for either constipation or diarrhea. It is very important to monitor for signs and symptoms of local or systemic infections (redness, swelling, foul drainage, fever, increased white blood cell count). The skin is inspected for bruising, bleeding, or trauma. Sensation in the extremities is evaluated. The nurse asks if sexual dysfunction has been a problem and obtains a description of the difficulty.

It is helpful to determine what the patient knows about chronic renal failure, its treatment, and self-care measures. Reasons are documented if the patient is unable to carry out usual activities of daily living.

NURSING DIAGNOSIS. Specific nursing diagnoses vary based on the individual patient assessment. Many diagnoses and interventions discussed under acute renal failure also apply to the patient with chronic renal failure. The emphasis in this section is on the common problems experienced by the patient in chronic failure. Nursing diagnoses may include the following:

- **Fluid Volume Excess** related to fluid retention
- **Altered Nutrition: Less than Body Requirements** related to anorexia, nausea, vomiting, stomatitis, dietary restrictions
- **Sensory Perceptual Alterations** related to effects of uremia on the nervous system
- **Ineffective Individual Coping** related to multiple life changes
- **Situational Low Self-Esteem** related to change in appearance, loss of kidney function, venous access devices, inability to fulfill usual roles and responsibilities
- **High Risk for Infection** related to impaired immune response, malnutrition, break in skin integrity
- **High Risk for Injury** related to coagulation disorder, impaired wound healing, bone demineralization, peripheral neuropathy
- **Constipation** related to inactivity, drug side effects, fluid restriction, electrolyte imbalances
- **Diarrhea** related to electrolyte imbalances, drug side effects
- **Sexual Dysfunction** related to fatigue, drug side effects, hormone deficiencies, altered self-image
- **Self-Care Deficit** related to lack of knowledge, confusion, anemia, fatigue

GOALS. Goals of nursing care for the patient with chronic renal failure include reduced fluid volume and absence of symptoms of heart failure, adequate food intake, improved mental status, effective coping, improved self-esteem, absence of infection, absence of injury, normal bowel elimination, satisfactory sexual function, and accomplishment of self-care.

INTERVENTIONS

Fluid Volume Excess. As renal failure progresses, the patient's ability to excrete excess fluids continually declines. In the early stages, diuretics may be used to treat fluid retention, but they are not used once dialysis is begun. Fluid intake may be restricted. Intravenous fluids, if ordered, are closely monitored. Antihypertensives may be needed to control blood pressure and digitalis to support cardiac function. Dosage adjustments are often needed because kidney failure affects the ability to excrete these drugs. The nurse administers medications, monitors for side effects, and teaches the patient how to take them after discharge. Dialysis is needed when conservative measures are no longer effective in managing fluid balance. Dialysis nurses have specialized education that is beyond the scope of this text.

Patients with fluid volume excess require comfort and safety measures. Edematous legs are easily injured and heal slowly. The nurse protects them from pressure or trauma. If cardiac failure and dyspnea develop, the patient is positioned with the head elevated to ease breathing. Cerebral edema causes confusion and decreasing consciousness. Safety measures must be taken to protect the confused or semiconscious patient from injury.

PHARMACOLOGY CAPSULE

Because drugs are excreted in the urine, people with impaired renal function are at risk for drug toxicity.

Altered Nutrition. Adequate nutrition can be a real challenge with the chronic renal failure patient. Anorexia, nausea, vomiting, and stomatitis interfere with food intake. In addition, sodium and protein restrictions make the diet less appealing. Measures to encourage food intake include frequent mouth care and small feedings. The nurse explains the importance of good nutrition to the patient and family. The dietitian can help the patient learn to cope with the diet. The person who prepares the patient's food at home is included in dietary instructions. Vitamin supplements are routinely ordered because of the dietary restrictions. The nurse administers the supplements and makes sure the patient knows how to take them at home. Weight is monitored to evaluate both fluid and nutritional status.

Sensory Perceptual Alterations. Renal failure affects both the central and the peripheral nervous systems. Cerebral edema and elevated metabolic wastes in the blood can cause confusion, slowed thought processes, lethargy, and loss of consciousness. The nurse protects confused patients and orients them to person, place, and time. Information is presented simply and repeated as needed. Sensory overload is avoided by reducing environmental stimuli and demands on the patient. For safety reasons, the patient is assigned a room close to the nurse's station. The bed is put in low position and the call bell is kept within reach.

The effects of renal disease on the peripheral nerves can lead to loss of sensation in the extremities (peripheral neuropathy). These patients are at risk for injury. The affected areas are inspected daily for any signs of injury. Pressure, ill-fitting shoes, or external heat or cold can cause serious injury before the patient is aware of it. The nurse teaches the patient about peripheral neuropathy and how to prevent injuries.

Ineffective Individual Coping. Patients with chronic renal failure often experience anxiety and fear. They face life-threatening illness, endure invasive treatments and procedures, and undergo radical changes in lifestyle. The nurse explores the patient's coping strategies and identifies factors that interfere with adjustment to renal disease. It helps for the patient to have a regular primary nurse so that a therapeutic relationship can develop. Nurses can help by talking to patients and helping them focus on the sources of their distress. It is important to be accepting of the patient's thoughts and feelings. Giving false reassurance or telling patients not to worry should be avoided. The nurse explains routines and procedures and provides practical advice on the management of everyday problems. Many patients benefit from talking to a mental health professional or attending support groups with people with similar problems. While encouraging patients to accept treatment, the nurse respects their rights to be informed and to refuse treatment.

Dialysis patients typically go through stages of adjustment. When dialysis is first started, they usually feel much better. They are encouraged and view dialysis positively. This might be described as a "honeymoon period." At this stage, the patient is most receptive to teaching. It is wise to take advantage of this opportunity to educate the patient.

After several months of treatment, patients tire of the routine. Depression and disappointment are common. Some cope by denying the need for treatment. They may omit medications or fail to keep appointments for follow-up. Nurses must be accepting of the patient but not the behavior at this stage. The nurse should confront the patient when ineffective coping behaviors are identified.

Eventually, most dialysis patients accept the need for ongoing treatment. They may try to resume their former levels of activity. At this point, nurses may need to guide them in realistic goal setting.

Situational Low Self-Esteem. The patient's self-esteem may suffer because of changes in body image and role performance. Nurses should encourage patients to talk about the changes they are experiencing and what they mean. Therapeutic communication and touch convey acceptance to patients. The nurse can help the patient with grooming to enhance appearance.

Patients are encouraged to examine their daily routines and look for ways to conserve time and energy. Sources of help and support need to be identified. Family functions may have to be redistributed. It is important for the patient to continue to have roles in the family and to be seen as a contributing family member.

High Risk for Infection. The patient needs to be protected from sources of infection. Chronic renal failure patients must avoid exposure to others with infections. The nurse teaches them how to take their own temperatures and instructs them to report signs of infection to the physician. Nurses set good examples by practicing good hand-washing and aseptic technique for invasive procedures.

High Risk for Injury. The patient is susceptible to injury for many reasons: impaired coagulation and wound healing, bone demineralization, and peripheral neuropathy. There is a danger of bleeding, fractures, and undetected bleeding. The nurse maintains a safe environment to prevent falls and bruises. Calcium, vitamin D, and phosphate binders are given as ordered to reduce loss of calcium from the bones. Ambulation is encouraged as another measure to maintain bone mass. Body parts that lack sensation must be assessed and protected.

Constipation. Constipation is a common problem with chronic renal failure because of inactivity, fluid restriction, electrolyte imbalances, and drug side effects. The nurse encourages activity within the patient's tolerance level. Stool softeners are often ordered to prevent constipation.

Diarrhea. Diarrhea may be caused by drugs or by anxiety. Liquid stools are measured and counted as fluid output. Antidiarrheals are given as ordered. Perianal care is given after each stool.

Sexual Dysfunction. Sexual dysfunction is attributed to both physical and emotional causes. Not all nurses are comfortable discussing sexual function with patients, but patients need to know that it is acceptable to express concerns. The nurse explains how kidney disease affects sexual function and explores what this means to the patient. Referral to a counselor who specializes in treatment of sexual dysfunction may be appreciated. Alternative means of sexual expression may enable the patient to continue to feel loved and to be intimate with another.

Self-Care Deficit. Chronic renal failure patients spend more time at home than they do in the hospital. Nurses need to prepare them for self-care. Topics to include in a teaching plan are how the kidneys work, the effects of renal disease, prescribed treatment, signs and symptoms of complications, significant signs and symptoms to report to the physician, and self-medication. The patient in dialysis is taught by an expert in that procedure.

EVALUATION. Criteria for evaluating the outcomes of nursing care are blood pressure within normal range; consumption of prescribed diet; alert and oriented mental status; patient's use of healthy coping strategies; positive statements of self-worth; normal body temperature and white blood cell count; lack of bruising, bleeding, fractures; regular, formed bowel movements without straining; patient's identification of satisfactory intimate relationship; and completion of activities of daily living within limitations imposed by renal failure and treatments.

RENAL TRANSPLANTATION

A patient's life expectancy on dialysis is seldom more than 12 years. The only alternative available is renal transplantation.

KIDNEY DONATION

A healthy kidney may be obtained from a live donor (usually a relative) or from a cadaver. The tissues of the donor and the recipient must match or the recipient will reject the new kidney. Matching is based on blood groups and human leukocyte antigens. When a kidney is obtained from a living related donor, the 1-year survival rate for transplantation is about 95 to 97%. Ninety percent of patients who receive transplants from cadavers are alive 1 year later. A national network maintains lists of people awaiting donor kidneys. When a cadaver kidney is available, the network tries to locate the best match for the kidney to improve the chances of success.

Kidney donors must be at least 18 years old, free of systemic disease or infection, have no history of cancer or renal disease, have normal renal function, and be without major medical problems. People over age 60 may be considered as candidates for donation on an individual basis. Unfortunately, many older people have advanced cardiac or respiratory disease that makes them ineligible.

Cadavers must meet the same criteria as living donors. Many people carry signed donor cards indicating willingness to have organs used for transplantation in the event of brain death. If brain death does occur, written permission is still sought from the family of the potential donor before organs are removed. The vital organs of the brain-dead person must be kept functioning until the kidney is removed.

PREOPERATIVE CARE

In some respects, preoperative care of the renal transplant recipient is like that of any other patient facing major surgery. General care of the surgical patient is described in Chapter 14. Steps are taken to prepare the patient mentally and physically for the procedure. The unique aspect of this situation is that the patient awaits an organ from another human being. If a relative is the donor, the surgery can be planned and both individuals emotionally prepared. Counseling is advised for both the donor and the recipient. The patient may be ambivalent about receiving a relative's organ. The gift of a kidney can restore health, but the recipient may feel guilty about asking a loved one to endure surgery and to give up an organ. The donor also faces the stress of surgery and a future with only one kidney. The donor also has to accept that the kidney could be rejected. Both face the threat of surgical complications.

If awaiting a cadaver kidney, the patient must face the idea that someone must die for a kidney to be available. These potential recipients are on call and must be ready to report to the hospital at any time.

The recipient and the donor have complete diagnostic work-ups to rule out other medical problems and to evaluate the function of the urinary tract. Normal function of both of the donor's kidneys must be affirmed. The recipient is given medications to bring blood pressure within normal limits. Immunosuppressant drugs are started to control the body's response to foreign tissue (i.e., the donated kidney) (see Table 36–5). The recipient may also be given a transfusion of the donor's blood, a measure that has been found to reduce rejection. If the recipient has severe hypertension or a UTI, bilateral nephrectomies may be done before the transplant. The patient is dialyzed shortly before the transplant.

Preoperative Nursing Care of the Renal Transplant Patient

ASSESSMENT. In the preoperative period, a complete assessment is done as outlined in Chapter 14. Before renal transplantation, the nurse assesses the patient's understanding of the surgery. Baseline vital signs are recorded. The nurse identifies any specific fears or questions that need to be addressed.

NURSING DIAGNOSIS. The primary nursing diagnoses specific to the renal transplantation patient are the following:

- **Fear** related to perceived threat of death
- **Knowledge Deficit** of surgical routines

GOALS. Goals of preoperative care are reduced fear and patient's knowledge of surgical routines.

INTERVENTIONS. To achieve these goals, the nurse acknowledges and encourages the patient to discuss concerns. Fear is accepted as understandable and natural. Factual information helps the patient cope by reducing the fear of the unknown. The nurse can involve the patient in planning and in self-care. When patients are active participants in their care, they feel less helpless and less anxious. It is somewhat difficult to teach the patient who is awaiting a cadaver kidney because one never knows when, or if, the transplant will take place. Preoperative teaching begins when the patient is identified as a candidate for transplantation. Information must be reinforced when the actual surgery is imminent.

EVALUATION. Criteria for evaluating the success of nursing interventions include verbalization of accurate information and statement of lessened fear and anxiety.

SURGICAL PROCEDURE

The donor kidney is removed from the live donor in an operating room and taken to an adjacent room where the recipient has been prepared to receive it. A cadaver kidney is removed under sterile conditions and transported to the hospital where the recipient is waiting. The donor kidney is placed in the recipient's abdomen and anastamosed (attached) to the bladder and to blood vessels (Fig. 36–15).

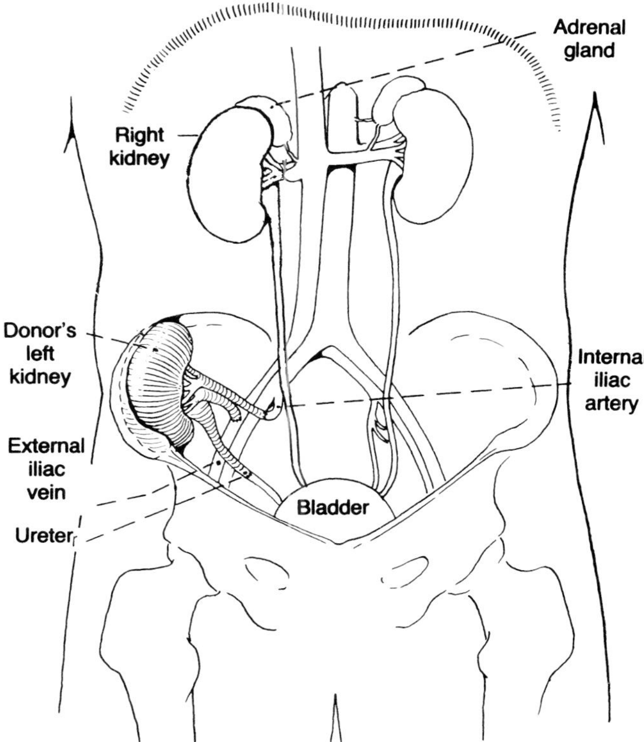

FIGURE 36–15

Kidney transplanted to right pelvis. (Adapted from Jacob, S. W., & Francone, C. A. [1989]. *Elements of anatomy and physiology* [2nd ed., p. 274]. Philadelphia: W. B. Saunders.)

Complications

Complications following renal transplantation include rejection, renal artery stenosis, hematomas, abscesses, and leakage of ureteral or vascular anastomoses. Rejection of the new organ by the recipient is a major problem with most tissue transplants. Rejection is characterized by fever, elevated blood pressure, and pain over the location of the new kidney. Three types of rejection can occur: hyperacute, acute, and chronic. Hyperacute rejection occurs within 48 hours after transplantation. It is not reversible, and the kidney must be removed. Acute rejection develops between 1 week and 2 years after transplant and is treated with increased immunosuppressant drugs. Chronic rejection develops and progresses slowly. Eventually, chronic rejection mimics chronic renal failure, and dialysis may become necessary.

Immunosuppressant drugs, begun preoperatively, are continued in the postoperative period to reduce the risk of rejection. These drugs include corticosteroids, antilymphocyte preparations, monoclonal antibodies, and T-cell suppressors. Examples of immunosuppressants, their actions and adverse effects, and nursing interventions are summarized in Table 36–6. They are called immunosuppressants because they inhibit the body's immune response to foreign tissue. This action is intended to prevent the donor kidney from being destroyed by the recipient's defenses. Unfortunately, the action of immunosuppressants also reduces the body's response to invasion by microorganisms. Therefore, patients who take these drugs are at increased risk for infection.

PHARMACOLOGY CAPSULE

Immunosuppressant drugs decrease the patient's ability to resist infection.

POSTOPERATIVE CARE

Postoperative Nursing Care of the Renal Transplant Patient

ASSESSMENT. General postoperative care is described in Chapter 14. This section emphasizes care that is unique to the renal transplant patient. Assessment of the renal transplant patient is similar to that of any surgical patient. It is especially important for the nurse to monitor fluid intake, urine output, weight changes, and vital signs.

NURSING DIAGNOSIS. Specific nursing diagnoses after renal transplantation may include

- **Altered Urinary Elimination** related to rejection of transplanted kidney, renal failure
- **Fluid Volume Deficit** related to diuresis, blood loss
- **High Risk for Infection** related to suppression of immune response
- **Knowledge Deficit** of immediate and long-term postoperative care
- **Anxiety** related to possibility of organ rejection

GOALS. Goals of nursing care are balanced fluid intake and output, normal blood pressure, absence of infection, patient's understanding of self-care measures, and reduced anxiety.

INTERVENTIONS. Immediately after surgery, the patient is taken to a special care unit for close monitoring. As with any surgical patient, the transplant patient is monitored for circulatory and respiratory complications. The patient is assisted with turning, coughing, deep breathing, and leg exercises. Pain control measures are instituted.

Altered Urine Elimination. The patient will have an indwelling catheter for up to a week to permit constant observation of urine output. Urine is pink to bloody initially, then gradually clears. The nurse maintains catheter patency at all times. The patient is monitored closely for signs that the transplanted organ is functioning: increasing urine output, normal blood pressure, decreasing BUN and serum creatinine, and stable weight.

If the patient is oliguric, a fluid challenge and diuretics are prescribed. In addition to the possibilities of renal failure and rejection, the nurse should be alert for signs and symptoms of cardiac failure related to fluid volume excess: dyspnea, edema, bounding pulse, and cardiac dysrhythmias.

Fluid Volume Deficit. Some patients have massive diuresis postoperatively. This may cause fluid volume deficit. With excessive fluid loss, the patient is at risk for electrolyte imbalances and decreased cardiac output. A thready pulse, low blood pressure, and poor tissue turgor suggest dehydration. The physician should be informed so that proper fluid replacement can be ordered. Serum electrolyte studies are ordered to identify specific imbalances.

High Risk for Infection. The immunosuppressant drugs that protect the new kidney also inhibit the body's ability to resist pathogens. The nurse must monitor the transplant patient carefully for signs and symptoms of infection: fever, elevated white blood cell count, cough, purulent wound drainage. Signs and symptoms may be very subtle despite a major infection. The nurse uses good hand-washing and aseptic technique when working with the patient. The patient is separated from others who have infections. The patient and family members are taught the importance of protecting the patient from exposure to infections. Prophylactic antibiotics are given as prescribed.

Knowledge Deficit. Patient teaching begins as soon as possible. The teaching plan includes drug therapy, diet, fluids, activity, and signs and symptoms of rejection and infection. Patients need to know what drugs are prescribed, why they are important, how to take them, what side effects to expect, and what effects to report to the physician. The physician prescribes any restrictions on diet, fluids, and activity. The nurse clarifies and reinforces these orders. It is critical that the patient knows how to recognize signs and symptoms of infection, rejection, and renal failure.

Anxiety. Anxiety may lessen as renal function improves, but the patient always lives with the possibility of rejection. The nurse recognizes this anxiety and accepts it as normal. It is helpful for the patient to talk about feelings and explore ways to deal with them. Some patients find comfort in a support group of people who have had similar experiences. Others may need referral to a mental health professional to help them deal with their stress constructively.

EVALUATION. Criteria for successful nursing interventions include urine output equal to fluid intake, normal pulse and blood pressure, normal body temperature and white blood cell count, accurate patient statement of self-care measures, and patient's statement of lessened anxiety.

Kidney function is vital to survival. Many urologic conditions can be prevented or treated fairly easily if detected early. Nurses can play a role in preventing or detecting many potentially serious urologic disorders. When kidney disorders are advanced, the nurse continues to play an important part in teaching and supporting patients.

NUTRITION CONCEPTS

- Renal failure results in an inability of the kidneys to excrete wastes and maintain fluid and electrolyte balance.
- In renal failure, the nutritional goal is to modify the diet so that the work of the kidneys is reduced.
- Fluid intake may be restricted to 1000 to 1500 ml per day for patients with renal disease.
- Sodium and potassium intake is restricted (including medications) in patients receiving dialysis to maintain electrolyte balance.
- Protein is restricted in patients with renal disease, and any protein ingested should be high in essential amino acids. Examples of these proteins are eggs, meat, poultry, fish, and milk products.
- Persons with renal calculi should increase fluid intake to maintain at least 2 liters of urine output daily and avoid foods leading to the formation of calculi.
- Calcium restriction is limited to certain types of renal calculi.

BIBLIOGRAPHY

Chernecky, C. C., Krech, R. L., & Berger, B. J. (1993). *Laboratory tests and diagnostic procedures.* Philadelphia: W. B. Saunders.

Dunetz, P. S. (1992). If your med-surg patient is on dialysis. *RN, 55*(9), 46–53.

Dunn, S. A. (1993). How to care for the dialysis patient. *American Journal of Nursing, 93*(6), 26–34.

Fischbach, F. (1988). *A manual of laboratory diagnostic tests* (3rd ed.). Philadelphia: W. B. Saunders.

Giddens, J. F., Vigil, G., & Sanchez, A. (1993). Risks and rewards of kidney transplant. *RN, 56*(6), 56–61.

Ignatavicius, D. D., & Bayne, M. V. (1991). *Medical-surgical nursing: A nursing process approach.* Philadelphia: W. B. Saunders.

Jacob, S. W., & Francone, C. A. (1989). *Elements of anatomy and physiology* (2nd ed.). Philadelphia: W. B. Saunders.

Jarvis, C. (1992). *Physical examination and health assessment.* Philadelphia: W. B. Saunders.

King, B. A. (1994). Detecting acute renal failure. *RN, 57*(3), 34–40.

Lewis, S. M. (1992). Nursing role in management: Acute and chronic renal failure. In S. M. Lewis & I. C. Collier (Eds.), *Medical-surgical nursing* (pp. 1221–1257). St. Louis: Mosby Year Book.

Lewis, S. M. (1992). Nursing role in management: Renal and urological disorders. In S. M. Lewis & I. C. Collier (Eds.), *Medical-surgical nursing* (pp. 1185–1220). St. Louis: Mosby Year Book.

Matteson, M. A., & McConnell, E. S. (1989). *Gerontological nursing.* Philadelphia: W. B. Saunders.

McConnell, E., & Lewis, L. W. (1990). Self test: Managing the patient with acute renal failure. *Nursing 92, 22*(3), 84–88.

Moore, S., Newton, M., Grant, E., & Keetch, D. (1993). Treating bladder cancer: New methods, new management. *American Journal of Nursing, 93*(5), 32–41.

Pollin, S., & DeLuca, E. (1992). How to use the new weapon against anemia. *RN, 55*(1), 36–38.

Tootla, J., & Easterling, A. D. (1992). Current options in bladder cancer management. *RN, 55*(4), 42–49.

Toto, K. H. (1992). Acute renal failure: A question of location. *American Journal of Nursing, 92*(11), 44–53.

Webber-Jones, J. E. (1991). Performing clean, intermittent self-catheterization. *Nursing 91, 21*(8), 56–64.

KEY CONCEPTS

1. The urinary system eliminates metabolic wastes in urine, stimulates red blood cell production, and maintains fluid, electrolyte, and acid-base balance.
2. Age-related changes in the urinary system include reduced ability to concentrate or dilute urine, nocturia, and decreased bladder capacity.
3. Urinary tract infections, the most common nosocomial infections, can lead to renal failure.
4. Inflammatory conditions of the urinary tract include cystitis (bladder inflammation), urethritis (urethral inflammation), glomerulonephritis (glomerular inflammation), and pyelonephritis (inflammation of the renal pelvis).
5. Cystitis may result from prolonged immobility, renal calculi, urinary diversion, and indwelling urinary catheters.
6. Urinary tract infections are treated with antibiotics, urinary tract antiseptics, analgesics, and antispasmodics.
7. Acute glomerulonephritis commonly follows a streptococcal respiratory infection and results in scarring of the glomeruli.
8. Patients with renal disorders are at risk for fluid volume excess, hypertension, and heart failure.
9. Management of renal disorders requires attention to pain management, fluid balance, activity intolerance, and patient education.
10. Urinary obstructions anywhere in the urinary tract can lead to hydronephrosis and kidney damage.
11. Urinary calculi, commonly called stones, form in the urinary tract and may move through the tract with the flow of urine.
12. Although most calculi pass spontaneously, some require surgical removal or disintegration by lithotripsy.
13. Nursing care of the patient with renal calculi focuses on pain management, monitoring urine

KEY CONCEPTS *(continued)*

output, maintaining fluid balance, and patient education.

14. Complications of urinary tract surgery include urinary tract and wound infection, atelectasis, paralytic ileus, and hemorrhage.
15. Renal tumors are often large before they are detected because early symptoms are subtle.
16. Cystectomy (bladder removal) requires urine to be diverted to a drainage collection system. Types of urinary diversion are ileal and sigmoid conduits, ureterosigmoidostomy, ureteroileosigmoidostomy, ureterostomy, and nephrostomy.
17. Nursing care after bladder surgery focuses on pain management, unobstructed urine flow, skin integrity, bowel function, and self-care.
18. Renal failure can result from hypotension, toxins, infections, impaired blood flow, trauma, and obstructions.
19. The four stages of acute renal failure are onset, oliguria, diuresis, and recovery.
20. Management of acute renal failure emphasizes fluid and dietary restrictions, restoration of fluid balance, waste elimination, and maintenance of cardiac output.
21. When 90 to 95% of kidney function is lost, the patient is considered to be in chronic renal failure.
22. Effects of chronic renal failure include fluid volume excess, hyperkalemia, hypocalcemia, hyperuricemia, and anemia.
23. Dialysis uses a semipermeable membrane to draw excess water, electrolytes, and wastes into a special solution called dialysate.
24. Renal transplantation is the only alternative to dialysis for the patient in end-stage renal disease.
25. Signs and symptoms of rejection of a transplanted kidney are fever, increased blood pressure, and pain over the location of the new kidney.

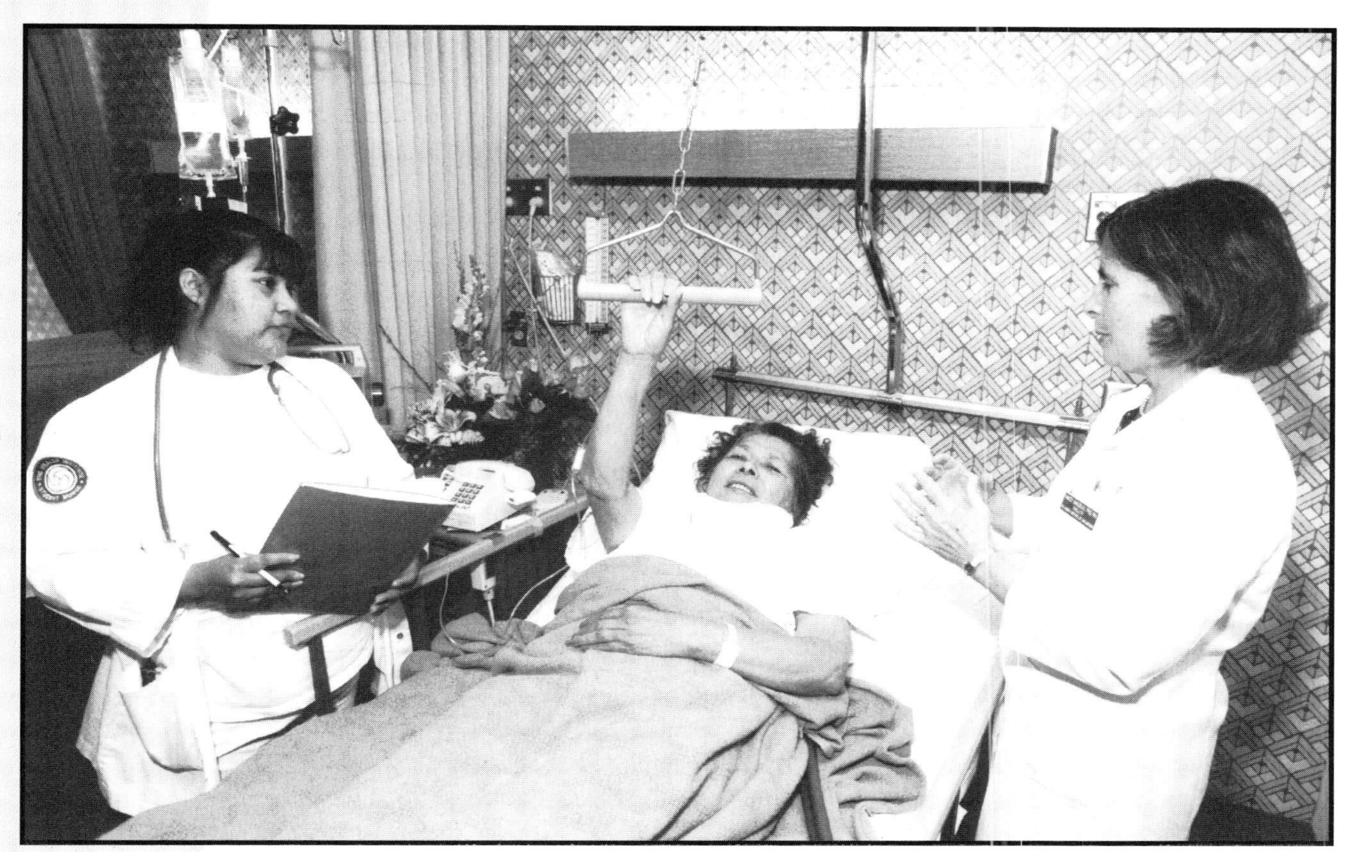

UNIT 11
Musculoskeletal Disorders

Dorothy Greene Jackson

CHAPTER 37

Connective Tissue Disorders

OBJECTIVES

1. Define connective tissue.
2. Describe the function of connective tissue.
3. Describe the characteristics and prevalence of connective tissue diseases.
4. Describe the diagnostic tests and procedures used for assessing diseases of connective tissue.
5. Discuss the drugs indicated for treatment of patients with connective tissue diseases.
6. Describe the pathologic basis for osteoarthritis (degenerative joint disease); rheumatoid arthritis; osteoporosis; gout; systemic lupus erythematosus; progressive systemic sclerosis; polymyositis; periarteritis nodosa; ankylosing spondylitis; polymyalgia rheumatica; Reiter's syndrome; Behçet's syndrome; and Sjögren's syndrome.
7. Identify the data to be collected in the nursing assessment of a patient with a connective tissue disorder.
8. Utilizing the nursing process, formulate a plan of care for a patient whose life has been affected by a connective tissue disease.

GLOSSARY

ANKYLOSIS Joint immobility

ARTHRALGIA Pain in a joint

ARTHROPLASTY Plastic repair of a joint

BOUCHARD'S NODES Enlarged proximal interphalangeal joints of the fingers

CREPITUS Crackling sound or sensation

DISCOID LUPUS Circular, scaly lesions with erythematous raised rim; occurs over scalp, ears, face, and areas exposed to sun

GONIOMETER Instrument used to measure joint range of motion

HEBERDEN'S NODES Protrusions of the distal interphalangeal finger joints; associated with osteoarthritis

HYPERURICEMIA Elevated level of uric acid in the blood

MYALGIA Muscle pain

PERIARTICULAR Around the joint

TOPHUS Deposit of sodium urate crystals under the skin (*plural* tophi)

VASCULITIS Inflammation of blood vessels

More than 37 million people in the United States have one or more connective tissue diseases. These rheumatoid disorders affect women more frequently than men, with no respect to racial group. For the most part, these diseases are long term and share a set of characteristic features. They are chronic and variable in nature; have a tendency to exacerbate or to go into remission with treatment; are very damaging to the immune system; and sometimes have a very unclear pathology. These diseases present a taxing challenge to the spirit and body of the patient. They have a compromising effect on the patient's lifestyle, self-image, employability, and hope for the future. The variability of symptoms and response to therapy makes treatment very difficult.

ANATOMY AND PHYSIOLOGY OF CONNECTIVE TISSUES

Connective tissues are defined as the extracellular compartments and components of the body that provide the body's structure and support. They bind together the cells, organs, and tissues and provide the framework for other cells. The major connective tissues are bone, blood, cartilage, ligaments, skin, and tendons.

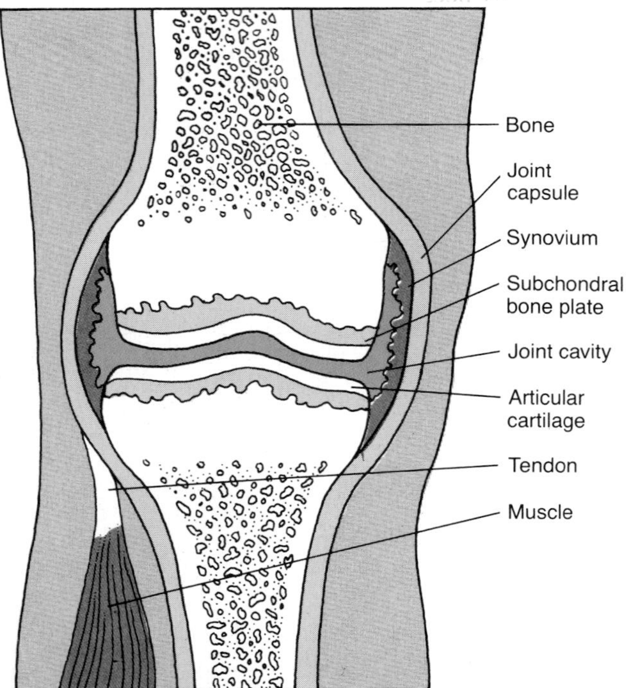

FIGURE 37-1

Major structures in a normal synovial joint. (From Ignatavicius, D. D., & Bayne, M. V. [1991]. *Medical-surgical nursing: A nursing process approach* [p. 720]. Philadelphia: W. B. Saunders.)

Bone

Bone is the hard tissue that makes up most of the skeletal system. The functions of the bones are support, protection, movement, and manufacture of blood cells.

Blood

Blood is a liquid type of connective tissue. As the main transport system of the body, it transports oxygen from the lungs to the body tissues, and carbon dioxide from the tissues to the lungs. Blood also contains cells that function in the body's defense and in blood clotting.

Cartilage

Cartilage is a specialized fibrous connective tissue. It provides firm but flexible support for the embryonic skeleton and part of the adult skeleton. Cartilage differs from bone in that its matrix has the consistency of a firm plastic or gristle-like gel. Cartilage cells are called chondrocytes and are located in tiny spaces that are distributed throughout the matrix.

Ligaments

Ligaments are strong, flexible fibrous bands of connective tissue that connect bones and cartilage and serve as support for muscles. Yellow ligaments and white ligaments have distinctively different functions. Yellow ligaments are elastic, located in the vertebral column, and allow for stretching. White ligaments, found in the knee, do not stretch but do provide stability.

Skin

The skin is the largest organ of the body. Its main function is that of protection. It provides the first line of defense against bacteria and injury. The skin also participates in regulation of body heat through perspiration, eliminates body wastes, receives sensory input, and is the site for production of vitamin D. Skin characteristics, including color, texture, and lesions, give clues to a person's general health status.

The skin is composed of two main layers, the epidermis and the dermis. The epidermis is the outermost layer of the skin that is nonvascular, meaning that it has no blood vessels. The dermis is composed of bundles of collagen fibers and elastic connective tissue that act to support blood vessels, sweat glands, sebaceous glands, and hair follicles.

Tendons

Tendons are composed of very strong, dense fibrous connective tissue. They are made in the shape of heavy cords that anchor muscles firmly to bones. One of the most prominent tendons is the Achilles tendon, which can be felt at the back of the ankle just above the heel.

JOINT STRUCTURE AND FUNCTION

The fact that joint problems are common manifestations of connective tissue disorders merits special attention. A joint is the site at which two or more bones of the body are joined. Joints permit motion and flexibility of the rigid skeleton. The only bone in the human body that does not articulate with at least one other bone is the hyoid bone, to which the tongue is attached. Classified on the basis of the extent of movement, joints include synarthroses (fixed joints), amphiarthroses (slightly movable joints), and diarthroses (freely movable joints). Synarthroses, such as those in the skull, allow no movement at all. An example of a slightly movable joint, an amphiarthrosis, is the juncture of the ulna and radius in the forearm. Diarthroses, such as those in the elbows, shoulders, fingers, hips, and knees, allow considerable movement.

Diarthroses are sometimes called synovial joints. They are encased in a fibrous capsule made of strong cartilage and lined with the synovial membrane. The synovial membrane is very smooth, permitting structures to move without friction. Ligaments are tough fibrous cords that bind the capsule. A smooth layer of cartilage also covers the ends of the bones, where it serves as a type of shock absorber. Synovial fluid fills and lubricates the space in the middle of the joint. Bursae are sacs of synovial fluid found in joints that also promote smooth articulation of joint structures.

AGE-RELATED CHANGES

Important changes in the connective tissue of the body occur with aging. Most of the changes that take place can have great functional significance. There is a loss of bone mass and bone strength. The progressive loss of bone mineral content during later adult life accounts for the decline in bone strength. This bone loss is probably the most characteristic aging change in the skeletal system. Age-related osteoporosis, loss of bone mass, is seen in older males and females.

Age-related joint changes include the following:

- Diminished viscosity (thickness) of synovial fluid.
- Degeneration of collagen and elastin cells.
- Fragmentation of fibrous structures in connective tissues.
- Outgrowths of cartilaginous clusters in response to continuous wear and tear.
- Formation of scar tissues and calcification in the joint capsules.
- Degenerative changes in the arterial cartilage that result in fraying and cracking.

These joint changes result in limited mobility and movement, increase the risk of musculoskeletal injury, and can lead to erosion of bone surfaces that are normally cushioned by cartilage.

Age-related changes that take place in the skin are quite apparent. There is evidence that most changes are due to internal and external conditions (most importantly, sun exposure) rather than to normal aging. Nevertheless, some common skin changes are seen in older people. The epidermis itself does not become thinner with age, but there is a large decrease in the density of the small interlocking projections (dermal papillae) that hold the dermis and epidermis together. The dermis becomes thinner with age owing to decreased collagen. These changes result in wrinkling and looseness that leaves the skin very susceptible to injury from shearing forces.

In the healthy older person, the blood volume and components do not change appreciably. Some sources document slight decreases in hemoglobin, hematocrit, lymphocyte and granulocyte counts, and platelet function, but these findings are often disputed by other sources. Red blood cell volume and life span, total blood volume, and platelet morphology are generally thought not to change significantly.

NURSING ASSESSMENT OF CONNECTIVE TISSUE STRUCTURES

HEALTH HISTORY

The nursing assessment of the person with a disorder of connective tissue relies heavily on the nurse's interviewing skills because the symptoms of these disorders vary with each individual. Since many of the signs and symptoms involving this group of structures are insidious, it may be helpful to have a family member present to assist the patient as historian. Patients with chronic conditions may come to accept their symptoms as a way of life and fail to report them to the nurse. The family member may help the nurse get a clear picture of how the changes in health have evolved.

Chief Complaint and History of Present Illness

The nurse determines why the patient is seeking health care. Complaints that should alert the nurse to possible problems related to connective tissue disorders are aches, pain, joint swelling, joint stiffness, generalized weakness, change in ability to work or to enjoy leisure activities, change in appearance that is significant to the patient, and change in ability to carry out activities of daily living.

Past Medical History

The nurse should ask about any previous acute or chronic health problems. The past health history gives information about the patient's prior state of health. The nurse asks questions about major childhood and adult illnesses, operations, and current medications and allergies. Certain illnesses may affect the connective tissue or musculoskeletal system directly or indirectly. The nurse asks about a history of tuberculosis, poliomyelitis, diabetes mellitus, gout, arthritis, rickets, infection of bones or joints, and neuromuscular disabilities.

IMMUNIZATIONS. The patient is asked about immunizations for polio and tetanus. Improper immunization can result in problems of the musculoskeletal system.

ACCIDENTS. Determining whether the patient has had a recent or past accident may be significant since it may relate to the patient's current problem. For example, a patient's current complaint of low back pain may be related to an injury of several years ago.

CURRENT MEDICATIONS. Many persons who have musculoskeletal problems are taking medications for the musculoskeletal problem or for other unrelated problems. The patient is questioned carefully regarding the use of prescription and over-the-counter drugs. The nurse records problems associated with the medication and whether or not the patient thinks the medication is effective. Allergies are also documented.

Family History

Certain disorders have a hereditary tendency. The nurse asks whether the patient or any relatives have had rheumatoid arthritis, degenerative arthritis, gout, or scoliosis because these have a tendency to occur in families.

Review of Systems

The review assesses the body systems for the presence of significant symptoms. Assessment of general health status determines the patient's perception of well-being. The nurse asks whether the patient has had fatigue, malaise, anorexia, weight loss, pain, stiffness, dysphagia, or dyspnea.

Functional Assessment

The patient's perception of the problem has great impact on his or her cooperation and participation in the therapy prescribed. A patient who thinks the treatment is ineffective may not cooperate fully. The following questions may be used to assess how the patient really feels about the condition:

- What effect has your problem had on the way you live?
- Have you had to modify your activities of daily living?
- How do you feel about the changes that you have had to make in the way you live?
- What have you found helpful in adapting to these changes?
- How do you carry out the treatment program prescribed by your physician?
- Has your treatment plan been effective for you?

Answers to the above questions will guide the nurse's approach in assisting the patient with his or her care and in helping the patient plan for future adjustments.

PHYSICAL EXAMINATION

The physical examination begins with measurement of vital signs and height and weight. Measurements must be compared with the patient's norms, if available. The nurse is alert for fever, tachycardia, tachypnea, and weight loss. Physical examination of the patient consists of a systematic inspection from head to toe, paying special attention to areas of concern as ascertained from the health history. For example, if the patient complained of pain in a particular joint, the nurse should concentrate on that area and compare it with the opposite body part.

The skin is inspected for color, rashes, lesions, scars, or any signs of falls or injuries. The nurse palpates for warmth, edema, and moisture. Joints are inspected for swelling and deformity and palpated for warmth, swelling, and tenderness. Joint pain and range of motion are assessed by asking the patient to move each extremity through the normal range of motion. During the movement, the nurse watches for signs of pain and listens for the crackling sound called crepitus. A more in-depth assessment of joint motion may be done by the physician or other advanced health care provider using an instrument called a goniometer. A goniometer measures the amount of bending or angles of the joints. Measurement of limb length and muscle strength also may be done. Lymph nodes are palpated for enlargement and tenderness.

The nursing assessment of the patient with a connective tissue disorder is outlined in Table 37–1.

TABLE 37–1
ASSESSMENT OF THE PATIENT WITH A CONNECTIVE TISSUE DISORDER

HEALTH HISTORY

Present illness: changes in movement, activities of daily living; areas of pain, swelling, or tenderness

Past medical history: tuberculosis, poliomyelitis, diabetes mellitus, gout, arthritis, rickets, neuromuscular disabilities

Family history: rheumatoid arthritis, degenerative arthritis (need for joint replacement surgery), gout, scoliosis, autoimmune disorders

Review of systems: pain or swelling in joints, limitation of movement, weakness, malaise, change in general appearance of skin

Functional assessment: past or recent injuries due to accidents or falls, use of assistive devices

PHYSICAL EXAMINATION

General survey: posture, balance, gait, skin condition

Joints: warmth, redness, swelling, tenderness, range of motion, function of hands

Skin: color, scars, bruising, warmth, swelling

Upper extremities: symmetry, swelling, tenderness, pain, range of motion, posture

Lower extremities: movement of hips, knees, and ankles; pain; skin condition

DIAGNOSTIC TESTS AND PROCEDURES

Diagnostic procedures used to diagnose connective tissue diseases are mainly laboratory studies of blood and urine and radiographic (x-ray) studies of the bones. Other useful measures are biopsy, arthroscopy, and ultrasound. A summary of commonly used diagnostic studies, including nursing interventions, is given in Table 37–2.

Laboratory Studies

A number of blood and urine studies may be helpful in diagnosing connective tissue disorders. Besides a complete blood count, the routine blood studies for evaluation for musculoskeletal disorders should include the erythrocyte sedimentation rate and the C-reactive protein. These are useful in determining whether the disorder is inflammatory or noninflammatory. Other blood studies are the VDRL (Venereal Disease Re-

TABLE 37–2
DIAGNOSTIC TESTS AND PROCEDURES FOR CONNECTIVE TISSUE DISORDERS

TEST/STUDY	PURPOSE/PROCEDURE	PATIENT PREPARATION	POSTPROCEDURE NURSING CARE
Blood Studies			
Erythrocyte sedimentation rate (ESR)	Measures rate at which red blood cells settle out of unclotted blood. Determines presence of inflammation. Approximately 5–10 ml of venous blood is collected. Results elevated in any inflammatory process, especially rheumatoid arthritis (RA), rheumatic fever. Decreased in degenerative arthritis. Normal values: norms vary with gender, age, and method used.*	Fasting *not* required. Tell patient that a blood sample will be drawn.	Apply pressure to venipuncture site. Assess site for bleeding.
Red blood cell count (RBC)	Assessment of number of circulating erythrocytes. Detection of blood dyscrasias; differentiation of anemias, leukemia, and thalassemia. Decreased in RA and systemic lupus erythematosus (SLE). Normal values: adult female, 4.0–5.5 ml/μL; adult male, 4.5–6.2 ml/μL.	Fasting *not* required. Tell patient that a blood sample will be drawn.	Apply pressure to venipuncture site. Assess site for bleeding.
White blood cell count (WBC)	Measures number of circulating leukocytes. Approximately 5–7 ml of venous blood is collected. Abnormal findings: increased in infection, tissue necrosis, inflammation. Sometimes decreased in SLE.	Fasting *not* required. Tell patient that a blood sample will be drawn.	Apply pressure to venipuncture site. Assess site for bleeding.
Rheumatoid factor (RF)	Determines the presence of antibodies. Present in approximately 80% of persons with RA. Normal values: qualitative, negative; quantitative, <1:20.	Fasting *not* required. Tell patient that a blood sample will be drawn.	Apply pressure to venipuncture site. Assess site for bleeding.
Creatinine	Assesses renal function. Small venous blood sample is collected. Elevated in SLE, systemic sclerosis, polyarteritis. Normal values: vary with gender, age, method used.*	Fasting *not* required. Tell patient that a blood sample will be drawn.	Apply pressure to venipuncture site. Assess site for bleeding.
Venereal disease research laboratory (VDRL) test	Measures antibodies to syphilis. Small sample of venous blood is collected. Sometimes decreased in SLE. Normal value: nonreactive.	Fasting *not* required. Tell patient that a blood sample will be drawn.	Apply pressure to venipuncture site. Assess site for bleeding.
C-reactive protein	Measures abnormal glycoprotein produced by liver during acute inflammation. Small venous blood sample is collected. Positive reading in active inflammation. Often positive for RA and disseminated lupus erythematosus. Normal value: qualitative, negative; quantitative, 68–8200 ng/ml or 20 mg/dl or <8 μg/ml.	Tell patient that a blood sample will be drawn. Restrict food and fluids for 4 hr.	Apply pressure to venipuncture site. Assess site for bleeding.

Table continued on following page

TABLE 37-2
DIAGNOSTIC TESTS AND PROCEDURES FOR CONNECTIVE TISSUE DISORDERS *Continued*

TEST/STUDY	PURPOSE/PROCEDURE	PATIENT PREPARATION	POSTPROCEDURE NURSING CARE
Antinuclear antibodies (ANA)	Measures presence of antibodies that react with a variety of nuclear antigens. Positive in SLE, RA, systemic sclerosis, Raynaud's disease, Sjögren's syndrome, necrotizing arteritis. Normal values: negative at 1:20 dilution.	Should fast 8 h prior to test. Venous blood sample collected. Instruct patient in fasting and to expect a blood sample to be drawn.	Apply pressure to venipuncture site. Assess site for bleeding.
Urine Studies			
24-hour urine for creatinine	Measures renal function. Also measures status of muscle diseases. In muscle diseases, amount of creatinine converted by muscle is decreased and amount excreted by kidneys is increased. A 24-hr urine specimen is collected. Discard the first morning specimen. Save rest of urine for 24 hr in a clean, refrigerated 3-L container with or without preservative. Include urine voided at end of 24-hr period. Normal values: corrected to 1.73 m^2 of body surface area.	Fasting *not* required. Explain procedure to patient.	None.
Urinary uric acid (24-hr collection)	Measures uric acid metabolism. Collect 24 hr urine specimen (as described above). Increased in gout, liver disease, chronic myelogenous leukemia, febrile illness. Normal values: adult female, 250–750 mg/24 hr; adult male, 250–800 mg/24 hr.	Fasting *not* required. Explain procedure to patient.	None.
Radiologic Studies			
Radiographs	Determine density, texture, and alignments of bone. Assess soft tissue involvement. Serve as a baseline assessment for what appears to be a chronic process.	Find out time required for procedure. Tell patient to expect to lie on an x-ray table or to stand next to a special device while films are taken. Before procedure, ask patient to remove any radiopaque objects, such as jewelry, that can interfere with results. No other preparation is needed.	None.
Ultrasound	Visualization of soft tissue produced by sound waves. Detects masses and fluid accumulation. A jelly-like substance is placed on skin to promote contact by metal probe.	No special preparation. Tell patient what to expect and that procedure is painless.	None.
Arthrogram	Examines soft tissue joint structures. Performed most commonly on shoulder or knee when a traumatic injury is suspected and determines presence of bone chips, torn ligaments, or other loose bodies within joint. Contrast medium (air or solution) is injected into joint to enhance visualization.	Question patient about allergy to contrast solution. Ask patient if there is allergy to seafood or iodine: if yes, advise radiologist. Tell patient that test may be uncomfortable, related to pressure at needle insertion site. May cause swelling for several days after test.	Instruct patient to refrain from strenuous activity after test for 12–24 hr. Joint may be wrapped.
Bone scan	Intravenous radioactive material that is taken up by bone is injected for visualization of entire skeletal system. Procedure detects malignancies, osteoporosis, osteomyelitis, and some fractures.	Tell patient that a small amount of radioactive material will be injected intravenously, after which a scanner will move slowly back and forth over body as patient lies on a stretcher. Procedure is painless except for venipuncture and may take 1 hr. Explain that no harm comes from radioactive isotopes, but it should not be given during pregnancy. Ask patient to empty bladder immediately before procedure for comfort and to prevent blocked view of pelvis.	No special precaution required for handling urine or stool.

TABLE 37-2

DIAGNOSTIC TESTS AND PROCEDURES FOR CONNECTIVE TISSUE DISORDERS *Continued*

TEST/STUDY	PURPOSE/PROCEDURE	PATIENT PREPARATION	POSTPROCEDURE NURSING CARE
Magnetic resonance imaging (MRI) scan	A noninvasive procedure that makes use of magnetic energy sources to view soft tissue. Patient lies on nonmagnetic scanning table that slides body into a giant cylindric magnet. A receiver coil measures energy created by this magnetic field. These measurements provide information regarding condition of tissue. Images produced by MRI are very clear and are useful in diagnosis of avascular necrosis, disk disease, tumors, osteomyelitis, and ligament tears.	Tell patient that procedure is painless and that he or she must lie motionless for 30 min or more. May induce claustrophobia; with newly designed equipment, videos are used for patients's viewing to reduce anxiety. Procedure may be contraindicated in patients who have cardiac pacemakers, or intracranial vascular aneurysm clips, because a magnetic field is used. Ask patient to remove any metallic objects such as jewelry. As more modern equipment becomes available, presence of metal on patient may not be a problem.	No special postprocedure care. Patient may express some discomfort because of lying still for more than 30 min. Implement comfort measures as appropriate.
Diskogram	Contrast medium injected directly into vertebral disk being examined. Leakage of medium may indicate herniated disk.	Same as arthrogram.	Same as arthrogram.
Tomogram	Body-section radiographs showing details of structures otherwise hidden by overlying radiopaque bone. Study focuses on tissue in a single plane while other surrounding tissue is blurred.	Patients who are claustrophobic may have some difficulty tolerating procedure as it requires lying for an hour in a cylindric scanner.	None.
Computed tomography (CT) scan	Scans the soft tissue and bones by use of both x-rays and computers. Determines presence of tumors or some spinal fractures. Procedure may take 30 min per body part.	Tell patient that procedure may be lengthy. Coordinate patient's activity so that a day of rest between other procedures is allowed.	Implement measures of comfort as appropriate.
Special Tests			
Skin biopsy	Confirms inflammatory connective tissue diseases such as lupus erythematosus or systemic sclerosis (scleroderma). May be done by several techniques, as described in Chapter 14.	Tell patient that there may be slight discomfort.	Keep biopsy site clean and dry with small adhesive bandage until scab develops.
Muscle biopsy	Procedure consists of microscopic examination of skeletal muscle obtained by surgical incision. May be performed under local or general anesthesia. Tissue reveals features of inflammatory reaction as in polymyositis or myopathic disease.	Explain procedure to patient.	Apply pressure dressing to affected area and keep immobilized for 12–24 hr.
Joint aspiration	Needle aspiration of synovial fluid from within joint cavity for examination or to remove excess fluid. Local anesthesia and aseptic technique are used. Procedure is useful in diagnosis of joint inflammation. Normal synovial fluid is straw colored and clear and has viscosity of oil. In inflammation, fluid is turbid and watery.	Tell patient that a local anesthetic is used to minimize discomfort. Procedure is usually done at bedside or in examination room.	Apply pressure dressing to joint. Instruct patient to rest joint for 8–24 hr. Document on patient's charts and report any leakage of blood or fluid.
Arthroscopy	A surgical procedure performed in operating room. Insertion of arthroscope allows visualization of joint cavity and structure. Used as treatment to remove damaged structures and as diagnostic test by collecting fluid for biopsy and detecting abnormalities of meniscus, cartilage, ligaments, or joint capsule.	Inform patient that procedure is performed in operating room under local or general anesthesia.	A sterile dressing is applied, then wrapped with compression dressing. Instruct patient to limit activity for a few days. Report any drainage of blood or fluid.

* Note: See agency laboratory manual. Results vary with different types of tests and may be reported in various units of measurement.

search Laboratory), rheumatoid factor, creatinine, and antinuclear antibodies tests. Urine may be tested for creatinine and uric acid levels. Fluids aspirated from joints may be studied to detect inflammation.

Radiologic and Imaging Studies

Radiologic studies include radiographs, ultrasound, arthrograms, bone scans, magnetic resonance imaging scans, diskograms, tomograms, and computer tomographic scans.

Other Diagnostic Tests and Procedures

In addition to laboratory and radiologic studies, diagnostic procedures may include biopsies of skin and muscle and arthroscopy.

COMMON THERAPEUTIC MEASURES

Management of the patient with a connective tissue disorder often requires a team approach that includes the patient, nurse, physician, social worker, physical therapist, and occupational therapist. Involving the patient in the care can help maintain the patient's individuality and emotional and psychological integrity. The common therapies employed in treating patients with connective tissue disorders are directed at reducing the inflammatory process, reducing the pain, and preserving the psychological integrity of the patient. Therapeutic measures may include physical therapy, modification of activities of daily living, patient education, drug therapy, and surgical intervention. Although none of these measures are curative, they can greatly enhance the patient's lifestyle and quality of life.

Physical therapy employs exercise and positioning to help preserve functional capability and minimize disability. Occupational therapy assists the patient to make adaptations in work and personal life that allow the maximal possible function.

Patient education emphasizes the significance and rationale for the therapeutic regimen. All members of the health care team must be sensitive to the inconvenience and discomfort the disease has caused the patient while assisting the patient in self-management principles. Community support groups can offer encouragement, information, and resources to the patient and the family. Drug therapy, including prednisone and nonsteroidal anti-inflammatory drugs (NSAIDs), are indicated for the inflammation (Table 37–3). Some patients respond positively to periarticular injections of glucocorticoids. Simple analgesics are given to reduce the pain; narcotics are rarely indicated.

Surgical management may be effective in some musculoskeletal disorders, such as degenerative joint disease and arthritis. Specific surgical interventions are discussed with the particular conditions.

A device that is used after some types of joint replacement surgery is the continuous passive motion (CPM) machine. This device moves the joints through a set range of motion at a set rate of movements per minute. The movement prevents formation of scar tissue and promotes flexibility of the new joint. The operative extremity may be placed in the CPM machine in the postanesthesia care unit or on the first postoperative day. The machine is used for specific intervals, and the time is gradually increased. The part of the machine that cradles the limb is padded to prevent pressure or abrasions. The nurse ensures that the machine settings are correct as ordered and that the limb is properly aligned. The machine is kept clean since it could be a source of contamination. Several types of CPM machines are illustrated in the section on total joint replacement.

DISORDERS OF CONNECTIVE TISSUE STRUCTURES

OSTEOARTHRITIS

Osteoarthritis (OA), also termed degenerative joint disease, is the most common form of arthritis. It is characterized by the degeneration of articular cartilage, hypertrophy of the underlying and adjacent bone, and mild inflammation of the surrounding synovium. It may be classified as primary or secondary. Primary OA has no known cause, but secondary OA may be associated with trauma, infection, or congenital deformities. The incidence of OA increases with age, with persons over 50 most affected. It is estimated that more than 100,000 people in the United States are unable to walk independently to and from the bathroom because of OA.

The patterns of clinical manifestations vary with ethnic background. For example, OA of the hips is more common among people who live in Japan and Saudi Arabia than among whites in the United States.

Osteoarthritis generally affects joints under pressure, especially the spine, fingers, knees, hips, and shoulders. People who are obese, have poor posture, or experience occupational stress are at greatest risk for the disease. The most common source of major disability is OA of the knee.

Pathophysiology

The pathophysiology of primary OA is obscure. Normally, the articular cartilage provides a smooth surface for one bone to glide over another. The cartilage transfers the weight of one bone to another so that the bones do not shatter. In OA, these functions are compromised because the basic structure of the cartilage is altered. Bone spurs develop owing to new bone growth. Despite the erosion of articular cartilage, inflammation is not a usual sign of this disease.

Signs and Symptoms

Many people with OA have no symptoms, but others have pain that ranges from mild to severe. The pain is what usually brings the patient to the physician. Pain is

TABLE 37-3

DRUGS USED TO TREAT CONNECTIVE TISSUE DISORDERS

DRUG	USE/ACTION	SIDE EFFECTS	NURSING INTERVENTIONS
Anti-inflammatory drugs Aspirin	Inhibit prostaglandin synthesis, resulting in decrease in pain and deformity; Anti-inflammatory. Antipyretic. Inhibits platelet aggregation (clumping).	GI upset. Ototoxicity. Bleeding due to anticoagulation.	Instruct patient to take with food or take enteric-coated aspirin. Report ringing in ears (tinnitus). Assess for bruising and bleeding.
Nonsteroidal anti-inflammatory drugs (NSAIDs) ibuprofin (Motrin, Rufen) Naproxen (Naprosyn) Carprofen (Rimadyl) Ketoprofen (Orudis)	Inhibit prostaglandin synthesis; reduce joint swelling, stiffness; analgesic and antipyretic properties.	GI irritation, nausea, vomiting, heartburn, GI bleeding (may be silent in elderly, detected only by gastrostomy), and ulceration.	Administer with food. May require frequent blood counts. Caution patient to refrain from driving or operating heavy equipment if drowsiness occurs.
Indole analogues Indomethacin (Indocin) Sulindac (Clinoril)	Analgesic anti-inflammatory effect. Inhibit prostaglandin synthesis. Indicated for severe ankylosing spondylitis, painful shoulders.	Gastric bleeding, headaches, dizziness, psychiatric disturbances.	Administer with food. Report any signs of bleeding (tarry stools, hematemesis) to physician.
Glucocorticoids Hydrocortisone (Cortef, Hydrocortone) Hydrocortisone sodium succinate (Solu-Cortef, cortisol) Cortisone acelate (Cortone) Prednisone (Deltasone) Prednisolone (Delta-cortef)	Suppress normal immune response and inflammation. Used in inflammatory diseases, allergic diseases.	Muscular weakness, nausea, anorexia, hypotension; sodium retention, hypokalemia; insomnia; nervousness; euphoria; rise in serum glucose. Increased susceptibility to infections. Osteoporosis.	Administer at scheduled times. Highest dose usually given early morning; lowest dose given later in day to mimic normal secretion in body. Stress to patient necessity of adhering to prescribed schedule. Remember glucocorticoids mask signs of infection. Observe for any unusual drainage, odors, and elevated temperatures. Must be tapered off rather than stopped abruptly.
Disease-altering drugs Carprofen (Rimadyl)	Prevent growth of cells. Regulate immune system. Counteract inflammation.	Skin rash, oral ulcers, respiratory difficulty, nausea and vomiting, diarrhea, hemorrhage, bone marrow depression (anemia, leukopenia, thrombocytopenia), hyperuricemia.	Assess oral mucous membrane for lesions, encourage to avoid alcohol as it causes toxic effect on liver, effects of drug toxicity increased by salicylates (aspirin), phenbutazone, and PABA. Monitor complete blood count platelets and liver and renal functions.
Antigout agents Allopurinol (Xyloprim)	Inhibit synthesis of uric acid.	Drowsiness. Toxicity: maculopapular rash, fever, chills, joint pain. Rarely: bone marrow depression, nausea, diarrhea, bone marrow depression.	Tell patient to drink 8–10 glasses of fluid daily to maintain output of at least 2000 ml/day. Assess urine for abnormal characteristics. Safety precautions if drowsy. Tell patient it takes several weeks for full effects. Assess and document response.
Probenecid (Benemid)	Increases urinary excretion of uric acid.	Headache, urinary frequency, GI distress. Rarely: anaphylaxis. Toxicity: maculopapular rash, fever, joint pain, leukopenia, GI distress. Urinary calculi (stones).	Assess allergies. Do not give with penicillin. Caution with renal impairment. Encourage fluid intake maintain output of at least 2000 ml/day. Tell patient it takes several weeks for full therapeutic effect.

GI, Gastrointestinal.

commonly associated with activity and is lessened while the patient is at rest. Along with pain in the affected joint, the patient with OA may complain of crepitus, stiffness, limitation of movement, mild tenderness, swelling, and deformity or enlargement of the joint (Fig. 37–2). Sometimes the symptoms subside for long periods of time and then return. The disease usually affects a single joint or only a few joints.

Medical Diagnosis

The diagnosis of OA is usually based on the history from the patient and radiographic studies. In the early stages of the disease, radiographs may be normal. In fact, there is a reported disparity between radiographic findings and symptoms. Although more than 90% of people over the age of 40 have some osteoarthritic changes on radiographs, only 30% of these have symptoms. Radiographic changes include narrowing of joint spaces, sclerosis of the subchondral bone, changes in the contours of the joints, cyst formation, and cartilage destruction.

Medical Treatment

There is no known cure for OA, but much can be done to make the patient more comfortable. The goals of patient therapy are to reduce the pain to a manageable level, to maintain as much mobility as possible, and to minimize disability. The course of the treatment is dictated by the individual patient's condition and response.

The medical treatment regimen includes drug therapy, surgery, education, and physical therapy. For some patients, diet and psychosocial interventions are indicated.

DRUG THERAPY. Although drug therapy is not curative, it can still be very helpful in relieving the patient's pain. Drugs that are effective are nonnarcotic analgesics, disease-modifying drugs, and glucocorticoids. Narcotics are rarely indicated. Often the pain in OA can be controlled with acetaminophen, NSAIDs, or a low dose of salicylates (aspirin). An advantage to using salicylates is that the cost is relatively low, but there is a risk of toxicity. It should be emphasized that symptoms of salicylate intoxication in the elderly may be atypical. Instead of the common gastrointestinal complaints or ototoxicity, the older person may exhibit confusion, slurring of speech, agitation, hyperactivity, or seizures.

NSAIDs may decrease pain and improve mobility in OA patients. These drugs are especially effective when the patient shows signs of inflammation such as warmth, swelling of joints, and erythema. Indomethacin also is effective, but the patient and family must be instructed about the gastrointestinal and neurologic side effects (Table 37–3). Attempts are being made to develop disease-altering drugs that affect the pathophysiology of OA. Although systemic glucocorticoids are not indicated for treatment of OA, beneficial effects have been shown with intra-articular injections.

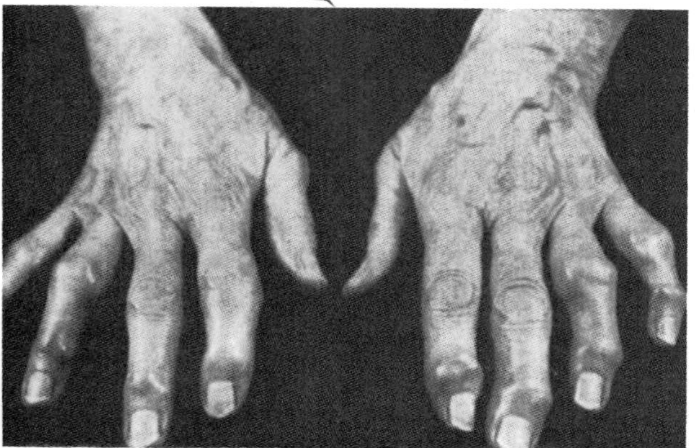

FIGURE 37–2

Bony nodules associated with osteoarthritis. (From the AHPA Arthritis Teaching Slide Collection, ©1980. Used with permission of the American College of Rheumatology.)

PHARMACOLOGY CAPSULE

Corticosteroids suppress the inflammatory response, so monitor the patient carefully for evidence of infection.

PHARMACOLOGY CAPSULE

Salicylate toxicity may be manifested by tinnitus or, in the elderly, by confusion, agitation, slurred speech, or seizures.

SURGICAL MANAGEMENT. Surgical management is usually reserved for persons with severe disease who respond poorly to nonsurgical modalities. Currently, the surgical treatment of choice for OA is total joint replacement (arthroplasty) (see Care Plan: The Patient with a Total Hip Replacement). The primary indication for total joint replacement is intractable pain. Total hip or knee arthroplasty usually relieves pain and restores function to the joint (Fig. 37–3).

PATIENT EDUCATION. Patient education is essential to enable the patient to live with OA.

PHYSICAL THERAPY. The physical therapy program employs measures to improve range of motion and to strengthen muscles. Most patients with OA benefit from such a program. Moist heat and occasionally cold can be used to help relieve pain and prepare the muscles and joints for exercise. Heat may be contraindicated in patients who have had arthroplasty or have metal prostheses because it may lead to deep thermal burns.

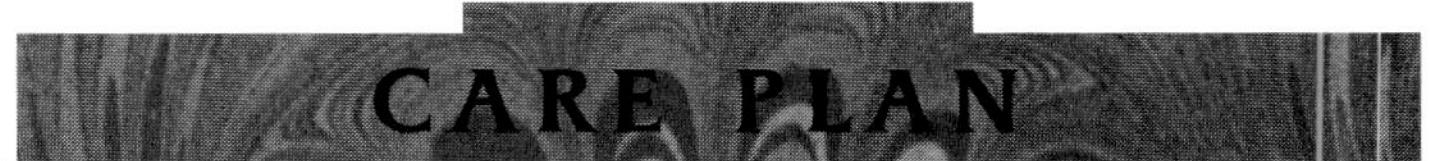

The Patient with a Total Hip Replacement

ASSESSMENT

Health History: Minnie Smith is a 74-year-old homemaker who has had osteoarthritis for 10 years with progressive loss of function in both hips. She had a left total hip replacement (arthroplasty) 2 days ago. Her past medical history reveals no other major health problems except poor vision. She lives with her daughter and helps with household chores, which gives her some satisfaction. Postoperatively, she is alert and participates in her exercises. The physical therapists assisted her out of bed for the first time this morning. She was somewhat weak but was able to walk a short distance.

Physical Examination: Vital signs: temperature, 98°F orally; pulse, 82; respiration, 16; blood pressure 148/66. Height, 5′9″. Weight, 162 lb. She is positioned on her right side with an abductor cushion in place. Breath sounds are clear on auscultation. Abdomen is soft, and bowel sounds are present. There is no bladder distention and no redness over bony prominences on back and left side. Warmth, color, and peripheral pulses are symmetric in both legs. She has good sensation in affected leg. The dressing on the surgical incision is dry and intact.

NURSING DIAGNOSIS	GOALS AND OUTCOME CRITERIA	INTERVENTIONS
Altered tissue perfusion (peripheral) related to deep vein thrombosis, decreased mobility, and surgical trauma.	The patient will have adequate circulation in the affected extremity as evidenced by warmth, normal color, and palpable pulses.	Assess neurologic and circulatory status. Check vital signs at least every 4 hours. Report and document any abnormalities. Observe for excess swelling or bleeding at operative site. Assist with exercises as prescribed by physical or occupational therapist. Document and report any change in condition of skin at operative site and pressure areas.
High risk for injury related to unsteady gait.	The patient will experience no falls during hospitalization.	Assist patient in and out of bed. Place call light in easy reach. Check frequently for patient's need to toilet and need for change of position. Provide assistive devices as ordered.
High risk for injury related to subluxation (dislocation) of joint prosthesis due to improper position, movement, or activity.	The patient will maintain proper alignment and demonstrate absence of signs of prosthesis dislocation: sudden severe pain, abnormal position.	Instruct patient to keep legs slightly abducted. May place pillows between legs to achieve abduction while supine and during turning. Turn only to unaffected side. Tell patient not to cross legs, put on own shoes, socks, or stockings for 2 months. Assess for pain and loss of function. Make home health referral if needed to facilitate transition to home setting.
High risk for infection related to break in skin integrity from surgical hip replacement procedure.	The patient will be free of infection during hospitalization and at discharge from hospital.	Encourage fluids and activity when appropriate. Observe for change in mental status or confusion in elderly, which may be first signs of infection. Keep in mind that previous administration of prednisone may mask symptoms of infection. Turn at least every 2 hours from back to unaffected side only. Use aseptic technique for wound care. Offer fluids at least every 2 hours.

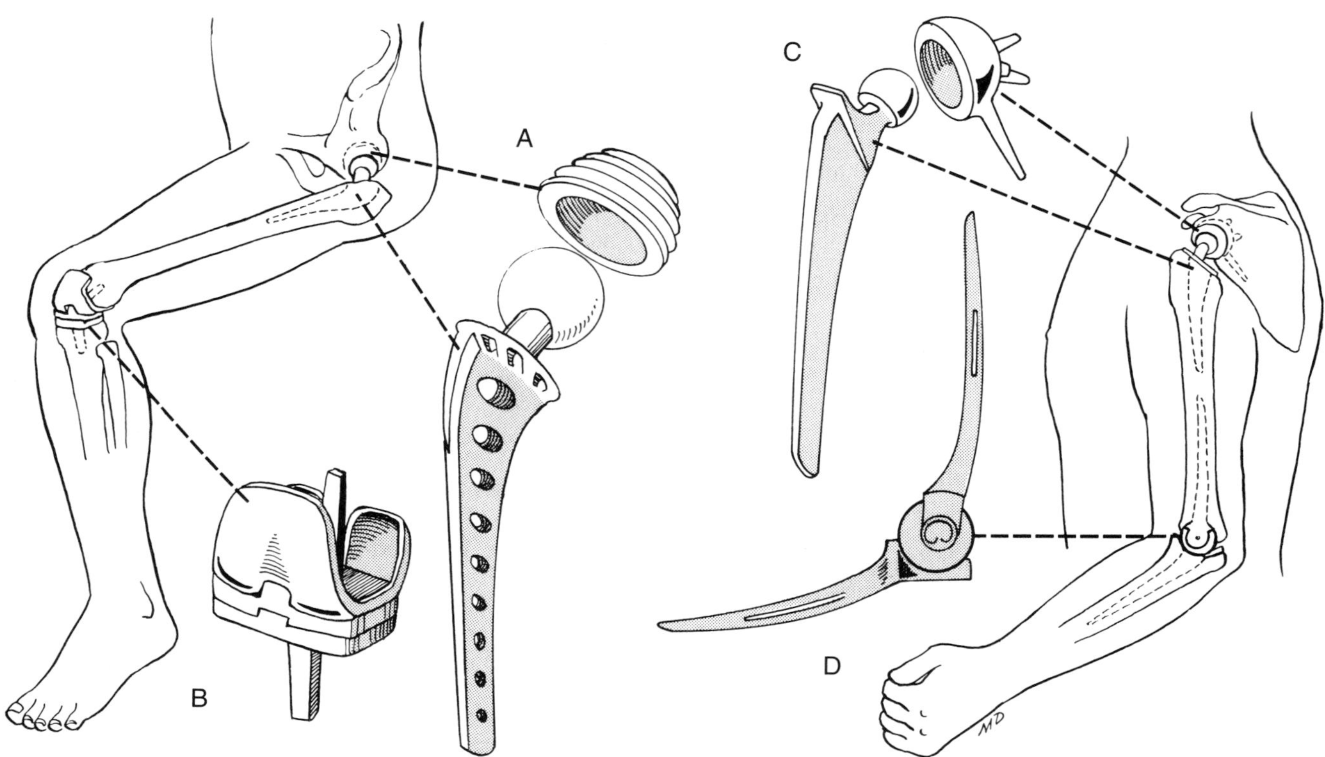

FIGURE 37-3

Total joint replacements. *A*, Hip; *B*, knee; *C*, shoulder; *D*, elbow. (From Black, J. M., & Matassarin-Jacobs, E. [1993]. *Luckmann and Sorensen's medical-surgical nursing: A psychophysiologic approach* [4th ed., pp. 603, 604]. Philadelphia: W. B. Saunders.)

Nursing Care of the Patient with Osteoarthritis

ASSESSMENT. General nursing assessment of the patient with a connective tissue disorder is summarized in Table 37–1. When a patient has OA, the nurse focuses on the movement and functions of the patient's joints and documents the location and severity of any problems. The health history focuses on how the disease affects the patient's mobility and ability to perform activities of daily living. Joints are handled and moved gently to minimize the patient's discomfort. The presence of the following signs and symptoms is carefully assessed: tenderness, swelling, limitations of movement, decrease in range of motion when compared to unaffected joints, and difficult gait.

NURSING DIAGNOSIS. Patients who have OA may have the following nursing diagnoses:

- **Pain** with motion related to loss of smooth joint surfaces
- **Impaired Physical Mobility** related to pain, limited range of motion
- **Ineffective Individual Coping** related to pain, discomfort, disability
- **Knowledge Deficit** of osteoarthritis management and self-care

GOALS. Goals of nursing care for the identified nursing diagnoses are pain relief, functional mobility, patient's adaptation to osteoarthritis, and patient's knowledge of disease management and self-care.

INTERVENTIONS

Pain. Good pain management can enable the patient to be more active and to have a better quality of life. Measures that protect the joint, discussed next under impaired physical mobility, help to minimize chronic pain. In addition, the nurse administers prescribed analgesics and anti-inflammatory drugs or instructs the patient in self-medication. Heat or cold treatments are carried out as ordered. The nurse monitors and documents the effects of interventions designed to relieve pain.

Impaired Physical Mobility. Impaired physical mobility can significantly interfere with the patient's ability to carry out usual activities in the home or work setting. Modification of daily activities and joint protection measures can help to maintain function. A regular program of exercise is recommended. The importance of balancing rest and activity to avoid overtiring is stressed. The household may need to be reorganized to reduce demands on the patient. Everyday tasks like dressing and bathing may be affected by the disorder. Clothing with Velcro closures rather than buttons and shoes that slip on are easier to manage if the patient's hands are affected. Bathroom grab bars, a seat in the shower, and a raised toilet seat may promote independence and safety for the patient with poor hip mobility. The patient is advised of the following:

- Maintain proper posture and body alignment.
- Identify those activities that take a long time to do or require assistance.
- Plan activities when help is available or when time is not a major concern and rest periods can be taken at intervals.
- Wear splints or support devices that rest or relieve painful, unstable joints.
- Push or slide heavy objects rather than pull them.
- Wear low heels to help decrease stress on the knee joints.
- Avoid stairs whenever possible.
- Sit rather than stand. Use high stools when sitting at a counter.
- Use higher chairs rather than low sofas.
- When arising from a chair, inch to the edge of the seat and then use the arm rests to push up from the seat.

Ineffective Individual Coping. The nurse provides an opportunity for the patient to discuss concerns about OA and its effects on lifestyle. The patient is asked to prioritize activities and is helped to plan how to continue those activities that are most valued. Practical suggestions about management of the condition help the patient to feel a sense of control and confidence in his or her ability to live with it.

Knowledge Deficit. The nurse determines what the patient already knows about OA and corrects any misconceptions. The patient teaching plan includes a general description of the nature of OA, pain management, coping measures, self-administration of prescribed medications, rest and modification of activities, resources for information (local chapter of the Arthritis Foundation), and incorporation of leisure and recreation into daily living.

EVALUATION. Criteria for evaluating the outcomes of nursing care for the patient with OA are patient's statement of reduced or relieved pain, relaxed expression; accomplishment of usual activities; positive statements about ability to manage; and patient's statements and demonstration of self-care and prescribed therapeutic measures.

Nursing Care Following Total Joint Replacement

Joints that can be replaced include the elbow, shoulder, phalangeal finger joints, hip, knee, and ankle. Preoperative care prepares the patient for the surgical procedure and the postoperative period. The nurse and the physical therapist may instruct the patient in postoperative exercises. The patient and family are advised of postoperative limitations and encouraged to plan for adapting the home and work environment as needed. General nursing care of the surgical patient is discussed in Chapter 14. This section describes the postoperative nursing care needs of the patient who has had a joint replacement. Surgeon orders or protocols are usually very specific for each type of joint surgery. Common postoperative measures for specific procedures are presented in Table 37–4.

ASSESSMENT. Routine postoperative care is covered in Chapter 14 and includes assessment of vital signs, level of consciousness, intake and output, respiratory and neurovascular status, urinary function, bowel elimination, wound condition, and comfort. After total joint replacement, the nurse specifically monitors circulation and sensation in the affected extremity. The need for assistance with activities of daily living is determined.

NURSING DIAGNOSIS. Nursing diagnoses after total joint replacement may include the following:

- **Pain** related to tissue trauma
- **High Risk for Injury** related to improper alignment, dislocated prosthesis, weakness
- **Impaired Physical Mobility** related to immobilization, pain, weakness
- **Altered Peripheral Tissue Perfusion** related to trauma, hemorrhage, thrombi, compression of blood vessels
- **High Risk for Infection** related to invasive procedure, prosthesis placement
- **Anxiety** or **Fear** related to outcome of procedure
- **Knowledge Deficit** of postoperative self-care

TABLE 37–4

GUIDELINES FOR NURSING CARE AFTER REPLACEMENT OF SPECIFIC JOINTS

HIP REPLACEMENT

1. Do not flex hip more than 90 degrees.
2. Avoid flexion adduction and internal rotation.
3. Place a large pillow between legs when turning, when supine, and when lying on unaffected side.
4. Advise patient not to cross legs or feet and not to put on own shoes, socks, or stockings for 6 wk to 2 mo, as directed by surgeon.
5. Apply leg abductor splints as ordered.
6. Do not turn on operative side unless specifically ordered by surgeon.
7. Have patient sit in a chair that has arms to facilitate rising without extreme hip flexion.
8. Arrange for a raised toilet seat to allow toileting without extreme hip flexion.
9. Permit weight bearing as ordered, depending on type of prosthesis used and whether cement was used.
10. Exercise unaffected extremities to maintain strength.

KNEE REPLACEMENT

1. Encourage quadriceps-setting exercises and straight leg lifts beginning postoperative day 2–5, as ordered.
2. Use passive motion machine as ordered; check alignment and settings.
3. Monitor weight bearing with walker or crutches as ordered.

FINGER REPLACEMENT

1. Elevate affected hand.
2. Assess sensation and warmth in affected fingers.
3. Apply splints during sleep as ordered.
4. Reinforce exercises taught by physical therapist—must be continued for 10–12 wk.
5. Advise patient not to lift heavy objects with affected hand.

GOALS. Goals for the listed nursing diagnoses are pain relief, absence of injury, improved physical mobility without complications of immobility, normal circulation to affected extremity, absence of infection, reduced anxiety and fear, and patient's knowledge of self-care.

INTERVENTIONS

Pain. The nurse assesses the patient's pain, describing its location, nature, and severity. Surgical pain is expected, but the patient may also have pain in other joints. Analgesics are administered as ordered, and the effects are assesed and documented. The patient is repositioned as permitted. The nurse may use massage, relaxation techniques, imagery, or other strategies described in Chapter 16 to help the patient deal with the pain. Sudden severe pain in the surgical area is reported to the surgeon since it may signal prosthesis dislocation. Uncontrolled pain may make the patient reluctant to participate in rehabilitation measures. The administration of analgesics 30 minutes to 1 hour before painful exercises may improve patient participation.

High Risk for Injury. Prosthetic joints can become dislocated if they are not maintained in proper alignment. For example, after hip replacement, the affected leg must be kept in a position of abduction to prevent dislocation. Splints or traction may be used as ordered to maintain the desired position. Progressive exercises are usually prescribed and may be done by the physical therapist. As the patient's activity is increased, the nurse teaches and reinforces precautions. The patient is taught to recognize signs and symptoms of dislocation: pain in affected joint, loss of function, and shortening or deformity of the extremity (Fig. 37–4).

Impaired Physical Mobility. The degree of mobility impairment depends on which joints are affected as well as the patient's general physical state. In general, early mobility is encouraged. When mobility is severely impaired, the patient is at risk for pulmonary and circulatory complications, urinary retention, constipation, and skin breakdown. In addition, unused muscles weaken and unused joints stiffen. The nurse repositions the patient as allowed, carefully assessing for redness caused by circulatory impairment. The patient is coached and supported during coughing and deep breathing exercises and use of the incentive spirometer. Breaths sounds are auscultated to detect atelectasis or retained secretions. The abdomen is assessed for bladder or bowel distention. Intravenous fluids are administered as ordered until the patient takes adequate oral fluids. Stool softeners and laxatives are also given as ordered.

The patient may have self-care deficits related to mobility impairments or restrictions. The nurse identifies activities the patient cannot do alone and provides appropriate assistance. As the patient progresses, the nurse encourages increasing independence. Rehabilitation re- patient participation in the prescribed exercise The patient may need reassurance that the d should be exercised (Fig. 37–5). The pa- exercises better if there is adequate pain

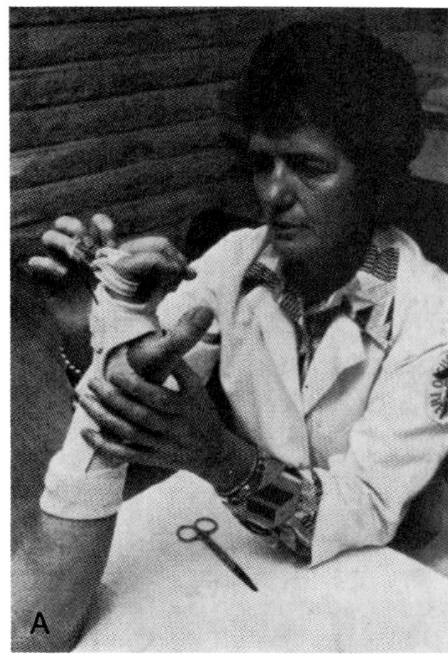

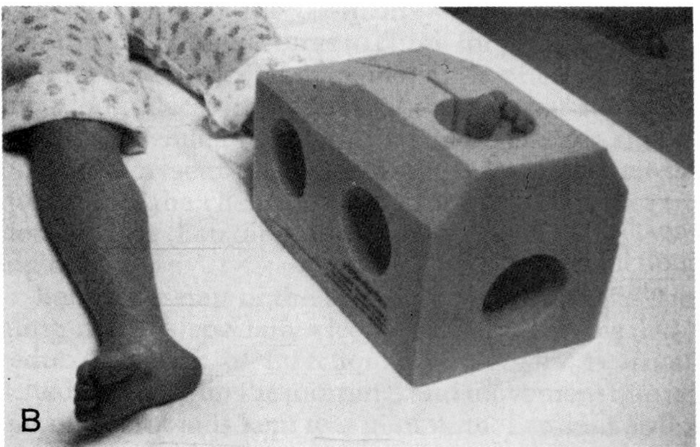

FIGURE 37-4

Devices used to maintain desired joint positions after total joint replacement surgery include a dynamic splint used after finger implants *(A)* and a cradle boot used after hip replacement *(B)*. (*A*, from the AHPA Arthritis Teaching Slide Collection, © 1980. Used with permission of the American College of Rheumatology; *B* courtesy of Span America Corporation.)

control. A CPM machine may be used to reduce scar tissue formation and improve range of motion (Fig. 37–6).

Altered Peripheral Tissue Perfusion. Body areas distal to the operative joint are monitored for circulatory adequacy by assessing warmth, color, and peripheral pulses. Splints, dressings, and antiembolic stockings also can restrict circulation and must be checked for proper positioning. To reduce the risk of deep vein thrombosis in the legs, pillows and pads should not be placed under the legs. Signs and symptoms of deep vein thrombosis include tenderness, swelling, redness, firm palpable blood vessels called cords, and positive Homans's sign (pain behind the knee or in the calf when the foot is dorsiflexed). The nurse determines the specific exercises

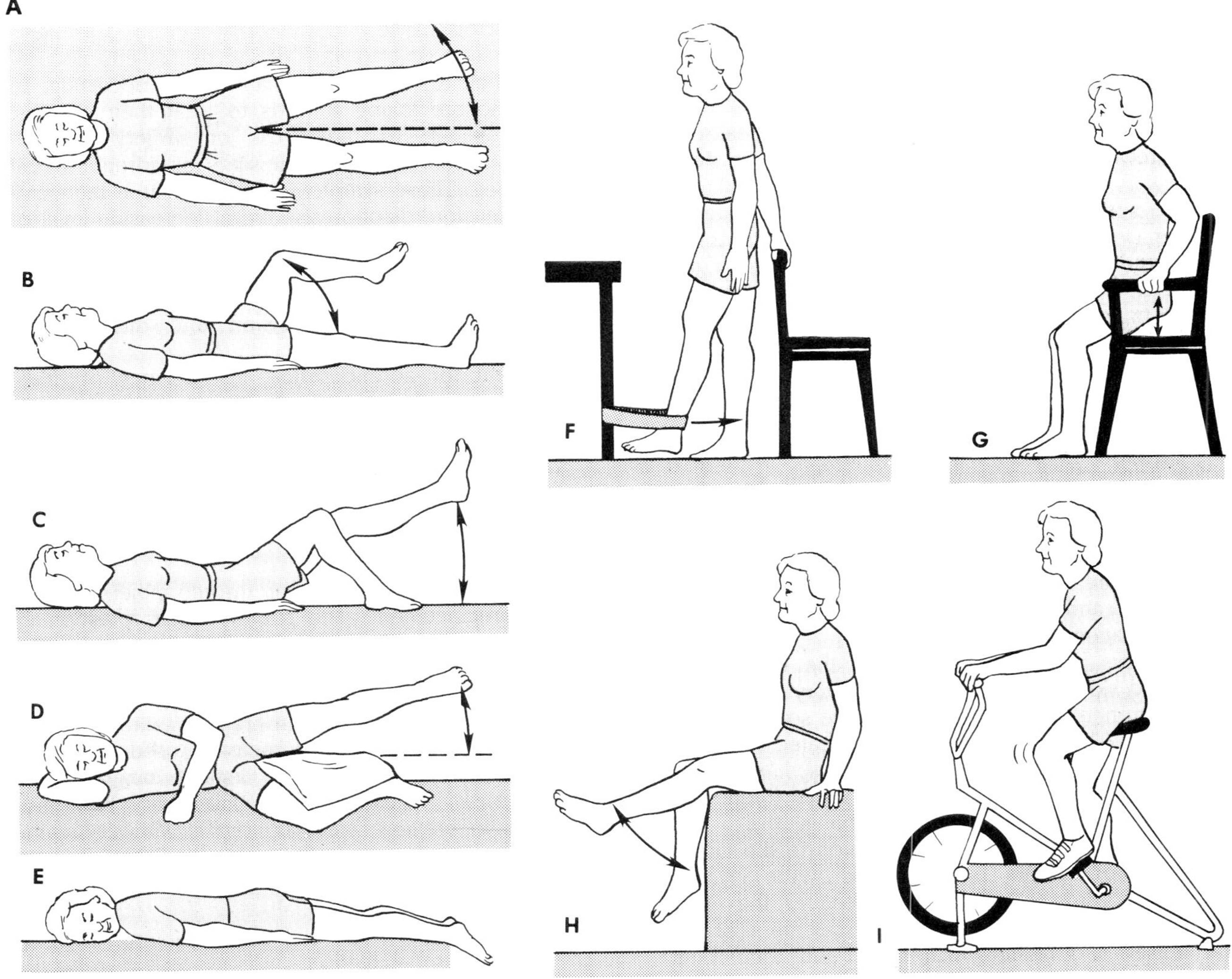

FIGURE 37-5

Rehabilitation exercises after total hip replacement. *A*, Lie on back and gently swing leg away from body and return it to midline. *B*, While supine, raise hip and knee as shown. *C*, While supine, keep the leg straight and raise it. *D*, Lie on unoperated side and raise operated leg straight up toward the ceiling. *E*, Lying prone to stretch muscles that flex the hip. *F*, Put a resistive material like rubber tubing on the ankle of the operated leg, secure it to a sturdy object, and try to pull the leg back to midline. *G*, Use the arms to raise self from the chair seat. *H*, In a sitting position, raise and lower the leg. *I*, Use the stationary bicycle—an exercise prescribed late in the rehabilitation program. (From Black, J. M., & Matassarin-Jacobs, E. [1993]. *Luckmann and Sorensen's medical-surgical nursing: A psychophysiologic approach* [4th ed., p. 608]. Philadelphia: W. B. Saunders.)

that may be done based on physician's orders and protocols. For example, after hip replacement, the patient should flex and extend the toes, feet, and ankles hourly to promote venous return.

The patient is at risk for hemorrhage after joint replacement. The nurse checks the dressings for increasing bleeding, monitors vital signs for tachycardia and hypotension, and observes for restlessness and anxiety. Wound drainage in suction devices is inspected and measured at least every 8 hours. There is also a risk of fat embolus, which can produce signs of local or cerebral blood vessel occlusion: petechial hemorrhage of upper chest and conjunctiva, fat globules in the urine, headache, irritability, confusion, loss of consciousness.

Pressure caused by edema or constrictive dressings can cause nerve damage, which may be manifested by anesthesia or paresthesia. Therefore, the nurse monitors sensation distal to the joint and reports symptoms of impairment to the surgeon. Dressings, stockings, and splints are checked to be sure that they are not too tight.

Ambulation is supervised until the patient is steady and clearly understands the limitations. The environment is kept free of clutter.

High Risk for Infection. The patient's temperature is monitored for elevations that may reveal infections. The surgical wound is assessed for redness, swelling, warmth, and foul drainage. The nurse uses strict sterile technique when handling the wound, drains, or dressings.

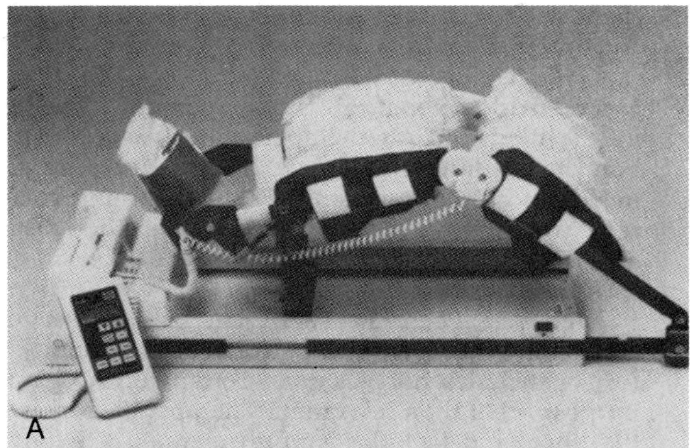

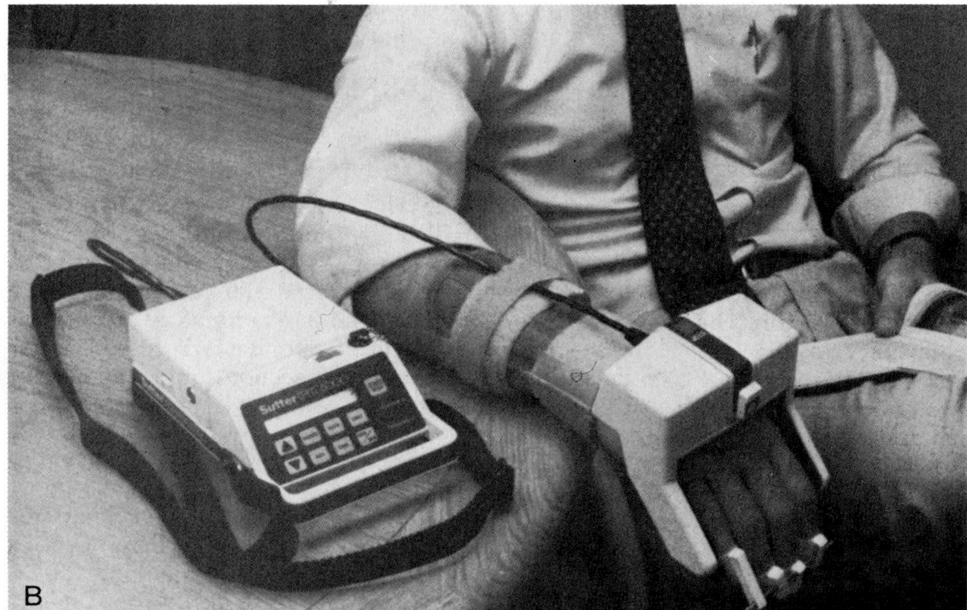

FIGURE 37-6

Continuous passive motion machines prevent scar formation and promote flexion. *A*, A continuous passive motion (CPM) machine for use after total knee replacement: note the sheepskin padding. *B*, A CPM machine in use after finger implant surgery. (Courtesy of Sulter Corporation.)

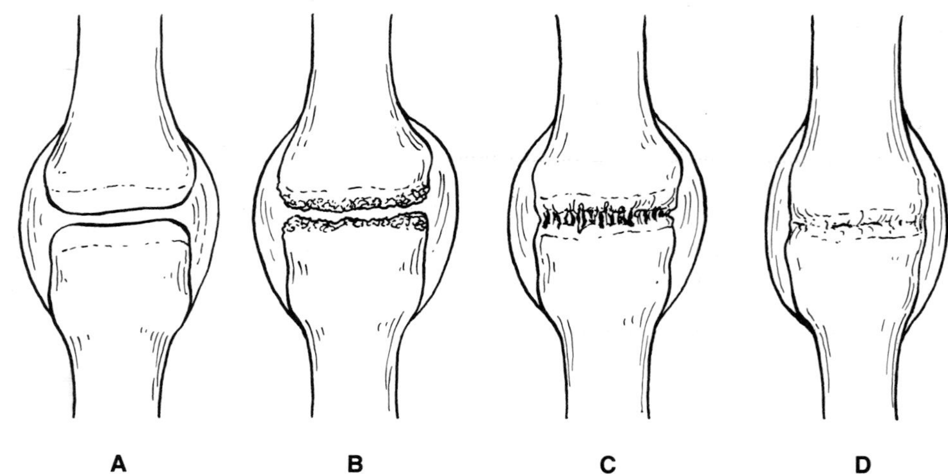

FIGURE 37-7

Pathologic changes in the joint with rheumatoid arthritis. Inflammation begins in the synovium and eventually results in fibrous immobilization of the joint. (From Black, J. M., & Matassarin-Jacobs, E. [1993]. *Luckmann and Soren-* *dical-surgical nursing: A* *ologic approach* [4th Philadelphia: W. B.

Wound dressings must be kept clean and dry. Antimicrobials are administered as ordered. The patient is instructed in hand washing and wound care.

Anxiety or Fear. Total joint replacement is usually done after conservative treatments have failed to maintain joint mobility. The patient is typically hopeful but anxious about the outcome of the surgery. The nurse tells the patient what to expect, explains procedures and equipment, and offers to answer questions. Responding promptly to the patient's needs and checking on him or her frequently are reassuring.

Knowledge Deficit. From admission to discharge, the patient is instructed in self-care. Specifics depend on which joint was replaced, but all patients need to know (1) what activities are permitted and contraindicated, (2) directions for drug therapy, (3) wound care, (4) signs and symptoms that should be reported to the surgeon, and (5) when to return for follow-up care. Referrals may be made for a home health nurse to assist the patient.

EVALUATION. Criteria for evaluating nursing care are patient's statement of pain relief and relaxed expression; continuous proper alignment of operative joint; increasing patient mobility without excess fatigue or injury; vital signs consistent with patient's norms, symmetric warmth and color of extremities; absence of fever or increasing wound redness; patient's statement of reduced anxiety and calm manner; and patient's description of self-care measures and restrictions.

RHEUMATOID ARTHRITIS

Rheumatoid arthritis (RA) is a chronic, progressive inflammatory disease. Although it is a systemic disorder, RA is characterized by its effect on synovial joints. The disease has a peak onset in people 20 to 40 years of age and is more common in women than in men. It affects an estimated 1 to 3% of the population in the United States. The course of the disease is variable, ranging from minimal symptoms to severe debilitation.

Pathophysiology

There is no single known cause for RA. Proposed explanations include immunologic processes, a virus, genetic predisposition, and hormonal factors. The onset of the disease is characterized by inflammation of the synovial tissue in joints. The synovial tissues hold the lubricating fluid of the joints. In RA, the synovium thickens and fluid accumulates in the joint space. Vascular granulation tissue, called pannus, forms in the joint capsule and breaks down cartilage and bone. Fibrous tissue invades the pannus, converting it first to rigid scar tissue and finally to bony tissue. These changes result in ankylosis (loss of joint mobility) (Fig. 37–7).

Signs and Symptoms

The most common symptom of RA is pain in the affected joints, aggravated by movement. Morning stiffness lasting more than 1 hour is almost always a feature of RA, unlike in osteoarthritis, in which stiffness is relieved within minutes. Other symptoms include weakness, easy fatigability, anorexia, weight loss, muscle aches, and tenderness, warmth, and swelling of the affected joint.

The distal interphalangeal and metacarpophalangeal joints are most often affected. The wrist, elbow, knee, and ankle are other possible areas affected. Rheumatoid nodules, which are subcutaneous nodules over bony prominences, also may be present (Fig. 37–8). Joint changes are usually symmetric, meaning that the disease tends to affect the same joints in both extremities simultaneously.

Any organ of the body may be affected by RA. If blood vessels are affected, they become inflamed, a

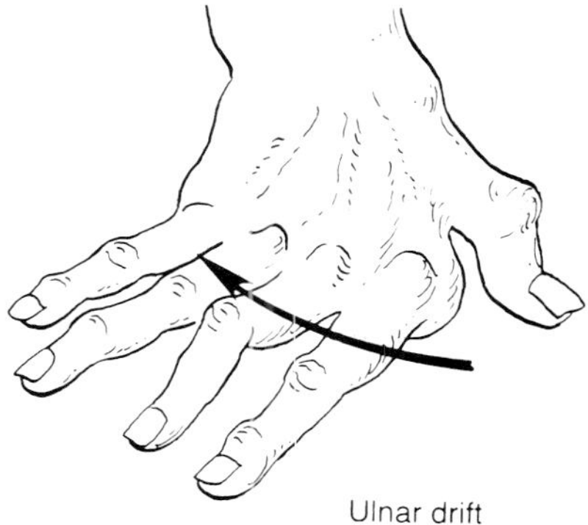

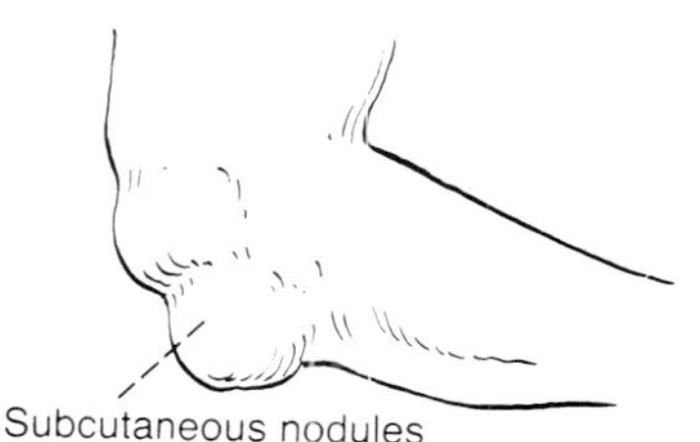

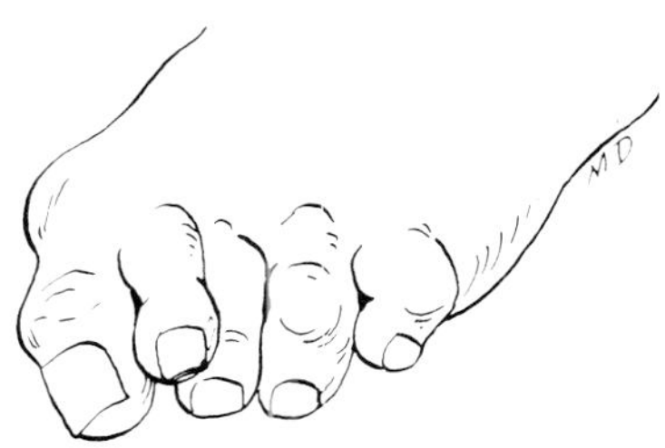

FIGURE 37–8

Common changes in the elbows, hands, and feet with rheumatoid arthritis. (Modified from Black, J. M., & Matassarin-Jacobs, E. [1993]. *Luckmann and Sorensen's medical-surgical nursing: A psychophysiologic approach* [4th ed., p. 597]. Philadelphia: W. B. Saunders.)

condition called vasculitis. With vasculitis, blood supply to body organs is impaired, with possible ischemia or infarction of affected organs. Ischemic lesions of the skin are brownish spots most often seen around the nail beds. Large lesions that tend to ulcerate may appear on the legs. Secondary effects on bone can cause osteoporosis, making the bones susceptible to fractures. The disease may produce inflammatory changes in the tissues of the heart, lungs, kidneys, and eyes. Pleural effusions and pulmonary fibrosis can lead to respiratory impairment or pulmonary hypertension and eventual heart failure.

Some patients with RA develop clusters of symptoms, including Sjögren's syndrome, Felty's syndrome, or Caplan's syndrome. Sjögren's syndrome is characterized by dry mouth, dry eyes, and dry vagina. Felty's syndrome, which consists of enlarged liver and spleen and neutropenia, is less commonly seen. Caplan's syndrome occurs most often in coal miners and asbestos workers and is marked by rheumatoid nodules in the lungs.

Medical Diagnosis

The diagnosis of RA is supported by a comprehensive history and physical examination, laboratory findings, and radiographic changes. There is no single test to diagnose RA, but groups of tests and radiographic findings may help to confirm the disorder. See Table 37–2 for common studies for connective tissues disorders.

The presence of rheumatoid factor does not establish the diagnosis of RA; however, its presence may confirm a diagnosis in persons who have other supportive clinical factors. The C-reactive protein and erythrocyte sedimentation rate, although not specific, also help support the diagnosis in patients with other suggestive symptoms.

The primary purpose of radiographs is to detect changes brought about by RA and to determine the usefulness of disease-modifying drugs or surgery.

Medical Treatment

The treatment of RA involves an interdisciplinary approach, including medicine, nursing, physical therapy, occupational therapy, and social services. In addition to drug therapy, the following supportive treatments may be employed: rest, splinting to reduce motion that aggravates the inflamed joints, orthotic devices to support deformed joints, and assistance in modifying activities of daily living.

Drug therapy is aimed at controlling the local inflammatory process. Aspirin and other NSAIDs may provide symptomatic relief. If symptoms are not relieved, disease-modifying drugs may be prescribed. Disease-modifying drugs, such as gold compounds, D-penicillamine, antimalarials, and sulfasalazine, can induce remission or significant clinical improvement for weeks or even months at a time. Glucocorticoids, although effective in reducing the inflammatory process, are the last choice owing to their adverse side effects. Cytotoxic drugs (cyclophosphamide [Cytoxan]) are another class of drugs that may provide some relief to patients with RA (see Table 37–3 for commonly used drugs to treat connective tissue disorders.)

Surgical management of RA is reserved for those patients with severe pain and deformities. Arthroplasties including total joint replacements can be done. The most successful procedures are those performed on the knees and hips (see the section on osteoporosis).

PHARMACOLOGY CAPSULE

Aspirin prolongs bleeding time, so patients must be monitored for bruising and bleeding.

Nursing Care of the Patient with Rheumatoid Arthritis

ASSESSMENT. The general assessment of the patient with a connective tissue disorder is summarized in Table 37–1. When a patient has RA, the nurse includes assessment for pain, swelling, tenderness, limitation of movement, decreased ability to perform activities of daily living (dressing, grooming, eating, toileting), fatigue, and joint deformities.

NURSING DIAGNOSIS. The following are common nursing diagnoses for a patient with RA:

- **Pain** related to swelling and tenderness
- **Activity Intolerance** related to fatigue
- **Ineffective Individual Coping** related to embarrassment, inability to do activities independently
- **Social Isolation** related to physical impairment and poor body image
- **Knowledge Deficit** of RA, its treatment, and self-care

GOALS. Goals of nursing care for the patient with RA include reduced pain, improved tolerance for activity, effective coping, continued social contacts, and patient's knowledge of RA, its treatment, and self-care.

INTERVENTIONS

Pain. Chronic pain imposes a terrible burden on the patient. Measures to control pain include application of heat or cold and administration of medications as ordered. A warm shower, on arising, may relieve morning pain and stiffness. Maintaining a program of exercise and rest also can help to manage joint pain. Care of the patient with pain is discussed in Chapter 16.

Activity Intolerance. The nurse and the patient plan activities around periods of rest and activity. Assistance is provided as needed with getting in and out of bed and going to the bathroom. Patients who are severely disabled may need help with all activities of daily living. If needed, the nurse helps the patient change positions and assists with meals. The patient's response to activity is monitored to detect tachycardia, dyspnea, or muscle weakness. Physical therapy may be ordered, and the nurse supports the patient's prescribed therapy program.

Ineffective Individual Coping. Developing a trusting, collaborative relationship is a prerequisite for the nurse to assist and plan care that is meaningful to the patient. The nurse visits the patient often and initiates conversations to explore concerns, answer questions, and plan care. The patient's strengths are emphasized, and previously used coping skills are explored. Some patients respond to their physical and functional losses with demanding behavior that others see as manipulative. Caregivers must recognize this as an attempt to maintain some control in their lives. An important part of coping is learning to maintain maximal possible independence despite the crippling effects of RA. Adaptations in the home and workplace and the use of appropriate assistive devices can promote independence and an improved sense of well-being. Since a chronic illness affects the family as well as the patient, the nurse reaches out to the family, offering information, encouragement, problem solving, and resources. Information should be provided about community resources such as the local chapter of the Arthritis Foundation. A referral may be made to a home care agency to help the patient learn to manage better at home.

Social Isolation. Physical deformities that impair function evoke a great sense of loss in the RA patient. Resulting depression, irritability, and feelings of helplessness can have a devastating effect on the patient's interpersonal relationships. In addition, patients who take glucocorticoids often have mood swings, which makes their behavior unpredictable. These emotional changes may discourage visits from staff and from family. The nurse needs to visit the patient often so that he or she does not feel isolated and lonely. Family and friends may need help understanding the patient's irritability and mood swings. The nurse emphasizes the importance of their continued support to the patient. The patient is encouraged to identify social activities that are appropriate and to remain involved to the extent possible.

Knowledge Deficit. The teaching plan should include information about the disease process, drug therapy, rest and activity, and signs and symptoms that should be reported to the physician (increasing activity intolerance, dyspnea).

EVALUATION. Criteria for goal achievement for the patient with RA are patient's statement of reduced pain, relaxed expression; performance of small tasks without needing a rest period; patient's identification of ways to deal with physical changes; identification of at least one social opportunity that can be maintained; and patient's statement of self-care measures.

OSTEOPOROSIS

Pathophysiology

Bone is constantly being formed and absorbed. Until adolescence, bone formation exceeds bone absorption. The processes remain equal through the twenties, but, beginning around age 30, bone absorption surpasses bone formation. Loss of trabecular bone, the innermost layer, occurs first. The loss of cortical bone, the hard outer shell, begins later in life. The loss of cortical bone begins earlier and progresses faster in women than in men. The net result is loss of bone mass, which makes the patient susceptible to fractures. Common sites of fractures due to osteoporosis are the wrist, vertebrae, and hip. This age-related process without apparent underlying medical causes is one type of osteoporosis (primary osteoporosis). Another type (secondary osteoporosis) is loss of bone mass due to factors other than age, such as hyperparathyroidism or long-term therapy with corticosteroids or heparin.

Risk Factors

Many factors appear to increase the risk of osteoporosis. At greatest risk are elderly females who have small frames, are white or of Northern European heritage, and who have fair skin and blond or red hair. Other risk factors are removal of both ovaries, physical inactivity, inadequate calcium or vitamin D intake, and excessive use of cigarettes, caffeine, and alcohol. A number of disorders, such as Cushing's disease and type II diabetes mellitus, also seem to be associated with osteoporosis.

Signs and Symptoms

Signs and symptoms of osteoporosis may include back pain, fractures, loss of height due to vertebral compression, and kyphosis. Bone deterioration in the jaw can cause dentures to fit poorly.

Medical Diagnosis

Bone mass can be measured using a technique called absorptiometry. Absorptiometry is a quick, painless radiologic procedure that measures the amount of bone tissue in the hip and spine. Blood studies are usually normal for primary osteoporosis, but a battery of tests may be ordered to rule out possible causes of secondary osteoporosis. Radiographs detect bone fractures but do not reveal decreased bone density until there is loss of 30 to 50% of the bone mass. A bone specimen may be obtained for study from the iliac crest.

Medical Treatment

There is no cure for osteoporosis, but medical treatment aims to prevent fractures and stimulate bone formation. It is believed that regular exercise slows bone loss and improves strength, balance, and reaction time, thereby reducing the risk of falls and fractures. The incidence or severity of the disorder may be reduced by identifying high-risk people and taking steps to promote healthy bone development. It is generally accepted that calcium supplementation and estrogen replacement for postmenopausal women slow bone loss. The recommended elemental calcium intake is 1000 mg per day for premenopausal women and for postmenopausal women who are on estrogen replacement therapy. Postmenopausal women who are not on estrogen replacement therapy require 1500 mg of calcium daily. The only contraindication to supplementary calcium is a history of kidney stones. Estrogen replacement is controversial, and the patient should discuss the issue with her physician. Physical therapy may be consulted to develop an appropriate exercise program for the patient.

Nursing Care of the Patient with Osteoporosis

ASSESSMENT. The nursing assessment of the patient with a connective tissue disorder is summarized in Table 37–1. When a patient has osteoporosis, the nurse specifically assesses the patient's diet, calcium intake, and exercise plan. A history of cancer of the reproductive system is noted. The patient's height is measured and compared with previous measurements. The patient's posture is described.

NURSING DIAGNOSIS. When a patient has osteoporosis, the nursing diagnoses may include the following:

- **High Risk for Trauma** related to loss of bone strength
- **Pain** related to fractures, pressure on nerves due to vertebral compression
- **Knowledge Deficit** of measures to promote bone formation and prevent bone loss

GOALS. Goals for the patient with osteoporosis are absence of trauma, pain relief, and patient's understanding of preventive and treatment measures.

INTERVENTIONS

High Risk for Trauma. The nurse monitors the patient's ability to carry out activities of daily living. Assistance is provided if necessary. Ambulatory patients are advised to wear good supportive shoes. Canes or walkers are provided to improve balance if needed. The environment is kept free of hazards that might cause the patient to fall. Personal articles are placed within the patient's reach. In the home setting, an assessment is done to identify possible hazards, and steps are taken to provide a safer environment. The nurse should also do a screening of gross visual acuity. In order to maneuver safely, the patient must be able to see. If indicated, an eye examination is recommended.

Pain. The nurse obtains a complete description of the patient's pain. Analgesics may be administered as ordered, but the nurse also uses nonpharmacologic interventions as described in Chapter 16. Some patients, especially those with vertebral compression, may have chronic pain that is difficult to manage. The nurse may suggest referral to a pain clinic. The effects of pain management strategies are documented.

Knowledge Deficit. Content to be included in a teaching plan for the patient with osteoporosis is the importance of adequate dietary calcium and vitamin D, the calcium supplementation recommended by the physician, the need to limit intake of alcohol and caffeine, the value of exercise, and the need for safety precautions to avoid falls and fractures.

EVALUATION. Criteria for evaluating the outcomes of nursing interventions are performance of daily activities without falls or injuries, patient's statement of reduced pain and relaxed expression, and patient's verbalization of content taught and intent to follow instructions.

GOUT

Gout is a systemic disease characterized by the deposition of urate crystals in the joints and other body tissues. There are two forms of gout: primary gout, in which uric acid is elevated due to a metabolic disorder, and secondary gout, in which uric acid is elevated owing to another disease process. Primary gout is more prevalent among men than women, with a peak incidence in people in their forties and fifties. The primary form of the disorder is inherited.

Pathophysiology

Gout is characterized by an excess of uric acid in the blood, referred to as hyperuricemia. Hyperuricemia is related either to an excessive rate of uric acid production or to decreased uric acid excretion by the kidneys. Features of gout may include (1) increased serum urates; (2) recurring acute attacks of arthritis; (3) the clumping of urate clusters around the joints of the extremities, causing crippling deformities; (4) renal disease involving blood vessels and interstitial tissues; and (5) uric acid kidney stones.

Signs and Symptoms

The onset of acute gout cannot be ignored by the patient. The onset is abrupt, usually occurring at night. The patient is suddenly afflicted with severe, crushing pain that cannot bear even the light touch of bed sheets. The joint commonly affected is that of the great toe. The attack may be precipitated by trauma, diuretics, increased alcohol consumption, or high purine diet (food high in proteins). The symptoms usually disappear within a few days, and joint function is completely restored.

Other symptoms may include fever and the appearance of tophi, which are deposits of sodium urate crystals under the skin (Fig. 37–9). Infection may develop if the skin breaks open. Kidney stones develop in about 20% of patients with gout.

Medical Diagnosis

Since not all patients with gout have hyperuricemia, measurement of uric acid is not specific for a diagnosis of gout. The presence of tophi or urate crystals, or both, in synovial fluid usually indicates chronic gout.

Medical Treatment

Drug therapy provides effective treatment for acute gout. Colchicine is no longer the drug of choice because

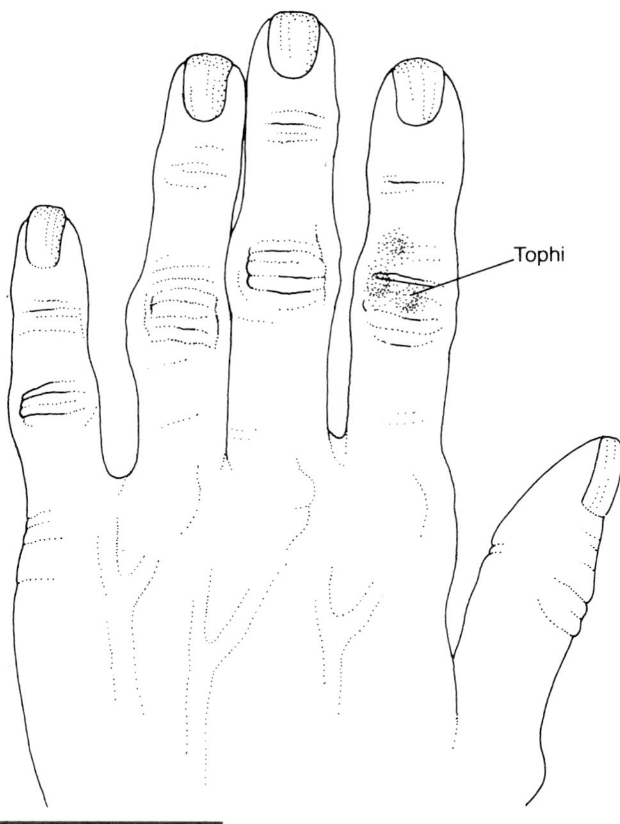

FIGURE 37-9

Tophi: nodules typical of gout. (From Ignatavicius, D. D., & Bayne, M. V. [1991]. *Medical-surgical nursing: A nursing process approach* [p. 707]. Philadelphia: W. B. Saunders.)

of its adverse effects on the gastrointestinal system. Nevertheless, colchicine may be given at hourly intervals until the acute symptoms ease or until the patient develops nausea and vomiting. Other drugs effective in abating symptoms are indomethacin and NSAIDs (Table 37–3). If the patient does not respond to these drugs, parenteral glucocorticoids may be prescribed. Drugs used to inhibit uric acid synthesis include allopurinol (Zyloprim) and probenecid (Benemid).

PHARMACOLOGY CAPSULE

Patients on antigout drugs need to maintain urine output of at least 2000 ml per day to reduce the risk of urinary calculus formation.

Nursing Care of the Patient with Gout

ASSESSMENT. Complete assessment of the patient with a connective tissue disorder is summarized in Table 37–1. The patient with gout should be specifically assessed for pain, joint swelling, tophi, uric acid stones, fever, and a history of trauma, injury, or surgery.

NURSING DIAGNOSIS. Common nursing diagnoses for the patient with gout include the following:

- **Pain** related to joint inflammation
- **Impaired Physical Mobility** related to painful joint movement
- **Altered Urinary Elimination** related to urate kidney stones
- **Knowledge Deficit** of gout, its treatment, and self-care measures

GOALS. Goals of nursing care for the patient with gout include reduced pain, improved mobility, normal urine output without symptoms of renal stones, and patient's knowledge of the disease, how it is treated, and self-care measures.

INTERVENTIONS

Pain. Nursing care to decrease discomfort includes elevation of the affected extremity, administration of prescribed medications, and avoidance of pressure on the area. Hot or cold packs may be ordered. Splints or bandages may be used to immobilize the affected joint.

Impaired Physical Mobility. Bedrest is usually recommended during the acute period. The nurse provides assistance with activities of daily living as needed. When ambulation is permitted, the patient is advised to protect affected joints from trauma by wearing supportive, firm shoes and by keeping walking pathways clearly lighted and free of obstacles that might easily cause falls.

Altered Urinary Elimination. When the serum uric acid level is elevated, the excess acid is excreted in the urine, where it may form uric acid stones. Urinary stones can obstruct urine flow from the kidney, causing renal damage. To prevent this complication, the patient is advised to consume at least eight glasses of fluid daily unless contraindicated. Drugs may be prescribed to make the urine alkaline since uric acid stones precipitate in acid urine. During hospitalization, intravenous fluids may be given. The nurse monitors urine intake and output. Signs and symptoms of urinary stones (pain in the flank, lower abdomen, or genitals; fever; hematuria; decreased urine output) are reported to the physician promptly.

Knowledge Deficit. The nurse instructs the patient in measures to prevent or decrease future attacks. The diet should be low in purines. Foods to be avoided include meat, fish, fowl, spinach, lentils, mushrooms, peas, and asparagus. Alcohol also is discouraged. The dietitian should be consulted to help the patient plan a well-balanced diet. Patients are also usually taught to maintain a high fluid intake to reduce the risk of uric acid stone formation in the urinary tract. The importance of adhering to the prescribed drug regimen is explained, and information is provided about dosage, schedule, and side effects.

The patient is encouraged to report early joint or urinary symptoms to the physician promptly. Severe attacks may be averted if treatment is begun soon after symptoms develop.

EVALUATION. Overall, the goals of treatment for gout are to reduce the number of gouty attacks and to prevent renal complications. Criteria for measuring achievement of the specific goals identified are patient's verbalization that affected joint is free of pain; patient's planning a diet low in purine and stating intent to lower alcohol consumption; absence of flank or abdominal pain and absence of hematuria; and patient's description of appropriate self-care measures.

SYSTEMIC LUPUS ERYTHEMATOSUS

Systemic lupus erythematosus (SLE) is a chronic inflammatory disease of unknown cause. It is classified as an autoimmune disease, meaning that it is characterized by an immune system that has gone haywire. Antibodies are produced that destroy the body's own organs, such as the skin, heart, kidneys, and brain. Systemic lupus erythematosus, as defined by Goldfinger and Corron (1992), gives a vivid portrayal of the character of the disease: "No disease more dramatically illustrates the body's capacity to turn on itself than systemic lupus erythematosus."

It is believed that viral infections and heredity are predisposing factors for SLE. The disease affects populations in urban areas more than those in rural locales. It is estimated to affect 1 in 2100, with a high incidence among black females, Latinos, and Asians. The course of SLE is variable as it may be acute and episodic followed by periods of remissions.

Pathophysiology

It appears that people with SLE become immune to the body's different tissues. Abnormal antibodies are produced that destroy the organs. The initial response to the antibodies is inflammation. Immune complexes form in the serum and affect organs by direct invasion or by causing inflammation of blood vessels (vasculitis) that supply the organs. With vasculitis, blood flow decreases, depriving tissue of oxygen. The effects on specific body tissues include damage to the joints, kidneys, heart, lungs, and central nervous system. Renal, cardiac, and central nervous system complications can be fatal.

Signs and Symptoms

Signs and symptoms of SLE vary depending on the organ affected and the individual patient. Symptoms are mild in some people, devastating in others. Common symptoms include fatigue, malaise, dry scaly skin, raised butterfly-shaped rash over the nose and cheeks, pain and decreased mobility of joints, myalgia (muscle pain), fever, anorexia, weight loss, tachycardia, chest pain, abdominal pain, and enlarged lymph nodes.

Medical Diagnosis

There is no specific test for SLE, so diagnosis is based on the history and physical examination along with blood and urine studies. The best screening test is the blood test for antinuclear antibodies, which is elevated with SLE. Routine blood testing may also detect anemia, leukopenia (decreased white blood cells), lymphopenia (decreased lymphocytes), and thrombocytopenia (decreased platelets). The urinalysis may show microscopic hematuria and proteinuria.

Medical Treatment

There is no cure for SLE. The treatment is symptomatic and supportive. The patient is included in the development of the treatment plan. The goal of treatment is to manage the inflammation. Aspirin and other NSAIDs may reduce mild symptoms, but glucocorticoids, antimalarial drugs, and cytotoxins may be necessary. Topical steroid creams are often helpful for skin lesions.

Nursing Care of the Patient with Systemic Lupus Erythematosus

ASSESSMENT. The general assessment of the patient with a connective tissue disorder is summarized in Table 37–1. When a patient has SLE, the health history includes a complete description of the symptoms that caused the patient to seek medical attention. The family medical history is noted, especially a history of autoimmune diseases. In the past medical history, the nurse assesses exposure to viral infections and past serious illnesses. If the patient is on medications, including any for SLE, the drug name and dose are recorded. The review of systems documents pain; joint stiffness or swelling; rash; photosensitivity or vision disturbances; vertigo; nausea, vomiting, or diarrhea; decreased urine output; and hematuria. The functional assessment determines the extent to which symptoms are interfering with the patient's life. Sources of stress, coping strategies, and sources of support are noted. The physical examination focuses on the presence of a rash, especially across the nose and cheeks, and joint swelling and stiffness.

NURSING DIAGNOSIS. Nursing diagnoses for the patient with SLE may include the following:

- **Fatigue** and **Activity Intolerance** related to arthralgia and weakness
- **Impaired Skin Integrity** related to rash
- **Pain** related to joint inflammation
- **Body Image Disturbance** related to change in physical appearance and in role performance
- **Altered Nutrition: Less than Body Requirements** related to anorexia, fatigue, inflamed mucous membranes
- **Altered Urinary Elimination** related to renal complications
- **Knowledge Deficit** of SLE and its management

GOALS. Goals of nursing care for the patient with SLE are absence of excessive fatigue, intact skin, reduced pain, improved body image, maintenance of desirable weight, absence of urinary complications, and patient's knowledge of SLE and its management.

INTERVENTIONS

Fatigue, Activity Intolerance. In counseling the patient, the nurse helps identify activities that cause fatigue and encourages the patient to seek assistance as needed. Rest periods are incorporated into the daily schedule at appropriate times, but excessive rest is discouraged as it tends to permit joints to become stiffer. One cause of fatigue is anemia. If the patient is anemic, supplemental iron may be administered as ordered.

Impaired Skin Integrity. The skin rash may involve the face and the extremities. The patient is discouraged from applying powders or chemicals to the affected areas. Topical corticosteroids may be applied as ordered. Cool baths may be soothing to the inflamed skin. The patient is advised to avoid excessive exposure to sunlight, ultraviolet light, or fluorescent light.

The mucous membranes of the mouth also may become inflamed. Gentle mouth care is provided to avoid trauma to the painful tissue.

Pain. The nurse assesses the patient's comfort and identifies types and sites of pain. The patient with SLE may have headaches and joint pains. Analgesics and anti-inflammatories are administered as ordered. Nursing interventions for arthritis, a common development with SLE, are described under osteoarthritis and rheumatoid arthritis.

Body Image Disturbance. The nurse explores the patient's thoughts and feelings about the changes brought on by SLE. It may be helpful to ask the patient how he or she thinks the changes will affect his or her life. Coping strategies can then be identified to deal with the anticipated problems. Stress-reduction techniques are especially important because stress is thought to be a factor in triggering exacerbations. Since patients with chronic diseases sometimes feel helpless and inadequate, they are encouraged to be active participants in their care and to be as independent as possible.

Changes in appearance and loss of function typically result in a grief response. Patients need the nurse's kindness and support while adapting to these losses. A mental health professional, spiritual counselor, or support group may be helpful. The Lupus Foundation of America is a useful resource.

Altered Nutrition: Less than Body Requirements. Depression, pain, anxiety, inflamed oral mucous membranes, and joint dysfunction may affect the patient's appetite and ingestion of food. A pleasant mealtime environment with other people makes eating more enjoyable. Assistive devices such as large-handled utensils are easier to hold with stiff fingers. If the mouth is inflamed, the diet may require adjustment to eliminate irritating foods and fluids. Body weight is monitored to assess nutritional adequacy. The dietitian should be consulted if intake remains poor.

Altered Urinary Elimination. Renal function is monitored in the patient with SLE because kidney involvement may lead to renal failure. Urinary symptoms that may be distressing to the patient include nocturia, dysuria, and incontinence. Nocturia may be reduced by voiding before bedtime and reducing fluid intake in the evening. To reduce the risk of urinary tract infection, good perineal care is emphasized. Females are taught to clean the perineal area from front to back after elimination. Dysuria should be reported to the physician as it suggests infection of the urinary tract. Declining urine output may be due to renal failure and must be reported promptly. Care of the patient with renal failure is discussed in Chapter 36.

EVALUATION. Criteria for evaluating the outcomes of nursing interventions include performance of usual activities without excessive fatigue, intact skin with decreasing inflammation, patient's statement of decreased pain, positive statements about self, stable body weight, absence of urinary symptoms (burning, frequency, nocturia), and patient's descriptions of SLE and its treatment.

PROGRESSIVE SYSTEMIC SCLEROSIS (SCLERODERMA)

Progressive systemic sclerosis (PSS) is commonly called scleroderma. It is a chronic, multisystem disease of unknown origin that draws its name from the characteristic hardening of the skin. Other organs affected include the blood vessels, gastrointestinal tract, lungs, heart, and kidneys. The course of the disease varies among individuals, depending on the severity of involvement in the internal organs. There are approximately 100,000 to 200,000 cases of PSS in the United States. The onset of disease is usually between 30 and 50 years of age, with more women than men affected. Death may occur due to infection or cardiac or renal failure.

There are two types of PSS: progressively fatal PSS and CREST syndrome. Progressively fatal PSS is characterized by thickening of the skin and systemic effects. CREST syndrome consists of five symptoms: *c*alcinosis (calcium deposits in the tissues), *R*aynaud's phenomenon (vascular spasms), *e*sophageal dysfunction, *s*clerodactyly (scleroderma of the digits), and *t*elangiectasis (dilated superficial blood vessels).

Pathophysiology

Progressive systemic sclerosis is thought to be the result of primary vessel injury or dysfunction of the immune system. The manifestations of the disease follow a chain of events from inflammation to degeneration of tissues that results in decreased elasticity, stenosis, and occlusion of vessels.

Signs and Symptoms

The signs and symptoms of PSS reflect problems of the blood vessels, skin and joints, and internal organs. Common manifestations are Raynaud's phenomenon; symmetric painless swelling or thickening of the skin; taut, shiny skin; morning stiffness; frequent reflux of gastric acid; difficulty swallowing; weight loss; difficulty breathing; pericarditis; and renal insufficiency.

Medical Diagnosis

A complete history and physical examination may lead the physician to suspect fibrotic changes in the skin, lungs, heart, or esophagus. A positive antinuclear antibodies test, elevated erythrocyte sedimentation rate, and increased serum muscle enzymes support the diagnosis.

Medical Treatment

Even though there is no cure for PSS, treatment with high doses of steroids or immunosuppressants may bring about remission. Additional aims of treatment are management of symptoms and prevention of complications. Treatment includes physical therapy to maintain joint mobility and preserve muscle strength. Esophageal reflux may be treated with drugs to decrease the acidity of gastric secretions and periodic dilation of the esophagus and other measures, such as small, frequent feedings and elevation of the head of the bed.

The management of Raynaud's phenomenon is aimed at elimination of anything that causes vasospasm: smoking, cold environmental temperature, and vasoconstricting drugs.

Various drugs can be used to treat the symptoms of PSS. D-Penicillamine is used to decrease skin thickening and reduce the severity of visceral organ involvement. Antihypertensives are used to control hypertensive crisis, and anti-inflammatory drugs can be used to control joint pain and stiffness.

Nursing Care of the Patient with Progressive Systemic Sclerosis

ASSESSMENT. The general assessment of the patient with a connective tissue disorder is summarized in Table 37–1. When a patient has PSS, the health history specifically includes information about pain and stiffness in the fingers and intolerance for cold. The review of systems identifies signs and symptoms suggestive of cardiovascular, respiratory, renal, and gastrointestinal problems.

The physical examination assesses for skin rash, loss of wrinkles on the face, limitations of joint range of motion, muscle weakness, and dry mucous membranes. The hands are carefully inspected for contractures of the fingers and for color changes or lesions on the fingertips.

NURSING DIAGNOSIS. The nursing diagnoses for patients with PSS are similar to those of patients with other connective tissue diseases. The following are the major diagnoses:

- **Impaired Skin Integrity** related to thickening of tissues
- **Self-Care Deficits** related to pain, contractures of fingers, discomfort
- **Pain** related to swelling and stiffness, vasospasm
- **Social Isolation** related to poor self-concept
- **Altered Nutrition: Less than Body Requirements** related to esophageal dysfunction
- **Knowledge Deficit** related to scleroderma, medical management, and self-care

GOALS. The goals of nursing care are optimum skin integrity, independent self-care activities, reduced pain, improved socialization, adequate nutrition, and patient's knowledge of disease and self-care.

INTERVENTIONS

Impaired Skin Integrity. The skin is kept clean and dry. Protective clothing is provided as needed to maintain warmth and reduce skin discomfort. Cool baths with mild soaps followed by skin lotions may be soothing. A quiet environment also may decrease skin discomfort. Meticulous mouth care is warranted to prevent oral lesions. Anti-inflammatory drugs are administered as ordered. Practices that trigger vasospasm, such as exposure to cold and smoking, should be avoided.

Self-Care Deficit. The patient is encouraged to participate in self-care as much as possible. The nurse monitors the patient's tolerance for activity and provides assistance as needed. Activities are scheduled to prevent overtiring. The patient is permitted to pace himself or herself and should not attempt to do too much.

Pain. The patient with PSS usually has chronic joint pain and episodes of severe pain in the hands and feet associated with Raynaud's phenomenon. Measures to treat joint pain are described under rheumatoid arthritis. During acute episodes of Raynaud's phenomenon, the patient may be unable to tolerate anything touching the affected skin. A bed cradle can be used to keep the linens off the feet. Room temperature is adjusted to prevent chilling, which could provoke vasospasm. Other causes of vasospasm are smoking and severe stress.

Social Isolation. Swelling of the hands and facial changes create a "bird-like" appearance that may cause the patient to withdraw from social interactions (Fig. 37–10). The nurse can explore the patient's concerns about the altered appearance and help the patient anticipate how to deal with various social situations. The nurse demonstrates acceptance of the patient by expressing concern and using touch.

Altered Nutrition: Less than Body Requirements. If the patient has esophageal involvement, smaller, more frequent meals may be better tolerated. A relaxing environment before and after meals is helpful. Spicy foods, alcohol, and caffeine are restricted because they stimulate gastric secretions. Antacids and histamine$_2$ receptor blockers may be given as ordered to neutralize gastric acid and reduce the risk of esophagitis and ulceration

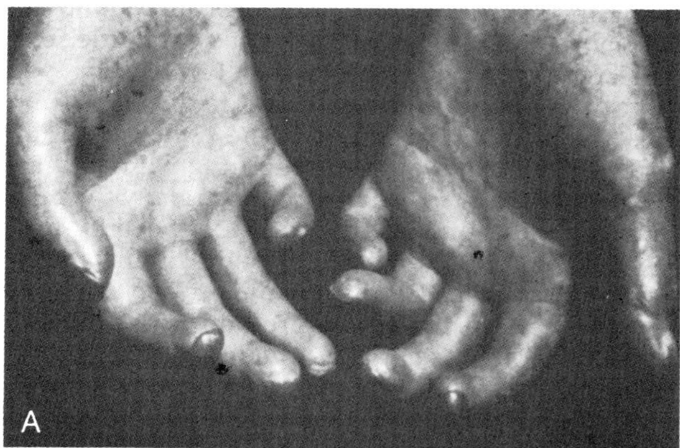

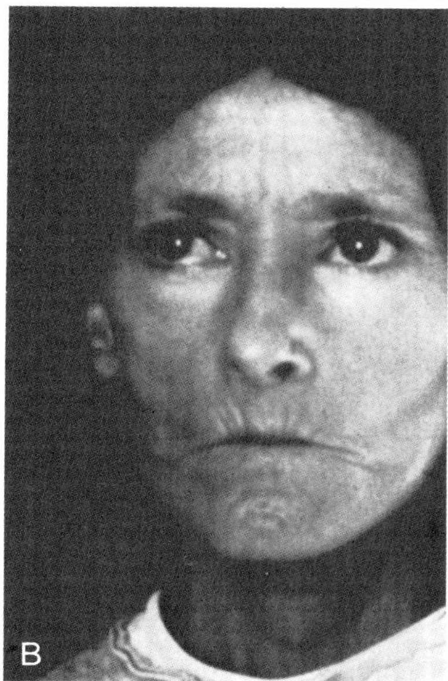

FIGURE 37-10
The patient with scleroderma. *A*, Edema of the hands and fingers. *B*, Typical facial appearance. (From the AHPA Arthritis Teaching Slide Collection, © 1980. Used with permission of the American College of Rheumatology.)

caused by esophageal reflux. After meals, the head should remain elevated for 1 to 2 hours to discourage reflux. The patient's weight should be monitored to assess adequacy of nutritional intake.

Knowledge Deficit. Patient teaching with PSS includes the nature of the disease, measures to prevent episodes of Raynaud's phenomenon, measures to maintain good nutrition and prevent esophageal reflux, signs and symptoms that should be reported to the physician, and self-medication.

EVALUATION. Criteria for evaluating the outcomes of nursing interventions include warm, intact skin with normal color; accomplishment of self-care activities without excessive fatigue; patient's statement of reduced pain and relaxed expression; increased socialization; stable body weight and absence of epigastric pain; and patient's statement of disease process and self-care measures.

POLYMYOSITIS

Polymyositis is a relatively rare acute or chronic inflammatory disease that primarily affects the skeletal muscle. The term *polymyositis* is applied to the condition when there is no skin involvement, and *dermatomyositis* is used when there is a characteristic skin rash. There is no known cause for polymyositis, but it is frequently seen in patients with scleroderma, rheumatoid arthritis, vasculitis, systemic lupus erythematosus, or Sjögren's syndrome.

Pathophysiology

The major activity producing pathology in polymyositis is infiltration of inflammatory cells causing destruction of muscle fibers. Inflammation of tissues surrounding blood vessels is an outstanding pathologic feature of the disease.

Signs and Symptoms

The primary symptom of polymyositis is muscle weakness reflected in inability to do normal activities like climbing stairs, raising the arms over the head, and turning over in bed. Other symptoms are Raynaud's phenomena and joint pain and inflammation. Patients with dermatomyositis typically have periorbital edema (swelling around the eyes) as well. The onset may be abrupt or slow.

Medical Diagnosis

The diagnosis is established by the presence of proximal muscle weakness, positive muscle biopsy for muscle degeneration, elevated muscle enzymes, and myopathic electromyographic changes.

Medical Treatment

Drug therapy includes high-dosage glucocorticosteroids such as prednisone and chemotherapeutic agents such as methotrexate. Supportive treatment centers around the right combination of rest and exercise to prevent contractures. This is difficult because range of motion exercises may aggravate the condition.

Nursing Care of the Patient with Polymyositis

Since polymyositis is seen in conjunction with other connective tissue diseases, the reader should refer to earlier sections of the chapter for applicable nursing interventions.

PERIARTERITIS NODOSA

Periarteritis nodosa (PAN) is also referred to as polyarteritis nodosa. The disease is a form of systemic necrotizing vasculitis. Vasculitis, characterized by inflammation and damage to blood vessels, is present in nearly all connective tissue diseases. In necrotizing vasculitis, the medium-sized muscular arteries are involved, and the condition results in fibrinoid necrosis of the entire thickness of the blood vessel wall.

Pathophysiology

The pathophysiology of PAN is characterized by a necrotizing inflammation of the small and medium-sized arteries. The consequences of the disease include narrowed vessel lumen, thrombosis, infarction of tissue supplied by the vessel, and, sometimes, hemorrhage. The disease can affect multiple systems. The severity of PAN is related to the location of the vessels involved and the degree of ischemia produced.

The disease is rare and has a progressive course marked by intermittent flare-ups. It affects men more than women; the average age of onset is 45 years. Death usually results from renal, gastrointestinal, or cardiovascular complications.

Signs and Symptoms

The onset of PAN is usually insidious. No single pattern of symptoms is seen. The major symptoms are usually fever and weight loss. Other characteristic features of the disease include skin lesions, hypertension, joint swelling, malaise, abdominal pain, change in urinary pattern, anemia, ischemia of the fingers, pleuritis, and symptoms of renal, gastrointestinal, and cardiac involvement.

Medical Diagnosis

Signs and symptoms and laboratory findings of PAN are nonspecific, making an accurate diagnosis very difficult. Biopsy of tissue shows vasculitis. Other laboratory findings include excessively increased erythrocyte sedimentation rate, elevated leukocyte count, and anemia, none of which are specific for PAN.

Medical Treatment

The treatment of PAN is similar to that of systemic lupus erythematosus. Signs and symptoms of the affected organs should be assessed and treated as appropriate. Drug therapy may include antihypertensives, diuretics, corticosteroids (prednisone), methotrexate, and cyclophosphamide. There is usually no need for surgical intervention.

Nursing Care of the Patient with Polyarteritis Nodosa

Nursing care of patients with PAN is like that provided for patients with systemic lupus erythematosus.

OTHER CONNECTIVE TISSUE DISEASES

Other connective tissue diseases described here are ankylosing spondylitis, polymyalgia rheumatica, Reiter's syndrome, and Behçet's syndrome.

Ankylosing Spondylitis

Ankylosing spondylitis (AS) is an inflammatory disease of unknown origin that primarily affects the vertebral column, causing spinal deformities. Early symptoms most commonly appear in males younger than age 40. The first symptom of AS is usually a dull aching pain in the buttock. Other features of the disease include low back morning stiffness of a few hours duration that improves with activity. The pain returns after long periods of inactivity. The patient may also complain of fatigue. There is evidence that AS is linked to the HLA-B27 antigen. The most common complications of the disease are spinal fractures, iritis (inflammation of the iris), and arthritis. Despite the chronic discomfort of AS, most patients do not experience disabling symptoms. The disease is treated with NSAIDs and physical therapy.

Polymyalgia Rheumatica

Polymyalgia rheumatica occurs in women over age 50 and is characterized by stiffness and pain in the shoulders and hips. Pain at night and morning stiffness are common features of the condition. Getting out of bed is a difficult task for patients with this disease. Patients also have anemia and muscle atrophy and weakness. Administration of NSAIDs is usually beneficial.

Reiter's Syndrome

Reiter's syndrome is a connective tissue disease characterized by a triad of arthritis, urethritis, and conjunctivitis. The disease has familial tendencies and is linked to the HLA-B27 antigen. The disease results from exposure to venereal disease or dysentery. Treatment consists of NSAIDs and physical therapy.

Behçet's Syndrome

Behçet's syndrome is a chronic syndrome involving oral ulceration, genital ulceration, and uveitis resulting from arthritis, vasculitis, synovitis, meningitis, phlebitis, and gastrointestinal ulcers. The most persistent symptom is ulceration of the mouth, which appears in clusters on the mucous membranes of the cheeks, tongue, palate, and pharynx. Recurrent, painful lesions also appear on the penis, scrotum, vulva, cervix, or vagina. The cornerstone of treatment for Behçet's syndrome is corticosteroid therapy.

Sjögren's Syndrome

Sjögren's syndrome is an inflammatory disease that obstructs secretory ducts, resulting in dryness of the eyes, mouth (xerostomia), and vagina. The disease is often seen in combination with rheumatoid arthritis. Treatment includes artificial tears, artificial saliva, and perineal hygiene. Treatment with steroids may bring symptomatic relief.

Connective tissue provides the body's support, structure, and framework. The major connective tissues are

NUTRITION CONCEPTS

- A diet high in calcium (1000 to 1500 mg per day) and vitamin D (100 to 500 mg per day) is important for the prevention of osteoporosis.
- Two servings of milk per day provide 75% of the recommended daily allowance for calcium.
- A well-balanced diet, including foods high in vitamin E and zinc, is recommended for persons with rheumatoid arthritis.
- A weight-loss program for persons with osteoarthritis helps to reduce stress on weight-bearing joints.

bone, blood, cartilage, ligaments, skin, and tendons. Diagnostic tests for diseases of connective tissue are nonspecific. A complete history and physical examination combined with laboratory findings and radiographs help to confirm a specific diagnosis. Drugs used to treat connective tissue are mainly NSAIDs and, with much discretion, glucocorticoids.

The pathology and etiology of connective tissue diseases are not always obvious. The courses of these diseases are variable in nature, depending on the individual patient and organs affected. The major pathogenesis is that of autoimmune response with the body turning on itself. Generally, treatment is symptomatic and provides no cure. An interdisciplinary approach enhances the optimum outcome for the patient.

BIBLIOGRAPHY

Arking, R. (1991). *Biology of aging: Observations and principles.* Englewood Cliffs, NJ: Prentice Hall.

Black, J. M., & Matassarin-Jacobs, E. (1993). *Luckmann and Sorensen's medical-surgical nursing: A psychophysiologic approach* (4th ed.) Philadelphia: W. B. Saunders.

Bullock, L. B., & Rosendahl, P. P. (1992). *Pathophysiology: Adaptations and alterations in function* (3rd ed.). Philadelphia: J. B. Lippincott.

Carpenito, L. J. (1993). *Nursing diagnosis: Application to clinical practice* (5th ed.). Philadelphia: J. B. Lippincott.

Fong, E., Scott, A., Ferris, E., & Skelley, E. (1993). *Body structure and function* (8th ed.). Albany: Delmar.

Goldfinger, S. E., & Corron, P. (1992). Systemic lupus erythematosus: A bodily betrayal. *Harvard Health Letter, 17,* 3–5.

Guyton, A. C. (1991). *Textbook of medical physiology* (8th ed.). Philadelphia: W. B. Saunders.

Ignatavicius, D. D., & Bayne, M. V. (1991). *Medical-surgical nursing: A nursing process approach.* Philadelphia: W. B. Saunders.

Jacob, S. W., & Francone, C. A. (1989). *Elements of anatomy and physiology* (2nd ed.). Philadelphia: W. B. Saunders.

Kelly, W. N., Harris, E. D., Jr., Ruddy, S., & Sledge, C. B. (1993). *Textbook of rheumatology* (4th ed.) (Vol. 2). Philadelphia: W. B. Saunders.

Krane, S. M., & Harris, E. D., Jr. (1992). Crystal-induced joint disease. In *Scientific American medicine: Sec. 15. Rheumatology: Vol. 3* (pp. 1–15). New York: Scientific American, Inc.

Krane, S. M., & Harris, E. D., Jr. (1992). Rheumatoid arthritis. In *Scientific American medicine: Sec. 15. Rheumatology: Vol. 3* (pp. 1–20). New York: Scientific American, Inc.

Kuhn, M. M. (1991). *Pharmacotherapeutics: A nursing process approach* (2nd ed.). Philadelphia: F. A. Davis.

Maricic, M. J. (1993). Therapy of osteoporosis. In R. Bressler & M. D. Katz (Eds.), *Geriatric pharmacology.* New York: McGraw-Hill.

Maskowitz, R. W., Howell, D. S., Goldberg, V. M., & Mankin, H. J. (Eds.). (1992). *Osteoarthritis diagnosis and medical surgical management* (2nd ed.). Philadelphia: W. B. Saunders.

Miller, C. (1990). *Nursing care of older adults: Theory and practice.* Glenview, IL: Foresman Scott/Little Brown.

Phipps, W. J., Long, B. C., Woods, N. F., & Cassmeyer, V. L. (Eds.). (1991). *Medical-surgical nursing: Concepts and clinical practice* (4th ed.). St. Louis: Mosby Year Book.

Rakel, R. E. (Ed.). (1992). *Conn's current therapy.* Philadelphia: W. B. Saunders.

Robinson, D. R. (1988). Systemic lupus erythematosus. In *Scientific American medicine: Sec. 15. Rheumatology: Vol. 3* (pp. 1–15). New York: Scientific American, Inc.

Robinson, D. R. (1990). Polymyositis. In *Scientific American medicine: Sec. 15. Rheumatology: Vol. 3* (pp. 1–9). New York: Scientific American, Inc.

Robinson, D. R. (1991). Osteoarthritis. In *Scientific American medicine: Sec. 15. Rheumatology: Vol. 3* (pp. 1–9). New York: Scientific American, Inc.

Robinson, D. R. (1992). Scleroderma. In *Scientific American medicine: Sec. 15. Rheumatology: Vol. 3* (pp. 1–13). New York: Scientific American, Inc.

Thibodeau, G., & Anthony, C. P. (1988). *Structure and function of the body.* St. Louis: Times Mirror/Mosby College Publishing.

Wilson, J. D., Braunwald, E., Isselbacher, K. J., Petersdorf, R. G., Facui, A. S., & Root, R. K. (Eds.). (1991). *Harrison's principles of internal medicine* (12th ed.). New York: McGraw-Hill.

Wyngaarden, J. B., Smith, L. H., Jr., & Bennett, J. C. (Eds.). (1992). *Cecil textbook of medicine* (18th ed.). Philadelphia: W. B. Saunders.

KEY CONCEPTS

1. The major connective tissues are bone, blood, cartilage, ligaments, skin, and tendons.
2. Age-related changes in connective tissue can have a significant impact on function and quality of life.
3. Osteoarthritis is characterized by degeneration of articular cartilage, hypertrophy of underlying and adjacent bone, and inflammation of surrounding synovium that leads to pain with joint movement.
4. Osteoarthritis may be treated with drug therapy,

KEY CONCEPTS *(continued)*

education, physical therapy, modification of daily activities, and surgery.

5. Nursing care of the patient with osteoarthritis focuses on chronic pain, impaired physical mobility, ineffective individual coping, and knowledge deficit.
6. Total joint replacements can be done on the elbow, shoulder, phalangeal finger joints, hip, knee, and ankle.
7. Nursing care after total joint replacement addresses pain, high risk for injury, impaired physical mobility, altered peripheral tissue perfusion, high risk for infection, anxiety and fear, and knowledge deficit.
8. Rheumatoid arthritis, a chronic, progressive inflammatory disease that leads to deformity and loss of joint mobility, is treated with drug therapy, supportive treatments, and modification of activities of daily living.
9. Gout, a systemic disease characterized by the deposition of urate crystals in the joints and other body tissues, usually responds to drug therapy that lowers the serum uric acid level.
10. Systemic lupus erythematosus (SLE) is a chronic inflammatory disease that may affect the joints, skin, kidneys, heart, lungs, and central nervous system.
11. Nursing care of the patient with SLE focuses on fatigue and activity intolerance, impaired skin integrity, pain, body image disturbance, altered nutrition, altered urinary elimination, and knowledge deficit.
12. Progressive systemic sclerosis (PSS), commonly called scleroderma, is characterized by thickening of the skin and may affect the blood vessels, gastrointestinal tract, lungs, heart, and kidneys.
13. Nursing care for the patient with PSS addresses impaired skin integrity, self-care deficits, pain, social isolation, altered nutrition, and knowledge deficits.
14. Less common connective tissue disorders are polymyositis, periarteritis nodosa, ankylosing spondylitis, polymyalgia rheumatica, Reiter's syndrome, Behçet's syndrome, and Sjögren's syndrome.
15. Most connective tissue disorders are chronic and, though there is no specific cure, can be improved with symptomatic treatment.

Mary Ann Matteson

CHAPTER 38

Fractures

OBJECTIVES

1. Identify the various types of fractures.
2. Describe the five stages of the healing process.
3. Discuss the major complications of a fracture, including infection, fat embolism, and compartment syndrome.
4. Compare the types of medical treatment for fractures, particularly reduction and fixation.
5. Describe common therapeutic measures for fractures, including casts, traction, crutches, walkers, and canes.
6. Discuss the nursing care of a patient with a fracture.
7. Describe specific types of fractures, specifically hip fracture, Colles' fracture, and pelvic fracture.

GLOSSARY

BONE REMODELING Process in which immature bone cells are gradually replaced by mature bone cells

CLOSED OR SIMPLE FRACTURE Fracture in which the broken bone does not break through the skin

CLOSED REDUCTION OR MANIPULATION Nonsurgical realignment of the bones to their previous anatomic position using traction, angulation, or rotation, or a combination of these

COMPARTMENT SYNDROME Serious complication of a fracture caused by internal or external pressure to the affected area, resulting in decreased blood flow, pain, and tissue damage

COMPLETE FRACTURE Fracture in which the break extends across the entire bone, dividing it into two separate pieces

DELAYED UNION Fracture healing does not occur in the normally expected time

FAT EMBOLISM Condition in which fat globules are released from the marrow of the broken bone into the blood stream, migrate to the lungs, and cause pulmonary hypertension

Glossary continued

FIXATION Procedure done during the open reduction surgical procedure to attach the fragments of the broken bone together when reduction alone is not feasible

FRACTURE Break or disruption in the continuity of a bone

INCOMPLETE FRACTURE Fracture in which the bone breaks only part way across, leaving some portion of the bone intact

NONUNION Failure of a fracture to heal

OPEN OR COMPOUND FRACTURE Fracture in which the fragments of the broken bone break through the skin

OPEN REDUCTION Surgical procedure in which an incision is made at the fracture site, usually on patients with open (compound) or comminuted fractures, to cleanse the area of fragments and debris

REDUCTION Process of bringing the ends of the broken bone into proper alignment

STRESS FRACTURE Fracture caused by either sudden force or prolonged stress

A fracture is defined as a break or disruption in the continuity of a bone. With a fracture, injury to surrounding soft tissue also occurs, depending on the location and severity of the break.

All fractures are either complete or incomplete. A complete fracture is one in which the break extends across the entire bone, dividing it into two separate pieces. An incomplete fracture is one in which the bone breaks only part way across, leaving some portion of the bone intact.

CLASSIFICATION OF FRACTURES

Fractures may be classified as open or closed, depending on the type and extent of soft tissue damage. A closed or simple fracture is one in which the broken bone does not break through the skin. In an open or compound fracture, the fragments of the broken bone break through the skin. Open fractures have three grades of severity:

Grade I: least severe injury with minimal skin damage.
Grade II: moderately severe injury with skin and muscle contusions (bruises).
Grade III: most severe injury (wound larger than 6–8 cm) with skin, muscle, blood vessel, and nerve damage.

Fractures may also be classified by their cause. For example, a stress fracture is caused by either sudden force or prolonged stress. Stress fractures are frequently related to athletic endeavors such as track or basketball. A pathologic fracture occurs because of a pathologic condition in the bone, such as a tumor or disease process, that causes a spontaneous break. Figure 38–1 illustrates common types of fractures.

ETIOLOGY AND RISK FACTORS

Fractures are most commonly caused by trauma to the bone, especially as a result of automobile accidents and falls. Bone disease such as bone cancer also can lead to a fracture. Hip fractures in the elderly are usually associated with falls. Risk factors for hip fractures include osteoporosis, advanced age, white race, use of psychotropic drugs, and being female.

In adults, the bones most commonly fractured are the ribs. Fractures of the femur are most common in young and middle-aged adults, and hip and wrist fractures are most common in the elderly. More than 200,000 hip fractures occur each year in the United States, and the number is rising. Most people with fractured hips must be hospitalized, resulting in an overall estimated cost of more than $7 billion.

FRACTURE HEALING

A bone begins to heal as soon as an injury occurs. New bone tissue is formed to repair the fracture, resulting in a sturdy union between the broken ends of the bone. Healing occurs in the following five stages:

1. *Hematoma formation.* Immediately after a fracture, bleeding occurs, along with edema. In 48 to 72 hours, a clot or hematoma forms between the two broken ends of the bone.
2. *Cellular proliferation.* The hematoma that surrounds the fracture does not resorb like hematomas in other parts of the body. Instead, other tissue cells enter the clot, and granulation tissue forms. The granulation tissue then forms a collar around each end of the broken bone, gradually becoming firm and forming a bridge between the two ends.
3. *Callus formation.* By the end of the first week after injury, the granulation tissue changes into a callus formation. Callus is made up of cartilage, osteoblasts (bone cells that form new bone), calcium, and phosphorus. The callus is larger than the diameter of the bone and serves as a temporary splint.
4. *Ossification.* Within 2 to 3 weeks after the break, a permanent bone callus, known as "woven bone," forms. It is during this stage that the ends of the broken bone begin to "knit."
5. *Consolidation and remodeling.* Consolidation occurs when the distance between bone fragments decreases and eventually closes. During remodeling, the immature bone cells are gradually replaced by mature bone cells. The excess bone is naturally chiseled away by stress to the affected part from motion, exercise, and weight bearing. The bone then takes on its original shape and size (Fig. 38–2).

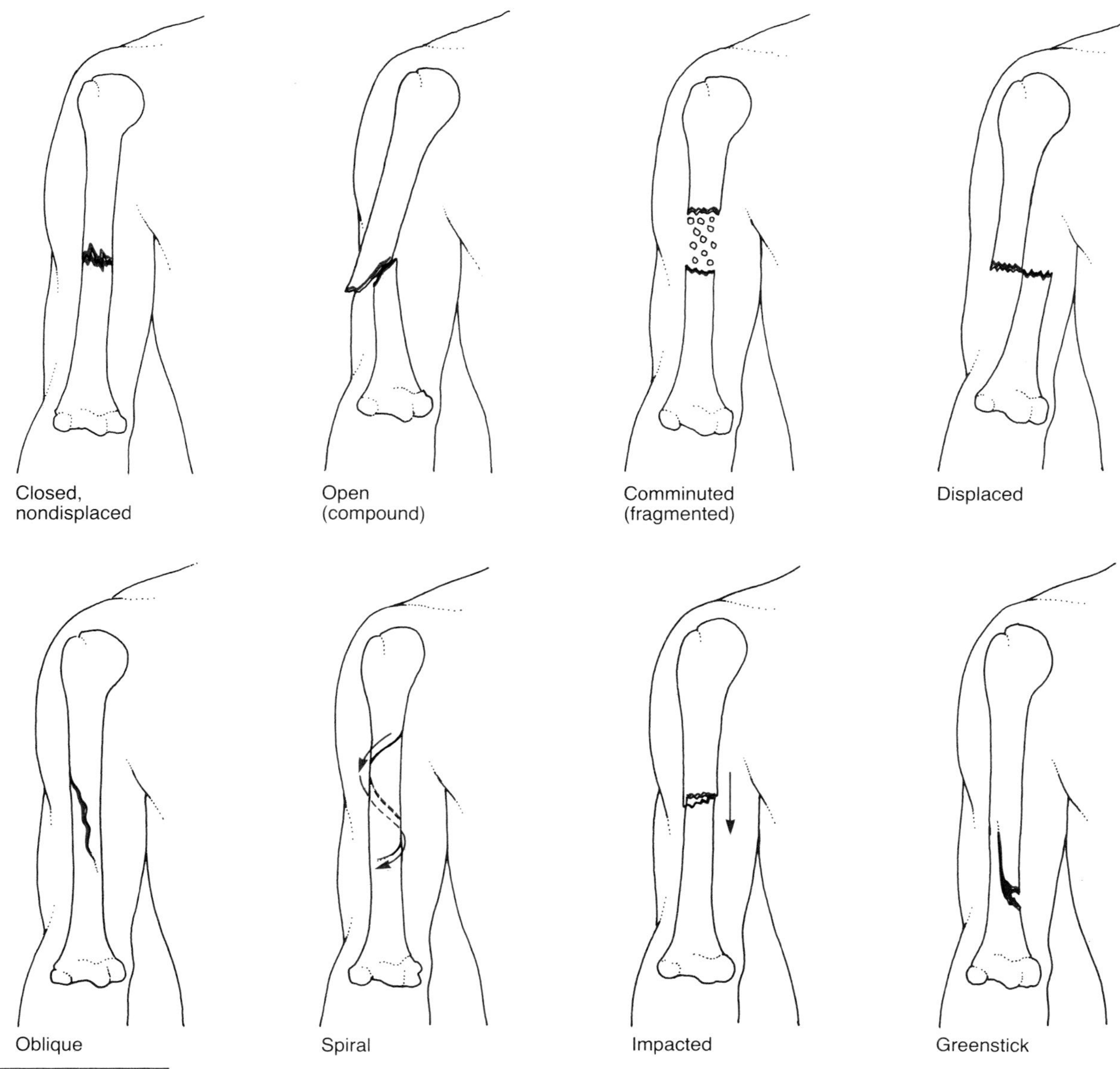

FIGURE 38-1

Common types of fractures. (From Ignatavicius, D. D., & Bayne, M. V. [1991]. *Medical-surgical nursing: A nursing process approach* [p. 781]. Philadelphia: W. B. Saunders.)

Healing is affected by many factors, such as age, location of the fracture, and blood supply to the area. Healing time for fractures increases with age, and it may take six times as long for the same type of fracture to heal in an older person as it does in an infant.

When fracture healing does not occur in the normally expected time, it is called a delayed union. If a fracture never heals, it is called a nonunion. Delayed union or nonunion may be caused by inadequate immobilization or excess movement, poor alignment of the bone fragments, infection, or poor nutrition.

When there is nonunion of a fracture, an electromagnetic device may be used to stimulate bone growth. The stimulation may be internal or external and is done up to 10 hours a day for 3 to 6 months. Although the procedure is time consuming, it can prevent further surgery and bone grafting.

COMPLICATIONS

Complications of a fracture can delay or impede healing or can even be life threatening. Complications include infection, fat embolism, and compartment syndrome.

INFECTION

Infections associated with fractures result from contamination of the open wound or indwelling hardware

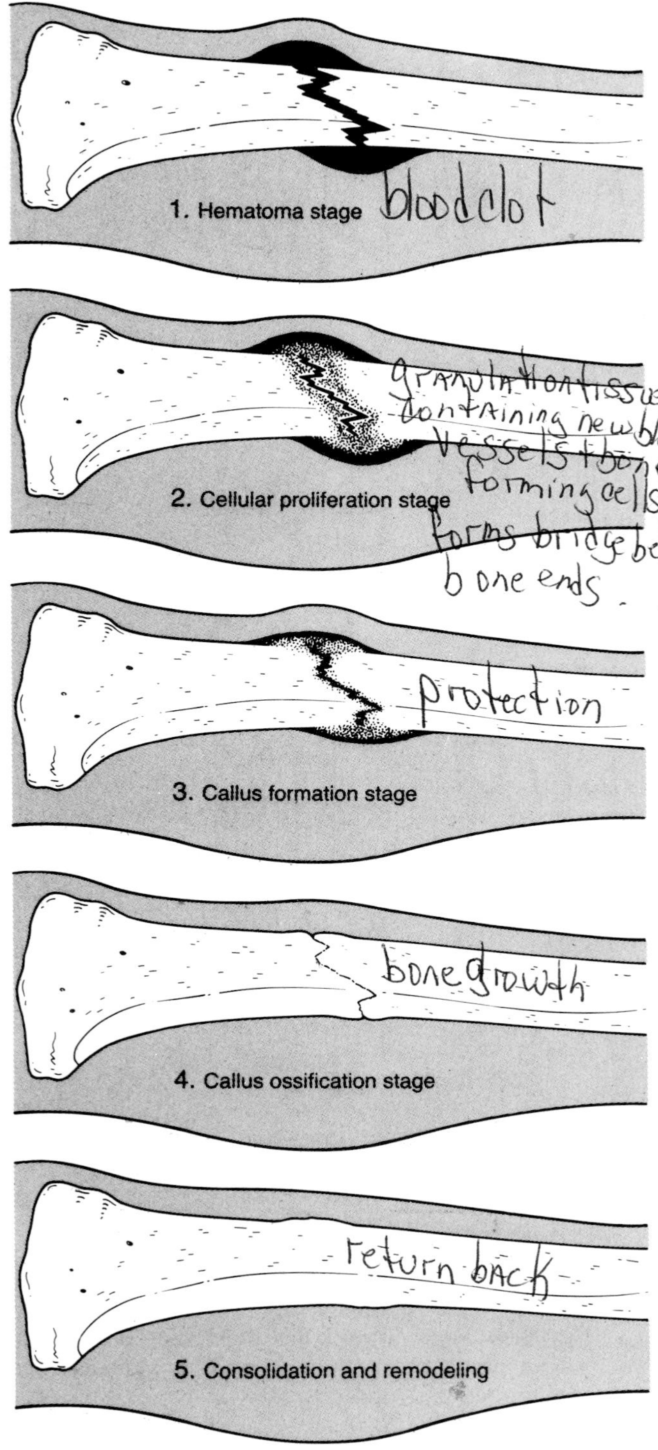

FIGURE 38-2

Stages of fracture healing. (From Black, J. M., & Matassarin-Jacobs, E. [1993]. *Luckmann and Sorensen's medical-surgical nursing: A psychophysiologic approach* [4th ed., p. 1918]. Philadelphia: W. B. Saunders.)

used to repair the broken bone. Any infection can lead to delayed union of the bone fragments. Osteomyelitis (infection of the bone) most commonly occurs after an open fracture and surgical repair. In deep, grossly contaminated wounds, gas gangrene may develop.

FAT EMBOLISM

Fat embolism is a condition in which fat globules are released from the marrow of the broken bone into the blood stream. Once the fat droplets enter the circulation, they migrate to the lungs. Because they are too large to pass through the pulmonary circulation, they lodge in the capillaries, break down into fatty acids, and produce pulmonary hypertension. The condition can be fatal.

Fat embolism syndrome is most commonly associated with fractures of the long bones, multiple fractures, and severe trauma. It occurs 24 to 48 hours after injury, most often in young men aged 20 to 40 and in older adults aged 70 to 80. An older patient with a hip fracture is at highest risk.

Respiratory distress is the first sign of a fat embolism, followed by tachycardia (rapid heartbeat), tachypnea (rapid breathing), fever, confusion, and decreased level of consciousness. Another characteristic feature is petechiae, a measle-like rash over the neck, upper arms, chest, or abdomen. Treatment of fat embolism consists of bedrest, gentle handling, oxygen, fluid replacement with intravenous fluids, and corticosteroids.

COMPARTMENT SYNDROME

Compartment syndrome is a serious complication that results from internal or external pressure to the affected area. Compartments are located in the muscles of the extremities. They are enclosed spaces made up of muscle, bone, nerves, and blood vessels wrapped by a fibrous membrane. Internal pressure is caused by bleeding or edema into a compartment; external pressure is caused by a cast or tight dressing. When there is bleeding or edema into a compartment, there is nowhere for the drainage to go because it is trapped in the space. The increased fluid puts pressure on the tissues, nerves, and blood vessels, so blood flow is decreased, resulting in pain and tissue damage. External pressure also can cause decreased blood flow to the area.

Although compartment syndrome is relatively rare, it is a serious condition and can create an emergency situation. Within 4 to 6 hours after the onset of compartment syndrome, irreversible muscle damage can occur. In 24 to 48 hours, the limb can become useless.

A primary symptom of compartment syndrome is pain, especially with touch or movement, that cannot be relieved with narcotic analgesia. Other signs and symptoms are edema, pallor, weak or unequal pulses, cyanosis, tingling, numbness, paresthesia, and, finally, severe pain. As noted earlier, paresis can result if the condition is not treated within 24 hours.

The goal of treatment is to relieve pressure. When there is internal pressure, a surgical fasciotomy, which consists of making linear incisions in the fascia, may be done to relieve pressure on the nerves and blood vessels. For external pressure, the cast or dressings are removed and replaced.

SIGNS AND SYMPTOMS

Signs and symptoms of a fracture depend on the type and location of the break. Some fractures have so few clinical manifestations that they can be detected only radiologically. The most common signs and symptoms are swelling, bruising, pain, tenderness, loss of normal function, and abnormal mobility. Table 38–1 lists various signs and symptoms of fractures and their causes.

DIAGNOSTIC TESTS AND PROCEDURES

The most common diagnostic tests used to confirm the presence of a fracture are various radiologic studies. Standard x-ray films are used first to reveal bone disruption, deformity, or malignancy. A computed tomographic scan may be used to detect fractures of complex structures, such as the hip and pelvis, or compression fractures of the spine. A bone scan may be useful for detecting small bone fractures or fractures caused by stress or disease. Diagnostic tests for fractures are the same as those for connective tissue disorders described in Table 37–2.

TABLE 38–1
SIGNS AND SYMPTOMS OF FRACTURES AND THEIR CAUSES

Deformity. Strong muscle pull may cause bone fragments to override; therefore, alignment and contour changes occur, such as (1) angulation, rotation, limb shortening; (2) bone depression; or (3) altered curves in the injured site, especially when compared with the opposite site.
Swelling. Edema may appear rapidly from localization of serous fluid at the fracture site and extravasation of blood into adjacent tissues.
Bruising (ecchymosis). From subcutaneous bleeding.
Muscle spasm. Involuntary muscle contraction near the fracture.
Tenderness. Over fracture site due to underlying injuries.
Pain. Immediate severe pain at the time of injury. Following injury, pain may result from muscle spasm, overriding of the fractured ends of the bone, or damage to adjacent structures.
Impaired sensation (numbness). May occur from nerve damage or nerve entrapment from edema, bleeding, or bony fragments.
Loss of normal function. May result from instability of the fractured bone, pain, or muscle spasm. Paralysis may be caused by nerve damage.
Abnormal mobility. Movement of a part that is normally immobile, due to instability when long bones are fractured.
Crepitus. Grating sensations or sounds felt or heard if the injured part is moved. Crepitus results from broken bone ends rubbing together.
Hypovolemic shock. May result from blood loss or other injuries.

From Black, J. M., & Matassarin-Jacobs, E. (1993). *Luckmann and Sorensen's medical-surgical nursing: A psychophysiologic approach* (4th ed., p. 1919). Philadelphia: W. B. Saunders.

MEDICAL TREATMENT

The goals of medical treatment for a fracture are to realign the bone fragments, establish a sturdy union between the broken ends of the bone, and restore function. The most common therapeutic techniques to accomplish these goals are closed and open reduction and internal and external fixation.

REDUCTION

Reduction is the process of bringing the ends of the broken bone into proper alignment. Closed reduction or manipulation is a nonsurgical realignment of the bones to their previous anatomic position. No surgical incision is made; however, the procedure can be painful, and general or local anesthesia may be given. Closed reduction may be done by using traction, angulation, or rotation, or a combination of these (Fig. 38–3). After reduction of a fracture, a radiograph is taken, and a cast is usually applied.

Open reduction is a surgical procedure in which an incision is made at the fracture site. It is usually carried out on patients with open (compound) or comminuted fractures to cleanse the area of fragments and debris.

PHARMACOLOGY CAPSULE

Effective pain management of a fracture is essential for mobilization and healing.

FIXATION

Fixation is an attempt to attach the fragments of the broken bone together when reduction alone is not feasible because of the type and extent of the break. Fixation is done during the open reduction surgical procedure. Internal fixation includes the use of rods, pins, nails, screws, or metal plates to align bone fragments and keep them in place for healing (Fig. 38–4). Figure 38–5 illustrates an open reduction and internal fixation of a fractured femur in which a nail is used to maintain alignment. Internal fixation promotes early mobilization and is often preferred for older adults who have brittle bones that may not heal properly or may suffer the consequences of immobility.

External fixation is similar to internal fixation, but the pins in the bone are attached to an external frame (Fig. 38–6). When there is extensive soft tissue damage or infection, external fixation allows easier access to the site and facilitates wound care. In addition, the device allows for early ambulation and mobility while relieving pain. Pin-track infection occurs in approximately 10% of patients with external fixation. Pin care is extremely important to prevent the migration of organisms along the pin from the external skin to the internal bone. Patients

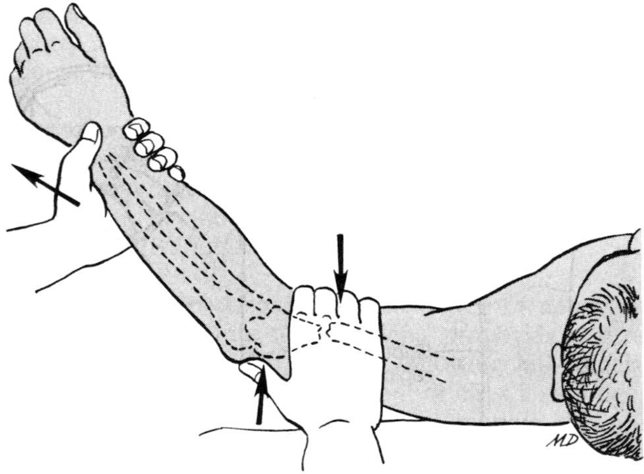

FIGURE 38-3

Closed (manipulative) reduction to realign a fracture of the arm. (From Black, J. M., & Matassarin-Jacobs, E. [1993]. *Luckmann and Sorensen's medical-surgical nursing: A psychophysiologic approach* [4th ed., p. 1923]. Philadelphia: W. B. Saunders.)

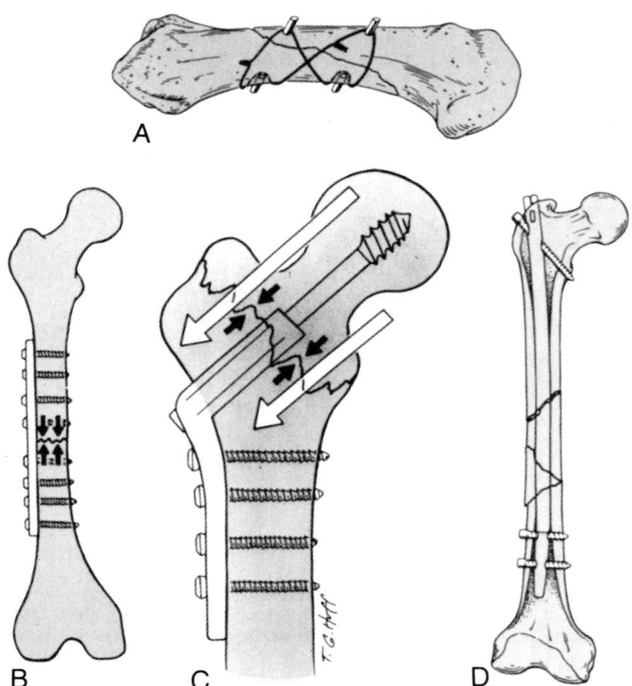

FIGURE 38-4

Examples of different types of internal fixation devices. *A*, Tension band wiring technique using Kirschner wires for fracture of a phalanx; *B*, compression plate to the lateral aspect of the femur; *C*, sliding hip screw; *D*, static locked intramedullary nail fixed to both proximal and distal fragments of the femur. (From Browner, B. D., Jupitor, J. B., Levine, A. M., & Trafton, P. G. [1992]. *Skeletal trauma* [pp. 253, 254, 942, 1551]. Philadelphia: W. B. Saunders.)

should be taught to do their own pin care and watch for signs of infection as soon as they are able.

COMMON THERAPEUTIC MEASURES

CASTS

Casts are used for external fixation of extensive fractures and fractures of the extremities. They hold the bone in alignment while allowing enough movement to other parts of the body to carry out activities of daily living. Types of materials used for a cast are plaster of Paris, fiberglass, thermoplastic resins, thermolabile plastic, and polyurethane.

Plaster of Paris consists of anhydrous calcium sulfate embedded in gauze. It is often preferred because it is the least expensive type of cast to use. After applying well-fitting stockinette, the gauze is immersed in water and wrapped around the affected part. The stockinette must not be too tight because it may cause circulation impairment. Stockinette that is too loose can wrinkle and result in pressure sores. The strength of the cast is determined by the number of layers of wrapped gauze and the technique of application.

Initially the wet cast is hot, and the heat generated may cause edema of the underlying tissues from the increased circulation. In a short period of time, the cast becomes damp and cool, and it dries after about 24 to 72 hours, depending on the size and location. When the cast is dry and strong, it can withstand weight bearing and other stresses. The underlying stockinette covers the edges of the cast to prevent scratching and irritation from the rough plaster. Sometimes a "window" is cut into the cast over the fracture site to allow access to the wound.

Fiberglass is a newer type of synthetic material used for casts that is lighter and has a shorter drying time than plaster of Paris. Drying time is 10 to 15 minutes, and the cast can withstand weight bearing 30 minutes after application. Sometimes physicians choose to use plaster of Paris casts on lower extremities for heavier weight bearing and fiberglass casts on upper extremities.

Other types of synthetic materials are thermolabile plastic (Orthoplast) and thermoplastic resins (Hexcelite). They are heated in warm water and molded to fit the torso or extremity. Polyurethane is formed from chemically treated polyester and cotton fabric. The fabric is immersed in cool water to start the chemical process for wrapping.

The four main groups of casts are (1) upper extremity, (2) lower extremity, (3) cast brace, and (4) body or spica cast. Examples of various types of casts are shown in Table 38–2. An upper extremity cast is used for breaks in the shoulder, arm, wrist, and hand. A patient who is wearing an arm cast should keep the arm elevated above the head when lying in bed to prevent swelling. The arm is kept in a sling for support when the patient is up and around.

Lower extremity casts are used for breaks in the upper and lower leg, ankle, and foot. A leg cast is used

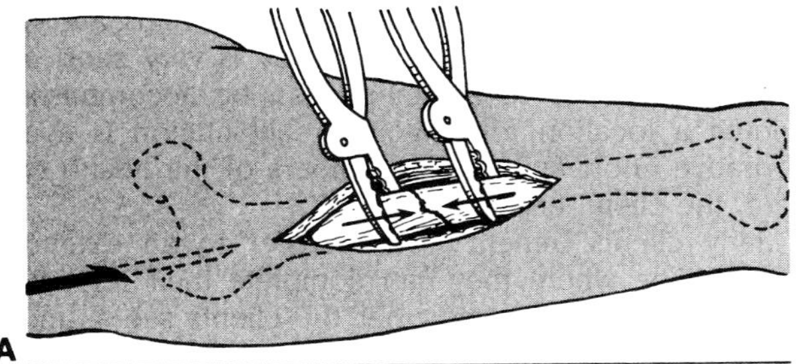

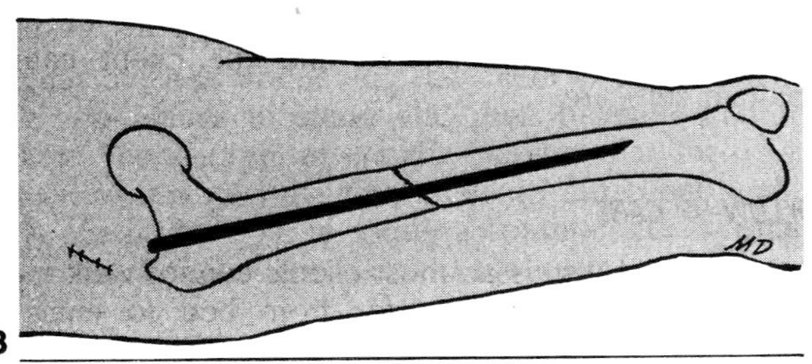

FIGURE 38-5

Open reduction and internal fixation of a fractured shaft of femur. *A*, Fractured bone ends are realigned by open reduction. Nail is inserted through the femur. *B*, Fractured bone ends are secured in the correct position with a nail. (From Black, J. M., & Matassarin-Jacobs, E. [1993]. *Luckmann and Sorensen's medical-surgical nursing: A psychophysiologic approach* [4th ed., p. 1928]. Philadelphia: W. B. Saunders.)

to allow mobility and may be used with crutches. A cast shoe or rubber walking pad protects the cast and prevents falls. The affected leg should be elevated on several pillows during the first few days after the break to prevent swelling.

After an adequate amount of healing has taken place and edema has subsided, cast braces may be used for injury to the knee. A cast brace supports the affected part while allowing the knee to bend. This is accomplished by applying a cast above and below the knee and connecting them with a hinge.

Body or spica casts are used when a fracture is located somewhere in the trunk of the body. A body cast encircles the trunk, whereas a spica cast encases the trunk plus one or two extremities. Body or spica casts severely limit mobility and may cause complications related to lack of movement, such as skin breakdown, respiratory problems, constipation, and joint contractures. In addition, a condition known as cast syndrome, in which a patient may have feelings of claustrophobia, may occur. Signs and symptoms of cast syndrome include anxiety; increased blood pressure, pulse, and respirations; nausea; vomiting; and abdominal distention from paralytic ileus.

Clients with casts should be instructed to *avoid* (1) getting the cast wet, (2) removing any padding, (3) inserting any foreign object inside the cast, (4) bearing weight on a new cast for 48 hours, and (5) covering the cast with plastic for prolonged periods. Swelling, discoloration of toes or fingers, pain during motion, and burning or tingling under the cast should be reported to a health care provider.

TRACTION

Traction exerts a pulling force on a fractured extremity to provide alignment of the broken bone fragments. It is also used to prevent or correct deformity, decrease muscle spasm, promote rest and exercise, and maintain the position of the diseased or injured part.

Traction may be applied directly to the skin (skin traction) or attached directly to a bone (skeletal traction) by means of a metal pin or wire. An example of skin traction is Buck's traction with a Velcro boot (Fig. 38–7). It is used for hip and knee contractures, muscle spasms, and alignment of hip fractures. Skin traction weight is no more than 5 to 10 pounds to prevent injury to the skin.

Skeletal traction provides a strong, steady, continuous pull and can be used for prolonged periods of time. Examples of skeletal traction are Crutchfield's traction and a halo vest, in which tongs are inserted into either side of the skull (see Fig. 27–9). Heavier weights can be used with skeletal traction, usually from 15 to 30 pounds. Crutchfield's traction and a halo vest are used for reduction and immobilization of fractures of the cervical or high thoracic vertebrae.

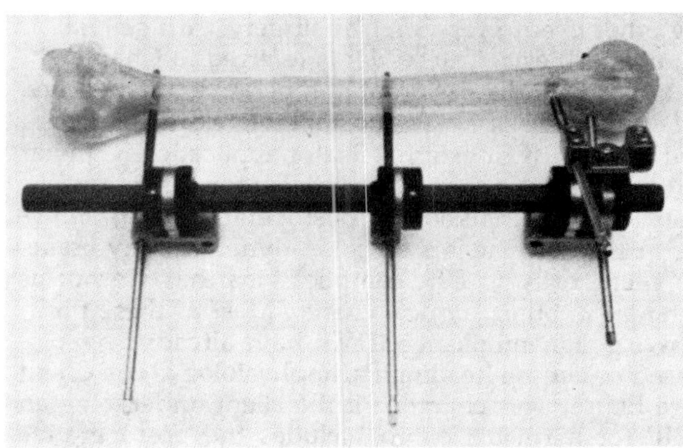

FIGURE 38-6

Hex-Fix external fixation system for tibial fracture. (Courtesy of Smith & Nephew Richards, Inc.)

TABLE 38-2
CAST TYPES AND COMMON USES

TYPE	ILLUSTRATION	BODY PART COVERED	COMMON USES
Short leg cast	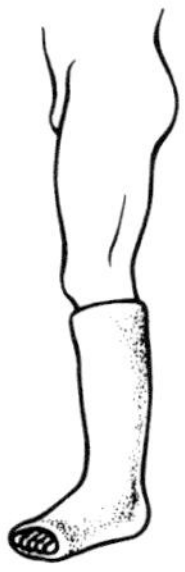	Foot to below knee	Fracture of foot, ankle, or distal tibia or fibula Severe sprain or strain Postoperative immobilization following open reduction and internal fixation Correction of deformity, such as talipes equinovarus
Leg cylinder cast	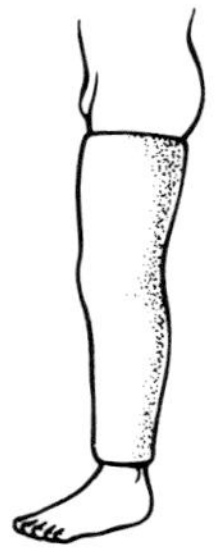	Ankle to upper thigh	Fracture or dislocation of knee Soft tissue injury to knee Postoperative immobilization following tibial valgus osteotomy Correction of varus or valgus deformity of knee
Long leg cast	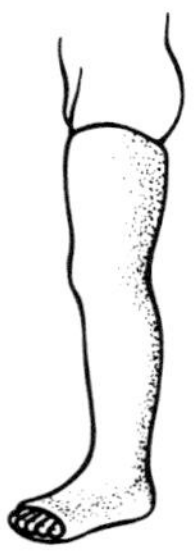	Foot to upper thigh	Fracture of distal femur, knee, or lower leg Soft tissue injury to knee or knee dislocation Postoperative immobilization following arthrodesis of knee
Unilateral hip spica cast	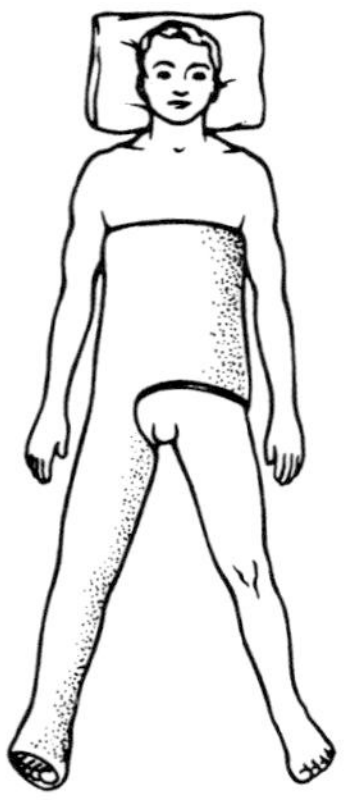	Entire leg and trunk to waist or nipple line	Fracture of femur Postoperative immobilization following open reduction and internal fixation Correction of deformity, such as congenital soft tissue injury following dislocation of hip

TABLE 38-2
CAST TYPES AND COMMON USES *Continued*

TYPE	ILLUSTRATION	BODY PART COVERED	COMMON USES
Bilateral long leg hip spica cast		Entire leg bilaterally to waist or nipple line	Fractures of femur, acetabulum, or pelvis Postoperative immobilization following open reduction and internal fixation
Short arm cast		Hand to below elbow	Fracture of hand or wrist Postoperative immobilization following open reduction and internal fixation
Long arm cast		Hand to upper arm	Fracture of forearm, elbow, or humerus Postoperative immobilization following open reduction and internal fixation

Modified from Maher, A. B., Salmond, S. W., & Pellino, T. A. (1994). *Orthopedic nursing* (pp. 279–280). Philadelphia: W. B. Saunders.

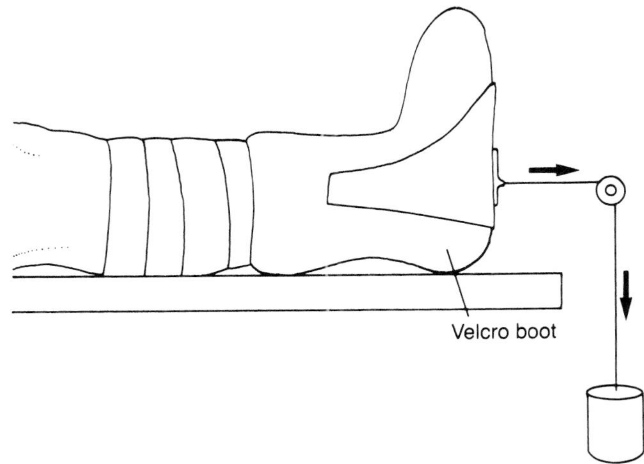

FIGURE 38-7
Buck's traction with Velcro boot, commonly used for hip fractures. (From Ignatavicius, D. D., & Bayne, M. V. [1991]. *Medical-surgical nursing: A psychophysiologic approach* [p. 795]. Philadelphia: W. B. Saunders.)

Traction may involve complications, such as impaired circulation, inadequate fracture alignment, skin breakdown, and soft tissue injury. As noted earlier, pin-track infection and osteomyelitis can occur with skeletal traction.

CRUTCHES

Crutches are used to increase mobility and assist with ambulation after a fracture of the lower extremity. Success in crutch walking is dependent on many factors, including the patient's motivation, age, interests and activities, and ability to adjust to the crutches. Crutch use requires good upper body strength, so it may not be appropriate for elderly or medically compromised patients.

In most cases, a physical therapist measures the patient for proper fit and instructs the patient in crutch-walking techniques. The nurse helps to reinforce the instructions and evaluate whether the crutches are being used properly. A properly fitting crutch should reach to three fingerbreaths below the axilla to avoid pressure on the axilla when walking. This type of pressure could result in temporary or permanent numbness in the hands. When walking, the patient's weight should be put on the hand grips. The hand grips are adjusted so that the elbow is flexed no more than 30 degrees when standing in the tripod position, which is the basic crutch stance (Fig. 38–8).

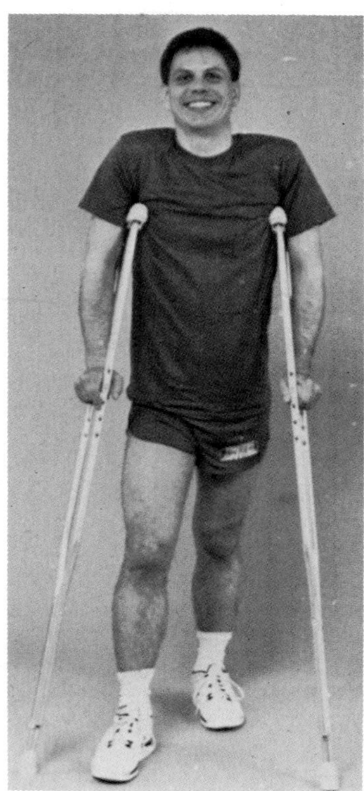

FIGURE 38-8
Tripod position. (From Maher, A. B., Salmond, S. W., & Pellino, T. A. [1994]. *Orthopedic nursing* [p. 326]. Philadelphia: W. B. Saunders.)

Gait Patterns

Several types of gait patterns are used with crutches. The type of gait used depends on the severity of the patient's disability and the patient's physical condition, trunk strength, upper and lower extremity strength, and balance. All of the gaits begin with the tripod position.

The five types of gait patterns used with crutches are

1. *Two-point gait:* Advance crutch on one side at the same time as the opposite foot. Used with partial weight-bearing limitations and with bilateral lower extremity prostheses.
2. *Three-point gait:* Advance both crutches and the foot of the affected extremity, followed by the foot of the unaffected extremity. Requires strength and balance. Used for partial or non–weight bearing on the affected leg.
3. *Four-point gait:* Advance the right crutch, then the left foot, then the left crutch, then the right foot. Used if weight bearing is allowed and one foot can be placed in front of the other.
4. *Swing-to gait:* Advance both crutches together, then lift both legs to the area behind the crutches. Feet and crutches form a tripod.
5. *Swing-through gait:* Advance both crutches together, then lift both legs past the crutches. Used when there is adequate muscle power and balance in the arms and legs.

When getting into a sitting position, the patient walks up to the chair, turns using the crutches, and backs up until the unaffected leg touches the seat of the chair. One hand then grips both crutches by the hand grips, and the crutches are placed on the unaffected side. The patient bends at the waist, places the affected side's hand on the seat, moves the affected leg forward, and lowers onto the seat slowly (Fig. 38–9*A* and *B*). To get up from a sitting position, the patient pushes off against the chair with the hand of the affected side and pushes down with the other hand, which is holding both crutches by the hand grips.

Going up and down stairs is challenging with crutches. When climbing stairs, the unaffected leg goes up the step first while the body is supported by the crutches. The full body weight is transferred to the unaffected leg, followed by movement of the crutches and the affected leg to the step. When descending stairs, the affected leg and the crutches move down one step followed by the affected leg. Therefore, when climbing stairs, the "good" leg goes first, and when descending stairs, the "bad" leg goes first.

WALKERS

A walker is used for support and balance, usually by older clients. A modified swing-to gait is used with a walker so that the walker is pushed or lifted forward followed by the legs. Rather than lifting both legs forward together, as with crutch walking, one foot is brought forward at a time.

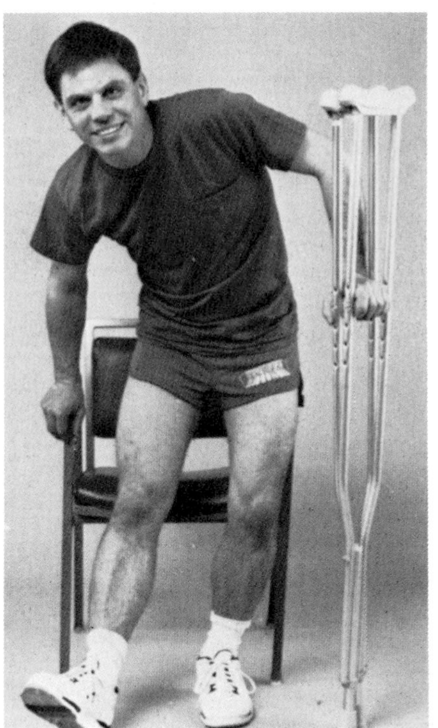
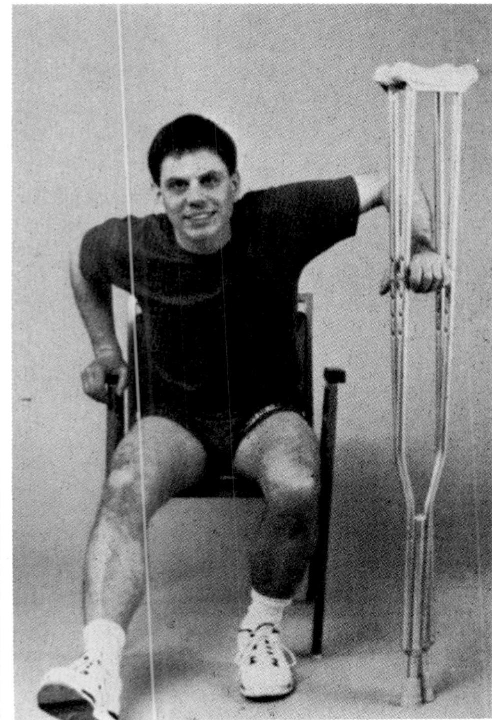

FIGURE 38-9
Stand to sitting with crutches. (From Maher, A. B., Salmond, S. W., & Pellino, T. A. [1994]. *Orthopedic nursing* [p. 327]. Philadelphia: W. B. Saunders.)

CANES

Canes are used to provide minimal support and balance and to relieve pressure on weight-bearing joints. The cane is placed on the unaffected side, and the top of the cane is even with the patient's greater trochanter. The elbow should be flexed at approximately 30 degrees (Fig. 38–10). Two-point or four-point gaits are used with a cane. The cane should be held close to the body on the unaffected side and advanced with the affected leg. When walking, it is better to lift the cane rather than slide it along to prevent catching the cane tip and tripping or falling.

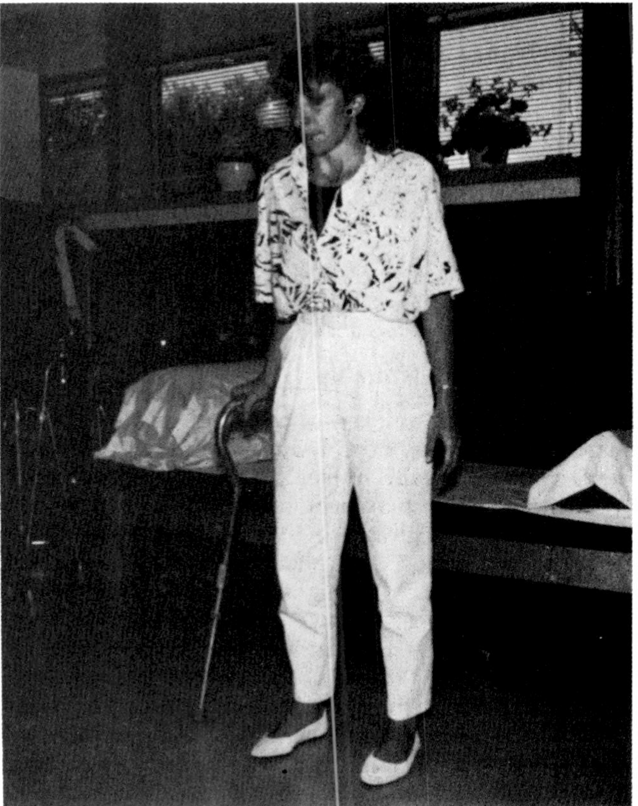

FIGURE 38-10
Using a cane to ambulate. Note that the top of the cane is parallel to the greater trochanter of the femur. (From Ignatavicius, D. D., & Bayne, M. V. [1991]. *Medical-surgical nursing: A nursing process approach* [p. 801]. Philadelphia: W. B. Saunders.)

NURSING CARE OF THE PATIENT WITH A FRACTURE

Once the initial emergency treatment and medical management of a patient with a fracture have taken place, nursing care becomes very important. The focus of nursing care is on preventing complications and restoring the patient to independent function. (See Care Plan: The Patient with a Fracture and Chapter 13 for emergency care.)

ASSESSMENT

Health History

Even after the initial medical care has been given and the fracture has been set, it is helpful to gain data regarding the cause, type, and extent of the injury. This information is important so that the nurse can observe for complications or other injuries that may have been

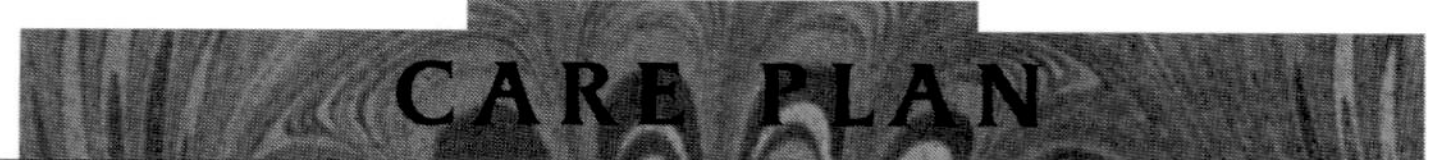

The Patient with a Fracture

ASSESSMENT

Health History: A 69-year-old female was admitted for a Colles' fracture in the left wrist 2 days ago. Before the injury, she lived alone and cared for herself. She was active, alert, and independent. Since the fracture repair, she has complained of pain over the area of the break but has had no signs of infection. Her physician is ready to discharge her to her home.

Physical Examination: Vital signs: temperature, 97.4°F orally; pulse, 98 with slight irregularity; respiration, 20; blood pressure, 165/95. Height, 5′3″. Weight, 132 lb. She is alert, oriented to time, place, and person. She needs assistance with activities of daily living (ADL), particularly bathing, dressing, and toileting. A cast is on her left arm from below the elbow to the fingers.

NURSING DIAGNOSIS	GOALS AND OUTCOME CRITERIA	INTERVENTIONS
Pain related to bone fracture, edema, soft tissue damage, muscle spasm.	The patient will have relief from pain as evidenced by absence of verbal complaints, anxiety, and moaning or wincing.	Provide adequate pain relief using medications and other comfort measures such as positioning and massage.
Altered tissue perfusion (peripheral) related to decreased blood flow caused by injury.	The patient will have adequate tissue perfusion as evidenced by satisfactory color in areas distal to the fracture, adequate capillary refill, and adequate sensation.	Relieve edema by elevating the affected limb above the patient's head while she is lying in bed and applying cold for brief periods of time; encourage patient to wiggle fingers and toes to increase circulation to the area.
High risk for infection related to disruption of skin integrity, bone trauma, soft tissue damage.	The patient will remain free from infection as evidenced by absence of redness, swelling, drainage, and fever.	Use strict aseptic technique for dressing changes, wound irrigations, and pin care; observe wounds for signs of infection; use isolation precautions and administer antibiotics as ordered if infection develops.

overlooked during the emergency situation. The patient, family members, or witnesses should be asked about the events leading up to the accident and exactly what happened during the accident. In addition, symptoms associated with the injury should be assessed, including a description of the type and extent of pain, the presence of numbness or tingling or both, the loss of motion and sensation, and the complaint of muscle spasms.

The number and types of prescription and over-the-counter medications should be assessed to determine whether they played any role in the development of the fracture or will affect the recovery and rehabilitation. It is also helpful to find out about other medical problems that either may have been related to the cause of the fracture, such as a pathologic fracture, or may have an affect on healing. The patient's occupation and usual roles and responsibilities are determined, and the effects of the injury on usual activities may be discussed.

Physical Examination

Because fractures usually involve some type of accidental injury, the nurse should be on the alert for signs of serious complications, such as head, thoracic, and abdominal injuries. In addition, the patient should be examined for associated tissue trauma, such as bleeding, bruising, and lacerations.

When inspecting the fracture area, the nurse observes for deviations in bone alignment. The limb may appear to be out of correct shape or deformed. The length of the extremity may change, usually becoming shorter. The skin over the fracture is inspected for lacerations, bruising, or swelling.

The affected extremity is always compared with the unaffected extremity. Neurovascular checks in the areas distal to the wound should be done to compare circulation and sensation. Skin color is a good indication of

The Patient with a Fracture *(Continued)*

NURSING DIAGNOSIS	GOALS AND OUTCOME CRITERIA	INTERVENTIONS
Impaired physical mobility related to pain and treatment modalities for fracture.	The patient will maintain as much mobility as possible as evidenced by independence in ADL and absence of secondary complications.	Encourage regular movement, including passive or active range of motion exercises; provide gait training with mobility aids to promote mobility and independence; reinforce activity and exercise program for the patient.
High risk for impaired skin integrity related to injury and immobility.	The patient will maintain skin integrity as evidenced by intact skin.	Move the patient around as soon as possible after fracture has been treated; use proper positioning and frequent turning.
Activity intolerance related to prolonged immobility.	The patient will maintain tolerance to activity as evidenced by participation in activities without weakness or excessive tiring.	Encourage range of motion exercises, resistance exercise of the unaffected extremities, and, when possible, ambulation; encourage participation in ADL and recreational activities; have rest periods between activities to preserve strength.
Knowledge deficit related to lack of experience with the use of immobilization devices (e.g., casts, traction, splints) or mobilization devices (e.g., crutches, walkers, canes).	The patient will display knowledge of immobilization and mobilization devices as evidenced by their proper use.	Teach the patient interventions that promote bone and tissue healing; teach patient to recognize signs and symptoms of complications that should be reported to a physician; instruct the patient in the use of equipment, assistive devices, and techniques to assist with ADL.

circulation to the extremity, and pallor indicates poor circulation. Pulse rate and intensity are assessed, as well as capillary refill in the nails. Capillary refill is observed by applying pressure to the nail and checking the speed of blood return to the area. Sensation is determined by pinprick, especially in the web space between the first and the second toes or between the thumb and the forefinger.

NURSING DIAGNOSIS

Common nursing diagnoses for the patient with a fracture may include the following:

- **Pain** related to bone fracture, edema, soft tissue damage, or muscle spasm
- **Altered Tissue Perfusion** (peripheral) related to decreased blood flow caused by the injury
- **High Risk for Infection** related to disruption of skin integrity, bone trauma, and soft tissue damage
- **Impaired Physical Mobility** related to pain and treatment modalities for the fracture
- **High Risk for Impaired Skin Integrity** related to injury and immobility
- **Activity Intolerance** related to prolonged immobility
- **Knowledge Deficit** related to lack of experience with the use of immobilization devices (e.g., casts, traction, splints) or mobilization devices (e.g., crutches, walkers, canes)

Additional nursing diagnoses may include **Altered Nutrition: Less than Body Requirements** related to additional metabolic need for healing of bone and soft tissues; **Constipation** related to prolonged immobility; **Self-Care Deficit** related to pain and immobility; **Ineffective Individual Coping** related to prolonged immobility, hospitalization, or altered lifestyle; **Sleep Pattern Disturbance** related to pain, immobility; and **Diversional Activity Deficit** related to immobility.

GOALS

The general goals for the care of a patient with a fracture are to promote healing and rehabilitation and to prevent complications. Specific goals are pain relief, adequate tissue perfusion, absence of infection, improved physical mobility, normal skin integrity, improved activity tolerance, and proper use of therapeutic devices.

INTERVENTIONS

PAIN. All fractures are painful. The degree of pain experienced depends on the extent and type of injury and the pain tolerance of the patient. The primary method of pain relief is immobilization of the affected part. Analgesic medications and muscle relaxants also are used. Other methods of pain relief include repositioning, massage, and diversion. General pain management is discussed in more detail in Chapter 16.

PHARMACOLOGY CAPSULE

To be most effective, pain medications should be administered before the pain becomes severe or gets out of control.

PHARMACOLOGY CAPSULE

Pain medication may be successfully administered by oral, intramuscular, intravenous, or epidural routes.

ALTERED TISSUE PERFUSION. Factors that cause impaired peripheral tissue perfusion are soft tissue injury resulting from trauma, fracture fragments, hemorrhage, edema, and positioning. The treatment of the fracture also can interfere with peripheral circulation, including moving or splinting the fracture, manipulation during reduction, and application of a cast, a splint, traction, or a brace.

Neurovascular checks (pulse, skin color, capillary refill, sensation) are made routinely by the nurse to ensure that circulation is adequate. For patients at risk for impaired tissue perfusion, the nurse may elevate the affected part above the head, apply cold to minimize edema, and encourage finger and toe movement. If a cast is too tight, it may be cut or replaced.

HIGH RISK FOR INFECTION. Disruption of skin may occur with a fracture, and, when there is open reduction with external fixation, the potential for infection always exists. Infection can cause delayed healing and postpone rehabilitation. Strict aseptic technique should be used for dressing changes, wound irrigations, and pin care. Wounds should be observed for signs of infection, such as drainage, redness, swelling, and heat, and the patient's temperature is monitored for fever. If an infection develops, isolation precautions are implemented and antibiotics are prescribed. Infection is discussed more completely in Chapter 9.

IMPAIRED PHYSICAL MOBILITY. Interventions for immobility are aimed at promoting independence and preventing related complications. Patients may experience anxiety and powerlessness when their activity is restricted because of the enforced immobilization related to traction, casts, or other equipment. In addition, they may experience secondary complications of immobility, such as deep vein thrombosis, pulmonary embolism, contractures or muscular atrophy, skin breakdown, and gastrointestinal problems, especially constipation. Older individuals are particularly vulnerable to the effects of immobility.

All patients with fractures should be encouraged to engage in regular movement of some kind. Passive or active range of motion exercises are helpful for both bedridden and ambulatory patients. Gait training with crutches, walkers, and canes promotes mobility and independence. A physical therapist usually works out an activity and exercise program for patients recovering from fractures, and the role of the nurse is to reinforce and encourage patients to carry out the program. More discussion of immobility is in Chapter 19.

HIGH RISK FOR IMPAIRED SKIN INTEGRITY. Skin integrity may be impaired as a result of the injury itself or the treatment of the injury. A compound fracture causes a break in the skin, and soft tissue injury occurs with almost every kind of fracture. Treatment measures such as immobilization or devices such as casts or traction may cause pressure to areas of the skin and result in pressure sores. In addition, the improper use of equipment can cause pressure to certain areas of the skin. Individuals who are at highest risk for skin breakdown are older adults, people with preexisting conditions, such as diabetes mellitus, and people whose general condition was poor before the injury.

To prevent skin breakdown, patients should begin moving around as soon as possible after the fracture has been treated. Proper positioning and frequent turning are essential for the prevention of skin breakdown. Guidelines for proper positioning are listed in Table 38–3.

ACTIVITY INTOLERANCE. With prolonged immobility, individuals become weaker and their ability to participate in activities diminishes. Patients should be encouraged to keep their strength up by carrying out range of motion exercises, resistance exercises of the unaffected extremities, and, when possible, ambulation. Participation in activities of daily living and recreational activities also is helpful. Rest periods between activities help to preserve strength.

KNOWLEDGE DEFICIT. Patients who have never been injured or who have never suffered a fracture usually have little knowledge about how to manage after the fracture has been medically treated. They need to be taught about the types of medical and nursing interventions that will be carried out to promote bone and tissue healing. Patients need to learn to recognize signs and symptoms of complications that should be reported to a physician. In addition, they must be instructed in the use of equipment, assistive devices, and techniques to assist with activities of daily living.

TABLE 38-3
TIPS ON POSITIONING

FRACTURE	POSITIONING
Cervical spine	Before treatment—supine, immobilize neck with sandbags or Philadelphia collar Turn with head well supported
Thoracic spine	Position of comfort
Lumbar spine	Avoid high sitting positions, logroll
Pelvis	Stable fracture or after fixation—turn to side *opposite* fracture Unstable—do not turn
Hip	Before surgical treatment—turn *toward* fracture (avoid dislocation or further displacement of fragments) with pillows between legs Postoperative—turn away from fracture until comfortable enough to turn on operative side, pillows between legs Arthroplasty—maintain abduction at all times with abduction pillow or regular pillows between legs
Shoulder/humerus	Elevate head of bed to comfort Turn to side opposite fracture
Forearm/foreleg	Elevate distal portion of extremity higher than heart

From Maher, A. B., Salmond, S. W., & Pellino, T. A. (1994). *Orthopedic nursing* (p. 281). Philadelphia: W. B. Saunders.

Teaching should take place in the hospital immediately after the fracture is treated to prepare for the patient's discharge to the home. Patients and family members must be assessed for their readiness and ability to learn. If patients are unable to care for themselves independently at home, assistance from formal agencies such as home health or social services may be needed. Areas to be assessed for home care needs include ability to carry out activities of daily living, mobility, mental status, and skilled nursing needs.

PHARMACOLOGY CAPSULE

When patients administer their own pain medication, they are more in control and more able to manage their pain successfully.

EVALUATION

Criteria for evaluating the outcomes of nursing interventions are patient's verbalization of pain relief; absence of moaning, wincing, and the like; normal color, capillary refill, and sensation in affected area; absence of swelling, drainage, and fever; independence in activities of daily living and absence of complications (pressure sores, constipation, contractures, atelectasis); intact skin without redness; participation in exercise without excessive tiring; and patient's demonstration of correct use of therapeutic devices.

MANAGEMENT OF SPECIFIC FRACTURES

FRACTURE OF THE HIP

Hip fractures most commonly occur in older adults, especially older women. Most hip fractures are located in the femoral neck and intertrochanteric regions (Fig. 38–11). The most common cause is a fall on a hard surface; however, it is thought that many fractures in older individuals result from decreased bone mass or brittle bones associated with osteoporosis. Signs and symptoms of a hip fracture are history of a fall, severe pain and tenderness in the region of the fracture site, a shortened externally rotated hip, and soft tissue trauma.

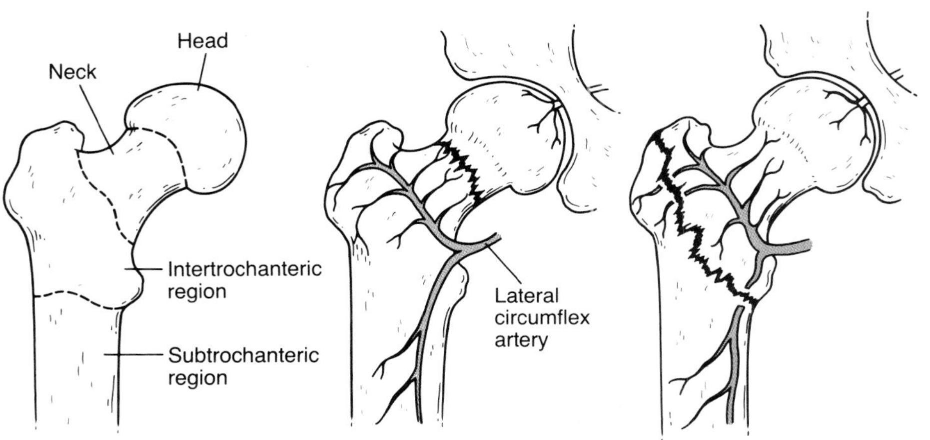

FIGURE 38-11
A, Normal proximal end of femur; *B*, intracapsular fracture of femur; *C*, intertrochanteric fracture. (Modified from Black, J. M., & Matassarin-Jacobs, E. [1993]. *Luckmann and Sorensen's medical-surgical nursing: A psychophysiologic approach* [4th ed., p. 1924]. Philadelphia: W. B. Saunders.)

Medical Diagnosis

The diagnosis of hip fracture is confirmed by radiography. Other diagnostic tests may be obtained in preparation for surgery, such as complete blood count, urinalysis, and electrocardiogram.

Medical Treatment

Traction and surgical repair are the standard treatments for hip fracture. For older patients, surgical repair of the fracture is often the treatment of choice because it allows them to move around sooner and results in fewer complications related to immobility. Traction may require 12 to 16 weeks of immobilization for healing. Patients may be on bedrest at home if family members are able to care for them. They may begin sitting in a chair in 2 to 3 days and then progress to ambulation with a walker. Weight bearing on the affected side is limited to 10% initially and then gradually increased as tolerated.

Nursing Care of the Patient with a Hip Fracture

ASSESSMENT. Patients with a hip fracture are assessed in the same way as patients with other types of fractures. They should be assessed for pain, impaired peripheral circulation on the affected side, complications of immobility, skin breakdown, and ability to carry out activities of daily living. Older patients are particularly prone to developing delirium after a broken hip, and so mental status and problem behaviors related to confusion should be noted.

NURSING DIAGNOSIS, GOALS, AND EVALUATION. General nursing diagnoses, goals, and evaluation for the patient with a fracture have already been presented. The special needs of the patient with a hip fracture are discussed here.

INTERVENTIONS. Nursing interventions are geared toward relieving pain, promoting mobility and independence, and preventing complications. Older patients have special nursing care needs because of their vulnerability to complications of immobility and confusion. Pain management is of utmost importance. Confused patients may not be able to tell the nurse the extent or degree of their pain, and many times they may be undermedicated. Problem behaviors such as agitation, trying to climb out of bed, pulling out intravenous or other tubes, and alterations in sleep patterns may be related to pain. Other comfort measures, such as repositioning, body massage, and diversional activities, enhance the effect of medications.

Proper body alignment is extremely important in preventing injury to the fracture area after it has been medically treated. Patients should be turned carefully (and frequently) from side to side, and the affected hip should not be flexed more than 90 degrees. Patients should use an elevated toilet seat, sit in a supporting chair with a straight back and seat, and avoid crossing their legs.

COLLES' FRACTURE

Colles' fracture is a break in the distal radius (wrist area) (Fig. 38–12). Colles' fractures frequently occur in older adults, particularly older women, when an outstretched hand is used to break a fall. The major signs and symptoms are pain and swelling in the area of the injury and a characteristic displacement of the bone in which the wrist has the appearance of a dinner fork. The most frequent complication is impaired circulation in the area resulting from edema.

Medical Diagnosis

Diagnosis is confirmed by the characteristic bone deformity of the wrist and radiography.

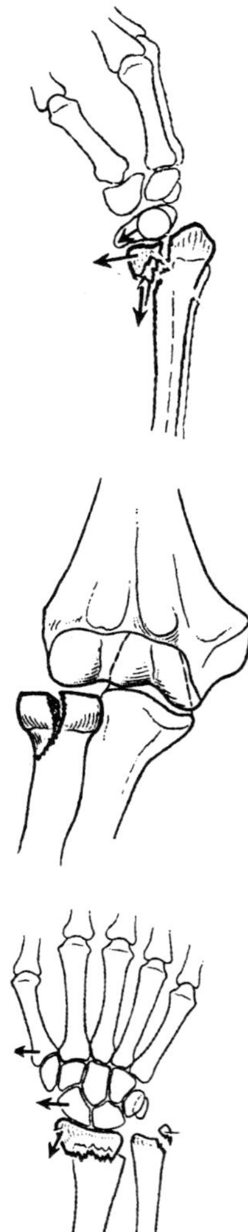

FIGURE 38–12
Colles' fracture. (Modified from Maher, A. B., Salmond, S. W., & Pellino, T. A. [1994]. *Orthopedic nursing* [p. 713]. Philadelphia: W. B. Saunders.)

Medical Treatment

Colles' fractures are managed by closed reduction or manipulation of the bone and immobilization by either a splint or a cast. The elbow is immobilized as well to prevent misalignment.

Nursing Care of the Patient with a Colles' Fracture

ASSESSMENT. Patients should be assessed for pain and swelling following medical treatment of the fracture.

NURSING DIAGNOSIS, GOALS, AND EVALUATION. General nursing diagnoses, goals, and evaluation for the patient with a fracture have already been presented. The special needs of the patient with a Colles' fracture are discussed here.

INTERVENTIONS. Interventions are aimed at relieving pain and preventing or reducing edema. The extremity should be supported and protected and can be elevated on a pillow during the first few days. Patients are encouraged to move their fingers and thumb to promote circulation and reduce swelling, and to move their shoulder to prevent stiffness and contracture. In addition, patients should be taught proper cast care.

FRACTURE OF THE PELVIS

Although pelvic fractures account for a small percentage of total fractures (3%), next to head injury, they are the second leading cause of death from trauma. Motor vehicle accidents are the most common cause of pelvic fractures in young adults, and falls are the main cause in older adults. The extent of the injury can range from minimal in a non–weight-bearing fracture to severe in a weight-bearing fracture. Internal trauma, such as laceration of the colon, hemorrhage, or rupture of the urethra or bladder, often accompanies a pelvic fracture. The patient may demonstrate local swelling, tenderness, bruising, and deformity.

Medical Diagnosis

As with other fractures, the diagnosis and severity of the injury are confirmed by radiography.

Medical Treatment

Medical treatment depends on the severity of the fracture. A less severe non–weight-bearing fracture is usually treated with bedrest on a firm mattress or bed board for a few days to 6 weeks. A more severe weight-bearing fracture may require a pelvic sling, skeletal traction, a double hip spica cast, or external fixation. Because of the high risk of internal trauma, the health care team continually observes the patient so that specific injuries can be treated immediately. They check for the presence of blood in the urine and stool and watch the abdomen for any signs of rigidity or swelling.

Nursing Care of the Patient with a Pelvic Fracture

ASSESSMENT. Patients are observed for signs of bleeding, swelling, infection, thromboembolus, and pain.

NURSING DIAGNOSIS, GOALS, AND EVALUATION. General nursing diagnoses, goals, and evaluation for the patient with a fracture have already been presented. The special needs of the patient with a pelvic fracture are discussed here.

INTERVENTIONS. Interventions consist of alleviating pain, promoting mobility, and preventing complications. Extreme care should be taken when handling patients to prevent displacement of the fracture fragments. The patients are turned only under orders of a physician. Back care can be carried out when the patient is raised from the bed using the trapeze or with adequate assistance from others. Weight bearing is restricted until healing is complete.

NUTRITION CONCEPTS

- Calcium in the diet and calcium supplements are recommended for helping to prevent fractures due to osteoporosis in older age.
- Prolonged immobilization, which is often required after multiple fractures, contributes to the loss of calcium and protein.
- To promote healing after a fracture, caloric and protein requirements increase.
- To achieve optimal bone healing, excessive amounts of calcium, along with vitamin D, are recommended.
- Supplemental feedings that are high in calories, protein, and calcium, such as milk shakes, may be served between meals to promote healing.

BIBLIOGRAPHY

Allan, D. J. (1993). Adding food for thought: Structuring nutritional support for elderly trauma patients. *Professional Nurse, 8*(10), 632, 634, 636–637.

Bailey, M. M., & Michalski, J. (1992). Close-up on Colles' fracture. *Nursing, 22*(10), 47.

Barden, R. M., & Sinkora, G. L. (1991). Bone stimulators for fusions and fractures. *Nursing Clinics of North America, 26*(1), 89–103.

Belinsky, J. D. (1993). Acetabular fracture: ORIF . . . open reduction internal fixation. *Orthopedic Nursing, 12*(1), 42–45, 48–50.

Blair, J. E. Z. (1991). Colles' fracture. In F. F. Rogers-Seidl (Ed.), *Geriatric nursing care plans* (pp. 172–176). St. Louis: Mosby Year Book.

Cummings, J. (1991). Managing the patient with fractured femur, part 1. *Nursing Standard,* *5*(25, Tissue Viability), 11–13.

Cummings, J. (1991). Managing the patient with fractured femur, part 2. *Nursing Standard,* *5*(36, Tissue Viability), 11–13.

Cummings, J. (1991). Managing the patient with fractured femur, part 3. *Nursing Standard,* *5*(50, Tissue Viability), 11–13.

Dunwoody, C. J. (1991). Pelvic fracture patient care: Reflections on the past, implications for the future. *Nursing Clinics of North America,* *26*(1), 65–72.

Dykes, P. C. (1993). Minding the five Ps of neurovascular assessment. *American Journal of Nursing,* *93*(6), 38–39.

Edwards, K. P. (1993). Orthopedic trauma: Pelvic fracture. *Today's OR Nurse,* *15*(4), 24–28.

Egan, M., Warren, S. A., Hessel, P. A., & Gilewich, G. (1992). Activities of daily living after hip fracture: Pre- and postdischarge. *Occupational Therapy Journal of Research,* *12*(6), 342–356.

Evans, B. (1993). Nurse-aid management of fractures, part 1. *British Journal of Nursing,* *2*(8), 432–436.

Evans, B. (1993). Nurse-aid management of fractures, part 2. *British Journal of Nursing,* *2*(9), 483–487.

Maher, A. B., Salmond, S. W., & Pellino, T. A. (1994). *Orthopedic nursing.* Philadelphia: W. B. Saunders.

Mandzuk, L. L. (1991). External pinsite care: A review of the literature and nursing practice. *CONA Journal,* *13*(1), 10–15.

Reuben, J. D. (1991). Rehabilitation of the fracture patient. *Hospital Practice,* *26*(Suppl. 1), 46–48.

Ruda, S. C. (1991). Common ankle injuries in the athlete. *Nursing Clinics of North America,* *26*(1), 167–180.

Ruhl, J. M. (1991). Pelvic trauma. *RN,* *54*(7), 50–55.

Smrcina, C. M. (1991). Stress fractures in athletes. *Nursing Clinics of North America,* *26*(1), 159–166.

Sneed, N. V., & VanBree, K. M. (1990). Treating ununited fractures with electricity: Nursing implications. *Journal of Gerontological Nursing,* *16*(8), 26–31, 36–37.

KEY CONCEPTS

1. A fracture is a break or disruption in the continuity of a bone, usually causing injury to surrounding soft tissue.
2. Open or compound fractures have three grades of severity, ranging from least severe injury with minimal skin damage to most severe injury with skin, muscle, blood vessel, and nerve damage.
3. Fractures of the femur are most common in young and middle-aged adults, and hip and wrist fractures are most common in the elderly.
4. Fractures are usually caused by trauma to the bone, especially as a result of automobile accidents and falls.
5. Risk factors for hip fractures include osteoporosis, advanced age, white race, use of psychotropic drugs, and being female.
6. The most common signs and symptoms of a fracture are swelling, bruising, pain, tenderness, loss of normal function, and abnormal mobility.
7. Bone healing occurs in five stages: (1) hematoma formation, (2) cellular proliferation, (3) callus formation, (4) ossification, and (5) consolidation and remodeling.
8. Healing time for fractures increases with age, and it may take six times as long for the same type of fracture to heal in an older person as it does in an infant.
9. Complications of a fracture include infection, fat embolism, and compartment syndrome.
10. The goals of medical treatment for a fracture are to realign the bone fragments, establish a sturdy union between the broken ends of the bone, and restore function.
11. The most common therapeutic techniques used to treat a fracture are closed and open reduction and internal and external fixation.
12. Casts are used for external fixation of extensive fractures and fractures of the extremities.
13. Traction provides alignment of the broken bone fragments, prevents or corrects deformity, decreases muscle spasm, promotes rest and exercise, and maintains the position of a diseased or injured part.
14. Crutches increase mobility and assist with ambulation after a fracture of the lower extremity.
15. A walker is used for support and balance, usually by older patients.
16. Canes provide minimal support and balance and relieve pressure on weight-bearing joints.
17. The focus of nursing care for a fracture is on preventing complications and restoring the patient to independent function.

Dianne Murray Rudolph

CHAPTER 39

Amputations

OBJECTIVES

1. Identify clinical indications for amputations.
2. Describe different types of amputations.
3. Discuss medical and surgical management of the amputation patient.
4. Identify appropriate nursing interventions during the preoperative and postoperative phases of care.
5. Use the nursing process to develop a plan of care for the amputation patient.

GLOSSARY

AMPUTATION Removal of a limb, part of a limb, or an organ; may be done by surgical means or in an accident

AMPUTEE Individual who has undergone an amputation

CLOSED AMPUTATION Amputation in which a limb or part of a limb is removed and surgically closed

CONGENITAL AMPUTATION Deformity or absence of a limb or limbs occurring during fetal development in the uterus

GANGRENE Necrosis or death of tissue, usually due to a deficient or absent blood supply; may result from inflammatory processes, injury, arteriosclerosis, frostbite, or diabetes mellitus

GUILLOTINE AMPUTATION Type of amputation in which a limb or portion of a limb is severed from the body and the wound is left open; a type of open amputation

OPEN AMPUTATION Amputation that is left open; usually done in cases of infection or necrosis

PHANTOM LIMB Illusion, following an amputation of a limb, that the limb still exists; the sensation that pain exists in removed limb is called phantom limb pain

REPLANTATION Surgical reattachment of an organ to its original site; reimplantation

Glossary continued

STAGED AMPUTATION Amputation that is done over the course of several surgeries; usually done to control the spread of infection or necrosis

STUMP Refers to the distal portion of an amputated limb

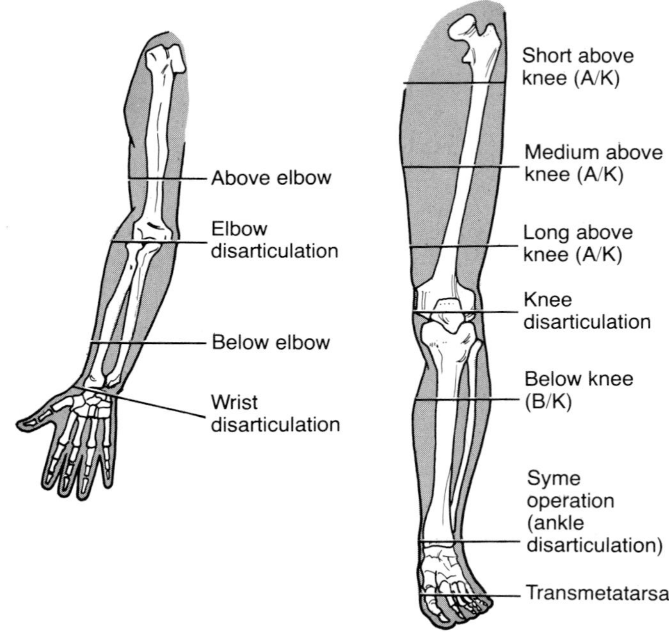

FIGURE 39-1
Common sites of amputation in the upper and lower extremities.

Derived from the Latin word meaning "cutting around," the term *amputation* refers to the surgical removal of body limbs or parts of limbs. Amputations have been performed since the beginning of mankind, according to findings by archaeologists. Ancient amputations were originally performed to remove gangrenous or damaged limbs; they were also performed for ritual sacrifice, punishment, exorcism of evil spirits, and, in some cases, beautification.

In the past two decades, many advances have been made in surgical amputation and replantation (limb reattachment) techniques, prosthetic devices (artificial limbs), and rehabilitation programs. This has allowed many amputees to remain active and productive despite their disabilities. There are an estimated 400,000 amputees in the United States alone, with an annual increase of 5%. The vast majority of these have had lower extremity amputations.

AMPUTATION

Amputation can occur through the joint or the bone itself. Disarticulation is the term for an amputation through the joint. The general site of the amputation is described by the joint nearest to it. For example, the removal of the lower leg at the middle of the shin or calf is called a below-knee amputation. Some of the most common sites of amputation can be seen in Figure 39–1.

INDICATIONS AND INCIDENCE

Conditions or situations that lead to the need for an amputation can generally be grouped into four categories: trauma, disease, and tumors. In addition, congenital defects account for a fourth category of amputation, situations in which a limb is missing at birth.

Trauma

In some serious accidents, part or all of a limb may be removed. This is often referred to as a traumatic amputation. In other situations, the limb may be damaged enough to require surgical removal. Common types of accidents and injuries leading to amputation include those involving motorcycles and automobiles, farm machinery, firearms and explosives, electrical equipment, power tools, and frostbite. Trauma tends to be the most common reason for upper extremity amputations. Because these accidents are typically occupational hazards, the victims are usually younger males.

Disease

Vascular diseases can lead to the need for amputation. In these cases, blood supply to the tissues is inadequate and the tissues become deprived of oxygen and other important nutrients. Without these nutrients, necrosis or death of the tissue occurs. Some examples of diseases leading to impaired circulation are peripheral vascular disease, diabetes mellitus, and arteriosclerosis. These problems can also be complicated by infection because wounds sustained to limbs without a good blood supply do not heal well and gangrene can set in quickly. Since circulation problems are more common among the elderly and in the lower extremities, affected individuals tend to be 60 years of age or more.

Tumors

Amputations may also be performed for tumors. These are usually tumors of the bone and can be very large and invasive. They typically result in amputations and disarticulation that involve an entire limb, such as a whole arm or leg. Primary bone tumors occur most frequently in adolescents but can occur at any age. Approximately one third of these individuals are 11 to 20 years of age.

Congenital Defects

In some situations, a limb or part of a limb may be absent or deformed at birth. These are sometimes called congenital amputations. They are a result of changes that occur while the fetus is developing in the uterus such that the infant is born with a missing, deficient, or abnormal limb. Sometimes surgery is performed in order to convert a deformed limb into a more functional one that can be fitted with a prosthetic device.

DIAGNOSTIC TESTS AND PROCEDURES

The types of diagnostic studies done for a patient requiring amputation depend on the underlying disease or injury. For example, in a patient with an infection, blood is drawn for a white blood cell count. An elevated white blood cell count (≥10,000) indicates infection.

Table 39–1 lists examples of diagnostic findings associated with some of the contributing factors in amputations.

Vascular Studies

Vascular studies may be done for a patient with compromised circulation, such as in trauma or vascular disease. Angiography is a procedure that involves the injection of a radioactive dye into blood vessels that are then viewed under x-rays to determine their patency.

Plethysmography

Plethysmography is the use of a noninvasive device that gives general information about the volume of blood flow to an extremity. Another name for this procedure is pulse volume recording.

Thermography

Thermography involves the use of a device that records heat present in various parts of the body. Relatively hot or cold spots are revealed, indicating the amount of blood flow to that part of the body. Cool spots generally indicate a decreased blood flow as compared to warm.

Transcutaneous Doppler Recordings

Transcutaneous Doppler recordings (ultrasound) use sound waves to determine the presence of pulses in the extremities. This is much more sensitive than using the fingertips to try to palpate a pulse.

Transcutaneous Po_2

Transcutaneous Po_2 is a measurement of the partial pressure or amount of oxygen present at the skin surface. In patients with impaired circulation, this measurement can be greatly diminished.

Biopsy

In patients with tumors, a biopsy is often done to determine the nature of the tumor. A biopsy involves the removal of a small portion of tissue that is examined for malignancy.

TABLE 39–1
DIAGNOSTIC STUDIES

UNDERLYING PROBLEM	STUDIES	FINDINGS
Infection	WBC count, assessment of skin and tissues	Redness, swelling, pus/exudate at site, elevated WBC
Peripheral vascular disease	Arteriography	Occluded vessels
	Plethysmography	Decreased blood flow
	Doppler (ultrasound)	Decreased/absent peripheral pulses
	Transcutaneous Po_2	Decreased Po_2, cool, clammy, mottled skin
Limb deformity	Assessment of limb function, motor, and sensation	Dysfunctional limbs, impaired sensory and motor function
Trauma	Physical examination	Dirt/debris in wounds, necrosis, burned areas
	Doppler	Decreased/absent pulses
	Arteriography	Loss of blood vessel patency, damaged vessels, and bleeding into viable tissues, cool and mottled skin
Tumor	Assessment and biopsy	Pervasive tumor growth into and around joint, loss of function and sensation distal to tumor

WBC, White blood cell.

MEDICAL AND SURGICAL TREATMENT

The management of amputations requires both medical and surgical approaches by the physicians involved in the care of the patient who requires an amputation.

Medical Treatment

The medical care of the patient requiring an amputation involves the appropriate treatment and control of the underlying diseases. For example, the diabetic with poor circulation to the lower extremities needs to work toward good control of diabetes by means of diet and medications. Patients with peripheral vascular disease may be encouraged to stop smoking or to regulate their diets. The patient who has experienced trauma may have to be stabilized with measures that will maintain his or her heart rate and blood pressure within a normal range. Some physicians may prescribe medications such as aspirin or pentoxifylline (Trental) to improve blood flow.

Surgical Treatment

Amputation is recommended only when other options are not possible or have failed. In an effort to avoid amputation, the physician may perform angioplasty or surgical bypass of obstructed vessels.

Surgical management of the patient is aimed at performing an amputation at the lowest level that will still preserve healthy tissue and favor wound healing. The surgeon chooses one of two basic types of surgical procedures, depending on the condition of the extremity and the reason for the surgery. These two types are closed amputations and open amputations.

CLOSED AMPUTATIONS. Closed amputations are usually performed in order to create a weight-bearing stump, which is especially important for lower extremity amputations. In this procedure, a long skin flap with soft tissue and muscle are positioned over the severed end of the bone and sutured in place. The sutures are usually placed so that they are not in a position to bear the full weight of the patient. This technique has many variations. A more common method is the posterior flap technique, which is illustrated in Figure 39–2.

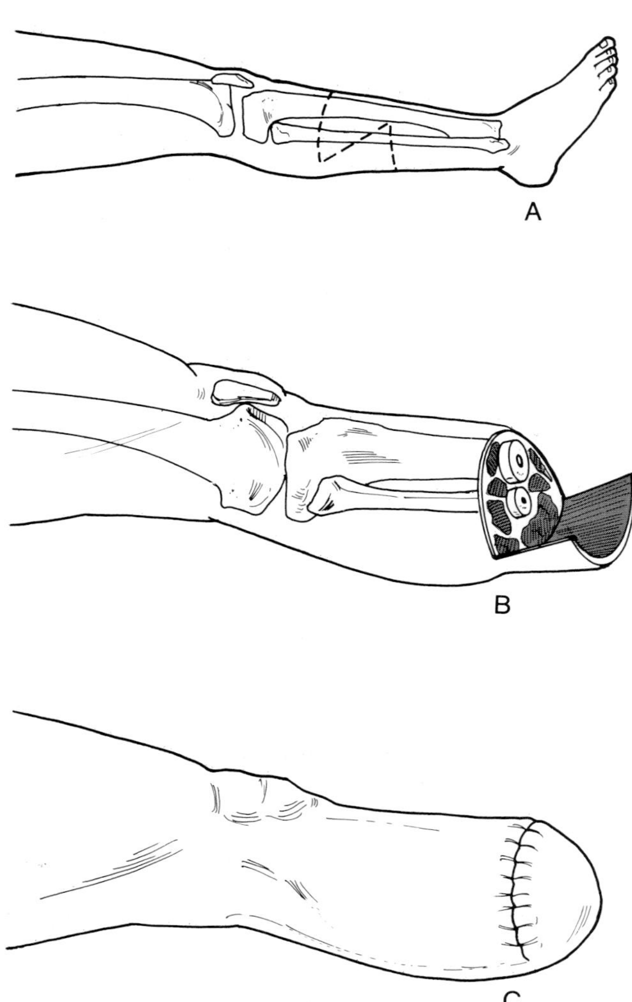

FIGURE 39–2

One of the most commonly performed closed amputations is the posterior flap technique. *A*, Skin incisions are outlined for the procedure. *B*, A myofascial flap is created using muscle and skin. *C*, The wound is closed and sutured.

OPEN AMPUTATIONS. In open amputations, the severed bone or joint is left uncovered by a skin flap. This type of amputation is required when an actual or potential infection exists, as in the case of gangrene or trauma. The wound is left open for 5 to 10 days, sometimes longer, and can be closed surgically when infection no longer poses a problem. Another term for this procedure is a staged or guillotine amputation.

COMPLICATIONS

A large number of complications are associated with amputations, including hemorrhage and hematoma, necrosis, wound dehiscence, gangrene, edema, contracture, pain, and infection. A list of these complications and contributing factors can be found in Table 39–2.

NURSING CARE OF THE PATIENT HAVING AMPUTATION SURGERY

Preoperative Nursing Care

Management of the patient having an amputation involves the use of the nursing process to assess the patient's physical and psychological status, plan care according to prioritized needs, implement care according to carefully considered strategies, and evaluate whether the patient's needs were met. Nursing care of the amputation patient is based on a preoperative phase and postoperative phase. Routine preoperative and postoperative care is detailed in Chapter 14. This section focuses on the specific needs of the patient having an amputation (see also Care Plan: The Patient with an Upper Extremity Amputation). Preoperative nursing assessment

TABLE 39–2

COMPLICATIONS OF AMPUTATION

Hematoma and hemorrhage	Bleeding into tissue in and around stump due to inadequate hemostasis.
Necrosis	Tissue destruction and death due to ongoing disease; requires surgical débridement or revision, or both.
Wound dehiscence	Opening of suture line due to early removal of sutures or falling; requires reclosure.
Gangrene	Death of tissue associated with inadequate blood supply and bacterial destruction of tissue; requires reamputation.
Edema	Swelling and discomfort in stump due to dependent position or incorrect wrapping; requires elevation and rewrapping.
Contracture	Flexion of joints with loss of range of motion due to prolonged elevation or immobilization of extremities. May be prevented by frequent position changes and range of motion exercises.
Pain	Extreme sharp pain at incision site due to scar formation on nerve fibers (neuroma); may require surgical treatment.
Infection	Redness, warmth, swelling, and exudate formation at stump site due to invasion of tissues by pathogens. May require antibiotics and surgical drainage.

of the patient having an amputation is summarized in Table 39–3.

Preoperatively, the patient needs to prepare both physically and psychologically for an impending amputation.

ASSESSMENT. The patient undergoing an amputation should be systematically and thoroughly assessed.

Health History. It is important for the nurse to document the conditions that resulted in the need for an amputation (diseases such as diabetes mellitus or peripheral vascular insufficiency, traumatic injuries, neoplasms, and birth defects) and to focus on stabilization and control of ongoing problems. A complete health history is obtained, including information on the patient's past medical and surgical histories. Examples of this type of information are previous surgeries, illnesses, hospitalizations, and accidents. Preexisting cardiovascular problems are noted because hypertension, coronary artery disease, congestive heart failure, and cardiac murmurs or defects can greatly affect the patient's ability to tolerate surgery and to recover successfully. The nurse also determines whether the patient has ever had phlebitis, varicosities, thrombosis, emboli, or stasis ulcers in either the affected or the unaffected extremities.

TABLE 39–3

ASSESSMENT OF THE PATIENT HAVING AN AMPUTATION

HEALTH HISTORY

Chief complaint and history of present illness: Condition or incident leading to amputation
Past medical history: Previous illnesses, surgeries, hospitalizations, trauma; hypertension, coronary artery disease, congestive heart failure, cardiac murmurs or defects, phlebitis, varicosities, thrombosis, emboli, stasis ulcers, diabetes mellitus
Family history: Diabetes mellitus, hypertension, vascular diseases
Review of systems:
- Pain: Nature, location, severity, precipitating factors, alleviating factors
- Sensation: Loss or change, abnormal, perception of heat and cold
- Skin color
- Leg ulcers
- Sexual dysfunction

Functional assessment:
- Usual diet and fluid intake
- Intake of salt and alcohol
- Use of tobacco
- Exercise, rest, and sleep habits
- Occupation, roles, and responsibilities
- Coping strategies
- Fears and concerns

PHYSICAL ASSESSMENT

Height and weight
Vital signs
Skin: Color, texture, temperature, turgor, lesions
Peripheral pulses: Presence, quality, symmetry
Capillary refill
Sensation
Mental status: Level of consciousness, emotional state
Cognition: Ability to follow directions

A family history of relevant disorders, including diabetes, hypertension, and vascular diseases, also is addressed.

The nurse systematically assesses signs and symptoms that relate to the vascular condition or other chronic and acute problems. Significant signs and symptoms are pain (location, severity, type, precipitating factors, alleviating factors), loss of sensation or abnormal sensations, intolerance of local heat or cold, color changes in the extremities, leg ulcers, and sexual dysfunction.

Important data in the functional assessment are usual diet and fluid intake, intake of salt and alcohol, and use of tobacco. Exercise and rest and sleep habits are described, as are the effects of the current symptoms on the patient's usual activities. The nurse also identifies the patient's occupation and responsibilities to determine how the amputation will affect that aspect of his or her life.

A review of the patient's psychosocial background may offer insight as to how the patient will tolerate treatments and procedures. Information related to how the patient copes with stress may help the nurse in planning care in order to minimize excess anxiety and fear. The patient about to undergo an amputation will undoubtedly have a number of fears and concerns about the surgical procedure, the loss of a body part, the potential loss of independence, and pain and disfigurement. Encouraging open discussion may help alleviate many of these concerns.

Physical Examination. A total physical assessment should be performed, placing special attention on the neurologic, cardiovascular, and integumentary systems. The nurse begins with measurement of height and weight and vital signs to document obesity and hypertension. Throughout the examination, the patient's skin is assessed for color, texture, temperature, and turgor. The overall color, condition, and temperature of the skin are good indicators of blood supply to the extremities. Cool or cold, clammy, mottled skin that is pale or cyanotic may indicate a poor blood supply. Additionally, there may be open areas on the skin such as lesions or ulcers with or without drainage. Wounds to the extremities are common when blood supply is inadequate.

The peripheral pulses are palpated for presence, quality, and symmetry. If pulses are not palpable, the nurse can use a Doppler ultrasound device to assess them. Capillary refill also is assessed. Capillary refill can be tested by applying pressure to the nail bed of a finger or toe until it blanches (turns white). When the pressure is released, the nail bed normally regains its normal pink color within 3 seconds. In extremities with a diminished supply of blood, capillary refill may take 5 seconds or longer. Sensation is assessed by asking the patient to identify touch on the extremities. Experienced examiners may evaluate the patient's ability to sense sharp, dull, warm, and cold stimuli.

Assessing the patient's mental and emotional status and general cognitive abilities is important in order to determine the patient's understanding of the nature of

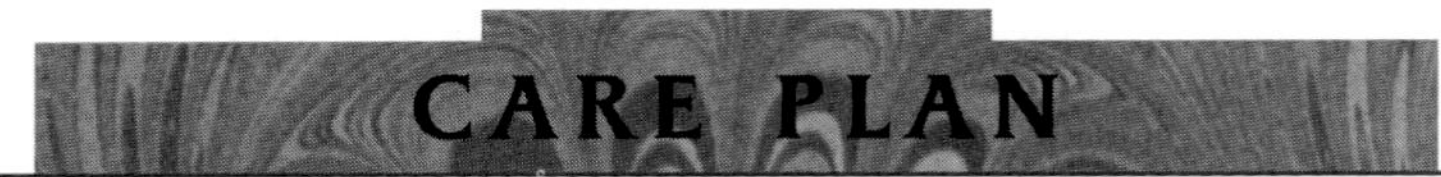

CARE PLAN

The Patient with an Upper Extremity Amputation

ASSESSMENT

Health History: Mr. Girard Blue is a 32-year-old African American male. As a result of an industrial accident, he sustained an injury that required amputation of his right forearm and hand just below the elbow. Mr. Blue's right hand was his dominant hand. He has had no other serious physical injuries or illnesses. He is a machinist who is a senior employee in his department. He is married and the father of three children. His wife is a housewife who has never worked outside the home.

Physical Examination: Mr. Blue is lethargic but responds to commands. Vital signs: temperature, 98.2°F orally; pulse, 80; respiration, 16; blood pressure, 126/68. A bulky dressing is in place in the stump of the right arm. The dressing is dry and intact. A Jackson-Pratt drain is in place, and the receptacle contains approximately 30 ml sanguineous fluid. Intravenous fluids are infusing into the left arm.

NURSING DIAGNOSIS	GOALS AND OUTCOME CRITERIA	INTERVENTIONS
Decreased cardiac output related to blood loss.	The patient's blood volume will remain normal as evidenced by stable vital signs, urine output equal to fluid intake, and absence of restlessness or frank bleeding.	Assess dressing and drain for steady or increasing bleeding. Monitor vital signs and intake and output. Observe behavior. Report signs of bleeding to surgeon. Reinforce dressing, apply pressure, and elevate stump if bleeding apparent.
Pain related to surgical incision, trauma, edema.	The patient will state pain is relieved and will appear more relaxed.	Assess pain nature, location, and severity. Administer analgesics as ordered. Provide comfort measures such as back rub, distraction, imagery. Inform surgeon if pain not relieved.
High risk for infection related to surgical wound, traumatic injury.	The patient will remain free of infection as evidenced by normal body temperature and absence of foul drainage, excessive redness, warmth, or edema.	Monitor temperature for elevation. Assess dressing for foul drainage. When dressing is removed, inspect stump for excessive redness, warmth, or edema. Handle dressing and stump using universal precautions. Teach the patient good hygiene to decrease the risk of infection. Administer antimicrobials as ordered.
Impaired skin integrity related to incision.	The patient's stump will heal completely.	Keep the stump dressing smooth and snug to mold the stump for future prosthesis use. Use caution not to impair blood flow. Check the stump for irritation or signs of pressure. Maintain elevation as ordered to minimize edema and pressure on suture line. Apply cold to stump dressing as ordered. After the first week, massage the stump as ordered to promote circulation.
Sensory-perceptual alteration related to phantom limb sensations.	The patient will report phantom limb sensations if they occur.	Tell the patient that these sensations sometimes follow amputation. Notify the surgeon. Advise the patient that several therapies are available for treatment of this condition.
High risk for injury related to loss of part of limb, weakness.	The patient will identify activities requiring adaptation for injury and will avoid dangerous activities.	Help the patient identify usual activities that cannot be safely done without the dominant hand. Discuss strategies to adapt activities or to learn to use the left hand. Consult rehabilitation specialist.

An Upper Extremity Amputation Patient *(Continued)*

NURSING DIAGNOSIS	GOALS AND OUTCOME CRITERIA	INTERVENTIONS
Self-care deficit related to loss of part of limb, inability to carry out activities of daily living.	The patient will accomplish self-care with minimal assistance from others.	Assist the patient with self-care but encourage increasing effort on his part. Praise efforts. Organize environment to facilitate self-care. For example, place bedside objects on the patient's left.
Anxiety related to perceived threat of disability.	The patient will verbalize concerns about injury.	Explore the patient's fears and anxiety. Encourage the patient to talk about the loss. Express concern but not pity. Request services of mental health or spiritual counselor if the patient desires. Include family in care, and explore their needs as well.
Ineffective individual coping related to overwhelming injury.	The patient will demonstrate realistic goal setting and express intent to participate in rehabilitation program.	Explain the importance of proper stump care in preparing for rehabilitation. Consult social worker to assist patient in obtaining rehabilitation services.
Body image disturbance related to loss of body part.	The patient will express feelings about loss of the hand and will consider strategies to improve function and appearance.	Gradually encourage the patient to take more responsibility for care of the stump. Counsel family members to demonstrate acceptance of the injury and not to promote excessive dependence. Discuss ways to conceal the loss if the patient desires. Facilitate meeting with prosthetist to discuss cosmetic and functional options.
Knowledge deficit of therapy, self-care.	The patient will verbalize personal role in recovery and rehabilitation.	Teach the patient to care for the stump and any prosthesis: 1. Wash stump with soap and water daily, rinse, and dry. 2. Inspect stump daily for irritation, redness, edema. 3. Keep prosthetic socket and stump sock clean and dry. 4. Do not apply lotions, powders, or creams except as prescribed by the physician. 5. If stump is red or irritated, temporarily remove the prosthesis and see the physician. 6. Prosthesis will require periodic adjustments.

his or her illness and its implications. The patient's ability to understand the treatment and care will allow him or her to participate and comply more readily. This in turn will allow a more timely recovery.

NURSING DIAGNOSIS. On the basis of information gathered from interviewing and assessing the preoperative patient, a number of nursing diagnoses can be generated. Common diagnoses include the following:

- **Anxiety** related to anticipated change in body image, anticipated change in function
- **Anticipatory Grieving** related to expected loss of body part and function
- **Knowledge Deficit** of surgical routines, postoperative course, rehabilitation

GOALS. Although a large number of potential goals can be established for the patient preoperatively, those related to the identified diagnoses are decreased anxiety, patient's expression of feelings about impending loss of body part, and patient's knowledge of routines and procedures, including identification of potential outcomes.

INTERVENTIONS

Anxiety. Emotional support is important throughout all phases of care of the patient with an amputation. The patient needs time to prepare psychologically and emotionally for the surgery. The nurse encourages the patient to express thoughts and concerns about the impending amputation. The nurse accepts the patient's responses. The patient is allowed to express anger or to cry without being judged or given false reassurances.

Anticipatory Grieving. The nurse recognizes that the loss of a limb or part of a limb as well as the loss of functional abilities is stressful. Most patients experience a period of grief and mourn over this loss. Grief experienced before the loss actually occurs is called anticipatory grief. The patient may be concerned about altered physical appearance as well as loss of function. The nurse explores the patient's expectations and fears about these changes. The patient is gently encouraged to focus on what he or she will be able to do despite physical limitations. Allowing patients to grieve is an important part of their recovery and rehabilitation. Nursing care of the grieving patient is discussed in Chapter 22.

Knowledge Deficit. The nurse provides and reinforces information that the patient receives regarding the reason for the amputation, prosthetic devices, and rehabilitation. The nurse also ensures that the patient understands that he or she may experience phantom limb sensations. This is a common experience for amputees in which sensations are perceived in the limb that has been removed. Patients need to be aware of this so that they will not be fearful or distressed if phantom sensations occur after surgery. Some patients experience these sensations for months to years after surgery, and others have them for the rest of their lives.

In some situations, the surgeon who performs the amputation may request a preoperative visit by a prosthetist. A prosthetist creates and supervises the use of a prosthesis. He or she explains the type of device to be used as well as the process of fitting the patient and providing instructions on its use.

Exercises are another important part of the preoperative phase. Either a physical therapist or a nurse works with the patient to teach some basic exercises to increase overall strength. Upper body training for a patient with a lower extremity amputation is important because he or she will need to use the arms to assist with transfers and to use crutches more easily in the early postoperative phase. The nurse also demonstrates the use of transfer techniques such as moving from bed to chair and encourages the patient to practice crutch walking.

EVALUATION. Criteria for successful nursing interventions are patient's statement of reduced anxiety, calm demeanor; patient's verbalization of feelings about loss; and patient's description of routines, procedures, and expected outcomes.

Postoperative Nursing Care

The postoperative phase begins immediately after the surgical amputation and includes immediate postoperative care as well as planning for the long-term rehabilitation that is necessary for these patients.

Priorities for the postoperative patient are based on three distinct needs. First, the patient needs to remain as pain free as possible, especially during the immediate postoperative period. Second, mobility needs to be maintained by learning to ambulate as soon as possible after surgery. This will be an especially big challenge for lower extremity amputees. Third, he or she needs to remain free from the many potential complications that can occur in amputees. The most common postoperative problems for patients with amputations are hemorrhage, edema, infection, and pain.

ASSESSMENT. Vital signs are assessed frequently in the first 48 hours postoperatively to detect early signs of problems. The dressing also is assessed frequently for any oozing. Some nurses try to monitor the amount of oozing by marking the stained area on the dressing with a pen, although this is a very rough assessment of bleeding. Sometimes the dressing is dry, but blood is draining around the dressing and under the patient. If a drain receptacle is present, the color and amount of the drainage is noted. The drainage should gradually decrease in amount and lighten in color. The patient's temperature is assessed for elevations that may indicate infection. The nurse also notes any foul or unpleasant odor from the stump dressing. After the dressing is removed, the stump is inspected for edema. The nurse also assesses the patient's pain, including type, location, and severity. Other aspects of postoperative assessment are detailed in Chapter 14.

NURSING DIAGNOSIS. The nursing diagnoses most commonly associated with amputation in the postoperative period include the following:

- **Decreased Cardiac Output** related to blood loss
- **Pain** related to surgical incision, scar formation on severed nerve
- **High Risk for Infection** related to surgical wound
- **Impaired Skin Integrity** related to presence of incision, advanced age, decreased mobility
- **Sensory Perceptual Alteration** related to phantom limb sensations
- **High Risk for Injury** related to loss of a limb or part of a limb, weakness, debilitation
- **Impaired Physical Mobility** related to loss of a limb or part of a limb
- **Activity Intolerance** related to prolonged bedrest, weakness
- **Self-Care Deficit** related to loss of limb or part of a limb, inability to carry out activities of daily living
- **Anxiety** or **Fear** related to perceived threat of disability, death
- **Ineffective Individual Coping** related to inadequate support system, use of inappropriate coping mechanisms
- **Body Image Disturbance** related to loss of a body part

- **Knowledge Deficit** of postoperative procedures and therapy

GOALS. Postoperative goals following an amputation are normal blood volume, reduced pain, absence of infection, well-healed wound, patient's understanding of phantom limb sensation, freedom from falls or injuries, restored mobility, improved activity tolerance, improved self-care, reduced anxiety, effective coping, improved body image, and patient's knowledge of procedures and therapies.

INTERVENTIONS

Decreased Cardiac Output. Hemorrhage is the greatest danger in the postoperative period. Hemorrhage may be detected by observations of excessive bleeding or by detection of changes in vital signs. Vital signs should be checked frequently. Restlessness and increasing pulse and respiratory rates may be early signs of hemorrhage. Hypotension and cyanosis are late signs.

A portable wound suction system, such as a Hemovac or a Jackson-Pratt drain, may be placed to collect drainage. The dressing and the bed linens under the patient are checked. Bright red bleeding, either from the drains or the dressing itself, is *not* normal. If this is observed, the nurse applies a pressure dressing over the existing dressing, elevates the extremity (also called a stump), and notifies the surgeon immediately. A large blood pressure cuff may be placed at the bedside for emergency use as a tourniquet.

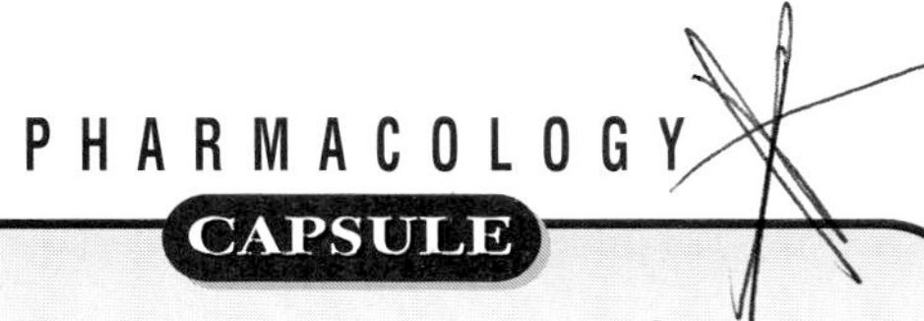

Watch for bleeding when patients are taking anticoagulants.

Pain. Postoperatively, the patient has incisional pain that is treated with prescribed pain medications, usually narcotic analgesics. Sometimes a sympathectomy is done during the amputation to prevent pain. A second source of pain may be a neuroma, which is a scar formation on a severed nerve. These can cause a great deal of sharp, severe pain and require excision by the surgeon. The nurse assesses the effects of analgesics and notifies the physician if pain relief is not achieved. Pain management is discussed in detail in Chapter 16.

High Risk for Infection. Aseptic techniques when handling the stump, the dressing, and the drains help reduce the risk of infection. The nurse monitors for signs and symptoms of infection. The incision should be dry, intact, and only slightly red. Infection is suspected if a foul or unpleasant odor comes from the stump dressing, if the patient has a sudden temperature elevation, or if the stump is red, excessively warm, or edematous. Laboratory results also may detect an elevated white blood cell count. Treatment for infection may include antibiotics, hot packs, and incision and drainage of the infected stump. In severe cases, the infection may cause further tissue damage and require reamputation at a higher level.

Impaired Skin Integrity. The care of the stump depends on the overall condition of the patient and the type of prosthesis. If the amputation is closed, there is some type of compression dressing with elastic bandages and, in some cases, a plaster cast. The stump is bandaged to promote healing and to shrink and shape the stump to a tapered, round, smooth end that will fit the prosthesis. The bandage should be wrapped smoothly with even, moderate tension to all parts of the stump. The stump can be rewrapped as needed to maintain pressure. It is very important to avoid a tourniquet-like effect caused by pulling the bandage too tightly or unevenly. Figure 39–3 illustrates the correct bandaging of a stump.

The stump is inspected frequently for irritation and edema. Edema in the stump is most common during the first 24 hours postoperatively. To minimize this, a heavy cast or pressure dressing is applied in surgery. The stump should be elevated by raising the foot of the bed. Pillows can be placed under a below-knee amputation, although continuous use of pillows is discouraged because it can cause contractures of hip. For the same reason, the patient is positioned in low Fowler's rather than high Fowler's position. If ordered, ice bags can be applied to the stump. When using ice, it should be for brief periods of time to prevent the risk of cold injuries.

After the fifth to seventh postoperative day, the stump can be massaged to promote circulation.

Sensory Perceptual Alteration. As mentioned earlier, phantom limb sensation is common. It tends to lessen with activity, weight bearing, and exercise. Phantom limb pain, however, is uncommon. It is often described as a burning, stinging, or crushing pain. If the patient reports such pain, the nurse should notify the surgeon. Treatment for this type of pain may include whirlpool, massage, injection of the stump with an anesthetic, or transcutaneous electric nerve stimulation (or TENS). A properly fitting dressing helps some patients.

High Risk for Injury. The patient must learn to function without the amputated limb. He or she must also learn to compensate for the lost extremity in unexpected ways such as maintaining balance in sitting and standing positions. After lower extremity amputation, safe mobility is a priority. The nurse reinforces proper use of assistive devices (crutches, walkers) as taught by the physical therapist. The nurse also encourages and assists the patient to do exercises to strengthen remaining limbs. The environment is kept free of clutter to prevent tripping. Patients with upper limb amputations must learn adaptations to perform activities of daily living. Everyday activities such as cooking may result in injury. The occupational therapist helps the patient learn to perform these tasks safely.

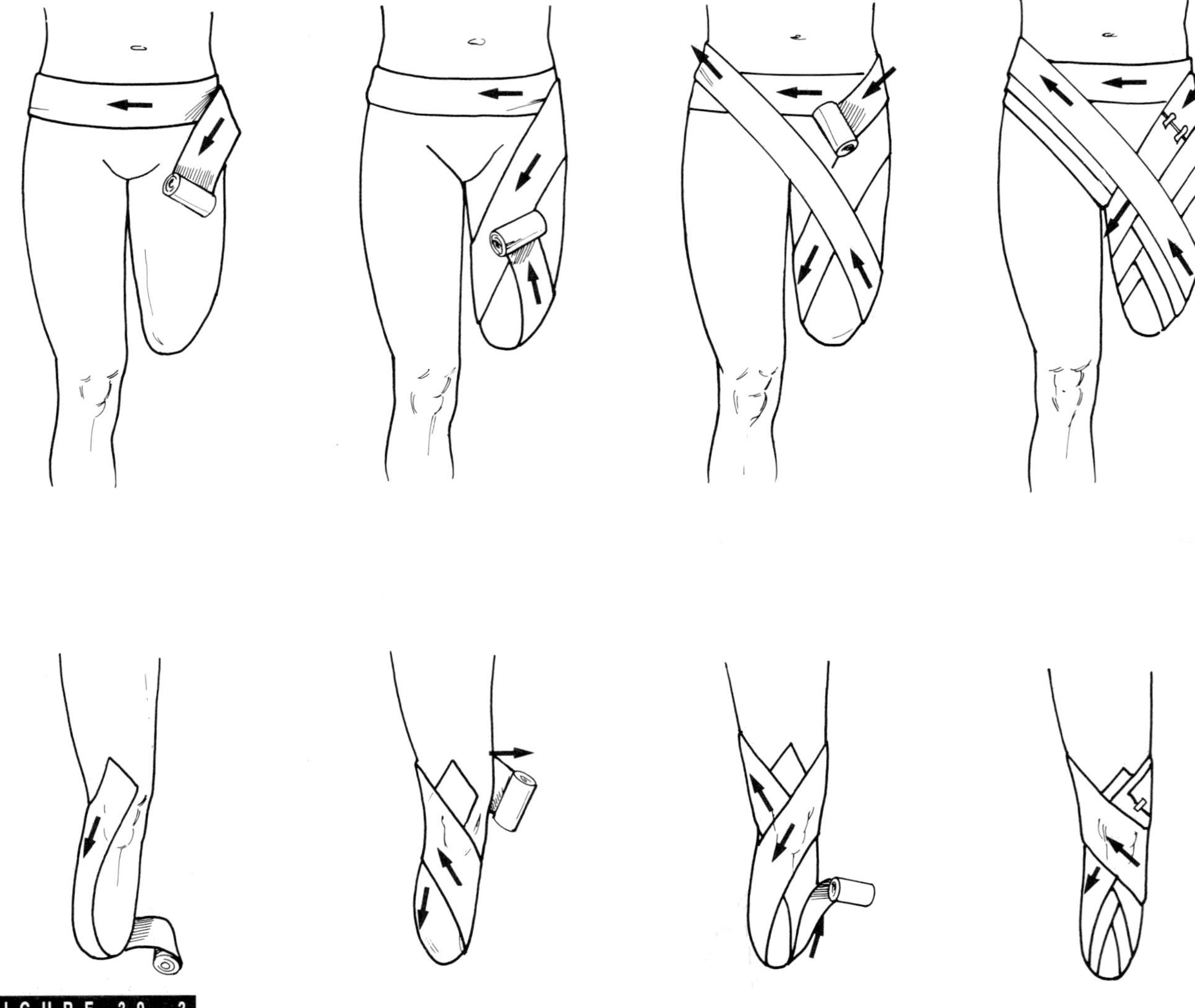

FIGURE 39-3
The proper technique for wrapping a lower extremity stump.

Impaired Physical Mobility. An exercise program is usually initiated by a physical therapist. An important goal is the prevention of contractures. These are most common in the knee, hip, and elbow. The patient may be instructed to lie prone (if tolerable) with the head turned away from the affected side for 30 minutes three or four times a day. Traction, trochanter rolls, and a firm mattress may keep the body in alignment while the patient is in bed. An overbed trapeze may be ordered for patients with lower extremity amputations to facilitate moving back and forth between the bed and the chair. Prolonged abduction of the hip (as when propped on a pillow) should be avoided. Prolonged sitting can lead to hip and knee contractures. Active and passive range of motion exercises also are an important part of maintaining mobility and preventing debilitation.

The patient may have either an immediate or a delayed prosthetic fitting, depending on the individual. An immediate fitting allows the patient to become accustomed to weight bearing, ambulation, and balance shortly after surgery. A delayed fitting is usually performed in above-knee amputations, bilateral extremity amputations, or cases of infection in which an open amputation has been performed. The appropriate time frame for a prosthesis in these situations depends on the healing of the stump and the overall condition of the patient. A general goal for weight bearing of a lower extremity amputation is about 3 months. When the stump has healed satisfactorily, the patient is fitted for a prosthesis. A suitable choice for a prosthesis is based on the site of the amputation and the age, intelligence, health, motivation, occupation, and financial status of the patient.

Activity Intolerance. The effects of surgery and bedrest may adversely affect the patient's tolerance for any type of sustained activity. It is extremely important for the nurse to plan care in order to avoid too much patient exertion. Encouraging the patient to resume his or her preoperative level of activity too soon can impair physical and psychological healing. A typical activity order is for the patient to be assisted out of bed two or three times on the first postoperative day for 1 hour at a time. Over the next few days, the patient with a lower extremity amputation is usually encouraged to remain out of bed for longer periods and to begin to practice ambulation gradually. This may initially involve only a few steps, but these will gradually be increased over time. The patient's level of activity and the rate at which he or she regains endurance depend on many individual factors.

Self-Care Deficits. During the immediate postoperative period, the nurse assists the patient to perform activities of daily living as needed. Gradually, the patient is guided to adapt to the lost limb and encouraged to become more independent. Patients feel less helpless when they regain the abilities to provide self-care.

Anxiety, Fear, and Ineffective Individual Coping. The nurse provides opportunities for patients to talk about their concerns. It may be helpful to explore how the patient's usual coping strategies can be employed in this situation. Effective coping strategies are encouraged and supported. The nurse identifies inappropriate behaviors and attempts to help the patient find alternatives. Referral to a local amputee support group may be helpful.

As mentioned earlier, it is important to expect the patient to experience a grieving process, especially if the amputation is traumatic.

Body Image Disturbance. The patient may have difficulty looking at and caring for the affected extremity. It takes time for the patient to incorporate the change into his or her body image. The nurse encourages the patient to talk about the change and what effects it will have. The nurse and therapist emphasize ways to adapt to the loss and, if the patient wishes, to conceal it. The patient is gradually encouraged to participate more in care of the stump. Family and friends are counseled to support the patient and not to encourage excessive dependence.

Knowledge Deficit. Patient instruction for stump care is extremely important. Teaching includes the following information:

1. Wash the stump with soap and water every night. Rinse and dry skin thoroughly. Use a mirror to observe the entire stump and especially the incision. Check for irritation, redness, and edema. Expose the stump to air when possible.
2. The prosthetic socket (the opening in which the stump is seated) and the stump sock must both be kept clean. Stump socks should be hand washed, rinsed well, and dried flat. A clean sock should be used every day. It is a good idea to have several socks so that there is time for the socks to dry between washings. A mended sock should not be worn because a seam is irritating and creates pressure.
3. Avoid wearing shoes with uneven heels because it will change the weight distribution of the stump. This can lead to irritation and possible skin breakdown.
4. Do not use lotions, ointments, or powders unless prescribed by the physician.
5. Discontinue use of the prosthesis if redness or irritation develops on the stump. Have the area checked before resuming use of the prosthesis.
6. The stump may shrink in size for up to 2 years after surgery. This will require some adjustment of the prosthesis. Annual visits to the prosthetist are recommended. (More frequent adjustments are necessary for children as their stump grows in size with them.)
7. The prosthesis also requires special care. Each day, wipe the inside of the socket with a damp, soapy cloth, then remove the soap with a clean, damp cloth. Dry the socket thoroughly.
8. Consult a prosthetist if there are any problems with the prosthesis. Do not attempt to make adjustments yourself.

EVALUATION. In order to ensure that patients are reaching their goals, the nurse needs to evaluate their progress on a frequent basis. In this way, the nurse can determine whether interventions are appropriate for the specific patient or require some revision. Criteria for successful nursing interventions are normal pulse and blood pressure; patient's statement of pain relief, relaxed expression; absence of fever, purulent drainage, redness; well-healed incision; patient's verbalization of understanding of phantom limb sensation; freedom from bruises or fractures associated with injury; return to maximum mobility; performance of activities of daily living without fatigue; resumption of independent self-care; patient's statement of reduced anxiety and calm demeanor; patient's caring for stump without distress; and patient's demonstration of stump care and rehabilitation exercises.

THE ELDERLY AMPUTEE

The elderly patient with an amputation may have some additional needs that should be taken into consideration when planning and providing care. For example, when constructing a teaching plan for the elderly, it should be kept in mind that the healthy older person is completely capable of learning but often requires smaller units of information, more repetition, and more time. The nurse should skip unnecessary details and make sure that during the teaching process patients with glasses or hearing aids have them in place.

It is also important to clearly explain phantom sensations to the elderly. Some may not wish to report phantom sensations or phantom pain for fear of seeming foolish. By reminding the elderly patient that phantom sensations are not uncommon or bizarre, the nurse can eliminate fear or anxiety that these sensations can cause.

Many elderly have one or more chronic health problems. This factor should be taken into account in choosing a prosthetic device. A patient with diabetes, for example, is prone to circulation problems and poor wound healing and may require a prosthesis with extra padding or support. Poor vision and decreased sensation may keep the older person from recognizing complications.

Because many elderly have decreased appetites, their nutritional status may be poor. Emphasizing higher calorie and higher protein intake is essential to prevent problems and to maintain strength.

It is important when providing psychosocial support to remember that the loss of a limb or part of a limb can be especially difficult in the elderly. This is because many elderly have had to deal with other losses in their lives, such as loss of loved ones, loss of independence, and loss of income associated with retirement. Older people may lack confidence that they can adapt and gain strength.

If the patient is unable to participate fully in his or her care, one or more family members should be instructed along with the elderly patient. Home health nursing services may be arranged to facilitate adaptation in the home setting and to monitor for complications. Empathy, patience, and respect are essential in approaching elderly patients.

REPLANTATION

In some amputation injuries, a type of surgical technique called replantation may be performed. This generally involves the use of a microscope and highly specialized instruments to reanastomose or reconnect blood vessels and nerve fibers in a severed limb. The limb is then sutured into its correct anatomic position. Recent advances in microsurgical techniques and preservation of severed limbs have made this technique increasingly successful. Replantation surgery is most likely to be performed for amputations through the hand or wrist. Amputated thumbs are reattached whenever possible because of the thumb's importance in total hand function. In a severely injured hand in which two or more fingers are detached, an attempt is made by the surgeon to restore as many fingers as possible.

INDICATIONS

A number of factors are taken into consideration by the surgeon before performing replantation surgery—for example, the type of injury and location. An attempt to reattach the hand or severed fingers is usually made owing to the functional importance of the hand. Amputations above the wrist do not lend themselves as readily to replantation because of the extensive tissue, muscle, and bone damage accompanying the injury. A large muscle mass injury involves a great amount of tissue damage. Severely traumatized tissue can become ischemic, leading to death of the tissues and loss of the replanted limb. Severe crushing injuries or avulsion injuries in which the limb is mutilated also are not appropriate for replantation. In general, the greater the muscle mass injury, the less likely that replantation is possible.

Another factor that is considered in deciding whether to attempt replantation is the length of warm or cold ischemia time.

EMERGENCY CARE

Proper handling of amputated parts is extremely important for successful replantation. Current preservation techniques include wrapping the amputated parts in a clean cloth saturated with normal saline or Ringer's lactate solution. These parts are then placed in a sealed plastic bag that is placed in ice water. Direct contact between the amputated part and the ice can lead to further tissue damage and cell death. Partially amputated parts should remain attached to the patient and also should be kept cool if possible. Extra care should be taken to avoid detaching any parts since even small connections increase the chances for successful repair.

The patient may require treatment for shock due to blood loss. This may include intravenous fluids and blood products. Blood loss from the stump may be minimized by using a clean, dry dressing, which can be reinforced as needed. Tourniquets should not be used unless absolutely necessary as they can cause ischemia of the stump.

NURSING CARE OF THE PATIENT HAVING REPLANTATION SURGERY

Preoperative Nursing Care

ASSESSMENT. General preoperative care of the replantation patient includes careful assessment of hemodynamic status, close monitoring of vital signs, and inspection of the stump (or dressing) for bleeding. Pain at the site of the injury and at other locations is assessed. Fluid intake and output are measured and recorded. The patient's emotional status is noted, and the nurse assesses understanding of the preoperative activities and postoperative routines. Sources of support are documented.

NURSING DIAGNOSIS. Nursing diagnoses for the patient facing replantation surgery may include the following:

- **Decreased Cardiac Output** related to decreased blood volume
- **Fear** related to severe injury or possible failure of replantation
- **Anxiety** related to lack of knowledge of surgical routines
- **Pain** related to tissue trauma

GOALS. Preoperative goals for the replantation patient are normal blood volume, decreased fear, decreased anxiety, and decreased pain.

INTERVENTIONS. The nurse administers intravenous fluids and blood as ordered. If the dressing becomes saturated with blood, the nurse reinforces the dressing. Continued or excessive bleeding is reported to the physician. Even though preparations for replantation are hurried, the nurse is sensitive to the patient's fear and anxiety. The patient's feelings are accepted. Brief, simple explanations are provided. Analgesics, if ordered, are administered for pain.

EVALUATION. Criteria for evaluating goal achievement are normal blood pressure, pulse, and urine output; patient's statement of decreased fear and anxiety, calmer expression; and patient's statement of pain reduction or relief, more relaxed manner.

Postoperative Nursing Care

Routine postoperative care is discussed in detail in Chapter 14. This section emphasizes the special needs of the replantation patient.

ASSESSMENT. Postoperative assessment includes monitoring vital signs, intake and output, and level of consciousness. An essential aspect of care after replantation is hourly neurovascular assessment of the replanted limb. A Doppler device or pulse oximeter may be used to evaluate circulation. A baseline documentation of circulatory status is obtained on arrival to the unit. These include color, capillary refill, turgor, temperature, and sensation. Signs of arterial occlusion are pale or blue color, slow capillary refill, shriveled appearance, and coolness. Signs of venous congestion are cyanosis, rapid capillary refill, edema, and warmth. The nurse also assesses the limb for edema because massive edema often accompanies replantation.

NURSING DIAGNOSIS. Nursing diagnoses for the replantation patient may include the following:

- **Altered Tissue Perfusion** related to trauma, edema, compensatory vasoconstriction
- **Pain** related to tissue trauma
- **Body Image Disturbance** related to disfigurement, loss of function
- **Knowledge Deficit** of therapeutic measures and self-care

GOALS. Nursing goals after replantation are adequate circulation in replanted limb, pain relief, improved body image, and patient's knowledge of therapeutic measures and self-care.

INTERVENTIONS. Measures to promote circulation to the replanted limb include elevation of the limb and "microvascular precautions." Elevation of the limb promotes venous and lymphatic drainage. Care is taken not to elevate the limb above the level of the heart as this may impair arterial flow. Several soft pillows or a stockinette connected to an intravenous pole may help to achieve this. Microvascular precautions include avoidance of any substances or conditions that contribute to blood vessel spasm or constriction. The patient is encouraged to abstain from nicotine and caffeine-containing products for 7 to 10 days postoperatively. A strict ban on cigarette smoking should be enforced. In addition, room temperature is maintained at 80°F to prevent compensatory vasoconstriction of the peripheral tissues in response to cold. Tight or restrictive gowns or pajamas also are discouraged. The nurse explains the importance of these measures to the patient and family.

The physician may order intravenous low molecular weight dextran (dextran 40), aspirin, or heparin to reduce the risk of thrombosis. The nurse administers the drugs as ordered and monitors for adverse effects.

Inadequate arterial blood flow is a medical emergency. The surgeon is notified immediately, and the patient is prepared for a return to surgery. In some facilities, venous congestion is treated with leeches. Leeches are attached to a selected area of the replanted limb. The saliva of these worms contains an anticoagulant, a local vasodilator, and a local anesthetic. The leech extracts excess blood, reducing venous congestion.

The nurse provides the patient an opportunity to discuss thoughts and feelings about the replantation, disfigurement, and loss of function. It may take a while before the patient is able to look at and touch the replanted limb. The nurse supports the patient and demonstrates acceptance of him or her. The nurse's comfort with handling the limb can help the patient feel accepted. The rehabilitation team works with the patient to restore maximum possible function.

If the replantation is not successful, the limb is surgically removed. This represents a significant loss to the patient. The nurse must recognize this loss and support the patient.

Other essential aspects of care include routine postoperative measures such as frequent position changes, pulmonary toilet, and pain management.

EVALUATION. Criteria for evaluating achievement of goals are presence of warmth, normal skin color, and

NUTRITION CONCEPTS

- A nutritional assessment should be made preoperatively for patients undergoing surgical amputation, especially in older, immobilized, or chronic alcoholic patients.
- Patients undergoing surgical amputation should be well hydrated; intravenous fluids may be given if oral fluids are not tolerated.
- Surgical amputation is accompanied by a stress response, resulting in an increased need for calories and protein for healing.
- Dietary supplements such as Sustacal or Ensure may be needed for patients whose intake of regular foods is inadequate for healing.
- Patients are encouraged to become mobile as soon as possible after an amputation to prevent loss of calcium and protein.
- Dietary choices high in protein, zinc, and vitamin C promote wound healing.

arterial pulses in the replanted limb; patient's statement of pain relief; patient's statements reflecting acceptance of altered appearance or function; and patient's verbalization of microvascular precautions.

BIBLIOGRAPHY

Jarvis, C. (1992). *Physical examination and health assessment.* Philadelphia: W. B. Saunders.

Mulvey, M. A., & Sharma, P. K. (1991). Traumatic amputation. *RN, 54*(9), 26–30.

Nicholas, J. J., Robinson, L. R., Schulz, R., Blair, C., Aliota, R., & Hairston, G. (1993). Problems experienced and perceived by prosthetic patients. *Journal of Prosthetics and Orthotics, 5*(1), 36–39.

Nissen, S. J., & Newman, W. P. (1992). Factors influencing reintegration to normal living after amputation. *Archives of Physical Medicine and Rehabilitation, 73*(6), 548–551.

Rounsaville, C. (1992). Phantom limb pain: The ghost that haunts the amputee. *Orthopedic Nursing, 11*(2), 67–71.

Ruda, S. C. (1992). Nursing role of management: Musculoskeletal problems. In S. C. Lewis & I. C. Collier (Eds.), *Medical-surgical nursing: Assessment and management of clinical problems* (3rd ed.). St. Louis: Mosby Year Book.

Rybarczyk, B. D., Nyenhyuis, D. L., Nicholas, J. J., Schulz, R., Alioto, R. J., & Blair, C. (1992). Social discomfort and depression in a sample of adults with leg amputations. *Archives of Physical Medicine and Rehabilitation 73*(12), 1169–1173.

Shlafer, M. (1993). *The nurse, pharmacology, and drug therapy* (2nd ed.). Redwood City, CA: Addison-Wesley.

Strangio, L. (1991). Leeches: When bleeding is exactly what you want. *RN, 54*(9), 31–33.

Wainwright, S. T., & Bacon, E. S. (1993). Traumatic amputation. *Nursing 93, 23*(10), 33.

Williamson, V. C. (1992). Amputation of the lower extremity: An overview. *Orthopedic Nursing, 11*(2), 55–65.

KEY CONCEPTS

1. Amputation is the surgical removal of body limbs or parts of limbs.
2. Conditions or situations that can lead to an amputation include trauma, disease, tumors, and congenital problems.
3. The medical management of patients who have amputations involves the appropriate treatment and control of underlying diseases such as diabetes mellitus and peripheral vascular disease.
4. Complications of amputation include hemorrhage, hematoma, necrosis, wound dehiscence, gangrene, edema, contracture, pain, and infection.
5. Preoperatively, the patient needs to prepare physically and psychologically for an impending amputation.
6. Postoperative nursing care focuses on decreased cardiac output, pain, high risk for infection, impaired skin integrity, sensory-perceptual alterations, high risk for injury, impaired physical mobility, activity intolerance, self-care deficit, anxiety or fear, ineffective individual coping, body image disturbance, and knowledge deficit.
7. In some amputation injuries, replantation (reattachment) may be possible.
8. To preserve a body part for possible replantation, the part should be wrapped in a clean cloth saturated with normal saline or Ringer's lactate solution and placed in a sealed plastic bag that is immersed in ice water.
9. Nursing care of the replantation patient addresses altered tissue perfusion, pain, body image disturbance, and knowledge deficit.

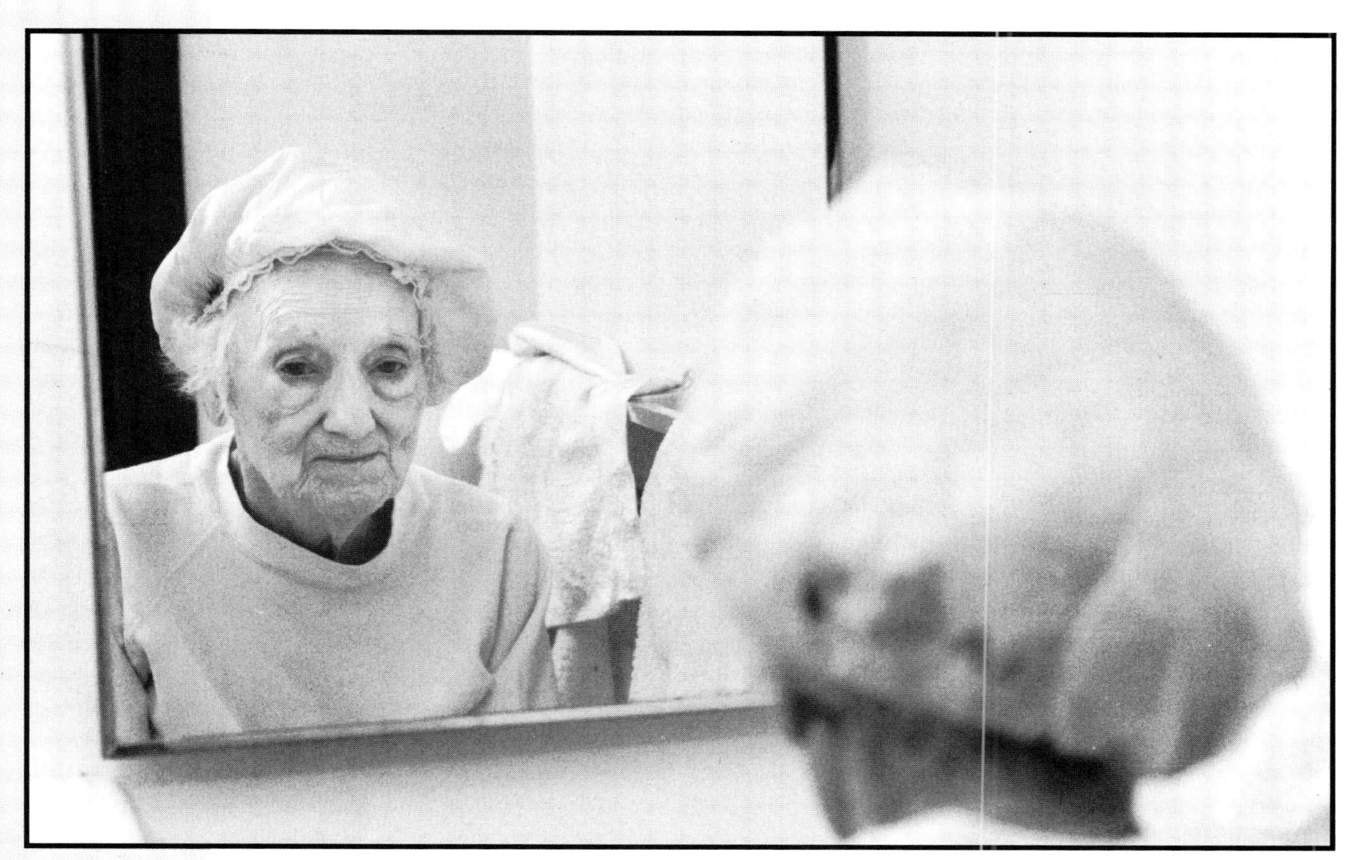

UNIT 12
Endocrine Disorders

Adrianne Linton

CHAPTER 40

Thyroid and Parathyroid Disorders

OBJECTIVES

1. Identify nursing assessment data related to the functions of the thyroid and parathyroid glands.
2. Describe tests and procedures used to diagnose disorders of the thyroid and parathyroid glands and identify nursing responsibilities relevant for each.
3. Describe the pathophysiology, signs and symptoms, complications, and treatment of hyperthyroidism, hypothyroidism, hyperparathyroidism, and hypoparathyroidism.
4. Develop nursing care plans for patients with disorders of the thyroid or parathyroid glands, including assessment, nursing diagnoses, goals, interventions, and evaluation criteria.

GLOSSARY

CHVOSTEK'S SIGN Spasm of the facial muscles when the facial nerve is tapped; indicative of hypocalcemia

CRETINISM Permanent mental and physical retardation caused by congenital deficiency of thyroid hormones

EXOPHTHALMOS Protrusion of the eyeballs associated with hyperthyroidism

GOITER Enlargement of the thyroid gland, causing the neck to appear swollen

GOITROGEN Substance that suppresses thyroid function

LARYNGOSPASM Spasmodic closure of the larynx

MYXEDEMA Facial edema that develops with severe, long-term hypothyroidism; sometimes used as a synonym for hypothyroidism

NODULE Small mass of tissue that can be palpated

PAROTIDITIS Inflammation of the parotid (salivary) gland; most commonly called parotitis

TETANY Steady muscle contraction; caused by hypocalcemia

THYROIDITIS Inflammation of the thyroid gland

Glossary continued

THYROTOXICOSIS Excessive metabolic stimulation caused by elevated thyroid hormone level

TROUSSEAU'S SIGN Carpopedal spasm following compression of the nerves in the upper arm; a sign of hypocalcemia

THE THYROID GLAND

ANATOMY AND PHYSIOLOGY OF THE THYROID GLAND

The thyroid gland is located in the lower portion of the anterior side of the neck. It consists of two lobes that are slightly to either side of the trachea and connected in front of the trachea by a narrow bridge of tissue called the isthmus (Fig. 40–1).

The thyroid gland plays a major role in regulating the body's rate of metabolism and growth and development. When the metabolic rate falls, the hypothalamus stimulates the pituitary gland to secrete thyroid-stimulating hormone (TSH). This hormone in turn stimulates the thyroid gland to secrete hormones that affect the production and use of energy.

The hormones produced by the thyroid gland are thyroid hormone, triiodothyronine, and calcitonin. Each of these is known by several names. Thyroid hormone is also called thyroxine, tetraiodothyronine, or T_4. Triiodothyronine is referred to as T_3. Both thyroxine and triiodothyronine increase the body's metabolic rate. Calcitonin, or thyrocalcitonin, plays a role in regulating the serum calcium level. It is secreted when serum calcium levels are high to limit the shift of calcium from the bones into the blood.

AGE-RELATED CHANGES IN THYROID FUNCTION

With age, there is an increase in nodules and small, firm goiters. Levels of T_4 remain about the same in the healthy older person, but levels of T_3 more often decline. Thyroid conditions are often overlooked in the elderly because signs and symptoms may be subtle and attributed to the aging process.

NURSING ASSESSMENT OF THE THYROID GLAND

Thyroid disorders may escape detection until they are rather severe because the symptoms are often vague. Periodic assessment of the patient with a thyroid disorder is necessary to evaluate the response to treatment.

HEALTH HISTORY

The health history is taken to obtain a thorough description of the patient's reason for seeking medical care and to elicit other data that may be related to the immediate problem. Information about the patient's energy level is important in assessing thyroid function since fatigue may be found with hypothyroidism or hyperthyroidism. The nurse asks if the patient is aware of any changes in sleep patterns, personality, mental function, or emotional state. Because thyroid hormones affect the metabolic rate, patients may have unexplained weight changes. In the review of systems, the nurse assesses menstrual cycles in women, changes in sexual function, hydration (thirst, changes in urine output, tissue turgor, moisture of mucous membranes), bowel elimination pattern, and tolerance of heat and cold.

PHYSICAL EXAMINATION

The nurse begins the physical examination by taking the patient's vital signs and measuring height and weight. Vital signs are important because they reflect the metabolic rate. Thyroid disorders may cause increases or decreases in pulse, respirations, blood pressure, and temperature and irregular heart rhythms. The

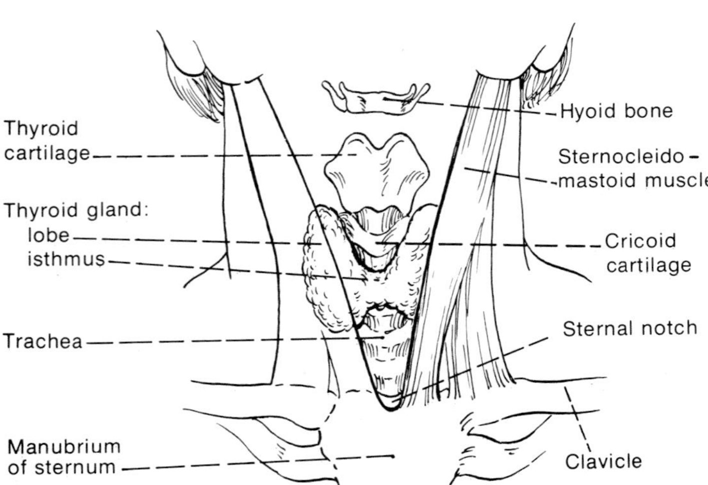

FIGURE 40-1

The thyroid gland. (From Black, J. M., & Matassarin-Jacobs, E. [1993]. *Luckmann and Sorensen's medical-surgical nursing: A psychophysiologic approach* [4th ed., p. 1764]. Philadelphia: W. B. Saunders.)

TABLE 40-1
ASSESSMENT OF THE PATIENT WITH A THYROID DISORDER

HEALTH HISTORY
Present illness: Fatigue, weight changes, mental-emotional changes
Past medical history: Recent surgery or trauma, radiation of the head or neck, recent and current medications, history of thyroid or renal disorders
Review of systems: Fatigue, changes in hair or skin, voice changes, palpitations, edema, constipation or diarrhea, polyuria, nervousness, weight loss, temperature intolerance, excessive perspiration, changes in libido or sexual performance
Functional assessment: Sleep disturbances, usual dietary intake, anorexia, ability to cope with stress

PHYSICAL EXAMINATION
Vital signs: Abnormal heart rate and rhythm, blood pressure changes, tachypnea
Height and weight
Skin: Changes in moisture, temperature, and texture
Hair: Changes in texture
Eyes: Exophthalmos
Neck: Enlargement
Hands: Tremor

nurse inspects and palpates the skin for moisture, temperature, and texture. In the head and neck examination, the hair texture should be noted. The eyes are examined for exophthalmos (bulging). The neck is inspected for enlargement typical of goiter. The hands are observed for tremor. Nurses with advanced physical examination skills may palpate the neck for thyroid enlargement or nodules.

Key components of the nursing assessment of the patient with a thyroid disorder are outlined in Table 40–1.

DIAGNOSTIC TESTS AND PROCEDURES

Diagnostic studies of the thyroid gland include laboratory blood tests and studies employing radioactive iodine. Table 40–2 summarizes the use of each test and identifies nursing implications.

The most useful tests of thyroid function are measurements of serum T_3, T_4, and TSH. These tests re-

TABLE 40-2
DIAGNOSTIC TESTS AND PROCEDURES FOR THYROID DISORDERS

TEST/STUDY	PURPOSE/PROCEDURE	PATIENT PREPARATION AND POSTPROCEDURE CARE
Serum T_3 (triiodothyronine) Serum T_4 (thyroxine)	Serum T_3 and T_4 measurements detect abnormal levels of thyroid hormones. Elevated T_3 seen with Graves' disease, toxic adenoma, and toxic nodular goiter. T_4 elevated with hyperthyroidism or excessive thyroid hormone replacement. T_3 and T_4 decreased with hypothyroidism.	No preparation except to explain need for venipuncture. Medications may be withheld before blood is drawn. After blood sample is drawn, assess for oozing. Apply small dressing.
Serum TSH (thyroid stimulating hormone)	Detects increases seen with hypothyroidism and decreases seen with hyperthyroidism.	Tell patient a blood sample will be drawn. After venipuncture, assess for oozing. Apply small dressing.
Radioactive iodine uptake test	Radioactive iodine is given orally. After specified time, an instrument (scintillator) is used to measure amount of ^{131}I taken up by thyroid gland. Uptake is high with hyperthyroidism; low with hypothyroidism. The procedure is painless.	Patient should be asked about pregnancy, in which case radiation is contraindicated. Advise patient that radiation dose is small and will not harm others. Tell patient what to expect. For 24 hours after test, patient should wash hands with soap and water after voiding. If caregiver discards urine, gloves should be worn. Afterward, gloves should be washed, removed, and the bare hands washed. Pregnant caregivers should avoid patient contact for 24 hours.
Thyroid scan	^{131}I or ^{123}I is given orally. After specified time, a scanner is used to detect pattern of uptake by thyroid gland. Can help determine whether nodules are benign or malignant and detect other abnormalities.	Tell patient what to expect: If ^{131}I is used, patient will be given isotope in liquid form and will return to radiology 24 hr later for scan. With ^{123}I, scan is done after 3–6 hr. During scan, patient will have to lie still on back for ~20 min. For 1 week before test, patient should not consume iodine. Iodine is in radiographic dyes, some oral contraceptives, weight-control drugs, multivitamins, all thyroid drugs, and some food, especially seafood. Postprocedure care same as for radioactive iodine uptake test.
TRH (thyroid releasing hormone) stimulation test	Assesses the response of the pituitary to TRH. Helps differentiate types of hypothyroidism. TRH normally increases after TRH given intravenously. Several blood samples must be drawn.	Tell patient that a drug will be given intravenously, then several blood samples will be drawn. Assess venipuncture site for oozing. Apply small bandage.

quire no special preparation. An overnight fast is advised before blood is drawn to measure calcitonin. The thyroid-releasing hormone (TRH) stimulation test measures the blood level of TSH after administration of TRH. This test shows whether thyroid hormone abnormalities are caused by a disorder of the thyroid gland itself or by altered production of stimulating hormones by the hypothalamus or the pituitary.

The thyroid gland uses iodine to manufacture hormones. Therefore, radioactive iodine (^{131}I or ^{123}I) is useful for diagnostic purposes because it concentrates in the thyroid. The amount of iodine taken up by the thyroid is measured to assess the activity level of the gland.

Following the patient's ingestion of radioactive iodine, a specialized instrument called a scintillator is used to scan the area of the thyroid gland. It creates a picture of the gland based on the distribution of the iodine. The picture aids in diagnosing cancer because the patterns of iodine concentration in normal and malignant tissue are different. Since a low dose of radiation is used for diagnostic purposes, the patient poses no danger to others.

DISORDERS OF THE THYROID GLAND

HYPERTHYROIDISM

Hyperthyroidism is abnormally increased production of thyroid hormones. Several forms of hyperthyroidism occur. The most common types are Graves' disease and multinodular goiter. The cause of Graves' disease is unknown but is thought to be a combination of genetic and environmental factors. The presence of thyroid-stimulating antibodies in the blood of people with Graves' disease suggests an autoimmune process. Graves' disease most often develops in young women. Whether the patient has treatment or not, the condition tends to have periods of remission and exacerbation. Some patients who have Graves' disease eventually develop hypothyroidism.

Multinodular goiter occurs most often in females in their fifties and sixties. It is most likely to develop in people who have had goiter for a number of years. Hyperthyroidism in this case is caused by small thyroid nodules that secrete excess thyroid hormone and cause hyperthyroidism. The nodules can be benign or malignant. Symptoms of hyperthyroidism are usually less severe with multinodular goiter than with Graves' disease.

Signs and Symptoms

The signs and symptoms of hyperthyroidism are caused by an increased metabolic rate and can range from mild to severe. Weight loss and nervousness may be the only symptoms in patients with a mild form of the disease. In more severe cases, the patient's history may reveal restlessness, irritable behavior, sleep disturbances, emotional lability, personality changes, and fatigue. Weight loss, even when eating well, is common. Many patients report poor tolerance of heat and excessive perspiration. Changes in menstrual and bowel patterns may occur. Examination findings may include fine tremors of the hands, flushed skin, exophthalmos, and swelling of the neck. Exophthalmos is more common with Graves' disease than with nodular goiter (Fig. 40–2).

Excess thyroid hormones stimulate the heart, causing tachycardia, increased systolic blood pressure, and sometimes atrial fibrillation. The heart rate may be as rapid as 160 beats per minute. Even during sleep, the pulse may remain above 80 beats per minute.

Complications

If untreated, hyperthyroidism may lead to thyrotoxicosis. Thyrotoxicosis is excessive stimulation caused by elevated thyroid hormone levels that produce dangerous tachycardia and hyperthermia. There is a risk of heart failure. The patient is restless and agitated and may lapse into a coma. Thyrotoxicosis is a medical emergency. Fortunately, modern treatment of hyperthyroidism has made this complication rare.

Medical Diagnosis

Elevated serum T_3 or T_4 measurements, or both, are generally suggestive of hyperthyroidism. Measurement

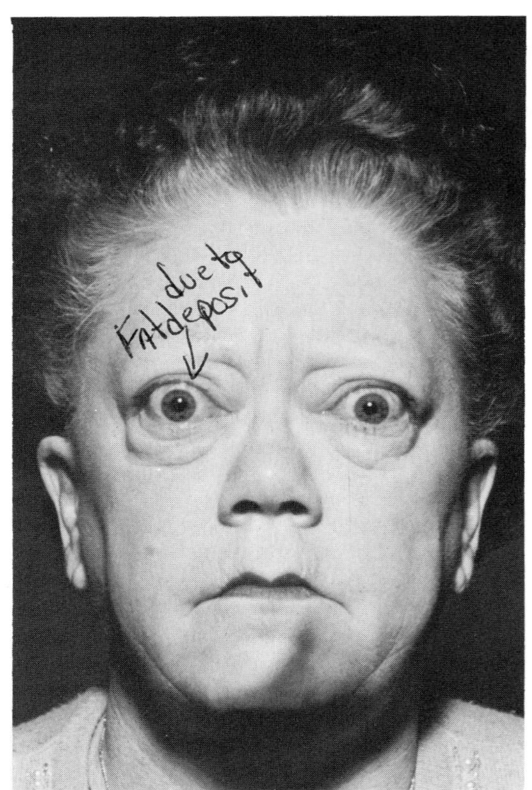

FIGURE 40–2
This patient has exophthalmos, bulging eyes, associated with Graves' disease. (From Jacob, S. W., & Francone, C. A. [1989]. *Elements of anatomy and physiology* [2nd ed., p. 151]. Philadelphia: W. B. Saunders.)

of thyroid-stimulating antibodies is useful in specifically diagnosing Graves' disease. Other laboratory tests may be done to determine whether the pituitary production of TSH is normal.

Medical Treatment

Three methods are used to treat hyperthyroidism: drug therapy, surgery, and radiation therapy. In addition, beta-adrenergic blockers like propranolol (Inderal) may be given to relieve some of the cardiovascular symptoms associated with hyperthyroidism.

DRUG THERAPY. Hyperthyroidism may be treated initially with antithyroid drugs. Antithyroid drugs block the synthesis, release, or activity of thyroid hormones. The two classes of drugs that are commonly used as antithyroid drugs are thioamides and iodides. These drugs are effective in treating hyperthyroidism, but their effects are temporary. They are often used to lower the level of hormones in the blood before surgery. This process reduces the risk of bleeding and lowers the danger of releasing large amounts of thyroid hormones into the blood stream during surgery. When a patient is on drugs that interfere with thyroxine secretion, the nurse should monitor for symptoms of hypothyroidism (cold intolerance, edema, and weight gain).

PHARMACOLOGY CAPSULE

Patients on antithyroid drugs must be monitored for hypothyroidism.

Thioamides. Examples of thioamides are propylthiouracil (PTU) and methimazole (Tapazole). It usually takes several weeks before the effects of thioamides are noticeable. The drug may be given for months or years. It is hoped that a remission will occur, allowing the drug to be discontinued. A disadvantage of thioamides is that they can cause agranulocytosis, a condition in which the production of neutrophils is suppressed. Without adequate neutrophils, the patient is unable to resist infection. Any signs of infection, such as sore throat or fever, should be reported to the physician immediately.

Iodides. Iodides are useful because iodine inhibits the production of thyroid hormones. The most popular forms used to treat hyperthyroidism are Lugol's solution (5% iodine and 10% potassium iodide) and saturated solution of potassium iodide (or SSKI). Iodides may bring some relief within 24 hours, but it takes several weeks for maximum effect. The effect does not last as long as that of thioamides.

Iodine solutions can cause discoloration of the teeth and gastric upset. These effects are minimized if the iodine solution is mixed with milk and sipped through a straw. Signs of iodine toxicity include swelling and irritation of the mucous membranes and increased salivation.

PHARMACOLOGY CAPSULE

Iodine solutions can stain the teeth! They should be mixed with milk and sipped through a straw.

RADIOACTIVE IODINE. Radioactive iodine (^{131}I) can be used alone or with antithyroid drugs to treat hyperthyroidism. It quickly accumulates in the thyroid gland, causing destruction of thyroid tissue. The resulting decrease in thyroid hormone production is not evident for several months. Meanwhile, beta-adrenergic blockers can be given to control symptoms.

The radiation dose used to treat hyperthyroidism does not pose a threat to others. It should not be used during pregnancy, however, as it will affect the thyroid gland of the fetus. Side effects of the treatment are minimal. Inflammation of the thyroid gland (thyroiditis) and the parotid glands (parotiditis) may occur. Parotiditis causes the mouth to be dry and irritated. Hypothyroidism may develop years after treatment. Drugs used to treat thyroid disorders are summarized in Table 40–3.

Surgical Treatment

Graves' disease is often treated by removing most of the thyroid gland. This procedure is called a subtotal thyroidectomy. As mentioned earlier, patients are commonly given antithyroid drug therapy for several weeks before surgery. Before these drugs were commonly used, patients often had dramatic postoperative responses due to the escape of thyroid hormones into the blood stream during surgery. This severe episode of hyperthyroidism, called thyroid storm or thyroid crisis, is potentially fatal.

Nursing Care of the Nonsurgical Patient with Hyperthyroidism

Most patients with hyperthyroidism are treated as outpatients. Therefore, the nurse in the community or clinic setting may need to help the patient learn to adapt until treatment brings relief.

ASSESSMENT. Complete assessment of the patient with a thyroid disorder is summarized in Table 40–1. For the patient with hyperthyroidism, the nursing assessment begins with assessment of relevant data, including activity tolerance, heat and cold tolerance, bowel elimination pattern, appetite, weight changes, and food intake. The nurse can also assess the patient's mental-emotional state, adaptation to the condition, and understanding of the treatment. Vital signs and height and weight are recorded.

NURSING DIAGNOSIS. Nursing diagnoses for the hyperthyroid patient may include the following:

- **Sleep Pattern Disturbance** related to metabolic imbalance
- **Hyperthermia** related to increased metabolic energy production

TABLE 40-3

DRUGS USED TO TREAT THYROID CONDITIONS

DRUG	USE/ACTION	SIDE EFFECTS	NURSING INTERVENTIONS
Thyroid hormone replacement drugs Dessicated thyroid (thyroid USP) Levothyroxine (Synthroid) Liothyronine (Cytomel) Liotrix (Euthroid)	Treat hypothyroidism and thyroiditis. Increase metabolic rate.	Overdose produces irritability, insomnia, nervousness, tachycardia, diarrhea, weight loss. Elderly patients develop toxicity more readily.	Low doses of one or more preparations given initially. Dosage gradually increased and patient maintained on one preparation. Hypothyroid patients usually require lifelong therapy. Patient teaching needed. Monitor pulse and blood pressure of elderly patients. Withhold and notify physician if pulse>100. Thyroid preparations interact with many other drugs, including digitalis, estrogen, beta blockers, hypoglycemics, and anticoagulants.
Antithyroid drugs Thioamides (methimazole [Tapazole], propylthiouracil [PTU])	Treat hyperthyroidism by interfering with formation of thyroid hormones.	Adverse reactions: agranulocytosis, rash, thrombocytopenia, skin discoloration, fever, headache, drowsiness, diarrhea, nausea, vomiting.	Avoid use during pregnancy. Monitor patient for bleeding due to decreased platelets and prothrombin, signs of liver toxicity (jaundice, abdominal pain), agranulocytosis (fever, sore throat, malaise), and hypothyroidism (weight gain, fatigue). Teach patient to report any of these signs and symptoms. Safety precautions if drowsy. Encourage patient to adhere to drug prescription and to keep follow-up appointments.
Iodides Strong iodine solution (Lugol's solution) Saturated solution of potassium iodide (SSKI)	Reduce size and vascularity of thyroid gland in hyperthyroidism. May be used alone or prior to surgery for hyperthyroidism.	Excess iodine: fever, rash, oral lesions, metallic taste. Diarrhea, parotitis, hypothyroidism.	Dilute liquids in water, fruit juice, or milk. Reduce unpleasant taste and tooth staining by using a straw. Monitor for symptoms of excess iodine. Give SSKI after meals.
Beta-adrenergic blockers Propranolol (Inderal)	Reduce tachycardia, tremor, and anxiety associated with hyperthyroidism.	Bradycardia, hypotension, decreased blood glucose, bronchial constriction.	Assess vital signs. Caution with asthmatics or diabetes mellitus patients.
Radioactive iodine Sodium iodide ^{131}I and ^{123}I	Concentrates in thyroid tissue for diagnostic scans. Higher therapeutic dose destroys thyroid tissue in hyperthyroidism and in thyroid malignancies.	Diagnostic dose: none. Therapeutic dose: nausea, vomiting.	Diagnostic dose usually requires no radiation precautions except precautions with urine for 24 hr after the test. (See Table 40–2). Therapeutic dose requires isolation measures. Monitor patient for signs of hypothyroidism (fatigue, weight gain).

- **Altered Nutrition: Less than Body Requirements** related to increased energy production
- **Decreased Cardiac Output** related to excessive thyroid hormone stimulation
- **High Risk for Injury** to the eyes related to exophthalmos
- **Diarrhea** related to excessive thyroid hormone stimulation
- **Knowledge Deficit** of hyperthyroidism and its treatment

GOALS. Goals of nursing care include lessening of fatigue, comfort in the environment, adequate intake of nutrients, normal vital signs, absence of corneal injury, formed stools, and ability to manage self-care.

INTERVENTIONS. Nursing care focuses on helping the patient cope with hyperthyroidism until the condition is corrected. The nurse monitors drug therapy and also teaches the patient about any long-term self-care.

Sleep Pattern Disturbance. Despite fatigue and weakness, the hyperthyroid patient often feels restless and has trouble sleeping. The patient's day should be arranged to allow periods of rest. Food and fluids containing caffeine should be avoided. Bedtime rituals may be helpful in preparing for sleep. A restful environment and a soothing back rub encourage relaxation. Sedatives may be ordered to promote sleep.

In addition to physical rest, patients need emotional rest. The patient and the family may be able to cope better if they understand the reason for the patient's irritability and nervousness. Patients need to recognize stressful situations and avoid them.

Hyperthermia. Owing to their high metabolic rate, hyperthyroid patients usually have some heat intolerance. They tend to feel too warm even when others are comfortable. Only light clothing may be needed. The environmental temperature should be adjusted as much as possible for comfort. A private room allows the patient more freedom to select the room temperature. If the patient perspires heavily, frequent bathing and clothing changes will help promote comfort.

Altered Nutrition: Less than Body Requirements. Despite a normal dietary intake, the patient may not be meeting the increased caloric needs. Daily weights are suggested to monitor nutritional adequacy. A diet high in calories, vitamins, and minerals is recommended. Depending on the severity of the condition, the patient may need additional full meals or between-meal snacks. Some patients require as many as 4000 to 5000 calories daily to maintain body weight. The physician may order supplementary vitamins. Additional fluids may be needed to replace fluids lost through increased insensible loss.

Decreased Cardiac Output. The patient's pulse and blood pressure should be measured at intervals. Drugs should be given as ordered to counteract the stimulant effects of the elevated thyroid hormones. Signs of heart failure include tachycardia, tachypnea, dyspnea, confusion, and edema. Elderly patients should be assessed often since they are more susceptible to cardiovascular stress with thyroid disease. Any signs of heart failure should be reported immediately. Medical treatment of heart failure usually includes oxygen, intravenous fluids, sedative and cardiac drugs, and a hypothermia blanket.

High Risk for Injury. Exophthalmos is a condition in which deposits of fat and fluid behind the eyeballs make them bulge outward (Fig. 40–2). Both eyes are usually affected. If the condition is severe, the eyelids do not cover the eyeball. The eyeball is not kept moist and is susceptible to injury. It may be necessary to tape the lids shut. Raising the head of the bed at night and limiting salt intake may be helpful.

The patient with exophthalmos has a startled appearance. This may make the person self-conscious and embarrassed. Dark glasses will help to conceal the eyes. For these patients, altered body image is an important additional nursing diagnosis. It is reassuring for the patient to know that the condition usually goes away after treatment of hyperthyroidism.

Diarrhea. If the patient develops diarrhea, electrolyte imbalances and skin irritation may result. Antidiarrheal medications should be given as ordered, and the effect monitored. Thorough perianal cleansing after each stool reduces the risk of skin breakdown.

Knowledge Deficit. Patients with hyperthyroidism need to understand the nature of the illness and the need for continued supervision. If they are taking their own medications, they need to recognize the importance of taking them as directed. The patient should also be told how to recognize hypothyroidism because it can be caused by antithyroid treatment.

EVALUATION. Evaluation of nursing care is based on patient's statements of improved restfulness and comfort; stable or increased weight; vital signs within normal limits, absence of signs and symptoms of heart failure (dyspnea, edema); absence of eye pain or excessive tearing; formed stools; patient's ability to describe hyperthyroidism and its treatment correctly; and patient's performance of self-care activities.

Nursing Care of the Patient Having a Thyroidectomy

General care of the surgical patient is discussed in Chapter 14. This section covers the special needs of the thyroidectomy patient.

ASSESSMENT

Preoperative. The preparation of the patient undergoing thyroid surgery is essentially the same as for any major surgery. The nurse should assess the patient's knowledge about surgery and what to expect before and after the procedure. Nursing diagnoses may include those listed earlier for hyperthyroidism, but the condition is usually brought under control before surgery is scheduled. In addition, knowledge deficits should be identified and addressed. The goals of preoperative teaching are patient understanding of the usual preoperative and postoperative procedures and decreased anxiety.

Teaching is the primary preoperative nursing intervention. In addition to usual preoperative routines (nothing by mouth, skin preparation, etc.), the patient is told to expect a dressing on the front of the neck. To avoid straining the neck incision, the patient should learn to support the head when rising. This can be demonstrated preoperatively (Fig. 40–3).

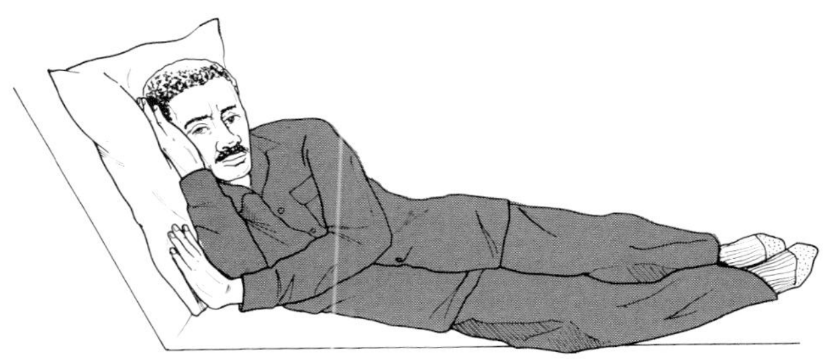

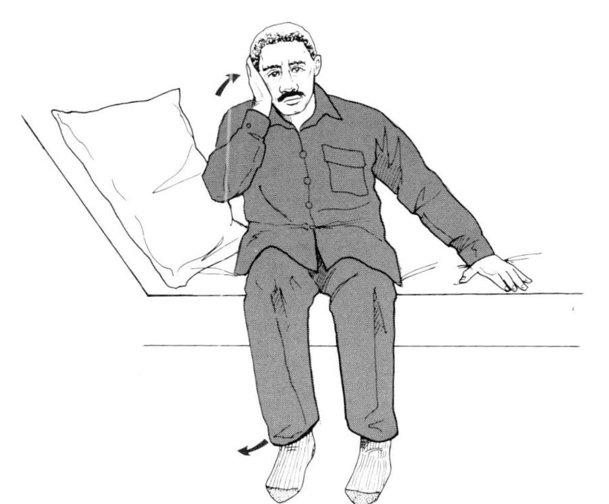

FIGURE 40–3
To avoid straining the neck incision, the thyroidectomy patient supports the head when rising.

To evaluate the effectiveness of preoperative teaching, the nurse can ask patients to repeat the information presented. Patients can also be asked to return demonstrations of activities such as deep breathing and supporting the head during position changes.

Postoperative. The patient usually recovers quickly from a thyroidectomy and may be discharged in 2 or 3 days. Rare but serious complications are airway obstruction, recurrent laryngeal nerve damage, hemorrhage, and tetany. One other complication, thyroid crisis, is generally prevented by preoperative treatment with antithyroid drugs.

Immediately after thyroidectomy, it is especially important to assess respiratory status, level of consciousness, wound drainage or bleeding, voice quality, comfort, and neuromuscular irritability.

NURSING DIAGNOSIS. Possible nursing diagnoses for the thyroidectomy patient include the following:

- **Ineffective Airway Clearance** related to airway obstruction, laryngeal nerve damage, tetany
- **Decreased Cardiac Output** related to blood loss, heart failure secondary to thyroid crisis
- **Body Image Disturbance** related to surgical scar
- **Knowledge Deficit** of self-care and long-term management of condition
- **Pain** related to tissue trauma
- **High Risk for Infection** related to impaired skin integrity

GOALS. Goals of nursing care after thyroidectomy are normal respirations with patent airway, normal cardiac output, improved body image, patient's knowledge of self-care and management of thyroid condition, pain relief, and absence of signs and symptoms of infection.

INTERVENTIONS

Ineffective Airway Clearance. Turning and deep breathing are recommended to prevent respiratory complications, as with any other surgical patient. The surgeon may not want the patient to cough, however, because of possible stress on the suture line.

It is especially important to monitor the rate and ease of respirations after thyroidectomy. Respiratory distress can result from compression of the trachea or from a spasm of the larynx due to nerve damage or hypocalcemia. Before the patient returns from surgery, suction equipment, a laryngoscope, an endotracheal tube, oxygen, and an emergency tracheotomy tray should be at the bedside. The head of the bed should be elevated to decrease edema. Pillows are used to prop and support the head in order to avoid stress on the suture line.

Because of the location of the thyroidectomy incision, edema or bleeding can cause pressure on the trachea. Signs and symptoms of poor oxygenation due to airway obstruction or blood loss include restlessness, increasing pulse and respiratory rates, and dyspnea. Without prompt intervention, the patient could die.

The laryngeal nerve innervates the vocal cords. If it is damaged during surgery, vocal cord paralysis can occur. Paralysis of both cords may cause spasms (laryngospasm) that close the airway. An emergency tracheotomy is needed to restore the airway. Signs of laryngeal nerve damage are hoarseness and inability to speak. This is more severe than the usual hoarseness most people have after general anesthesia. The patient is asked to respond verbally to simple questions to determine voice quality.

Before the parathyroid glands were understood, patients having thyroidectomies often developed unexplained muscle contractions and respiratory difficulty that sometimes led to death. Eventually, it was determined that the symptoms were caused by lack of parathyroid hormone. Surgeons are now careful to locate and spare the small parathyroid glands. Occasionally, however, the parathyroid glands are injured or accidentally removed during thyroidectomy.

Without parathyroid hormone, the serum calcium level falls, causing tetany. Muscle contractions begin as twitches around the mouth and eyes. The face, fingers, and toes begin to tingle. The patient may have painful "cramps," including the classic carpopedal spasm of the hands (Fig. 40–4). The most serious effect of hypocalcemia is spasm of the larynx. As the larynx closes, the patient has difficulty breathing and can suffocate. Cardiac dysrhythmias and seizures also can occur.

Tetany is treated with calcium salts given intravenously or orally. The condition usually improves as the injured parathyroid glands recover. Rarely is hypoparathyroidism permanent. If it is, lifetime treatment is required as described later in this chapter.

Decreased Cardiac Output. The nurse should assess the dressing and the vital signs frequently to detect bleeding. Since the dressing is on the front of the neck, blood might flow under the dressing to the back of the neck. The nurse must check behind the patient's neck and upper back to detect this.

Thyroid crisis can develop when large amounts of thyroid hormone enter the blood stream during surgery. About 12 hours after surgery, the patient shows signs of severe hyperthyroidism (tachycardia, cardiac arrhythmias, vomiting, fever, and confusion). It must be treated

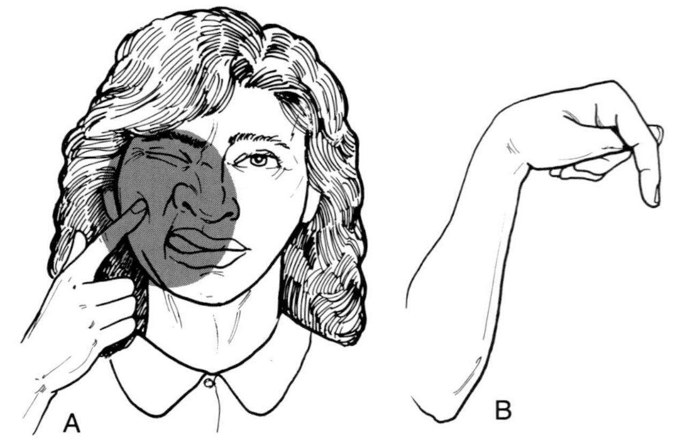

FIGURE 40–4

Signs of hypocalcemia: *A*, Chvostek's sign; *B*, Trousseau's sign (carpopedal spasm).

promptly or the patient will die as a result of heart failure. Early detection of thyroid crisis requires careful monitoring of vital signs during the first postoperative day. The risk of thyroid crisis is reduced if serum hormone levels are reduced preoperatively with medications.

Treatment consists of intravenous sodium iodide and corticosteroids, cardiac drugs, sedatives, oxygen, and a hypothermia (cooling) blanket.

Body Image Disturbance. The patient may be worried about the appearance of the surgical scar. Thyroidectomy incisions follow the natural contours of the neck. Once the scar fades, it is usually not noticeable. Meanwhile, it is easy to conceal the fresh scar with clothing.

Knowledge Deficit. Lifelong replacement of thyroid hormones is necessary after total thyroidectomy. If part of the thyroid gland is left (subtotal thyroidectomy), it should eventually regenerate and produce adequate hormones. These patients are somewhat hypothyroid at first, but replacement therapy is not recommended. Giving thyroid hormone interferes with the regeneration of thyroid tissue.

Pain. The postoperative patient's comfort level should be frequently assessed. Analgesics are ordered for pain and should be given promptly. Position changes and back rubs enhance the effects of prescribed analgesics.

High Risk for Infection. Any time the skin is disrupted, the potential for infection exists. The nurse should practice good hand washing and use aseptic technique when handling dressings. The patient should also be told to avoid touching the fresh incision and to report any signs and symptoms of infection (fever, increasing wound redness and swelling, and foul drainage). The incision is also protected from strain and possible dehiscence by supporting the neck when arising and reclining.

EVALUATION. Criteria for evaluating the effectiveness of nursing care following thyroidectomy include normal respiratory rate and effort, normal pulse and blood pressure, patient's verbalized acceptance of scar, patient's demonstration of self-care, patient's statement of pain relief, and absence of fever, wound drainage, redness, or swelling.

HYPOTHYROIDISM

Hypothyroidism is the result of inadequate secretion of thyroid hormones. It is seen in infants, children, and adults. Hypothyroidism during infancy causes permanent retardation of physical and mental development (cretinism) if not treated early (Fig. 40–5). The effects in adults can be quite serious but are generally reversible with treatment. The term myxedema is sometimes used for hypothyroidism. Myxedema actually refers to facial edema that develops with severe, long-term hypothyroidism (Fig. 40–6). Not all hypothyroid patients have myxedema.

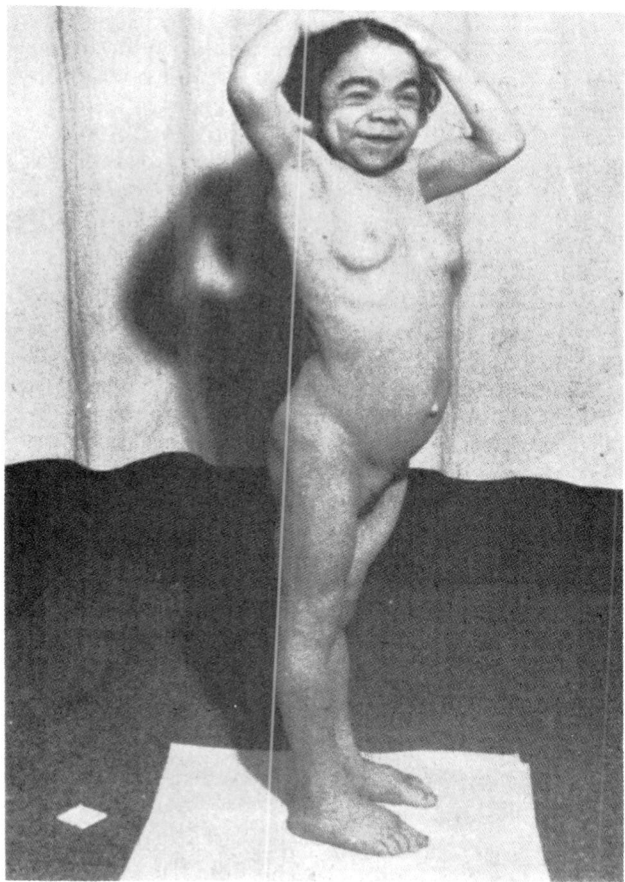

FIGURE 40-5
Cretinism is a condition of permanent physical and mental retardation resulting from untreated hypothyroidism in infancy. (From Ignatavicius, D. D., & Bayne, M. V. [1991]. *Medical-surgical nursing: A nursing process approach* [p. 1571]. Philadelphia: W. B. Saunders.)

Etiology and Risk Factors

Hypothyroidism has many causes. It may be the result of atrophy of the thyroid gland after years of Graves' disease of thyroiditis. Deficiency of TSH lowers the secretion of thyroid hormones even though the thyroid gland itself remains normal. Some foods and drugs act as goitrogens, meaning that they suppress thyroid hormone production. Examples of foods that are goitrogens are soybeans, turnips, and rutabagas. Goitrogenic drugs are often used to treat hyperthyroidism, as discussed earlier. These drugs are propylthiouracil, methimazole, and iodine. Of course, patients who have had their entire thyroid or pituitary glands surgically removed also will be hypothyroid.

Signs and Symptoms

The signs and symptoms of hypothyroidism are generally the opposite of those of hyperthyroidism (Table 40–4). The onset is usually gradual. In hypothyroidism, the metabolic rate slows, often causing weight gain even

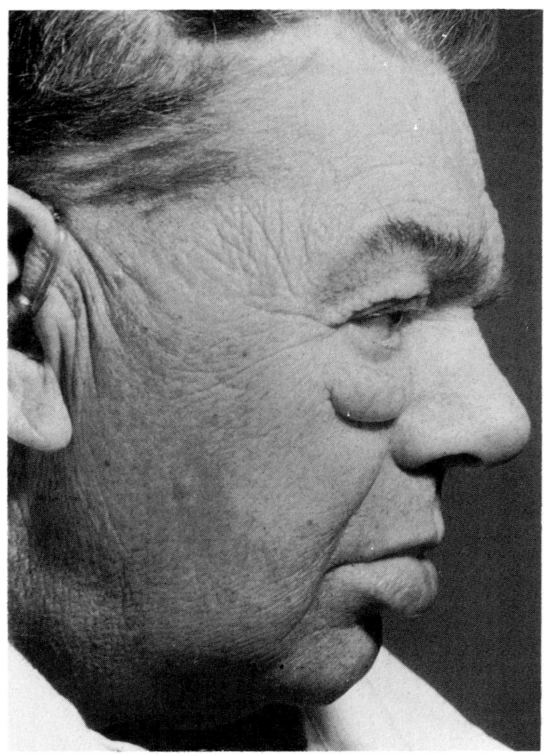

FIGURE 40-6
Typical appearance of the patient with myxedema. (From Jacob, S. W., & Francone, C. A. [1989]. *Elements of anatomy and physiology* [2nd ed., p. 151] Philadelphia: W. B. Saunders.)

with decreased food intake. Hypothyroid patients commonly report lethargy, forgetfulness, and irritability. They may experience frequent headaches, constipation, menstrual disorders, numbness and tingling in the arms and legs, and intolerance to cold. The pulse tends to be slow, and dyspnea may be present.

Examination may reveal swelling of the lips and eyelids; dry, thick skin; bruising; thin, coarse hair; and hoarseness. Generalized nonpitting edema and facial edema may be present. The patient may seem slow, depressed, or apathetic. Pallor may be present, associated with anemia.

Medical Diagnosis

Hypothyroidism is diagnosed based on the laboratory determination of T_3, T_4, and TSH. A TRH stimulation test also may be ordered. Levels of T_3 and T_4 are usually low with hypothyroidism. Measures of TSH levels and response to TRH enable the physician to determine whether the basic problem is in the thyroid gland, the pituitiary, or the hypothalamus.

Complications

Severe, untreated hypothyroidism can progress to myxedema coma. Infection, trauma, excessive chilling, and some drugs (narcotics, sedatives, tranquilizers) may precipitate myxedema coma in a hypothyroid patient. The main signs of this life-threatening condition are hypothermia, hypotension, and hypoventilation.

PHARMACOLOGY CAPSULE

Narcotics, sedatives, and tranquilizers can precipitate potentially fatal myxedema coma in a severely hypothyroid patient.

Hypothyroidism is treated with hormone replacement therapy. Natural and synthetic forms of thyroid hormones are available. The natural form is thyroid extract obtained from animal tissue. Examples of the synthetic form are levothyroxine (Synthroid) and liothyronine (Cytomel). Hypothyroid patients usually require lifelong replacement therapy. They should be monitored periodically to evaluate the response to therapy.

A patient with heart disease may have difficulty adapting to a sudden increase in metabolic rate. For that reason, replacement therapy for elderly patients or those with heart disease is usually started with a low dose and gradually increased. If these patients have any chest pain once therapy is started, the physician should be notified immediately.

Nursing Care of the Patient with Hypothyroidism

Hypothyroidism does not usually require hospitalization, but it may be detected when patients are hospitalized for other reasons (see Care Plan: The Patient with Hypothyroidism).

ASSESSMENT. Table 40–1 summarizes the general assessment of the patient with a thyroid disorder. Assessment of the patient with hypothyroidism should include measurement of vital signs and weight. In addition, the nurse should assess activity and temperature tolerance, voice quality, bowel elimination pattern, and changes in weight and dietary intake. The skin is assessed for edema, texture, and moisture. Level of consciousness and emotional state should be noted. The nurse also assesses the patient's understanding of hypothyroidism and its treatment.

NURSING DIAGNOSIS. The following nursing diagnoses are examples that apply to many hypothyroid patients:

- **Activity Intolerance** related to decreased metabolic energy production
- **Altered Nutrition: More than Body Requirements** related to intake greater than metabolic needs
- **Hypothermia** related to cold intolerance
- **Constipation** related to decreased peristalsis
- **High Risk for Impaired Skin Integrity** related to dryness and edema

TABLE 40-4

COMPARISON OF SIGNS AND SYMPTOMS OF HYPOTHYROIDISM AND HYPERTHYROIDISM

SYSTEM	HYPOTHYROIDISM	HYPERTHYROIDISM
Integumentary	Coarse, dry skin and hair	Smooth, moist skin
	Thick nails	Silky hair
		Diaphoresis
Musculoskeletal	Muscle aches and pains	
	Weakness	Weakness
	Slow movements	
Cardiovascular	Bradycardia	Tachycardia
	Dysrhythmias	Dysrhythmias
	Hypotension	Palpitations
		Systolic hypertension
	Anemia	Angina
	Capillary fragility	
Respiratory	Hypoventilation	Increased respiratory rate
	Dyspnea	Dyspnea
Gastrointestinal	Anorexia	Increased appetite
	Nausea and vomiting	Increased bowel sounds
	Constipation	Diarrhea
	Weight gain	Weight loss
Neurologic	Apathy	Nervousness and irritability
	Lethargy	Insomnia
	Slowed mental function	Personality change
	Depression	Agitation
	Slow speech	Inability to concentrate
	Paresthesias	Fine tremor of fingers and tongue
	Decreased tendon reflexes	Hyperreflexia
Reproductive	Females	Females
	Amenorrhea or prolonged menses	Menstrual irregularities
	Infertility	
	Decreased libido	Decreased libido
	Males	Males
	Decreased libido	Decreased libido
	Impotence	Impotence
		Gynecomastia
Other	Cold intolerance	Heat intolerance
	Decreased body temperature	Increased body temperature
	Facial puffiness or coarseness	Exophthalmos
	Thick tongue	Goiter
	Nonpitting edema of hands and feet	
	Sensitivity to central nervous system depressants	Sensitivity to central nervous system stimulants

- **Decreased Cardiac Output** related to cardiovascular changes secondary to hypothyroidism
- **Altered Thought Processes** related to decreased cerebral oxygenation
- **Body Image Disturbance** related to altered physical appearance, altered thought processes, lack of energy
- **Self-Care Deficit** related to fatigue, lack of knowledge of the effects and treatment of hypothyroidism

GOALS. Goals of nursing care for the hypothyroid patient include improved activity tolerance, adequate nutrition, improved cold tolerance, normal stools, intact skin, normal cardiac output, mental alertness, adaptation to symptoms, and ability to care for self.

INTERVENTIONS

Activity Intolerance. The hypothyroid patient lacks energy and tires easily. The schedule should be arranged to allow for rest periods. Ideally, sedatives and barbiturates should not be given as they may cause excessive sedation. If they are given, lower dosages are recommended and the patient's respirations and level of consciousness must be monitored.

Altered Nutrition: More than Body Requirements. Despite having a poor appetite, the patient may have had a weight gain. Weekly weights are helpful in evaluating the effects of hormone replacement therapy. Calorie reduction may be prescribed for the patient who is overweight. A balanced diet should still be encouraged.

Hypothermia. Cold intolerance is a very uncomfortable effect of hypothyroidism. The patient should be provided extra clothing and blankets as needed. The room temperature can be maintained at a level comfortable to the patient. This is easier to manage if the patient has a private room. Once thyroid replacement is initiated, the cold intolerance will gradually improve.

Constipation. Constipation is a common problem. Until the hypothyroidism is corrected, measures must be taken to promote normal elimination. Adequate

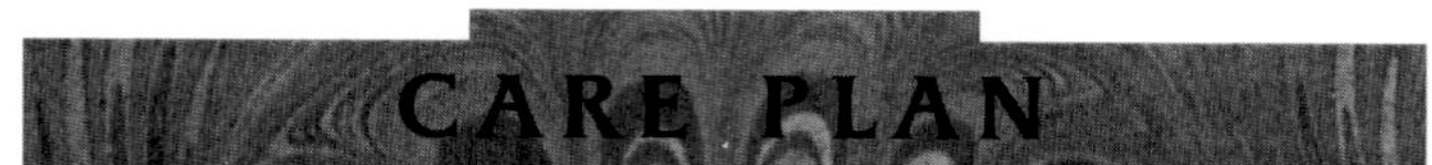

The Patient with Hypothyroidism

ASSESSMENT

Health History: Margie Frances is a 53-year-old woman who comes to the physician's office complaining of fatigue and irritability. Her symptoms have gradually worsened and are now interfering with her work as an executive secretary. She reports that her health has generally been good, with only one hospitalization for an appendectomy 7 years ago. The review of systems reveals frequent headaches, anorexia, constipation, menstrual irregularity, numbness and tingling in the legs, and intolerance to cold. She has noticed a 10-pound weight gain over the last 6 months without a change in diet or exercise.

Physical Examination: Vital signs: temperature, 97°F orally; pulse, 56; respiration, 18; blood pressure, 90/60. (Her record indicates that her previous blood pressure was 128/76 and pulse was 74.) Height, 5′5″. Weight, 155 lb. She is oriented but lethargic. Her hair is coarse, and her skin is dry.

NURSING DIAGNOSIS	GOALS AND OUTCOME CRITERIA	INTERVENTIONS
Activity intolerance related to decreased metabolic energy production.	The patient will perform activities of daily living without excess fatigue.	Advise patient to schedule additional rest periods until condition improves. Assure her that these symptoms are temporary.
Altered nutrition: greater than body requirements related to intake greater than metabolic needs.	The patient's weight will stabilize within 2 pounds of her usual 145 pounds.	Weigh during each office visit. Encourage balanced diet. Tell her that weight should normalize when condition is corrected.
Hypothermia related to cold intolerance.	The patient will report adequate warmth and increased tolerance of cool temperatures.	Adjust room temperature for patient comfort. Provide adequate covering during physical examination.
Constipation related to decreased peristalsis.	The patient will have regular bowel movements passed without difficulty.	Encourage increased fluid intake, high-fiber diet with fresh fruits and raw vegetables. Instruct in taking stool softeners if advised by physician. Encourage gradual increase in physical activity as tolerance improves.

fluids, dietary fiber, and physical activity all help reduce constipation. Stool softeners may be indicated if other measures do not solve the problem.

High Risk for Impaired Skin Integrity. Dry skin found with hypothyroidism is prone to breakdown. Lotions and creams applied liberally help maintain moisture and control itching. The frequency of bathing can be reduced to prevent additional drying of the skin.

Decreased Cardiac Output. Patients who have uncorrected hypothyroidism for a long time develop atherosclerosis and heart disease. The nurse monitors these patients for any signs and symptoms of heart failure, such as dyspnea and increasing edema. After hormone replacement therapy is begun, there is some risk of excessive cardiac stimulation. The patient should be told that any chest pain should be reported promptly. The pulse should be monitored to detect potentially serious changes in rhythm or rate.

Altered Thought Processes. Mental dullness and depression can significantly affect the patient's life. The nurse should explain that these symptoms are related to hypothyroidism and that correction of hypothyroidism usually results in marked improvement. (An exception is the individual who has cretinism caused by untreated hypothyroidism during fetal development or early infancy. The mental retardation of cretinism is not reversible.) Until mental function improves, the nurse should be careful not to demand too much of the patient. Teaching should be broken into small units and reinforced at intervals.

Body Image Disturbance. The puffy, apathetic look and weight gain associated with hypothyroidism can be

The Patient with Hypothyroidism *(Continued)*

NURSING DIAGNOSIS	GOALS AND OUTCOME CRITERIA	INTERVENTIONS
High risk for impaired skin integrity related to dryness and edema.	The patient's skin will remain intact, and usual moisture will be restored.	Advise to decrease bathing frequency and to use moisturizing creams or lotions. Advise to avoid scratching.
Decreased cardiac output related to cardiovascular changes secondary to hypothyroidism.	The patient's cardiac output will improve as evidenced by improved stamina, regular pulse between 60 and 100, and absence of dyspnea.	Monitor for tachycardia, hypertension, and dysrhythmias after hormone replacement therapy is begun. Be alert for signs and symptoms of heart failure (dyspnea, edema).
Altered thought processes related to decreased cerebral oxygenation.	The patient will report improved mental functioning and will appear less lethargic.	Explain that mental slowness is related to hypothyroidism and that will improve with treatment. Do not overload patient with information. Teach only critical information initially and supplement with written information. Ask her how her work expectations could be adjusted to accommodate her symptoms temporarily.
Body image disturbance related to impaired mentation, lack of energy.	The patient will acknowledge that functional problems are caused by hypothyroidism and that improvement is expected with treatment.	Explore patient's concerns about effects of condition on her functioning. Explain that skin and hair changes are reversible.
Self-care deficits related to fatigue, lack of knowledge of effects and treatment of hypothyroidism.	The patient's activities of daily living will be accomplished with only normal fatigue.	Ask patient to consider her daily activities and set priorities to decrease demands on her energy. Encourage rest periods during day. Delay difficult or strenuous tasks until condition improves.

very distressing to the patient. The nurse should be accepting of the patient's concerns but encourage good grooming and attention to appearance. The patient can be told that treatment will gradually eliminate these changes.

Self-Care Deficit. The hypothyroid patient can expect to need hormone replacement therapy for life. The nurse should explain this and stress the need for periodic medical evaluation. The name, dosage, and adverse effects of the prescribed drug therapy are explained. The patient should also be taught the symptoms of hyperthyroidism that might occur with excessive hormone replacement (tachycardia, weight loss, nervousness).

EVALUATION. Criteria for successful nursing interventions are patient's report of feeling rested; stable or decreased weight; absence of complaints of coldness; regular stools without discomfort; intact, moist skin; absence of signs and symptoms of circulatory failure (dyspnea, dysrhythmias); orientation to person, place, and time; attention to appearance and grooming; and demonstrated ability to care for self.

GOITER

Goiter is the term used to describe enlargement of the thyroid gland. Enlargement may be due to simple goiter, thyroid nodules, or thyroiditis.

Simple Goiter

Thyroid enlargement with normal thyroid hormone production is called simple goiter (Fig. 40–7). Causes include iodine deficiency and long-term exposure to goitrogens. The gland may enlarge to compensate for

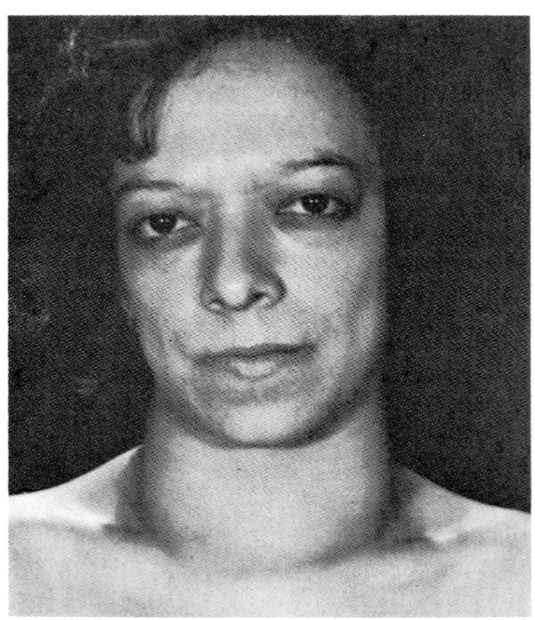

FIGURE 40–7

Goiter. (From Wilson, J., & Foster, D. [1985]. *Williams textbook of endocrinology* [7th ed., p. 1563]. Philadelphia: W. B. Saunders.)

hypothyroidism. Sometimes the enlarged gland produces excess hormones, making the patient hyperthyroid.

The type of treatment depends on the degree of enlargement and level of thyroid hormone production. If enlargement is mild and hormones are normal, no intervention is required. Some patients need hormone replacement therapy. Surgery is indicated if there is pressure on the trachea or esophagus or if the condition is disfiguring.

Nodules

Multinodular goiter is discussed under hyperthyroidism. As noted, nodules can be benign or malignant. A scan using radioactive iodine permits the physician to determine whether cancer is present. Nodular goiters are usually surgically removed. In benign conditions, only the nodule may be removed.

THYROID CANCER. Thyroid cancer is not common, but it can be fatal. In the early stages, the only sign may be a nodule that can be felt on the thyroid gland. Later, if the cancer spreads, enlarged lymph nodes will be felt in the neck. The patient may not show dramatic changes in thyroid hormone levels. Total thyroidectomy is the usual treatment. Nursing care of the thyroidectomy patient is covered under hyperthyroidism. If the malignancy has spread beyond the thyroid gland, a radical neck dissection may be indicated. Care of the patient with a radical neck dissection is discussed in Chapter 49.

Surgery may be followed with radioactive iodine treatment to destroy any remaining tissue that might harbor malignant cells. This is the same type of iodine used in diagnostic studies, but a larger dose is used. The patient needs to be isolated and on radiation precautions. Body fluids must be handled carefully as they will be contaminated. The care of the patient receiving internal radiation therapy is discussed in Chapter 23.

The patient will be alarmed at the diagnosis of cancer. He or she may find some comfort in knowing that the 5-year survival rate for thyroid cancer is among the highest of all types of cancer. Long-term care after thyroid cancer includes management of hypothyroidism and monitoring for recurrence. Scans using radioactive iodine are sometimes ordered at intervals to detect the presence of any remaining cancerous tissue.

THE PARATHYROID GLANDS

ANATOMY AND PHYSIOLOGY OF THE PARATHYROID GLANDS

The parathyroid glands are four small glands usually located on the back of the thyroid gland (Fig. 40–8). Occasionally, some glands are found in the mediastinum as well. Even though they are typically embedded in the thyroid, the parathyroids function independently. They secrete only one hormone, but it is a vital one. Parathyroid hormone, or parathormone (PTH), plays a critical role in regulating the serum calcium level.

Calcium is an essential component of strong bones and plays a vital role in the functions of nerve and muscle cells. When the serum calcium level falls, PTH is secreted. Parathormone increases the absorption of calcium from the intestines, transfers calcium from the bones to the blood, and signals the kidneys to conserve calcium. Generally, calcium retention by the kidney is balanced by phosphate loss. Figure 40–9 depicts the action of PTH.

NURSING ASSESSMENT OF THE PARATHYROID GLANDS

When assessing the patient who has a parathyroid disorder, the nurse focuses on skeletal and neuromuscular function.

HEALTH HISTORY

When taking the health history, the nurse asks if the patient has noticed any change in mental-emotional status, such as memory problems, irritability, or personality changes. A history of musculoskeletal problems, including weakness, skeletal pain, backache, and muscle twitching or spasms, also should be assessed. It should be noted if the patient has experienced urinary frequency, polyuria, urinary calculi (stones), or constipation. A past medical history of head or neck radiation, renal calculi, or chronic renal failure is documented. Medications, including calcium and vitamin D supplements are listed.

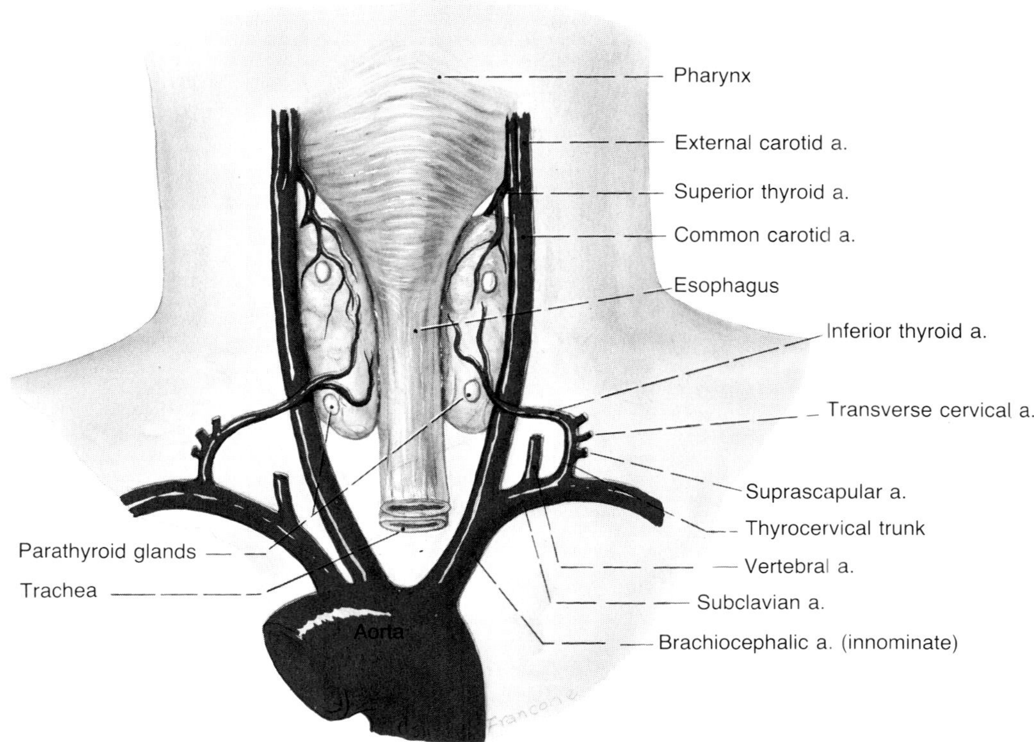

FIGURE 40-8

Posterior view of the neck and thyroid gland, showing the approximate location of the parathyroid glands. (Adapted from Jacob, S. W., & Francone, C. A. [1989]. *Elements of anatomy and physiology* [2nd ed., p. 152]. Philadelphia: W. B. Saunders.)

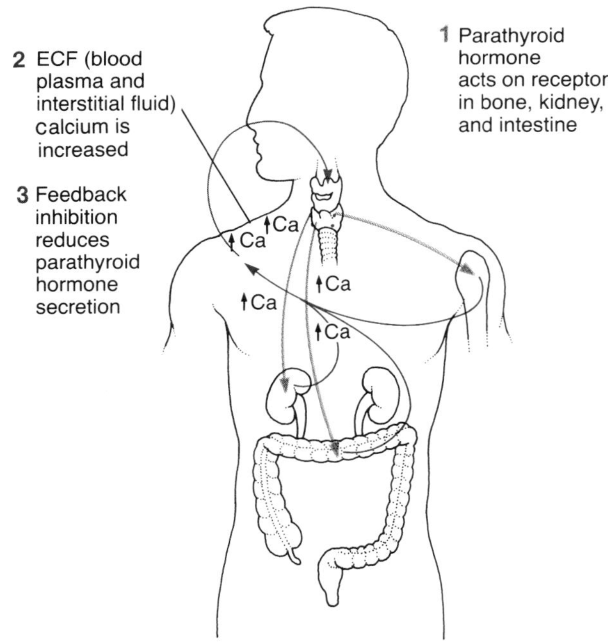

FIGURE 40-9

Physiologic actions of parathormone. ECF, extracellular fluid. (Adapted from Ignatavicius, D. D., & Bayne, M. V. [1991]. *Medical-surgical nursing: A nursing process approach.* [p. 1576]. Philadelphia: W. B. Saunders.)

PHYSICAL EXAMINATION

Important data in the physical examination include heart rate and rhythm, blood pressure, respiratory effort, muscle strength, muscle twitching, and hair and skin texture. Simple tests are used to elicit Chvostek's sign and Trousseau's sign, which are both indicative of hypocalcemia. Chvostek's sign is a spasm of the facial muscle when the face is tapped over the facial nerve. Trousseau's sign is a carpopedal spasm that occurs when a blood pressure cuff is inflated above the patient's systolic blood pressure and left in place for 2 to 3 minutes (see Fig. 40–4).

Nursing assessment of the patient with a parathyroid disorder is outlined in Table 40–5.

DIAGNOSTIC TESTS AND PROCEDURES

The diagnosis of parathyroid disorders is based on blood and urine studies and skeletal radiographs. Blood tests include measurements of calcium, phosphate, creatinine, uric acid, magnesium, alkaline phosphatase, and PTH. The presence of parathyroid antibodies also may be identified through blood studies. A 24-hour urine specimen may be collected to determine how much calcium is being excreted in the urine.

If sufficient calcium has been drawn from bones, de-

TABLE 40-5

ASSESSMENT OF THE PATIENT WITH A PARATHYROID DISORDER

HEALTH HISTORY

Present illness: Changes in mental-emotional status, neuromuscular symptoms

Past medical history: Head or neck radiation, renal calculi, chronic renal failure, recent and current medications, including calcium and vitamin D supplements

Review of systems: Fatigue, irritability, muscle tremors or spasms, bone pain, urinary frequency, polyuria, constipation or diarrhea, depression, personality changes

PHYSICAL EXAMINATION

Vital signs: Dysrhythmias, hypertension or hypotension

Skin and hair: Changes in moisture and texture

Urologic: Flank pain

Musculoskeletal: Weakness, tremors

Neurologic: Abnormally active or depressed reflexes, irritability, headache, confusion, positive Chvostek's sign, positive Trousseau's sign

mineralization will be apparent on radiographs. Bone cysts and tumors may be found. A dental examination may be done to detect changes in the teeth consistent with parathyroid dysfunction. An electrocardiogram also may be ordered because calcium imbalances can cause alterations in the electrical activity in the heart.

DISORDERS OF THE PARATHYROID GLANDS

HYPERPARATHYROIDISM

The secretion of excess PTH is called hyperparathyroidism. It is most often caused by a tumor called an adenoma. Tumors can be benign or malignant. Other factors that may stimulate excess PTH secretion are vitamin D deficiencies, malabsorption, chronic renal failure, and elevated serum phosphate. Individuals who receive a kidney transplant after having been on dialysis for a long time may become hyperparathyroid.

The most notable effect of hyperparathyroidism is elevation of serum calcium (hypercalcemia). High levels of PTH cause calcium to shift from the bones into the blood stream. Excess PTH also promotes retention of calcium and loss of phosphate by the kidneys. If untreated, severe demineralization of bone tissue occurs. Bones can become brittle, resulting in serious fractures. The high level of calcium in the urine can lead to the formation of urinary calculi. Obstruction of the urinary tubules by calculi can quickly lead to severe kidney damage. The effects of hyperparathyroidism on the heart can cause dysrhythmias and hypertension.

Signs and Symptoms

Since hyperparathyroidism usually develops gradually, symptoms are vague at first. The patient may report weakness, lethargy, depression, anorexia, and constipation. Other findings might include mental and personality changes, cardiac arrhythmias, weight loss, and urinary calculi. Additional signs and symptoms of hyperparathyroidism are outlined in Table 40–6.

Medical Diagnosis

The diagnosis of hyperparathyroidism is based primarily on blood and urine studies. Typical findings include elevated serum calcium and decreased serum phosphate, elevated PTH, and elevated 24-hour urine calcium. Skeletal radiographs reveal bone demineralization if the condition is severe. Sometimes the condition

TABLE 40-6

COMPARISON OF SIGNS AND SYMPTOMS OF HYPOPARATHYROIDISM AND HYPERPARATHYROIDISM

SYSTEM	HYPOPARATYHYROIDISM	HYPERPARATHYROIDISM
Musculoskeletal	Fatigue Weakness Cramps Twitching	Poor muscle tone Weakness Bone pain Demineralization Fractures
Urinary	Frequency	Polyuria Renal calculi
Cardiovascular	Decreased cardiac output Dysrhythmias	Hypertension Dysrhythmias
Nervous	Hyperactive reflexes Memory impairment Depression Anxiety Irritability Personality changes Confusion Numbness and tingling of hands and feet and around mouth	Depressed reflexes Decreased mental function Depression Mood swings Confusion Coma Poor coordination
Gastrointestinal	Abdominal cramps	Anorexia Nausea and vomiting Constipation
Integumentary	Dry skin Brittle nails	Moist skin

is not recognized until the patient has a spontaneous fracture.

Medical Treatment

If a tumor is causing hyperparathyroidism, it is usually removed surgically. In some cases, more than one gland is removed. The surgeon attempts to leave some parathyroid tissue to prevent hypoparathyroidism. This can be a complicated procedure because some parathyroid glands may be located in the mediastinum. If the condition is mild or the patient is not a good candidate for surgery, medical treatment is aimed at lowering the serum calcium level. The patient is instructed to maintain a high fluid intake. Calcium intake may be restricted. Sodium and phosphorus replacements also may be ordered.

DRUG THERAPY. Several drugs can be used to treat hyperparathyroidism. Plicamycin (Mithracin), gallium nitrate (Ganite), and calcitonin (Calcimar) inhibit the release of calcium from bones. Because plicamycin has severe toxic effects, it is generally reserved for patients with metastatic parathyroid cancer. When it is necessary to lower the calcium level quickly, an infusion of normal saline is often prescribed. Furosemide (Lasix) may be given to promote the excretion of calcium in the urine. Propranolol also is useful in reducing PTH secretion. Drugs used to treat parathyroid disorders are described in Table 40–7.

PHARMACOLOGY CAPSULE

Furosemide (Lasix) is a diuretic that promotes the excretion of calcium in the urine.

TABLE 40-7
DRUGS USED TO TREAT PARATHYROID CONDITIONS

DRUG	USE/ACTION	SIDE EFFECTS	NURSING INTERVENTIONS
Calcium salts Calcium chloride Calcium gluconate	Correct calcium deficiency due to hypoparathyroidism.	Overdosage can cause hypercalcemia: weakness, hypertension, dysrhythmias, polyuria, bone pain.	Serum calcium levels should be monitored. Notify physician of signs of hypercalcemia.
Vitamin D Calcitrol Dihydrotachysterol Ergocalciferol	Promotes calcium absorption from digestive tract.	Overdosage can cause hypercalcemia: weakness, hypertension, dysrhythmias, polyuria, bone pain.	Serum calcium levels should be monitored. Notify physician of signs of hypercalcemia.
Diuretics Furosemide (Lasix)	Promote excretion of excess calcium in hyperparathyroidism.	Fluid and electrolyte imbalances: metabolic alkalosis, hypovolemia, dehydration, hyponatremia, hypokalemia. Dizziness, headache, tinnitus, hyperglycemia.	Monitor intake and output, serum calcium and potassium levels, pulse, blood pressure, blood glucose.
Parathormone	Short-term treatment of hypoparathyroidism.	Overdosage can cause hypercalcemia: weakness, hypertension, dysrhythmias, polyuria, bone pain.	Available only for parenteral use.
Calcitonin (Calcimar, Cibacalcin)	Treats hypercalcemia caused by hyperparathyroidism.	Nausea, vomiting, injection-site reactions, facial flushing, anaphylaxis.	Monitor for tachycardia due to hypocalcemia. Sensitivity test should be done before giving; have epinephrine, antihistamines, and oxygen available. Tell patient that flushing is temporary. Teach self-medication. Encourage adequate fluid intake.
Etidronate disodium (Didronel)	Reduces serum calcium level in hyperparathyroidism.	Diarrhea, nausea, metallic taste, bone pain, and tenderness. Hypocalcemia: weakness, muscle spasms.	Dividing dose through the day may control diarrhea. Advise that metallic taste is temporary.
Plicamycin (Mithracin)	Treats hypercalcemia by inhibiting release of calcium from bones.	Hypocalcemia: weakness, muscle spasms. Hypokalemia, thrombocytopenia, leukopenia, bleeding, drowsiness, depression, anorexia, nausea, vomiting.	Reserved for patients with metastatic parathyroid cancer because of severity of toxic effects. Monitor for bleeding. Avoid injections. Apply pressure to venipuncture sites for 10 min. Assess for signs of infection. Discontinue if extravasation occurs.
Gallium nitrate (Ganite)	Reduces serum calcium level in hypercalcemia.	Hypotension, nausea and vomiting, decreased serum calcium and bicarbonate, increased BUN and creatinine.	Administer intravenously with normal saline. Monitor serum electrolytes, blood pressure, CBC, and urine output.

Nursing Care of the Patient with Hyperparathyroidism

ASSESSMENT. When caring for the hyperparathyroid patient, the nurse should assess vital signs, urine output, weight, muscle strength, bowel elimination, and digestive disturbances.

NURSING DIAGNOSIS. The following nursing diagnoses commonly apply to patients with hyperparathyroidism. Since the disorder can vary in severity, nursing diagnoses must be based on individual assessments.

- **Activity Intolerance** related to weakness and fatigue
- **High Risk for Injury** related to weakness and decreased bone mass
- **Altered Urinary Elimination** related to presence of renal calculi
- **Constipation** related to altered intestinal motility
- **Altered Thought Processes** related to hypercalcemia
- **Altered Nutrition: Less than Body Requirements** related to nausea and vomiting
- **Knowledge Deficit** of self-care to manage condition

GOALS. Goals of nursing care for the hyperparathyroid patient include improved activity tolerance, absence of injuries (fractures), normal urinary output, regular bowel elimination, improved mental-emotional status, adequate nutritional intake, and patient's knowledge of self-care practices.

INTERVENTIONS

Activity Intolerance and High Risk for Injury. The nurse assesses the patient's ability to perform self-care safely and provides help as needed. The environment should be evaluated for any safety hazards, and corrective measures taken. Care should be planned to allow for periods of rest. The patient can be assured that weakness and fatigue are caused by the parathyroid disorder and will improve as the condition is corrected.

Altered Urinary Elimination. Since hypercalcemia can cause urinary calculi and serious kidney damage, the patient's intake and output should be accurately recorded. Decreasing urine output; sharp pain in the flank (kidney area), lower abdomen, or genitalia; and hematuria are consistent with urinary calculi and should be reported to the physician. A high fluid intake, sometimes as much as 4000 ml per day, may be ordered. Urine output and vital signs must also be monitored when large volumes of fluid are administered. The elderly and people with heart disease are at risk for fluid volume excess and congestive heart failure. Of course, patients with cardiac or renal disease may be unable to tolerate this much fluid. Urine may be strained and examined for crystals or calculi. A low-calcium diet and urine acidifiers may be ordered to decrease the risk of calculi formation.

Constipation. Bowel movements should be charted, including frequency and characteristics of stools. Constipation can often be managed with adequate fluids and fiber in the diet. If these measures are not effective, the physician may order stool softeners. It is especially important to monitor bowel elimination in the elderly. Illness, inactivity, and multiple medications combine to increase their risk of constipation and even fecal impaction.

Altered Thought Processes. The nurse and others need to recognize that irritability, personality changes, and depression are common with hyperparathyroidism. Patients and their families appreciate knowing that these symptoms improve with treatment.

Altered Nutrition: Less than Body Requirements. Measures should be taken to control nausea and vomiting if present. If the patient's intake is poor, periodic weights should be taken to detect inadequate nutrition. Small feedings may be better tolerated. The nurse provides a pleasant mealtime environment.

Knowledge Deficit. Patient teaching focuses on helping the patient understand the condition and how it is treated. The teaching plan should include drug therapy, diet, fluids, and signs and symptoms of complications.

POSTOPERATIVE CARE. Following parathyroidectomy, the patient requires care like that of any surgical patient, as detailed in Chapter 14. Two potential complications specific to parathyroidectomy are airway obstruction and hypocalcemia. When the patient has a neck incision, accumulated fluid and blood in the surgical site can compress the trachea, causing airway obstruction. The nurse monitors the respiratory rate and effort and the pulse rate. Increasing pulse and respiratory rates, especially accompanied by restlessness, suggest inadequate oxygenation. The physician should be notified of any indications of respiratory distress. An emergency tracheotomy tray is kept at the bedside in the event of acute obstruction.

A second possible cause of airway obstruction is related to severe hypocalcemia. The nurse should be alert for tetany, a symptom of hypocalcemia, caused by the postoperative decrease in parathyroid hormones. A tingling sensation around the mouth and in the fingers is an early symptom of tetany. It may progress to severe muscle spasms or cramps and even to laryngospasm. Calcium and other electrolytes will be monitored closely in the postoperative period. The nurse should promptly inform the physician of signs of tetany or abnormal electrolyte values. Tetany is treated with oral or intravenous calcium supplements. Treatment of hypocalcemia is discussed in detail under hypoparathyroidism.

The patient's incision will be on the front of the neck or upper chest, or both, and will probably be covered with a bulky dressing. As with the thyroidectomy patient, this patient's suture line should be protected from stress. The patient should be shown how to support the head when changing positions (see Fig. 40–3). The nurse should assess the dressing and the back of the patient's neck for bleeding. Elevating the patient's head helps reduce swelling.

EVALUATION. Evidence of successful nursing interventions includes patient's ability to increase activity without undue fatigue, absence of injuries, urine output equal to fluid intake, regular passage of soft stools, patient's report of improved mental-emotional status, maintenance of body weight, and patient's ability to assume self-care.

HYPOPARATHYROIDISM

Hypoparathyroidism is a deficiency of PTH. It is an uncommon condition most often due to accidental removal of or damage to parathyroid glands during surgery. Inadequate secretion of PTH leads to hypocalcemia. Severe hypocalcemia can progress to convulsions and respiratory obstruction due to spasms of the larynx. Laryngospasm can be fatal.

Signs and Symptoms

Assessment of parathyroid function is most important after thyroid surgery. Trauma or accidental removal of one or more parathyroid glands may lead to symptoms of hypoparathyroidism as discussed under thyroidectomy.

Signs and symptoms of hypocalcemia are painful muscle cramps, fatigue and weakness, tingling and twitching of the face and hands, mental and emotional changes, dry skin, and urinary frequency. With severe hypocalcemia, the patient may have difficulty breathing and cardiac dysrhythmias.

Medical Diagnosis

The diagnosis of hypoparathyroidism is based on patient signs and symptoms and blood studies. Typical findings include low serum calcium, elevated serum phosphate, low urine calcium and sometimes low serum magnesium. Two classic signs of hypocalcemia that support a diagnosis of hypoparathyroidism are Chvostek's sign and Trousseau's sign.

Medical Treatment

Acute hypoparathyroidism is sometimes treated with parenteral PTH. Severe hypocalcemia is treated with intravenous calcium salts.

On a long-term basis, the patient with chronic hypoparathyroidism is treated with oral calcium salts and vitamin D. Aluminum hydroxide also may be ordered with meals to reduce the absorption of phosphates in the intestines. Lowering serum phosphate levels tends to raise serum calcium levels. Chronic hypoparathyroidism that is normally well controlled may be affected when the patient is under severe stress or is very ill. If the patient is unable to take oral calcium, hypocalcemia can develop quickly. Temporary intravenous calcium may be needed.

PHARMACOLOGY CAPSULE

Lifelong calcium supplementation is required to treat chronic hypoparathyroidism.

Nursing Care of the Patient with Hypoparathyroidism

ASSESSMENT. Assessment of the hypoparathyroid patient is summarized in Table 40–5.

NURSING DIAGNOSIS. Nursing diagnoses for the hypoparathyroid patient include the following:

- **High Risk for Injury** related to hypocalcemia
- **Decreased Cardiac Output** related to dysrhythmias and heart failure secondary to hypocalcemia
- **Knowledge Deficit** related to requirement for long-term self-care

GOALS. Goals of nursing care for the hypoparathyroid patient are absence of injury, normal cardiac output, and patient's knowledge of management of hypoparathyroidism.

INTERVENTIONS. The nurse administers drugs as ordered for hypoparathyroidism and hypocalcemia. When administering calcium salts intravenously, the nurse monitors the infusion site carefully. Since the leakage of calcium salts into the body tissues causes inflammation, the infusion site must be changed if extravasation occurs. The nurse frequently assesses the patient for signs and symptoms of calcium imbalances. Hypocalcemia may appear as a result of inadequate calcium supplementation. Hypercalcemia can result from excessive calcium intake.

If there has been any recent seizure activity or the patient shows severe neuromuscular irritability, seizure precautions should be taken. Any signs of respiratory distress may suggest laryngospasm and should be reported to the physician immediately. The pulse and blood pressure are monitored to detect dysrhythmias and heart failure. Cardiac irregularities, edema, and dyspnea are reported to the physician.

Patients with chronic hypoparathyroidism need to be taught signs and symptoms of calcium imbalances and given self-medication instructions. They should be advised to carry medical identification cards to alert health care providers to the disorder in the event of an emergency.

EVALUATION. Criteria for successful nursing interventions are absence of muscle spasms and respiratory distress, normal pulse and blood pressure, and accurate patient's statement of self-care measures.

Most thyroid disorders are treated easily and cause minimal disruption of patients' lives. Undiagnosed or poorly controlled disorders, however, can significantly impair a patient's well-being. The nurse can play an important role in detecting signs and symptoms of thyroid imbalances and in teaching patients how to manage their conditions. Parathyroid disorders are relatively rare but can be life threatening. The nurse's ongoing assessment, administration of prescribed treatments, and patient teaching are vital.

NUTRITION CONCEPTS

- Lack of iodine is associated with the development of a goiter (enlargement of the thyroid gland) in adults and cretinism in infants.
- Iodized salt is the best way to obtain an adequate amount of iodine in the diet.
- Another important source of iodine is saltwater seafoods.
- Parathormone, secreted by the parathyroid gland, and thyrocalcitonin, secreted by the thyroid gland, maintain serum calcium levels.

BIBLIOGRAPHY

Black, J. M., & Matassarin-Jacobs, E. (1993). *Luckmann and Sorensen's medical surgical nursing: A psychophysiologic approach* (4th ed.). Philadelphia: W. B. Saunders.

Caine, R. M., & Bufalino, P. M. (1991). *Nursing care planning guides for adults* (2nd ed.). Baltimore: Williams & Wilkins.

Chernecky, C. C., Krech, R. L., & Berger, B. J. (1993). *Laboratory tests and diagnostic procedures.* Philadelphia: W. B. Saunders.

Haas, L. B. (1992). Nursing assessment: Endocrine systems. In S. M. Lewis & I. C. Collier (Eds.), *Medical-surgical nursing* (3rd ed., pp. 1258–1281). St. Louis: Mosby Year Book.

Haas, L. B. (1992). Nursing role in management: Endocrine problems. In S. M. Lewis & I. C. Collier (Eds.), *Medical-surgical nursing* (3rd ed., pp. 1319–1355). St. Louis: Mosby Year Book.

Hodgson, B. B., Kizior, R. J., & Kingdon, R. T. (1993). *Nurse's drug handbook.* Philadelphia: W. B. Saunders.

Ignatavicius, D. D., & Bayne, M. V. (1991). *Medical-surgical nursing: A nursing process approach.* Philadelphia: W. B. Saunders.

Jarvis, C. (1992). *Physical examination and health assessment.* Philadelphia: W. B. Saunders.

Johnson, J. L., & Felicetta, J. V. (1992). Hypothyroidism: A comprehensive review. *Journal of the American Academy of Nurse Practitioners, 4*(4), 131–138.

Matteson, M. A., & McConnell, E. S. (1989). *Gerontological nursing.* Philadelphia: W. B. Saunders.

Shlafer, M., & Marieb, E. N. (1989). *The nurse, pharmacology, and drug therapy.* Redwood City, CA: Addison-Wesley.

Sugino, K., Mimura, T., Toshima, K., Iwabuchi, H., Kitamura, Y., Kawano, M., Ozaki, O., & Ito, K. (1993). Follow-up evaluation of patients with Graves' disease treated by subtotal thyroidectomy and risk factor analysis for post-operative thyroid dysfunction. *Journal of Endocrinological Investigation, 16*(3), 195–199.

KEY CONCEPTS

1. Thyroxine, tetraiodothyronine, and calcitonin are hormones produced by the thyroid gland that affect metabolic rate, growth and development, and serum calcium regulation.
2. Hyperthyroidism is the abnormally increased production of thyroid hormones that may be treated with antithyroid drugs, surgery, or radiation therapy.
3. Nursing care of the hyperthyroid patient may address sleep pattern disturbance, hyperthermia, altered nutrition, decreased cardiac output, high risk for injury, diarrhea, and knowledge deficit.
4. Nursing care after thyroidectomy is concerned with ineffective airway clearance, decreased cardiac output, body image disturbance, knowledge deficit, pain, and high risk for infection.
5. Hypothyroidism is inadequate secretion of thyroid hormones that is treated with hormone replacement therapy.
6. Nursing care of the hypothyroid patient addresses activity intolerance, altered nutrition, hypothermia, constipation, high risk for impaired skin integrity, decreased cardiac output, altered thought processes, body image disturbance, and self-care deficits.
7. Goiter is enlargement of simple goiter, thyroid nodules, or thyroiditis that may require treatment with hormone replacement therapy or surgery, or both.
8. The parathyroid glands secrete parathormone, which regulates the serum calcium level.
9. Hyperparathyroidism raises the serum calcium level and may cause bone demineralization and obstruction of kidney tubules.
10. Nursing care of the patient with hyperparathyroidism focuses on activity intolerance, high risk for injury, altered urine elimination, constipation, altered thought processes, altered nutrition, and knowledge deficit.
11. Hypoparathyroidism, a deficiency of parathormone that sometimes follows thyroidectomy, causes the serum calcium level to fall, producing neuromuscular irritability that can progress to seizures, cardiac dysrhythmias, and laryngospasm.
12. Nursing diagnoses for the hypoparathyroid patient are high risk for injury, decreased cardiac output, and knowledge deficit.

Phyllis Karmels
Gayleen Ienatsch

CHAPTER 41

Diabetes Mellitus and Hypoglycemia

OBJECTIVES

1. Describe the role of insulin in the body.
2. Explain the pathophysiology of diabetes mellitus and hypoglycemia.
3. Describe the signs and symptoms of diabetes mellitus and hypoglycemia.
4. Demonstrate knowledge of tests and procedures used to diagnose diabetes mellitus and hypoglycemia.
5. Verbalize treatment of diabetes mellitus and hypoglycemia.
6. Explain the difference between insulin-dependent diabetes mellitus and non–insulin-dependent diabetes mellitus.
7. Differentiate between insulin shock and diabetic ketoacidosis.
8. Describe the treatment of a patient experiencing insulin shock and diabetic ketoacidosis.
9. Describe the complications of diabetes mellitus.
10. Develop a care plan for a patient diagnosed with diabetes mellitus or hypoglycemia.
11. Develop a care plan for a patient diagnosed with ketoacidosis.

GLOSSARY

ENDOGENOUS Internally produced or caused by internal factors

EUGLYCEMIA Normal blood glucose level

GLYCOSURIA Presence of glucose in the urine

HYPOGLYCEMIA Abnormally low level of glucose in the blood

KETOACIDOSIS Metabolic acidosis related to accumulated ketone bodies in the blood

KETONE BODIES Products of fatty acid metabolism

LIPOATROPHY Decreased subcutaneous fat mass

LIPOHYPERTROPHY Increased subcutaneous fat mass

MACROVASCULAR Pertaining to the large blood vessels

MICROVASCULAR Pertaining to the small blood vessels (i.e., arterioles, capillaries, and venules)

NEPHROPATHY Kidney disease

NEUROPATHY Pathologic changes in the peripheral nervous system

POLYDIPSIA Excessive thirst

POLYPHAGIA Excessive food ingestion

POLYURIA Excessive urine output

RETINOPATHY Disease of the retina of the eye

DIABETES MELLITUS

Symptoms of diabetes mellitus (DM) have been reported in the literature throughout history. Not until the early twentieth century did medicine discern the cause of diabetes, as a result of an experiment in which the pancreata of several sheep were removed. These sheep became diabetic. Through this experiment, insulin and its role in the body were discovered. Insulin was made available for use in humans in 1921. Prior to this date, young diabetics were placed on a high-protein diet until they went into acidosis and died, usually a short time after the onset of the disease. In the United States today, DM is a major health problem and a leading cause of death by disease, killing more than 150,000 people annually.

PATHOPHYSIOLOGY

Diabetes mellitus is a heterogeneous collection of symptoms characterized by the body's inability to utilize glucose. It is also a disorder of protein and fat metabolism resulting from an imbalance between the availability of insulin and insulin requirements.

Insulin is a hormone produced by the beta cells in the islets of Langerhans located in the pancreas. This hormone is released into the body in response to carbohydrate ingestion.

Two different types of DM occur; insulin-dependent diabetes mellitus (IDDM) and non–insulin-dependent diabetes mellitus (NIDDM). The absence of endogenous insulin characterizes IDDM, whereas a diminished or inadequate amount of insulin to meet daily requirements characterizes NIDDM.

The more severe form of the disease is IDDM. It was formerly known as type I diabetes mellitus or juvenile-onset diabetes mellitus. Insulin-dependent diabetes usually occurs in juveniles and young adults, but it can also occur in middle-aged and older adults. Affected individuals are usually dependent on daily insulin injections for the rest of their lives.

The less severe form of the disease is NIDDM, or type II diabetes mellitus, in that the pancreas does have some functioning beta cells. In some instances, body tissues may exhibit a decreased response to insulin, or specific receptor sites may become insensitive to insulin. These patients may have to take insulin when first diagnosed in order to get their serum glucose levels down to normal, but their disease may then be controlled by diet and exercise alone or by one of the several hypoglycemic agents that are available today.

Role of Insulin

Table 41–1 summarizes the role of insulin in the body and the effects of insulin deficiency. Insulin stimulates the active transport of glucose into the cells. When insulin is absent, glucose cannot enter most cells, so it remains in the blood stream. The blood then becomes thick with glucose, which increases its osmolality. This increased osmolality stimulates the thirst centers in an effort to dilute the glucose. Thus, the patient experiences polydipsia, or excessive thirst. The increased fluid does not pass into body tissues because of the high serum osmolality. The kidneys, in an effort to reduce the glucose concentration, increase urine output. This activity is called polyuria. Because the cells of the body are not able to use carbohydrates, the body uses fat stores for heat and energy, resulting in weight loss. Tissue breakdown and wasting (burning of lean body mass) send hunger signals to the hypothalamus. The patient experiences excessive hunger, or polyphagia. Unfortunately, the patient cannot utilize the extra food and loses weight despite the increase in appetite and food ingestion.

TABLE 41–1
INSULIN: ACTIONS AND EFFECTS OF DEFICIENCY

INSULIN
- Increases the transport of glucose into the resting muscle cell.
- Regulates the rate at which carbohydrates are used.
- Promotes the conversion of glucose to glycogen.
- Inhibits the conversion of glycogen to glucose.
- Promotes fatty acid synthesis.
- Spares fat.
- Inhibits the breakdown of adipose tissue.
- Inhibits the conversion of fats to glucose.
- Stimulates protein synthesis in the tissues.
- Inhibits the conversion of protein into glucose.

LACK OF INSULIN
- Stimulates the conversion of glycogen to glucose.
- Permits fat stores to break down.
- Increases triglyceride storage in the liver.
- Halts the storage of proteins.
- Causes protein to be dumped into the blood stream.

List compiled by Phyllis Karmels.

Insulin increases the transport of glucose into resting muscle cells, which are nearly impermeable to glucose in the absence of insulin. Note that during heavy exercise, muscle fibers are highly permeable to glucose even in the absence of insulin. Therefore, exercise is very important in the regulation of serum glucose levels.

Insulin regulates the rate at which glucose is metabolized for energy. Even though the pancreas constantly secretes small amounts of insulin, the output of insulin is increased shortly after food is eaten. The greater the insulin response to carbohydrate ingestion, the faster the carbohydrates are metabolized. This phenomenon is often seen in children. They seem to get a burst of energy shortly after eating a piece of candy. This response can occur within a few seconds to a few minutes.

Insulin promotes the conversion of glucose to glycogen, which is stored in the liver. Conversely, insulin inhibits the conversion of glycogen to glucose. More than half of the glucose consumed in a meal is stored in the liver. Lack of insulin stimulates the conversion of glycogen to glucose for use by the body.

Insulin promotes fatty acid synthesis and the conversion of fatty acids into fat, which is stored as adipose tissue. Insulin also spares fat by inhibiting the breakdown of adipose tissue. The presence of insulin increases the rate of glucose utilization, inhibits the mobilization of fat, and inhibits the conversion of fats to glucose.

Lack of insulin permits fat stores to break down and encourages a great increase in the amount of triglycerides to be stored in the liver. The liver can store up to one third of its weight as fat. Increases in fatty acids in the liver cause as much as threefold increase in the production of lipoproteins. This increase promotes the development of atherosclerosis, which explains why people with DM have a high incidence of cardiovascular disease.

Insulin stimulates protein synthesis in tissues but, by the same token, inhibits the conversion of protein into glucose. This works by permitting the entry of amino acids into cells, which enhances the rate of protein formation while preventing the degradation of proteins. Lack of insulin halts the storage of proteins and causes large amounts of amino acids to be dumped into the blood stream. The presence of high levels of plasma amino acids explains why diabetics are at risk for developing gout. This protein wasting leads to extreme weakness as well as to poor organ functioning. Some organs of the body do not depend on insulin for the transport of glucose into them. They are the brain and nerve cells, the lens of the eye, the heart, and exercising muscles.

ETIOLOGY

Some researchers attribute the cause of IDDM as being genetic, immunologic, or environmental (such as viruses). To date, researchers have been unable to isolate a diabetic gene. The tendency for DM to run in families is possibly due to a genetic predisposition or tendency. The tendency for this disease is found in families with the human leukocyte antigen.

One explanation for the sudden onset of diabetes in the young, which may account for this genetic tendency, may be an immune system gone haywire (Fig. 41–1). Our bodies are guarded by an elaborate and extensive immune system. Initially, a microbe and its antigen enter the blood stream and encounter white blood cells called macrophages, which have antigen receptors on their surfaces. These antigen receptors steer the antigens to lymphocytes, which have antigen-specific receptors. When a specific antigen is present, it activates the immune response. The lymphocytes begin producing custom-made antibodies against the antigens, at the same time signaling other types of cells in the immune system to attack the invaders. The lymphocytes and the antibodies are unable to destroy the foreign cells independently without the help of phagocytes and complement cells. This group of cells is selective in identifying and destroying foreign protein. Unfortunately, this part of the immune system can become a renegade faction and turn on its own healthy cells. It is this autoimmune malfunction that can cause complete destruction of the islets of Langerhans in the pancreas, creating IDDM. Islet cell antibodies are identified in more than 80% of all people at the onset of IDDM.

RISK FACTORS

According to the American Diabetes Association, the following groups of people are at risk for diabetes:

- People who are overweight.
- People with a family history of diabetes.
- People who are 40 years of age and older.
- Blacks (have a 33% higher risk for NIDDM).
- Latinos (have a >300% higher risk for NIDDM).
- Native Americans (have a 33–50% higher risk for NIDDM).

COMPLICATIONS

Long-Term Complications

Epidemiologic studies have established that the duration of DM and poor glycemic control are the best correlates of the severity of complications. These complications affect almost every organ of the body. They are generally classified as microvascular, macrovascular, or neuropathic.

MICROVASCULAR COMPLICATIONS

Microvascular changes are unique to DM and are identical in both IDDM and NIDDM patients. These changes cause problems in the eyes and kidneys. Changes in the small blood vessels that impair the exchange of nutrients, gases, and wastes characterize microvascular complications. Neuropathy is sometimes

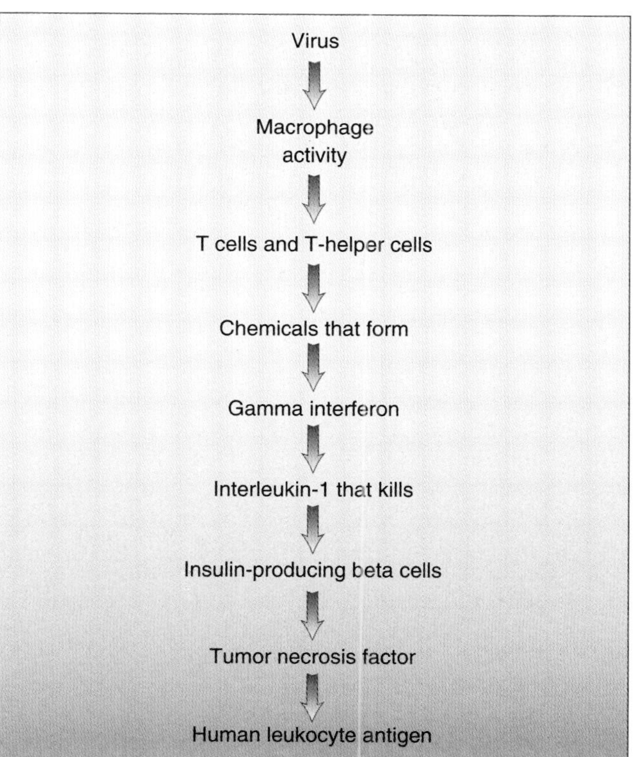

FIGURE 41–1

Possible immunologic cause of diabetes mellitus.

classified with microvascular complications but is discussed separately here.

Retinopathy. The exact cause and pathogenesis of diabetic retinopathy have not been defined. One theory is that it results from retinal hypoxia. Features of diabetic retinopathy include increased capillary permeability and a thickened basement membrane due to leakage of the blood vessels. When there is hemorrhaging into the vitreous, it becomes cloudy and vision is lost. Reabsorption of the blood may cause scarring, which allows pulling on the retina, causing it to detach. Signs and symptoms of impending eye problems are the presence of spots, called floaters, and seeing cobwebs or experiencing sudden visual changes. Patients with either NIDDM or IDDM must be counseled to have frequent eye examinations so that the ophthalmologist can detect early changes in the eye and prevent further deterioration and possible blindness.

Nephropathy. Persons with diabetes account for a large percentage of patients with end-stage renal disease. About one quarter of patients entering dialysis each year or waiting for kidney transplants are diabetics. NIDDM patients often have symptoms of renal disease within 10 years after diagnosis, whereas patients with IDDM often have symptoms within 15 to 20 years. In a patient with DM, the kidneys have an increased workload due to polyuria. High concentrations of glycosuria contribute to thickening of the basement membranes of the kidney. Increased permeability of the glomeruli permits serum proteins to be lost in the urine. The kidney's filtering mechanism is overworked, causing the pressure in these blood vessels to rise. Elevated pressure in the renal vessels, over a period of years, destroys the filtering ability of the kidney. Signs and symptoms of kidney failure include persistent proteinuria, elevated blood pressure, and oliguria or anuria. Diagnosis is made based on laboratory values (see Chapter 36).

MACROVASCULAR COMPLICATIONS. Some experts have theorized that chronic hyperglycemia as a result of poor serum glucose control plays an important role in the premature development of atherosclerosis in patients with DM. The accelerated atherosclerotic changes in the person with diabetes are called macrovascular complications. However, recent research indicates that it is the elevated insulin levels circulating in the blood that play a role in the development of atherosclerosis. Atherosclerotic plaque development occurs earlier and is more severe and more extensive in diabetics than in nondiabetics. The atherosclerosis involves the peripheral, carotid, cerebral, and coronary blood vessels. It is postulated that circulating insulin affects the endothelium of blood vessels, permitting lipids to be easily deposited on the cell walls of the blood vessels. Individuals with DM who have mild hyperlipemia often demonstrate a more rapid development of atherosclerosis than nondiabetics who have moderate to high levels of lipidemia. These changes in the blood vessels often lead to coronary artery disease or cerebral vascular accidents.

Peripheral vascular disease may cause occlusive vascular disease in the lower extremities. Signs and symptoms may include diminished pedal pulses and claudication (pain in the calf, back, or buttocks while walking). When arteries in the lower extremities become totally blocked, gangrene may develop, necessitating subsequent amputations of toes or limbs.

Treatment for macrovascular disease is directed toward weight loss and exercise. With weight loss, circulating insulin levels decrease and insulin uptake improves. As a result of aerobic exercise, insulin receptor sites increase and exogenous insulin levels decrease. Exercise, in conjunction with weight loss, serves to reduce the amount of exogenous insulin needed by the body. When insulin needs are lessened or eliminated, the diabetic's risk for macrovascular disease is reduced.

NEUROPATHIC COMPLICATIONS. Neuropathy is related to poor glucose control and to the effects of circulatory impairment on nerve tissue. It affects about 13% of all diabetics. Patients who have had DM for more than 25 years have a 50% chance of experiencing neuropathies. Several different types of neuropathies can occur. Subacute mixed motor and sensory neuropathy affects both the motor and the sensory nerves and often improves with better control of plasma glucose. Chronic sensory neuropathy, however, does not improve with better control of DM. The patient complains of tingling, numbness, burning, or sharp pains that are usually worse in the legs or arms. These pains are often worse at night or after ingesting alcoholic beverages. Sometimes the pain is relieved by walking. On examination, there is a symmetric, patchy loss of light touch. The patient has difficulty distinguishing between hot and cold sensations. Because the patient has diminished sensorimotor awareness, an unsteady gait develops that may lead to falls and injuries.

Autonomic neuropathy is evident in the form of gustatory sweating (sweating after eating) following a meal containing cheese or spicy foods. Gastrointestinal problems, such as diarrhea or slow stomach emptying, also may develop. Cardiovascular involvement may be seen as postural hypotension resulting in falls, dysrhythmias such as tachycardia, or a fixed heart rate that does not change with vigorous exercise.

The patient may have urinary symptoms such as an atonic bladder, which is seen as retention with overflow in the absence of prostatic obstruction. Sexual problems such as impotence are not uncommon.

Diabetic amyotrophy (loss of muscle size) causes pain in the muscles of the pelvic girdle and thighs. This pain may be so severe that it interferes with activity and sleep. The muscles look wasted, and fasciculation (involuntary twitching, or contraction of muscle fibers) may be visible under the skin. These contractions do not cause movement.

THE DIABETIC FOOT. Foot problems in the diabetic may be caused by an impaired nerve supply, impaired blood supply, or a combination of both. When the nerve supply is impaired but blood flow is adequate, the foot is warm and pink. Good pulses can be felt, but sensation is impaired. Because of this phenomenon, the patient may have an ulcer or necrotic area and be unaware of the problem.

If the blood supply is impaired but the nerve function is adequate, the foot is cold. When the foot is raised, it turns pale. When the foot is lowered, it becomes red. No pulses can be palpated, but sensation is normal.

Neuropathic ulcers can result from injury to the foot in three ways:

- Mechanical irritation such as that caused from rough shoe linings or amateur attempts at shaving calluses or cutting toenails.
- Burns caused from a hot-water bottle, sitting too close to a fire or radiator, or other heat exposure.
- Chemical irritation caused from substances such as salicylic acid, found in many corn plasters.

If the patient can neither see nor feel his or her feet, an unnoticed injury may fester. A neglected callus may become inflamed. Blood and fluid can collect beneath the lesion, which may become infected. An abscess may form that ruptures to form an ulcer. The best treatment is prevention. Listed in Table 41–2 are "dos and don'ts" regarding foot care.

PREVENTING LONG-TERM COMPLICATIONS. The landmark Diabetes Control and Complications Trial found that intensive treatment of IDDM patients delayed the onset or slowed the progress of diabetic retinopathy, nephropathy, and neuropathy. The trial evaluated the effects of tight control of blood glucose levels with multiple daily insulin injections or programmable insulin pumps. Patients were closely monitored and treated by a team of diabetes experts. The authors believe that patients with NIDDM would probably benefit from tight control as well.

Emergency Complications

KETOACIDOSIS. Diabetic ketoacidosis is a life-threatening emergency caused by a lack of insulin or inadequate amounts of insulin. This results in disorders in the metabolism of carbohydrates, fats, and proteins. Signs and symptoms are nausea, vomiting, abdominal pain, constipation, blurred vision, air hunger (seen as Kussmaul's respirations, or rapid and deep respirations), polydipsia, polyuria, tachycardia, dehydration, and hypothermia. The patient with ketoacidosis has high serum glucose levels (>300 mg/dl); ketonuria, with total serum ketone concentration exceeding 3 mmol per liter; and acidosis, with pH less than 7.3 or bicarbonate level less than 15 mEq per liter. The patient may or may not be comatose.

Death can result if prompt medical care is not instituted. The National Diabetes Data Group indicates that 10% of all deaths of persons with DM, as recorded on death certificates, result from ketoacidosis. It is most likely to occur when DM is undiagnosed, when the patient eats too much food and does not take enough insulin, when the uncontrolled IDDM patient exercises too vigorously, or when the patient experiences stress linked to illness, infection, surgery, or emotions. Treatment is aimed at correction of the three main problems: dehydration, electrolyte imbalance, and acidosis.

TABLE 41–2

"DOS AND DON'TS" REGARDING FOOT CARE

DO

Examine your feet daily with a mirror that magnifies images. Look for blisters, cuts and scratches.
Notify your physician if you notice any blisters, scratches, or cuts.
Check between the toes.
Wear white socks. If there is any drainage, it will show up on white socks.
Wash feet daily, rinse well, and dry carefully, especially between the toes.
Inspect the insides of your shoes for foreign objects, torn linings, and rough or sharp points.
Wear socks to bed if your feet are cold.
Lubricate dry feet with baby oil after bathing but do not put the oil between the toes.
Buy shoes that are comfortable at the time of purchase.
Buy shoes made of leather. Check with your physician regarding running shoes or sneakers.
See your physician regularly. Have him or her examine your feet and make sure that he or she knows the status of your diabetes.
Wear wool socks and fleece-lined boots to protect your feet from the cold in winter.

DON'T

Smoke.
Take very hot or cold baths or showers.
Soak feet in hot water.
Use heating pads or hot-water bottles.
Walk barefoot, even in the house.
Walk on hot surfaces such as sidewalks or sandy beaches.
Remove corns or calluses yourself. See a podiatrist for their removal.
Secure bandages with adhesive tape.
Wear garters. Instead, wear well-fitting pantyhose or socks.
Wear stockings with seams.
Wear stockings that have been darned or mended.
Wear socks or stockings that have not been washed since worn last.
Wear shoes without stockings.
Wear sandals with thongs between the toes.
Cross your legs or ankles.

Adapted from Levin, M. E. (1990). Diabetic foot lesions: Pathogenesis and management. *Journal of Enterostomal Therapy, 17*(7), 32.

Dehydration. The patient with ketoacidosis may have lost a large volume of fluid as the result of vomiting, diarrhea, polyuria, and hyperventilation. The first need is to replace the fluid to aid the kidneys in getting rid of excess glucose. The physician usually orders a solution of normal saline to run at 500 to 1000 ml per hour for several hours. If the patient has hypertension or hypernatremia or is at risk for congestive heart failure, the order may be given for 45% saline solution instead of normal saline. After several hours, the physician may reduce the rate to 200 or 300 ml for several more hours.

Electrolyte Imbalance. The electrolyte of primary concern is potassium. With ketoacidosis, a loss of potassium from body stores occurs that is decreased further by fluid loading and subsequent diuresis. Insulin administration also enhances the movement of potassium from the extracellular compartment into the cells. Replacement of potassium is vital because hypokalemia can lead to severe cardiac dysrhythmias. Large doses of potassium may be required even though the serum potassium level is normal at the onset of treatment because the plasma level will drop during treatment. Since potassium is irritating to the veins and a potassium drip must be carefully regulated, it is better to run the bottle of intravenous fluid containing potassium by the piggyback method at a prescribed rate, which will be slower than the hydration rate.

PHARMACOLOGY CAPSULE

When a patient is given insulin to treat diabetic ketoacidosis, monitor for hypokalemia because insulin causes potassium to move from the extracellular fluid into the cells.

Acidosis. Acidosis occurs because ketone bodies accumulate as the result of the breakdown of fats for energy when insulin is absent or insufficient. The presence of insulin inhibits the breakdown of fats, thus preventing ketone body accumulation. Acidosis is treated with the slow intravenous infusion of insulin. When the serum glucose level reaches 250 to 300 mg per dl, the intravenous fluid is changed to dextrose solution. The intravenous insulin drip must be continuous until subcutaneous insulin can be given, or else ketoacidosis may return and be worse than on admission. The serum glucose levels are normal several hours before the serum bicarbonate levels return to normal. When the glucose levels are normal but the serum bicarbonate levels are still abnormal, the insulin drip must be maintained and glucose levels corrected, with more glucose added to the intravenous fluid to cover the insulin. Normal levels of glucose *do not* mean that the acidosis has been corrected. The insulin drip must be maintained until the serum bicarbonate is 15 to 18 mEq per liter. When the patient can eat and take subcutaneous insulin and all laboratory values are normal, the insulin drip may be discontinued.

HYPEROSMOLAR NONKETOTIC COMA. Hyperosmolar nonketotic coma is a condition in which a patient goes into a coma from extremely high glucose levels (≥2000 mg/dl) but there is no evidence of elevated ketones. Apparently, the patient's pancreas produces just enough insulin to prevent the breakdown of fatty acids and the formation of ketones but not enough insulin to prevent hyperglycemia. Hyperglycemia, which causes the increased osmolality, affects the sensorium, causing the patient to lapse into a coma. This may be the first sign that the patient is diabetic. The basic biochemical defect is the lack of effective insulin. The patient's persistent hyperglycemia causes osmotic diuresis, resulting in the loss of fluid and electrolytes. To maintain osmotic equilibrium, fluid shifts from the intracellular fluid space to the extracellular space. The patient experiences hyperglycemia, dehydration, and hypernatremia. Patients in hyperosmolar nonketotic coma do not experience gastrointestinal symptoms nor do they experience Kussmaul's respirations because they lack significant lactic acid levels. These patients often tolerate polyuria and polydipsia for weeks before seeking treatment. This condition may also be brought about by total parenteral nutrition or dialysis because solutions that contain large amounts of glucose are given to the patient but do not go through the digestive system to trigger pancreatic release of insulin.

MEDICAL DIAGNOSIS

The diagnosis of diabetes is based on serum glucose levels. The normal fasting serum glucose levels are between 80 and 120 mg per dl. Nonfasting glucose levels of greater than 140 mg per dl are a cause for further investigation. A patient is considered to have DM if he or she meets one or more of the following criteria:

- A fasting glucose level of 140 mg per dl or greater on at least two occasions
- A random glucose level of 200 mg per dl or greater
- The presence of the classic symptoms of DM: polyphagia (excessive hunger), polydipsia (excessive thirst), polyuria (excessive urinary output), and weight loss without dieting
- A fasting glucose level of less than 140 mg per dl plus a sustained elevated plasma glucose level during at least two oral glucose tolerance tests

Impaired Glucose Tolerance Test

Impaired glucose tolerance is indicated by a glucose tolerance test that shows the presence of moderately high glucose levels; that is, levels that are between normal levels and diabetic levels. These moderately high glucose levels may increase until the patient has overt diabetes, or they may decrease until the patient has normal glucose levels. However, in many cases they may remain unchanged.

The diagnosis of impaired glucose tolerance is based on a fasting serum glucose level of less than 140 mg per dl and a 2-hour postprandial (after a meal) level equal to or greater than 140 mg per dl but less than 200 mg per dl with one intervening value equal to or greater than 200 mg per dl.

Oral Glucose Tolerance Test

The oral glucose tolerance test is performed when a patient is suspected of having DM. The literature advises that the patient consume a diet composed of 150 to 300 grams of carbohydrates for 3 days prior to the test. Some physicians tell their patients to eat their normal diet. The night before the test, the patient is instructed to fast after midnight. On the morning of the test, a sample of blood is drawn for a fasting serum glucose test. The patient is then given a drink (glucola) containing 75 grams of carbohydrates and instructions to remain quiet. This drink is quite sweet and should be served very cold in order to deaden the taste buds. In certain situations, the glucose can be given by the intravenous route, but this method is not as accurate as the oral route. Blood is then drawn at 30 minutes and 1 hour after the ingestion of glucose. Following these two samples, blood is drawn at hourly intervals until the test is completed. Most physicians order either a 3-hour or a 5-hour oral glucose tolerance test. Because blood must be drawn several times, it may be best to insert a heparin lock into the vein at the time blood is obtained for the fasting blood sugar. This will eliminate the need to puncture the skin more than once.

MEDICAL TREATMENT

The goals of managing diabetes are to help the patient remain euglycemic (having normal blood glucose) while meeting energy needs and achieving ideal body weight for age, sex, and body build. Ideal body weight for females can be calculated by assigning 100 pounds for the first 5 feet of height. For each additional inch, 5 pounds should be added. For example, a woman with an average body build who is 5 feet 5 inches tall should weigh 125 pounds. The ideal body weight for a man of medium build would be calculated at 106 pounds for the first 5 feet of height and 6 pounds for each additional inch. For example, a man who is of medium build and is 5 feet 11 inches tall should weigh 172 pounds.

To determine obesity, the percentage of ideal body weight is calculated. If a person is 110 to 129% of ideal body weight, he or she is considered overweight. A person who is 130 to 199% of ideal body weight is considered obese. A person who is 200% or greater of ideal body weight is considered morbidly obese.

Dietary Management

To maintain weight, calories are calculated based on 28 calories per kg of body weight. To reduce weight, the caloric intake is calculated based on 15 to 20 calories per kg of body weight. To arrive at weight in kilograms, the weight in pounds is divided by 2.2. If a woman weighs 110 pounds, her weight in kilograms would be 55 kg. To maintain her weight, she would need to consume 1540 calories daily.

The American Diabetes Association recommends that carbohydrates compose 55 to 60% of the total calories daily. These calories should be evenly distributed throughout the day to avoid fluctuations in serum glucose levels.

It is recommended that protein represent 12 to 20% of the caloric intake. The American Diabetes Association cautions that greater than 20% of the daily intake of calories in protein may be associated with an increase in glomerular filtration rate. Sustained increases in glomerular filtration rate cause renal and retinal vasodilation, leading to renal damage and retinopathy.

Fat should represent 30% or less of the daily total caloric intake. Ten percent or less of these fat calories should come from saturated fats such as animal fats, egg yolks, coconut oil, palm kernel oil, palm oil, and hydrogenated vegetable oils. Another 10% of total fat calories should come from polyunsaturated fats such as are found in corn oil, safflower oil, and most nuts. The rest of the fat should come from monounsaturated fats such as those found in peanut oil, olive oil, canola oil, sesame oil, and avocado. Cholesterol should not exceed 300 mg per day. Sodium should not exceed 3000 mg per day and may be modified for medical reasons.

Elevated serum cholesterol and triglyceride levels are often associated with NIDDM, increasing the risk of cardiovascular disease. Research in the past several years has indicated that replacing some of the allotted fat calories with calories from carbohydrates and fiber has a positive effect on the lipid profile. The exception is the patient who has glucose intolerance. The addition of water-soluble fibers in the daily diet may lower total cholesterol and low-density lipoprotein levels by a significant margin. In addition, the lower fat intake permits increased insulin binding to receptor sites, resulting in insulin sparing. Foods containing soluble fibers include oatmeal, rice, dried beans, oat bran, lentils, squash, whole wheat breads, and some fruits.

The potential glucose-lowering effect of fiber in the diet may be due to the slower rate of glucose absorption from the gastrointestinal tract. When fiber is added to the diet, it should be done gradually. A sudden addition of fiber to the diet may reduce the amount of glucose available for the exogenous insulin or hypoglycemic agent taken by the patient and may result in hypoglycemic episodes. The 1986 Exchange List for Meal Planning is a very good guide for adding fiber to the diet.

The nondiabetic can plan meals based on the four main food groups:

- Bread/cereal/starches
- Milk/cheese
- Meat/poultry/fish
- Fruit and vegetables

For the patient who has diabetes, fruit and vegetables are not interchangeable. The exchange list for diabetics consists of six food groups:

- Bread/starches
- Fruit
- Vegetables, type 1 and type 2
- Meat
- Milk/dairy
- Fat

Foods included in one list are similar in calories, protein, fat, and carbohydrates to other lists and may be exchanged to add variety to meals. For example, two bread exchanges are equal to a bagel or a plain bun such as a hot dog roll. Exchanges for a variety of foods are published in several books that are available to the public. In addition, food companies often include the exchanges on the packaging of their frozen dinners and other products.

It is important to include ethnic foods, when appropriate, in order to encourage compliance with the diet. For example, a taco made with hamburger meat, browned and drained well, with grated skim milk cheese, lettuce, and a diced tomato may include the following:

- One bread exchange
- One or two meat exchanges (depending on amount)
- One vegetable exchange

- One milk exchange
- One fat exchange

It is important to teach the patient to read labels when purchasing packaged or canned foods. Patient teaching should include sample menus composed of as many favorite foods as possible. For help with this aspect of teaching, the hospital or extended care facility dietitian is a good resource and should be consulted. The home health nurse can reinforce teaching at home.

Exercise

Exercise is a very effective treatment adjunct to improve insulin sensitivity. A single episode of exercise results in a dramatic decrease in serum glucose. The exercising muscle does not need insulin to utilize glucose. Furthermore, the exercising muscle utilizes glucose at 20 times the rate of a muscle at rest. Research suggests that exercise is quite effective in controlling plasma glucose levels in persons with glucose intolerance or with moderate NIDDM. Exercise affects IDDM patients differently than those with NIDDM. In NIDDM patients, exercise not only lowers plasma glucose levels, it makes insulin receptor sites more sensitive to insulin.

Much of the morbidity and mortality in NIDDM patients occurs because of increased atherosclerosis, which accompanies long-term diabetes and which places the patient at greater risk than the general population for stroke and cardiovascular disease. Exercise is known to produce more favorable low-density lipoprotein levels, serum glucose levels, blood pressure levels, some blood coagulation parameters, and decreased triglyceride levels. However, exercise must be accompanied by an appropriate diet in order to have long-term beneficial results in the general population. This is especially true in the diabetic population.

For the NIDDM patient, aerobic exercise produces the most therapeutic effect. The patient should exercise nonstop for 30 to 60 minutes three to four times a week. Warm-up and cool-down exercises are recommended prior to exercise, such as stretching and walking prior to jogging. The best aerobic exercises are walking, swimming, bicycle riding, and jogging. Eventually, the NIDDM patient who adheres to a sound diet and exercise regimen will be able to decrease the amount of exogenous insulin or hypoglycemic agents needed.

For the IDDM patient, exercise can be dangerous. When exercising, the liver may release more glucose than is metabolized and, in effect, actually raise the blood sugar. If the pancreas is not producing insulin, the body will mobilize free fatty acids, causing ketone bodies to form. In this manner, exercise will increase the hazard of ketosis in IDDM patients.

Both IDDM and NIDDM patients should shun exercise if their serum glucose levels are 300 mg per dl or greater. The circulating insulin may be inadequate to ensure glucose uptake. Another problem could be that exercise may utilize too much glucose, leaving an excess of insulin in the blood stream, which could cause a hypoglycemic episode.

IDDM patients need to take some precautions, including avoiding injecting insulin in an area that is exercised during a workout, such as the leg prior to walking or jogging, and ensuring that exercise does not coincide with peak insulin activity. Finally, they should eat a snack before or during exercise to prevent hypoglycemia.

Insulin Therapy

All IDDM patients need insulin injections, and some NIDDM patients may need insulin at times. Insulins are classified by their onset of action, peak action, or duration of action. Insulins are also designated as beef, pork, or beef-pork; semisynthetic human; or biosynthetic human. Because of differences in amino acid structure, insulins vary in antigenicity (the ability to provoke an antibody response). Circulating antibodies bind with insulin and delay its effects. High antigenicity in an insulin causes it to be released more slowly. Thus, a long-acting insulin such as protamine zinc insulin is released very slowly and lasts up to 36 hours in the body. Regular insulin has a low antigenicity and is released 30 to 60 minutes after injection (Fig. 41–2).

PHARMACOLOGY CAPSULE

Regular insulin acts rapidly; NPH has an intermediate duration, and protamine zinc and Ultralente insulin are long acting. Be sure to administer the correct type!

CONCENTRATIONS. Insulins are available in varying concentrations. The insulin with the lowest concentration, U-40, meaning 40 units of insulin per ml, is rarely used today. The insulin U-100 has a concentration of

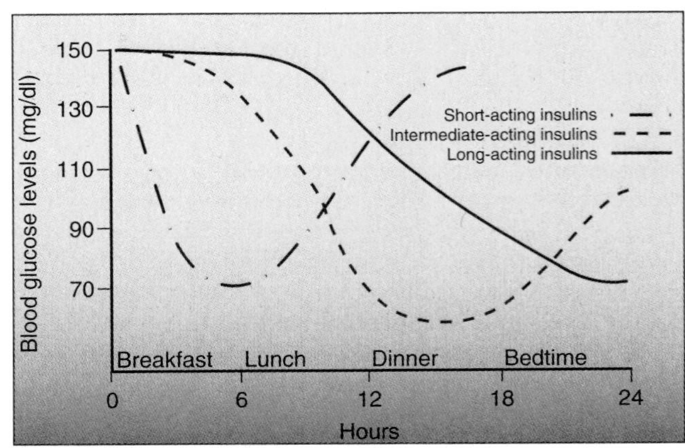

FIGURE 41–2

Effect of insulin on blood glucose levels. (Adapted from American Diabetes Association. [1992]. *Teaching standards for diabetes mellitus* [5th ed.]. Austin, TX: American Diabetes Association, Texas Affiliate, Inc.)

100 units of insulin per ml, and U-500 has 500 units of insulin per ml. The latter is used for patients who are insulin resistant. Patients who have been on pork or beef insulin for a period of time build up antibodies and require increasing amounts of insulin to overcome resistance and to be effective. Human insulin has less immunogenic effect than animal insulins, and the patient does not need as high a dose of insulin to be effective.

The starting dose of insulin for IDDM patients is usually between 0.5 and 1 units per kg of body weight per day. The prescription for insulin, including times, types, and amounts, is written to mimic the action of a normal pancreas. The pancreas secretes minute amounts of insulin continuously. After the ingestion of a meal, the pancreas pours a bolus of insulin into the system. The physician prescribes a long-acting or an intermediate-acting insulin, which releases insulin slowly into the body to keep glucose levels fairly even. At mealtimes, the body requires a bolus of insulin to prevent too rapid a rise in glucose. For this reason, regular insulin is prescribed prior to a meal. Most diabetics who are insulin dependent are controlled with a combination of regular insulin and long-acting or intermediate-acting insulin. The long-acting and intermediate-acting insulins have protein (Lente) or protamine zinc, respectively, added to slow their release.

Many physicians use the one-fifth rule for prescribing insulin. In the morning, the patient takes two fifths of the day's supply in an intermediate-acting insulin such as NPH. In addition, the patient takes one fifth of the daily requirement of insulin as regular insulin. The latter will cover breakfast glucose. Because the NPH will peak at lunchtime, the patient will not need regular insulin for this meal. At suppertime, the patient will take one fifth of the daily insulin requirement in the form of an intermediate-acting insulin and one fifth of regular insulin to cover supper carbohydrates. The patient then needs a snack before retiring to cover the evening NPH insulin peak. Thus, a patient who is prescribed 50 units of insulin a day would take it as follows:

A.M.: 20 units of NPH insulin
10 units of regular insulin
P.M.: 10 units of NPH insulin
10 units of regular insulin

INSULIN MIXING. Following are directions for mixing insulins:

1. Get out both bottles of insulin. The regular insulin will have a large R on the label.
2. Have alcohol wipes ready.
3. Check the physician's orders.
4. Make sure the patient's meal tray is on the unit.
5. To prevent bubbles, roll (do not shake) the bottle of longer-acting insulin. Insulin will normally appear cloudy except for regular insulin, which is clear.
6. Wipe tops of both bottles with alcohol wipes.
7. Draw up the proper amount of air for the longer-acting insulin and inject it into that bottle.
8. Next, draw up the proper amount of air for the regular insulin and inject it into that bottle.
9. Withdraw the prescribed amount of regular insulin.
10. After removing the needle from the bottle, draw 1/10 ml of air into the syringe. Prepare the top of the longer-acting insulin again and withdraw the prescribed amount of this insulin.
11. Change needles if the original needle becomes dulled and administer the insulin.

PHARMACOLOGY CAPSULE

When mixing regular and longer-acting insulins, draw the regular insulin into the syringe first.

INSULIN INJECTION. The following are suggested rotation sites:

- The outer area of the upper arm.
- The abdomen just above and below the waist (except a 2-inch circle directly around the navel).
- The upper area of the buttocks, just in back of the iliac.
- The front of the thigh on the outer aspect, about 4 inches down from the torso and 4 inches above the knee (Fig. 41–3).

Site rotation helps prevent lipohypertrophy (swelling or lumps) or lipoatrophy (hollowing or pitting of the subcutaneous tissue). Patients with the latter problem should see a physician regarding changing the insulin to human insulin (Humulin). In some cases, injecting these sites with their prescribed daily human insulin has resolved the problem. Since lipohypertrophy interferes with the absorption of insulin, these areas should be avoided as injection sites.

The absorption rate of insulin varies with different body sites. The rate of absorption from the abdomen is about 50% faster than from the thighs. For this reason, some experts recommend rotating sites within one anatomic area rather than moving among all areas. Heat and massage increase the absorption rate. Another event that increases the rate of absorption is exercise. If insulin is injected into the thigh prior to exercise such as jogging, the absorption rate is greatly increased.

INSULIN PUMP. The insulin pump is composed of a battery-driven syringe with a long piece of tubing (usually made of Teflon) that is attached to a needle, which is placed subcutaneously in an appropriate part of the anatomy (Fig. 41–4). The syringe usually contains a 3-day supply of insulin, which gives the patient a steady trickle of insulin throughout the day and a bolus of insulin at mealtimes. In this manner, the unit mimics the pancreas. The patient calculates the bolus based on self-monitored blood glucose levels. Every 3 days, the syringe, the needle, and the tubing are replaced.

An advantage of the insulin pump is that patients do not have to use intermediate- or long-acting insulins, with their uncertain peaks and valleys. Other advantages are that it gives the patient more flexibility regarding

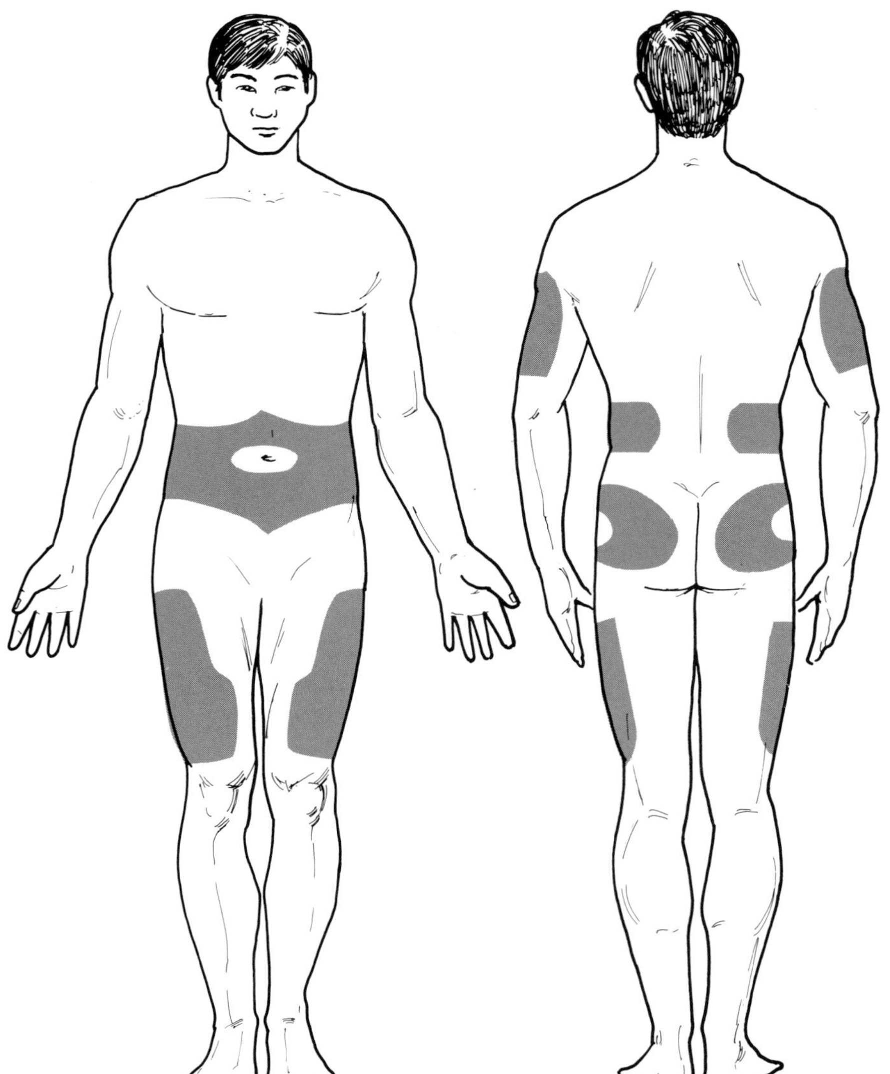

FIGURE 41–3
Injection sites. (From American Diabetes Association. [1986]. *Teaching standards for diabetes mellitus* [4th ed., p. 48]. Austin, TX: American Diabetes Association, Texas Affiliate, Inc., Capital Area Chapter.)

mealtimes, travel, and exercise. Some disadvantages of the pump are that the battery may die, the tubing may become occluded, the needle may become clogged, or infection may occur at the site of insertion. The pump is also a constant reminder that the patient has diabetes, and it often is visible to others, which may have some bearing on a negative body image. In order to use the pump, the patient must undergo intensive education and be willing to self-monitor blood glucose levels several times a day while on pump therapy. Some medical insurance companies do not cover the cost of the pump or pump therapy, which makes the cost prohibitive to many diabetics.

Oral Hypoglycemic Agents

When diet and exercise fail to control diabetes, that is, NIDDM diabetics are unable to restore euglycemia or serum glucose levels are below 300 mg per dl, the physician usually prescribes an oral hypoglycemic agent. It should be noted that if the serum glucose level rises above 300 mg per dl, insulin may be prescribed until the blood glucose levels are back below 300 mg per dl. Oral hypoglycemic drugs are sulfonylureas, which lower blood sugars by stimulating the pancreas to secrete more insulin. The drugs also have the effect of improving insulin action inside the cell and lowering glucose production by the liver.

Two principal groups of oral hypoglycemic agents exist (Table 41–3). These are first- and second-generation sulfonylureas. They are equally effective in controlling serum glucose. If a patient becomes resistant to first-generation drugs, he or she may be switched to a second-generation drug. The second-generation drugs have fewer side effects and are not as likely to react with other medications taken by the patient. Drugs with a long half-life are contraindicated in elderly diabetics because these patients do not metabolize drugs rapidly. When oral hypoglycemic agents are ordered for the elderly patient, usually one of two is prescribed. They are

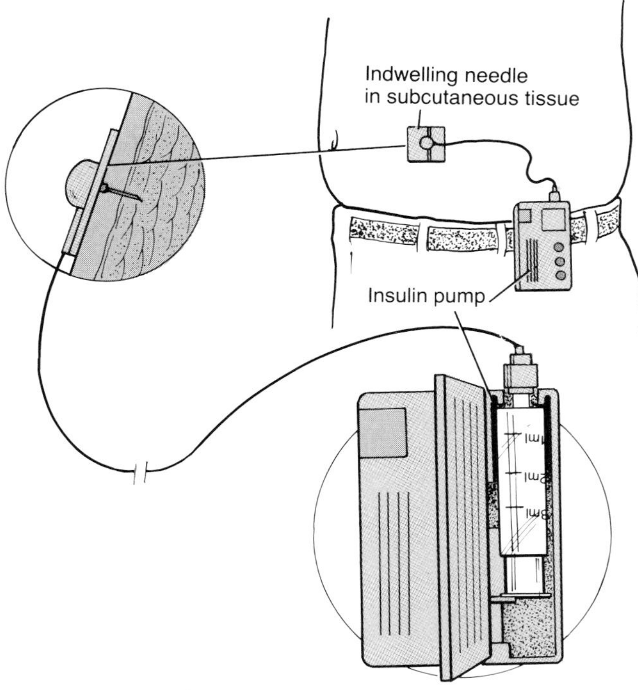

FIGURE 41-4

An insulin pump in use. (Adapted from Black, J. M., & Matassarin-Jacobs, E. [1993]. *Luckmann and Sorensen's medica'-surgical nursing: A psychophysiologic approach* [4th ed., p. 1785]. Philadelphia: W. B. Saunders.)

glipizide (Glucotrol), which must be taken on an empty stomach, and glyburide (DiaBeta, Micronase).

The problem with first-generation drugs is that they bind to protein sites in competition with aspirin, phenytoin (Dilantin), and sulfinpyrazone (Anturane). Although the second-generation drugs are also protein bound, they do not interfere with the binding mechanism or metabolism of other agents, and they are usually metabolized by the liver into inert compounds.

Decreased renal function in the elderly makes them more prone to hypoglycemia—a compelling reason for avoiding long-acting drugs. Chlorpropamide (Diabinese, Glucamide) is the worst drug choice for the very elderly patient because of its 60-hour duration of action and hepatic conversion to active metabolites.

Tolbutamide (Orinase) has the shortest duration of action of the sulfonylureas, 6 to 12 hours. This makes it a good choice for a patient with hepatic insufficiency. But, because it is a first-generation drug, it may not be the drug of choice for a patient taking other medications.

Use of oral agents in the treatment of DM involves a risk of hypoglycemia. To minimize this risk, the patient is placed on the lowest dose possible of a short-acting or an intermediate-acting drug with instructions, and the nurse ensures that the patient understands the importance of eating regularly.

Approximately 30 to 40% of patients with NIDDM fail to respond to oral hypoglycemic agents. Another 10% cease to respond after a period of successful treatment. These patients have to go on an insulin regimen. Some of them may have to take one dose of insulin in the morning and then may be able to control serum glucose for the rest of the day with sulfonylureas. A variety of combination regimens (using oral agents and insulin) are being studied.

Newly diagnosed NIDDM patients may be placed on insulin to get their plasma glucose levels within normal limits. They are then placed on a diet and exercise program with or without oral hypoglycemic agents to maintain euglycemia.

Self-Monitoring of Blood Glucose

Patients who require insulin injections need to self-monitor blood glucose levels in order to regulate their

TABLE 41-3

CHARACTERISTICS OF SULFONYLUREA AGENTS

Generic Name	Brand Name	Daily Dosage Range (mg)	Duration of Action (hr)	Comments
First-Generation Sulfonylureas				
Tolbutamide	Orinase	500–3000	6–12	Metabolized by liver to an inactive product; given two to three times a day
Acetohexamide	Dymelor	250–1500	12–18	Metabolized by liver to active metabolite; given one to two times a day
Tolazamide	Tolinase	100–1000	12–24	Metabolized by liver to both active and inactive products; given one to two times a day
Chlorpropamide	Diabinese	100–500	60	Metabolized by liver (~70%) to less active metabolites and excreted intact (~30%) by kidneys; can potentiate antidiuretic hormone action; given once a day
Second-Generation Sulfonylureas				
Glipizide	Glucotrol	5–40	12–24	Metabolized by liver to inert products; given one to two times a day
Glyburide	DiaBeta, Micronase	2.5–20	16–24	Metabolized by liver to mostly inert products; given one to two times a day

Compiled by Phyllis Karmels.

diet, exercise, and insulin regimens to remain euglycemic and lead as near to normal lifestyles as possible.

The self-monitoring of blood glucose levels is seen as the greatest breakthrough in managing diabetes since the advent of insulin. It plays a decisive role in normalizing these levels, thus reducing the complications of long-term DM.

One of several methods of self-monitoring may be used. Most of them require a drop of blood taken from the side of the finger and placed on a reagent strip. After a specified length of time, the blood is wiped or rinsed off and the color change is compared with a color chart provided by the manufacturer that indicates the serum glucose level. If the patient has a problem distinguishing colors, this method may not be appropriate.

Some newer methods require the use of a meter. The patient inserts the reagent strip with its drop of blood in the meter. In less than a minute, the serum glucose level appears on a monitor. Factors that may affect the use of these meters include cost, comfort with technology, fine motor coordination, intellectual ability, and willingness to use the meter. In managing the pregnant diabetic, whose glucose levels may change hourly, self-monitoring is a useful tool. It is also a must in managing unstable diabetics and individuals who are prone to hypoglycemic episodes without warning and to ketoacidosis or to abnormal renal glucose thresholds.

Glycosylated Glucose Levels

Determination of glycosylated hemoglobin (HbA_{1c}) or fructosamine levels every 2 to 3 months is an essential check of glycemic control. The HbA_{1c} levels reflect glucose levels over the past few months, whereas the fructosamine levels reflect those over several weeks. When glucose levels are elevated, a certain percentage of the glucose molecules bind to the hemoglobin on the red blood cell. If the patient has ingested a lot of carbohydrates, a high percentage of glucose adheres to the red blood cell. The glucose stays on the cell for the life of the cell, which is about 3 months. By drawing HbA_{1c} or fructosamine levels, the physician is able to determine how compliant the patient has been regarding carbohydrate intake. It also allows patients who monitor their blood glucose levels at home to determine how well their methods of control are working.

Complications of Therapy

HYPOGLYCEMIA. The major complication of insulin therapy is hypoglycemia. If a person injects too much insulin, does not eat enough, or exercises too vigorously, serum glucose levels may suddenly drop. The signs and symptoms of hypoglycemia are shakiness, nervousness, irritability, tachycardia, anxiety, lightheadedness, hunger, tingling or numbness on the lips or tongue, nightmares, and crying out during sleep. Glucose levels between 50 and 70 mg per dl are considered moderate hypoglycemia for most diabetics. However, some diabetics have been known to have serum glucose levels below 50 mg per dl and not to experience the signs and symptoms of hypoglycemia.

If treatment is delayed, a second set of symptoms may appear (caused by a shortage of glucose to the brain). However, if the glucose levels are falling rapidly, they may be the first signs of hypoglycemia. These include sleepiness, anger, stubbornness, sadness, lack of coordination, blurred vision, nausea, headaches, strange behavior, confusion, delirium, seizures, and unconsciousness.

Treatment. To treat hypoglycemia, the patient is given one of the following:

- 120 ml or one half glass of undiluted orange or apple juice
- 90 ml of a cola-type soft drink
- 4 tablespoons of a light or dark corn syrup
- 4 tablespoons of jelly or jam
- Five or six pieces of hard candy
- One or two glucose tablets

The IDDM patient should always carry, or keep near at hand, glucagon injectable. If the patient is unable to swallow, an injection of glucagon, intramuscularly or subcutaneously, should be given. The patient should be given an additional treatment of some form of glucose in 10 to 15 minutes. To prevent rebound hypoglycemia when the episode of hypoglycemia occurs in the evening, or if it will be an hour or more until the next meal, the patient should be given one slice of cheese and a slice of bread or other form of complex carbohydrate.

INSULIN SHOCK. When a patient goes into insulin shock, oral liquids or foods should not be given. A 50-ml bolus of 50% dextrose is ordered by the physician, to be given by the intravenous route. The patient may be placed on an intravenous drip of 10 or 20% dextrose in water. If the patient is not in the hospital and is unable to swallow, a solution of 2 tablespoons of honey or light or dark corn syrup dissolved in 4 ounces of tap water may be instilled in the rectum. It should be given slowly and the buttocks held together after instillation to facilitate absorption.

SOMOGYI EFFECT. Too much insulin can actually cause hyperglycemia. The Somogyi effect is a rebound response that occurs in the presence of too much insulin. The stress caused by hypoglycemia triggers the body's ability to mobilize its forces in times of stress for the purpose of maintaining homeostasis. The body can overreact and boost the serum glucose levels to the point of hyperglycemia. This response soon wears off, and the serum glucose levels return to normal. However, hyperglycemia can be induced by insulin and is associated with a strong antagonistic response to insulin, which the layperson tries to overcome by giving himself or herself more insulin. It occurs when a patient is unaware that serum glucose levels are low and gives the next scheduled dose of insulin, or when a patient experiences an episode of hyperglycemia and takes too much insulin to compensate.

The low serum glucose induced by too much insulin triggers the release of epinephrine, which can stimulate the liver to release glycogen and deplete its stores of glucose so that fats are mobilized for energy and to make more glucose. The dynamic combination of low blood glucose and epinephrine also stimulates the pituitary to release growth hormone and adrenocorticotropic hormone. The latter stimulates the release of glucocorticoids, which stimulate the liver to make glucose from proteins. This glucose molecule is impervious to insulin. Furthermore, epinephrine, adrenocorticotropic hormone, cortisol, glucagon, and growth hormone conserve vital nutrition by inhibiting glucose use in the peripheral cell. Thus, by increasing insulin, the patient sets up a vicious cycle that can be cured only by gradually decreasing the amount of exogenous insulin by 2 or 3 units every 3 or 4 days until the rebound hyperglycemia is brought under control.

NURSING CARE OF THE PATIENT WITH DIABETES MELLITUS

Assessment

A complete assessment may have to be delayed until the patient is stable (see Care Plan: The Patient with Insulin-Dependent Diabetes Mellitus). Patients admitted with a diagnosis of ketoacidosis are assessed for ketonuria, Kussmaul's respirations, orthostatic hypotension, hypertension at times, nausea, vomiting, and lethargy or loss of consciousness. The nurse is also alert for indications of hyperosmolar nonketotic coma (decreased level of consciousness, polyuria, and polydipsia in the absence of ketosis). The hypoglycemic patient is assessed for tachycardia, anxiety, trembling, and decreasing level of consciousness. In each of these situations, the nurse attempts to determine the following:

- Type of diabetes
- Hypoglycemic agents: name, dosage, when last dose was taken
- Food and fluid intake for the last 3 days
- Relevant laboratory values: blood pH, bicarbonate levels, electrolytes, and osmolality and urine osmolality

HEALTH HISTORY. When the patient's condition has stabilized, a more complete assessment is done. The health history is focused on the signs and symptoms of chronic hyperglycemia and possible complications. It also elicits physical and psychosocial factors that may have an impact on the patient's capacity to learn and perform self-care activities.

Chief Complaint and History of Present Illness. During the patient interview, the patient is asked to describe the signs and symptoms that prompted him or her to seek medical care. That is, did the patient experience any of the following: polyphagia, polydipsia, polyuria, unexplained weight loss, dryness of skin, vaginal itching, or sores that were slow in healing? The nurse needs to know the blood glucose levels and presence or absence of urine ketones if this information is available.

Past Medical History. If the patient is known to have DM, the nurse inquires about the type and duration. The name and dosage of the prescribed hypoglycemic agent is recorded, noting when it was last taken. If the patient monitors blood glucose or urine ketones, the nurse asks about the type of equipment used, the testing schedule, and recent test results.

The nurse documents a history of circulatory, cardiac, or renal problems. Previous hospitalizations and surgeries are recorded. If the client is female, the nurse takes an obstetric history, including number of pregnancies, if any, outcomes of all pregnancies, and birth weights of full-term infants. For patients who had gestational diabetes, the nurse determines whether insulin was required or whether diet and exercise maintained adequate control. Other important data to collect are immunization records and allergies.

Family History. The nurse assesses the patient for family history of DM, heart disease, or stroke.

Review of Systems. The review of symptoms begins by asking about the patient's general health. The nurse then asks if the patient has noticed changes in skin moisture or turgor. To detect possible changes in the eyes associated with DM, the nurse inquires whether the patient has had floaters (dark spots that cross the field of vision), diplopia (double vision), or blurred vision or has seen white halos around objects. Significant abdominal symptoms to be assessed are diarrhea, abdominal bloating, and gas. Problems passing or holding urine are documented. The nurse also determines whether the patient has any pain in the legs and, if so, when the pain occurs. Numbness in the extremities also is recorded. Last, the nurse asks if the patient has experienced changes in mental alertness or seizures.

Functional Assessment. The functional assessment explores factors that can affect the patient's ability to perform self-care, including literacy, financial resources such as health insurance, and family support. The patient is asked to describe the usual pattern of activity and rest. A typical 24-hour dietary history is recorded. The nurse also explores the impact of DM on the patient's life, including self-concept, social relationships, and employment.

PHYSICAL EXAMINATION. The patient is assessed head to toe using inspection, auscultation, palpation, and percussion. In the general survey, the nurse notes the patient's level of consciousness, posture and gait, and apparent well-being. Vital signs, including blood pressure, and height and weight measurements are taken. The skin is inspected throughout the examination for color, warmth, turgor, and the presence of poorly healed lesions.

The trained examiner inspects the eye grounds for evidence of diabetic retinopathy or cataracts. The vision assessment is important because visual defects may affect the patient's ability to read vital medication instructions or labels. Gross visual acuity may be assessed by having the patient read available print. Snellen's test and other, more sophisticated measures also may be used to

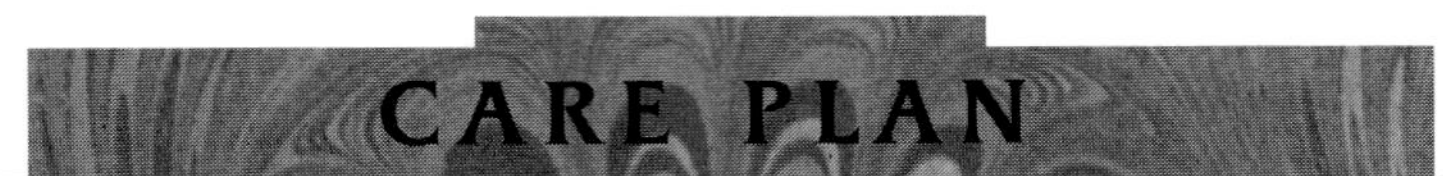

CARE PLAN
The Patient with IDDM

ASSESSMENT

Health History: Myra Frieberger is a 17-year-old female who has recently been diagnosed with insulin-dependent diabetes mellitus (IDDM). She was hospitalized to begin her insulin therapy and stabilize her blood glucose. She sought medical attention because of persistent thirst and increased urination. She has no other health problems but has had frequent upper respiratory infections the last few years. The review of systems reveals periodic blurred vision, itching, increased appetite, weight loss of 7 pounds in 3 months, and fatigue.

Physical Examination: Vital signs: temperature, 98.4°F orally; pulse, 88; respiration, 14; blood pressure, 92/58. Height, 5′2″. Weight, 107 lb. Physical findings are all within normal limits.

NURSING DIAGNOSIS	GOALS AND OUTCOME CRITERIA	INTERVENTIONS
Altered health maintenance related to lack of knowledge of diabetes management.	The patient will correctly describe IDDM and its treatment. Patient will demonstrate self-medication, meal planning, and understanding of management of exercise and drug effects.	Explain the physiology of glucose metabolism, signs and symptoms of ketoacidosis, and hypoglycemia. Teach to perform self-monitoring of blood glucose and urine ketone testing and how to interpret results. Explain insulin types, actions, and administration. Have patient practice insulin injection. Explain relationship between diet, exercise, insulin, and blood glucose. Obtain dietary consult regarding diet. Monitor food intake and replace food not eaten with substitute identified by dietitian.
Noncompliance related to monetary, personal, or family pattern disruption.	The patient will express intent to adhere to prescribed regimen of care.	Request patient education by certified diabetes educator if available. If not, present information in a positive manner and in small units. Identify barriers to adhering to regimen. Determine resources and sources of support. Have patient repeat aspects of care and consequences of nonadherence to program. Acknowledge difficulty in making major changes in eating and activity patterns and in administering self-injections. Identify community resources such as the local chapter of the American Diabetes Association. Teach the patient and family members to recognize and respond to hypoglycemia and ketoacidosis.
Fluid volume deficit related to altered urine output.	The patient will maintain normal blood volume as evidenced by normal tissue turgor, pulse, and blood pressure.	Stress the importance of drinking at least eight glasses of water daily. Point out that excessive urine output may indicate hyperglycemia. Assess hydration, including tissue turgor, mucous membrane moisture, and vital signs.
High risk for injury related to adverse effects of drugs, increased susceptibility to infection.	The patient's blood glucose will remain within goal range established by physician. The patient will state measures to reduce risk of infection and will identify symptoms that should be reported to physician.	Teach patient to recognize signs and symptoms of hypoglycemia: shakiness, nervousness, irritability, tachycardia, anxiety, lightheadedness, hunger, tingling or numbness of lips and tongue. Instruct to take concentrated sugar if hypoglycemia occurs, followed by a complex carbohydrate (milk, bread) to prevent rebound hypoglycemia. The patient should contact the physician if ill and unable to take food or fluids. Caution the patient that

The Patient with IDDM *(Continued)*

NURSING DIAGNOSIS	GOALS AND OUTCOME CRITERIA	INTERVENTIONS
		impaired sensation could develop in the extremities and that healing of injuries may be impaired. Encourage to avoid trauma and to inspect the feet daily to detect any injuries.
Activity intolerance related to metabolic imbalance.	The patient will perform usual activities of daily living and carry out planned exercise program without excess fatigue.	An exercise regimen is built into the plan of care. Exercise must be done as part of a regular routine. Tell the patient to avoid injecting insulin into a body area that will be affected by exercise soon after the injection. Patient should not exercise during peak insulin activity, and should eat a snack before or during exercise to avoid hypoglycemia.
Sensory-perceptual alterations (visual) related to abnormal serum glucose.	The patient will report correction of blurred vision.	Advise the patient that blurred vision may be due to hyperglycemia. Encourage annual ophthalmic examination to detect vision changes or problems.
Altered thought processes related to abnormal serum glucose.	The patient will continue to be alert and fully oriented.	Monitor the patient's mental status. Recognize confusion as sign of abnormal serum glucose. Tell the patient and family that mental changes are best treated with sugar. If the patient does not improve, the blood glucose should be measured and medical attention must be enlisted.
Ineffective individual coping related to diagnosis, dietary restrictions, altered body image, anxiety, and fear.	The patient will identify concerns about living with diabetes mellitus and plan strategies for dealing with it.	Encourage the patient to express feelings about diabetes and to ask questions. Assure the patient that most regular activities can be resumed. Identify the patient's strengths and resources. Explore knowledge about diabetes and any misconceptions. Tell the patient that childbearing must be carefully monitored but that it is a future option. Offer support groups if available.

evaluate the function of the eyes. During the examination of the head and neck, the nurse assesses the patient's breath for a sweet, fruity odor common with ketoacidosis.

The feet receive special attention. The nurse inspects for blisters, lesions, pallor, discoloration, and edema. Both ankles and feet are palpated simultaneously for warmth and pedal pulses.

Neurologic integrity is assessed by testing gait, balance, and motor coordination. This is important because patients who have problems walking or feeding themselves will have problems manipulating syringes and glucose monitors. The patient is also assessed for the ability to perceive hot and cold, sharp and dull sensations, and the presence or absence of pain, especially in the lower extremities, or for any other neurologic deficits that may impair the ability to understand and perform self-care.

Assessment of the patient with DM is outlined in Table 41–4.

Nursing Diagnosis

Nursing diagnoses for diabetes and hypoglycemia may include the following:

- **Altered Health Maintenance** related to lack of knowledge of dietary management of glucose or a faulty metabolism, nausea and vomiting, imbalance between food intake and activity expenditure

TABLE 41-4
ASSESSMENT OF THE PATIENT WITH DIABETES MELLITUS

HEALTH HISTORY
Present illness: Polydipsia, polyuria, polyphagia, unexplained weight loss, dry skin, vaginal itching, delayed healing, blood glucose, urine ketones
Past medical history: Previous diagnosis of diabetes mellitus: type, onset. Drug therapy: drug name, dosage, time last dose taken. Blood glucose monitoring: type equipment used, testing schedule, recent test resutls. Circulatory, cardiac, or renal problems. Previous hospitalizations. Obstetric history: number of pregnancies, outcomes, birth weights, gestational diabetes. Immunization. Allergies.
Family history: Diabetes, heart disease, stroke
Review of systems: Changes in skin moisture or turgor; changes in vision; diarrhea, abdominal bloating, gas; urine retention or incontinence; pain, tingling or numbness in extremities; changes in mental status; seizures
Functional assessment: Literacy, financial resources, usual activity and rest pattern, diet, personal impact of diabetes on life

PHYSICAL EXAMINATION
General survey: Level of consciousness, posture and gait, well-being
Vital signs: Tachycardia, hypertension, hypotension, Kussmaul's respirations
Height and weight: Present and usual
Skin: Color, warmth, turgor, lesions
Eye: Changes in eye grounds, acuity
Mouth: Sweet, fruity breath odor
Lower extremities: Blisters, lesions, color, edema, pulses
Neurologic: Gait and balance; motor coordination; perception of temperature, touch, and pain

- **Noncompliance** related to monetary, personal, family pattern disruption
- **Fluid Volume Excess** or **Deficit** related to alterations in urine output
- **High Risk for Injury** related to adverse effects of drugs, diminished alertness, increased susceptibility to infection
- **Activity Intolerance** related to altered tissue perfusion, decreased mobility
- **Chronic Pain** related to neuropathy
- **Sensory Perceptual Alterations** (visual, auditory, tactile) or impaired skin integrity related to neurologic and circulatory changes
- **Altered Thought Processes** related to abnormal blood glucose, metabolic imbalances
- **Ineffective Individual Coping** related to diagnosis, dietary restrictions, altered body image, sexual dysfunction, anxiety, fear

This is not an exhaustive list as many other nursing diagnoses may be made if a patient has temporary or chronic complications associated with DM. The nurse individualizes the care plan based on the assessment. Management of emergencies is discussed under complications.

Goals

The overall goals for the patient with DM are maintenance of electrolyte balance and blood glucose levels within normal limits of 80 to 120 mg per dl, achievement of optimal weight, and ability to manage own diabetes. Specific goals for the identified nursing diagnoses are knowledgeable self-care; adherence to prescribed treatment regimen; normal blood volume; normal blood glucose and absence of infection; regular exercise; pain reduction; lack of injury, intact skin; mental alertness and orientation; and effective coping.

Interventions

Immediate nursing care of the patient with DM is geared toward urgent needs and complications. After urgent needs are met, nursing care focuses on teaching the patient to manage DM as described in the following interventions.

ALTERED HEALTH MAINTENANCE. Patient education requires that the patient understand the physiology of glucose metabolism and the signs and symptoms of ketoacidosis, hyperosmolar nonketotic coma, and hypoglycemia. The patient must be taught how and when to monitor blood glucose levels and test for urine ketones, how to interpret the results, and the appropriate actions to take based on the results. If using a glucometer, the nurse explains and demonstrates calibration and operation of the device, collection of blood samples, and disposal of lancets or needles. The teaching plan also prepares the patient for self-medication as prescribed. Drug names, dosages, actions, and adverse effects are presented. If insulin is prescribed, proper techniques for drawing up and injecting insulin are demonstrated and site rotation is explained. The nurse explains how adjustments in insulin or diet and exercise are made to maintain blood glucose levels at 80 to 120 mg per dl. The nurse not only provides verbal instruction but also allows the patient to handle equipment and demonstrate skills. The patient is advised to consult the physician or pharmacist before taking new medications because many medications interact with hypoglycemic drugs.

PHARMACOLOGY CAPSULE

Many drugs can affect blood glucose. For example, beta blockers lower the blood glucose and hydrochlorothiazide raises it.

A dietitian should be consulted regarding diet, and the nurse reinforces nutritional information. During hospitalization, food intake is recorded. Details of medical and dietary management are presented earlier in this chapter.

The nurse ideally presents small units of content in each teaching session. Unfortunately, there may be time only to provide the patient with "survival skills" during a brief or busy hospitalization. Therefore, verbal instructions should be accompanied by written material and information about local resources such as the hospital's certified diabetes educator and the local chapter of the

American Diabetes Association. Office nurses, community health nurses, and home health nurses also may participate in teaching the patient with DM.

NONCOMPLIANCE. When a patient has had diabetes education but does not follow the prescribed plan, the nurse explores possible barriers to compliance. Some patients may think the program is too hard to follow and not even try. Others may think complications are inevitable and that treatment will not really make a difference. Another reason for noncompliance is lack of financial resources for drugs, supplies, and a balanced diet. Nursing interventions depend on the reasons for noncompliance. They are designed to provide practical help, support, and encouragement.

The nurse teaches family members how to support and help the family member with diabetes. The family should be treated as integral members of the health care team. It is especially important to include in the diet teaching the person who does the shopping and cooking. A referral to social services is necessary if the patient cannot afford syringes and insulin. A referral to a community health nurse for follow-up teaching and monitoring also is recommended.

FLUID VOLUME EXCESS OR DEFICIT. The patient should be taught how to ascertain the difference between normal urinary output and oliguria or polyuria. The nurse stresses the importance of drinking at least eight glasses of water a day.

HIGH RISK FOR INJURY. The nurse advises the patient to keep necessary immunizations current. The patient is taught to recognize the signs and symptoms of infection and is instructed to see a physician immediately if they occur.

On sick days, insulin or hypoglycemic agents should be taken as usual and blood and urine tested for glucose and ketones, respectively. Glucose levels greater than 300 mg per dl or ketonuria should be reported to the physician. Insulin-dependent patients may need insulin coverage. If nausea and vomiting are present, the patient may need soft foods or liquids in place of solid foods. Nausea, vomiting, and diarrhea are reported to the physician at once because extreme fluid loss may be dangerous. Inability to retain fluids may result in hospitalization.

ACTIVITY INTOLERANCE. An exercise regimen can be designed with the hospital rehabilitation department. "All things in moderation" is the best rule of thumb. Lack of exercise or too vigorous activity just before bedtime may contribute to sleeplessness. Details about the effects of exercise on blood glucose and activity recommendations are discussed earlier in this chapter.

PAIN. Lower extremity pain due to long-term complications may necessitate the use of pain medication to maintain comfort. The nurse documents pain, administers medications as ordered, and evaluates effects of analgesics. If the patient is discharged with analgesics, the nurse explains how the medication is to be taken and any significant side effects such as drowsiness.

SENSORY PERCEPTUAL ALTERATIONS. The nurse instructs the patient on the importance of having yearly eye examinations. The patient should inform the ophthalmologist of the diagnosis of DM. If the patient has impaired vision, audiotapes, special reading materials, and special devices for preparing and administering insulin may be needed.

If the patient has a hearing problem, the nurse gives directions while facing the patient at eye level and speaks clearly. The patient should be asked to repeat or demonstrate instructions to make sure that they were heard correctly.

Alterations in tactile sensations may result in burns or frostbite. The patient and the family need to be aware of these alterations. The patient may need instruction to use sunscreen and warm clothing as appropriate when outdoors in extreme weather. Indoors, the patient is cautioned about the possibility of burns when using heating pads or electric blankets or when working around a hot stove or sitting next to a hot radiator.

The patient or someone else should examine the patient's feet daily for signs of trauma. Injuries or blisters should be seen promptly by a physician. Foot care for the diabetic is summarized in Table 41–2.

When taking a bath, the temperature of the bath water should be measured with a bath thermometer. The temperature should not exceed 43°C (109.4°F). Tissue may be burned before the patient is aware of the excessive heat.

ALTERED THOUGHT PROCESSES. Altered thought processes, including confusion, irritability, anger, and decreased level of consciousness, may be due to hypoglycemia or ketoacidosis. The family should be taught to recognize mental changes as abnormal and to give the patient orange juice or to use one of the interventions for hypoglycemia given earlier in this chapter. If that fails to correct the symptoms, a blood glucose level should be measured and the urine tested for ketones. If the blood sugar is greater than 300 mg per dl or if ketones are present, the patient or family should contact the physician.

INEFFECTIVE INDIVIDUAL COPING. Patients are encouraged to express their feelings regarding diabetes and to ask for help or advice when needed. Every effort is made to encourage them to resume normal activities and to continue their usual social activities. Patients can be helped to identify their strengths and weaknesses. The nurse helps patients explore coping strategies for managing areas of concern. For example, the nurse can demonstrate how favorite foods can be incorporated into a diet plan.

One source of stress to some patients is altered sexual function. The nurse listens to the patient's concerns and encourages consultation with the physician on the matter. Altered sexual function may be due to diabetes, but there may also be other causes. Some diagnostic procedures may be done to assess impotence. If impotence is found to be physiologic and not reversible, the physician can offer the male patient some surgical options, as discussed in Chapter 44. The nurse may encourage the patient to discuss the importance of sexual intercourse and to consider alternative means of sexual expression. Patients and their partners may wish to seek counseling from therapists with expertise in sexual dysfunction.

Patients may be anxious about the long-term effects of diabetes and how it will affect their lives. They may be overwhelmed by what they need to learn for self-care. They may also be fearful about lifestyle changes, self-medication, adverse drug effects, and possible complications. The nurse encourages patients to express these concerns so that they can be addressed (see Care Plan: The Patient with Non–Insulin-Dependent Diabetes Mellitus). Talking with other people who are coping successfully with diabetes can have positive effects.

PHARMACOLOGY CAPSULE

Patient teaching for self-medication cannot be done at the last minute. Supplement teaching with written material and information about outpatient resources.

Evaluation

Criteria for evaluating the outcomes of nursing interventions are patient's statement of correct diabetes self-care measures as presented in teaching plan; patient's verbalized understanding of and intent to adhere to treatment regimen; patient's correct description of fluid needs and of the significance of polyuria and oliguria; patient's statement of correct measures to take when sick; patient's ability to discuss the relationship between exercise, diet, and diabetic medications; patient's statement of pain reduction or relief; patient's verbalization of appropriate self-care measures in relation to vision, foot care, and safety; patient's description of significant mental changes and related measures; and patient's verbalization of feelings about diabetes and expressed willingness to use resources for help with problems.

HYPOGLYCEMIA

PATHOPHYSIOLOGY

Hypoglycemia may result from causes other than the pharmacologic treatment for DM. Regulation of blood glucose depends on insulin levels, available glucagon, and the secretion of catecholamines, growth hormone, and cortisol. Hypoglycemia may occur if abnormalities in these regulators are present. Hypoglycemia is defined as a syndrome that develops when the blood glucose level falls to less than 45 to 50 mg per dl. Symptoms can occur at different blood levels according to individual tolerances.

The causes of hypoglycemia may be divided into three categories: exogenous, endogenous, and functional. Summaries of each of these three categories are presented in Tables 41–5 to 41–7. Exogenous hypoglycemia results from outside factors acting on the body to produce a low blood glucose. These include insulin, oral hypoglycemic agents, alcohol, or exercise. Endogenous hypoglycemia occurs when internal factors cause an excessive secretion of insulin or an increase in the metabolism of glucose. These conditions may be related to tumors or genetics. Functional hypoglycemia may be a result of, for example, gastric surgery, fasting, or malnutrition. Alimentary hypoglycemia occurs in a patient who has undergone gastric surgery. The gastric contents empty rapidly, resulting in an increased glucose absorption. Excessive insulin production occurs, causing the hypoglycemia. In impaired glucose tolerance hypoglycemia, there is an excessive response of insulin to glucose. Spontaneous reactive hypoglycemia has received much publicity by the lay and medical communities alike. Symptoms occur as a result of an extreme insulin response to ingesting foods containing carbohydrates. Verification of low blood glucose levels needs to be demonstrated for the diagnosis to be accepted.

SIGNS AND SYMPTOMS

Signs and symptoms of hypoglycemia may vary according to how quickly the blood glucose levels are falling. When the levels fall rapidly, epinephrine, cortisol, glucagon, and growth hormone are secreted by the body in an attempt to increase glucose levels. Symptoms that result include weakness, hunger, diaphoresis, tremors, anxiety, irritability, headache, pallor, and tachycardia. The symptoms of a blood glucose level that falls over several hours are associated with the central nervous system since the brain depends on glucose for its functions. These symptoms include confusion, weakness, dizziness, blurred or double vision, seizure, and, in severe cases, coma.

MEDICAL DIAGNOSIS

The diagnosis of hypoglycemia can be made by using a variety of diagnostic procedures, depending on the cause. Fasting blood glucose, oral glucose tolerance test, intravenous glucose tolerance test, and prolonged fasting are among those used. The diagnosis should be based on the (1) presence of symptoms, (2) documentation of symptoms at the time the symptoms occur, and (3) improvement of these symptoms with treatment. These three criteria are known as Whipple's triad.

MEDICAL TREATMENT

Treatment of hypoglycemia is dependent on the cause of the problem. In an unconscious patient, hypoglycemia should be suspected until it is ruled out. Glucose should be administered by the intravenous route, with 50 ml of a 50% solution given immediately. In patients with a milder form of hypoglycemia, the treatment is consumption of 5 to 10 grams of some form of carbohydrate. If the patient's condition does not improve, another 10 grams of carbohydrate should be given after 10 minutes. Giving more than 10 grams initially may lead

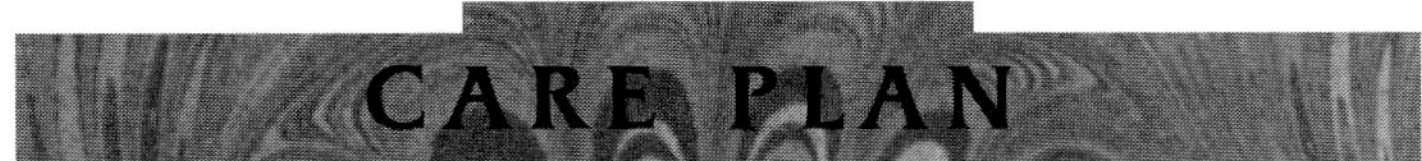

The Patient with NIDDM

ASSESSMENT

Health History: Mrs. Maria Garcia, an 80-year-old Latino, was seen in her physician's office and diagnosed with non–insulin-dependent diabetes mellitus (NIDDM). A referral has been made to a home health agency. The assessment was done in the patient's home. She is three blocks from a grocery store, which also has a pharmacy. Her physician prescribed glyburide (Micronase), 2.5 mg daily before breakfast. Mrs. Garcia sought medical treatment for fatigue, weight loss (10 lb in 2 months), and symptoms of a urinary tract infection. Mrs. Garcia has a history of hypertension, which is treated with verapamil, and venous insufficiency. When asked, she states she has had some problems with her vision and vaginal pruritus. She reports that her appetite is very good, so she could not understand why she was losing weight. Her usual diet is primarily Mexican-American food, but she reports trying not to eat "too much fat." She expresses concern that a diabetic diet will be too expensive, since she only has Social Security income. She said that her father died of a heart attack at age 57, and her mother died at age 73 from kidney failure. One of her brothers has diabetes mellitus, one is deceased from heart disease, and a third is alive and well at age 70. Mrs. Garcia says her symptoms have interfered with performance of usual daily activities and that she is getting up frequently during the night to void, which has affected the quality of her rest. She is a widow who lives alone. She has four adult children, but only one lives in the same city and visits her mother on weekends.

Physical Examination: Vital signs: temperature, 97°F, orally; pulse, 86; respiration, 16; blood pressure, 160/95. Patient is alert and oriented. Her skin is dry, and tissue turgor is poor. She has kyphosis and walks slowly. Heart and breath sounds are normal; 2+ edema in both legs. Popliteal pulses are weak; pedal pulses are not palpable. Skin is dark around the ankles. Feet are cool. Capillary return in toenails is 4 seconds. Toenails are unevenly cut. There is a reddened area on one heel, but she says it is not painful.

NURSING DIAGNOSIS	GOALS AND OUTCOME CRITERIA	INTERVENTIONS
Altered health maintenance related to lack of knowledge of dietary management of NIDDM, drug therapy, and self-monitoring.	The patient will demonstrate the ability to adhere to prescribed diet and drug therapy and to monitor blood glucose.	Assess the patient's understanding of her condition and treatment and explore her attitude toward managing NIDDM. Assess gross visual acuity and assist her to get an eye examination and corrective lenses as needed. Contact local Lions Club if she cannot afford prescribed lenses. Design a teaching plan to explain key aspects of care. Emphasize skills needed immediately: how to take medications, what foods to avoid, and how to recognize and treat hypoglycemia. If home blood glucose monitoring is prescribed, practice the process with the patient and evaluate her ability to perform the test and interpret the results. Develop a plan with the patient to cover additional topics (exercise, foot care) on each visit. Supplement teaching sessions with written or pictorial material. Provide large print reading matter if appropriate. Identify resource people and services in the community, which might include the local chapter of the American Diabetes Association, a community-based Certified Diabetes Educator, and group classes sponsored by various health care facilities. Offer Spanish language materials.
Noncompliance related to financial limitations and transportation for food, drugs,and medical care.	The patient will adhere to her prescribed diet and drug therapy.	Assess any barriers the patient perceives to adhering to her prescribed diet and drug therapy. If there are financial problems, consult a social worker to determine what assistance is available. If

Care Plan continued on following page

The Patient with NIDDM *(Continued)*

NURSING DIAGNOSIS	GOALS AND OUTCOME CRITERIA	INTERVENTIONS
		transportation and shopping are difficult, explore how daughter can help or provide information about public transportation available for the elderly and the disabled. Provide dietary information that incorporates Mexican dishes. Discuss the advantages of using senior nutrition programs or Meals-on-Wheels to provide some meals and ease the burden of food preparation. Monitor weight and blood glucose to assess effects of treatment.
High risk for injury related to adverse effects of drugs, circulatory impairment, decreased sensation, and increased susceptibility to infection.	The patient will take measures to reduce the risk of injury associated with hypoglycemia, inadequate circulation, and diminished sensation; the patient will remain free of fever.	Explain the importance of eating properly while on oral medications that lower the blood glucose. Describe the related signs and symptoms, and advise the patient to consume a glucose source such as sweetened orange juice to reverse hypoglycemia. Stress the importance of contacting the physician if ill and unable to take oral food and fluids. Explain how diabetes affects the blood vessels and nerves, making the extremities especially vulnerable to injury. Emphasize the importance of protecting the feet from injury by wearing properly fitting shoes and keeping the nails trimmed correctly. She should be told to avoid heating pads and to test bath water with a bath thermometer. Advise her to have foot care done by a physician or other specialist (see Table 41–2). Assess the feet on each visit. Explain that people with diabetes are more susceptible to infection and must avoid exposure to others who have active infections.
Activity intolerance related to fatigue, venous insufficiency, circulatory impairment.	The patient will resume previous level of activity without excessive fatigue.	Assess energy level. Explore usual day and discuss ways to conserve energy.
Ineffective individual coping related to diagnosis of serious chronic illness that requires alterations in daily life.	The patient will demonstrate effective coping with diagnosis of diabetes.	Encourage patient to share her thoughts and feelings about having diabetes and her ability to deal with it. Assure her that many older people learn to manage quite well and that resources are available to help her. Communicate with her frequently until her confidence increases. Let her know how she can reach ready sources of information.

TABLE 41-5
EXOGENOUS CAUSES OF HYPOGLYCEMIA

EXOGENOUS CAUSE	PREDISPOSING FACTORS	OCCURRENCE
Insulin	Intentional or accidental overdose; may be combined with inadequate food intake, usually increased exercise, decrease in insulin requirement, or potentiating medications	Most frequent cause of hypoglycemia
Oral hypoglycemia agents	Intentional or accidental overdose; may be combined with inadequate food intake, increased exercise, or potentiating medications	Frequent cause of hypoglycemia
Alcohol	Particularly likely in chronically malnourished or acutely food-deprived individuals	Occurs within 6–36 hr of ingesting moderate to large amounts of alcohol
Other agents	Salicylates, hypoglycins, pentamidine, perhexilin	Common in children <2 yr of age
Exercise	Increased duration and intensity of exercise increases glucose uptake and normally decreases insulin secretion	Occurs with both insulin and sulfonylurea administration and intense exercise but may be unpredictable in onset

From Gray, P. D., & Ludwig-Beymer, P. (1990). Alterations of hormonal regulation. In K. L. McCance & S. E. Huether (Eds.), *Pathophysiology: The biologic basis for disease in adults and children* (pp. 594–643). St. Louis: C. V. Mosby.

to rebound hyperglycemia. In terms of food exchanges, one bread exchange contains 15 grams of carbohydrate, one fruit exchange contains 10 grams of carbohydrate, and one milk exchange contains 12 grams of carbohydrate.

Prevention of hypoglycemia by diet is an important treatment component. The diet is directed by the underlying cause. If the cause is related to an overreaction of insulin to carbohydrate ingestion, a low-carbohydrate, high-protein diet is frequently ordered. Restriction of carbohydrates to 100 grams or less per day is recommended. Simple sugars are avoided, and complex carbohydrates are encouraged. Since no significant increase in blood glucose is noted with protein ingestion, a high-protein diet is recommended. The remaining calories in the diet are obtained from fat. Because the carbohydrates are restricted, the calories required from fat are high. Patients may tolerate smaller, more frequent meals. Alcohol should be avoided.

NURSING CARE OF THE PATIENT WITH HYPOGLYCEMIA

Assessment

History taking is especially important in the diagnosis of hypoglycemia. The nurse describes the present illness, which may include the following symptoms: shakiness, nervousness, irritability, tachycardia, anxiety, lightheadedness, hunger, tingling or numbness of the lips or tongue, nightmares, and crying out during sleep. The past medical history determines whether the patient has or has had DM, previous gastric surgery, abdominal cancer, or adrenal insufficiency. Medications are recorded, paying particular attention to hypoglycemic agents. The names of hypoglycemic agents, prescribed dose, and time last dose was taken are noted. The functional assessment elicits information about current diet, exercise, and alcohol intake. Important aspects of the

TABLE 41-6
ENDOGENOUS CAUSES OF HYPOGLYCEMIA

ENDOGENOUS CAUSE	PREDISPOSING FACTORS	OCCURRENCE
Organic hypoglycemia	Insulinoma	Uncommon neoplasm of beta cells of islets of Langerhans
	Nesidioblastosis and beta-cell hyperplasia	Rare disease causing persistent hypoglycemia of infancy
Extrapancreatic neoplasms	May be mesenchymal tumors, hepatomas, adrenocortical carcinomas, gastrointestinal tumors, lymphomas, or leukemias	Rare; most common in adults 40–70 yr of age
Inborn errors of metabolism	Hereditary fructose intolerance	Rare autosomal recessively inherited inborn error of metabolism
	Fructose-1,6-disphosphatase deficiency	Rare autosomal recessive disease
	Galactosemia	Autosomal recessive disease; hypoglycemia less common than in fructose intolerance
	Phosphenolpyruvate carboxykinase deficiency	Reported in a few infant cases
	Inborn errors in glycogen metabolism, leucine sensitivity	Reported in von Gierke's disease, Hers' disease, and type IXb glycogen storage disease

From Gray, P. D., & Ludwig-Beymer, P. (1990). Alterations of hormonal regulation. In K. L. McCance & S. E. Huether (Eds.), *Pathophysiology: The biologic basis for disease in adults and children* (pp. 594–643). St. Louis: C. V. Mosby.

TABLE 41-7
FUNCTIONAL CAUSES OF HYPOGLYCEMIA

DYSFUNCTION	PRECIPITATING FACTORS	OCCURRENCE
Alimentary hypoglycemia	Rapid dumping of carbohydrates into upper small intestine	Post gastrectomy
Spontaneous reactive hypoglycemia	Syndrome with symptoms such as diaphoresis, tachycardia, tremulousness, headache, fatigue, drowsiness, and irritability	Rarely diagnosed throughout the world; widely diagnosed in US, prompting American Diabetes Association and Endocrine Society to issue statement that entity is probably overdiagnosed
Alcohol-promoted reactive hypoglycemia	Drinking on an empty stomach	More common with drinks containing both alcohol and glucose or saccharin (e.g., beer; gin and tonic; rum and cola; whisky and ginger ale)
Posthyperalimentation hypoglycemia	Rapid discontinuation of total parenteral alimentation	Easily prevented
Endocrine deficiency states	Glucocorticoid deficiency	A danger for any person with adrenal insufficiency
	Growth hormone deficiency	Particularly during a prolonged fast
	Catecholamine deficiency	Possible cause in children
Severe liver deficiency	Insufficient glucose output by liver	Fasting hypoglycemia
Lack of body stores for protein, fat, and carbohydrates	Profound malnutrition	Frequent; also found with relative frequency in kwashiorkor
Prolonged muscular exercise	Metabolism of energy-producing substances	Occurs if exercise is too prolonged or severe or if nutritional intake and carbohydrate stores are insufficient
Functional or transient hypoglycemia in infancy	Transient neonatal hypoglycemia	Occurs in 10% of live births during first 3 days of life
	Maternal diabetes	Due to beta-cell hyperplasia and possibly relative hypoglucagonemia
	Erythroblastosis fetalis	Frequently associated with erythroblastosis fetalis
	Leucine-induced hypoglycemia	Generally in infants <6 mo of age; severe hypoglycemia attacks may occur postprandially or after short periods of fasting
	Ketotic or ketogenic hypoglycemia	One of most common forms of hypoglycemia in childhood, occurs after food deprivation in children 1–8 yr old; generally, spontaneous recovery before age 10
	Maple sugar urine disease	Frequent in those with maple sugar urine disease
	Adrenal hyporesponsiveness	Found in children born small for dates, after complicated pregnancy

From Gray, P. D., & Ludwig-Beymer, P. (1990). Alterations of hormonal regulation. In K. L. McCance & S. E. Huether (Eds.), *Pathophysiology: The biologic basis for disease in adults and children* (pp. 594–643). St. Louis: C. V. Mosby.

physical examination include general behavior, appearance, pulse, and blood pressure.

Nursing Diagnoses

Nursing diagnoses for the hypoglycemic patient may include the following:

- **Knowledge Deficit** of management of hypoglycemia
- **High Risk for Injury** related to episodes of dizziness and weakness
- **Impaired Adjustment** related to effects of illness or lifestyle

Goals

Goals of nursing care for the patient with hypoglycemia are patient's ability to explain and demonstrate self-care, absence of injury, and patient's adjustment to hypoglycemia.

Interventions

KNOWLEDGE DEFICIT. Patient education is a priority after a confirmed diagnosis in order to prevent future occurrences. Patients should be taught to recognize the signs and symptoms and to treat them promptly. The nurse advises the patient of factors that may trigger hypoglycemic episodes, such as foods, medications, alcohol, fasting, and exercise. Basic concepts of the diet described earlier need to be stressed and reinforced. A referral for a consultation with a registered dietitian may be helpful for the patient. As a patient educator, the nurse can be very influential in promoting self-monitoring and treatment of hypoglycemia before it causes serious consequences.

HIGH RISK FOR INJURY. The hypoglycemic patient is at risk for injury as a result of weakness and dizziness.

NUTRITION CONCEPTS

- Diet is an essential component in the management of both insulin-dependent and non–insulin dependent/diabetes mellitus.
- The goal of the diabetic diet is to maintain plasma glucose at as near to the normal physiologic range as possible.
- A person with insulin-dependent diabetes mellitus should coordinate insulin administration with mealtime patterns.
- A person with non–insulin-dependent diabetes should spread food intake throughout the day and eat consistently every day.
- Caloric intake in a diabetic diet depends on the individual needs of the patient and is divided as follows: 12 to 20% protein, 55 to 60% carbohydrates, and less than 30% fat.

The nurse is alert for signs and symptoms of hypoglycemia. Serum glucose levels are monitored. Carbohydrates are administered as prescribed by the physician. Until the episode passes, the patient should be kept in bed with the siderails up and the call button nearby. The patient is advised not to get up unassisted.

IMPAIRED ADJUSTMENT. Emotional support for the patient with hypoglycemia is necessary during both diagnosis and treatment. The nurse prepares the patient for diagnostic tests and tells the patient what to expect. Once the diagnosis is made, the nurse explores the patient's feelings and concerns. The nurse supports the patient in learning to incorporate management of hypoglycemia into his or her lifestyle. The patient is guided to anticipate problem situations and possible solutions.

Evaluation

Criteria for evaluating the outcome of the nursing goals are patient's ability to describe self-care measures, absence of falls or injuries as a result of hypoglycemic episodes, and patient's statement of ability to adjust to prescribed regimen.

BIBLIOGRAPHY

American Diabetes Association. (1986). *Teaching standards for diabetes mellitus* (4th ed.). Austin, TX: Author.

American Diabetes Association. (1988). *Diabetes facts and figures*. Alexandria, VA: Author.

American Diabetes Association. (1988). *Who we are, what we do*. Alexandria, VA: Author.

American Diabetes Association. (1989). What is diabetes? *Diabetes 89, 38*, 2.

American Diabetes Association. (1990). Exercise and NIDDM. *Diabetes Care, 13*, 785–789.

American Diabetes Association. (1990). Eye care guidelines for patients with diabetes mellitus. *Diabetes Care, 13*, 14–15.

American Diabetes Association. (1990). Office guide to diagnosis and classification of diabetes mellitus and other categories of glucose intolerance. *Diabetes Care, 13*, 3–4.

American Diabetes Association. (1992). *Diabetes: Texans at risk*. Austin, TX: Author.

American Diabetes Association. (1993). *Implications of the diabetes control and complications trial*. Alexandria, VA: Author.

Ball, N. A., Stempien, L. M., Pasupuleti, D. V., & Wertsch, J. J. (1989). Radial nerve palsy: A complication of walker usage. *Archives of Physical Medicine Rehabilitation, 70*, 236–238.

Bonheim, R. (1982). The pump. *Diabetes Forecast, 35*(5), 22–26.

Brunner, L. S., & Suddarth, D. S. (1992). *Textbook of medical-surgical nursing* (7th ed.). Philadelphia: J. B. Lippincott.

Campbell, R. K. (1989). Clinical use of insulin: Side effects and dosing factors (Pt. II). *Journal of Practical Nursing, 39*, 22–31.

Christman, C., & Bennett, J. (1987). Diabetes: New names, new test, new diet. *Nursing 87, 17*(1), 34–41.

Cox, H. C., Hinz, M. D., Lubno, M. A., Newfield, S. A., Ridenour, N. A., & Sridaromont, K. (1989). *Clinical applications of nursing diagnosis*. Philadelphia: F. A. Davis

Deakins, D. A. (1994). Teaching elderly patients about diabetes. *American Journal of Nursing, 94*(4), 38–43.

Diabetes update 93. (1993). *Nursing 93, 23*(8), 59–61.

Drass, J., Muir, J., Boykin, P., Baker, K., Turek, J., & Schaffer, A. (1990). Caring for the diabetic patient who takes insulin. *Nursing 90, 20*(5), 98–102.

Drass, J. (1992). What you need to know about insulin injections. *Nursing 92, 22*(11), 40–43.

Forbes, K., & Stokes, S. A. (1984). Saving the diabetic foot. *American Journal of Nursing, 84*, 884–888.

Galuk, D. L. (1990). Adult education for the patient with diabetes mellitus. *Advancing Clinical Care, 5*(3), 33–35.

Gambert, S. R., Morley, J. E., Morrow, L. A. (1990). When diabetes strikes the old old. *Patient Care, 24*, 106–118.

Graham, S., & Morley, M. (1984). What 'footcare' really means. *American Journal of Nursing, 84*, 889–891.

Gray, P. D., & Ludwig-Beymer, P. (1990). Alterations of hormonal regulation. In K. L. McCance & S. E. Huether (Eds.), *Pathophysiology: The biologic basis for disease in adults and children* (pp. 594–643). St. Louis: C. V. Mosby.

Guthrie, D. W., & Guthrie, R. A. (1990). Approach to management. *The Diabetes Educator, 16*, 401–406.

Hahn, K. (1990). Teaching patients to administer insulin. *Nursing 90, 70*(4), 120–122.

Haire-Joshu, D., Flavin, K., & Clutter, W. (1986). Contrasting type I and type II diabetes. *American Journal of Nursing, 86*, 1240–1243.

Hernandez, C. G. (1989). The pathophysiology of diabetes mellitus: An update. *The Diabetes Educator, 15*, 162–169.

Hollander, P., Castle, G., Joynes, J. O., & Nelson, J. (1993). Helping patients manage intensified insulin regimens. *Nursing 93, 23*(10), 48–52.

Hoops, S. (1990). Renal and retinal complications in insulin-dependent diabetes mellitus: The art of changing the outcome. *The Diabetes Educator, 16*, 221–233.

Juvenile Diabetes Foundation. (1988). Basic causes of diabetes: Genetics and immunology. *Juvenile Diabetes Foundation International Countdown, 9*(1), 8–12.

Juvenile Diabetes Foundation. (1988). Complications: Kidney, retinopathy, neuropathy, the heart and circulation. *Juvenile Diabetes Foundation International Countdown, 9*(1), 14–28.

Juvenile Diabetes Foundation. (1988). Overview: Search and research. *Juvenile Diabetes Foundation International Countdown, 9*(1), 7.

Juvenile Diabetes Foundation. (1991). Diabetes and pregnancy: Healthy moms and babies. *Juvenile Diabetes Foundation International Countdown, 12*(3), 10–21.

Juvenile Diabetes Foundation. (1991). Prediction & prevention: Solving one mystery . . . struggling with others. *Juvenile Diabetes Foundation International Countdown, 12*(4), 6–13.

Juvenile Diabetes Foundation. (1991). Treatment & technology: Next wave science. *Juvenile Diabetes Foundation International Countdown, 12*(4), 16–20.

Juvenile Diabetes Foundation. (1992). Fitness: Just do it! *Juvenile Diabetes Foundation International Countdown, 13*(1), 18–24.

Juvenile Diabetes Foundation. (1992). Fitness: Why work out? *Juvenile Diabetes Foundation International Countdown, 13*(1), 6–16.

Juvenile Diabetes Foundation. (1992). Looking ahead: Cosmic crystals. *Juvenile Diabetes Foundation International Countdown, 13*(2), 14–17.

Juvenile Diabetes Foundation. (1992). Research in action: Twins unveil secrets of diabetes. *Juvenile Diabetes Foundation International Countdown, 13*(2), 18–23.

Juvenile Diabetes Foundation. (1992). Treatment & technology: Designer insulins. *Juvenile Diabetes Foundation International Countdown, 13*(3), 14–19.

Kelly, J. U., & Kelly, T. (1991). Insulin-dependent diabetes: Its effect on the surgical patient. *Association of Operating Room Nurses, 54*(1), 61–68.

Kestel, F. (1993). Using blood glucose meters: What you and your patient need to know. *Nursing 93, 23*(3), 34–39.

Levin, M. E. (1990). Diabetic foot lesions: Pathogenesis and management. *Journal of Enterostomal Therapy, 17*(7), 29–34.

Lodewick, P. A. (1987). Choosing a doctor. *Diabetes Forecast, 40*(10), 20–22.

Lumley, W. A. (1988). Controlling hypoglycemia and hyperglycemia. *Nursing 88, 18*(8), 34–41.

Lumley, W. A. (1989). Recognizing and reversing insulin shock. *Nursing 89, 19*(9), 34–42.

Macheca, M. K. K. (1993). Diabetic hypoglycemia: How to keep the threat at bay. *American Journal of Nursing, 93*(4), 26–30.

Massouh, S. R., Steele, T. M., Alseth, E. R., & Diekmann, J. M. (1989). The effect of social learning intervention on metabolic control of insulin-dependent diabetes mellitus in adolescents. *The Diabetes Educator, 15*(6), 518–521.

Murray, R. (1993). Home before dark. One nurse's experience with diabetic neuropathy. *American Journal of Nursing, 93*(11), 36–40.

Narins, B. (1986). A primer on insulin therapy. *Diabetes Forecast.*

Nelson, R. L. (1985). Hypoglycemia: Fact or fiction? *Mayo Clinic Proceedings, 60,* 844–850.

O'Connell, K. A., Hamera, E. K., Schorfheide, A., & Guthrie, D. (1990). Symptom beliefs and actual blood glucose in type II diabetes. *Research in Nursing and Health, 13,* 145–151.

Roberta, P. L. (1990). Diabetic nephropathy: Causes, complications, and considerations. *Critical Care Nursing Clinics of North America, 2*(1), 55–66.

Roberts, A. (1990). Systems of life no. 184. Senior systems—Diabetes in late life, part 49. *Nursing Times, 86*(24), 61–64.

Robinson, C. H., Lawler, M. R., Chenoweth, W. L., & Garwick, A. E. (1990). *Normal and therapeutic nutrition* (17th ed.). New York: Macmillan.

Russo, A. (1990). Cardiovascular disease risk factor reduction and the occupational health nurse. *American Association of Occupational Health Nurses, 38,* 419–459.

Sabo, C. E., & Michael, S. R. (1989). Diabetic ketoacidosis: Pathophysiology, nursing diagnosis, and nursing interventions. *Focus on Critical Care, 16*(1), 21–28.

Siarkowski-Amer, K., & Pidgeon, V. (1991). Documentation of discharge teaching before and after use of a discharge teaching tool. *Journal of Pediatric Nursing, 6,* 296–301.

Steil, C., & Deakins, D. (1992). Oral hypoglycemics: What you and your patient need to know. *Nursing 92, 22*(11), 34–39.

Steil, C. F. (1990). Today's insulins: What you and your patient need to know. *Nursing 90, 20*(8), 34–40.

Tietyen, J. (1987). Diet, cardiovascular disease, and diabetes. *The Diabetes Educator, 13*(4), 415–416.

Tietyen, J. (1993). Tight metabolic control reduces threat of diabetic complications. *Nursing 93, 23*(8), 15–16.

Tonino, R. P. (1990). Diabetes education: What should health care providers in long-term nursing care facilities know about diabetes? *Diabetes Care, 13*(2), 55–59.

Travis, L. B. (1985). *An instructional aid on insulin-dependent diabetes mellitus* (7th ed.). Galveston, TX: The University of Texas Medical Branch.

Ulrich, S. P., Canale, S. W., & Wendell, S. A. (1986). *Nursing care planning guides: A nursing diagnosis approach.* Philadelphia: W. B. Saunders.

Weakland, B. S. (1993). Administering insulin through an indwelling catheter. *Nursing 93, 23*(11), 58–61.

Wikblad, K. F. (1991). Patient perspectives of diabetes care and education. *Journal of Advanced Nursing, 16,* 837–844.

Wolfson, A. B. (Ed.). (1990). *Endocrine and metabolic emergencies.* New York: Churchill Livingstone.

Wozniak, L. (1988). Your teaching plan: The key to controlling type II diabetes. *RN, 51*(8), 29–33.

Zeman, F. J. (1991). *Clinical nutrition and dietetics* (2nd ed.). New York: Macmillan.

KEY CONCEPTS

1. Diabetes mellitus is a condition characterized by insulin deficiency that impairs metabolism.
2. Diabetes mellitus is managed with diet, exercise, and insulin or oral hypoglycemic agents.
3. The major complications of diabetes mellitus are ketoacidosis, hyperosmolar nonketotic coma, vascular changes, and neuropathy.
4. Ketoacidosis causes dehydration, electrolyte imbalance, and metabolic acidosis and is treated with fluid and electrolyte replacement and insulin.
5. Hyperosmolar nonketotic coma is loss of consciousness due to extremely high serum glucose without ketoacidosis.
6. The major complications of insulin therapy are hypoglycemia, insulin shock, and hyperglycemia (Somogyi effect).

7. Nursing care of the patient with diabetes mellitus focuses on altered health maintenance, noncompliance, fluid volume excess or deficit, high risk for injury, activity intolerance, chronic pain, sensory-perceptual alterations, altered thought processes, and ineffective individual coping.
8. Hypoglycemia (low serum glucose) in the absence of diabetes mellitus can be caused by pancreatic tumors, adrenal insufficiency, liver disease, and pituitary disorders, but sometimes no specific cause is identified.
9. When hypoglycemia is attributed to an overproduction of insulin due to carbohydrate ingestion, a low-carbohydrate, high-protein diet with smaller meals may control the condition.
10. Nursing care of the nondiabetic who has hypoglycemia focuses on knowledge deficit, high risk for injury, and impaired adjustment.

CHAPTER 42

Dianne Murray Rudolph

Adrenal and Pituitary Disorders

OBJECTIVES

1. Identify nursing assessment data relevant to the function of the adrenal and pituitary glands.
2. Describe the tests and procedures used to diagnose disorders of the adrenal and pituitary glands and identify nursing considerations relevant for each.
3. Describe the pathophysiology and medical treatment of adrenocortical insufficiency, excess adrenocortical hormones, hypopituitarism, diabetes insipidus, and pituitary tumors.
4. Develop a nursing care plan for patients with selected disorders of the adrenal and pituitary glands.

GLOSSARY

ACROMEGALY Disease of middle-aged adults resulting from overproduction of growth hormone by the anterior pituitary

ADDISON'S DISEASE Disease resulting from a deficiency of adrenocorticotropic hormone caused by destruction or dysfunction of the adrenal glands

ADRENALINE Epinephrine; a powerful vasoactive substance produced by the medulla or adrenal gland in times of stress or danger

ANDROGENS Hormones produced by the adrenal cortex, the testes, and the ovaries that stimulate the development of male characteristics

CATECHOLAMINES Chemicals (dopamine, epinephrine, norepinephrine) released at sympathetic nerve endings in response to stress

CUSHING'S DISEASE Disease caused by the hypersecretion of glucocorticoids due to excessive release of adrenocorticotropic hormone by the pituitary

CUSHING'S SYNDROME Disorder resulting from excessive glucocorticoids in the body as a result of tumor or hypersecretion of the pituitary or by prolonged administration of large doses of exogenous steroids

DIABETES INSIPIDUS Disease caused by inadequate secretion of antidiuretic hormone by the posterior portion of the pituitary

ENDOCRINE GLAND Ductless gland that produces an internal secretion discharged into the lymph or blood stream and circulated to all parts of the body

ESTROGENS Hormones produced by the ovaries, adrenal glands, and fetoplacental unit in females that are responsible for the sexual development and maturation of females

GIGANTISM Disease caused by excessive growth hormone in children and young adolescents resulting in excessive proportional growth

GLUCOCORTICOID Class of adrenocortical hormones that affect protein and carbohydrate metabolism and help protect the body against stress

HYPOPHYSECTOMY Surgical removal of all or part of the pituitary gland

MINERALOCORTICOID Type of hormone secreted by the adrenal cortex and involved in the regulation of fluid and electrolyte levels in the body

SYNDROME OF INAPPROPRIATE ANTIDIURETIC HORMONE Disorder caused by excess antidiuretic hormone production; symptoms include decreased urination, edema, and fluid overload

Virtually every cell in the human body is affected by the endocrine system. The endocrine system is a complex communication network composed of glands and glandular tissue that make, store, and secrete chemical messengers called hormones. Hormones affect target organs and body tissues via the blood stream. The endocrine glands are depicted in Figure 42–1.

Another class of glands are the exocrine glands. The exocrine glands pass secretions through ducts or tubes that empty outside the body or into the lumen or opening of other organs. Examples of this type of gland are sweat glands and the portion of the pancreas that secretes digestive enzymes.

HORMONE FUNCTIONS AND REGULATION

The term *hormone* was coined in 1905. It is derived from the Greek word meaning "I arouse to activity." This definition is appropriate because hormones are generally released in response to the body's needs. Hormones are responsible for important functions related to reproduction, fluid and electrolyte balance, host defenses, responses to stress and injury, energy metabolism, and growth and development. The overall mission of the endocrine system is to maintain homeostasis. Homeostasis is the maintenance of physiologic stability despite the constant changes that occur in the environment. A hormone is a substance composed of amines, peptides, or steroids. These substances bind to receptors located inside the cell nucleus or on the cell membrane of target organs or tissues. These receptors are specific for certain kinds of hormones. When the hormones bind with receptors, they exert their effects on the organ or tissue.

Regulation of endocrine activity is controlled by mechanisms, called feedback mechanisms, that either stimulate or inhibit hormone synthesis and secretion. Feedback mechanisms are triggered by blood levels of a particular substance. This substance may be a hormone or other chemical compound regulated by a hormone. Feedback may be either positive or negative (Fig. 42–2).

In negative feedback, high levels of a substance inhibit hormone synthesis and secretion, whereas low levels stimulate hormone synthesis and secretion. A simple example of this is the household thermostat. As the environmental temperature rises, the production of heat is decreased or stopped; however, as the temperature drops, heat production increases. In positive feedback, high levels of a substance stimulate hormone synthesis and secretion, whereas low levels inhibit this process.

Regulation of hormone production and activity varies with the time of day. Humans and most other animals have a circadian or diurnal rhythm. This rhythm is based on a 24-hour cycle, during which hormone synthesis and secretion are at their slowest rate during the early morning hours and at their highest rate during the evening hours.

THE PITUITARY GLAND

ANATOMY AND PHYSIOLOGY OF THE PITUITARY GLAND

The pituitary gland, also called the hypophysis, is a structure that weighs about 0.6 gram and is located in the sella turcica, a small indentation in the sphenoid bone located on the base of the brain. It is connected to the hypothalamus by the infundibular (hypophyseal) stalk. The pituitary gland is small and oval and has a diameter of approximately 1 cm. It consists of two parts or lobes (Fig. 42–3). The larger of the two lobes, which accounts for 70 to 80% of the gland's weight, is the anterior lobe. The anterior lobe is also called the adenohypophysis. The hormones of the anterior pituitary and their actions are as follows:

1. Growth hormone (GH) or somatotropic hormone: stimulates the growth and development of bones, muscles, and organs.

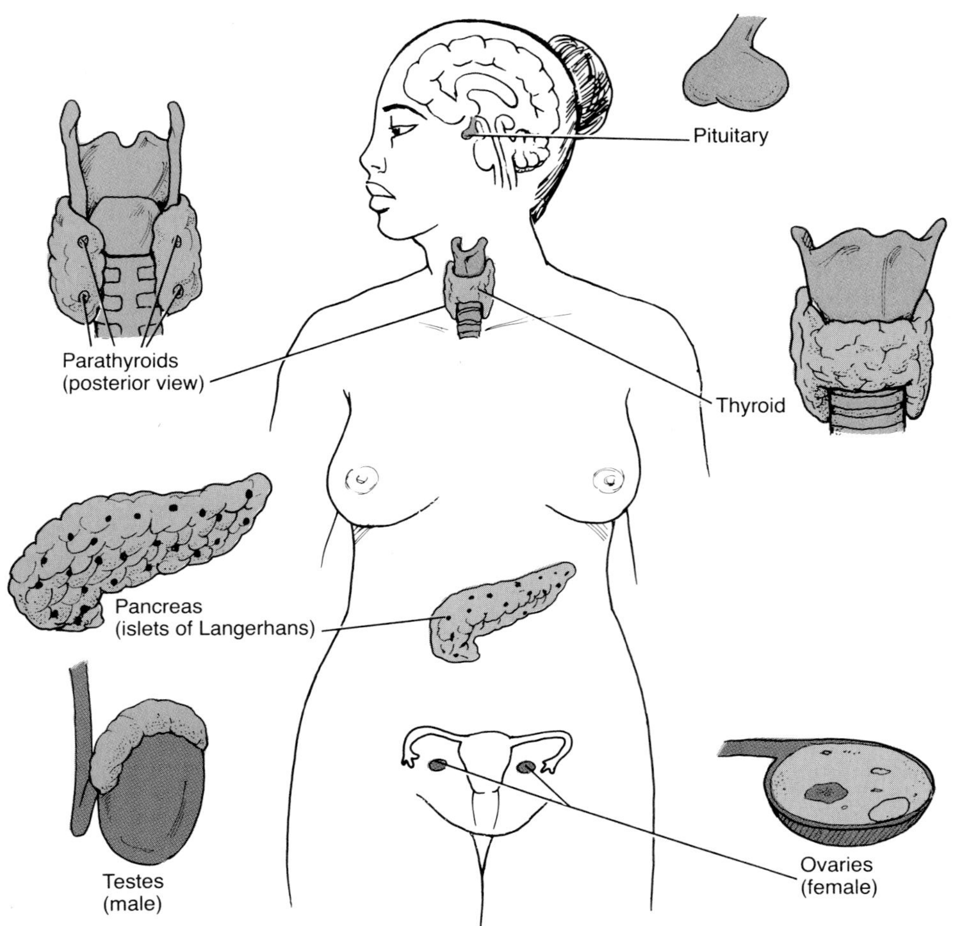

FIGURE 42-1

The endocrine system. The organs of the endocrine system include the pituitary gland, thyroid gland, parathyroid glands, adrenal glands, pancreas, testes (in the male), and ovaries (in the female).

2. Adrenocorticotropic hormone (ACTH): controls the growth, development, and function of the cortex of the adrenal glands; controls release of glucocorticoids and adrenal androgens.
3. Thyroid-stimulating hormone (TSH) or thyrotropic hormone: controls the secretory activities of the thyroid gland.
4. Follicle-stimulating hormone (FSH): stimulates the development of the eggs in the ovary of the female and sperm production in the male.
5. Luteinizing hormone (LH): controls ovulation or egg release in the female and testosterone production in the male.
6. Prolactin (PRL) or lactogenic hormone: stimulates breast milk production in the female.
7. Melanocyte-stimulating hormone: promotes pigmentation.

The smaller lobe of the pituitary is also known as the posterior pituitary because of its location in the sella turcica behind the anterior lobe. It is sometimes referred to as the neurohypophysis. The hormones of the posterior pituitary and their actions are as follows:

1. Antidiuretic hormone (ADH) or vasopressin: causes the reabsorption of water from the renal tubules of the kidney. By doing so, water excretion from the body in the form of urine is decreased.
2. Oxytocin: causes contractions of the uterus in labor and the release of breast milk.

NURSING ASSESSMENT OF THE PITUITARY GLAND

HEALTH HISTORY

Present Illness

Some problems related to pituitary function that may bring the patient to seek medical care are slowed or accelerated growth, visual disturbances, headache, and changes in urine output, appearance, skin, and secondary sex characteristics.

Past Medical History

The nurse inquires about a history of brain tumors, pituitary surgery, head trauma, central nervous system infection, vascular disorders, chronic renal failure, hypothyroidism, and disease of the pancreas, liver, or bone.

Family History

A family history of diabetes insipidus is documented.

Review of Systems

The nurse asks about the patient's general health state and notes fatigue, weakness, restlessness, or agitation. The patient is asked about skin moisture and body hair distribution. Significant sensory changes to note are blurred vision and diplopia (double vision). Both males and females are asked about changes in the breasts. The nurse also assesses the presence of chest pain, constipation, polyuria, changes in genitalia, sexual dysfunction, joint pain, abnormal sensations, edema, seizures, and intolerance of heat or cold.

Functional Assessment

The functional assessment elicits sleep disturbances, usual diet, and effects of symptoms on the person's self-concept and usual activities.

PHYSICAL EXAMINATION

The patient's vital signs and height and weight are measured. The skin is palpated for moisture and edema.

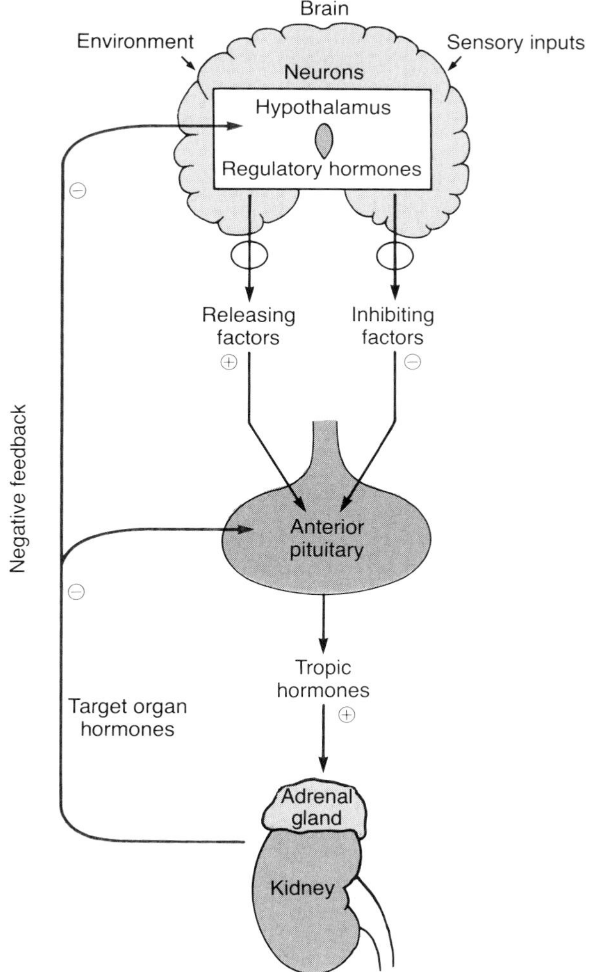

FIGURE 42-2
The feedback system of the hypothalamus, pituitary, and target glands. (Redrawn from Ignatavicius, D. D., & Bayne, M. V. [1991]. *Medical-surgical nursing: A nursing process approach* [p. 1514]. Philadelphia: W. B. Saunders.)

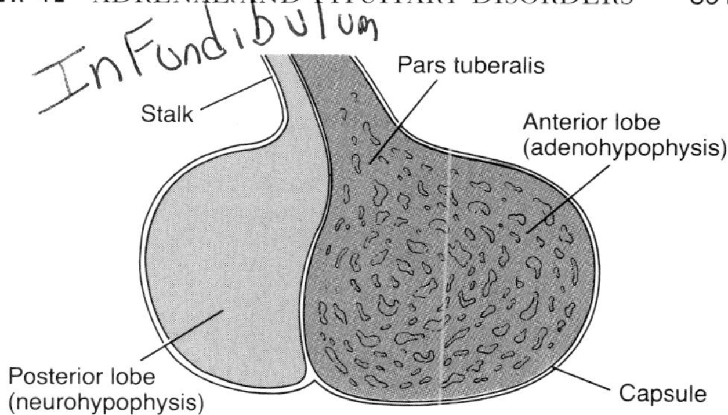

FIGURE 42-3
The two parts of the pituitary gland. (From Ignatavicius, D. D., & Bayne, M. V. [1991]. *Medical-surgical nursing: A nursing process approach* [p. 1514]. Philadelphia: W. B. Saunders.)

The head and face are inspected for thickened lips, broad nose, and prominent forehead and jaw. Visual acuity is tested. The breasts are inspected for enlargement (in males), atrophy (in females), and discharge. The extremities are inspected and palpated for edema. Joint range of motion is assessed, and crepitus is noted. Reflexes are tested for slowness of response. The male patient's genitalia are inspected for loss of hair and palpated for testicular atrophy. The nursing assessment of the patient with a pituitary disorder is outlined in Table 42–1.

TABLE 42-1
ASSESSMENT OF THE PATIENT WITH A PITUITARY DISORDER

HEALTH HISTORY

Present illness: Slowed or accelerated growth, change in urine output, change in appearance, change in secondary sex characteristics
Past medical history: Brain tumors, pituitary surgery, head trauma, central nervous system infection, vascular disorders, chronic renal failure, hypothyroidism, diseases of the pancreas, liver, or bone
Family history: Diabetes insipidus
Review of systems: Fatigue, restlessness, agitation, skin moisture and hair distribution, vision disturbances, changes in breasts, chest pain, constipation, polyuria, changes in genitalia, sexual dysfunction, joint pain, abnormal sensations, edema, seizures, intolerance of heat or cold
Functional assessment: Sleep pattern, usual diet, effects of disease on self-concept and daily life

PHYSICAL EXAMINATION

General survey: Body proportion, behavior, mental-emotional state
Vital signs
Height and weight
Skin: Moisture and edema
Head and face: Thickened lips, broad nose, prominent forehead and jaw
Neck: Jugular venous distention
Eyes: Visual acuity
Breasts: Enlargement, discharge
Extremities: edema, range of motion, crepitus
Neurologic: Slow reflexes
Genitalia: Loss of pubic hair, testicular atrophy

Age-Related Changes

In the healthy older person, pituitary function remains adequate. There may be increased secretion of ADH, which could contribute to decreased ability to concentrate urine and lead to dehydration.

DIAGNOSTIC TESTS AND PROCEDURES

Radiographic Studies

Conventional radiographs and computed tomographic (CT) scans may indicate the presence of a pituitary or cranial tumor. Cerebral angiography, in which a radiopaque dye is injected into the cerebral arteries, may indicate the presence of aneurysms or arteriovenous malformations. Vascular anomalies can interfere with the supply of blood in the brain and lead to pituitary damage.

Laboratory Studies

Since hormones are circulated in very small quantities, tests to identify normal levels must be sensitive and precise. The radioimmunoassay is a commonly performed test that identifies whether adequate levels of hormones are present. This test is based on antigen-antibody displacement reactions. A known amount of antibody and a radioactively labeled hormone are placed in a tube with an unlabeled hormone. The labeled and unlabeled hormones act as antigens and compete for binding sites on the antibody. As the concentration of the unlabeled hormone increases, it displaces the labeled hormone. The unlabeled hormone is then measured against a control.

A similar type of test, which uses enzyme-labeled hormones instead of radioactively tagged hormones, is the enzyme-linked immunoabsorbent assay (or ELISA). This is also thought to be an accurate test for levels of hormones in the blood.

Hormone reserve activity also can be measured using a number of "suppression" or "stimulation" tests. In these cases, an agent that stimulates or suppresses hormonal function is introduced into the body and hormone levels are measured. The response of target glands to stimulation helps the physician determine whether a deficiency is caused by failure of the target organ or dysfunction of the hypothalamic-pituitary regulatory mechanisms.

A glucose tolerance test for GH suppression may be done by administering a standard amount of glucose (100 grams or 0.5 gram/kg body weight) intravenously and measuring serial blood glucose levels for 120 minutes. The rationale is that the glucose will suppress GH levels via a negative feedback process. In normal patients, GH levels will fall less than 5 ng per ml. In patients with hyperpituitarism, large decreases in GH occur. This constitutes a positive result.

Additional information about diagnostic tests and procedures for pituitary disorders is presented in Table 42–2.

DISORDERS OF THE PITUITARY GLAND

Dysfunction of the pituitary gland can result from a problem in the gland itself or from a problem in the hypothalamus. The hypothalamus is an organ in the brain that secretes factors that can directly inhibit or stimulate the pituitary (see Fig. 42–2). Pituitary pathology is usually manifested by excess or deficient production and secretion of a specific hormone. These hormone imbalances lead to disorders that can be manifested in a variety of ways, including changes in physical appearance, emotional state, mental status, metabolism, and homeostatic mechanisms essential for survival. The pituitary disorders that are discussed in this chapter are hyperpituitarism, hypopituitarism, diabetes insipidus, and syndrome of inappropriate antidiuretic hormone.

HYPERPITUITARISM

Etiology

Hyperpituitarism is a pathologic state caused by excess production of one of the anterior pituitary hormones. Growth hormone, the substance responsible for the growth and development of the body's muscles, bones, and other tissue, is one of the hormones most prone to being produced in excess. Excess GH can be a result of hypothalamic dysfunction, hyperplasia of the anterior pituitary, or tumor formation. Overproduction of GH can lead to gigantism or acromegaly.

The most common factor in hyperpituitarism is the presence of a pituitary adenoma. An adenoma is a benign tumor composed of epithelial tissue. It may vary in size and invasiveness. Those that are larger than 10 mm are called macroadenomas; those that are smaller than 10 mm are called microadenomas. Adenomas tend to occur most commonly in young women in their teens through early thirties. Pituitary adenomas that secrete hormones may cause amenorrhea, galactorrhea (abnormal milk secretion), hyperthyroidism, and Cushing's syndrome in addition to gigantism or acromegaly.

Another function of GH, in addition to tissue growth, is the mobilization of stored fat for energy. As a result of lipolysis of body adipose, levels of free fatty acids are elevated in the blood stream. This can stimulate the development of atherosclerosis, which causes coronary artery disease and cerebrovascular disease over time. Growth hormone also antagonizes insulin and interferes with its effects, thus leading to hyperglycemia and possibly diabetes.

GIGANTISM. Gigantism occurs in early childhood or puberty while the long bones of the body are still growing. The long bones consist of epiphyses, which are the end portions of the bone, and a diaphysis, which is the middle or shaft of the bone. Toward the end of puberty or in early adulthood, the line between these structures seals or closes, thus preventing further growth. Before the epiphyseal plates on the ends of these bones close, the diaphysis or long shaft of the bone may continue to

TABLE 42-2

DIAGNOSTIC TESTS AND PROCEDURES FOR PITUITARY DISORDERS

TEST/STUDY	PURPOSE/PROCEDURE	PATIENT PREPARATION	POSTPROCEDURE NURSING CARE
Cerebral CT scan	Uses x-rays to create images of internal structures. Detects tumors, edema, structural abnormalities. Patient lies still on stretcher while circular scanner moves around head. Clicking sounds are heard, but no sensations are felt.	Remove jewelry and hairpins. Tell patient what to expect. If contrast medium to be used, assess sensitivity to iodine and seafood and inform radiologist.	No special aftercare needed. If contrast medium used, assess for side effects: nausea, vomiting, headache.
Cerebral angiogram	Contrast medium is injected into an artery. Radiographs are taken to study cerebral blood flow and blood vessels. General anesthesia needed for patients who cannot cooperate.	Signed consent required. Tell patient importance of lying still and that there may be burning sensation when contrast medium injected. Remove jewelry and hairpins from head.	Pressure applied to arterial puncture site for 15 min. Assess for bleeding afterward. Immobilize extremity as ordered. Bedrest 12–24 hr. Neurologic checks hourly 4 times, then every 4 hr 20 times.
Glucose tolerance test	Fasting blood glucose measured. IV or oral glucose solution given. Blood samples taken to measure glucose levels at specified intervals. Detects diabetes mellitus and hyperpituitarism.	Tell patient what to expect. Enforce NPO.	Check venipuncture site. Apply bandage if needed. Provide ordered diet.
Dexamethasone suppression tests	Baseline serum and urine cortisol are measured. For overnight test, a low dose of dexamethasone is given usually around 11 P.M. and a blood sample is drawn for cortisol level at 8 A.M. Alternative tests are the low-dose test and high-dose test, with various schedules for obtaining blood and urine specimens. Cortisol is increased with adrenal hyperplasia, Cushing's syndrome, oat cell lung cancer. Decreased with histoplasmosis and tuberculosis.	Tell patient what to expect. Explain 24-hr urine collection, if ordered.	Send blood samples to lab within 30 min. Apply dressing to venipuncture site. Check for bleeding.
Pituitary hormone levels: LH, FSH, GH, ACTH, TSH, prolactin	Detect elevations or deficiencies of pituitary hormones. Generally require only a blood sample.	Check agency manual for any special preparation. Tell patient what to expect.	Check venipuncture site. Apply dressing. Check for bleeding.
Hypertonic saline test	Stimulates release of ADH. Evaluates ADH secretion to detect diabetes insipidus (DI). A water load is given to the patient followed by an infusion of hypertonic saline. Urine output and specific gravity are measured hourly.	Tell patient what to expect. Give directions for urine collection.	No special aftercare needed.
Fluid deprivation	Patient is kept NPO for specified time. Vital signs; urine output, specific gravity, and osmolality; and body weight are measured hourly. Aqueous vasopressin given SQ, and hourly measurements continued. Detects changes in specific gravity and osmolality. Decreases with primary and secondary DI. No response with nephrogenic DI.	Explain test to patient. Administer ordered medication and collect designated specimens.	No special aftercare needed.

CT, Computed tomographic; IV, intravenous; NPO, nothing by mouth; LH, luteinizing hormone; FSH, follicle-stimulating hormone; GH, growth hormone; ACTH, adrenocorticotropic hormone; TSH, thyroid-stimulating hormone; ADH, antidiuretic hormone; SQ, subcutaneously.

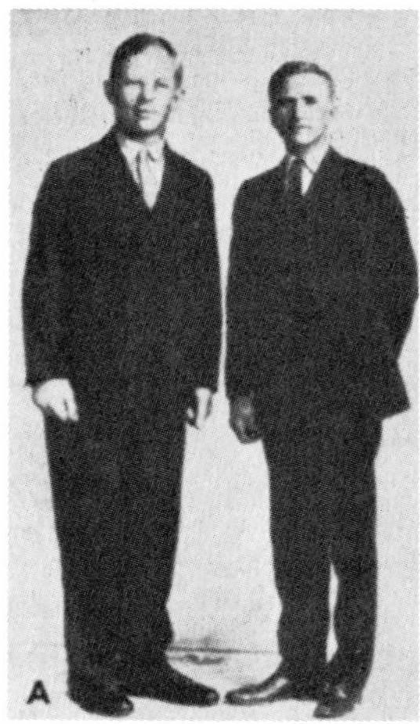

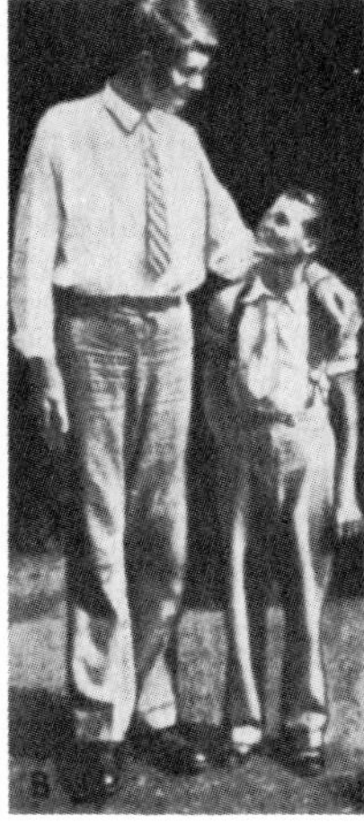
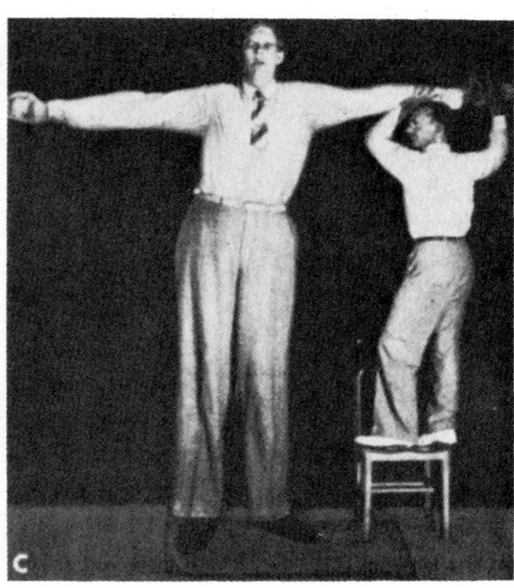

FIGURE 42–4
Clinical features of growth hormone excess. Robert Wadlow, nicknamed "The Alton Giant," weighed 9 pounds at birth but grew to 32 pounds by 6 months of age. By his first birthday, he weighed 62 pounds. He died at age 22 due to complications from cellulitis of the feet. At the time of his death, he was 8 feet, 11 inches tall and weighed 475 pounds. (*A* and *B* from Fadner, F. [1944]. *Biography of Robert Wadlow.* Courtesy of Bruce Humphries, Publishers. *C,* Courtesy of C. M. Charles and C. M. MacBryde.)

grow to great lengths when stimulated by excess GH. The growth in these bones is usually proportional and may cause individuals to reach heights of up to 8 feet and weights of over 300 pounds. These people tend to have multiple health problems and often die in early adulthood. A photograph of an individual with gigantism is shown in Figure 42–4.

ACROMEGALY. Acromegaly, although rare, is more common than gigantism. Symptoms appear later in life, typically in individuals in their thirties or forties, and affect both males and female equally. In these people, excess GH production occurs after epiphyseal closure. The closed epiphyses prevent longitudinal growth of the bones. Instead, bones increase in thickness and width.

Signs and Symptoms

Visual deficits are common in hyperpituitarism and may be the first symptom of a problem. Visual problems are most often a result of pressure on optic nerves where they are joined near the pituitary gland. Physical features of the disease include enlargement of the hands, feet, paranasal and frontal sinuses, and deformities of the spine and mandible. Additionally, soft tissues may become enlarged, especially the tongue, skin, liver, and spleen. This may in turn lead to speech impediments, coarse or distorted facial features, and abdominal distention. People with acromegaly may also experience diaphoresis, oily skin, peripheral neuropathies, degeneration of the joints, and proximal muscle weakness.

In addition to the features described, patients with gigantism and acromegaly initially present with increased strength, progressing rapidly to complaints of weakness and fatigue. The examiner may also detect organomegaly, hypertension, dysphagia, and a deep voice due to hypertrophy of the larynx. Some patients experience elevated levels of prolactin, which may present as galactorrhea (milk production) in females and hypogonadism in males. A dramatic example of acromegaly is presented in Figure 42–5.

Medical Diagnosis

The diagnosis of hyperpituitarism is based on a number of data sources, including physical assessment, radiographic studies, and laboratory findings.

RADIOGRAPHIC STUDIES. Radiographic films of the skull may show a large sella turcica and increased bone density. Enhanced CT scans using a water-soluble dye or magnetic resonance imaging may be performed in order to locate and evaluate potential intra- or extracellular lesions or tumor formation. Angiography may also be of use to rule out any vascular abnormalities such as aneurysms or arteriovenous malformations.

LABORATORY STUDIES. As mentioned earlier, in hyperpituitarism only one pituitary hormone is usually produced in excess, such as GH, prolactin, or ACTH. Pathologic conditions producing elevated levels of luteinizing hormone or follicle-stimulating hormone are extremely rare. In suspected cases of hyperpituitarism, levels of anterior pituitary hormones are measured. Elevation of any levels requires further evaluation and follow-up. It is normal for LH and FSH to be slightly elevated in postmenopausal women. A glucose tolerance test may be ordered. A large drop in the GH level is characteristic of hyperpituitarism.

Dexamethasone suppression tests are used to rule out problems related to dysfunction of the adrenal glands (discussed in detail under Adrenal Disorders).

Medical Treatment

Typically, the patient with hyperpituitarism that is manifested as acromegaly or gigantism has skeletal changes and disfigurement that cannot be reversed with treatment. Radiation therapy is sometimes used to treat tumors that produce excess GH, but overall response is slow and numerous complications, such as hypopituitarism, optic nerve damage, and visual defects, can occur.

DRUG THERAPY. One drug commonly prescribed for patients with hyperpituitarism is bromocriptine (Parlodel). Bromocriptine activates dopamine receptors in the central nervous system and inhibits the release of prolactin and GH, thus decreasing serum levels of these substances. Bromocriptine may be used in conjunction with radiotherapy or alone. Bromocriptine is usually administered on a daily basis, beginning at a dosage of 1.25 to 2.5 mg per day for 3 days. The dosage is then increased by 1.25 to 2.5 mg every 3 to 7 days until an optimum response is attained and serum levels of GH or prolactin, or both, decrease. Some patients may require dosages of 30 mg per day in order to achieve an effect. Some of the most common side effects of this drug are headache, dizziness, drowsiness, confusion, nausea, vomiting, dry mouth, and urticaria.

Octreotide acetate (Sandostatin) also may be prescribed to suppress the secretion of GH. Common side effects of octreotide acetate are nausea, vomiting, diarrhea, abdominal pain, and pain at the injection site. Since this drug also suppresses insulin secretion, the patient's blood glucose must be monitored. Blood pressure and weight are monitored to detect fluid retention.

Table 42–3 provides additional information about drugs used to treat hyperpituitarism.

PHARMACOLOGY CAPSULE

Drugs used to treat gigantism and acromegaly decrease hormone secretion bui do not reverse the existing skeletal effects of the condition.

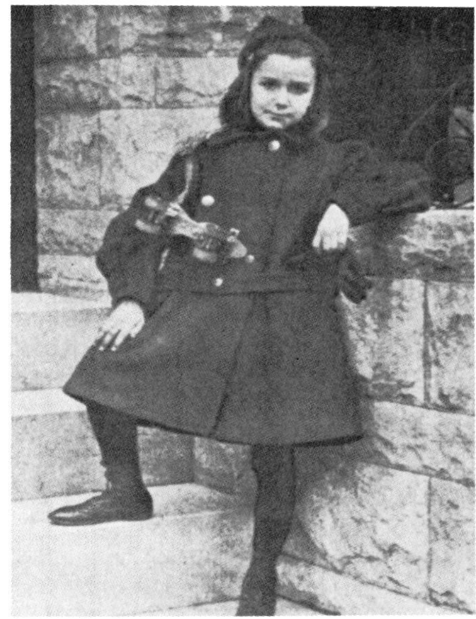
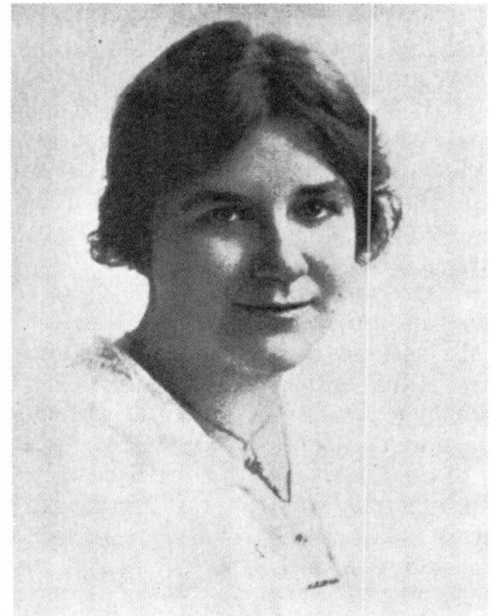
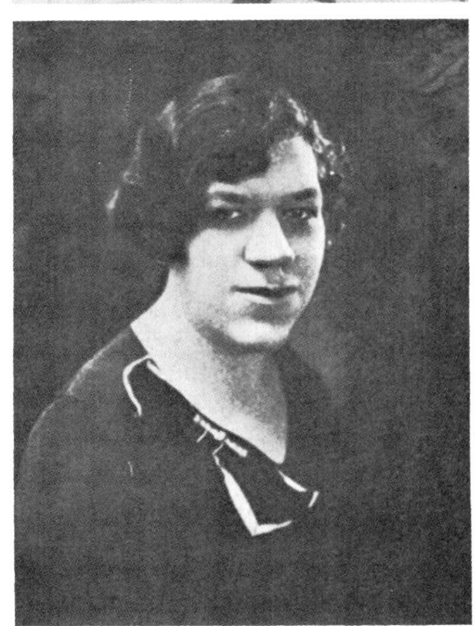
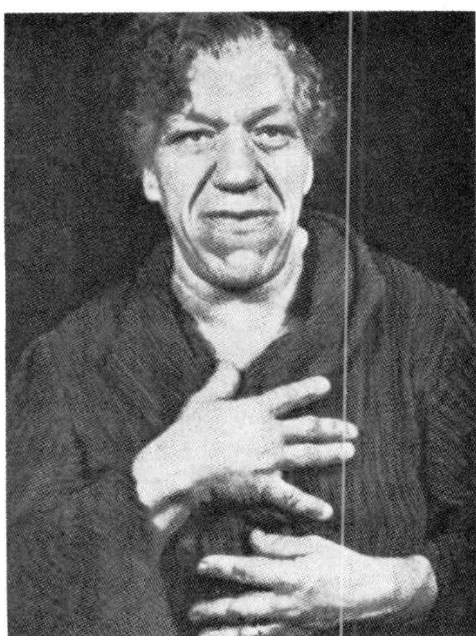

FIGURE 42–5
The progression of acromegaly. A series of photos of the same person over the course of her lifetime depicts the physical changes that occur. The woman was affected after reaching maturity. (From Mendeloff, A., & Smith, D. E. [Eds.]. [1956]. Acromegaly, diabetes, hypermetabolism, proteinuria and heart failure. Clinical Pathological Conference. *American Journal of Medicine, 20,* 133.)

TABLE 42-3
DRUGS USED TO TREAT PITUITARY DISORDERS

DRUG	USE/ACTION	SIDE EFFECTS	NURSING INTERVENTIONS
Lypressin (Diapid) nasal spray Desmopressin (DDAVP) nasal spray		Rhinorrhea, nasal congestion, nasal irritation, headache. Rarely, dyspnea, hypertension, coronary vasoconstriction.	Monitor BP, pulse, intake and output, nasal irritation. Check serum electrolyte results. Teach how to use intranasal inhaler: hold bottle upright, place nozzle in nostril while sitting up, spray prescribed number of times, do not inhale medication.
Bromocriptine (Parlodel)	Inhibits release of prolactin from anterior pituitary. Suppresses lactation. Restores ovulation. Treats acromegaly.	Nausea, vomiting, constipation, hypotension, anorexia, headache, nasal stuffiness, vasoconstriction. Rarely, visual disturbances, confusion.	Safety measures if dizzy. Monitor BP. Record bowel movements and stool consistency. Assess effects. Teach patient to rise slowly to standing position.
Octreotide acetate (Sandostatin)	Suppresses secretion of growth hormone.	Nausea, vomiting, diarrhea, headache, flushing, edema, dizziness, altered blood glucose.	Monitor weight, BP, pulse, respirations, urinary output. Assess for edema. Refrigerate ampules. Discard if discolored or contains visible particles.
Levothyroxine (Synthroid) Liothyronine (Cytomel)	Increases metabolic rate. Treats hypothyroidism.	With excessive dosage: weight loss, palpitations, tachycardia, nervousness, headache, hypertension.	Give oral dose at same time each morning. Reconstitute IV form immediately before giving.

IM, Intramuscular, intramuscularly; BP, blood pressure; IV, intravenous.

Surgical Management

For patients diagnosed with pituitary tumors, the surgical removal of the adenoma or of the pituitary itself (hypophysectomy) is the treatment of choice. A transsphenoidal approach is the most commonly used surgical method. A transsphenoidal hypophysectomy is a microsurgical procedure performed under general anesthesia with the patient in the semi-Fowler position. An incision is made at the inner aspect of the upper lip through the maxillary bone, and the sella turcica is entered through the sphenoid sinus (Fig. 42–6). After the gland or a portion of it is removed, a small piece of adipose tissue is harvested from the abdomen and is used to pack the dura mater (one of the meningeal layers) to prevent leakage of cerebrospinal fluid (CSF). An absorbent gauze or similar dressing is used to pack the nasal passages, and an external nasal dressing is applied to keep the packing in place.

An earlier surgical approach, called a transfrontal craniotomy, is sometimes used if a tumor is especially large or is invading other structures. This is a more invasive procedure that involves the removal of a portion of the frontal bone of the skull. The cranial vault is then entered, and structures superior to the pituitary gland are displaced in order to reach it. This involves manipulation of the meningeal layers and the frontal and temporal lobes of the cerebrum as well as the optic nerve. As a result, the risk of complications and brain damage is great.

Nursing Care of the Patient with Hyperpituitarism

Education and emotional support are vital components in the nursing care of the patient with hyperpituitarism. Patients presenting with hyperpituitarism need to know that many body changes, such as visual disturbances and visceral enlargement, are not reversible. Surgical treatment is aimed only at preventing further symptoms and complications.

ASSESSMENT. Assessment of the patient with a pituitary disorder is summarized in Table 42–1. When a patient has gigantism or acromegaly, areas that merit

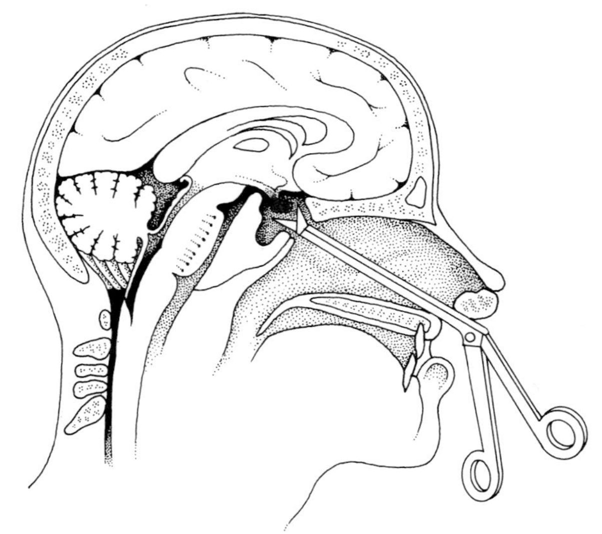

FIGURE 42-6
The transsphenoidal surgical approach to the pituitary gland. (From Ignatavicius, D. D., & Bayne, M. V. [1991]. *Medical-surgical nursing: A nursing process approach* [p. 1537]. Philadelphia: W. B. Saunders.)

special attention are energy level, height and weight, vital signs, contours of the face and skull, visual acuity, speech, voice quality, and abdominal distention. If surgical intervention is planned, the nurse determines what the patient knows and expects.

NURSING DIAGNOSIS. Nursing diagnoses for the patient with hyperpituitarism may include the following:

- **Body Image Disturbance** related to changes in physical appearance
- **Self-Care Deficit** related to lack of knowledge of condition, treatment, and expected outcomes

GOALS. Goals of nursing care are adjustment to physical changes and ability of patient to manage own treatment with realistic expectations.

INTERVENTIONS. The nurse demonstrates acceptance of the patient and provides opportunities for the patient to share feelings and concerns. The patient is encouraged to pay attention to grooming. If he or she has difficulty adjusting, a referral to a support group or mental health professional may be appropriate.

Important nursing considerations for patients on bromocriptine include teaching patients about side effects, to take medication with food in order to minimize gastrointestinal upset, and not to drive. Monitoring of liver function tests also is important because the drug may be hepatotoxic in high concentrations.

EVALUATION. Evaluation of patient care is based on patient's verbalization of feelings and adjustment to changes and on patient's description of self-medication and management of side effects.

If the patient has surgery, general pre- and postoperative care is provided, as described in Chapter 14. This section describes specific nursing care of the patient having pituitary surgery. The patient may be admitted to an intensive care unit for the first 24 hours after surgery owing to the risk of a number of complications.

Postoperative Nursing Care of the Patient with Hyperpituitarism

ASSESSMENT. During the postoperative period, frequent and thorough assessment of neurologic status and vision is important. Particular attention is given to level of consciousness, pupil size and equality, vital signs, and intake and output. The patient is asked to place his or her chin to the chest to assess for nuchal rigidity (severe head or neck pain associated with meningeal inflammation). Changes in assessment findings that may reflect edema due to the manipulation of tissues or intracranial bleeding are decreasing alertness, slow pupil response to light, and decreased or asymmetric muscle strength.

Strict documentation of intake and output and measurement of specific gravity are important because these patients are at risk for diabetes insipidus or possibly syndrome of inappropriate antidiuretic hormone. These disorders are discussed in detail later in this chapter.

Inspection of nasal packing for drainage is important because CSF leaks may sometimes occur. Any clear, colorless drainage is documented and brought to the attention of the surgeon. A bedside test can be done with a testing strip to detect whether drainage is CSF. Since CSF has a high glucose content, the CSF tests positive for glucose. Cerebrospinal fluid leaks are often resolved with rest; however, excessive or continued leakage may require surgical intervention.

Monitoring the patient for signs and symptoms of infection also is an important aspect of nursing care. Elevations in white blood cell counts, sudden rises in temperature, headache, or nuchal rigidity may be indications of meningitis (inflammation of the meninges, the protective layer of membranes that cover the brain and spinal cord).

NURSING DIAGNOSIS. Specific nursing diagnoses after pituitary surgery may include the following:

- **Knowledge Deficit** of surgical pre- and postoperative care and routines
- **Sensory Perceptual Alterations** (visual) related to tissue trauma and swelling
- **Pain** related to tissue trauma
- **Altered Mucous Membrane** related to surgical incision
- **Fluid Volume Excess** or deficit related to abnormal ADH production
- **High Risk for Infection** related to impaired tissue integrity
- **High Risk for Injury** related to disruption of packing

GOALS. Goals of nursing care for the surgical patient are patient's knowledge of surgical routines and self-care, early detection of visual disturbances, pain relief, healed surgical incision, normal fluid balance, absence of infection, and absence of CSF drainage.

INTERVENTIONS. The nurse orients the patient to the environment and explains all procedures. Drugs are given as ordered to replace pituitary hormones. When the patient is well enough, the nurse provides information about drug therapy and self-medication. The patient who has a complete hypophysectomy requires hormone replacements for the rest of his or her life. Replacement therapy typically includes glucocorticoids and thyroid medication (see Adrenal Disorders for a more detailed discussion of glucocorticoids). The immediate postoperative period is uncomfortable since the nasal packing remains in place for 2 to 3 days and the patient is forced to breathe through the mouth. The presence of a "moustache" dressing may also make the patient feel uncomfortable or embarrassed. Frequent mouth care increases comfort. Analgesics are administered as ordered, and the effects are assessed. Intravenous fluids are administered as ordered, and urine output is monitored.

In order to prevent dislodgment of the fat pad or adipose graft at the surgical site, the patient is instructed to avoid any activities that can cause a Valsalva maneuver. Coughing, straining, vomiting, or sneezing can create enough intracranial pressure to disrupt the surgical site and cause CSF leakage or even bleeding.

Stool softeners and laxatives may be ordered to prevent straining. Incentive spirometry, instead of coughing, and deep-breathing exercises help maintain pulmonary function without increasing intrathoracic and intracranial pressure. Lifting heavy objects and bending from the waist are avoided. Patients are instructed to avoid these activities at home for 2 to 3 months after surgery.

The nurse notifies the surgeon of signs of complications: visual disturbances, fluid retention or diuresis, clear fluid drainage from the nose, and fever.

EVALUATION. Criteria for evaluation of nursing care are patient's verbalization of treatment and self-care, visual acuity consistent with patient's norms, patient's statement of pain relief and relaxed expression, healed incision, balanced fluid intake and output with normal skin turgor, normal body temperature and white blood cell count, and absence of CSF fluid drainage.

HYPOPITUITARISM

Etiology and Pathophysiology

When inadequate secretion of GH occurs during preadolescence, a syndrome called dwarfism may result. Dwarfism is defined as attainment of a maximum height that is 40% below normal. In addition, chronic diseases associated with inadequate growth may be present. The causes of dwarfism may be hereditary or may be related to damage to the anterior portion of the pituitary gland. The anterior pituitary may be damaged by necrosis following hemorrhage, trauma, infection, radiation, or autoimmune disorders. Inadequate secretion of GH or an inability of the target organs to respond to GH is generally considered to be the major cause. In rare instances, hypothalamic dysfunction can lead to dwarfism as well. It is important to note that while an actual or relative deficiency of GH may exist, other anterior pituitary hormones also may be deficient.

If growth has been completed and some pathologic process impairs the function of the pituitary, a syndrome known as panhypopituitarism can occur. In this situation, all hormones of the anterior pituitary are usually affected. There are a number of causes for panhypopituitarism, which are identified as follows:

1. Sheehan's syndrome: shock and hypotension during the postpartum period can lead to infarction of the pituitary gland.
2. Tumors of the pituitary gland itself or cranial tumors that impinge on the pituitary.
3. Chronic recurrent infections.
4. Total or subtotal ablation of the pituitary as a result of trauma, surgery, or radiation therapy.
5. Suppression of pituitary tropic hormones by excess target gland hormones (such as is seen in patients on prolonged corticosteroid therapy).

Signs and Symptoms

The manifestations of hypopituitarism depend on the stage of life when the deficiency occurs and which hormones are deficient. In dwarfism, which occurs early in life, the individual is remarkably short in stature, sometimes as short as 36 inches, but with proportionate physical characteristics. These individuals often have delayed or absent sexual maturation. There is a greater frequency of mental retardation than in the population at large. Dwarfs also have an accelerated pattern of aging and thus have a shorter life span, by as much as 20 years, than the general population.

When a state of panhypopituitarism exists, a syndrome called Simmonds' cachexia is present. The patient has muscle and organ wasting and disruptions of both digestion and metabolism. Decreased muscle and organ size is attributed to decreased GH. An absence of ACTH affects the individual's ability to effectively cope with stress. (See section on adrenal hypofunction later in this chapter.) This in turn affects the ability of the individual to metabolize glucose, and hypoglycemia may result. Since thyroid-stimulating hormone is depleted, the thyroid is unable to produce thyroid hormone. A lack of thyroid hormone produces a state referred to as myxedema or hypothyroidism. In myxedema, insufficient thyroid hormone is available for normal metabolism and thermogenesis or heat production. Consequently, these individuals are potentially unable to maintain a normal basal metabolic rate or body temperature.

If there is a lack of melanocyte-stimulating hormone, decreased pigmentation of the skin occurs. This results in extreme pallor. Finally, with the absence of gonadotropins, gonads may become atrophied. In both males and females, there may be loss of libido, decreased body hair, and sexual dysfunction, and, in females, amenorrhea (absence of menstruation). General signs and symptoms may include fatigue, weakness, malaise, cold intolerance, and lethargy. Again, the type and degree of symptoms depend on specific hormones affected.

Medical Diagnosis

A diagnosis of dwarfism or panhypopituitarism is based on the health history, physical examination, and diagnostic tests. In cases of dwarfism, the physical examination findings are fairly diagnostic. Diagnostic tests and procedures may include conventional radiographs and CT scans to detect pituitary or cranial tumors. Cerebral angiography may be ordered to detect malformed blood vessels. Serum levels of pituitary hormones may be measured as well.

Medical Treatment

Deficient hormones are replaced as needed depending on the specific deficiencies of the patient. Deficiency of thyroid-stimulating hormone necessitates thyroid replacement with drugs such as levothyroxine (Synthroid) or liothyronine (Cytomel), usually for the rest of the individual's life. Gonadotropin deficiency requires lifetime therapy. To produce or maintain libido, secondary sexual characteristics, and well-being, males should also receive testosterone and females should also receive estrogen. In patients for whom childbearing is desirable, follicle-stimulating hormone and luteinizing hormone are administered to both males and females.

Growth hormone replacement is necessary in children but not in adults. In most instances, GH is administered until the individual reaches a height of 5 feet. A new development, the production of biologically active human growth hormone by recombinant DNA technology, may make treatment more effective. If a tumor is causing hypopituitarism, surgery is the treatment of choice. (See Surgical Management under Hyperpituitarism earlier in this chapter). Table 42–3 provides additional information about drug therapy for hypopituitarism.

PHARMACOLOGY CAPSULE

Biologically active human growth hormone is now available for treatment of growth hormone deficiency.

Nursing Care of the Patient with Hypopituitarism

ASSESSMENT. The general assessment of the patient with a pituitary disorder is summarized in Table 42–1. The nurse should be thorough in taking a history and in performing a physical assessment of the patient with hypopituitarism. Throughout the assessment, the nurse is alert for changes in mental acuity, emotional stability, and affect. The health history documents the patient's general sense of well-being, energy level, and appetite. In reviewing the system, the patient is asked about changes in skin texture, body temperature, hair, and libido. The nurse determines the patient's usual activities and whether there has been any difficulty carrying out those activities.

In the physical examination, height and weight are measured and compared with previous measurements. The hair is inspected for distribution, texture, and thickness. The skin and nails are inspected and palpated for color, texture, and moisture. The development of secondary sex characteristics, including axillary and pubic hair, genital maturity, breast development, and onset of menarche, is documented.

NURSING DIAGNOSIS. A list of nursing diagnoses that may apply to the patient with hypopituitarism follows:

- **Body Image Disturbance** related to lack (or loss) of secondary sex characteristics
- **Sexual Dysfunction** related to hormone deficiency
- **Altered Nutrition: More or Less than Body Requirements** related to hormone imbalance
- **Fluid Volume Deficit** related to hormone deficiency, impaired homeostasis
- **Knowledge Deficit** of condition, treatment, and self-care

GOALS. Goals of nursing care for the patient with hypopituitarism are improved body image, enhanced sexual development and function, adequate nutrition, normal fluid balance, and patient's knowledge of the disorder, treatments, importance of lifelong therapy, and self-monitoring.

INTERVENTIONS. Patient education is the most important aspect of nursing care since disturbances in body image, sexual function, nutritional status, and fluid balance can all be improved if the patient understands and follows the prescribed therapy. Meanwhile, the nurse acknowledges the patient's feelings and encourages expression of concerns. Referral to a mental health counselor is appropriate if the patient has difficulty dealing with the effects of the disease. A significant amount of patient and family teaching is essential for them to understand hypopituitarism and to participate in the treatment plan. The teaching plan should include the following:

- Pituitary functions.
- Effects of hormone deficits in relation to patient signs and symptoms.
- Prescribed therapy, including effects of drugs, drug dosage, and importance of lifelong replacement. (See Table 42–8)
- Symptoms of excessive or inadequate hormone replacement, and appropriate actions.
- Need for follow-up care.
- Need for a medical alert bracelet or necklace so that the disease can be quickly recognized in an emergency. A card should also be carried that lists prescribed drugs and dosages and the physician's name and phone number.

EVALUATION. Criteria for evaluating goal achievement are patient's making positive statements about self and taking measures to improve appearance; development of secondary sex characteristics and satisfying sexual function; body weight normal for height; normal skin turgor, pulse, and blood pressure; and patient's verbalization of disease effects, treatment, self-care, and intent to continue therapy and to keep follow-up appointments.

DIABETES INSIPIDUS

Disorders of the posterior pituitary or neurohypophysis are directly related to deficient or excess ADH production. Another name for ADH is vasopressin. Antidiuretic hormone normally functions by allowing the renal tubules of the nephron to reabsorb water. The amount of ADH secreted is proportional to the amount of water retained by the kidney. Increased ADH release causes increased water retention. This results in increased intravascular volume and decreased urine output. Two disorders are associated with dysfunction of the neurohypophysis: diabetes insipidus (DI) and syndrome of inappropriate antidiuretic hormone (SIADH). Diabetes insipidus is the more common of the two disorders.

Etiology

Diabetes insipidus is related to a deficit in production and synthesis of ADH. It can be caused by a number of factors. Thus, DI is classified as nephrogenic, primary, secondary, or drug related. Nephrogenic DI is an inherited defect in which the renal tubules of the kidney do not respond to ADH, resulting in inadequate water reabsorption by the kidneys. In this case there are sufficient amounts of ADH, but the kidneys do not respond to them appropriately. In primary DI, there is a defect in the posterior pituitary gland related to familial or idiopathic causes. Secondary DI is typically the result of hypothalamic tumors, head trauma, infection, surgical procedures (hypophysectomy), or metastatic tumors originating in the lung or breast. Secondary DI can also be triggered by a cerebrovascular accident, aneurysm, or intracranial bleed. Drug-related DI is typically caused by lithium carbonate (Eskalith) or demeclocycline (Declomycin), which affect the kidney by inhibiting its response to ADH.

Pathophysiology

Antidiuretic hormone deficiency or an inability of the kidneys to respond to ADH results in the excretion of large volumes of very dilute urine, a symptom referred to as polyuria. The distal tubules and collecting ducts do not reabsorb excess water. Massive diuresis occurs, resulting in increased plasma osmolarity, which stimulates the osmoreceptors. The osmoreceptors in turn relay information to the cerebral cortex, causing the person to feel thirsty. Increased thirst serves as a compensatory mechanism in that it causes the individual to increase water ingestion. Unfortunately, this compensatory mechanism cannot keep up with the demand for water, and diuresis continues. Massive dehydration ensues, which leads to decreased intravascular volume, hypotension, and circulatory collapse. This is accompanied by neurologic changes such as a decreased level of consciousness and severe electrolyte imbalances. Electrolyte imbalances contribute to circulatory collapse by causing arrhythmias and impaired contractility of the heart. If left untreated, severe cases of DI can lead to cardiac arrest and death.

Signs and Symptoms

Common signs and symptoms of DI are massive diuresis, dehydration, and thirst. Dehydration is characterized by hypotension, tachycardia, dizziness, decreased skin turgor, weakness, and possible fainting episodes. Additional findings include malaise, lethargy, and irritability. An irregular heartbeat may be detected.

Medical Diagnosis

The diagnosis of DI is made primarily on the basis of the health history and physical examination and laboratory findings. A history of any known etiologic factors, such as surgery, infection, injury, or medication ingestion, should be noted.

The loss of free water is apparent in laboratory studies of blood and urine. An initial diagnosis of DI is made on the basis of a 24-hour urine output of greater than 4 liters of fluid, without food or fluid restrictions. Patients with DI can excrete up to 30 liters per day, depending on the severity of the ADH deficiency or relative deficiency. Because the urine is very dilute, the specific gravity is also extremely low (< 1.005) and the osmolarity of the urine is decreased (50–200 osm/kg). Additional studies used to diagnose DI are listed in Table 42–2.

Medical Treatment

The management of DI is geared to controlling the signs and symptoms of the disease and possibly reversing the cause of the syndrome. Intravenous fluid volume replacement and vasopressors are often required to maintain adequate blood pressure. Treatment also includes a variety of pharmacologic therapies. A list of these agents can be found in Table 42–3. Most of these agents act by augmenting existing ADH or replacing it. Short-term therapy is usually managed with subcutaneous injections of aqueous vasopressin. This is usually indicated in situations in which the cause of DI is reversible, such as infection- or medication-related DI. Individuals on long-term therapy are placed on nasal spray, which may be required for life. This long-term therapy may be necessary after hypophysectomies or other surgical procedures.

PHARMACOLOGY CAPSULE

Adverse effects of vasopressin administered as a nasal spray are mucous membrane ulcers, chest tightness, and upper respiratory infections.

Nursing Care of the Patient with Diabetes Insipidus

ASSESSMENT. A complete history of the patient's symptoms, medical history, and drug history should be obtained. The nurse monitors for thirst, change in urine appearance or volume, dizziness, weakness, fainting, and palpitations. The physical examination focuses on the symptoms of DI. The nurse assesses hydration, including skin turgor, moisture of mucous membranes, pulse rate and quality, blood pressure, and mental status. Records of intake and output, daily weights, and urine specific gravities are maintained to detect potential problems.

NURSING DIAGNOSIS. Depending on the patient's diagnosis and symptoms, a number of nursing diagnoses may apply. A list of potential nursing diagnoses follows:

- **Anxiety** related to physical symptoms and diagnosis
- **Body Image Disturbance** related to altered function
- **Fluid Volume Deficit** related to excessive urine output (DI)
- **Activity Intolerance** related to fatigue and weakness
- **Knowledge Deficit** of management of symptoms and treatment modalities

GOALS. Important goals for the patient may include reduced anxiety, adaptation to physical changes, normal fluid balance, improved ability to participate in activities of daily living, and understanding of medical treatments and medications.

INTERVENTIONS. The patient with a pituitary disorder may be experiencing mild to moderate symptoms or may be critically ill. Specific nursing care largely depends on the disorder, the severity of the symptoms, and the needs identified in the nursing assessment.

Anxiety, Body Image Disturbance. The patient who is able must be allowed adequate time to ventilate feelings and discuss the disorder. Changes in body function can be very disturbing. The nurse assures the patient that some changes can be controlled with proper treatment. The nurse must be alert to the patient's emotional status and provide support and make referrals as necessary.

Fluid Volume Deficit. Intake and output are carefully measured. When the urine output is excessive, as in DI, the physician may order measurement of output at 15- to 30-minute intervals. Adequate hydration is essential, and intravenous fluid replacements are administered as ordered. Oral intake is encouraged, with the prescribed amount based on the volume of urinary output. In addition, the patient is weighed at least once daily to identify significant weight loss secondary to water loss. In situations in which the patient is experiencing an excessive fluid loss, exogenous ADH is administered (Table 42–3). The nurse should be well versed in administration, side effects, and contraindications associated with the use of these agents.

Activity Intolerance. Extreme fatigue or muscle weakness can interfere with the patient's ability to participate in activities of daily living, such as hygiene and grooming. The functional ability of these individuals should be assessed on a frequent basis, and the amount of assistance required should be addressed in the patient's care plan.

Knowledge Deficit. If treatment involves the use of various pharmacologic agents, the patient needs in-depth information about the medication schedule, drug effects and related side effects, and proper use of nasal sprays. The importance of adhering to dosage strength and schedule is emphasized. A thorough teaching plan for patients with pituitary disorders also addresses the importance of maintaining adequate food and fluid intake and regular, frequent monitoring of weights. Marked changes in weight should be reported to the physician. Some patients are taught to use hydrometers to measure urine specific gravity. Keeping office or clinic appointments is emphasized because these patients require ongoing assessments to identify any changes in pituitary function. The patient is also instructed to schedule activities and regular rest periods to avoid excessive fatigue.

Patients with lifelong requirements for ADH replacement therapy need in-depth instruction in order to enhance compliance with this therapy. The nurse informs the patient of the risks associated with the prolonged use of nasal sprays, such as ulceration of mucous membranes, chest tightness, upper respiratory infections, and respiratory problems secondary to the inhalation of these products. Patients are instructed to report signs that may indicate the need for additional treatment, such as increased urine output, thirst, weight loss, and general feelings of malaise or weakness.

EVALUATION. Evaluation of nursing care for the patient with a pituitary disorder is directed at determining goal achievement and making changes as needed for the individual patient. The following outcome criteria are used to evaluate goal achievement: patient's statement that anxiety is reduced or markedly diminished; patient's demonstration or verbalization of acceptance of body image changes; fluid output equal to intake, normal blood pressure, and stable weight; accomplishment of daily activities without excess fatigue; and patient's demonstration of symptom management and self-medication.

SYNDROME OF INAPPROPRIATE ANTIDIURETIC HORMONE

Etiology

This syndrome is characterized by a water imbalance related to an increase in ADH synthesis or secretion, or both. Factors that may cause or contribute to the development of SIADH include brain trauma, surgery, tumors, or infection; some drugs, including vasopressin, general anesthetic agents, oral hypoglycemics, and tricyclic antidepressants; some pulmonary diseases; hypothyroidism; lupus erythematosus; and some types of cancer, including oat cell bronchiogenic carcinoma, duodenal cancer, and pancreatic cancer.

Pathophysiology

When ADH is elevated despite normal or low serum osmolality, the kidneys retain fluid. Plasma volume expands, causing the blood pressure to rise. Body sodium is diluted (hyponatremia), and the patient develops water intoxication.

Signs and Symptoms

The main symptoms of SIADH initially reflect the effects of hyponatremia and water retention: weakness, muscle cramps or twitching, anorexia, nausea, diarrhea, irritability, headache, and weight gain without edema. When the central nervous system is affected by water intoxication, the level of consciousness deteriorates and the patient may have seizures or lapse into a coma.

Medical Diagnosis

The diagnosis of SIADH is confirmed by laboratory tests of serum and urine electrolytes and osmolality. Radiographic studies of the brain and lungs also may be done to detect causative factors.

Medical Treatment

The treatment is intended to correct the cause, if possible, and promote elimination of excess water. Fluids are restricted and sodium chloride given. Diuretics, demeclomycin (a drug that increases water excretion), and hypertonic enemas may be ordered (Table 42–3).

Nursing Care of the Patient with SIADH

ASSESSMENT. The health history assesses the presence of anorexia, nausea, vomiting, diarrhea, headache, irritability, and muscle cramps and weakness. A history of cancer, pulmonary disease, nervous system disorders, hypothyroidism, or lupus erythematosus is recorded. If the patient is taking any prescription drugs, they are noted. The nurse monitors the patient's vital signs, weight, intake and output, and urine specific gravity. The skin is palpated for moisture and edema. Muscle strength is tested by having the patient grip the nurse's hands and push and pull against resistance. Seizures and muscle weakness, twitching, or cramps are documented. Mental status is assessed by determining the patient's level of consciousness and orientation.

NURSING DIAGNOSIS. The primary nursing diagnoses for the patient with SIADH are the following:

- **High Risk for Injury** related to water intoxication, cerebral edema, confusion
- **Fluid Volume Excess** related to excess ADH secretion
- **Knowledge Deficit** of management of chronic SIADH

GOALS. The goals for the primary nursing diagnoses are absence of injury, normal fluid balance, and patient's knowledge of SIADH and its treatment.

INTERVENTIONS

High Risk for Injury. If the patient becomes confused, the nurse takes measures to ensure safety, including putting the bed in low position and checking on the patient frequently.

Fluid Volume Excess. The patient is positioned flat or with no more than a 5-degree elevation of the head as ordered to reduce progressive cerebral edema. The physician is advised of declining neurologic status or weight gain in excess of 2 pounds per day. The nurse enforces fluid restrictions, which may be as little as 500 ml per 24 hours. The restriction is explained to the patient and family. Fluids are spaced over waking hours to reduce thirst and feelings of deprivation. Oral fluids are served in small containers to create the illusion of volume. Frequent mouth care is encouraged.

Knowledge Deficit. Although SIADH is usually temporary, it may not resolve during hospitalization, and the nurse must teach the patient how to manage the condition at home. The teaching plan includes the nature of the condition, signs and symptoms of water intoxication, medical management, and self-medication.

EVALUATION. Criteria for successful nursing interventions are absence of seizures and injuries, fluid output equal to intake, and patient's description of condition and long-term management.

THE ADRENAL GLANDS

ANATOMY AND PHYSIOLOGY OF THE ADRENAL GLANDS

The adrenal glands are a pair of small, highly vascularized, triangular-shaped organs. They are located in the retroperitoneal cavity on the superior poles of each kidney, lateral to the lower thoracic and upper lumbar vertebrae. Each gland weighs approximately 4 grams and measures 3.3 cm in length. The adrenal gland itself is composed of two parts: an outer portion called the cortex and an inner portion called the medulla. The cortex and medulla have very different, independent functions (Fig. 42–7).

MEDULLA

The medulla constitutes one tenth of the gland and contains sympathetic ganglia (groups of nerve cell bodies) with secretory cells. Stimulation of the sympathetic nervous system causes the medulla to secrete two types of catecholamines: norepinephrine (noradrenaline) and epinephrine (adrenaline). Both of these substances act as neurotransmitters. They are released into the circulation and transported to target organs or tissues, where they exert their effects by binding to adrenergic receptors. The effects of the catecholamines vary depending on the specific receptor in the cell membrane of the target. There are two types of receptors: α-adrenergic and β-adrenergic. These are further classified as α_1, α_2, β_1, and β_2 receptors. Norepinephrine binds to α-adrenergic receptors, whereas epinephrine affects primarily β-adrenergic receptors. Table 42–4 describes the specific effects of these catecholamines. The major function of these substances is maintenance of homeostasis and adaptation to stress, as characterized by the "fight or flight response."

CORTEX

The adrenal cortex, which comprises 90% of the adrenal gland, is the outer portion of the gland. This is the portion that is considered to be a part of the endocrine system. The cortex is essential for maintenance of many life-sustaining physiologic activities. The cells of the cortex are organized into three distinct layers or zones. Proceeding from the outermost to innermost layers, they are the zona glomerulosa, zona fasciculata, and zona reticularis. The hormones synthesized and secreted by the cortex are known as steroids and consist of mineralocorticoids, glucocorticoids, and androgens or estrogens.

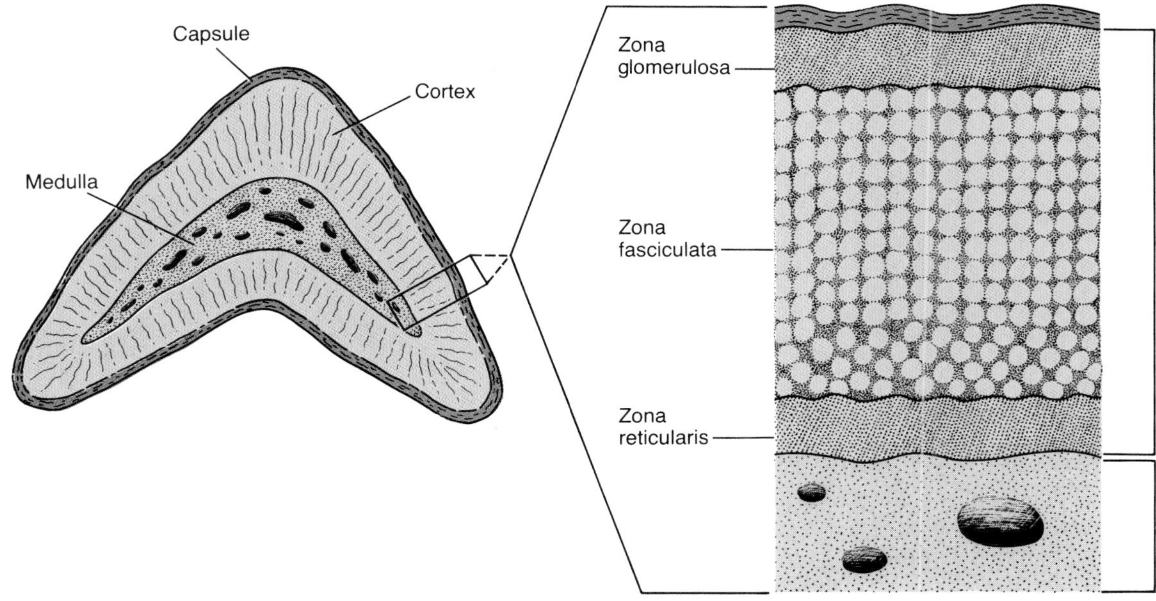

FIGURE 42-7
The structure of the adrenal glands. The adrenal cortex consists of three layers: the zona glomerulosa, the zona fasciculata, and the zona reticularis. (Modified from Ignatavicius, D. D., & Bayne, M. V. [1991]. *Medical-surgical nursing: A nursing process approach* [p. 1518]. Philadelphia: W. B. Saunders.)

FUNCTION OF THE ADRENAL GLANDS

MINERALOCORTICOIDS

The zona glomerulosa produces mineralocorticoids, the most abundant of which is aldosterone. Mineralocorticoids play a key role in maintaining an adequate extracellular fluid volume. Aldosterone functions at the renal collecting tubule to promote the reabsorption of sodium and the excretion of potassium by the kidney. The secretion of aldosterone is regulated by several factors: serum levels of potassium, the renin-angiotensin mechanism, and ACTH.

TABLE 42-4
RECEPTORS AND EFFECTS OF ADRENAL MEDULLARY HORMONES ON SELECTED ORGANS AND TISSUES

ORGAN OR TISSUE	RECEPTOR	EFFECT
Heart	β	Positive chronotropic action Positive inotropic action
Blood vessels	α	Vasoconstriction (except in cardiac and skeletal muscles)
	β_2	Vasodilation
Gastrointestinal tract	α, β	Increased sphincter tone; decreased motility
Kidney	β_2	Increased renin release
Bronchioles	β_2	Relaxation; dilation
Bladder	α	Sphincter contractions, urinary retention
	β_2	Relaxation of detrusor muscle
Skin	α	Increased sweating, piloerection
Adipose tissue	β	Increased lipolysis
Liver	α	Increased gluconeogenesis and glycogenolysis
Pancreas	α	Decreased glucagon and insulin release
	β	Increased glucagon and insulin release
Eyes	α	Dilation of pupils

RENIN

Renin is produced by the juxtaglomerular cells of renal afferent arterioles. Its release is stimulated by a decrease in extracellular fluid volume. Any factor that can cause this decrease (blood or fluid loss, sodium depletion, or changes in body position or posture) can stimulate renin release. Renin acts on plasma proteins to release angiotensin I, which is catalyzed in the lung to angiotensin II. Angiotensin II stimulates the secretion of aldosterone, which results in sodium and water retention. Retention of sodium and water preserves or increases extracellular fluid volume and subsequently increases blood pressure. This compensatory mechanism plays a very important role in maintaining intravascular volume in shock states.

GLUCOCORTICOIDS

The glucocorticoids are produced by the zona reticularis and zona fasciculata. The most abundant and potent of the glucocorticoids is cortisol. Approximately 92% of circulating cortisol is bound to transcortin (a corticosteroid-binding globulin). Free cortisol (~8%) binds with receptors in the cytoplasm and nuclei of target cells. Cortisol has a permissive effect on other physiologic processes, meaning that the glucocorticoid must be present in order for other processes, such as catecholamine activity and excitability of the myocardium, to occur. Functions of the glucocorticoid include control of carbohydrate, lipid, and fat metabolism, regulation of anti-inflammatory and immune responses, and control of emotional states. The maintenance of these physiologic mechanisms is accomplished in the following ways:

- Maintenance of glucose levels by increasing hepatic gluconeogenesis and by inhibiting peripheral glucose use.
- Increased lipolysis and release of glycerol and free fatty acids.
- Increased protein catabolism.
- Degradation of collagen and connective tissue.
- Increased number of polymorphonucleocytes released from bone marrow.
- Increased anti-inflammatory effects due to migration of inflammatory cells to sites of injury.
- Maintenance of behavioral and cognitive functions.

SEX HORMONES

Adrenal androgens are another class of steroids produced in the zona fasciculata and zona reticularis of the adrenal cortex. Their primary function is masculinization in males. Other sex hormones include estrogen and progesterone. In males, these substances contribute little to reproductive maturation. In females, however, estrogens are supplied by both the ovaries and the adrenal glands. In postmenopausal women, the adrenal cortex is the primary source of endogenous estrogen.

NURSING ASSESSMENT OF THE PATIENT WITH AN ADRENAL DISORDER

HEALTH HISTORY

Present Illness

Symptoms of adrenal dysfunction that may cause the patient to seek medical attention include decreased energy, mental changes (depression, anxiety, nervousness, confusion), sexual dysfunction, gastrointestinal disturbances, and abnormal skin pigmentation. The nurse elicits a thorough description of the chief complaint.

Past Medical History

Aspects of the past medical history that may be significant include radiation to the head or abdomen, intracranial surgery, and recent and current medications.

Review of Systems

The patient's perception of his or her general well-being is assessed. The nurse asks about changes in skin color, especially bronzed or smoky pigmentation, and increased facial hair in women. Changes in weight and appetite are noted. Symptoms that may be related to adrenal dysfunction are headache, lightheadedness with position changes, muscle weakness, nausea, vomiting, abdominal pain, anorexia, menstrual dysfunction, and impotence.

Functional Assessment

The functional assessment documents usual dietary and activity patterns and disruptions in lifestyle.

PHYSICAL EXAMINATION

The patient's height, weight, and vital signs are measured. The blood pressure is taken when the patient is reclining and after the patient has moved to an upright position to detect a significant drop. Patient responses and ability to follow instructions are noted. The skin is inspected for a bronzed or smoky pigmentation (especially in surgical scars, the skin over the knuckles, in skin folds, and the areola), bruising, petechiae, vitiligo (loss of pigmentation), and pallor. The face of the female patient is inspected for excess facial hair. The oral mucous membranes are inspected for color changes. The anterior thorax is inspected for fat pads under the clavicles, and the posterior thorax for the "buffalo hump." Obesity of the trunk is noted. The breasts are examined for striae and darkening of the areola. The nurse inspects the abdomen for striae, and the extremities for muscle wasting and edema. During examination of the external genitalia the nurse assesses for atrophy, hair loss, and appropriateness for age.

Assessment of the patient with an adrenal disorder is summarized in Table 42–5.

TABLE 42–5
ASSESSMENT OF THE PATIENT WITH AN ADRENAL DISORDER

HEALTH HISTORY

Present illness: Decreased energy, mental changes, sexual dysfunction, gastrointestinal disturbances, abnormal skin pigmentation

Past medical history: Radiation to head or abdomen, intracranial surgery, recent and current medications

Review of systems: General well-being, bronzed or smoky skin color, increased facial hair in females, headache, lightheadedness with position changes, muscle weakness, nausea, vomiting, abdominal pain, anorexia, menstrual dysfunction, impotence

Functional assessment: Changes in height and weight, changes in diet, salt craving, disruption of lifestyle by symptoms

PHYSICAL EXAMINATION

Height and weight

Vital signs

Mental status

Skin: Smoky or bronzed pigmentation prominent on surgical scars, knuckles, in skin folds, areola; bruising, petechiae, vitiligo, pallor

Head and face: Excess facial hair

Mouth: Color change of oral mucous membranes

Thorax: Supraclavicular fat pads, "buffalo hump"

Trunk: Obesity

Breasts: Striae, darkening of areola

Abdomen: Striae

Extremities: Muscle wasting, edema

Genitalia: Atrophy, loss of hair, appropriate development for age

Age-Related Changes

Under normal circumstances, adrenal function remains adequate in the older person. Some patients have a decline in cortisol secretion, but this is balanced by a decrease in cortisol metabolism such that blood levels remain normal. Secretion of aldosterone and plasma renin activity decline with age. This causes the ability to conserve sodium and to adapt to position changes to be less efficient.

DIAGNOSTIC TESTS AND PROCEDURES

Since only two deviations from normal adrenal function are covered here, the appropriate diagnostic tests and procedures are discussed with each condition.

DISORDERS OF THE ADRENAL GLANDS

ADRENAL HYPOFUNCTION

Etiology

Adrenal insufficiency may be classified as either primary or secondary. Primary adrenal insufficiency, which is also called Addison's disease, is frequently due to a destructive disease process that results in deficiencies of cortisol and aldosterone. The most common cause of Addison's disease is idiopathic atrophy, an autoimmune disease in which adrenal tissue is destroyed by antibodies formed by the patient's own immune system. Other causes of Addison's disease are tuberculosis, hemorrhage related to anticoagulant therapy, fungal infections (histoplasmosis, coccidioidomycosis), acquired immunodeficiency syndrome (AIDS), metastatic cancer, gram-negative sepsis (Waterhouse-Friderichsen syndrome), adrenalectomy, adrenal toxins, and abrupt withdrawal of exogenous steroids.

Secondary adrenal insufficiency is a result of dysfunction of the hypothalamus or pituitary (decreased corticotropin, ACTH), which leads to decreased androgen and cortisol production. Unlike primary adrenal insufficiency, in which all steroids are affected, aldosterone may or may not be affected. Causes of secondary adrenal insufficiency include pituitary tumors, postpartum necrosis of the pituitary (Sheehan's syndrome), hypophysectomy, radiation therapy, pituitary or intracranial lesions, or high-dose, long-term glucocorticoid treatment, which suppresses the adrenal glands' intrinsic activity.

Pathophysiology

Insufficiency of adrenocortical steroids causes defects associated with the loss of mineralocorticoids and glucocorticoids. Impaired secretion of cortisol results in decreased gluconeogenesis and decreased liver and muscle glycogen. This in turn causes decreased supplies of available glucose and hypoglycemia. In addition, the glomerular filtration rate of the kidneys and gastric acid production by the parietal cells of the stomach both slow significantly. The cumulative effects of these processes cause decreased urea nitrogen excretion, irritability, anorexia, weight loss, nausea, vomiting, and diarrhea.

Decreased levels of aldosterone alter the clearance of potassium, water, and sodium by the kidney. Potassium excretion is decreased, and hyperkalemia may occur. Since hyperkalemia promotes hydrogen ion retention, metabolic acidosis also can occur. Sodium and water excretion accelerates and causes potential problems, such as hypovolemia and hyponatremia.

Other manifestations of adrenal insufficiency may include progressive weakness, lethargy, unexplained abdominal pain, and malaise. Skin hyperpigmentation, particularly in sun-exposed areas, pressure points, joints, and creases of the body, is another possible sign. It is most likely due to increased secretion of a beta-lipoprotein or a melanocyte-stimulating hormone, which is released by a part of the pituitary. This is a direct result of hypocortisolism and a lack of negative feedback.

If adrenal androgen levels are lowered, a decrease or loss of body, axillary, and pubic hair can occur. In prepubescent individuals, facial, pubic, and axillary hair may fail to grow entirely. The severity of these symptoms is linked to the degree of hormone deficiency. This lack of secondary sex characteristics tends to be seen in primary adrenal insufficiency rather than in secondary adrenal insufficiency.

ACUTE ADRENAL CRISIS (ADDISONIAN CRISIS). Patients with either primary or secondary adrenal insufficiency are at risk for episodes of acute adrenal crisis, also called addisonian crisis, which is a life-threatening emergency. This is typically the result of a sudden marked decrease in available adrenal hormones. Precipitating factors are adrenal surgery, pituitary destruction, abrupt withdrawal of steroid therapy (often a result of a patient unwittingly stopping medications), and stress. Any factor that causes stress in the individual can initiate a crisis. Examples of stressors include infection, illness, trauma, and emotional or psychiatric disturbances. Manifestations of an addisonian crisis include symptoms of mineralocorticoid and glucocorticoid deficiency but are more severe: hypotension, tachycardia, dehydration, confusion, hyponatremia, hyperkalemia, hypercalcemia, and hypoglycemia. If left untreated, fluid and electrolyte imbalances can lead to circulatory collapse, cardiac arrhythmias, cardiac arrest, coma, and death. The management of an addisonian crisis is given in Table 42–6.

Medical Diagnosis

LABORATORY STUDIES. In addition to the presence of various clinical signs and symptoms, the diagnosis of Addison's disease is made on the basis of a variety of laboratory findings, which include a low serum cortisol level, decreased fasting glucose, decreased sodium, and increased potassium and blood urea nitrogen. Additionally, 24-hour urine tests may be performed. This type of testing reflects steroid secretion over a 24-hour period and is the most accurate measurement of steroid secretion, which varies with the diurnal rhythm. Urinary 17-hydroxycorticosteroids also are sometimes measured

TABLE 42-6
EMERGENCY CARE: ACUTE ADRENAL CRISIS

INTERVENTION	RATIONALE
1. Before initiating treatment, obtain complete blood count and electrolyte, blood urea nitrogen, and plasma cortisol levels as ordered by physician.	1. To establish a baseline and obtain data for diagnosis and treatment.
2. Give an initial dose of hydrocortisone (Solu-Cortef), 100–300 mg IV; then infuse 100 mg/8 hr as ordered by physician.	2. To provide a loading dose and maintenance infusion. The output of adrenal glucose is 300 mg/24 hr. The half-life of IV hydrocortisone is 60–90 min; 100 mg/8 hr is needed to avoid a relapse.
3. Give concomitant doses of hydrocortisone, 50 mg IM every 12 hr as ordered by physician.	3. To ensure constant source of glucocorticoids in case of IV failure (infiltration, infusion phlebitis).
4. After resolution of crisis, adjust dosage of medications as ordered by physician: a. Give oral glucocorticoids. b. Decrease dosage of oral glucocorticoids over several days as maintenance levels are reached. c. Give supplemental mineralocorticoids as glucocorticoid dosage is tapered.	4. To ensure adequacy of mineralocorticoid activity with minimal glucocorticoid dose.
5. Provide emotional support to patient and family.	5. To minimize excess anxiety and fear during a crisis period.

IV, Intravenously, intravenous; IM, intramuscularly.
Adapted from Ignatavicius, D. D., & Bayne, M. V. (1991). *Medical-surgical nursing: A nursing process approach* (p. 1545). Philadelphia: W. B. Saunders.

as an indicator of glucocorticoid metabolites and are specific for this category of steroids. Androgen metabolites can be determined by measurement of 17-ketosteroids. Both of these substances are low or borderline low in adrenal hypofunction. A list of drugs that interfere with urine tests for 17-hydroxycorticosteroids and 17-ketosteroids is presented in Table 42–7.

An ACTH stimulation test is necessary for a definitive diagnosis of hypoadrenalism. One common technique used in this test is the administration of a synthetic dose

TABLE 42-7
DRUGS THAT INTERFERE WITH URINE TESTS FOR 17-HYDROXYCORTICOSTEROIDS AND 17-KETOSTEROIDS

Acetaminophen	Medroxyprogesterone
Acetazolamide	Meperidine
Acetylsalicylic acid	Metyrapone
Amphetamines	Mitotane
Ascorbic acid	Morphine
Barbiturates	Nalidixic acid
Calcium gluconate	Oral contraceptives
Carbon disulfide	Paraldehyde
Chloral hydrate	Penicillin
Chlordiazepoxide	Pentazocine
Chlorthalidone	Perphenazine
Colchicine	Phenobarbital
Corticotropin	Phenothiazines
Cortisone	Phenylbutazone
Dexamethasone	Phenytoin
Diazepam	Promazine
Digoxin	Propoxyphene
Diphenhydramine	Quinidine
Erythromycin	Quinine
Estrogens	Reserpine
Fructose	Secobarbital
Glutethimide	Spironolactone
Hydralazine	Testosterone
Iodides	Vitamin K

Adapted from Ignatavicius, D. D., & Bayne, M. V. (1991). *Medical-surgical nursing: A nursing process approach* (p. 1552). Philadelphia: W. B. Saunders.

of ACTH (cosyntropin), which is given intramuscularly. Plasma cortisol levels are measured at onset of administration and at 30 minutes and 60 minutes after administration. In primary adrenal insufficiency, the cortisol response is absent or markedly decreased. In secondary insufficiency, there is a decrease in serum cortisol levels; however, it is not as significant a decrease as in cases of primary insufficiency. An adjunctive test that may be performed during ACTH stimulation is the eosinophil count. The eosinophil count drops 60 to 90% after the administration of ACTH in normal patients, but, in patients with Addison's disease, there is little or no change in the number of circulating eosinophils. If a glucose fasting test is performed, the serum glucose does not rise as high as it would in normal patients and returns to a fasting level more rapidly.

ELECTROCARDIOGRAM. Alterations in electrolyte levels are often reflected as deviations in the normal electrocardiogram, or ECG. For example, hyperkalemia will result in peaked T waves, a widened QRS interval, and an increased PR interval.

RADIOGRAPHIC STUDIES. Skull films, arteriograms, and CT scans may be performed in order to rule out causative factors in secondary adrenal insufficiency. These are of use in identifying intracranial lesions that may be impinging on the pituitary, aneurysms, or other defects. An abdominal CT scan may depict atrophy of the adrenal glands and identify a possible cause of primary insufficiency.

Medical Treatment

The mainstay of treatment of patients with Addison's disease is replacement therapy with glucocorticoids and mineralocorticoids. Glucocorticoids, such as cortisone, are typically divided into doses: two thirds of a daily dose is taken in the morning and one third in the evening. The rationale for this dosage schedule is based on human hormonal variations, in which glucocorticoids normally peak in the early morning and are at their lowest level in the evening. Mineralocorticoids, such as fluorocortisone, are typically given in the afternoon or evening. Table 42–8 details this type of replacement therapy.

Secondary adrenal insufficiency is treated with glucocorticoids, but mineralocorticoids are usually unnecessary.

PHARMACOLOGY CAPSULE

Addison's disease is treated with glucocorticoids given in divided doses to mimic the body's normal hormonal cycles.

Nursing Care of the Patient with Addison's Disease

ASSESSMENT. Assessment of the patient with an adrenal disorder is summarized in Table 42–5 (see also Care Plan: The Patient with Addison's Disease). Details of the health history that are especially relevant are the presence of weight loss, salt craving, nausea and vomiting, abdominal cramping and diarrhea, muscle weakness and aches, poor stress response, decreased libido, and amenorrhea. During the physical examination, the nurse is alert for pale skin with bronzed areas, emaciation, sparse body hair, poor skin turgor, hypotension, muscle wasting, irritability, and confusion. Nursing care of the patient with acute episodes of Addison's disease requires frequent reassessment, monitoring of fluid and electrolyte levels, and measurement of daily weights.

TABLE 42–8
DRUGS USED TO TREAT ADRENAL DISORDERS

DRUG	USE/ACTION	SIDE EFFECTS	NURSING INTERVENTIONS
Glucocorticoids Cortisone acetate (Cortone Acetate) Prednisolone (Delta-Cortef, Prelone) Prednisolone acetate (Econopred) Hydrocortisone (Cortef)	Stimulate formation of glucose, promote storage of glucose as glycogen, affect fluid and electrolytes, increase hemoglobin, anti-inflammatory. Used to treat adrenal insufficiency.	Hypokalemia, hypocalcemia, nausea and vomiting, edema, hypertension, increased risk of infection, hyperglycemia, muscle wasting, osteoporosis, ulcer development, acne, pathologic fractures. May cause death if suddenly discontinued.	Monitor weight, intake and output, BP, blood glucose. Assess for edema. Protect from sources of infection. Report signs of infection even if subtle. Assess for hypocalcemia: muscle weakness and twitching. Assess for hypokalemia: muscle weakness and tingling, cardiac dysrhythmias, irritability. Protect from falls and possible fractures. Give oral drugs with food or milk. Many patients with adrenal insufficiency manage with only glucocorticoid replacement; others require mineralocorticoids also. Instruct patient to take on prescribed schedule, not to discontinue suddenly, and to carry drug ID card.
Mineralocorticoids Fludrocortisone (Florinef)	Stimulate reabsorption of sodium and excretion of potassium and hydrogen ions in renal tubules. Used to treat adrenal insufficiency.	Hypokalemia, nausea and vomiting, edema, hypertension, increased risk of infection, muscle weakness, depression, mood swings, dizziness, impaired wound healing, ulcers.	Monitor weight, intake and output, BP, blood glucose, serum electrolytes. Protect from infection. Assess for hypokalemia. Explain effects of drug on emotional state. Give with food or milk. Do not discontinue suddenly. Tell patient to carry drug identification card. Do not take with aspirin.
Adrenocortical cytotoxic agents Mitotane (Lysodren)	Suppress adrenocortical function.	Nausea and vomiting, diarrhea, lethargy, dizziness, hypouricemia, hearing and vision disturbances, BP changes, dyspnea.	Monitor BP. Report infections or trauma so drug can be temporarily discontinued. Tell patient not to have immunizations without physician approval and to avoid contact with people who have recently had polio vaccine. Increase fluid intake and monitor uric acid.
Antifungal agents Ketoconazole (Nizoral)	Fungistatic. Suppresses adrenocortical function.	Nausea and vomiting, pruritus, diarrhea or constipation, GI bleeding, lethargy, adrenocortical insufficiency, headache, dizziness. Occasionally, thrombocytopenia, hemolytic anemia, hepatotoxicity.	Monitor stools. Administer antipruritics or apply topical agents as ordered. Safety measures if dizzy or drowsy. Monitor liver function tests and assess for pale stools, dark urine, fatigue, and anorexia. Avoid alcohol.

BP, Blood pressure; GI, gastrointestinal.

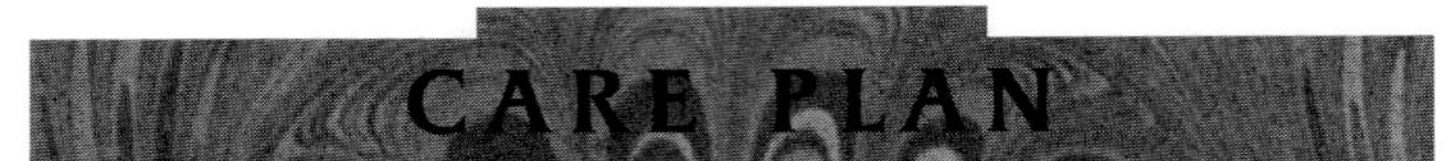

The Patient with Addison's Disease

ASSESSMENT

Health History: Ronald Damon, a 52-year-old white man, is admitted with Addison's disease. He considers himself healthy but has had some joint pain in his knees. He had an appendectomy in 1975. The patient complains of weight loss, anorexia, weakness, and darkening of the skin on his face and arms. His usual weight is 170 pounds. He has had bouts of nausea, vomiting, and diarrhea accompanied by vague abdominal pain. The patient is a salesman and reports that his symptoms are making it difficult for him to keep up with his work. He is embarrassed about the change in his skin color.

Physical Examination: Vital signs: blood pressure, 110/80 (sitting) and 88/42 (standing); pulse, 102 with slight irregularity; respiration, 20; temperature, 98°F orally. Height, 5′8″. Weight, 155 lb. The patient is oriented but somewhat lethargic. The skin on his face and arms and his abdominal scar is darkly pigmented. His body hair is sparse. The patient's oral mucous membranes are slightly dry.

NURSING DIAGNOSIS	GOALS AND OUTCOME CRITERIA	INTERVENTIONS
Impaired tissue perfusion related to electrolyte imbalance, fluid volume deficit, and cardiac arrhythmias.	The patient will have improved tissue perfusion as evidenced by warm, dry skin, strong peripheral pulses, and fluid intake equal to fluid intake.	Monitor for signs and symptoms of inadequate tissue perfusion: confusion, disorientation, tachycardia, hypotension, apical-radial pulse deficit, fluid output exceeding intake. Administer intravenous fluids (normal saline, plasma expanders) and vasopressors, as ordered. Monitor for hyperkalemia: weakness, paresthesia, and dizziness. Report evidence of inadequate tissue perfusion or hyperkalemia to physician.
High risk for injury related to acute adrenal insufficiency, impaired stress response, postural hypotension.	The patient will remain free of injury due to hypotension, shock, or falls.	Monitor for postural hypotension. If the patient has dizziness with position changes, instruct him to exercise his legs before rising, to rise slowly, and to call for help when getting out of bed. Administer fluids and hormones as ordered.
Alteration in nutrition: less than body requirements related to impaired metabolism, inability to ingest sufficient nutrients, and lack of interest in eating.	The patient will be adequately nourished as evidenced by weight within 5 pounds of baseline.	Weigh daily to monitor fluid balance and nutritional status. Request dietary consult for patient education and so that food preferences can be respected. Provide high-protein, low-carbohydrate diet as ordered. Tell the patient salt may be used freely. Provide a pleasant atmosphere for meals. Report signs of hypoglycemia: headache, trembling, tachycardia, sweating.
Fatigue related to fluid, electrolyte, and glucose imbalances.	The patient will report lessened fatigue.	Explain medically prescribed activity limitations. Plan care to allow for periods of rest. Discuss energy conservation after discharge.
Body image disturbance related to changes in appearance and function.	The patient will adapt to altered physical appearance and function as evidenced by efforts to improve appearance and positive comments about self.	Explore how the patient feels about skin changes. Discuss strategies to deal with changes: long sleeves, avoidance of excess sunlight, scheduling work with rest periods. Encourage attention to grooming. Compliment efforts.

The Patient with Addison's Disease *(Continued)*

NURSING DIAGNOSIS	GOALS AND OUTCOME CRITERIA	INTERVENTIONS
Knowledge deficit of long-term glucocorticoid therapy.	The patient will correctly explain the disease, its treatment, and medication therapy and will state intent to adhere to prescribed regimen.	Implement teaching plan, to include the following: 1. Wear a medical alert tag and carry emergency kit with dexamethasone. 2. Take glucocorticoid in divided doses in morning and afternoon with food. 3. Increase medication dosage as ordered when under stress. 4. Notify physician or go to emergency room if unable to take oral medications for more than 24 hours. 5. Lifelong therapy and monitoring are needed. 6. Report signs and symptoms of inadequate and excessive hormone replacement.

NURSING DIAGNOSIS. Nursing diagnoses for the patient with Addison's disease may include the following:

- **Impaired Tissue Perfusion** related to electrolyte imbalance, hypovolemia, cardiac dysrhythmias
- **High Risk for Injury** related to acute adrenal insufficiency, impaired physiologic response to stress, postural hypotension
- **Altered Nutrition: Less than Body Requirements** related to impaired metabolism, inability to ingest sufficient nutrients, lack of interest in eating
- **Fatigue** related to fluid, electrolyte, and glucose imbalances
- **Body Image Disturbance** related to changes in appearance and function
- **Knowledge Deficit** of long-term glucocorticoid replacement therapy

GOALS. Goals of nursing care for the identified nursing diagnoses are improved tissue perfusion, absence of injury or signs of shock, adequate nutrition, improved stamina, adaptation to physical changes, and patient's knowledge of self-medication.

INTERVENTIONS

Impaired Tissue Perfusion. The nurse monitors for signs and symptoms of inadequate tissue perfusion: confusion, disorientation, tachycardia, hypotension (including postural changes), apical-radial pulse deficit, general weakness and malaise, and output greater than intake. Intravenous normal saline, plasma expanders, and vasopressors are administered as ordered to maintain blood volume. The patient is at risk for hyperkalemia, so the nurse monitors serum electrolytes and assesses for weakness, paresthesia, dizziness, and electrocardiogram changes. These signs and symptoms of hyperkalemia are reported to the physician.

High Risk for Injury. The nurse assesses the patient for postural hypotension and other signs of hypovolemia. The patient who has dizziness with position changes is instructed to call for help when getting out of bed to prevent falls. Exercising the legs before standing promotes venous return and may minimize the drop in blood pressure.

Sudden profound weakness with postural hypotension is characteristic of acute addisonian crisis and will lead to shock and death if not corrected. Fluid replacement and hormones are administered as ordered to treat addisonian crisis.

Altered Nutrition. The patient is weighed daily to monitor fluid balance, but weight changes also provide information about the adequacy of the patient's diet. If nutrition is a problem, the dietitian should be consulted. The prescribed diet is usually high protein, low carbohydrate. Salt may be used liberally since patients with Addison's disease tend to lose sodium. The patient's food preferences should be respected as much as possible. The mealtime atmosphere should be conducive to eating.

Hypoglycemia may develop as a result of decreased cortisol secretion. Frequent rest periods are encouraged to avoid depletion of glycogen stores. Meals should be taken regularly, and between-meal snacks may be advised to maintain blood glucose. The nurse monitors for and teaches the patient symptoms of hypoglycemia: headache, tachycardia, trembling, sweating. Periodic laboratory studies are done to assess nitrogen balance, liver function, and serum albumin, glucose, electrolytes, blood urea nitrogen, and creatinine.

Fatigue. The nurse explains any prescribed activity limitations to the patient. Specific rest periods are planned to conserve energy. Assistance with activities of daily living is provided as needed. If the patient is on bedrest, the nurse intervenes to prevent complications of immobility as described in Chapter 19.

Body Image Disturbance. The nurse explores the patient's reaction to the physical changes experienced. Strategies to cope with changes are discussed. When the patient's condition has stabilized, the nurse encourages attention to grooming and compliments the patient's efforts.

Knowledge Deficit. Care of the patient with a chronic disease requires in-depth education and advice and information related to stress management. It is critical that the patient understand Addison's disease and know how to recognize the effects of the disease as well as the effects of overmedication. Written material is provided to supplement the teaching sessions. The teaching plan should include the following:

1. Lifelong cortisol replacement therapy will be required.
2. Take glucocorticoids as ordered in divided doses, one dose in the morning and the other in the afternoon.
3. Take glucocorticoids with food.
4. Increase the dosage as directed by the physician if you have severe emotional stress or increased physical demands, including pregnancy, surgery, or an acute illness.
5. If you are unable to take your oral medicine for more than a day, notify your physician or go to an emergency room so that you can be given your medication by injection.
6. Always wear a medical alert tag and carry an emergency kit with a dose of dexamethasone to be administered in the event of acute addisonian crisis.

EVALUATION. Criteria for goal achievement for the patient with Addison's disease are warm, dry skin with strong peripheral pulses; blood pressure within patient's norms and absence of faintness with position changes; weight within 5 pounds of patient's baseline; patient's statement of lessened fatigue; patient's efforts to improve appearance and positive comments about self; patient's verbalization of disease process, treatment, and medication regimen with stated intent to adhere to prescribed regimen.

ADRENAL HYPERSECRETION (CUSHING'S SYNDROME)

Etiology

Hypersecretion of the adrenal cortex may result in the production of excess amounts of corticosteroids, particularly glucocorticoid. The condition that results from excessive cortisol is called Cushing's syndrome. An overproduction of adrenocortical hormones may result from endogenous (internal) causes as well as from exogenous (external) causes.

Endogenous causes include corticotropin-secreting pituitary tumors, a cortisol-secreting neoplasm within the adrenal glands and excess secretion of corticotropin by a carcinoma of the lung or other tissues. Excessive production of ACTH because of a pituitary tumor is called Cushing's disease.

The single exogenous cause of Cushing's syndrome is prolonged administration of high doses of corticosteroids. This is the most common cause of Cushing's syndrome. The incidence of Cushing's syndrome caused by disease is infrequent, affecting females eight times more often than males. Approximately 25% of cases of Cushing's syndrome are due to adrenal tumors.

Pathophysiology

Clinical manifestations of Cushing's syndrome affect most body systems and are related to excess levels of circulating corticosteroids. In some instances, signs and symptoms of mineralocorticoid and androgen excess may appear; however, signs and symptoms of glucocorticoid excess usually predominate.

Hyperadrenalism produces marked changes in the personal appearance of the affected individual, including obesity, facial plethora (redness), hirsutism, menstrual disorders, hypertension of varying degrees, and muscle wasting of the extremities. Additional findings can be delayed wound healing and mood disturbances such as irritability, anxiety, insomnia, and irrational behavior. The hallmark findings that lead to a diagnosis of Cushing's syndrome are the following:

- A combination of truncal obesity and protein wasting. Protein wasting is evidenced by slender extremities and very thin and friable skin
- Facial fullness or a "moon face"
- Purple striae on the abdomen, breasts, buttocks, or thighs
- Osteoporosis (a significant finding in premenopausal women)
- Hypokalemia of uncertain etiology

A visual example of these findings is depicted in Figure 42–8.

Medical Diagnosis

In addition to physical signs and symptoms, some laboratory and radiographic findings may be useful in determining a diagnosis.

LABORATORY STUDIES. Abnormal laboratory findings include polycythemia, hypokalemia, hypernatremia, hyperglycemia, leukocytosis, glycosuria, and elevated levels of plasma cortisol.

The overnight dexamethasone test also is used as an initial screening for Cushing's syndrome. Patients are instructed not to take any medications for 2 days since certain drugs such as phenytoin and phenobarbital can interfere with results. At midnight on the first day of testing, the patient receives 1 mg of oral dexamethasone. The following morning, the plasma cortisol levels are measured. A normal finding is a serum level of less than 5 mg per dl. If the level is higher, additional testing is performed. A dexamethasone suppression test using a low dose may be given to confirm the findings of the overnight dexamethasone suppression test. For

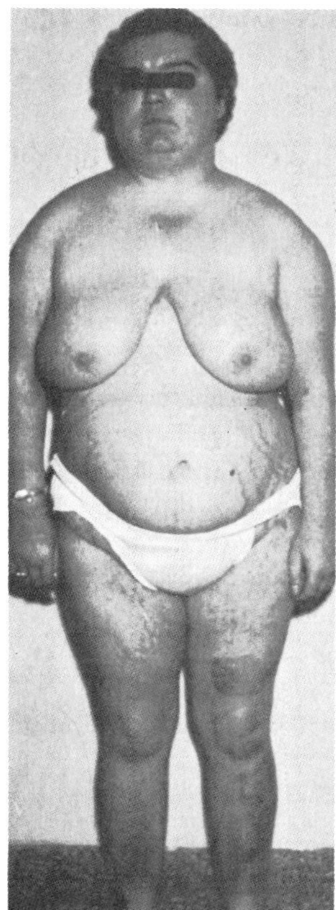
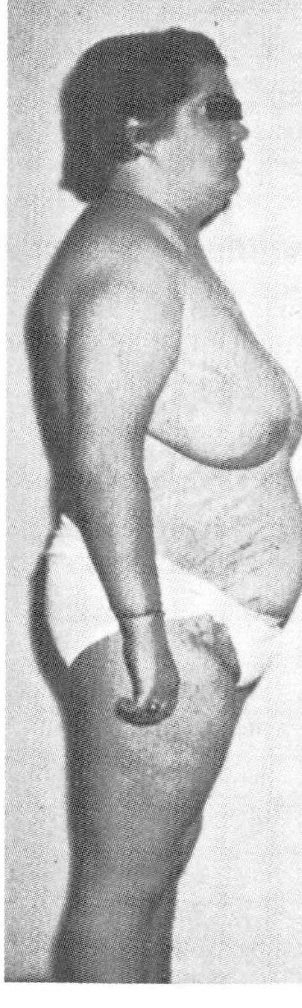

FIGURE 42-8
Cushing's syndrome. Clinical manifestations in the patient with Cushing's syndrome. (From Bondy, P. K., & Rosenberg, L. E. [1980]. *Metabolic control and disease* [8th ed.]. Philadelphia: W. B. Saunders.)

these tests, the patient is again instructed to avoid certain medications (Table 42–7) and to avoid excess stress. On day 1 of the test, a baseline 24-hour urine sample is collected. Dexamethasone is then administered in doses of 0.5 mg every 6 hours, and 24-hour urine collections are taken on day 2 and again on day 3. The urine is tested for 17-ketosteroids, 17-hydroxycorticosteroids, creatinine, and free cortisol. In normal patients, the cortisol and 17-hydroxycorticosteroid levels are suppressed. If these levels are not suppressed (as compared to the baseline sample), the test is repeated using a high dose of dexamethasone (2 mg every 6 hours).

RADIOGRAPHIC STUDIES. If a tumor is suspected as a causative factor in Cushing's syndrome, a CT scan and magnetic resonance imaging may be done to localize the site of the tumor. Radiographic films may depict osteoporosis of the spinal column, especially in females.

Medical Treatment

Depending on the specific individual and the etiology of the disease, a combination of therapies may be employed. These include drug therapy, radiation, and surgery. If the condition is caused by administration of synthetic glucocorticoids, the physician may gradually withdraw them. The majority of patients affected with hyperadrenalism due to a tumor undergo surgical intervention.

DRUG THERAPY. In situations in which it is not feasible for the patient to undergo surgery, certain agents that interfere with ACTH production or adrenal hormone synthesis may be administered. One example is mitotane (Lysodren), a cytotoxic substance that is used as a palliative treatment for inoperable adrenal tumors. Agents that interfere with cortisol production include aminoglutethimide (Cytadren), metyrapone (Metopirone), and ketoconazole (Nizoral). Metyrapone is also used in combination with mitotane for enhanced effects. Trilostane (Modrastane) is another agent that acts as an enzyme inhibitor and has recently been used, although its effectiveness has not been established. There is a risk of acute adrenal crisis when patients are on drugs that suppress adrenal function. In addition, the drugs must be promptly discontinued if trauma or shock occurs because the patient's ability to adapt is diminished. Table 42–8 provides additional information about drug therapy.

PHARMACOLOGY CAPSULE

Drugs that suppress adrenal function can lead to acute adrenal crisis and must be promptly discontinued if shock or trauma occurs.

RADIATION. In some cases, radiation therapy is used for pituitary adenomas that secrete excessive quantities of ACTH. Radiation can be administered either externally or internally. Internal radiation involves the use of a transsphenoidal implantation of a radioactive material that remains in place for a specified period of time. Radiation therapy is not always effective and can destroy healthy tissue. If radiation therapy is being used to treat a patient with a pituitary adenoma, the nurse should be alert for any significant changes in the patient's neurologic status, such as a complaint of headache or a change in mentation or pupillary responses. In addition, the patient may experience side effects associated with radiation therapy. These include alopecia (hair loss) and dry, red, or irritated skin. It is essential that the nurse reviews these conditions with the patient and educates him or her about these effects.

Surgical Management

The surgical treatment of hyperadrenalism depends on the specific cause of the disorder. For example, if adrenal hypersecretion is due to a pituitary adenoma that is producing ACTH, a transsphenoidal hypophysectomy is performed (see surgical management under hyperpituitarism earlier in this chapter). If adrenal adenoma or carcinoma is the cause of the adrenal hypersecretion, an adrenalectomy (removal of the adrenal gland) is performed. If only one gland is removed, the procedure is referred to as a unilateral adrenalectomy; the removal of both of the glands is called a bilateral adrenalectomy. An adrenalectomy may be performed in situations in which drug and radiation therapy are unsuccessful. Patients who are undergoing a unilateral adrenalectomy can expect to require replacement therapy for up to 2 years after surgery. A bilateral adrenalectomy necessitates the need for lifelong replacement of both glucocorticoid and mineralocorticoids.

Nursing Care of the Patient with Cushing's Syndrome

ASSESSMENT. Initial assessment of the patient with Cushing's syndrome includes a detailed history and physical examination. Specific information about the onset of symptoms, prior treatments, drug allergies, and current medications is obtained. Depending on the severity of the disorder and the number of symptoms present, a number of nursing diagnoses may be applicable. The complete nursing assessment of the patient with an adrenal disorder is summarized in Table 42–5.

NURSING DIAGNOSIS. The most appropriate nursing diagnoses for the majority of the individuals with Cushing's syndrome include the following:

- **High Risk for Infection** related to high serum cortisol levels
- **Altered Thought Processes** related to fluid and electrolyte imbalance
- **High Risk for Impaired Skin Integrity** related to changes in skin and connective tissue and edema
- **High Risk for Injury** (fracture) related to osteoporosis
- **Body Image Disturbance** related to changes in physical appearance and function
- **Knowledge Deficit** of disease, drug therapy, diet, and self-care

GOALS. Goals for nursing care of the patient with Cushing's syndrome are absence of infection, absence of thought disturbances, preserved skin integrity, absence of fractures, adaptation to altered body image, and patient's knowledge of disease, treatment, and self-care.

INTERVENTIONS

High Risk for Infection. Exposure to individuals with infections should be avoided owing to the patient's decreased resistance to infection. Minor symptoms, such as a low-grade fever (99.5°F or higher), sore throat, or aches, can indicate the onset of a potentially serious infection. Any symptoms indicative of a cold or other problem should be brought to the attention of the physician.

Altered Thought Processes. Personality changes often accompany adrenal disorders. When they do occur, they should be discussed with both the patient and the family. Understanding that mood swings are a part of this disorder may help the patient and family cope more effectively. If the emotional changes, particularly depression, become severe, the patient should be carefully monitored, and a psychiatric referral may be necessary.

High Risk for Impaired Skin Integrity. The skin of the patient with Cushing's syndrome is extremely fragile. The nurse inspects the skin daily to detect early signs of pressure or injuries. The patient with limited mobility is assisted to change positions at least every 2 hours. Bed linens are kept clean and dry. The patient is advised to wear shoes when out of bed to reduce the risk of foot injuries. During transfers and position changes, caregivers must be careful to prevent trauma to the skin.

High Risk for Injury. Since fractures occur very easily, the patient with Cushing's syndrome must be protected from falls or trauma. The bed is kept in low position, and the call button within reach. If the patient is very weak or confused, the siderails are raised. The nurse instructs the patient to call for assistance when getting in and out of bed.

Body Image Disturbance. Bruises, abnormal fat distribution, and hirsutism may cause embarrassment to the patient. The nurse provides an opportunity for the patient to share thoughts and concerns about these changes. If they are distressing, the nurse can suggest clothing to conceal them. Patients are encouraged and assisted to be well groomed. Females may choose to shave or to use depilatories to remove unwanted hair. The nurse can reassure the patient that physical changes generally improve gradually after medical or surgical treatment.

Knowledge Deficit. Patient teaching must include an explanation of adrenal function and the effects of Cushing's syndrome. The nurse explains the need to avoid exposure to infections and what signs and symptoms are to be reported to the physician. The nurse also emphasizes that mood swings are common and are part of the disease process. The patient must understand the importance of continuing drug therapy under medical supervision. Drug names and dosages are reviewed as well as adverse effects. Supplementary written material should be provided. Dietary instructions usually include guidelines for a low-calorie diet with sufficient protein and calcium. The dietitian should be consulted for patient education.

EVALUATION. Evaluation of nursing care is based on the patient's success in reaching those goals established in planning his or her care. Specific criteria for achievement of the identified goals are normal body temperature and white blood cell count; stable mood and patient's denial of depression; intact skin with minimal bruising; no skeletal trauma or fractures; patient's efforts to improve appearance; and patient's description of syndrome, treatment, and self-care, including diet and self-medication.

Nursing Care of the Adrenalectomy Patient

General nursing care of the surgical patient is discussed in Chapter 14. This section addresses the specific needs of the adrenalectomy patient.

PREOPERATIVE CARE. Preoperative care of the patient undergoing an adrenalectomy involves assessing for and correcting any existing electrolyte imbalances. The prevention of infections in these susceptible patients is maintained through strict hand washing and observance of asepsis. Preoperative education involves a discussion of glucocorticoid replacement therapy, including dosage, side effects, and complications.

POSTOPERATIVE CARE. Following adrenalectomy, patients are sent to an intensive care unit for at least 1 to 2 days for close observation and assessment. During this period, the nurse monitors the vital signs for signs and symptoms of impending shock, which may be evident as hypotension, a weak or thready pulse, decreased urinary output, and changes in level of consciousness. Pulse and blood pressure may be unstable for 24 to 48 hours postoperatively, and vasopressors may be needed to maintain blood pressure in the immediate postoperative period.

A nursing diagnosis specific to the adrenalectomy patient is the potential for injury related to addisonian crisis as a result of the sudden decrease in adrenal hormone secretion. The nurse assesses for signs and symptoms of acute adrenal insufficiency: vomiting, weakness, hypotension, joint pain, pruritus, and emotional disturbances. Fluid and electrolytes are closely monitored and intravenous fluids prescribed to restore or maintain balance. High doses of cortisol are given intravenously during and for several days after surgery to enable the patient to deal with the physical stress of surgery. The dosages are adjusted on the basis of the blood pressure, blood glucose, serum electrolytes, and serum cortisol levels. Later, glucocorticoids are administered orally.

Since the patient's resistance to infection is lowered, the nurse is especially careful to protect the patient by using strict aseptic technique for wound care and invasive procedures. Signs of infection may be very subtle.

Pain or discomfort is assessed at frequent intervals and treated with narcotic analgesics. The effects of treatment are observed and documented. To minimize the risk of pulmonary complications, such as stasis of secretions and pneumonia, the patient is instructed to turn, cough, deep breathe, or use an incentive spirometer if ordered.

PHEOCHROMOCYTOMA

A pheochromocytoma is a tumor, usually benign, of the adrenal medulla that causes secretion of excessive catecholamines. Patients with a pheochromocytoma exhibit episodes of hypertension, hypermetabolism, and hyperglycemia. Other signs and symptoms include severe headaches, pallor, pupil dilation, orthostatic hypotension, and blurred vision. Episodes may be triggered by emotional distress, exercise, manipulation of the tumor, postural changes, and major trauma, including surgery.

The condition is treated by surgical removal of the tumor. Preoperatively, the surgeon attempts to normalize vital signs and stabilize the patient's fluid status. The nurse monitors cardiovascular status and prepares the patient for surgery as detailed in Chapter 14. Postoperative nursing care is the same as that described for the patient having an adrenalectomy.

NUTRITION CONCEPTS

- Patients with Cushing's syndrome may experience sodium and water retention.
- Reducing sodium intake can decrease edema and related weight gain with Cushing's syndrome.
- Early symptoms of Addison's disease may include anorexia, nausea, vomiting, diarrhea, and weight loss, resulting in impaired nutrition.
- Patients with diabetes insipidus usually experience excessive thirst or urination, so they must drink liquids almost continuously to avoid dehydration and hypovolemic shock.

BIBLIOGRAPHY

Agana-Defensor, R. (1992). Pheochromocytoma: A clinical review. *Clinical Issues in Critical Care Nursing, 3*(2), 309–318.

Blissitt, P. A. (1992). Pituitary tumor, hypophysectomy, and diabetes insipidus. *Journal of Post Anesthesia Nursing, 7*(3), 209.

Cagno, J. M. (1989). Diabetes insipidus. *Critical Care Nurse, 9*(6), 86–93.

Chernecky, C. C., Krech, R. L., & Berger, B. J. (1993). *Laboratory tests and diagnostic procedures.* Philadelphia: W. B. Saunders.

Chipps, E. (1992). Transsphenoidal surgery for pituitary tumors. *Critical Care Nurse, 12*(1), 30–39.

Epstein, C. D. (1991). Fluid volume deficit for the adrenal crisis patient. *Dimensions of Critical Care Nursing, 10*(4), 210–217.

Gumowski, J., Proch, M., & Kessler, C. A. (1992). Endocrinopathies of hyperfunction: Cushing's syndrome and aldosteronism. *Clinical Issues in Critical Care Nursing, 3*(2), 331–349.

Haas, L. B. (1992). Nursing role in management: Endocrine problems. In S. M. Lewis & I. C. Collier (Eds.), *Medical-surgical nursing* (3rd ed.). St. Louis: Mosby Year Book, pp. 1319–1355.

Handerhan, B. (1992). Recognizing adrenal crisis. *Nursing 92, 22*(4), 33.

Hartshorn, J., & Hartshorn, E. (1988). Pharmacology update: Vasopressin in the treatment of diabetes insipidus. *Journal of Neuroscience Nursing, 20*(1), 58–59.

Hodgson, B. B., Kizior, R. J., & Kingdon, R. T. (1993). *Nurse's drug handbook.* Philadelphia: W. B. Saunders.

Ignatavicius, D. D., & Bayne, M. V. (1991). *Medical-surgical nursing: A nursing process approach.* Philadelphia: W. B. Saunders.

Jarvis, C. (1992). *Physical examination and health assessment.* Philadelphia: W. B. Saunders.

Johnson, J. L. (1991). Tuberculous Addison's disease. *Postgraduate Medicine, 90*(6), 139–140

Lindaman, C. (1992) SIADH: Is your patient at risk? *Nursing 92, 22*(6), 60–63.

Loriaux, T. C. (1993). Nursing care of clients with adrenal, pituitary, and gonadal disorders. In J. M. Black & E. Matassarin-Jacobs (Eds.), *Luckmann and Sorensen's medical-surgical nursing* (4th ed.) (pp. 1837–1862). Philadelphia: W. B. Saunders.

Matteson, M. A., & McConnell, E. S. (1989). *Gerontological nursing.* Philadelphia: W. B. Saunders.

Miell, J., Wasif, W., McGregor, A., Butler, J., & Ross, R. (1991). Life threatening hypercalcemia in association with addisonian crisis. *Postgraduate Medical Journal, 67*(790), 770–772.

Montoli, A., Colussi, G., & Minetti, L. (1992). Hypercalcemia in Addison's disease. *Journal of Internal Medicine, 232*(6), 535–540.

Patterson, L. M., & Noroian, E. L. (1989). Diabetes insipidus versus syndrome of inappropriate antidiuretic hormone. *Dimensions of Critical Care Nursing, 8*(4), 226–234.

Poe, C. M., & Taylor, L. M. (1989). Syndrome of inappropriate antidiuretic hormone: Assessment and nursing implications. *Oncology Nursing Forum, 16*(3), 373–381.

Schultz, P. N. (1989). Hypopituitarism in patients with a history of irradiation to the head and neck area: Diagnosis and implications for nursing. *Oncology Nursing Forum, 16*(6), 823–826.

Shlafer, M., & Marieb, E. N. (1989). *The nurse, pharmacology, and drug therapy.* Redwood City, CA: Addison-Wesley.

Sonino, N., Boscaro, M., Paoletta, A., Mantero, F., & Ziliotto, D. (1991). Ketoconazole treatment in Cushing's syndrome: Experience in 34 patients. *Clinical Endocrinology, 35*(4), 347–352.

Stuckey, P., & Waters, H. (1988). Oncology alert for the home care nurse: Syndrome of inappropriate antidiuretic hormone. *Home Healthcare Nurse, 6*(6), 26–30.

Tabarin, A., Navarranne, A., Geurin, J., Corcuff, J. B., Parneix, M., & Roger, P. (1991). Use of ketoconazole in the treatment of Cushing's disease and ectopic ACTH syndrome. *Clinical Endocrinology, 34*(1), 63–69.

Tobin, M. V., Aldridge, S. A., Morris, A. I., Belchetz, P. E., & Gilmore, I. T. (1989). Gastrointestinal manifestations of Addison's disease. *American Journal of Gastroenterology, 84*(10), 1302–1305.

Wanke, L. A. (1991). *Ketoconazole therapy of hyperadrenocorticalism* (Drugdex Vol. 78). Portland, OR: Micromedix, Inc.

Yucho, C., & Suddaby, P. (1991). David could have died of thirst, yet he never felt thirsty . . . diabetes insipidus. *Nursing 91, 21*(7), 42–45.

KEY CONCEPTS

1. The endocrine system secretes hormones, chemical messengers that affect target organs and body tissues.
2. Endocrine activity is regulated by feedback mechanisms that either stimulate or inhibit hormone synthesis and secretion.
3. Pituitary hormones affect growth, fluid and electrolyte balance, metabolism, ovulation, milk production, uterine contractions, and skin pigmentation.
4. Pituitary and adrenal function generally remain adequate in older people.
5. Hyperpituitarism, caused by excess anterior pituitary hormones, leads to gigantism or acromegaly.
6. Hyperpituitarism is treated with drugs (bromocriptine, octreotide acetate) or surgery to remove the tumor or the entire pituitary (hypophysectomy).
7. Treatment of hyperpituitarism can prevent further changes and complications, but existing body changes are not reversible.
8. Dwarfism is the result of inadequate growth hormone.
9. Panhypopituitarism is a deficiency of all anterior pituitary hormones and is treated with replacement hormones.
10. Diabetes insipidus, caused by a deficit in antidiuretic hormone, results in massive diuresis and is treated with vasopressin.
11. Syndrome of inappropriate antidiuretic hormone, caused by excess antidiuretic hormone, results in fluid retention and is treated with diuretics, demeclocycline, and hypertonic enemas.
12. The adrenal medulla secretes the catecholamines epinephrine and norepinephrine, which promote adaptation to stress.
13. The adrenal cortex secretes steroids in the form of mineralocorticoids, glucocorticoids, and androgens or estrogens.
14. Primary adrenal insufficiency, called Addison's disease, causes hypoglycemia, hyperkalemia, hyponatremia, and hypovolemia and requires lifelong replacement of glucocorticoids and mineralocorticoids.
15. Acute adrenal crisis is a life-threatening emergency caused by a sudden marked decrease in adrenal hormones that can lead to circulatory collapse and death.
16. Cushing's syndrome results from hypersecretion of cortisol, a glucocorticoid, or from prolonged administration of corticosteroids.
17. Cushing's syndrome is characterized by polycy-

themia, hypokalemia, hyperglycemia, leukocytosis, and glycosuria.

18. Cushing's syndrome is treated with drug therapy, radiation, and hypophysectomy or adrenalectomy.
19. Nursing care for the patient with Cushing's syndrome is concerned with high risk for infection, altered thought processes, high risk for impaired skin integrity, high risk for injury, body image disturbance, and knowledge deficits.
20. All chronic pituitary and adrenal conditions require patient teaching to enable the patient to manage the condition by taking medications properly and recognizing the need for medical intervention.
21. A pheochromocytoma is an adrenal tumor that increases secretion of catecholamines, causing hypertension, hypermetabolism, and hyperglycemia.

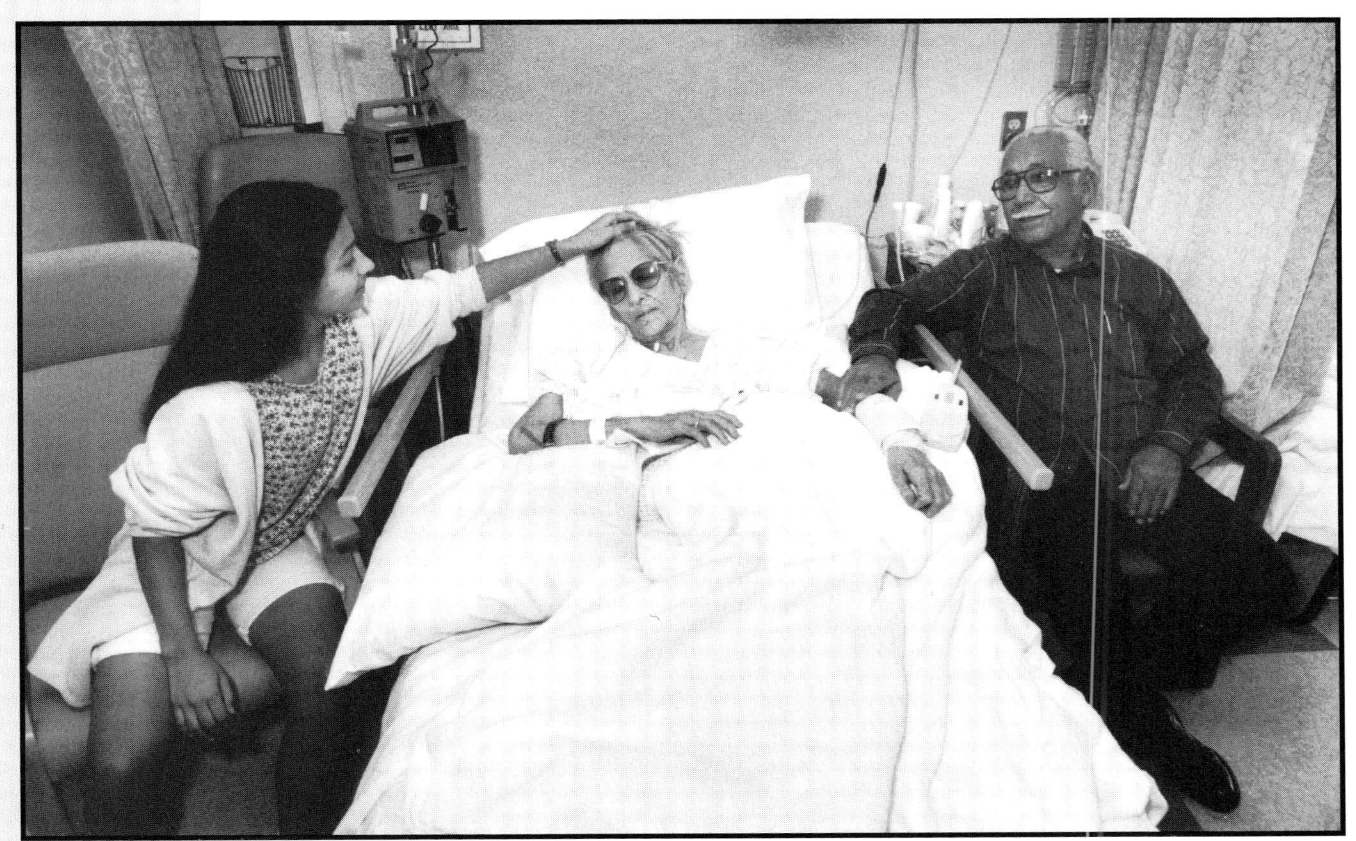

UNIT 13
Reproductive Disorders

Pauline Lee

CHAPTER 43

Female Reproductive Disorders

OBJECTIVES

1. List data to be collected when assessing the female reproductive system.
2. Describe the nursing interventions for women who are having diagnostic tests and procedures for reproductive system disorders.
3. Identify the nursing interventions associated with douche, cauterization, heat therapy, and topical medications used to treat disorders of the female reproductive system.
4. Explain the pathophysiology, signs and symptoms, complications, diagnostic procedures, and medical or surgical treatment for selected disorders of the female reproductive system.
5. Apply the nursing process to plan care for the patient with common disorders of the female reproductive system.
6. Describe the nursing interventions for the patient who is menopausal.

GLOSSARY

CYSTOCELE Herniation of the urinary bladder into the vagina

DYSMENORRHEA Painful menstruation

DYSPAREUNIA Difficult or painful sexual intercourse in women

DYSPLASIA Abnormal cells

ENDOMETRIOSIS A condition in which endometrial tissue is located abnormally outside the uterus

HYSTERECTOMY Surgical removal of the uterus

MASTITIS Inflammation of breast tissue

MENARCHE Age at which the first menstrual period occurs

MENOPAUSE Cessation of menstruation

MENORRHAGIA Menstrual periods characterized by profuse or prolonged bleeding

METRORRHAGIA Bleeding or spotting between menstrual periods

RECTOCELE Herniation of part of the rectum into the vagina

Glossary continued

RETROVERSION Bending backward of an entire organ

SALPINGO-OOPHORECTOMY Surgical excision of a fallopian tube and ovary

VAGINITIS Inflammation of the vagina

VULVITIS Inflammation of the vulva

The female reproductive system includes external and internal genitalia and the breasts. The term *vulva* refers to the external genitalia, which comprise the mons pubis, labia majora, labia minora, clitoris, urethral opening, and vaginal opening (Fig. 43–1). Also included in the vulva are Bartholin's glands on both sides of the posterior edge of the vaginal opening and Skene's glands just inside the urethral opening. The perineum is the area between the posterior junction of the labia minora and the anus. Internal genitalia include two ovaries, two fallopian tubes, the uterus, and the vagina (Fig. 43–2).

ANATOMY AND PHYSIOLOGY OF THE FEMALE REPRODUCTIVE SYSTEM

EXTERNAL GENITALIA

The mons pubis is a pad of fatty tissue that covers and protects the symphysis pubis. The labia majora are extensions of the fatty tissue that cover and protect inner vulvar structures and that extend from the mons pubis to the perineum. The mons and outer surfaces of the labia majora become covered with hair during the puberty period. The inner folds of the labia majora are smooth and moist.

The labia minora are thin folds of smooth skin that form a hood, called the prepuce, over the clitoris and that extend inside the labia majora to the posterior edge of the vagina, where they form a fold called the fourchette. The labia minora are richly endowed with sebaceous glands, nerves, and blood vessels, all of which respond to psychological and tactile stimulation. The labia minora may be entirely covered by the labia majora or may protrude between the outer labia.

The clitoris is a small cylindric structure that corresponds to the male penis and is composed of erectile tissue with sensory nerve endings that are responsive to psychological and tactile stimuli. The visible portion of the clitoris is called the glans.

The urethral (urinary) meatus is below the clitoris. The openings of Skene's glands are located on both sides of the urinary meatus.

The vaginal opening, the introitus, is partially or entirely covered by a thin fold of tissue called the hymen. The hymen may be intact, distended, or ruptured. The size of the introitus varies from very small to large and gaping. Bartholin's glands, located at the posterior aspects of the introitus, secrete lubrication fluid. Their openings seldom are visible.

INTERNAL GENITALIA

The vagina is a canal that extends from the vulva to the uterus. Its thin, muscular walls are rugated, meaning arranged in transverse ridges or folds. This structure has the ability to expand and to lengthen to accept entrance of an erect penis and to provide an exit for a term fetus. The mucous membranes of the vaginal walls secrete lubricating fluid that interacts with bacteria to maintain an acid range pH and to serve as a self-cleansing mechanism.

The uterus is a firm, muscular organ that is pear shaped and hollow. Its lower segment is called the cervix, or neck. The end of the cervix extends into the upper aspect of the vagina. The os is the opening of the cervix into the vagina. The inner lining of the uterus is called the endometrium. The upper segment of the uterine body, or corpus, is called the fundus. The fundus is the site of insertion of the fallopian tubes.

The two fallopian tubes are thin, hollow, cilia-lined, tubular structures that extend laterally from the uterus. The fallopian tubes terminate in funnel-shaped ends that partially surround the ovaries and that receive the ovum from the ovary. The fallopian tubes serve as passages for ova from the ovaries and for sperm that travel from the vagina, through the cervical os, into the uterine body, and into the tubes. Fallopian tubes also serve

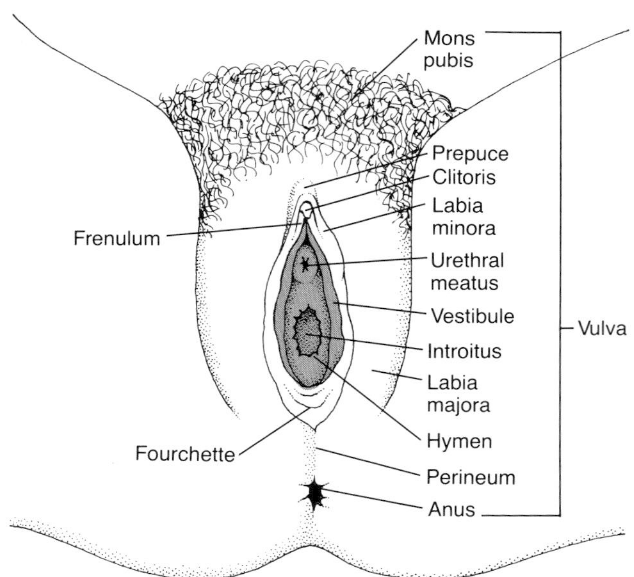

FIGURE 43-1

External female genitalia. (Modified from Ignatavicius, D. D., & Bayne, M. V. [1991]. *Medical-surgical nursing: A nursing process approach* [p. 1628]. Philadelphia: W. B. Saunders.)

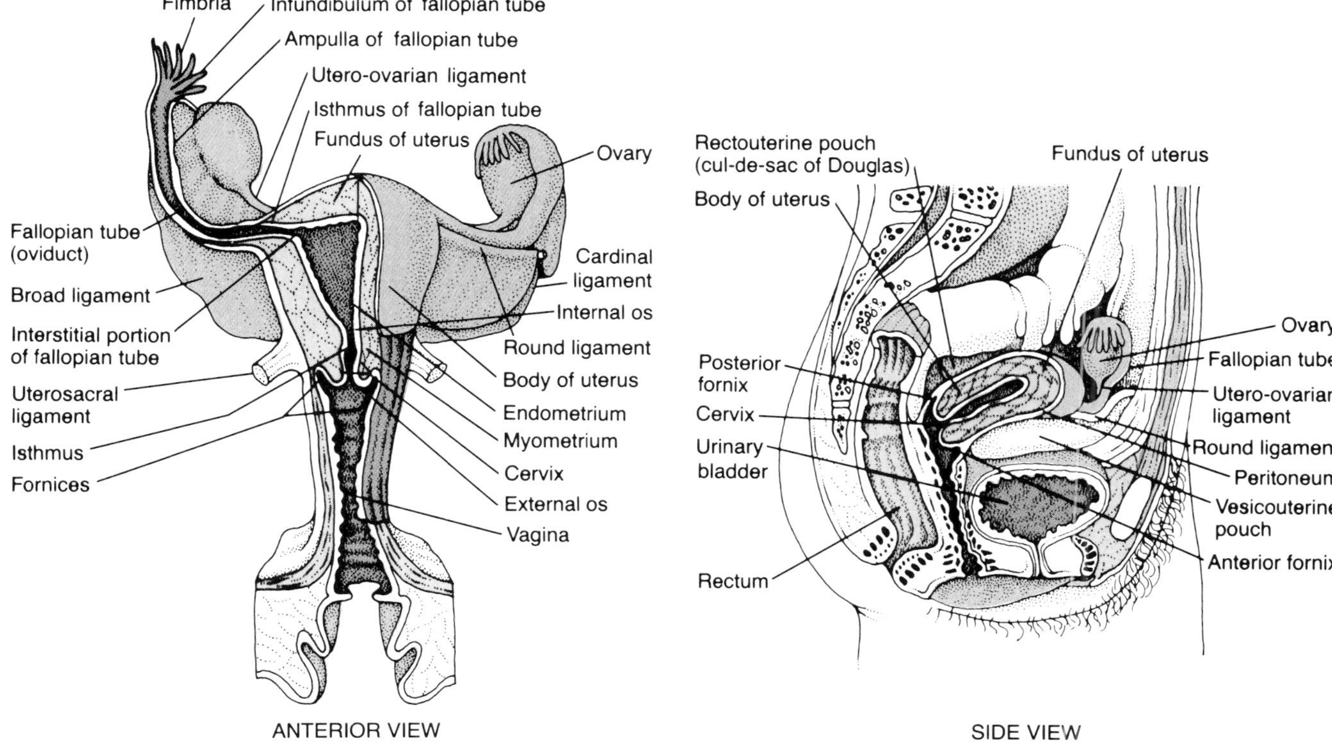

FIGURE 43–2

Internal female genitalia. (Modified from Ignatavicius, D. D., & Bayne, M. V. [1991]. *Medical-surgical nursing: A nursing process approach* [p. 1629]. Philadelphia: W. B. Saunders.)

as the site of fertilization, where sperm and ovum meet and unite.

The ovaries correspond to the male testes and are almond-shaped, paired structures, one on each side of the uterus. Ovarian functions include maturation and release of ova (ovulation) and secretion of hormones: estrogens, progesterone, androgens, and relaxin.

It is important to note that the communication through the female reproductive tract, intended to serve as a route for reproduction, also serves as a route for infectious organisms to travel from the vulva or vagina to the pelvic cavity.

BREASTS

Although they are not directly involved in the reproductive process, female breasts are addressed as accessories to reproduction because of their function: to nourish the infant after birth. Breast structure is illustrated in Figure 43–3. The inner structure is composed of glandular and ductal tissue, fibrous tissue, and fat. (The fat is responsible for the majority of the wide variations in breast sizes and shapes.) The breast is divided into several lobes, and each lobe is divided into lobules. Lobules contain many hollow, grape-shaped alveoli that produce milk when stimulated by the pituitary hormone prolactin. Ducts carry milk from the lobules, through the lobes, to the opening in the nipple.

The nipple with its surrounding areola is a pigmented structure located at the midline of each breast. The openings of the lactiferous ducts permit expression of breast milk. Small, round sebaceous glands called Montgomery's tubercules are visible under the skin of the areolae and produce a lubricating secretion that protects nipple tissue. It is important to note that secretion of milk or any other discharge should be reported, as it may be abnormal.

MENSTRUAL CYCLE

The menstrual cycle, or female reproductive cycle, consists of the ovarian cycle and the uterine cycle. It results from a complex interaction (Fig. 43–4) involving the hypothalamus, the anterior lobe of the pituitary gland, and the ovary. The interaction causes the ovary to release a mature ovum (ovulation) and prepares the uterine lining to receive and to nourish the ovum if it is fertilized during its journey through the fallopian tube. If the ovum is not fertilized, the menstrual cycle begins with the onset of menstruation. Menstruation is the vaginal discharge of a mixture of the blood and other fluids and tissue formed in the lining of the uterus to receive the fertilized ovum.

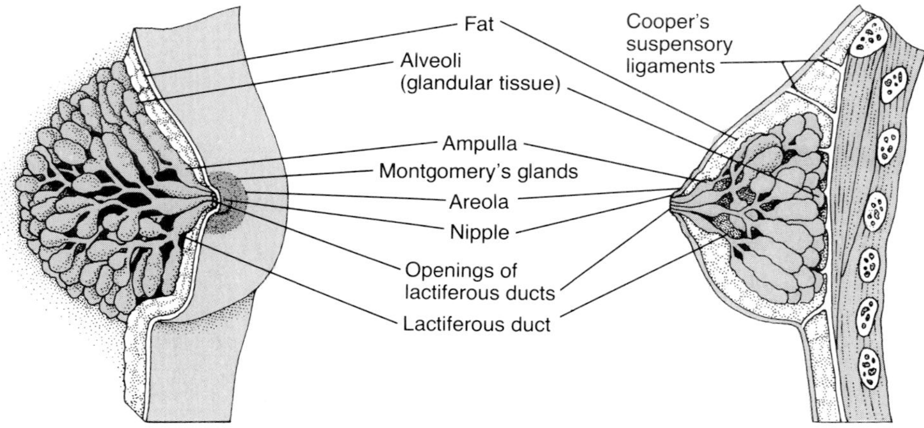

FIGURE 43-3

Structure of the mature female breast. (From Ignatavicius, D. D., & Bayne, M. V. [1991]. *Medical-surgical nursing: A nursing process approach* [p. 1634]. Philadelphia: W. B. Saunders.)

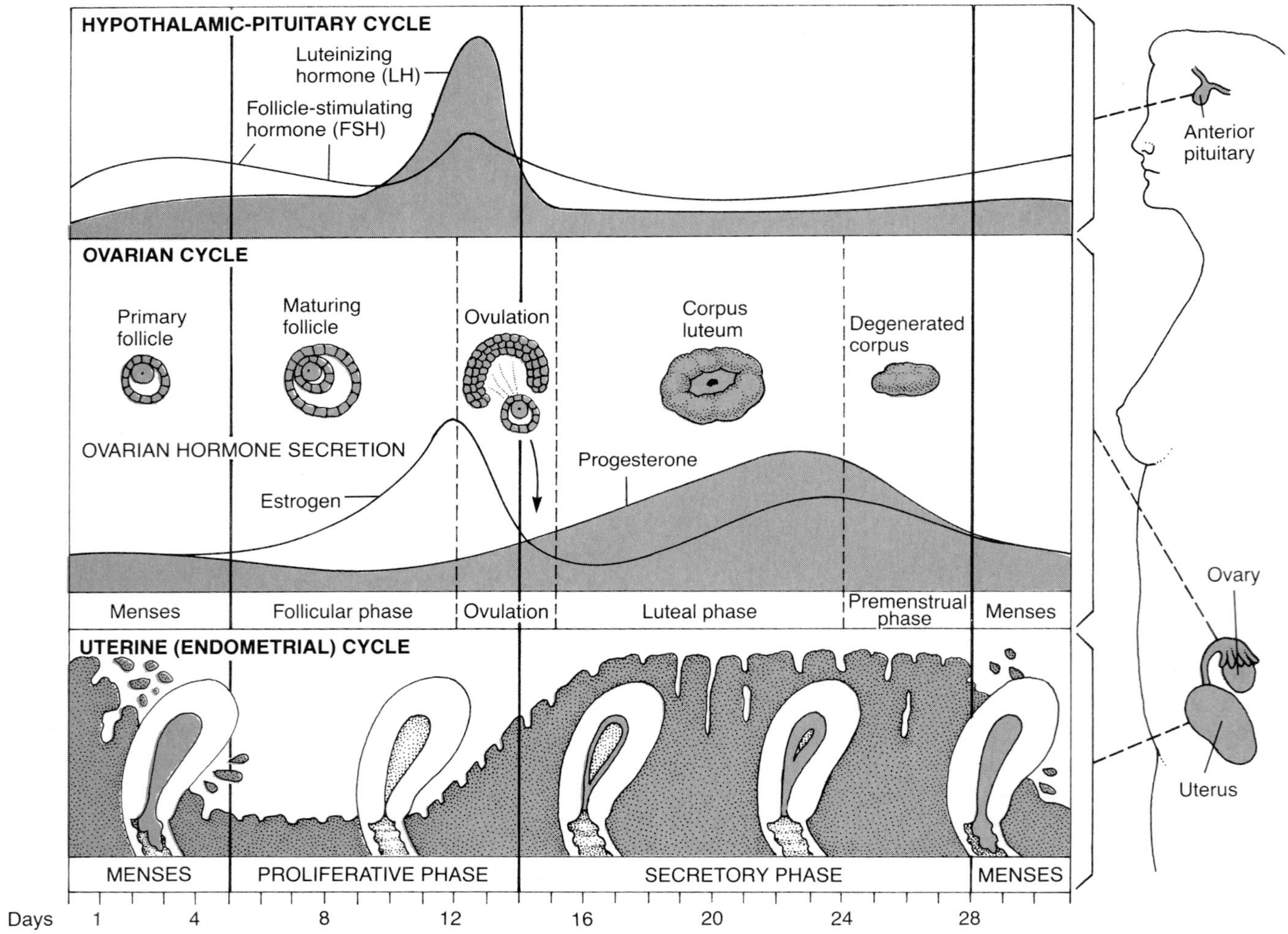

FIGURE 43-4

Interrelationships of the events of the menstrual cycle. (From Ignatavicius, D. D., & Bayne, M. V. [1991]. *Medical-surgical nursing: A nursing process approach* [p. 1632]. Philadelphia: W. B. Saunders.)

The length of the menstrual cycle averages 28 to 30 days, but the range may be 21 to 35 days and may be affected by various factors such as stress, physical activity, and illness. Regardless of the length of the cycle, the progression is the same:

1. Menstruation (day 1 through days 4–7)
2. Maturation of an ovarian follicle with subsequent rupture and release of an ovum in response to follicle-stimulating hormone and luteinizing hormone from the anterior pituitary (days 1–14 in a 28-day cycle)
3. Production of estrogen (days 6–14) by the maturing follicle and of progesterone (days 15–26) by the corpus luteum formed from the ruptured follicle
4. Preparation of the uterine lining for implantation of the fertilized ovum, stimulated by estrogen and progesterone from the follicle and corpus luteum (days 6–26)
5. Fertilized ovum implants in uterine lining and secretes human chorionic gonadotropin, which maintains the corpus luteum and estrogen-progesterone levels; menstruation does not occur (day 14)
6. Unfertilized ovum does not implant; absence of human chorionic gonadotropin causes corpus luteum to degenerate, which in turn causes a drop in estrogen-progesterone levels and necrosis of the uterine lining (days 27–28). The necrotic lining sheds as menstrual flow and begins another cycle at day 1

NURSING ASSESSMENT OF THE FEMALE REPRODUCTIVE SYSTEM

HEALTH HISTORY

It often is the nurse's responsibility to collect and record information from patients experiencing reproductive disorders. The policy of the work setting directs the nurse's role in collection of information.

Whether the nurse's responsibility is limited or extensive, the nurse begins the interview with a brief explanation of the purpose for the questions that will be asked. The basic assessment begins with the patient's reason for the visit to the physician's office or the clinic or the hospital. In addition to a general physical and psychosocial health history, the nurse may obtain from the patient a menstrual history and an obstetric and gynecologic history.

Chief Complaint and History of Present Illness

"What is the reason for your visit?" is an opening question that allows the patient not only to describe in her own terms the reason for the visit but also to include related information that may give direction for the questions that follow. The nurse's assessment includes the patient's knowledge about her reproductive health. If the reason for the visit is an existing problem, the nurse includes a brief history of the problem. Related signs and symptoms, their onset, frequency, and effect on the patient's normal functioning should be included in the problem history.

Past Medical History

MENSTRUAL HISTORY. Direct questions are used to gather initial information for the basic menstrual history. Included are the age at which menstruation began (menarche), the date of the onset of the last menstrual period, the usual number of days between the onset of one period and the onset of the next, the total amount of menstrual flow, the usual number of days of menstrual flow per period, and the use of tampons.

"Many women experience problems with their periods. What problems have you noticed?" is a questioning technique that implies acceptance of a wide variety of problems and that invites the patient to provide additional relevant information. Problems commonly reported include spotting or frank bleeding between periods, abdominal pain at the time of ovulation, abdominal cramping or pain before or during periods (or both), and premenstrual mood changes.

For women who have stopped menstruating owing to menopause, the nurse records the age at which menstruation was last experienced as well as related details, such as whether menopause occurred naturally or resulted from surgery, chemotherapy, or radiation therapy. Information should be included about menopausal symptoms or about prescribed or over-the-counter medication taken to relieve menopausal symptoms.

OBSTETRIC-GYNECOLOGIC HISTORY. "How many times have you been pregnant?" is an appropriate opening question for the obstetric history. If the response indicates that the woman has been pregnant, further questioning provides additional information to be recorded: number of term and preterm births, number of living children, number of abortions (spontaneous or induced), number of multiple pregnancies (e.g., twins, triplets). Blood type and Rh factor and a history of rubella or rubella immunization are noted. Terms related to obstetric history are *gravidity* and *parity*. Gravidity refers to the total number of pregnancies. Parity refers to the number of pregnancies that terminated after 20 weeks of gestation, considered the "age of viability." Parity may be recorded according to a number of different codes that use from one- to five-digit numbers. Each institution provides direction on how parity is to be coded for obstetric histories.

The gynecologic history addresses current and former problems related to the reproductive system, the endocrine system, and the lower urinary tract. Examples of such problems are infections and sexually transmitted diseases, cysts and tumors, structural and functional abnormalities, infertility, and stress incontinence.

Family History

The nurse records a family history of diabetes mellitus, cancer, complications of pregnancy, occurrence of multiple pregnancies, genetic disorders, or congenital anomalies.

Review of Systems

The nurse records as much information as the patient is able to recall regarding symptoms and treatment. Commonly reported symptoms are pain, itching, burning, vaginal bleeding between periods or after menopause, heavy or prolonged bleeding with periods, vaginal discharge, and urinary frequency or urgency. When the patient reports such problems, the nurse asks questions related to the degree of each problem and to any prescribed or self-selected measures taken to relieve each problem.

Functional Assessment

The functional assessment includes a diet history, use of dietary supplements including calcium and iron, exercise pattern, sexual history, and occupational exposure to potential teratogens.

PHYSICAL EXAMINATION

The physical examination begins with the general survey noting the patient's appearance, facial expression, and any obvious signs of distress. Vital signs and height and weight are measured. The skin color, texture, and moisture are assessed. The breasts are inspected for dimpling and abnormal skin texture. The patient is instructed to lean forward and the examiner observes for asymmetry when leaning forward. The patient is asked about changes from usual contours. All breast tissue is palpated for thickening or lumps (see Breast Self-examination in next section). The abdomen is inspected for distention and palpated for tenderness. The legs are inspected for swelling and palpated for tenderness. The presence of Homans's sign is assessed to detect possible thrombophlebitis. Nurses with advanced training may do the pelvic examination, but it is more commonly performed by the physician. Therefore, it is discussed in detail under Diagnostic Tests and Procedures. Basically, the examiner is assessing the external genitalia for lesions, lumps, swelling, and discharge. The vagina and uterine cervix are inspected for lesions, growths, discharge, and redness. The vagina, abdomen, and rectum are palpated for abnormalities. Assessment of the female reproductive system is summarized in Table 43–1.

Pelvic Examination

The pelvic examination allows inspection and palpation of external and internal reproductive structures to identify deviations from normal, to provide information for medical diagnoses, and to collect specimens for laboratory analysis.

The patient assumes the lithotomy position, with buttocks at the edge of the table, hips and knees flexed, and feet in stirrups. Many women report that the position is unpleasant because of the sense of vulnerability that they experience. The nurse can help to decrease this effect by delaying positioning until just before the examination begins, by careful draping to preserve modesty, and by verbal and nonverbal patient supportive measures. Physical discomfort associated with use of the stirrups may be decreased by covering them with thick footlets or by encouraging the patient to keep socks or shoes on.

The pelvic examination is divided into three parts: (1) visual inspection and palpation of the external genitalia, (2) visual inspection of the vagina and uterine cervix

TABLE 43–1

ASSESSMENT OF THE FEMALE REPRODUCTIVE SYSTEM

HEALTH HISTORY

Present illness: Reason for visit, related signs and symptoms, onset and frequency of symptoms, effects on normal functioning

Past medical history:

- Menstrual history: Age at menarche, date of onset of last menstrual period, duration of menstrual period, amount of menstrual flow, use of tampons, pain, bleeding between periods, premenstrual mood changes. If menopausal: age at which menopause occurred, whether menopause was natural or surgical, related symptoms, medications taken to relieve symptoms
- Obstetric and gynecologic history: Number of pregnancies, number of term and preterm births, number of living children, number of abortions (spontaneous and induced), number of multiple pregnancies, past problems with reproductive organs, infertility, stress incontinence, history of rubella or rubella immunization, frequency of breast self-examination

Family history: Diabetes, cancer, complications of pregnancy, genetic disorders, multiple pregnancies, congenital anomalies

Review of systems: Pain, itching, burning, vaginal bleeding between periods or after menopause, heavy or prolonged bleeding with periods, vaginal discharge, urinary frequency or urgency

Functional assessment: Diet, use of dietary supplements including calcium and iron, exercise pattern, sexual history, occupational exposure to potential teratogens

PHYSICAL EXAMINATION

General survey: Appearance, facial expression, obvious distress

Vital signs

Height and weight

Skin: Texture, moisture, color

Breasts: Dimpling, texture changes in skin, asymmetry when leaning forward, changes from usual contours, changes in texture, lumps, nipple discharge

Extremities: Homans's sign, temperature, swelling, tenderness

Abdomen: Contour, distention, tenderness

Pelvic examination:

- External genitalia: Appearance, lesions, lumps, swelling, discharge
- Vagina and uterine cervix: Appearance, lesions, growths, discharge, redness
- Rectal examination

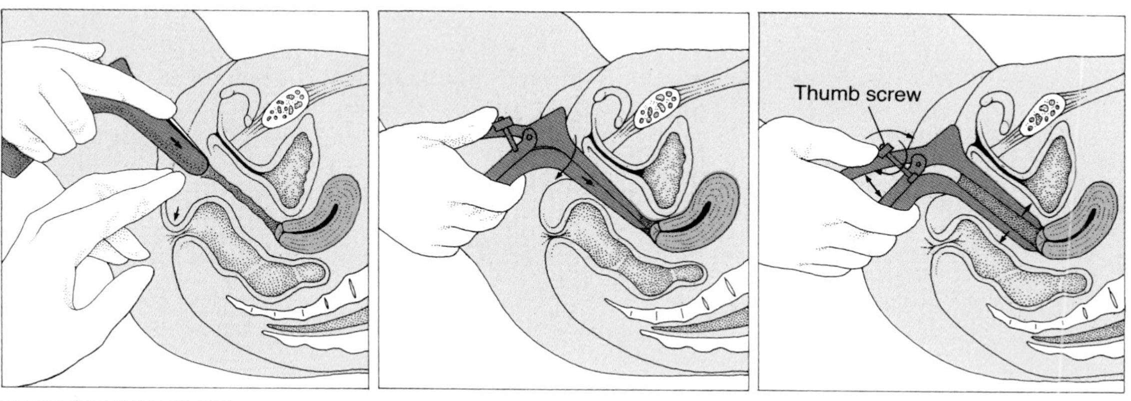

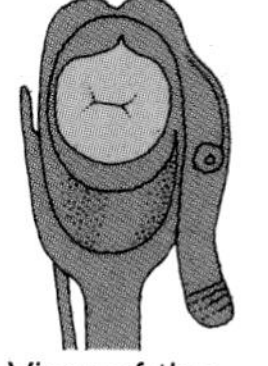

FIGURE 43-5

Internal examination of the cervix. (From Ignatavicius, D. D., & Bayne, M. V. [1991]. *Medical-surgical nursing: A nursing process approach* [p. 1644]. Philadelphia: W. B. Saunders.)

after introduction of a plastic or metal speculum (Fig. 43–5), and (3) bimanual palpation of the vagina and abdomen. The latter procedure may be performed with two fingers of one gloved hand in the vagina (Fig. 43–6) or with one finger in the vagina and one finger in the rectum (Fig. 43–7) and the other hand on the abdomen to allow compression of internal structures between the two hands. The final step is a rectal examination with a gloved finger.

Discomfort varies among women. Some women report no discomfort other than feelings of pressure; other women report pain. One common discomfort is related to a cold speculum. The nurse can prevent this by warming the speculum in water or by wrapping the packaged speculum in the folds of a heating pad. Supportive measures include talking to the patient and directing breathing and relaxation techniques to relieve pain and tension.

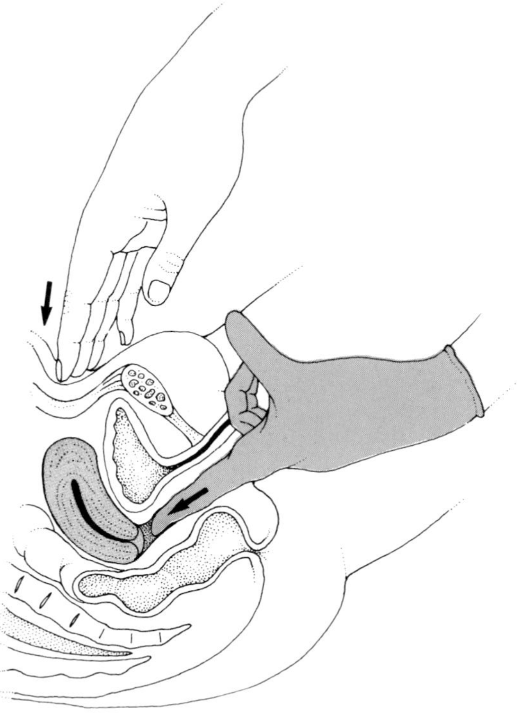

FIGURE 43-6

Bimanual pelvic examination. (From Ignatavicius, D. D., & Bayne, M. V. [1991]. *Medical-surgical nursing: A nursing process approach* [p. 1645]. Philadelphia: W. B. Saunders.)

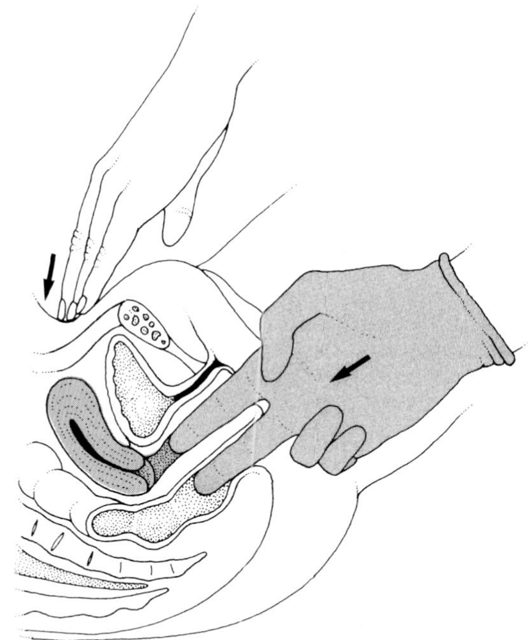

FIGURE 43-7

Bimanual rectovaginal examination. (From Ignatavicius, D. D., & Bayne, M. V. [1991]. *Medical-surgical nursing: A nursing process approach* [p. 1645]. Philadelphia: W. B. Saunders.)

Following the pelvic examination, the patient is assisted to assume a sitting position and to get off the table. She should be provided with tissues to wipe the perianal area and, if possible, an adhesive panty liner to absorb lubricant as it is expelled from the vagina.

DIAGNOSTIC TESTS AND PROCEDURES

Most diagnostic tests and procedures are performed by the physician or by the nurse practitioner. The responsibilities of the nurse usually focus on patient instruction regarding the procedure, preparation of the patient, support of the patient throughout the tests and procedures, and assistance to the physician or nurse practitioner. Regardless of the test or procedure to be performed, the nurse provides anticipatory guidance by telling the patient what to expect. The nurse checks the institution's procedure manual for specific preparations and assistant's responsibilities for each test or procedure.

Smears and Cultures

Collection of specimens for laboratory analysis is one of the purposes of the pelvic examination (Fig. 43–8). Institutional policy directs the nurse to the necessary equipment and the care of slides for each specimen. The well-prepared nurse will have extra equipment available for the collection of specimens other than those originally anticipated. During inspection and palpation of external and internal structures, the physician or nurse practitioner may detect deviations from the normal that require further inspection.

Specimens are collected routinely for a Papanicolaou (Pap) smear for detection of cervical cancer and other abnormal cervical cells (dysplasia). Additional specimens may be collected for identification of suspected infections such as herpes, chlamydia, and gonorrhea.

Endometrial and Cervical Biopsies

Endometrial biopsies generally are performed for three reasons: (1) to assess the endometrium for readiness to accept and nourish a fertilized ovum, (2) to indirectly assess corpus luteum function in cases of suspected infertility, and (3) to diagnose uterine cancer. The nurse's responsibilities are similar to those for a pelvic examination and collection of specimens for smears and cultures. The physician or nurse practitioner dilates the cervix and scrapes tissue specimens from the endometrium. The procedure may cause cramping so severe that an anesthetic is necessary.

Cervical biopsies are performed to diagnose suspected cervical cancer. There are two types of biopsy: multiple punch and conization. Multiple punch biopsies are done in physician's offices or outpatient clinics. Because several specimens are obtained by punching out small samples of cervical tissue, the process is usually painful. The nurse's responsibilities are similar to those for endometrial biopsies. The supportive nurse directs the patient in the use of breathing and relaxation techniques to minimize discomfort.

The cone biopsy is invasive surgery and requires admission to an outpatient surgery facility or a hospital.

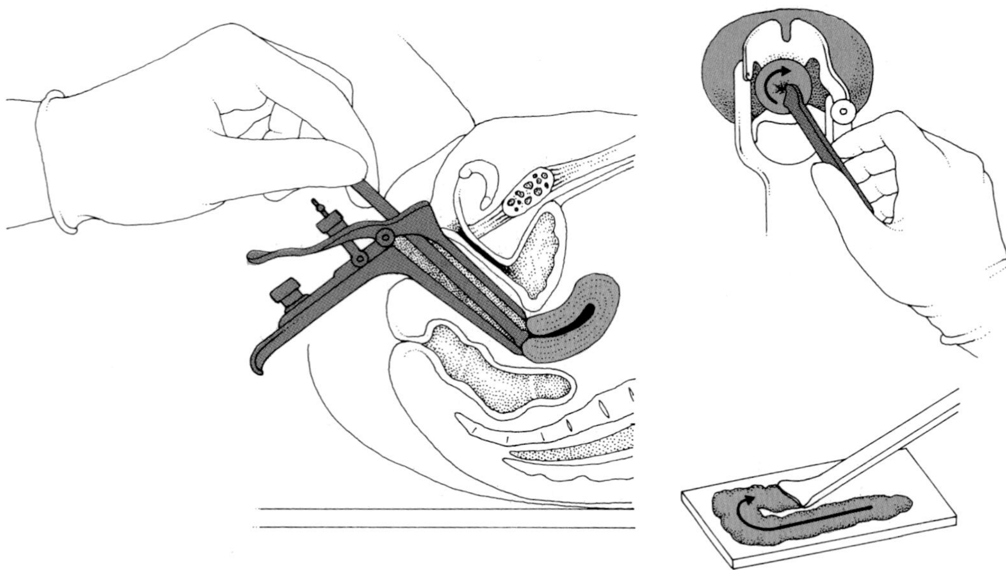

FIGURE 43-8

Procedure for obtaining specimens for cervical smear or culture. (Modified from Ignatavicius, D. D., & Bayne, M. V. [1991]. *Medical-surgical nursing: A nursing process approach* [p. 1648]. Philadelphia: W. B. Saunders.)

Under general anesthesia, a large amount of cervical tissue is removed. Although the cone biopsy is rarely used for diagnosing cancer, its advantage lies in its potential both to diagnose and to remove cancerous tissue.

Colposcopy

The physician or nurse practitioner uses an instrument called a colposcope to inspect the cervix under magnification and to identify abnormal and potentially cancerous tissue. Colposcopy is commonly done before cervical biopsies. Preparation of the patient and nursing care are similar to those for a pelvic examination.

Culdoscopy

A culdoscopy (Fig. 43–9) is an invasive surgical procedure usually performed with light sedation and local anesthetic on an outpatient basis. When utilized by a physician who has developed the skill to perform it safely, the culdoscopy is viewed as the simplest mechanism for direct visualization of the female pelvic cavity. With the patient in the knee-chest position, the physician inserts the culdoscope through a small incision in the posterior vagina. The culdoscope enables the physician to examine the patient's uterus and adnexa (uterine appendages, ovaries, fallopian tubes), to identify ectopic pregnancy or pelvic masses, to identify some causes of infertility or pain, and to obtain tissue specimens.

The nurse's responsibilities are similar to those for other outpatient procedures, with details specified by institutional policies. Scrupulous asepsis must be maintained. Many women consider the knee-chest position not only physically uncomfortable but especially embarrassing or humiliating. The empathetic nurse assures the patient that she will be draped throughout the procedure and is conscientious about following through with that assurance. When the procedure is completed, the nurse helps the patient get out of the knee-chest position without exposure. The patient is advised that she may experience shoulder pain caused by air entering the pelvic cavity during the procedure. The nurse also reassures the patient that the incision will close and heal without sutures but that nothing should be inserted in the vagina (e.g., no vaginal intercourse, douching, or tampons) for the period of time specified by the physician.

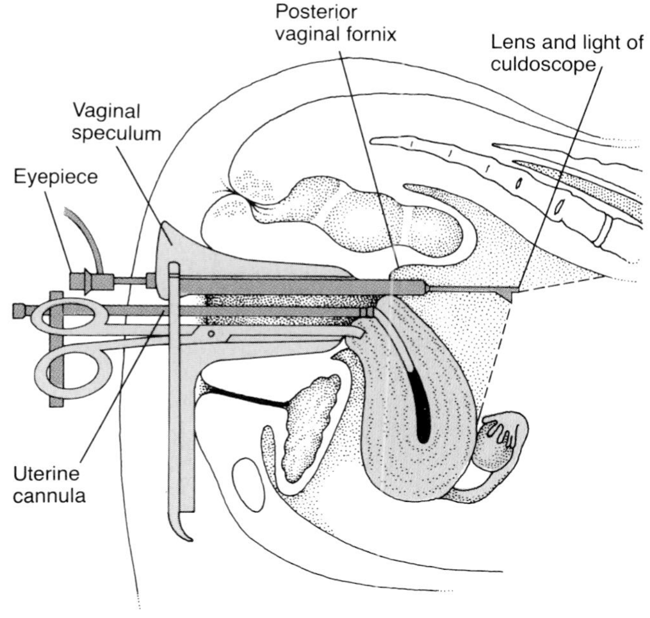

FIGURE 43-9

Culdoscopy. (From Ignatavicius, D. D., & Bayne, M. V. [1991]. *Medical-surgical nursing: A nursing process approach* [p. 1654]. Philadelphia: W. B. Saunders.)

Laparoscopy

A laparoscopy (Fig. 43–10) is an invasive surgical procedure that may be performed under local anesthesia on an outpatient basis or under general anesthesia in an outpatient surgical facility or a hospital. The physician uses an instrument called a laparoscope to visualize abdominal organs and to perform minor surgery such as a tubal ligation. The laparoscope is inserted through a small abdominal buttonhole incision. Instruments may be inserted through the laparoscope itself or through a small second incision. Before insertion of the laparoscope, a small quantity of gas is injected into the abdomen to create a pocket in which to insert the laparoscope and to allow a clear view of the organs. This gas eventually is absorbed but in the immediate postoperative period tends to cause shoulder pain or pain below the rib cage or both. The nurse should inform and reassure the patient that the discomfort is expected and is temporary.

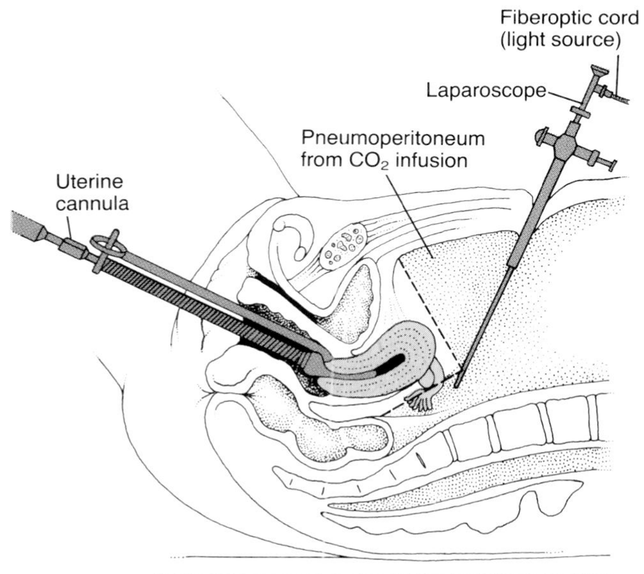

FIGURE 43-10

Laparoscopy. (From Ignatavicius, D. D., & Bayne, M. V. [1991]. *Medical-surgical nursing: A nursing process approach* [p. 1655]. Philadelphia: W. B. Saunders.)

Dilation and Curettage

The major purpose of dilation and curettage (D&C) is diagnostic, but it also may serve as treatment for some conditions. The D&C is generally considered to be the diagnostic test of choice when uterine cancer is suspected and is more thorough than is the endometrial biopsy. It is used to diagnose causes of abnormal uterine bleeding and is effective as a treatment if it removes the tissue that causes the bleeding. Although the D&C traditionally was performed under general anesthesia in a hospital setting, today most D&Cs can be performed under local anesthesia in the physician's office or outpatient clinic.

Preparation and positioning is similar to that used for the pelvic examination. As for all procedures, institutional policy directs the nurse's role and responsibilities.

The D&C is performed in two steps. The first is dilation of the cervix by insertion of a series of progressively larger rods. The second step is endometrial curettage, which is scraping the entire area of uterine lining. The scraped tissue sample is removed by vacuum aspiration (suction). The tissue samples are prepared for laboratory analysis according to institutional procedures.

Mammography

The mammogram is a radiologic test used to detect breast cysts or tumors, especially those not palpated on physical examination. It is recommended by the American Cancer Society that baseline mammograms be performed on women between the ages of 35 and 39. Subsequent tests should be done every 1 to 2 years for women 40 to 49 years of age and annually for women age 50 and older. The test takes only a few minutes and is performed by a trained technician. For the procedure, each breast is compressed in a mammography machine, and two views are taken of each breast, one from above and one from the side. The film is developed immediately and is often "read" by a radiologist before the patient leaves the setting. Most mammograms are done in settings that do not routinely employ nurses. However, the nurse needs to be familiar with the process so that anticipatory guidance can be provided for the patient.

Breast Self-Examination

Through regular monthly breast self-examination (BSE), the patient is in the best position to recognize changes from her normal findings. Every female patient who has begun to menstruate should know how to perform a BSE accurately.

The BSE should be performed at the same time each month: at the end of the menstrual period for menstruating females or on the same date each month for women who have ceased menstruating. The nurse's responsibilities include teaching the importance of BSE, demonstrating the examination, and evaluating the patient's ability to perform a return demonstration on herself.

The BSE begins with inspection of the breasts while sitting or standing before a mirror. The patient observes for changes in her breasts as she assumes four positions: (1) arms relaxed at the sides, (2) arms held straight above her head, (3) hands pressed against waist or hips with elbows brought forward, and (4) leaning forward. She observes for any changes from the previous BSE: for dimpling, puckering, or texture changes of skin; for elevation or enlargement of one breast when she leans forward or when she brings elbows forward in the third position; and for new other differences between the breasts.

The second step of the BSE is palpation of the breasts and the axillary area. The position of choice is for the patient to lie on the back with a folded towel under the shoulder of the breast to be examined. The arm on the same side is raised above the head. The examining hand should be lotioned or powdered to help the fingers move smoothly over the skin. Fingers are positioned flat against the skin, and moved to cover the entire breast area in one sliding motion. Firm pressure is used, beginning at the nipple and traveling in a circular track around and around the breast until the breast has been covered. Areas to be covered extend from the midaxillary line, to the sternum, and to the top and bottom boundaries. The process is repeated on the opposite side.

Some practitioners prefer to begin at the midaxillary line and palpate the breast tissue in a vertical stripping pattern. The fingers travel up and down in closely spaced strips without leaving the skin surface until the entire breast has been palpated.

Women with small breasts may examine their breasts while showering. This method is less acceptable for women with larger breasts because it does not allow the breasts to flatten for thorough palpation. Any changes in breast texture, particularly any lumps, and any nipple discharge should be reported as soon as possible to the physician or nurse practitioner.

Although many women learn to perform BSE from reading magazines or pamphlets, it has been observed that women perform the examination more accurately when they have received direct instruction and demonstration and when they have returned the demonstration for correction of technique.

Breast Biopsy

When breast changes are discovered, a breast biopsy is considered to determine the reason for the change. Biopsy is the only method of diagnosing breast cancer.

The physician decides which diagnostic procedures are appropriate. Breast biopsies for palpable small lumps can be performed under local anesthesia on an outpatient basis (Fig. 43–11). A needle may be used to aspirate fluid from cysts. Solid masses require a surgical approach to obtain a specimen of the questionable tissue or to remove the mass. Biopsies of large masses are performed under general anesthesia in a hospital setting. All removed tissue and aspirated fluid are sent to the laboratory for analysis. Decisions for further treatment are based on biopsy reports.

The patient admitted to the health care setting for a breast biopsy requires a great deal of supportive care.

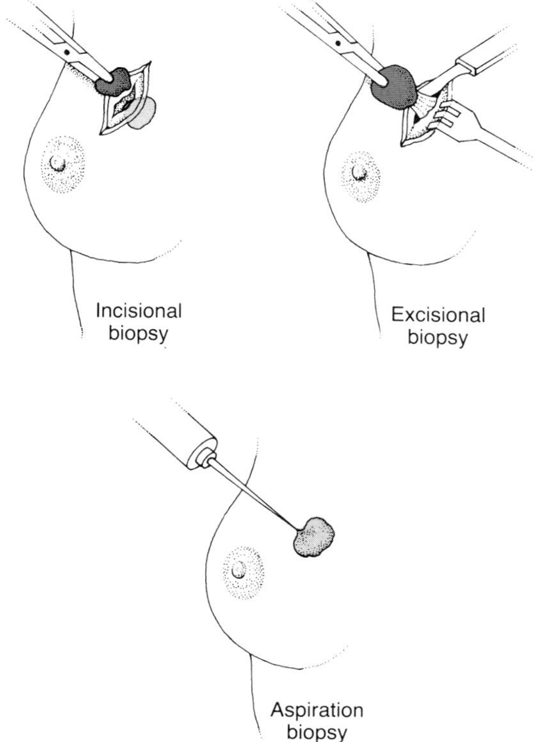

FIGURE 43-11

Breast biopsy techniques. (From Ignatavicius, D. D., & Bayne, M. V. [1991]. *Medical-surgical nursing: A nursing process approach* [p. 1657]. Philadelphia: W. B. Saunders.)

She needs an opportunity to talk about her fears, and she needs a thorough explanation of what she can expect during the preoperative, operative, and postoperative periods. Physical care will be directed by the physician and by institutional policies and procedures.

Information about diagnostic tests and procedures is summarized in Table 43-2.

COMMON THERAPEUTIC MEASURES

DOUCHING

Douching is a procedure used to flood the vagina with fluid to which a wide variety of cleansing or perfumed agents are added. Douching is not recommended for regular hygiene, because it washes away some of the elements that maintain the normal acidic pH. The acidic environment helps the vagina maintain its self-cleansing properties, and to fight off invading organisms.

Douching is potentially dangerous, because it may force tissue and microorganisms up into the uterus. In addition, cleansing and perfumed agents added to the douche solution may cause allergic or irritant reactions. Contrary to common belief, douching is not an effective contraceptive practice.

Douching may be ordered by the physician or nurse practitioner to wash the vagina with a bactericidal solution in preparation for surgery, radiation therapy, or other treatment. If ordered, the nurse prepares the douche solution, using exact measures of prescribed ingredients, and administers the douche according to institutional policy and procedure.

Because it is also the nurse's responsibility to teach the patient about appropriate vaginal hygiene, the nurse can teach while the douche is administered. Points to be addressed are the following:

- The external genitalia should be washed with plain soap and water at least once a day.
- The genital area should be kept clean and dry.
- Cotton panties should be worn.
- Douching should never be done unless it is ordered by the physician or nurse practitioner.

CAUTERIZATION

Cauterization is a method of deliberate tissue destruction through use of heat, electricity, or chemicals. The physician or nurse practitioner may cauterize small growths or polyps during the pelvic examination. Necessary equipment and supplies are usually listed in the agency procedure manual.

APPLICATION OF HEAT

Application of heat is utilized as a therapeutic treatment for many reproductive system conditions and disorders. Both dry and moist heat are used to relieve pain, to increase blood flow and metabolism to promote healing and pus formation, and to stimulate rupture of abscesses. Because potential damage is associated with excessively high temperature and with conditions such as impaired circulation, edema, and bleeding disorders, any form of heat must be used judiciously.

Dry heat in the form of a hot water bottle, a disposable chemical pack, an electric heating pad, or an aquathermia pad (K-pad) may be applied to the breasts or abdomen to relieve pain and to enhance circulation. The commonly recommended temperature range for most of these devices is 40 to 56°C (115–125°F). Institutional policy dictates the exact temperature to set. Duration of application time is dictated by institutional policy or by physician's order. Although the exact procedure for each method varies among institutions, key points when applying dry heat are the following:

1. A physician's order is required.
2. The skin must be protected by using a barrier between the device and the skin.
3. The patient's response must be monitored.
4. The dry heat source temperature must be maintained in the appropriate range.

Moist heat in the form of hot compresses and sitz baths is employed for the same general purposes as is dry heat. Hot compresses are particularly useful for heat application to small areas such as the vulva or perineum. Depending on the treatment purpose, the acceptable

TABLE 43-2
THE FEMALE REPRODUCTIVE SYSTEM: DIAGNOSTIC TESTS AND PROCEDURES

TEST	PURPOSE/PROCEDURE	PATIENT PREPARATION	POSTPROCEDURE NURSING CARE
Pelvic examination	Visual inspection and palpation of external genitalia, visual inspection of vagina and uterine cervix, bimanual palpation of vagina and abdomen, and rectal examination. Permits identification of abnormalities and collection of specimens for analysis or study.	Explain the examination to the patient. Assist the patient to assume the lithotomy position immediately before the examination. Maintain draping for privacy. Warm the vaginal speculum with warm water or wrap it in a heating pad. Encourage relaxation.	Assist the patient to assume a sitting position and get down from the examining table. Offer tissues to wipe the perineal area and a panty liner to absorb lubricant as it drains.
Smears and cultures	Secretions are obtained for laboratory study for a variety of purposes. The Papanicolaou smear uses cervical cells to detect abnormalities including cervical cancer. Pathogens that cause herpes, chlamydia, gonorrhea, and other infections may be identified.	Specimens may be obtained during the pelvic examination. Appropriate equipment should be on hand for the anticipated tests. Proper handling of specimens is essential for accurate studies.	Specimens are prepared, labeled, and sent to the laboratory. Used supplies are disposed of properly.
Biopsies: Endometrial, cervical, and breast	Samples of endometrial tissue may be used to study fertility and to detect cancer. Cervical biopsies are done to detect cervical cancer. Breast biopsies are done to diagnose breast cancer. Fluid may be aspirated with a needle from fluid-filled cysts. Lumpectomy or mastectomy may follow immediately if malignant cells are found.	Explain the procedure to the patient. For endometrial and cervical biopsies, assist her to assume the lithotomy position, using drapes to maintain privacy. Guide the patient in breathing and relaxation exercises during the procedure, which is painful. Breast biopsies may be done under local or general anesthesia. Patient may be very anxious about outcome and possible need for surgery or other treatment.	Same as pelvic examination for endometrial and cervical biopsies. After breast biopsy, check incision for bleeding. Safety precautions if sedated. Provide opportunity for her to express fears. Identify sources of support.
Colposcopy	A colposcope is used to inspect the cervix under magnification to identify potentially abnormal tissue. Usually done before cervical biopsy.	Same as pelvic examination.	Same as pelvic examination.

temperature range for hot compresses is 40.5 to 46.0°C (105–115°F).

Sitz baths provide heat to the perianal area to relieve pain, to cleanse the area, to promote healing or drainage, or to stimulate urination. As implied by the name, the patient sits in warm water that may be in a special tub or in a disposable plastic device that fits on the rim of a regular toilet bowl. A continuous flow of fresh temperature-controlled warm water is provided by the plumbing apparatus of the sitz bath tub and by a suspended plastic water bag with tubing extended to the disposable device. Water temperature is maintained within the 38 to 46°C (100–115°F) range, the treatment is employed for a maximum of 25 minutes, and the patient is monitored closely for signs of faintness, shock, or severe pain. Hypotension may be caused by dilation of large pelvic blood vessels; therefore, the patient should not be left alone. Disposable devices usually are taken home by the patient, so it is the nurse's responsibility to give detailed instructions on their use.

TOPICAL MEDICATIONS

Medications for application to the vulva or vagina are in the forms of creams and suppositories. Because mucous membranes are both delicate and highly vascular, the nurse must use caution to avoid injury and to observe for systemic effects related to the high absorption capability of the tissue. The application hand should be gloved for protection of both patient and nurse. Whether inserted with finger or applicator, a suppository is positioned with a down and backward motion into the vagina of the supine woman. Cream is administered through an applicator packaged with the cream. The patient is directed to maintain the supine position for at least 15 minutes after application of either medium, to allow the medication to be dispersed throughout the vagina and to be absorbed. The medication is left in the vagina but will dribble out over time, so the patient should use a sanitary pad to protect underclothing from staining. Drugs commonly used to treat disorders of the female reproductive system are listed in Table 43–3.

DISORDERS OF THE FEMALE REPRODUCTIVE SYSTEM

UTERINE BLEEDING DISORDERS

Pathophysiology

Normal menstrual patterns vary widely in length of cycles (21–40 days), duration of menstruation (2–8 days), and amount of blood loss (40–100 ml). Irregular bleeding patterns in both spacing and amount are common in the first 2 years after the onset of menarche and in the 5-year period before menopause. Deviations from the normal cycles are viewed as uterine bleeding disorders. Two of the most common abnormal bleeding patterns, metrorrhagia (bleeding or spotting between menstrual periods) and menorrhagia (menstrual periods characterized by profuse or prolonged bleeding), are addressed in Table 43–4. Amenorrhea is the absence of menses.

Etiology and Risk Factors

Both metrorrhagia and menorrhagia are symptoms of underlying factors, rather than being specific definable conditions in themselves. Underlying causes for each vary widely. Common causes include hormonal dysfunction, both benign and malignant tumors, coagulation disorders, systemic diseases, use of some contraceptives, endometrial hyperplasia, inflammatory processes, and systemic diseases. The amount of blood loss varies with the type of disorder. Causes of amenorrhea include pregnancy; excessive weight loss, physical activity, or stress; pituitary, hypothalamic, thyroid, or adrenal disorders; ovarian failure; and uterine abnormalities.

Medical Diagnosis and Treatment

The diagnosis of uterine bleeding is based on the health history and physical examination as well as

TABLE 43–3
DRUGS USED TO TREAT DISORDERS OF THE FEMALE REPRODUCTIVE SYSTEM

DRUG	USE/ACTION	SIDE EFFECTS	NURSING INTERVENTIONS
Ovarian Hormones			
Conjugated estrogens (Premarin)	Used to replace natural hormones after menopause, treat (palliatively) advanced breast cancer, and treat osteoporosis caused by estrogen deficiency. Stimulates endometrial growth and thickening. Enhances bone formation. Depresses beta-lipoprotein and cholesterol plasma levels.	Breast tenderness, breakthrough bleeding, vaginal candidiasis, headache, dizziness, depression, elevated blood pressure, thromboembolism, nausea, skin hyperpigmentation, and decreased glucose tolerance. Increased risk of endometrial cancer, especially in postmenopausal women who take estrogens continuously for a year or more.	Advise patients to report signs of: 1. Thromboembolism: calf pain or swelling, chest pain, numbness, visual disturbances. 2. Cardiovascular problems: weight gain, edema. 3. Liver disorders: abdominal pain, jaundice. 4. Breast lumps. 5. Vaginal bleeding. Encourage smoking cessation because smoking increases risk of adverse effects. Take with evening meal to reduce nausea. Reinforce physician's instructions re dosage, schedule. Contraindicated with known or suspected breast cancer, undiagnosed vaginal bleeding, past or current thromboembolism.
Progesterone	Promotes secretory function in endometrium. Influences contractile activity of the uterus. Used to treat uterine bleeding, some types of amenorrhea, and premenstrual syndrome (PMS). Palliative treatment of endometriosis and some cancers. Used with estrogens as oral contraceptives.	Breakthrough bleeding, amenorrhea, breast tenderness, edema, pruritus, increased blood pressure, thromboembolism, depression, photosensitivity.	Monitor weight and blood pressure. Assess for pruritus. Tell patient to report signs of circulatory impairment: swelling, numbness, pain in calf or thigh. Advise to avoid excessive sun exposure. Assess mental state. Contraindicated with history of thromboembolism, undiagnosed vaginal bleeding, liver dysfunction, cerebral hemorrhage.

Table continued on following page

TABLE 43-3
DRUGS USED TO TREAT DISORDERS OF THE FEMALE REPRODUCTIVE SYSTEM *Continued*

DRUG	USE/ACTION	SIDE EFFECTS	NURSING INTERVENTIONS
Androgens Danazol (Danocrine)	Inhibits production of pituitary gonadotropins. Used to treat endometriosis and fibrocystic breast disease.	Acne, oily skin and hair, hirsutism, edema, weight gain, nervousness, deepening of the voice, decreased breast size, muscle cramps, sleep disorders.	Monitor weight and blood pressure. Assess for signs of liver dysfunction: jaundice, abdominal pain, light colored stools. Explain side effects to patient. Contraindications: undiagnosed vaginal bleeding; severe cardiovascular, renal, or hepatic disorders.
Gonadotropin-releasing Hormone Leuprolide acetate (Lupron)	Initially increases and then decreases testosterone levels. Used to treat endometriosis and advanced prostatic cancer.	Hot flashes, edema, decreased libido, dizziness, headache, nausea, constipation or diarrhea. Symptoms associated with prostatic cancer may worsen at first, then subside.	Discard if discolored or precipitate forms. Use only diluent provided to reconstitute. Administer immediately after reconstituting. Ask about possibility of pregnancy before giving. Tell patient to expect hot flashes but state that they usually decrease over time. Contraindicated during pregnancy—may cause abortion.
Oral Contraceptives	Suppresses ovulation to prevent pregnancy.		
Estrogen-progestin combinations (Ortho-Novum, Norinyl, Loestrin, Ovral) Progestin only (Norplant system)		Nausea, vomiting, headache, edema, weight gain, breast tenderness. Increased risk of thromboembolism (especially among smokers).	Reinforce instructions for self-medication. Monitor weight. Tell patient to report signs of circulatory impairment: swelling, pain, numbness in an extremity. Contraindicated during pregnancy and with a history of thromboembolism, myocardial infarction, cerebral vascular disease. Follow manufacturer's instructions if a dose is missed.
Estrogen only (diethylstilbestrol)	Prevents implantation of fertilized ovum. Used as emergency postcoital contraceptive; must be given within 24 hr after intercourse.	Severe nausea and vomiting.	
Ovulatory Stimulant and Fertility Drugs	Stimulate or mimic actions of natural pituitary gonadotropins.	All can result in multiple births.	
Clomiphene citrate (Clomid)		Hot flashes, breast tenderness, nausea, vomiting, visual disturbances, headache, depression, fatigue, reversible hair loss, weight gain, dizziness, ovarian enlargement. Contraindicated with liver dysfunction, pregnancy, abnormal bleeding.	Safety precautions if dizzy or has visual disturbances. Stop drug and contact physician if visual disturbances occur. Tell patient to report vaginal bleeding or weight gain signifying ovarian hyperstimulation, in which case, monitor fluid status, weight, and possible signs of internal bleeding. Tell patient to avoid sexual intercourse with ovarian enlargement because of possible rupture.
Menotropins (Pergonal)		Pain and irritation at injection site. Ovarian enlargement and abdominal distention. Rarely, flu-like symptoms: nausea, vomiting, fever.	Reconstitute with sterile saline and administer immediately.
Urofollitropin (Metrodin)	Stimulates ovarian follicular growth. Used to treat selected patients who have not responded to clomiphene citrate.	Same as menotropins.	

TABLE 43-4
UTERINE BLEEDING DISORDERS

DISORDER	ETIOLOGY	SIGNS AND SYMPTOMS	MEDICAL TREATMENT
Metrorrhagia	1. Ovulation	Spotting occurs with regularity 14 days before menses.	None—this is regarded as a normal deviation.
	2. Intrauterine contraceptive device	Intermittent spotting between menses	None if bleeding is not severe and if other causes are ruled out. Monitor serum hemoglobin; if low, iron supplements prescribed. Remove intrauterine device if bleeding is severe.
	3. Oral contraceptive use	Irregular spotting	Patient directed to take pill at same time each day.
		Early cycle spotting	Estrogenic potency of oral contraceptive increased.
		Late cycle spotting	Progestational potency of oral contraceptive increased.
	4. Trauma; introduction of foreign objects	Sudden onset of frank bleeding or spotting	Foreign object removed. Tissue damage repaired.
	5. Vaginitis, cervicitis	Spotting, combined with vaginal discharge characteristic of infectious organism	Vaginal examination; culture and Papanicolaou smear to identify underlying cause; cause treated as warranted.
	6. Ectopic or molar pregnancy	Spotting or frank bleeding, in addition to symptoms specific to molar pregnancy, ectopic pregnancy	Ultrasonography and laboratory tests (serum human chorionic gonadotropin level) done. Surgical removal of products of conception.
	7. Reproductive tract pathology: • Endocervical polyps • Cervical eversion • Cervical dysplasia • Endometriosis • Salpingitis • Ovarian cyst • Benign neoplasm • Malignant neoplasm	Spotting or frank bleeding, in addition to other symptoms characteristic of specific pathology	Diagnostic procedures and treatment specific to identified pathologic condition: hormone therapy, antimicrobial or other drug therapy, surgery.
Menorrhagia	1. Intrauterine contraceptive device	For all: By definition, profuse or prolonged bleeding during menstruation, in addition to other symptoms characteristic of specific etiology	Substitution of intrauterine device with structural incorporation of progesterone (Progestasert-T) or discontinuation or removal of intrauterine device, with substitution of alternate contraceptive method. Use of PGSIs may be effective in reducing menstrual blood loss. Treatment for remaining etiologies is specific for each underlying cause.
	2. Hormonal disturbances		Determination of hormone status is critically important before hormone therapy or other drug therapy is initiated. Endometrial hyperplasia may be diagnosed and treated by dilation and curettage. For women past childbearing age, hysterectomy may be performed.
	3. Benign neoplasm		Benign tumors may be left alone and monitored.
	4. Malignant neoplasm		Malignant tumors require a combination of surgical and medical interventions.
	5. Inflammatory process		Specific cause is treated.
	6. Systemic diseases		Specific cause is treated.

PGSI, Prostaglandin synthesis inhibitor.

various diagnostic tests and procedures. Colposcopy, biopsy, and cauterization, as well as laboratory analyses of blood components, hormone levels, and tissue specimens or smears, provide diagnostic information. Because anemia may result from excessive bleeding, hemoglobin concentration and hematocrit levels are usually measured as well. The treatment of amenorrhea depends on the cause and whether pregnancy is desired by the patient.

Nursing Care of the Patient with Uterine Bleeding

The nurse works closely with the primary caregiver to provide assistance with data collection, diagnostic examinations and procedures, and collection of specimens for laboratory analyses.

ASSESSMENT. Complete assessment of the female patient with a disorder affecting the reproductive system is summarized in Table 43–1. When a patient has metrorrhagia or menorrhagia, it is especially important to document the menstrual history.

NURSING DIAGNOSIS. The primary nursing diagnoses for the patient with metrorrhagia or menorrhagia are the following:

- **Knowledge Deficit** of condition and treatment
- **Anxiety** related to unknown cause of menorrhagia, metrorrhagia

GOALS. The goals of nursing care are patient's knowledge of condition and treatment and reduced anxiety.

INTERVENTIONS

Knowledge Deficit. When the course of treatment has been selected, it may be the nurse's responsibility to teach the patient her role in the treatment process and to make sure that the patient is able to follow through appropriately.

Anxiety. The nurse is a source of emotional support for the patient, who often is fearful or anxious about the unidentified cause of abnormal bleeding. Because the underlying causes of abnormal uterine bleeding may be relatively simple and easily treatable or complex and life threatening, the nurse must be able to offer support to help patients cope with all eventualities. Supportive measures such as encouraging the patient to express her feelings, use of touch, and listening convey to the patient the nurse's concern. Generally it is the nurse's responsibility to provide information regarding procedures to be done. Explanations should be given in terms the patient can understand with avoidance of technical vocabulary and medical jargon.

EVALUATION. The criteria for evaluating goal achievement are the patient's description of the condition and treatment and the patient's statement of reduced anxiety.

INFECTIONS

Infections of the female reproductive tract affect the patients both physiologically and psychologically. Physiologic effects range from short-term reversible changes to long-term changes that result in infertility. Potential psychological effects are numerous. Changes in relationships, feelings of distrust toward sexual partners, shame, embarrassment, diminished self-esteem are but a few.

The majority of infections covered in this chapter not only *can* be but often *are* transmitted through sexual intercourse. In addition, the causative organisms often are those associated with sexually transmitted diseases (STDs) as covered in Chapter 45. However, this chapter focuses primarily on the effects of the microorganisms on the female reproductive tract and on subsequent medical and nursing intervention rather than on the disease processes themselves.

Because of their association with sexuality and sexual function, many women view reproductive tract infections as threats or insults to their self-images. They may react with guilt, embarrassment, denial, defensiveness, or a combination of these that cause them to delay seeking diagnosis and treatment. Others are coping with infertility problems that result from infectious processes. Any nurse who interacts with women experiencing reproductive tract infections or their sequelae must employ sensitivity, tact, and an absolutely nonjudgmental approach.

VULVITIS AND VAGINITIS

Pathophysiology

Inflammation of the vulva is called vulvitis. Depending on the causative agent, vulvitis may be viewed as an infection, as a local manifestation of a general skin disease, as a reaction to a chemical irritant or allergen, or as a normal consequence of the aging process. Regardless of its cause, the most common characteristics of vulvitis are inflammation and usually intense pruritus of the vulva and perianal region.

Vaginitis is similar to vulvitis and is characterized by a local inflammatory response to many of the same factors that result in vulvitis: infection, chemical irritants, allergens, and the aging process. Vaginitis differs from vulvitis primarily because with vaginitis there is a significant vaginal discharge.

Etiology and Risk Factors

As implied earlier, vulvitis and vaginitis are caused by a number of factors that precipitate an inflammatory response. The two most common causes of infection are *Candida albicans* (fungus, or yeast infection) and *Trichomonas vaginalis* (protozoal infection). Both most commonly infect the vagina and produce characteristic vaginal discharges that are irritating to the vulva and vagina. The discharge associated with *C. albicans* has a distinctive odor and a cottage cheese–like appearance; the discharge associated with *T. vaginalis* is profuse, frothy, and yellow-gray in color and has a fishy odor. Both can be transmitted sexually, although yeast infections often are associated with disruption of the normal vaginal flora or with diabetes mellitus. Other microorganisms may serve as sources of infection: streptococci, staphylococci, and intestinal tract organisms are common offenders.

Generalized skin diseases that may be manifested in the vulva include psoriasis and inflammation of sweat glands. When lesions of these diseases occur in the vulva, the constant moist state intensifies the inflammation and subsequent itching.

Vulvar reactions to chemical irritants are common. The vulva is exposed to a wide variety of chemicals that may act as irritants and thus elicit an inflammatory response; the response often extends into the vagina. Perfumed soaps, scented toilet tissue and perineal pads, feminine hygiene sprays, laundry detergent residues, and spermicides are a few examples of common irritants.

Poison ivy is an example of a reaction to an allergen that may affect the vulva. Estrogen deficiency associated with the aging process frequently results in nonpathogenic vulvitis and vaginitis due to a combination of tissue atrophy and decrease of acid vaginal secretions that normally maintain optimal mucous membrane conditions.

Signs and Symptoms

Regardless of the cause, signs and symptoms include local swelling, redness, and itching. Infectious agents may cause specific signs and symptoms that aid in identification of the offending organisms.

Complications

Ascending infection (infection that moves through the vagina to internal structures) is a potential complication of vulvitis and vaginitis. Infection confined to the lower reproductive tract seldom poses a threat to life or fertility.

Medical Diagnosis

Diagnosis is based on the patient's report of subjective symptoms and on inspection of the vulva and vagina. Discharge specimens may be collected to aid in identification of specific microbes if microbial infection is suspected.

Medical Treatment

Treatment specific to the causative agent is initiated and may include topical antifungal creams, oral antiprotozoal agents or antibiotics, vaginal suppositories to reestablish normal vaginal flora, topical or systemic estrogen replacement therapy, improved diabetes control, and discontinued use of offending chemical agents. Treatment of symptoms includes frequent cleansing with neutral agents; wearing of cotton panties, cotton-crotched pantyhose, and nonconstricting clothing; and heat in the form of sitz baths and perineal irrigations. The patient is cautioned to refrain from scratching the itching tissues to avoid further mechanical trauma and infection, to avoid sexual intercourse, or to use condoms during the course of treatment. The woman's sexual partner or partners may be treated for some infections to avoid reinfection.

Nursing Care of the Patient with Vulvitis or Vaginitis

Vulvitis and vaginitis usually are diagnosed and treated on an outpatient basis. Because treatment usually is administered by the patient herself, the nurse may be responsible for making sure that the patient understands all self-care instructions necessary for treatment and for reinforcing other instructions given by the physician or nurse practitioner. General nursing care of patients with reproductive tract infections is addressed in Table 43–5.

BARTHOLIN'S GLAND ABSCESS (BARTHOLINITIS)

Pathophysiology

Owing to their location on either side of the vaginal introitus, Bartholin's glands are vulnerable to a wide variety of infectious microorganisms. The resultant edema and pus formation occlude the duct of the affected gland and form an abscess.

Etiology and Risk Factors

Bacteria, mycoplasmas, and protozoa are transmitted from the gastrointestinal tract, vulva, or vagina to the Bartholin gland duct. Commonly cultured organisms include normal intestinal bacterial flora, *Staphylococcus aureus, Streptococcus, T. vaginalis, Neisseria gonorrhoeae,* and *Mycoplasma homines.* The organisms are often introduced through improper perineal hygiene.

Signs and Symptoms

Perineal pain is the symptom that most commonly motivates the woman to seek medical assistance. In addition to discomfort, presenting signs and symptoms include fever, labial edema, fever, chills, malaise, and purulent discharge.

Complications

Without proper treatment, bartholinitis may progress from a local infection to a systemic infection.

Medical Diagnosis

Visual inspection reveals a swollen, often reddened, mass on the affected side of the vaginal introitus. Gentle palpation causes pain, tenderness, or both. If there is exudate, a specimen may be processed for culture and sensitivity testing. Because causative microorganisms include those responsible for transmission of STDs, the patient is usually screened for these (see Chapter 45).

TABLE 43-5
CARE OF PATIENTS WITH REPRODUCTIVE TRACT INFECTIONS

PATIENT PROBLEM	NURSING INTERVENTIONS
Denial, embarrassment, related to questions about infection	Convey acceptance of patient. Use tact in eliciting information about hygiene and sexual practices: • All products applied on or near the vulva or in the vagina: feminine hygiene products "love" potions, i.e., flavored or scented lubricants, massage oils • Anal contact with penis, fingers, or other objects before contact with vulva or vagina • Number of sexual partners; accessibility to partners if treatment of them is indicated
Knowledge deficit regarding treatment	Explanation and teaching about use of creams, jellies, suppositories: • Purpose • Position for application or insertion • Application or insertion method • Postinsertion position • Care of equipment, i.e., applicator • Use of tampon or perineal pad to hold medication in place Instructions about perineal hygiene: • Frequent washing with neutral soap • Thorough rinsing with irrigating device • No douching unless specifically ordered • No commercial perineal deodorants • Frequent change of underpants (preferably cotton) • Sitz baths to relieve pain, itching • Wiping perineal-anal area from front to back; one stroke per tissue • Complete full course of prescribed drug therapy

Medical Treatment

Conservative treatment consists of oral analgesics and moist heat in the form of frequent sitz baths or hot wet packs. The moist heat serves two functions: pain relief and facilitation of spontaneous rupture and drainage of the abscess. Surgical incision and drainage of the abscess may be elected by the physician. More aggressive treatment with broad-spectrum antibiotics is indicated if symptoms of systemic infection are present.

Nursing Care of the Patient with Bartholinitis

Basic nursing assessment and interventions are outlined in Table 43–1. The nurse provides the instruction appropriate to help the patient comply with the treatment ordered by the primary health care provider. Tactful instruction in basic perineal hygiene principles is in order if the evidence indicates that inappropriate or inadequate practices are being followed. Basic practices include soap-and-water cleansing at least once daily and wiping the perineal area with a clean tissue from front to back following urination or defecation.

CERVICITIS

Pathophysiology

Cervicitis is inflammation of the cervix that may be acute or chronic. Although cervicitis is usually due to an infectious process associated with STDs, the inflammation may be associated with physical or chemical trauma.

Etiology and Risk Factors

Cervicitis is caused by a variety of agents: infectious organisms, scraping of cells for diagnostic tests, cryosurgery, use of vaginal tampons, or medications, childbirth, postmenopausal decreased estrogen levels, and use of oral contraceptives.

Signs and Symptoms

Cervicitis is usually asymptomatic, although it may cause pain, visible vaginal discharge, bleeding, or dysuria. Unsuspected cervicitis may be evident on pelvic examination or detected by routine Pap smears. On inspection via speculum, the cervix appears swollen and reddened; bleeding may be precipitated by gentle touch alone. Mucopurulent discharge and vesicular or ulcerated lesions most often are associated with STDs.

Complications

Cervicitis itself is considered to be a relatively benign condition. However, if the causative agent is an infection, the infection may ascend through the reproductive tract and cause pelvic inflammatory disease (PID). Certain microorganisms that cause cervicitis also alter the vaginal pH and exert a spermicidal effect that results in infertility.

Medical Diagnosis and Treatment

Cervicitis may be diagnosed on the basis of the pelvic examination or results of the Pap smear. Treatment depends on the causative agent(s). Infections are treated by systemic or topical medications appropriate to the identified organisms. Cervicitis related to menopause is treated with topical or oral estrogens. Additional treatment options include topical application of acidic preparations in the form of douches or jellies, cauterization with silver nitrate, and cryosurgery or laser surgery.

Nursing Care of the Patient with Cervicitis

Cervicitis usually is diagnosed and treatment is prescribed in outpatient settings: physicians' offices and clinics. Treatment is administered by the primary health care provider, by another practitioner on referral, or by the client herself. Nursing care is limited to assisting with assessment procedures, client support, and teaching the client to carry out the prescribed treatment and posttreatment procedures.

PHARMACOLOGY CAPSULE

Instruct patients to complete the full course of antimicrobial therapy to treat infections.

MASTITIS

Pathophysiology

Mastitis is an infection-induced inflammation of breast tissue in the lactating woman. Historically, early postpartum mastitis epidemics were common among women who delivered in hospitals and who were hospitalized for the then-usual 10 or more days. With today's short hospital stays, mastitis is associated not with hospitalization but rather with a combination of ineffective breast-feeding techniques that result in poor drainage of mammary ducts and alveoli, lowered resistance to infection due to stress and fatigue, and exposure of breast tissue to infection-causing organisms.

Etiology and Risk Factors

S. aureus is the microorganism most commonly associated with mastitis; *Escherichia coli* and streptococci also may serve as the agents of infection. The nipple serves as the portal of entry for the organism. Cracked nipples are especially susceptible. A common method of organism transmission is failure to wash the hands before touching the nipples.

Signs and Symptoms

Mastitis is usually confined to one breast and may be asymptomatic except for breast tenderness and low-grade (and often unsuspected) fever. The infection therefore may be undetected if frequent breast-feeding empties breast ducts and alveoli and if the woman's natural immune response prevents proliferation of the infectious process. In symptomatic mastitis, the causative organism invades the breast connective tissue or the lobes and ducts and stimulates an inflammatory response that results in localized pain, fever, tachycardia, general malaise, and headache. The affected breast tissue feels hard and warm on palpation; the skin over the infected area is reddened.

Complications

Untreated symptomatic mastitis may result in abscess formation as the sepsis becomes localized. Enlargement of axillary lymph nodes also may result.

Medical Diagnosis and Treatment

Diagnosis is based on presenting symptoms. Symptomatic mastitis is unmistakable. If there is a purulent discharge from the nipple, a specimen can be collected for culture and sensitivity testing. However, treatment is initiated based on the symptoms alone and consists primarily of immediate and aggressive antibiotic therapy.

Symptoms are managed by frequent emptying of the breast, heat application, rest, and administration of an analgesic. The question of whether to empty the breast by breast-feeding or by artificial pumping is a controversial one. Proponents of breast-feeding contend that the infant already has been exposed to the causative organism and therefore is not likely to be further jeopardized. Others insist that breast-feeding be discontinued temporarily until antibiotic therapy is completed. There are many broad-spectrum antibiotics that are tolerated well by both mother and infant. This is significant because the antibiotic or antibiotics taken by the mother will be present in her breast milk.

If an abscess forms, treatment is the same as for mastitis, with the possibility of surgical excision and drainage of the abscess and a longer period of antibiotic therapy.

Nursing Care of the Patient with Mastitis

The most effective nursing intervention is the prevention of mastitis.

ASSESSMENT. The nurse assesses the breast-feeding woman's knowledge of measures to prevent mastitis. The patient's temperature is taken, and the breasts are assessed for pain, tenderness, warmth, hardness, and purulent discharge from the nipple.

NURSING DIAGNOSIS. The primary nursing diagnoses for mastitis are the following:

- **High Risk for Injury** related to possible abscess formation
- **Knowledge Deficit** of mastitis prevention and treatment

GOALS. The goals of nursing care are recovery without complications and patient's knowledge of measures to prevent or treat mastitis.

INTERVENTIONS

High Risk for Injury. If mastitis or breast abscess occurs, nursing intervention is directed toward reinforcement of the prescribed treatment. The teaching plan emphasizes completion of antibiotic therapy in the specified time frame, reporting of continued or additional symptoms, demonstration of methods of heat application, correction of breast-feeding techniques if indicated, administration of analgesics, and institution of efficient time management to increase rest periods.

Knowledge Deficit. The commonly addressed points in breast-feeding education are those that also prevent the infectious process from occurring:

- Frequent breast-feeding with complete emptying of the breasts
- Scrupulous handwashing before handling breasts
- Avoidance of cracked nipples by making certain that the infant's lips and gums are around the areola and not on the nipple itself; breaking suction before removing the nipple from the infant's mouth; cleansing with plain water to prevent chemical trauma from soap, alcohol, and other drying agents; and leaving milk on nipples and exposing them to the air or a heat lamp after breast-feeding
- Wearing of supportive but nonconstrictive bra
- Importance of rest, nutrition, and fluids
- Identification of early symptoms of breast infection and prompt reporting of symptoms to health care provider

EVALUATION. Criteria for evaluating the effects of interventions are the absence of fever, pain, redness, and purulent drainage and the patient's statement and demonstration of preventive measures.

PELVIC INFLAMMATORY DISEASE

Pathophysiology

Pelvic inflammatory disease is an infectious process that may affect any or all structures in the pelvic portion of the reproductive tract and peritoneal cavity. It is called an ascending infection because causative organisms migrate from the portal of entry at the vulva or vagina or at any point in the tract where organisms are introduced. Migration is facilitated by the unbroken continuity of the moist and organism-hospitable environment that is characteristic of the tract.

Pelvic inflammatory disease is a major female reproductive health problem and a major cause of infertility in the United States. The infectious process results in scarring and adhesions in the fallopian tubes that can cause total or partial obstruction. Total obstruction results in infertility. Partial obstruction often results in ectopic pregnancy, which is the implantation of the fertilized ovum in a site other than the uterus, usually in the fallopian tube or the pelvic cavity. Unfortunately, the incidence of PID is particularly high in the adolescent population.

Etiology and Risk Factors

Because the majority of PID cases are caused by sexually transmitted organisms, PID is generally classified as an STD syndrome. *N. gonorrhoeae, Chlamydia trachomatis,* and *M. hominis* are recognized as the organisms most associated with PID. Chlamydia is thought to be the most commonly occurring STD and the one most often responsible for PID. As such, it is often implicated in infection of the fallopian tubes (salpingitis) and is considered to be the primary cause of ectopic pregnancy and infertility associated with tubal obstruction.

However, non-STD organisms also have been identified as causative agents. Staphylococcal, streptococcal, and other aerobic and nonaerobic organisms have been cultured from women with PID. Sources of non-STD–associated PID include contaminated hands or instruments during gynecologic surgery, childbirth, abortion, pelvic examinations, and the like. Women with compromised resistance to infection and women who are poorly nourished are particularly prone to developing non-STD–associated PID.

Intrauterine devices used for contraception have been identified as being heavily associated with the incidence of PID. Partially because of this association, only one brand of intrauterine device is now manufactured or used in the United States.

The risk of PID increases as the number of sexual partners increases. This factor is most applicable to PID caused by organisms implicated in STDs.

Vaginal douching also is considered to be a possible risk factor associated with PID. It is thought that the propulsive force of the fluid used in douching may assist migration of microorganisms from the vagina throughout the cervical os (opening) into the uterus and hence into the fallopian tubes and pelvic cavity.

Signs and Symptoms

Pelvic inflammatory disease may be a "silent" infection with no discernible presenting symptoms. As a result, it may remain undiagnosed and untreated while causing damage to pelvic structures. Symptomatic PID may appear with either gradual onset of dull, steady, low abdominal pain or sudden, severe abdominal pain, chills, and fever. Other symptoms may include dysuria, irregular bleeding, a foul-smelling vaginal discharge that may cause inflammation and excoriation (abrasion) of the vulva, and dyspareunia (pain with sexual intercourse).

Symptomatic PID is much more likely to be diagnosed and treated than is asymptomatic PID. In many instances evidence of PID is first discovered during surgery for ectopic pregnancy, blocked fallopian tubes, ovarian abscess, or other pelvic disorders.

Complications

The risk of complications of PID increases with each repeated infection. Common effects of PID include ectopic pregnancy, infertility, and chronic abdominal discomfort. Without prompt diagnosis and aggressive treatment, infection of the entire peritoneal cavity (peritonitis) and systemic septic shock also are potential complications.

Medical Diagnosis

Medical diagnosis is based on presenting symptoms and the pelvic examination. Definitive diagnosis is made on the basis of the isolation of the causative organism or organisms by culture. Sonography, laparoscopy, and culdocentesis are additional diagnostic procedures that may be employed.

Medical Treatment

Treatment for PID includes rest; application of heat via warm compresses, heating pad, or sitz baths; and administration of analgesics and a combination of broad-spectrum antibiotics. Depending on the severity and extent of the infection, antibiotics are administered intramuscularly, orally, or both on an outpatient basis or intravenously on an inpatient basis. The woman is cautioned to avoid sexual intercourse for the duration of treatment. If the causative organism is thought to have been transmitted sexually, the woman's sexual partner or partners should be treated to avoid repeated infection.

Nursing Care of the Patient with Pelvic Inflammatory Disease

ASSESSMENT. Nursing assessment of the woman with a disorder of the reproductive system is summarized in Table 43–1. Preparation of the patient for physical examination includes anticipatory guidance, positioning and draping, and emotional support (see Table 43–5). The nurse simultaneously assists the physician or nurse practitioner and provides support for the patient. Precautions to avoid transmission of infection to self and others are summarized in Table 43–6 and should be taught to the patient.

TABLE 43-6

PRECAUTIONS TO AVOID REPRODUCTIVE TRACT INFECTION

- Maintain optimum general health: adequate nutrition and sleep, good stress management.
- Cleanse perianal area daily with neutral soap followed by thorough rinsing; no other products unless ordered by health care provider.
- Wipe perianal area with one front-to-back swipe per tissue.
- Avoid sharing of any equipment (including washcloths) used for perianal or vaginal hygiene.
- Change perineal pads or tampons frequently during menses even when flow is slight. Increase soap-and-water cleansing to at least twice per day.
- Inspect genitalia of partner before intercourse or other contact with perianal area. Avoid contact if any lesions or discharge are noted. The same precautions should be followed for any part of the partner's anatomy, e.g., mouth, hands, fingers, that will contact perianal area during sexual encounter.
- Wash with soap and water the penis, hands, other objects that contact anus before contact with vulva or vagina.
- Use condoms with spermicidal cream or jelly for penis–vulva-vaginal contact when monogamous relationship is not well established.
- Avoid intercourse during treatment for reproductive tract infection. Use condom if intercourse cannot be avoided.

NURSING DIAGNOSIS. The primary nursing diagnoses for the patient with PID are the following:

- **Pain** related to inflammation
- **Impaired Skin Integrity** related to infectious drainage
- **Knowledge Deficit** of treatment and prevention of reinfection

GOALS. The goals of nursing care are pain relief, absence of skin excoriation, and patient's knowledge and performance of measures to treat or prevent PID.

INTERVENTIONS. Whether performed or supervised by the nurse in the acute care setting or performed by the patient herself at home, care of the patient with PID includes bedrest with limited activity, application of heat as ordered, administration of antibiotics as ordered, and observing for and reporting signs and symptoms of the side effects of antibiotics.

Pain. Prescribed analgesics are administered for pain control. Additional pain relief measures are discussed in Chapter 16. The nurse monitors and reports on the efficacy of analgesics.

Impaired Skin Integrity. If perineal pads are needed for collection of vaginal discharge, they are changed frequently. The nurse should note the character, amount, color, and odor of vaginal discharge. Frequent perineal cleansing is done with mild soap and water, followed by rinsing, and patting dry. The vulva is inspected for signs of inflammation or excoriation, and the temperature is monitored and recorded.

Knowledge Deficit. The nurse also plays a significant role in the primary prevention of PID and in fostering early diagnosis and treatment of reproductive tract infections so that they do not result in PID. Primary prevention includes measures to reduce risk factors. All women should practice good reproductive tract hygiene habits. When teaching the sexually active woman with multiple partners or with a single partner with unknown sexual history, the following points are included:

- Avoidance of sexual intercourse without protective mechanical and chemical barriers, for example, condom, diaphragm, vaginal sponge, spermicidal vaginal jelly or cream
- Recognition of signs and symptoms of common STDs
- Prompt medical diagnosis and treatment of STDs or other suspected reproductive tract infections
- Routine yearly pelvic examination by a physician or nurse practitioner, with cultures made for detection of *N. gonorrhoeae, C. trachomatis,* and other organisms.
- Routine inspection of the sexual partners' genitalia for signs of infection before each contact for sexual intercourse

EVALUATION. Criteria for evaluating the outcomes of nursing interventions are patient's statement of pain relief, intact skin without excessive redness or edema, and patient's verbalization of instructions and statement of intent to follow prescribed measures.

BENIGN GROWTHS

ENDOMETRIOSIS

Pathophysiology

Endometrial tissue that lines the uterus responds to hormonal influences during the menstrual cycle. During menstruation, small amounts of menstrual fluid are ejected through the fallopian tubes into the pelvic cavity (retrograde menstruation) rather than through the cervical os into the vagina. In some women, the endometrial cells deposited in the pelvic cavity implant themselves on any or all structures within the cavity and continue to respond to menstrual cycle hormonal stimulation. The result is the periodically painful and potentially destructive condition called endometriosis.

In women with endometriosis, the ectopic (out of place) endometrial tissue behaves in the pelvic cavity as it does in the uterus: it proliferates and then bleeds if fertilization of the ovum does not occur. As a result, more and more endometrial cells attach to pelvic structures. These cell clusters, called implants, are sometimes referred to as chocolate cysts because of their color. The implants can migrate to other areas of the body, possibly transported by blood or lymph. Whatever the site of implantation may be, bleeding by endometrial tissue causes inflammation and pain in the areas of cell implantation. The number of implants gradually increases, creating multiple sites of inflammation and pain. In response to the inflammation, fibrous tissue forms that results in scarring and adhesions (Fig. 43–12).

Etiology and Risk Factors

Although it is known that almost all women experience retrograde menstruation to some degree, it is not known why some women develop endometriosis and others do not. Several theories have been explored; one is that endometriosis may be linked to a defect in the immune system of its victims. Although the exact cause has not been identified, it is widely recognized and documented that a genetic predisposition exists: Incidence and severity are greatest in women with relatives who have endometriosis.

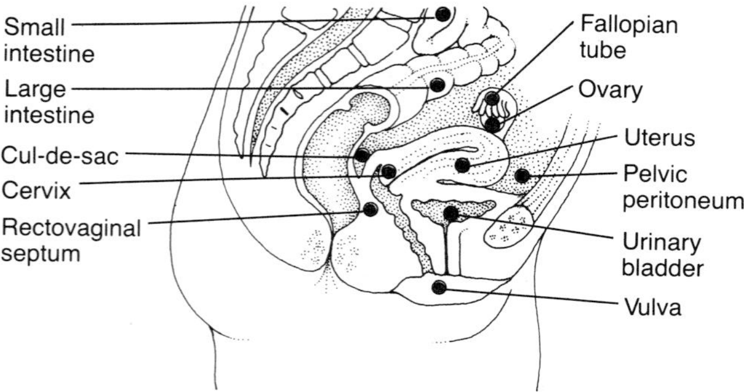

FIGURE 43-12

Common sites of endometriosis. (From Ignatavicius, D. D., & Bayne, M. V. [1991]. *Medical-surgical nursing: A nursing process approach* [p. 1695]. Philadelphia: W. B. Saunders.)

Signs and Symptoms

As noted previously, the major symptom is pain, although some women are asymptomatic. Because the uterine endometrial tissue is bleeding simultaneously, pain appears as dysmenorrhea and may extend to a feeling of general pelvic heaviness. Additional symptoms include pain with defecation, dyspareunia, and abnormal bleeding. Infertility may be a sign of endometriosis when adhesions affect uterine position or fallopian tube patency, movement, or both.

Complications

The most common complication of endometriosis is constriction of pelvic structures by endometriosis-related adhesions. Constriction of the bowel, ureters, or both may cause partial or complete obstruction within the affected structure, creating a medical emergency.

Medical Diagnosis

Excision of endometrial implants via laparoscopy provides specimens for laboratory analysis and is the primary diagnostic procedure for endometriosis. Ultrasonography may be employed as a preliminary diagnostic tool to determine the presence of pelvic masses.

Medical Treatment

Medical management includes the use of analgesics to relieve pain. The most commonly used drug for pharmacologic treatment of endometriosis is danazol (Danocrine), a synthetic androgenic steroid that inhibits gonadotropin excretion, resulting in amenorrhea and atrophy of intrauterine and ectopic endometrial tissue. Many women find the common side effects of danazol to be unacceptable: masculinizing characteristics such as voice deepening, hirsutism (excess hair growth), clitoral enlargement, and skin changes and menopausal symptoms such as hot flushes, vaginal atrophy, and dryness.

PHARMACOLOGY CAPSULE

Androgens have masculinizing effects on females.

Oral contraceptives may be prescribed to cause pseudopregnancy, because pregnancy is known to inhibit endometrial proliferation, thereby relieving symptoms.

PHARMACOLOGY CAPSULE

Oral contraceptives are contraindicated in a woman with a history of cardiovascular disease, cerebrovascular disease, or thrombophlebitis.

Surgical management is commonly employed and includes laparoscopy both for diagnosis and removal of endometrial implants via resection, electrocauterization, or laser excision. Because it is difficult to visualize and remove all implants and because the underlying cause of endometrial migration continues to exist, such surgery does not constitute a permanent cure and may need to be repeated at intervals. Total abdominal hysterectomy with bilateral salpingo-oophorectomy may be performed to achieve permanent suppression of estrogenic stimulation to endometrial tissue. However, estrogen replacement therapy is not an option to relieve menopausal effects for these women as long as endometrial implants remain, because the implants continue to respond to the estrogen and symptoms return.

Nursing Care of the Patient with Endometriosis

Endometriosis is usually treated on an outpatient basis, so nursing care is limited unless the patient is admitted for surgery. Perhaps the most significant nursing intervention is validation that pain is real and guidance in the identification of measures that effect pain relief (see Chapter 16). The office or clinic nurse may be involved in patient teaching. Patient teaching is based on the treatment method selected by the physician and patient and includes anticipatory guidance and treatment-specific instructions. Because periodic bleeding of all endometrial sites may cause anemia, teaching should include symptoms of anemia and the need for dietary or supplemental vitamin and mineral therapy. Preoperative and postoperative nursing care of the patient who has had a hysterectomy is addressed in the nursing care plan. (see Care Plan: The Patient with a Hysterectomy).

CYSTS

A cyst is a closed sac-like structure that is lined with epithelium and that contains fluid, semisolid, or solid material. Cysts are classified as neoplasms and may be benign or malignant; the majority are benign. There are a vast number of benign cysts; they are named for and contain material specific to the structures from which they are formed. The most common ovarian and breast cysts are covered individually in the sections that follow.

FOLLICULAR OVARIAN CYSTS

Etiology and Risk Factors

The follicular ovarian cyst forms when the dominant follicle fails to rupture and release its ovum and thus continues to grow. A cyst occasionally is formed in response to ovarian hyperstimulation by fertility drugs.

Signs and Symptoms

Unless the cyst is unusually large, the follicular cyst is asymptomatic. If the cyst reaches the maximum lemon size, the patient may complain of pelvic heaviness or congestion and an aching feeling.

Complications

Although rare, the cyst may rupture and bleed into the pelvic cavity, which causes severe and sudden abdominal pain.

Medical Diagnosis and Treatment

Most follicular cysts disappear spontaneously without treatment within two to three menstrual cycles. A cyst may be palpated during a pelvic examination. Its size and location are noted and the examination repeated in 6 to 10 weeks. If the cyst continues to be present or is enlarged, laparoscopy may be employed to examine and remove the cyst or drain it by needle aspiration.

CORPUS LUTEUM OVARIAN CYSTS

Etiology and Risk Factors

Although less common than follicular cysts, corpus luteum cysts tend to be more clinically significant because they are associated with more complications. The corpus luteum cyst forms after ovulation and is characterized by excessive bleeding into the luteal cavity and by increased progesterone secretion. Use of fertility drugs is associated with ovarian hyperstimulation and formation of multiple cysts.

Signs and Symptoms

Delay in onset of the menstrual period is the initial symptom, followed by menstrual irregularities in amount and duration of flow. The patient may complain of dull, aching pelvic pain or cramping.

Complications

The corpus luteum cyst usually disappears spontaneously. However, the cyst may rupture and hemorrhage into the pelvic cavity, causing a degree of pain related to the amount of bleeding. Symptoms may be similar to those associated with ectopic pregnancy or acute appendicitis.

Medical Diagnosis and Treatment

The cyst is palpated as a small, tender mass on the affected ovary. If severe abdominal pain exists, a pregnancy test should be done to rule out ectopic pregnancy. Visualization of the cyst may be accomplished by laparoscopic or culdoscopic examination if diagnosis is questionable. Usually no treatment is indicated once the diagnosis is certain.

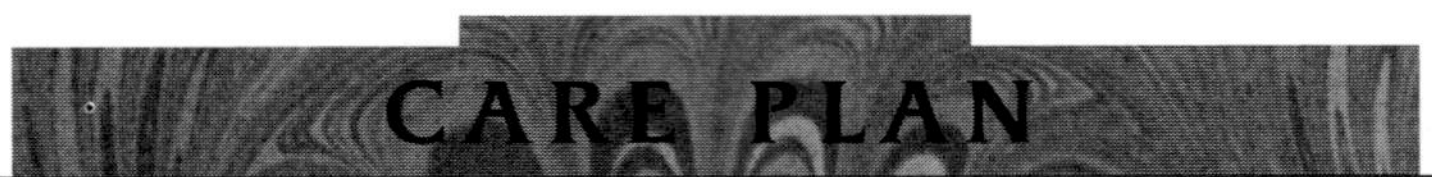

The Patient with a Hysterectomy

ASSESSMENT

Health History: Marcia Hudson, a 42-year-old married woman, is a secretary with a diagnosis of uterine fibroid tumors. She has been pregnant three times and has three living children, two boys and one girl, all of whom are teenagers still living at home. Her menstrual periods have been regular, with onset every 30 days and lasting for 6 days. She describes menstrual flow as heavy. She states that she saturates six to eight heavy duty pads and six to eight super tampons per 24 hours for the first 3 days of each period, after which flow tapers off and she can manage the remainder of each period with four to six tampons per 24 hours. Her last period ended 6 days ago. She describes her health as excellent, with the exception of the uterine tumors that were diagnosed when she was 33 years old. She is admitted for a total abdominal hysterectomy with bilateral salpingo-oophorectomy. This will be her first experience with surgery.

Physical Examination: Vital signs: temperature 97.8°F orally; pulse, 72; respiration, 18; blood pressure, 116/74. Lungs clear on auscultation. Weight: 116 pounds. Height: 5′3.5″. Alert. Skin color medium tan; nailbeds pink with rapid capillary refill. Appears to be in good physical condition: body is firm with little evidence of adipose tissue and with excellent muscle tone; abdomen firm but protruding, appears about 5 months pregnant.

Laboratory: Urinalysis, complete blood count: All reports indicate no deviation from normal ranges except for hemoglobin (Hgb) concentration 10.4 gm/dl (normal 11–16 gm/dl) and hematocrit 30% (normal 31–43%). Mrs. Hudson has been typed and crossmatched for two units of whole blood "on hold" for surgery.

NURSING DIAGNOSIS	GOALS AND OUTCOME CRITERIA	INTERVENTIONS
Preoperative Nursing Diagnoses		
Self-esteem disturbance related to perceived potential changes in femininity, effect on sexual relationship.	The patient will verbalize understanding of expected changes in anatomy and physiology and of ability to resume a satisfying sexual relationship with husband after recovery from surgery.	Explain that: 1. The only expected noticeable effects of loss of uterus and ovaries will be cessation of menstrual periods and ability to become pregnant, in addition to cessation of symptoms for which she is seeking surgery. 2. She may experience vaginal numbness for a short period of time. 3. Many women experience improved libido and sexual satisfaction after hysterectomy; sexual spontaneity may increase with lack of need for contraception. 4. Although penile or vaginal intercourse should not be resumed until at least 6 weeks following surgery, oral sex and masturbation to orgasm are safe. 5. Positions for sexual intercourse should avoid pressure on the abdominal incision for as long as incisional tenderness persists. 6. Orgasmic contractions of the uterus will no longer be present; this change of uterine sensation is noted by some but not by most women. 7. Estrogen replacement therapy (ERT) will avoid atrophy of vagina and decreased lubrication associated with removal of ovaries.

The Patient with a Hysterectomy *(Continued)*

NURSING DIAGNOSIS	GOALS AND OUTCOME CRITERIA	INTERVENTIONS
Knowledge deficit related to information or misinterpretation of effects of ERT.	The patient will verbalize understanding of potential side effects of ERT and of strategies to minimize side effects.	Explain that: 1. The dosage of estrogen replacement may be adjusted for optimum therapeutic effect; she should report any concerns to her gynecologist. 2. Estrogen may increase fluid retention, which may make one "feel fat." Dietary control of sodium intake will reduce tendency for fluid retention. 3. Gradual resumption of presurgical physical activity and a well-balanced diet should maintain weight and fitness at presurgical levels.
Postoperative Nursing Diagnoses (See Chapter 14 for general postsurgical diagnoses and care)		
Altered tissue perfusion related to reduction of cellular components necessary for delivery of oxygen, hypovolemia, reduction of blood flow, intraoperative trauma.	The patient will have adequate oxygenation of tissues as evidenced by a pulse rate of 66–80, respiration rate of 12–20, stable skin color, alert mental status, negative Homans's sign.	Monitor pulse, respiration, and blood pressure rates and auscultate respirations on schedule according to institutional policy. Assist patient to turn, deep breathe, cough on schedule; assist with incentive spirometer if ordered. Monitor skin color and temperature, and capillary refill, including lower extremities. Instruct and assist with foot and leg exercises while confined to bed; encourage and assist with ambulation when allowed. Assess ability to answer questions appropriately. Check for Homans's sign by dorsiflexing foot; report positive sign (calf pain) to physician. If elastic hose are ordered, make sure they are applied and removed according to schedule when patient is in bed and at all times when out of bed; instruct patient about self-application. Monitor lab reports. Report to appropriate person any deviations from normal ranges. Medicate with analgesics to maximize comfort status.
High risk for fluid volume deficit related to postoperative bleeding.	The patient will maintain adequate fluid volume, balanced fluid intake and output, moist mucous membranes, stable pulse and blood pressure.	Check abdominal dressing and perineal pad at least every hour for the first 12 hr; report any drainage observed on dressing, excessive vaginal bleeding. Should saturate less than one perineal pad per hour. Compare fluid intake (intravenous, oral) with urinary output (indwelling catheter collection bag or voided); report discrepancies. Monitor intravenous infusion; carry out related responsibilities according to institutional policy. Encourage oral fluid intake when allowed. Check mucous membranes for moisture; offer frequent mouthwashes during nothing by mouth status. Monitor pulse and blood pressure, compare with baseline levels; report deviations from acceptable ranges.

Care Plan continued on following page

The Patient with a Hysterectomy *(Continued)*

NURSING DIAGNOSIS	GOALS AND OUTCOME CRITERIA	INTERVENTIONS
Urinary retention related to surgical manipulation, local tissue edema, temporary sensory or motor impairment.	Patient will empty bladder completely at regular intervals without catheterization.	Assist patient to bathroom or commode; use bedpan only if absolutely necessary. Assist patient to assume comfortable position. Provide privacy but remain within calling distance. If patient is unable to void without assistance, employ assistive measures: run water in sink or shower, pour warm water over perineum. Teach or assist patient to perform perineal hygiene at least every 8 hr: wash vulva with warm, soapy water, rinse with warm water from irrigating apparatus; rinse perineum after every voiding. Measure and record urine output; note color, clarity, odor of urine. Palpate for bladder fullness above symphysis pubis to assess for urinary retention. If patient is unable to void or is retaining urine, allow her to rest for 30 minutes and repeat attempt for spontaneous voiding. Follow orders for intermittent catheterization or repeat insertion of indwelling catheter if patient is unable to void a sufficient quantity. Continue to monitor and to assist with voiding until patient consistently empties her bladder without assistance.
Colonic constipation related to weakening of abdominal musculature, abdominal pain, decreased physical activity, dietary changes, environmental changes.	Patient will have bowel movement on or before the fourth day after surgery.	Auscultate abdomen for bowel sounds, palpate for distention. Insert rectal tube as ordered, if appropriate. When oral intake is allowed, administer antiflatulent if ordered; teach patient self-administration if allowed. Encourage early and frequent ambulation. Encourage oral intake of fluids, especially of fruit juices. Assess for nausea and vomiting; administer antiemetic if nausea and vomiting are present. Follow protocol for diet; encourage selection of high-fiber goods when patient is allowed options. Administer stool softener or laxative if ordered. Assist patient to splint abdomen while attempting to pass feces. Report inability to have a bowel movement within the allotted time period.

DERMOID OVARIAN CYSTS

Etiology and Risk Factors

A dermoid cyst is a germ cell neoplasm that is composed of tissue from the three embryonic germ cell layers and thus may contain remnants of tissue peculiar to any body structures. Fat, hair, teeth, cartilage, and nerve tissue are the most commonly identified constituents of these cysts. The cyst usually arises from the ovary on a pedicle (stalk).

Signs and Symptoms

When small in size, the dermoid cyst is asymptomatic. Pelvic heaviness or aching is associated with a large cyst; the cyst may be 10 cm or more in diameter. If there is torsion (twisting) of the pedicle, pain may be moderate with gradual twisting to extremely severe with sudden twisting.

Complications

A small number (3–5%) of dermoid cysts become malignant. Because there are multiple cell types within the cystic structure, there is a broad range of potential malignancies that may develop.

Medical Diagnosis and Treatment

A dermoid cyst is palpated as a dense, firm mass during pelvic examination. Depending on pedicle length, the mass may be found some distance from the ovary to which it is attached. A pregnancy test should be done to rule out ectopic pregnancy. Radiographic examination may be ordered to visualize teeth in the mass, which would provide a definitive diagnosis. Any dermoid cyst should be removed surgically because of the potential for the development of malignancy.

BREAST CYSTS

The vast majority of palpable breast lumps are round freely movable, benign cysts. Cysts may be soft or firm, depending on whether they contain fluid or semisolid matter. Breast cysts are generally classified under the term *fibrocystic diseases*, which is a misnomer because the condition is not really a disease but an exaggerated response to hormonal influence. Cysts may alternately enlarge during the premenstrual period and shrink from the onset of menstruation until the next ovulation during any period.

Etiology and Risk Factors

The most commonly identified cause is ovarian estrogen secretion. Additional contributing factors may be stress and caffeine.

Signs and Symptoms

Small cysts tend to be asymptomatic; their presence may be unrecognized and unsuspected until they become large enough to be detected by palpation. If small cysts are numerous, the breasts have a lumpy "cottage cheese" consistency on palpation. Varying degrees of pain may occur between ovulation and menstruation.

Complications

Although controversial as a theory, some fibrocystic subtypes are considered precancerous.

Medical Diagnosis

Palpation, mammography, and ultrasonography are noninvasive methods of preliminary diagnosis. If cysts are determined by sonography to be fluid filled, many physicians prefer to observe them over time rather than aspirating their contents. Other physicians prefer to aspirate the contents for laboratory study. To make a definitive diagnosis and to rule out cancer, surgical biopsy is indicated for cysts that are not fluid filled, when aspirated fluid is bloody, or if cyst characteristics change over time.

Medical Treatment

Treatment is generally palliative rather than curative in nature. Oral analgesics, application of heat, and caffeine restriction are commonly recommended. Vitamin and hormonal therapy may be employed. The most aggressive form of hormone therapy approved by the U.S. Food and Drug Administration is danazol (Danocrine), which decreases secretion of estrogen. Although danazol is known to cause side effects unacceptable to many women, the dose used to treat fibrocystic disease is low enough to avoid the effects for most women. The most aggressive form of surgical treatment is mastectomy, which occasionally is an option selected by women who undergo repeated surgical biopsies.

Nursing Care of the Patient with Ovarian or Breast Cysts

For women with ovarian or breast cysts, nursing intervention focuses on teaching. The patient should be instructed to keep a diary of symptoms detailing when they occur and any factors that may be associated with the symptoms. Teaching is specific to the prescribed therapy.

FIBROID TUMORS (MYOMAS, LEIOMYOMAS)

Pathophysiology

Uterine fibroid tumors are both benign and common. It is predicted that at least 25% of all women will develop fibroid tumors during their reproductive periods, with an apparent increased likelihood among African-American women. Fibroid tumors grow slowly during the reproductive years but tend to atrophy after the onset of menopause.

Etiology and Risk Factors

Although the exact cause is unknown, it is widely thought that fibroid tumors form and grow in response to stimulation by estrogen, primarily estradiol. Human growth hormone and human placental lactogen may also promote the tumors' development and growth.

Signs and Symptoms

Fibroid tumors may be asymptomatic, but the most common symptoms are menstrual irregularities: menorrhagia and dysmenorrhea. Discomfort from pressure on pelvic structures and dyspareunia (painful sexual intercourse) may be associated with a large tumor. For some women, the initial hint that "something is wrong" is the gradual enlargement of the lower abdomen, which may be mistaken for pregnancy.

Complications

A very large fibroid tumor may compress the urethra, obstructing urine flow and causing secondary hydronephrosis. More common complications include infertility, crowding and malpositioning of the fetus during pregnancy, and degenerative changes related to interruption of blood supply.

Medical Diagnosis

On pelvic examination, the uterus is found to be enlarged and distorted. A pregnancy test, Pap smear analysis, and complete blood count should be done to rule out other conditions.

Medical Treatment

Many women require no treatment, and their tumors atrophy following menopause. Methods of contraception are limited by fibroid tumors: intrauterine devices are contraindicated, the estrogen in oral contraceptives may stimulate growth of the tumors, and diaphragms may be uncomfortable. For women who desire to become pregnant, some gynecologic surgeons perform myomectomy (removal of the tumor alone), usually by laser surgery. For tumors that are very large or that are associated with complications, hysterectomy is the usual surgery of choice.

Nursing Care of the Patient with Fibroid Tumors

The nurse assists the physician or nurse practitioner with diagnostic procedures and provides support to the patient. Women tend to equate the word tumor with malignancy. Therefore, the nurse may need to give repeated reassurance that the fibroid tumor is benign. If the practitioner elects a conservative approach of monitoring tumor growth, the patient may need reassurance that this approach is commonly used (see Care Plan: The Patient with a Hysterectomy).

UTERINE DISPLACEMENT

CYSTOCELE AND RECTOCELE

Pathophysiology

Cystocele and rectocele are vaginal disorders caused by weakness of supportive structures between the vagina and bladder (cystocele) or the vagina and rectum (rectocele). They typically occur together. Herniation of the bladder and rectum through the vaginal wall is visible and palpable on vaginal examination. Although small cystoceles and rectoceles may cause no problems, larger herniations may cause problems with emptying of both bladder and bowel. Stress incontinence, incomplete bladder emptying, difficulty with expulsion of fecal matter collected in the area of herniation, and incontinence of gas or liquid feces are typical problems reported.

Etiology and Risk Factors

During pregnancy and childbirth, the pubococcygeal muscle that provides the structural support of the pelvic floor may be weakened. Repeat pregnancies result in further weakening.

Signs and Symptoms

Symptoms other than the already described common bladder and bowel problems include dyspareunia, lower back and pelvic discomfort, and recurrent bladder infections.

Medical Diagnosis and Treatment

Diagnosis is made on the basis of inspection and palpation. Treatment of small cystoceles and rectoceles may be limited to pelvic floor (Kegel) exercises, which improve the tone of the pubococcygeal muscle. Surgical intervention via anterior colporrhaphy and posterior colporrhaphy (A&P repair) to tighten the vaginal wall has long been the treatment of choice for larger or symptomatic cystoceles and rectoceles. However, nurse researchers who utilize noninvasive methods based on pelvic floor exercises report long-term success rates comparable to those found with colporrhaphy.

Nursing Care of the Patient with Cystocele and Rectocele

ASSESSMENT. Assessment of the patient with a disorder of the reproductive system is outlined in Table 43–1. When a patient has uterine displacement, the nurse also records problems related to urinary and bowel function. If surgery is planned, the patient's understanding of the procedure and the pre- and postoperative care and the patient's concerns are assessed.

NURSING DIAGNOSIS. Nursing diagnoses with cystocele and rectocele may include the following:

- **Stress Incontinence** related to pelvic muscle weakness
- **Constipation** related to collection of feces in herniated bowel
- **Sexual Dysfunction** related to painful intercourse
- **High Risk for Infection** related to incomplete bladder emptying

After surgical intervention, additional nursing diagnoses are the following:

- **Pain** related to tissue trauma
- **High Risk for Injury** related to infection and stress on surgical incisions
- **Knowledge Deficit** of postoperative self-care

Goals

Goals of nursing interventions are urinary continence, normal bowel elimination, satisfying sexual practices, and absence of urinary tract infections. Additional goals for the surgical patient are reduced pain, wound healing without disruption or infection, and patient's knowledge of self-care.

INTERVENTIONS. Nursing interventions vary depending on the medical treatment.

Stress Incontinence. For conservative treatment via pelvic floor exercise, the nurse teaches this simple exercise: The patient alternately contracts the pubococcygeal muscle, as if interrupting a stream of urine, and then relaxes the muscle. The exercise should be repeated several times in succession, several times a day. It can be done in any position and at any time, including while standing in line and while waiting for traffic lights to change. (The exercise is also viewed as a preventive measure adopted in early adulthood to maintain optimum pelvic floor muscle support throughout life.)

Constipation. For the patient who reports problems with expelling feces, teaching by the nurse includes directions regarding the necessity for maintaining soft stool consistency and regular bowel elimination. Dietary support focuses on frequent ingestion of fluids and a wide variety of high-fiber foods such as fruits, vegetables, and grains. Regular administration of bulk stool softener may be necessary.

Sexual Dysfunction. For the patient for whom colporrhaphy is employed as treatment, preoperative nursing care includes anticipatory guidance regarding the impending surgery and postsurgical period and carrying out the physician's orders. The patient may be fearful of painful intercourse postoperatively or may be concerned about the effects of surgery on sexual function. The nurse explains that intercourse should be delayed for a prescribed period of time for healing to occur. No permanent impairment of sexual function is expected.

High Risk for Infection. Preoperative orders commonly include a vaginal douching with an antibacterial solution, a cleansing enema, and a perineal shave. Postsurgical nursing care is directed at prevention of infection and protection of the suture line. Perineal care is provided at regular intervals. In addition to incisional infections, the patient is at risk for urinary tract infections. An indwelling urethral or suprapubic catheter commonly is left in place for several days to keep the bladder empty and thus to prevent strain on sutures and to let local edema subside. The patient is instructed to report urinary frequency, burning or foul odor, which suggests infection of the urinary tract.

Pain. Postoperative perineal care is similar to that employed after vaginal delivery: cleansing of the perineum at regular intervals, initial application of cold to reduce pain and swelling, and subsequent application of heat via sitz baths and heat lamps. In addition to these comfort measures, analgesics may be administered as ordered because postoperative pains may be severe. The nurse assesses the effects of comfort measures and notifies the physician of unrelieved pain.

High Risk for Injury. A low-residue diet reduces fecal bulk, and stool softeners are administered to prevent straining during defecation after surgery. Adequate fluids and ambulation are encouraged.

Knowledge Deficit. Discharge teaching focuses on the patient's responsibility for continued self-care as ordered by the physician; reinforcement of instructions regarding diet, medications, and activity restrictions; avoidance of sexual intercourse until permission is given by the physician; and reassurance that expected loss of vaginal sensation is temporary and will resolve after a few months.

EVALUATION. Criteria for evaluating the outcomes of nursing interventions (with medical treatment) are improved bladder control, regular bowel movements without straining, patient's statement of the lack of pain during intercourse, and normal body temperature without pain on urination. For the surgical patient, additional outcomes are patient's statement of pain relief; intact surgical incisions without increasing redness or purulent drainage; and patient's statement of postoperative self-care.

UTERINE PROLAPSE

Uterine prolapse is a condition in which the uterus descends into the vagina from its usual position in the pelvis (Fig. 43–13). Descent is rated as first degree if the cervix is above the vaginal introitus, second degree if the cervix protrudes from the introitus, and third degree if the vagina is inverted and both the cervix and the body of the uterus protrude from the introitus. If the vagina inverts, it carries with it the adjacent bladder and rectum. Although uterine prolapse can occur in women who have never been pregnant, it is most common in postmenopausal women who have had multiple pregnancies.

Etiology and Risk Factors

Cardinal ligaments support the uterus in its anatomic position. The ligaments may be congenitally weak or may become stretched during pregnancy or injured during childbirth, resulting in weakening of support. As the woman ages, other supportive structures and uterine walls tend to relax, resulting in some degree of uterine prolapse.

Signs and Symptoms

Dyspareunia, a feeling of pelvic heaviness and pressure, and backache are commonly reported symptoms. Cystocele and rectocele usually accompany uterine prolapse.

Complications

In second-degree and third-degree prolapse, the protruding uterine portion is subject to trauma and may become eroded and necrotic.

Medical Diagnosis

Second-degree and third-degree prolapse are readily detected by visual inspection. First-degree prolapse is diagnosed through pelvic examination, although early first-degree prolapse may escape detection as the uterine descent is resolved by assuming the supine position.

Medical Treatment

Vaginal hysterectomy with anterior and posterior colporrhaphy is the most common surgical treatment for uterine prolapse. For the woman who desires to preserve childbearing capability, it is possible to shorten the supportive ligaments surgically and return the uterus to the correct anatomic position.

Prolapse

Grade I — The uterus bulges into the vagina, but the cervix does not protrude through the entrance to the vagina.

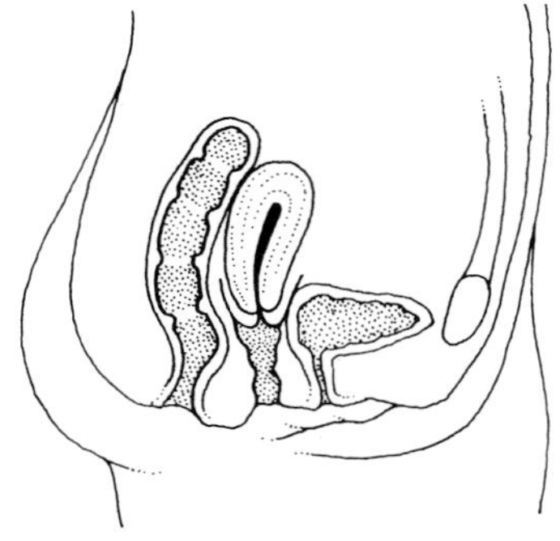

Grade II — The uterus bulges further into the vagina, and the cervix protrudes through the entrance to the vagina.

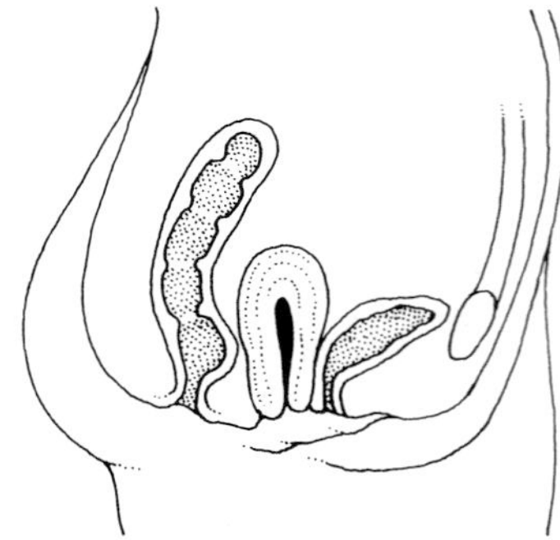

Grade III — The body of the uterus and the cervix protrude through the entrance to the vagina. The vagina is turned inside out.

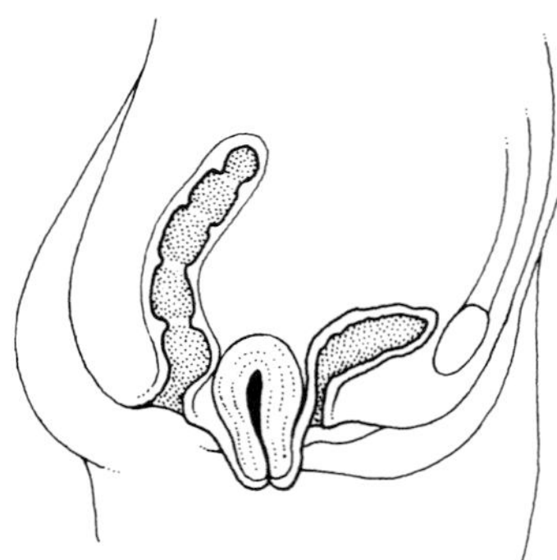

FIGURE 43-13

Uterine prolapse. (From Ignatavicius, D. D., & Bayne, M. V. [1991]. *Medical-surgical nursing: A nursing process approach* [p. 1705]. Philadelphia: W. B. Saunders.)

For women who are poor surgical risks or who refuse surgical treatment, pessaries may be used. A pessary is inserted to elevate the uterus. However, pessaries must be removed, cleaned, and replaced frequently. If pessaries are not maintained or are fitted improperly, they may act as irritants and cause tissue erosion, malignant tissue changes, or both.

Nursing Care of the Patient with Uterine Prolapse

ASSESSMENT. Nursing assessment of the patient with a disorder of the reproductive system is outlined in Table 43–1. When the patient has uterine prolapse, the nurse documents related symptoms. If the prolapsed uterus is visible, the nurse notes any signs of trauma or tissue breakdown.

NURSING DIAGNOSIS. Nursing diagnoses for the patient with second-degree or third-degree prolapse commonly include the following:

- **Body Image Disturbance** related to interference with daily activities
- **Sexual Dysfunction** related to abnormal uterine position
- **High Risk for Injury** related to trauma to the exposed uterus
- **Knowledge Deficit** of self-care

GOALS. Goals of nursing care are improved body image, satisfying sexual function, absence of uterine trauma, and patient's knowledge of self-care.

INTERVENTIONS. The nurse serves as a source of emotional support and information for the patient. Nursing care depends on the treatment selected. Proper use of a pessary can reduce the risk of uterine trauma. When a pessary is the treatment of choice, the nurse must provide detailed instructions regarding the necessity for frequent examination by a physician or nurse practitioner, for reporting pessary-related discomfort to the health care provider, and for pessary care. Although some primary health care providers prefer to remove, clean, and replace pessaries themselves, capable patients can be taught to do this themselves.

EVALUATION. Criteria for evaluating the outcomes of nursing interventions are positive patient remarks about self and ability to manage uterine prolapse, absence of traumatic injury or signs of infection, and patient's description of self-care.

RETROVERSION AND RETROFLEXION: ANTEVERSION AND ANTEFLEXION

The uterus is normally positioned at a 45-degree angle anterior to the vagina, with the cervix pointed downward toward the posterior vaginal wall (Fig. 43–14). Displacement from the normal position may be a normal congenital variation or may be related to a number of other factors (Fig. 43–15). Posterior displacement may be retroversion or retroflexion. Retroversion is a backward tilt of the uterus with the cervix pointed downward toward the anterior vaginal wall. With retroflexion, the body of the uterus bends backward on itself. Anterior displacement may be anteversion of anteflexion. Anteversion is the forward tilt of the uterus at a sharper angle to the vagina. With anteflexion the uterus bends forward on itself.

Etiology and Risk Factors

Weakening and stretching of the round, broad, and uterosacral ligaments and weakened pelvic floor musculature related to childbearing are the most common causes of uterine displacement. Other causes include surgical trauma, pelvic tumors, PID and endometriosis.

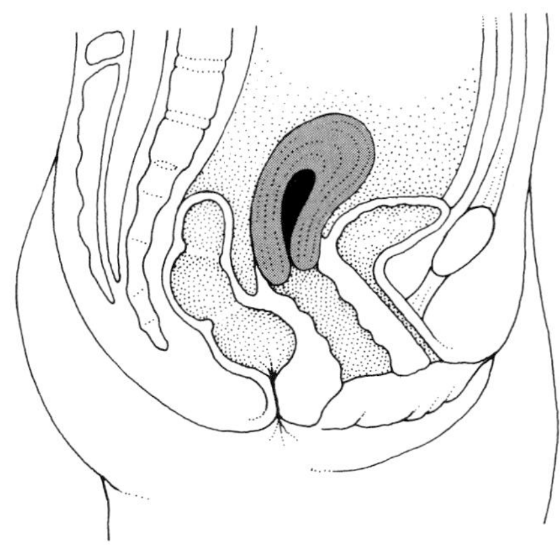

FIGURE 43-14
Normal position of the uterus. (From Ignatavicius, D. D., & Bayne, M. V. [1991]. *Medical-surgical nursing: A nursing process approach* [p. 1703]. Philadelphia: W. B. Saunders.)

Signs and Symptoms

Most uterine displacement is asymptomatic, although dyspareunia and low back pain may be noted with retroversion.

Complications

Difficulty with conception has been associated with uterine displacement, particularly with retroversion. However, most complications are now thought to be associated with an underlying pathology (e.g., endometriosis, PID) rather than with displacement itself.

Medical Diagnosis and Treatment

The pelvic examination reveals uterine displacement. Treatment is seldom employed, although some women find relief from backache by assuming a knee-chest position. Kegel exercises may be employed to strengthen the pelvic floor muscular support system. Pessaries are rarely used to regain or achieve normal uterine position.

Nursing Care of the Patient with Retroversion and Retroflexion; Anteversion and Anteflexion

The nurse's role is usually limited to history taking and providing information. If a pessary is used, however, the nurse provides instructions similar to those described under uterine prolapse.

VAGINAL FISTULAS

Vaginal fistulas are abnormal passageways between the vagina and other pelvic organs. A fistula between the vagina and the urinary bladder is called a vesicovaginal fistula; a urethrovaginal fistula is located between the urethra and the vagina. Both of these fistulas permit urine to flow into the vagina. A rectovaginal fistula is located between the vagina and the rectum and permits flatus and feces to pass into the vagina. Urine or fecal matter in the vagina can lead to severe vaginal vulvar irritation and infection. Vaginal fistulas can often be diagnosed on the basis of the health history and physical examination. Dye may be injected into the vagina and radiographs made to locate the fistula.

Surgical correction is often needed, although some small fistulas close spontaneously. Surgery may be delayed until the infection and inflammation have subsided. Preoperatively, the patient is instructed in perineal hygiene and measures to control odor. Fluid intake is encouraged to reduce the risk of infection. The physician may prescribe sitz baths and deodorizing douches. Excessive pressure must be avoided with douching to prevent forcing the fluid through the fistula. Perineal pads are needed but must be changed frequently, and perineal care should be done every 4 hours.

After repair of a urinary fistula, the patient will have a urinary catheter that must be kept patent. Fluids are encouraged to promote urine output and to prevent occlusion of the catheter. After repair of a rectovaginal fistula, the patient is initially put on a liquid, low-residue diet to delay the need for a bowel movement so the

Minor Displacements

Retroversion — The uterus *tilts posteriorly,* and the cervix rotates anteriorly.

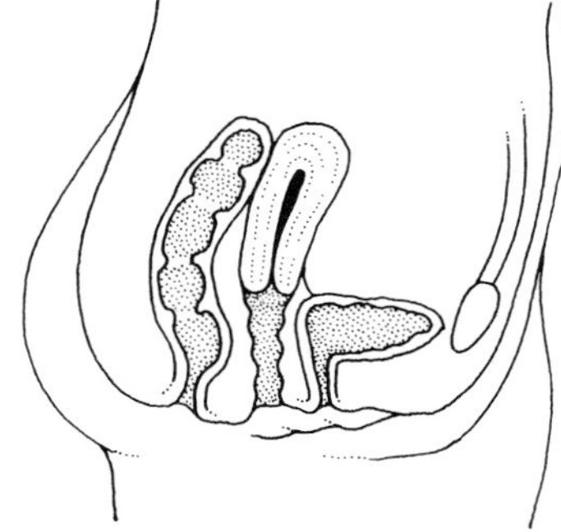

Retroflexion — The uterus *bends posteriorly.*

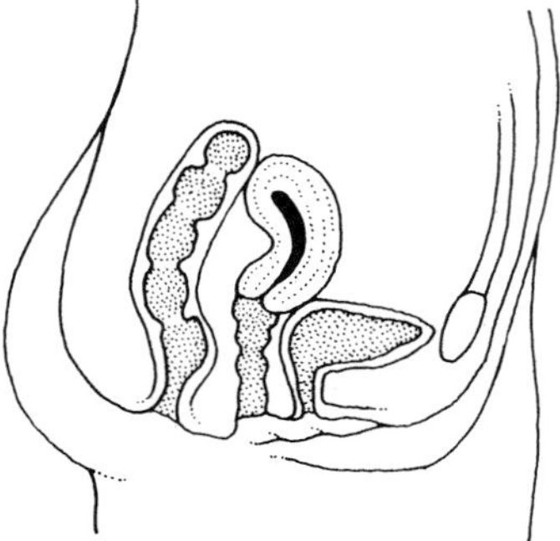

Anteversion — The uterus *tilts anteriorly.*

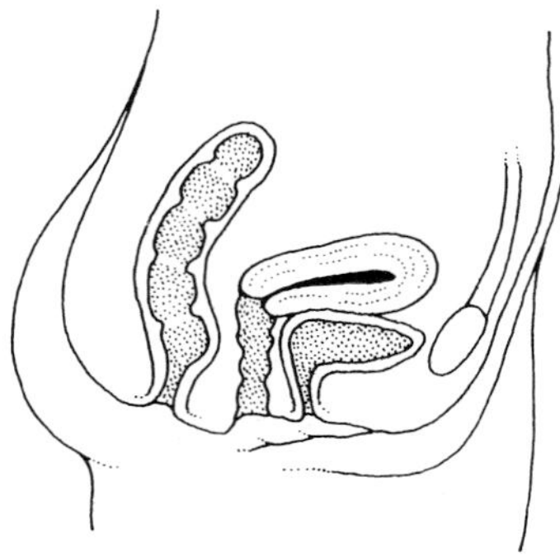

Anteflexion — The uterus *bends anteriorly.*

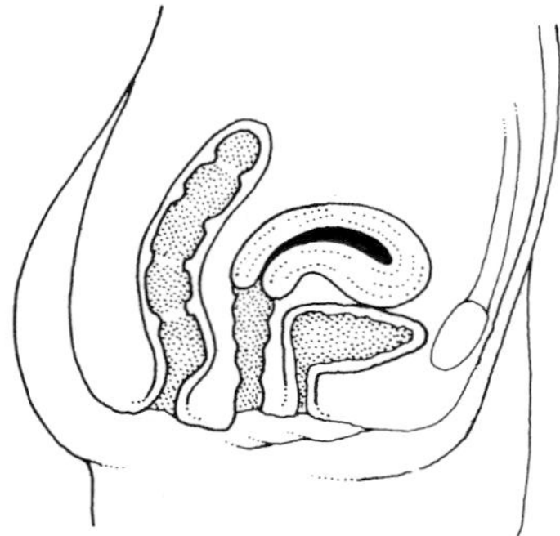

FIGURE 43-15

Abnormal uterine positions. (From Ignatavicius, D. D., & Bayne, M. V. [1991]. *Medical-surgical nursing: A nursing process approach* [p. 1704]. Philadelphia: W. B. Saunders.)

surgical site can heal. After several days, stool softeners and laxatives may be ordered to promote bowel elimination. Enemas are contraindicated as they may disrupt the sutured area. Unfortunately, surgical correction is not always successful.

CANCER

A diagnosis of cancer of the female reproductive system can produce a multifaceted psychological impact. For example, cancer implies threats to personal survival, sexual relationships, family integrity, and one's concept of self as a female. The nurse plays a potentially significant role in assisting the patient to cope successfully with decision making, treatment methods and their effects, the inevitable grieving process, and reactions of family members and friends.

BREAST CANCER

Breast cancer is the most prevalent form of cancer in American women: the current prediction is that one of every eight or nine women will develop breast cancer at some point in her life. Regular monthly BSE is identified as the single best initial step toward detection of breast cancer in its early stage, with prompt diagnosis and treatment producing a 5-year survival rate greater than 90%. Although it is estimated that 80% of breast lumps prove to be benign, those that are malignant must be identified and treated aggressively to prevent invasion of surrounding tissue, metastasis to distant structures, and death.

The three major types of breast cancer according to the type of cells undergoing malignant changes are ductal, lobular, and nipple. Malignant growths usually are singular and unilateral, and they can be found in any part of the breast. However, nearly one half of all malignant breast tumors are located in the upper outer quadrant, and nearly one fourth are located in the nipple-areolar complex. Most malignant lumps are painless and are palpated as firm, irregularly shaped, and fixed to underlying structure or skin. However, they may possess characteristics similar to those associated with benign lumps: soft or semifirm, symmetric in shape with discrete borders, and freely movable. Therefore, no lump should be ignored because it "feels" benign. Prompt evaluation is vital and may include tissue examination of cells obtained by needle aspiration or surgical biopsy.

Etiology and Risk Factors

Although no cause has been identified for breast cancer, statistical evidence indicates the existence of several risk factors:

- Gender: female
- Family history: mother or sister diagnosed with breast cancer
- Race: white
- Age: 45 and older
- Duration of menstruating life stage (menarche to menopause): early menarche, late menopause
- Age at first childbirth: older age
- Body build: obese
- Breast tissue density: increased density
- History of malignancy: breast, thyroid, colon, reproductive tract
- Radiation exposure: females during puberty or soon after menarche
- The relationship of fat intake and premenopausal exercise to breast cancer is being studied.

The risk of developing breast cancer for the woman who has multiple risk factors rises as the number of factors rise. However, it is important to remember that approximately 70% of women diagnosed with breast cancer have none of these known risk factors.

A great deal of research has focused on the suspected association between breast cancer and female sex hormones, androgens, and thyroid hormone. Results have been both inconclusive and contradictory. Statistics indicate that oophorectomy may reduce the potential for breast cancer development, particularly when surgery is performed before age 35. Researchers continue to attempt to discover both causes and risk factors, with ability to cope with stress and diet among the many possible factors currently being studied.

Breast cancer is staged according to the tumor-node-metastasis classification explained in Chapter 23. The four stages are summarized in Figure 43–16.

Signs and Symptoms

Painless breast tissue thickening or lump is the initial sign, palpated during BSE or visualized by mammogram. Most late symptoms are associated with the tumor's invasion of surrounding tissues: dimpling of the skin, nipple discharge, nipple or skin retraction, edema, dilated blood vessels, ulceration, and hemorrhage. Dry, patchy nipple skin is suggestive of Paget's disease, an uncommon cancer of the nipple and areola. Chest pain may be associated with metastasis to the lung.

Complications

Infiltration of adjacent breast and axillary tissue and metastasis to distant sites are the major complications of advanced breast cancer.

Medical Diagnosis

Diagnosis includes routine screening methods and follows specific guidelines:

- Physical examination every 3 years until age 40, every year after age 40
- Baseline mammogram by age 40, followed by repeat mammogram every 1 to 2 years from age 40 to 49, every year beginning at age 50
- Sonogram or magnetic resonance imaging scan for questionable mammogram readings
- Biopsy of suspicious tissue for histologic analysis

Stage I
Tumor smaller than 2 cm, with 0 lymph nodes positive for cancer and no metastases evident

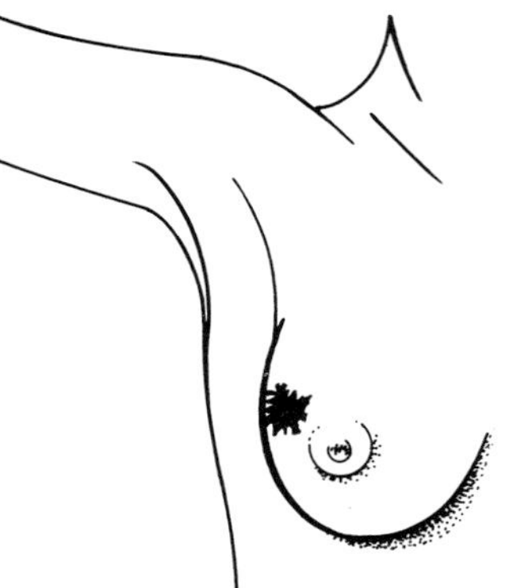

Stage II
Tumor 2–5 cm, with 0–1 lymph nodes positive for cancer and no metastases evident

Stage III
Tumor larger than 5 cm, with 0 lymph nodes positive for cancer and no metastases evident

Tumor smaller than 2 cm, with axillary lymph nodes positive for cancer cells and no metastases evident

Tumor 2–5 cm, with axillary lymph nodes positive for cancer cells and no metastases evident

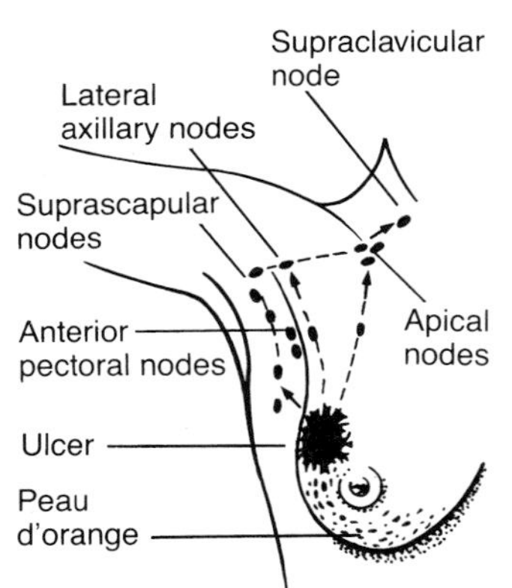

Stage IV
Tumor of any size, with or without lymph nodes positive for cancer cells and distant metastases present

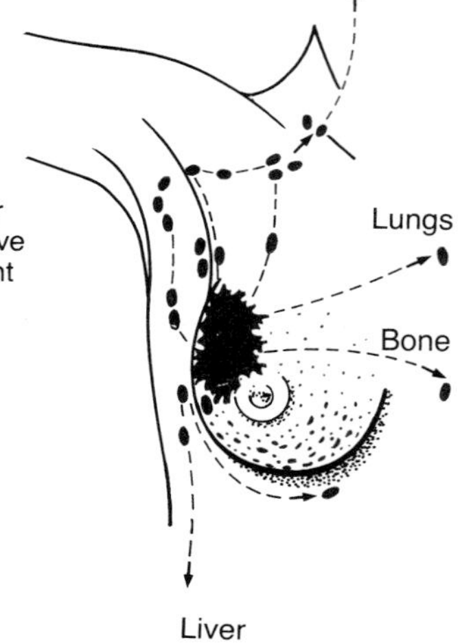

FIGURE 43-16
Stages of breast cancer. (From Ignatavicius, D. D., & Bayne, M. V. [1991]. *Medical-surgical nursing: A nursing process approach* [pp. 1670–1671]. Philadelphia: W. B. Saunders.)

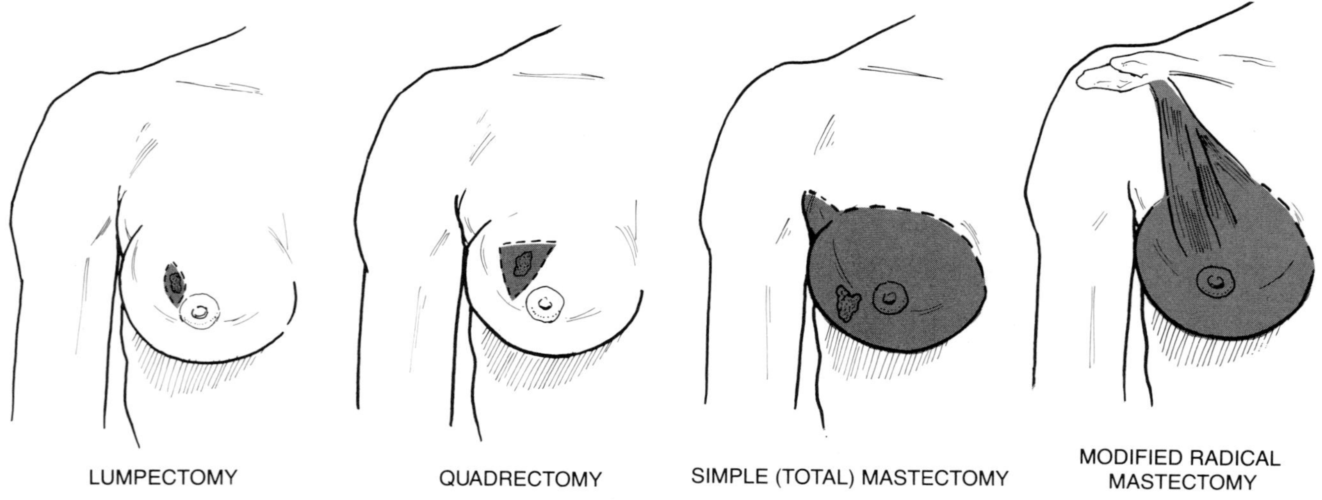

FIGURE 43-17
Options in surgical management of breast cancer.

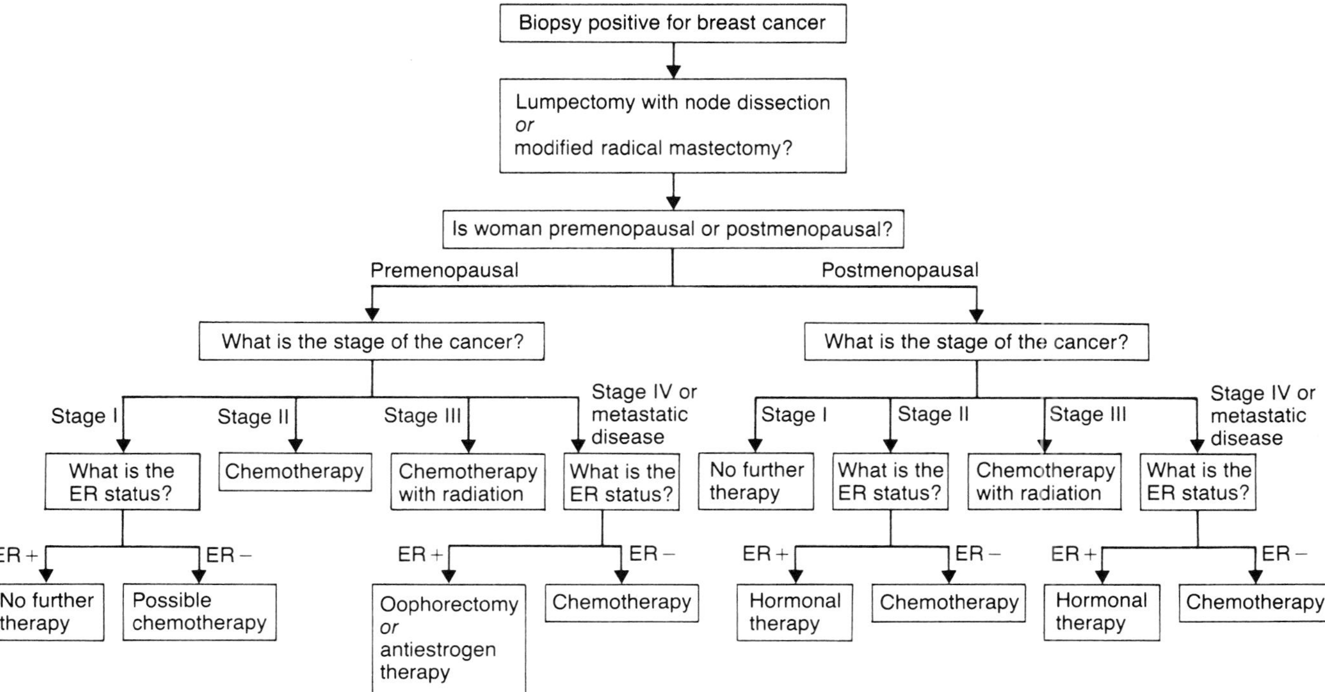

FIGURE 43-18

Treatment considerations and approaches after diagnosis of breast cancer. ER, Estrogen receptor. (From Ignatavicius, D. D., & Bayne, M. V. [1991]. *Medical-surgical nursing: A nursing process approach* [p. 1673]. Philadelphia: W. B. Saunders.)

Medical Treatment

Once tissue examination confirms the malignancy, the patient and her physician consider surgical options that ideally are based on the type, size, and extent of the cancerous growth. Women are playing increasingly active roles in the decision-making process and may "shop" for surgeons with whom they can agree on the selected surgical method. An oncologist may serve as a consultant in the decision-making process. Surgical options range from lumpectomy to radical mastectomy. Lumpectomy is removal of the tumor with a margin of surrounding healthy tissue but with preservation of most of the breast. Radical mastectomy is removal of all breast tissue, overlying skin, axillary lymph nodes, and underlying pectoral muscles. A variation of radical mastectomy adds removal of the internal mammary lymphatic chain. The four most commonly employed options are depicted in Figure 43–17. Additional treatment options depend on a number of factors, as outlined in Figure 43–18.

After the selected surgery is completed, the removed nodes are examined for evidence of cancer, and at this point the cancer is staged. Another critical factor is determined: whether the cancer cells are estrogen receptors (ER+) or nonreceptors (ER−). If cells are ER+, indicating that the tumor needs estrogen for growth, the drug tamoxifen citrate may be prescribed. Tamoxifen is a synthetic nonsteroidal antiestrogen that blocks circulating estrogen from reaching the receptor cells. Researchers also employ the drug in studies directed toward primary prevention of malignancy in selected women identified as being at high risk for development of breast cancer.

Once surgery is completed, the oncologist plays an increasingly dominant role in continued management of care. Chemotherapy, hormone therapy, radiation therapy, or a combination of these may or may not be employed. Most physicians routinely follow lumpectomy with radiation therapy, even though evidence indicates that all malignant cells were removed. The radiation therapy is used because studies indicate that small metastases without nodal involvement are possible. See Chapter 23 for discussion of chemotherapy and radiotherapy.

Many women elect breast reconstruction following modified radical or radical mastectomy. Reconstruction is performed by a plastic surgeon and may be initiated immediately after the mastectomy and before closure of the wound, or it may be delayed. Reconstruction usually begins with implantation of a tissue expander placed under the pectoralis muscle. Periodic injections of small amounts of normal saline are made into the expander until the expander creates a space the size of the prosthesis that will replace the expander in a future surgical procedure. Other reconstruction methods employ transfer of tissue from other areas of the patient's own body, including the abdomen and back.

Nursing Care of the Patient with Breast Cancer

Nurses provide direct patient care throughout every phase of care from preliminary data collection to diagnostic procedures, immediate pre- and postsurgical treatment, and further oncologic treatment. The nurse-patient contact period may be lengthy.

ASSESSMENT. Nursing assessment of the patient with breast cancer is particularly critical. Nursing assessments are focused on physical manifestations of disease, physical and psychological responses to treatments, review of all body systems, presence of pain, psychosocial factors, and level of knowledge. In the immediate postoperative period, the nurse monitors the patient's vital signs, the wound dressings and drainage, and the arm on the affected side for edema.

NURSING DIAGNOSIS. Care of the surgical patient is covered in Chapter 14, and care of the patient who has cancer is covered in Chapter 23. Additional specific nursing diagnoses for the mastectomy patient are the following:

- **Body Image Disturbance** related to altered appearance, loss of breast, or perceived loss of attractiveness
- **High Risk for Injury** related to lymphedema secondary to excision of lymph nodes
- **Knowledge Deficit** of self-care and resources

Goals

Goals of nursing care after mastectomy are improved body image, absence of injury to the affected arm, and patient's understanding of self-care and resources.

INTERVENTIONS

Body Image Disturbance. The breasts are an important component of the woman's self-image. To many women, loss of breast represents loss of femininity. Even with immediate reconstruction, the breasts do not look completely normal. The patient may see herself as sexually unattractive and fear rejection by her sexual partner. These feelings are superimposed on the fear created by a diagnosis of cancer. The nurse gently explores how the patient is feeling about the surgery and encourages her to express her concerns. It is critical to be accepting of the patient whose feelings may surface in a variety of ways including anger, denial, and depression. From the early postoperative period, the patient is encouraged to attend to her appearance. Information is provided about breast prostheses and clothing designed for women who have had mastectomies. If the patient has chemotherapy, hair loss may also contribute to her body image disturbance. Strategies and resources for the cancer patient with a body image disturbance are discussed in Chapter 23.

High Risk for Injury. A radical mastectomy includes the removal of lymph nodes in the axilla on the affected side. Because lymph nodes normally play a role in returning tissue fluid to the blood stream, their removal can result in lymphedema (the accumulation of fluid in the affected area). An important aspect of postoperative care after mastectomy is directed toward preventing and minimizing lymphedema in the arm on the affected side. Intervention includes the following:

1. Elevation of the arm to a height above the level of the heart
2. Blood pressure cuff placed on the arm on the unaffected side, *never on the affected side*
3. No venipuncture or parenteral fluid administration in the affected arm
4. No deodorant application to or shaving of the axilla on the affected side
5. Frequent measurement of affected arm circumference; immediate reporting of increase
6. Frequent and progressive exercise of the arm on the affected side; encouragement of the patient to use the arm for as many exercises of daily living as possible

The patient is positioned alternately on her unaffected side and her back, observing regular postoperative care as described in Chapter 16. If the nipple has been grafted to another site for preservation for future reconstruction, it is treated as a secondary surgical site. Orders are written for specific postoperative care of the nipple. Routine assessment of the grafted nipple includes hourly observation for bleeding and signs of infection or necrosis (pallor, cyanosis, coolness).

Knowledge Deficit. Arrangements are usually made for visits from a representative of the American Cancer Society's Reach for Recovery program. The representatives are volunteers who have experienced breast cancer themselves and who have learned to cope successfully with diagnosis, treatment, and related stressors. They assist the patients by providing teaching, anticipatory guidance, and emotional support.

Patient teaching should have begun preoperatively, but must be reinforced postoperatively. Content to cover includes signs and symptoms of infection, wound care, arm exercises, prevention of lymphedema, resources, and (if appropriate) management of effects of chemotherapy or radiotherapy. With the patient's permission, her significant other is included in the teaching process. This provides an opportunity for the partner to understand the patient's experience, to demonstrate support, and to participate in her recovery.

EVALUATION. In addition to routine postoperative outcomes, evaluation criteria after mastectomy include patient's demonstration of comfort with the new body image, absent or minimal lymphedema, and patient's demonstration of self-care and use of resources.

CERVICAL CANCER

Cervical cancer is a generally slow-growing malignancy. For patients who have regular pelvic examinations and Pap smears, cervical cancer is usually diagnosed and treated in its early stage. Advanced cervical cancer may invade such surrounding structures as pelvic side walls, bowel, and bladder. On inspection, the affected cervical tissue in advanced cancer tends either to resemble a cauliflower in shape and texture or to appear as an ulcerated lesion that bleeds easily.

Research indicates that most cervical cancer is associated with microbes such as some strains of human papillomavirus and herpes simplex virus. Thus, cervical cancer is considered by many medical scientists to be an STD.

Etiology and Risk Factors

Although the exact relationship between cervical cancer and microorganisms that cause STDs is unknown, the link is strongly supported by research. Another research-supported link applicable to relatively few women is in utero exposure to diethylstilbestrol. Additional factors associated with cervical cancer are cigarette smoking, initial sexual intercourse in early adolescence, multiple sexual partners, and dietary deficiencies in folic acid and in vitamins A and C. There is no evidence that family history or the patient's menstrual history increases the risk of cervical cancer. Although cervical cancer formerly was thought to be linked with sexual intercourse with uncircumcised males, current research does not support this.

Signs and Symptoms

Early cervical cancer is asymptomatic. Advanced cancer may also be asymptomatic or may be associated with blood-tinged or frank bloody vaginal discharge, menstrual irregularities, or bleeding after intercourse.

Complications

Invasion of cervical cancer into adjacent structures causes site-related symptoms such as pain, backache, and bleeding. Anemia due to chronic bleeding may develop.

Medical Diagnosis

Cervical cancer is often first suspected when a positive Pap smear result reveals atypical cells. Tissue specimens obtained by multiple punch biopsy, endocervical curettage, or conization are studied for microscopic evidence of malignancy. Cervical cancer is staged according to the extent of invasion, with stage 0 signifying limitation to the cervical epithelium and stage IVB indicating metastasis to distant organs.

Medical Treatment

Treatment depends on the stage of the tumor and on various general health factors. Localized carcinoma (in situ) may be treated with laser destruction, cryosurgery, or conization alone; total hysterectomy may be performed if childbearing is not desired.

Invasive cancer is treated with radiation, surgery, or both. Radiotherapy may be external or internal. If the therapy is internal, a sealed source is placed in the vagina. The container is left in place for a specified period of time depending on the total radiation dosage prescribed. Because placement and subsequent maintenance of placement are critical to effectiveness of the therapy, the patient is immobilized as much as possible for the duration of the treatment. Radiotherapy and related nursing care is discussed in detail in Chapter 23.

If surgery is elected, the extent of surgery depends on the extent of invasion. It ranges from radical hysterectomy (removal of the uterus, fallopian tubes, upper third of the vagina, and usually the ovaries) to total pelvic exenteration (removal of the uterus, ovaries, fallopian tubes, vagina, bladder, urethra, descending colon, rectum, anal canal, and pelvic lymph nodes; see Fig. 43–18). Nursing care of the patient with cervical cancer is discussed at the end of the section on Cancer.

OVARIAN CANCER

Although the incidence of ovarian cancer is relatively low compared with that of other cancers, the mortality rate of ovarian cancer is the highest of all female reproductive system cancers. The high mortality rate is due to the fact that ovarian cancer is asymptomatic and usually grows for an extended period of time before it is diagnosed. For well over half of the women with ovarian cancer, their tumors are bilateral, meaning abnormal cell growth occurs in both ovaries.

More than half of ovarian cancers are diagnosed around the time of menopause, with the remaining cases divided evenly between women younger than age 40 and women older than age 60. The ovary may also be a target site for metastasis from other primary cancer sites, resulting in secondary ovarian cancer.

Because ovarian cancer is rarely found in women who have had children or who have used oral contraceptives, birth control pills often are prescribed as a preventive measure even for women for whom pregnancy is not a possibility. Prophylactic bilateral oophorectomy (surgical removal of the ovaries) is a more drastic preventive measure employed for women identified as high risk candidates for ovarian cancer.

Etiology and Risk Factors

No specific causes have been found for ovarian cancer. However, risk factors include family history of ovarian cancer; personal history of ovarian cancer; personal history of ovarian dysfunction or of breast, endometrial, or colorectal cancer; nulliparity (has not produced a viable offspring); and either early menarche or late menopause. Exposure to such carcinogens as asbestos and talc and ingestion of animal fats have been identified as possible risk factors by some researchers. However, additional studies are needed to determine whether a cause-effect relationship exists.

Signs and Symptoms

Ovarian cancer is asymptomatic in its early stage. Symptoms of even advanced ovarian cancer tend to be vague and nonspecific; they usually are thought to be related to a number of other possible conditions before ovarian cancer is considered. Abdominal pain and bloating, abnormal uterine bleeding, gastrointestinal tract symptoms such as flatulence, and urinary tract complaints may be reported. In extremely advanced cancer, ascites may be noted.

Complications

Ovarian cancer metastasizes widely via direct invasion, peritoneal fluid, and the lymphatic and venous systems.

Medical Diagnosis

Palpable tumors are discovered by pelvic and rectal examinations. The findings of bilateral masses is a particularly significant finding, because most benign ovarian masses are unilateral. Computed tomography and ultrasound may be used as diagnostic tools. Blood may be drawn for a CA-125 serum marker test, which if elevated above 35 units per ml indicates the presence of an antigen associated with ovarian epithelial cancer. However, an exploratory laparotomy should be done as soon as possible to directly visualize the tumor or tumors and to obtain tissue for definitive diagnosis and for staging and grading of the malignancy.

For early diagnosis, ovarian cancer should be considered as a possibility for all women, especially those women identified as high-risk candidates, who present with virtually any symptoms of reproductive tract problems. Some practitioners advocate screening of blood serum for CA-125, although the test is not specific for ovarian cancer.

Medical Treatment

Treatment depends on the staging of the tumor or tumors. Stage 1 tumors, in which tumor growth is confined to the ovary, are surgically removed via total abdominal hysterectomy and bilateral salpingo-oophorectomy. Chemotherapy, radiotherapy, or both usually are used after surgery. More advanced tumors generally are treated palliatively with total abdominal hysterectomy and bilateral salpingo-oophorectomy followed by chemotherapy and radiotherapy to shrink remaining tumor tissue and thus to relieve pressure and pain associated with metastases to the peritoneum, omentum, bowel, and distant sites. Regardless of the stage and prognosis for survival, CA-125 may be monitored to assess the progress or regression of tumor growth. Nursing care of the patient with ovarian cancer is discussed at the end of the section on Cancer.

VULVAR CANCER

Cancer of the vulva is the most rare but also the most visible of the cancers of the female reproductive system. It may appear as a visible and palpable lump on the vulva or as a deviation from the normally pink, moist mucosa. The lesion may be scaly; red, white, or irregularly pigmented; edematous; serosanguineous or frank bloody discharge. The most common site is the labia majora.

Malignant melanoma may be manifested in the vulva, although the vulva is a rare site for this form of cancer. Its incidence is highest in postmenopausal women; symptoms are similar to those of more common vulvar cancers.

Etiology and Risk Factors

No definite causes have been identified for vulvar cancer, but it may be related to STDs, particularly human papillomavirus.

Signs and Symptoms

The most commonly reported symptom is pruritus (itching). Pain and bleeding are additional symptoms.

Complications

Although cancer of the vulva generally remains localized, it may become invasive if not discovered and treated. Invasion may be to adjacent structures or may be in the form of metastases to distant sites via the lymphatic system.

Medical Diagnosis

Preliminary diagnosis is made through palpation of a mass or by visualization of tissue that appears suspicious. Biopsy is necessary for definitive diagnosis.

Medical Treatment

Treatment depends on the extent to which the malignant cells have spread. For localized lesions, conservative removal of the malignant tissue by laser surgery may be employed. For wider, deeper, or invasive lesions, radical surgical removal through vulvectomy and bilateral dissection of groin lymph nodes or through pelvic exenteration may be necessary. Chemotherapy, radiation therapy, or both may follow surgery. Nursing care of the patient with vulvar cancer is discussed at the end of the section on Cancer.

VAGINAL CANCER

The vagina seldom is the primary site for cancer; rather it is the site for the extension of cancer that originates in the vulva, cervix, or endometrium. Except for young women whose vaginal cancers are associated with intrauterine exposure to diethylstilbestrol, vaginal cancer most commonly is found in postmenopausal women.

The 5-year survival rate for women treated for in situ vaginal cancer approaches 100%. However, its in situ stage is relatively short compared with that of other reproductive tract malignancies; invasion of adjacent tissues is common unless the cancer is detected and treated early. Because early diagnosis most often is made on the basis of a Pap smear report rather than on visualization of suspicious epithelium or symptoms, a strong argument can be supported for yearly Pap smears for postmenopausal women and for women at no risk for cervical cancer because of posthysterectomy status. Metastasis is facilitated by the presence of numerous lymph nodes in the area.

Etiology and Risk Factors

No definite cause has been identified for vaginal cancer. As already described with other cancers in the vulva, vagina, and cervix, researchers have identified the following risk factors: sexually transmitted diseases (syphilis, herpes virus type 2, human papillomavirus), previous diagnosis of cervical or vulvar cancer, previous radiation therapy, and intrauterine exposure to DES.

Signs and Symptoms

In its early and most easily treated form, vaginal cancer usually is asymptomatic. Later symptoms include a burning sensation, vaginal discharge that may have a foul odor, dyspareunia (painful intercourse), spotting after intercourse, and vaginal bleeding. Pelvic pain usually is associated with invasion of adjacent structures.

Complications

Invasion of adjacent structures and metastasis are the most common complications of vaginal cancer that is epithelial in nature. The prognosis is poor for vaginal malignant melanoma, with an extremely low five-year survival rate.

Medical Diagnosis and Treatment

Most cases are detected during inspection of the vagina and by routine Pap smears. Definitive diagnosis is made via colposcopy and biopsy of suspicious areas followed by tissue studies. Treatment of vaginal cancer depends on the extent of invasion. In situ (localized) cancer may be treated relatively simply by local laser surgery or cryosurgery. More radical treatment is indicated if the cancer is more invasive. Possible treatments employed either singly or in combination include topical chemotherapy, internal or external radiotherapy, partial or total vaginectomy, and pelvic exenteration.

Nursing Care of the Patient with Cancer of the Cervix, Ovaries, Vulva, or Vagina

The patient with cancer of the cervix, ovaries, vulva, or vagina presents multiple challenges. She has been diagnosed with a life-threatening condition and with a condition whose treatment very often constitutes a threat not only to her self-concept as a woman but also to her ability to function sexually. Treatments beyond local excision of affected tissue may result in disfigurement or in anatomic changes that hinder penile-vaginal intercourse, or in both. Nursing care focused on psychosocial needs is as critical as is care focused on physical needs.

ASSESSMENT. Complete assessment of the patient with a disorder of the female reproductive system is summarized in Table 43–1. When the patient has or may have cancer, the health history documents signs and symptoms and possible risk factors. When reviewing the systems, the nurse describes changes or problems that may be related such as fatigue, pain, and bowel or bladder dysfunction. Effects of the symptoms on the normal functioning are explored. The nurse assesses the patient's concerns about the condition and may find anxiety, fear, depression, anger, or withdrawal. The patient may express fear of the diagnosis of cancer as well as fear of the prescribed treatments. A complete physical examination should be done. The physician or nurse practitioner performs a pelvic examination that may reveal lesions, masses, and lymph node enlargement.

NURSING DIAGNOSIS. Nursing diagnoses for the patient with cancer of the cervix, ovaries, vulva, or vagina may include the following:

- **Anxiety** and **Fear** related to threat to health and lack of knowledge about the cancer and prescribed treatment
- **Body Image Disturbance** related to change in body appearance or function
- **Altered Sexuality Patterns** related to physical and emotional effects of cancer of the reproductive system
- **Ineffective Family Coping** related to lack of knowledge, situational crisis, role changes, or patient preoccupation with self
- **High Risk for Injury** (to patient and others) related to effects of radiotherapy, chemotherapy

GOALS. Goals of nursing care for the identified nursing diagnoses are reduced anxiety and fear, improved body image, satisfactory sexual patterns, appropriate family-patient interactions, and absence of injury resulting from treatment.

INTERVENTIONS

Anxiety and Fear. The woman needs encouragement and permission to ventilate her reaction to the diagnosis and treatment. The nurse should listen carefully to determine any knowledge deficits or misconceptions and to provide information as appropriate. Anticipatory guidance is particularly important.

Body Image Disturbance. The patient may be distressed if there is a change in appearance or function caused by the cancer or the treatment. Loss of reproductive capacity can be especially painful for women who still wish to bear children. The nurse can gently explore the patient's response to the situation and encourage her to express her thoughts. Patients who are severely disturbed should be offered the benefit of a mental health professional or spiritual counselor. Measures to improve the appearance should be encouraged, and the patient's positive efforts praised. Management of alopecia (hair loss) associated with cancer therapy is discussed in Chapter 23.

Altered Sexuality Patterns. Realistic expectations for future sexual functioning should be discussed and should focus both on sexual practices that will not be possible on a temporary or permanent basis and on alternative sexual practice that may be explored. Paramount in nursing intervention is an accepting attitude toward sexuality in general and toward any specific sexual practices acceptable to the patient and her partner or partners.

Ineffective Family Coping. The family or identified support system should be included in care. The family needs to understand the effects of the cancer and the treatments. They also need to appreciate the patient's need for support and for assistance during therapy and recovery. Members of the household are encouraged to consider ways to reduce demands on the patient. In addition, the nurse must be sensitive to the needs of family members who may fear losing a loved one. Inclusion of the woman's sexual partner or partners is particularly critical if alteration in sexual expression is expected after treatment.

High Risk for Injury. Physical care of the patient varies with the prescribed treatment and is based on physician's orders, institutional policies and procedures, and nursing diagnoses. General guidelines for the care of the patient who is having radiotherapy are covered in Chapter 23.

Internal radiation poses a nursing challenge. If a sealed radiation source is to be implanted in the vagina, an indwelling urinary catheter is inserted first. An applicator that will contain the radiation source is inserted into the vagina while the patient is in the operating room. The placement is checked by radiograph and is maintained by vaginal packing. The radiation source may be placed in the applicator before the applicator is inserted, or it may be placed in the applicator after the patient is transferred to her room and positioned in bed. Radiation dosage is determined and ordered by a radiologist; the duration of implantation is based on the total dosage but generally ranges from 24 to 72 hours.

The patient poses a source of radiation exposure to anyone within a radius of several feet, so usual radiation precautions are in force. For each nurse who is allowed to care for the patient, exposure should not exceed a total of 30 minutes per 24 hours. Visitors are screened according to protocol; those cleared to visit should be instructed to remain outside a 6-foot radius of the patient and to limit the duration of visits according to policy.

The patient is assigned a private room for the duration of internal radiotherapy. Strict bedrest must be enforced to prevent dislodgment of the applicator; movement is restricted to cautious turning from side to side. The fact that radiation therapy may precipitate nausea, vomiting, and diarrhea; that movement must be restricted; and that total time for nursing care is restricted makes care particularly challenging. The nurse needs to be exceptionally well organized and able to anticipate and to intervene rapidly and effectively. For example, judicious administration of antiemetics, tranquilizers, and antidiarrheal medications may moderate radiation side effects and thus facilitate patient comfort, maintenance of applicator position, and efficiency of nursing care time.

Effects on local tissue by the radioactive material produce a profuse, malodorous vaginal discharge that is largely absorbed by the packing and thus cannot be controlled with cleansing. A room deodorizer may be partially effective in making the odor tolerable. Following removal of the packing and applicator at the conclusion of therapy, a cleansing vaginal douche is administered, and the patient is free to resume activities normal for her. She is no longer a source of radiation exposure. Transfer of the patient to another room should be considered to remove her from a noxious environment and to allow housekeeping personnel to clean and air the room.

Care of the patient admitted for a pelvic exenteration is exceptionally complex and is beyond the scope of this textbook. An expert nursing staff is essential to provide the emotional support and physical care demanded for this patient.

EVALUATION. Achievement of nursing goals is determined by the patient's statement of reduced anxiety and fear with calm manner, positive patient statements about self and efforts to maintain or improve appearance, patient's discussion of effects of disease or treatment on sexuality and coping strategies, family demonstration of support and positive coping, and maintenance of application position and adherence of patient and others to radiation precautions.

INFERTILITY

Fertility impairment, or infertility, generally is defined as the inability to conceive within 1 year of regular unprotected sexual intercourse or as the ability to conceive but inability to deliver a live infant. Infertility is categorized as primary infertility if the woman has never conceived or if the man has never impregnated a woman. Secondary infertility refers to the woman who has conceived at least one time but either is not able to deliver a viable infant or is not able to conceive again. An estimated 17% of American couples want to produce children but are unable either to conceive or to deliver live infants. Of those couples, treatment enables approximately 60% to conceive and carry pregnancies to term. The remaining 40% of couples represent sterility that is not amenable to treatment.

In recent years, the entertainment and news media have provided mechanisms for the frank discussion of components of infertility: causes, psychosocial effects, and treatments. Associated problems and treatments have been described by professional health care providers and scientists, and personal accounts have been given by affected individuals. For many, the acceptance of infertility as a topic for public discussion has removed the stigma of infertility as a source of shame and embarrassment, myths have been debunked, and lay and professional people are becoming more knowledgeable about the subject. As a result, infertility has become a major subspecialty of gynecology, and infertility researchers have developed highly sophisticated and effective diagnostic techniques and treatments.

Etiology and Risk Factors

Research indicates that approximately 40% of infertility is attributable to female factors, 40% to male factors, and the remaining 20% either to a combination of male and female factors or to unknown factors. Conception depends on the interaction of a number of factors, broadly categorized as follows:

- Timing and techniques used for sexual intercourse

  Impregnation of the ovum by the sperm must occur

within 24 hours after ovulation. Intercourse should be scheduled for every other day around ovulation time to optimize the potential for fertilization of the ovum.

Semen should be deposited deeply in the vagina, in close proximity to the cervical os. Although a sperm from semen deposited outside the vagina (i.e., in the vulva or anus) is known to be able to reach and to penetrate the ovum, extravaginal deposition of semen does not facilitate conception for couples with infertility problems.

- Production and release of a healthy ovum by the female and of both healthy and numerous (approximately 200,000,000 per ejaculate) sperm by the male.
- Anatomically and physiologically correct female and male reproductive conduit systems.

  Female: patent fallopian tubes with active fimbriated ends, uterine endometrium prepared for reception and implantation of a fertilized ovum.

  Male: epididymis temperature that maintains viability of sperm during storage, patent seminiferous tubules, and vas deferens with enervated musculature.
- Biochemical compatibility between female vaginal-cervical-fallopian environment and male ejaculate.

Other than faulty timing or technique for sexual intercourse, both of which are easily corrected through patient education, causes related to the remaining factors are exceptionally numerous. As has been mentioned previously, untreated or inadequately treated STDs potentially impair fertility by altering anatomy, physiology, and patency of the reproductive tracts of either or both partners.

Additional identified influences on conception include dysfunction of any part of the hypothalamic-pituitary-endocrine system, malnutrition or obesity, smoking, drug and alcohol use, exposure to toxic chemicals or radiation, nervous system disorders that affect motility of the male and female reproductive conduit structures, and male practices that maintain above-normal epididymal temperature (i.e., wearing tight underwear and pants, frequent and prolonged immersion in hot water or sauna).

Medical Diagnosis

Diagnosis is based on data obtained from exhaustive psychosocial and physical health and sexual health histories of both partners. If the histories provide clues that may explain possible detriments to fertility, such as poor timing or techniques of sexual intercourse or habitual epididymal exposure to high temperatures, further diagnostic attempts may be delayed until the couple has had time to remediate the potential problem or problems. If such simple factors are not identified, history taking is followed by systematic, comprehensive physical examinations and laboratory tests.

The male partner usually is the initial focus of diagnostic procedures because tests for diagnosis of male-associated infertility problems are generally easier, less invasive, less expensive, and (unlike a complete female fertility work-up) not cycle dependent. A semen specimen for analysis is collected by masturbation after a period of sexual abstinence that approximates the male's average frequency interval for intercourse. The specimen is then assessed for volume and for sperm count, morphology (shape), duration of viability, motility, and liquefaction. A second specimen is examined if variations from normal are found in any of the values. He may be referred to a urologist or endocrinologist for further diagnosis and possible treatment of persistent seminal variations (see Chapter 46).

Further diagnostic work on the female partner may be delayed when male problems are identified. However, if the history or physical examination data or both yield evidence of female-related fertility problems, the work-up may proceed simultaneously with male diagnosis and treatment.

Evaluation of the female partner includes a battery of tests, most of them dependent on timing related to her menstrual cycle. Thus, scheduling of each test is critical. Basal body temperature monitoring and recording of detailed data related to menstruation, cervical mucous characteristics, sexual intercourse, and duration of sleep are done daily by the woman. In addition to data from the basal body temperature record, serum progesterone levels and endometrial biopsy provide data related to ovulation, cervical patency, and adequacy of the endometrium for ovum implantation.

If findings from the basal body temperature, serum progesterone level, and endometrial biopsy indicate normal hormonal functions, a postcoital test is done immediately before ovulation. The couple has intercourse the evening or morning before the scheduled test. A specimen of cervical mucus is aspirated from the cervix by the physician or nurse practitioner. The characteristics of the mucus are assessed by gross inspection and by microscopic examination. The examiner is looking for the clear, elastic mucus necessary to facilitate the progression of semen through the cervix. Abnormal consistency of the mucus may block progression of the semen beyond the cervical os. The examiner also inspects the specimens for number and motility of sperm. If a previous test of the male's semen indicated normal motility and viability of sperm but the postcoital test indicates nonviabile sperm, this suggests that the cervical mucus is not conducive to maintenance of sperm survival, perhaps because of an antigen-antibody response to the semen.

Determination of uterine and fallopian tube patency and physical assessment of the peritoneal cavity are accomplished by invasive procedures: hysterosalpingography, laparoscopy, and culdoscopy. Ultrasonography may be employed for additional assessment.

Women are considered to be sterile and thus are not candidates for infertility diagnosis and treatment if they have congenital reproductive tract anomalies than cannot be corrected by surgery. Absence of one or more reproductive tract structures is also untreatable.

Medical Treatment

Treatment for infertility is related to diagnostic findings. A brief overview of specific problems and related treatments is presented in Table 43–7.

TABLE 43-7

OVERVIEW OF COMMON CAUSES OF FEMALE INFERTILITY AND RELATED MEDICAL TREATMENT

ETIOLOGY	MEDICAL TREATMENT
Anovulation, associated with:	Administration of:
• Delayed follicular maturation	• Clomiphene citrate (Clomid)
• Hypogonadotropin secretion	• Menotropins (Pergonal)
• Hypothalamic-pituitary dysfunction	• Gonadotropin-releasing hormone
• Elevated prolactin level	• Bromocriptine mesylate (Parlodel)
• Hypothyroidism	• Thyroid-stimulating hormone
Ovarian tumors	Surgical excision
Poor quality midcycle cervical mucus	Conjugated estrogens (Premarin) therapy
Inadequate endometrial development	Progesterone therapy
Endometriosis	Danazol therapy Gamete intrafallopian transfer
Reproductive tract infections	Antimicrobial therapy
Tubal construction	Hysterosalpingogram Surgical excision
Sperm-inhospitable cervical mucus	Therapeutic intrauterine insemination In vitro fertilization
Immunologic reaction to sperm	Use of condoms to reduce antibody titer, followed by unprotected intercourse at time of ovulation only In vitro fertilization

PHARMACOLOGY CAPSULE

Ovulatory stimulants can cause ovarian hyperstimulation with possible rupture of the enlarged ovary.

Nursing Care of the Patient with an Infertility Disorder

When working with a patient who is being treated for infertility, the nurse must be skilled in history data collection, infertility-related support procedures, patient education, patient advocacy, and providing both physical and emotional support.

ASSESSMENT. Assessment of the female reproductive system is summarized in Table 43–1. Dealing with infertility requires skillful and compassionate assessment skills.

NURSING DIAGNOSIS. Nursing diagnoses for the infertile patient may include the following:

- **Situational Low Self-Esteem** related to inability to conceive or feeling of failure
- **Altered Sexuality Patterns** related to structured efforts to conceive or loss of spontaneity
- **Ineffective Individual Coping** related to unmet expectations or feelings of loss
- **Knowledge Deficit** of diagnostic and treatment procedures

GOALS. Goals of nursing care for the infertile patient are improved self-esteem, acknowledgment of the effects of the situation on one's sexual relationship, effective coping, and patient's knowledge of diagnostic and treatment procedures.

INTERVENTIONS. Fertility tests and treatments are generally done on an outpatient basis. For the woman who undergoes the process, her relationship with the nurse in the outpatient setting usually is prolonged, and contacts are frequent.

Situational Low Self-Esteem. Invasion of personal privacy is by necessity greater in fertility diagnosis and treatment than in any other condition. The nurse gently explores the feelings of the patient and her partner about their difficulty conceiving. An open, empathetic attitude is vital if the patient is to be open. Support groups or professional counselors may help the couple to maintain self-esteem.

Altered Sexuality Patterns. The most intimate details of her sexual relationship with her partner are elicited, and diagnostic and treatment procedures repeatedly violate the desire for modesty. Lovemaking becomes scheduled rather than spontaneous.

Ineffective Individual Coping. The nurse may be the only person with whom the woman shares her psychological reactions to the diagnosis of infertility and her subsequent emotional highs and lows throughout diagnosis and treatment. The nurse therefore plays a critical role in assisting the patient to cope with infertility. The patient is given the opportunity to discuss her thoughts and feelings about infertility, and to explore coping strategies.

Knowledge Deficit. The needs of her sexual partner must be considered as well, and he should be included in patient teaching. Patient teaching includes information about diagnostic procedures, treatments, causes of infertility, and resources.

EVALUATION. Criteria for evaluating the outcomes of nursing care are positive expressions about self, discussion of ways to maintain a satisfying sexual relationship, identification of healthy coping strategies, and patient's verbalization of diagnostic and treatment procedures.

MENOPAUSE

Menopause is the cessation of menstruation that marks the end of a woman's reproductive capacity. Natural menopause is part of normal aging, but surgical menopause results from removal of the ovaries. Natural menopause occurs gradually and may permit better adaptation than surgical menopause, which suddenly eliminates the source of natural estrogen. Diminished ovarian function associated with aging causes ovulation to cease and estrogen production to decline. The onset of menopause may begin as early as age 35 but is more common between ages 40 and 55. With natural menopause, the woman's first sign may be menstrual irregularity. Menstrual periods tend to be spaced farther apart and the amount of bleeding gradually diminishes. The entire process from earliest signs to complete cessation of menstruation usually is 2 years or less. A woman is said to be menopausal when she has not had a menstrual period for 1 year. Some women experience a surgical menopause brought on by the surgical removal of the ovaries. Unless estrogen replacement is begun promptly, the patient develops the signs and symptoms of menopause more rapidly.

Signs and Symptoms

The signs and symptoms of menopause may include hot flashes—a warm feeling caused by vasodilation that affects the face, neck, and upper body. Hot flashes are typically accompanied by perspiration and sometimes a feeling of faintness. Other common symptoms are vaginal dryness, insomnia, joint pain, headache, and nausea. Without estrogen, the uterus becomes smaller, the vagina shortens, and vaginal tissues become drier. Breast tissue may lose its firmness, and pubic and axillary hair become sparse. Supporting pelvic structures relax, causing some women to have stress incontinence. There may be significant loss of bone mass leading to fragile bones, a condition called osteoporosis. Some women report emotional instability, irritability, and depression, but the impact of menopause on a woman is very individualized. Some grieve for the loss of reproductive capacity, and some feel a loss of femininity and sexual attractiveness. Others welcome the end of menstrual periods and no longer having to worry about the risk of pregnancy.

Medical Treatment

Unless contraindicated, menopausal symptoms can usually be treated with hormone replacement. A typical treatment for the patient who still has her uterus and ovaries is the prescription of cyclic estrogen and progesterone. A conjugated estrogen is taken for 25 days, followed by a form of progesterone for 10 days. The addition of progesterone decreases the risk of endometrial cancer related to estrogen therapy. Oral drug therapy is most commonly used, but a transdermal form of the drug is also available and is preferred by some. The transdermal drug is delivered by an adhesive bandage–like patch. Estrogen creams and suppositories may be used to relieve vaginal dryness. Estrogen replacement is contraindicated with a history of certain types of cancer, undiagnosed uterine bleeding, or thromboembolism. Some physicians advise postmenopausal women to take calcium supplements to reduce the risk of osteoporosis.

NUTRITION CONCEPTS

- Long-term dieting is associated with amenorrhea and reduced fertility.
- Factors that may interfere with optimal nutrition for women of childbearing age include lack of resources, lack of nutrition knowledge, self-imposed dietary restrictions, and genetic idiosyncrasies.
- High dietary fat intake has been linked to breast cancer.

Nursing Care of the Menopausal Patient

ASSESSMENT. Assessment of the woman with a disorder of the reproductive system is summarized in Table 43–1. When a woman has menopausal symptoms, the nurse documents them and explores how the patient is coping with this significant life change.

NURSING DIAGNOSIS. The primary nursing diagnosis for the menopausal patient is usually knowledge deficit of the effects of menopause and management of signs and symptoms.

GOAL. The goal of nursing care is patient's understanding of menopause and its management.

INTERVENTIONS. The nurse assesses the patient's understanding of menopause and how she feels about it. The patient may need reassurance that her symptoms and responses are normal and common. If drug therapy is used, the nurse instructs the patient regarding self-medication. Patients on estrogen must be cautioned to report any signs of circulatory disorders (numbness, pain in calf, shortness of breath) to the physician immediately. Additional information about drug therapy is summarized in Table 43–3. The patient who cannot or chooses not to take hormone therapy needs additional assistance to cope with the symptoms of menopause. Women who wish to prevent "menopausal" pregnancy should utilize a reliable form of contraception for at least 1 year following cessation of menses.

EVALUATION. Successful nursing intervention is marked by the patient's accurate description of her prescribed drug therapy and symptoms that should be reported to the physician.

BIBLIOGRAPHY

Bernhard, L. (1990). Gynecological conditions and sexuality. In C. I. Fogel & D. Lauver (Eds.), *Sexual health promotion* (pp. 436–458). Philadelphia: W. B. Saunders.

Bernstein, J., Brill, M., Levin, S., & Seibel, M. (1992). Coping with infertility. *NAACOG's Clinical Issues in Perinatology and Women's Health, 3*(2), 335–342.

Bishop, K. R., Dougherty, M., Mooney, R., Gimotty, P., & Williams, B. (1992). Effects of age, parity, and adherence on pelvic muscle response to exercise. *Journal of Obstetric, Gynecologic, and Neonatal Nursing, 21*(5), 401–406.

Bobak, I. M., & Jensen, M. D. (1993). *Maternity and gynecologic care: The nurse and the family* (5th ed.). St. Louis: C. V. Mosby.

Bolander, V. R. (1994). *Sorensen and Luckmann's basic nursing: A psychophysiologic approach* (3rd ed.). Philadelphia: W. B. Saunders.

Cohn, S. D. (1991). Delay in diagnosis of breast cancer: A professional liability risk. *Journal of Nurse Midwifery, 36*(1), 74–79.

Cook, M. J. (1993). Perimenopause: An opportunity for health promotion. *Journal of Obstetric, Gynecologic, and Neonatal Nursing, 22*(3), 223–228.

Corney, R. C., Everett, H., Howells, A., & Crowther, M. (1992). The care of patients undergoing surgery for gynaecological cancer: The need for information, emotional support and counselling. *Journal of Advanced Nursing, 17*(6), 667–671.

Davis, D. C., & Dearman, C. N. (1991). Coping strategies of infertile women. *Journal of Obstetric, Gynecologic, and Neonatal Nursing, 20*(3), 221–228.

Derwinski-Robinson, B. (1990). Infertility and sexuality. In C. I. Fogel & D. Lauver (Eds.), *Sexual health promotion* (pp. 291–304). Philadelphia: W. B. Saunders.

Doenges, M. E., & Moorhouse, M. F. (1992). *Application of nursing process and nursing diagnosis: An interactive text.* Philadelphia: F. A. Davis.

Doenges, M. E., & Moorhouse, M. F. (1993). *Nurse's pocket guide: Nursing diagnoses with interventions* (4th ed.). Philadelphia: F. A. Davis.

Doenges, M. E., Moorhouse, M. F., & Geissler, A. C. (1993). *Nursing care plans: Guidelines for planning and documenting patient care* (3rd ed.). Philadelphia: F. A. Davis.

Dondero, T., & Lichtman, R. (1990). The breasts. In R. Lichtman & S. Papera (Eds.), *Gynecology: Well-woman care* (pp. 141–171). East Norwalk, CT: Appleton & Lange.

Dulaney, P. E., Crawford, V. C., & Turner, G. (1990). A comprehensive education and support program for women experiencing hysterectomies. *Journal of Obstetric, Gynecologic, and Neonatal Nursing, 19*(4), 319–325.

Dunn, M. E. (1990). Sexual health. In R. Lichtman & S. Papera (Eds.), *Gynecology: Well-woman care* (pp. 427–434). East Norwalk, CT: Appleton & Lange.

Earnest, V. V. (1993). *Clinical skills in nursing practice* (2nd ed.). Philadelphia: J. B. Lippincott.

Edge, V., & Miller, M. (1994). *Women's health care.* St. Louis: C. V. Mosby.

Frank, D. I. (1990). Factors related to decisions about infertility treatment. *Journal of Obstetric, Gynecologic, and Neonatal Nursing, 19*(2), 162–167.

Goode, C. J., & Hahn, S. J. (1993). Oocyte donation and in vitro fertilization: The nurse's role with ethical and legal issues. *Journal of Obstetric, Gynecologic, and Neonatal Nursing, 22*(2), 106–111.

Gossage, J. (1990). Early-stage breast cancer: How nurses help. *American Journal of Nursing, 90*(11), 31.

Hahn, S. J., Butkowski, C. R., & Capper, L. L. (1994). Ovarian hyperstimulation syndrome: Protocols for nursing care. *Journal of Obstetric, Gynecologic, and Neonatal Nursing, 23*(3), 217–226.

Haller, K. B. (1991). One out of every nine women . . . *Journal of Obstetric, Gynecologic, and Neonatal Nursing, 20*(6), 438.

Harper, D. C. (1990). Perimenopause and aging. In R. Lichtman & S. Papera (Eds.), *Gynecology: Well-woman care* (pp. 405–424). East Norwalk, CT: Appleton & Lange.

Henley, J. D., Kratzer, S. S., Seo, I. S., & Davis, T. (1993). Endometriosis of the small intestine presenting as a protein-losing enteropathy. *American Journal of Gastroenterology, 88*(1), 130–133.

Ignatavicius, D. D., & Bayne, M. V. (1991). *Medical-surgical nursing: A nursing process approach.* Philadelphia: W. B. Saunders.

Ingle, R. (1990). Cancer and sexuality. In C. I. Fogel & D. Lauver (Eds.), *Sexual health promotion* (pp. 313–324). Philadelphia: W. B. Saunders.

Jackson, V. (1990). The fallopian tubes. In R. Lichtman & S. Papera (Eds.), *Gynecology: Well-woman care* (pp. 273–281). East Norwalk, CT: Appleton & Lange.

Jackson, V. (1990). The uterus. In R. Lichtman & S. Papera (Eds.), *Gynecology: Well-woman care* (pp. 261–272). East Norwalk, CT: Appleton & Lange.

James, C. A. (1992). The nursing role in assisted reproductive technologies. *NAACOG's Clinical Issues in Perinatology and Women's Health, 3*(2), 328–334.

Jarvis, C. (1992). *Physical examination and health assessment.* Philadelphia: W. B. Saunders.

Jossens, M. O. R., & Sweet, R. L. (1993). Pelvic inflammatory disease: Risk factors and microbial etiologies. *Journal of Obstetric, Gynecologic, and Neonatal Nursing, 22*(2), 169–178.

Kaufman, R. H., & Hammill, H. A. (1992). Vaginitis. *NAACOG's Clinical Issues in Perinatology and Women's Health, 3*(2), 115–125.

Keating, C. E. (1992). The role of the expanded function nurse in fertility preservation. *NAACOG's Clinical Issues in Perinatology and Women's Health, 3*(2), 293–300.

Knobf, M. T. (1990). Early-stage breast cancer: The options. *American Journal of Nursing, 90*(11), 28–30.

Lauver, D., & Rubin, M. (1991). Women's concerns about abnormal Papanicolaou test results. *Journal of Obstetric, Gynecologic, and Neonatal Nursing, 20*(2), 154–159.

Lichtman, R. (1990). The cervix. In R. Lichtman & S. Papera (Eds.), *Gynecology: Well-woman care* (pp. 249–259). East Norwalk, CT: Appleton & Lange.

Lichtman, R. (1990). The well-woman gynecologic interview. In R. Lichtman & S. Papera (Eds.), *Gynecology: Well-woman care* (pp. 19–28). East Norwalk, CT: Appleton & Lange.

Lichtman, R., & Duran, P. (1990). The vulva and vagina. In

R. Lichtman & S. Papera (Eds.), *Gynecology: Well-woman care* (pp. 173–201). East Norwalk, CT: Appleton & Lange.

Lindell, M. E., & Olsson, H. M. (1990). Personal hygiene in external genitalia of healthy and hospitalized elderly women. *Health Care for Women International, 11*(2), 151–158.

Lindow, K. B. (1991). Premenstrual syndrome: Family impact and nursing implications. *Journal of Obstetric, Gynecologic, and Neonatal Nursing, 20*(2), 135–138.

Lyke, E. M. (1992). *Assessing for nursing diagnosis: A human needs approach.* Philadelphia: J. B. Lippincott.

Mason, E. (1991). Medical causes of abnormal vaginal bleeding. *NAACOG's Clinical Issues in Perinatal and Women's Health Nursing, 2*(3), 322–327.

McCance, K. L., & Huether, S. E. (1994). *Pathophysiology: The biologic basis for disease in adults and children* (2nd ed.). St. Louis: C. V. Mosby.

Mitchell, E. S. (1991). The elusive premenstrual syndrome. *NAACOG's Clinical Issues in Perinatal and Women's Health Nursing, 2*(3), 294–303.

Murata, J. M. (1990). Abnormal genital bleeding and secondary amenorrhea: Common gynecological problems. *Journal of Obstetric, Gynecologic, and Neonatal Nursing, 19*(1), 26–36.

Murphy, P. A. (1990). Laboratory testing. In R. Lichtman & S. Papera (Eds.), *Gynecology: Well-woman care* (pp. 41–54). East Norwalk, CT: Appleton & Lange.

Nettles-Carlson, B. (1989). Early detection of breast cancer. *Journal of Obstetric, Gynecologic, and Neonatal Nursing, 18*(5), 373–381.

Norwood, S. L. (1990). Fibrocystic breast disease: An update and review. *Journal of Obstetric, Gynecologic, and Neonatal Nursing, 19*(2), 116–121.

Pace-Owens, S. (1989). Gamete intrafallopian transfer (GIFT). *Journal of Obstetric, Gynecologic, and Neonatal Nursing, 18*(2), 93–97.

Papera, S. (1990). The physical and pelvic examinations. In R. Lichtman & S. Papera (Eds.), *Gynecology: Well-woman care* (pp. 29–39). East Norwalk, CT: Appleton & Lange.

Porth, C. M. (1994). *Pathophysiology: Concepts of altered health states* (4th ed.). Philadelphia: J. B. Lippincott.

Potter, S. G. (1990). Infertility. In R. Lichtman & S. Papera (Eds.), *Gynecology: Well-woman care* (pp. 441–450). East Norwalk, CT: Appleton & Lange.

Sackett, C. (1990). Genitourinary conditions and sexuality. In C. I. Fogel & D. Lauver (Eds.), *Sexual health promotion* (pp. 407–435). Philadelphia: W. B. Saunders.

Sampselle, C. M. (1990). Changes in pelvic muscle strength and stress urinary incontinence associated with childbirth. *Journal of Obstetric, Gynecologic, and Neonatal Nursing, 19*(5), 371–377.

Shulman, J. F. (1990). Bleeding disorders. In R. Lichtman & S. Papera (Eds.), *Gynecology: Well-woman care* (pp. 355–365). East Norwalk, CT: Appleton & Lange.

Sneed, N. V., Edlund, B., & Dias, J. K. (1992). Adjustment of gynecological and breast cancer patients to the cancer diagnosis: Comparisons with males and females having other cancer sites. *Health Care for Women International, 13*(1), 11–22.

Stern, C. (1990). Body image concerns, surgical conditions, and sexuality. In C. I. Fogel & D. Lauver (Eds.), *Sexual health promotion* (pp. 498–516). Philadelphia: W. B. Saunders.

Sullivan, N. (1990). Dysmenorrhea. In R. Lichtman & S. Papera (Eds.), *Gynecology: Well-woman care* (pp. 345–353). East Norwalk, CT: Appleton & Lange.

Swehla, M. (1990). Identifying and validating nursing diagnoses in a gynecologic ambulatory-care setting. *Journal of Obstetric, Gynecologic, and Neonatal Nursing, 19*(5), 439–447.

Toback, B. M. (1992). Recent advances in female infertility care. *NAACOG's Clinical Issues in Perinatal and Women's Health Nursing, 3*(2), 313–319.

Ulrich, S. P., Canale, S. W., & Wendell, S. A. (1994). *Medical-surgical nursing care planning guides* (3rd ed.). Philadelphia: W. B. Saunders.

Walker, M., & Wond, D. L. (1991). A battle plan for patients in pain. *American Journal of Nursing, 91*(6), 32–36.

Williamson, M. L. (1992). Sexual adjustment after hysterectomy. *Journal of Obstetric, Gynecologic, and Neonatal Nursing, 21*(1), 42–47.

KEY CONCEPTS

1. The female reproductive system includes external and internal genitalia and the breasts.
2. Common therapeutic measures for the female reproductive system include douche, cauterization, heat application, and topical medications.
3. Two common uterine bleeding disorders are metrorrhagia (bleeding or spotting between menstrual periods) and menorrhagia (menstrual periods characterized by profuse bleeding).
4. The primary nursing diagnoses for the patient with a uterine bleeding disorder are knowledge deficit of condition and treatment and anxiety related to unknown cause of bleeding.
5. Effects of reproductive tract infections may include infertility, changes in relationships, feelings of distrust toward sexual partners, shame, embarrassment, and diminished self-esteem.
6. Because most infections are treated on an outpatient basis, the nurse's primary role is patient education for prevention and treatment.
7. Benign growths of the female reproductive system include cysts of the breasts and ovaries and endometriosis.
8. The primary nursing diagnoses for the patient with endometriosis, a disorder marked by the growth of endometrial tissue outside the uterus, are pain and knowledge deficit.
9. Cysts are sac-like structures that contain fluid, semisolid, or solid material, and are usually benign.
10. Fibroid tumors (myomas, leiomyomas) are benign but may have to be removed because they can compress abdominal structures and lead to infertility, crowding, and malpositioning of the

KEY CONCEPTS *(continued)*

fetus during pregnancy and degenerative changes related to interruption of blood supply.

11. Herniation of the bladder (called cystocele) or rectum (rectocele) into the vagina can disrupt urinary and bowel function and is often corrected surgically.
12. Nursing diagnoses after surgery for correction of a cystocele or rectocele may include altered urinary elimination, high risk for injury and pain.
13. Uterine prolapse, the descent of the uterus into the vagina, may be treated with corrective surgery or vaginal hysterectomy.
14. Abnormal uterine positions include retroversion (backward tilt), retroflexion (uterine body bends backward), anteversion (forward tilt), and anteflexion (uterine body bends forward); these conditions rarely require treatment.
15. Breast cancer is the most prevalent form of cancer in American women, with a 5-year survival rate of more than 90% when detected early.
16. After mastectomy, nursing diagnoses may include high risk for injury, impaired physical mobility, high risk for infection, body image disturbance, and altered sexuality patterns.
17. Cervical cancer can be detected early by regular pelvic examinations and Pap smears; prompt treatment is usually curative.
18. Ovarian cancer has the highest mortality rate of all female reproductive system cancers because it is asymptomatic in the early stages.
19. Nursing diagnoses for the patient with cancer of the reproductive system may include anxiety and fear, body image disturbance, altered sexuality patterns, ineffective family coping, and (if treated with radiotherapy) high risk for injury.
20. Infertility, the inability to produce viable offspring, can sometimes be treated medically or surgically.

Beverly F. Halter

CHAPTER 44

Male Reproductive Disorders

OBJECTIVES

1. Describe major structures and functions of the normal male reproductive system.
2. Identify data to be collected when assessing a patient with a disorder of the male reproductive system.
3. Discuss commonly used diagnostic tests and procedures and nursing implications of each.
4. Identify common therapeutic measures and nursing implications of each when patients are treated for disorders of the male reproductive system.
5. For selected disorders of the male reproductive system, explain the pathophysiology, signs and symptoms, complications, medical diagnosis, and medical treatment.
6. Apply the nursing process to design a care plan for a patient with a disorder of the male reproductive system.

GLOSSARY

EJACULATION Reflexive expulsion of semen from the male urethra

EMISSION Involuntary discharge of semen

EPIDIDYMITIS Inflammation of the epididymis

ERECTION Swelling and rigidity of the penis

HEMATOCELE Accumulation of blood in the tunica vaginalis, which is the membrane that lines the front and sides of the testis and the epididymis

HYDROCELE Accumulation of clear fluid in the scrotum along the spermatic cord

IMPOTENCE Inability to achieve and maintain an erection for sexual intercourse

INFERTILITY Inability to conceive and produce viable offspring

PROSTATECTOMY Removal of all or part of the prostate gland

PROSTATITIS Inflammation of the prostate gland

SMEGMA Sebaceous secretion found beneath the foreskin

Glossary continued

SPERMATOCELE A cystic mass on the epididymis that contains fluid and spermatozoa

STERILE Free of microorganisms; infertile

ANATOMY AND PHYSIOLOGY OF THE MALE REPRODUCTIVE SYSTEM

ANATOMY

The male reproductive system consists of the scrotum, testes, epididymis, vas deferens, seminal vesicles, prostate gland, ejaculatory duct, internal urethra, and penis (Fig. 44–1).

Scrotum

The scrotum is a thin sack on the outside of the body composed of involuntary muscle that encloses the testicles in separate compartments. The scrotum contracts into thick folds during fear, anger, arousal or cold, drawing the testes close to the body for protection and insulation. On warm days the scrotal muscles relax and hang free of the body. Sweat glands may be activated to cool the glands and maintain a testicular temperature that is below body temperature.

Testes

The two testes (testicles) are composed of numerous highly coiled seminiferous tubules, and their two main functions are the production of sperm and sexual hormones. They develop in the embryo about the seventh week of gestation and begin producing small amounts of testosterone. Secretion of this male hormone results in the development of other male reproductive organs and causes the testes to descend into the scrotum during the last 2 months of gestation. Around 10 to 13 years of age, during puberty, the increased production of testosterone results in the production of sperm and the development of body hair, muscle mass, and other secondary sex characteristics (Fig. 44–2).

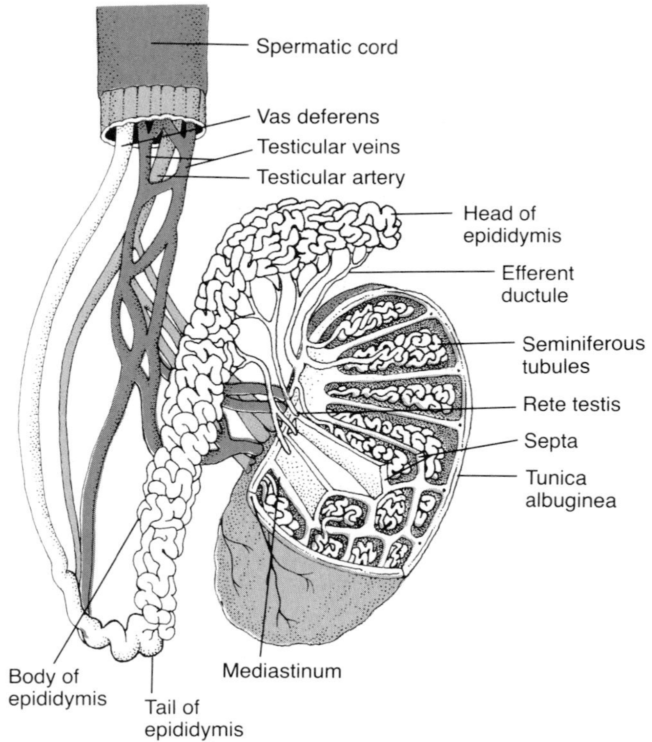

FIGURE 44–2

Basic structures of the scrotum. (From Ignatavicius, D. D., & Bayne, M. V. [1991]. *Medical-surgical nursing: A nursing process approach* [p. 1637]. Philadelphia: W. B. Saunders.)

Epididymis

New sperm move from the testicles through the epididymis, a coiled tubule almost 20 feet long that rests along the top and side of the testes. This passage may

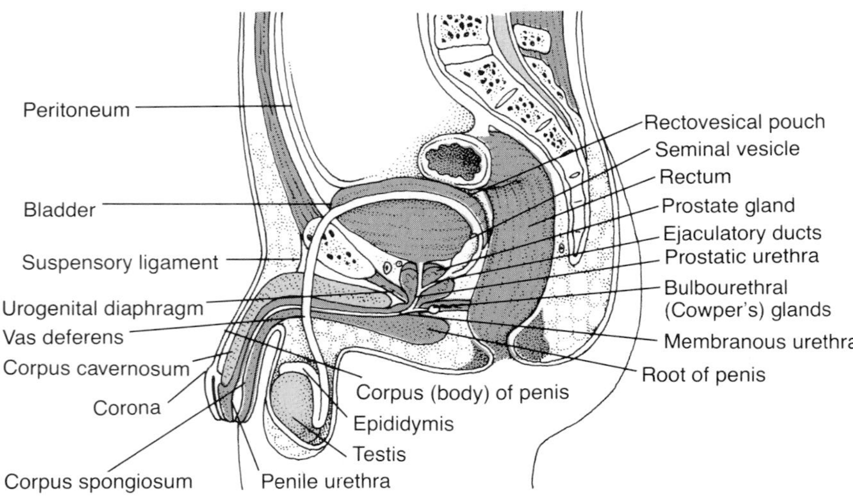

FIGURE 44–1

Male reproductive system. (From Ignatavicius, D. D., & Bayne, M. V. [1991]. *Medical-surgical nursing: A nursing process approach* [p. 1637]. Philadelphia: W. B. Saunders.)

take several days and allows the sperm to mature and develop the capability for motility and fertilization (see Fig. 44–2).

Vas Deferens

As mature sperm leave the epididymis, they enter the vas deferens, tubes of secretory ducts that leave the scrotum, pass through the abdominal wall into the pelvic cavity, and propel sperm into the urethra. The vas deferens serve as the primary storage sites for sperm and contribute to the fluid content of semen (see Fig. 44–2).

Seminal Vesicles

The seminal vesicles are secretory glands composed of twisted tubes located on the posterior surface of the bladder. They produce a mucoid fluid that constitutes about 60% of the volume of the semen and provides nutrients and hormones important for motility and successful fertilization (Fig. 44–3).

Prostate Gland

The prostate is a walnut-sized secretory gland that produces a thin, milky, alkaline liquid that enhances the motility and fertility of the sperm. It surrounds the neck of the urinary bladder and the first inch of the urethra (see Fig. 44–3). The prostate has no function other than a reproductive one.

Cowper's Glands

Cowper's glands (bulbourethral glands) are pea-sized structures that secrete a clear mucus into the urethra. The secretion contributes little to semen volume but provides lubrication during sexual arousal.

Urethra

The urethra extends from the bladder to the urinary meatus at the end of the penis. The vas deferens and the seminal vesicles come together to form the ejaculatory duct that passes through the prostate and empties into the internal urethra. The sperm and fluids from the vas deferens, seminal vesicles, and prostate are propelled through the ejaculatory duct into the penile urethra during ejaculation. Although the urethra serves to empty urine from the bladder and provide outflow for semen during ejaculation, urine and semen are never in the urethra at the same time.

Penis

The external penis in its flaccid state is a round soft cylinder of spongy tissue ending in an acorn-shaped tip known as the glans. The glans has a sensitive ridge at its base called the corona that gives rise to a hood or foreskin in uncircumcised men that can be rolled back to expose the glans. About one half of the penis extends within the body toward the anus and attaches to the pelvis. Two corpora cavernosa lie on the upper side of the penis. These erectile chambers provide a huge surface area for the inflow of blood and blood storage, which results in expansion of the penis during sexual arousal, called an erection. The corpus spongiosum on the underside of the penis surrounds the urethra and supplies blood to the glans (Fig. 44–4).

PHYSIOLOGY

Spermatogenesis

Sperm are produced in the seminiferous tubules of the testes from about age 13 throughout the remainder of life. Testosterone is believed to set in motion the

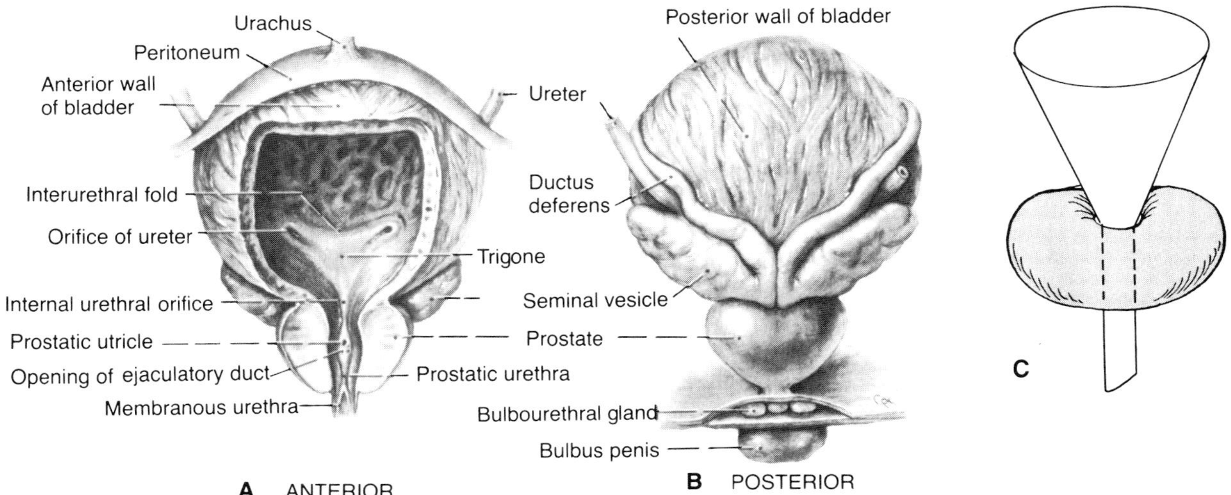

FIGURE 44-3

A and *B*, Anterior and posterior views of the prostate gland. *C*, Diagrammatic representation of the anatomic position of the prostate gland. It surrounds the urethra at the base of the bladder. (*A* and *B* from Jacob, S. W., & Francone, C. A. [1989]. *Elements of anatomy and physiology* [2nd ed.]. Philadelphia: W. B. Saunders; *C* from Black, J. M., & Matassarin-Jacobs, E. [1993]. *Luckmann and Sorensen's medical-surgical nursing: A psychophysiologic approach* [4th ed., p. 2082]. Philadelphia: W. B. Saunders.)

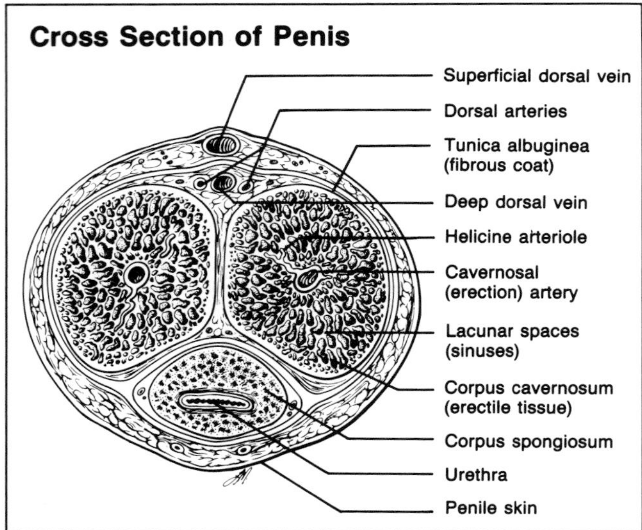

FIGURE 44-4

Cross section of the penis. (Reprinted by permission of the Putnam Publishing Group from Goldstein, I., & Rothstein, L. [1990]. *The potent male* [p. 12]. Los Angeles: The Body Press. Copyright © 1990 by Price Stern Sloan, Inc., and Irwin Goldstein and Larry Rothstein.)

division of germinal cells into spermatocytes that develop into sperm, a process that may take 75 days.

The cooling function of the scrotum is essential for spermatogenesis. An increase in testicular temperature may cause degeneration of some of the cells of the seminiferous tubules; it may also contribute to sterility.

Cryptorchidism, or failure of the testicles to descend from the abdomen into the cooler scrotum, may result in sterility. Incomplete or partial descent of the testicles may be resolved by surgical assistance before maturity, but if fetal testes are abnormally formed and do not secrete enough testosterone to cause the testicles to descend into the scrotum, surgical intervention is unlikely to be successful. The tubular epithelium of testes that remain in the warm abdomen degenerates completely and is incapable of producing sperm.

Erection

For the penis to become erect, it must have a high-pressure supply of arterial blood, relaxation of the smooth muscle tissue of cavernosal arterioles, and a functioning blood storage mechanism to keep the blood in the penis long enough for sexual function. The blood pressure in the flaccid corpus cavernosa is about 6 to 8 mm Hg, very low when compared with the 120/90 blood pressure in the arm or cavernosal artery.

During sexual arousal parasympathetic nerves release neurotransmitters that cause the relaxation of the cavernosal arteriole walls. This allows the relatively high pressure arterial blood to flood the sinuses of the erectile chambers, increasing the blood volume of the penis to eight to 10 times the flaccid volume and raising the cavernosal blood pressure to approximately the same as that in the arteries.

The blood storage mechanism for the penis is unique. The cavernosal artery is buried deep in the erectile chambers, causing them to fill from the inside. The venules that drain blood from the erectile chambers are near the surface and are compressed against the outer coat of the chambers during engorgement. The elastic limitations of this covering severely decrease the drainage of blood from the chamber sinuses and maintain the erection. After stimulation ceases or ejaculation occurs, sympathetic nerves release constricting neurotransmitters that narrow the arteriole walls and decrease the inflow of blood. As the cavernosal pressure decreases, drainage increases and the penis returns to a flaccid state.

Emission and Ejaculation

The male sex act culminates in emission and ejaculation. Emission is the result of sympathetic stimulation leaving the spinal cord at L1 and L2. The pudendal nerve communicates with the spinal cord at S2 and S3 and affects motor responses for ejaculation. Physical stimulation of internal and external sex organs initiates contractions of the vas deferens that expel sperm into the internal urethra. There they mix with prostatic and seminal fluids and are propelled forward through the penile urethra. The filling of the urethra excites nerves in the sacral region of the spinal cord to initiate rhythmic muscular contractions of the internal genital organs, pelvis, and body trunk and results in ejaculation of semen.

Although psychic stimulation is not essential to the male sex act, it is an enhancing factor and should be considered in the physiology. Experience, culture, and self-development influence the impact of visual, fantasy, and dream stimulation on sexual sensation and nocturnal erections and emissions.

AGE-RELATED CHANGES IN THE MALE REPRODUCTIVE SYSTEM

Normal aging produces several changes in the male reproductive system. Testosterone production continues throughout life after puberty but decreases rapidly after the age of 50, as demonstrated in Figure 44–5. This phenomenon has been called the male climacteric and may be associated with symptoms of hot flashes, suffocation, and psychic disorders similar to those of menopause. These symptoms may be relieved by the administration of testosterone and other androgens.

Many men believe they are too old for sex, and when this belief is supported by functional decline, they may lose interest or become depressed. Men in their late forties and early fifties may be slower to arouse and have a longer refractory period between erections, but in a healthy male spermatogenesis and the ability to have erections lasts a lifetime. Changes in lifestyle related to alcohol consumption, dietary habits, exercise, and the complexities of managing chronic conditions such as hypertension and diabetes and multiple medication therapies also contribute to loss of function and satisfactory sexual activities.

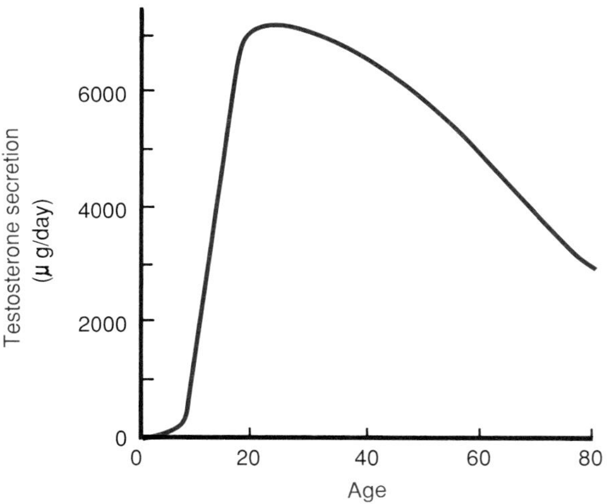

FIGURE 44-5
Testosterone secretion by age. (From Guyton, A. C. [1991]. *Textbook of medical physiology* [8th ed., p. 892]. Philadelphia: W. B. Saunders.)

NURSING ASSESSMENT OF THE MALE REPRODUCTIVE SYSTEM

Assessment of the male reproductive system should provide information about changes in health status, sexual function, and sexual relationships, as well as the patient's knowledge level and ability for self-care. This information may be obtained by interview, inspection, and palpation. The extent of the nursing assessment of the male reproductive system depends on the nurse's education, experience, and role in the setting. This section describes a complete nursing assessment, although some aspects may be performed only by an examiner with advanced training.

The interview and physical assessment may be particularly difficult for some male patients because of health beliefs, the need for privacy, or defensiveness about behaviors. It is important to allow the patient to tell his own story and maintain as much control over the environment and experience as possible. Establishing a comfortable relationship with the patient is most successful if open-ended questions are used, questions beginning with "why" are avoided, and sensitive questions are left until later in the interview. It is helpful to empathize with the patient and gently pin him down about details, but it is very important to avoid making comments that imply how he should or should not feel or behave, come to conclusions too early, or bias his story by adding professional opinion.

HEALTH HISTORY

Present Illness

The health history begins with a detailed description of the current problem. The nurse should be alert to descriptive terms and body language used by the patient during the interview. These methods of communicating may yield valuable information about the patient's health care attitudes, his ability to cope with disease, and the quality or intensity of specific symptoms. Complaints may include pain, weight loss, infertility, impotence, alteration in self-image, scrotal masses, penile discharge, or skin lesions. If the symptoms are acute, detailed information about the onset and development of the problem, activities related to the symptoms, and descriptors such as pain scales are important. If the problem is a chronic one, the nurse determines what made the patient seek help at this time and what his expectations for care are.

Past Medical History

The past medical history helps to link the current problem with previous symptoms, injuries, diseases, surgeries, or allergies and the treatments or medications prescribed for them. The nurse questions the patient about his management of chronic health problems such as diabetes, thyroid or pituitary dysfunction, cardiovascular disease, neurologic injury or disease, and addictive behavior. Trauma to the groin or perineum may have implications for diseases of the urethra or penile circulation, so the nurse inquires about childhood injuries or accidents. Spinal cord injuries must also be described because the level of the injury dictates specific types of sexual dysfunctions.

Patients who are reluctant to discuss what may be considered by many to be the most private part of their lives and selves may also be hesitant to do regular self-examinations or comply with recommended self-care regimens. Thoughtfully planned questioning provides clues about knowledge deficits and patient participation in health management. This information is important in developing plans for care that include the patient and his family or significant other and require their cooperation.

Family History

Exploration of the family history should include information about the age and health or age at death of parents, grandparents, and siblings. In addition, a family history is taken to document occurrence of cancer, diabetes, hypertension, stroke, and blood disorders such as sickle cell anemia and hemophilia.

Review of Systems

Review of all systems with a focus on male reproductive system disorders should begin with an assessment of general health state. Questions about changes in appetite, weight, exercise or activity level, and management of daily self-care should reveal general changes in health status that are affected by the reproductive system.

The nurse asks the patient about changes in the skin that include lesions, drainage, bleeding, itching, or pain. If the patient has itching or pain, the nurse should inquire whether it is intermittent or continuous, whether it has any relationship to specific activities or time, descriptors such as stinging or aching, and degree of intensity on a scale of one to 10.

Review of the circulatory and pulmonary systems provides information about edema and dyspnea. The relationship of these symptoms or problems to work and normal activity should be established.

Symptoms of possible endocrine dysfunction are important because undiagnosed or poorly managed endocrine disorders may have a direct and devastating impact on sexual function, sterility, and self-image for the male patient. The nurse should ask questions about fatigue, nervousness, the ability to tolerate heat or cold, polyphagia, polydipsia, polyuria, heat or cold intolerance, and medications taken for pituitary or thyroid conditions.

PHARMACOLOGY CAPSULE

The health history should document medications the patient is taking because many drugs, including a number of antihypertensives, can impair sexual function.

Review of the musculoskeletal and nervous systems should include questions about weakness, paralysis, coordination problems, joint pain or stiffness, mood changes, and depression.

Functional Assessment

The functional assessment includes information about diet, usual activities, sleep and rest, medications, and use of tobacco, alcohol, and illicit drugs. Sources of stress and coping strategies are documented. The nurse who has been able to establish a therapeutic relationship with the patient should also cover the interest level and satisfaction of sexual relationships. Questions may include the frequency of intercourse, the ability to have and maintain an erection, the desire and ability to have children, and the relationship of sexual function to self-image.

PHYSICAL EXAMINATION

Physical examination of the male reproductive system can be accomplished by inspection and palpation. Sharing normal findings, maintaining eye contact, involving the patient in the examination, and using an unhurried manner increase the comfort level of the patient. The bladder should be emptied before the examination and urine collected if a specimen is needed. Gloves are worn to examine the genitalia.

The nurse measures the patient's height, weight, and vital signs and observes his general appearance. The skin is inspected for lesions or discolorations and the breasts for gynecomastia (enlargement). For the examination of the genitalia, the patient may be supine with the legs slightly spread or standing. Pubic hair distribution is observed. It should be diamond-shaped across the symphysis pubis, cover the base of the penis, and spread along the inner thighs. The lower abdomen and groin are palpated for masses. The skin of the external organs and perineum should be warm, dry, and free of lesions, edema, and odor.

Penis

The normal flaccid penis is semisoft and straight. The size, shape, and appearance are documented. It is palpated for nodules, swelling, and lesions. If the patient is uncircumcised, the foreskin is retracted to observe the glans (Fig. 44–6). Normally there is a small amount of white, thick, odoriferous smegma between the glans and the foreskin. The urethral meatus should be at the tip of the penis. Gently squeezing the glans opens the meatus so it can be observed for signs of irritation, infection, or discharge. If there is any discharge from lesions or the urethra, a specimen should be collected for culture.

Scrotum

The skin of the scrotum should be slightly darker in color, wrinkled, and loose. Because the scrotum is close to the body and may not be well ventilated, it is important to look for irritation from heat and moisture, fungal infections, abscesses, and parasites.

The right and left sides of the scrotum are palpated for the testes, epididymis, and vas deferens. It is normal for the testes to retract temporarily when the scrotum is touched or cooled; they will reappear with relaxation. The left testicle hangs lower than the right, and both should be oval in shape, smooth, and firm and without

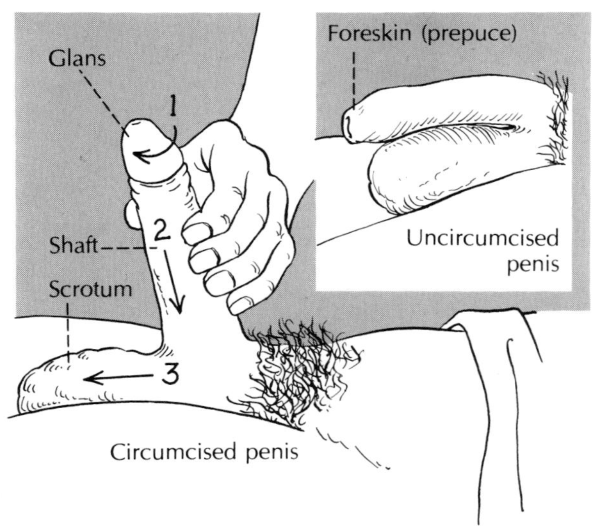

FIGURE 44-6
Circumcised and uncircumcised penis. (Adapted from Black, J. M., & Matassarin-Jacobs, E. [1993]. *Luckmann and Sorensen's medical-surgical nursing: A psychophysiologic approach* [4th ed., p. 2113]. Philadelphia: W. B. Saunders.)

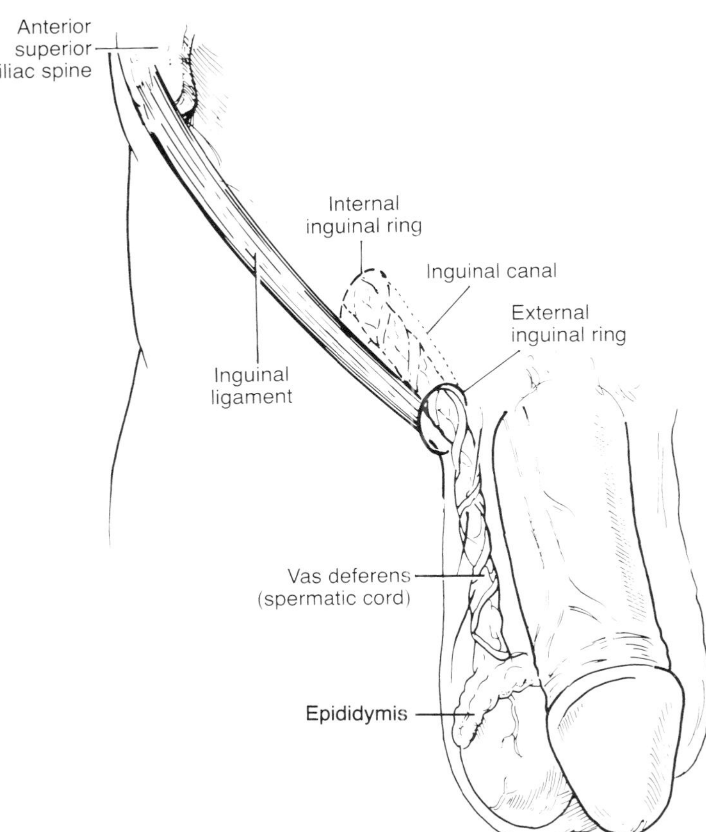

FIGURE 44–7

Location of epididymis and vas deferens. (From Black, J. M., & Matassarin-Jacobs, E. [1993]. *Luckmann and Sorensen's medical-surgical nursing: A psychophysiologic approach* [4th ed., p. 2079]. Philadelphia: W. B. Saunders.)

masses or tenderness. It is important, especially in the young patient, to note that there are two testes. Older patients may have smaller, softer testes. Lack of a testicle should be reported to the physician.

The epididymis lies on the superior end of each testicle and extends downward on the posterior surface. When palpated with the thumb and forefinger it should feel soft and tender but without swelling or hardening. The vas deferens begins at the lower pole of each testicle and extends upward toward the inguinal canal. It is a small cord-like structure that feels firmer than the epididymis (Fig. 44–7). It should show no thickening or asymmetry.

Discovery of thickening, nodules, masses, or asymmetric conditions can be further investigated by shining a light through the scrotum in a darkened room (Fig. 44–8). If the mass is filled with serous fluid, the light makes a red glow. If the mass is solid like a hematoma or tumor, no light passes through it, making it appear as a dark shadow.

Examination for protrusion of the bowel through the inguinal wall or canal (hernia) should be done while the patient is standing. The lower abdomen, groin, and upper scrotal area are inspected for bulges while the patient stands quietly and again when straining as if to have a bowel movement. The practitioner with advanced training is able to palpate inguinal hernias by reaching

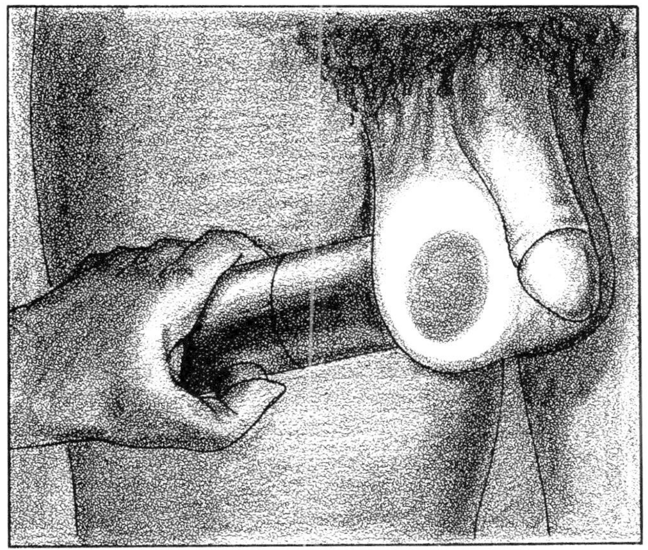

FIGURE 44–8

Transillumination of the scrotum. (From Black, J. M., & Matassarin-Jacobs, E. [1993]. *Luckmann and Sorensen's medical-surgical nursing: A psychophysiologic approach* [4th ed., p. 2080]. Philadelphia: W. B. Saunders.)

up through the scrotum into the inguinal canal. Abnormal findings should be noted and referred to a physician.

The advanced practitioner or physician also examines the prostate gland by inserting the examining finger through the anus toward the anterior wall of the rectum. The normal prostate lies 2 to 5 cm beyond the rectal sphincter and feels smooth, rubbery, and firm. Increased firmness and enlargement of the prostate gland may indicate benign hypertrophy, a tender boggy feeling may be the result of chronic prostatitis, and a hard prostate may be malignant. Should prostatic massage be necessary, the examiner should be prepared to collect meatal secretions for culture or microscopic examination.

The skin of the perineum is darker than the skin on the buttocks and should be intact. The anal area has more coarse skin and is moist and without hair. The area is inspected for lesions, irritation, inflammation, fissures, abscesses, and dilated veins (hemorrhoids). The patient is asked to bear down, and the anus is reinspected for rectal prolapse or internal hemorrhoids. The advanced practitioner or physician examines the anal canal with the index finger to assess for resistance, bleeding, sphincter tone, nodules, or polyps. A stool specimen may be tested for occult blood if it is necessary.

The assessment of the male reproductive system is summarized in Table 44–1.

TABLE 44–1
ASSESSMENT OF THE MALE REPRODUCTIVE SYSTEM

HEALTH HISTORY

Present Illness: Pain, weight loss, infertility, impotence, scrotal mass, penile discharge, lesions
Past Medical History: Previous injuries, diseases, or surgeries
- chronic illnesses: Diabetes mellitus, cardiovascular disease, addictive behavior
- Allergies
- Current medications

Family History: Diabetes, hypertension, stroke, blood disorders, cancer
Review of Systems:
General health state: Changes in appetite, weight, activity, self-care
- Skin: Lesions, drainage, bleeding, itching, pain
- Cardiovascular: Edema
- Respiratory: Cough, dyspnea
- Endocrine: Fatigue, heat or cold intolerance, nervousness

Nervous: Paralysis
Genitourinary: Changes in urination or urine characteristics
Sexual function: Interest in sexual relationship, frequency of intercourse, impotence, desire to have children, effect of sexual function on self-image
Functional Assessment
- Usual day: Occupation, home roles and responsibilities, diet, rest
- Use of tobacco and alcohol
- Stressors and coping strategies
- Sexual relationships

PHYSICAL EXAMINATION

Vital signs
General appearance of genitalia: Skin lesions or discoloration, hair distribution
Penis: Size, shape, skin lesions, discharge, position of urinary meatus, nodules, swelling
Scrotum: Color, edema, irritation, presence of testicles, testicular tenderness or masses
Inguinal hernia
Prostate: Size, texture, masses
Perineum: Color, lesions
Anus: Lesions, irritation, inflammation, fissures, abscesses, hemorrhoids, prolapse

DIAGNOSTIC TESTS AND PROCEDURES

Diagnostic tests and procedures for male reproductive system disorders include laboratory studies, radiologic studies, and imaging procedures.

Laboratory Studies

SEMEN ANALYSIS. Analysis of the semen may be done to assess male fertility or to document sterilization after a vasectomy. The analysis may include gross evaluation of semen for volume, thickness, color, and pH and microscopic evaluation of the sperm for count, motility, shape, and ability to penetrate cervical mucus. More sophisticated testing can also determine the presence of serum antibodies and genetic abnormalities.

The patient is instructed to abstain from sexual activity for 3 to 5 days and then collect a semen specimen in a clean container. Patients are discouraged from prolonged abstinence as it may result in diminished quality and motility of the sperm. If the patient is unable to collect the specimen in the physician's office or laboratory by masturbating, it may be collected at home by using a plastic condom or coitus interruptus. Rubber condoms should not be used because the powders and lubricants used in their manufacture may be spermicidal. The specimen should be kept at room temperature, protected from heat or cold, and brought to the lab within 1 hour after collection.

Sperm count varies from day to day and should be repeated for data to be reliable. Men with very high or very low counts are often infertile and should be evaluated for pituitary, thyroid, adrenal, or testicular dysfunctions.

ENDOCRINOLOGIC STUDIES. The endocrine system secretes hormones directly into the blood that regulate metabolism, growth, stress response, and reproduction (gonadotropins). Serum levels of these hormones can be obtained from blood drawn from the patient without special preparation.

Luteinizing hormone is secreted by the anterior pituitary gland and causes stimulation of special cells (Leydig's) in the testes to produce testosterone. As testosterone is produced, a negative feedback system reduces the amount of luteinizing hormone secreted by the pituitary. Below normal levels of testosterone result in abnormally high levels of serum luteinizing hormone. This indicates an effort by the pituitary to stimulate Leydig's cells and return testosterone levels to normal.

Prolactin, another hormone excreted by the anterior pituitary gland, is closely related to luteinizing hormone and is known to have a potentiating effect on testosterone production. In some patients, when endocrine function is in question, serum prolactin levels may be tested. Secretion of prolactin is controlled by a negative feedback system. Above normal levels of prolactin may be caused by a benign pituitary tumor and result in gynecomastia in the male patient.

Follicle-stimulating hormone is secreted by the anterior pituitary gland and causes stimulation of cells (Sertoli's) in the seminiferous tubules of the testes to complete the formation (spermiation) and maturation of sperm. Oversecretion of follicle-stimulating hormone is prevented and a constant level of sperm production is maintained by the negative feedback system. Below normal levels of sperm result in increased secretion of follicle-stimulating hormone from the pituitary gland and high serum levels of follicle-stimulating hormone. Spermatogenesis results in decreased excretion of follicle-stimulating hormone and normal serum levels.

Testosterone is secreted by Leydig's cells in the interstitium of the testes. Below normal levels of testosterone may be the result of hypothalamus or pituitary dysfunction or seminiferous tubule destruction. High levels of testosterone are produced in newborn male infants, males after puberty, and in the presence of testicular tumors that develop from Leydig's cells. Lower serum levels of testosterone may be expected as the male patient ages.

TUMOR MARKERS. Tumor markers are substances found in the serum of cancer patients. When used in conjunction with other diagnostic tools, they can be helpful in diagnosing cancer, estimating the degree of cancer development, predicting the effect of treatment, and monitoring the effect of treatment on the cancer or the return of cancer after treatment. There is no special preparation for these tests.

GENERAL LABORATORY STUDIES. Urinalysis provides information about infection of the genitourinary tract, presence or degree of control of diabetes, and kidney function. Samples should be clean catches unless the patient is unable to collect them without contamination. If appropriate instruction is given for collection, there is no need for other patient preparation. If the patient is unable to properly clean himself, cannot see well enough, or is not able to understand the instructions, it may be necessary to obtain a specimen by catheterization.

Blood studies may include a complete blood count to establish baseline data and provide information in forming a diagnosis when anemia or bone metastases are suspected. Alkaline phosphatase and serum calcium may also be ordered because they rise with metastasis to bone (Table 44–2). Acid phosphatase may also be ele-

TABLE 44-2
LABORATORY TESTS FOR MALE REPRODUCTIVE DISORDERS

TEST	REFERENCE VALUES	CONDITION IN WHICH LEVELS ARE ALTERED
Hematologic Tests (CBC)		
Hemoglobin	14–18 gm/dl	↓ In anemia, nonspecific, may indicate malignancy
Hematocrit	40–50%	↓ In anemia, nonspecific, may indicate malignancy
Leukocytes (WBC)	4800–11,000 mm^3	↓ In metastatic disease to bone
Neutrophils	54–62%	↓ In bone marrow depression
Lymphocytes	25–30%	↓ In bone marrow depression
Eosinophils	1–3%	↓ In bone marrow depression
Platelets	150,000–300,000 mm^3	↓ In bone marrow depression
Blood/Serum Tests		
Acid phosphatase	0.11–0.60 mU/ml	↑ In metastatic prostate cancer
Alkaline phosphatase	20–90 mU/ml	↑ In cancer of bone or bone metastasis, liver cancer
Calcium	9.0–11.0 mg/dl	↑ In bone metastasis
Tests for Tumor Markers		
AFP	<10 ng/ml	↑ In nonseminomatous testicular cancer
CEA	0–2.5 ng/ml nonsmokers <3.0 ng/ml smokers	↑ Prostate cancer
HCG	0–5 IU/L	↑ In germ cell testicular cancer
Prostatic acid phosphatase	0.26–0.83 U/L	↑ In metastatic prostate cancer
PSA	0–4 ng/ml	↑ In prostate cancer

CBC, Complete blood count; WBC, white blood cells; AFP, alpha-fetoprotein; CEA, carcinoembryonic antigen; HCG, human chorionic gonadotropin; PSA, prostatic-specific antigen.

Adapted from Black, J. M., & Matassarin-Jacobs, E. (1993). *Luckmann and Sorensen's medical-surgical nursing: A psychophysiologic approach* (4th ed., pp. 496–497). Philadelphia: W. B. Saunders.

vated with prostate cancer and with bone metastasis. Prostatic-specific antigen may also be elevated with cancer of the prostate. Thyroid function studies may be done in patients with erectile dysfunctions. Low thyroid hormone may result in loss of libido; high thyroid hormone may cause impotence. No special preparation for these tests is usually necessary. Blood glucose levels may be drawn when diabetes mellitus is a concern, and patients should be fasting for the test. The venipuncture site should be observed for bleeding and dressed with a small pressure bandage on completion of sample collection.

Radiologic Studies

Computed tomography may be used in assessing metastatic testicular and prostatic tumors. The patient lies on a movable table for 45 minutes. If contrast dye is used, it is important to ask the patient about allergies. The procedure is painless unless dye is given, which sometimes causes a burning sensation. Patients may also experience nausea, vomiting, flushing, itching, or a bitter taste. Some patients may require mild sedation if they have tendencies to be claustrophobic and become agitated during the test.

Imaging Procedures

Ultrasound may be used to examine scrotal masses or define prostatic lesions. Examination of the prostate is done via the rectum and should be explained to the patient. An enema may be ordered to eliminate gas and feces. In this procedure high-frequency sound waves are bounced off tissue and form an electronic picture that can differentiate tissue textures. The procedure is painless and requires only cooperation from the patient.

Radionucleotide imaging may be done to assess testicular abnormalities such as torsion, tumors, abscesses, epididymitis, or hydroceles. Radioactive substances are injected intravenously or given orally and are distributed throughout the body for use like any other element. Scans trace the substance to organs and tissues that have increased concentrations of the isotopes owing to abnormal tissue metabolism. It is important to ask the patient about allergies and reassure him that the dose of radiation is so small that no cell destruction will occur. There is a waiting period after the initial dose to allow for distribution of the radioisotope, then the patient is asked to lie still while the scanner measures and records data. Restless or agitated patients may require sedation.

A summary of diagnostic tests and procedures is presented in Table 44–3.

DISORDERS OF THE MALE REPRODUCTIVE SYSTEM

INFECTIONS AND INFLAMMATORY CONDITIONS

Infections of the male reproductive system may be caused by bacteria, viruses, protozoa, fungi, and ectoparasites that can be acquired through sexual contact. Sexually transmitted diseases are covered in Chapter 45. The most common inflammatory conditions are prostatitis and epididymitis. Orchitis is rare but important because it can cause sterility.

Prostatitis

Prostatitis is inflammation of the prostate gland. It may be caused by bacterial infection, but when no pathogens can be detected the condition is classified as nonbacterial prostatitis. Signs and symptoms of acute inflammation are prostate swelling, warmth, and tenderness. The patient may also have dysuria, frequency, hematuria, and foul-smelling urine. Patients with chronic inflammation may have minimal symptoms or just malaise.

Acute prostatitis is treated with antimicrobials, analgesics, and sitz baths. The patient is advised to increase fluid intake and to rest. Stool softeners may be prescribed to prevent constipation, which is especially painful with prostatitis. Catheterization is avoided as it may cause further infection, but it is needed if the patient cannot void. Chronic prostatitis is treated much like acute prostatitis. Sometimes long-term, low-dose antimicrobial therapy is used. The physician may massage the prostate to express congested prostatic fluid. Nonbacterial prostatitis is primarily treated symptomatically with analgesics, anti-inflammatory agents, and sitz baths. Short-term antimicrobial therapy may be prescribed.

Most patients with prostatitis are treated as outpatients, but hospital admission may be indicated if a high fever is present or if catheterization or parenteral antimicrobial therapy is needed. The nurse assesses the patient's comfort and administers analgesics and other treatments as ordered. If the patient is discharged with medications, instructions and information about the drugs are provided.

Epididymitis

Epididymitis, inflammation of the epididymis, may be caused by infections, trauma, or the reflux of urine from the urethra through the vas deferens. Signs and symptoms are painful scrotal edema, nausea, vomiting, chills, and fever. Epididymitis is treated with bedrest, ice packs, sitz baths, analgesics, antibiotics, anti-inflammatory drugs, and scrotal support. If the condition is associated with a sexually transmitted infection, the patient's sexual partner requires antibiotic therapy as well.

Nursing care involves assessment of temperature, edema, and comfort. Prescribed treatments are carried out and the effects documented. A bridge made of tape and gauze or a rolled towel can be placed across the patient's thighs while in bed to elevate the scrotum. This helps to reduce pain.

Orchitis

Orchitis is inflammation of one or both testes. It may be related to trauma or to infections such as mumps, pneumonia, or tuberculosis. Signs and symptoms of orchitis include fever, tenderness, and swelling of the af-

TABLE 44-3

THE MALE REPRODUCTIVE SYSTEM: DIAGNOSTIC TESTS AND PROCEDURES

TEST/STUDY	PURPOSE/PROCEDURE	PATIENT PREPARATION	POSTPROCEDURE NURSING CARE
Mumps test	Determines whether a person is susceptible or resistant to the mumps virus. An antigen is injected intradermally, marked with a waterproof pen, and examined after 48 hr to detect immune response.	Inform the patient that an injection will be given under the skin to determine if he has resistance to mumps. He must not wash off the marking, and must return in 48 hr to have the results "read."	To read the test, examine the site for redness and swelling after 48 hr. A red area larger than 10 mm in diameter is called "positive" and indicates susceptibility to mumps. A negative reaction indicates resistance.
Cystoscopy	A lighted instrument is inserted through the urethra to visualize the urethra, bladder, and prostatic urethra. May detect prostatic hypertrophy.	Routine preoperative measures are indicated (consent form, skin scrub, food restriction). Antibiotics may be prescribed. Inform the patient the procedure is done in a special room under sterile conditions. Local anesthetic is instilled in the urethra and an intravenous sedative is given.	Measure urine output for 24 hr. Urine will be pink tinged. Report excessive bleeding or inability to void promptly. Encourage fluids when voiding well. Burning and hesitancy are common for several days. Give antibiotics as ordered.
Smears and stains	A small amount of material is prepared on a slide for microscopic identification of pathogens. A urethral smear is done to detect sexually transmitted diseases. A sterile swab is inserted into the urethra. The urethra is gently scraped to obtain a specimen. The physician may massage the prostate to increase the organisms in the urethra. Specimens may also be obtained from the anal canal and pharynx.	Explain process of specimen collection to patient.	Body fluids and instruments exposed to them should be handled with universal precautions. If antimicrobials are ordered, collect the specimen for culture before beginning the antimicrobials. Prepare specimens and send to laboratory.
Cultures	Cultivation of organisms obtained from a source being tested. Permits identification of pathogens. Susceptibility to various antimicrobials can be determined.	Explain specimen collection process.	Prepare specimens according to laboratory protocol. Send to laboratory.
Serum acid phosphatase	Detects elevations associated with metastatic prostate cancer and many other conditions. Used to assess effects of treatment for prostate cancer.	Inform patient that a venous blood sample will be drawn.	Assess venipuncture site for hematoma.
Semen analysis	Examination of a semen specimen to assess male fertility or to document sterilization after vasectomy.	Instruct patient to abstain from sexual activity 3–5 days, then collect specimen in a clean container. Rubber condoms should not be used. Specimen should be kept at room temperature and brought to the lab within 1 hr after collection.	No special care needed.
Endocrinologic studies: luteinizing hormone, prolactin, follicle-stimulating hormone, testosterone	Assesses the level of hormones that play a role in sexual development, function, or both.	Tell patient that a venous blood sample will be drawn.	Assess venipuncture site for oozing or hematoma. Apply small dressing.

Table continued on following page

TABLE 44-3
THE MALE REPRODUCTIVE SYSTEM: DIAGNOSTIC TESTS AND PROCEDURES *Continued*

TEST/STUDY	PURPOSE/PROCEDURE	PATIENT PREPARATION	POSTPROCEDURE NURSING CARE
Tumor markers: serum prostatic-specific antigen	Detects increases that may be associated with prostatic cancer, prostatic hypertrophy, cirrhosis, osteoporosis, and a number of other conditions.	Patient should fast for 8 hr before the test. Tell patient a venous blood sample will be drawn.	Assess venipuncture site for oozing or hematoma. Apply small dressing.
Computed tomography	Creates images of internal structures. Used to assess testicular and prostatic tumors. Contrast dye may be injected intravenously.	Assess allergy to iodine. Tell patient he will lie on a movable table while a machine moves around him. There are no sensations unless dye is injected. Some patients react to dye with nausea, vomiting, flushing, itching, or bitter taste. Claustrophobic patients may need mild sedation.	No special postprocedure care is required. If dye is injected, the patient is encouraged to drink fluids to flush the dye from the body.
Ultrasonography	Uses sound waves to create images of internal structures. Used to study the prostate for enlargement or lesions.	Tell the patient the procedure is painless, but that an instrument is inserted into the rectum to study the prostate. Patient instructions usually include drinking 4 glasses of water 1 hr before the test. The patient should not void until the test is completed.	No special care is needed.
Radionucleotide imaging procedures	Uses radioactive substances injected intravenously or given orally followed by imaging to assess testicular abnormalities: torsion, tumors, abscesses, epididymitis, hydrocele.	Assess allergies and inform radiologist. Reassure patient that radiation dose is low and does not cause cell destruction. The patient receives the isotope, waits a specified period of time, and then is scanned.	Fluids are encouraged to promote elimination of the isotope.

fected testicle and scrotal redness. The inflammation can lead to reduced fertility or, as previously mentioned, to sterility. Orchitis is treated with analgesics, antipyretics, bedrest, scrotal support, and local heat to the scrotum. Nursing care includes pain management, assistance with activities of daily living, patient teaching, and anxiety reduction.

BENIGN PROSTATIC HYPERTROPHY

Benign prostatic hypertrophy (BPH) is enlargement of the prostate gland. It is a common age-related change. The exact cause is unknown, but researchers are trying to find links to hormonal alterations, diet, chronic inflammation, heredity, and racial factors.

Signs and Symptoms

Signs and symptoms of BPH include decreasing size and force of the urinary stream, inability to empty the bladder, frequency, hematuria, and urinary retention. Factors that may trigger retention are alcohol, infections, delayed voiding, bedrest, narcotics, antihistamines, and chilling.

Medical Diagnosis

Benign prostatic hypertrophy is diagnosed on the basis of results from the rectal examination, laboratory and radiographic studies, endoscopy, ultrasound, catheterization for residual urine, and sometimes urodynamic testing (see Chapter 36). A urine specimen and prostatic secretions are obtained and examined for evidence of infection.

Medical Treatment

Conservative measures can be taken to decrease urinary retention. Classifications of drugs that may be prescribed to treat BPH and related symptoms include testosterone-ablating agents, testosterone-sparing agents, and alpha-adrenergic blocking agents (Table 44–4).

Drugs that suppress prostatic tissue growth by decreasing testosterone levels are called testosterone-ablating agents. Examples are diethylstilbestrol and flutamide (Eulexin). Finasteride (Proscar) is a testosterone-sparing agent that reduces the size of the prostate without lowering circulating testosterone levels. Alpha-adrenergic agents like phenoxybenzamine hydrochloride (Dibenzyline) are used to relax smooth muscle in the bladder neck and prostate, thereby reducing obstruction to urinary flow.

Measures that stimulate release of prostatic fluid and reduce symptoms include sexual intercourse, hot sitz baths, and prostatic massage. If there is evidence of prostatitis, antimicrobials may be prescribed.

Surgical Treatment

Surgical intervention is usually advised if complete urinary obstruction develops, evidence of existing or impending renal damage exists, the patient has repeated urinary tract infections, or significant bleeding occurs.

TYPES OF PROSTATECTOMY. The most widely used surgical procedure is the transurethral prostatectomy (resection of the prostate), in which obstructing portions of the gland are cut away through a resectoscope inserted into the urethra. Resected tissue is then irrigated from the bladder. Sometimes a patient absorbs a significant amount of the irrigating fluid, placing him at risk for fluid volume excess. There is no external incision. A catheter is required for a day or two. Because the entire gland is not removed, the remaining tissue can continue to grow and obstruction may recur.

A suprapubic prostatectomy is performed through the bladder by way of a low abdominal incision. It may be selected when the prostate is very large or when there are also bladder abnormalities that require surgical correction. Convalescence is longer than with a transurethral prostatectomy, and some patients develop incontinence or impotence. A retropubic prostatectomy employs a low abdominal incision but, unlike a suprapubic prostatectomy, the surgeon does not enter the bladder but rather opens the front of the prostate. Although the risk is small, some men develop incontinence, impotence, or both. A perineal prostatectomy requires an incision between the scrotum and the anus to gain access to the prostate. Radical prostatectomy is discussed in the section on prostatic cancer. New procedures employ freezing, laser incision, and placement of stents to prevent obstruction of urine flow. Balloon dilation is controversial.

Postoperatively, the patient may have a urethral catheter, bladder irrigation, or a suprapubic catheter.

COMPLICATIONS. Depending on the type of prostatectomy, the patient is at risk for urinary infection and incontinence, impotence, hemorrhage, urinary leakage, and inflammation of the pubic bone. Retrograde ejaculation may occur, meaning that semen enters the bladder instead of being ejected through the penis. The semen is then voided later with urine. This is not harmful to the patient but does render him sterile.

Nursing Care of the Patient with Benign Prostatic Hypertrophy

ASSESSMENT. Assessment of the patient with BPH includes a complete description of urinary symptoms:

TABLE 44-4
DRUGS USED TO TREAT DISORDERS OF THE MALE REPRODUCTIVE SYSTEM

DRUG	USE/ACTION	SIDE EFFECTS	NURSING INTERVENTIONS
Testosterone Methyltestosterone (Metandren) Fluoxymesterone (Halotestin) Testosterone cypionate in oil (DEPO-Testosterone)	Treats hormone deficiency caused by developmental disorders, testicular diseases, or removal of testicles.	Retention of water, sodium, potassium, and chloride. Jaundice, gastrointestinal distress. Increased effects of anticoagulants and oral hypoglycemics.	Assess for hypertension and edema. Intramuscular injections should be given deeply into the gluteus muscle using the Z-track technique.
Estrogen Products Chlorotrianisene (Tace) Estrone (Theelin Aqueous) Ethinyl estradiol (Estinyl)	Treats prostate cancer.	Fluid retention. Nausea and vomiting. Temporary breast enlargement (gynecomastia) and impotence in males. Contraindicated with thrombophlebitis or clotting disorders.	Monitor blood pressure and weight. Rotate vials of injectable suspension to mix. Inject into large muscle mass.
Testosterone-Ablating Agents Diethylstilbestrol (DES) Flutamide (Eulexin)	Palliative therapy for inoperable cancer of the prostate.	Anorexia, nausea, gynecomastia, hypertension.	Monitor blood pressure and weight. DES: monitor blood glucose, and be alert for signs of thrombosis. Eulexin: protect from infection since resistance is lowered.

frequency, urgency, hesitancy, change in stream size or force, and nocturia. The presence of pain or hematuria is documented. The lower abdomen is palpated to detect bladder distention. If ordered, the patient may be catheterized after voiding to measure residual urine.

NURSING DIAGNOSIS. Nursing diagnoses may include:

- **Altered Urinary Elimination** related to obstruction
- **Fear** related to invasive diagnostic and therapeutic procedures
- **Knowledge Deficit** of condition, treatment, and self-care

GOALS. Goals for these diagnoses are absence of bladder distention, reduced fear, and patient's knowledge of condition, treatments, and self-care.

INTERVENTIONS

Altered Urine Elimination. The patient is instructed to void promptly when the urge is felt and to space fluid intake throughout the day rather than consuming large amounts of liquids at one time. Fluid restriction is *not* recommended as it increases the risk of urinary tract infection. The patient should avoid drinking alcohol and taking antihistamines commonly found in cold remedies.

PHARMACOLOGY CAPSULE

Common nonprescription drugs, including many cold remedies, may cause urinary retention in the patient with prostatic hypertrophy.

If the patient is unable to void and the bladder becomes distended, the physician should be notified. Catheterization is performed as ordered, but the nurse may have difficulty passing the catheter because of the enlarged prostate. If the catheter does not pass easily, it is never forced. The physician is informed, and the procedure is usually done by a urologist using special instruments.

Fear. The nurse explores the patient's fears and provides information about anticipated procedures and effects.

Knowledge Deficit. Patient teaching should include normal anatomy and physiology of the male reproductive system, effects of BPH, measures to prevent urinary retention, signs and symptoms of infection and obstruction, and self-medication if appropriate.

EVALUATION. Evidence of effective nursing interventions requires urine output approximately equal to fluid intake, absence of bladder distention on palpation; patient statement that fear is reduced, calm demeanor; and patient description of condition, treatment, and self-care measures and stated intent to follow prescribed regimen.

Nursing Care of the Prostatectomy Patient

Detailed care of the surgical patient is presented in Chapter 14. This section emphasizes the specific needs of the postoperative prostatectomy patient (see Care Plan: The Patient with a Prostatectomy).

ASSESSMENT. When the patient returns to the nursing unit, vital signs are taken and compared with preoperative measurements. Urinary catheters are checked for patency and positioned for proper drainage. Urine is inspected for color and amount. Irrigating fluids are hung and regulated to flow at the prescribed rate. Intravenous fluids are checked, and the rate of flow is regulated. The patient's comfort level is assessed.

NURSING DIAGNOSIS. Common nursing diagnoses after prostatectomy are the following:

- **High Risk for Fluid Volume Deficit** related to hemorrhage
- **Pain** related to tissue trauma and bladder spasms
- **High Risk for Infection** related to invasive procedures of the urinary tract and surgical incision
- **High Risk for Injury** related to obstructed urine flow, excessive absorption of irrigating fluids, trauma to the urinary sphincter
- **Sexual Dysfunction** related to removal of prostate, retrograde ejaculation, possible neurologic injury
- **Situational Low Self-Esteem** related to anticipated alteration in sexual function
- **Knowledge Deficit** of postoperative routines and self-care

GOALS. Goals for the identified nursing diagnoses are normal fluid volume; pain relief; absence of infection; absence of complications due to obstruction, water intoxication, or sphincter injury; management of sexual dysfunction; improved self-esteem; and patient's knowledge of routines and self-care.

INTERVENTIONS

High Risk for Fluid Volume Deficit. The nurse inspects urine, dressings, and wound drainage for excess bleeding. Blood in the urine is expected for several days after a prostatectomy, but bleeding with clots can lead to hemorrhage and must be reported to the physician immediately. Restlessness and increasing heart rate are early signs of fluid volume deficit. Measures to control bleeding include surgical intervention and application of pressure to the prostatic area. To apply pressure, the physician may inject additional fluid into the balloon that anchors the indwelling catheter. The catheter is then pulled so that the balloon fits tightly against the neck of the bladder, and various forms of traction are used, including taping the catheter to the thigh. This traction may be maintained for several hours or more and then released by the physician.

Pain. Pain after prostatectomy may be associated with urinary obstruction, bladder spasms, and surgical trauma. If urine is not draining freely, the tubing is repositioned and milked or irrigated according to agency

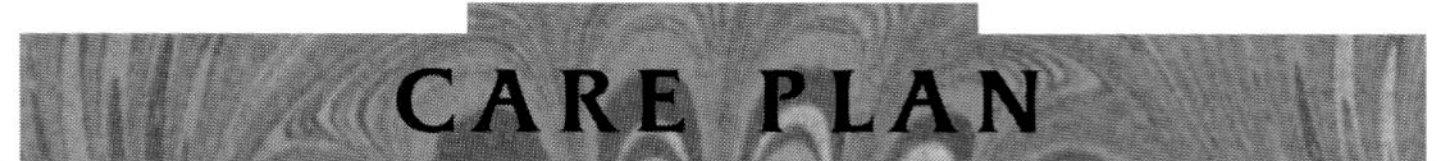

CARE PLAN

The Patient with a Prostatectomy

ASSESSMENT

Health History: Mr. Mark Alan is a 77-year-old retired radio announcer who has had a transurethral prostatectomy this morning. He returned to the nursing unit 3 hours ago. He complains of genital pain and states that he feels like he needs to empty his bladder. He appears tense and is clenching the siderails.

Physical Assessment: Vital signs: temperature, 98°F orally; pulse, 84; respiration, 18; blood pressure 122/70. Alert and oriented. Breath sounds clear to auscultation. Intravenous fluids infusing at 100 ml per hour. Three-way Foley catheter in place, taped to inner thigh, and draining freely into collection bag. Irrigation fluid set at the prescribed flow rate. Urine is pink, not viscous. Several clots observed in bag. Output approximately equal to fluid intake.

NURSING DIAGNOSIS	GOALS AND OUTCOME CRITERIA	INTERVENTIONS
High risk for fluid volume deficit related to hemorrhage.	The patient will have balanced fluid intake and output without signs of hypovolemia: tachycardia, decreased urine output, hypotension, restlessness.	Monitor urine for excessive bleeding: thick, bright blood with clots. Assess for signs of hypovolemia. Be sure traction is maintained on catheter by keeping tape in place until surgeon removes it. Maintain flow of irrigating fluid as ordered. If urine flow decreases or bladder distention is detected, irrigate the catheter as ordered. Inform surgeon if unable to irrigate or urine output remains low.
Pain related to tissue trauma and bladder spasms.	The patient will verbalize relief from pain and will appear more relaxed.	Check tubing to be sure urine is draining freely. If not, reposition the tubing and milk or irrigate it as ordered or per agency policy. Notify surgeon immediately if unable to clear tubing. Administer analgesics and antispasmodics as ordered. Reposition patient. Give back rub. Use distraction. Assess effects of pain relief interventions.
High risk for infection related to invasive procedures of the urinary tract or catheterization.	The patient will remain free of infection as evidenced by normal body temperature, normal white blood cell count, and absence of confusion or cloudy, foul urine.	Use strict aseptic techniques when handling the urinary drainage system. Keep closed system intact. Monitor temperature and urine characteristics. Report fever (greater than 101°F), confusion, cloudy or foul urine.
High risk for injury related to obstructed urine flow, excessive absorption of irrigating fluids, or trauma to urinary sphincter.	The patient will have no injuries as evidenced by continuous urine flow and absence of signs of fluid volume excess: hypertension, bradycardia, weakness, seizures.	Maintain flow of isotonic irrigating fluid as ordered. Monitor output and assess bladder for distention. Monitor vital signs. Report signs of fluid volume excess to surgeon. Administer stool softeners as ordered to prevent constipation. Encourage fluid intake when able.
Sexual dysfunction related to removal of prostate or retrograde ejaculation.	The patient will correctly describe the physiologic effects of prostatectomy.	Be open to patient's questions about effects of surgery on sexual function. Reinforce preoperative teaching that impotence is not common after transurethral prostate resection. Retrograde ejaculation may occur but is not harmful. Offer to include sex partner in teaching. Be sensitive to possible feelings about loss of masculinity. Patient may demonstrate some anger or sadness related to a sense of loss.

Continued on following page

The Patient with a Prostatectomy *(Continued)*

NURSING DIAGNOSIS	GOALS AND OUTCOME CRITERIA	INTERVENTIONS
Knowledge deficit of postoperative routines or self-care.	The patient will demonstrate understanding of postoperative exercises and procedures.	Support and encourage patient to turn and deep breathe at least every 2 hr. Explain catheter and irrigation system. Tell him that some blood is normal the first few days after surgery. Encourage early ambulation as soon as permitted and explain benefits of activity to recovery. Before discharge, advise to restrict strenuous activity and heavy lifting (more than 20 lb) for 4 to 6 weeks. If he will go home with a catheter, discuss catheter care.

policy. Antispasmodics such as oxybutynin chloride (Ditropan), belladonna and opium suppositories or propantheline bromide (Pro-Banthīne) are usually effective in relieving bladder spasms. Analgesics may be administered as ordered. The nurse should also employ nonpharmacologic interventions such as repositioning, back rubs, and relaxation exercises.

High Risk for Infection. To reduce the risk of infection, strict aseptic technique is used when handling urinary drainage, wound drains, and dressings. Closed urinary drainage systems should be kept intact to prevent introduction of pathogens. Wound care is done in accordance with the physician's orders or the agency's policy. The nurse monitors for signs of infection, including temperature greater than 38.3°C (101°F), purulent wound drainage, and confusion in elderly patients.

High Risk for Injury. Urinary obstruction and bladder distention can lead to renal complications (hydronephrosis), infection, and increased bleeding. Therefore, it is critical to maintain urine flow. If urine flow ceases, the bladder is assessed for distention. If the bladder is distended, the irrigating fluid is temporarily turned off and the bladder irrigated as ordered. If the nurse cannot clear the tubing, the surgeon must be notified immediately. After the catheters are removed, the nurse must continue to monitor output because edema or scarring may occur and obstruct the urethra.

Another possible complication is water intoxication caused by absorption of irrigating fluid in addition to intravenous fluids. For that reason, isotonic fluids rather than pure water are used for irrigation. Manifestations of hypervolemia are hypertension, bradycardia, weakness, and seizures.

If the urinary sphincter is damaged, the patient may have urinary incontinence. In most cases, control can be improved with perineal exercises and in some cases drug therapy or even surgery. For additional information, see Chapter 21 (Incontinence).

Sexual Dysfunction, Situational Low Self-Esteem. Alterations in sexual function that may distress the patient include sterility, retrograde ejaculation, and impotence. These concerns should be discussed with the physician before surgery. Impotence is not common after surgical treatment of BPH, but if it does occur the patient may need counseling as described later in this chapter. There is no treatment for retrograde ejaculation, but the nurse can reassure the patient that it is not harmful. All of these alterations can threaten the patient's self-image and self-esteem. The nurse must be sensitive to the patient's feelings of loss and need to assert a masculine image. With the patient's permission, his sex partner should be included in teaching and counseling.

Knowledge Deficit. The postoperative teaching plan provides information about the effects of prostatectomy, signs and symptoms of complications that should be reported, self-medication, perineal exercises, and activity restrictions. The patient is encouraged to maintain a fluid intake of at least eight glasses each day. Stool softeners and a high-fiber diet may be prescribed to prevent constipation and straining, which could lead to bleeding. If he is discharged with a catheter, he must be taught how to care for it. Ambulation is encouraged, but strenuous activity and heavy lifting (more than 10 pounds) should be avoided for 3 weeks.

EVALUATION. Criteria for evaluating the outcomes of nursing interventions are balanced fluid intake and output and stable vital signs consistent with patient's norms; patient's statement of pain relief, relaxed expression; absence of fever and foul drainage or urine; freely flowing urine, normal blood pressure and mental state; patient's statement of understanding of sexual dysfunctions and appropriate resources; positive statements about self by patient; and patient's description or demonstration of self-care activities and limitations.

IMPOTENCE (ERECTILE DYSFUNCTION)

The most devastating and obvious functional change for the male may be the onset of impotence, which is the inability to produce and maintain an erection for sexual intercourse. An adequate erection requires intact neurologic capability to initiate the erection process, vigorous and unimpeded inflow of blood to fill the

TABLE 44-5
SUMMARY OF SYMPTOMS, CAUSES, AND TREATMENTS OF IMPOTENCE

TYPE OF IMPOTENCE	SYMPTOMS*	CAUSES	TREATMENTS
Failure to initiate	Inability to initiate (develop) an erection	Nerve damage due to disease or injury; stress, anxiety, or other psychological problems; hormonal disorders	Sex therapy, hormonal therapy, vacuum constriction device, penile injections, penile implant
Failure to fill†	Erections develop slowly and may not be sufficiently rigid for intercourse or masturbation except sometimes after extended foreplay or stimulation; sleep erections or erections on awakening may appear more rigid	Arterial blockage(s) due to atherosclerosis, aging, or injury	Sex therapy, vacuum constriction device, revascularization surgery (arterial bypass surgery), penile implant
Failure to store†	Erections poorly maintained and not rigid enough for intercourse or masturbation	Abnormal storage due to stress, aging, injury, or any process that causes erectile tissue to stiffen and not expand enough to compress subtunical venules	Sex therapy, vacuum constriction device, penile injections, venous ligation surgery, crural plication surgery, penile implant

* Changes in erections (in rigidity or sustaining capability or both) must occur with morning erections, during masturbation, and during intercourse for a period of 6 months to a year before the patient is considered in need of treatment for impotence.

† Failure-to-fill impotence and failure-to-store impotence often occur together as the result of a disease process, atherosclerosis, or aging.

Reprinted by permission of the Putnam Publishing Group from Goldstein, I., & Rothstein, L. (1990). *The potent male* (p. 39). Los Angeles: The Body Press. Copyright © 1990 by Price Stern Sloan, Inc., and Irwin Goldstein and Larry Rothstein.

corpus cavernosa, and a leakproof storage mechanism for maintaining the erection (Table 44–5).

Contributing Factors

A number of vascular, neurologic, endocrine, and psychogenic factors may cause or contribute to impotence.

VASCULAR DISORDERS. Arteriosclerosis is the hardening of an artery due to injury to the endothelial lining of the vessel and eventual scarring. The scarring narrows the artery and may reduce blood flow through the narrowed area. Localized cavernosal artery damage in the perineum between the scrotum and anus may result from physical injury to the pelvis, falls on the crossbar of a bicycle, horseback riding, or other blows. This type of injury may damage the artery to such an extent that scarring limits the inflow of blood, compromising ability to fill.

Atherosclerosis is the hardening or stiffening of an arterial wall due to systemic rather than localized insults. High cholesterol levels, smoking, excessive alcohol consumption, illicit drug use, and inadequate exercise contribute to disease processes that cause atherosclerosis.

ENDOCRINE DISORDERS. Diabetes mellitus is a systemic disease characterized by glucose intolerance. When too little insulin is produced or the insulin produced is ineffective, the result is high blood glucose levels and disturbances of fat and protein metabolism. Patients with diabetes mellitus are at risk for impotence due to atherosclerosis and autonomic neuropathy.

Studies have shown that approximately 50% of diabetic men, regardless of type of treatment, develop impotence, making diabetes the most common cause of impotence. Diabetes is believed to interfere with blood supply to the penis when arterial walls lose flexibility, or distensibility, as a result of hardening of the arteries (atherosclerosis). Atherosclerosis is a common part of the aging process but may be accelerated in the diabetic.

Autonomic neuropathy in patients with diabetes affects the ability of nerves to relax the smooth muscle surrounding the tiny sinuses (lacunar spaces) of the erectile chambers. Without decreased muscle tone and expansion of the sinuses, adequate filling with blood for an erection may not be possible.

Effective management of diabetes mellitus is always desirable for general good health, but maintenance of strict blood glucose has not been shown to reduce the incidence of impotence. Although the primary cause of impotence related to diabetes mellitus is physiologic, the psychological reaction to the problem is an important factor. Cognitive behavioral therapy may be used to teach the patient to manage negative thinking.

Vascular surgery to clear blocked arteries is not usually recommended for diabetic patients because they frequently have complicating problems with nerves, cells, erectile tissue, and blood vessels throughout the penis.

Penile implants (Fig. 44–9) may be recommended for patients with problems of failure to initiate (nerve damage) or artery damage (failure to fill), which are problems of the diabetic. As many as one third of penile implant patients are diabetic.

Papaverine self-injection (Fig. 44–10) is indicated as a treatment for failure to initiate or fill and has had wide acceptance by patients. Patients require training for self-injection and must have hand dexterity, adequate vision, and absence of obesity.

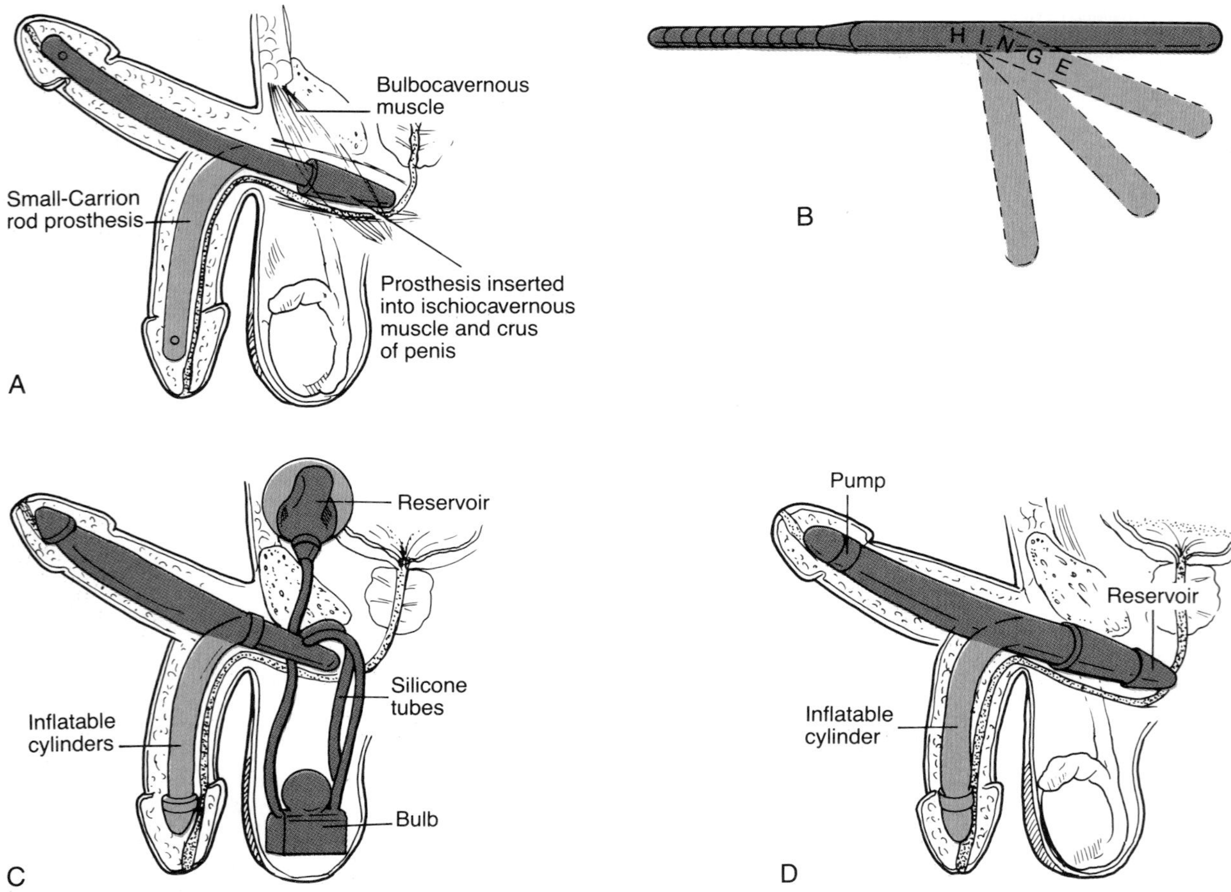

FIGURE 44-9

Penile prostheses. *A*, Small-Carrion prosthesis; *B*, Flexi-rod semirigid implant; *C*, inflatable prosthesis; *D*, self-contained prosthesis. (From Black, J. M., & Matassarin-Jacobs, E. [1993]. *Luckmann and Sorensen's medical-surgical nursing: A psychophysiologic approach* [4th ed., p. 2091]. Philadelphia: W. B. Saunders.)

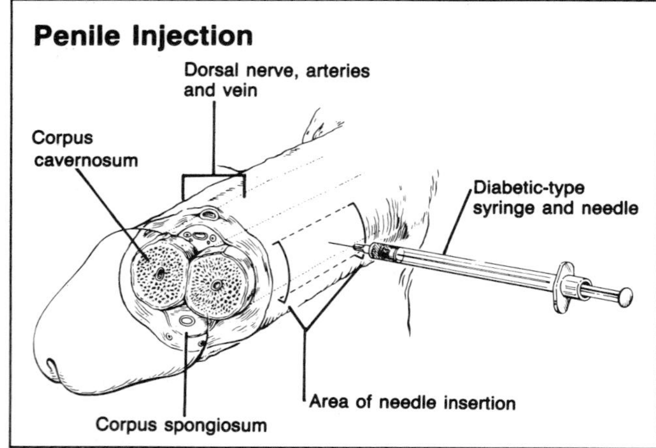

FIGURE 44-10

Penile injection. (Reprinted by permission of the Putnam Publishing Group from Goldstein, I., & Rothstein, L. [1990]. *The potent male* [p. 119]. Los Angeles: The Body Press. Copyright © 1990 by Price Stern Sloan, Inc., and Irwin Goldstein and Larry Rothstein.)

NEUROLOGIC DISORDERS. Spinal cord injuries and other neurologic disorders may cause impotence. If communication between the spinal cord and the penis remains intact, the penis becomes erect with direct stimulation. For the penis to remain erect, smooth muscle relaxation is necessary and in some way is reliant on communication between the brain and the spinal cord. The more complete the injury and the lower the injury, the more likely it is for potency to be affected, even though higher injuries tend to cause more paralysis and loss of sensation.

Treatment of impotence related to spinal cord injuries or neurologic disorders such as multiple sclerosis may include papaverine injections, vacuum constriction devices, or penile implants. Medications used to treat a variety of conditions may cause or contribute to impotence. Drugs used to reduce high blood pressure (antihypertensives) are the most likely to interfere with erection. If systemic hypertension is accompanied by blockages and stiffening in artery walls of the penis, antihypertensives that lower the blood pressure in all the arteries of the body may reduce the blood pressure in penile arteries to the extent that failure to fill occurs. Digoxin, which is used to treat heart conditions, may increase levels of estrogen and decrease levels of testosterone, medications for stomach ulcers such as cimetidine may decrease libido, anticancer drugs may decrease libido, and anticholinergics and antihistamines may block neurotransmitters that cause relaxation of smooth muscle.

Treatment for impotence related to these drugs' side effects may include changes in drugs or dosage but should never be undertaken without the consultation and supervision of a physician. Counseling or sex therapy, vacuum constriction devices, penile injections, or penile implants may be appropriate for these patients.

PSYCHOLOGICAL FACTORS. The psychological aspects of impotence are extremely important and should be included in the medical history. Psychogenic impotence is often the result of anxiety about performance. Problems may arise with aging, sexual beliefs or behavior, communication patterns or relationships with sex partners, changes in lifestyle, changes in medications, or chronic or poorly managed disease processes. The resultant anxious state may initiate the release of neurotransmitters that cause constriction of smooth muscle tissue in the penis and its arteries, reducing inflow and increasing outflow of blood from the penis, leaving it flaccid. Sex therapy that includes behavior modification techniques may be able to restore potency.

Interventions

HORMONE THERAPY. Testosterone replacement for men with low hormone levels may be recommended for decreased desire and failure to initiate.

VACUUM CONSTRICTION DEVICES. Vacuum constriction devices may be prescribed for failure to initiate, fill, or store or for psychogenic causes (Fig. 44–11). The flaccid penis is slipped into a cylinder, then the patient squeezes a pump that removes all of the air from the space in the cylinder around the penis, creating a vacuum that draws blood into the penis. When the erection has been achieved, a rubber ring is slipped off the bottom of the cylinder onto the penis near the base, trapping the blood safely for up to about 30 minutes. Allowing air to enter the cylinder allows the cylinder to be removed.

SELF-INJECTION THERAPY. Self-injection therapy may be recommended for failure to initiate, fill, or store or for psychogenic causes. Papaverine is injected with a small needle into the erectile chambers with relatively little pain (see Fig. 44–10). Most patients achieve an erection within 10 to 15 minutes that usually lasts about 30 to 60 minutes. Papaverine acts on smooth muscle to relax artery walls and erectile tissue, increasing blood flow into the penis. Papaverine is often mixed with phentolamine, which acts to block constriction of erectile tissue, making it possible to sustain the erection.

REVASCULARIZATION. Revascularization may be recommended for patients with blocked arteries. It is

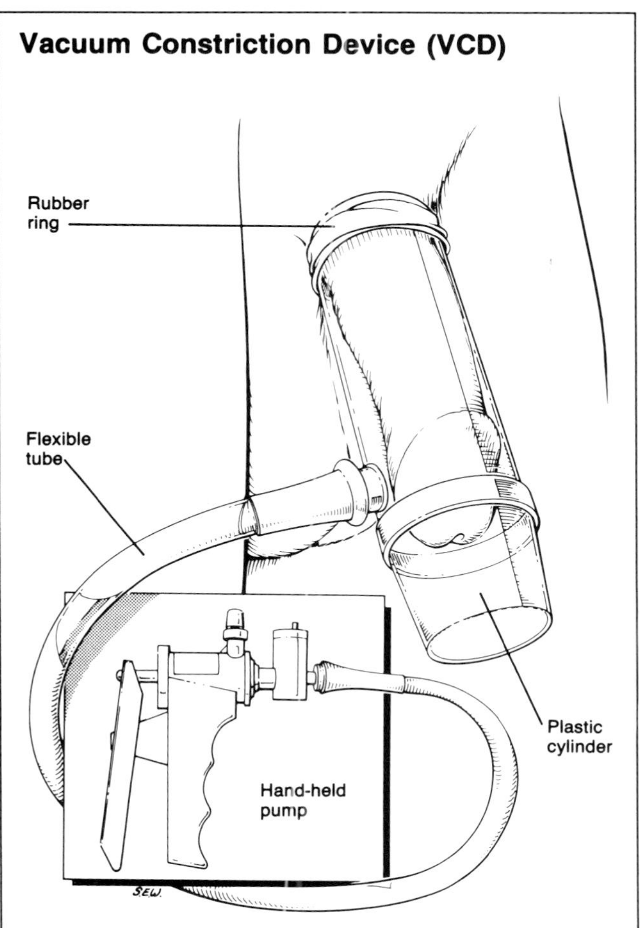

FIGURE 44–11

Vacuum constriction device. (Reprinted by permission of the Putnam Publishing Group from Goldstein, I., & Rothstein, L. [1990]. *The potent male* [p. 170]. Los Angeles: The Body Press. Copyright © 1990 by Price Stern Sloan, Inc., and Irwin Goldstein and Larry Rothstein.)

important to evaluate how the blockage affects both the flow of blood into the penis and the extent to which it can be stored to maintain an erection. Arteries that block inflow are bypassed. Veins that are causing excessive drainage are removed (excision) or tied off (ligation). In addition the tunica surrounding the erectile tissue may be tightened (plication). The increased pressure on veins caused by swelling of the erectile tissue against the tunica during erection decreases leakage and maintains the erection.

PENILE IMPLANTS. Penile implants (see Fig. 44–9) may be prescribed for patients with failure to initiate, failure to fill or store when they are not good candidates for revascularization, and for some patients with psychogenic problems that are not appropriate for or responsive to counseling or sex therapy. Semirigid implants are silicon cylinders placed in the erection chambers that keep the penis firm at all times but without increasing in circumference. Some models are inflexible and create problems concealing the erection, but others are flexible enough that they can be bent downward and the erection more easily concealed. Hydraulic implants have cylinders that can be inflated by squeezing a pump in the scrotum or at the end of the penis behind the glans. The pumping action causes the cylinders to fill with fluid from a reservoir in the abdomen or the scrotum. These implants more nearly duplicate the natural states of flaccidity and erection.

Nursing Care of the Patient with Impotence

ASSESSMENT. The nursing assessment of the impotent male includes a health history that elicits information about frequency of intercourse and ability to enjoy sexual relations. Impotence may be the first sign of diabetes mellitus, so complete exploration of general health and family history of diabetes is important. Surgeries, injuries, illness, cancer, and medications used regularly should also be included. Descriptions of home life, daily activities, diet, use of alcohol and illicit drugs, exercise habits, and lifestyle, as well as health care beliefs, interpersonal relationships, capability for self-care, age, physical condition, and educational needs, should also be included.

NURSING DIAGNOSIS. Specific nursing diagnoses vary with the cause and treatment of impotence, but general nursing diagnoses often include the following:

- **Sexual Dysfunction** related to impotence
- **Situational Low Self-Esteem** related to impaired sexual function
- **Knowledge Deficit** of factors contributing to impotence and measures to improve sexual function

GOALS. Goals of nursing care for the patient with sexual dysfunction include improved sexual function or satisfying alternatives to sexual intercourse, improved patient self-esteem, and patient's understanding and management of impotence.

INTERVENTIONS. The management of impotence requires sensitivity and knowledge. When the patient and the nurse have a therapeutic relationship, the patient may choose to share his concerns with the nurse. The nurse listens and is careful not to dismiss the issue as unimportant. Factual information and resources can be provided. Nurses who are not well-informed about impotence should refer patients to counselors with training in this area.

EVALUATION. Criteria for measuring the success of interventions for impotence are patient's statement of improved function or satisfaction with alternatives, patient makes more positive comments about self, and patient describes factors contributing to his impotence and treatment or coping measures.

PEYRONIE'S DISEASE

Peyronie's disease is the development of a hard, nonelastic, fibrous tissue (plaque) just under the skin of the penis of men between 45 and 70 years of age. The plaque develops as a result of an injury that causes inflammation and scarring of the tunica surrounding the corpora cavernosa. Loss of elasticity of the tunica results in decreased ability to fill during an erection and failure to store because of low pressure on the veins against the covering of the erectile tissue. The plaque is usually located on the dorsal midline surface of the penis and results in an upward bending of the penis during erection that may be painful and interfere with successful vaginal penetration (Fig. 44–12).

Medical Treatment

Treatment of Peyronie's disease may include topical or oral medications with vitamin E, oral aminobenzoic acid, radiation, steroidal anti-inflammatory drugs, enzymes that dissolve collagen, ultrasound, surgical removal, and penile implants. The choice of treatment depends on the size of the plaque and the curvature and the resultant degree of dysfunction.

PRIAPISM

Priapism is a prolonged penile erection that is not related to sexual desire. Priapism may be caused by injury to the penis, sickle cell crisis, medications such as antipsychotics and antidepressants, antihypertensives, anticoagulants, alcohol, marijuana, and papaverine injections. Priapism due to the inability to drain blood from

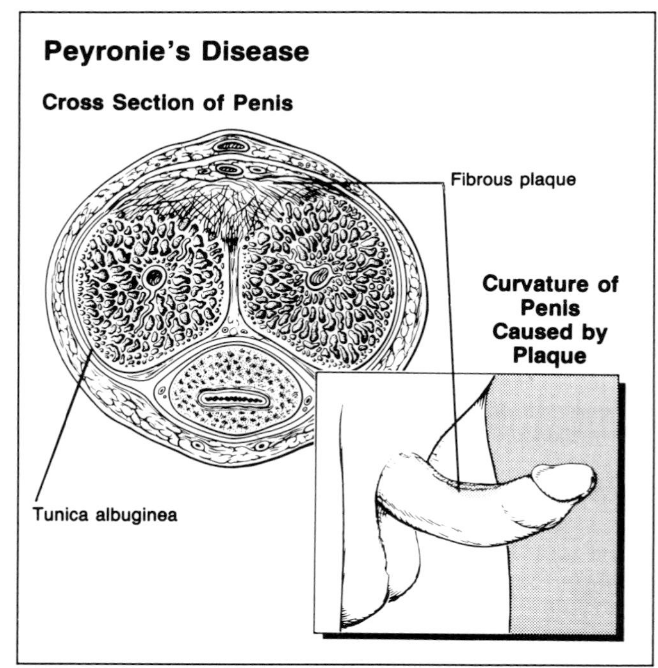

FIGURE 44-12
Peyronie's disease. (Reprinted by permission of the Putnam Publishing Group from Goldstein, I., & Rothstein, L. [1990]. *The potent male* [p. 152]. Los Angeles: The Body Press. Copyright © 1990 by Price Stern Sloan, Inc., and Irwin Goldstein and Larry Rothstein.)

the erectile tissue can reduce artery flow to the penis so greatly that oxygenated blood cannot reach penile tissue. This erection may be very painful and constitutes an emergency situation, as circulation to the penis and ability to void are compromised. Failure to resolve the problem within 12 to 24 hours may result in ischemia, gangrene, fibrosis, and impotence. Priapism due to a blunt blow to the groin or penis that lacerates an artery may cause bleeding into the erectile tissue, causing continuous filling until the artery is repaired or the bleeding is stopped.

Medical Treatment

Treatment of storage priapism may include discontinued use of offending drugs and correction of neurologic or coagulation problems. Immediate removal of blood may be accomplished by aspirating blood from the erectile chambers or injecting drugs that cause contraction of smooth muscle, inhibiting inflow of blood and allowing outflow. Failure of these efforts may result in emergency surgery.

Nursing care must be particularly sensitive to the embarrassment this patient may experience. Understanding of the condition and provision of comfort measures for pain are important.

PHIMOSIS

Normally the penile foreskin can be retracted, exposing the glans. Inflammation under the foreskin, often associated with poor hygiene, causes edema that may prevent retraction of the foreskin. This condition, called *phimosis*, is treated with antimicrobials and proper cleansing. Circumcision is sometimes recommended. Uncircumcised men need to retract the foreskin for cleaning as part of daily hygiene.

INFERTILITY

Infertile is a term used to describe couples who have had unprotected intercourse over a 12-month period and have been unable to become pregnant. Research data over the past 20 years has shown that in approximately 30% of the cases significant pathology is found in the male alone and in approximately 50% of the cases the male is at least partially the cause of failure to conceive. The female partner most often brings the problem to the attention of a physician and may do so after a significant level of anxiety and apprehension has already been established. Research has also shown that long durations of infertility increase the chances of ultimate infertility. Considering these facts, work-up of the male partner should not be delayed.

Etiology and Risk Factors

Causes of infertility include infections, cryptorchidism, testicular torsion, varicocele, and vasectomy.

INFECTIONS. Destruction of the seminiferous tubular epithelium results in failure or reduced ability to produce sperm. Mumps in the adult male or pubescent male may result in acute orchitis and epididymitis accompanied by fever and debilitating pain, bilateral swelling, and redness of the testicles. If damage to seminiferous epithelium occurs, the testes will be reduced to subnormal size after recovery. Other viral infections such as tuberculosis, pneumonia, and syphilis may affect the testes, but none of them is as dramatic as mumps in the acute phase, and loss of testicular mass may appear to be more gradual.

Genitourinary tract infections can cause infertility in males. *Chlamydia trachomatis* is sexually transmitted and is most prevalent in young adults with multiple sex partners. The infection is most frequently limited to the urethra and causes varying degrees of painful urination and discharge. Progressive infection may include the epididymis and prostate gland. *Neisseria gonorrhoeae* is the most common urethral infection in the United States. It is sexually transmitted and may cause severely painful urination and a purulent discharge. Ascending infections to the epididymis may result in decreased fertility.

CRYPTORCHIDISM. Cryptorchidism is defined as any testes located outside a dependent scrotal position. It is a common congenital condition found in approximately 30% of preterm male infants and 1.0 to 3.4% of full-term male infants (Fig. 44–13). Although the condition may occur as a result of genetic disorders, the cause is usually unknown and may be related to an endocrine or a mechanical defect, an inherent testicular disorder, or a combination of several factors. Damage to the seminiferous epithelium and the resulting decrease or loss of spermatogenesis is caused by excessive temperatures of the testes in the abdominal cavity.

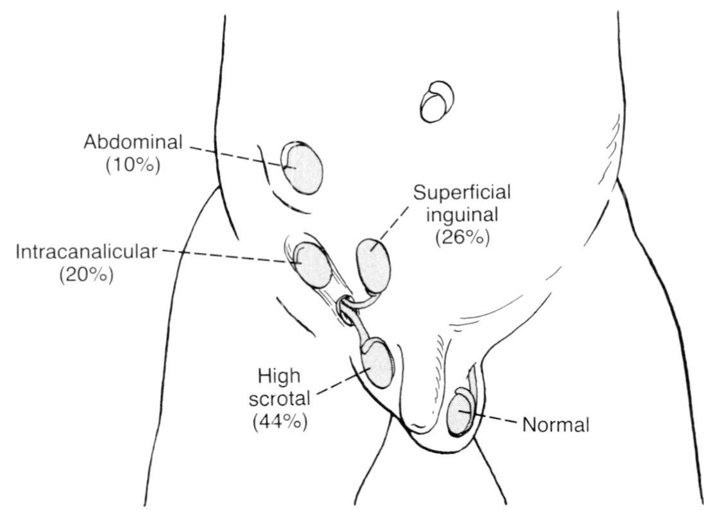

FIGURE 44–13

Common sites of undescended testicles. (From Black, J. M., & Matassarin-Jacobs, E. [1993]. *Luckmann and Sorensen's medical-surgical nursing: A psychophysiologic approach* [4th ed., p. 2112]. Philadelphia: W. B. Saunders.)

Medical Treatment. Correction must occur within the first 18 months to give the best chance for fertility. Men with undescended testes have a 10 to 30 times higher incidence of testicular cancer, even if corrected, than men whose testes descend normally. If the testes are within the normal path but do not descend or cannot be pulled into the scrotum, they do not usually respond to hormonal therapy and require surgical intervention. Whether medical or surgical therapy is indicated, it is recommended after the first birthday and before the second birthday. Untreated bilateral cryptorchidism results in sterility; unilateral cryptorchidism may result in lowered sperm count, but spermatogenesis continues and initiation of a pregnancy may occur without difficulty.

The problem of testes that retract as a result of overactive muscles usually appears about age 3 to 6 years and will respond to hormonal therapy by spontaneously descending at or before puberty.

TESTICULAR TORSION. Testicular torsion occurs unilaterally when the testicle is mobile and the spermatic cord twists, cutting off the blood supply to the testicle (Fig. 44–14). It is an acute surgical emergency requiring immediate release of the torsion or removal of the testicle. It most commonly occurs in adolescents and usually occurs when the scrotum is warm and relaxed but may occur for no apparent reason. Symptoms are nausea and vomiting and intense pain. When testicular torsion is corrected, lowered sperm counts and infertility may follow as a result of reduced spermatogenesis from the ischemic insult. There is sometimes collateral effect on the healthy testicle. After the testicle that underwent torsion is removed, sperm counts are normal.

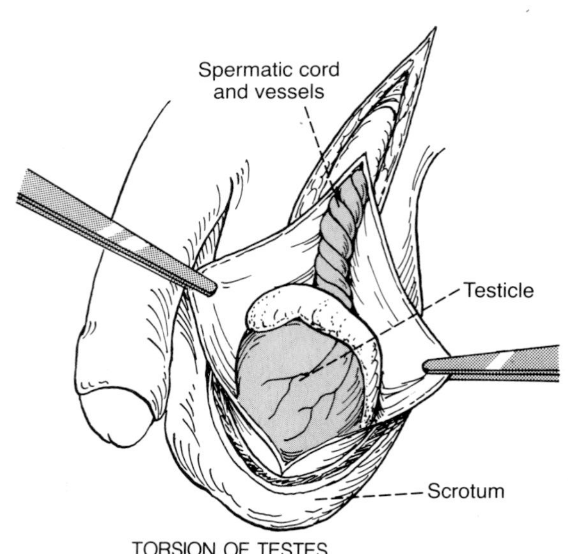

FIGURE 44–14

Torsion of the testes. (Adapted from Black, J. M., & Matassarin-Jacobs, E. [1993]. *Luckmann and Sorensen's medical-surgical nursing: A psychophysiologic approach* [4th ed., p. 2111]. Philadelphia: W. B. Saunders.)

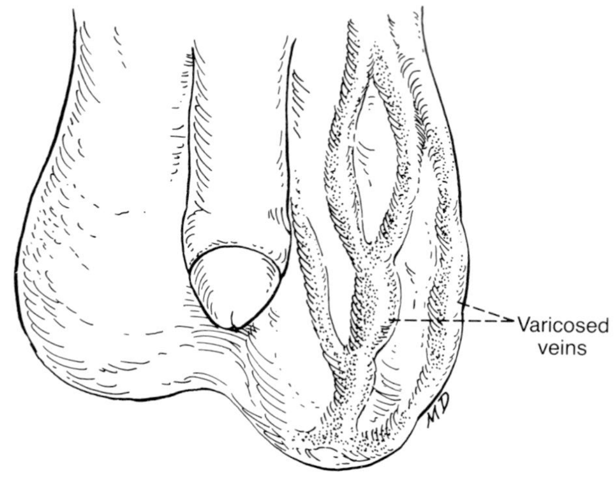

FIGURE 44–15

Varicocele. (Adapted from Black, J. M., & Matassarin-Jacobs, E. [1993]. *Luckmann and Sorensen's medical-surgical nursing: A psychophysiologic approach* [4th ed., p. 2111]. Philadelphia: W. B. Saunders.)

VARICOCELE. A varicocele is a lengthening and enlargement of the scrotal portion of the venous system that drains the testicle (Fig. 44–15). Varicoceles are caused by the incompetence or absence of valves in the spermatic venous system, which allows pooled blood and the resulting increased hydrostatic pressure to dilate the veins. The left testicle is the most frequent site, but bilateral or right-sided varicoceles do occur. Affected testicles may be smaller in size and may have reduced spermatogenesis. Although the pathophysiologic effect of a varicocele on fertility is still debated, hyperthermia is the most widely accepted explanation. On examination of the testes, large varicoceles may be visible through the scrotal skin as a bluish discoloration. Small varicoceles may be palpable only when the patient is asked to bear down. Treatment includes scrotal support or surgical ligation and is indicated when fertility is thought to be affected. Varicoceles may reappear after surgery, and fertility or the ability to conceive may or may not improve.

VASECTOMY. Vasectomy is the surgical removal of a portion of the vas deferens (Fig. 44–16). Although sperm are no longer found in the semen after the procedure, the ability for erection, ejaculation, and successful intercourse remains intact. Vasectomy is usually an outpatient procedure, done in the physician's office or an outpatient clinic. There may be postoperative pain or swelling that can be managed with application of an ice bag, mild analgesics, and scrotal support. The patient can resume intercourse as soon as he feels comfortable, but it is important that he use other methods of birth control until analysis of the semen determines that there is a complete absence of sperm. The patient can expect

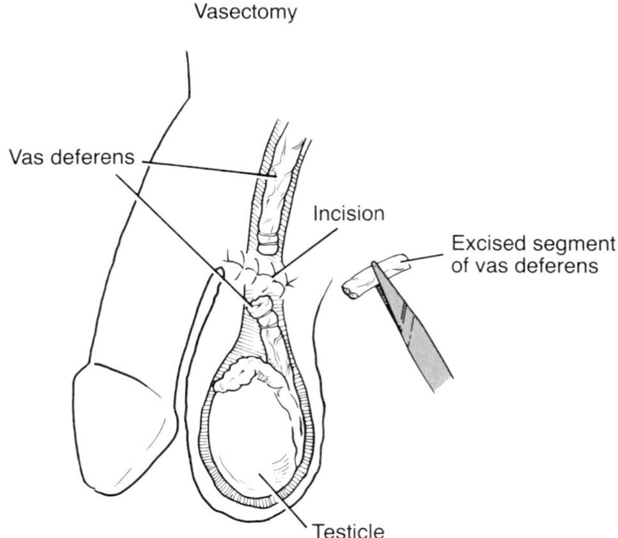

FIGURE 44-16

Vasectomy. (From Black, J. M., & Matassarin-Jacobs, E. [1993]. *Luckmann and Sorensen's medical-surgical nursing: A psychophysiologic approach* [4th ed., p. 2112]. Philadelphia: W. B. Saunders.)

the analysis to be done after about 15 ejaculations following the vasectomy.

Nursing care of the vasectomy patient should include preoperative teaching about the procedure itself and the resultant infertility. Although vasectomy can sometimes be successfully reversed, it should be considered permanent. The nurse should be sensitive to the readiness of the male patient to undergo this procedure. Fears related to postoperative loss of sexual function and development of cancer may cause anxiety in some men, even though they desire the procedure. Acceptance and reassurance are important.

PENILE CANCER

Cancer may be the most frightening diagnosis for any patient. Cancer of the male reproductive system may arouse the worst fears about sexual dysfunction, disfigurement, and self-esteem in men, especially in young adults or adolescents.

Penile cancer is relatively rare and occurs exclusively in uncircumcised men who have had chronic irritation and poor hygiene. The cancer may appear as dry, wartlike, painless growths on the penis that do not respond to antibiotic therapy. They can be removed surgically if treated in early stages. Advanced stages of growths may ulcerate and involve the foreskin and penile shaft and require extensive resection or amputation as well as resection of nearby lymph nodes.

TESTICULAR CANCER

Testicular germ cell carcinoma occurs most often in young men between the ages of 18 and 34 years of age. The three established risk factors for this type of cancer are cryptorchidism, white race, and previous testicular cancer. Patients most frequently present with hard, painless tumors (Fig. 44–17). Diagnosis is often delayed because patients do not seek medical help.

Early Detection

Self-examination and early diagnosis offer the highest chance of finding low-stage disease and subsequent cure. Increased awareness of the need for self-examination is an important part of health education for men. Although men are used to touching their genitals, they may not feel comfortable examining themselves. Self-examination includes monthly examination of the penis, scrotum, and perineal area. The patient should use a mirror to visualize areas that he cannot see and look for any changes from normal such as swelling, lumps, tenderness, lesions, asymmetry, discoloration, or discharge. The examination is best done after a warm bath or shower when he is warm and the scrotum is relaxed. The scrotum should be held in the palm of his hands with the index and middle fingers on the underside of the testicle and the thumb on top (Fig. 44–18). Each testicle is palpated between the thumbs and forefingers of both hands, rolling the testicle between the fingers. The left testicle usually is lower than the right. The testicles are egg shaped and should feel firm but not hard and smooth without lumps. The epididymis located on the top and posterior side of each testicle feels soft and spongy; the spermatic cords are smooth, firm, tubular structures that run upward from the testicles on the back side.

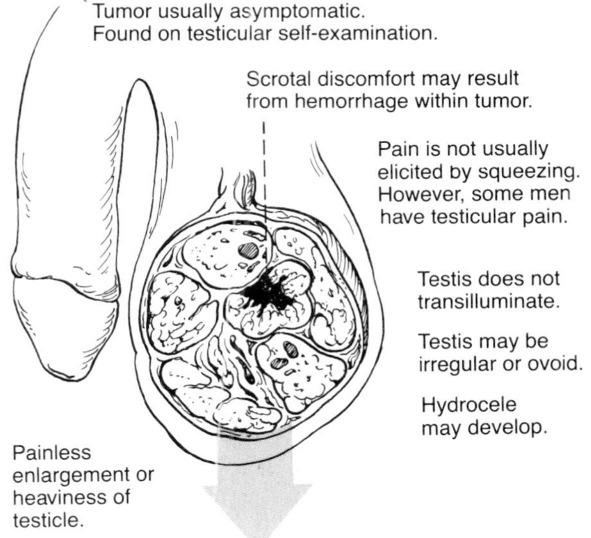

FIGURE 44-17

Characteristics of testicular tumors. (From Black, J. M., & Matassarin-Jacobs, E. [1993]. *Luckmann and Sorensen's medical-surgical nursing: A psychophysiologic approach* [4th ed., p. 2109]. Philadelphia: W. B. Saunders.)

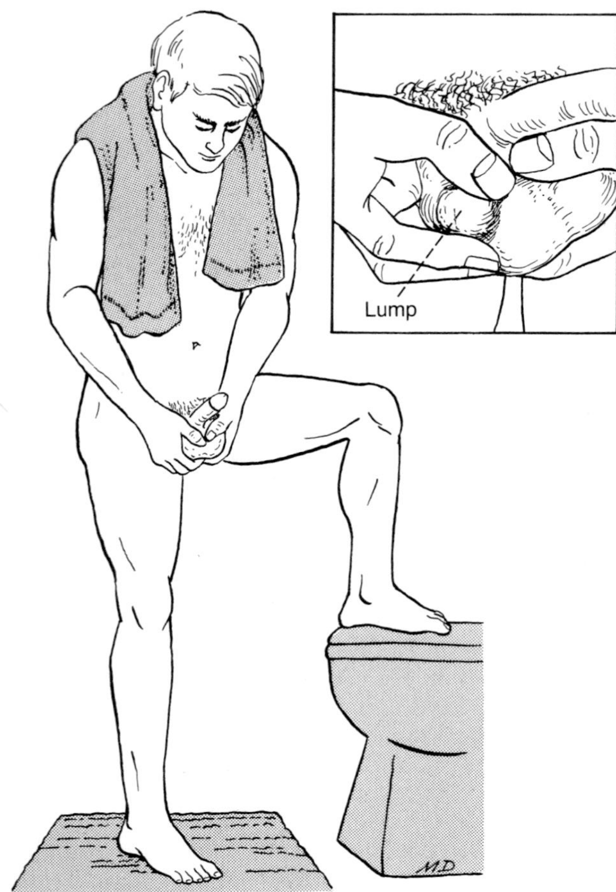

FIGURE 44-18

Testicular self-examination. (From Black, J. M., & Matassarin-Jacobs, E. [1993]. *Luckmann and Sorensen's medical-surgical nursing: A psychophysiologic approach* [4th ed., p. 2085]. Philadelphia: W. B. Saunders.)

Medical Diagnosis

Diagnosis of testicular cancer is confirmed by removal of the affected testis (orchiectomy), leaving the other testicle intact and preserving fertility when possible. The diagnosis may be supported by elevated tumor markers, and testicular ultrasound. If there is doubt of the diagnosis or no primary site is obvious, surgical exploration is done.

Medical Treatment

Treatment for testicular cancer is designed according to the type of cancer and the stage. Seminoma is a radiosensitive malignant tumor of the testes that is thought to arise from sexually undifferentiated embryonic cells. Stage I seminoma is defined as being confined to the testes or extending into the epididymis, scrotum, or spermatic cord without lymph node involvement. After removal of the testis, radiotherapy to the pelvic region is usual and results in a 95% cure rate. Relapsed patients may be treated successfully with chemotherapy. Follow-up includes monitoring tumor markers and radiographic examinations of lymph nodes for a period of 5 years from diagnosis.

Treatment of stage I nonseminomatous tumors is controversial. These tumors were once thought to be of different origin than seminoma but are now believed to have the same germ cell origin and be part of a continuum of differentiation or organized development. They are less sensitive to radiotherapy and require larger doses for tumor control. Subsequent gastrointestinal and bone marrow complications may adversely affect any follow-up chemotherapy. Removal of retroperitoneal lymph nodes is effective but may cause loss of ejaculation and infertility. Chemotherapy is effective with relapses, and the cure rate is near 100%. Follow-up for these patients includes monitoring serum tumor markers and chest radiographs.

Nursing Care of the Patient with Testicular Cancer

Nursing care of the surgical patient is covered in Chapter 14, and care of the patient who has cancer is discussed in Chapter 23. Therefore, this section only covers aspects of nursing care specific to the patient with testicular cancer.

ASSESSMENT. The nursing assessment of the male reproductive system is outlined in Table 44–1. When a patient has testicular cancer, the nurse also assesses fears or concerns related to the effects of surgery and other treatment.

NURSING DIAGNOSIS. Nursing diagnoses for the patient with testicular cancer may include the following:

- **Anxiety** related to the diagnosis of cancer and the anticipation of side effects of treatments
- **Pain** related to surgical incision
- **Altered Urinary Elimination** related to the effects of anesthesia and abdominal surgery
- **High Risk for Injury** (shock, infection, fluid and electrolyte imbalances) related to surgery
- **Constipation** related to diminished or absent peristalsis caused by bowel manipulation during surgery
- **Situational Low Self-Esteem** related to potential loss of reproductive capacity
- **Knowledge Deficit** of disease, treatment, and self-care

GOALS. Goals of nursing care for the patient being treated for testicular cancer include reduced anxiety; pain relief; absence of excess bleeding or infection and normal fluid balance; normal urine elimination; normal bowel elimination; improved self-esteem; and patient's knowledge of disease, treatment, and self-care.

INTERVENTIONS

Anxiety. From the time cancer is suspected, the patient faces threats to self-image and self-esteem that can be very anxiety producing. The nurse must be sensitive to the patient's fears of altered sexual function, loss of fertility, stressful treatments, and the threat of a potentially fatal disease. The nurse can help the patient through active listening, provision of information, and referrals for counseling if needed. The patient may wish to have a significant other included in interactions with the nurse and other health professionals.

Pain. There is no pain in the early stages of testicular cancer. If the disease is advanced or if the patient has surgery or radiotherapy, pain may be a problem. The nurse assesses the pain and takes steps to treat it promptly. Analgesics may be appropriate, but the nurse can also employ other pain control techniques such as mental imagery and relaxation exercises (see Chapter 16).

Altered Urinary Elimination. Some patients with testicular cancer have radical retroperitoneal lymph node dissections. These patients have extensive surgical incisions and usually require intensive nursing care initially. As with any major abdominal surgery, the patient is at risk for shock, infection, bowel and bladder dysfunction, and fluid and electrolyte imbalances. Shock can result from fluid loss and effects of anesthesia during the lengthy surgery. Vital signs and fluid intake and output are measured and evaluated. The patient's electrolytes are monitored, and intravenous fluids are ordered to maintain fluid and electrolyte balance. He is likely to have a urinary catheter and a nasogastric tube attached to suction.

Constipation. The abdomen is assessed for bowel or bladder distention.

Situational Low Self-Esteem. The patient may or may not be rendered sterile as a result of the treatment employed. Radical surgery results in sterility but does not impair erection and orgasm. After radiotherapy, the patient's sperm count typically declines at first but usually returns to normal by 2 to 3 years after treatment is completed. The effects of chemotherapy on fertility vary with the drug used. The nurse can help the patient formulate questions for the physician about the effects of specific treatments on sexual function and fertility. If sterility is anticipated, the patient should be counseled preoperatively about the possibility of banking sperm for future use. Because this type of cancer commonly affects young men, the potential to father a child at a later date may be very important to them.

Knowledge Deficit. Teaching is essential to prepare the patient for treatment. The teaching plan should include the type of therapy prescribed, side effects, management of side effects, and available resources.

EVALUATION. Criteria for evaluating the effects of nursing interventions are patient's statement of reduced anxiety and calm demeanor; patient's statement of reduced pain and relaxed manner; vital signs consistent with patient's preoperative readings, oral temperature less than 38.3°C (101°F), electrolytes within normal ranges, and fluid output approximately equal to intake; absence of bladder distention; absence of bowel distention; positive remarks about self; and patient's accurate description of condition, treatment, side effects, management of side effects, and self-care.

PROSTATIC CANCER

Cancer of the prostate is found in postmortem examination of 30% of men over the age of 50, and the incidence increases steadily each decade to 100% of men in the tenth decade. Although the cause is unknown, genetic tendency, exposure to chemical carcinogens, viruses, gonorrhea with concurrent exposure to a virus, high-fat diet, late puberty, frequent intercourse, multiple sex partners, and high fertility have all been studied in relation to cancer of the prostate.

Medical Diagnosis

Prostatic tumors are usually adenocarcinomas that begin in the periphery of the posterior lobe. Lesions are typically slow growing and confined to the prostatic capsule, but younger men tend to have very aggressive tumors. Prostatic tumors may go undetected until the disease is advanced and there are metastases to bone or liver. Large tumors may cause bladder outlet obstruction, rectal pressure, stool changes, painful defecation, or painful ejaculation. Early diagnosis is important, and patients may be encouraged to have annual rectal digital examinations and blood tests after reaching 40 years of age. Diagnosis may include rectal examination, transrectal ultrasound, serum tumor markers, laboratory screening tests, radiographs, radionucleotide imaging, and needle aspiration or biopsy.

Medical Treatment

Treatment of prostatic cancer is controversial because of the difficulty staging tumors and the unpredictable biologic behavior of the disease. However, the discovery of prostatic-specific antigen as a tumor marker has allowed earlier identification and treatment of prostatic cancer. Prostatic-specific antigen is a product of prostatic tissue. One of the most important uses of the measurement of this antigen is the follow-up of patients after treatment because persistent or rising levels indicate advancing or recurrent tumor growth.

Localized tumors may be treated surgically or with radiation therapy. Radical prostatectomy includes removal of the prostate gland, the outer capsule, the seminal vesicles, sections of the vas deferens, and sometimes a portion of the bladder neck. Most operations include removal of pelvic lymph nodes to check for metastasis. The surgical approach may be perineal or retropubic, the advantage of the latter being that it permits autonomic nerve sparing technique, which preserves erectile function in 70% of patients. The urinary incontinence that occurs in 10 to 15% of men having radical prostatectomy usually subsides within 6 months for 85 to 90% of the patients.

Radiation therapy is an alternative therapy that gives equal results for about 10 years, after which 20% of the tumors recur. Radiation can be delivered by external beam directly on the tumor or by implanting seeds of radioactive gold, iodine, or iridium in the prostate through hollow needles inserted under anesthesia.

Hormonal therapy is used to eliminate androgenic effect, which aids tumor growth.

Nursing Care of the Patient with Prostatic Cancer

Nursing care of male patients should include thorough investigation of risks for cancer and emphasis on the importance of early diagnosis. Careful assessment of the family history of cancer and the medications that the mother may have taken during pregnancy to prevent pregnancy or miscarriage is important. Additional details of the assessment of the male reproductive system are summarized in Table 44–1. If the patient has surgery, nursing care is similar to that described earlier in this chapter under benign prostatic hypertrophy. Nursing care of the patient with cancer is presented in Chapter 23, and care of patients having urologic surgery is covered in Chapter 36.

BIBLIOGRAPHY

Anthony, C. A., & Thibodeau, G. A. (1979). *Textbook of anatomy and physiology* (10th ed.). St. Louis: C. V. Mosby.

Black, J. M., & Matassarin-Jacobs, E. (1993). *Luckmann and Sorensen's medical-surgical nursing: A psychophysiologic approach* (4th ed.). Philadelphia: W. B. Saunders.

Bostwick, D. G. (Ed.). (1990). *Pathology of the prostate.* New York: Churchill Livingstone.

Bullock, B., & Rosendahl, P. P. (1988). *Pathophysiology: Adaptations and alterations in function* (2nd ed.). Boston: Scott, Foresman & Co.

Catalona, W. J., Coffey, D. S., & Karr, J. P. (1989). *Clinical aspects of prostate cancer: Assessment of new diagnostic and management procedures.* New York: Elsevier.

Fonkalsrud, E. W., & Mengel, W. (1981). *The undescended testis.* Chicago: Year Book Medical Publishers.

Gehring, P. (1991). Physical assessment begins with a history. *RN, 11,* 27–31.

Glezerman, M., & Jecht, E. W. (Eds.). (1984). *Varicocele and male infertility II.* Berlin: Springer-Verlag.

Goldstein, I., & Rothstein, L. (1990). *The potent male.* Los Angeles: The Body Press.

Guyton, A. C. (1991). *Textbook of medical physiology* (8th ed.). Philadelphia: W. B. Saunders.

Horwich, A. (1991). *Testicular cancer: Investigation and management.* Baltimore: Williams & Wilkins.

Lederer, J., Marculescu, G., Mocnik, B., & Seaby, N. (1990). *Care planning pocket guide* (3rd ed.). Redwood City, CA: Addison-Wesley Nursing.

Lipshultz, L. I., & Howards, S. S. (1991). *Infertility in the male* (2nd ed.). St. Louis: Mosby Year Book.

Luckmann, J., & Sorensen, K. C. (1980). *Medical-surgical nursing: A psychophysiologic approach* (2nd ed.). Philadelphia: W. B. Saunders.

Martin, F. L. (1990). When the solution is a prosthesis. *RN, 3,* 32–35.

Newling, D. W., & Jones, W. G. (Eds.). (1990). *Prostate cancer and testicular cancer* (EORTC Genitourinary Group Monograph No. 7). New York: John Wiley & Sons.

Ostchega, Y., & Culnane, M. (1985). Tumor markers: Key pieces to your cancer patient's clinical picture. *Nursing 85, 9,* 48–51.

Pagana, K., & Pagana, T. (1982). *Diagnostic testing and nursing implications.* St. Louis: C. V. Mosby.

Pagana, K., & Pagana, T. (1986). *Laboratory and diagnostic tests.* St. Louis: C. V. Mosby.

Rajfer, J. (1990). *Common problems in infertility and impotence.* Chicago: Year Book Medical Publishers.

Reznichek, C., & Reznichek, R. (1990). The problem most men won't talk about. *RN, 3,* 28–32.

Spark, R. F. (1988). *The infertile male.* New York: Plenum Medical Book Co.

KEY CONCEPTS

1. The male reproductive system consists of the scrotum, testes, epididymis, vas deferens, seminal vesicles, prostate gland, ejaculatory duct, internal urethra, and penis.
2. Prostatitis is an inflammation of the prostate gland that is treated with antimicrobials, analgesics, and sitz baths.
3. Epididymitis is an inflammation of the epididymis that is treated with bedrest, ice packs, sitz baths, analgesics, antibiotics, and scrotal support.
4. Benign prostatic hypertrophy, enlargement of the prostate gland that may lead to obstruction of the urethra, may be treated with drugs or surgical intervention.
5. Nursing care after prostatectomy addresses high risk for fluid volume deficit, acute pain, high risk for infection, high risk for injury, sexual dysfunction, situational low self-esteem, and knowledge deficit.
6. Impotence, the inability to achieve or maintain an erection adequate for sexual intercourse, may be treated with psychological intervention, hormone therapy, vacuum constriction devices, self-injection therapy, revascularization, or penile implants.
7. Nursing care of the impotent patient may focus on sexual dysfunction, situational low self-esteem, and knowledge deficit.
8. Peyronie's disease is the formation of fibrous tissue in the penis that causes it to bend upward during erection, creating pain and interfering with vaginal penetration.

9. Priapism is prolonged penile erection not related to sexual desire that requires emergency treatment to prevent ischemia, gangrene, fibrosis, and impotence.
10. Infertility, the inability to become pregnant despite unprotected intercourse over a 12-month period, is due to male pathology alone in approximately 30% of all cases.
11. Causes of infertility include infections, cryptorchidism, testicular torsion, varicocele, and vasectomy.
12. Cancer of the male reproductive system may affect the penis, testicles, or prostate gland.
13. Nursing care of the patient with testicular cancer focuses on anxiety, acute pain, high risk for injury, altered urine elimination, constipation, situational low self-esteem, and knowledge deficit.
14. Other disorders affecting the male reproductive system are hydrocele, hematocele, spermatocele, prostatodynia, phimosis, and paraphimosis.

CHAPTER 45

Kenn M. Kirksey
Esperanza V. Joyce

Sexually Transmitted Diseases

OBJECTIVES

1. List infectious diseases classified as sexually transmitted diseases.
2. Explain why the nurse's approach is important when dealing with patients who have sexually transmitted diseases.
3. Identify therapeutic communication strategies.
4. Describe tests used to diagnose sexually transmitted diseases and the nursing considerations associated with each.
5. Explain why sexually transmitted diseases must be reported to the health department.
6. For selected sexually transmitted diseases, describe the pathophysiology, signs and symptoms, complications, and medical treatment.
7. List information to be included when teaching patients how to prevent sexually transmitted diseases.
8. List nursing considerations when a patient is on drug therapy for a sexually transmitted disease.
9. Identify data to be collected when assessing a patient with a sexually transmitted disease.
10. Develop a nursing care plan for a patient with a sexually transmitted disease.

GLOSSARY

CERVICITIS Inflammation of the cervix (narrow, lower end of the uterus)

CHANCRE A papule that breaks down into a painless ulcer at the site of entry of the organism that causes syphilis

HIV POSITIVE A condition in which the blood has antibodies for the human immunodeficiency virus (HIV), meaning the individual has been infected with this virus

LATENT Dormant; during the latency period of a disease, there are no signs or symptoms of the disease

OPPORTUNISTIC INFECTION An infection caused by an organism that usually does not cause a disease but becomes pathogenic when body defenses are impaired

PELVIC INFLAMMATORY DISEASE An infection of the ovaries, fallopian tubes, and pelvic area

SEXUALLY TRANSMITTED DISEASE A disease that can be transmitted by intimate genital, oral, or rectal contact

VAGINITIS Inflammation of the vagina; can be caused by chemical irritants, dryness, estrogen deficiency, or infectious agents

Sexually transmitted diseases (STDs) continue to be a serious public health problem in the United States despite medical advances. These diseases that are usually spread during sexual activity may occur again and again and can produce serious and permanent consequences. Annually, more than 10 million Americans are infected and more than 100,000 women are left sterile. Eighty-five percent of the cases involve people between the ages of 15 and 30.

Perhaps the high incidence of STDs can be attributed to people ignoring the symptoms because of lack of knowledge about the diseases and to increasing sexual activity, especially among young people. Unfortunately, some people who are aware of the risk of STDs resist taking preventive measures. Infected people do not always inform their sexual partners, so the disease continues to be passed on. Also, symptoms are sometimes not easily noticed, so STDs are undetected and spread and invade other parts of the body.

Nursing implications for the care of patients diagnosed with STDs must focus on the delivery of the same quality of care that is given to patients with any other diagnoses. Some nurses are uncomfortable about caring for patients with STDs. Perhaps an increase in knowledge of the diseases, modes of transmission, types of treatment, and follow-up care will increase acceptance of the patient.

In this chapter, specific diseases are discussed followed by a general discussion of nursing care appropriate for all patients with STDs.

DIAGNOSTIC TESTS AND PROCEDURES

The primary measures used to diagnose STDs are serologic tests and studies of smears and cultures.

SEROLOGIC TESTS

Serologic tests may be ordered to detect infections with hepatitis A, B, or C; syphilis; human immunodeficiency virus (HIV); herpes simplex; and cytomegalovirus. These tests are designed to detect infectious diseases by measuring antigens or antibodies in the blood. Many factors can cause inaccurate results, especially with older tests. Agency laboratory procedures specify the patient preparation for specific tests.

SMEARS AND CULTURES

Patients with gonococcal, chlamydial, herpes simplex, *Trichomonas*, or yeast infections often have discharge from the vagina or penis. This discharge, as well as exudate from lesions, can be collected and studied to determine the exact infecting organism. For females, the sample may be collected from the vagina or from the cervix. The procedure varies with the type of organism suspected. To collect a sample from a male patient, a swab or a special loop may be used. The person who collects the sample wears gloves and treats the sample as a potential source of infection. The sample may be submitted for microscopic examination or for culture and sensitivity tests.

REPORTING SEXUALLY TRANSMITTED DISEASES

Confirmed cases of certain STDs must be reported to the local public health department. The patient is asked to name sexual contacts. Those individuals are contacted and advised that they have been exposed to the disease and encouraged to seek medical evaluation. The purpose of this process is to identify and treat infected individuals so that transmission of the disease can be slowed.

SPECIFIC SEXUALLY TRANSMITTED DISEASES

GONORRHEA

Gonorrhea is one of the most commonly reported STD in the United States. In young adults between the ages of 20 and 24, gonorrhea accounts for the highest number of cases of STD. In children between the ages of 10 and 14 more than 10,000 cases are reported annually. The bacterium that causes this disease is *Neisseria gonorrhoeae.* This organism lives in warm, moist areas of the body such as the cervix and the urethra. Gonorrhea can be found in the penis, cervix, throat, and anus. There is a high incidence of rectal gonorrhea among homosexual and bisexual males. The presence of bacteria in the throat is common among individuals who perform oral sex (fellatio) on an infected partner. Gonorrhea is transmitted through direct sexual contact. It is not picked up from toilet seats, doorknobs, or towels.

Signs and Symptoms

More than half of all gonococcal infections are without symptoms. If present, they are usually more easily detected in males. Symptoms generally appear 3 days to 3 weeks after sexual contact with an infected partner. Males often present with whitish- or greenish-colored discharge from the penis and often complain of a burning sensation during urination. Females may experience vaginal discharge, a burning sensation during urination, abdominal pain, or abnormal menstruation. Symptoms generally disappear after a few weeks, but if untreated the bacteria remain in the body and the person remains highly infectious. Areas affected by gonorrhea may include the pharynx, rectum, urethra, prostate, epididymis, uterus, and fallopian tubes.

Complications

If untreated, gonorrhea can cause sterility in both sexes and infections that may lead to damage to heart tissue and joints. Males may complain of pain that initially involves the penis but can spread to the entire groin area. In females, pelvic inflammatory disease (PID) is an infection of the ovaries, fallopian tubes, and pelvic area and is a frequent complication of gonorrhea.

Medical Diagnosis

Diagnosis requires a complete physical examination as well as laboratory analysis of secretions from infected body parts.

Medical Treatment

Treatment with ceftriaxone sodium (Rocephin) and doxycycline calcium (Vibramycin) or tetracycline cures most cases of gonorrhea quickly and safely. Penicillin is not used as much as it once was because many organisms have developed resistance to it. Erythromycin ophthalmic ointment may be ordered for the newborn to prevent eye infection caused by exposure to gonococci during delivery. Patients should be instructed to follow up with a physician to be sure the treatment was effective. Additional information about drug therapy for gonorrhea is provided in Table 45–1.

PHARMACOLOGY CAPSULE

Follow-up examination is essential after antimicrobial therapy to be sure the infection has been eradicated.

TABLE 45–1
DRUGS USED TO TREAT SEXUALLY TRANSMITTED DISEASES

DRUG	USE/ACTION	SIDE EFFECTS	NURSING INTERVENTIONS
Antibiotics			
1. Penicillin G (Bicillin, Pfizerpen, Crysticillin)	Effective against organisms that cause gonorrhea and syphilis	Nausea; vomiting; diarrhea; pain at injection site; anaphylaxis; Jarisch-Herxheimer reaction: headache, fever, chills, diaphoresis, tachycardia, muscle and joint pain	Inquire about allergy to penicillin. Withhold drug and inform physician if allergic to penicillin. Scratch test may be ordered to assess allergy. Check drug insert for preparation of injection. Give by deep injection in large muscle. Do not pause during injection—needle may clog. Massage site. Have patient wait 30 min after injection in case there is allergic reaction. Tell patient Jarisch-Herxheimer reaction may occur beginning about 12 hr after injection and lasting about 12 hr. Assure patient it is not harmful and requires no treatment. Encourage patient to return for all three injections 1 week apart.
2. Tetracycline hydrochloride (Achromycin, Panmycin, Tetracyn)	Effective against organisms that cause gonorrhea, syphilis, and chlamydia	Nausea, vomiting, diarrhea, pain at injection site, allergic reactions, discoloration of developing teeth	Ask about allergies before giving. Withhold and inform physician if allergic to tetracycline. Contraindicated in pregnancy and lactation. Check patient's medication list for possible interactions. Oral form given with full glass of water. No milk, calcium, or antacids within an hour before or after ingestion of drug.
3. Erythromycin (E-Mycin, Ilosone, Erythrocin Stearate)	Effective against organisms that cause chlamydia, syphilis, and gonorrhea; ophthalmic ointment used in newborn to prevent eye infection	Nausea, vomiting, diarrhea, phlebitis at infusion site, allergic reactions, hepatitis, ototoxicity	Assess allergies; if allergic to erythromycin, withhold and inform physician. Report tinnitus or jaundice. Give oral drug on empty stomach with full glass of water—no fruit juice.
4. Ceftriaxone sodium (Rocephin)	Effective against organism that causes gonorrhea	Nausea, vomiting, headache, dizziness, and (rarely) bleeding. Allergic reactions including anaphylaxis in patients allergic to cephalosporins or penicillin. Nephrotoxicity with high doses or renal disease. Superinfections: diarrhea, candidiasis. Intravenous route: thrombophlebitis. Intramuscular route: pain, induration at injection site.	Assess allergies to cephalosporins and penicillin. If present, withhold and notify physician. Monitor intravenous site for pain, red streak. Monitor stools for diarrhea. Report vaginal or anal itching. Assess for bruising, bleeding.
5. Doxycycline (Vibramycin)	Effective against organisms that cause gonorrhea, granuloma inguinale, syphilis, and lymphogranuloma venereum	Anorexia, nausea, vomiting, diarrhea, dysphagia, fungal infections, anaphylaxis, increased intracranial pressure, photosensitivity; rarely: rash, urticaria, hemolytic anemia	Assess allergies to tetracycline and to sulfites. Monitor food intake and stools. Assess blood pressure and level of consciousness. Report genital or anal itching. Give with full glass of water. Advise patient to complete course of therapy.

TABLE 45-1

DRUGS USED TO TREAT SEXUALLY TRANSMITTED DISEASES *Continued*

DRUG	USE/ACTION	SIDE EFFECTS	NURSING INTERVENTIONS
Antibiotics			
6. Trimethoprim with sulfamethoxazole (Bactrim, Septra)	Used to treat urinary tract infections and *Pneumocystis carinii* infections	Rash, pruritus, nausea, vomiting, unpleasant taste, epigastric distress, photosensitivity, thrombocytopenia, neutropenia, anemia, leukopenia; rarely: anaphylaxis, elevated blood urea nitrogen and creatinine	Assess for itching, rash, fever, sore throat, bleeding. Tell patient to avoid excessive sun exposure. Can be taken with food if gastrointestinal upset occurs.
Antifungals			
Clotrimazole (Gyne-Lotrimin, Mycelex)	Effective against yeast that causes vaginal candidiasis	Vaginal burning and irritation with vaginal use; nausea, with lozenges; hepatitis	Do not use with abdominal pain, fever, or foul discharge. Tell patient to contact physician if no improvement after 3 days. Instruct patient to let lozenge dissolve—don't chew or swallow whole. Apply creams with gloved hand. Show patient how to use applicator. Advise to wear perineal pad to protect clothing. Do not double up if a dose is missed.
Miscellaneous Anti-infectives			
1. Metronidazole (Flagyl)	Effective against organism that causes *Trichomonas* infection	Headache, dizziness, nausea, vomiting, abdominal pain, anorexia, diarrhea, skin irritation, peripheral neuropathy, leukopenia, severe reaction with alcohol	Give with food or milk. Do not double up if a dose is missed. Tell patient to avoid alcohol. Advise to have sex partner treated at same time. Safety precautions if dizziness occurs. Monitor fluid status because drug contains sodium. Urine may be dark. Monitor blood cell counts.
2. Azithromycin (Zithromax)	Effective against the organism that causes chlamydial urethritis and cervicitis	Diarrhea, nausea, vomiting, abdominal pain, vaginitis; dysrhythmias if given with Seldane	Caution if patient has liver impairment. Assess allergies. Withhold if allergic to macrolides and notify physician. Do not give with antacids. Give 1 hr before meals or 2 hr after meals.
3. Pentamidine isethionate (Pentam 300)	An antiprotozoal that is used to treat *P. carinii*—an opportunistic organism that often causes infection in people with AIDS; routes: intramuscular, intravenous, inhalation	Elevated serum creatinine, leukopenia, thrombocytopenia, hypoglycemia, nausea, anorexia, renal damage, bronchospasm; pain and sterile abscess at intramuscular site; phlebitis with intravenous infusion	Inhalation contraindicated with asthma or history of anaphylactic reaction to any drug. Monitor blood pressure, pulse, blood glucose. Check intramuscular and intravenous sites. Assess appetite and food intake. Watch for dyspnea.
Antivirals			
1. Acyclovir (Zovirax)	Decrease frequency and severity of genital herpes infections; is not curative	Dizziness, headache, diarrhea, nausea, vomiting, renal failure, seizures	Ointment applied with gloved finger. Do not double up if an oral dose is missed. Tell patient drug is not curative. Condoms should be used during sexual contact, and sexual contact should be avoided when lesions are present.
2. Didanosine (Videx)	Used to treat infection with human immunodeficiency virus in combination with or instead of zidovudine	Rash, inflammation of oral mucous membranes, fever, and (rarely) pancreatitis	Assess skin and mouth. Good oral hygiene. Monitor temperature. Report nausea, vomiting, abdominal pain.
3. Foscarnet sodium (Foscavir)	Treats cytomegalovirus retinitis in AIDS patients	Fever, nausea, vomiting, diarrhea, abnormal kidney function, bone marrow suppression, changes in blood pressure, seizures, bronchospasm, urinary retention in addition to a number of other side and adverse effects	Monitor electrolytes. Record intake and output. Safety precautions if seizures occur. Monitor vital signs and blood cell counts. Encourage adequate fluids.

TABLE 45-2
GONORRHEA

SIGNS/SYMPTOMS	POSSIBLE COMPLICATIONS	MEDICAL TREATMENT	NURSING CONSIDERATIONS
Male			
1. Thick urethral discharge (purulent green or yellow)	Epididymitis Urethritis	Collect specimen for culture Rocephin, Vibramycin, penicillin, or tetracycline	Instruct the patient that all sexual partners should also be treated. Instruct patient to take complete prescription of the drug (if receiving tetracycline) even if symptoms have disappeared. Abstinence or condom use must be stressed.
2. Swelling and redness of the meatus 3. Urinary urgency and dripping	Infections of Cowper's and Tyson's glands		
Female			
1. Increased, foul-smelling vaginal discharge	Infertility	Same as male patients. Streptomycin may also be used if the other drugs do not relieve symptoms.	Counsel on potential complications.
2. Dysuria (difficulty urinating)	Urethral and labial infection		
3. Abnormal or painful menstruations	Risk of tubal pregnancy		
4. Vulval soreness	Pelvic inflammatory disease (PID); septicemia		
5. Peritonitis 6. No complaints 7. Fever 8. Backache 9. Lower back pain, usually involving only one side			

Nursing care of the patient with gonorrhea and other STDs is covered later in this chapter. Table 45–2 summarizes information related to the signs and symptoms of gonorrhea, the possible complications, the medical treatment, and the nursing considerations.

SYPHILIS

Syphilis is caused by a microscopic organism, a spirochete called *Treponema pallidum.* The organism is generally transmitted by sexual contact but can also be spread through breaks in the skin. It can also be passed through the placenta, causing an infant to be born with the disease (congenital syphilis).

Signs and Symptoms

Signs and symptoms change throughout the course of the disease. If untreated, syphilis progresses through four stages: primary, secondary, latent, and late.

PRIMARY STAGE. A typical lesion, called a *chancre,* is the first sign of syphilis. The chancre is generally first noticed 1 to 12 weeks after contact. During the primary stage, a reddish papule appears where the organism entered the body, usually the genitals, anus, or mouth. Within a week, the papule becomes a painless, red ulcer. Lymph nodes in the area of the chancre may be enlarged but are not tender. The chancre may last from 1 to 5 weeks. When it disappears, patients may erroneously assume they are cured. In fact, the infecting organism has moved into the blood.

SECONDARY STAGE. The secondary stage occurs 1 to 6 months after contact. Symptoms may include a rash on the extremities, chest or back, palms of the hands, and soles of the feet. Pustules often develop that contain highly contagious material. Fever, sore throat, and generalized aching are also seen in this stage. The patient is contagious during the first and second stages.

LATENT STAGE. The latent stage in which there are no symptoms follows the secondary stage. Although there are no symptoms, the organisms are invading the major organs. The disease is not spread by sexual contact during the latent stage but may be transmitted by blood exposure. It is generally 3 years after contact before late syphilis develops, although it may be decades.

LATE STAGE. Signs and symptoms of late syphilis include arthritis; numbness of the extremities; ulcers of the skin and internal organs; and pain due to damage to the heart, blood vessels (especially the aorta), spinal cord, or brain.

Complications

The patient with syphilis may develop severe neurologic problems and blindness and may even die. Syphilis can also be passed from mother to fetus. Fortunately, congenital syphilis can be cured easily if it is detected early.

Medical Diagnosis

Diagnosis requires a physical examination and a blood test to detect the presence of the organism. Tests for syphilis include screening and confirmation tests. Two screening tests are the venereal disease research laboratory (VDRL) test and the rapid plasma reagin (RPR) test. Both detect a protein that appears in the blood when a person has syphilis. Screening tests can be inaccurate because other factors can cause false positive reactions. Also, the tests are not effective until antibodies for *T. pallidum* are present in the blood. This may not occur until 3 to 4 weeks after exposure.

Other tests that specifically detect *T. pallidum* are needed to confirm the disease. They are the fluorescent treponemal antibody absorption test and the microhemagglutination test.

Medical Treatment

The treatment of choice for syphilis is penicillin unless contraindicated. Information about drug therapy for syphilis is presented in Table 45–1. The patient should be told to make a follow-up appointment with a physician to see if the treatment was effective. The patient is advised not to engage in sexual activity until 1 month after completing treatment for primary or secondary syphilis.

Nursing care of the patient with syphilis and other STDs is covered later in this chapter. Table 45–3 summarizes the signs and symptoms of syphilis, possible complications, medical treatment, and nursing implications.

CHLAMYDIAL INFECTION

Chlamydial infection is thought to be the most common STD in the United States. It affects approximately 10 million people annually. The symptoms are similar to those seen with gonorrhea. It is sometimes labeled *nongonococcal urethritis.* The infecting organism is a virus-like bacterium called *Chlamydia trachomatis,* which infects both men and women. This disease is transmitted by contact with the mucous membranes in the mouth, eyes, urethra, vagina, or rectum.

Signs and Symptoms

Symptoms are noticed more by men, and include penile discharge, which is initially thin and then becomes creamy later. This symptom is generally noted 1 to 3 weeks after infection. Another common complaint

TABLE 45-3
SYPHILIS

SIGNS/SYMPTOMS	POSSIBLE COMPLICATIONS	MEDICAL TREATMENT	NURSING CONSIDERATIONS
Primary Syphilis 1. Chancre (round ulcer with well-defined margin); lesion is thickened, rubbery, and painless. If untreated, the lesion persists only for 3 to 6 weeks and then heals. 2. Regional lymphadenopathy: enlarged lymph nodes only in the area of the chancre. **Secondary Syphilis** 1. Sore throat 2. Malaise 3. Rash 4. Fever 5. Weight loss 6. Headaches 7. Musculoskeletal pain 8. Patchy hair loss 9. Pustules of face or feet 10. Generalized lymphadenopathy **Latent Syphilis** No signs or symptoms **Late Syphilis** 1. Generalized papules and tumors 2. Paresis 3. Ataxia 4. Psychosis	Prompt, effective treatment can result in complete recovery without complications. Otherwise complications may include: 1. Arthritis 2. Bursitis 3. Osteitis 4. Liver enlargement 5. Heart disease 6. Meningitis 7. Central nervous system disorders	Benzathine penicillin given intramuscularly in a single dose that is divided into two injections given in each buttock. *or* Procaine penicillin given intramuscularly daily for 8–12 days. *or* If unable to take penicillin, oral doxycycline or tetracycline is used.	Ensure that ordered blood studies are done: VDRL, RPR, FTA-AB. Assess for transient fever, flu-like symptoms, malaise. Provide rest periods. Wear gloves to assess the skin and mucous membranes. Inspect skin changes, lesions. Provide medications. After administration of parenteral antibiotics, observe patient for 30 min for allergic reactions, such as rash, fever, or chills. Have emergency drugs on hand in the event of anaphylaxis. When penicillin is administered, warn the patient to expect Jarisch-Herxheimer reaction. Instruct in self-medication if taking oral drugs. Advise patient to notify sexual partners and to avoid sexual contacts until cured. Stress importance of keeping follow-up medical appointment to assess effectiveness of treatment.

VDRL, Venereal Disease Research Laboratory; RPR, rapid plasma reagin; FTA, fluorescent treponemal antibody absorption.

among males is painful or frequent urination. Females may experience vaginal discharge and lower abdominal pain. Some patients have no symptoms.

Complications

If left untreated, chlamydial infection can result in sterility in both sexes. The sperm ducts can become inflamed and blocked. In females, PID can block the fallopian tubes. Newborns of infected women may have eye damage or infant pneumonia. The silver nitrate drops used at birth do not prevent eye damage associated with chlamydial infection. Therefore, erythromycin ophthalmic ointment is recommended because it is effective against chlamydial infection as well as gonorrhea.

Medical Diagnosis and Treatment

Diagnosis is based on sexual history and the results of laboratory studies. A *Chlamydia* antigen test is used to screen for chlamydial infection. The most accurate test, however, is the cell tissue culture.

The infection is treated with tetracycline, doxycyline (Vibramycin), or erythromycin. Other antimicrobials may also be administered because patients with chlamydial infection may have gonorrhea as well. The culture should be repeated 4 to 7 days after treatment to confirm successful treatment. The patient is advised to avoid all sexual contact (genital, oral, anal) until a cure has been achieved.

PHARMACOLOGY CAPSULE

Review the patient's complete drug profile. Azithromycin dihydrate (Zithromax) interacts with many other common drugs.

Nursing care of the patient with chlamydial infection and other STDs is discussed later in this chapter.

HERPES SIMPLEX

The herpes virus was first discovered many centuries ago. Several different types of the virus are easily passed from person to person. The virus that causes cold sores *(herpes febrilis)* was first described in 100 A.D. and is transmitted through contact with open lesions, usually on the lips or inside the mouth. Prevention strategies generally focus on avoidance of direct contact (kissing) and good hand-washing technique when caring for infected persons.

The incidence of genital herpes (herpes simplex virus, or HSV) has been on the rise since the 1960s. Herpes simplex virus is generally transmitted by sexual contact. Vaginal or anal intercourse and oral-genital contact are the primary transmission modes, but HSV can certainly be transferred by hand contact.

Signs and Symptoms

Symptoms of herpes infection include painful, itching sores on or around the genitals approximately 2 to 20 days after infection. These symptoms last about 2 to 3 weeks. A rash may appear first, followed by small blisters that eventually ulcerate. People often complain of flu-like symptoms and a burning sensation during urination. Herpes simplex virus may recur and is frequently precipitated by anxiety.

Complications

There is an increased risk of cervical cancer in women who have HSV. Babies of infected women are also at high risk for brain damage or death. Premature births and miscarriages are high among women with HSV. An infected woman should be taught to have Papanicolaou smears annually to detect cervical cancer early. If she is pregnant, she should be supervised closely by a physician. Obstetricians recommend cesarean sections for infected women who have active lesions to decrease the risk of transmission to the baby. New diagnostic procedures allow the physician to detect active disease more accurately than in the past.

Medical Diagnosis and Treatment

A diagnosis of HSV may be suspected on the basis of the appearance of genital lesions. Laboratory tests are used to confirm the diagnosis. Exudate from lesions can be examined under a microscope and cultured to reveal the virus. An antibody test called the Herp-Check can detect active herpes. The Herp-Check results are available in only 4 hours. It is used to assess for active infections during pregnancy. If negative results are obtained near the time of delivery, the physician may permit a vaginal delivery rather than requiring a cesarean section.

There is no cure for HSV, but the antiviral drug acyclovir (Zovirax) may be helpful in minimizing symptoms. This drug may be taken orally or applied topically.

Nursing care of the patient with HSV and other STDs is discussed later in this chapter. Table 45–4 summarizes the signs and symptoms of HSV infections, possible complications, medical treatment, and nursing considerations.

TRICHOMONIASIS

Trichomoniasis is a form of vaginitis that infects an estimated 1 million people each year. It is caused by the protozoan parasite *Trichomonas vaginalis* and is usually sexually transmitted. The parasite can survive for hours, however, on damp cloths and clothing.

Signs and Symptoms

Women complain of a frothy, yellowish vaginal discharge that has a foul odor. Vaginal irritation and itching may also be present. Although the incidence of trichomoniasis is less in males, it can certainly occur. Men usually have few or no symptoms.

TABLE 45-4
HERPES

SIGNS/SYMPTOMS	POSSIBLE COMPLICATIONS	MEDICAL TREATMENT	NURSING CONSIDERATIONS
Painful genital lesions Burning during urination	Localized infections Risk of infecting baby on delivery	Treatment is basically symptomatic —sitz baths Acyclovir may be useful in minimizing symptoms; however, there is no cure for herpes	Ensure that patient notifies sexual contacts. Inform the patient that virus can survive on objects such as towels. Assist in decreasing patient's anxiety by allowing patient to verbalize feelings. Instruct patient to avoid sexual contact when lesions are present. Use condoms at other times.

Medical Diagnosis and Treatment

The organism may be detected by microscopic study of vaginal discharge or urine (in males). The discharge can also be cultured to reveal the organism.

Metronidazole (Flagyl) is the drug of choice for treating trichomoniasis. It is important that both sexual partners be treated at the same time to avoid reinfection.

Nursing care of the patient with trichomoniasis and other STDs is covered later in this chapter.

CONDYLOMATA ACUMINATA

Condylomata acuminata, or venereal warts, are caused by the human papilloma virus. They generally affect the genital and anal regions of both men and women. Transmission of the virus is by vaginal, anal, or genital contact with an infected person. There have been incidents of transmission from persons who had no visible signs of infection. The incubation period usually ranges from 3 weeks to 8 months.

Signs and Symptoms

Males generally present with warts on the glans, foreskin, urethral opening, penile shaft, or scrotum. These lesions may be single or multiple. In females, warts generally appear in or around the vulva, vagina, cervix, perineum, anal canal, and urethra. Less often, the lesions are seen on the labia and deep within the vaginal canal and endocervix. In homosexual and bisexual men and women who engage in anal intercourse, warts are common in the anal area.

Condylomata warts are generally pink or red and soft, with a cauliflower-like appearance. Multiple warts can become so large that they obstruct the vaginal opening or rectal canal. Genital warts tend to grow large if they are located in an area that is kept moist by vaginal or urethral discharge. Pregnancy can stimulate venereal warts to grow very large. The reason for this rapid growth is unknown.

Medical Diagnosis

Diagnosis is usually made on the basis of a simple observation of the warts. A biopsy of the lesions is necessary to make a definitive diagnosis.

Medical Treatment

Cryotherapy, using liquid nitrogen or solid carbon dioxide, may be used to "freeze" the warts. Other treatments are destruction with the carbon dioxide laser, cautery (burning of tissue), and surgical excision. None of these methods has proved totally effective in all cases. The incidence of recurrence is very high.

Nursing care of the patient with condyloma warts as well as other STDs is discussed later in this chapter.

BACTERIAL VAGINOSIS

Bacterial vaginosis caused by *Gardnerella vaginalis* was previously called nonspecific vaginitis. The signs and symptoms are genital irritation and itching, a thin gray discharge, and a "fishy" odor. The infection is diagnosed by microscopic examination of the discharge fluid and by culture. The condition is treated with metronidazole (Flagyl). The patient is advised not to consume alcohol while taking metronidazole, to avoid intercourse while being treated, and to use condoms to prevent recurrence.

HUMAN IMMUNODEFICIENCY VIRUS INFECTION

Many diseases causing illness or death have plagued Americans, but it is likely that none of these has had the profound medical, social, economic, and psychological effects as has acquired immunodeficiency syndrome (AIDS). This syndrome is a disorder of the immune system caused by HIV. Human immunodeficiency virus gradually destroys T4 lymphocytes, which are essential for resisting pathogens. As the number of T4 lymphocytes declines, the patient becomes increasingly susceptible to opportunistic infections. An opportunistic infection is one that thrives when the immune system is impaired. Many manifestations of AIDS can be attributed to these infections, but others such as severe wasting are not well understood.

Persons with AIDS are sometimes treated as outcasts because the disease is communicable and fatal and is seen more commonly in homosexuals and intravenous drug users. It is estimated that 1 million Americans are infected. Most are unaware that they are carriers. The incidence of HIV infection in the United States is currently doubling every 8 to 10 months. The National AIDS Hotline (1-800-342-2437) reported more than 361,000 cases of AIDS in the United States in 1993 and more than 220,000 deaths. Females constitute the fastest growing group of people with AIDS in the United States.

Human immunodeficiency virus infection is included here because it is often transmitted sexually and requires precautions similar to those used against other STDs. Advanced AIDS, however, is discussed with disorders of the immune system in Chapter 10.

Modes of Transmission

Human immunodeficiency virus is passed from person to person primarily through sexual contact. Other means of transmission include sharing intravenous needles, exposure to HIV-contaminated blood products and body fluids, and from mother to child during the perinatal period. Individuals at highest risk of infection are homosexual or bisexual men and intravenous drug users. The primary risk factors for women are injecting recreational intravenous drugs, having multiple sex partners, and having sexual contact with high-risk partners. Previously, recipients of blood and blood products such as hemophiliacs were at high risk for HIV infection. Blood is carefully screened today for the presence of the virus, and thus the risk of infection via blood products has been greatly reduced.

Signs and Symptoms

It is sometimes years after exposure before any sign of illness appears. Early symptoms include fever, night sweats, anorexia, and weight loss. A variety of other symptoms may eventually occur that are associated with opportunistic infections acquired because of impaired immune function. The most common infection seen in persons with AIDS is *Pneumocystis carinii* pneumonia. For many women, vaginal candidiasis is the first symptom of HIV infection. In these patients, the candidiasis is often resistant to topical antifungals but responsive to ketoconazole (Nizoral) or fluconazol (Diflucan). Skin lesions such as herpes zoster, warts, and dermatitis may also be seen. Kaposi's sarcoma is a type of skin cancer previously seen primarily in elderly men. The incidence of Kaposi's sarcoma has increased dramatically in younger people as a result of AIDS.

Medical Diagnosis

Serologic tests are most often used to detect the presence of HIV. They include a screening test known as the enzyme-linked immunosorbent assay (ELISA), the Western blot test, and the latex agglutination test. The ELISA detects the presence or absence of an immune response to HIV infection. If the test is positive, the ELISA is generally repeated. In the event the second ELISA is positive, a Western blot test is performed. This test is highly accurate when performed and analyzed by expert technicians. Although the Western blot is more accurate, its tremendous cost makes the ELISA the usual examination of choice. The latex agglutination test can be done in the home and provides results in 5 minutes. New tests continue to be developed, so the nurse consults laboratory personnel about unfamiliar tests and the nursing responsibilities associated with each.

People who test positive for the virus are considered to be infectious. They should be counseled to abstain from sexual activity or to use a condom. It is generally believed that infected patients will test positive within 12 months after exposure, but this area continues to be studied.

The role of the nurse in counseling HIV patients merits special attention. Such counseling in itself carries a number of legal pitfalls. If not recognized, these legal aspects can expose both the nurse and the health care institution to legal liability for their collective actions. To help reduce the liability of counseling, the following guidelines should be followed:

1. Ensure that all available information is given to the patient.
2. Advise of the purpose of HIV testing.
3. Explain that a positive test result means a person has been exposed to the HIV virus but does not mean a person has AIDS.
4. Explain that a positive test result does not indicate that a person will develop AIDS.
5. Inform people whose test result was negative for HIV that negative results do not necessarily mean they have not been infected with the HIV virus. The physician will probably advise retesting if the exposure occurred less than 12 weeks before the initial test.
6. People who test positively should be told that there can be false positive and false negative results.

Medical Treatment

There is no cure for HIV infection, but there are drugs that often slow the progress of the disease. Zidovudine (AZT, Retrovir) is the most widely used drug. The best time to start Zidovudine is under study, but it may be prescribed when the T4 level drops below 500 mm^3. Other drugs being used for HIV infections are zalcitabine (Hivid) and didanosine (Videx). Drugs used to prevent or treat opportunistic infections include pentamidine (Pentam), trimethoprim-sulfamethoxazole (Bactrim, Septra), and foscarnet sodium (Foscavir). Information about these drugs is presented in Table 45–1.

PHARMACOLOGY CAPSULE

Drugs used to treat HIV infections are not curative, so the patient must continue to take precautions to prevent transmission of the virus to others.

Prevention

The best way to prevent transmission of HIV is to abstain from sexual contact. Use of condoms greatly reduces the risk of transmission of HIV during sexual contact but certainly is not 100% safe. Condoms can tear or break or may be ineffective owing to improper use. Patients should be taught to use latex condoms correctly and water-based lubricants like K-Y jelly.

INFECTION CONTROL GUIDELINES. The Centers for Disease Control and Prevention has devised infection control guidelines that originally were meant to be used when working with persons infected with HIV. Because infected people cannot always be identified, the precautions are now required for all patients. Gloves are recommended when handling any body fluid. Masks, gowns, and goggles should be worn when the possibility of blood splattering (multiple trauma victims) is anticipated. Needles must be handled with extreme caution. They should not be bent or recapped. Puncture-proof containers are used for the disposal of all sharps, including needles. If an accidental spill of a body fluid occurs, it should be cleaned with a dilute solution of chlorine bleach. This is believed to inactivate the HIV virus on contact.

PATIENT TEACHING. Nursing care of the patient with an HIV infection or other STD is covered later in this chapter. When a patient has an HIV infection, patient teaching is critical. The teaching responsibilities may be shared by the physician and the nurse. The plan must include the following:

1. Explain how the infection is transmitted and how to reduce the risk of transmission.
   A. Reduce the number of sexual partners.
   B. Do not share needles.
   C. Do not donate blood, plasma, or body tissue.
   D. Follow guidelines for safe sex.
   E. Notify sexual or needle-sharing partners of positive HIV status.
   F. Advise females of the risk of transmission to the fetus. Therefore, the possibility of pregnancy deserves careful consideration.
2. Tell the patient to report for periodic blood tests to monitor T4 lymphocytes.
3. Explain the prognosis with an HIV infection: the infection cannot be cured, but the onset of AIDS may be delayed with drug therapy and a healthy lifestyle.
4. Provide information regarding sources of support and additional education.

Information provided must be current, complete, and consistent with standards of care. Checklists help the nurse ensure that all important points have been covered with the patient. Results of HIV testing are kept strictly confidential. The best guidelines are those issued by the Centers for Disease Control and Prevention.

This chapter has addressed only the needs of the HIV positive patient. The needs of the patient who exhibits the signs, symptoms, or complications that indicate the presence of AIDS are even more complex and are discussed in Chapter 10.

NURSING CARE OF THE PATIENT WITH A SEXUALLY TRANSMITTED DISEASE

ASSESSMENT

Assessment of the male and female reproductive systems is discussed in Chapters 43 and 44 and outlined in Tables 43–1 and 44–2. When a patient has an STD, certain aspects of that assessment are especially important (see Care Plan: The Patient with Gonorrhea).

Health History

The nurse must take a thorough history and also identify high-risk behaviors. A discussion of sexual behavior can be awkward for the nurse and the patient. Before nurses can deal with patients' sexuality, they must be aware of their own feelings and values. Privacy is essential for the patient interview. Questions about sexuality are addressed in a straightforward manner. The nurse must keep in mind that many patients lack scientific knowledge about the reproductive system and sexual activity. The patient may use some words that are considered crude by professionals, but the nurse is careful not to embarrass or shame the patient.

HISTORY OF PRESENT ILLNESS. The history begins by exploring the present illness that prompted the patient to seek medical care. With an STD, common reasons include pain, fever, lesions, or genital discharge. The nurse obtains a thorough description of the signs and symptoms, including onset, duration, and severity.

PAST MEDICAL HISTORY. In the assessment of past health, the nurse is alert for serious conditions or chronic illnesses. It is especially important to document hemophilia. The obstetric history may be significant as well. If the patient is of childbearing age, the date of the last menstrual period is documented. Recent and current medications are recorded and drug allergies noted.

REVIEW OF SYSTEMS. The review of systems elicits potentially significant signs and symptoms, including weight change; fever; weakness; fatigue; skin rashes or lesions; oral lesions; dysuria; whether the patient is sexually active; pain, lesions, or lumps in the genitals; vaginal or penile discharge; sexual contact with a person known to have an STD; altered sexual functioning; and history of blood transfusions.

FUNCTIONAL ASSESSMENT. Relevant aspects of the functional assessment include frequency and variety

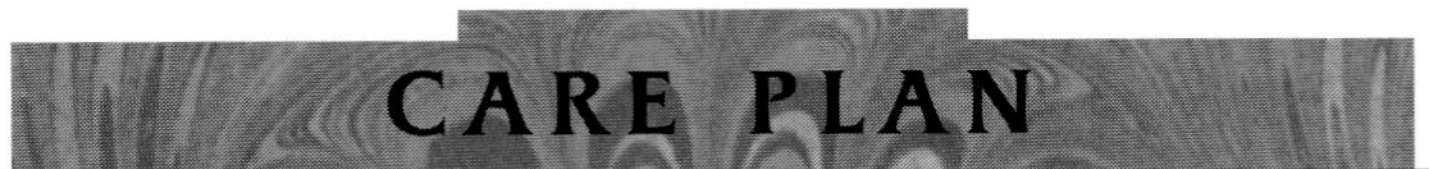

CARE PLAN

The Patient with Gonorrhea

ASSESSMENT

Health History: Miss Carrie Singleton is a 23-year-old teacher who came to the physician's office because of painful urination, abdominal pain, and vaginal discharge of 3 days' duration. She has had no serious illnesses or injuries. She has had 2 sexual partners in the last 6 months, with her most recent contact 2 weeks ago when a condom was not used. The patient expresses concern about STDs and AIDS. States she cannot believe she was "so stupid" and is very embarrassed about these symptoms.

Physical Examination: The physical examination findings are all normal except the genital and pelvic examination. The vaginal tissues are red and edematous with a whitish discharge. A smear was taken for examination and revealed a gonococcal infection. Antimicrobial therapy was prescribed.

NURSING DIAGNOSIS	GOALS AND OUTCOME CRITERIA	INTERVENTIONS
Impaired tissue integrity and pain related to infection and inflammation.	The patient will report decreased pain, and redness and discharge will diminish.	Tell the patient the symptoms should improve with treatment. Mild analgesics may be needed as ordered. Sitz baths may be soothing.
High risk for injury related to disease process.	The patient will report for follow-up examination and remain free of signs and symptoms of complications.	Explain that persistent infection can lead to sterility and affect the heart and joints. Emphasize the importance of returning for an examination to ensure successful treatment.
Anxiety related to possible complications of gonorrhea or stigma of STD.	The patient will express reduced anxiety and will be calm.	Provide opportunity to talk. Help her focus on the source of anxiety. For example, if she doesn't know what to expect, information is needed. If she is trying to decide how to discuss the condition with her significant others, help her solve the problem. Assure her that proper treatment is usually effective and prevents complications.
Self-esteem disturbance related to diagnosis.	The patient's self-image will improve as evidenced by positive comments about self.	Be accepting and nonjudgmental. Assure her that she has done the right thing by seeking medical attention.
Knowledge deficit of disease process, treatment, or prevention of future infections.	The patient will verbalize importance of treatment, complications of untreated infection, and measures to prevent future infections.	Explore her understanding of gonorrhea. Provide information as needed. Emphasize use of condoms in sexual contacts to reduce risk of future infections with gonorrhea or other STDs. Assess drug allergies before giving antimicrobials. Explain self-medication dosage, side effects, and adverse effects.

of sexual behaviors, intravenous drug use, and past infections with sexually transmitted diseases. In addition, the nurse determines whether the patient may be classified as an at-risk-patient because age (e.g., adolescent experimenting with sexuality), sexual preference (male homosexual or bisexual), or habits (drug use) place him or her at a higher risk for acquiring an STD. Occupation may also be significant if the patient comes into contact with potentially infected body fluids. Health care providers at risk for exposure include nursing personnel, physicians, emergency medical technicians, operating room technicians, housekeepers in health care facilities, and medical laboratory technicians.

Physical Examination

The nurse begins the physical examination by inspecting the patient's skin for rashes and lesions. During the head and neck examination, the mouth is inspected for lesions. The neck is palpated for enlarged lymph nodes. The abdomen is inspected for distention and palpated for tenderness. Depending on the setting and the nurse's education, the nurse may examine the genitals or assist the physician or nurse practitioner in the examination. The examiner wears gloves to examine the genitals. A good light source is essential for thorough inspection. In the male patient, the examiner notes the general appearance of the penis, scrotum, and anal area. Any skin breaks, rashes, or redness is noted.

The nurse prepares the female patient for a pelvic examination. While the patient is on the examination table, the genitalia and the perianal area are inspected. The labia are separated and inspected for skin breaks, redness, or rashes. If a vaginal examination is to be done, the nurse ensures that the speculum and other supplies are ready. The speculum is warmed and lubricated before insertion into the vagina. Tissue and fluid specimens may be taken, including tissue scrapings for a Papanicolaou smear. The nurse is often responsible for preparing the specimen and sending it to the laboratory.

If a discharge is present, its color, amount, and consistency are documented. Specimens may be collected for laboratory study. The patient is instructed not to void before collection of the specimen because urine may wash off the evidence. The specimen is handled as infective material, prepared according to agency procedures, labeled, and sent to the laboratory.

Assessment of the patient with an STD is outlined in Table 45–5.

TABLE 45-5

ASSESSMENT OF THE PATIENT WITH A SEXUALLY TRANSMITTED DISEASE

HEALTH HISTORY

Present illness: Pain, fever, lesions, genital discharge

Past medical history: Serious conditions, chronic conditions, hemophilia, obstetric history, date of last menstrual period, recent and current medications

Review of systems: Weight change, fever, weakness, fatigue, skin rashes or lesions, oral lesions, dysuria, whether sexually active, sexual contact with a person known to have a sexually transmitted disease, sexual dysfunction, history of blood transfusions

Functional assessment: Frequency and variety of sexual behaviors, intravenous drug use, past sexually transmitted diseases, sexual preference, occupational exposure to infective material

PHYSICAL EXAMINATION

General survey: Distress, lethargy

Skin: Rashes, lesions

Mouth: Lesions

Abdomen: Distention, tenderness

Genitals: General appearance; lesions; rashes; redness; color, amount, odor, and consistency of discharge

NURSING DIAGNOSIS

The following nursing diagnoses may apply to the patient with a sexually transmitted disease:

- **Impaired Skin Integrity** related to lesions, rash
- **Pain** related to lesions, inflammation
- **High Risk for Injury** related to disease process, potential adverse effects of drugs
- **Anxiety** related to possible effects of STD, reaction of partner
- **Self-Esteem Disturbance** related to diagnosis of STD
- **Impaired Social Interactions** related to presence of communicable disease, social stigma
- **Altered Sexuality Patterns** related to fear of transmission, impaired skin integrity
- **Ineffective Individual Coping** related to stigma associated with STD, shame, anger
- **Knowledge Deficit** of disease process, mode of transmission, treatment, and prevention
- **Noncompliance** with treatment and precautions related to lack of knowledge, denial, anger

GOALS

Goals of nursing care for the patient with an STD are restored tissue integrity, pain relief, freedom from additional injury, reduced anxiety, improved self-image, resumption of social activity, knowledge of safe sexual practices, effective coping, knowledge of treatment and prevention of an STD, and adherence to prescribed treatment and limitations.

INTERVENTIONS

IMPAIRED SKIN INTEGRITY. The patient's skin should be assessed on a daily basis. Changes in lesions are documented. Orders for treatments including topical medications and sitz baths are carried out. Temperature is measured at regular intervals to detect fever that may accompany acute infection. Soiled clothing and bed linens are handled in accordance with agency policy.

PAIN. Some STDs are painless, but patients may have pain associated with pelvic infection, oral lesions, or rectal lesions. The lesions of HSV are especially painful. The nurse assesses the severity of the patient's pain and provides analgesics as ordered. Topical medications, ice packs, or warm compresses are also applied according to the physician's orders.

HIGH RISK FOR INJURY. Untreated STDs can lead to serious complications such as PID and sterility. The patient with AIDS is at high risk for secondary infections because of impaired immune function. Infected patients also pose a threat to their sexual partners. An STD may be passed to the fetus in utero or transmitted during delivery. Therefore, it is important for the patient to receive the entire course of prescribed therapy. The nurse also stresses the importance of notifying sexual contacts so that they can be tested and treated as well if necessary.

Drug therapy itself has the potential for injury. Before administering medications, the nurse assesses the patient's allergies. When injections are given to an outpatient, the patient is asked to remain for 30 minutes afterward in case an allergic reaction occurs. Emergency drugs including epinephrine, corticosteroids, and diphenhydramine hydrochloride (Benadryl) must be readily available. Information about drugs commonly used to treat STDs is presented in Table 45–1.

ANXIETY. People may be anxious about the outcome of treatment and the potential complications of the disease. Anxiety may be heightened by the stigma associated with having contracted an STD, and the patient may feel ashamed. The nurse encourages the patient to verbalize fears and frustrations, provides accurate information, and teaches the patient how to avoid reinfection and how to avoid infecting others.

SELF-ESTEEM DISTURBANCE. The patient's self-esteem may suffer because of a diagnosed STD. The patient is encouraged but not forced to talk about the effects of the disease on self-concept. The nurse tries to guide the patient to focus on his or her positive attributes. If the patient's self-esteem remains low despite nursing intervention, a referral to a mental health counselor may be suggested.

IMPAIRED SOCIAL INTERACTIONS. A diagnosis of STD can be very distressing to the patient who may fear rejection by others. The patient may be angry at the person who transmitted the infection and may be concerned about infecting others. Because STDs must be reported to public health authorities, who attempt to trace all sexual contacts, the patient may also fear reprisals. One way the nurse can help is by demonstrating acceptance of the patient through kindness and touch.

ALTERED SEXUALITY PATTERNS. Patients with STDs may experience sexual dysfunction related to fear of transmission, the presence of lesions, or anxiety. In addition, precautions that should be taken to prevent transmission of the disease may require changes in sexual practices. In general, sexual activity should be avoided until the infection is cured. Chronic infections (e.g., HSV and HIV) require permanent alterations in sexual activity. The nurse explores the importance of sexual activity to the patient. The patient's feelings are accepted in a nonjudgmental way. The nurse explains that emotions and sexual function are closely related and that dysfunction may be overcome by dealing with the emotional reactions to the disease. For persistent dysfunction, the nurse may advise the patient to discuss the problem with the physician. A referral to a therapist who specializes in sexual dysfunction may be made. The patient is encouraged to communicate openly with the sexual partner about the difficulties experienced. Alternative means of sexual expression (other than intercourse) may be suggested. Table 45–6 compares the relative safety of various sexual practices.

TABLE 45-6

COMPARATIVE SAFETY OF VARIOUS SEXUAL PRACTICES TO PREVENT TRANSMISSION OF DISEASE

SAFE
- Mutual masturbation
- Closed-mouth kissing
- Body massage
- Use of own sex devices or toys

POSSIBLY SAFE
- Opened-mouth kissing
- Vaginal or anal intercourse with properly used condom
- Oral sex with properly used condom

UNSAFE
- Vaginal or anal intercourse without condom
- Oral sex without condom
- Oral/anal contact
- Insertion of hand into vagina or rectum followed by ejaculation
- Ingestion of urine or semen
- Contact with blood

From Lewis, S. M., & Rickert, B. D. (1992). Altered immune response. In S. M. Lewis & I. C. Collier (Eds.), *Medical-surgical nursing* (p. 156). St. Louis: Mosby Year Book.

INEFFECTIVE INDIVIDUAL COPING. Ineffective individual coping may be related to guilt, shame, anger, actual or anticipated rejection, or a combination of these. Behaviors associated with ineffective coping include failure to adhere to the prescribed treatment, failure to exercise precautions to prevent spread or reinfection of the disease, reports of chronic anxiety or depression, and complaints of inability to cope. The patient with an HIV infection also must deal with the poor prognosis and often with inadequate personal support. The nurse shows support for the patient by being sensitive, courteous, and nonjudgmental. Inappropriate behaviors are pointed out. The patient is encouraged to evaluate his or her lifestyle and the effects of inappropriate behavior. The nurse may refer patients who have herpes simplex and HIV infections to support groups. A spiritual counselor may also be contacted if the patient desires.

KNOWLEDGE DEFICIT. Patient teaching is essential for effective treatment and prevention of future infections. The nurse explains to the patient what causes the infection, how it is transmitted, how it can be prevented, and why treatment and follow-up care are important. Key points to teach the patient with an STD are the following:

1. Be sure to complete the prescribed antibiotics and return so the physician can determine whether the treatment was effective.
2. Sexually transmitted diseases are transmitted by sexual contact. Avoid sexual contact with high-risk individuals: people who have had multiple sex partners, prostitutes, and those with known HIV or hepatitis B infections.

3. Patients are generally advised to avoid sexual activity until the condition is cured. If the patient does engage in sexual activity, condoms are recommended.

4. Condoms should be worn for all genital contact, not just intercourse.

5. People who have sexual contact with high-risk individuals, people they do not know well, or persons who do not use condoms should have periodic medical examinations.

6. Patients with condylomata are advised to use condoms. Females should have annual Papanicolaou smears, as they are at increased risk of cervical cancer.

7. Patients with HSV infections should abstain from sexual activity when lesions are present. Condoms should be used at other times. It is important for the patient to realize that there are periods of remission, but the condition is chronic. Females are also advised to have annual Papanicolaou smears, as they are at increased risk of cervical cancer.

8. Patients with HIV infections must understand that the infection is not curable but that medical treatment may delay the development of AIDS. They must also be told that precautions must be taken to prevent infecting sexual partners even though the patient may not have signs and symptoms of disease. Because HIV is transmitted through body fluids, the HIV-positive person cannot donate blood.

Condom Use. Many people do not know how to use condoms correctly. At this time, only male condoms are in common use, although female condoms are now available. Key points to stress about condom use are the following:

1. Condoms do not provide 100% protection against disease transmission.
2. Latex condoms are preferred because some pathogens can pass through natural membrane condoms.
3. Protect condoms from heat and sunlight to keep them from deteriorating.
4. Do not use condoms that are brittle, discolored, or in damaged packages.
5. Use only water-based lubricants because other lubricants can cause the condom to break. Spermicides may be used.
6. To put a condom on, hold it by the tip and unroll it onto the penis. Leave a space of about 1 inch at the tip for semen.
7. Withdraw the penis carefully after ejaculation to keep the condom from slipping off and spilling the contents and to avoid unprotected contact.
8. Always discard used condoms for sanitary disposal.

NONCOMPLIANCE. Knowledge does not guarantee compliance, but patients cannot comply unless they understand what they need to do to care for themselves. The nurse provides information about the disease and its treatment in terms the patient can understand. If the patient can read, supplementary written material is advised. The importance of completing the course of therapy and returning for follow-up are stressed, as are complications associated with untreated disease. The nurse evaluates the patient's understanding of the material covered and explores any barriers that might prevent the patient from following the instructions.

EVALUATION

Criteria for evaluating whether nursing goals have been met are healed, intact skin; patient's report of pain reduction; absence of complications; patient's report of reduced anxiety, calm manner; increased positive comments about self; patient's stated satisfaction with social interactions; patient's statement of no unsafe sexual activity; patient's statement of improved ability to cope; patient's correctly repeating content of teaching plan; and evidence of compliance (reduced evidence of disease, return for follow-up appointments).

NUTRITION CONCEPTS

- Malnutrition is common in patients with AIDS.
- Patients with AIDS often use alternative nutritional therapies to bolster immune function, such as megadoses of vitamins, restrictive diets, and herbal remedies.
- The goal of nutritional interventions in patients with AIDS is to identify and correct nutritional deficiencies.
- For patients with dyspnea related to pulmonary infections, small, frequent, highly nutritious meals are recommended.
- Patients with dementia or neurologic dysfunction may need to be encouraged or reminded to eat; some individuals may need to be fed.

BIBLIOGRAPHY

Anastasi, J. K. (1992). Identifying the skin manifestations of HIV. *Nursing 92, 22*(11), 58–61.

Black, J. M., & Matassarin-Jacobs, E. (1993). *Luckmann and Sorensen's medical-surgical nursing: A psychophysiologic approach* (4th ed.). Philadelphia: W. B. Saunders.

Clinical news: AIDS FILE. (1991). *American Journal of Nursing, 91*(11), 13.

Deglin, J. H., Vallerand, A. H., & Russin, M. M. (1991). *Davis's drug guide for nurses* (2nd ed.). Philadelphia: F. A. Davis.

Editors. (1993). To tell or not to tell. *Nursing 93, 23*(3), 50–53.

Hodgson, B. B., Kizior, R. J., & Kingdon, R. T. (1993). *Nurse's drug handbook.* Philadelphia: W. B. Saunders.

Kelly, P. (1992). Counseling patients with HIV. *RN, 55*(2), 54–58.

Kelly, P. J., & Holman, S. (1993). The new face of AIDS. *American Journal of Nursing, 93*(3), 26–32.

Lewis, S. M., & Collier, I. C. (1992). *Medical-surgical nursing* (3rd ed.). St. Louis: Mosby Year Book.

Lippman, H. (1992). HIV and professional ethics: Nurses speak out. *RN, 55*(6), 28–33.

Meyer, C. (1991). Nursing and AIDS: A decade of caring. *American Journal of Nursing, 91*(12), 26–31.

Meyer, C. (1991). New drugs: The class of 1991. *American Journal of Nursing, 91*(12), 40–43.

Nettina, S. L. (1990). Syphilis: A new look at an old killer. *American Journal of Nursing, 90*(4), 68–70.

Pugliese, G. (1992). Universal precautions: Now they are the law. *RN, 55*(9), 63–69.

Shlafer, M. (1993). *The nurse, pharmacology, and drug therapy* (2nd ed.). Redwood City, CA: Addison-Wesley.

Stroud, S., & Dyer, J. (1991). Fluconazole protects AIDS patients against recurrent meningitis. *American Journal of Nursing, 91*(8), 45.

Tannenbaum, I. (1993). Women and HIV. *RN, 56*(5), 34–41.

Touchstone, D. M., & Davis, D. D. (1992). Consider chlamydia. *RN, 55*(2), 32–36.

Ungvarski, P. J. (1992). AIDS patients under attack. *RN, 55*(11), 36–45.

Weaver, K. (1991). Reversible malnutrition in AIDS. *American Journal of Nursing, 91*(9), 24–31.

KEY CONCEPTS

1. Gonorrhea is the most commonly reported STD in the United States, but it often has no symptoms even though it can lead to damage to the heart and joints as well as to PID.
2. Syphilis, if untreated, progresses through four stages with eventual damage to the cardiovascular and nervous systems, the skin, and the joints.
3. Chlamydia affects 10 million people in the United States and can result in sterility in both sexes.
4. Newborns of women with gonorrhea or chlamydia may acquire eye infections during birth.
5. Herpes simplex virus can be transmitted by sexual contact, but unlike most other STDs, it can also be transmitted by hand contact.
6. Because HSV increases the risk of cervical cancer in infected women, they are advised to have annual Papanicolaou smears.
7. Condlyomata acuminata, or "genital warts," are caused by a virus and have a high rate of recurrence despite drug therapy, cryotherapy, cautery, and surgical or laser excision.
8. Infection with HIV causes AIDS, which gradually destroys T4 lymphocytes, leaving the patient unable to resist opportunistic infections.
9. Human immunodeficiency virus is transmitted through exposure to body fluids, and there is no cure for the infection.
10. Most STDs respond to antimicrobial agents except HSV, which is minimized but not cured by acyclovir sodium (Zovirax), and HIV, which may be slowed by drugs like zidovudine (AZT).
11. The best way to prevent transmission of STDs is to abstain from sexual contact, but use of condoms during sexual contact reduces the risk as well.
12. Universal precautions prescribe specific protective measures to be taken when working with people who have infections that can be transmitted through body fluids.
13. Nursing care of patients with STDs may address impaired skin integrity, pain, high risk for injury, anxiety, self-esteem disturbance, impaired social interactions, altered sexuality patterns, ineffective individual coping, knowledge deficit, and noncompliance.
14. Patient teaching is essential for patients with STDs and should include information about drug therapy and other treatment options, disease transmission, abstinence during treatment, and preventive measures.

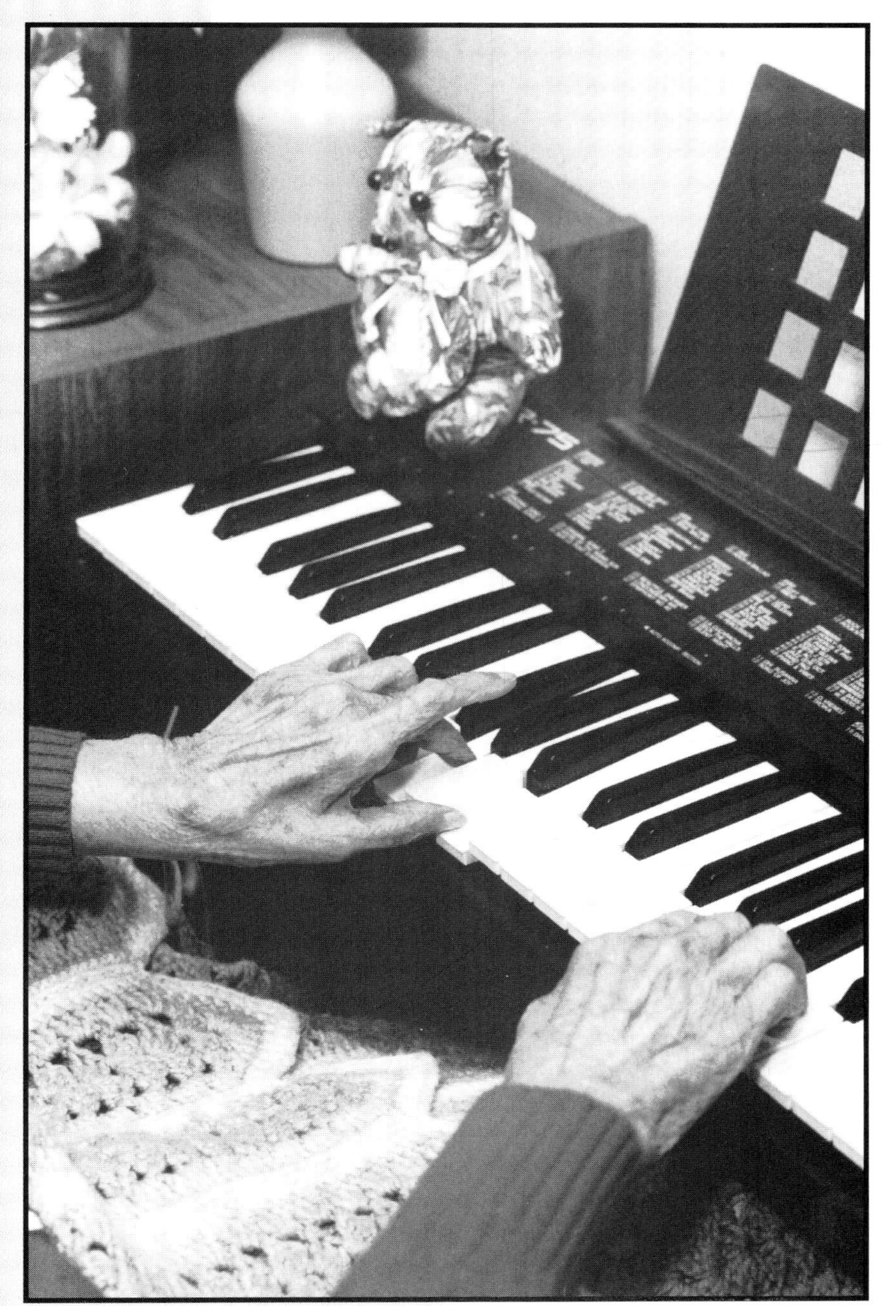

UNIT 14

Integumentary Disorders

Adrianne Linton

CHAPTER 46

Skin Disorders

OBJECTIVES

1. Describe the structure and functions of the skin.
2. List the components of the nursing assessment of the skin.
3. Define terms used to describe the skin and skin lesions.
4. Explain the tests and procedures used to diagnose skin disorders.
5. Explain the nurse's responsibilities regarding the tests and procedures for diagnosing skin disorders.
6. Explain the therapeutic benefits and nursing considerations for patients who receive dressings, soaks and wet wraps, phototherapy, and drug therapy for skin problems.
7. For selected skin disorders, describe the pathophysiology, signs and symptoms, diagnostic tests, and medical treatment.
8. Apply the nursing process to plan care for the patient with a skin disorder.

GLOSSARY

ACNE Inflammatory skin disorder characterized by comedones, pustules, and cysts

ACROCHORDON Small, soft, raised lesion (skin tag)

ANGIOMA Benign tumor composed of blood vessels

DÉBRIDE To remove debris, including necrotic tissue

DERMATITIS Inflammation of the skin

INTERTRIGO Skin inflammation where two skin surfaces touch

KERATOLYTIC Capable of dissolving keratin, the outer surface of the epidermis

LENTIGO Pigmented spot on sun-exposed skin (plural *lentigines*)

NEVUS Mole (plural *nevi*)

PEMPHIGUS Chronic autoimmune condition characterized by blisters on the face, back, chest, groin, and umbilicus

Glossary continued

PRURITUS Itching

PSORIASIS Skin condition characterized by scaly lesions and caused by rapid proliferation of epidermal cells

ANATOMY AND PHYSIOLOGY OF THE SKIN

The skin is an organ that covers the body surface. The anatomy of the skin is illustrated in Figure 46–1. It is composed of two distinct layers: the epidermis and the dermis. The epidermis is the outermost layer that covers the dermis. The base of the epidermis continually produces new cells to replace those at the surface. Epidermal cells produce melanin, a dark pigment, that helps determine the color of the skin. Strong ultraviolet light, like sunlight, stimulates the production of melanin. The dermis is strong connective tissue that contains nerve endings, sweat glands, and hair roots. The dermis is well supplied with blood vessels, causing the skin to redden when surface vessels are dilated. Subcutaneous tissue is beneath the dermis.

The hair, nails, and sebaceous glands are appendages (or derivatives) of the skin. The hair root is located in a tube in the dermis called a hair follicle. The arrector muscles of the hair (arrectores pilorum), located around the hair follicles, can contract, causing the hairs to stand erect and the skin to take on a "goose-flesh" appearance. Also around the hair follicles are sebaceous glands that secrete an oily substance called sebum. Sweat glands, found in most parts of the skin, secrete water through the skin surface that contains salts, ammonia, amino acids, lactic acid, ascorbic acid, uric acid, and urea.

FUNCTIONS OF THE SKIN

The functions of the skin are protection, body temperature regulation, secretion, sensation, and synthesis of vitamin D. In addition, the blood vessels of the skin can serve as a blood reservoir.

PROTECTION. The skin performs its protective function by shielding underlying tissues from trauma and pathogens and by preventing excess loss of fluids from those tissues. A second type of protective function is fulfilled by antigen-presenting cells in the skin that respond when foreign substances are introduced into the skin.

TEMPERATURE REGULATION. The skin participates in temperature regulation by altering the diameter of surface blood vessels and through sweating. To dissipate heat, the blood vessels dilate. As the blood flows close to the body surface, heat is lost through the surface. To retain heat, blood vessels constrict and heat loss is minimized. Sweating helps cool the body because heat is lost as sweat evaporates from the skin.

SECRETION. Sweat is one skin secretion; sebum is another. Sebum coats the skin, creating an oily barrier that holds in water. Sweat promotes loss of body heat through evaporation and plays a minor role in excretion of wastes.

SENSATION. The skin is heavily endowed with sensory receptors for touch, pressure, pain, and temperature. When these sensory receptors are stimulated, nerves convey messages to the brain for interpretation.

SYNTHESIS OF VITAMIN D. Ultraviolet rays in sunlight activate a substance in the skin that is eventually converted into vitamin D.

BLOOD RESERVOIR. The skin contains an extensive blood vessel network that can store as much as 10% of the body's total blood volume. Constriction of these superficial blood vessels shunts blood to vital organs when needed.

AGE-RELATED CHANGES IN THE SKIN

Changes in the skin are probably the most readily recognized of all signs of physical aging. Wrinkling of the skin occurs as a result of thinning of the skin layers and degeneration of elastin fibers. Dryness and pruritus (itching) are common. Skin often becomes paler as people age because the number of cells that produce melanin decrease. Many skin lesions are more common in the elderly. They include the following:

1. Lentigines: pigmented spots on sun-exposed areas; they are commonly called "liver spots," although they have nothing to do with the liver.
2. Senile purpura: large purplish bruises that resolve very slowly; they can result from minor trauma.
3. Senile angiomas: bright-red papules.
4. Seborrheic keratoses: waxy, raised lesions; they are flesh-colored to dark brown or black and variously sized from small and nearly flat to large and prominent.
5. Acrochordons (skin tags): small, soft, raised lesions; they are flesh-colored or pigmented.

Color Plate II illustrates some age-related changes in the skin.

The risk of premalignant and malignant skin lesions also increases with age. These are discussed along with other pathologic conditions later in this chapter.

By age 50, about half of all people have some gray hair. Men commonly begin to lose some hair from the scalp in their thirties, and, by the time they are 80, many men are almost bald. Scalp hair thins in women as well but generally less obviously. Many older women and men have an increase in facial hair. Men may also have increased hair in the nares, eyebrows, or helix of the ear. In addition to aging changes in the skin and hair, the nails flatten and become dry, brittle, and discolored.

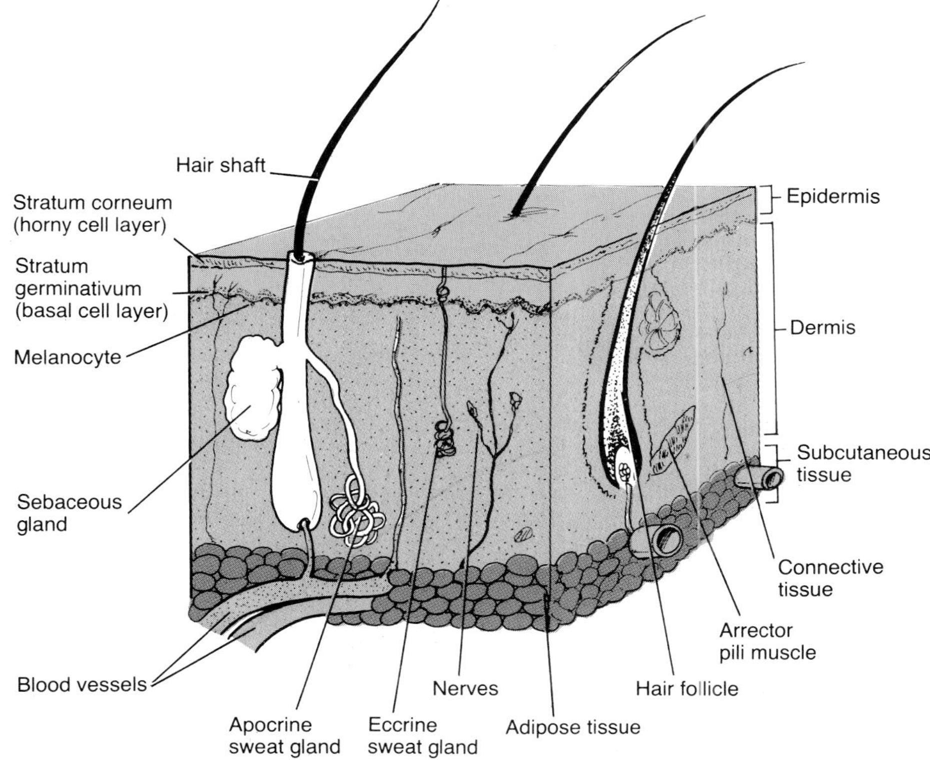

FIGURE 46-1
Anatomy of the skin.

NURSING ASSESSMENT OF THE SKIN

HEALTH HISTORY

Chief Complaint and History of Present Illness

When a patient has a skin disorder, the chief complaint may be discomfort, pruritus, color changes, lesions, hair loss, or abnormal hair growth. The nurse takes a history of the present illness, describing the onset of the condition and any precipitating factors. The progression of symptoms and changes in the distribution or appearance of lesions may be helpful in the diagnostic process.

Past Medical History

The past medical history documents previous skin diseases or problems, current and recent medications (including nonprescription drugs), and allergies. In addition to skin diseases, conditions that may have skin manifestations include diabetes mellitus, cancer, kidney failure, thyroid disease, liver disease, and anemia.

Review of Systems

The review of systems includes additional data that may be related to the skin problem: change in skin color or pigmentation, change in a mole, sores that have been slow to heal, itching, dryness or scaliness, excessive bruising, rashes, lesions, hair loss, unusual hair growth, changes in nails. The review of systems must be complete because many disorders cause changes in the skin. Specific signs and symptoms may be associated with circulatory, respiratory, renal, hepatic, gastrointestinal, and endocrine conditions.

Functional Assessment

Because the functional assessment can provide important clues to skin problems, the nurse records the patient's past and present occupations, exposure to chemicals or other irritants, skin care habits, and extent of sun exposure. Recent changes in the work or living environment are noted. The nurse also inquires about current stresses and sources of anxiety.

PHYSICAL EXAMINATION

Assessment of the skin is done throughout the physical examination. The nurse inspects the skin, noticing the color and variations in pigmentation. Sun-exposed areas are typically darker than protected areas. Dilated blood vessels and angiomas are noted. Table 46–1 describes variations in skin color and the significance of each. Nevi (moles) are carefully inspected for irregularities in shape, pigmentation, and ulcerations or changes in surrounding skin. The nevi are palpated for tenderness. Lesions should be measured and reported in centimeters. If there is a rash, the nurse describes the location, distribution, and characteristics. If there is any drainage, the color, amount, and odor are noted. Terms used to describe skin lesions are defined in Table 46–2 and illustrated in Figure 46–2.

TABLE 46-1
VARIATIONS IN SKIN COLOR

COLOR CHANGE	DESCRIPTION	CAUSES
Pallor	White or pale in light-skinned people. Yellowish brown in brown-skinned people. Ashen in black-skinned people. May be evident in mucous membranes, lips, and nail beds as well as skin.	Vasoconstriction due to acute anxiety or fear, cold, some drugs, cigarette smoking. Edema.
Erythema	Bright red.	Increased local blood flow due to inflammation, fever, or emotions such as embarrassment or anger.
Cyanosis	Bluish.	Inadequate oxygenated blood in the tissue due to anemia, respiratory disorders, or cardiovascular disorders.
Jaundice	Golden or greenish yellow.	Reflects increased bilirubin in the blood due to liver disease or destruction of red blood cells.

TABLE 46-2
COMMON SKIN LESIONS

LESION	CHARACTERISTICS	EXAMPLES
Macule	Distinct flat area with color different from surrounding tissue	Freckle, petechia, hypopigmentation
Papule	Any raised, solid lesion with clearly defined margins; <1 cm in diameter	Mole, wart
Vesicle	Raised, fluid-filled cavity <1 cm in diameter	Herpes simplex, herpes zoster
Pustule	Raised, well-defined cavity that contains pus	Acne, impetigo
Patch	Macule >1 cm	Vitiligo
Plaque	Combined papules that form a raised area >1 cm in diameter	Psoriasis
Nodule	Raised, solid lesion >1 cm in diameter; may be hard or soft and may extend deeper into dermis than papule	Fibroma, xanthoma
Wheal	Superficial, irregular swelling caused by fluid accumulation	Allergic response, insect bite
Tumor	Firm or soft lesion that extends deep into dermis; may be firm or soft	Lipoma, hemangioma
Bulla	Thin-walled, fluid-filled chamber >1 cm in diameter	Blister
Crust	Thick, dried exudate remaining after vesicles rupture	Impetigo, weeping ezcematous dermatitis
Scale	Dry or greasy skin flakes	Psoriasis, seborrheic dermatitis, eczema
Fissure	Distinct linear crack extending into dermis	Cheilosis, tinea pedis
Erosion	Shallow, superficial depression	
Ulcer	Depression deeper than erosion, may bleed	Pressure ulcer, chancre
Excoriation	Abrasion caused by scratching	Scratching with insect bites, scabies, dermatitis
Nevus (mole)	Flat or raised, color darker than surrounding skin	
Cyst	Fluid-filled cavity in dermis or subcutaneous tissue	Sebaceous cyst

The skin is palpated for temperature, moisture, texture, thickness, edema, mobility, and turgor. Assessment of mobility and turgor is illustrated in Figure 46–3.

The nurse inspects the hair for color, distribution, and oiliness and palpates to determine the texture. The scalp is inspected for scaliness, infestations, and lesions.

The fingernails and toenails are inspected for shape and contour. The nurse notes the color of the nail bed and assesses capillary refill by applying pressure to cause blanching and then releasing the pressure. The color should return to normal within 3 to 5 seconds. The angle of the nail base is assessed to detect clubbing of the nails (see Fig. 28–6).

The nursing assessment of the patient with a skin disorder is outlined in Table 46–3.

DIAGNOSTIC TESTS AND PROCEDURES

Potassium Hydroxide Examination

The potassium hydroxide (or KOH) examination is used in combination with a culture to diagnose fungal infections of the skin, hair, or nails. A scraping is taken from the affected area or from a nail clipping and examined microscopically. No special care is needed except an explanation to the patient.

Tzanck's Smear

Tzanck's smear is used to diagnose viral skin infections. The lesion is washed and then opened, and a sample of fluid is taken from the bottom of the lesion. The sample is smeared on a slide and examined microscopically. No special care is needed except an explanation to the patient.

Scabies Scraping

When a skin lesion is thought to be caused by scabies, the top of a lesion is excised with a scalpel. The sample is then examined microscopically for mites, eggs, or feces excreted by mites. The procedure is briefly uncomfortable, but anesthesia is not necessary.

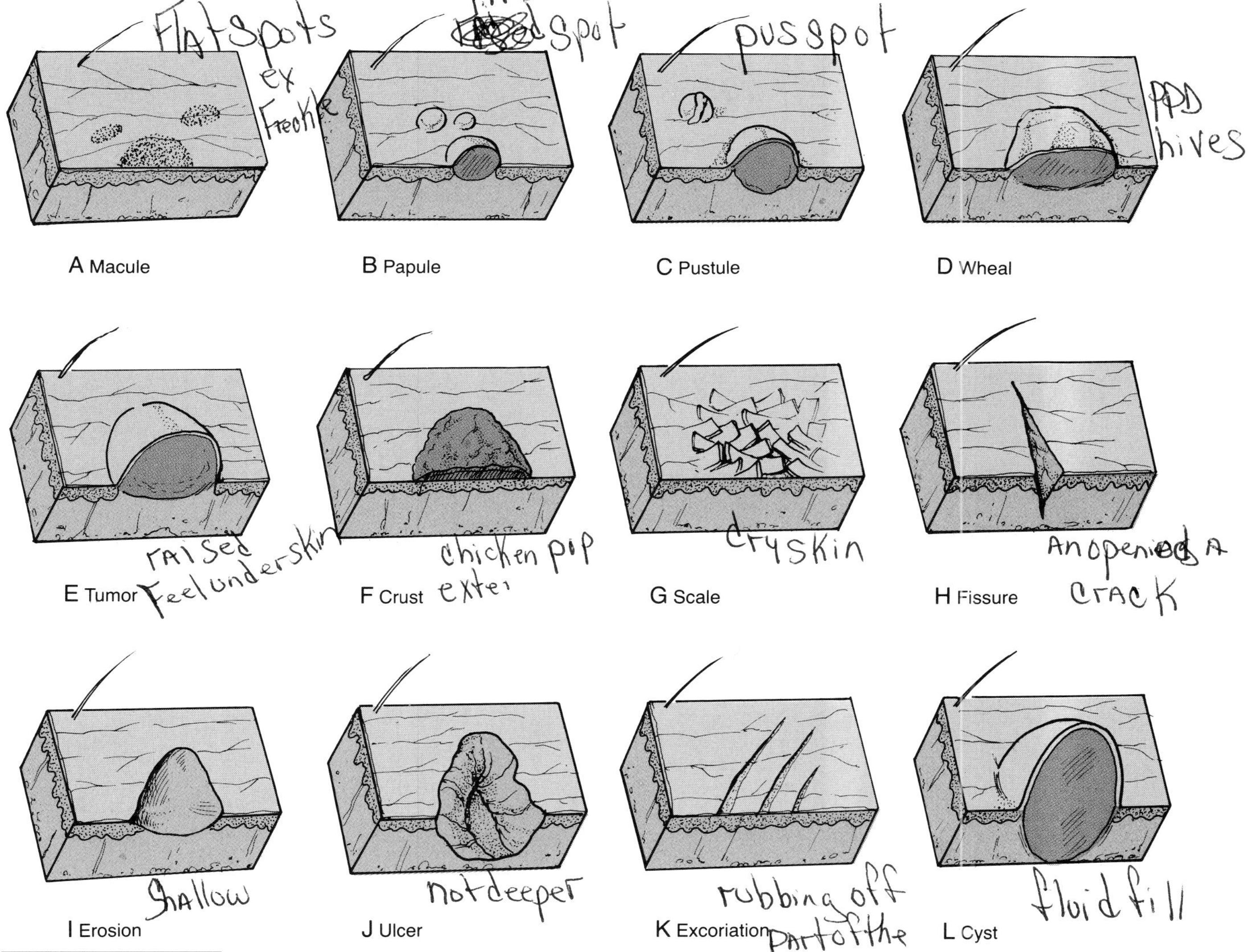

A Macule B Papule C Pustule D Wheal

E Tumor F Crust G Scale H Fissure

I Erosion J Ulcer K Excoriation L Cyst

FIGURE 46-2
Skin lesions.

Wood's Light Examination

In a Wood's light examination, the patient's skin is inspected under black light in a darkened room. This technique permits careful examination of pigmentation and may reveal superficial skin infections.

Patch Testing for Allergy

Skin inflammation may represent an allergic response to some substance. To identify allergens, common irritants are applied to the skin and covered with special patches. The patches are left in place, and then the skin

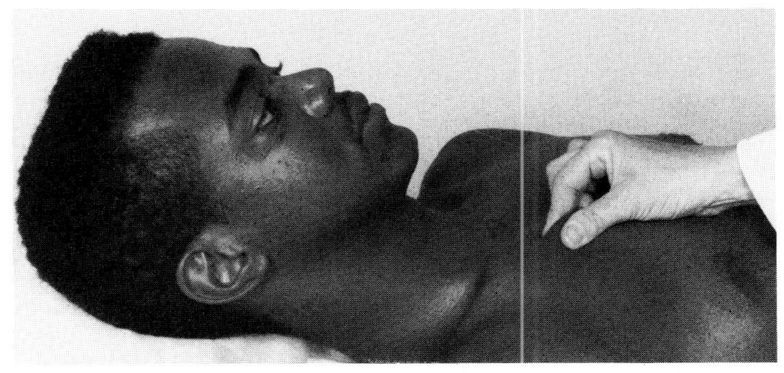

FIGURE 46-3
Skin mobility is determined by assessing how easily a large fold of skin is pinched up. Skin turgor is evaluated by observing how quickly the fold returns to the previous position. (From Jarvis, C. [1992]. *Physical examination and health assessment* [p. 238]. Philadelphia: W. B. Saunders.)

TABLE 46-3

ASSESSMENT OF THE PATIENT WITH A SKIN DISORDER

HEALTH HISTORY

Chief complaint or history of present illness: Pruritus, skin color changes, lesions, hair loss, abnormal hair growth

Past medical history: Skin diseases or problems, drug therapy, allergies, chronic illnesses: diabetes mellitus, cancer, kidney failure, thyroid disease, liver disease, anemia

Review of systems: Change in skin color or pigmentation, change in a mole, sores that heal slowly, itching, dryness or scaliness, excessive bruising, changes in nails

Functional assessment: Occupation, exposure to chemicals or other irritants, skin care habits, extent of sun exposure, dietary habits

PHYSICAL EXAMINATION

Skin: Color, pigmentation, dilated blood vessels, angiomas, nevi, lesions, rash, drainage, temperature, texture, moisture, thickness, edema, mobility, turgor, scars

Hair: Color, distribution, oiliness, texture, nits

Scalp: Scaliness, lesions

Nails: Shape, contour, color of nail bed, blanching with pressure, capillary refill, angle of nail base

reactions are "read" at specified intervals. The sites are examined for erythema, papules, and vesicles that have developed as a result of contact with the allergen. Assessment and treatment of allergies are explained in detail in Chapter 10.

Biopsy

A biopsy is the removal of tissue for microscopic examination. There are three types of skin biopsies: shave, punch, and surgical excision (Fig. 46–4). For a shave biopsy, the skin is cleansed and the specimen obtained with a scalpel or other specialized instrument. The shave biopsy is no deeper than the dermis. Bleeding is usually minimal and controlled with pressure, cautery, or chemicals. A punch biopsy is performed with a circular tool that cuts around the lesion, which is then lifted up and severed. Pressure or chemicals usually control bleeding, but suturing may be needed to close the site. Shave and punch biopsies obtain relatively shallow specimens. For deep specimens, surgical excision biopsy is indicated. Sutures are required to close the defect left by the procedure.

When a biopsy is scheduled, the physician may advise the patient to avoid aspirin for 48 hours before the procedure to reduce bleeding. The patient is told the purpose of the biopsy and what to expect. After the procedure, the site is inspected for bleeding. Direct pressure is applied if necessary. If sutures are used, the patient is instructed to return on a specified date for suture removal. The nurse or physician also tells the patient how and when he or she will learn the results of the biopsy.

COMMON THERAPEUTIC MEASURES

Dressings

Dressings are used to protect healing wounds and to retain surface moisture to promote healing. Specific dressings and wound healing are discussed in Chapter 9.

Soaks and Wet Wraps

Soaks and wet wraps are used to soothe, soften, and remove crusts, debris, and necrotic tissue. Warm water is used, and various agents may be added for specific skin conditions. A wet wrap may be applied to a single affected area or to the entire body. It is usually covered by a dry dressing and left in place for 15 to 20 minutes. Unless débridement is intended, the wet dressing is moistened again before removal. Otherwise, healthy tissue may adhere to the dry material and be traumatized. After a soak, the treated area is dried gently. Topical medications may then be applied as ordered.

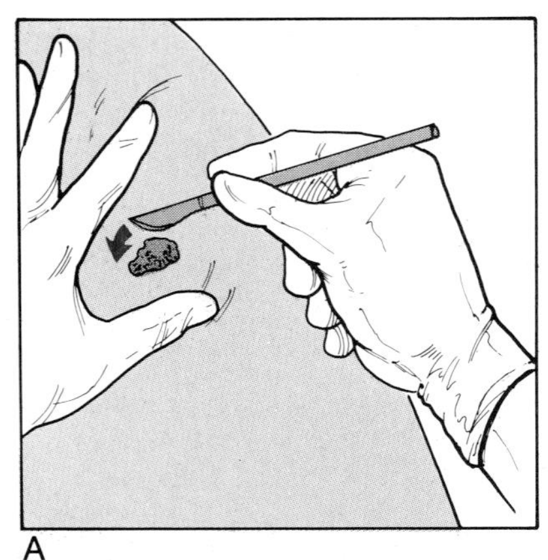

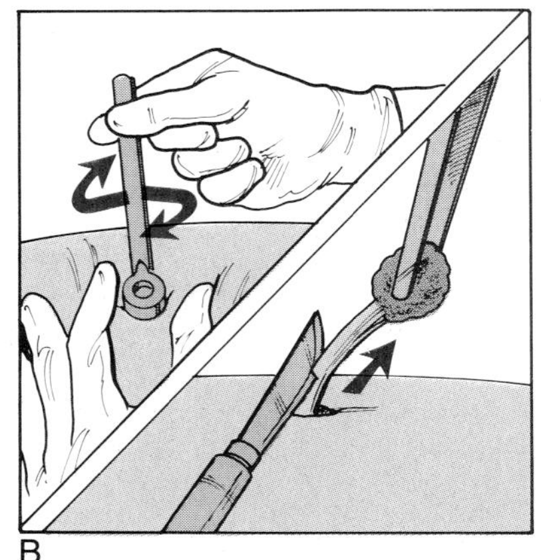

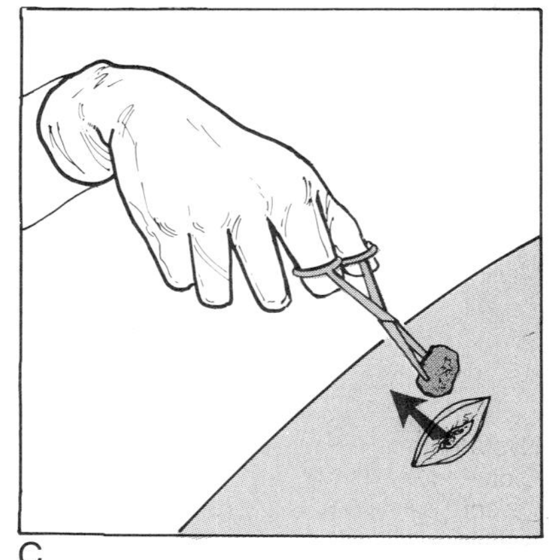

FIGURE 46-4

Types of biopsy procedures: *A*, Shave; *B*, punch; *C*, surgical excision. (*A* and *B* redrawn from Black, J. M., & Matassarin-Jacobs, E. [1993]. *Luckmann and Sorensen's medical-surgical nursing: A psychophysiologic approach* [4th ed., p. 1952]. Philadelphia: W. B. Saunders.)

Phototherapy

Phototherapy is the use of ultraviolet light in combination with photosensitive drugs to promote shedding of the epidermis. Types of ultraviolet light are A, B, and C. Phototherapy may be employed in the treatment of psoriasis, vitiligo, and chronic eczema. It is contraindicated in patients with a history of herpes simplex infection, skin cancer, cataracts, and lupus erythematosus because it aggravates these conditions. After phototherapy, the patient may have pruritus and dry skin. The nurse assesses for signs and symptoms of phototoxicity (redness, vesicles, pain).

GOECKERMAN REGIMEN. The Goeckerman regimen is a type of phototherapy specifically used to treat psoriasis and atopic dermatitis. The patient first bathes in a tar emulsion bath. Then a topical tar product is applied, and the patient is exposed to ultraviolet light.

PHOTOCHEMOTHERAPY (PUVA). PUVA is a treatment that uses a combination of oral or topical 8-methoxypsoralen and ultraviolet A (long-wave ultraviolet light). It is used to treat vitiligo, psoriasis, and cutaneous T-cell lymphoma. For 8 hours prior to and following the treatment, the patient is instructed to wear sunscreen, protective clothing, and dark glasses to decrease exposure to other sources of ultraviolet light.

Drug Therapy

A number of topical and oral drugs are used to treat skin disorders and skin manifestations of other conditions. Topical drugs include keratolytics, antipruritics, emollients, lubricants, sunscreens, tars, anti-infectives, glucocorticoids, antimetabolites, antihistamines, antiseborrheic agents, and vitamin A derivatives. Examples of selected drug classifications and their actions, side effects, and nursing interventions are presented in Table 46–4.

For topical application, drugs are combined with various substances in forms called vehicles. Topical medication vehicles include powders, lotions, aerosols, gels, creams, and ointments.

TABLE 46–4
DRUGS USED TO TREAT DISORDERS OF THE SKIN

DRUG	USE/ACTION	SIDE EFFECTS	NURSING INTERVENTIONS
Keratolytics Benzoyl peroxide Salicylic acid Sulfur Coal tar	Dissolve keratin and slow bacterial growth. Used to treat acne and psoriasis.	Excessive dryness, irritation, scaling, edema, photosensitivity.	Advise patient to avoid excessive sun exposure. Assess effects.
Topical anti-infectives Bacitracin Polysporin Erythromycin Clindamycin Meclocycline	Destroy microorganisms. Used to treat skin infections.	Contact dermatitis. Allergy (rare): itching, burning, anaphylaxis.	Assess allergies before applying. Apply as prescribed after allergy ruled out. Report itching, burning, rash, redness.
Silver sulfadiazine (Silvadene)	Bactericidal. Used to prevent and treat wound infection with serious burns.	Rash, pruritus, burning, pain. Rare: nephritis, anorexia, GI distress, headache, joint pain. Can cause blood dyscrasias, hepatitis, nephrosis, hypoglycemia.	Apply to clean burn surface with gloved hand. Cover burn completely and continuously. Monitor renal and hepatic function. Monitor vital signs, CBC, serum glucose.
Antiviral agents Acyclovir (Zovirax)	Interfere with viral replication. Used to treat infections caused by HSV types 1 and 2 and herpes zoster. Not curative but may reduce severity and duration of symptoms.	Topical form: burning, stinging, pruritus. Oral form: nausea and vomiting. IV form: phlebitis, rash, urticaria, hypotension, hematuria, diaphoresis. Rare: confusion, agitation, seizures. Nephrotoxicity with high IV doses.	Assess allergies. Monitor closely if patient has renal impairment. Measure intake and output. Monitor infusion site for redness. Monitor neurologic status. Use gloved finger to apply ointment. Encourage adequate fluid intake.
Topical antifungal agents Nystatin Clotrimazole Oxiconazole Naftifine	Effective against fungi. Used to treat fungal infections.	Irritation, erythema, burning, rash. Abdominal cramps and cystitis with vaginal preparations.	Apply as directed. Do not apply occlusive dressings without order.
Topical anti-inflammatories Hydrocortisone Triamcinolone Fluocinolone	Reduce inflammation in various skin disorders.	Itching, erythema, irritation. Severe allergic reactions rare.	Do not apply occlusive dressing without order. Apply sparingly and rub in thoroughly.

Table continued on following page

TABLE 46-4
DRUGS USED TO TREAT DISORDERS OF THE SKIN *Continued*

DRUG	USE/ACTION	SIDE EFFECTS	NURSING INTERVENTIONS
Vitamin A derivative Tretinoin (Retin-A)	Reduces formation of comedones. Increases mitosis of epithelial cells. Used to treat acne.	Stinging, erythema, scaling expected. Allergy rare. Occasionally severe erythema, blistering.	Tell patient not to use with keratolytics. Do not apply to eyes, mouth, angles of nose. Patient should avoid sun exposure, use sunscreen. If dryness excessive, decrease frequency of use.
Isotretinoin (Accutane)	Decreases size of sebaceous glands. Decrease sebum production. Used to treat severe acne.	Excessive dryness of skin, nose, mouth. Conjunctivitis, vomiting, elevated serum triglycerides, bone or joint pain, muscle aches. Rare: hepatitis, inflammatory bowel disease, depression. Contraindicated during pregnancy: can cause major deformities.	Tell patient to expect symptoms to worsen at first, then improve. Do not use topical acne drugs at same time. Report severe GI symptoms. Avoid sun exposure owing to photosensitivity. Explain importance of avoiding pregnancy 1 mo before, during, and 1 mo after therapy. Recommend two reliable forms of contraception to be used simultaneously.
Pediculicides and scabicides Lindane (Kwell) Crotamiton (Eurax) Permethrin (Nix)	Kill parasites and their eggs. Used to treat pediculosis (lice) and scabies (mite) infestations.	Skin and eye irritation. Systemic effects with excessive use.	Follow directions specifically. Avoid contact with eyes. Most products are effective with one application, but a repeat treatment may be recommended. Clothing and bed linens must be treated to prevent reinfestation.
Antipsoriatics Anthralin Tar (Estar gel)	Used to treat psoriasis.	Anthralin: erythema, inflamed eyes, staining. Tar: skin irritation, photosensitivity, staining.	Protect skin and clothing from preparations that stain. Most have unpleasant odor.
Photosensitivity drug Methoxsalen (Oxsoralen)	Decreases proliferation of epidermal cells in psoriasis.	Nausea, headache, vertigo, rash, pruritis, burning and peeling of skin. Can cause anemia, leukopenia, thrombocytopenia, ulcerative stomatitis, bleeding, alopecia, cystitis.	Encourage patient to return for periodic blood tests as ordered and to report easy bruising or excessive bleeding.

GI, Gastrointestinal; CBC, complete blood count; HSV, herpes simplex virus; IV, intravenous.

DISORDERS OF THE SKIN

PRURITUS

Pruritus is simply itching. It is a symptom rather than a disease but is very common with many skin and systemic disorders. Therefore, an overview of pruritus is presented here.

Etiology and Risk Factors

The sensation of itching is not completely understood, but it may be triggered by touch, temperature changes, emotional stress, and chemical, mechanical, and electrical stimuli. The severity of the response to stimulation is enhanced by emotional stress, anxiety, and fear.

Pruritus is a prominent symptom with psoriasis, dermatitis, eczema, and insect bites. It may also be present with the following systemic conditions: urticaria, some cancers, renal failure, diabetes mellitus, thyroid disorders, liver disease, and anemia.

Medical Treatment

When the cause of pruritus is known, treatment is directed at correcting the cause. Measures that may help control the symptom include stress management and avoidance of known irritants, sudden temperature changes, and alcohol, tea, and coffee. Lubricants in the bath water and emollients applied after bathing also may help. Medications that are often ordered for pruritus include corticosteroids, antihistamines, and local anesthetics. In some situations, antidepressant and antiserotonin drugs may be ordered.

Nursing Care of the Patient with Pruritus

ASSESSMENT. When a patient has pruritus, the nurse assesses the patient's symptoms and obtains a history that may help determine the cause. The history of the current illness is important since pruritus may be just one symptom of a condition that requires attention. Possible contributing factors to be documented include exposure to irritants, drug therapy, and past medical history.

NURSING DIAGNOSIS. The most common nursing diagnoses when a patient has pruritus are the following:

- **High Risk for Impaired Skin Integrity** related to scratching
- **Knowledge Deficit** of prevention or management

GOALS. The goals of nursing care for the identified nursing diagnoses are intact skin and patient's knowledge of prevention and self-care measures.

INTERVENTIONS. The specific interventions vary with the cause of pruritus. If the patient has dry skin, application of lubricants or emollients may be helpful. Lotion can usually be applied to unbroken skin without a physician's order. If topical or systemic drugs are ordered, the nurse applies them or instructs the patient in their use. The skin is inspected daily to determine the effects of the treatments. The nurse discusses possible causes of pruritus and encourages the patient to avoid them.

EVALUATION. Criteria for evaluating the outcomes of nursing interventions are absence of skin abrasions and patient's statement of correct self-care measures and verbalization of decreased pruritus.

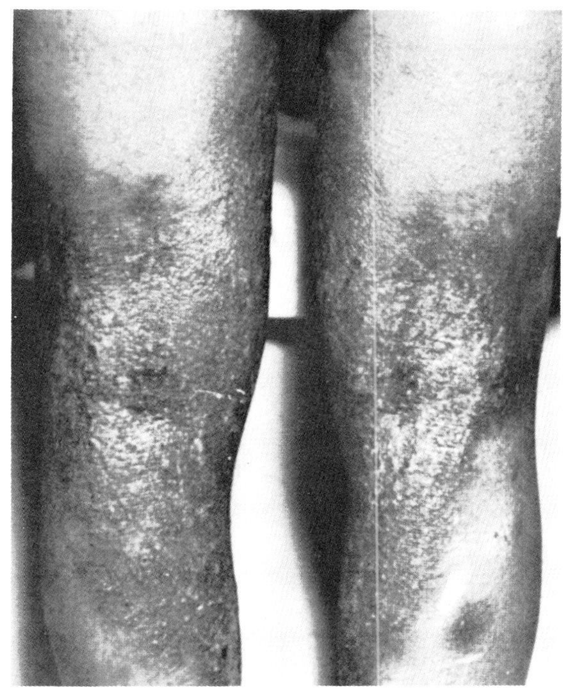

FIGURE 46-5

Atopic dermatitis in the popliteal areas. (From Domonkos, A. N., Arnold, H. L., & Odom, R. B. [1982]. *Andrews' diseases of the skin* [7th ed., p. 78]. Philadelphia: W. B. Saunders.)

INFLAMMATORY CONDITIONS AND INFECTIONS

ATOPIC DERMATITIS (ECZEMA)

Etiology and Risk Factors

Atopic dermatitis, also called eczema, is characterized by abnormally dry, itchy skin that becomes inflamed and is prone to infections. The condition may be chronic and lead to thickening and discoloration of the affected skin (Fig. 46–5).

Medical Diagnosis

A medical diagnosis of atopic dermatitis is based primarily on the health history and physical examination. Other procedures that might be done to confirm the diagnosis are skin biopsy, serum immunoglobulin E levels, and cultures to diagnose secondary infections. If allergy is suspected as a cause of dermatitis, the physician may perform allergy tests to identify allergens.

Medical Treatment

Soaks and occlusive dressings may be ordered to restore moisture to the skin. Topical medications used to treat atopic dermatitis include occlusives, moisturizers, corticosteroids, and tar preparations. Systemic drugs that may be ordered are antibiotics, antihistamines, and corticosteroids. Treatment of allergic disorders is detailed in Chapter 10.

Nursing Care of the Patient with Atopic Dermatitis

ASSESSMENT. Assessment of the patient with a skin disorder is summarized in Table 46–3. When the patient has atopic dermatitis, the nurse specifically inquires about known allergies and bathing practices (frequency, water temperature, use of soaps) to identify possible contributing factors. The physical examination includes assessment of the skin for moisture and abrasions.

NURSING DIAGNOSIS. Nursing diagnoses for the patient with atopic dermatitis may include the following:

- **Impaired Skin Integrity** related to excessive dryness, scratching
- **High Risk for Infection** related to break in skin, decreased resistance to infection
- **Body Image Disturbance** related to lesions
- **Knowledge Deficit** of self-care practices to prevent and treat dermatitis

GOALS. Nursing goals for the identified diagnoses are improved skin integrity, absence of skin lesions and infection, improved body image, and patient's knowledge of self-care practices.

INTERVENTIONS

Impaired Skin Integrity. Measures that decrease itching and moisturize the skin help to maintain skin integrity. The patient is encouraged to maintain the room temperature at 68 to 75°F with 45 to 55% humidity. The patient is also instructed to avoid possible irritants. New clothing should be washed before wearing. Mild detergent should be used for laundry, and clothes rinsed twice. Open-weave, loose clothing is recommended. Moisturizers and sunscreens are advised. If drugs are ordered for pruritus, the nurse administers them or instructs the patient in self-medication. Skin integrity and hydration are assessed on an ongoing basis.

High Risk for Infection. Any break in the skin presents a portal for pathogens. The nurse inspects the skin and reports new lesions to the physician. The temperature is monitored for elevation that may reflect a systemic infection. The patient is taught the importance of protecting the skin from trauma. If scratching is a problem, the fingernails need to be cut short and kept smooth. Gloves or mittens may help prevent traumatic scratching during sleep or in the confused person. Antibiotics are administered as ordered.

Body Image Disturbance. The nurse demonstrates acceptance of the patient's appearance through attentive care and touch. The patient and family are taught that dermatitis is not contagious and is not caused by poor hygiene. The nurse may ask the patient about concerns that he or she has about the skin disorder. If the patient is very stressed, the nurse explores coping strategies that may help.

Knowledge Deficit. Patient teaching includes facts about dermatitis: causes, contributing factors, and treatment. Measures to protect the skin and decrease inflammation are explained. If drugs are ordered, the nurse reinforces the instructions and advises the patient of any specific consideration for the specific drug.

EVALUATION. Criteria for goal achievement are intact, moist skin; absence of fever, decreasing redness, and drainage; positive patient statements about self; and patient's statement of correct self-care measures.

CONTACT DERMATITIS

Contact dermatitis is an inflammatory condition caused by contact with a substance that triggers an allergic response. Allergic and immune disorders are addressed in Chapter 10.

SEBORRHEIC DERMATITIS

Etiology and Risk Factors

Seborrheic dermatitis is a chronic inflammatory disease of the skin caused by excess production of sebum. It usually affects the scalp, eyebrows, eyelids, lips, ears, sternal area, axillae, umbilicus, groin, gluteal crease, and area under the breasts. Seborrheic dermatitis of the scalp is called dandruff. Areas affected by this condition may have fine powdery scales, thick crusts, or oily patches. Scales may be white, yellowish, or reddish. Pruritus is common. The condition is aggravated by emotional stress.

Medical Diagnosis

Diagnosis of seborrheic dermatitis is based on data obtained in the health history and physical examination.

Medical Treatment

Seborrheic dermatitis of the scalp is treated with medicated shampoos used two or three times a week. Appropriate shampoos are those that contain selenium sulfide (Selsun), tar, zinc pyrithionate, or resorcin. Some corticosteroid solutions also may be prescribed. Sites other than the scalp may be treated with corticosteroid creams and topical antibiotics.

Nursing Care of the Patient with Seborrheic Dermatitis

Although seborrheic dermatitis does not require inpatient treatment, it is a common condition that the nurse encounters among patients hospitalized for other reasons.

ASSESSMENT. The assessment includes determination of symptoms and identification of treatments being used. The affected areas are inspected for scales and crusts.

NURSING DIAGNOSIS. The primary nursing diagnosis for seborrheic dermatitis is knowledge deficit of treatment. Patients with severe cases may also experience body image disturbance since the condition may affect the appearance.

GOALS. The goal of nursing care is patient's knowledge of measures to relieve symptoms. For the patient who has a body image disturbance, the goal is improved patient appearance and improved body image.

INTERVENTIONS. The nurse explains the condition and reinforces the physician's instructions for treatment. Measures to relieve pruritus, as described earlier in this chapter, may be suggested. The nurse assesses the patient's concerns about the condition and emphasizes that seborrheic dermatitis can be controlled with treatment. Acceptance of the patient is demonstrated by genuine interest and use of touch.

EVALUATION. The criterion for determining goal achievement is patient's verbalization of appropriate treatment. To evaluate improved patient appearance and improved body image, the nurse observes for decreasing signs of the condition and for statements reflecting a positive view of self.

PSORIASIS

Etiology and Risk Factors

Psoriasis is characterized by bright-red lesions that may be covered with silvery scales (Fig. 46–6). The condition, caused by rapid proliferation of epidermal cells, is usually chronic, with cycles of exacerbations and remissions. Psoriasis may affect a limited area or may be extensive. Some people have systemic effects of the disease, such as psoriatic arthritis.

Medical Diagnosis

Psoriasis is diagnosed by the presence of the characteristic lesions.

Medical Treatment

Patients with mild psoriasis are usually treated with topical medications: tar derivatives, corticosteroids, and keratolytics. Anthralin (Anthra-Derm) may be used to remove heavy scales. It is applied to the lesions without contact with normal skin. After a specified period of time, the medication is removed with tissues. The patient removes the residue by showering or bathing. The medication must be handled carefully since it stains hair, skin, fingernails, furniture, and bathroom fixtures. Some preparations are now available that do not stain (Estar gel). More severe psoriasis may be treated with whole-body radiation, etretinate (Tegison), or methotrexate.

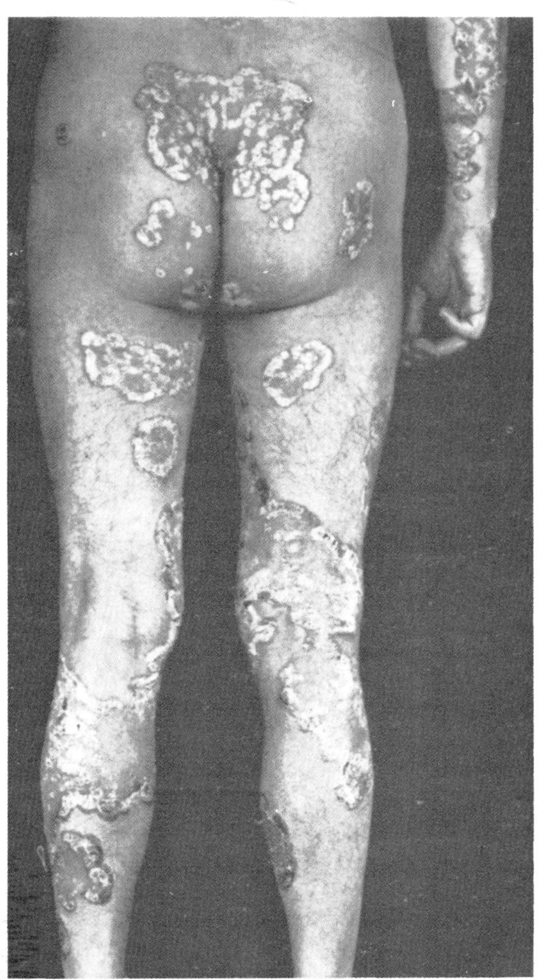

FIGURE 46-6

Psoriasis. (From Domonkos, A. N., Arnold, H. L., & Odom, R. B. [1982]. *Andrews' diseases of the skin* [7th ed., p. 226]. Philadelphia: W. B. Saunders.)

PHARMACOLOGY CAPSULE

Caution patients that anthralin (Anthra-Derm) can stain normal skin, hair, fingernails, furniture, and bathroom fixtures.

Nursing Care of the Patient with Psoriasis

ASSESSMENT. Assessment of the patient with psoriasis includes a description of symptoms and identification of treatments being used (see Care Plan: The Patient with Psoriasis). The affected areas are inspected for lesions and scales. Joint pain or stiffness is documented since the condition may cause arthritis. The functional assessment explores the impact of psoriasis on the patient's everyday life and the coping strategies used.

NURSING DIAGNOSIS. Nursing diagnoses for the patient with psoriasis may include the following:

- **Knowledge Deficit** of condition, treatment
- **Body Image Disturbance** related to lesions and scales on skin
- **Social Isolation** related to embarrassment about skin lesions

GOALS. The goals of nursing care are patient's knowledge of measures to relieve symptoms, improved body image, and maintenance of social contacts.

INTERVENTIONS

Knowledge Deficit. The focus of nursing care for the patient with psoriasis is patient education. The patient and family need to know that the condition is not contagious and usually responds to treatment. The nurse teaches the patient about the prescribed medications and treatments. The patient is told to report signs of secondary infection (fever, purulent discharge, increased redness) to the physician. The nurse also encourages adequate rest, good nutrition, and stress management.

Body Image Disturbance. The patient is given the opportunity to express feelings about psoriasis and the effects on his or her life. The nurse demonstrates acceptance of the patient's appearance and the feelings that are expressed. Learning to manage the condition

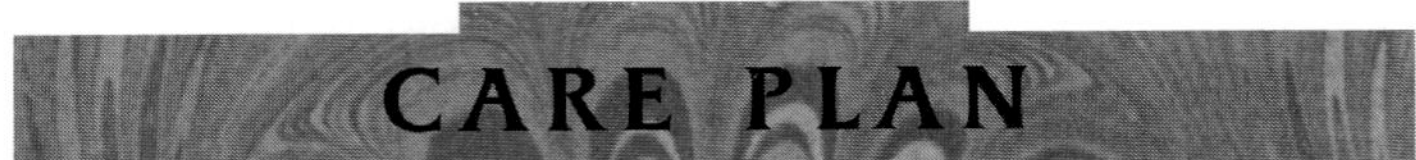

The Patient with Psoriasis

ASSESSMENT

Health History: Mike Pickell is a 45-year-old police officer. He came to the physician's office because of a "rash" on his trunk. He reports that he is in good health and has had no major injuries or illnesses except a left knee injury sustained in a fall as a teenager. He is taking no medications but is allergic to penicillin. He is alarmed at the "rash" and is afraid it might spread and that it might be something serious. The physician diagnoses psoriasis. Mr. Pickell is divorced and enjoys socializing, especially dancing. He is concerned about how people might react to his condition.

Physical Examination: Vital signs: temperature, 98.2°F orally; pulse, 84; respiration, 16; blood pressure, 144/88. Height, 5′10″. Weight, 164 lb. He is alert and oriented but mildly anxious. The skin on the face and extremities is normal. Bright-red lesions with silvery scales are distributed over the anterior and posterior chest, abdomen, buttocks, and hands. Heart and breath sounds are normal. The abdomen is soft, with bowel sounds present in all four quadrants. There is full range of motion of all joints with crepitation in left knee. Peripheral pulses are strong and symmetric. The extremities are warm and dry.

NURSING DIAGNOSIS	GOALS AND OUTCOME CRITERIA	INTERVENTIONS
Knowledge deficit of psoriasis, treatment.	The patient will correctly describe psoriasis and prescribed treatment measures.	Explain that psoriasis typically has periods of exacerbation and remission, that it is not contagious, and that symptoms can be improved with treatment. Explain the prescribed treatment, including proper application of topical medications and side and adverse effects of drug therapy. For oral drugs, provide information about schedule as well as adverse and side effects. Tell the patient signs of secondary infection (fever, purulent drainage, increased redness) that should be reported to the physician. Encourage patient to plan for adequate rest and to eat a balanced diet. Explore stress management strategies. Refer to mental health counselor if needed. Supplement teaching plan with written material.
Body image disturbance related to lesions and scales on skin.	The patient's body image will improve as evidenced by positive statements about self.	Demonstrate acceptance of the patient by eye contact and touch. Be aware of personal reaction to lesions. Encourage patient to share feelings about condition. Help the patient feel "in control" by providing information about management of psoriasis.
Social isolation related to embarrassment about skin lesions.	The patient will continue social activities and identify strategies to deal with social situations.	Explore how the patient thinks others will react to his condition. Role-play strategies to use in social situations. Encourage continued activity. Emphasize expected improvement.

can help the patient feel more hopeful, realizing that remission will occur.

Social Isolation. The patient is encouraged to maintain social contacts and to plan strategies to deal with exacerbations without undue stress.

EVALUATION. Criteria for evaluating the outcomes of nursing interventions are patient's descriptions of proper self-care, patient's efforts to improve appearance and positive remarks about self, and patient's continued involvement in social activities.

INTERTRIGO

Etiology and Risk Factors

Intertrigo is inflammation of the skin where two skin surfaces touch. Sites commonly affected are the axillae, abdominal skin folds, and area under the breasts. The inflamed skin is often the site of *Candida albicans* ("yeast") infections.

Medical Diagnosis and Treatment

The medical diagnosis is based on the site and appearance of the inflamed skin, and the presence of *C. albicans* is confirmed by potassium hydroxide examination and culture of skin scrapings. If the skin is not broken, it can be washed with water twice daily. The area is then rinsed and patted dry. Talc or cellulose powder may be applied. Cornstarch is contraindicated because it supports the growth of *C. albicans.* For severe inflammation, a topical corticosteroid may be ordered.

Nursing Care of the Patient with Intertrigo

ASSESSMENT. Intertrigo is fairly common among patients in long-term care facilities. The nurse investigates complaints of pain, irritation, or redness in body folds. Body temperature is monitored to detect possible infection. Susceptible areas (axillae, groin, beneath breasts, abdominal skin folds) are inspected daily.

NURSING DIAGNOSIS. Nursing diagnoses for the patient with intertrigo include the following:

- **High Risk for Impaired Skin Integrity** related to inflammation
- **High Risk for Infection** related to moist environment, broken skin

GOALS. Goals of nursing care for the patient with intertrigo are improved skin integrity and absence of signs and symptoms of infection.

INTERVENTIONS. Areas where skin surfaces are in close contact must be kept clean and dry. Topical medications (antifungals and corticosteroids) are applied as ordered. Increasing redness and tenderness, fever, and broken skin are reported to the physician.

EVALUATION. The criteria for evaluating the outcomes of nursing interventions are intact skin without redness and absence of fever, pain, or edema.

FUNGAL INFECTIONS

Etiology and Risk Factors

Humans are susceptible to a number of fungal infections. Superficial infections of the skin and mucous membranes caused by fungi include tinea pedis (athlete's foot), tinea manus (hand), tinea cruris (groin), tinea corporis (scalp), tinea barbae (beard), and candidiasis, which can affect the skin, mouth, vagina, gastrointestinal tract, and lungs.

The organisms that cause tinea infections take advantage of trauma in moist, warm tissue. Some organisms can be spread through direct contact or by inanimate objects. Lesions vary but may be scaly patches with raised borders. Pruritus is a common symptom of tinea. Tinea capitis, tinea corporis, and tinea pedis are rather easily spread by sharing contaminated objects.

Candidiasis, commonly called a yeast infection, is caused by *C. albicans.* Patients at risk for candidiasis include those who are pregnant, malnourished, immunosuppressed, or taking antibiotics or oral contraceptives. People with diabetes mellitus are also at risk for this disease. Common sites affected are the mouth, vagina, and skin. The skin around an ostomy site also is susceptible to candidiasis owing to the constant moisture there. Infections of the mucous membranes are manifested as red lesions with white plaques. Skin infections with *C. albicans* are seen as moist red lesions. The lesions are often found in folds of body tissue (see Intertrigo).

Medical Diagnosis

Fungal infections are usually diagnosed on the basis of the history and physical examination but may be confirmed by microscopic examination of skin scrapings using a potassium hydroxide wet mount preparation.

Medical Treatment

Fungal infections are treated with antifungal powders and creams. Wet compresses and keratolytics may be ordered to soften scales with some tinea infections. Oral candidiasis is treated with nystatin in the form of mouthwash or lozenges or amphotericin B.

Nursing Care of the Patient with a Fungal Infection

ASSESSMENT. The nursing assessment identifies conditions that might make a person susceptible to fungal infections: diabetes mellitus, malnutrition, and immunosuppression. Antibiotic therapy, another risk factor, is noted. During the physical examination, the nurse inspects the skin and mucous membranes for lesions. Creamy white lesions that can be scraped off easily are characteristic of oral candidiasis.

PHARMACOLOGY CAPSULE

Antibiotic therapy eliminates the microorganisms that normally control fungal growth, making the patient susceptible to fungal infections.

NURSING DIAGNOSIS. Nursing diagnoses for a patient with a superficial fungal infection may include the following:

- **Body Image Disturbance** related to skin lesions
- **Altered Oral Mucous Membrane** related to oral candidiasis
- **Knowledge Deficit** of prevention, causes, and treatment of fungal infections

GOALS. Goals for nursing care of the patient with a fungal infection are improved body image, healthy oral mucous membranes, and patient's knowledge of prevention, causes, and treatment of specific infection.

INTERVENTIONS

Body Image Disturbance. The nurse must be sensitive to the patient's reaction to a skin infection. Visible lesions may be embarrassing to the patient. If the genitalia are affected, the patient may think the symptoms are due to a sexually transmitted disease. The nurse explains the cause of the infection, how it is treated, whether it is contagious, and how transmission and reinfection can be avoided. The affected areas of the skin are kept as clean and dry as possible. A cool environment helps by reducing perspiration. Eradication of candidiasis infections in bedridden patients can be especially challenging. The patient must be repositioned frequently to permit evaporation of moisture. The thighs can be separated by using a pillow between the knees, and a folded cloth may be placed beneath pendulous breasts. Prescribed medications are administered, or the patient is taught self-medication.

Altered Oral Mucous Membrane. The nurse instructs the patient with oral candidiasis in the proper use of prescribed medications. Mouthwashes may be swished to coat all oral surfaces before swallowing. Lozenges should be dissolved in the mouth. If the patient wears dentures, they should be soaked in an antifungal solution.

Knowledge Deficit. Patients with tinea infections are advised to avoid sharing personal items such as hairbrushes and clothing. They should also dry thoroughly after bathing and wear absorbent underwear and socks.

EVALUATION. Criteria for evaluating the outcomes of nursing care for a patient with a fungal infection include absence of skin lesions and patient's positive statements about appearance, absence of oral lesions, and patient's description of self-care measures to treat infection and prevent reinfection.

ACNE

Etiology and Risk Factors

Acne is a skin condition that affects the hair follicles and sebaceous glands. It is characterized by comedones (whiteheads and blackheads), pustules, and cysts. These lesions most often develop on the face, neck, and upper trunk.

Acne lesions develop when androgenic hormones cause increased sebum production and bacteria proliferate, causing hair follicles to become blocked and inflamed. Despite popular opinion, acne is not caused by fatty foods, chocolate, or poor hygiene. Acne commonly begins in adolescence and may last into adulthood. Most cases are mild, but serious cases with extensive inflammation can cause permanent scarring.

Medical Diagnosis

Acne is diagnosed on the basis of the health history and physical examination findings.

Medical Treatment

Treatment varies with the severity of the condition. Mild cases may respond very well to topical medications, including antibiotics, benzoyl peroxide, or tretinoin (Retin-A). If these agents do not adequately control acne, oral antibiotics (usually tetracycline or erythromycin) may be given over a period of several months. Estrogen may also be prescribed to counteract the effects of androgenic hormones. If acne is severe and unresponsive to all of these treatments, isotretinoin (Accutane) may be prescribed.

PHARMACOLOGY CAPSULE

Isotretinoin (Accutane) can cause severe fetal deformities. Therefore, females who take the drug must avoid pregnancy until at least 1 month after therapy has been completed.

Nursing Care of the Patient with Acne

ASSESSMENT. The nurse assesses the patient's concerns and knowledge about acne. Any treatments being used are documented. All medical conditions and medications are documented since some contribute to or aggravate acne. The skin is assessed to determine the extent and severity of the condition.

NURSING DIAGNOSIS. Nursing diagnoses that may apply to the patient with acne include the following:

- **Body Image Disturbance** related to comedones, pustules, and cysts
- **Knowledge Deficit** of causes and treatment of acne

GOALS. Goals of nursing care for the patient with acne are improved body image and appropriate self-care.

INTERVENTIONS
Body Image Disturbance. When working with a person who has acne, the nurse provides support and information. Since acne almost always affects the face, most patients with moderate or severe acne suffer body image disturbances. The nurse is sensitive to this concern and encourages the patient to see a dermatologist for treatment. This condition can be very harmful to the patient's self-esteem and should not be dismissed as a minor problem.

Knowledge Deficit. The causes of acne are explained as well as the many myths about the disease. The patient is assured that acne does not reflect poor hygiene but that cleanliness does reduce the risk of infections. Picking or squeezing lesions is discouraged since it may force infected material deeper into the follicle. Harsh cleansers and vigorous scrubbing have no therapeutic value.

Prescribed drugs are explained, and any adverse effects are discussed. Patient teaching is especially important if isotretinoin is used. Isotretinoin is an oral medication that has a drying effect on the skin. The patient is told to expect the condition to worsen initially and then begin to improve. Patients must be informed that the drug is teratogenic, meaning it is harmful to a developing embryo. Therefore, contraception must be used if the patient is sexually active while taking the drug.

EVALUATION. Criteria for successful nursing interventions are decreased lesions and patient's expression of improved body image, and patient's verbalization and demonstration of correct skin care and self-medication.

HERPES SIMPLEX

Etiology and Risk Factors

The herpes simplex virus (HSV) causes an infection that begins with itching and burning and progresses to the development of vesicles that rupture and form crusts (Color Plate III). Sites most often infected by the virus are the nose, lips, cheeks, ears, and genitalia. Oral HSV lesions are commonly called cold sores or fever blisters. There are two types of HSV. Infections on the face and upper body are generally caused by HSV type 1; genital infections are usually caused by HSV type 2. Patients typically have repeated outbreaks and remissions. Herpes simplex virus can be transmitted by direct contact. Genital infection is therefore considered a sexually transmitted disease and is discussed in detail in Chapter 45.

Medical Diagnosis

Diagnostic tests used to identify herpes infections include Tzanck's smear and viral culture.

Medical Treatment

Herpes simplex infections are treated with acyclovir (Zovirax), an antiviral drug that is not curative but may hasten healing. Analgesics and topical anesthetics may be prescribed for pain.

Nursing Care of the Patient with Herpes Simplex

Nursing care is primarily patient education about the nature of the herpes simplex infection and its treatment and prevention. The nurse emphasizes that the condition is contagious and tends to recur. Prevention of sexually transmitted herpes simplex is discussed in Chapter 45.

ASSESSMENT. The health history describes the development of the herpetic lesions. Contacts with people known to be infected are documented. A complete medical history is taken with particular attention to disorders or medications that might suppress the immune response. The physical examination includes a careful inspection of the lesions. Gloves are worn to avoid direct contact with lesions.

NURSING DIAGNOSIS. Nursing diagnoses for the patient with a nongenital HSV infection may include the following:

- **Pain** related to lesions
- **Ineffective Individual Coping** related to anticipated recurrent lesions, embarrassment
- **Knowledge Deficit** of cause, transmission, and treatment of HSV type 1 infections

GOALS. Goals of nursing care for the identified nursing diagnoses are pain relief, effective coping, and patient's knowledge of cause, transmission, and treatment of HSV type 1 infection.

INTERVENTIONS
Pain. Patient reports of pain are documented. Analgesics and topical anesthetics are administered as ordered, or the patient is instructed in self-medication. Compresses saturated with astringent solutions such as Burow's solution may be applied to the lesions as ordered.

Ineffective Individual Coping. The nurse explores the patient's knowledge and concerns about HSV type 1. The lesions on the face may be especially distressing because they are so obvious. The nurse demonstrates acceptance of the patient's feelings and provides factual information to enable the patient to cope with the condition.

Knowledge Deficit. Topical and oral acyclovir may be ordered. The nurse instructs the patient in use of the drug. It must be stressed that HSV remains in a dormant state in the body after the initial infection. Periodic recurrences are expected and may be triggered by stresses, including emotional distress, fever, trauma, sunburn, or fatigue. The patient may be able to identify "personal triggers" and try to avoid or minimize them. Recurrent episodes are typically less severe than the initial one.

To prevent transmission of the infection to others, the patient is advised to avoid oral contact while the lesions are present. The patient should exercise good hand washing and avoid picking at the lesions. Immunosuppressed patients are especially susceptible to herpes infections and must be protected from infected people.

PHARMACOLOGY CAPSULE

Acyclovir (Zovirax) does not cure herpes infections. Patients can transmit the infection as long as the lesions are present despite antiviral therapy.

EVALUATION. Criteria for evaluating the outcomes of nursing interventions are patient's statement of pain relief and relaxed expression, patient's statement of ability to cope with condition, and patient's description or demonstration of self-care and measures to prevent transmission of the infection.

HERPES ZOSTER

Etiology and Risk Factors

Herpes zoster infection is commonly called shingles. It is caused by the same organism that causes chickenpox. The first symptoms of shingles are pain, itching, and heightened sensitivity along a nerve pathway, followed by the formation of vesicles in the area. When the skin is affected, crusts form (Color Plate IV). When the mucous membranes are affected, ulcers develop. The lesions typically last about 2 weeks. The infection is contagious to people who have not had previous exposure to the virus.

The elderly are especially susceptible to complications, which include postherpetic neuralgia, trigeminal herpes zoster (affecting the facial and acoustic nerves), and ophthalmic involvement. With postherpetic neuralgia, pain and itching may persist for years. Immunosuppressed people are at greater risk for herpes zoster infections and may have very serious systemic complications.

Medical Diagnosis

Diagnosis of herpes zoster infection can usually be made on the basis of the health history and physical examination findings. The diagnosis can be confirmed by Tzanck's smear or a viral culture of material from a lesion.

Medical Treatment

Herpes zoster infection is treated with oral or intravenous acyclovir. Wet dressings soaked in Burow's solution may be ordered to loosen crusts, decrease oozing, and soothe the affected areas. Pain may be treated with analgesics and sedatives. Systemic corticosteroids may also be given to decrease the risk of herpetic neuralgia.

Nursing Care of the Patient with Herpes Zoster

ASSESSMENT. The nurse records the history of the patient's present illness. A complete medical history is taken to identify conditions or treatments that might cause the patient to have reduced immune response. The extent to which the symptoms are affecting the patient's life is explored. If this is a recurrent infection, the patient's understanding of the condition is assessed. The physical examination includes inspection of the lesions and documentation of distribution and appearance.

NURSING DIAGNOSIS. Nursing diagnoses for the patient with herpes zoster may include the following:

- **Impaired Skin Integrity** related to lesions
- **Pain** related to lesions, inflammation, or postherpetic neuralgia
- **Ineffective Individual Coping** related to long-term pain associated with postherpetic neuralgia

GOALS. Goals of nursing care for the patient with herpes zoster may include intact skin without vesicles, pain relief, and effective individual coping.

INTERVENTIONS

Impaired Skin Integrity. The lesions are inspected daily. Cool medicated compresses may be applied and antipruritic agents administered as ordered.

Pain. The nurse administers analgesics and antiviral medications as ordered or instructs the patient in self-medication.

Ineffective Individual Coping. Emotional support is especially important for the patient who has chronic pain. Management of chronic pain is discussed in detail in Chapter 16. To promote healing, prevent transmission, and support coping, the nurse provides information about herpes zoster: cause, course, treatment, and communicability. The nurse advises the patient that the condition is communicable to people who have never been exposed to chickenpox.

EVALUATION. Criteria for evaluating the effects of nursing interventions are absence of vesicles and pruritus, patient's statement of pain relief, and patient's identification of strategies to cope with acute and chronic symptoms.

OTHER INFECTIONS

A number of skin infections can occur in addition to those discussed in this chapter. They are impetigo, folliculitis, furuncles, carbuncles, erysipelas, cellulitis, and warts (Color Plate V). Information about these infections is presented in Table 46–5.

TABLE 46-5
ADDITIONAL SKIN INFECTIONS

INFECTION	CAUSE	SIGNS AND SYMPTOMS	TREATMENT
Impetigo	Streptococcus A	Vesicle or pustule that ruptures, leaving a thick crust	Antibiotic therapy: erythromycin or dicloxacillin
Folliculitis	*Staphylococcus aureus*	Inflamed hair follicles with white pustules	Warm compresses, topical antibiotics
Furuncle (boil)	*S. aureus*	Inflamed skin and subcutaneous tissue with deep, inflamed nodules	Warm compresses, topical antibiotics
Carbuncle	*S. aureus*	Clustered, interconnected furuncles	Systemic antibiotics, incision and drainage
Erysipelas	β-Hemolytic group A streptococcus	Round or oval patches that enlarge and spread. Redness, swelling, tenderness, warmth	Systemic antibiotics, usually penicillin
Cellulitis	Usually *Streptococcus pyogenes*	Local tenderness and redness at first, then malaise, chills, and fever. Site becomes more erythematous. Nodules and vesicles may form. Vesicles may rupture, releasing purulent material.	For *S. pyogenes,* penicillin, a cephalosporin, or vancomycin. Other antibiotics for other organisms identified by culture
Verruca (wart)	Human papillomavirus	At first, small shiny lesions. They enlarge and become rough.	Electrical current to destroy lesion followed by removal with curette, cryotherapy (freezing), topical medications

INFESTATIONS

Lice and scabies infestations are described in Table 46–6 and illustrated in Figures 46–7 and 46–8.

PEMPHIGUS

Pemphigus is a chronic autoimmune condition in which bullae (blisters) develop on the face, back, chest, groin, and umbilicus. The blisters rupture easily, releasing a foul-smelling drainage. Potassium permanganate baths may be ordered to soothe the affected areas, reduce odor, and decrease the risk of infection. Treatments may include corticosteroids, immunosuppressives, and plasmapheresis. Patients with extensive skin loss require the same care as burn patients (see nursing care section under burns later in this chapter).

CANCER

Skin cancers include actinic keratosis, basal cell carcinoma, squamous cell carcinoma, melanoma, and cutaneous T-cell lymphoma (Color Plate VI). They are most common among light-skinned people who have had repeated sun exposure. Kaposi's sarcoma is mentioned here as well because it is manifested by skin lesions. The reader is referred to Chapter 23 for detailed nursing care of the patient with cancer.

Skin cancers may be suspected because of the lesion appearance and location. The diagnosis is confirmed by microscopic examination of cells obtained from the excised lesion or a tissue sample obtained by biopsy.

TABLE 46-6
INFESTATIONS OF THE SKIN

INFESTATION	CAUSE	SIGNS AND SYMPTOMS	TREATMENT
Scabies	*Sarcoptes scabiei,* sometimes called "itch mite"	Thin, red lines on skin. Itching	Topical scabicide applied and repeated 1 wk later. Clothing and bed linens washed in hot water or dry cleaned
Lice	*Pediculus humanus* or *Phthirus pubis*	Itching of hairy areas of body (head, pubis). Nits (eggs) seen as tiny white particles attached to hair shafts	Head lice: pediculicide shampoo applied to dry hair, then hair combed with fine-toothed comb to remove nits and dead lice. Treat brushes and combs too. Body or pubic lice: apply pediculicide lotion as directed. For both sites, wash clothing and bed linens in hot water or have dry cleaned. Usually need to treat all members of household. Assure patient that infestations are common and not caused by unsanitary living conditions

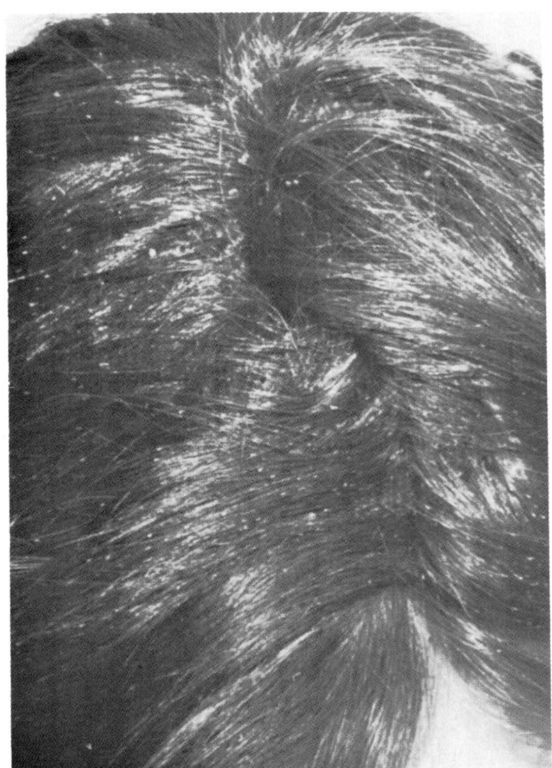

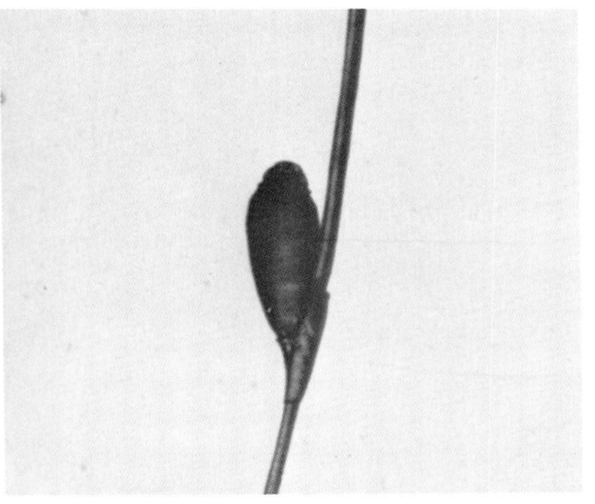

FIGURE 46-7

Pediculosis. *A*, Appearance of nits on scalp hair. *B*, Nit (egg) attached to hair shaft. (From Domonkos, A. N., Arnold, H. L., & Odom, R. B. [1982]. *Andrews' diseases of the skin* [7th ed., pp. 555, 557]. Philadelphia: W. B. Saunders.)

ACTINIC KERATOSIS

Etiology and Risk Factors

Actinic keratosis is actually a precancerous lesion most often found on the face, neck, forearms, and backs of the hands—all areas exposed to sunlight. They are most common among elderly white people. Actinic keratosis may appear as a raised or flat lesion of irregular shape. There is typically a hard scale on the lesion that may shed and reappear (see Color Plate VI).

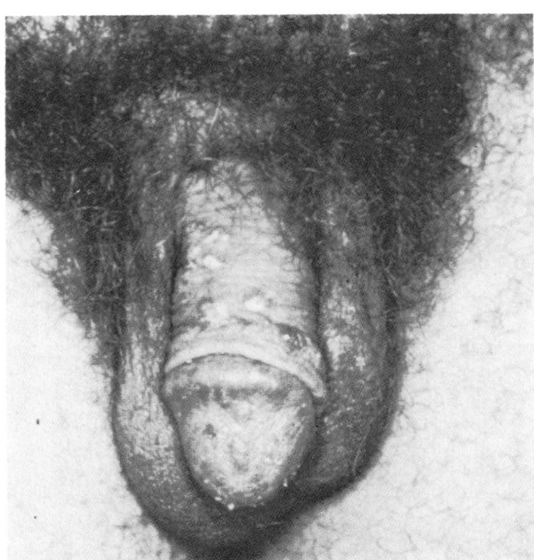

FIGURE 46-8

Scabies in an adult. (From Domonkos, A. N., Arnold, H. L., & Odom, R. B. [1982]. *Andrews' diseases of the skin* [7th ed., p. 566]. Philadelphia: W. B. Saunders.)

Medical Treatment

A number of treatments for actinic keratosis exist, including drug therapy, cryotherapy, electrodesiccation, and surgical excision. The drug of choice for actinic keratosis is 5-fluorouracil (5FU). Cryotherapy is the use of liquid nitrogen to freeze and destroy the lesion. The procedure may cause a blister to form but is only slightly painful. Electrodesiccation is the use of electrical current to destroy the lesion, which is then scraped off. The patient is given a local anesthetic. Surgical excision may be done in several ways, and the patient may or may not have sutures.

BASAL CELL CARCINOMA

Basal cell carcinomas usually begin as painless, nodular lesions that have a pearly appearance (see Color Plate VI). They are thought to be related to sun exposure. Basal cell carcinomas grow slowly and rarely metastasize. Nevertheless, they should be removed because they can cause local tissue destruction. Basal cell carcinomas are excised or destroyed in the same way as actinic keratoses.

SQUAMOUS CELL CARCINOMA

Squamous cell carcinomas may appear as scaly ulcers or raised lesions. There are usually no clear lesion margins (see Color Plate VI). They often develop on the lips and in the oral cavity. Squamous cell carcinomas are most often caused by overuse of tobacco and alcohol. Unlike basal cell carcinomas, they grow rapidly and metastasize. Treatment may include surgical excision, chemotherapy, and radiotherapy.

MELANOMA

A malignant melanoma arises from the pigment-producing cells in the skin. It is the most serious form of skin cancer because it is fatal if it metastasizes. Melanomas can be found anywhere on the body, not just sun-exposed areas. Typical melanomas have irregular borders and uneven coloration (see Color Plate VI). Many are very dark, but they may be lighter in color. They usually begin as a tan macule that enlarges. Malignant melanomas are removed surgically. A technique called Mohs' surgery is employed, in which microscopic tissue samples are studied to determine the margins of the malignancy. This approach is meant to avoid leaving malignant tissue around the excised lesion. A wide area around a melanoma is usually excised.

CUTANEOUS T-CELL LYMPHOMA

Cutaneous T-cell lymphoma is also called mycosis fungoides. It is characterized by the migration of malignant T cells to the skin. At first it may resemble eczema, but tumors then form and ulcerate. The patient has exacerbations and remissions until the inevitable fatal episode. Signs and symptoms include pruritus, eversion of the eyelids, and thickening of the skin of the soles of the feet and palms of the hands.

Treatment may include topical medications, phototherapy, photophoresis, radiotherapy, and chemotherapy. Skin moisturizers, topical steroids, and topical nitrogen mustard may be prescribed. Phototherapy involves exposing the patient to ultraviolet B waves. Photophoresis is a process by which small amounts of blood are removed, irradiated, and returned to the patient. The total body may be treated with electron beam therapy, sometimes in combination with chemotherapy.

KAPOSI'S SARCOMA

Kaposi's sarcoma is a malignancy of the blood vessels. It is manifested by red, blue, or purple macules accompanied by pain, itching, and swelling. The lesions appear first on the legs and then on the upper body, face, and mouth. They enlarge to form large plaques that may drain. Kaposi's sarcoma may be seen in patients with human immunodeficiency virus infection, but it is not confined to this group. Treatment results have not been encouraging but may include excision of the local lesion and chemotherapy or radiotherapy.

DISORDERS OF THE NAILS

The two major conditions affecting the nails are infections (fungal or bacterial) and inflammation caused by ingrown nails. Infections are usually indicated by redness, swelling, and pain around the margin of the nail. They are treated with warm soaks and topical or systemic anti-infectives. Incision and drainage may be necessary.

An ingrown toenail causes painful inflammation at the distal corner of the nail. It is usually caused by trimming the nail too short at the corners or wearing shoes that are too tight on the toes. The ingrown nail should be protected from pressure as it grows out. Warm soaks may be soothing. Sometimes surgical excision of the ingrown portion of the nail is needed.

Nursing Care of the Patient with a Nail Disorder

Nail disorders do not often require inpatient care unless there are complications. However, nurses may be the first to detect nail problems and often teach patients how to prevent or treat them.

ASSESSMENT. The health history documents the diagnoses of diabetes mellitus or peripheral vascular disease. The physical examination includes inspection of the nails for redness, swelling, or pain. The extremities are inspected for color and lesions and palpated for warmth and peripheral pulses.

NURSING DIAGNOSIS. Nursing diagnoses for the patient with a nail disorder may include the following:

- **High Risk for Injury** related to improper nail trimming, poor peripheral circulation
- **Knowledge Deficit** of proper nail care and treatment of nail disorders

GOALS. Goals for the identified nursing diagnoses are absence of injury related to the nail disorder and patient's demonstration of proper nail care and treatment of disorders.

INTERVENTIONS. Nurses need to teach patients how to trim their nails correctly and the importance of proper-fitting shoes. Toenails should be cut straight across and even with the end of the toe. Patients with peripheral vascular disease or diabetes mellitus must be taught to inspect their feet daily and to seek medical attention for any abnormality. A seemingly minor foot infection can have drastic consequences, including amputation, for the patient with poor circulation. If the patient cannot care for the feet adequately, a referral to a podiatrist should be sought.

EVALUATION. Criteria for evaluating the effects of nursing interventions are properly trimmed nails without evidence of inflammation and patient's demonstration of correct self-care measures.

BURNS

Burns are tissue injuries caused by heat that is produced or results from contact with flame, flash, scalding liquids, hot objects, chemicals, electricity, or radiation. Burns are a leading cause of accidental death despite improved survival rates attributed to tremendous advances in the care of burn patients.

Emergency treatment of the burn patient is discussed in Chapter 13. Acute care of seriously burned patients is an advanced specialty that is beyond the scope of this book; therefore, this section provides a limited discussion of nursing care of the patient after reaching a medical facility.

Classification of Burns

Burns are classified by the size and depth of the tissue injury. Extent is often defined as the percentage of body surface area affected. To describe depth, a burn is classified as partial thickness or full thickness, depending on the layers of tissue injured.

BURN SIZE. Burn size may be estimated using the rule of nines or the Lund and Browder method.

Rule of Nines. The rule of nines estimates the percentage of body surface area burned. Areas of the body are assigned percentage values of nine or multiples of nine (Fig. 46–9). The percentages are totaled to estimate burn size. For example, if one arm and one leg are burned, the burn size is estimated as 27%.

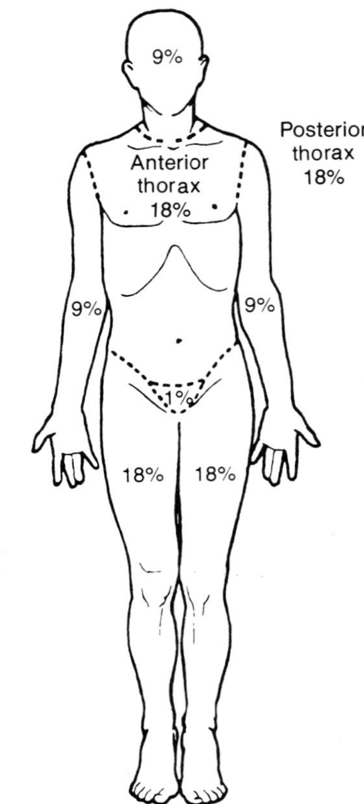

FIGURE 46–9

Rule of nines. (From Black, J. M., & Matassarin-Jacobs, E. [1993]. *Luckmann and Sorensen's medical-surgical nursing: A psychophysiologic approach* [4th ed., p. 1989]. Philadelphia: W. B. Saunders.)

Lund and Browder Method. The Lund and Browder method also estimates the percentage of body surface burned, but the body is divided into smaller segments. Different percentages are assigned to body parts depending on the patient's age (Fig. 46–10). This is more accurate than the rule of nines because it accounts for differences in body proportions. For example, the head of an infant is 19% of the total body surface area, whereas the head of an adult is only 7% of the total body surface area.

BURN DEPTH. Partial-thickness burns are sometimes called first- or second-degree burns. A burn affecting only the epidermis is a superficial (first degree) burn. A burn that affects the epidermis and the dermis is a superficial or deep partial-thickness (or second degree) burn, depending on the tissues affected. Burns that extend into even deeper tissue layers are called full-thickness (or third degree) burns (Fig. 46–11).

Superficial Burns. A superficial burn, like a sunburn, is pink to red and painful.

Superficial Partial-Thickness Burns. Superficial partial-thickness burns are painful and usually appear blistered or "weepy" and pale to red or pink. A severe sunburn can be a superficial partial-thickness burn.

Deep Partial-Thickness Burns. A deep partial-thickness burn is characterized by large, thick-walled blisters or by edema and weeping, cherry red, exposed dermis. It is painful and sensitive to cold air.

Full-Thickness Burns. Full-thickness burns involve the epidermis, dermis, and underlying tissues, including fat, muscle, and bone. Full-thickness burns typically appear dry, feel leathery, and may be red, white, brown, or black. The burned tissue usually lacks sensation.

BURN SEVERITY. Burn severity is based on size, depth, location, age, general health status, and mechanism of injury. The American Burn Association criteria for a major burn in an adult are the following:

1. Burn size: 25% or more body surface area for people under age 40; 20% or more body surface area for people over age 40.
2. Disfiguring or disabling injuries to the face, eyes, ears, hands, feet, or perineum.
3. High-voltage electrical burn injury.
4. Inhalation injury.
5. Major trauma in addition to the burn.

Pathophysiology of Burn Injury

LOCAL EFFECTS. Burn-injured tissue releases chemicals that cause increased capillary permeability. The more permeable capillaries permit plasma to leak into the tissues. Injury to cell membranes permits excess sodium to enter the cell and allows potassium to escape

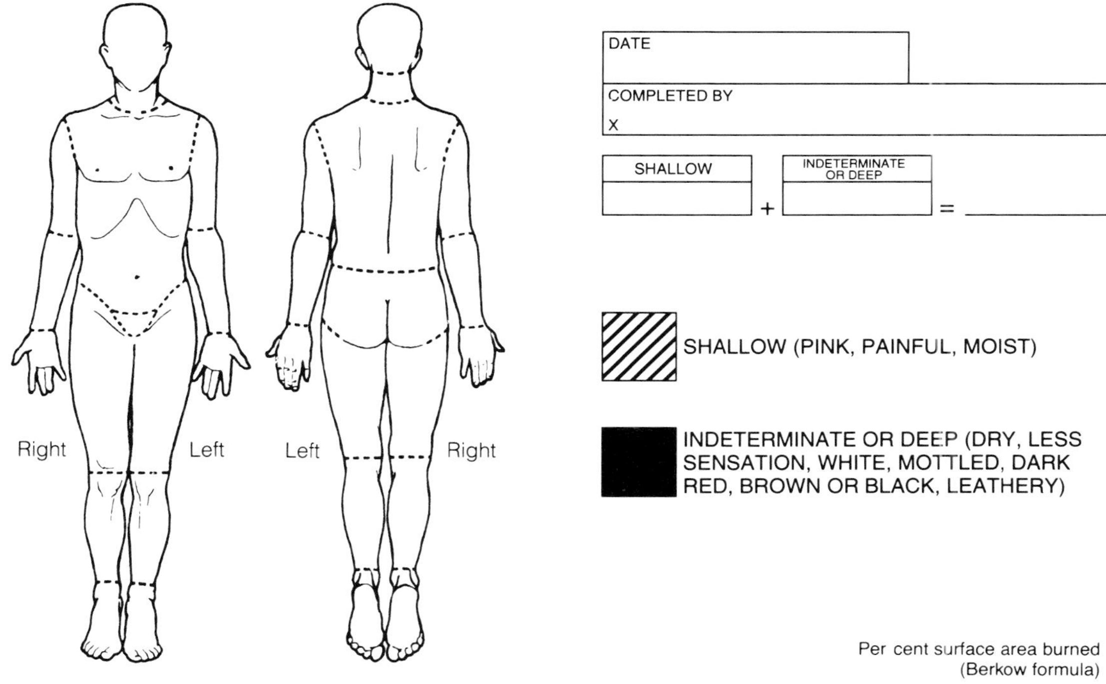

AREA	1 YEAR	1 to 4 YEARS	5 to 9 YEARS	10 to 14 YEARS	Y 15 YEARS	ADULT	SHALLOW	INDETERMINATE OR DEEP
Head	19	17	13	11	9	7		
Neck	2	2	2	2	2	2		
Ant. Trunk	13	13	13	13	13	13		
Post.Trunk	13	13	13	13	13	13		
R. Buttock	2½	2½	2½	2½	2½	2½		
L. Buttock	2½	2½	2½	2½	2½	2½		
Genitalia	1	1	1	1	1	1		
R. U. Arm	4	4	4	4	4	4		
L. U. Arm	4	4	4	4	4	4		
R. L. Arm	3	3	3	3	3	3		
L. L. Arm	3	3	3	3	3	3		
R. Hand	2½	2½	2½	2½	2½	2½		
L. Hand	2½	2½	2½	2½	2½	2½		
R. Thigh	5½	6½	8	8½	9	9½		
L. Thigh	5½	6½	8	8½	9	9½		
R. Leg	5	5	5½	6	6½	7		
L. Leg	5	5	5½	6	6½	7		
R. Foot	3½	3½	3½	3½	3½	3½		
L. Foot	3½	3½	3½	3½	3½	3½		
TOTAL								

FIGURE 46-10

Lund and Browder method of estimating body surface area burned. (From Black, J. M., & Matassarin-Jacobs, E. [1993]. *Luckmann and Sorensen's medical-surgical nursing: A psychophysiologic approach* [4th ed., p. 1990]. Philadelphia: W. B. Saunders.)

into the extracellular compartment. These shifts in fluids and electrolytes cause local edema and a decrease in cardiac output. Fluid evaporates through the wound surface, further contributing to the declining blood volume. Eighteen to 36 hours after a burn injury, capillary permeability begins to normalize and reabsorption of edema fluid begins. Cardiac output returns to normal and then increases to meet increased metabolic demands.

SYSTEMIC EFFECTS. Serious burns can have widespread effects on body functions.

Fluid Balance. The shift of plasma proteins from the capillaries may result in hypoproteinemia, which draws fluid from the blood stream to the extracellular tissue. This shift causes decreased blood volume and generalized edema in the early postburn period. Blood is

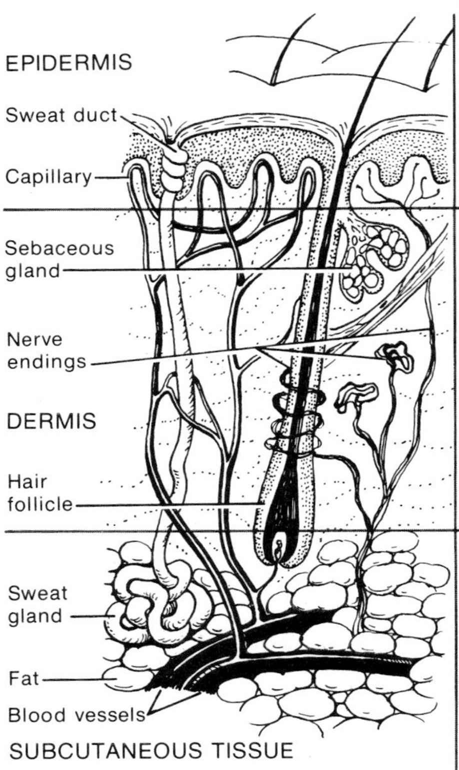

EPIDERMIS
Sweat duct
Capillary
Sebaceous gland
Nerve endings
DERMIS
Hair follicle
Sweat gland
Fat
Blood vessels
SUBCUTANEOUS TISSUE

	APPEARANCE	SENSATION	COURSE
SUPERFICIAL BURN	Mild to severe erythema; skin blanches with pressure	Painful Hyperesthetic Tingling Pain eased by cooling	Discomfort lasts about 48 hours Desquamation in 3–7days
PARTIAL-THICKNESS BURN	Large thick-walled blisters covering extensive area (vesiculation) Edema; mottled red base; broken epidermis; wet, shiny, weeping surface	Painful Sensitive to cold air	Superficial partial-thickness burn heals in 14–21 days Deep partial-thickness burn requires 21–28 days for healing Healing rate varies with burn depth and presence or absence of infection
FULL-THICKNESS BURN	Variable, e.g., deep red, black, white, brown Dry surface Edema Fat exposed Tissue disrupted	Little pain Insensate	Full-thickness dead skin suppurates and liquefies after 2–3 weeks Spontaneous healing impossible Requires removal of eschar and subsequent split- or full-thickness skin grafting Hypertrophic scarring and wound contractures likely to develop without preventive measures

FIGURE 46-11

Burn classification by depth. (From Black, J. M., & Matassarin-Jacobs, E. [1993]. *Luckmann and Sorensen's medical-surgical nursing: A psychophysiologic approach* [4th ed., p. 1989]. Philadelphia: W. B. Saunders.)

shunted from the kidneys to compensate for the fluid volume deficit, and urine output falls. These fluid shifts, if not corrected, result in decreased tissue perfusion and decreased cardiac output that may lead to hypovolemic shock.

As the capillaries recover and edema fluid is reabsorbed, the patient's blood volume increases. If kidney function is adequate, urine output increases to prevent hypervolemia.

Gastrointestinal Function. Blood flow to the intestines decreases, and the patient may develop an ileus. Some patients develop stress ulcers, sometimes called Curling's ulcers, after severe burns. They are, therefore, routinely treated with antacids and H_2 blockers.

Immune System. Because immunity is depressed after a serious burn, the patient is less able to resist infection. The loss of the protective skin barrier also puts the patient at risk for infection.

Respiratory System. The burn patient may suffer inhalation injuries, including carbon monoxide poisoning, smoke poisoning, and thermal damage. Inhalation injury occurs with flame burns or from being trapped in an enclosed space filled with smoke.

Inhalation injury is suspected if the patient has facial burns, redness and swelling of the pharynx, restlessness, cough, dyspnea, or sooty sputum. Carbon monoxide displaces oxygen on hemoglobin, so the blood is unable to transport oxygen to the tissues. The patient shows signs of hypoxia and dies if the condition if not corrected. See Chapter 13 for additional discussion of carbon monoxide poisoning. Smoke poisoning is the result of inhaling combustion byproducts. Thermal damage to the lower airway is rare but can happen if the patient was unconscious or inhaled live steam. With inhalation injury, the patient develops pulmonary edema that may progress to adult respiratory distress syndrome.

Stages of Burn Injury

Care of the burn patient is often described in terms of three stages: emergent, acute, and rehabilitation. The emergent stage begins with the injury and ends when fluid shifts have stabilized. The acute stage begins with fluid stabilization. Some sources mark the end of the acute stage when all but 10% of the burn wounds are closed, but others define the acute stage as extending until all wounds are closed. The rehabilitation stage follows the acute stage and lasts as long as efforts continue to promote improvement or adjustment. There is some overlap between the acute and rehabilitation stages because nursing care in the acute stage can significantly affect the potential for rehabilitation.

Medical Treatment in the Emergent Stage

In the emergency department, the staff first assesses airway, breathing, and circulation and then determines whether the patient has injuries in addition to the burn. If inhalation injury is suspected, oxygen therapy is started. Intravenous lines are established to begin fluid resuscitation and to provide emergency vascular access. An indwelling urinary catheter and a nasogastric tube are usually inserted. Blood is drawn for baseline laboratory studies (hematocrit, electrolytes, blood gases if indicated). Tetanus prophylaxis may be administered. Pain is assessed and analgesics are ordered. The wound is then cleaned, débrided, and inspected.

Once the initial care is completed, the patient with serious burns is transferred to a burn specialty care unit or a critical care unit. Intravenous fluid therapy is an essential aspect of care during the first few days of burn treatment. Several formulas are used to select the volumes and solutions to be administered. Volume is based on the patient's weight and extent of injury. For the first 24 hours, intravenous fluids may consist of various combinations of electrolyte, colloid, and dextrose solutions. Some formulas prescribe only electrolyte solutions in the first 24 hours. For the second 24 hours, volume is usually decreased based on urine output. Fluids then consist of different combinations of electrolyte, colloid, and dextrose solutions. Some formulas omit electrolyte solutions in the second 24 hours.

In addition to fluids, medical care may include mechanical ventilation, antibiotic therapy, and surgical procedures.

Wound Care

Wound care after a burn injury is intended to promote healing, prevent infection, control heat loss, retain function, and minimize disfigurement. Burn wounds may be treated by the open or closed method. The method of wound care is based, in part, on the state of the wound. The open method involves the use of topical antimicrobials but no dressings. Open care is less restrictive and simpler than closed care but does provide greater opportunity for loss of fluid and heat through the wound surface. Closed care employs the use of topical medications covered by dressings. For clean partial-thickness wounds that will heal without grafting, temporary wound coverings are often employed. Temporary wound coverings include amniotic membranes, grafts from cadavers or pigs, and a number of synthetic materials that promote wound healing or protect donor or graft sites. Grafted areas in need of protection are often covered by temporary wound coverings as well. Donor sites are also treated with a variety of products, including fine-mesh gauze and synthetic and biosynthetic products.

DÉBRIDEMENT. A partial-thickness burn may blister, peel, and heal with minimal long-term effects. A full-thickness burn, however, is often covered by a thick, leathery layer of burned tissue (eschar) that shelters microorganisms and inhibits healing. Eschar must be removed before healing can take place. Débridement is the removal of debris and necrotic (dead) tissue from a wound. In the case of a burn wound, débridement includes removal of eschar. Débridement may be accomplished by mechanical means (using scissors and forceps), surgical excision, or the use of enzymes. Enzymatic débridement is the use of topical medications containing enzymes capable of dissolving necrotic tissue. These substances are applied directly to the wound but should not be applied to wounds that communicate with major body cavities or to exposed nerves. Enzymatic agents may cause pain and bleeding.

SKIN GRAFTING. A burn wound may be covered using the patient's own skin, called an autograft. The graft is usually taken from the thigh or buttocks using a tool called a dermatome. The thickness of the graft determines whether it is a split-thickness or a full-thickness graft. If a thin layer of skin is used, it is considered a split-thickness graft. A split-thickness graft may be a sheet graft (an intact section of skin) or a meshed graft. A meshed graft has multiple tiny slits that allow the skin to be stretched to cover a larger area. The slits also allow for wound exudate to be absorbed by the cover dressing. Grafts vary in size, with the smallest being "pinch" and "postage stamp" grafts. Larger grafts may be needed to cover all or part of the burn.

For very deep burns and burns of the face, neck, or hands, a full-thickness graft may be preferred. A full-thickness graft includes skin and subcutaneous tissue and provides better cosmetic results. Another type of full-thickness graft is a pedicle or flap graft in which one end of a section or tube of donor tissue is sutured to the recipient site while another section remains attached to the donor site. This type of graft continues to receive blood from the donor site. Once the graft "takes" or attaches to the recipient site, the pedicle or flap is cut free from the donor site.

After grafting, the recipient site is inspected for bleeding under the graft that could interfere with survival of the graft. The area is immobilized for 3 to 7 days to permit attachment of the graft to the wound base. Splints, traction, and restraints may be used for immobilization. After an autograft, the patient's donor site requires care as well. The donor site is usually covered with fine-mesh gauze or synthetic dressings and bandages. The dressings are usually left in place until the epithelium has regenerated.

SCARRING. Burn scars can be reduced by the use of pressure dressings in the early stages of care followed by the use of custom-fitted garments that apply continuous pressure. These garments are worn 23 hours a day and may be prescribed for as long as 2 years (Fig. 46–12).

Nursing Care of the Patient with Burn Injury

ASSESSMENT. When the patient is stabilized, a complete assessment should be done. As priorities change, the nurse adds relevant data.

Health History. The history of the present illness describes the circumstances surrounding the burn injury. The past medical history documents any chronic diseases, surgeries, or hospitalizations. Medications and allergies are identified. The family history is not specific to burn injuries but is taken to alert the nurse to other problems. The review of systems detects current problems with each body system. The functional assessment describes the patient's habits and lifestyle, roles and responsibilities, stressors, and coping strategies.

Physical Examination. The physical examination begins with vital signs. The nurse is alert for abnormalities that suggest hypoxia (restlessness, tachypnea), fluid volume excess (bounding pulse, hypertension), fluid volume deficit (tachycardia, hypotension), hypovolemia (hypotension, tachycardia), or infection (fever, tachycardia). Height and weight are measured if the patient is stable enough to be weighed.

Throughout the examination, the nurse inspects the skin for burn wounds and other lesions. Wound color and the presence of eschar are noted. Intact skin is palpated for temperature and turgor. Chest expansion is observed, and the lungs are auscultated for wheezing, stridor, or atelectasis. The apical pulse is auscultated for rate and rhythm. The abdomen is assessed for active bowel sounds and distention. The extremities are inspected for injury and deformity. Range of motion assessment may be delayed if an extremity is immobilized.

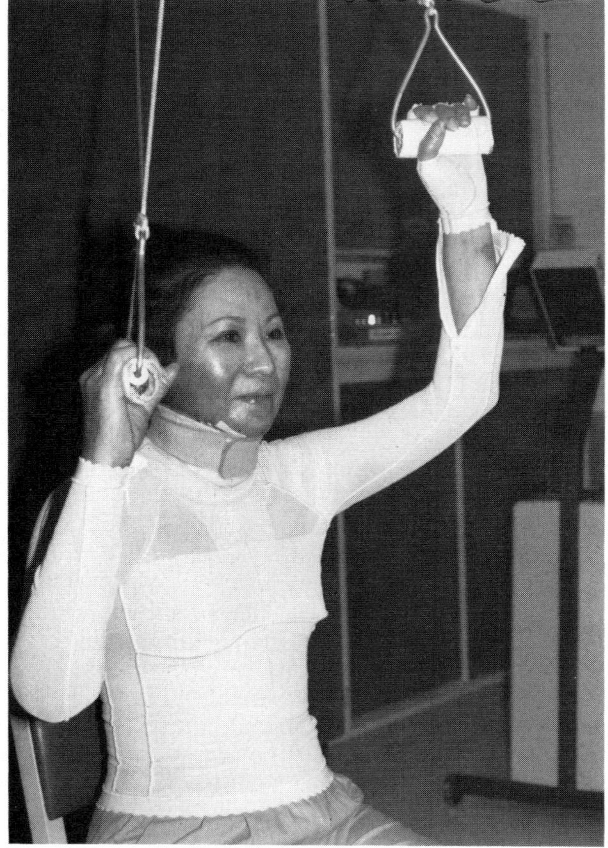

FIGURE 46–12

Antiscar pressure garment minimizes the hypertrophic scarring that is common after burn injuries. (From Black, J. M., & Matassarin-Jacobs, E. [1993]. *Luckmann and Sorensen's medical-surgical nursing: A psychophysiologic approach* [4th ed.]. Philadelphia: W. B. Saunders.)

NURSING DIAGNOSIS. Depending on the severity and type of burn, nursing diagnoses for the patient with burns may include those listed here. The first two are most likely to occur in the emergent stage; the remaining diagnoses may be made in the emergent, acute, or rehabilitation stage.

- **Decreased Cardiac Output** related to hypovolemia secondary to shift of fluid from vascular to extracellular compartment
- **Fluid Volume Excess** related to increased capillary permeability
- **Pain** related to tissue trauma of burn injury
- **High Risk for Infection** related to loss of protective skin barrier
- **Hypothermia** related to impaired heat-regulating ability of injured skin
- **Altered Nutrition: Less than Body Requirements** related to increased metabolic demands
- **Impaired Physical Mobility** related to contractures, therapeutic immobilization, pain
- **Ineffective Individual Coping** related to possible disfigurement, dysfunction, fear of death
- **Ineffective Family Coping** related to uncertain outcome, fear of patient death, and altered family function
- **Knowledge Deficit** of recovery from burn injuries or patient role in rehabilitation

GOALS. Goals of nursing care for the burn patient are normal cardiac output, normal fluid balance, pain relief, absence of infection, normal body temperature, adequate nutritional intake, adaptation to physical limitations, effective patient coping, effective family coping, and patient's knowledge of recovery process and rehabilitation.

INTERVENTIONS

Decreased Cardiac Output. The risk of decreased cardiac output is greatest in the emergent stage when fluid has shifted from the blood to the extracellular compartment. If blood volume is not maintained, the patient's blood pressure falls and tissue perfusion is impaired. To monitor cardiac output, the nurse assesses the patient's vital signs and fluid intake and output. Signs of decreased cardiac output include hypotension, tachycardia, and decreased urine output. Inadequate tissue perfusion may be manifested by cool, pale or cyanotic skin, restlessness, and confusion. Intravenous fluids are administered as ordered with close, continuous monitoring of fluid status.

Fluid Volume Excess. Fluid volume excess may result from the retention of fluid in the extracellular compartment. As capillary permeability returns to normal and fluid is reabsorbed, the patient's blood volume increases. If the patient's kidneys can eliminate the excess fluid efficiently, the patient suffers no ill effects from the increasing blood volume. There is a risk, however, that the patient's circulatory system may be unable to adapt to the increased volume. This puts the patient at risk for heart failure.

The nurse monitors the patient's vital signs for hypertension, dyspnea, and full, bounding pulse. Urine output is measured and compared with fluid intake. Intravenous fluids are administered as ordered and monitored closely.

Pain. Partial-thickness wounds are typically very painful. Full-thickness burns lack sensation because of the destruction of the superficial nerves. However, burns are often uneven in depth, so patients with full-thickness burns often have pain as well. The burn patient is given narcotic analgesics as necessary, as ordered. Analgesics are usually given before painful wound care. If given orally, the medication should be given 45 minutes before the procedure. If given intravenously, it is given 5 to 10 minutes ahead of time. The intramuscular route is not routinely used until fluid shifts have stabilized because absorption is less reliable. Nonsteroidal anti-inflammatory drugs also may be prescribed. Pain is aggravated by anxiety, so the nurse includes patient teaching and reduction of fear and anxiety in the management of pain. Additional nursing measures for pain are described in Chapter 16.

High Risk for Infection. The burn patient, with loss of protective skin, is at great risk for infection. The nurse routinely monitors for signs of local infection (pus, foul odor, increased redness) and systemic infection (fever, increased white blood cell count). Infection can come from the staff, visitors, the environment, and the patient's own body. Specific infection-control measures vary with the agency. Strict hand washing should be practiced by the patient and all who enter the room. Body hair around wounds is usually shaved or cut to prevent wound contamination. The eyebrows are *not* shaved because, if shaved, they tend to grow back in a disorganized pattern. Wound care is carried out as ordered or according to routines of the specialty care unit.

Hypothermia. Loss of heat through the burn wound surface places the patient at risk for hypothermia (low body temperature). The patient's tympanic or rectal temperature is monitored to detect declining body temperature. The room is kept warm, and external heat sources are used as needed. The nurse attempts to limit body surface area exposure during wound care. Body heat loss may be greater if the patient is on an air-fluidized bed, so the temperature of the bed must be carefully monitored.

Altered Nutrition: Less than Body Requirements. Healing of a large burn wound requires considerable energy. It is, therefore, critical that nutrition be provided to meet the increased metabolic demands. The nurse consults with the dietitian about the patient's nutritional needs and preferences. Regular meals may need to be supplemented with between-meal feedings. Patient teaching emphasizes the need for increased intake during the recovery period. The nurse tries to create an environment conducive to eating and encourages the patient to eat all food served. Assistance with meals is provided if needed. Some patients require tube feedings or total parenteral nutrition to meet their calorie needs.

Impaired Physical Mobility. Patients with burns may have restrictions on their mobility imposed by the injury or the treatment. The hazards of immobility, including pressure sores, joint contractures, pneumonia and atelectasis, constipation, and urinary infections, are covered in Chapter 19. The nurse monitors range of motion in affected joints and performs passive or active exercises unless contraindicated. It is essential that injured limbs be kept in functional positions as much as possible (Fig. 46–13). Unaffected joints also must be exercised to maintain flexibility and strength. Impaired mobility may interfere with the patient's ability to participate in his or her own care. The nurse assesses self-care deficits and provides assistance as needed. As the patient moves toward recovery, the rehabilitation

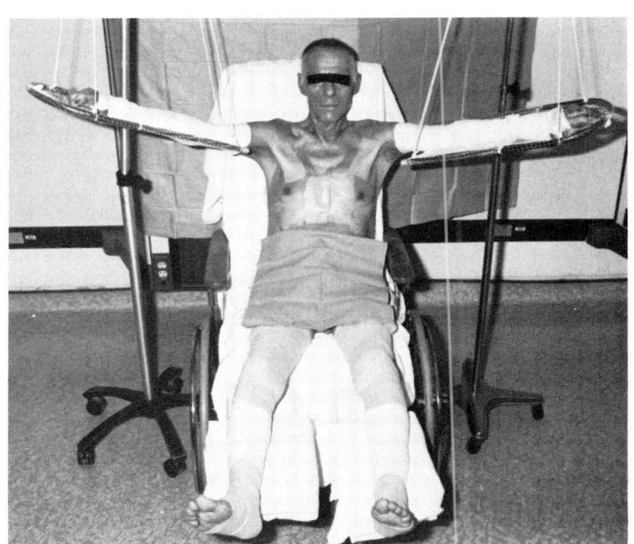

FIGURE 46–13
Therapeutic positioning. This patient's arms are extended to prevent flexion contractures. Pressure dressings on legs prevent edema and minimize scarring. (From Black, J. M., & Matassarin-Jacobs, E. [1993]. *Luckmann and Sorensen's medical-surgical nursing: A psychophysiologic approach* [4th ed.]. Philadelphia: W. B. Saunders.)

team helps the patient adapt self-care activities for permanent injuries.

Ineffective Individual Coping. Severe burns can result in disfigurement and loss of function. The patient faces a long and difficult recovery period. The emotional responses of the burn patient are often like those of any grieving person: shock, disbelief, withdrawal, denial, regression, depression, and anger. The nurse demonstrates acceptance of the patient regardless of the emotional state. Opportunities are provided for the patient to express his or her thoughts and feelings. The patient may find it helpful to talk to a clinical nurse specialist, counselor, or spiritual adviser. Some patients find support groups helpful in learning to live with their injuries. The patient is encouraged to identify and use coping strategies that have been effective in the past. If effective coping strategies are employed, the patient eventually incorporates the physical and functional changes into a new body image.

Ineffective Family Coping. A serious burn injury that may require months or years of therapy has a tremendous impact on the family. The nurse must include significant others in the patient's care. When the family arrives after the injury, the physician or clinical nurse advises them of the patient's injuries, what to expect when they see the patient, and what is being done for the patient. The family should be offered an opportunity to talk with a social worker, clinical nurse specialist, counselor, or spiritual adviser.

Knowledge Deficit. When the patient is acutely ill, patient teaching consists of telling the patient what is being done, why, and what to expect. As the patient stabilizes, the teaching plan should include infection control, nutritional needs, prevention of complications of immobility, pain management, protection of grafts, measures to conceal scars and improve appearance, adaptive devices to compensate for disabilities, and rehabilitation plans.

EVALUATION. Criteria for evaluating goal achievement are normal pulse and blood pressure; absence of edema; patient's statement of pain reduction; absence of foul odor or drainage and fever; rectal temperature of 98.6°F or higher; stable weight; minimal contractures, clear breath sounds, bowel movement at least every 2 to 3 days; positive patient statements about the future; positive family statements about the future; and patient's verbalization of content covered in teaching plan and demonstration of understanding content.

CONDITIONS TREATED WITH PLASTIC SURGERY

Plastic surgery includes aesthetic (cosmetic) and reconstructive procedures. Aesthetic surgical procedures are performed to improve appearance, whereas reconstructive procedures are done to correct abnormalities. In addition to usual surgical approaches, methods employed in plastic surgery may include use of flaps and grafts, skin expansion, implants, liposuction, and microvascular surgery.

AESTHETIC SURGERY

In general, aesthetic surgery alters a body feature that is structurally normal but perceived by the patient as unattractive. Examples of aesthetic surgery are rhytidectomy, blepharoplasty, chin implants, rhinoplasty, abdominoplasty, breast augmentation, and breast reduction. A rhytidectomy, commonly called a face-lift, is done to remove facial wrinkles and tighten sagging tissue. A blepharoplasty is the removal of excess tissue around the eyes. It is usually an aesthetic procedure but may be done to improve function if droopy eyelids impair vision. Chin implants are done by placing a prosthesis to correct a receding chin. A rhinoplasty alters the shape or size, or both, of the nose. In an abdominoplasty, excess skin and adipose tissue are removed and the abdominal muscles are tightened. Breast augmentation is breast enlargement, which may be performed to increase the size of both breasts or to improve breast symmetry. A variety of techniques have been used for breast augmentation. The most common procedure has been to implant a silicone rubber implant filled with saline or silicone gel. There is considerable concern at this time about the effects of possible leakage of filler substances into the body. Breast reduction decreases breast size and may be requested to improve appearance or body proportion or to eliminate discomfort associated with excessively large breasts. Liposuction is the removal of excess adipose tissue with a suction device, most commonly used on the thighs, abdomen, arms, and buttocks.

RECONSTRUCTIVE SURGERY

A number of procedures may be classified as reconstructive. Reconstructive surgery may be done to repair disfiguring scars, restore body contours after radical surgery like mastectomy, eliminate benign lesions such as birthmarks, restore features damaged by trauma or disease, and correct developmental defects.

NURSING CARE OF THE PATIENT HAVING PLASTIC SURGERY

When working with people who are having plastic surgery, nurses must be aware of their own biases and feelings. Nurses who view cosmetic procedures as vain or frivolous may have difficulty being supportive of patients who choose to have these procedures done. Many factors may motivate people to have aesthetic surgery. Physical appearance is a component of body image and may affect self-esteem. Some people believe that a change in appearance will benefit their personal or professional lives. A person who is very self-conscious about a physical feature can benefit immensely from aesthetic surgery. It is important that the nurse not judge the patient's motivation for seeking surgery. It is also important to be alert to the patient's unrealistic expectations for the surgical outcome.

Although each procedure may require some specific nursing interventions, this section addresses general nursing care for the patient having plastic surgery. Some specific procedures, complications, and nursing care are presented in Table 46–7.

Preoperative Nursing Care

Many of these procedures may be done in day surgery or short-stay surgical units. Therefore, patient preparation emphasizes teaching for self-care. Initial teaching may be done by the physician, office nurse, or staff nurse.

ASSESSMENT

Health History. The nurse documents the patient's description of the problem being treated with plastic surgery and what the patient expects the procedure to accomplish. The past medical history records all previous surgeries as well as any serious illnesses. It is especially important to note conditions that might affect wound healing, such as diabetes mellitus, circulatory disorders, and impaired blood coagulation. A thorough review of systems is done, with special attention to the surgical area. If a blepharoplasty is being done, visual acuity is tested and documented. The functional assessment describes the patient's lifestyle and usual activities, which may require some temporary modification after plastic surgery.

TABLE 46-7
COMPLICATIONS OF COMMON PLASTIC SURGERY PROCEDURES

PROCEDURE	DESCRIPTION	COMPLICATIONS
Rhytidectomy (face-lift)	Removal of excess skin and tissue from face	Hematoma, hemorrhage, temporary or permanent facial nerve damage, infection, bruising, edema, skin necrosis, hair loss
Blepharoplasty	Removal of bulging fat and excess skin around eye	Hematoma, ectropion, corneal injury, visual loss (rare), infection (rare)
Rhinoplasty	Removal of excess cartilage and tissue from nose with correction of septal defects if indicated	Hematoma, hemorrhage, bruising, edema, infection, septal perforation, minor skin irritation
Breast augmentation	Insertion of breast-shaped synthetic implants	Hematoma, hemorrhage, infection, phlebitis, capsule formation
Breast reduction	Excision of excessive breast tissue and skin	Hematoma; hemorrhage; infection; fat necrosis; wound dehiscence; necrosis of nipple, areola, and skin flap

Data from Cuzzell, J. Z. (1991). Interventions for clients with skin disorders. In D. D. Ignatavicius & M. V. Bayne (Eds.), *Medical-surgical nursing: A nursing process approach* (p. 1205). Philadelphia: W. B. Saunders; and Black, J. M., & Matassarin-Jacobs, E. (1993). *Luckmann and Sorensen's medical surgical nursing: A psychophysiologic approach* (4th ed., p. 2030). Philadelphia: W. B. Saunders.

Physical Examination. The routine preoperative physical examination is performed as described in Chapter 14. The condition that is being treated is described. Most plastic surgeons have preoperative photographs made to document the condition. The nurse may take the photographs and must be sensitive to the patient's discomfort or embarrassment.

NURSING DIAGNOSIS. Nursing diagnoses before plastic surgery may include the following:

- **Anxiety** related to uncertain outcome, anticipated change in appearance, surgical procedure
- **Knowledge Deficit** of surgical routines and procedures, postoperative routines, and self-care

GOALS. The goals of preoperative nursing care are reduced anxiety and patient's knowledge of pre- and postoperative care.

INTERVENTIONS

Anxiety. The nurse assesses the patient's anxiety by observing for nervousness, trembling, increased pulse, and difficulty concentrating. The nurse can share such observations and ask how the patient feels about the planned surgery. Anxiety may be reduced by encouraging the patient to express concerns, acknowledging that these feelings are normal, and providing information about what to expect.

Knowledge Deficit. The nurse assesses the patient's perception of the procedure and its outcome. Surgical pre- and postoperative procedures and self-care are discussed. The patient is advised whether swelling, bruising, and scars are expected in the immediate postoperative period. Generally, patients have been told not to take drugs that prolong bleeding time, including aspirin, before surgery. Smoking is discouraged since nicotine causes vasoconstriction, which can interfere with healing. The patient may be instructed to scrub the surgical area at intervals before the procedure. Specific teaching depends on the exact procedure and the surgeon's orders or agency's protocol.

EVALUATION. Criteria for evaluating the success of nursing interventions are patient's statement of reduced anxiety, absence of trembling, tachycardia, or tense expression; and patient's statements of expected outcomes, surgical routines, and postoperative self-care.

Postoperative Nursing Care

Routine postoperative nursing care is detailed in Chapter 14. This section emphasizes special considerations when a patient has plastic surgery.

ASSESSMENT. The patient may have had general, regional, or local anesthesia. Vital signs are monitored, and level of consciousness is assessed. Dressings are inspected for drainage or bleeding but are not removed. Some dressings, such as those used after rhinoplasty, may serve as splints, so they must not be disturbed. Flaps and grafts are observed for color and evidence of fluid accumulation and palpated for warmth. If drains are present, the contents are inspected and measured each shift. The fluid should gradually lighten from sanguineous (red) to serosanguineous (pink) to serous (pale yellow). The patient's comfort level also is monitored.

NURSING DIAGNOSIS. Nursing diagnoses after plastic surgery may include the following:

- **Pain** related to tissue trauma
- **High Risk for Infection** related to surgical incision
- **High Risk for Injury** related to inadequate circulation to grafted tissue, pressure created by edema or implants, nerve damage
- **High Risk for Fluid Volume Deficit** related to effects of liposuction
- **Body Image Disturbance** related to altered appearance
- **Knowledge Deficit** of postoperative self-care

GOALS. Goals of nursing care after plastic surgery are reduced pain, absence of infection, adequate tissue perfusion, normal fluid balance, healthy body image, and patient's knowledge of postoperative self-care.

INTERVENTIONS

Pain. Minor procedures such as blepharoplasty usually cause minimal pain, but major procedures such as grafting or abdominoplasty can be very painful. Pain is treated with analgesics as ordered. Aspirin is usually not ordered because it prolongs bleeding time. The nurse employs comfort measures also, such as positioning, relaxation, and imagery, to decrease pain. After surgery on the face or head, the head of the bed is usually elevated and cold compresses ordered to decrease swelling. The effects of interventions are assessed and documented. Increasing pain or pain that is not responsive to treatment must be reported to the physician.

High Risk for Infection. The nurse monitors for signs and symptoms of infection, but these are unlikely to be seen during a brief hospitalization. The patient must therefore be instructed to report increasing redness, swelling, drainage, or fever. The nurse and patient must exercise good hand washing before any contact with the incisions, flaps, or grafts. Antimicrobial drugs are given as ordered. Some plastic surgeons order topical antimicrobials applied to the incisions. After rhytidectomy, the patient is usually not permitted to shampoo the hair for several days to avoid contamination of the incisions.

High Risk for Injury. After plastic surgery, the nurse assesses the affected tissues for adequate circulation. Grafts rely on blood flow in underlying tissue to supply nutrients and oxygen and to remove wastes. Therefore, grafts must be protected from trauma and pressure. Pallor, cyanosis, and coolness in a graft suggest inadequate circulation and must be reported to the surgeon immediately. If fluid accumulates under the graft, it separates the graft from the underlying tissue, depriving it of oxygen and nutrients. Therefore, swelling or blisters must be reported to the surgeon, who may remove the accumulated fluid with a small-gauge needle and syringe.

Rhytidectomy poses a risk of injury to the facial nerve, which is manifested by facial asymmetry. If asymmetry is observed, the nurse notifies the surgeon immediately. The patient may be returned to surgery in an effort to relieve the pressure on the nerve and prevent permanent damage. After blepharoplasty, the patient's visual status is monitored. Although the risk is slight, the eye could be injured during the procedure.

The patient who has had an abdominoplasty must protect the operative site by remaining in a flexed position for a specified period of time. The bed is positioned so that the head and knees are elevated to reduce stress on the suture line. When out of bed, the patient must continue the flexed position. The patient is gradually permitted to straighten up.

Following breast augmentation, the patient is monitored for bleeding, infection, and altered sensation. The patient is also at risk for capsule formation, in which scar tissue gradually encloses the implant, causing the breast to become hard and misshapen. The surgeon may advise the patient to massage the breast to reduce the risk of capsule formation. This procedure involves pushing each breast up, to the side, and toward the center of the chest, holding each position to the count of 10. For a period specified by the surgeon, the patient should avoid raising the arms above the head.

High Risk for Fluid Volume Deficit. Patients who have liposuction are at risk for hypovolemia due to excessive fluid loss. Intravenous fluids may be ordered postoperatively, and oral fluids are usually encouraged when the patient is fully alert. Vital signs are monitored for tachycardia and hypotension associated with fluid volume deficit.

Body Image Disturbance. In the immediate postoperative period, the patient often has edema and bruising as well as visible incisions. The nurse assures the patient that these effects will gradually resolve. The nurse can explore measures to conceal the evidence of trauma, but

NUTRITION CONCEPTS

- Vitamin A is essential for healthy skin.
- Food sources of vitamin A are liver, pumpkin, sweet potatoes, carrots, spinach, broccoli, cantaloupe, and apricots.
- Food allergies can cause atopic dermatitis.
- Skin changes associated with malnutrition include cracked skin, dermatitis, xerosis (dry skin), purpura, and petechiae (purple or red spots).

no makeup should be applied to surgical incisions until they are well healed.

Knowledge Deficit. In preparing for discharge, the nurse provides verbal and written instructions for self-care. The following topics must be included: drug therapy (names of drugs ordered, schedule), wound care, signs and symptoms of infection, activity restrictions, and measures to prevent complications.

EVALUATION. Criteria for evaluating the outcomes of plastic surgery include patient's statement of pain relief; absence of fever, foul drainage, increasing redness and edema; normal tissue warmth and color, normal neuromuscular function; normal vital signs, intake equal to output; patient's expression of understanding healing process and of satisfaction with outcomes; and patient's description of details of postdischarge care.

BIBLIOGRAPHY

Anastasi, J. K., & Rivera, J. (1992). Identifying the skin manifestations of HIV. *Nursing 92, 22*(11), 58–61.

Black, J. M., & Matassarin-Jacobs, E. (1993). *Luckmann and Sorensen's medical surgical nursing: A psychophysiologic approach* (4th ed., p. 2030). Philadelphia: W. B. Saunders.

Calistro, A. (1993). Burn care basics and beyond. *RN, 56*(3), 26–31.

Chernecky, C. C., Krech, R. L., & Berger, B. J. (1993). *Laboratory tests and diagnostic procedures.* Philadelphia: W. B. Saunders.

Cuzzell, J. Z. (1990). Clues: Pain, burning, and itching. *American Journal of Nursing, 90*(7), 15–16.

Cuzzell, J. Z. (1991). Interventions for clients with skin disorders. In D. D. Ignatavicius & M. V. Bayne (Eds.), *Medical-surgical nursing: A nursing process approach* (p. 1205). Philadelphia: W. B. Saunders.

DeWitt, S. (1990). Nursing assessment of the skin and dermatologic lesions. *Nursing Clinics of North America, 25*(1), 235–245.

Dodson, J. M., DeSpain, J., Hewett, J. E., & Clark, D. P. (1991). Malignant potential of actinic keratoses and the controversy over treatment. *Archives of Dermatology, 127,* 1029–1031.

Domonkos, A. N., Arnold, H. L., & Odom, R. B. (1982). *Andrews' diseases of the skin* (7th ed.). Philadelphia: W. B. Saunders.

Drake, L. A., Ceilley, R. I., Cornelison, R. L., Dobes, W. A., Dorner, W., Goltz, R. W., Lewis, C. W., Salasche, S. J., Turner, M. L., Graham, G. F., et al. (1992). Guidelines of care for basal cell carcinoma. *Journal of the American Academy of Dermatology, 26*(1), 117–120.

Flory, C. (1992). Skin assessment. *RN, 55*(6), 22–26.

Guyton, A. C. (1991). *Textbook of medical physiology* (8th ed.). Philadelphia: W. B. Saunders.

Hodgson, B. B., Kizior, R. J., & Kingdon, R. T. (1993). *Nurse's drug handbook.* Philadelphia: W. B. Saunders.

Jarvis, C. (1992). *Physical examination and health assessment.* Philadelphia: W. B. Saunders.

Kaplan, R. P. (1991). The aging skin. *Geriatrics, 17*(8), 59–67.

Kurban, R. S., & Kurban, A. K. (1993). Common skin disorders of aging: Diagnosis and treatment (review). *Geriatrics, 48*(4), 30–31, 35–36, 39–42.

Marks, R. (1991). The role of treatment of actinic keratoses in the prevention of morbidity and mortality due to squamous cell carcinoma. *Archives of Dermatology, 127,* 1031–1033.

Matteson, M. A., & McConnell, E. S. (1989). *Gerontological nursing.* Philadelphia: W. B. Saunders.

McMahon, R. (1991). The prevalence of skin problems beneath the breasts of in-patients. *Nursing Times, 87*(39), 48–51.

Phillips, W. G. (1992). Pruritus. *Postgraduate Medicine, 92*(7), 34–46, 53, 56.

Proper, S. A., Rose, P. T., & Fenske, N. A. (1990). Non-melanomatous skin cancer in the elderly: Diagnosis and management. *Geriatrics, 45*(7), 57–65.

Ries, W. R., Aly, A., & Vrabec, J. (1990). Common skin lesions of the elderly. *Otolaryngologic Clinics of North America, 23*(6), 1121–1139.

Robertson, D. R., & George, C. F. (1990). Treatment of post herpetic neuralgia in the elderly. *British Medical Bulletin, 46*(1), 113–123.

Schmader, K. E., Studenski, S., MacMillan, J., Grufferman, S., & Cohen, H. J. (1990). Are stressful life events risk factors for herpes zoster? *Journal of the American Geriatrics Society, 38*(11), 1188–1194.

Schmidtling, R. E., Gordon, S. I., & Davenport, B. B. (1992). Treating pressure ulcers with a myocutaneous flap. *Nursing 92, 22*(7), 58–61.

Shlafer, M. (1993). *The nurse, pharmacology, and drug therapy* (2nd ed.). Redwood City, CA: Addison-Wesley.

Skewes, S. M. (1994). No more bed baths! *RN, 57*(1), 34–35.

Tortora, G. J., & Grabowski, S. R. (1993). *Principles of anatomy and physiology* (7th ed.). New York: Harper Collins College Publishers.

KEY CONCEPTS

1. The functions of the skin are protection, body temperature regulation, secretion, sensation, synthesis of vitamin D, and blood storage.
2. The skin assessment may detect skin disorders and systemic disorders that affect the skin.
3. Pruritus (itching) is a symptom rather than a disease that is treated by correction or removal of the underlying cause, skin moisturizers, and drugs such as antihistamines, corticosteroids, and local anesthetics.
4. Atopic dermatitis (eczema) is abnormally dry, itchy skin that is treated with moisturizers, antihistamines, antibiotics, and corticosteroids.
5. Seborrheic dermatitis is a chronic inflammatory disease of the skin caused by increased sebum production that is treated with medicated shampoos for the scalp and topical corticosteroids and antibiotics for other body sites.

KEY CONCEPTS *(continued)*

6. Psoriasis, characterized by bright-red lesions with silvery scales, may require treatment with keratolytics, radiation, and antipsoriatics.
7. Fungal infections, including tinea pedis, tinea manus, tinea cruris, tinea corporis, tinea barbae, and candidiasis, are usually treated with antifungal drugs.
8. Acne, which is characterized by comedones, pustules, and cysts primarily on the face, neck, and upper trunk, may be treated with topical medications, oral antibiotics, estrogen, and vitamin A derivatives.
9. The herpes simplex virus types 1 and 2, which cause outbreaks of vesicles that rupture and form crusts, is treated with acyclovir, an antiviral drug that hastens healing but is not curative.
10. Herpes zoster infection (shingles) causes pain and itching along a nerve pathway and may respond to acyclovir.
11. Common nursing diagnoses for the patient with an infectious or inflammatory skin disorder include impaired skin integrity, pain, high risk for (secondary) infection, body image disturbance, social isolation, and knowledge deficit.
12. Lice and scabies are tiny parasites that may infest the hair and skin, causing intense itching.
13. Pemphigus is a chronic autoimmune condition in which fragile bullae develop and rupture, spilling a foul drainage.
14. Skin cancers include actinic keratoses, basal cell carcinomas, squamous cell carcinomas, melanomas, and cutaneous T-cell lymphoma.
15. The two major conditions affecting the nails are infections and inflammation caused by ingrown nails.
16. Burns are classified by size and depth of the tissue injury.
17. Serious burns affect not only the skin but also fluid balance, gastrointestinal function, respiratory function, and the immune system.
18. The three stages of burn injury are emergent, acute, and rehabilitation.
19. Wound care after burn injury is intended to promote healing, prevent infection, control heat loss, retain function, and minimize disfigurement.
20. Nursing care of the burn patient may address decreased cardiac output, fluid volume excess, acute pain, high risk for infection, hypothermia, altered nutrition, impaired physical mobility, ineffective individual coping, ineffective family coping, and knowledge deficit.

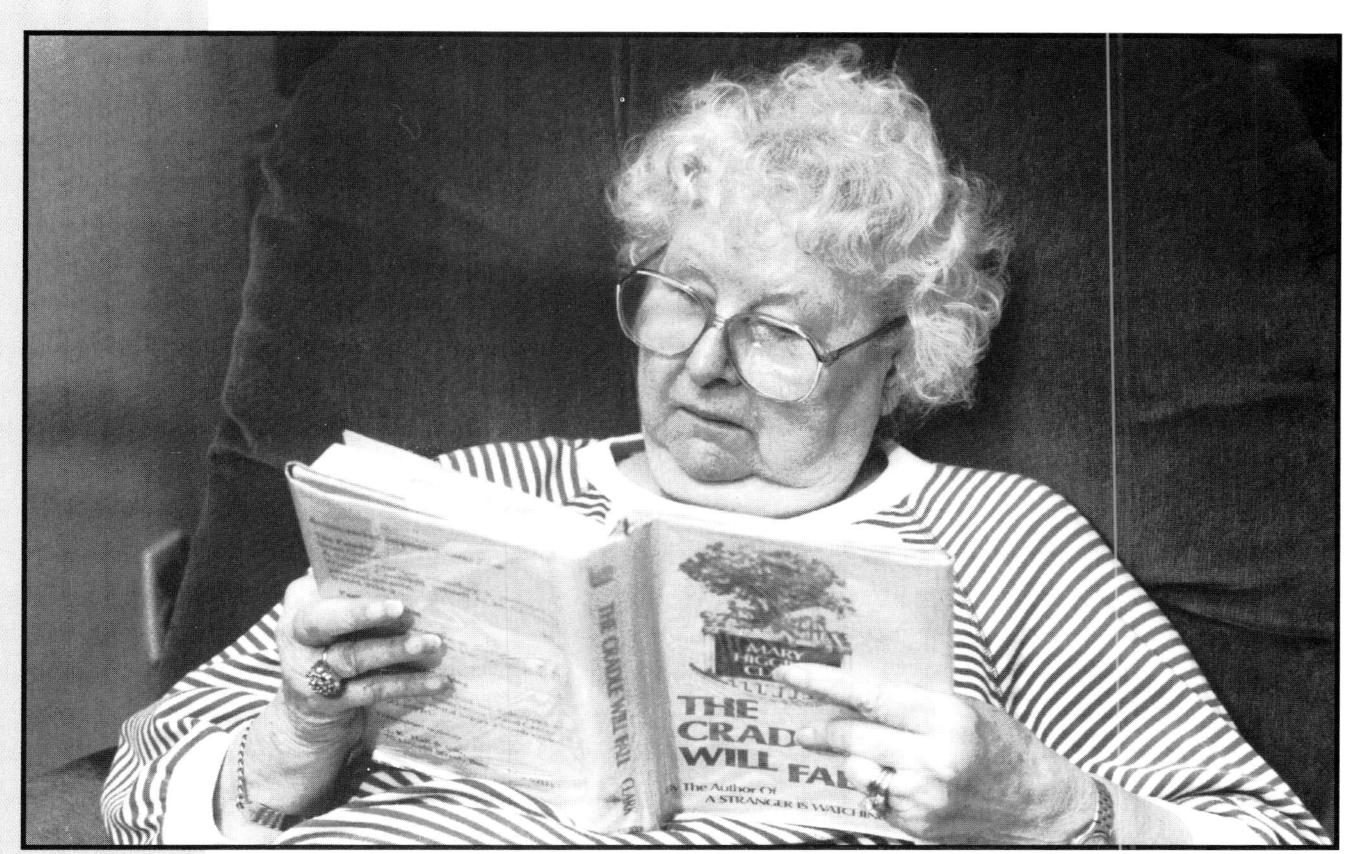

UNIT 15

Disorders of the Eyes, Ears, Nose, and Throat

Adrianne Linton

CHAPTER 47

Eye and Vision Disorders

OBJECTIVES

1. Identify the data to be collected in the nursing assessment of the eye and vision.
2. Identify the nursing responsibilities for patients having diagnostic tests or procedures to diagnose eye disorders.
3. Describe the nursing care of patients who require common therapeutic measures for eye disorders: irrigation, application of ophthalmic drugs, and surgery.
4. Describe the pathophysiology, signs and symptoms, diagnosis, and treatment of selected eye conditions.
5. Apply the nursing process to plan care for the patient with an eye disorder.

GLOSSARY

ASTIGMATISM Error of refraction caused by uneven curvature of the cornea or lens; causes visual distortion

CATARACT Clouding or opacity of the normally transparent lens within the eye; causes blurred vision and objects to take on a yellowish hue

CONJUNCTIVITIS Inflammation of the membrane lining the eyelids and the eyeball

CYCLOPLEGIC Agent that paralyzes the ciliary muscle so that the eye does not accommodate

ECTROPION In relation to the eyelid, outward turning of the lid

ENTROPION In relation to the eyelid, inward turning of the lid

ENUCLEATION Removal of an intact organ, such as the eyeball

Glossary continued

HYPEROPIA Farsightedness; ability to see distant objects better than near objects

KERATITIS Inflammation of the cornea

MIOTIC Agent that causes the pupil to constrict

MYDRIATIC Agent that causes the pupil to dilate

MYOPIA Nearsightedness; ability to see near objects better than distant objects

PRESBYOPIA A visual impairment associated with older age in which the lens becomes more rigid and less able to change shape, resulting in a decreased ability to focus on near objects

REFRACTION Bending of light rays

TONOMETRY Measurement of pressure such as intraocular pressure

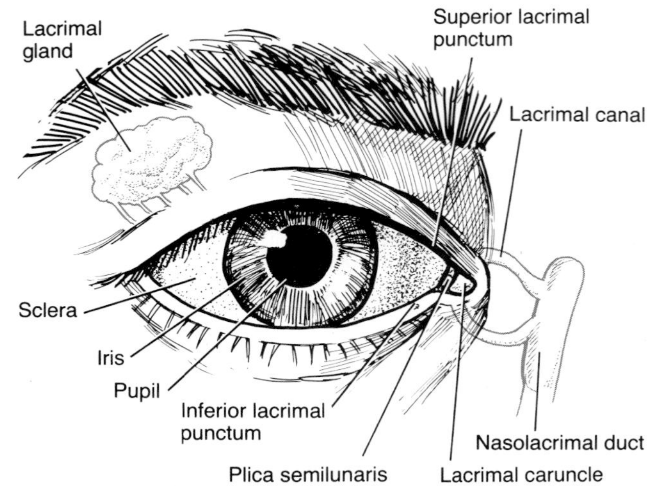

FIGURE 47-1
External parts of the visual system.

It has been said that the eye is the window to the world. Indeed, vision plays an extremely important part in everyday life. It enables people to move about freely, to avoid danger, and to appreciate physical beauty. The eyes are also credited with conveying (or betraying!) one's emotions and communicating trust. Romantics speak of gazing into the eyes of a loved one.

In the United States, more than 11 million people have some vision impairment. For most people, loss of vision is perceived as a most tragic event. Nurses can play important roles in the prevention of vision loss, treatment of disorders of the eye, and rehabilitation of people with vision disturbances.

ANATOMY AND PHYSIOLOGY OF THE EYE

The eyeball is the primary structure involved in seeing. Several structures in addition to the eyeball serve to make up the visual system. The external structures of the visual system include the eyelids, eyelashes, conjunctiva, cornea, sclera, and extraocular muscles. These structures are illustrated in Figure 47–1.

EXTERNAL STRUCTURES

The external structures of the visual system serve to protect and move the eyeball. The eyelids and eyelashes protect the eye by keeping it moist and shielding it from foreign substances. The lids are lined with a mucous membrane called the palpebral conjunctiva. The membrane continues from the inner eyelid margins to form a pocket around the eye, and then covers the sclera up to the margin of the iris. The portion of the membrane that covers the anterior sclera is the bulbar conjunctiva.

Lacrimal glands located above the eyes secrete tears into the eyes through lacrimal ducts in the upper eyelids. Spontaneous blinking (about 15 times a minute) bathes the eyeballs in tear fluid. Tear fluid provides oxygen and some nutrients to the cornea. Normally, the fluid drains from the eye through the lacrimal sac into the nose. With excessive tear production, tears run from the eyes. Increased tear production occurs with trauma, irritation, or emotional distress. Decreased tear production occurs to some extent with aging. Severe deficiencies in tear fluid cause "dry eyes," making the cornea susceptible to injury.

Normal vision requires the eyes to move together. The simultaneous movement of both eyes in the same direction is called conjugate movement. Eye movements are coordinated by three cranial nerves and six extraocular muscles.

THE EYEBALL

The eyeball consists of three layers of tissue: the sclera, the choroid, and the retina (Fig. 47–2).

Sclera

The sclera is the tough outer layer of the eyeball. It is mostly white except for the clear cornea over the iris. The cornea is covered by a protective membrane called the conjunctiva.

Choroid

The middle choroid layer makes up the iris and ciliary muscle at the front of the eye. The colored part of the eye, the iris, is actually a muscle. The hole in the center of the iris is the pupil. The iris contracts and relaxes to control the amount of light entering the eye. Dim light or severe stress causes the iris to contract. This makes the pupil dilate, or enlarge. Bright light causes the iris to relax, leaving the pupil constricted. The choroid is rich in blood vessels that deliver nourishment to the retina in the back of the eye.

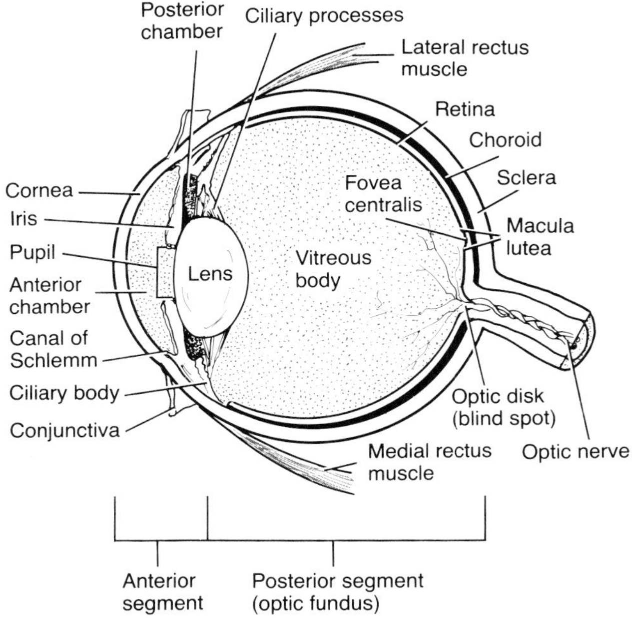

FIGURE 47-2
Internal structures of the eye.

Retina

The retina is the inner lining of the eyeball. It is composed of two layers. The pigmented layer is between the choroid and the sensory layer. The pigmented layer receives nutrients and oxygen from the choroid and supplies the sensory layer.

The area at the back of the eye contains light-sensitive receptors called rods and cones. Rods are most important for vision in dim light. Cones are used for daylight vision and color perception. The area of sharpest vision on the retina is the macula. Because the macula has no blood vessels, it depends on the choroid for nourishment.

Optic Nerve

The optic nerve enters the back of the eyeball. This nerve sends visual messages to the brain for interpretation. When the eye is examined with an ophthalmoscope, the part of the optic nerve that can be seen is referred to as the optic disk.

Fluid Chambers

ANTERIOR CHAMBER. Within the eyeball are two chambers separated by the lens. The anterior chamber is located between the iris and the cornea. It is filled with aqueous humor, a clear, watery fluid. Aqueous humor is produced in the ciliary body. It flows over the lens, through the pupil, and out through the trabecular meshwork into the canal of Schlemm. The canal of Schlemm returns the fluid to the venous circulation. The flow of aqueous humor is illustrated in Figure 47–3.

The function of aqueous humor is to moisturize and nourish the lens and cornea. The production and drainage of the fluid from the eye must be balanced to maintain normal pressure within the eye.

POSTERIOR CHAMBER. The larger posterior chamber behind the lens is filled with vitreous humor. Vitreous humor is a clear, gelatinous material that helps hold the retina in place.

Lens

The lens is a transparent structure behind the iris. It is attached to the ciliary muscle. The ciliary muscle relaxes and contracts to change the shape of the lens. This process, called accommodation, permits the eye to focus on objects at different distances. To focus on a near object, the ciliary muscle contracts, making the lens curve. For distance, the muscle relaxes, making the lens flatter.

VISUAL PATHWAY

As light enters the eye, it passes through the transparent cornea, aqueous humor, lens, and vitreous humor. These structures are called refractive media. They refract (bend) horizontal and vertical light rays so that the light rays focus on the retina.

On the retina, the light rays reflected from the image are reversed and upside down. Images are carried as impulses through the optic nerve. At the optic chiasm, fibers from the left field from each eye join to form the left optic tract. Fibers from the right field of each eye

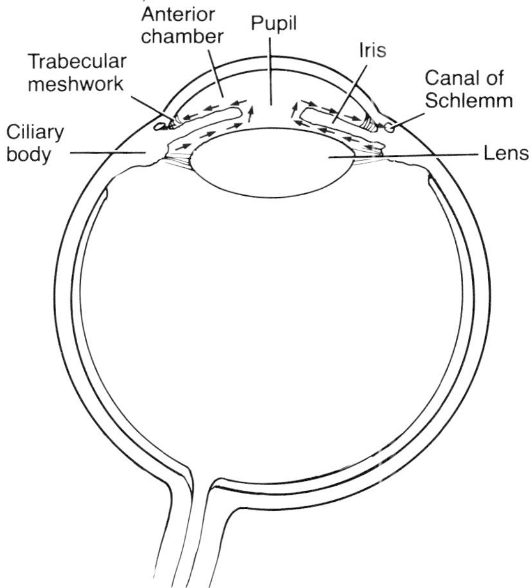

FIGURE 47-3
The flow of aqueous humor through the eye. Fluid is produced by the ciliary body. It flows through the pupil into the anterior chamber and out through the trabecular meshwork and the canal of Schlemm.

join to form the right optic tract. Images are transmitted to the brain by way of the optic tracts (Fig. 47–4).

AGE-RELATED CHANGES IN THE EYE

As people age, typical changes occur in the structures and function of the eye. The skin around the eye becomes wrinkled and looser. The eyelids usually have some excess tissue; this is not important unless it interferes with vision. The amount of fat around the eye decreases, permitting the eyeball to sink deeper into the orbit. Tear secretion diminishes, and the cornea loses sensitivity. A grayish ring may be seen around the outer margin of the iris. This ring is called the arcus senilis. There is some disagreement about the significance of the arcus senilis. It may be related to elevated serum lipid levels. It does not affect vision. The pupil is generally smaller in the older person and responds somewhat more slowly to light.

Vision changes associated with age are related to changes in the lens and the ciliary muscle. The lens becomes less elastic, more dense, opaque, and yellow. These changes have several significant effects. First, light passing through the lens scatters, causing the patient to be sensitive to glare. The second, more important effect is that the ability to focus is impaired. This farsightedness (hyperopia) in older people is called presbyopia. This is the reason most older people have to wear glasses for reading or other close work. Some older people report seeing specks moving across the field of vision. These dark spots, called floaters, are actually bits of debris in the vitreous.

Despite the age-related changes in the eye, most older people retain adequate vision for daily activities.

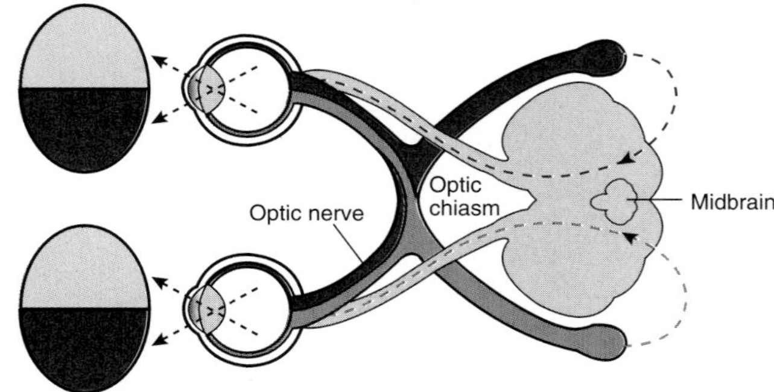

FIGURE 47–4

The visual pathway. (Adapted from Jarvis, C. [1992]. *Physical examination and health assessment* [pp. 314–315]. Philadelphia: W. B. Saunders.)

NURSING ASSESSMENT OF THE EYE

HEALTH HISTORY

History of Present Illness

When assessing specific eye complaints, the nurse records changes in vision, including blurred vision, diplopia (double vision), spots, floaters, flashes of light, tunnel vision, altered color perception, halos around lights, blind spots (scotomata), and loss of part of the visual fields. If the patient reports pain, the nurse inquires about its location and nature (sharp, stabbing, aching). Sensitivity to light, called photophobia, is documented. Drainage might be described as tears, purulent discharge, or crusting of the eyelids or eyelashes. The patient is asked to describe the type of discharge. The nurse also notes if the patient complains that the eyes feel dry and irritated. Another complaint that might prompt the patient to seek medical attention is redness or swelling of the lids, eyes, or periorbital area (around the eyes).

Past Medical History

People tend to assume that changes in vision are caused by problems in the eye or related structures. Although this is often true, visual disturbances can also be associated with many other conditions. Therefore, it is important to obtain a good history of past medical problems from the patient who reports with vision problems. Conditions to be alert for include the following:

- **Diabetes.** Elevated blood glucose can cause temporary blurring of vision. Permanent changes in the retina associated with diabetes can cause blindness.
- **Neurologic disorders.** Brain tumors, head injuries, and strokes are examples of conditions that may impair vision. Effects may be blurred vision, diplopia, inability to move eyes, or loss of part of the visual fields.
- **Thyroid disease.** Hyperthyroidism may cause exophthalmos (bulging eyes).
- **Hypertension.** Hypertension can cause changes in the blood vessels of the eye, eventually leading to vision loss.

Any eye injury or previously diagnosed eye disease is noted, including date of last examination and treatment.

A current medication history also is important in assessing vision problems. Some drugs can cause temporary or permanent changes in visual acuity and color vision. Others may contribute to the development of cataracts or glaucoma. Drugs that are especially likely to be related to vision disturbances are digitalis, corticosteroids, indomethacin, and sulfisoxazole.

Family History

The family history includes any known eye diseases as well as a history of arteriosclerosis, diabetes, and thyroid disease.

Functional Assessment

The functional assessment documents the patient's occupation, roles, and usual activities. The nurse is alert for activities that might pose a risk to the eyes.

PHYSICAL EXAMINATION

The physician performs a complete examination, including inspection of the inner eye. The nurse, however, can inspect the external eye, assess response of the pupil to light, and evaluate gross visual acuity. If abnormalities are suspected, the nurse informs the physician or advises the patient to seek medical evaluation.

The nurse first examines the eyelids for redness, drainage, and position. The lids should cover the eyeball completely when closed. When the eyes are open, the lower lid should be at the level of the iris. The upper lid should barely cover the upper margin of the iris. The lids should fit closely to the eyeball, and the eyelashes should not turn toward the eye. Any crusting or drainage on the lids or the lashes is described.

The eyeball is inspected for color and moisture. The sclera should be clear white. Excessive redness may be due to irritation or inflammation. A yellow color, called icterus, is associated with liver dysfunction.

The pupils are assessed for size, equality, and reaction to light. Pupils that are unequal, dilated, or do not respond to light suggest neurologic problems. Some medications can also affect pupil characteristics. Accommodation is tested by having the patient focus on the nurse's finger held at a distance, and then having the patient watch the finger as it is slowly moved toward the patient's nose. The pupil should constrict and the eyes converge.

Visual acuity is commonly tested using the Snellen chart (Fig. 47–5). The Snellen chart has rows of progressively smaller letters. From a distance of 20 feet, the patient reads down the chart until more than two mistakes are made on a single line. Each eye is tested separately and then together. The lines are numbered 20 over 200, 100, 70, 50, 40, 30, 25, 20, and 15. The findings are reported as the last line the person could read with no more than two errors. That is, if the person read the 20/30 line with one error, but made three errors on the 20/25 line, the vision would be recorded as 20/30 in the eye tested. This means that the person could read at 20 feet what a person with normal vision could read at 30 feet. Nurses may use the Snellen chart for vision screening in clinic and office settings. In the hospital, it may be more practical to simply ask the patient to read available print. This provides the nurse with some practical measure of visual acuity.

Some nurses learn to assess visual fields, extraocular movements, and the corneal reflex. There are also several tests used to detect strabismus.

When assessing the eyes, the nurse is alert for the signs of trouble listed in Table 47–1. If any of these are present, the patient is referred to the physician for evaluation. The nursing assessment of the patient with an eye disorder is summarized in Table 47–2.

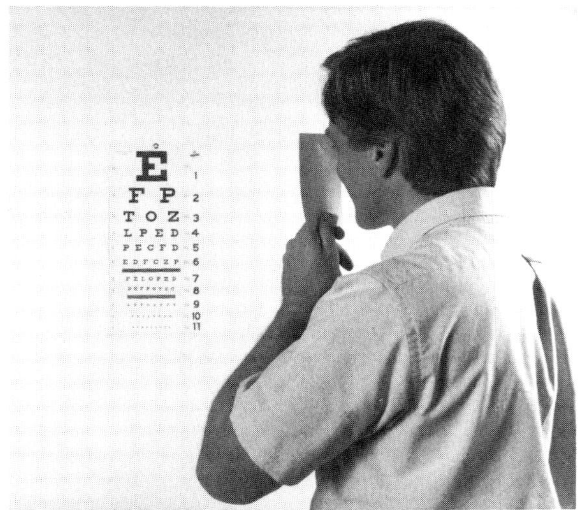

FIGURE 47–5
The Snellen chart is used to measure visual acuity. (From Jarvis, C. [1992]. *Physical examination and health assessment* [p. 321]. Philadelphia: W. B. Saunders.)

TABLE 47–1
SIGNS OF POSSIBLE EYE PROBLEMS

- Particular trouble adjusting to a dark room
- Squinting or blinking due to unusual sensitivity to light or glare
- Change in color of iris
- Red-rimmed and crusted or swollen eyelids
- Inflamed or red eyes
- Recurrent pain in or around eyes
- Sudden loss of vision in one eye
- Sudden hazy or blurred vision
- Flashes of light or showers of black spots
- Halos or rainbows around light
- Curtain-like loss of vision
- Loss of peripheral or side vision

Data from "Signs of Possible Eye Trouble in Adults" (pamphlet), the Texas Society to Prevent Blindness.

TABLE 47–2
ASSESSMENT OF THE PATIENT WITH AN EYE DISORDER

HEALTH HISTORY

Present illness: Changes in vision, symptoms of eye disorders: pain, photophobia, drainage, dryness, irritation, redness, swelling

Past medical history: Diabetes, neurologic disorders, thyroid disease, hypertension, previously diagnosed eye disease or injury, date of last eye examination, current medications (specifically digitalis, corticosteroids, indomethacin, sulfonamides)

Family history: Known eye diseases, arteriosclerosis, diabetes, thyroid disease, arthritis

Functional assessment: Occupation, roles, usual activities, changes required by eye problems

PHYSICAL EXAMINATION

Eyelids: Redness, drainage, position, closure, crusting, inversion or eversion

Eyeball: Color, moisture

Pupils: Size, equality, reaction to light, accommodation

Visual acuity: Measured with Snellen's chart, gross acuity

Visual fields

Extraocular movements

Corneal reflex

Inner eye: Ophthalmoscopic examination of anterior chamber, lens, vitreous, and fundus (inner surface of retina)

DIAGNOSTIC TESTS AND PROCEDURES

Several professionals are trained to assess and treat conditions of the eye. The nurse should understand the differences between these individuals. An ophthalmologist is a physician with specialized training in diagnosing and treating eye conditions. The ophthalmologist prescribes corrective lenses for refractive errors as well as treats other eye conditions with medications and surgery. An optometrist is trained to diagnose errors of refraction and to prescribe corrective lenses. An optician fills prescriptions written by an ophthalmologist or optometrist and fits the prescribed lenses.

Diagnostic tests and procedures for disorders of the eye are described in Table 47–3.

OPHTHALMOSCOPIC EXAMINATION

The ophthalmoscopic examination involves using an ophthalmoscope (Fig. 47–6) to examine the lens, vitreous humor, retina, and optic disk. A solution such as phenylephrine 2.5% may be instilled in the eye first to dilate the pupil. This permits a better view of the inner eye. A darkened room also causes the pupil to dilate.

The examiner studies the cornea, lens, and vitreous for opacities. The blood vessels at the back of the eye (called the fundus) are inspected for evidence of dis-

TABLE 47–3
DIAGNOSTIC TESTS AND PROCEDURES FOR DISORDERS OF THE EYE

TEST/STUDY	PURPOSE/PROCEDURE	PATIENT PREPARATION	POSTPROCEDURE NURSING CARE
Ophthalmoscopy	Ophthalmoscope used to look through pupil to see inner eye. Allows diagnosis of abnormalities of retina, optic disk, and blood vessels.	Cycloplegic medication may be ordered to dilate pupil and prevent accommodation. Room is darkened during examination.	If pupils are dilated, advise patient of need for sunglasses.
Refraction	Identifies refractive errors and corrective lens needed. A refractor contains various lenses on rotating wheels. Patient looks through refractor as lenses are changed. Examiner determines which lens produces best visual acuity.	Explain procedure to patient.	If pupils are dilated, advise patient of need for sunglasses until pupil returns to normal.
Tonometry	The Schiotz tonometer is a hand-held instrument that is placed on cornea. It measures intraocular pressure. Another, more accurate procedure uses biomicroscope to measure pressure. Pneumotonometer is an instrument that measures intraocular pressure by emitting a puff of air toward cornea.	For procedures in which an instrument touches cornea, anesthetic drops are ordered. Patient needs to remain still during procedure.	Patient should be advised not to rub eyes for 15 min after procedure. This is to prevent trauma to eye when sensation is absent.
Fluorescein angiography	A dye (fluorescein) is injected into a vein in hand or arm. A series of pictures of blood vessels in eye is then taken. This permits diagnosis of abnormalities of vessels and retina.	Cycloplegic medication is ordered to dilate pupil. Patient is seated with chin on a chin rest. A bright blue light flashes as pictures are taken. This may cause some discomfort as well as visual disturbance that lasts several minutes after test. Flashing light can trigger seizure activity in patients with epilepsy.	Dye may cause a yellowish skin color for 6–24 hr. Urine may be greenish as dye is eliminated.
Visual fields	Identifies the area a person can see while looking straight ahead. Assessed by comparing fields patient can see with those seen by a "normal" examiner. Patient and examiner sit facing each other. They cover opposite eyes. Examiner moves his or her hand out of line of vision and then brings it into expected line of vision in a specific pattern. Patient states when examiner's fingers are seen.	No preparation is needed.	No postprocedure care is needed.

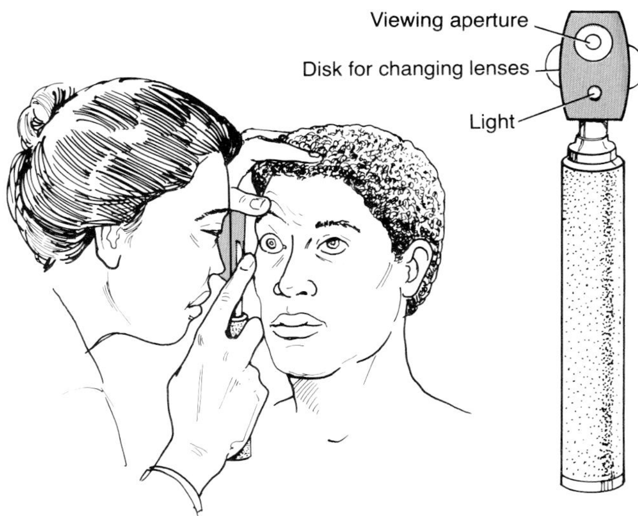

FIGURE 47–6

An ophthalmoscope is used to examine the inner structure of the eye.

ease. Degenerative changes of the retina may be observed.

The patient requires no special preparation for the ophthalmoscopic examination. If the pupils are dilated, the eyes will be very sensitive to light. Sunglasses will be needed when going into brightly lit areas. Visual acuity will be temporarily affected, so the patient may need to have someone drive him or her home after the examination.

REFRACTION

As light enters the eye, it passes through the aqueous humor, lens, and vitreous humor. The light rays bend so that they focus on the retina. This bending is called refraction. Refractive errors occur when the light does not bend properly. This causes alterations in vision, which are discussed in more detail later. Refraction is assessed by having the patient read a chart through a series of lenses. The patient identifies which lens permits the clearest image. This enables the examiner to detect refractive errors. The procedure requires no special preparation.

VISUAL FIELDS

Visual fields include the area a person can see while looking straight ahead without moving the head. Some conditions, such as glaucoma, retinal detachment, and certain neurologic abnormalities, cause loss of parts of the visual fields. Visual fields are assessed by comparing the patient's field of vision with that of a "normal" examiner (Fig. 47–7). No special equipment is required.

TONOMETRY

Tonometry is the measurement of pressure in the anterior chamber of the eye. Normal intraocular pressure is 12 to 21 mm Hg. Glaucoma is a condition in which the pressure in the eye is increased. Sustained pressure elevation causes progressive damage to the eye. If untreated, blindness results. In most cases, the patient has no symptoms. Therefore, routine measurement of intraocular pressure is important to detect abnormalities.

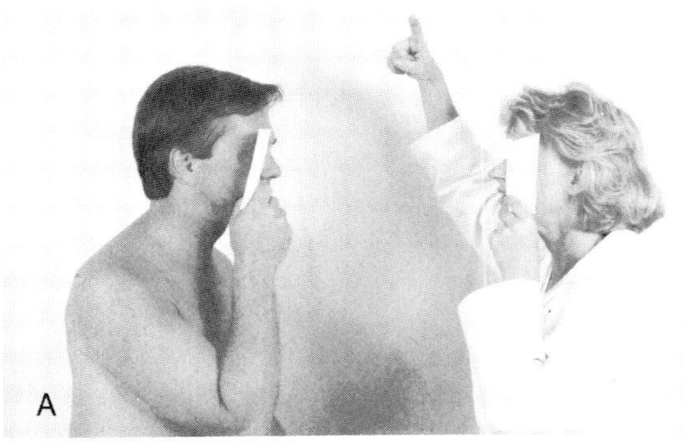

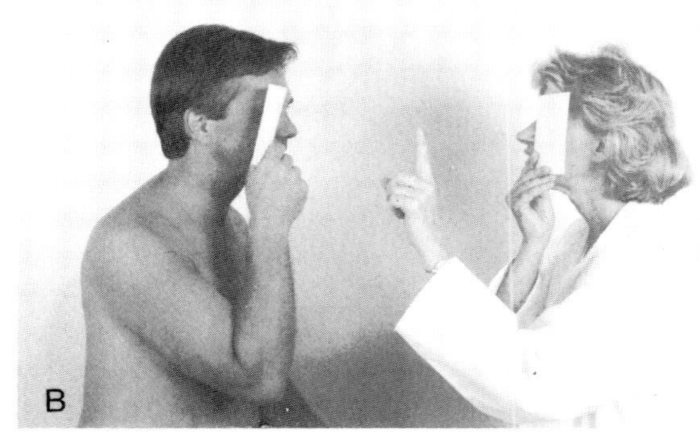

FIGURE 47–7

Assessment of visual fields. (From Jarvis, C. [1992]. *Physical examination and health assessment* [p. 322]. Philadelphia: W. B. Saunders.)

Several procedures are used to measure intraocular pressure. The Schiøtz tonometer, seen in Figure 47–8, is commonly used for this purpose. Another, more accurate procedure is called applanation. It is done with a slit-lamp microscope.

Both of these procedures require that the cornea be anesthetized. Proparacaine 0.5% (Ophthaine) is used for this purpose. Since the medication deadens the cornea, however, the patient must be told not to rub the eye for at least 15 minutes. Otherwise, the cornea might be accidentally scratched. The nurse explains that the patient needs to remain still and that the procedure is not painful.

The pneumotonometer is a hand-held instrument that directs a puff of air to the surface of the eye. It measures intraocular pressure by measuring resistance to the air.

OPHTHALMODYNAMOMETRY

In ophthalmodynamometry, a spring plunger is used to apply pressure to the sclera while the retinal vessels are observed with an ophthalmoscope. The instrument

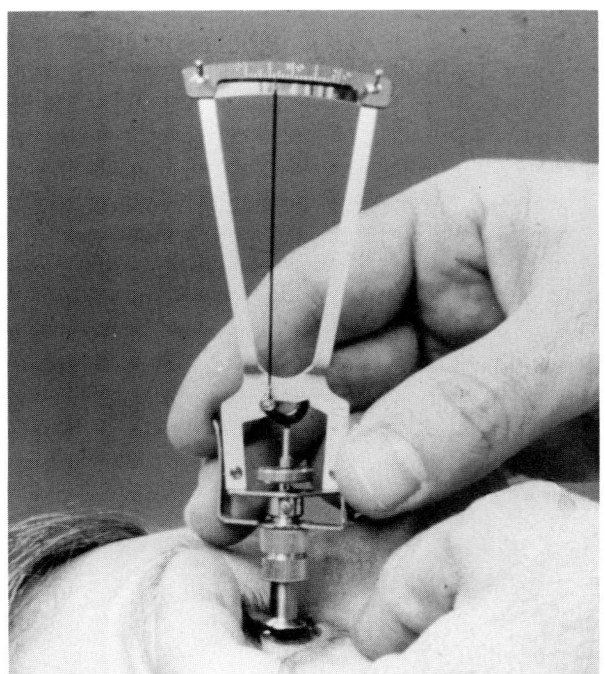

FIGURE 47-8

A Schiøtz tonometer measures intraocular pressure. (From Black, J. M., & Matassarin-Jacobs, E. [1993]. *Luckmann and Sorensen's medical-surgical nursing: A psychophysiologic approach* [4th ed., p. 842]. Philadelphia: W. B. Saunders.)

measures the approximate pressure in the blood vessels of the eye. Both eyes are assessed. Differences in pressure from one eye to the next reflect insufficiency of the carotid artery on the side with lower pressure.

MEASURES OF ELECTRICAL POTENTIAL

Since the retina is composed of nerve tissue, it has electrical potential that can be measured. This is useful in detecting retinal disorders, including retinitis pigmentosa, massive ischemia, widespread infection, and some chemical toxicities. Two procedures used to measure electrical potential are electroretinography and visual evoked response.

Electroretinography

In electroretinography, a contact lens is placed on the eye and exposed to a diffuse flash of light. The response of the retina is recorded. The patient must fix his or her gaze on a target and remain very still.

Visual Evoked Response

For visual evoked response, electrodes are placed on the patient's scalp, and each eye is stimulated. The electrical response is measured.

FLUORESCEIN ANGIOGRAPHY

To detect abnormal blood vessels or blood flow, fluorescein is injected intravenously and the retina is observed and photographed as the dye circulates (Fig. 47–9). Informed consent is required for this test. Some people are allergic to the dye, so diphenhydramine (Benadryl) may be given in advance. Nevertheless, emergency equipment is on hand in case of severe allergic response. The nurse can tell the patient to expect to hear the cameras operating and to see bright flashes of light. Some patients report a feeling of warmth, nausea, or vertigo. After the test, the patient needs to drink extra fluids to promote elimination of the dye. The patient is advised that the dye temporarily causes the urine to be yellow and may make the skin appear yellowish as well.

TOPICAL DYES

Topical dyes can be applied to the eye to detect abrasions of the cornea. Fluorescein is applied, followed by a saline rinse. The cornea is then examined. Dye permits scratches to be seen more readily.

IMAGING PROCEDURES

To obtain images of the eye for diagnostic purposes, the physician may order computed tomography scanning, ultrasonography, or magnetic resonance imaging.

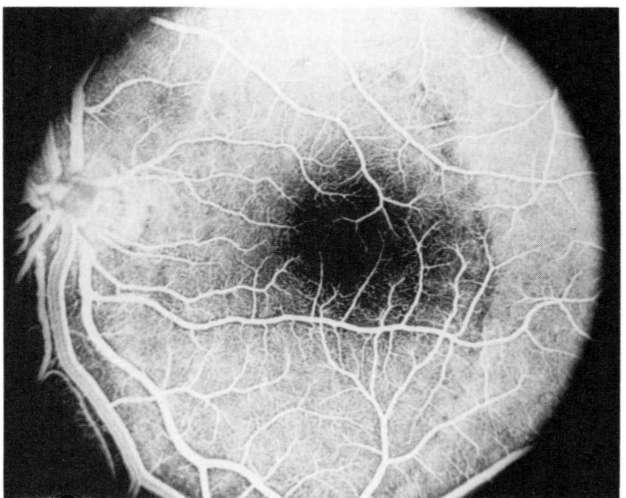

FIGURE 47-9

Fluorescein angiography permits visualization of the blood vessels of the eye to examine the inner structure of the eye. (From Black, J. M., & Matassarin-Jacobs, E. [1993]. *Luckmann and Sorensen's medical-surgical nursing: A psychophysiologic approach* [4th ed., p. 844]. Philadelphia: W. B. Saunders.)

COMMON THERAPEUTIC MEASURES

EYE IRRIGATION

Irrigations are done to remove irritating chemicals from the eye. Sterile normal saline is the best solution to use. Plain water also is acceptable, especially in emergencies. In the hospital or clinic setting, the physician sometimes orders irrigations with ophthalmic medications. Key points in irrigating the eye include the following:

1. Cleanse the eyelids and eyelashes.
2. Position the patient with the affected eye down so that contaminated fluid does not run into the unaffected eye.
3. Place a basin and waterproof pad to collect the fluid.
4. Gently direct the fluid into the lower conjunctival sac from the inner canthus (corner of the eye) to the outer canthus.
5. Do not touch the eye with the tip of the irrigating syringe.
6. Have the patient blink occasionally to move particles toward the lower conjunctival sac.

TOPICAL MEDICATIONS

A number of medications can be applied directly to the eye. These include miotics, mydriatics, anesthetics, cycloplegics, antibiotics, and anti-inflammatory drugs. Some systemic drugs also may be ordered, such as diuretics to treat glaucoma. Examples of ophthalmic drugs are included in Table 47–4.

The following are key points for the nurse to remember when administering topical eye medications:

1. Be *very* careful that only medications labeled for *ophthalmic* use are put in the eye!
2. Drops should be room temperature when administered. Rolling the bottle between the palms is a good way to warm the medication.
3. Tell the patient to tilt his or her head back and look at the ceiling. The head can be turned slightly so that excess medication runs out the outer canthus of the eyes and does not contaminate the opposite eye.
4. Gently pull the lower eyelid down to expose the conjunctival sac.
5. Brace the hand holding the medication and then drop the medication into the conjunctival sac without touching the eyelid with the container.
6. Tell the patient to close his or her eyes and move them as if looking around. This distributes the medication over the eye.
7. The nurse or the patient should apply gentle pressure to the lacrimal sac at the inner canthus of the eye for about 1 minute. This reduces the amount of the medication entering body fluids.
8. If more than one medication is being given, wait 5 minutes between each medication.

PHARMACOLOGY

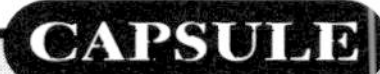

> Mydriatics dilate the pupils. Miotics constrict the pupils.

EYE SURGERY

A number of eye conditions are treated or corrected with surgery. Eye surgery may involve surgical incisions, the application of cold probes (cryotherapy), or the use of lasers. Individualized care plans must be developed based on the specific type of procedure done. Some general considerations, however, apply to most patients having eye surgery.

Preoperative Care

ASSESSMENT. Preoperative assessment and care are discussed in detail in Chapter 14. The preoperative assessment specifically focuses on the patient's emotional state, ability to perform self-care, and knowledge of surgical routines and outcomes. Most patients awaiting eye surgery are somewhat anxious. They may be fearful that the procedure will not be successful or that some complication will lead to blindness. The nurse determines whether there are any activity limitations. If the patient has poor vision, the type of help needed is documented. The nurse also notes the physician's orders for intravenous fluids or preoperative medications, or both. The patient's food and fluid intake is usually restricted from the evening before surgery to reduce the risk of nausea, vomiting, and aspiration after surgery.

NURSING DIAGNOSIS. Preoperative nursing diagnoses before eye surgery may include the following:

- **Anxiety** related to uncertain outcome, lack of knowledge about surgery and surgical routines
- **Self-Care Deficit** related to visual impairment

GOALS. The goals of preoperative nursing care are reduced anxiety, patient's understanding of surgical routines, and achievement of activities of daily living.

INTERVENTIONS

Anxiety. The nurse explores the patient's feelings about the surgery and provides information. Specific questions about the surgical procedure, risks, complications, or outcomes are referred to the physician. The nurse explains general surgical and postoperative routines.

Self-Care Deficit. The patient with vision impairment is oriented to the room. Objects are kept in one place, and the patient is advised of any new equipment or articles in the environment. Consent forms and other written material may need to be read to the patient.

EVALUATION. Criteria for effective nursing care are patient's statement of reduced anxiety and relaxed expression and completion of activities of daily living.

TABLE 47-4

DRUGS USED TO TREAT DISORDERS OF THE EYE

GENERAL NURSING CONSIDERATIONS

1. Advise patient to follow directions exactly.
2. If condition worsens or does not improve, physician should be notified.
3. If multiple ophthalmic drugs are ordered, wait 5 min between them.
4. After administering ophthalmic solutions, apply gentle pressure to lacrimal sac for about 1 min to decrease absorption and systemic effects.
5. Teach patient or family member correct technique for drug administration.
6. Emphasize to patients never to share eye medications.

DRUG	USE/ACTION	SIDE EFFECTS	NURSING INTERVENTIONS
Miotics	Primarily used to treat glaucoma.	See Table 47–5.	See Table 47–5.
Sympathomimetics Epinephrine bitartrate (Epitrate) Dipivefrin HCl (Propine) Phenylephrine (Neo-Synephrine)	Dilate pupil. Used in open-angle (chronic) glaucoma. Decreases corneal congestion. Controls hemorrhage.	Cardiac stimulation, headache, brow pain, allergy, worsening of acute (narrow-angle) glaucoma.	Sunglasses needed for 6 hr. Tell patient to report eye pain immediately—may be caused by increased intraocular pressure.
Antimuscarinics Atropine (Isopto Atropine) Homatropine (Isopto Homatropine) Scopolamine (Isopto Hyoscine) Cyclopentolate (Cyclogyl) Tropicamide (Mydriacyl)	Dilate pupil. Used before eye exams and for uveitis. Decrease lacrimal gland secretion. Cyclopentolate and tropicamide preferred for eye exam because of shorter duration of action.	Photophobia, inability to accommodate, corneal dryness and irritation.	Apply at ordered time before eye exam. If eye pain occurs, may indicate undetected glaucoma. Safety measures while pupils dilated, as vision is blurred. Artificial tears may be needed.
Antibiotics Gentamicin sulfate (Garamycin Ophthalmic) Erythromycin (Ilotycin) Polymyxin B sulfate (neomycin sulfate, bacitracin) Sulfonamides (Sulamyd Ophthalmic)	Treatment or prevention of eye infections.	Allergic reaction, conjunctivitis.	Screen for previous allergic reactions. Withhold drug and notify physician if allergic. Inspect eye and lids for increasing redness.
Antifungals Natamycin (Natacyn)	Effective against some fungal infections of eye.	Rarely: allergic reaction, conjunctival edema.	Advise patient to continue treatment as prescribed (usually 14–21 days). Notify physician if symptoms continue or if edema develops.
Antivirals Idoxuridine (Herplex) Vidarabine (Vira-A)	Treatment of herpes simplex keratitis.	Irritation, redness, edema, pain, itching, photophobia. Rarely: allergic reactions.	Advise sunglasses for sensitivity. Refrigerate.
Topical Anesthetics Proparacaine HCl (Ophthaine, Ophthetic) Tetracaine HCl (Pontocaine)	Block sensation in external eye for tonometry, removal of sutures or foreign bodies, some surgical procedures.	Stinging, irritation. Allergic reactions rare.	Do not use discolored solution. Caution patient not to touch or rub eye or insert contact lens until sensation returns.
Anti-inflammatory Agents Prednisolone acetate Prednisolone sodium phosphate Dexamethasone Fluorometholone	Prevent redness and swelling caused by inflammation due to causes other than bacterial infection.	Systemic effects possible if sufficient drug is absorbed, including fluid retention, nausea, mood swings, hypokalemia, and many others.	Apply pressure to lacrimal sac for 1–2 min after application to reduce absorption. Monitor blood studies.

Postoperative Care

ASSESSMENT. Postoperatively, the nurse assesses the patient's vital signs and level of consciousness as he or she recovers from anesthesia. The dressing, or the operative eye, is inspected for bleeding or drainage. The nurse also assesses patient comfort, including pain and nausea. If vision is impaired, the environment is assessed for safety hazards. Prior to discharge, the nurse determines the patient's understanding of and ability to administer prescribed medications.

NURSING DIAGNOSIS. Nursing diagnoses after eye surgery may include the following:

- **High Risk for Injury** related to pressure or trauma
- **Sensory Perceptual Alteration** (vision) related to disease process, trauma to the eye, patching

- **Pain** related to tissue trauma
- **Anxiety** related to temporary vision impairment
- **Knowledge Deficit** of self-care measures and usual postoperative course

GOALS. Goals of nursing care after eye surgery are absence of injury, adaptation to impaired vision, pain relief, reduced anxiety, and patient's knowledge of self-care.

INTERVENTIONS

High Risk for Injury. The physician may prescribe limitations on activity or position, or both. The head of the bed is usually elevated. The patient may be wearing a bulky dressing or a small eye patch. Either may be covered with a lightweight metal shield (Fig. 47–10). The dressing absorbs any drainage, and the shield protects the eye from rubbing. The patient is instructed not to try to rub the eye. The nurse checks the physician's orders to determine whether the dressing can be changed. Eye drops or ointments may be ordered. They may be different from those used before surgery. When an eye is patched, safety precautions must be taken to prevent injury.

An important aspect of the care of postoperative eye patients is to prevent increased intraocular pressure. The patient is cautioned against straining, leaning forward, lifting, and lying on the affected side. Since vomiting and retching raise intraocular pressure, nurses should treat nausea promptly.

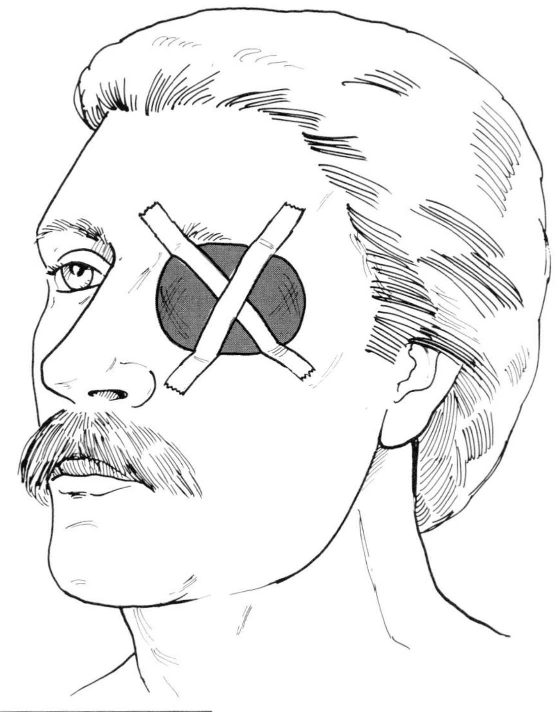

FIGURE 47–10

The shield protects the operative eye from pressure or rubbing.

Sensory Perceptual Alteration. Measures to assist the patient with visual impairment are discussed in detail in the section on nursing care of the visually impaired patient.

Pain. Although one might expect eye surgery to be painful, postoperative pain is usually mild to moderate. Mild analgesics may be given as ordered. If a patient reports severe pain, the physician should be notified.

Anxiety. Measures to reduce anxiety include explaining what is being done and why and encouraging the patient to express concerns and ask questions.

Knowledge Deficit. Eye patients are often discharged with some medications. The nurse provides careful directions and a written schedule for the medications. To assess the patient's ability to self-administer eye medications, the nurse can have the patient demonstrate the procedure before discharge. If necessary, a family member is instructed in administering the medications.

EVALUATION. Criteria for goal achievement after eye surgery are patient's avoidance of potentially harmful activities, adaptation of daily activities to vision impairment, patient's statement of reduced or absent pain, patient's statement of reduced anxiety and calm demeanor, and patient's demonstration of self-care.

PROTECTION OF THE EYES AND VISION

Maintaining adequate vision involves the prevention of injuries and the treatment of abnormalities. Nurses must be knowledgeable about the assessment and care of the eyes.

PATIENT TEACHING

Nurses can teach people how to care for their eyes in order to protect vision. Adults under the age of 40 should have their eyes examined every 3 to 5 years. After the age of 40, eye examinations should be done every 2 years and should include testing for glaucoma. This permits early detection and treatment of eye disorders.

Patients should be told to report sharp, stabbing eye pain or deep, throbbing eye pain. Other symptoms that should be reported to a physician are photophobia (sensitivity to light), blurred or double vision, loss of part of the visual fields, halos around lights, and floaters. Floaters are spots that appear to move across the field of vision. Some patients describe floaters as being like birds swooping past one's face. Other symptoms that require medical evaluation are burning sensations, itching, excessive tearing, and the presence of drainage from the eyes.

When there are symptoms of eye problems, patients should seek medical advice rather than trying home remedies. First aid for eye injuries is explained in Chapter 13.

Sometimes nurses have the opportunity to correct misconceptions that people have about vision. The following are some examples of misconceptions:

- Watching too much television or sitting too close to the television injures the eyes.
- Eating foods that contain large amounts of vitamin A improves vision.
- Eyes need to be rinsed regularly.

Prevention of Injuries

Injuries caused by foreign objects are a major cause of vision loss. Young children can be taught the danger of throwing or poking objects at the faces of playmates. Toys should be assessed for safety. Adult activities that produce sparks or cause fragments to be dispersed also cause injuries. Protective eyewear is advised for these potentially dangerous activities.

Basic Eye Care

The eyes are usually gently cleansed each time the face is washed. A clean cloth without soap should be used. The eye is washed from the inner canthus (near the nose) toward the outer canthus. Dry crusts on the eyelids and eyelashes can usually be wiped off. If necessary, the nurse can place a warm, damp cloth on the lids for several minutes to soften the crusts.

Routine eye rinses and drops are unnecessary for most people. Exceptions are people with inadequate tear production and those whose eyes do not close completely. Lubricating drops called "artificial tears" are available for those people. Sometimes, eye patches are applied or the lids are taped shut to prevent drying of the cornea.

IMPACT OF VISUAL IMPAIRMENT

Vision loss usually has significant impact on all areas of a person's life. Mild losses may require only some adaptations. More serious losses affect independence, mobility, employment, and interpersonal relationships. In addition, there is the loss of pleasure in seeing the people and things a person treasures.

The loss of vision triggers a grief response. People grieve for the lost function just as they might grieve following the death of a loved one. Reactions that are likely to follow loss of vision include shock, denial, anger, bargaining, and depression.

Factors that affect a person's response to this loss include personality, usual coping style, impact of vision loss on one's life, and the circumstances of the loss. If grief is resolved in a healthy manner, adaptation and acceptance eventually occur. People who have progressive loss of vision may experience anticipatory grief. Nursing care to help the person who is grieving is discussed in Chapter 22.

NURSING CARE OF THE VISUALLY IMPAIRED PATIENT

When people hear the word "blind," they think of someone who is unable to see. There are, however, degrees of visual impairment. Although some visually impaired people are unable to see at all, many others have partial vision. Therefore, medical literature is more likely to use terms such as "visual impairment" or "visually handicapped" rather than blind. Also, there may be a stigma attached to the word "blind." Some people automatically associate blindness with helplessness.

Trauma, disease, and some congenital defects account for visual handicaps throughout the life span. Some types of visual disturbances are more common in older people.

Those who work with the visually impaired need to be aware of their thoughts and feelings about visual handicaps. The nurse should demonstrate the attitude that people with visual impairments can be independent and productive. Sympathy or pity has no place in this situation because it encourages hopelessness and helplessness. The person needs help with some tasks but should still be treated as an adult.

The extent of vision loss determines the types of assistance that might be needed. Many people have visual problems that can be corrected with eyeglasses, drug therapy, or surgical treatment. When planning care, the nurse must consider whether the patient's condition is temporary, permanent, correctable, treatable, or progressive.

ASSESSMENT

The nursing assessment of the patient with an eye disorder is summarized in Table 47–2.

NURSING DIAGNOSIS

Common nursing diagnoses for patients with impaired vision may include the following:

- **Sensory Perceptual Alteration** (vision) related to altered reception, transmission, interpretation of visual stimuli
- **Ineffective Individual Coping** related to decreased independence, threat to body image, denial
- **Self-Care Deficit** (feeding, hygiene, grooming) related to perceptual impairment
- **Knowledge Deficit** of diagnosis and treatment of vision impairment

GOALS

Nursing goals when working with a patient with vision impairment are recognition and treatment of impairments, absence of injury; effective coping with vision loss; accomplishment of self-care; and patient's knowledge of diagnostic and therapeutic measures.

INTERVENTIONS

Sensory Perceptual Alteration

When a visually impaired person is admitted to the hospital, the nurse provides an orientation to the environment. The fact that the patient has visual impairment should be reflected on the nursing care plan. In addition, a sign may be posted to alert other caregivers and employees. Safety is a primary consideration for these patients. Measures to support the patient with impaired vision and to prevent injury include the following:

1. When you enter the room, announce your presence and introduce yourself to avoid startling or embarrassing the patient.
2. Speak before touching the patient to avoid frightening him or her.
3. Speak in a normal tone of voice. People tend to act as if those who cannot see cannot hear, so there is a tendency to raise one's voice when talking to the visually impaired.
4. Address the patient in the appropriate manner for his or her age and intellectual ability. Visual impairment is not associated with mental impairment.
5. Advise the patient what to expect during procedures.
6. Tell the patient when you leave the room.
7. Leave the bed in low position.
8. Place the call button in reach, and be sure the patient knows how to use it.
9. Keep doors either open or closed so that the ambulatory patient does not run into a partially closed door.
10. Eliminate meaningless noise from the environment as much as possible.
11. To lead a blind person, have him or her take your arm.

The environment significantly influences the visually impaired patient's ability to function. The environment should be safe and promote maximal independence. As already mentioned, orientation to the hospital room is especially important. The nurse makes sure the patient can use the call system, locate personal items, and use the bathroom. The patient is told if any new equipment or furniture is brought into the room. The pathways in the room are kept free of clutter.

For patients who are partially sighted, lighting is very important. Glare must be reduced because it actually interferes with vision. Windows should have adjustable shades, blinds, or sheers. Floors should not be highly polished (Fig. 47–11). Color can provide important cues to enable the partially sighted person to function. This is especially true of the older person whose color perception often changes. Older people perceive warm colors (red, orange, yellow) more accurately than cool colors (blue, green). Furniture color should be distinctly different from the color of floors and walls. Light switches, handrails, and steps marked with contrasting colors are easier to locate. Dishes and cups with colored rims facilitate self-feeding and reduce spills.

Ineffective Individual Coping

People who have lived with vision impairment usually have developed routines and strategies to cope with the situation. The nurse asks about such routines and maintains them as much as possible. If the patient uses assistive devices such as eyeglasses or magnifying glasses, the nurse makes sure they are available and encourages their use. The older person who becomes confused during hospitalization may show dramatic improvement when eyeglasses are provided.

Diversional activities are encouraged when appropriate. The patient with some vision may be able to enjoy reading with magnifiers or large-print reading material. "Talking books" are available without charge through the American Foundation for the Blind. Many bookstores now stock books on tape. Braille reading material and typewriters can be used by those who have been trained in this method. Braille uses arrangements of raised dots to represent letters. The reader reads the material by moving the fingertips over the characters. Not everyone is able to master reading Braille because of the sensitive touch needed. Community resources and rehabilitation centers offer ongoing services and assistance.

Self-Care Deficit

The nurse asks the patient what assistance is required instead of assuming that help is needed. Many patients are quite independent despite impaired vision. The nurse does not encourage dependence during hospitalization. To orient the patient to the location of foods, fluids, or other objects, their arrangement should be thought of as a clock face ("your meat is at 3 o'clock"). A consistent environment enables the patient to be more independent with less risk of injury. Furniture, personal effects, and equipment are not moved without patient consent.

Some visually impaired people have Seeing Eye dogs that enable them to move about more independently. These dogs are trained to guide their owners both inside and outside the home. They can generally go anywhere their owners go. Laws that restrict pets in public places usually do not apply to guide dogs. When the dogs are wearing their harnesses, they are working and should not be distracted by friendly strangers.

Knowledge Deficit

Patients with severe impairment should be referred to specialists in rehabilitation. They need to learn self-care activities, safe mobility, and strategies to carry out usual roles such as child care and occupational skills. Patients with diseases of the eye are taught any prescribed measures to cure or slow the progression of the disease.

EVALUATION

The outcomes of nursing interventions are evaluated by the following criteria: adherence to treatment plan and absence of injury such as falls or trauma, patient's

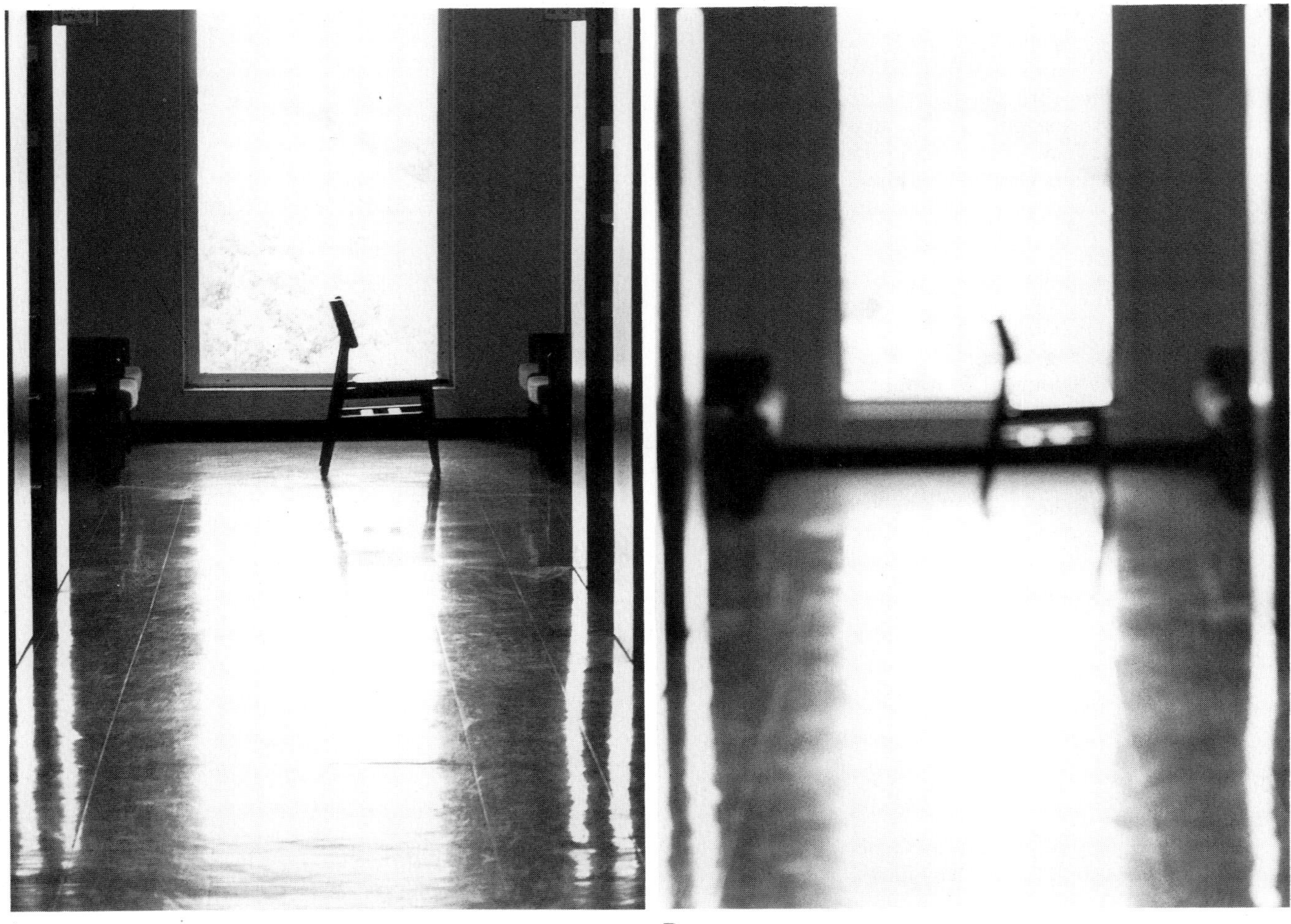

A B

FIGURE 47-11

Glare perceived by a person with normal vision *(A)* and an older person whose eyes have undergone age-related changes *(B)*. (From Matteson, M. A., & McConnell, E. S. [1988]. *Gerontological nursing* [p. 314]. Philadelphia: W. B. Saunders.)

efforts to learn to deal with visual impairment, maximum possible patient participation in care, and patient's statement of treatment regimen and demonstration of self-medication.

DISORDERS AFFECTING THE EYE OR VISION

EXTERNAL EYE DISORDERS

INFLAMMATION AND INFECTION

The eye is a potential site for infectious and inflammatory conditions. Because of the sensitivity of the eye, such disorders can cause considerable discomfort. Some may even threaten vision if not treated.

Blepharitis

Blepharitis is an inflammation of the hair follicles along the eyelid margin. It can be caused by bacteria, most often staphylococcus. Seborrheic blepharitis is found with seborrhea of the scalp and eyebrows.

Symptoms include itching, burning, and photophobia. Scales or crusts may be seen on the lid margins. The patient may complain that the eyelids are "glued" shut upon awakening.

Untreated blepharitis could lead to inflammation of the cornea or hordeolum (stye). The physician may prescribe an antibiotic ointment for the condition. The nurse should always be certain that any medication applied to the eye is an *ophthalmic* preparation. The eyelids can also be gently cleansed with baby shampoo solution.

Hordeolum

Hordeolum is commonly called a stye. It is a common acute staphylococcal infection of the eyelid margin. The affected area of the lid is red, swollen, and tender. The primary treatment is the application of warm, moist compresses several times a day. If a person has repeated infections, these may be related to staphylococcal infections at some other location on the body. The physician attempts to locate any other infections and may order the hordeolum treated with ophthalmic antibiotics.

Chalazion

Chalazion is an inflammation of the glands in the eyelids. Swelling prevents fluid from leaving the glands, causing them to become enlarged and tender. Warm compresses may bring some relief. The physician may order antibiotics if infection is present. Surgical removal of the gland is necessary if the condition persists.

Conjunctivitis

Conjunctivitis is an infection of the conjunctiva caused by bacteria or viruses. Bacterial conjunctivitis is commonly called pinkeye. It is characterized by redness of the conjunctiva, mild irritation, and mucopurulent drainage. The infection can be passed from one person to another. Infected persons should practice good hand washing and should avoid sharing washcloths. The condition usually clears up spontaneously, but antibiotics may be prescribed.

Viral conjunctivitis can be caused by herpes simplex virus type 1, herpes zoster virus, or adenoviruses. Viral infections are characterized by redness and drainage. The drainage in viral infections is watery rather than purulent. Round, raised areas that are white or gray in color may be seen on the conjunctiva. These areas are called follicles.

Viral infections tend to persist longer than bacterial infections. They are also more likely to produce severe eye damage. The medical management varies with the causative organism. Infections caused by herpes simplex virus type 1 are treated with idoxuridine (Stoxil, IDU) ointment or other topical medications. Corticosteroids are contraindicated with the herpes virus. If given in the presence of herpes simplex virus type 1, corticosteroids may contribute to deep corneal ulcers and other complications.

Other organisms that can cause conjunctivitis include chlamydia and fungi. These eye infections are more common in developing countries but are occasionally seen in the United States. They are treated with antimicrobial medications.

Keratitis

Keratitis is inflammation or infection, or both, of the cornea. The structure of the cornea makes it especially vulnerable to injury. The portion of the cornea in front of the pupil has no blood vessels because it must remain transparent. This means that it has no direct blood supply, making it vulnerable to infections.

Sources of infection include bacteria, viruses, and fungi. Also, chemical or mechanical injuries cause inflammation that may be followed by infection. If scar tissue forms, that portion of the cornea becomes cloudy and vision is impaired. Also, the infection can extend to the inner structures of the eye. Serious lesions can rupture if the eye is rubbed. Prompt treatment of keratitis, therefore, is very important to preserve vision.

Keratitis does not produce noticeable drainage, but it causes considerable pain. Medical treatment includes topical antibiotics and topical corticosteroids. Systemic antibiotics also may be ordered after culture and sensitivity results are obtained. Sometimes the physician injects antibiotics directly into the conjunctiva. Topical anesthetics are not used since the patient might accidentally cause additional injury to the anesthetized cornea. Eye pads are not used with keratitis because they provide a dark, damp environment for microorganisms to grow.

ENTROPION AND ECTROPION

Proper closure of the eyelids is important to protect the eye and keep the cornea moist. Entropion is a condition in which the lower lid turns in. Eyelashes rub against the eye, causing pain and possibly scratching the cornea. The eyelid can be gently everted (turned out) and taped to the cheek. Surgical correction is generally recommended.

Ectropion is a condition in which the lower lid droops and turns out. The eye does not close completely, causing it to become dry and irritated. The dry cornea is easily injured. Like entropion, ectropion requires surgical correction.

FOREIGN BODY

Everyone has experienced the discomfort of having a foreign body in the eye. Blinking and tearing usually wash small irritants from the eye. If the foreign body remains in the eye, the nurse everts the upper and lower lids as illustrated in Figure 47–12. If the object is clearly visible and does not appear to be embedded in the eye, the nurse may attempt to remove it. A sterile cotton swab is used to touch the object gently. If the object is not embedded, it usually clings to the swab and can be removed. Foreign bodies that are embedded in the eye should be removed only by a physician.

CHEMICAL SPILLS AND SPLASHES

Chemical spills and splashes are discussed in Chapter 13.

CORNEAL OPACITY

A healthy cornea is clear, allowing light to enter the pupil. When the cornea is injured by infection or trauma, scar tissue may form. The scar tissue is opaque, so light is unable to enter the eye. This causes varying degrees of vision impairment. The only treatment for corneal opacity is removal of the scarred cornea and replacement with a healthy cornea. The surgical procedure is called a keratoplasty.

Healthy corneas are obtained from donors shortly after death. This may be authorized by the donor prior

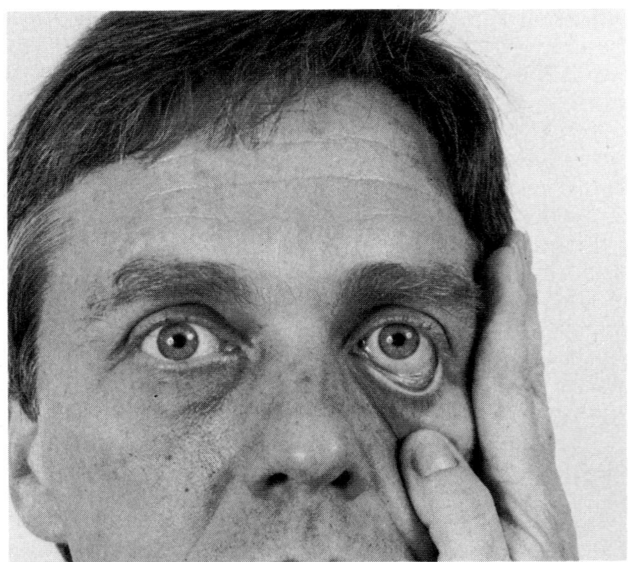

FIGURE 47-12

Eversion of the eyelid for inspection of the sclera and conjunctiva. (From Jarvis, C. [1992]. *Physical examination and health assessment* [p. 325]. Philadelphia: W. B. Saunders.)

to death or by the family. The entire eye is removed and preserved. Eye tissue is easier to preserve than other body tissues. This permits keratoplasty to be done as a scheduled procedure rather than as an emergency "on call" procedure. It can be done under local anesthesia. Preoperatively, eye drops may be ordered to either dilate or constrict the pupil. Usually, drops are used that constrict the pupil (miotics). Constriction of the pupil pulls the iris over the lens like a curtain and protects the lens during surgery. Sometimes, it is necessary to remove the lens as well as the cornea. Lens extraction is necessary if the lens is cloudy owing to injury or age-related changes. In this case, mydriatic drops are ordered preoperatively to allow access to the lens.

Three types of grafts are used in keratoplasty: penetrating, lamellar, and keyhole lamellar. The type of graft used depends on the extent of injury to the recipient's cornea. A penetrating graft consists of all layers of the cornea. A lamellar graft is only the superficial tissue layers of the cornea. A keyhole lamellar graft contains a section of the cornea and other underlying tissues.

During a keratoplasty, the surgeon first removes the patient's damaged cornea. An identical size graft is then taken from the donor eye and secured with very fine sutures, as seen in Figure 47–13. When a penetrating keratoplasty is done, the aqueous humor is lost from the anterior chamber of the eye. The surgeon replaces the fluid with a saline solution.

Nursing Care of the Patient Having Keratoplasty

Preoperative nursing care of the patient having eye surgery is discussed earlier. Postoperatively, the keratoplasty patient has an eye pad and a metal shield over the operative eye. Sometimes the other eye is temporarily patched as well. This is to reduce eye movement until the operative eye heals.

ASSESSMENT. The nurse assesses the dressing for drainage and asks if the patient is having any pain or nausea. After the dressing is removed, the eye is inspected for corneal opacity. The patient's visual acuity also is evaluated.

NURSING DIAGNOSIS. Routine nursing diagnoses after eye surgery are discussed earlier. In addition, the following nursing diagnoses may apply to the keratoplasty patient:

- **High Risk for Injury** related to activities that increase intraocular pressure
- **Pain** related to tissue trauma
- **Sensory Perceptual Alteration** (vision) related to inflammation, rejection of transplanted tissue
- **Knowledge Deficit** of usual postoperative course

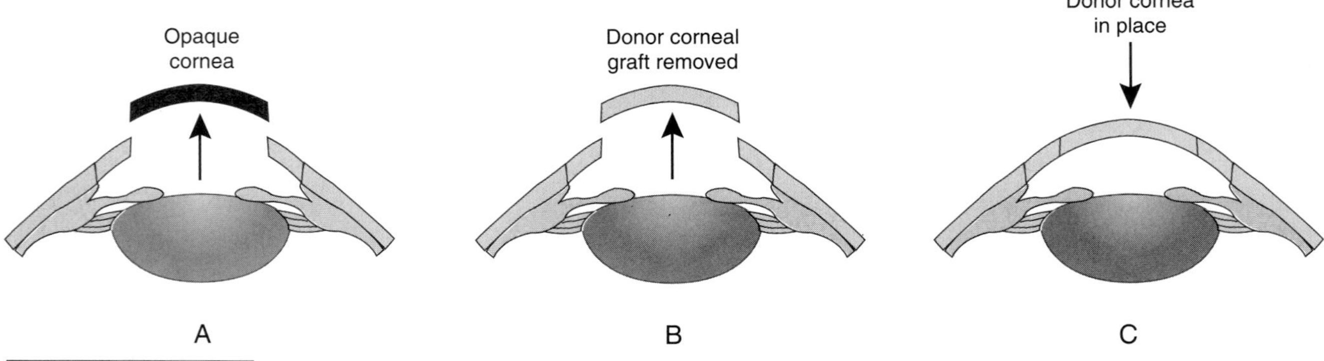

FIGURE 47-13

Keratoplasty. The damaged cornea is removed and then replaced with a corneal graft from a donor eye.

GOALS. Nursing goals specific to the keratoplasty patient are avoidance of behaviors that increase intraocular pressure, pain relief, adaptation to vision impairment, and patient's knowledge of usual postoperative course.

INTERVENTIONS

High Risk for Injury. The patient is cautioned to avoid any activities that increase pressure in the eye, including bending forward, lifting, straining at stool, and coughing. Nausea should be reported and treated promptly since vomiting raises intraocular pressure.

Pain. Some pain is expected after keratoplasty. The physician usually orders analgesics to be given as needed. Severe or increasing pain should be reported to the physician because it suggests increased intraocular pressure or infection.

Sensory Perceptual Alteration. Rejection of corneal grafts is not common, but it can happen. When rejection occurs, blood vessels appear in the cornea, and the cornea becomes cloudy. Corticosteroid drops are ordered to reduce inflammation and the risk of rejection. Other topical medications that are usually ordered are antibiotics to prevent infection and mydriatics to dilate the pupil.

Knowledge Deficit. Nurses and patients should realize that the grafted eye must heal just like any other body part that has undergone surgery. In the movies, the physician removes the dressing dramatically. The patient blinks a few times, and the world comes into focus. In reality, it takes a while before the patient's vision clears. The patient must be reassured that this is normal.

Prior to discharge, the nurse determines what medications the patient will be taking at home. The medications are reviewed with the patient, and the nurse demonstrates proper self-administration.

EVALUATION. Goal achievement is evaluated by avoidance of behaviors that increase intraocular pressure (bending forward, lifting, straining), prompt treatment of nausea; patient's statement of pain relief and relaxed expression; improvement in vision; and patient's statement of expected outcomes of surgery.

ERRORS OF REFRACTION

Light must pass through the cornea, aqueous humor, lens, and vitreous humor to reach the retina. These structures through which light passes are called refractive media. The term refraction refers to the bending of light rays so that these focus on the retina (Fig. 47–14). Abnormalities, called errors of refraction, occur when refractive media do not bend light rays correctly. Myopia, hyperopia, and astigmatism are common problems caused by variations in the structure of the eyeball. Figure 47–15 illustrates these variations and the type of correction required.

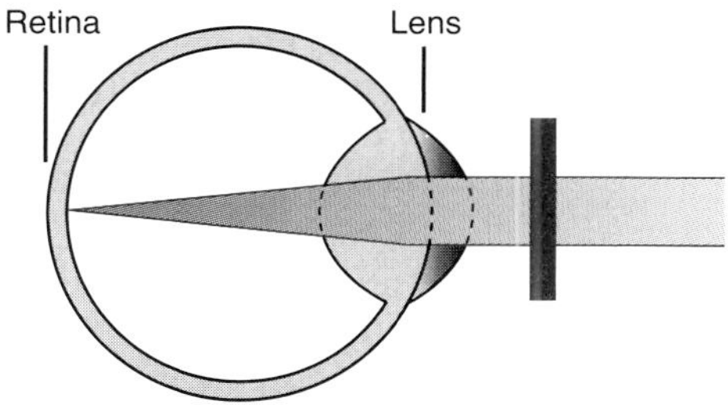

FIGURE 47–14
Normal vision. The lens bends the light rays so they focus directly on the retina.

TYPES OF ERRORS OF REFRACTION

Myopia

Myopia is the medical term for nearsightedness. In myopia, the lens is situated too far from the retina. Light rays come together to focus in front of the retina. People with myopia have difficulty seeing distant images clearly. It is often recognized in the early school years. Typically, the condition slowly progresses until adolescence. Nothing can be done to stop the changes. New glasses are usually needed about every 2 years.

Hyperopia

When the lens is too close to the retina, light rays come together behind the retina. This condition creates hyperopia, commonly known as farsightedness. The hyperopic person sees clearly in the distance but has difficulty focusing on close objects.

Astigmatism

When there are irregularities in the cornea or lens, astigmatism results. Most people have some degree of astigmatism. If the condition is mild, the lens can correct for the abnormality. If it is severe, however, vision is distorted and corrective lenses are needed. A person can have astigmatism with myopia or hyperopia.

Presbyopia

Presbyopia is another disorder that is classified with errors of refraction. Presbyopia is poor accommodation due to loss of elasticity of the ciliary muscles. Accommodation is the adjustment of the lens for near and distant vision. It is accomplished by contraction or relaxation of the ciliary muscles, which causes the lens to change shape.

Presbyopia is generally considered a normal age-related change. It most often develops after age 40. As it progresses, people may be observed holding reading material at arm's length. People who are already hyperopic tend to have presbyopia at an earlier age than other people. Myopic people are usually able to read small print by holding it close.

Corrective lenses are needed when the visual changes become bothersome. Bifocal lenses are often prescribed. Bifocals have two different lenses. The upper part of the

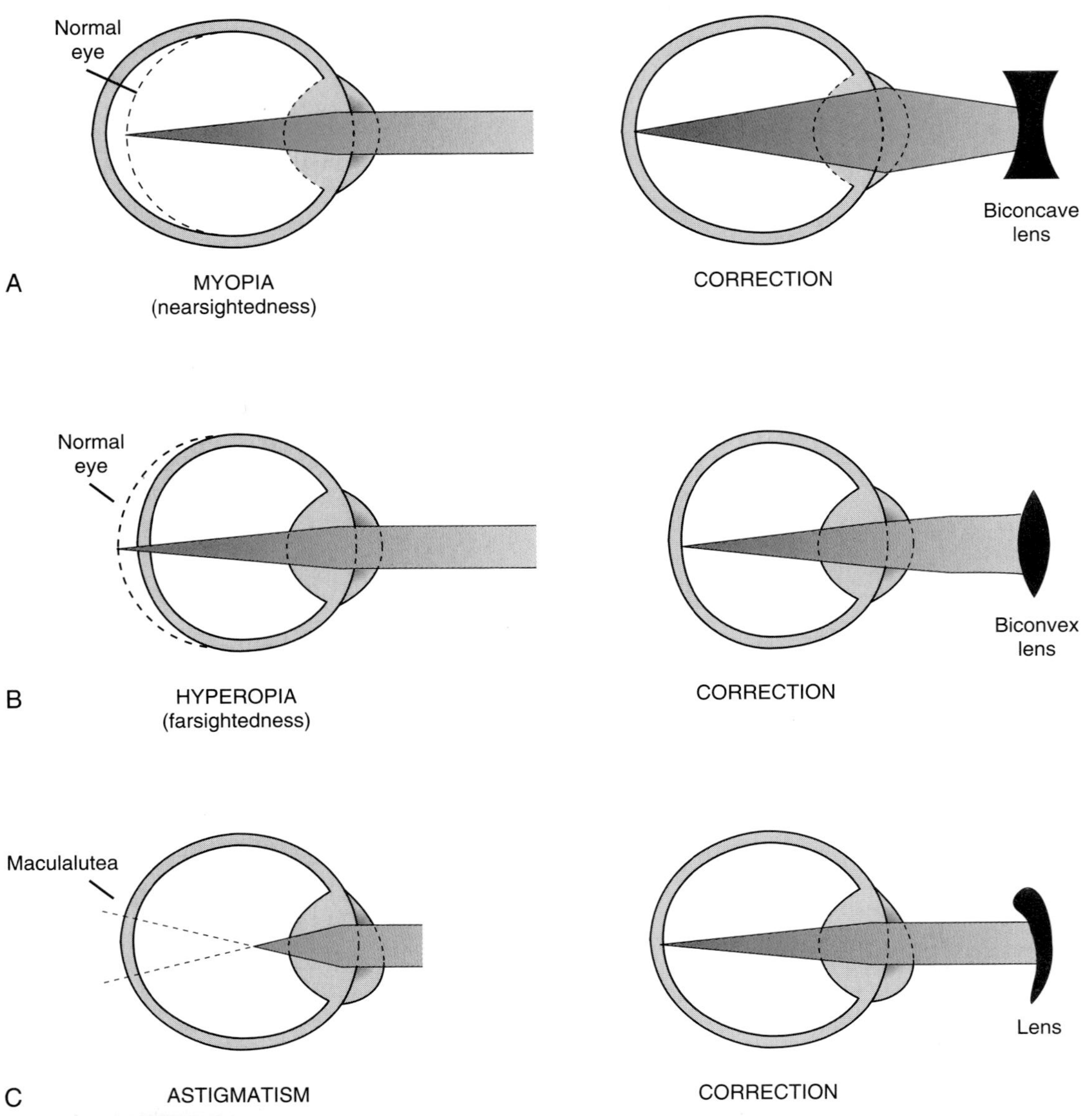

FIGURE 47-15

Errors of refraction. *A*, Myopia: Light rays converge before they reach the retina because the lens is too far from the retina. *B*, Hyperopia: Light rays converge beyond the retina because the lens is too close to the retina. *C*, Astigmatism: Uneven surfaces of the cornea bend light rays in a way that causes distortion of the image.

lens is used for distant vision, and the lower part is used for near vision. Trifocals have three lenses, for distant, closer, and near vision. Progressive lenses gradually blend the lens needed for seeing various distances. The wearer scans the lens to find the area needed for a particular task. Reading lenses must usually be changed every 2 to 3 years.

MEDICAL TREATMENT

The primary treatment of errors of refraction is the prescription of corrective lenses. Eyeglasses are most often used. The obvious advantage of eyeglasses is that they require no special skills to use. Disadvantages are heavy frames and dirty lenses.

Contact lenses are tiny plastic disks made to fit over the patient's cornea. The lenses float on the tear film over the cornea. The primary advantages of contact lenses are convenience and appearance. Disadvantages include cost, the need for training and dexterity to insert and remove the lenses, and that they are easily lost. Another important disadvantage is the risk of corneal injury.

Several types of contact lenses are available. Hard lenses were developed first. Hard lenses can be used to correct astigmatism. They must be removed from the eye at the end of the day to prevent damage to the cornea. Soft lenses can be worn longer than hard lenses and require a shorter period of adjustment. Gas-permeable lenses are made of materials that allow oxygen and carbon dioxide to pass through. This is important because the cornea exchanges gases through the tear film beneath the contact lens. Extended-wear contact lenses can be worn for as long as 2 weeks. For this reason, they may be prescribed for elderly patients who have cataract surgery. Extended-wear contact lenses are more expensive than other lenses. The patient is cautioned to follow the prescribed cleaning schedule. Disposable contact lenses can be worn for up to 1 week and are then discarded.

NURSING CARE OF THE PATIENT WITH ERRORS OF REFRACTION

Nursing responsibilities for the patient with errors of refraction are limited except to encourage periodic examinations and to know if the patient uses corrective lenses. In emergency situations, the nurse may have to remove contact lenses for the patient.

INTERNAL EYE DISORDERS

CATARACT

The lens is a clear, flexible structure encased in an elastic capsule. It is located behind the iris and changes shape to focus on images of various sizes. When the lens becomes opaque (cloudy) so that it is no longer transparent, it is called a cataract.

Causes

Cataracts may be congenital, traumatic, or degenerative. Congenital cataracts are those that are present at birth. Traumatic cataracts are caused by chemical, mechanical, heat, or radiation injury. Degenerative cataracts are more common with aging, but they occur earlier in people with diabetes or Down's syndrome.

Pathophysiology

The lens may become cloudy or opaque quickly or slowly. Injuries tend to cause opacity rapidly, whereas age-related opacity progresses slowly. As opacity increases, light is unable to enter the eye and vision becomes cloudy. Blindness eventually results if a cataract is untreated. With age, both eyes are usually affected, although they may not change at the same rate.

Signs and Symptoms

Signs and symptoms of cataracts include cloudy vision, seeing "spots" or "ghost" images, and floaters. The pattern of vision changes depends on the location of the developing cataract. A central cataract is located in the center of the lens. Patients with central cataracts may have fairly good peripheral vision. They may actually see better in dim light because the pupil dilates, allowing them to see around the cloudy center of the lens. Conversely, patients who have peripheral cataracts can see straight ahead but not to the side. As cataracts develop, people who were hyperopic to begin with may have temporary improvements in near vision. This is referred to as second sight.

Medical Treatment

The only treatment for cataract is removal of the lens. Cataract extraction is the most frequently performed eye operation in the United States. There are several types of cataract extraction, as illustrated in Figure 47–16. If the lens and capsule are removed, it is called an intracapsular cataract extraction (ICCE). For the extracapsular cataract extraction (ECCE), the lens is removed, leaving the capsule in place. The most common extracapsular procedure is phacoemulsification, in which sound waves are used to break up the lens. The lens fragments are then suctioned out. The ECCE is generally preferred because it permits the placement of an

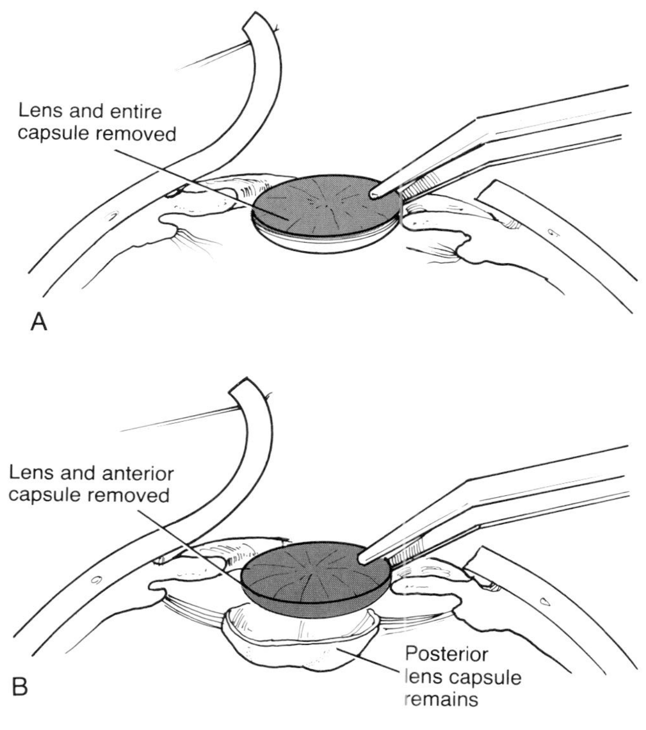

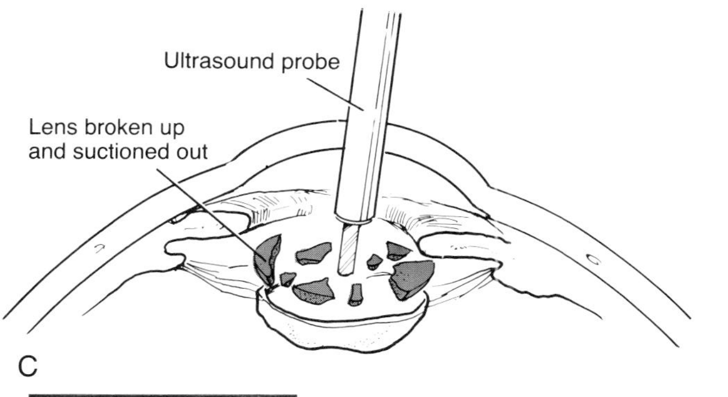

FIGURE 47-16

Methods of cataract extraction. *A*, Intracellular extraction; *B*, extracellular extraction; *C*, phacoemulsification.

artificial lens. The remaining capsule can become cloudy, causing vision to become blurred again. This can usually be corrected easily with laser treatment.

Cataract extraction is commonly done on an outpatient basis. Most patients tolerate the procedure well with just a mild sedative and local anesthesia. In some cases, general anesthesia may be preferred. Cataract surgery is generally considered safe even for the very old.

Complications

Complications that sometimes occur include leakage of vitreous humor, hemorrhage into the eye, and opening of the incision.

Lens Replacement

Once the lens has been removed, the eye is said to be aphakic. The patient is extra farsighted and unable to accommodate for changes in object size. Some type of artificial lens is needed for correction.

CATARACT EYEGLASSES. In the past, the only option for lens replacement was thick eyeglasses. They are heavy, unattractive, and leave the patient with poor peripheral vision. Cataract eyeglasses magnify objects so much that the patient also has poor depth perception. The result is that patients may misjudge distances. This causes difficulty in everything from eating to driving. Another disadvantage to the use of eyeglasses is that the patient must either have the lenses removed from both eyes or be blind in the unoperated eye. Otherwise, the strong magnification causes double vision.

CONTACT LENSES. Contact lenses overcome many disadvantages of eyeglasses, but they have drawbacks as well. Considerable dexterity is required to insert, remove, and care for contact lenses. This makes them impractical for some older patients. The main complication of contact lens use is corneal injury.

INTRAOCULAR LENSES. The invention of plastic lenses (Fig. 47–17) that can be implanted in the eye has been a tremendous advance for many cataract patients. This type of lens is called an intraocular lens. The intraocular lens may be implanted immediately after removal of the lens, or it may be done later. Complications of insertion include corneal edema, secondary glaucoma, lens displacement, and retinal detachment.

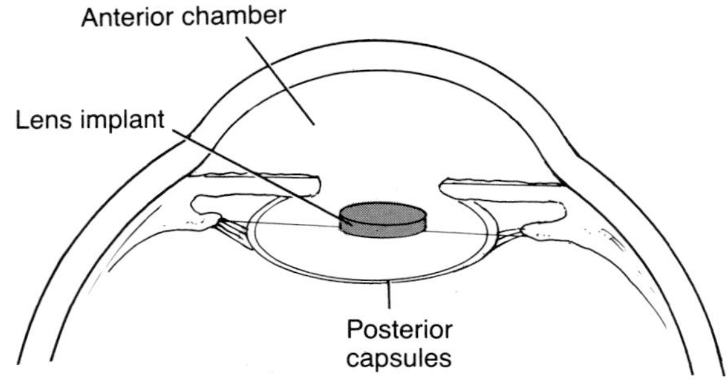

FIGURE 47–17
Intraocular lens in place after cataract extraction.

Nursing Care of the Patient with Cataracts

Cataract extractions are often done in day-surgery clinics. The nurse may have limited opportunity for patient and family teaching. Care of the patient having eye surgery is presented earlier in this chapter. This section emphasizes additional care specific to cataract surgery.

PREOPERATIVE CARE. Eye drops are often ordered at frequent intervals after cataract surgery. The orders must be followed exactly. Common drops used before cataract surgery are mydriatics, cycloplegics, and antibiotics. Mydriatics dilate the pupil, making it easier for the surgeon to access the lens. Cycloplegics temporarily paralyze the muscles of accommodation, keeping the eye still during the procedure. Antibiotics may be given to reduce the risk of infection.

POSTOPERATIVE CARE

Assessment. Following cataract surgery, the nurse assesses for pain and nausea. The patient is likely to return from surgery wearing a patch and shield over the operative eye. The nurse notes the presence of the patch and any apparent drainage. The patient's level of consciousness and orientation also are assessed (see Care Plan: The Patient Having Cataract Surgery).

Nursing Diagnosis. When the patient has cataract surgery, the primary nursing diagnoses are the following:

- **High Risk for Injury** related to increased intraocular pressure
- **Sensory Perceptual Alteration** related to vision impairment

Goals. The goals of nursing care are absence of injury from elevated intraocular pressure and adaptation to impaired vision.

Interventions

High Risk for Injury. Following cataract surgery, the most important thing is to prevent strain on the operative eye. The patient is cautioned not to rub the eye. The nurse can advise the patient to sleep on the unaffected side, not to lift more than 5 pounds, and to avoid bending forward. Stool softeners are administered as ordered to prevent straining at stool. If nausea occurs, it is treated promptly.

The nurse must always be aware of safety precautions after cataract surgery. When one eye is patched, the patient has limited peripheral vision. The "good" eye often has some degree of impairment as well. Medications may be ordered that cause blurred vision. To prevent injury, the nurse makes sure that the patient is familiar with the environment and knows how to use the

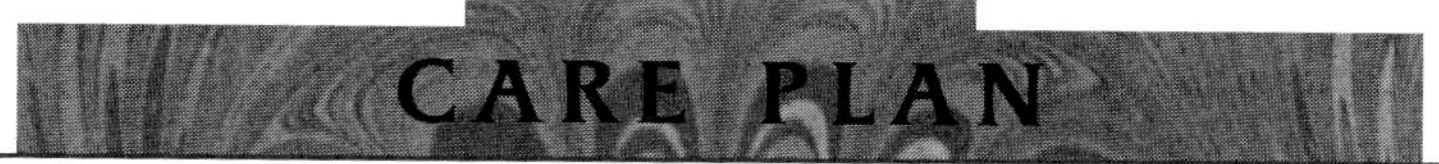

The Patient Having Cataract Surgery

ASSESSMENT

Health History: Mr. Don Dickson is a 72-year-old retired welder. He complained of cloudy vision that has become increasingly worse. He reported spots moving across his field of vision. Cataracts were diagnosed, with the right lens affected more severely than the left. Mr. Dickson had a right extracapsular cataract extraction under local anesthesia this morning in the outpatient surgery department. He says he has mild pain in the eye area at this time. His record reveals a history of myocardial infarction 5 years ago and surgery for prostate enlargement 6 months ago. Although he is retired, he works every day on his small farm. He lives with his wife and an adult daughter.

Physical Examination: Mr. Dickson is alert and oriented. Vital signs: temperature, 98°F orally; pulse, 88; respiration 18; blood pressure, 142/68. He is in semi-Fowler's position. An eye pad is in place over the right eye, protected with a metal shield. A small amount of clear drainage is noted seeping below the dressing.

NURSING DIAGNOSIS	GOALS AND OUTCOME CRITERIA	INTERVENTIONS
High risk for injury related to increased intraocular pressure (IOP), trauma.	The patient will avoid activities that increase IOP or impose stress on operative eye	Keep head of bed elevated. Instruct the patient not to rub the operative eye, strain, lean forward, or lie on the affected side. If nausea or vomiting, or both, occur, administer antiemetics immediately. Change damp pad as allowed. Administer eye drops (mydriatics, antimicrobials, and corticosteroids) as ordered. Encourage patient to take stool softeners as ordered to prevent constipation.
Sensory-perceptual alteration (visual) related to surgical trauma, lens removal, patching.	The patient will adapt to visual impairment and function in environment without injury.	Keep the bed in low position. Approach the left side. Place the call button on the left and instruct in use. Remove obstacles in the room. Assist with activities of daily living as needed.
Acute pain related to tissue trauma.	The patient will report decreased pain.	Assess pain. Notify the surgeon if severe (may indicate increased IOP). Administer analgesics as ordered and evaluate effects.
Anxiety related to temporary vision impairment, activity restrictions.	The patient will report decreased anxiety and will appear calm.	Explain what is being done and why. Explore feelings about surgery. Answer questions. Acknowledge fear of vision loss common with eye surgery. Respond to needs promptly.
Knowledge deficit of self-care, limitations, lens replacement.	The patient (and family member) will demonstrate instillation of medications and state limitations.	Explain limitations after discharge. No lifting over 5 pounds, bending forward, or straining until cleared by physician. Review procedure for eye drops and have patient or family member demonstrate instillation. Supplement verbal instructions with written information.

call button. The bed is kept in low position, and the environment kept free of obstacles.

Sensory Perceptual Alteration. Confusion sometimes occurs in the postoperative period, especially in the very elderly. The confused person may fail to follow safety precautions or may place strain on the operative eye. Therefore, the nurse monitors mental status and ensures that a caregiver is readily available.

Medications prescribed after cataract surgery usually include antibiotics and corticosteroids. Because the patient's vision is usually poor, the nurse may need to teach a family member or friend how to give the medications.

A mild analgesic is usually ordered as needed. Postoperative cataract patients should not have severe pain. If a patient complains of severe pain, the physician should be notified. Severe pain may indicate hemorrhage or rising pressure within the eye.

Evaluation. Criteria for evaluating the outcomes of nursing interventions are normal intraocular pressure without eye pain and patient's demonstration of self-care: maneuvering in the environment without injury, achievement of activities of daily living, and medication administration.

GLAUCOMA

Glaucoma is one of the leading causes of blindness in the United States. It occurs in infants, children, and adults. It is thought to affect 1% of Americans over the age of 60 and to account for 10% of all cases of blindness in the United States.

Pathophysiology

Normally, aqueous humor enters and leaves the anterior chamber so that intraocular pressure is maintained between 12 and 21 mm Hg. Glaucoma is a condition in which intraocular pressure is increased above normal. It can be caused by a number of changes that affect the flow of aqueous humor in the anterior chamber of the eye. It is most often caused by some interference with the outflow of aqueous humor. Although glaucoma may follow trauma, the exact cause is often unknown.

Excess pressure damages the back portion of the eye. It impairs blood flow to the optic nerve, resulting in vision impairment. Peripheral vision is lost first. The field of vision gradually narrows until the patient has tunnel vision. The patient who has tunnel vision can see only a small circle, as if looking through a tube or a tunnel. As the disease progresses, complete blindness eventually occurs. Vision may be restored if glaucoma is treated early. Otherwise vision loss is permanent.

Types of Glaucoma

The two types of glaucoma are open-angle glaucoma and angle-closure glaucoma. They are similar in that increased intraocular pressure is present in both, but they have some important differences. Both open-angle and angle-closure glaucoma are considered primary glaucomas. Increased intraocular pressure due to other conditions is called secondary glaucoma.

OPEN-ANGLE GLAUCOMA. Open-angle glaucoma is also called chronic glaucoma. It is more common than angle-closure glaucoma. Open-angle glaucoma results from some alteration that prevents the normal passage of aqueous humor through the trabecular meshwork. It is more common among blacks, people on corticosteroid therapy, and those with a parent or sibling who had the condition.

There are usually no signs and symptoms at first. Some patients complain of "tired eyes," occasional blurred vision, and halos around lights. Another clue may be the need for frequent changes in eyeglass prescriptions.

Open-angle glaucoma is usually treated first with drug therapy. The types of medications used include miotics, adrenergics, beta blockers, and carbonic anhydrase inhibitors. Miotics such as pilocarpine and carbachol constrict the pupil. This permits fluid to flow more easily through the angle where the iris meets the cornea and into the trabecular meshwork. A disadvantage of many currently used miotics is that they must be administered frequently. Some new preparations are being tested, including ocular inserts, that are effective for a longer period of time. These may eventually replace the preparations now in use.

Examples of adrenergic drugs used for glaucoma are epinephrine HCl (Epifrin) and dipivefrin HCl (Propine) eye drops. Adrenergics decrease intraocular pressure by decreasing the formation of aqueous humor and increasing its outflow.

Beta blockers are relatively new in the treatment of glaucoma. Timolol maleate (Timoptic) is an example of a beta blocker used topically for glaucoma. Timolol lowers intraocular pressure, but it is not known exactly how.

Carbonic anhydrase inhibitors such as acetazolamide (Diamox) reduce intraocular pressure by decreasing the production of aqueous humor. Carbonic anhydrase inhibitors and osmotic diuretics are given orally or parenterally. Additional information about drugs used to treat glaucoma is provided in Table 47–5.

Surgical intervention may be recommended when drugs do not reduce pressure adequately, the patient does not use prescribed drugs properly, or adverse reactions interfere with drug therapy. Surgical procedures for glaucoma include trabeculoplasty, trabeculectomy, and cyclocryotherapy. Trabeculoplasty may be tried first since it can be done under local anesthesia in an outpatient setting. The procedure involves the use of a laser to create multiple holes in the trabecular meshwork. This is intended to improve drainage of aqueous humor from the anterior chamber. If the procedure is successful, intraocular pressure falls over a period of time. Meanwhile, the physician usually has the patient continue using glaucoma medications.

A trabeculectomy creates a channel to allow aqueous humor to drain under the conjunctiva. If this procedure is not effective, cyclocryotherapy may be done. A cold probe, called a cryoprobe, is used to freeze part of the ciliary body. Freezing destroys some of the tissue, resulting in decreased production of aqueous humor.

ANGLE-CLOSURE GLAUCOMA. Angle-closure glaucoma is also called acute glaucoma. It accounts for only about 10% of all glaucomas. With angle-closure glaucoma, the flow of aqueous humor through the pupil is blocked. Pressure forces the iris forward, causing it to block the trabecular meshwork. There is a rapid rise in

TABLE 47-5

DRUGS USED TO TREAT GLAUCOMA

GENERAL NURSING CONSIDERATIONS

1. Teach patient or caregivers, or both, proper way to administer eye drops.
2. Recognize that failure to control intraocular pressure can result in permanent blindness.
3. *Avoid* corticosteroids, succinylcholine, and anticholinergics in glaucoma patients.
4. Ophthalmic solutions should be tightly capped and protected from light.
5. Ophthalmic solutions should not be used if they change color or other characteristics.
6. Be alert for systemic effects of ophthalmic drugs.

DRUG	USE/ACTION	SIDE EFFECTS	NURSING INTERVENTIONS
Agents That Decrease Formation of Aqueous Humor			
Carbonic anhydrase inhibitors Acetazolamide (Diamox) Dichlorphenamide (Daranide)		Increased urinary output. Potential hypokalemia. Possible allergic response in people who are allergic to sulfonamides. Tingling of fingers and toes (paresthesia). Itching. Sore throat, skin rash, and fever may suggest serious blood disorders.	Monitor intake and output. Assess for hypokalemia (pulse changes, mental status changes, muscle weakness, abdominal distention). Withhold and notify physician if allergic. Expect increased urine output. Provide access and assistance to toilet. Do not give at bedtime.
Osmotic diuretics	Treatment of acute (angle-closure) glaucoma. Preoperative preparation for glaucoma surgery.	Increased urinary output. Potential hypokalemia. Elevated blood glucose. Headache. Tissue necrosis due to infiltration of intravenous solution.	Record intake and output. Assess for hypokalemia (pulse changes, muscle weakness, mental status changes, abdominal distention). Monitor diabetics for elevated glucose. Monitor intravenous infusion. Stop infusion if infiltration suspected.
Mannitol (Osmitrol)			Mannitol may form crystals if cooled. If so, place vial in warm water until crystals dissolve. Cool to body temperature before administration.
Urea (Ureaphil)			Urea should be used within 24 hr after reconstitution. The rate of administration should be no more than 4 ml/min.
Beta-adrenergic blocking agents Timolol (Timoptic) Betaxolol (Betoptic)	Treatment of chronic (open-angle) glaucoma. Advantage: does not affect pupil or visual acuity. Often used in combination with other drugs.	Eye irritation. Possible systemic effects: bronchospasm, heart failure.	Contraindicated with asthma, heart failure. Monitor pulse, blood pressure, and respiration.
Direct Acting Miotics			
Parasympathomimetics	Initial treatment of acute and chronic glaucoma.	Myopia. Poor vision in dim light. Lacrimation (tearing). Systemic effects: change in pulse rate or rhythm, bronchospasm, decreased blood pressure, gastric distress, diarrhea, headache.	Advise patient to use caution for tasks requiring distant vision or vision in dim light. Antidote: atropine. Minimize systemic effects by applying pressure over lacrimal duct.

Table continued on following page

intraocular pressure. Pressure is often greater than 50 mm Hg. If the pressure is not lowered promptly, permanent blindness can result. Therefore, angle-closure glaucoma is considered a medical emergency. Unlike open-angle glaucoma, angle-closure glaucoma causes sudden, acute pain. Other signs and symptoms are blurred vision, halos around lights, nausea and vomiting, and headache on the affected side.

TABLE 47–5

DRUGS USED TO TREAT GLAUCOMA *Continued*

DRUG	USE/ACTION	SIDE EFFECTS	NURSING INTERVENTIONS
Pilocarpine (Ocusert therapeutic system)			Ocusert therapeutic system lasts 1 wk. There are few side effects, but it is more costly.
Carbachol (Isopto Carbachol)			Carbachol at first may cause aching of the eyes, brow pain, headache, light sensitivity, and blurred vision.
Acetylcholine (Miochol)	Acetylcholine is used primarily in operating room since effect lasts only about 10 min.		Acetylcholine comes in a two-compartment vial. It is reconstituted immediately before use.

The goal of medical treatment is to reduce the intraocular pressure quickly. Drugs used to treat angle-closure glaucoma include miotics, osmotic diuretics, and carbonic anhydrase inhibitors (see Table 47–5 for details). After the pressure has been lowered, surgery is usually recommended to prevent recurrence. Iridotomy is a surgical procedure in which a "window" is cut in the iris to permit aqueous humor to flow through the pupil normally. The procedure may be done on both eyes since the "healthy" eye is likely to develop similar problems in the future. There are two types of iridotomy: peripheral and keyhole.

Nursing Care of the Patient with Glaucoma

Nurses who work in acute care settings are most concerned with drug therapy and patient teaching for self-care.

ASSESSMENT. General assessment of the patient with an eye disorder is outlined in Table 47–2. Nurses who work in special clinics or units may also measure intraocular pressure as indicated. When a patient has glaucoma, the nurse also assesses patient knowledge of the disease and treatment and patient ability to carry out self-care.

NURSING DIAGNOSIS. The primary nursing diagnoses for the patient with glaucoma are the following:

- **High Risk for Injury** related to increased intraocular pressure
- **Fear** related to actual or potential loss of vision
- **Knowledge Deficit** of disease, treatment, complications
- **Pain** related to acute increase in intraocular pressure, inflammation caused by corrective procedures

If the patient has impaired vision, additional diagnoses may be appropriate. These are discussed in detail in the section on nursing care of the visually impaired patient.

GOALS. Nursing goals for the glaucoma patient are adherence to prescribed measures to reduce intraocular pressure, reduced fear, patient's knowledge of glaucoma and its management, and reduced pain.

INTERVENTIONS

High Risk for Injury. One of the most important things the nurse does to keep intraocular pressure within normal limits is to administer prescribed medications. The nurse must be extremely cautious in selecting and administering ophthalmic medications. Different medications are often ordered for the affected and the unaffected eye. The procedure for applying eye drops and ointments is described earlier.

Fear and Knowledge Deficit. The nurse must be sensitive to the patient's fears about glaucoma leading to blindness. The nurse emphasizes that adherence to prescribed drug therapy can usually control intraocular pressure and reduce the risk of complications. Since open-angle glaucoma is painless, the patient may not appreciate the need for ongoing treatment. The nurse stresses the importance of keeping regular appointments for evaluation of intraocular pressure. Unfortunately, noncompliance with drug therapy is a frequent nursing diagnosis with glaucoma. The nurse must remember (and teach the patient) that any drugs that dilate the pupil are contraindicated. Patients may not be aware that many nonprescription cold and allergy remedies contain chemicals that dilate the pupil. The physician or pharmacist should be consulted before taking any additional drugs.

Patients who have glaucoma should wear a bracelet to alert health care providers to the condition. They should keep their medications on hand at all times. When traveling, the glaucoma patient should keep spare medications in separate locations in case one is lost. It is helpful to have a wallet card stating the exact medication schedule in case the patient becomes ill and is unable to give this information.

Pain. Pain in acute glaucoma attacks is treated with drugs that reduce intraocular pressure. Analgesics may be given as ordered.

If the patient has surgery for glaucoma, postoperative care is similar to the general care after eye surgery described earlier. Monitoring intraocular pressure is especially important after glaucoma surgery. Postoperative pain can usually be treated with nonnarcotic analgesics. Increasing or unrelieved pain should be reported to the surgeon.

PHARMACOLOGY CAPSULE

Many drugs are contraindicated with glaucoma. Caution patients not to take nonprescription drugs without consulting their pharmacist or physician.

EVALUATION. Criteria for evaluating the outcomes of nursing interventions are normal intraocular pressure and unchanged visual fields, patient statement of feeling less fearful, patient description of and adherence to prescribed drug therapy, and patient statement of reduced pain.

RETINAL DETACHMENT

Pathophysiology

Retinal detachment is a separation of the sensory layer of the eyeball from the pigmented layer. It begins when a tear in the retina allows fluid to collect between the sensory and the pigmented layers. The fluid causes the two layers to separate. Separation deprives the sensory layers of nutrients and oxygen that are normally supplied by the blood vessels in the choroid. This leads to damage to the nerve tissue in the sensory layer and resultant partial or complete loss of vision. Retinal tears may occur spontaneously or as a result of trauma. They are more common in older people and in people with myopia.

Signs and Symptoms

Signs and symptoms of retinal detachment depend on the location and extent of the detachment. Patients may report seeing flashes of light or floaters. Vision may be cloudy. If the area of detachment is large, vision may be lost completely. Some patients say it seems as if a curtain has come down or across the line of vision (Fig. 47–18). This is very frightening to the patient.

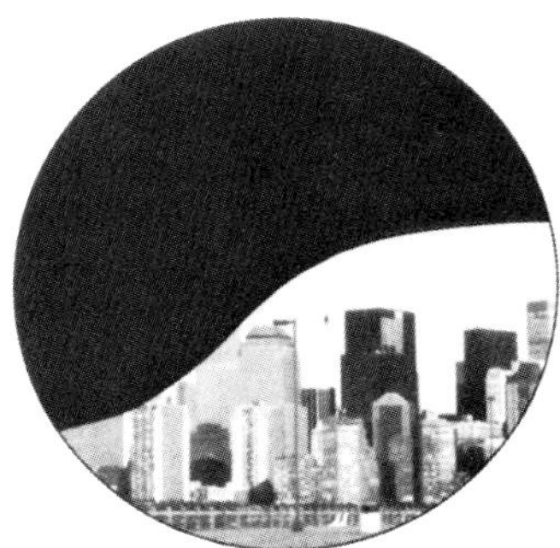

Detached Retina

FIGURE 47-18
Loss of partial field of vision due to retinal detachment. (Courtesy of the National Industries for the Blind, Wayne NJ.)

Medical Treatment

Special procedures are required to repair retinal detachments. Holes or tears must be sealed. Lasers are commonly used to do this. The intense light burns the detached portion of the retina. As the area heals, scar tissue forms that seals the tear. Cryotherapy also causes scar tissue to form, but it uses a cold probe applied to the eyeball beneath the tear. The cold radiates through the layers of tissue, freezing the torn tissue.

Scleral buckling is often done along with laser treatment or cryotherapy. The scleral buckle is a Silastic band that is secured around the eyeball under the sclera. Small pads are sutured under the band opposite the area of detachment. The band holds the pads in place. This procedure brings the layers of tissue back together by pressing from the outside. The band is left in place permanently (Fig. 47–19). The physician may inject an air bubble or some normal saline into the vitreous humor after the surgical procedure. The pur-

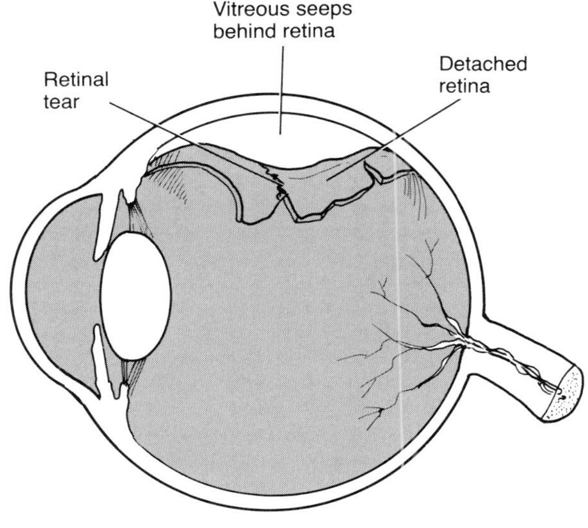

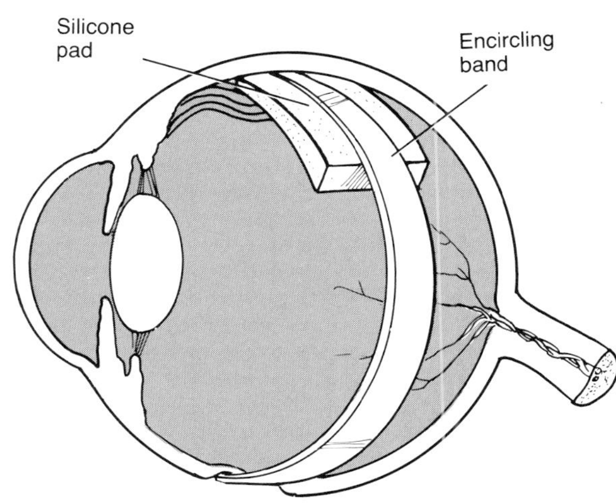

FIGURE 47-19
A, Retinal detachment; *B*, scleral buckle in place to treat retinal detachment.

pose of this is to apply internal pressure to the detached portion of the retina.

Sometimes tears cause bleeding into the vitreous. Significant amounts of blood in the vitreous interfere with vision. When this occurs, the physician may do a vitrectomy to remove the bloody tissue.

Nursing Care of the Patient with Retinal Detachment

In the preoperative period, many patients are very anxious. The nurse can encourage them to talk about their fears and to ask questions. Even though the procedure may be done under local anesthesia, oral intake may be restricted to reduce the risk of vomiting postoperatively. Intravenous fluids may be ordered.

Postoperative care is essentially the same as for other patients undergoing eye surgery, as described earlier in this chapter. Positioning orders may be very specific for these patients. If an air bubble has been injected, it will rise to the top of the eye. If the patient's detachment is in the back of the eye, a facedown position is necessary to keep the bubble in the right place. Saline will travel down rather than up, so the same patient would need to stay faceup if saline had been injected. The surgeon prescribes any activity limitations.

SENILE MACULAR DEGENERATION

The macula is the part of the retina that is responsible for central vision. As people age, changes in the eye cause the macula to degenerate. Both eyes are usually affected. The condition is progressive, causing central vision to get gradually worse (Fig. 47–20). Patients often report difficulty reading or doing close work. Peripheral vision remains intact. It is usually adequate to allow mobility in familiar settings.

Regular eyeglasses do not improve vision with macular degeneration. Special telescopic lenses may be helpful. Laser treatments may offer hope to some patients with macular degeneration. The nurse needs to help the patient and family members learn to cope with declining vision. The nursing care is like that described for patients with vision impairment.

ENUCLEATION

Some eye conditions are so serious that removal of the eyeball is the only treatment. Enucleation is the term used for removal of the eye. Conditions that may result in enucleation include injury, infection, sympathetic ophthalmia, and some glaucomas and malignancies.

During the surgical procedure, the eyeball is removed. A round device is placed in the cavity, and muscles are sutured over it. The conjunctiva is then sutured over the muscle. This procedure creates a foundation for the placement of a prosthesis in the future. The patient returns from surgery with a temporary shell called a conformer in the prosthesis base, which is covered with a pressure dressing. The nurse observes for excessive bleeding or increasing pain. Any temperature elevation should be reported. After the pressure dressing is removed, the physician may order wound care and topical medications.

About 1 month after the enucleation, a prosthesis can be fitted by an optician. The prosthesis is carefully made to look like the patient's natural eye. The patient must learn to insert, remove, and clean the prosthesis. Nurses should also know how to care for an eye prosthesis, as illustrated in Figure 47–21. To remove and clean a prosthesis, the nurse should do the following:

1. Wash hands thoroughly.
2. Gently depress and pull the lower lid down.
3. Allow the prosthesis to slip out over the lower lid.
4. Wash the prosthesis under running water, using the fingers to remove any debris.

If the prosthesis is to be stored, it should be placed in a container with normal saline or water. To reinsert the prosthesis, the nurse should do the following:

1. Raise the upper lid by pressing it up against the orbit.
2. Slip the top of the prosthesis under the orbit.
3. Pull the lower lid down so that the prosthesis can slip into place.

The patient's nursing care plan should always inform staff that the patient has a prosthesis.

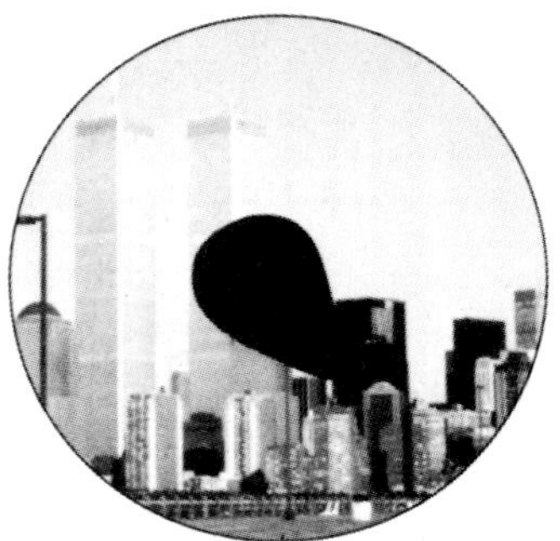

Macular Degeneration

FIGURE 47–20
Vision of the patient with macular degeneration. (Courtesy of the National Industries for the Blind, Wayne NJ.)

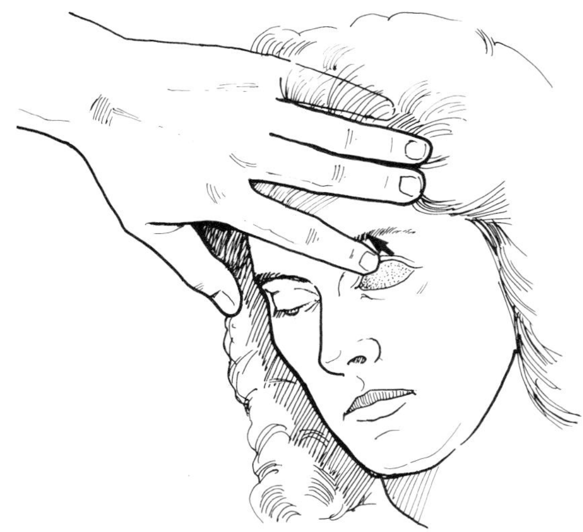

1 Lift the patient's upper lid using your nondominant hand.

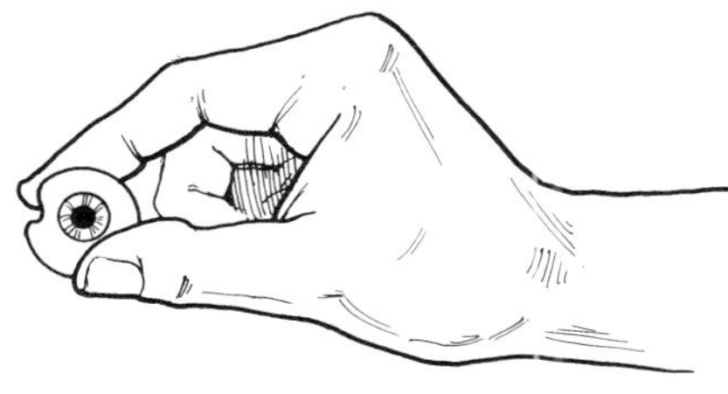

2 Place the prosthesis between the thumb and forefinger of your dominant hand. The notched end of the prosthesis should be closest to the patient's nose.

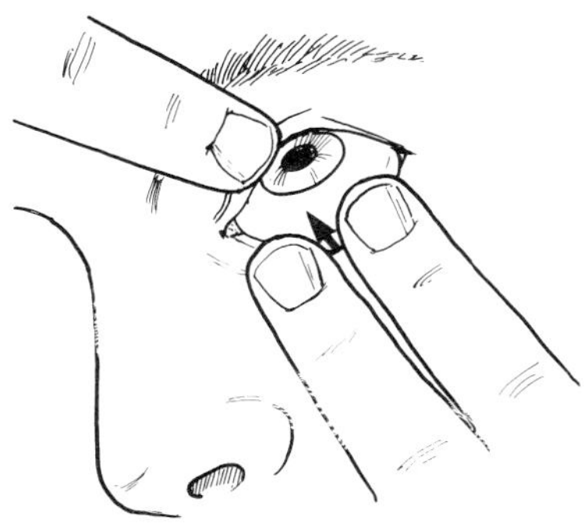

3 Insert the prosthesis with the top edge slipping under the upper lid. Continue until most of the iris is covered by the upper lid.

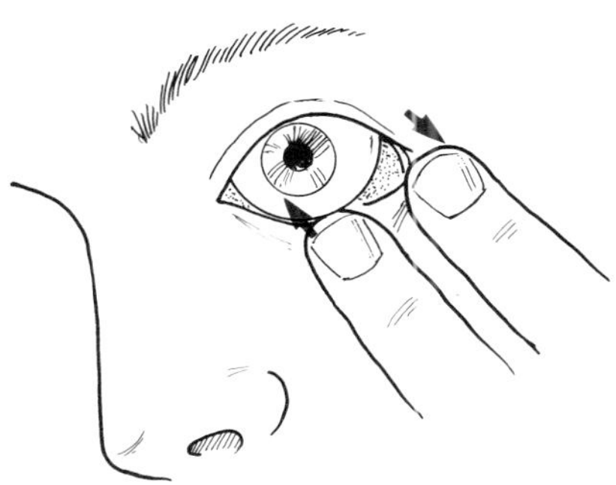

4 Gently release the upper eyelid.

Retract the lower lid slightly until the bottom edge of the prosthesis slips behind it.

A

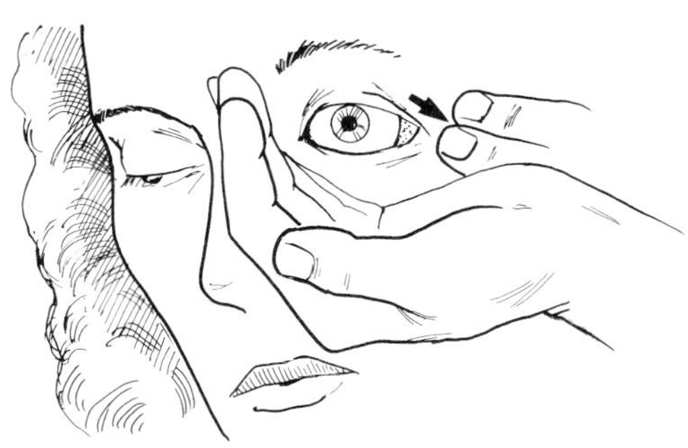

1 Place the palm of one hand on the cheek and pull the lower lid down and toward the side.

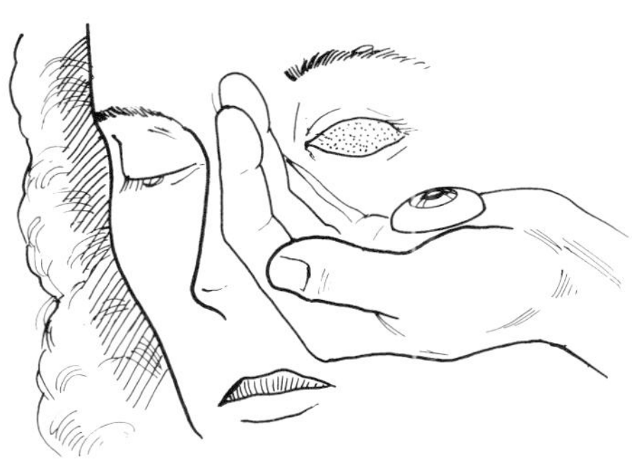

2 Allow the prosthesis to slide into the palm of your hand.

B

FIGURE 47-21

Insertion *(A)* and removal *(B)* of an eye prosthesis. (Adapted from Ignatavicius, D. D., & Bayne, M. V. [1991]. *Medical-surgical nursing: A nursing process approach* (pp. 1070–1071). Philadelphia: W. B. Saunders.)

BIBLIOGRAPHY

Black, J. M., & Matassarin-Jacobs, E. (1993). *Luckmann and Sorensen's medical-surgical nursing* (4th ed.). Philadelphia: W. B. Saunders.

Chernecky, C. C., Krech, R. L., & Berger, B. J. (1993). *Laboratory tests and diagnostic procedures.* Philadelphia: W. B. Saunders.

Deglin, J. H., Vallerand, A. H., & Russin, M. M. (1991). *Davis's drug guide for nurses* (2nd ed.). Philadelphia: F. A. Davis.

Faucher, D., Gunn, M., Morris, M., High, M., & Matto, M. (1993). Why some eye surgery patients are seeing dots. *Nursing 93, 23*(2), 41.

Fischbach, F. (1988). *A manual of laboratory diagnostic tests* (3rd ed.). Philadelphia: J. B. Lippincott.

Hodgson, B. B., Kizior, R. J., & Kingdon, R. T. (1993). *Nurse's drug handbook.* Philadelphia: W. B. Saunders.

Ignatavicius, D. D., & Bayne, M. V. (1991). *Medical-surgical nursing.* Philadelphia: W. B. Saunders.

Jarvis, C. (1992). *Physical examination and health assessment.* Philadelphia: W. B. Saunders.

Kee, J. L., & Hayes, E. R. (1993). *Pharmacology: A nursing process approach.* Philadelphia: W. B. Saunders.

Schremp, P. S., & Means, M. E. (1992). Nursing assessment: Vision and hearing. In S. M. Lewis & I. C. Collier (Eds.), *Medical-surgical nursing* (3rd ed., pp. 304–327). St. Louis: Mosby Year Book.

Schremp, P. S., & Means, M. E. (1992). Nursing role in management: Problems of vision and hearing. In S. M. Lewis & I. C. Collier (Eds.), *Medical-surgical nursing* (3rd ed., pp. 328–361). St. Louis: Mosby Year Book.

KEY CONCEPTS

1. Eleven million people in the United States have some vision impairment.
2. After eye surgery, nursing care addresses high risk for injury, sensory-perceptual alteration, acute pain, anxiety, and knowledge deficit.
3. Increased intraocular pressure must be controlled to prevent permanent vision loss.
4. Vision loss affects all aspects of a person's life: independence, mobility, employment, communication, and interpersonal relationships.
5. Common nursing diagnoses for patients with impaired vision include sensory-perceptual alterations, ineffective individual coping, self-care deficit, and knowledge deficit.
6. Infectious and inflammatory conditions of the eye include blepharitis, hordeolum, chalazion, conjunctivitis, and keratitis.
7. Entropion is inversion of the lower lid. Ectropion is eversion of the lower lid.
8. A foreign body embedded in the eye should be removed only by a physician.
9. Corneal opacity is treated with removal of the scarred cornea and replacement with a healthy donor cornea in a procedure called keratoplasty.
10. Errors of refraction include myopia, hyperopia, and astigmatism and are often correctable with corrective lenses.
11. An opaque lens, called a cataract, can be removed and vision restored with a lens replacement in the form of eyeglasses, contact lenses, or intraocular lenses.
12. Glaucoma, increased intraocular pressure, is a leading cause of blindness and is treated with drug therapy or surgery, or both.
13. Nursing care of the patient with glaucoma focuses on high risk for injury, fear, knowledge deficit, and pain.
14. Retinal detachment is separation of the sensory layer of the eyeball from the pigmented layer and can result in partial or complete loss of vision.
15. Treatment of retinal detachment may employ laser therapy, cryotherapy, scleral buckling, and vitrectomy.
16. Senile macular degeneration causes progressive loss of central vision but may be improved by laser treatment.
17. Enucleation is removal of the eyeball necessitated by injury, infection, sympathetic ophthalmia, and some glaucomas and malignancies.
18. After enucleation, a prosthesis can be used that restores the patient's normal appearance.

Adrianne Linton

CHAPTER 48

Ear and Hearing Disorders

OBJECTIVES

1. Identify the data to be collected when assessing a patient with a disorder affecting the ear, hearing, or balance.
2. Describe the tests and procedures used to diagnose disorders of the ear, hearing, or balance.
3. Explain the nursing considerations for each of the tests and procedures.
4. Explain the nursing involvement for patients receiving common therapeutic measures for disorders of the ear, hearing, or balance.
5. For selected disorders, describe the pathophysiology, signs and symptoms, complications, and medical or surgical treatment.
6. Write a nursing care plan for a patient with a disorder of the ear, hearing, or balance.
7. Identify measures the nurse can take to reduce the risk of hearing impairment and to detect problems early.

GLOSSARY

CERUMEN Waxy secretion in the external auditory canal; earwax

DIZZINESS Feeling of unsteadiness

EQUILIBRIUM State of balance needed for walking, standing, and sitting

OTALGIA Pain in the ear

OTIC Pertaining to the ear

OTOTOXIC Capable of injuring the eighth cranial (acoustic) nerve or other structures involved in hearing and balance

PRESBYCUSIS Hearing loss associated with aging

TINNITUS Ringing, buzzing, or roaring noise in the ears

TYMPANIC MEMBRANE Eardrum; the membrane that separates the external and middle portions of the ear

VERTIGO Sensation that one's body or one's surroundings are rotating

Approximately 1 in 1000 infants born in the United States has some hearing impairment. No one knows exactly how many adults are hearing impaired, but about half of those over age 75 have some hearing loss. Regardless of the numbers of people affected, the impact of hearing loss is certainly significant. Health care providers can reduce disability by teaching people how to prevent hearing loss and by helping to rehabilitate those who are impaired.

ANATOMY AND PHYSIOLOGY OF THE EAR

The ears are essential organs for hearing and for position sense. Position sense enables a person to know the position of body parts without looking. It is also necessary for equilibrium.

ANATOMY

The ear has three major sections: the external ear, the middle ear, and the inner ear (Fig. 48–1).

External Ear

AURICLE. The external ear includes the auricle and the external auditory canal. The auricle, also called the pinna, is the visible part of the ear. The parts of the auricle are labeled in Figure 48–2.

INNERVATION. Many nerves innervate the ear. This is the reason pain in the ear can sometimes be traced to disorders of the nose, mouth, or neck. Of special importance is the facial nerve (the seventh cranial nerve), which lies alongside the auditory canal. The facial nerve is protected in the canal by a thin bony covering. It exits from the skull just in front of the ear and branches across the face to control muscle movement.

LYMPH DRAINAGE. Lymph nodes located in front of, behind, and below the auricle drain the ear. In the presence of ear infections, they may become enlarged.

EXTERNAL AUDITORY CANAL. The external auditory canal extends from the external opening of the ear to the tympanic membrane. The tympanic membrane is commonly called the eardrum. The canal is lined with cells that secrete cerumen (earwax). The waxy secretion coats and protects the canal.

TYMPANIC MEMBRANE. The tympanic membrane at the end of the external auditory canal is shiny and pearl gray in color. Sound waves entering the external auditory canal cause the membrane to vibrate.

Middle Ear

BONES. The middle ear is an air-filled space in the temporal bone. It contains three small bones (ossicles): the malleus ("hammer"), the incus ("anvil"), and the stapes ("stirrup"). The job of these bones is to forward the sound waves transmitted by the tympanic membrane to the inner ear.

The malleus lies directly under the tympanic membrane. One portion of the malleus is attached to the membrane, and another portion is connected to the incus. The incus is connected to the stapes. The stapes has a footplate that fits into the oval window. The oval window, which opens into the vestibule, separates the middle ear from the inner ear. Sound waves are trans-

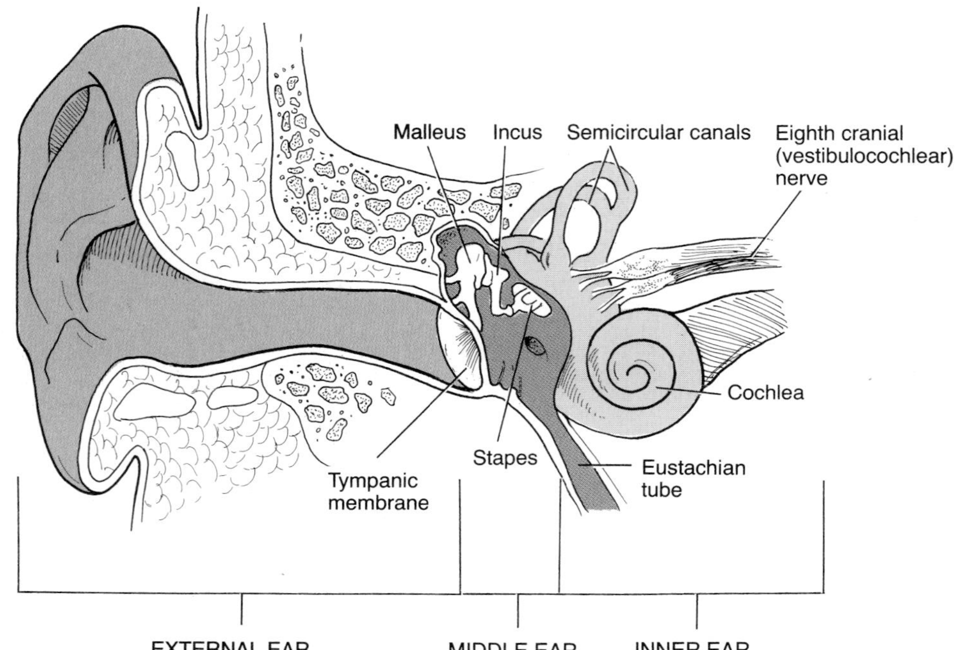

FIGURE 48–1
The ear has three major sections: the external ear, the middle ear, and the inner ear.

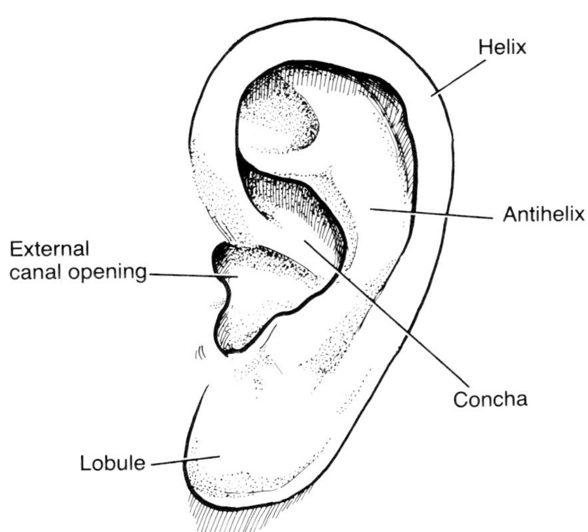

FIGURE 48-2
Parts of the auricle.

mitted from the tympanic membrane to the malleus, the incus, the stapes, and then to the oval window.

EUSTACHIAN TUBE. An important structure in the middle ear is the eustachian tube. The eustachian tube extends from the middle ear to the nasopharynx, as illustrated in Figure 48–3. It creates an air passage to the middle ear so that air pressure remains the same on both sides of the tympanic membrane.

MASTOID PROCESS. The mastoid process is the bony structure behind the auricle. The interior is made up of air cells that are directly connected to the middle ear. The mastoid process is very close to the brain.

Inner Ear

The inner ear consists of the membranous labyrinth and the bony labyrinth. The membranous labyrinth contains fluid called endolymph. Endolymph moves with changes in body position.

The parts of the bony labyrinth are the vestibule, semicircular canals, and cochlea. The oval window opens into the vestibule. Receptors in the vestibule monitor the position of the head to maintain posture balance. Receptors in the semicircular canals monitor changes in rate or direction of movement to maintain balance during movement. The cochlea is a coiled tube that looks like a snail. It contains the organ of Corti, which is the receptor end organ of hearing. The organ of Corti transmits stimuli from the oval window to the acoustic (auditory) nerve.

PHYSIOLOGY OF HEARING

The perception and interpretation of sound depend on a complex series of steps. A malfunction at any step can result in some type of hearing impairment. Figure 48–4 illustrates the steps involved in the hearing process.

AGE-RELATED CHANGES IN THE EAR

Changes occur in the external, middle, and inner ear with aging. Some changes have no functional signifi-

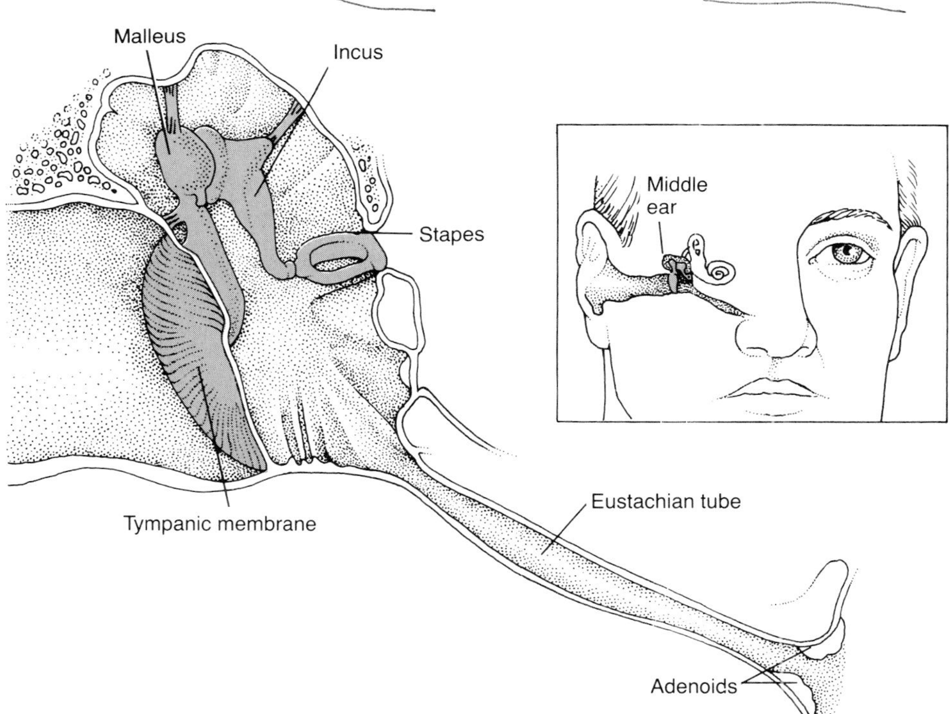

FIGURE 48-3
The eustachian tube extends from the middle ear to the nasopharynx. (From Ignatavicius, D. D., & Bayne, M. V. [1991]. *Medical-surgical nursing: A nursing process approach* [p. 1078]. Philadelphia: W. B. Saunders.)

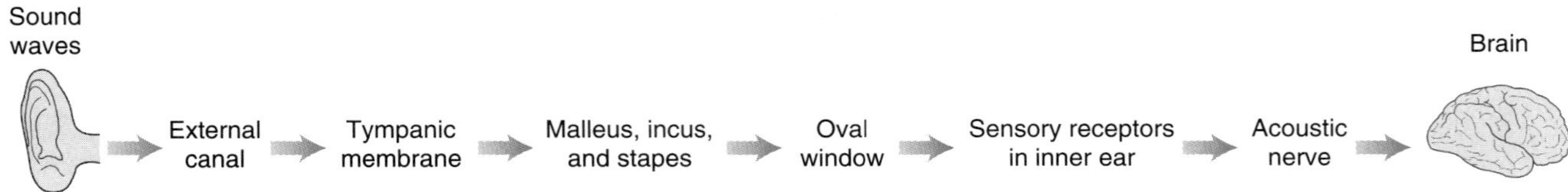

FIGURE 48-4
Physiology of hearing.

cance, but others can lead to serious problems with hearing or balance.

The skin of the auricle may become dry and wrinkled. Dryness of the external canal causes itching. Cerumen production declines, and the protective wax is drier. Hairs in the canal become coarser and longer, especially in males. The combination of dry cerumen and coarse hairs sometimes leads to obstruction of the canal. The eardrum thickens, and the bony joints in the middle ear degenerate somewhat. Surprisingly, these changes are not thought to impair hearing significantly.

Changes in the inner ear, however, affect sensitivity to sound, understanding of speech, and balance. Degenerative changes include atrophy of the cochlea, the cochlear nerve cells, and the organ of Corti. The result is that many older people have some degree of hearing loss, and some have problems with balance. The type of hearing loss most often associated with age is called presbycusis. Presbycusis is discussed later with other types of hearing impairments.

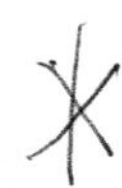

NURSING ASSESSMENT OF THE EXTERNAL EAR, HEARING, AND BALANCE

HEALTH HISTORY

The nursing assessment of the ear includes inspection of the external ear and evaluation of hearing and balance. If the patient's hearing impairment is severe, the nurse determines the usual means of communication. It may be necessary to call on a family member or a sign language interpreter or to use written communication during the assessment.

History of Present Illness

The nurse obtains a full description of any symptoms that may reflect problems with the ear, including changes in hearing acuity, pain, tinnitus, dizziness, vertigo, nausea, vomiting, and problems with balance. Changes in hearing acuity are reported, including the kind of change that occurred and whether it was sudden or gradual. The nurse asks the patient to describe the nature of the pain (e.g., sharp, throbbing, dull) and when it occurs. Pain in the ear is called otalgia. If tinnitus (ringing in the ears) is present, the type of sound heard is documented and described as continuous or intermittent. The presence of dizziness, vertigo, nausea, and vomiting are assessed, and the circumstances under which they occur are noted. The nurse also describes any problems with balance.

Past Medical History

The nurse asks about any previous acute or chronic ear problems. Acute conditions that may affect hearing or balance include sinus infections, dental problems, allergies, and upper respiratory infections. Chronic conditions that may be significant are hypertension, diabetes mellitus, and hypothyroidism. Recent surgical procedures on the ear or throat should be noted, as should a recent head injury.

Hearing impairments are often congenital (present at birth). One cause of hearing loss in an infant is rubella during the mother's pregnancy. Therefore, one assesses whether female patients have had rubella or have been immunized for the infection.

The medication history is important to identify any drugs taken that might be ototoxic. The term ototoxic means a drug can damage the eighth cranial nerve or the organs of hearing and balance. Examples of drugs that can have ototoxic effects are aspirin and aminoglycoside antibiotics. Ototoxicity is discussed more fully later. A family history of hearing loss also should be documented.

PHARMACOLOGY CAPSULE

Signs and symtoms of ototoxicity are tinnitus, hearing loss, dizziness, and ataxia.

Functional Assessment

The functional assessment determines exposure to excessively loud noise such as amplified music, firearms being used, or noisy machinery. The use of any assistive hearing devices is recorded.

PHYSICAL EXAMINATION

Some general observations of the patient give important clues about hearing and balance. The nurse observes how the patient responds to a normal voice. Patients who do not hear well use many adaptive behaviors. They may turn a "good ear" toward the speaker, ask people to repeat things, say "what?" frequently, or watch the speaker's mouth closely. The presence of a visible hearing aid also is noted. The patient's posture and balance while walking and sitting are observed.

External Ear

The position of the auricles is assessed. Normally, the top of the auricle is at about the level of the eye. The ears should be positioned symmetrically. The auricles are inspected for shape, lesions, and nodules. The auricles and the mastoid process are palpated for tenderness. Palpation in front of, below, and behind the ear may locate enlarged lymph nodes.

External Auditory Canal

A penlight is used to inspect the outer portion of the external auditory canal. The canal is inspected for any obvious obstructions or drainage. The only normal secretion in the canal is cerumen. It should be golden to brown in color and should not block the opening to the canal. If there is any drainage, the color, amount, and odor are recorded.

Some nurses are taught to use an otoscope to inspect the external canal and the tympanic membrane. The tympanic membrane should be shiny and pearl gray in color. The nursing assessment is outlined in Table 48–1.

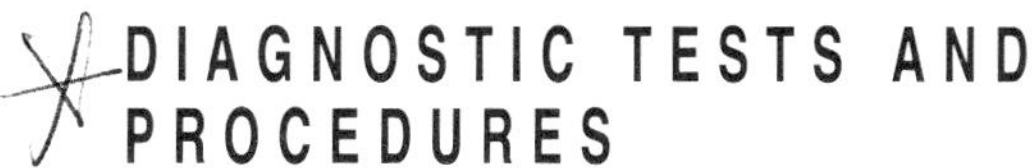

DIAGNOSTIC TESTS AND PROCEDURES

Several specialists handle different aspects of the diagnosis and treatment of hearing disorders. An otologist is trained to diagnose types of hearing loss. An audiologist carries out tests to determine whether a hearing aid will help a particular patient. If it is thought that a patient would benefit from a hearing aid, the audiologist also identifies the best kind of hearing aid. An otolaryngologist is a physician who specializes in diseases of the ears and throat.

Procedures and tests commonly used to diagnose disorders of the ear, hearing, and balance include the otoscopic examination, audiometry, the caloric test, electronystagmography, hearing acuity tests, and tuning fork tests. Radiographic examinations, especially the computed tomographic scan, may be used to study the mastoid bone, middle ear, and inner ear.

Diagnostic tests and procedures for patients with disorders of the ear, hearing, and balance are described in Table 48–2.

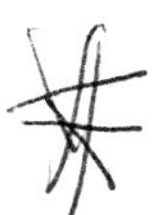

TABLE 48–1

ASSESSMENT OF PATIENTS WITH DISORDERS OF THE EAR, HEARING, AND BALANCE

HEALTH HISTORY

Present illness: Changes in the external ear, hearing acuity, or balance
Past medical history: Sinus infections, dental problems, allergies, upper respiratory infections, hypertension, diabetes mellitus, hypothyroidism, surgery on ear or throat, recent head injury, rubella and rubella immunization, recent and current medications
Family history: Hearing impairments
Review of systems: Pain in ear or throat, tinnitus, dizziness, vertigo, nausea, vomiting
Functional assessment: Exposure to excessively loud noise, use of hearing aid

PHYSICAL EXAMINATION

General survey: Response to normal voice, gait, posture, and balance
External ear: Position of auricles; lesions, tenderness, or nodules
Lymph nodes: Enlargement of lymph nodes in front of or behind ear
Mastoid: Tenderness
External auditory canal: Obstruction, lesions, drainage
Tympanic membrane: Redness, bulging

Otoscopic Examination

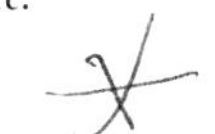

The otoscope is the instrument used to examine the external auditory canal (Fig. 48–5). In the past, otoscopic examinations were done only by physicians. Now nurses are learning to do this. The purpose of the otoscopic examination is to examine the external auditory canal and tympanic membrane. The examination permits diagnosis of inflammatory and infectious processes as well as obstructions of the external canal.

The following points should be remembered when using an otoscope:

1. Use the largest speculum that fits the ear canal easily.
2. For adult patients, pull the auricle up and back to straighten the canal, and then guide the speculum gently into the canal.
3. Steady the otoscope by resting the little finger against the patient's head, as illustrated in Figure 48–6.
4. Never force the speculum into the ear.
5. If the patient is unable to cooperate, have someone hold the head still during the examination.
6. Clean the speculum between patients and between ears on each patient.

Audiometry

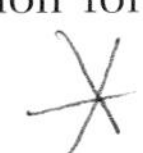

Audiometry is the assessment of the ability to hear simple sound waves. It requires a machine called an audiometer. Special training is needed to use the audiometer and to interpret test results. Nurses in some work settings learn to do these tests. The patient needs no special preparation for this test.

Caloric Test

The caloric test is used to diagnose disorders in the vestibular system or its central nervous system connections. The ear is irrigated with warm or cold water, and the patient is observed for reactions that suggest vestibular problems. A person with a labyrinth disorder responds with specific abnormal eye movements (nystagmus), vertigo, and nausea and vomiting. A person with vestibular disease has a decreased or absent response to the test.

Test results are altered by central nervous system depressants, barbiturates, and alcohol. The nurse should

TABLE 48-2
DIAGNOSTIC TESTS AND PROCEDURES FOR DISORDERS OF THE EAR, HEARING, AND BALANCE

TEST/STUDY	PURPOSE/PROCEDURE	PATIENT PREPARATION	POSTPROCEDURE NURSING CARE
Audiometry			
Pure tone audiometry	The patient's ability to hear a range of sounds is tested to detect hearing impairment.	Tell the patient test will be conducted in a sound-isolated room. The examiner will place earphones on the patient and introduce tones. The patient will be asked to identify when sounds are heard and when they disappear. A tuning fork will be placed near the patient's ear, and the patient will be asked when vibrating sound is heard and when it ceases. No other preparation is needed.	No special postprocedure care.
Speech audiometry	Measures ability to hear spoken words.	The patient listens to simple words through earphones and repeats the words that are understood. No special preparation.	No special postprocedure care.
Vestibular Tests			
Caloric test	The ears are irrigated with warm or cool water to help evaluate dizziness. The patient is then observed for nystagmus, nausea, vomiting, or dizziness.	The patient is told what to expect. The examiner is told if patient has had central nervous system depressants, alcohol, or barbiturates because they alter test response.	Assess nausea. Offer small amounts of clear liquids at first. Safety measures if dizzy.
Electronystagmography	Used to detect lesions in the vestibule.	Nothing by mouth for 3 hr before the test. Take eyeglasses to the test. Withhold medications as ordered. Tell the patient electrodes will be placed around the eyes. The patient will be asked to focus on specific targets. The ears will be irrigated. The patient will be turned in various positions in a special chair.	Assess for nausea. Offer small amounts of clear fluids at first. Safety precautions if dizzy.

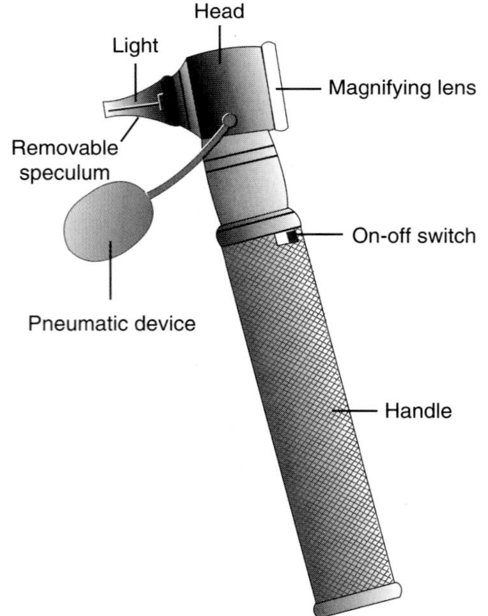

FIGURE 48-5
The otoscope is the instrument used to examine the external auditory canal.

inform the examiner if the patient has had any of these drugs prior to the examination.

Electronystagmography

Electronystagmography is used to detect lesions in the vestibule. Electrodes are placed around the eyes, and eye movements are measured as the patient focuses on specific targets, has the ears irrigated with warm and cool water, and is rotated and turned upside down.

The patient is usually allowed nothing by mouth for 3 hours before the test. Medications may be withheld on the physician's directions. Patients who normally wear eyeglasses are instructed to bring them to the test. After the test, the patient may report nausea and may vomit. If the patient is dizzy, appropriate safety precautions are taken.

Hearing Acuity Tests

Audiometry gives a precise measurement of hearing acuity. Other simple tests can be done by the nurse for a gross assessment of hearing. The whisper test can easily be done in any setting. The nurse stands 1 to 2 feet from the patient, facing away from him or her. The

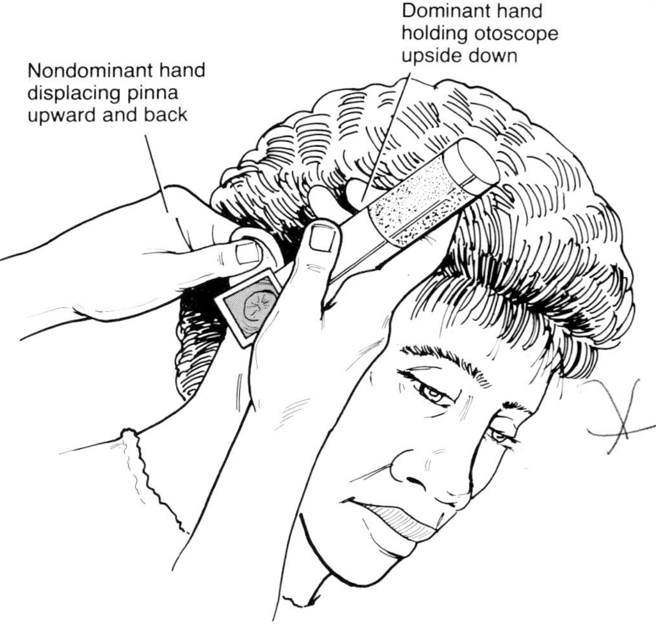

FIGURE 48-6
Correct technique for using an otoscope to examine the external auditory canal and the tympanic membrane.

patient occludes the ear on the opposite side. The nurse exhales and then speaks in a low whisper. The patient is asked to tell the nurse what was whispered. The words can be repeated louder until the patient is able to hear them. After assessing one ear, the nurse changes sides and assesses the other ear. This simple test gives the nurse an idea about the patient's general hearing ability.

Tuning Fork Tests

The Rinne and Weber tests use a tuning fork to assess the conduction of sound by air and by bone. This is useful in determining the nature of the hearing loss and in selecting the best treatment.

RINNE'S TEST. For the Rinne test, the examiner taps the tuning fork on the hand to activate it. The base of the tuning fork is then placed on the patient's mastoid bone. If the vibration is conducted through the bone, the patient hears a humming sound. When the sound is no longer heard, the fork is moved so that the tines of the tuning fork are near but not touching the ear canal. The patient is asked if he or she can hear the sound and, if so, to report when the sound disappears. This assesses the patient's ability to hear sound waves conducted through the air.

Normally, air conduction is better than bone conduction. Therefore, the patient should be able to hear the sound transmitted through air even after it can no longer be heard through bone. This normal finding is recorded as "AC > BC" (air conduction is greater than bone conduction). If bone conduction is greater than air conduction, the patient has a conductive hearing loss.

WEBER'S TEST. In the Weber test, the base of an activated tuning fork is placed on the midline of the skull. The patient is asked to identify the side in which the sound is loudest. With normal hearing in both ears, the sound is heard equally on each side. The sound is louder in an ear with conductive hearing loss and softer in an ear with sensorineural hearing loss.

COMMON THERAPEUTIC MEASURES

Problems of the ear and related structures sometimes require medications or surgery. Other therapeutic measures for problems of the ear include irrigations and the use of hearing aids. The nurse may encounter patients who are being treated by any of these measures.

EAR DROPS

Medications intended to be placed directly into the external ear canal are called otic drops, or simply ear drops. Ear drops may be ordered to treat infection or inflammation, to reduce pain, or to soften earwax. When administering ear drops, the nurse should keep the following points in mind:

1. Be sure to use an *otic* solution.
2. Warm the drops to body temperature by rolling the bottle between the palms.
3. Have the patient tilt the head so that the ear to be treated is positioned toward you.
4. Straighten the external auditory canal of an adult by pulling the auricle up and back. For a child, the auricle is pulled down and back.
5. Hold the dropper at the opening of the canal, but do not contaminate the tip by touching the skin.
6. Instruct the patient to keep the treated ear up for several minutes to keep the medication from leaking from the ear. Sometimes the physician orders a cotton ball to be placed loosely in the canal to keep the medicine in place.

Examples of commonly used otic medications are listed in Table 48–3.

PHARMACOLOGY CAPSULE

Medications intended to be administered into the external ear are called otic drugs.

IRRIGATION

Irrigation is the use of a solution to cleanse the external ear canal or to remove something from the canal. A

TABLE 48-3
DRUGS USED TO TREAT DISORDERS OF THE EAR, HEARING, AND BALANCE

DRUG	USE/ACTION	SIDE EFFECTS	NURSING INTERVENTIONS
Antibiotics Chloramphenicol (Chloromycetin Otic)	Broad-spectrum antibiotic used to treat infections of lining of external auditory canal.	Hypersensitivity: redness, rash, swelling, burning, pain.	If patient shows signs of hypersensitivity, withhold drug and notify physician.
Topical Corticosteroids Hydrocortisone combined with Neomycin sulfate and polymyxin B (Cortisporin Otic, Otocort) Polymyxin B (Otobiotic Otic) Neomycin and colistin (Coly-Mycin S Otic)	Treat inflammation, pruritus, and allergic response. Usually combined with antibacterial or antifungal drug.		Do not put in ear if tympanic membrane is perforated. Caution to avoid eye contact.
Antibacterial and Softening Agent Carbamide peroxide with glycerin (Debrox, Murine Ear Drops)	Soften earwax. Treat aphthous ulcers.	Redness, irritation, superinfection.	Contraindications: ear surgery, perforated tympanic membrane; ear drainage, redness, pain, or tenderness. Teach patient not to clean ear with cotton swabs, which force wax deeper into ear.
Drying Agents Boric acid in isopropyl alcohol (Ear-Dry, Swim Ear)	Dry external canal after swimming or bathing. Decrease risk of infection.		Instilled in external canal immediately after swimming or bathing. Contraindicated with perforated tympanic membrane.
Antiemetics Scopolamine (Transderm Scop) Dimenhydrinate (Dramamine) Diphenhydramine (Benadryl) Meclizine (Antivert) Chlorpromazine (Thorazine)	Prevent or treat nausea, vomiting, motion sickness.	Sedation, drowsiness, tremor, fever, tachycardia, hypotension, constipation, dry mouth.	Safety precautions for drowsiness. Monitor pulse and blood pressure. Monitor stools and urinary output. Mouth care.

common indication for irrigation is impacted cerumen. Impacted cerumen is dried earwax that blocks the canal. The nurse may perform the irrigation, if agency policy permits, or may assist with the procedure. The following key points should be remembered when irrigating an ear:

1. Select the correct solution as ordered by the physician.
2. Warm the solution to body temperature (95–105°F).
3. Have the patient sit up and hold an emesis basin under the ear to be irrigated.
4. Drape the shoulder under the basin.
5. Straighten the external canal of an adult by pulling the auricle up and back. For a child, pull the auricle down and back.
6. Select an irrigating syringe or bulb syringe with a tip that is smaller than the canal.
7. Direct the solution toward the top of the canal in a steady stream. The procedure can be repeated several times if needed.
8. Sometimes ear drops are ordered to soften impacted cerumen before irrigating.
9. Describe any substances rinsed out of the ear. If the impacted cerumen or foreign body does not wash out, inform the physician.
10. If the tympanic membrane (eardrum) is ruptured, the canal should *not* be irrigated because fluid could be forced into the middle ear.

HEARING AIDS

A hearing aid is a device that amplifies sound; that is, it makes sound louder. People with conductive hearing loss benefit the most from using a hearing aid. Those who have sensorineural or mixed losses may experience some benefit, but not as much.

Often it may take considerable persuasion from family and health care providers to get a hearing-impaired person to try a hearing aid. It may be helpful to point out the benefits of improved hearing in the patient's everyday life.

Hearing aids amplify all sounds, including background noise. This is especially annoying when a person first tries to use an aid. Patients are advised to wear the aid first in quiet settings. Once they learn to adjust the volume and tone comfortably, they can try it in noisy settings. It may take several months before a hearing aid feels comfortable.

The two basic types of hearing aids are bone conduction receivers and air conduction receivers. Bone conduction receivers are worn behind the ear against the skull. Air conduction receivers are worn in the external canal. An audiologist determines which type a patient needs.

Modern hearing aids use transistors, which allow the device to be very small. Small batteries are needed for them to work. The hearing aid requires some care. The ear mold (the part that fits into the ear) should be washed daily with soap and water and then dried. When not being worn, the aid should be turned off and stored in a protective case with the battery compartment open. Extra batteries should be kept on hand.

If the hearing aid is not working, the patient should first check to be sure it is turned on. If it is on, the ear mold should be checked to see if it needs cleaning. The next step is to check battery placement. If the battery is not inserted correctly, the hearing aid will not work. If the hearing aid has a cord, it should be checked to see if it is broken or unplugged. If these checks fail to locate the problem, the battery should be changed. If a new battery does not correct the problem, the cord can be changed. Should the hearing aid still not work, it should be returned to the dealer for service.

Nurses and other health care providers need to be familiar with hearing aids and how they work. The patient's nursing care plan should indicate that the patient usually wears a hearing aid. Confusion in some older patients might be avoided if the hearing aid is kept in place. The cost of hearing aids can range from $250 to $800 if both ears are involved. When patients are hospitalized, nurses should take care to prevent loss of these devices.

COCHLEAR IMPLANTS

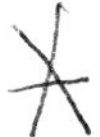

A cochlear implant may be recommended for people who cannot benefit from regular hearing aids. A cochlear implant allows the profoundly deaf to recognize some environmental sounds, such as sirens, doorbells, and telephones.

The cochlear implant consists of a microphone, a processor, a transmitter, and a receiver. The microphone, at ear level, picks up sounds that are amplified by the processor. The sound, in the form of magnetic signals, is transmitted electronically to the receiver. The receiver is surgically implanted behind the ear. Electrodes attached to the receiver stimulate nerve fibers in the cochlea to produce sound. Several months of training are needed to learn to tell sounds apart. Therefore, candidates for the cochlear implant must be highly motivated and carefully screened.

SURGERY ON THE EAR AND RELATED STRUCTURES

Many ear disorders are treated surgically. Nursing care of patients having specific surgical procedures is discussed with the appropriate pathophysiology. However, some general measures apply to most patients after surgery on the ear.

Nursing Care of the Patient Having Ear Surgery

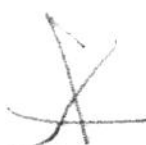

Preoperatively, the nurse assesses the patient's understanding of the procedure and surgical routine as well as the anxiety level. Knowledge deficit and anxiety are typical nursing diagnoses. The nurse corrects knowledge deficits by supplying needed information about the preoperative and postoperative routines. If the patient is anxious, the nurse explores the specific concerns. Sometimes patient teaching and reassurance are sufficient to reduce anxiety. The physician should be notified if the patient is very anxious.

Immediate preoperative care usually includes having the patient remove any articles such as eyeglasses or hearing aids. The hearing-impaired person going to surgery may feel very helpless without the hearing aid. The nurse can notify the operating room staff and ask if the patient can wear the hearing aid to the surgical suite. A note should be placed on the front of the chart to alert caregivers of the patient's hearing impairment and to the presence of a hearing aid.

Criteria for effective preoperative nursing care are patient description of surgical routine and expectations and patient statement of reduced anxiety accompanied by a calm manner.

Postoperative nursing care follows.

ASSESSMENT. In the postoperative period, the nurse assesses the patient for pain, nausea, dizziness, and fever. The wound dressing is inspected for drainage. Drainage color, odor, and amount are documented.

NURSING DIAGNOSIS. After ear surgery, nursing diagnoses may include the following:

- **Pain** related to tissue trauma or edema
- **High Risk for Injury** related to dizziness or vertigo
- **High Risk for Impaired Skin Integrity** related to pressure in the ear or delayed wound healing
- **High Risk for Infection** related to surgical incision
- **Sensory Perceptual Alteration** (auditory) related to packing and edema in affected ear

GOALS. Goals of nursing care after surgery on the ear are pain relief, patient safety, wound healing, absence of infection, and effective communication until packing is removed.

INTERVENTIONS

Pain. The nurse determines the nature of the patient's pain and has the patient rate the pain on a scale from 1 to 10, with 10 being the worst pain imaginable. Surgical pain usually requires analgesics for several days. In addition, the nurse uses measures such as positioning and massage to promote relaxation.

High Risk for Injury. Dizziness and vertigo are common after surgery on the ear. Dizziness is a feeling of unsteadiness, whereas vertigo is the sensation that one's body or the room is spinning. Vertigo is often triggered by sudden movements, so the patient is advised to move slowly and carefully. The patient is instructed to call for help when getting up the first few times. The nurse assists as long as dizziness is a problem. Siderails are raised, and the bed is left in low position.

High Risk for Impaired Skin Integrity. The ear is frequently packed and covered with a dressing. A drain may be in place. The packing is removed only by the physician. A specific position may be ordered postoperatively. If drainage is being encouraged, the patient is most likely positioned on the affected side. If the procedure includes a graft on the tympanic membrane, however, the patient is usually positioned on the unaffected side.

Straining is contraindicated because it increases pressure in the ear. The patient should avoid nose blowing, coughing, and sneezing; however, if these are unavoidable, the mouth should be kept open to relieve pressure. Stool softeners may be ordered to prevent constipation and straining. Ear surgery, like any other type of surgery, creates a wound that must heal. Healing requires a balanced diet with adequate protein and vitamin C.

High Risk for Infection. Measures are taken to reduce the risk of postoperative infection. The patient is advised to avoid crowds and people with colds for several weeks. The ear canal should be kept dry for 2 to 4 weeks as instructed by the physician. Shampooing is usually not allowed for 2 weeks, although it is restricted longer in some cases.

Sensory Perceptual Alteration. While the affected ear is packed, the patient's hearing in that ear is impaired. If the patient does not hear well in the unaffected ear, the nurse must devise appropriate means of communication. It is best to plan this with the patient preoperatively.

EVALUATION. Criteria for evaluating the effects of nursing care after surgery on the ear are patient's statement of pain relief, absence of injury associated with dizziness or vertigo, patient's performance of measures to prevent pressure in the ears, absence of fever, and evidence of effective communication.

HEARING LOSS

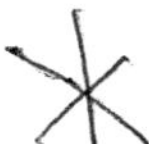

TYPES OF HEARING LOSS

Hearing loss covers a range from inability to hear sounds of a certain pitch to inability to hear any sounds at all. Millions of Americans have some degree of hearing impairment. Hearing losses are classified into categories. The categories of hearing loss discussed here include conductive, sensorineural, mixed, and central.

Conductive Hearing Loss

Conductive hearing loss results from interference with the transmission of sound waves from the external or middle ear to the inner ear. Factors that may cause conductive hearing loss include obstruction of the external canal or eustachian tube and otosclerosis. Otosclerosis is a condition in which the stapes in the middle ear does not vibrate.

Patients who have conductive hearing loss hear better in noisy settings than in quiet settings. They do not speak loudly because bone conduction allows them to hear their own voices.

Most conditions that cause conductive hearing loss are treatable. Obstructions can generally be removed. Otosclerosis can be treated surgically with a procedure called a stapedectomy. This condition is discussed in more detail later. Hearing aids are usually helpful for patients with conductive hearing loss.

Sensorineural Hearing Loss

Sensorineural hearing loss is sometimes called nerve deafness. It is a disturbance of the neural structures in the inner ear or the nerve pathways to the brain. Sensorineural hearing loss may be congenital, but it can also be caused by noise trauma, aging, Meniere's syndrome, ototoxicity, diabetes, and syphilis.

Patients with sensorineural hearing loss can hear sounds but have difficulty understanding speech. They often complain that speech sounds muffled. This type of hearing loss cannot be corrected. Hearing aids may help by amplifying the sound, but it still sounds muffled.

Mixed Hearing Loss

Mixed hearing loss is a combination of conductive and sensorineural losses. Treatment of any reversible problems often results in improvement of mixed hearing loss.

Central Hearing Loss

Central hearing loss is due to some problem in the central nervous system. The patient either cannot perceive or cannot interpret sounds that are heard.

SIGNS AND SYMPTOMS

Most hearing loss progresses over time. Patients may not readily recognize the losses. They may complain that their hearing is fine but that others are mumbling. There are many behaviors that should lead the nurse to suspect hearing loss. The patient may lean toward the speaker or turn one ear toward the speaker. The patient with a hearing loss may fail to follow directions, speak while others are speaking, or turn the radio or television up very loud. Irritability and even hostility are not unusual. Some people become very suspicious of others because they cannot hear what others are saying. Hearing loss often has no other symptoms. Otalgia (ear pain), dizziness, and tinnitus (ringing in the ears) may be present with certain types of disorders.

THE IMPACT OF HEARING IMPAIRMENT

People with obvious physical disabilities generally receive some consideration and understanding from strangers. People who have hearing impairments may not be treated as well.

Those who had impairments in early childhood usually have speech difficulties. If speech is not clear, others may assume the patient is intellectually impaired. Sadly, the phrase "deaf and dumb" has been used to refer to people who neither hear nor speak. This term is understandably offensive to the hearing-impaired person. The term "deaf" is not offensive but suggests a total inability to hear. "Hearing impairment," on the other hand, implies a range of abilities.

It is interesting that most people accept the use of eyeglasses fairly easily, but they are often resistant to using a hearing aid. There is a tendency to deny one's hearing loss. When a person refuses to admit to a hearing loss, family members and others may stop trying to communicate. The hearing-impaired person may alienate those who would like to be close and supportive.

People with severe hearing impairment probably suffer the most severe social isolation of those with sensory disorders. Nurses can help by educating the public about hearing loss. A teaching plan should include the following points:

1. Many types of hearing loss are correctable, or at least capable of being improved.
2. Hearing is not related to intelligence.
3. There is no reason to be ashamed of a hearing impairment.
4. Some measures can be taken to reduce the risk of certain types of hearing loss.
5. All women of childbearing age should be immunized for rubella to prevent one form of congenital hearing impairment.

ADAPTATIONS TO HEARING LOSS

Some hearing impairments can be corrected. If not, the patient and family need to learn to cope with the loss. For many people, hearing aids produce at least some improvement in hearing. Many patients read lips and observe body language closely to enhance understanding of spoken messages.

Sign language uses a universal set of hand signals. It provides a very effective means of communicating as long as there are others who know how to use it. Unfortunately, most nurses are not trained in this skill.

Several electronic devices are available to serve the hearing impaired. Telephones can be adapted to send and receive written messages. Earphones are readily available for use with radios, stereos, and televisions. These allow the hearing-impaired person to adjust the volume as needed. They also reduce environmental noises. Some television channels provide closed captioned programming, in which a written script is shown on the bottom of the screen. For the patient who does not speak, small hand-held computers called personal communicators print out messages typed by the user.

For many years, guide dogs have been used to help people with visual impairments. A similar intervention is being tried with dogs trained to assist the hearing impaired. These dogs are taught to recognize common sounds (doorbell, telephone, smoke alarm, crying baby) and to get the attention of the owner.

NURSING CARE OF THE PATIENT WITH IMPAIRED HEARING

Assessment

Assessment of the patient with impaired hearing is summarized in Table 48–1.

Nursing Diagnosis

Common nursing diagnoses for patients with hearing impairments may include the following:

- **Impaired Verbal Communication** related to inability to hear
- **Social Isolation** related to inability to communicate verbally
- **Ineffective Individual Coping** related to altered social interaction, threat to body image, or denial
- **Knowledge Deficit** of prevention, diagnosis and treatment of hearing impairment, and resources for adaptation

Goals

Nursing goals when working with a hearing impaired person are effective communication, participation in social activities, effective coping with permanent hearing impairment, and knowledge of prevention and treatment of hearing impairment.

Interventions

IMPAIRED VERBAL COMMUNICATION. Many techniques are available to improve communication with the hearing impaired. The nurse can use these approaches and teach others to use them as well. When working with a hearing-impaired patient, the nurse should use the following guidelines:

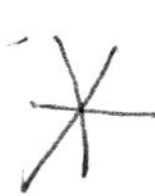

1. Be sure the patient knows you are present. Try to move into the patient's line of vision before touching him or her.
2. Find out the patient's usual means of communication, and be sure he or she has access to any assistive devices.
3. Speak slowly and distinctly.
4. Be sure the patient can see your face clearly. Do not turn away while speaking.
5. Do not eat, smoke, or chew gum if the patient reads lips.
6. Provide adequate lighting directed *toward* your face. A strong light behind you creates a glare and makes it hard to see your features.
7. Lower your voice tone.
8. Assess the patient's ability to hear a normal voice tone. The volume can be increased a little if needed, but shouting simply distorts the message. People who wear hearing aids often complain that everyone shouts at them.

9. If the patient has a "good ear," speak toward that side.

10. Amplify your voice, if necessary, by using a rolled-up sheet of paper or a stethoscope. To use the stethoscope, put the earpieces in the patient's ears and speak into the bell.

11. Help patients follow spoken messages by informing them of the topic to be addressed.

12. Use short sentences or phrases.

13. Use body language to support the verbal message.

14. Have a writing pad or "magic slate" available. Use it if the patient cannot understand you or if you do not understand the patient.

15. Try to validate patient understanding by encouraging feedback and assessing whether directions are followed.

16. When a hearing-impaired patient is hospitalized, be sure a call button is provided, but remind staff that the patient cannot use the intercom.

SOCIAL ISOLATION. The preceding guidelines may improve communication with the hearing-impaired person. The most important thing the nurse can do, however, is to have a positive attitude toward trying to communicate with the patient. Genuine interest and attention encourage the patient to express himself or herself in whatever way is possible.

When other people seem hurried or annoyed, they discourage the patient's attempts to communicate. Some patients withdraw from social interactions. They may become isolated and depressed. The nurse encourages the patient to learn new communication methods. The patient is taught how to use assistive devices. Information is provided about community resources for the hearing impaired. The nurse explores the type of activities that are satisfying to the patient and encourages continued involvement. The physician should be advised if the patient becomes increasingly sad or withdrawn. Counseling with a mental health professional may be suggested.

INEFFECTIVE INDIVIDUAL COPING. The way people cope with hearing loss varies with the individual. Some deny the problem for as long as possible; others deliberately learn everything they can about treatments and adaptive strategies. The nurse should recognize that both of these behaviors are responses to a stressful situation. It is important to explore the patient's feelings about hearing loss. If the patient is anxious, the nurse may employ stress-reduction techniques (relaxation exercises, massage, meditation). The patient who denies hearing loss is often resistant to teaching, so he or she may not take advantage of opportunities to deal with the problem effectively.

KNOWLEDGE DEFICIT. Most people with hearing impairment have some hearing ability. The nurse can emphasize measures to reduce the risk of additional impairment. The patient is advised to seek prompt treatment of any symptoms of infection (fever, pain in the ear, drainage). Hearing protection is recommended in excessively noisy settings. Patients taking ototoxic drugs (e.g., aspirin) are told to contact the physician if hearing acuity worsens or tinnitus develops. If ear drops or irrigations are ordered, the nurse demonstrates the procedure and reinforces the physician's orders. Patients also need instruction in the use of hearing aids, as described in the next section.

Evaluation

Criteria for effective nursing interventions include validation of effective communication by the patient and the nurse, patient's participation in social activities, patient's taking steps to adapt to hearing loss, and patient's statement of preventive and therapeutic measures.

DISORDERS AFFECTING HEARING AND BALANCE

EXTERNAL EAR AND CANAL

Foreign Bodies and Cerumen

Occasionally, foreign bodies get into the external ear canal. Most small objects can be flushed from the ear by gentle irrigation. Insects can be killed by instilling a small amount of mineral oil or alcohol. They can then be flushed from the canal. An alternative method is to hold a flashlight near the auricle. Since insects are often attracted to light, they may move out of the canal.

One of the most common causes of obstruction of the external ear canal is impacted cerumen. The patient is not always aware of the obstruction but may complain of hearing loss or tinnitus. When a large amount of hardened cerumen is present, the physician may order ear drops to soften the cerumen before irrigation. It may be necessary to repeat the procedure several times before all cerumen is removed. If the foreign body or cerumen is not removed by irrigation, the physician can use ear forceps or a cerumen spoon to remove it.

NURSING CARE OF THE PATIENT WITH IMPACTED CERUMEN. Nurses, especially in long-term care facilities, need to inspect the ear canal routinely for impacted cerumen. The dry cerumen may be gold to dark brown. Sometimes it fills the entire canal. If both ears are affected, the patient has some degree of hearing impairment.

In this situation, the primary nursing diagnosis is sensory perceptual alteration related to obstruction of the external auditory canal. The nursing goal is restored hearing. The nurse reports the findings to the physician and carries out orders for ear drops. Irrigations may be done by the physician or the nurse if policy permits. Successful interventions are evaluated by examining the canal and documenting the absence of obstructions.

Infection and Inflammation

Infection or inflammation of the lining of the external ear canal is called external otitis or "swimmer's ear." It may be caused by scratching or cleaning the ear with sharp objects. Swimming can lead to otitis by washing out protective cerumen, which leaves the lining of the external canal susceptible to injury. When infection is present, it is often caused by staphylococcus or streptococcus.

SIGNS AND SYMPTOMS. The most characteristic symptom of external otitis is pain that increases when the auricle is pulled. Other symptoms can include pain, dizziness, fever, and drainage. Drainage may be purulent or blood tinged.

MEDICAL TREATMENT. Topical antibiotics and corticosteroids are ordered to treat external otitis. If the external canal is obstructed by edema, the physician may insert an ear wick through the blocked canal. An ear wick is a long piece of gauze that extends out of the ear canal. Medication placed on the external portion of the ear wick soaks the gauze and distributes the medication in the canal. Pain is treated with aspirin or codeine. Any drainage from the ear should be treated as infected material and handled carefully.

NURSING CARE OF THE PATIENT WITH EXTERNAL OTITIS. External otitis is typically treated on an outpatient basis, so nursing care is limited. The nurse's assessment includes inspection of the external canal and evaluation of pain. Nursing diagnoses are acute pain related to inflammation and knowledge deficit of treatment and prevention of external otitis. Goals of nursing care are pain relief and patient knowledge of treatment and prevention of the condition.

Oral analgesics and topical corticosteroids and antibiotics are given as ordered to treat pain and to reduce inflammation and infection. The nurse may administer the prescribed drops or teach the patient to do so. Since it is awkward to put drops into one's own ear, the nurse may want to teach a family member how to do it also. The nurse also teaches patients to prevent external otitis by not using sharp instruments to clean the auditory canal and by avoiding suspected irritants such as hair spray and earphones. Ear plugs may be advised while swimming. The physician may instruct the patient to use a drying agent (Ear-Dry) after swimming or bathing.

Criteria for effective nursing interventions are patient statement of pain relief and patient's correct description of treatment and prevention of external otitis.

Furuncle

A furuncle is an inflamed area in the external auditory canal caused by infection of a hair follicle. The area is very painful to the touch. Hearing may be impaired if swelling blocks the canal. A ruptured furuncle releases fluid that may drain from the canal. Treatment includes systemic and topical antibiotics (with an ear wick if needed). If the condition does not improve, the physician may incise and drain it. Nursing care of the patient with a furuncle is like that for external otitis.

MIDDLE EAR

Conditions of the middle ear are serious because of the risk of complications, including permanent hearing loss and involvement of the inner ear.

Otitis Media

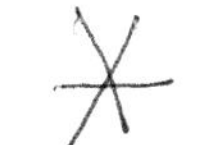

Otitis media is an infection of the middle ear. There are several types of otitis media. Acute otitis media and chronic otitis media are sometimes called suppurant or purulent otitis media because of the presence of purulent material. In serous otitis media, sterile fluid accumulates behind the tympanic membrane. It can precede or follow acute otitis media. Adhesive otitis media may develop if fluid remains in the middle ear. It is characterized by thickening and scarring in the middle ear structures.

ACUTE OTITIS MEDIA. Acute otitis media usually develops with colds. Edema leads to blockage of the eustachian tubes. Fluid accumulates in the middle ear, causing painful pressure on the tympanic membrane. The tympanic membrane may rupture, resulting in scarring and subsequent hearing loss. The patient frequently has a fever and complains of headache. Acute otitis media is more common in children than in adults.

Medical Treatment. Antibiotics are usually prescribed for acute otitis media. Sometimes myringotomy is performed. Myringotomy is the creation of a small opening in the tympanic membrane to reduce pressure and allow fluid to drain. If infection is eliminated, the tympanic membrane should heal without permanent damage.

CHRONIC OTITIS MEDIA. Chronic otitis media is characterized by hearing loss and continuous or intermittent drainage. The condition is usually not painful. On examination, the eardrum is usually perforated (ruptured) or shows signs of a healed perforation. An audiogram may detect some conductive hearing loss if the bones in the middle ear have been damaged by the chronic infection.

Possible complications of chronic otitis media include mastoiditis, meningitis, labyrinthitis, cholesteatoma, and hearing impairment.

Mastoiditis. Since the middle ear is directly connected to the air cells in the mastoid bone, infection in the middle ear can extend into the mastoid bone. And since the brain lies next to the mastoid bone, the infection can spread there as well. Signs and symptoms of mastoiditis include mastoid swelling (directly behind the ear) and soreness, headache, malaise, and an elevated white blood cell count. There may be thick, purulent drainage from the ear. Mastoiditis is very serious because it can lead to a brain abscess, meningitis (inflammation of the covering of the brain), or paralysis of the facial muscles.

Labyrinthitis. Labyrinthitis is inflammation of the labyrinth. It produces disturbances in both hearing and balance. Labyrinthitis is discussed later.

Cholesteatoma. A cholesteatoma is a growth in the middle ear. When the tympanic membrane is perforated around the margin where it attaches to the ear canal, epithelial cells grow into the middle ear. The cells form a ball of tissue that grows and that may damage the facial nerve and the labyrinth. A cholesteatoma must be removed surgically.

Medical Treatment. Chronic otitis media is treated with systemic antibiotics and irrigations to remove debris. If the tympanic membrane does not heal, tympanoplasty may be done to repair it. The procedure may be done through the ear canal or through an incision behind the auricle. Sometimes grafts of the patient's tissue are used to repair the tear. Tissue may be taken from the external canal or the temporalis muscle. After the graft is placed, the middle ear is filled with Gelfoam, and a cotton ball is put in the external ear to hold the graft in place.

If the infection has extended to the mastoid bone, a mastoidectomy is often done at the same time. A mastoidectomy can be modified (simple) or radical. In a modified procedure, infected mastoid tissue is removed but the middle ear is left intact. In a radical mastoidectomy, all the structures in the middle ear are removed. The radical procedure is not done now as often as it was in the past.

Nursing Care of the Patient Having Mastoidectomy. General care of the patient having surgery on the ear is discussed earlier in this chapter. Preoperatively, the emphasis is on patient teaching and reduction of anxiety. Primary considerations after surgery on the middle ear include comfort, safety, prevention of infection, and prevention of pressure on the tympanic membrane. Nursing diagnoses, goals, and interventions in relation to these problems also are described earlier. Nausea is another common problem after middle ear surgery. An emesis basin is kept nearby. The physician usually orders antiemetics to be given as needed for nausea. If the patient vomits frequently, there is a risk of fluid volume deficit. The nurse monitors intake and output and gives intravenous fluids if ordered.

The type of dressing varies. It may be small and placed over the auricle. If the surgeon entered through the mastoid bone, however, it is a large head dressing with a drain. The nurse inspects the dressing and describes any drainage but does *not* disturb or remove the dressing.

Otosclerosis

Otosclerosis is a hereditary condition in which an abnormal growth causes the footplate of the stapes to become fixed. The fixed stapes cannot vibrate, so sound waves cannot be transmitted to the inner ear. The effect of this abnormality is a conductive hearing loss. If the disease also involves the inner ear, the patient has sensorineural hearing loss as well. The condition affects both ears but may progress faster in one ear than in the other.

Otosclerosis is most common in young, white females. The onset is usually in the late teens or early twenties. During pregnancy it progresses at a faster rate.

SIGNS AND SYMPTOMS. The primary symptom of otosclerosis is slowly progressive hearing loss in the absence of infection. In the early stages, the patient may report tinnitus. The Rinne test reveals bone conduction to be greater than air conduction.

MEDICAL TREATMENT. Hearing aids are useful if the patient has only conductive hearing loss. The most common treatment is a surgical procedure called stapedectomy. The physician advises the patient of the surgical risks, including complete hearing loss, infection, prolonged vertigo, and damage to the facial nerve. Stapedectomy is done under local anesthesia. The stapes is removed and replaced with a prosthesis. A tissue graft taken from the patient is placed over the oval window. The physician puts packing in the ear canal at the completion of the stapedectomy. A small dressing is then placed over the ear. When the graft heals, hearing is restored in most patients.

Postoperatively, bedrest may be ordered for several days and drugs prescribed to control nausea and vertigo. Usually, the patient is allowed to lie on the back or the unaffected side, but specific position restrictions may be ordered.

NURSING CARE OF THE PATIENT HAVING STAPEDECTOMY. Care of the patient having ear surgery is detailed earlier in this chapter. In addition to the usual preoperative teaching, the patient should be told that hearing is usually worse immediately after stapedectomy but gradually improves over about 6 weeks.

Postoperatively, the nurse is concerned with pain relief, safety, prevention of infection, and avoidance of pressure in the ear. Nursing diagnoses, goals, and interventions related to these problems are discussed earlier. Since pressure can cause the graft to separate, it is especially important that the patient not do anything that increases pressure in the ear. After stapedectomy, nausea, vomiting, and vertigo are common.

The packing in the ear should not be disturbed. The physician removes it about 1 week after the surgery. After the dressing and packing are removed, the patient is usually advised to keep the ear dry for at least 2 weeks. Swimming and showering are usually not permitted for about 6 weeks.

The patient should avoid contact with people who have colds. A balanced diet and adequate rest are needed for tissue healing and resistance to infection. Vertigo may persist after discharge, and the nurse helps the patient plan for assistance with activities of daily living. It is important for the nurse to reinforce that hearing improvement is gradual.

INNER EAR

Labyrinthitis

Labyrinthitis is inflammation of the labyrinth. It may be acute or chronic. Acute labyrinthitis generally follows an acute upper respiratory infection, acute otitis media, pneumonia, or influenza. It can also be an adverse effect of some drugs. One type of labyrinthitis is suppurative labyrinthitis. It is an inner ear infection that usually follows an upper respiratory infection, ear infection, or ear surgery. Repeated episodes of labyrinthitis may lead to Meniere's disease.

SIGNS AND SYMPTOMS. Signs and symptoms of labyrinthitis include vertigo, nausea, vomiting, headache, photophobia, and anorexia. A typical episode lasts 3 to 6 weeks. Additional symptoms of suppurative labyrinthitis are tinnitus and hearing loss.

MEDICAL TREATMENT. Labyrinthitis is treated with antiemetics and supportive care until it resolves. Antibiotics are prescribed if infection is present.

NURSING CARE OF THE PATIENT WITH LABYRINTHITIS. During an acute episode of labyrinthitis, the nurse assesses the patient's symptoms. Intake and output, daily weights, and food intake are monitored if there is persistent vomiting.

Nursing Diagnosis. The primary nursing diagnoses are the following:

- **High Risk for Injury** related to vertigo
- **Altered Nutrition: Less than Body Requirements** related to anorexia and nausea
- **High Risk for Fluid Volume Deficit** related to vomiting
- **Anxiety** related to acute illness

Goals. Goals of nursing care for the patient with labyrinthitis are safety, adequate nutrition, normal hydration, and reduced anxiety.

Interventions. Safety is a major concern for the patient with vertigo. The patient is assisted and supervised when out of bed. Antiemetics are given as prescribed for nausea and vomiting. If vomiting persists, the patient is at risk for developing fluid and electrolyte imbalances (hypokalemia, fluid volume deficit), and intravenous fluids may be needed. The patient needs reassurance that the condition resolves in time.

Evaluation. Criteria for evaluating nursing care include absence of falls or injury, stable weight and vital signs, equal intake and output, and patient's statement of reduced anxiety.

Meniere's Disease

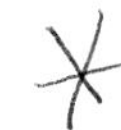

Meniere's disease is a disorder of the labyrinth. More than 2 million Americans are thought to have attacks of Meniere's disease. It is most common in men over the age of 60. The cause is unknown, but the symptoms are related to an accumulation of fluid in the inner ear. Some things that have been found to trigger attacks include alcohol and nicotine, stress, and certain stimuli such as bright lights and sudden movements of the head.

SIGNS AND SYMPTOMS. Some patients with Meniere's disease have more serious symptoms than others. Acute attacks occur at regular intervals. During an acute attack, the classic symptoms are hearing loss and vertigo. The hearing loss is unilateral, meaning that only one ear is affected. Tinnitus accompanies acute attacks. It is heard as a low buzzing sound that sometimes becomes a roar. Hearing usually improves between attacks, but some loss of low-frequency sounds may remain. Patients who have had many attacks may eventually have permanent hearing loss.

Vertigo is a sensation of movement that causes dizziness and nausea. Patients may say that the room seems to be spinning or that they feel like they are spinning. A feeling of fullness and pressure in the ear often precedes a vertigo attack. Attacks may last several minutes to several hours. They tend to become progressively more severe and more frequent. Sudden movement during an attack of vertigo can cause vomiting.

MEDICAL DIAGNOSIS. Diagnosis of Meniere's disease is based on the history and physical findings. The patient describes hearing and balance disturbances as described above. When the caloric test or electronystagmography is done, the patient with Meniere's disease has a severe attack of vertigo. An audiogram often reveals a loss of the ability to hear low-frequency sounds.

Meniere's disease is actually diagnosed by ruling out other conditions that can cause similar symptoms. Therefore, the physician is likely to order a number of radiographs and other tests to detect any neurologic, allergic, or endocrine disorders.

MEDICAL TREATMENT. Meniere's disease may be treated medically or surgically. Drugs prescribed during an acute attack include atropine, epinephrine, diazepam (Valium), antihistamines, antiemetics, anticholinergics, and vasodilators. Drugs may also be prescribed between attacks in an attempt to reduce their frequency and severity. Diuretics may be used in addition to the drugs previously listed.

A low-sodium diet seems to increase the length of time between attacks by reducing edema in the inner ear. If moderate sodium restriction is not effective, the patient may be put on a strict sodium-free diet.

Surgical Treatment. Surgery is usually advised only when all other measures have failed. Surgical procedures work by draining excess fluid from the inner ear or by cutting the part of the acoustic nerve that controls balance. The incision may be inside or behind the ear. In general, surgical procedures pose some risk for permanent hearing loss.

Potential complications of surgery for Meniere's disease include infection, hearing loss, loss of cerebrospinal fluid, and damage to the seventh cranial nerve. The leakage of cerebrospinal fluid may occur with procedures that require opening of the skull. Cerebrospinal fluid is clear and thin in consistency. The seventh cranial nerve is the facial nerve. It controls the movement of certain muscles of the face. It is located very close to the ear canal. Surgical procedures in and around the ear can result in trauma to the facial nerve.

NURSING CARE OF THE PATIENT WITH MENIERE'S DISEASE

Assessment. The nurse inquires about the pattern of acute attacks (see Care Plan: The Patient with Meniere's Disease). Substances or stimuli that trigger the

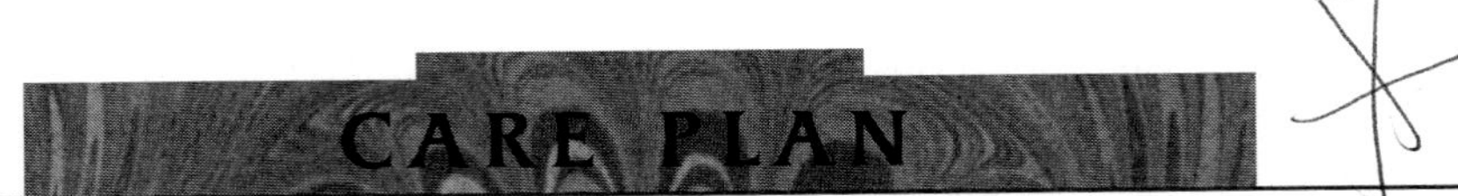

The Patient with Meniere's Disease

ASSESSMENT

Health History: Mr. Javier Riojas is a 62-year-old Latino who has had repeated episodes of nausea, hearing loss, and vertigo over the past year. His attacks last 2 to 3 hours, during which he is completely incapacitated. His wife brought him to the emergency department after he vomited repeatedly and seemed very weak. His health history reveals repeated urinary tract infections but no other serious illnesses or injuries. He is an accountant who has his own business.

Physical Examination: Vital signs: Oral temperature, 98°F; pulse, 88; respiration, 16; blood pressure, 136/82. Mr. Riojas appears acutely ill and unable to sit or stand. Physical findings are normal except for mild hearing loss. The physician diagnoses Meniere's disease.

NURSING DIAGNOSIS	GOALS AND OUTCOME CRITERIA	INTERVENTIONS
High risk for injury related to vertigo.	The patient will have no injuries during acute episodes.	Assist the patient to bed and allow him to remain still. Raise siderails and put the bed in low position. Place the call button in reach and caution the patient not to try to get up unassisted. Darken the room and keep it quiet. Postpone nonessential care. Provide a urinal for voiding. When the attack subsides, assist the patient out of bed until he is no longer dizzy.
High risk for fluid volume deficit related to vomiting.	The patient's fluid and electrolyte status will be balanced as evidenced by vital signs consistent with patient's norms, moist mucous membranes, and normal tissue turgor.	Give antiemetics as ordered. An emesis basin is provided. After vomiting, it is promptly emptied, cleaned, and returned. Administer intravenous fluids as ordered.
Anxiety related to acute illness, disruption of usual lifestyle.	The patient will state that anxiety is reduced and will appear more relaxed.	Be available, but let patient lie quietly. When the patient is able to talk, explore how the condition affects his life and how he can deal with it. Provide antiemetics promptly. Tell him that the condition can usually be improved with treatment.
Knowledge deficit of management of condition.	The patient will describe measures to manage acute attacks and to reduce frequency of attacks.	Explain drugs to patient, including dosage, schedule, side and adverse effects, and information that should be reported to the physician. If sodium restriction is prescribed, explain that some patients benefit from the restriction. Request dietary consult if special diet ordered.

episodes are noted. Specific symptoms (nausea, vomiting, vertigo, and tinnitus) are documented. The nurse determines how the condition affects the patient's life, what the patient knows about the disease, and what coping mechanisms are used.

Nursing Diagnosis. Nursing diagnoses for the patient with Meniere's disease may include the following:

- **High Risk for Injury** related to vertigo
- **High Risk for Fluid Volume Deficit** related to vomiting
- **Anxiety** related to acute illness or disruption of usual lifestyle
- **Knowledge Deficit** of management of Meniere's disease

Nursing Goals. Goals of nursing care for the patient with Meniere's disease are safety, normal fluid and electrolyte balance, reduced anxiety, and knowledge of self-care.

Interventions. Safety is a major concern. Attacks come on suddenly and can be dangerous in many circumstances. Fortunately, many people can recognize an aura, or peculiar feeling, that precedes an attack. They should know to seek safety promptly when an aura occurs. If driving, the patient should pull over and stop the car as soon as possible. During an acute attack in the hospitalized patient, the patient is allowed to remain still. The room is darkened and quiet. Nonessential care such as bathing is postponed. Medications are given promptly for nausea and vomiting, and an emesis basin is kept close by. An intravenous infusion may be ordered to provide fluids or medications, or both. After the symptoms subside, the patient should be assisted when getting up until dizziness goes away.

Patients with Meniere's disease may be anxious about the condition and the limitations it imposes. The nurse encourages the patient to share concerns and helps the patient learn how to manage the condition.

Patients with Meniere's disease need to know how to reduce their symptoms. The nurse should advise outpatients about taking their prescribed medications and how to manage side effects. They should also be advised to avoid alcohol and tobacco since these substances affect fluid in the inner ear. Other substances that should be restricted include caffeine and decongestants.

Avoidance of stimuli that tend to bring on attacks is advised. Patients should avoid noisy places and bright lights. They should also be told not to bend over with the head down or turn the head side to side.

If the patient has surgery for Meniere's disease, postoperative care is dependent on the exact procedure. The nurse should carefully check the physician's orders for position and activity limitations. General nursing care is concerned with safety, comfort, and detection of complications. The first few days after surgery, the patient's symptoms are usually severe. Antiemetics are ordered to control nausea and vomiting. Nonessential care should be delayed until the patient tolerates movement. Patients should be assisted when getting up and walking until they are able to walk steadily. The call button should always be within reach. It is not unusual for these patients to be dizzy for several days and unsteady for several weeks.

The nurse assesses for facial nerve damage by having the patient smile and show his or her teeth. If the facial nerve is damaged, the muscles on the affected side do not respond and the patient's face is not symmetric. Any evidence of facial nerve damage should be reported to the surgeon immediately. Nerve damage may not be permanent if treated promptly.

Evaluation. Criteria for successful nursing interventions include absence of injury, equal intake and output with moist mucous membranes and normal vital signs, patient's statement of reduced anxiety, and patient's statement of self-care measures.

Presbycusis

Although many older people hear very well, about half of those over age 75 have some difficulty hearing. Presbycusis is the term used to describe hearing loss associated with aging. It is the result of changes in one or more parts of the cochlea. The extent of the disability depends on the location of the changes in the cochlea.

SIGNS AND SYMPTOMS. People with presbycusis may hear well in quiet surroundings but hear poorly in noisy places. Some patients deny that they do not hear well. They may blame others for not speaking clearly.

MEDICAL DIAGNOSIS AND TREATMENT. A thorough hearing evaluation is indicated for the older person whose hearing seems to be declining. Many people have the mistaken idea that hearing loss in the elderly is inevitable and not treatable. In fact, many patients with presbycusis do benefit from hearing aids. If a hearing aid is recommended, the patient needs to learn how to use and care for it, as described earlier. Hearing aids are helpful but are not the only way to improve communication. The patient needs to be willing to tell others how they can more easily be understood. The patient can also practice and improve listening skills.

In addition to hearing aids, other electronic devices are available to improve hearing. These are described earlier and include phone amplifiers and personal earphones for radios and televisions.

NURSING CARE OF THE PATIENT WITH PRESBYCUSIS. Nursing assessment, diagnosis, goals, and interventions for the patient with impaired hearing are described earlier. In addition, nurses need to educate people about hearing loss and aging. They can also work to overcome the resistance that many people have to admitting hearing loss. Once the problem has been diagnosed, nurses can help the patient adapt and learn to use supportive devices.

Ototoxicity

Ototoxicity is damage to the ear or eighth cranial nerve caused by specific chemicals, including some drugs. Common ototoxic drugs are salicylates (aspirin) and aminoglycoside antibiotics. These and other ototoxic drugs that pose a threat to hearing are listed in Table 48–4. Ototoxicity can range from reversible tinnitus to permanent hearing loss. Hearing, balance, or both may be affected. The primary symptom of ototoxicity with salicylates is tinnitus, which disappears when the drug is discontinued. Aminoglycosides, on the other hand, cause permanent hearing loss. The extent depends on the drug dosage and how long it was given. Patients who have poor renal function are at special risk for ototoxicity since drugs are excreted more slowly. This increases the likelihood of toxicity.

NURSING CARE OF THE PATIENT WITH OTOTOXICITY. The primary nursing responsibilities are early detection and prevention of progressive hearing loss caused by ototoxic drugs. To reduce the risk of ototoxicity, the nurse should be familiar with these drugs. Patients are instructed to report hearing loss, tinnitus, or problems with balance. Such symptoms are reported promptly to the physician. The nurse also

TABLE 48-4
OTOTOXIC DRUGS

Antibiotics
Aminoglycoside
- Amikacin sulfate (Amikin)
- Gentamicin sulfate (Garamycin)
- Kanamycin sulfate (Kantrex)
- Neomycin sulfate
- Streptomycin sulfate
- Tobramycin sulfate (Nebcin)

Erythromycin
- Erythromycin estolate (Ilosone)
- Erythromycin ethylsuccinate (Pediamycin)
- Erythromycin stearate (Erythrocin)
- Erythromycin lactobionate (Erythrocin)

Tetracycline
- Minocycline (Minocin)

Vancomycin

Diuretics
Furosemide (Lasix)
Ethacrynic acid (Edecrin)

Antiarrhythmics
Quinidine

Anti-inflammatories/Analgesics
Aspirin
Ibuprofen (Motrin)
Indomethacin (Indocin)

Antineoplastics
Bleomycin (Blenoxane)
Cisplatin (Platinol, CDDP)
Dactinomycin (actinomycin D)
Mechlorethamine (nitrogen mustard, nitrogen)

teaches patients that aspirin is not a harmless drug. The nurse monitors the urine output of patients on ototoxic drugs because low urine output may mean the potentially toxic drug is excreted slowly, increasing the risk of toxicity. Low urine output is reported to the physician. The nursing care plan alerts all staff to the potential for ototoxicity.

Disorders that impair hearing or balance can have a profound effect on a person's life and well-being. The nurse plays an important role in the prevention, early detection, and treatment of hearing and balance disturbances.

BIBLIOGRAPHY

Aantaa, E. (1991). Treatment of acute vestibular vertigo. *Acta Oto-Laryngologica Supplement, 479,* 44–47.

Black, J. M., & Matassarin-Jacobs, E. (1993). *Luckmann and Sorensen's medical surgical nursing: A psychophysiologic approach* (4th ed.). Philadelphia: W. B. Saunders.

Caine, R. M., & Bufalino, P. M. (1991). *Nursing care planning guides for adults* (2nd ed.). Baltimore: Williams & Wilkins.

Chernecky, C. C., Krech, R. L., & Berger, B. J. (1993). *Laboratory tests and diagnostic procedures.* Philadelphia: W. B. Saunders.

Colletti, V., & Fiorino, F. G. (1991). Effect of sodium fluoride on early stages of otosclerosis. *American Journal of Otology, 12*(3), 195–198.

Doenges, M. E., & Moorhouse, M. F. (1993). *Nurse's pocket guide* (4th ed.). Philadelphia: F. A. Davis.

Gherini, S., Horn, K. L., Causse, J. B., & McArthur, G. R. (1993). Fiberoptic argon laser stapedectomy: Is it safe? *American Journal of Otology, 14*(3), 283–289.

Ghonim, M. R. (1992). Cochlear function after stapedectomy. *Journal of Oto-Rhino-Laryngology and Its Related Specialties, 54*(3), 148–151.

Haas, L. B. (1992). Nursing assessment: Endocrine systems. In S. M. Lewis & I. C. Collier (Eds.), *Medical-surgical nursing* (3rd ed.) (pp. 1258–1281). St. Louis: Mosby Year Book.

Haas, L. B. (1992). Nursing role in management: Endocrine problems. In S. M. Lewis & I. C. Collier (Eds.), *Medical-surgical nursing* (3rd ed.) (pp. 1319–1355). St. Louis: Mosby Year Book.

Harris, J. P., & Keithley, E. M. (1993). Inner ear inflammation and round window otosclerosis. *American Journal of Otology, 14*(2), 109–112.

Hodgson, B. B., Kizior, R. J., & Kingdon, R. T. (1993). *Nurse's drug handbook.* Philadelphia: W. B. Saunders.

Huang, T. S., & Lin, D. D. (1991). Surgical treatment of chronic otitis media and Meniere's syndrome. *Laryngoscope, 101*(8), 900–904.

Ignatavicius, D. D., & Bayne, M. V. (1991). *Medical-surgical nursing: A nursing process approach.* Philadelphia: W. B. Saunders.

Jarvis, C. (1992). *Physical examination and health assessment.* Philadelphia: W. B. Saunders.

Johnson, E. W. (1993). Hearing aids and otosclerosis. *Otolaryngologic Clinics of North America, 26*(3), 491–502.

Lesinski, S. G., & Newrock, R. (1993). Carbon dioxide lasers for otosclerosis. *Otolaryngologic Clinics of North America, 26*(3), 417–441.

Linthicum, F. H., Jr. (1993). Histopathology of otosclerosis. *Otolaryngologic Clinics of North America, 26*(3), 335–352.

Magnusson, M., Padoan, S., Karlberg, M., & Johansson, R. (1991). *Acta Oto-Laryngologica Supplement, 485,* 120–122.

Matteson, M. A., & McConnell, E. S. (1989). *Gerontological Nursing.* Philadelphia: W. B. Saunders.

McPhee, J. R., Gordon, M. A., Ruben, R. J., & Van de Water, T. R. (1993). Evidence of abnormal stromelysin mRNA expression in suspected carriers of otosclerosis. A possible molecular marker. *Archives of Otolaryngology, 119*(10), 1108–1116.

Moffatt, D. A., Toner, J. G., Baguley, D. M., & Hardy, D. G. (1991). Posterior fossa vestibular neurectomy. *Journal of Laryngology and Otology, 105*(12), 1002–1003.

Nedzelski, J. M., Chiong, C. M., Fradet, G., Schessel, D. A., Bryce, G. E., & Pfleiderer, A. G. (1993). Intratympanic gentamicin instillation as treatment of unilateral Meniere's disease: Update of an ongoing study. *American Journal of Otology, 14*(3), 278–282.

Nedzelski, J. M., Schessel, D. A., Bryce, G. E., & Pfleiderer, A. G. (1992). Chemical labyrinthectomy: Local application of gentamicin for the treatment of unilateral Meniere's disease. *American Journal of Otology, 13*(1), 18–22.

Oberascher, G., Albegger, K., Gruber, W., & Baselides, P. (1992). Otosclerosis—diagnosis and therapy. *Wiener Medizinische Wochenschrift, 142*(20–21), 474–481. (From *Medline,* March 1994, Abstract No. 93142395.)

Plath, P., Lenart, R., Matschke, R. G., & Kruppa, E. (1992). Long term results of stapedectomy and stapedotomy. *HNO, 40*(2), 52–55.

Rizer, F. M., & Lippy, W. H. (1993). Evolution of techniques of stapedectomy from the total stapedectomy to the small fenestra stapedectomy. *Otolaryngologic Clinics of North America, 26*(3), 443–451.

Santos, P. M., Hall, R. A., Snyder, J. M., Hughes, L. F., & Dobie, R. A. (1993). Diuretic and diet effect on Meniere's disease evaluated by the 1985 Committee on Hearing and Equilibrium guidelines. *Otolaryngology—Head and Neck Surgery, 109*(4), 680–689.

Shlafer, M., & Marieb, E. N. (1989). *The nurse, pharmacology, and drug therapy.* Redwood City, CA: Addison-Wesley.

Stahle, J., Friberg, U., & Svedberg, A. (1991). Long-term progression of Meniere's disease. *Acta Oto-Laryngologica Supplement, 485,* 78–83.

Tanioka, H., Zusho, H., Machida, T., Sasaki, Y., & Shirakawa, T. (1992). High resolution MR imaging of the inner ear: Findings in Meniere's disease. *European Journal of Radiology, 15*(1), 83–88.

Telischi, F. F., & Luxford, W. M. (1993). Long term efficacy of endolymphatic sac surgery for vertigo in Meniere's disease. *Otolaryngology—Head and Neck Surgery, 109*(1), 83–87.

KEY CONCEPTS

1. About half of all adults over age 75 have some hearing loss.
2. Common nursing diagnoses after ear surgery include acute pain, high risk for injury, high risk for impaired skin integrity, high risk for infection, and sensory-perceptual alterations.
3. Hearing losses are classified as conductive, sensorineural, mixed, or central.
4. Adaptations for the hearing impaired include sign language, electronic devices, television closed captioning, personal communicators, and trained dogs.
5. Nursing care of the patient with hearing impairment addresses impaired verbal communication, social isolation, ineffective individual coping, and knowledge deficit.
6. Cerumen (earwax) can become impacted and obstruct the external ear canal, causing pain and hearing impairment.
7. External otitis, infection and inflammation of the external ear canal, is treated with topical antibiotics and corticosteroids.
8. Otitis media, infection of the middle ear, can cause permanent hearing loss and inner ear problems.
9. Otosclerosis is a condition in which the stapes becomes fixed, causing a conductive hearing loss and sometimes sensorineural hearing loss.
10. Hearing aids are useful if the patient has only conductive hearing loss.
11. Labyrinthitis, which is inflammation of the labyrinth, causes vertigo and nausea and may be treated with antiemetics and antibiotics.
12. Meniere's disease, characterized by attacks of hearing loss and vertigo, may be treated with drug therapy, low-sodium diet, or surgical intervention, or a combination of these.
13. Nursing care of the patient with Meniere's disease may address high risk for injury, high risk for fluid volume deficit, anxiety, and knowledge deficit.
14. Presbycusis is hearing loss associated with aging that may be improved with a hearing aid.
15. Ototoxicity is damage to the eighth cranial nerve that may range from tinnitus to permanent hearing loss.

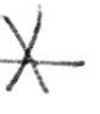

CHAPTER 49

Adrianne Linton

Nose, Sinus, and Throat Disorders

OBJECTIVES

1. Describe the nursing assessment of the nose, sinuses, and throat.
2. Identify nursing responsibilities for patients undergoing tests or procedures to diagnose disorders of the nose, sinuses, or throat.
3. Describe the nurse's role when the following common therapeutic measures are instituted for disorders of the nose, sinuses, or throat: administration of topical medications, irrigations, humidification, suctioning, tracheostomy care, and surgery.
4. Explain the pathophysiology, signs and symptoms, complications, and medical or surgical treatment of selected disorders of the nose, sinuses, and throat.
5. Apply the nursing process to plan care for patients with disorders of the nose, sinuses, or throat.

GLOSSARY

AEROSOL Solid or liquid particles suspended in a gas

ALLERGEN Substance capable of initiating an allergic or hypersensitivity response

ANTIHISTAMINE Drug that blocks the effects of histamine, a body chemical that causes allergic symptoms

CORYZA Discharge from the nasal mucous membranes

DECONGESTANT Agent that reduces swelling, especially of the nasal mucous membranes

EPISTAXIS Nosebleed

LARYNGECTOMY Surgical removal of the larynx

LARYNGITIS Inflammation of the larynx

POLYP Growth that protrudes from a mucous membrane

RHINITIS Inflammation of the nasal mucous membrane

SINUSITIS Inflammation of the paranasal sinuses

TONSILLITIS Inflammation of the tonsils

The nose and throat provide passageways to the respiratory and digestive tracts. In addition, they provide routes for drainage of the sinuses and are essential for normal voice production.

Many common conditions affect the nose, sinuses, and throat. Most are not life threatening, but they can cause considerable aggravation and loss of productivity. The most serious conditions of the nose, sinuses, and throat are hemorrhage and malignancy.

ANATOMY AND PHYSIOLOGY OF THE NOSE, SINUSES, AND THROAT

NOSE

The nose can be divided into internal and external sections. The external nose is made up of bone, cartilage, and mucous membrane. Only the upper one third of the external nose has a bony skeleton. The remainder is shaped by cartilage (Fig. 49–1).

The internal nose is divided by the nasal septum, a thin wall that creates two passages. The openings on each side of the septum are the nares. The outermost portion of the internal nose, called the vestibule, is covered by skin that contains nasal hairs. The rest of the interior is lined with mucous membrane. The internal nose is well supplied with blood by branches of the internal and external carotids.

A layer of mucus covers the membrane. The mucus traps inspired particles and moisturizes dry air. Mucus also protects the airway because it is acidic and contains an enzyme that destroys most bacteria. Cilia sweep particles that are trapped in the mucus toward the throat to be swallowed.

Olfactory cells line the roof of the nasal cavity. These are specialized sensory cells that detect odors and relay information about odors to the brain by way of the first cranial nerve (the olfactory nerve).

The side walls of the internal nose have folds of tissue called turbinates. Turbinates are projections that increase the surface area that inspired air crosses. As air swirls over the turbinates, it is quickly warmed to body temperature. The turbinates also contain openings through which secretions drain from the sinuses.

SINUSES

The sinuses are spaces in the bones of the skull. They are lined with mucous membrane and filled with air. The sinuses produce mucus that drains into the nasal cavity. They also act as sound chambers for the voice, and they reduce the weight of the skull. The sinuses around the nose are called the paranasal sinsues. They include the maxillary, frontal, ethmoid, and sphenoid sinuses. There are pairs of sinuses on either side of the face (Fig. 49–2).

THROAT

The throat, or pharynx, extends from the back of the nasal cavities to the esophagus. It provides passageways from the nose and mouth to the digestive and respiratory tracts. Figure 49–3 illustrates the structures in the throat.

The eustachian tubes that originate in the middle ear open into the nasopharynx. These tubes serve as pressure vents to prevent excessive pressure from building up in the middle ear.

Other important structures in the throat are the tonsils and adenoids. Tonsils and adenoids are masses of lymphatic tissue that guard against bacterial invasion of the respiratory and digestive tracts.

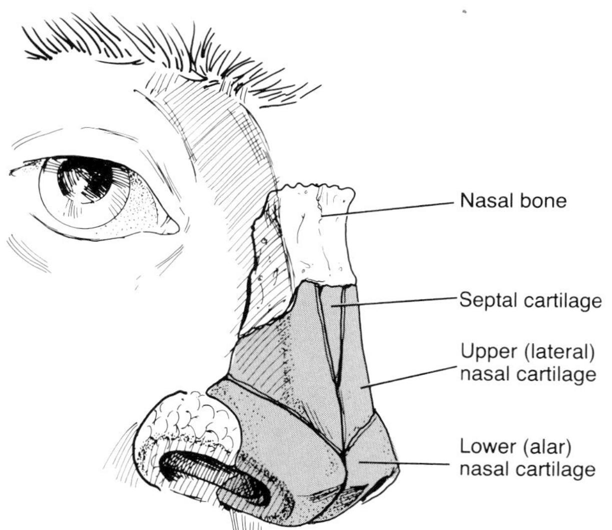

FIGURE 49–1

The upper one third of the external nose has a bony skeleton. The remainder is shaped by cartilage.

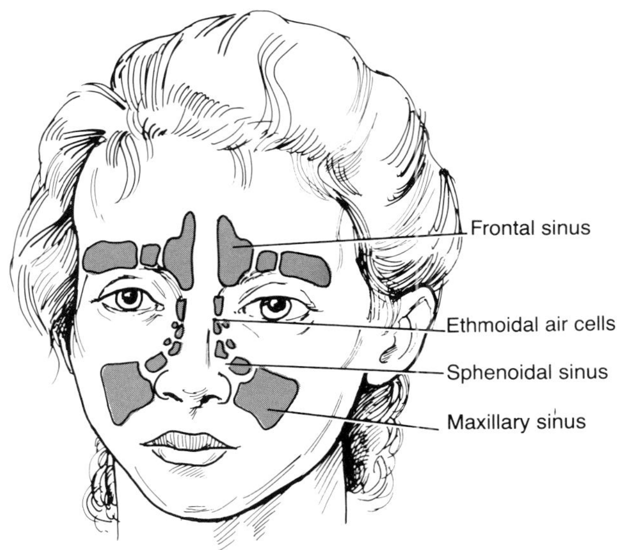

FIGURE 49–2

The paranasal sinuses.

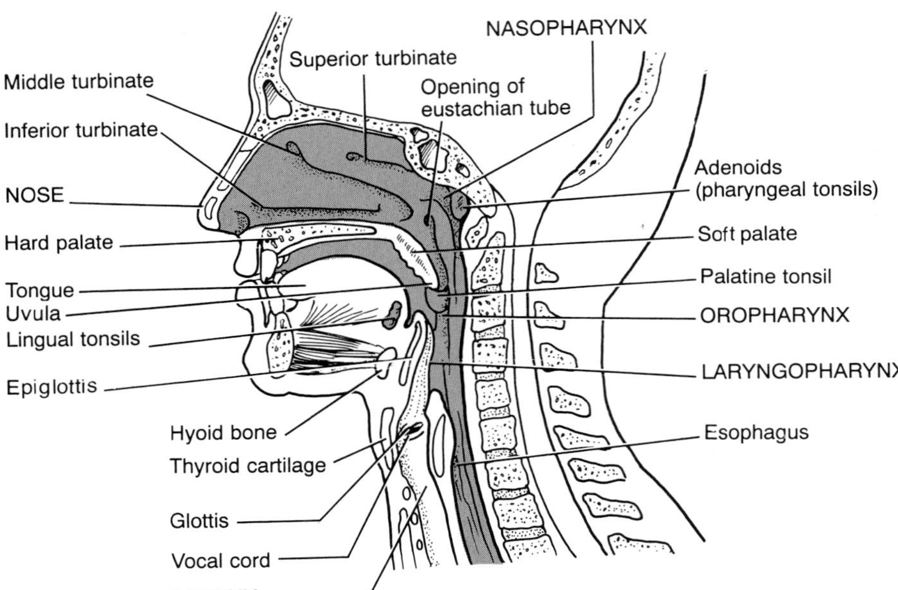

FIGURE 49-3
The nose and throat.

The larynx is the passageway between the throat and the trachea. The larynx is commonly referred to as the voice box. Two bands of tissue, the vocal cords, stretch across the interior of the larynx. The cords tighten and relax, producing different pitch sounds, as air moves through them. The sounds produced are modified and refined by the oral, nasal, and sinus cavities.

The epiglottis lies on top of the larynx. It is a flap that works like a trapdoor, closing during swallowing to prevent food and fluid from entering the airway.

NURSING ASSESSMENT OF THE NOSE, SINUSES, AND THROAT

HEALTH HISTORY

Patients often seek medical attention for symptoms that affect the nose, sinuses, and throat.

Chief Complaint and History of Present Illness

The nurse can aid in diagnosing and evaluating these conditions by collecting and recording a detailed description of the patient's complaints.

Past Medical History

The past medical history should assess previous streptococcal infection, known allergies, and current and recent medications.

Review of Systems

The review of systems assesses for the presence of nasal discharge (amount, color), obstruction, bleeding, sneezing, snoring, throat pain or soreness, hoarseness, aphonia (loss of voice), and earache. An altered sense of smell and the presence of facial pain also should be assessed.

PHYSICAL EXAMINATION

The nurse's examination of the nose and sinuses is generally confined to inspection of the external nose and palpation over the paranasal sinuses. The nurse inspects the external nose for size, shape, color, and lesions. If any drainage is present, the amount, color, and consistency are observed. The nurse listens for any abnormal breath sounds and notes whether the patient is breathing through the nose or the mouth. Patency of the nostrils is assessed by gently closing one naris at a time and instructing the patient to breathe through the other naris.

The sinuses are assessed indirectly. Palpation over the frontal and maxillary sinuses may reveal tenderness or pain. Transillumination is a procedure in which a special light is shone into the patient's mouth. The amount of light reflected through the sinuses reveals whether the cavities are filled with air, as they should be, or with fluid.

Examination of the throat is primarily an inspection of the throat at the back of the oral cavity. The mucous membranes and the tonsils are inspected for redness, swelling, drainage, or lesions. Inspection and palpation of the neck may reveal enlarged lymph nodes.

Additional physical examination may be done by the physician or a nurse with advanced preparation. A nasal speculum and a lighted scope are used to observe the mucosa of the nasal cavity. Observations should include color, drainage, and the presence of foreign bodies. The sense of smell is assessed by asking the patient to identify common scents like coffee and rubbing alcohol. Assessment of the nose, sinuses and throat is summarized in Table 49–1.

AGE-RELATED CHANGES

As a person ages, the nose gets longer and tends to droop somewhat. Nasal obstruction is more common because of the softening of the cartilage of the external nose. The mucous membrane becomes thinner and produces less mucus. Some older people report having a watery or "runny" nose when eating spicy or hot foods. Drugs used to treat nasal congestion or discharge can have serious side effects for the older patient. Older people on such drugs should be monitored for confusion, urinary retention, sedation, hypotension, fainting, and problems with coordination.

Epistaxis (nosebleed) is more common in older people, especially in those taking anticoagulants to slow blood clotting. If posterior nasal packing is needed to control bleeding, the older person is at greater risk for airway obstruction.

There is a decline in the sense of smell as people age. This may be due to neurologic changes but is probably aggravated by exposure to irritants such as cigarette smoke. The implications of decreased sense of smell in the elderly are significant. The older person may fail to detect smoke or gas in the home or may neglect personal hygiene owing to failure to notice body odors.

The tissues of the larynx are drier and less elastic in the older person. Some people complain of a constant tickling sensation that causes them to clear the throat frequently. Hard candies or lozenges may help by stimulating the production of saliva.

A weakened esophageal sphincter may allow gastric contents to flow back into the throat when the patient lies down. This is very irritating and may cause a burning sensation in the larynx. Elevating the head of the bed during sleep often relieves the problem.

TABLE 49-1

ASSESSMENT OF THE NOSE, SINUSES, AND THROAT

HEALTH HISTORY

Chief complaint and history of present illness: Nasal discharge, obstruction, bleeding; upper airway symptoms: sneezing, snoring; pain or soreness in the throat or face; change in voice; earache

Past medical history: Allergies, medications, history of streptococcal infections

Review of systems: Amount and color of nasal discharge; nasal obstruction; blood in nasal discharge or sputum; sneezing; snoring; throat pain or soreness; hoarseness; aphonia; earache; altered sense of smell; facial pain

PHYSICAL EXAMINATION

External nose: size, shape, lesions, drainage (color, amount, consistency)

Abnormal breathing sounds

Mouth breathing

Palpation of paranasal sinuses: Tenderness, pain

Patency of nares

Nasal mucosa: Color, drainage, foreign bodies

Transillumination of sinuses: Air, fluid

Throat: Inspection of mucous membranes and tonsils for redness, swelling, drainage, or lesions

Palpation of neck for enlarged lymph nodes

Ability to recognize common odors

DIAGNOSTIC TESTS AND PROCEDURES

Conditions of the nose, sinuses, and throat are diagnosed by cultures, measures of antibodies, and procedures to visualize internal structures.

Throat Culture

Throat cultures are done to isolate and identify infective organisms. A throat culture is usually done when streptococcal sore throat ("strep throat") is suspected. The procedure can also be used to screen for carriers of *Neisseria meningitidis* or diphtheria. Carriers harbor the organisms without showing evidence of the disease.

A throat culture requires no special preparation except an explanation. If the physician orders the culture and antibiotics at the same time, the culture specimen should be obtained before the antibiotics are begun.

Kits are available to collect and contain the specimen. The kit consists of a sterile swab or applicator and a tube of culture medium. To obtain the specimen, good lighting is essential. The patient's head must be tilted back and the tongue depressed with a tongue blade. The swab is rotated firmly but gently over the back of the throat, tonsils, and any obvious lesion. The swab should not touch any other area of the mouth. Patients often gag or cough, so the nurse should stand to one side or wear a mask (Fig. 49–4).

The swab is immediately placed in the tube of culture medium. Many commercial kits have an ampule of medium that must be broken to release the liquid. The directions on the kit should be followed carefully. The tube containing the specimen should be sent to the

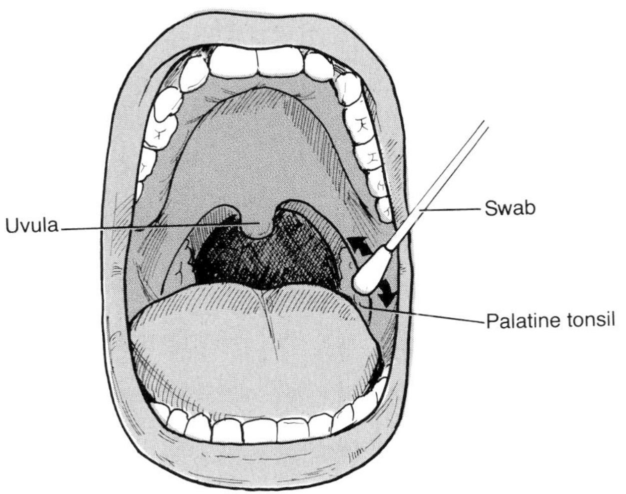

FIGURE 49-4
Throat culture technique.

laboratory promptly. If there is a delay of more than an hour, the tube should be refrigerated. The laboratory request form that accompanies the specimen should note any recent antibiotic therapy and the suspected organism, if known. No special care is necessary after collecting a specimen for culture. The results are reported in 24 to 48 hours.

Laryngoscopy

Laryngoscopy is the inspection of the larynx to aid in diagnosis of abnormalities or to remove foreign bodies. A laryngoscopy may be either direct or indirect. In the direct procedure, the physician uses a fiberoptic laryngoscope (a flexible lighted tube). An indirect procedure uses mirrors to visualize the larynx. Contrast media are sometimes instilled to outline the structures in the larynx. A tissue specimen may be taken for examination.

The patient is not allowed food or oral fluids for several hours before laryngoscopy. Drugs to decrease secretions and to relax the patient may be ordered. Any allergies to local anesthetics, iodine, or contrast media should be clearly noted on the patient's chart and identification band. The test is explained to the patient, who is encouraged to ask questions and express concerns.

Following the procedure, the patient takes nothing by mouth until the gag reflex returns. The vital signs and respiratory status are monitored according to agency protocol. A sore throat is common after this procedure. The physician may order lozenges or gargles. The patient is discouraged from talking, coughing, or clearing the throat for several hours after the procedure.

COMMON THERAPEUTIC MEASURES

NOSE DROPS

Some drugs are given by the nasal route, primarily to decrease nasal congestion and obstruction. Many over-

TABLE 49-2
DRUGS USED TO TREAT DISORDERS OF THE NOSE, SINUSES, AND THROAT

DRUG	USE/ACTION	SIDE/EFFECTS	NURSING INTERVENTIONS
Topical Anesthetics Benzocaine Cocaine Lidocaine	Anesthetic effect on skin and mucous membranes.	Allergy, sensitization, rash, burning, stinging. When sprayed on throat, can decrease gag reflex and cause dysphagia. If absorbed, lidocaine can cause drop in pulse and blood pressure. Cocaine can cause excitement and stimulation.	Inspect treated areas for side effects. Assess gag reflex before giving oral fluids or food. Monitor pulse, blood pressure, and mental status.
Anti-infectives	Kill or suppress growth of microorganisms.	Nausea, vomiting, diarrhea, superinfections. Anaphylaxis if allergic.	Instruct patient to complete course of therapy as ordered. Report diarrhea or signs of new infections. Check allergies before giving drug.
Antipyretics Aspirin Ibuprofen	Reduce body temperature; used to treat fever. Analgesic effects.	Aspirin: high risk for allergy in patients with nasal polyps, asthma, or both; prolonged bleeding time; gastric irritation; ototoxicity. Possible Reye's syndrome if given with viral infections. Ibuprofen: gastric irritation, ototoxicity, prolonged bleeding time, nephrotoxicity.	Aspirin for history or high risk for allergy. Watch for bleeding. Don't give with other anticoagulants. Report tinnitus, vertigo, hearing loss to physician. Tell patient not to use with possible viral infections. Ibuprofen: Assess for bleeding, tinnitus, vertigo, hearing loss, gastric discomfort. Take with full glass of water. Do not take with other drugs that prolong bleeding time.
Narcotic Analgesics	Reduce pain.	Drowsiness; decreased pulse, blood pressure, respirations; constipation; urinary retention; nausea and vomiting; pupil constriction.	Monitor vital signs and level of consciousness. Withhold if respirations below 12/min. Assess elimination. Safety precautions.

the-counter topical decongestants are available. Occasional use is not thought to be harmful, but frequent use is believed to damage the protective mechanisms in the nose. This increases the likelihood of additional obstruction and infection.

Drugs used to treat conditions of the nose, sinuses, and throat include sympathomimetics, anticholinergics, antihistamines, antipyretics, analgesics, anesthetics, and anti-infectives. Examples of these drugs, their uses and side effects, and nursing interventions are presented in Table 49–2.

To administer nose drops, the patient may be sitting or lying down, but the head must be tilted back so that the solution flows into the back of the nose. The nurse gently pushes the tip of the nose upward. The dropper is placed at the opening of the nostril and squeezed to deliver the prescribed amount of medication. The dropper should not touch the nose. The patient should keep his or her head tilted back for several minutes. The patient may report feeling medication run down the throat. A tissue should be provided for any nasal drainage or expectorated solution. Unused solution in the dropper should be discarded, not returned to the bottle.

Some medications are available as sprays. Many sprays have pumps that administer metered doses. These require that the pump be depressed several times before using to fill the dose chamber. These are administered by holding the head upright, inserting the tip into the nostrils, and pumping two or three times. The patient should then inhale deeply through the nose.

PHARMACOLOGY CAPSULE

Chronic use of nasal decongestant sprays may damage the protective mechanisms of the nose.

TABLE 49–2

DRUGS USED TO TREAT DISORDERS OF THE NOSE, SINUSES, AND THROAT *Continued*

DRUG	USE/ACTION	SIDE/EFFECTS	NURSING INTERVENTIONS
Sympathomimetics Phenylephrine	Decongestion, vasoconstriction.	Increased pulse and blood pressure, dysrhythmias, angina, nausea, vomiting, urinary retention. Contraindicated with monoamine oxidase inhibitors.	Monitor vital signs, especially in patients with heart disease, hypertension, urinary dysfunction, diabetes, and hyperthyroidism.
Anticholinergics Atropine Scopolamine	Decrease salivary and respiratory secretions.	Side and adverse effects vary with dosage but may include dry mouth, constipation, drowsiness, blurred vision, mydriasis, urinary hesitancy, tachycardia. May cause dizziness in the elderly.	Safety precautions if dizzy or drowsy. Contraindicated in narrow-angle glaucoma and acute hemorrhage. Monitor pulse, urine output, bowel elimination. Oral hygiene.
Antihistamines Diphenhydramine (Benadryl) Clemastine Fumarate (Tavist) Terfenadine (Seldane) Astemizole (Hismanal)	Block effect of histamine. Used to treat allergic reactions and prevent motion sickness.	Dry mouth, anorexia, tinnitus, urinary retention or frequency, drowsiness, increased or decreased pulse. Some patients experience nervousness, stimulation, sleep disturbances. Astemizole has caused serious cardiac dysrhythmias in some people.	Oral hygiene. Assess pulse, appetite, voiding. Safety precautions if drowsy. Give with food if it causes gastric distress, except astemizole, which should be given on an empty stomach. Monitor pulse for dysrhythmias with astemizole.
Glucocorticoids *Nasal inhalers* Beclomethasone (Beconase, Vancenase) Flunisolide (Nasalide) *Oral inhalers* Beclomethasone (Beclovent, Vanceril) Flunisolide (Aerobid) Triamcinolone acetonide (Azmacort)	Decrease bronchial and nasal inflammation. Decrease mucus production.	Decreased resistance to infection. Burning and dryness of nose and throat with nasal inhaler. Oral fungal infection with oral inhaler. Tachycardia, dizziness, headache, cough, unpleasant taste in mouth.	Teach patient how to use inhaler and stress prescribed frequency of use. Advise to take on schedule and not to make up missed doses. Rinse mouth after using oral inhaler.

NASAL IRRIGATION

Nasal irrigation is the washing of secretions from the nasal cavity. The procedure is not common but may be done on occasion. Normal saline at 100°F is usually used for the irrigation. The physician specifies which nostril to irrigate first.

The following are key points to remember when doing a nasal irrigation:

1. The patient should be sitting, leaning forward over a basin or sink.
2. Advise the patient to breathe through the mouth and not to swallow.
3. The container holding the irrigating fluid should not be more than 8 inches above the nose.
4. The irrigating nozzle is inserted into one nostril.
5. Allow the solution to flow in one nostril and out the other.
6. Document the procedure, patient response, and characteristics of the returned fluid.
7. Keep the patient in a warm place for at least an hour after the procedure.

THROAT IRRIGATION

A throat irrigation washes out the throat. It is done to treat congestion or pain. Like nasal irrigation, it is not commonly done. The following are key points to remember when irrigating the throat:

1. The patient is seated, leaning forward over a basin or sink.
2. The irrigating solution is usually normal saline, warmed to 115°F.
3. The fluid container is held or hung 12 inches above the mouth.
4. The stream of irrigating solution is moved around to reach different areas of the throat.
5. The patient must hold his or her breath while the solution is flowing. Therefore, it is generally best to let the patient control the flow of the fluid.
6. The flow can be turned on and off for comfortable breathing.

A throat irrigation requires no special preparation except a clear explanation. After the procedure, the nurse removes the basin and makes the patient comfortable. The procedure, patient response, and characteristics of returned fluid are then documented.

HUMIDIFICATION

The inspiration of dry air is uncomfortable, causes loss of body fluid, and can contribute to upper airway infections. Mouth breathing, necessitated by nasal obstruction, bypasses the turbinates that normally moisturize inspired air. A variety of devices are available to increase the humidity of inspired air.

Room humidifiers work in one of two ways: by creating an aerosol or by creating steam. Aerosols dispense tiny droplets of water into the room. Steam humidifiers increase humidity by distributing vaporized water (steam).

Because steam production requires raising water to the boiling point, there is little danger of steam humidifiers becoming contaminated. Aerosol humidifiers, however, are easily contaminated. Therefore, sterile distilled water should be used with aerosol units. Plain distilled water is acceptable with steam units.

With any type of room humidifier, the fluid reservoir should be checked and refilled regularly. Daily cleaning reduces the risk of bacterial contamination. Patients who use humidifiers at home should be shown how to care for the devices. Patients who use tap water in home units can clean them with a solution of one cup of white vinegar in one gallon of water. They are also advised not to inhale aerosol directly from units that do not contain sterile water.

Following nasal or sinus surgery, a bedside room humidifier may be ordered. A more effective option is a face tent or aerosol mask.

Patients who have tracheostomies inspire air directly into the trachea. Until the airway adjusts to this situation, humidification is essential to prevent excessive drying of the mucosa and secretions. If a tracheostomy tube is in place, aerosol nebulizers are used. For patients who have open stomas with tubes, tracheostomy masks with adjustable oxygen are used.

SUCTIONING

Suctioning is done to remove secretions from the upper airway. It is especially important for patients who cannot clear their upper airways effectively. Depending on the site of the secretions, the nurse may need to suction the oral cavity, the oropharynx, the nasopharynx, or the trachea.

Suctioning should be done only when there is evidence that it is necessary. Signs that indicate a need for suctioning include increased heart and respiratory rates, restlessness, and noisy expiration. Patients with tracheostomies also need suctioning when mucus is apparent in the tracheostomy tube. An indication for suctioning when a patient is on a ventilator is increased peak airway pressure.

Suctioning is not done unless indicated because it can cause complications, including hypoxia, tissue trauma, infection, vagal stimulation, and bronchospasm. The following are key points to remember when suctioning a patient:

1. Use sterile procedure.
2. Use water-soluble, rather than oil-based, lubricant to avoid getting oil into the respiratory tract.
3. Oxygenate the patient before suctioning.
   a. If able, the patient should take three deep breaths.
   b. Other patients should be ventilated with 100% oxygen for 30 seconds to 3 minutes by manual resuscitator or by oxygen mask.
4. During insertion of the catheter, the vent should be open so that suctioning does not occur.
5. As the catheter is withdrawn, rotate it and apply suction intermittently.
6. Removal of the catheter and suctioning should not

take more than 15 seconds. Holding your breath while suctioning the patient helps remind you not to suction too long.
7. Rinse the catheter by suctioning normal saline through it.
8. Oxygenate the patient again after suctioning.
9. If the patient has a tracheostomy, 2 to 3 ml of sterile distilled water may be instilled in the stoma (take the needle off the syringe!) before suctioning.
10. With a cuffed tracheostomy tube, the oropharynx and trachea are suctioned before deflating the cuff.
11. Document respiratory status before and after suctioning.

TRACHEOSTOMY CARE

In addition to suctioning, the tracheostomy requires care to maintain cleanliness and protect the integrity of the surrounding skin. In the early postoperative phase, the nurse does this care for the patient. The patient with a permanent tracheostomy should begin to participate as soon as he or she is able. The nurse can start the teaching process by placing a mirror so that the patient can see and by enlisting the patient's assistance.

A procedure manual should be consulted for details, but the following are key points to remember when doing tracheostomy care:

1. Use universal precautions.
2. Suction the tracheostomy before removing the old dressings.
3. Don sterile gloves to remove and clean the inner cannula.
4. Use a sterile solution of half hydrogen peroxide and half sterile water to clean the inner cannula.
5. Rinse and dry the inner cannula before reinserting it into the outer cannula.
6. Cleanse the stoma and surrounding skin with the peroxide and water solution, rinse with sterile water, and pat dry.
7. Be careful not to get solution into the stoma.
8. Change tracheostomy ties if soiled. If an assistant is not available, leave the old ties in place until the new ties are secure.
9. Replace the tracheostomy dressing with a precut pad or with a gauze pad folded as illustrated in Figure 49–5. Do not *cut* a pad because fibers will get into the stoma.
10. Tie the ties at the side of the neck in a square knot (not a bow).
11. Document the procedure and observations, including the appearance of the stoma, surrounding skin, and secretions.

NASAL SURGERY

Nasal surgery may be indicated for various obstructions, injuries, and chronic infections. Specific nursing care needs are discussed under individual disorders of the nose and sinuses, but general considerations are summarized here.

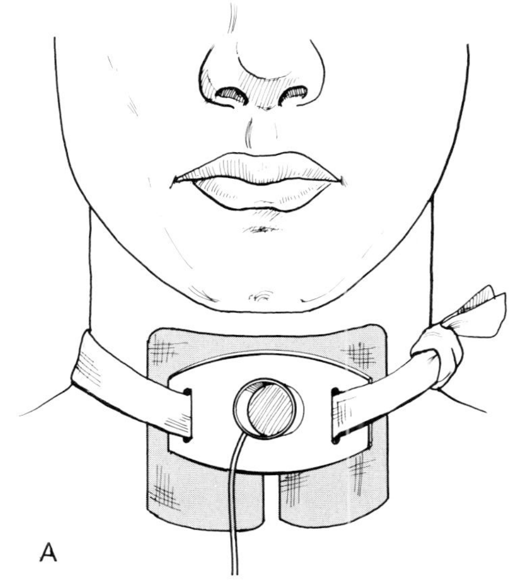

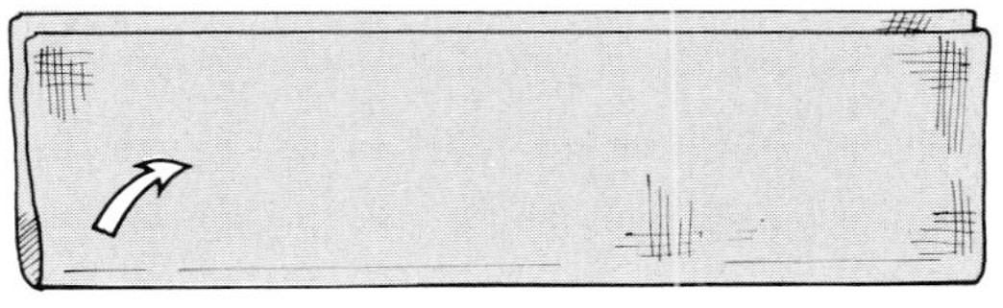

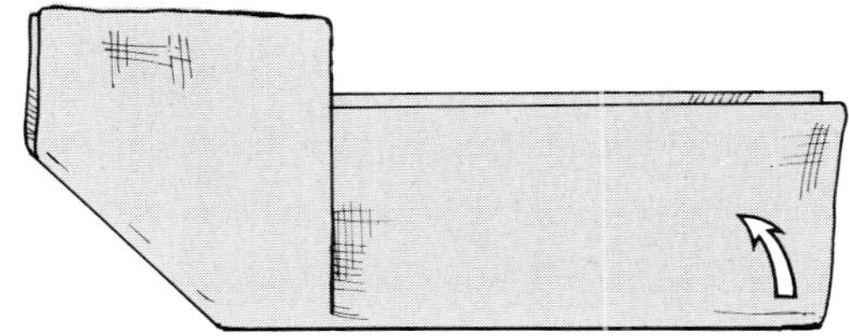

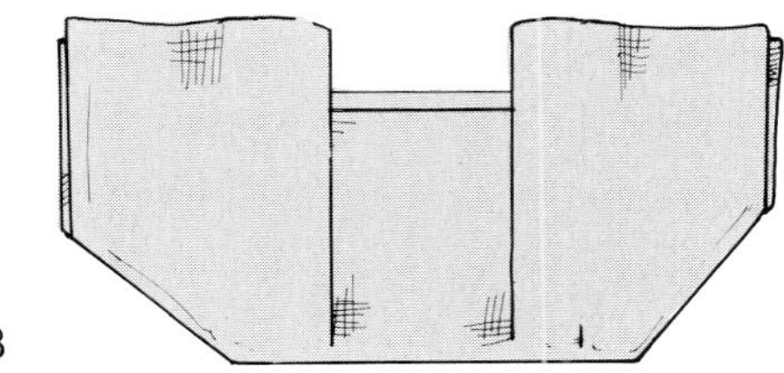

FIGURE 49–5
Precut dressings or a folded gauze pad can be used around the tracheostomy. *A*, A precut gauze dressing in place. *B*, Gauze square: Open the square once and fold it in half the long way *(top)*. Turn up one end of the dressing as shown *(middle)*. Turn up the other end to make a "U" shape *(bottom)*.

Nursing Care of the Patient Having Nasal Surgery

Preoperative care is discussed in detail in Chapter 14. Postoperative nursing care is as follows.

ASSESSMENT. After nasal surgery, the nurse assesses for pain, pressure, anxiety, and dyspnea. The patient's vital signs are monitored to detect signs of hypovolemia (tachycardia, restlessness, tachypnea, hypotension). Temperature is taken to detect fever associated with infection. Patients often have nasal packing in place with a moustache dressing (Fig. 49–6) to absorb drainage. The nurse notes the number of dressings saturated and the frequency of changes. The back of the throat is checked for bleeding. The nurse is alert for frequent swallowing, which may be a response to bleeding into the throat. Vomitus and stool are inspected for signs of blood (bright red or "coffee ground" emesis and red, maroon, or black stools).

NURSING DIAGNOSIS. Common nursing diagnoses for the patient who has had nasal surgery may include the following:

- **High Risk for Fluid Volume Deficit** related to blood loss from vascular nasal passageways
- **Pain** related to tissue trauma, edema, or packing
- **Impaired Gas Exchange** related to airway obstruction
- **Body Image Disturbance** related to facial bruising

GOALS. Goals of nursing care after nasal surgery are normal fluid volume, reduced pain, normal oxygenation, and acceptance of temporarily altered appearance.

INTERVENTIONS

High Risk for Fluid Volume Deficit. The nasal cavity has an extensive blood supply, so there is a risk of hemorrhage after nasal surgery. To reduce the risk of bleeding, the nurse advises the patient not to do anything that increases pressure in the nose. This includes blowing the nose and straining. Laxatives or stool softeners may be ordered to prevent straining due to constipation. The patient should not take any products containing aspirin because aspirin interferes with coagulation.

The physician is notified of indications of excessive bleeding: frequent, steady saturation of dressings with blood; increased pulse and respirations; restlessness; decreased blood pressure; frequent swallowing; hematemesis (blood in vomitus), and melena (dark stools associated with blood in stool).

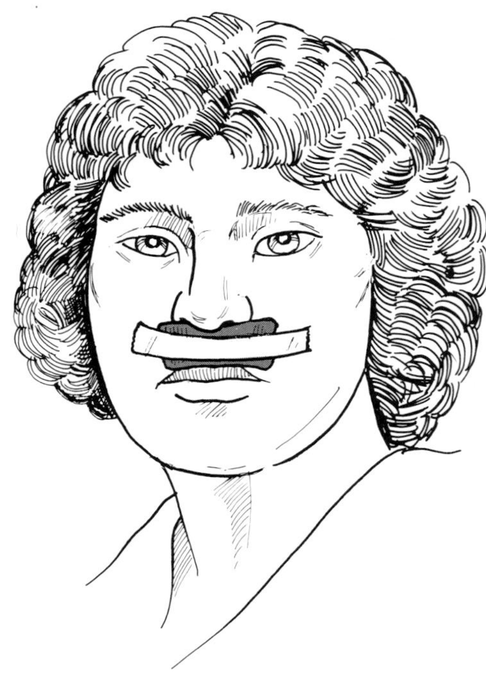

FIGURE 49–6
The moustache dressing absorbs nasal drainage. The nurse changes it as needed.

Pain. Following nasal surgery, some nasal pain is expected because of the trauma and swelling. Elevating the head of the bed helps to control swelling. Analgesics are administered and ice packs applied as ordered. Cold decreases pain by decreasing swelling. Other sources of discomfort after nasal surgery are dry mouth and sore throat. Frequent mouth care and, when allowed, oral fluids are soothing.

Impaired Gas Exchange. Nasal packing is often used after nasal or sinus surgery, often with a moustache dressing in place on the upper lip to absorb drainage. Only the physician removes the packing, but the nurse can change the moustache dressing as needed.

Nasal packing, especially posterior packing, can interfere with breathing. The patient is positioned in semi-Fowler's position with the head flat against the bed.

When the nasal cavity is packed, the patient breathes through the mouth. A humidifier helps decrease dryness of the mucous membranes. Frequent oral hygiene also is comforting. Because of the nasal packing, the patient will hear a sucking sound when swallowing. He or she can be reassured that this is normal. It is also common for patients to have poor appetites when the packing is present.

Body Image Disturbance. Some types of nasal surgery tend to cause "black eyes." The application of cool compresses to both eyes may reduce or prevent this effect. The nurse reassures the patient that this effect is temporary but is sensitive to any patient distress about it.

EVALUATION. Criteria for goal achievement are pulse and blood pressure consistent with patient's usual readings, decreasing signs of bleeding; patient's statement of pain relief; normal respiratory effort and rate consistent with patient's norms; and patient's acknowledgment that facial discoloration is temporary.

DISORDERS OF THE NOSE, SINUSES, THROAT, AND LARYNX

DISORDERS OF THE NOSE AND SINUS

SINUSITIS

Sinusitis is inflammation of the sinuses, most often the maxillary and frontal sinuses. The most common causative organisms are staphylococcus and streptococcus. The infection usually spreads from the nasal passages into the sinuses.

Sinusitis can be acute or chronic. Acute sinusitis follows obstruction of the flow of secretions from the sinus. Causes of acute sinusitis include allergic rhinitis, deviated septum, nasal polyps, tumors, airborne pollutants, and inhaled drugs such as cocaine. Chronic sinusitis is a permanent thickening of the mucous membranes in the sinuses following repeated infections.

Signs and Symptoms

Patients with sinusitis generally report pain or a feeling of heaviness over the affected area. They may report purulent drainage from the nose. When the maxillary sinuses are affected, the pain may seem like a toothache. Headache is common, especially in the morning. Fever may be present, and the white blood cell count may be elevated.

Complications

Although most patients recover without serious effects, sinus infections can be dangerous. Chronic sinusitis may follow acute sinusitis. Other potential complications are meningitis, brain abscess, osteomyelitis, and orbital cellulitis. The possibility of brain infection exists because the sinuses are located in the skull. Serious neurologic complications should be suspected if the patient develops a high fever, vomiting, chills, seizures, or blurred vision.

Medical Treatment

Several medications may be used to treat sinusitis. Antibiotics are prescribed for acute sinusitis. Other drugs that may be ordered for symptomatic relief include decongestants, analgesics, antipyretics, antihistamines, and mucolytics.

Warm, moist packs applied to the face can promote drainage and reduce pain. Other measures to reduce pain by promoting drainage include increased fluid intake and use of a humidifier. Sinus irrigation is sometimes done by the physician.

Surgical Treatment

Chronic sinusitis is sometimes treated surgically. Surgery may correct the underlying problem, remove the thickened membrane, or enlarge the opening through which secretions drain. Underlying problems that might be treated surgically include deviated septum, nasal polyps, and hypertrophy of turbinates.

The type of surgery employed for chronic maxillary sinusitis is the Caldwell-Luc procedure. This procedure involves making an incision in the upper gum line above the teeth. An opening is made between the affected sinus and the nose. This allows secretions to drain, relieving the pressure. The cavity is packed, and the packing is left in place for 48 hours. It is removed by the physician. Following the Caldwell-Luc procedure, swelling, bruising, and numbness are normal. The numbness usually lasts several weeks. The patient should be advised not to blow the nose, wear dentures, or chew on the affected side until permitted by the physician (usually about 2 weeks).

The Caldwell-Luc procedure is the most common type of sinus surgery, but others are used, depending on which sinuses are affected. One procedure for the frontal sinuses uses abdominal fat to fill the drained sinus cavity.

Nursing Care of the Patient Having Sinus Surgery

Nursing care after sinus surgery is essentially the same as that described earlier for nasal surgery. If abdominal fat is used to fill the sinus cavity, the patient will also have a small abdominal incision that requires attention.

NASAL POLYPS

Nasal polyps are swollen masses of sinus or nasal mucosa and connective tissue that extend into the nasal passages. They tend to grow, and they eventually obstruct the nasal airway. Polyps resemble white grapes in size and shape. Most patients have multiple polyps. The exact cause is unknown, but patients often have a history of allergic rhinitis or infections. Patients who have nasal polyps, asthma, and aspirin allergy are said to have triad disease.

The size of the polyps may be reduced by removing allergens or treating the allergic response. Surgical removal under local anesthesia is, however, often necessary. Unfortunately, nasal polyps tend to recur. Sometimes sinus surgery such as the Caldwell-Luc procedure or ethmoidectomy is done in an effort to limit new growths.

Nursing Care of the Patient Having Nasal Polyp Surgery

Nursing care after surgery for nasal polyps is like that described earlier for nasal surgery. This procedure is often done in an outpatient surgical facility, so patient teaching prior to discharge is especially important. The patient is advised not to take aspirin because it increases the risk of bleeding and because some of these patients are allergic to aspirin.

ALLERGIC RHINITIS

Allergic rhinitis, or "hay fever," is a common condition. It is classified as acute (seasonal) or chronic (perennial).

Pathophysiology

Allergic rhinitis follows exposure to a substance, called an allergen, that causes an allergic response. An allergic response is a reaction to the release of chemicals, including histamine, that cause vasodilation and increased capillary permeability. Fluid leaks from the capillaries, causing swelling of the nasal mucosa. Occasionally, these changes are triggered by overuse of decongestant nose drops or sprays.

Acute allergic rhinitis is most often due to exposure to pollens. It typically lasts several weeks, resolves, and does not return until the offending pollens reappear. The chronic form is more likely due to allergens that are continuously in the environment, such as house dust and animal dander. Symptoms may be consistent or intermittent, depending on the frequency of exposure.

Signs and Symptoms

Signs and symptoms of allergic rhinitis include nasal obstruction, sneezing, clear nasal discharge, frontal headache, and itchy, watery eyes. The nasal mucosa is often pale, but it can be red or bluish.

Medical Diagnosis

Diagnosis is made on the basis of a detailed history. With chronic symptoms, the patient may be instructed to keep a diary describing all episodes. This can help identify possible allergens.

Medical Treatment

The patient may also be referred to an allergist for further evaluation. The allergist injects or scratches the skin using solutions of common allergens. The allergens are applied in a specific pattern so that the patient's reaction to them can be assessed individually. Desensitizing injections may be advised to decrease the patient's reaction to the offending allergens. Patients often call these injections "allergy shots." The injections are composed of dilute solutions of the allergens to which the individual reacts. The strength of the solution is gradually increased as the patient's tolerance grows. In a sense, this process causes the body to get used to the allergen so that it no longer reacts with an allergic response. Another outcome of allergy testing is that it identifies substances that the patient should avoid.

The drugs used to treat allergic rhinitis are primarily antihistamines and decongestants. Many such medications are available without a prescription. In general, these products should be used only on a short-term basis. Patients are advised to consult with a physician or a pharmacist about the most appropriate over-the-counter drugs.

Nursing Care of the Patient with Allergic Rhinitis

Patients with allergic rhinitis are usually treated as outpatients. The nurse who works in a clinic or physician's office may need to reinforce teaching about desensitization and drug therapy.

ACUTE VIRAL CORYZA

Acute viral coryza, known as the common cold, can be caused by any of some 30 viruses. It is contagious and spread by droplet infection.

Signs and Symptoms

Signs and symptoms of the common cold are well known to most people. They usually consist of fever, fatigue, nasal discharge, and sore throat.

Complications

The infection usually runs its course in about a week. Complications that sometimes develop include otitis media, sinusitis, bronchitis, and pneumonia. Complications are more common in people with poor resistance.

Medical Treatment

Medical management of the common cold is primarily directed at relief of symptoms. Drug therapy includes antihistamines, decongestants, and antipyretics. Patients often expect to receive antibiotics. The nurse can inform them that antibiotics are not effective against infections caused by viruses. Inappropriate use of antibiotics promotes the development of resistant strains of bacteria.

Prevention

Prevention of the common cold is best accomplished by avoidance of people with colds. People with colds are most contagious during the first 2 or 3 days after symptoms appear. The very young, the very old, and those with weakened immune systems should especially be protected from exposure.

Nursing Care of the Patient with Acute Viral Coryza

Nursing care in relation to the common cold is primarily educating the public about prevention and teaching about drugs prescribed for treatment. The patient should be encouraged to rest and to drink plenty of fluids.

TUMORS

Signs and Symptoms

Tumors sometimes develop in the nasal passages and sinuses. They can be benign or malignant. The primary symptom is nasal obstruction. Either one or both sides may be affected. Another sign suggestive of a tumor is a bloody discharge from one nasal passage.

Carcinomas of the external nose are more common than those of the nasopharynx. They are more common in men, usually between the ages of 50 and 70. The lesions typically begin as small, painless ulcers that do not heal. External nasal tumors are usually either basal cell or squamous cell carcinomas. Squamous cell carcinomas are more dangerous because they grow faster and tend to metastasize early. Basal cell carcinomas grow more slowly, but they can still be fatal if not removed.

Medical Diagnosis

A diagnosis is made by taking a biopsy sample of the tumor or removing the entire tumor for examination. The earlier a malignancy is detected and treated, the better the chances of survival. Unfortunately, carcinomas in the nasopharynx tend to metastasize to the neck, liver, and lungs fairly early. Therefore, a patient with persistent nasal obstruction or bleeding should be examined by a physician.

Medical Treatment

Treatment of nasal malignancies usually consists of some combination of surgery, radiation therapy, and chemotherapy. Surgical procedures may be extensive and disfiguring, depending on the site and extent of the cancer. Reconstructive surgery or prostheses may be needed.

Benign tumors do not metastasize but are likely to be removed because they can still obstruct the nasal passages.

Nursing Care of the Patient with Nasal Cancer

The general nursing care of patients undergoing nasal surgery is discussed earlier. A diagnosis of cancer has special implications for the nurse. The patient may be especially anxious and fearful of disfigurement or even death. The nurse must be supportive and encourage the patient to ask questions and express concerns. Nursing care of the patient with cancer is discussed in detail in Chapter 23.

DEVIATED NASAL SEPTUM

The nose is divided into two passages by a cartilaginous wall called the septum. In most adults, the septum is slightly deviated, meaning it is off center. Minor deviations cause no symptoms and require no treatment. Major deviations, however, can obstruct the nasal passages and block sinus drainage. The patient may complain of headaches, sinusitis, and epistaxis (nosebleeds).

Surgical Treatment

Septal deviations are corrected by a surgical procedure called a submucosal resection or nasal septoplasty. The procedure is usually done under local anesthesia. An incision is made in the nasal mucosa, and the displaced bone and cartilage are removed. The mucosa is repositioned, and the nasal passage is packed with petrolatum gauze. The physician removes the packing after 24 to 48 hours.

COMPLICATIONS. The two major complications of submucosal resection are tears of the septum and saddle deformity. Saddle deformity is collapse of the bridge of the nose caused by removal of excessive support tissue or by contraction of the surgical scar.

Nursing Care of the Patient with Deviated Nasal Septum

Nursing care of the patient having nasal surgery is described earlier.

EPISTAXIS

The nose has an abundant blood supply that permits it to bleed easily. The medical term for a nosebleed is epistaxis. Problems that may lead to bleeding include trauma, clotting disorders, dryness, inflammation, and hypertension.

First Aid

When epistaxis occurs, the patient should sit down and lean forward. Direct pressure should be applied for 3 to 5 minutes, as illustrated in Figure 13–10, unless the patient has had a traumatic injury to the face.

Facial trauma suggests a possible nasal fracture, and direct pressure may do more harm. An ice pack or a cold compress can be applied to the nose whether or not facial trauma has occurred. Once the bleeding stops, the patient should be advised not to blow the nose for several hours, as this may trigger renewed bleeding.

Medical Treatment

If bleeding continues, medical attention is needed. The physician tries to identify the bleeding site and may treat it with silver nitrate or electric cautery. If cautery is used, the patient is given a local anesthetic.

If bleeding is not controlled, the next step is direct pressure to the nasal cavity. Two methods used to do this are placement of a nasal balloon catheter and placement of nasal packing.

NASAL BALLOON CATHETER. A nasal balloon catheter may be passed into the nasal cavity by the physician. The balloon is then inflated to apply pressure to the blood vessels. Smaller balloons anchor the catheter in place. Several different types of nasal catheters with single or double cuffs are available. Figure 49–7 shows a nasal balloon catheter in place.

NASAL PACKING. The physician may pack the anterior or posterior nasal cavity, or both. Posterior nasal packing is more complicated and requires close patient monitoring. One method of packing the posterior nasal

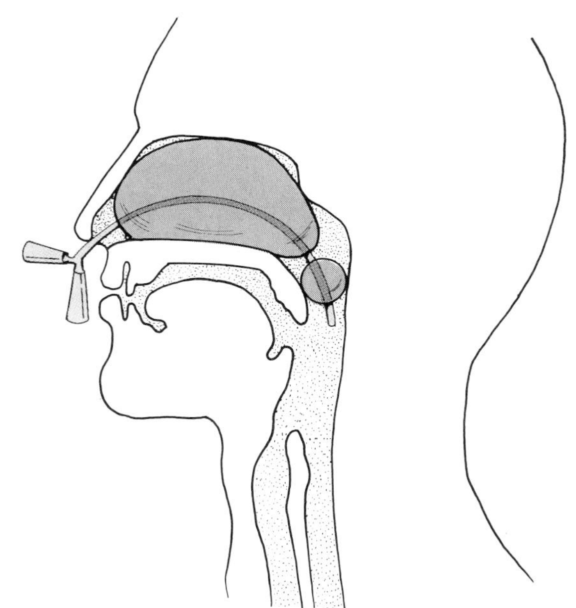

FIGURE 49-7
A nasal balloon catheter in place.

cavity is described here. Catheters are passed into the nostrils and pulled out through the mouth. Two strings are tied to the catheters and to a rolled pad. A third string is attached to the pad. As the catheters are pulled back out the nostrils, the pad is pulled into place in the posterior nasal cavity. An anterior pack is placed over the nares and secured with the two strings that are tied to the catheter. The third string remains attached to the packing. The loose end of the third string is brought out of the mouth and taped to the cheek. Figure 49–8 illustrates this procedure.

Complications. Complications related to posterior packing include infection, blockage of the eustachian tube, and airway obstruction. Posterior packing is usually left in place for 48 to 96 hours. The bulky posterior pad can depress the soft palate, causing airway obstruction. If the packing should slip out of place, it could block the airway.

Nursing Care of the Patient with Epistaxis

ASSESSMENT. Severe epistaxis is an emergency, so the nurse collects only priority data until the patient is stabilized. The priority assessment when a patient has severe epistaxis is for evidence of uncontrolled bleeding and excessive blood loss. The nurse inspects the nose and back of the throat for obvious bleeding and observes for frequent swallowing. The patient's level of consciousness and vital signs are monitored to detect signs of hypovolemia (restlessness, tachycardia, tachypnea, hypotension). Allergies and major illnesses are documented.

Once a nasal balloon catheter or nasal packing is in place, the nurse assesses for early signs of infection and airway obstruction (dyspnea, anxiety, tachycardia). The nurse also asks the patient about pain in the nose, pharynx, or ears.

NURSING DIAGNOSIS. Nursing diagnoses for the patient with epistaxis may include the following:

- **Decreased Cardiac Output** related to hypovolemia secondary to hemorrhage
- **Anxiety** related to threat of excessive bleeding or unpleasant procedures
- **High Risk for Injury** related to pressure (of packing, balloon) and possible airway obstruction
- **High Risk for Infection** related to presence of nasal packing

GOALS. Goals of nursing care for the patient with epistaxis are normal cardiac output, reduced anxiety, absence of complications of balloon or packing, and absence of infection.

INTERVENTIONS

Decreased Cardiac Output. Throughout the period of care for epistaxis, the nurse monitors for signs of continued and excessive blood loss. Signs and symptoms of hypovolemia are reported to the physician immediately.

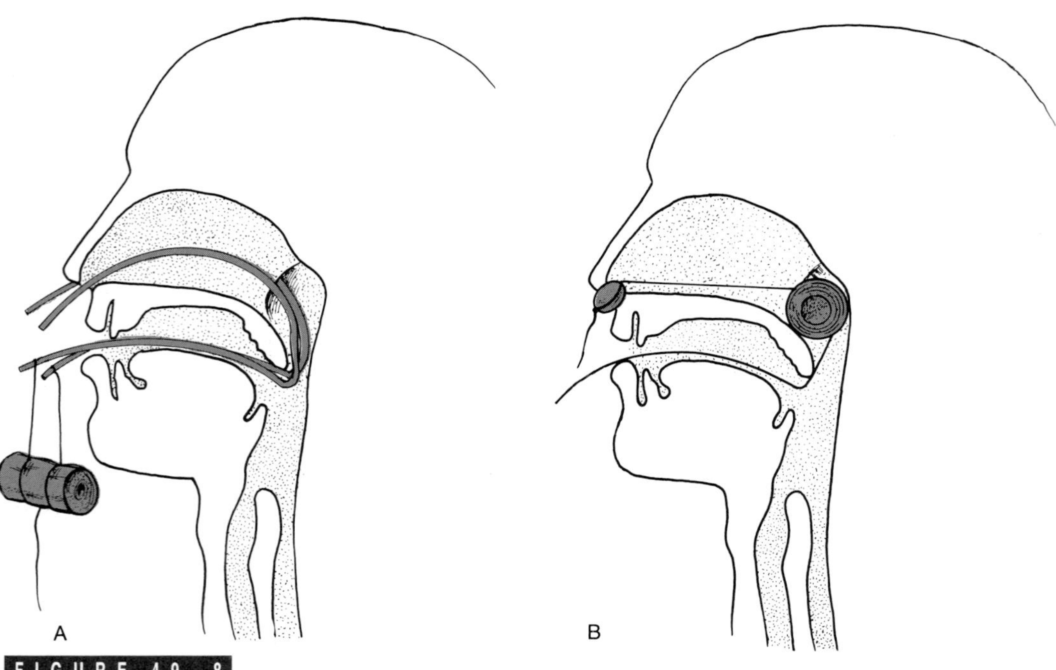

FIGURE 49–8

Posterior nasal packing. *A*, Catheters inserted through the nares and out the mouth are tied to a pad. *B*, The catheters are pulled back out the nose, pulling the pad into place.

PHARMACOLOGY CAPSULE

Patients who are prone to bleeding are generally advised to avoid aspirin because it inhibits platelet aggregation.

Anxiety. When a nasal balloon or packing is used, the nurse supports the patient and assists the physician during placement of the device. The patient is probably frightened by the visible blood and needs calm reassurance.

High Risk for Injury and Infection. After the catheter is inserted and the balloon inflated, it will be taped in place. Since the balloon can depress the soft palate and impair breathing, the nurse checks the patient's respiratory status frequently. The placement of the catheter also should be checked at least every 4 hours. Anchor cuffs should be deflated for 10 minutes every 24 hours as ordered or according to agency policy. The nurse must be careful to deflate the correct bulb.

Patients are usually hospitalized while nasal packing is in place. Frequent mouth care is needed because the patient must breathe through the mouth. It is also important to monitor the patient's temperature for elevation, which may indicate infection of the nasopharynx. If the posterior packing slips out of place, it could block the airway. If the airway is obstructed by the packing, the strings holding the anterior pad must be cut and the packing pulled out with the third string that is taped to the cheek.

Under normal circumstances, the physician removes the packing. The nurse assists by supporting the patient in a sitting position and providing an emesis basin to receive the packing. The patient should be draped to protect the clothing. Once the packing is removed, the patient appreciates mouth care.

EVALUATION. Criteria for goal achievement are normal pulse and blood pressure, no visible bleeding; patient calm, able to cooperate; respiratory rate of 12 to 20 without distress; and no fever.

DISORDERS OF THE THROAT

PHARYNGITIS

Pharyngitis is inflammation of the mucous membranes of the throat, or pharynx. It usually occurs along with acute rhinitis or sinusitis and is more common in late fall and spring. Pharyngitis is usually caused by a virus but is sometimes caused by bacteria. It can also follow exposure to irritating substances in the environment.

Signs and Symptoms

Signs and symptoms of pharyngitis are dryness, pain, dysphagia (difficulty swallowing), and fever. The throat appears red, and the tonsils may be enlarged.

TABLE 49-3
COMPARISON OF VIRAL AND BACTERIAL PHARYNGITIS

CHARACTERISTIC	VIRAL	BACTERIAL
Onset of symptoms	Gradual Rhinorrhea Headache Mild hoarseness	Abrupt Dysphagia Joint and muscle pain Malaise
Temperature	Mild elevation	>101°F
Diagnosis	CBC: normal Culture: negative	CBC: abnormal Culture: positive
Complications	Rare	Occur in 1–3%; can be glomerulonephritis, rheumatic fever, otitis media, sinusitis, mastoiditis

Viral and bacterial pharyngitis differ in several respects. Table 49–3 shows the key features of each. Compared with viral pharyngitis, bacterial pharyngitis has a more abrupt onset and is characterized by abnormal blood cell counts, fever greater than 101°F, and muscle and joint pain.

Additional signs of infection associated with beta-hemolytic streptococcus are a strawberry red tongue, vomiting, and a rash.

Complications

Patients with bacterial pharyngitis are more likely to have serious complications than those with viral pharyngitis. The most important complications are acute glomerulonephritis and rheumatic fever. If acute glomerulonephritis develops, it usually appears 7 to 10 days after the throat infection. When rheumatic fever develops, it generally appears 3 to 5 weeks after the initial infection.

Medical Diagnosis

Pharyngitis is diagnosed on the basis of the patient history and physical examination. A more specific diagnosis of viral or bacterial pharyngitis is made after the results of a throat culture and a complete blood count are obtained.

Medical Treatment

Pharyngitis is treated with rest, fluids, analgesics, and throat gargles or irrigations. Bedrest is often recommended as long as the patient has a fever. If the patient's oral intake is low, intravenous fluids may be ordered. A soft or liquid diet may be ordered because of painful swallowing. A humidifier also may be ordered to increase moisture in the room air.

The physician often orders antibiotics, usually penicillin or erythromycin, while awaiting the results of the throat culture. The culture specimen should be taken before the antibiotics are started. When the culture results are reported, the antibiotic is discontinued if there is no evidence of bacterial growth. If bacterial infection is confirmed, the antibiotic is usually continued until 48 hours after all signs and symptoms disappear. A usual course of antibiotic therapy is 10 days.

Prevention

To reduce the risk of pharyngitis, people with poor resistance should avoid others with upper respiratory infections. Measures that help to maintain resistance to throat infections include good nutrition, adequate rest, avoidance of chilling, and avoidance of inhaled irritants. People who have pharyngitis are contagious in the early stages and should avoid contact with susceptible persons.

Nursing Care of the Patient with Pharyngitis

ASSESSMENT. Mild pharyngitis is usually treated on an outpatient basis, so nursing interventions are limited. Assessment should document the presence of throat pain, dysphagia, muscle and joint pain, nausea and vomiting, and rash. The patient's temperature is taken, and the throat is inspected for redness and enlarged tonsils.

NURSING DIAGNOSIS. The primary nursing diagnosis for the patient with pharyngitis is knowledge deficit of treatment and importance of follow-up care.

GOALS. The goal of nursing care is patient's understanding of the treatment and of the need to have follow-up care.

INTERVENTIONS. The nurse reinforces the physician's directions for drug therapy, if ordered. The importance of completing prescribed antibiotics is stressed. Patients are encouraged to take 2000 to 3000 ml of fluids daily unless contraindicated. Fluids must be increased cautiously in the elderly because they do not adjust well to sudden changes in blood volume. Patients are advised that they are contagious at first and should not be exposed to people with poor resistance. A follow-up appointment is usually scheduled, and the patient is advised to contact the physician if a rash or strawberry red tongue develops within the next 2 months.

EVALUATION. The criteria for goal achievement is patient's verbalization of self-care measures, including drug therapy and symptoms that should be reported, and making and keeping a follow-up appointment.

TONSILLITIS

Tonsillitis is inflammation of the tonsils and other lymphatic tissue in the throat. It is most common in children but often more severe in adults. Low resistance seems to invite tonsillitis.

Causes

Tonsillitis is usually a bacterial infection, but it is sometimes due to a virus. Common causative organisms include streptococcus, staphylococcus, *Haemophilus influenzae*, and pneumococcus. The infection is contagious and is spread by food or airborne routes. Most cases run their course in 7 to 10 days. A person may have repeated infections that respond to treatment or have a chronic infection.

Signs and Symptoms

A patient with tonsillitis usually reports a sore throat, difficulty swallowing, fever, chills, muscle aches, and headache. If swollen tissue blocks the eustachian tubes, there may also be pain in the ears. Offensive breath odor is often present with chronic infection.

The tonsils are typically enlarged and red. Purulent drainage or yellowish or white patches may be seen on the tonsils. Lymph nodes in the neck may be tender and enlarged.

Medical Diagnosis

To diagnose tonsillitis, the physician will probably order a complete blood count, throat culture and sensitivity and a test for infectious mononucleosis. An elevated white blood cell count suggests a bacterial infection. The culture and sensitivity identify the pathogenic organisms present and what antibiotics are likely to be effective. A chest radiograph also may be ordered to assess for respiratory complications.

Medical Treatment

The medical treatment of tonsillitis usually includes a course of antibiotic therapy for 7 to 10 days. Analgesics and anesthetic lozenges may be prescribed for pain, and antipyretics for fever. Warm saline gargles or irrigations may be ordered to decrease swelling and remove drainage. Rest and adequate fluids promote recovery and decrease the risk of complications.

Complications

A peritonsillar abscess may develop with tonsillitis caused by streptococcus. A peritonsillar abscess is an infection of the tissue surrounding the tonsil. The affected side is very painful, and the patient has difficulty swallowing, talking, and opening the mouth. The immediate treatment is drainage of the abscess. Once the acute infection has subsided, tonsillectomy is performed.

Surgical Treatment

Tonsillectomy, removal of the tonsils, was once considered routine childhood surgery. Current thinking is that the tonsils play an important protective role as part of the immune system and should be retained if possible.

Tonsillectomy is generally recommended under the following conditions:

- Repeated tonsillitis in a year, especially if caused by beta-hemolytic streptococcus.
- Presence of a peritonsillar abscess.
- Malignancy of the tonsil.

- Airway obstruction by enlarged tonsils or adenoids.
- Evidence that the patient is a carrier of the diphtheria organism.
- Hearing loss associated with otitis media due to enlarged tonsils.

If surgery is indicated, it is usually delayed until the patient's temperature returns to normal. Even though tonsillectomy is a common procedure, it should not be considered minor. The usual procedure is a tonsillectomy and adenoidectomy. The adenoids are usually removed because they are almost always infected when the tonsils are. If only the adenoids are infected, an adenoidectomy alone may be done. In adult patients, these procedures may be done under local or general anesthesia.

Nursing Care of the Patient Having Tonsillectomy

Preoperative nursing care is discussed in detail in Chapter 14. The nurse completes the surgical checklist, reinforces teaching, answers questions, and administers preoperative medications as ordered. Postoperative nursing care is as follows (see also Care Plan: The Patient Having Tonsillectomy).

ASSESSMENT. In the immediate postoperative phase, the patient's responsiveness and vital signs are monitored frequently. They are usually checked every 5 minutes until stable, then every 15 minutes for an hour, and hourly for the remainder of the first 24 postoperative hours. Drainage from the mouth or vomited fluid is inspected for blood. Blood-tinged drainage is normal at first but should gradually decrease. The nurse notes excessive swallowing, which may indicate bleeding. Respiratory effort and skin color are assessed to evaluate oxygenation. Pain and dysphagia are evaluated.

NURSING DIAGNOSIS. Nursing diagnoses for the postoperative tonsillectomy patient may include the following:

- **Decreased Cardiac Output** related to excessive bleeding
- **Ineffective Airway Clearance** related to bleeding, edema, or effects of anesthesia
- **Pain** related to tissue trauma
- **Knowledge Deficit** of postoperative and postdischarge care

GOALS. Goals of nursing care after tonsillectomy are normal cardiac output, adequate oxygenation, reduced pain, and patient's knowledge of postoperative self-care.

INTERVENTIONS. The two major problems that may develop in the postoperative phase are hemorrhage and respiratory distress.

Decreased Cardiac Output. The nurse continually monitors for signs of excessive bleeding. Increased pulse rate and restlessness are early signs of hypovolemia. To reduce the risk of bleeding, the patient is reminded not to cough or clear the throat. If suctioning is needed, it is done very gently since it may cause further bleeding. Once oral fluids are permitted, the patient should not use a straw. The sucking may dislodge the clots that form at the surgical site.

Ineffective Airway Clearance. A patient who has had local anesthesia is at less risk for respiratory complications than one who had general anesthesia. After local anesthesia, the tonsillectomy patient is positioned with the head of the bed elevated at a 45-degree angle. After general anesthesia, the bed should be flat and the patient positioned on the side or semiprone. This promotes drainage of fluid from the mouth that might otherwise be aspirated. Once the patient is fully awake, he or she may prefer a semi-Fowler's position.

Increased pulse rate, restlessness, and confusion may be early signs and symptoms of inadequate oxygenation. Cyanosis (bluish discoloration of the nail beds or lips) is a late sign of inadequate oxygenation.

Pain. Analgesics are ordered for pain. Ice collars may be applied to the neck to decrease swelling and pain. Intravenous fluids are usually ordered until the patient is able to take oral fluids well. A clear liquid diet is ordered first. Cold or frozen liquids are especially soothing after tonsillectomy.

Knowledge Deficit. Prior to discharge, the nurse advises the patient of measures to promote healing and prevent complications. The diet should be soft and high in protein and calories for about 10 days. Fluid intake should be 8 to 12 8-ounce glasses daily. Citrus juices are not recommended because they irritate the healing throat tissues.

To reduce the risk of bleeding, the patient should avoid strenuous activity or straining for 2 weeks. Aspirin should not be used because it impairs blood clotting. Smoking also is discouraged.

Earaches are common and are not cause for alarm. It is also normal for white patches to form over the tonsillectomy sites. This tissue is like a scab, and it will slough off. If any bleeding occurs after discharge, however, the physician should be informed.

EVALUATION. Criteria for goal achievement are pulse consistent with patient's norms, minimal bleeding; no restlessness, normal skin color, easy respirations; patient's statement of pain relief; and patient's verbalization of postoperative self-care.

DISORDERS OF THE LARYNX

LARYNGITIS

Laryngitis is inflammation of the larynx. It may occur alone, or it may accompany other upper respiratory infections. A number of factors may lead to laryngitis. Upper respiratory infections, voice strain, smoking, alcohol ingestion, and inhalation of irritating fumes are all possible causes. Some patients have chronic laryngitis caused by prolonged exposure to irritants.

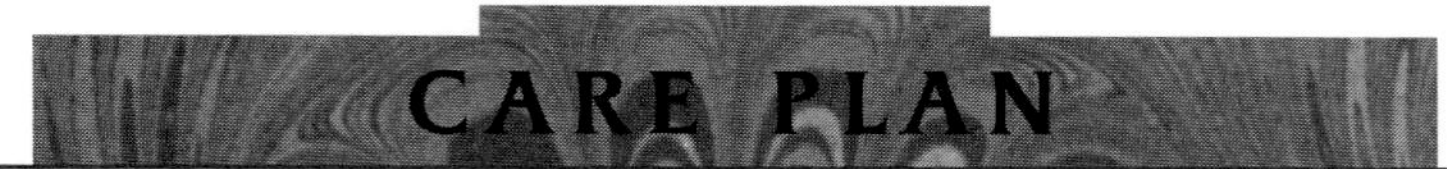

The Patient Having Tonsillectomy

ASSESSMENT

Health History: Miss Janice Morgan is a 20-year-old college student who has had tonsillitis three times this year, resulting in absences from school. Her symptoms included sore throat, dysphagia, fever and chills, muscle aches, and headache. She has had no other serious illnesses but was hospitalized overnight after an auto accident in 1991. She takes no medications except occasional acetaminophen for headache. She was admitted for tosillectomy, which was performed under local anesthetic this morning. She expressed the hope that it will relieve her recurrent illness. She clutches her throat and complains of throat pain.

Physical Examination: Miss Morgan is drowsy but responds appropriately. Vital signs: temperature, 98°F orally; pulse, 100; respiration, 18; blood pressure 110/88. She has expectorated a small amount of sanguineous drainage. Respiratory effort and breath sounds are normal. Intravenous fluids are infusing into the antecubital space of the left arm.

NURSING DIAGNOSIS	GOALS AND OUTCOME CRITERIA	INTERVENTIONS
Decreased cardiac output related to excessive bleeding.	The patient will maintain normal cardiac output as evidenced by vital signs consistent with preoperative readings, minimal visible bleeding, and absence of restlessness.	Assess for signs of excessive bleeding: tachycardia and restlessness. Advise the patient not to cough or clear throat. Inspect drainage for bleeding. Report continued or excessive bleeding to surgeon. When oral fluids are permitted, have patient sip from a glass or cup rather than using a straw.
Ineffective airway clearance related to bleeding, edema, effects of anesthesia.	The patient will maintain a patent airway as evidenced by clear breath sounds and respiratory rate of 12 to 20.	Position on one side till fully alert. Elevate head of bed 45 degrees. Monitor for signs and symptoms of inadequate oxygenation: tachycardia, restlessness. Auscultate breath sounds. Suction gently as needed to clear secretions from airway.
Acute pain related to tissue trauma.	The patient will state that pain is relieved and will appear more relaxed.	Administer analgesics as ordered. Apply ice collar as ordered. Give cold or frozen liquids when permitted. Provide simple explanations and reassurance.
Knowledge deficit of postoperative care.	The patient will describe postoperative self-care.	Prior to discharge, teach the following: 1. Consume soft, high-protein, high-calorie diet for 10 days. Omit rough foods. 2. Drink 8 to 12 8-ounce glasses of fluids daily. No citrus juices. 3. Avoid strenuous activity or straining for 2 weeks. 4. No aspirin. 5. Earaches are common. 6. White patches normally form over tonsillectomy sites. 7. Report any bleeding to the physician.

Signs and Symptoms

Symptoms of laryngitis include hoarseness, cough, and scratchy or painful throat. The patient may report "losing" his or her voice. This absence of sound production is called aphonia, and it occurs in varying degrees. Changes in the voice may be permanent after long periods of chronic inflammation.

Medical Diagnosis

Diagnosis of laryngitis is based primarily on the patient's history and symptoms. The physician may use a laryngeal mirror to examine the larynx for color, edema, and growths such as polyps and tumors. With laryngitis, the vocal cords appear red and swollen. If an upper respiratory infection is suspected, a throat culture may be done to determine the pathogen and best treatment.

Medical Treatment

Treatment of acute laryngitis is primarily aimed at reducing irritation of the larynx. Voice rest is advised, meaning that the patient is to rest the larynx by not talking. An important aspect of treatment for chronic laryngitis is removal of the irritant.

Nursing Care of the Patient With Laryngitis

Patients with laryngitis rarely require hospitalization, but nurses in other settings may teach people how to prevent and treat the condition.

ASSESSMENT. The assessment of the patient with laryngitis begins with a history of the problem. The nurse documents the severity of the condition, how long it has persisted, and any factors that seem to aggravate or precipitate it. Information about the patient's occupation and hobbies may provide some clues to the cause of the laryngitis. The patient's temperature is taken and respiratory status assessed to detect possible infection.

NURSING DIAGNOSIS. The two primary nursing diagnoses for the patient with laryngitis may include the following:

- **Impaired Verbal Communication** related to aphonia or prescribed voice rest
- **Knowledge Deficit** of treatment and prevention of laryngitis

GOALS. The goals of nursing care for the patient with laryngitis are effective nurse-patient communication and patient's understanding of measures to prevent and treat the condition.

INTERVENTIONS. When voice rest is prescribed, the nurse explains to the patient that it allows the larynx to heal. Meanwhile, an alternative means of communication must be established. A pad and pencil or "magic slate" is provided for written communication. A sign over the bed is needed to advise staff and visitors that the patient should not speak. It is also a good idea to put a notice on the intercom at the nurse's station that the patient cannot (or should not) speak. This alerts staff to go to the patient's room rather than asking what is needed on the intercom.

The teaching plan emphasizes measures to promote comfort and reduce future episodes of laryngitis. Smoking is discouraged. The patient should remain in an environment with a constant temperature since sudden changes in temperature tend to aggravate laryngitis. If the air is very dry, a room humidifier reduces the discomfort of a dry nose and throat. Lozenges containing a topical anesthetic also may be ordered to soothe the irritation (Table 49–2).

When the patient has chronic laryngitis, the primary goal of treatment is to remove the irritant. If the patient smokes, he or she should be advised that stopping smoking is likely to improve the symptoms. Changes in the voice may be permanent after long periods of chronic inflammation.

The nurse can teach patients the types of irritants that lead to laryngitis. Patients need to recognize irritants in the home and workplace and know how to protect themselves from harm. If the patient is inclined to stop smoking, information about resources in the community can be provided. The American Cancer Society is a good source of information on how to stop smoking.

EVALUATION. Criteria for goal achievement are patient's expression that communication is satisfactory and patient's acknowledgment of measures to prevent and treat laryngitis.

LARYNGEAL NODULES

Laryngeal nodules are benign masses of fibrous tissue that result primarily from overuse of the voice, but they can also follow infections. Singers and public speakers are prone to develop nodules because of the strain they put on their voices. The only symptom is hoarseness.

Nodules are surgically removed under local or general anesthesia. The removal of nodules is usually fairly simple, but they may recur if the voice is again misused. After the procedure, the patient is placed on voice rest for several days. The nurse explains voice rest as described previously under laryngitis and emphasizes the need to avoid strain on the voice.

LARYNGEAL POLYPS

A laryngeal polyp is a swollen mass of mucous membrane attached to the vocal cord. It can cause continuous or intermittent hoarseness, depending on its location and attachment.

Heavy smokers may develop flabby masses of tissue on both vocal cords. A procedure called stripping of the vocal cords is necessary to treat this condition. Unless the patient continues smoking, the condition usually does not return. As with other vocal cord surgery, voice rest is prescribed for patients who have polyps removed.

CANCER OF THE LARYNX

Cancer of the larynx accounts for about 4% of all cancers. It causes over 3000 deaths each year and is increasing in frequency. Cancer of the larynx is most common in men aged 50 to 65.

Factors believed to predispose one to laryngeal cancer are exposure to smoke or other noxious fumes, alcohol consumption, vocal strain, and chronic laryngitis. Individuals who both smoke and use alcohol are at particularly high risk.

Malignant tumors can develop at various points throughout the larynx: above the glottis, on the vocal cords, or below the vocal cords. Most malignancies of the larynx are squamous cell carcinomas.

The cure rate is highest with tumors that are confined to the vocal cords. Unfortunately, malignancies in the larynx tend to spread fairly early. The most common site of metastasis is the lung. The more widespread the cancer is, the more difficult it is to treat.

Signs and Symptoms

Hoarseness is the primary symptom of cancer of the larynx. Some patients report throat discomfort or a sensation that there is a "lump" in the throat. Other signs and symptoms of laryngeal cancer are hemoptysis (blood in sputum), difficulty swallowing or breathing, and persistent cough, sore throat, or earache. Pain and anorexia leading to weight loss are usually later symptoms of the disease.

Prevention

The most important measure to reduce the risk of cancer of the larynx is for people to stop smoking and drinking alcohol. The public should also be educated to recognize the signs and symptoms of laryngeal cancer and seek prompt medical attention. Early treatment may be able to preserve the voice.

Medical Diagnosis

A diagnosis of cancer of the larynx is confirmed by study of a tissue sample obtained during a laryngoscopy. Other studies that are likely to be ordered include laboratory blood studies, radiographs, scans, and imaging procedures. Laboratory findings often seen with malignancies include decreased hemoglobin and hematocrit and elevated alkaline phosphatase. The nurse should remember that these changes can be due to causes other than cancer.

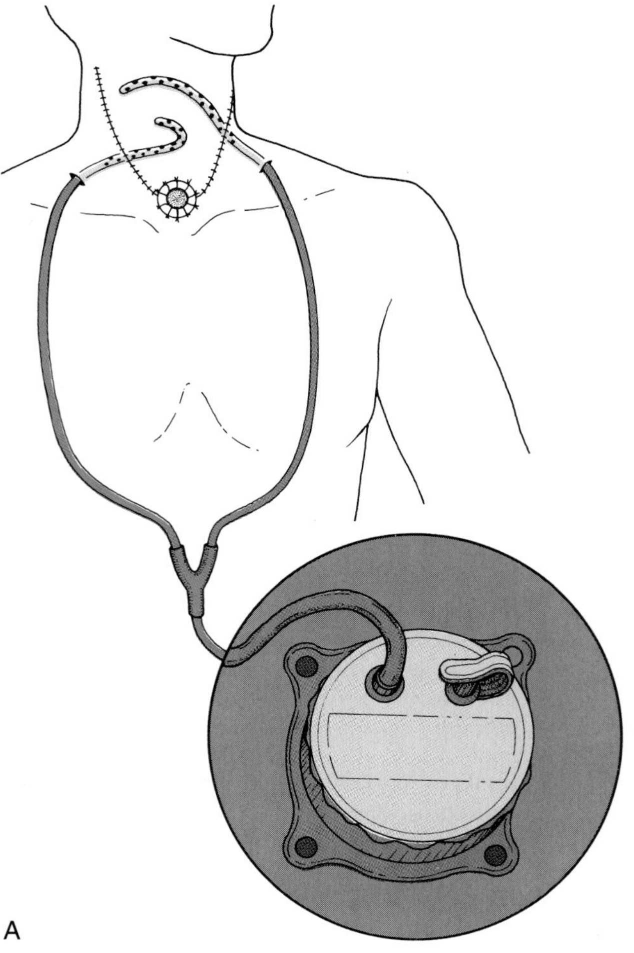

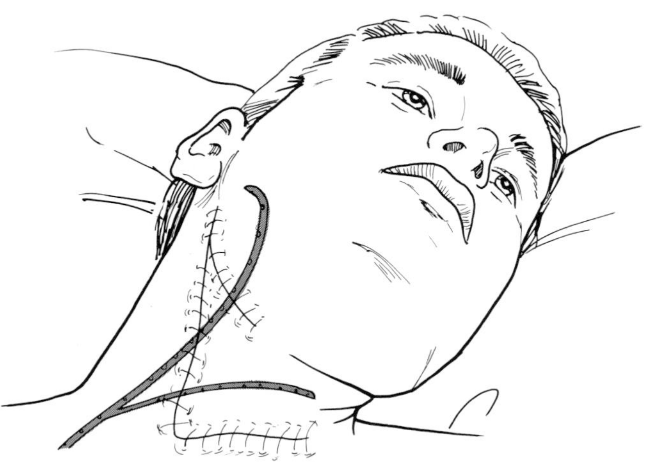

FIGURE 49-9

Surgical procedures for cancer of the larynx. *A,* Laryngectomy with tracheostomy and drains. (From Ignatavicius, D. D., & Bayne, M. V. [1991]. *Medical-surgical nursing: A nursing process approach* [p. 1969]. Philadelphia: W. B. Saunders.) *B,* Radical neck dissection.

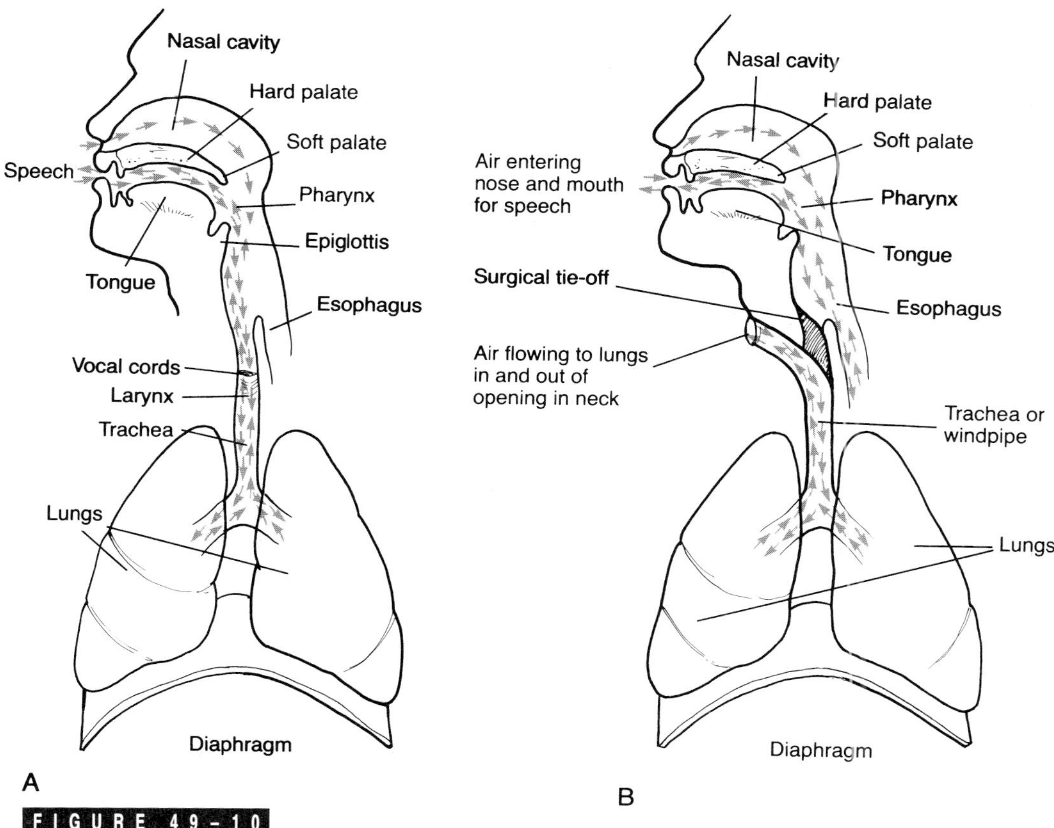

FIGURE 49–10
The throat before and after total laryngectomy. Arrows indicate the route of airflow.

Radiographs, computed tomographic scans, and magnetic resonance imaging are done to define the extent of the cancer. These studies give more detail about the primary site and help to locate metastases.

Medical Treatment

Treatment involves the use of surgery, radiotherapy, chemotherapy, or some combination of these. The diagnostic tests described above aid the physician in selecting the treatment of the patient with laryngeal cancer. Another important consideration is the patient's overall health state and ability to cope with the effects of specific treatments.

Radiotherapy alone can cure some small cancers that have not spread to surrounding tissues. In addition, radiation may be used before and after surgery. Chemotherapy is generally used along with radiation or surgery. Care of the patient undergoing radiotherapy or chemotherapy is discussed in Chapter 23.

Surgery

Surgical procedures for cancer of the larynx range from simple removal of the tumor to extensive procedures such as laryngectomy and radical neck dissection (Fig. 49–9). Laser surgery may be used alone or with radiotherapy for small tumors. A laryngectomy can be total or partial. Total laryngectomy causes permanent loss of the natural voice. Figure 49–10 illustrates air flow after laryngectomy.

Radical neck dissection is often done at the same time as laryngectomy, especially if lymph nodes are positive for cancer. Radical neck dissection is the excision of all nonessential structures on the affected side. The sternocleidomastoid muscle, jugular vein, submaxillary salivary gland, and surrounding soft tissue are removed. The spinal accessory nerve is cut, causing the shoulder to droop on the affected side. Figure 49–10 illustrates the appearance of the incisions present after total laryngectomy and radical neck dissection.

Nursing Care of the Patient Having Total Laryngectomy

General preoperative nursing care is discussed in Chapter 14. This section addresses the specific teaching needs of the patient facing surgery for laryngeal cancer. The nurse should try to find out which procedure will be done so that preoperative teaching can be individualized.

If the patient will lose the ability to speak, information about other means of communication should be available. The physician and speech therapist can advise the patient about appropriate alternatives. The anticipated loss of the voice can be very stressful to patients. The full impact may not actually hit them until later because the first concern is eliminating the cancer. The nurse should listen compassionately and be accepting of the patient's expressions of anger or despair. Some patients benefit from meeting a volunteer from an organization for people who have had laryngectomies. The patient should be consulted about this before a volunteer is invited.

The patient who will have a laryngectomy and radical neck dissection can expect to go to an intensive care unit for several days. This allows close monitoring and maintenance of a patent airway with the new tracheostomy. The patient should be advised in advance that this is routine and does not mean that anything has gone wrong. The nurse can also help prepare the patient to expect intravenous lines, wound drains, a feeding tube and, perhaps for a short time, a ventilator.

Postoperative care varies with the exact procedure done. Procedures include partial laryngectomy, supraglottic laryngectomy, and total laryngectomy. Nursing care of the patient with a total laryngectomy is presented in detail. The unique needs of the patient with a partial or supraglottic laryngectomy are identified.

A total laryngectomy involves removal of the entire larynx, vocal cords, and epiglottis as well as supportive tissues. The opening of the pharynx to the trachea is closed, and the tracheostomy is created by bringing the trachea to the opening in the neck. The upper airway is no longer connected to the lower airway. The patient breathes through the trachea. Figure 49–10 illustrates the changes with total laryngectomy. A radical neck dissection is often done because of the high risk of metastasis to the neck.

COMPLICATIONS. Complications of total laryngectomy with radical neck dissection include salivary fistula, carotid artery blowout, and tracheal stenosis.

A salivary fistula is a drainage pathway that forms when saliva leaks through a defect in the suture line in the pharynx. It usually closes spontaneously but sometimes requires surgical closure. Until the fistula closes, the patient must be fed through a nasogastric tube. Otherwise, whatever the patient eats leaks out the fistula.

Patients at highest risk for carotid artery blowout (rupture) are those who had radiation prior to surgery and developed a salivary fistula after surgery. Carotid blowout is an emergency that must be corrected surgically.

Tracheal stenosis is narrowing of the trachea that develops weeks or months after surgery. If the airway becomes obstructed, surgical correction is necessary.

The general nursing care of the postoperative patient is discussed in Chapter 14. This section addresses the special needs of the total laryngectomy patient.

ASSESSMENT. In the immediate postoperative period, the nurse's assessment focuses on oxygenation, circulation, and comfort. The patient's level of consciousness is documented. The nurse asks about pain and observes for signs of discomfort. Vital signs are measured at frequent intervals. Continuous electrocardiogram monitoring and pulse oximetry may also be used to assess oxygenation and circulation. Fluid intake and output are recorded, and the characteristics of wound drainage are documented.

Additional aspects of assessment after total laryngectomy are weight changes, ability to swallow, and effectiveness of alternate means of communication. The patient's response to the surgery, coping strategies used, and sources of support also are very important. During the rehabilitation phase, the nurse and other members of the health care team help the patient anticipate the effects of the surgery on everyday life and the adaptations that need to be made. The nurse also assesses the patient's readiness and ability to participate in self-care.

NURSING DIAGNOSIS. In addition to the general nursing diagnoses for the surgical patient discussed in Chapter 14, nursing diagnoses for the total laryngectomy patient may include the following:

- **Ineffective Airway Clearance** related to increased pulmonary secretions or weak cough
- **Anxiety** related to revised airway, uncertain outcome of cancer surgery, or threat to self-concept
- **Decreased Cardiac Output** related to excessive blood loss
- **Pain** related to tissue trauma
- **High Risk for Injury** related to excision of muscles in the neck or altered upper airway
- **Altered Nutrition: Less than Body Requirements** related to dysphagia or diminished sense of smell
- **Impaired Verbal Communication** related to surgical excision of larynx
- **Ineffective Individual Coping** related to loss of verbal communication or altered appearance
- **High Risk for Infection** related to altered airway or interrupted skin integrity
- **Knowledge Deficit** of self-care

GOALS. Goals of nursing care after total laryngectomy are adequate oxygenation and patent airway; reduced anxiety; adequate cardiac output; reduced pain; patient's knowledge of measures to protect incision and tracheostomy; adequate nutrition; effective communication; effective coping with body changes; absence of infection; and patient's performance of self-care.

INTERVENTIONS

Ineffective Airway Clearance. As previously emphasized, oxygenation status is assessed frequently. If the patient is on a ventilator, it is usually discontinued within a day after surgery. At first the patient has a laryngectomy tube in the tracheostomy. The laryngectomy tube is shorter and wider than a tracheostomy tube, but care of the two is essentially the same.

Since the new tracheostomy bypasses the upper airway, the respiratory tract has to adjust to a dramatic change. The mucous membranes respond to the unexpected trauma and irritation by increasing secretions. Because normal humidification is absent, the secretions tend to be drier than normal, making it more difficult to remove them from the airway.

The trachea and laryngectomy tube must be kept open at all times, or else the patient would suffocate. The nurse assesses the need for suctioning (increased pulse, restlessness, audible or visible mucus) and uses sterile technique to clear the airway as needed. Tracheostomy suctioning is reviewed earlier in this chapter. A procedure manual should be consulted for additional details.

Factors that affect respiratory status are positioning, fluids, and humidification. Semi-Fowler's or Fowler's position permits maximal lung expansion. Turning, coughing, and deep breathing prevent pooling of secretions in the lungs. Intravenous fluids and enteral feedings maintain hydration and nutrition. Good hydration helps to thin secretions. Two to 3 ml of normal saline can be instilled in the stoma prior to suctioning to loosen secretions. A tracheostomy collar is used to provide oxygen and humidification of inspired air.

Anxiety. The nurse should be sensitive to the patient's anxiety. A calm approach, attentive monitoring, and simple explanations help to reduce anxiety. The nurse must also remember to talk to the patient! There is a tendency to treat the patient who cannot speak as if he or she cannot hear either.

Decreased Tissue Perfusion. In the early postoperative period, the patient is at risk for excessive bleeding. Frequent monitoring of vital signs allows detection of indicators of hemorrhage, such as increasing pulse and respiratory rates and restlessness. Secretions also should be examined for excessive bleeding.

Drains are usually in place to remove excess fluid. The color of the drainage and the amount should be assessed. Over the first few postoperative days, the color should change from bright red to pink to clear or straw colored. The amount of drainage also should decrease steadily.

Pain. Analgesics are given as ordered postoperatively. Nurses may be surprised that the patient who has had a radical neck dissection may not seem to have much pain. Because the procedure is so extensive, many nerves are cut, so sensation is impaired. Some areas of numbness are permanent.

High Risk for Injury. The patient may be fearful of moving his or her head, especially after radical neck surgery. The nurse can help at first by placing a hand behind the patient's head when getting out of bed. The patient can also be shown to roll on one side and support the head while raising up from the bed.

The tracheostomy is open to the environment and must be protected from foreign substances. The patient is taught to avoid dusty places and to cover the tracheostomy loosely during shaving or haircuts. The patient cannot submerge the neck or allow bath water to splash into the trachea since the water would go directly into the airway.

Altered Nutrition. Nutrition is often a problem after laryngectomy. The patient's sense of smell is impaired because inspired air no longer goes through the nose. The patient may also have some difficulty swallowing because of tissue trauma around the surgical site. Nasogastric tube feedings are given initially. Oral fluids and foods are reintroduced gradually. Nursing measures to improve appetite should be employed, and the patient's weight should be monitored. Chapter 12 discusses nursing interventions for anorexia and for tube feedings.

Impaired Verbal Communication. A number of options exist for restoring some form of speech to the laryngectomy patient. The speech therapist and the physician will recommend appropriate methods.

Many patients are able to learn to use "esophageal speech." Air is swallowed and held in the upper esophagus. The patient then belches. The patient learns to control and use the air to produce sounds. The voice is deep but understandable. Considerable motivation and practice are needed to master esophageal speech. Patients and their families are likely to have periods of discouragement. The nurse can help by acknowledging their feelings and demonstrating patience.

A second option is the use of an artificial larynx. Several types of electronic devices are available that produce sound. One type is illustrated in Figure 49–11. The "voice," however, has a mechanical, computerized sound that tends to attract attention.

Some patients are candidates for laryngoplasty, a procedure performed during total laryngectomy. It is done to create a connection between the pharynx and the trachea. The patient is able to speak by occluding the tracheostomy with a finger. This procedure is not an option for all patients and is not always successful.

One final option for speech is the tracheoesophageal prosthesis. The surgeon creates a fistula between the trachea and the esophagus. A catheter is placed in the fistula until it heals. When the catheter is removed, a prosthesis is inserted into the fistula. Two prostheses that may be used are the Blom-Singer trapdoor prosthesis and the Panje voice button. The patient occludes the stoma with a finger during speech. A one-way valve allows air to flow only from the trachea to the esophagus (Fig. 49–12).

Those patients who are unable to use any form of speech must rely on written communication, gestures, or some assistive devices. A word board is a computerized device that enables the patient to select words that are "spoken" by the computer. A personal communicator produces a printed message that the patient enters on a keyboard.

It is especially important for the nurse to direct the laryngectomy patient to community resources. Organizations such as the Lost Chord Club or New Voice Club are the most useful because the members have had personal experiences with laryngectomies. The American Cancer Society can provide information about resources in the local community.

Ineffective Individual Coping. It has been said that language separates humans from animals. The perma-

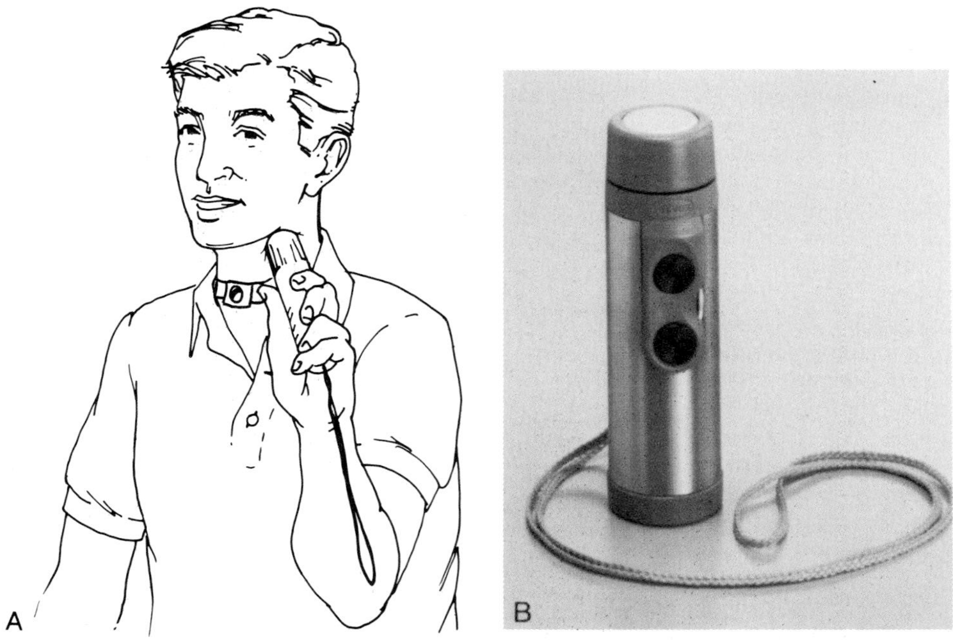

FIGURE 49-11
An external larynx. (*B,* Servox electrolarynx, distributed by Seimens Hearing Instruments, Inc., Piscataway, NJ.)

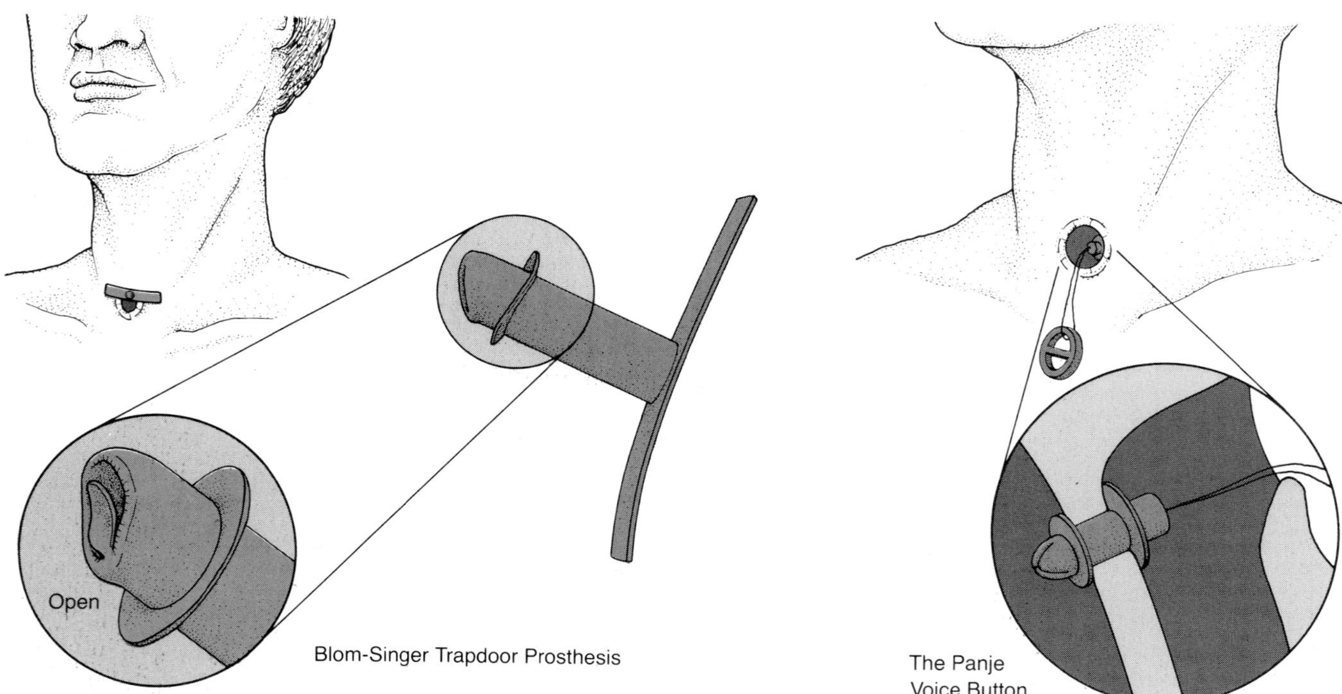

FIGURE 49-12
Tracheoesophageal prostheses. *Left,* Blom-Singer trapdoor prosthesis. *Right,* Panje voice button. (From Ignatavicius, D. D., & Bayne, M. V. [1991]. *Medical-surgical nursing: A nursing process approach* [p. 1970]. Philadelphia: W. B. Saunders.)

nent loss of the ability to communicate verbally is very traumatic. Patients who require laryngectomy usually have some time to prepare for this procedure in advance, but the actual event may still evoke a variety of emotional responses. Learning to live with a permanent tracheostomy and loss of the natural voice requires considerable adjustment. The patient may demonstrate behaviors typical of any loss situation: denial, anger, depression, bargaining, or acceptance. Depression may be reflected in withdrawal or refusal to learn about self-care and rehabilitative measures.

The nurse acknowledges the patient's feelings and gently urges participation in self-care and use of alternative means of communication. The patient who learns to care for the tracheostomy and to communicate effectively feels more confident of the ability to cope. Support groups can be especially helpful because the patient sees potential role models of successful adaptation to tracheostomy. The family also requires support, encouragement, and teaching.

High Risk for Infection. The tracheostomy permits unfiltered air to enter the respiratory tract. The effects are drying of the mucous membranes, increased secretions, and increased risk of infection. The nurse uses sterile technique during tracheostomy care. The patient is also protected from people who have respiratory infections.

Knowledge Deficit. As soon as the patient is able, the nurse encourages participation in self-care. At first, the patient might just be asked to hold some supplies. The nurse explains what is being done and why. Gradually, the patient should assume more responsibility for care of the tracheostomy. Even if the patient seems quite competent by discharge, a referral to a home health agency or visiting nurse association is recommended. The home care nurse helps the patient learn to adapt care to the home setting and to deal with various unanticipated problems. A family member or significant other should be taught tracheostomy care as well. Verbal teaching should be accompanied by written information for later use. The nurse should remember that people recall only a small percentage of what they hear.

EVALUATION. Criteria for goal achievement are respiratory rate of 12 to 20 without dyspnea, normal skin color; patient calm, affirms reduced anxiety; patient affirms reduced pain; patient's demonstration of protection of incision during movement and avoidance of introduction of foreign substances into the trachea; weight stabilized at admission weight; patient's indication of satisfaction with a means of communication; realistic plans made by patient; no fever, no purulent drainage or secretions; and patient's demonstration of self-care with minimal assistance.

Nursing Care of the Patient Having Supraglottic Laryngectomy

For patients who have cancer above the vocal cords, supraglottic laryngectomy and radical neck dissection are the usual procedures. These patients also have temporary tracheostomies. Cuffed tubes are used at first because of the danger of aspiration. These patients require oral and tracheal suctioning.

Nursing care of the patient having supraglottic laryngectomy is in many ways like that of the patient having total laryngectomy except that the tracheostomy is temporary, the voice is not lost, and swallowing is more problematic. Therefore, additional nursing interventions are indicated to maintain good nutrition. Enteral feedings may be needed for a long time, so the nurse can begin to instruct the patient in self-feeding. Some patients never regain the ability to swallow without aspirating, and total laryngectomy is recommended for them.

An example of a swallowing technique taught to these patients is the following:

1. Assume a sitting position.
2. Take a deep breath and hold it.
3. Place food on the back of the tongue with a spoon.
4. Swallow three times while holding the breath.
5. Cough. (Note: When the patient has a tracheostomy, any aspirated food or fluids may be ejected through the tracheostomy.)

The patient with a supraglottic laryngectomy is also at increased risk for aspiration pneumonia. The nurse should be alert for signs and symptoms of this complication: increased pulse and respiratory rates, dyspnea, cough, rales and rhonchi, fever, wheezing, and frothy pink sputum. A suction machine should be readily available.

Nursing Care of the Patient Having Partial Laryngectomy

If a patient has a partial laryngectomy, a temporary tracheostomy for 2 to 5 days can be expected. Intravenous fluids and enteral feedings will probably be ordered at first. Like patients with supraglottic laryngectomies, these patients have considerable difficulty swallowing when oral nourishment is resumed. In general, the nursing care is similar to that of the patient having a supraglottic laryngectomy. To prevent aspiration, the patient should be seated upright, with the head flexed slightly forward. Semisolids are often easier to manage than thin liquids. A suction machine should be on hand in case it is needed.

Many disorders of the nose, sinuses, and throat are common and self-limited. Persistent symptoms, however, may represent serious conditions, and the patient should be referred for medical evaluation. The nurse can play an important role in educating the public about the prevention of infections and malignancies of the head and neck.

BIBLIOGRAPHY

Alderfer, S. (1993). Common respiratory interventions. In J. M. Black & E. Matassarin-Jacobs (Eds.), *Luckmann and Sorensen's medical-surgical nursing: A psychophysiologic approach* (4th ed.) (pp. 941–992). Philadelphia: W. B. Saunders.

Chernecky, C. C., Krech, R. L., & Berger, B. J. (1993). *Laboratory tests and diagnostic procedures.* Philadelphia: W. B. Saunders.

Deglin, J. H., Vallerand, A. H., & Russin, M. M. (1991). *Davis's drug guide for nurses* (2nd ed.). Philadelphia: F. A. Davis.

Doenges, M. E., & Moorhouse, M. F. (1993). *Nursing diagnoses with interventions.* (4th ed.). Philadelphia: F. A. Davis.

Fischbach, F. (1988). *A manual of laboratory diagnostic tests* (3rd ed). Philadelphia: J. B. Lippincott.

Gallagher, M., & Kahn, C. (1990). Lasers: Scalpels of light. *RN, 53*(5), 46–52.

Hodgson, B. B., Kizier, R. J., & Kingdon, R. T. (1993). *Nurse's drug handbook.* Philadelphia: W. B. Saunders.

Ignatavicius, D. D., & Bayne M. V. (1991). *Medical-surgical nursing: A nursing process approach.* Philadelphia: W. B. Saunders.

Jarvis, C. (1992). *Physical examination and health assessment.* Philadelphia: W. B. Saunders.

Lockhart, J. S., & Bryce, J. (1993). Restoring speech with a tracheoesophageal puncture. *Nursing 93, 23*(1), 59–61.

Matteson, M. A., & McConnell, E. S. (1988). *Gerontological Nursing.* Philadelphia: W. B. Saunders.

Patten, B. C., & Holt, J. A. (1992). When your patient is allergic. *American Journal of Nursing, 92*(9), 58–61.

Potter, P. A., & Perry, A. G. (1992). *Fundamentals of nursing* (3rd ed.). St. Louis: C. V. Mosby.

Riley, M. A. K. (1987). *Nursing care of the client with ear, nose, and throat disorders.* New York: Springer Publishing Co.

Shlafer, M. (1993). *The nurse, pharmacology, and drug therapy* (3rd ed.). Redwood City, CA: Addison-Wesley.

Sigler, B. (1993). Nursing care of clients with upper airway disorders. In J. M. Black & E. Matassarin-Jacobs (Eds.), *Luckmann and Sorensen's medical-surgical nursing: A psychophysiologic approach* (4th ed.) (pp. 993–1020). Philadelphia: W. B. Saunders.

KEY CONCEPTS

1. Sinusitis is acute or chronic inflammation of the sinuses that can lead to meningitis, brain abscess, osteomyelitis, and orbital cellulitis.
2. Sinusitis is treated with drug therapy or with surgery to remove obstructions and to improve drainage.
3. Nasal polyps are masses of tissue extending from the sinuses into the nasal passage that can be surgically excised.
4. Allergic rhinitis, or "hay fever," is an allergic response to a substance that produces sneezing, nasal obstruction, clear nasal discharge, frontal headache, and itchy, watery eyes.
5. Allergic rhinitis may be treated with antihistamines and decongestants or with desensitizing injections of identified allergens.
6. Acute viral coryza, the common cold, is caused by a virus, is contagious, and is treated symptomatically with antihistamines, decongestants, and antipyretics.
7. Tumors of the nasal passages typically cause nasal obstruction requiring surgical excision.
8. Malignant tumors of the nasal passages and pharynx tend to metastasize early and may be treated with some combination of surgery, chemotherapy, and radiotherapy.
9. There are two kinds of carcinomas of the external nose: squamous cell carcinomas grow rapidly and tend to metastasize, and basal cell carcinomas grow more slowly and are less invasive.
10. A deviated nasal septum may obstruct the nasal passages and interfere with sinus drainage.
11. Surgical procedures for deviated nasal septum include nasal septoplasty and submucosal resection.
12. Epistaxis (nosebleed) can usually be controlled with external pressure but sometimes requires placement of a nasal balloon catheter.
13. Tonsillitis is more common in children but is more often severe in adults.
14. Tonsillitis may be treated with drug therapy, irrigations, or surgical excision.
15. Nursing care after tonsillectomy focuses on measures to counter decreased cardiac output, ineffective airway clearance, pain, and knowledge deficit.
16. Cancer of the larynx may be treated with surgery, radiotherapy, chemotherapy, or a combination of these.
17. After laryngectomy (removal of the larynx), the nurse addresses problems of ineffective airway clearance, anxiety, decreased cardiac output, pain, high risk for injury, altered nutrition, impaired verbal communication, ineffective individual coping, high risk for infection, and knowledge deficit.

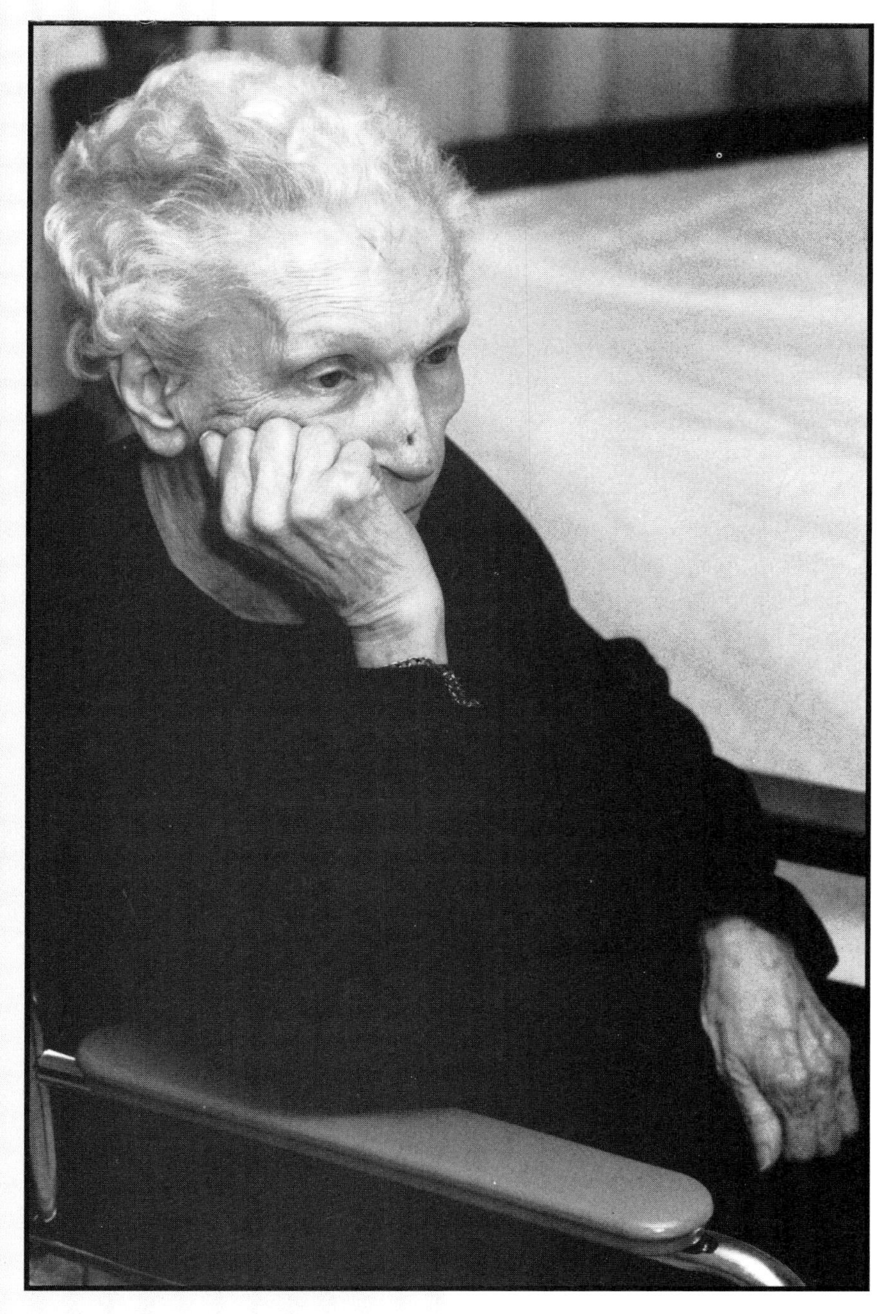

UNIT 16
Mental Health and Illness

Irma G. Aguilar
J. Gail Barry

CHAPTER 50

Psychological Responses to Illness

OBJECTIVES

1. Define mental illness.
2. Discuss a continuum for mental health and illness.
3. Discuss personality development from the psychoanalytic, social, behavioral, and cognitive perspectives.
4. Discuss the concepts of stress, anxiety, adaptation and homeostasis, and depression.
5. Identify some basic coping strategies (defense mechanisms).
6. Differentiate between conflict and motivation.
7. Discuss how age and cultural and spiritual beliefs affect an individual's ability to cope with illness.
8. Discuss the concepts of anxiety, fear, stress, loss, grief, hopelessness, and powerlessness in relation to illness.
9. Describe several factors that may precipitate adaptive or maladaptive coping behaviors in response to illness.
10. Discuss implementation of the nursing process to enhance a patient's mental health as the patient deals with the stresses of illness.

GLOSSARY

ADAPTATION The organism's attempt to return to homeostasis

ANXIETY A vague sense of impending doom or apprehension that appears to have no clearly identifiable cause

CONFLICT Psychological struggle that results when two incompatible possibilities occur at the same time

COPING STRATEGY An adaptive or maladaptive mental attitude, behavior, or both that is consciously or unconsciously perceived as helping to reduce stress, anxiety, or fear

CRISIS The point on the health continuum at which the individual moves toward illness and disequilibrium occurs

DEFENSE MECHANISM A conscious or unconscious mechanism used to relieve or diminish anxiety

DEPRESSION A mood of sadness; a withdrawal from usual commitments

EUSTRESS Stress that is perceived as helpful (e.g., graduation, vacation)

FEELINGS All emotional and physical responses and sensations

Glossary continued

HOPELESSNESS A condition of lack of hope, which may hinder action

MALADAPTIVE Attempts to cope using strategies that ultimately do not return the individual to homeostasis

MENTAL HEALTH CONTINUUM A model used to demonstrate the range of mental health on a line between health at one end and illness at the opposite extreme

SELF-ESTEEM The perception of self as having a sense of worth

STRESS Any physiologic or psychological tension that threatens a person's equilibrium

STRESSOR A factor that causes stress

Mental health is dependent on a great many factors, including perception, development, and stressors. Understanding mental health and the psychological response to illness requires that the nurse have an adequate knowledge of growth and development, adaptation, anxiety, and stress. Vulnerabilities differ throughout one's life span. Furthermore, cultural differences, community resources, the role of the family, and personal values may affect the adaptive capabilities of the individual. The patient and family may experience a wide range of normal feelings and emotions in response to illness. Nurses can promote adaptation and minimize maladaptive behaviors only if they are well versed in the expected range of emotions the individual may experience as a result of illness. Use of the nursing process provides a systematic approach for individualized care based on careful assessment combined with a knowledge of human behavior.

DEFINITION OF MENTAL HEALTH

Mental and physical health is an absence of dis-ease or dis-harmony within the holistic dimensions of mind-emotion, body-physiology, community-society, and soul-spirituality. Stressors can originate in any or all of these dimensions. The individual level of health is directly related to one's ability to adjust to a variety of internal and external stressors. Maslow proposed that human sickness and human health have a biologically based inner nature. He described and prioritized basic human needs for life, safety, and security; for belongingness and affection; for respect and self-respect; and for self-actualization. Healthy individuals, according to Maslow, possess several characteristics:

- An accurate perception of reality
- The ability to accept oneself and others
- The ability to be spontaneous
- The ability to solve problems
- A need for privacy
- Independence or autonomy
- The ability to express the self emotionally
- A frequency of "peak experiences"—happy moments that produce a sense of worthiness, hope, and love of life
- Identification with humankind
- The ability to maintain satisfactory relationships
- A sense of ethics
- Some sense of resistance to conformity

Mental health and illness can be viewed as a continuum, with mental health at one end and mental illness at the other end. At any given moment the individual is adapting to a variety of stessors in life from each of the dimensions of self—body-physiology, mind-emotion, community-society, and soul-spirituality—and subsequently may fall anywhere on this continuum.

STRESS

Stress is necessary for growth and development. Eustress is "good" stress—stress that is perceived as helpful, such as graduating from an educational program or taking a vacation. Distress, however, is defined as a stess perceived as harmful—the loss of a job or the death of a family member. Stress is caused by a stressor. A stressor can be anything that causes the individual stress, and adaptation to stress affects the whole organism. For example, a client who is immobilized lacks the stress of exercise, so that the muscles begin to atrophy, joints become rigid and inflexible, and so on until all the systems of the body are affected. With daily stress such as moderate exercise, muscles increase in mass, circulation improves, and joints become more flexible. So it is with mental health. The dimensions of the person—mind-emotion, body-physiology, community-society, and soul/spirituality—are not separate entities. These dimensions interact, resulting in the development of a unique human being. Mental health can be facilitated by mild stress, which increases one's repertoire of problem-solving behaviors. Mild stress produces mild anxiety and enables the patient to use energy focused exclusively on the problem. The result is successful problem solving. This in turn promotes self-esteem.

HOMEOSTASIS

Stress, response, and adaptation can be thought of as an individual's attempt to maintain homeostasis or equilibrium. If stressors are relatively mild and the person is able to respond and adapt, mental health is maintained. If, however, the person is overwhelmed by many stressors or does not have enough coping behaviors or problem-solving strategies to maintain equilibrium, illness or crisis may ensue. A crisis is the point at which the individual may move toward illness on the continuum. A crisis results in inner tension and anxiety, which may affect an individual's ability to function.

Illness (mental and physical) can be derived from all the dimensions: mind-emotion, body-physiology, community-society, and soul-spirituality. For example, some persons may be genetically predisposed to diabetes mellitus (body-physiology). If individuals grow up in families and cultures (community-society) in which exercise and diet are valued, the risk of developing diabetes may be decreased. If successful coping strategies have been acquired (mind-emotion), the body is subjected to less stress. An individual's perception of (soul-spirituality) any stressful life event may result in either well-being or disharmony (i.e., illness).

Similarly, depression can be related to a number of factors, including genetic predisposition, medication, neuroendocrine disturbances, and neurologic disorders. As with diabetes mellitus, there is a dynamic interplay within and between the holistic dimensions of each individual. If an individual who is genetically predisposed to depression grows up in a family in which maladaptive coping or poor problem-solving strategies are practiced, the individual may not be able to develop a repertoire of successful coping behaviors. If this individual is exposed to a severe stressor and does not believe he or she has the ability to cope, depression may result. The extent of the crisis depends on current resources of the individual (e.g., support systems, past coping strategies, and current health) counterbalanced by the number and severity of stressors.

THEORIES OF GROWTH AND DEVELOPMENT

Growth refers to the individual's gradual process of evolution from conception until death. As human beings move through sequential stages of development, they become increasingly complex. Individuals represent the expression of the totality of events up to any specific point in time. They are both the product and the totality of their perceived interactions with individuals as well as with their community and environment. Growth, then, refers not only to a change in physical size and structure, but to a process of development that becomes increasingly complex.

Theorists have attempted from varying perspectives to explain how personality develops. Most believe that the early experiences of a human provide the framework for all future references. Development is usually broken into stages that correspond to a specific age group. Developmental tasks are assigned to each of these stages.

The DSM-IV (*Diagnostic and Statistical Manual of Mental Health,* 4th ed., 1994) defines personality as "deeply ingrained patterns of behavior which include the way one relates to, perceives, and thinks about the environment and oneself" (p. 403). Nurses must have a knowledge base that includes the common stages of personality development to accurately assess behavioral responses in humans from infancy through old age.

FREUD'S THEORY OF PSYCHOANALYSIS

Sigmund Freud received his medical degree from the University of Vienna in 1881. Freud learned about a therapy called the "talking cure" from Josef Breuer, another Viennese physician. Through self-analysis and working with the theory of personality, Freud developed psychoanalysis, which he called both a method for treating emotionally disturbed people and a theory of personality.

Freud identified three components of the personality: id, ego, and superego.

ID (BEGINS AT BIRTH). As the baby experiences some degree of frustration and discomfort, the development of id occurs. The baby perceives pleasure or relief of distress when needs are met. The subjective reality of the id is the pursuit of pleasure and the relief or avoidance of pain. Freud believed that a person who acts impulsively, for example, to commit a rape, is under the influence of the id.

EGO (BEGINS AT 4 TO 6 MONTHS). It has been called the "rational self" or the reality principle. Its aim is to tolerate tension and postpone action until appropriate behavior can be invoked. The ego discovers or produces reality by thought, reason, and plan of action. Reality testing occurs as the ego carries out a plan of action until a suitable solution results. (In the case of hunger, the action is eating.) The ego is a mediator between the id and the superego. The ego decides what instincts (derived via the id) will be satisfied and how.

SUPEREGO (BEGINS AT 3 TO 6 YEARS). The superego is the moral or judicial branch of personality and can be equated to the person's moral code. The superego is the ideal or perfection rather than the reality (ego) or the pleasure (id). Between the ages of 3 and 6, the values and morals of the individual's caregivers are internalized. The superego functions to inhibit impulses of the id, to persuade the ego to substitute moralistic goals for realistic ones, and to strive for perfection.

Dynamics of Personality

Psychic energy (libido) is the kind used to operate the id, ego, and superego. This dynamic process involves a continuous exchange or transformation between psychic and bodily energy. An instinct is an inborn condition that is the principal source of bodily need or impulse. The aim of an instinct is to relieve tension or remove the bodily need. For example, hunger is an instinct that food (the object) relieves. Freud believed that an imbalance of energy among id, ego, and superego could result in internal conflict, which produces tension and anxiety.

Anxiety

Anxiety is a painful emotion that results from one's perception of danger. As people develop, they learn to cope with this painful emotion. The fight or flight response actually provides the physiologic ability for one to either fight or flee. Individuals continually regulate their behavior based on the level of perceived anxiety. When anxiety intensifies to an excessive level, perception of reality becomes solely focused on the crisis.

Defense Mechanisms

According to Freud, the ego may devise strategies or defense mechanisms to cope with anxiety. Defense mechanisms are used in an effort to diminish anxiety; however, when used excessively they can hinder the developing personality. Defense mechanisms used to protect against anxiety and internal conflict are the following:

- *Compensation*—an attempt to make up for real or imagined weakness. For example, an adolescent perceived as unattractive becomes an outstanding athlete.
- *Denial*—refusal to acknowledge a real situation. For example, a person who finds a suspicious lump in her breast does not keep appointments for a breast biopsy.
- *Displacement*—transferring feelings associated with one person or event to another that is considered less threatening. For example, a boy who is angry with a teacher comes home and yells at his dog.
- *Identification*—emulation of admirable qualities in another to enhance one's self-esteem. For example, a child dresses and uses mannerisms similar to those of a famous rock star.
- *Rationalization or intellectualization*—the use of logic, reasoning, and analysis to avoid unacceptable feelings. For example, a student fails to complete an assignment correctly and rationalizes subsequent feelings of incompetence by complaining about the objectives for the assignment.
- *Introjection*—internalizing or taking on the values and beliefs of another person. For example, a child takes on the values and beliefs of a parent.
- *Isolation*—the separation of emotion from an associated thought or memory. For example, a man appears apathetic as he discusses a fire fight in which he participated in Vietnam.
- *Projection*—unacceptable feelings or impulses are transferred to another. For example, a wife who is jealous of her husband accuses him of jealousy.
- *Reaction formation*—avoidance of unacceptable thoughts and behaviors by expressing opposing thoughts or behaviors. For example, a patient who unconsciously hates his father continuously tells the nurses how great his father is.
- *Regression*—withdrawing to an earlier level of development to benefit from the associated comfort levels. For example, a child starts sucking her thumb when her new baby brother comes home from the hospital.
- *Repression*—an unconscious defense mechanism in which unacceptable ideas, impulses, and memories are kept out of consciousness. For example, a woman cannot remember a sexual assault.
- *Sublimation*—the transformation of unacceptable impulses or drives (e.g., aggressiveness, anger, sexuality) into constructive or more acceptable behavior. For example, a person who has aggressive tendencies becomes a football star.
- *Suppression*—a conscious or voluntary inhibition of unacceptable ideas, impulses, and memories. For example, a child who fails an algebra class forgets to show his report card to his parents.
- *Undoing*—actually or symbolically attempting to cancel out an action that was unacceptable. For example, sprinkling salt over one's left shoulder to prevent bad luck after spilling salt on the table.
- *Substitution*—the individual replaces a highly valued, unattainable object with a less valued, attainable object. For example, the person who has a strong unconscious sexual attraction to a parent marries someone who resembles that parent.
- *Conversion*—an emotional conflict is turned into a physical symptom, which provides the individual with some sort of benefit (secondary gain). For example, the individual who witnesses a murder then experiences sudden blindness without an organic cause.

Defense mechanisms are adapted by the individual as protective measures to allow the ego relief from anxiety. One factor that enhances the development of ego is an environment with experiences that match the child's capacity to adapt. Ideally, defense mechanisms are shed and replaced by more realistic and efficient methods of adaptation as the individual matures.

Psychosexual Stages of Development

ORAL STAGE (BIRTH TO 18 MONTHS). The goal is to have immediate gratification (sense of comfort and satisfaction of needs). As the mother meets the needs of the infant, the child develops a sense of trust. Infants do not see themselves as being separate from the mother at this stage of development.

ANAL STAGE (18 MONTHS TO 3 YEARS). The goal at this stage of development is control and independence. At this time the child gains sphincter control over elimination. Freud believed that toilet training that was too rigid could cause a child to be "anal retentive" (and produce such traits as constipation and stubbornness).

PHALLIC STAGE (3 TO 6 YEARS). The goal of this stage is identification of sexual differences in genders. The Oedipus complex occurs when the child unconsciously desires the parent of the opposite sex. The conflict is resolved when the child identifies with the parent of the same sex.

LATENCY STAGE (6 TO 12 YEARS). The goal of this stage is learning and socialization. According to Freud, sexuality is dormant at this time in life.

GENITAL STAGE (13 TO 20 YEARS). During this stage the libidinal drive increases. Relationships evolve.

ERIKSON'S THEORY OF PSYCHOSOCIAL DEVELOPMENT

Erik Erikson in 1963 described eight stages associated with developmental tasks. According to this theory, each developmental task must be negotiated for continued emotional maturation.

TRUST VERSUS MISTRUST (BIRTH TO 18 MONTHS). Basic trust must be developed. Healthy future relationships are based on the successful completion of this stage. Basic needs must be met to establish trust.

AUTONOMY VERSUS SHAME AND DOUBT (18 MONTHS TO 3 YEARS). A sense of self-control and ability to delay gratification develops. During this stage the child seeks independence. Parents can promote self-confidence by allowing independent activities balanced with structure and limits.

INITIATIVE VERSUS GUILT (3 TO 6 YEARS). The development of the superego or conscience occurs. The child can initiate activities and take part in cooperative play.

INDUSTRY VERSUS INFERIORITY (6 TO 12 YEARS). The child learns about the culture's rules and regulations. A sense of self-confidence develops from intellectual experience.

IDENTITY VERSUS ROLE CONFUSION (12 TO 20 YEARS). The individual learns to view self as unique. Heterosexual relationships develop. Career choices are made.

INTIMACY VERSUS ISOLATION (20 TO 30 YEARS). An intimate relationship may develop that includes a lasting relationship to another person, cause, or institution.

GENERATIVITY VERSUS STAGNATION (30 TO 65 YEARS). The individual strives to achieve life goals.

EGO INTEGRITY VERSUS DESPAIR (65 YEARS TO DEATH). The task is to review one's life and find meaning from the events that were both positive and negative. This provides a sense of positive self-worth.

SULLIVAN'S THEORY OF INTERPERSONAL INTERACTION

Harry Stack Sullivan's theory of personality is based on his beliefs that the individual is a social being and that development evolves within the context of human interaction. Sullivan argued, in 1953, that all behavior is aimed at the relief of anxiety, which he defined as a feeling of emotional discomfort. Sullivan identified interpersonal needs associated with each stage of development:

INFANCY (BIRTH TO 18 MONTHS). Oral gratification relieves anxiety. Need: contact.

CHILDHOOD (18 MONTHS TO 6 YEARS). Anxiety is tolerated as the child learns to delay gratification. Need: participation in activities with adults.

JUVENILE (6 TO 9 YEARS). Peer relationships occur. Need: peers and acceptance.

PREADOLESCENCE (9 TO 12 YEARS). Same-sex relationships occur. Need: friendship and love.

EARLY ADOLESCENCE (12 TO 14 YEARS). Relationships with persons of the opposite sex begin; a sense of identity develops. Need: intimacy.

LATE ADOLESCENCE (14 TO 21 YEARS). Intimacy and relationships that are lasting develop. Self-identity is established. Need: heterosexual relationship.

PIAGET'S THEORY OF COGNITIVE DEVELOPMENT

Jean Piaget believed that human intelligence progresses through a series of stages that are related to age. He studied children extensively and postulated that four stages with major developmental tasks evolve, each with a higher level of logical organization.

SENSORIMOTOR (BIRTH TO 2 YEARS). Infants develop a sense of self. They become mobile and aware of the environment. Object permanence (the idea that an object or person will continue to exist even when no longer in sight) begins as soon as children are able to form a mental image.

PREOPERATIONAL (2 TO 7 YEARS). Children develop an understanding of symbolic gestures, including language. Children are egocentric, that is, they believe that they are at the center of the world. They cannot understand another's viewpoint at this stage of development.

CONCRETE OPERATIONS (6 TO 12 YEARS). Children learn to apply logic. Concepts such as reversibility and spatiality are developed (e.g., changing the shape of an object does not change the amount of the item).

FORMAL OPERATIONS (12 TO 15 YEARS AND OLDER). Children learn to think and reason in abstract terms. Cognitive maturity is achieved.

BEHAVIORAL THEORY

Behavioral theory is based on the idea that all behavior is learned response. Conditioning is one type of learning. An example of a conditioned response was demonstrated by Pavlov, who would ring a bell (stimulus) when feeding (reinforcement) his dog. The dog would salivate when the food was presented. The reflex response of salivation eventually occurred with the ringing of the bell only. Theorists such as B. F. Skinner, Albert Bandura, and Joseph Wople have based their theories on the idea that all behavior is learned and is a series of habitual responses to familiar stimuli.

MASLOW'S HIERARCHY OF NEEDS

According to Abraham Maslow, human beings attempt to achieve full human potential or self-actualization. Maslow, in 1968, assigned human needs from lower order (most basic) to higher order. Before an individual can achieve higher order needs (love and belonging, self-esteem), lower order needs (food, water, shelter, safety, security) must first be met (see Chapter 5).

KOHLBERG'S THEORY OF THE STAGES OF MORAL DEVELOPMENT

Lawrence Kohlberg focused on the child's development of morality. His theory maintains that morality evolves in much the same manner as cognition and is age-bound:

1. Level one: Limits are set externally. Children conform to those who are in authority.
2. Level two: External control gradually fades as children mimic what they perceive as the right thing to do based on the approval of others. This includes decisions based on the rules of society rather than on the approval of other individuals.
3. Level three: Morality is defined individually. Rigid adherence to laws becomes more flexible and takes into consideration individual circumstances.

PSYCHOLOGICAL RESPONSES TO ILLNESS

Responses to illness are as unique as the individuals who respond. Two people may experience a similar stressor, such as illness, and yet cope very differently. These individualistic responses may be based on such subjective experiences as self-concept, perception of threat to body image, or even spiritual and cultural values.

COPING WITH ILLNESS

Illness is seen by most people as a stressful, abnormal state. This stressful state may require that individuals draw from their inner resources. These resources may come from any or all of the following dimensions: mind-emotion, community-society, body-physiology, and soul-spirituality. For some, the inner strengths to be drawn from these various dimensions may be sufficient to cope effectively with illness. For others, however, the individual's ability to cope may be ineffective or maladaptive. This is where effective nursing intervention becomes essential.

The nurse's caring attitude is basic to helping the patient cope with illness. Through the trust gained from a therapeutic nurse-patient relationship, the patient-centered nurse will be able to assist the patient who is not capable of coping with the stresses precipitated by illness.

To assess an individual's potential for coping with an illness effectively, the nurse needs to understand how various factors can affect an individual's ability to cope: age, cultural beliefs, spirituality, self-concept, family and community resources, emotions, stress, fear, anxiety, loss, grief, and mourning.

Factors That Affect Coping with Illness

AGE. Age affects the coping ability of children and adults alike. The developmental process continues throughout the individual's life span. When illness interferes with that process, much stress may be experienced. Adults have a variety of roles that illness can alter. The individual may be in the midst of a successful career or a new marriage. Illness can be especially traumatic if the person is self-employed and has little or no health benefits. Hymovich and Hagopian found in 1992 that patients with cancer who were younger than 50 years of age experienced more frequent and more severe psychological problems than those older than 70. Nurses, in assessing the patient's ability to cope with illness, need to understand that regardless of age, illness in any individual's life is a stressful, disruptive experience. It not only disrupts the developmental process of the individual, but also has a traumatic impact on spouses, children, and other loved ones. The nurse plays an essential role in helping patients and their loved ones to cope.

CULTURAL BELIEFS. The holistic model is based on the premise that for individuals to be seen as unique entities, their cultural or ethnic background must be considered. This becomes especially important for the nurse who is trying to assess whether patients need assistance in coping with the stresses of illness. The nurse should understand that not all "minority" patients who look as if they belong to a specific cultural or ethnic group because of language, surname, or physical characteristics necessarily identify with any specific group. Effective nursing interventions can be made only after patients have been assessed as unique individuals, not as blacks or Latinos, males or females.

Culture is a system of symbols shared by a group of humans and transmitted by them to future generations. Culture brings organization and security to people's lives. It provides the underlying values and beliefs on which behavior is based. Culture can affect attitudes toward health and illness, diet and eating practices, reaction to pain, and values concerning death and dying. Ethnicity is a group's affiliation because of a shared language, race, and cultural values.

In helping patients cope with illness, nurses need to recognize that their own racial and cultural backgrounds may negatively affect their ability to do so. This is especially true if the patient's cultural values and the nurses' own values are in direct conflict with one another.

Before nurses suggest a plan of care they should ask themselves whether the nursing approach being suggested is relevant to the patient's individual needs. Does the nursing care help patients deal with their stress, or does it contribute to the stress? Nurses who state defensively that they give the same care to all patients may need assistance in understanding that effective care is individualized according to the patient's needs, values, and beliefs, not their own.

SPIRITUALITY. During the crisis of illness, patients may turn to their spiritual beliefs and values to find meaning in the experience. Patients who perhaps had not thought of themselves as being religious may suddenly have a need to speak to a spiritual counselor. Others, however, experience spiritual distress. They may feel that the crisis of illness was unfair, that God has betrayed them.

Spiritual distress can be characterized by the following: (1) Patients question the meaning of suffering or existence; (2) conflict exists between the patients' beliefs and their relationship with a deity; or (3) patients experience physical symptoms such as nightmares, sleep disturbances, and alterations in behavior and mood.

To assess whether spirituality is an asset or a liability to the patients' ability to cope with illness, nurses must understand that all individuals are experts about their own spiritual needs and paths. Nurses should allow patients to express their feelings in a therapeutic and nonjudgmental environment. More simply put, the nurse's role is to listen and to care. Effective therapeutic nursing interventions enhance the healing process by adding to the individual's self-concept.

SELF-CONCEPT. Self-concept refers to an organized set of thoughts about oneself and includes the type of person one is, how one relates to others, and one's significance in the family. Self-esteem develops from the people's own evaluations of their competence and of the value others place on them. Body image comprises physical and psychological experiences that influence how individuals perceive their own body.

Self-concept can be affected by changes in self-esteem as well as changes in body image. Patients' perception of these changes and their ability or lack thereof to cope with the changes may bring about stress, fear, and anxiety. Age and developmental levels can also have a direct bearing on a person's ability to cope. Age may directly affect the perception of self-esteem and body image. It is common knowledge that adolescents are especially vulnerable to changes in body image. Adolescents have a strong need to look like their peers. Any change in body image can be quite traumatic at this developmental stage. Adults can be just as vulnerable.

People who rely on their physical appearance or prowess to make a living, such as actors, models, or professional football players, are at high risk for not being able to cope well with the stress illness may impose on their body image and self-esteem. Their strengths and weaknesses have a direct bearing on how well they are able to cope with the threat that illness may have on their self-concept. Some patients, through their life experiences, may have developed coping styles that allow them to confront a problem; others may need to rely on other resources such as their family and or the community.

FAMILY AND COMMUNITY RESOURCES. The basic functions of the family are to provide for physical needs, give love, and strengthen the self-esteem of its members. Functional families may provide optimal support for a patient facing the stress of illness. However, the family's ability to provide support for the patient is dependent on the quality of relationships among its various members as well as its ability to access needed resources.

Because of increasing stresses on the family unit, many families are not able to provide as much support as the patient may need. The stress of illness of one of the family members may have a negative impact on a family that was already only marginally coping. Illness may have precipitated such stresses as a change in family roles, economic pressures, and geographic isolation that may make it difficult to access medical and other needed resources.

Many of the functions once provided by families are increasingly being assumed by social institutions within the community. Communities vary in their ability to assist their members just as families do. Some communities may be well equipped to assist the family unit with whatever needs it may have (e.g., financial, physical, legal, spiritual, emotional), whereas other communities may be less able to meet those very same needs. This is especially true if the patient lives in an impoverished, rural community. The nurse's knowledge of available resources can be invaluable to patients and families. Throughout the hospital stay, the nursing team must anticipate patients' needs on discharge. Putting patients in contact with a local, state, or national organization can be the very factor that keeps a family from succumbing to the pressures of a catastrophic illness.

EMOTIONS. When a serious illness occurs, patients and their families have many changes to adapt to. Some of these changes may involve permanent alterations in lifestyle, frequent visits to physicians' offices, frequent hospitalizations, financial problems, and increased social isolation. For those undergoing this crisis, the process of coping can be very difficult at best and at worst a seemingly impossible task.

The following section discusses a broad range of feelings and emotions that people may experience. Many of these feelings are normal and to be anticipated. However, there may be times when the coping methods being utilized by patients and families may be maladaptive. It is important for nurses to be able to differentiate adaptive coping mechanisms from those that are maladaptive.

Stress. The term *stress* is derived from the Latin word *stringer* which means "to draw tight." Stress is any physiologic or psychological tension that threatens a person's total equilibrium. Stress affects the whole person in all human dimensions. Prolonged or long-term stress is a serious threat to physical and emotional health. As the duration or intensity of stress or the number of stressors increases, a person's ability to adapt effectively is lessened.

Perceptions of stress and coping mechanisms are highly individualized. People subjected to prolonged stressors eventually became totally exhausted. Individuals who are not able to cope with stress adequately may experience a threat to their emotional well-being. They may find their perceptions of reality skewed, their ability to solve problems considerably less effective, and their stress consequently increased. In other words, without effective coping strategies, individuals can be caught in a vicious circle of ineffective coping mechanisms and increased stress that will stop only at the point of total exhaustion, which is death.

Nurses must learn to recognize individuals whose coping skills are ineffective and consequently who are caught in a downward spiral of debilitating exhaustion. Without effective nursing interventions to reverse this downward spiral, the ability to cope can be seriously impaired.

Fear. Fear and anxiety are often used interchangeably; however, fear generally refers to a specific threat and anxiety to a nonspecific one. The body's physiologic reaction to fear is the same as its response to anxiety. The person experiencing the crisis of illness has much to fear. There may be fear of pain, fear of financial ruin, fear of disfigurement, fear of the loss of self-esteem, and fear of not being able to return to a previous lifestyle.

Fears vary according to the developmental status and age of the individual. For example, toddlers may fear separation from their mothers, whereas adolescents may fear threats to their body image. Terminally ill patients may be struggling with fears of death and dying.

Nurses can be very helpful in assisting patients and families to cope with fear. Sometimes just allowing an opportunity to express fear helps to lessen the stress caused by fear. Providing information about tests or surgical procedures may empower clients to begin to cope with fear. However, too much information can also be very stressful. It is always better to provide only information that clients request.

Anxiety. Anxiety is a vague sense of impending doom or apprehension that appears to have no clearly identifiable cause. Anxiety is often an early response to illness. In the case of illness, the degree of anxiety may vary with the severity of the illness. Anxiety may lead to physical and psychological stress and may be caused by real or imagined fear resulting from loss.

Loss. Loss occurs when a person, object, or situation is changed so that its value is diminished or removed. An individual struggling with the crisis of a severe illness experiences the loss of many things: loss of life as it once was, loss of control, loss of a sense of worth, and loss of health. There are basically two kinds of loss: (1) actual loss and (2) anticipatory loss.

Actual loss can be recognized by others as well as by the patients. Examples of actual loss include loss of a limb or loss of a spouse. *Anticipatory loss* is a sense of loss that the patient may feel before the actual loss occurs. An example of anticipatory loss is loss of a spouse in the terminal stages of an illness.

A sense of loss can be a strong stressor that precipitates feelings of fear and anxiety. The fears associated with loss can be stressful enough to actually compromise the ability of an individual to recover from illness. One of the first psychological steps that must be taken to begin the process of coping is to permit oneself to experience the full emotional impact of the loss. This emotional response is known as grief or mourning.

Grief and Mourning. Grief is the subjective, emotional response that evolves from a sense of loss. Mourning is the process through which grief is faced and ultimately resolved or altered over time. Mourning occurs when a person is forced to relinquish original hopes. The process of mourning prepares the individual to reappraise values and to accept substitutions for hope.

The experience of loss is related to the individual's self-concept. The extent of loss depends on how strong the individual's sense of self is immersed with that which is lost.

Individuals experiencing grief may be under a great deal of stress, and stress may make them even more vulnerable to disease. They may become irritable and difficult to get along with. Sometimes they may experience a sense of guilt. Some people blame themselves for whatever they lost. They may perceive their illness and subsequent loss as a punishment from God for not having been a "better" person, a better parent, or a better spouse.

To alter the loss that grief causes, the self must change. The process of change is unique to each individual and each circumstance. One individual's need for change may require only a change in exercise and dietary habits. Another person's need for change may encompass a career, a lifestyle, or better strategies to cope with stress. Any changes in a person's life are stressful. The greater the change, the greater the resulting stress. To cope with stress, the individual may mobilize psychological resources known as coping mechanisms. Adaptive coping mechanisms can be an effective, therapeutic way of dealing with stress. Maladaptive coping behaviors, however, can be detrimental and decrease the ability to cope with illness.

COPING MECHANISMS AND STRATEGIES

Coping is the process of responding to stress or a potential stressor. Coping with stress basically refers to a self-regulatory process by which a person reduces or prevents the responses that would normally occur under stress. Coping strategies can be conscious or unconscious behaviors. Unconscious coping strategies are referred to as *defense mechanisms*. These mechanisms include such mental tactics as denial, repression, suppression, and the like. Conscious coping strategies are conscious, purposeful behaviors that are used to make an unfamiliar situation into one that is perceived as more controllable and predictable. Coping strategies and mechanisms vary from individual to individual. What all these behaviors have in common is that they are attempts to help people feel less stressed and anxious about their illness. Some of these methods provide only temporary relief, whereas others provide more permanent results. What is most important is that the nurse be able to identify and evaluate the effectiveness of these methods.

Some techniques that can be used to help patients cope are known as *relaxation techniques*. Relaxation techniques include such interventions as imagery, relaxation strategies, therapeutic touch, and music therapy. *Imagery* is the use of the imagination to develop sensory images that focus away from the stressful experience and emphasize other sensory experiences and pleasant memories. Relaxation techniques elicit the relaxation response. The positive effects of relaxation include reducing the effects of stress and decreasing anxiety. These techniques can provide clients with self-control during moments of stress. Relaxation techniques are taught only when patients are not in acute discomfort because the inability to concentrate makes the exercise ineffective. Relaxation techniques include biofeedback, meditation, yoga, and Zen practices. *Therapeutic touch* is a process by which the therapist acts as a channel for environmental and universal energy through the therapist's mental concentration.

Another coping mechanism that may be used is *music therapy*. Music can be an effective nursing intervention that helps the patient cope by enhancing the relaxation response and positive imagery. Musical selections should match a patient's mood and musical taste. Earphones with audio cassettes help the patient avoid annoying others and allow concentration on the music. This coping method provides only temporary relief of stress; however, use of such techniques can help to establish a therapeutic environment in which the nurse and patient can begin to discuss the real sources of patient concerns, fears, and anxieties.

Tapping into the spiritual dimension can also be a very effective way of coping with the stress of illness. As the nurse becomes more aware of the areas that affect the patient's spiritual dimension, the nurse and the patient can talk without using traditional religious language. For many patients, the opportunity to discuss beliefs about a higher power may be a very effective way of coping.

MALADAPTIVE COPING MECHANISMS AND STRATEGIES

In an effort to reduce the stress and anxiety that is precipitated by the crisis of an illness, an individual may sometimes engage in thinking patterns or behaviors that are ineffective or even self-destructive (Table 50–1). These ineffective coping mechanisms may evolve from a sense of helplessness or powerlessness.

Helplessness

Helplessness typically occurs when individuals have had repeated exposure to events they perceive as being uncontrollable. This leads to loss of motivation, feelings of despair or anxiety, and cognitive impairment. The individual may even begin to express anger as a means of diminishing feelings of helplessness. This anger may take the form of a personal attack on the nurse and the other caregivers. Helplessness can be prevented by allowing individuals to control as many events as possible within the constraints imposed by treatment and their energy level. The expression of anger is really not aimed at the nurse but is simply an attempt to cope with feelings of loss of control.

Powerlessness

Powerlessness can be defined as a feeling that one's actions cannot affect an outcome or that one lacks personal control over certain events or situations. According to Miller (1992), characteristics of powerlessness include (1) passivity; (2) nonparticipation in care and decision making; (3) dependence on others that may lead to anger, resentment, or guilt; and (4) verbal expression of loss of control over situations or outcomes.

When people are not ready to cope with the threat of illness, unconscious defense mechanisms of avoidance, such as denial, may be used. These avoidance defense mechanisms protect individuals from having to confront and deal with the threat of illness.

Denial

Denial is the subconscious blocking out of emotional experiences. Denial can take several forms: (1) verbal denial, (2) minimizing the severity of the illness, (3) displacing symptoms onto another organ, and (4) engaging in behaviors contrary to medical advice. The outcome of denial, as a coping strategy, may be positive or negative. Denial can lead to negative consequences if people fail to engage in appropriate problem-focused behaviors. Patients who claim that they were never afraid or insist that there is nothing wrong with them are engaging in denial. Denial is maladaptive when the patient's behavior interferes significantly with obtaining appropriate medical care. Arguing with patients about their denial only reinforces the inappropriate behavior.

When working with people in denial, a special effort should be made not to isolate them even though it may be uncomfortable having to care for an individual who denies he or she is ill. The nurse may need to allow the individual to deny the illness, while at the same time asking for cooperation. As the patient's trust in the nurse increases, he or she may be more able to lower unconscious defenses and begin to discuss true feelings of fear and anxiety. This will only occur after an effective, therapeutic nurse-patient relationship has been established.

In the next section the various steps of the nursing process are discussed to help the nurse assess and plan

TABLE 50–1

A SAMPLE PLAN FOR A PATIENT INEFFECTIVELY COPING WITH ILLNESS

NURSING DIAGNOSIS: Ineffective individual coping, related to patient's verbalization "I don't know if I can live through this."

GOAL: Patient will verbalize a feeling of being able to cope with illness by date of discharge.

INTERVENTIONS:

1. Give patient an opportunity to verbalize feelings of inadequacy by approaching patient care in an unhurried manner.
2. Assess patient's and family's knowledge of illness.
3. Establish several teaching sessions with the patient and family to empower the patient to begin self-care.
4. Implement stress reduction strategies (e.g., music therapy) to help patient cope with stressful moments.

EVALUATION: The patient will state that he or she feels more capable of dealing with the demands of the illness.

nursing interventions that will facilitate the patient's task of having to deal with the crisis of illness.

THE NURSING PROCESS IN ILLNESS

ASSESSMENT

An individual's ability to cope with an illness varies from moment to moment and from situation to situation. Therefore, it is essential that assessment be an ongoing process. Assessment of the following areas determines the effectiveness of individual coping strategies:

- Do individuals see themselves as effective in coping with their illness?
- What efforts have individuals made in seeking information about their situation?
- How skillful are individuals in caring for themselves?
- What resources do individuals believe are available to them in dealing with their illness?
- Do individuals effectively adhere to their medical regimen?
- Do individuals feel they have been able to keep a sense of normality in their life in spite of their illness?
- How have individuals and their families been able to cope with any role modification that the illness has brought about?
- Have individuals been able to maintain a sense of hope in spite of the demands of the illness?
- Do individuals feel that the important relationships in their life remain intact?

After problem areas have been identified, meaningful nursing diagnoses can be formulated.

NURSING DIAGNOSIS

The purpose of a nursing diagnosis is to formulate a plan of care that will supply effective nursing interventions to help patients achieve their desired goals. Patients and their families must be included in the process so that care plans are based on patients' values and perceptions of the problems rather than on those of the nurse. The following are suggested nursing diagnoses related to ineffective coping:

Ineffective Individual Coping related to

- verbalization of inability to cope or to ask for help
- inability to meet basic needs
- alteration in societal participation
- inappropriate use of defense mechanisms
- change in usual communication patterns
- destructive behavior toward self and others
- denial of obvious problems and weaknesses
- inability to admit impact of disease on life pattern

These examples serve only as a sample of potential areas that could possibly be identified as problems for patients. The formulation of nursing diagnoses can be successful only if it is a joint effort among nurse, patient, and family. Patients or family members need to agree that the identified problems are important ones if effective coping is to take place. This is especially true if a patient has a long-term or chronic illness.

NURSING GOALS, INTERVENTIONS, AND EVALUATION CRITERIA

The goal of nursing care is to help people manage and successfully cope with their illness. When effective coping strategies are used, patients can manage their illness and adapt to a new lifestyle that incorporates healthy behaviors and realistic goals. In addition, patients should emerge with a positive self-concept and self-esteem.

People with chronic, debilitating illnesses may have difficulty acquiring and maintaining coping skills for long periods of time. Individuals may be able to cope with their illness today, but tomorrow may bring a whole new set of challenges. This is especially true in terminal stages of illness when physical deterioration is on an accelerated course and every day brings new losses that need to be mourned and coped with.

Nursing interventions are based on identified patient problems (nursing diagnoses). Table 50–1 illustrates a sample nursing care plan for a client who is ineffectively coping with illness.

BIBLIOGRAPHY

Aguilera, D. C., & Messick, J. M. (1982). *Crisis intervention: Theory and methodology* (4th ed.). St. Louis: C. V. Mosby.

American Psychiatric Association. (1994). *Diagnostic and statistical manual of mental disorders* (4th ed.). Washington, D.C.: Author.

Bluementhal, J. A., Bradley, W., Kasl, S. V., Powell, L. H., & Taylor, C. B. (1989). Task force III: Assessment of psychological status in patients with ischemic heart disease. *Journal of American College of Cardiology, 14*(4), 1016–1042.

Castaglia, P. T., & Harbin, R. E. (1992). *Child health care. Process and practice.* Philadelphia: J. B. Lippincott.

Charmaz, K. (1980). *The social reality of death.* Reading, MA: Addison-Wesley.

Cook, J. S., & Fontaine, K. L. (1991). *Essentials of mental health nursing* (2nd ed.). Redwood City, CA: Addison-Wesley.

Cox, H. C., Hinz, M. D., Lubno, M. A., Newfield, S. A., Ridenour, N. A., & Sridarmont, K. L. (1989). *Clinical application of nursing diagnosis.* Philadelphia: F. A. Davis.

Dossey, B. M., Guzzetta, C. E., & Kenner, C. V. (1992). *Critical care nursing: Body-mind-spirit.* Philadelphia: J. B. Lippincott.

Downs, J. F. (1975). *Cultures in crisis* (2nd ed.). New York: Macmillan.

Erikson, E. (1968). *Childhood and society* (2nd ed.). New York: W. W. Norton.

Hall, C. S. (1979). *A primer of Freudian psychology.* New York: World Publishing.

Harvey, R. M. (1992). The relationship of values to adjustment in illness: A model for nursing practice. *Journal of Advanced Nursing, 17,* 467–472.

Hymovich, D. P., & Hagopian, G. A. (1992). *Chronic illness in children and adults: A psychosocial approach.* Philadelphia: W. B. Saunders.

Lazarus, R. S. (1966). *Psychological stress and the coping process.* New York: McGraw-Hill.

Lewis, S. M., & Collier, I. C. (1992). *Medical-surgical nursing: Assessment and management of clinical problems* (3rd ed.). St. Louis: C. V. Mosby.
Maslow, A. H. (1968). *Toward a psychology of being*. New York: Van Nostrand Reinhold Company.
McHaffie, H. E. (1992). Coping: An essential element of nursing. *Journal of Advanced Nursing, 17,* 933–940.
Miller, J. F. (1985). Inspiring. *American Journal of Nursing, 85,* 22–25.
Miller, J. F. (1992). *Coping with chronic illness: Overcoming powerlessness* (2nd ed.). Philadelphia: F. A. Davis.
Milliken, M. E. (1993). *Understanding human behavior*. Albany, N.Y.: Delmar Publishers.
Murray, R. B., & Zentner, J. R. (1979). *Nursing assessment and health promotion through the life span*. Englewood Cliffs, N.J.: Prentice-Hall.
Murray, R. B., & Zentner, J. R. (1979). *Nursing concepts for health promotion*. Englewood Cliffs, N.J.: Prentice-Hall.
Pender, N. J. (1987). *Health promotion in nursing practice* (2nd ed.). East Norwalk, CT: Appleton & Lange.
Piaget, J., & Inhelder, B. (1969). *The psychology of the child*. New York: Basic Books.
Potter, P. A., & Perry, A. G. (1991). *Basic nursing: Theory and practice* (2nd ed.). St. Louis: C. V. Mosby.
Rawlins, R. P., Williams, S. R., & Beck, C. K. (1993). *Mental health–psychiatric nursing*. St. Louis: Mosby Year Book.
Rogers, M. E. (1980). *The theoretical basis of nursing*. Philadelphia: F. A. Davis.
Rosdahl, C. B. (1985). *Textbook of basic nursing* (4th ed.). Philadelphia: J. B. Lippincott.
Selye, H. (1978). *The stress of life* (2nd ed.). New York: McGraw-Hill.
Spradley, B. W. (1990). *Community health nursing: Concepts and practices* (3rd ed.). Glenview, IL: Scott, Foresman/Little Brown Higher Ed.
Sullivan, H. S. (1953). *Interpersonal theory of psychiatry*. New York: W. W. Norton & Co.
Taylor, C., Lillis, C., & LeMone, P. (1989). *Fundamentals of nursing*. Philadelphia: J. B. Lippincott.
Townsend, M. C. (1993). *Psychiatric mental health nursing: Concepts of care*. Philadelphia: F. A. Davis.
Werner, E. E. (1979). *Cross-cultural child development: A view from the planet earth*. Monterey, CA: Brook/Cole.
Whaley, L. F., & Wong, D. L. (1991). *Nursing care of infants and children* (4th ed.). St. Louis: C. V. Mosby.

KEY CONCEPTS

1. Individuals' level of health is directly related to their ability to adjust to a variety of internal and external stressors.
2. Stress is necessary for growth and development.
3. A stressor is anything that causes the individual stress, and adaptation to stress affects the entire organism.
4. If individuals are overwhelmed by many stressors or do not have the coping behaviors or problem-solving strategies to maintain equilibrium, illness or crisis may ensue.
5. A crisis is the point at which the individual may move toward illness on the continuum between illness and health and can result in inner tension and anxiety, which may affect an individual's ability to function.
6. Growth refers to a process of development that becomes increasingly complex.
7. Three components of the personality identified by Freud are the id, the ego, and the superego.
8. Anxiety is a painful emotion that results from one's perception of danger, and individuals continually regulate their behavior based on the level of perceived anxiety.
9. Defense mechanisms are strategies used in an effort to diminish anxiety; however, when used excessively they can hinder the developing personality.
10. Behavioral theory is based on the idea that all behavior is a learned response.
11. Each person's response to illness is unique and is based on such subjective experiences as self-concept, perception of threat to body image, or spiritual and cultural values.
12. Illness produces a stressful state that requires individuals to draw from their innate resources or inner strengths.
13. Some people have enough inner strength to cope effectively with illness; others, however, may have ineffective or maladaptive coping abilities.
14. Factors that influence an individual's ability to cope with illness are age, cultural beliefs, spirituality, self-concept, family and community resources, and emotional responses to illness.
15. Specific emotional responses to illness include stress, fear, anxiety, loss, and grief and mourning.
16. Coping is the process of responding to stress or a potential stressor.
17. Coping strategies are conscious, purposeful behaviors that are used to make an unfamiliar situation into one that is perceived as more controllable and predictable.
18. Ineffective coping mechanisms may evolve from a sense of helplessness or powerlessness.
19. A nurse's caring attitude is basic to helping a client cope with illness.

CHAPTER 51

Sheila Kelly
June Schneberger

Psychiatric Disorders

OBJECTIVES

1. Describe the differences between social relationships and therapeutic relationships.
2. Describe key strategies in communicating therapeutically.
3. Describe the categories of the mental status examination.
4. Identify target symptoms and behaviors and side effects for the following types of medications: antianxiety, antipsychotic, and antidepressant drugs.
5. Summarize current thinking about the etiology of schizophrenia and the mood disorders.
6. For each of the following psychiatric disorders, identify key observations in relation to the categories of the mental status examination: anxiety disorders, schizophrenia, mood disorders, organic mental syndromes or disorders, and personality disorders.
7. For each of the following psychiatric disorders, identify primary nursing diagnoses, goals, and interventions: anxiety disorders, schizophrenia, mood disorders, organic mental syndromes or disorders, and personality disorders.

GLOSSARY

BIOLOGIC APPROACH Assumes that mental disorders are related to physiologic changes within the central nervous system

DENIAL A defense mechanism in which particular feelings or specific aspects of reality are excluded from awareness

DEPERSONALIZATION A state of feeling outside of oneself, watching what is happening as if it were to someone else

DISORDER A term used when a definite organic cause such as delirium or dementia is established for behaviors and symptoms (see syndrome)

EXTRAPYRAMIDAL EFFECTS Side effects of antipsychotic drugs on the portion of the central nervous system controlling involuntary movements

INTERPERSONAL APPROACH The patient learns new ways to behave in a therapeutic relationship built on trust

PROJECTION A defense mechanism in which one sees others as a source of one's own unacceptable thoughts, feelings, or impulses

PSYCHOANALYTIC APPROACH Based on the theory that people function at different levels of awareness (conscious to unconscious) and that ego defense mechanisms such as denial and repression are used to prevent anxiety

PSYCHOSIS A state in which a person's perception of reality is impaired, thereby interfering with the capacity to function and to relate to others

SENSORIUM Level of consciousness and orientation to time, place, person, and self

SYNDROME Refers to behaviors and symptoms (see disorder)

TARDIVE DYSKINESIA Frequently irreversible side effect of antipsychotic medication that develops after years of use; symptoms include involuntary movements of face, jaw, and tongue, leading to grimacing, jerky movements of upper extremities, and tonic contractions of neck and back

How people think about and explain mental health and mental illness has varied from one geographic location and culture to another and from one time period to another. For example, in early cultures, mental illness was thought to be caused by supernatural forces, and therefore people used rituals that appealed to these forces for help. In recent years, it has been thought that many factors contribute to the development of a mental illness, and many strategies for helping people with psychiatric disorders are available. Treatment settings vary from inpatient units to outpatient and residential settings; within these settings, many different treatment methods are available that range from individual therapy to group or family therapy to somatic treatments such as medication.

Nurses have the opportunity to work with patients with psychiatric disorders in settings specifically designated for that purpose. However, nurses also work with patients in other health care settings such as medical clinics or intensive care units who may have psychiatric difficulties along with their other health problems.

Nursing interventions are based on a number of different theoretical approaches, which are based on biologic, psychoanalytic, interpersonal, and cognitive behavioral theories. The *biologic* approach assumes that mental disorders are related to particular physiologic changes within the central nervous system. This approach dominates current thinking about psychiatric disorders. The *psychoanalytic* approach is based on the theory that (1) humans function at different levels of awareness, ranging from conscious to unconscious, and (2) people use ego defense mechanisms to prevent anxiety. Some important defense mechanisms are repression, denial, and projection. The *interpersonal* approach has three components: (1) anxiety is often communicated interpersonally, (2) the patient learns new ways of coping or maturing in a therapeutic relationship, and (3) the establishment of trust is an important first step in the nurse's work with patients. Key ideas from the *cognitive behavioral* approach are that behavior is learned, that behavior increases in response to positive consequences (positive reinforcement) or increases in response to the removal of negative stimuli (negative reinforcement), and that particular thoughts influence emotional states.

ESTABLISHING THERAPEUTIC RELATIONSHIPS

In caring for a patient with a psychiatric disorder, nurses establish therapeutic (as opposed to social) relationships (Table 51–1). A range of interpersonal strategies have been found to be particularly helpful in promoting the patient's comfort level with the nurse. They include being available, listening, clarifying, sharing observations, and accepting silence.

TABLE 51-1

THERAPEUTIC RELATIONSHIPS VERSUS SOCIAL RELATIONSHIPS

THERAPEUTIC	SOCIAL
1. Purpose is to benefit the patient.	1. Purpose is to benefit both participants in the relationship.
2. Relationship develops purposefully.	2. Relationship develops spontaneously.
3. Focus on personal and emotional needs of patient.	3. Focus on personal and emotional needs of both participants.
4. Helper has responsibility for evaluating the interaction and the changing behavior.	4. Participants are not formally responsible for evaluating their interaction.
5. Relationship has some boundaries (purpose, place, time) and a clear ending.	5. May or may not be clear boundaries and a clear ending.

Being Available

When with the patient, the nurse's attention should be directed completely to this other human being. Involvement in any other activity, such as reading a newspaper, which might be interpreted by the patient as lack of availability, should be avoided.

Listening

Nurses should be aware of their own thoughts and feelings. Their feelings are an important source of data because nurses may experience a wide range of feelings while interacting with patients. If they are aware of these feelings, they will be able to control their own response. Listening is done by experiencing the patient and by refraining from thinking of responses to the patient when the patient is speaking.

Clarifying

Asking questions may help patients clarify thoughts. For example, the nurse might state, "I'm not sure what you mean by 'the world is falling apart.'"

Sharing Observations

Patients benefit from knowing what nurses see and hear while listening. For example, the nurse might say, "You are saying that your life is falling apart and you are also smiling." This statement provides the patient with input that verbal and nonverbal behaviors are not congruent. Such input might lead to the patient's discovery of smiling as a coping mechanism.

Accepting Silence

Nurses must be comfortable with periods of silence. Silence enables patients to consider their own thoughts as well as the communication of the nurse.

NURSING ASSESSMENT OF THE PSYCHIATRIC PATIENT

A major feature of a complete health assessment of a psychiatric patient is the mental status examination. This examination is usually conducted as part of the admission process and throughout the treatment. It consists of observations regarding appearance, mood and affect, speech and language, thought content, perceptual disturbances, insight and judgment, sensorium, and memory and attention (Table 51–2). Each of the areas under examination includes specific descriptors that are addressed as a part of the mental status examination.

Nursing diagnoses, identified from health assessment data, are suggested for each major psychiatric disorder. Etiologies or related factors for each diagnosis have not been included in this chapter because there has been little agreement among mental health nursing investigators about them and they have not been approved by the North American Nursing Diagnosis Association.

MENTAL STATUS EXAMINATION

Appearance

The first step in a mental status examination is to observe how a person looks. The following observations should be made:

- Appearance in relation to stated age
- Appropriateness of clothing in relation to patient's particular peer group or subculture
- Personal hygiene
- Any unusual physical characteristics

Activity

A recent change in the patient's activity level (increase or decrease) should be assessed. Other types of activity that are observed include the following:

TABLE 51–2
COMPONENTS OF THE MENTAL STATUS EXAMINATION

Appearance	Age, clothing, personal hygiene, unusual physical characteristics
Activity	Recent change in activity level, hyperactivity, agitation, psychomotor retardation, repetitive mannerisms, stereotypes
Mood and affect	Happiness, sadness, worry; constricted or expanded feelings; intensity; lability; appropriateness
Speech and language	Mutism, paucity, pressured speech, tangential speech, blocking, loose associations, word salad
Thought content	Obsessions, compulsions, phobias, delusions
Perceptual disturbances	Illusions, hallucinations
Insight and judgment	Potential for suicide
Sensorium	Orientation to time, place, person; level of consciousness
Memory and attention	Remote and recent memory; attention; calculation
General intellectual level	Vocabulary; knowledge of current events; abstract thinking

- Hyperactivity, which is a level considerably above average purposeful activity
- Agitation, which is purposeless activity, such as wringing of hands, pacing, picking at clothing, foot tapping
- Psychomotor retardation, which is a decrease in movement, thinking, and speaking
- Repetitive movements that are part of a purposeful activity (mannerisms)
- Repetitive movements that are not part of purposeful activity (stereotypes)

Mood and Affect

Mood is a feeling state that a patient experiences over a long period of time. *Affect* is a briefly occurring feeling such as happiness, sadness, and worry. Feelings may be *constricted,* meaning that a person is experiencing very few feelings, or *expanded,* meaning that a person is experiencing a greater number of feelings than usual. The intensity of feelings may be increased or decreased (diminished). Feelings also may be stable or consistent rather than labile or rapidly changing.

The appropriateness of affect is another area that should be assessed. Appropriateness of affect is the degree of fit between the actual feelings and the way they are expressed. Inappropriate affect is the incongruence (poor fit) between the feelings appropriate to the situation and the way they are expressed (e.g., "My dog just died," she said with a smile).

Speech and Language

Assessment includes observations of speech and language. Characteristics of speech with a mental illness include *mutism* (not speaking), long pauses before responding, minimal or very little speech *(paucity),* and *pressured speech* (loud and insistent). *Tangential speech* may be noted, which means that a patient starts out toward a particular point but veers away and never reaches the point. *Blocking* may occur, which is stopping speaking before reaching the point. *Loose associations,* or a continual shifting from topic to unrelated topic, and *word salad,* or shifting topics to the point of incoherence, also may be noted.

Thought Content

Thought content includes the following areas of assessment:

- *Obsessions*—repetitious, unwanted thoughts
- *Compulsions*—actions repeatedly carried out in a specific manner that typically include washing, counting, or checking
- *Phobias*—unrealistic fears of specific objects or situations
- *Delusions*—false ideas not based on reality and not congruent with the patient's specific religious and cultural orientation

Obsessions and compulsions are often closely related.

Perceptual Disturbances

Perceptual disturbances may involve any one of senses such as vision, hearing, taste, touch, and smell. One type of perceptual disturbance is an *illusion,* in which a specific stimulus, like a spot on the wall, is misinterpreted (e.g., a spot is perceived as a bug). Another is a *hallucination,* which is a sensory experience that occurs without an external stimulus (e.g., a person sees nonexistent bugs crawling on the floor or feels nonexistent bugs crawling on the skin).

Insight and Judgment

Insight is a clear understanding of the significance of one's own symptoms and behavior, and *judgment* is the soundness of proposed actions in relation to one's particular background. Insight and judgment are often considered in relation to suicide potential. Suicide potential is assessed by asking questions about patients' thoughts about taking their own life, whether there is a specific plan to commit suicide and whether there are the means to carry out the plan. For example, if a man is thinking about killing himself with a gun, it should be determined whether a gun is available to him.

Sensorium

Assessment of sensorium focuses on orientation in terms of time, place, person, and self. This is done by asking the patient direct questions (e.g., "What time is it now?" or "What day is today?"; "Where are we now?"; "Tell me your name."). The patient's *level of consciousness* also is assessed. There are four levels of consciousness: (1) comatose, (2) stuporous, (3) drowsy, and (4) alert.

Memory and Attention

Remote memory (distant past) is assessed by comparing the patient's memory of past events with what is recalled by other reliable historians. *Recent memory,* or the ability to recall new information, is tested by asking the patient to learn three unrelated words and to recall these words 5 minutes later. A quick way to determine recent memory is to ask what was eaten at the previous meal. *Attention,* as well as ability to *calculate,* an aspect of general intellectual level, may be tested by asking the patient to subtract 7's from 100 or 3's from 20 or to spell a word like *world* backwards.

General Intellectual Level

The general intellectual level is assessed by determining the patient's vocabulary and knowledge of current events. For example, the patient is asked the name of the president of the United States and the name of the previous president. Abstract thinking is another area of general intellectual level. It is assessed by asking the patient to identify the common element of two objects such as a banana and an apple (e.g., "What do a banana and an apple have in common?") or asking the patient to interpret proverbs (e.g., "What does 'A rolling stone gathers no moss' mean?").

ANXIETY DISORDERS

A patient with an *anxiety disorder* either experiences the highly uncomfortable feeling of anxiety directly or experiences a symptom like compulsive hand washing that prevents or reduces the occurrence of anxiety. Common *physical* signs and symptoms of anxiety are increased heart rate, elevated blood pressure, sweaty palms, trembling, urinary frequency, diarrhea, a tight sensation in the chest, and difficulty breathing. *Psychological* manifestations often include irritability, restlessness, tearfulness, thought blocking, and lack of concentration.

Anxiety is experienced on various levels, ranging from mild to panic stages, depending on each person's subjective experience and ability to cope. Mild anxiety can be useful. It may motivate a person to take constructive action or focus attention on a particular task (such as concentrating on an examination). Moderate anxiety often is considered the optimal level for learning to take place. As anxiety progresses to severe or panic levels, however, an individual's ability to think clearly and to solve problems becomes progressively impaired. A person in a panic state may misperceive surrounding events altogether and may react impulsively by running or striking out. This may explain instances in which individuals jump from burning buildings in spite of imminent rescue.

All people experience anxiety. For most people, it is episodic and does not interfere greatly with day-to-day functioning. Even normally well-adjusted people can experience anxiety of panic proportions under significant stress. If anxiety persists at a high level for an extended period and causes significant interference with daily functioning, the person usually is determined to have an anxiety disorder. Examples of anxiety disorders are panic disorder, agoraphobia, obsessive-compulsive disorder, and posttraumatic stress disorder.

Panic Disorder

In *panic disorder,* the person experiences recurrent panic attacks, which are intense episodes of apprehension of variable length, at times to the point of terror, and are often accompanied by the feeling of impending doom. No triggering event can be identified. Severe physical symptoms of severe anxiety also are present. This disorder often is considered of biologic origins as it tends to run in families.

Agoraphobia

The person with *agoraphobia* is extremely fearful of situations outside the home from which escape may be difficult or in which help may be unavailable. Typically the person copes by avoiding the anxiety-producing situation, often becoming progressively reclusive and very dependent on family and friends.

Obsessive-Compulsive Disorder

Obsessive-compulsive disorder involves recurrent obsessions (thoughts) or compulsions (behaviors), or both, that produce distress and interfere with functioning. Obsessions frequently involve intrusive thoughts that a person cannot stop about unpleasant or violent acts, such as repeatedly imagining hurting a family member. Compulsive behaviors typically evolve as a way to reduce the anxiety experienced as a result of obsessive thoughts. Examples of compulsions are hand washing, counting, and checking (e.g., repeated checking to see whether the door is locked). The person experiencing obsessions and compulsions knows these thoughts and behaviors are not "normal" and often is embarrassed by them. However, if the compulsion is resisted, the anxiety that the individual experiences is too overwhelming to handle.

Research has found that neurochemical imbalances also may play a role in the origin of this disorder. Many people with obsessive-compulsive disorders have become symptom free once therapeutic levels of particular antidepressant drugs (selective serotonin re-uptake inhibitors such as Prozac) have been reached. This phenomenon suggests that the onset of the disorder may be physiologic, at least some of the time, rather than a response to some unresolved unconscious conflict as previously believed.

Posttraumatic Stress Disorder

Posttraumatic stress disorder is a cluster of symptoms experienced following a distressing event that is outside the range of normal events (e.g., watching one's family being murdered). Examples of symptoms include re-experiencing the trauma through repeated and intrusive recall of the event (at times as a flashback); avoiding situations that in some way remind the person of the event; feeling detached from other people; and having a heightened sense of arousal, which is experienced as difficulty falling asleep, hypervigilance, exaggerated startle, or a combination of these.

SOMATOFORM DISORDERS

An individual with one of the *somatoform* disorders experiences physical symptoms without having actual physiologic dysfunction. In other words, anxiety is thought to be converted into physical symptoms. Examples include conversion disorder and hypochondriasis.

Conversion Disorder

In *conversion disorder,* symptoms may include blindness, deafness, or paralysis of the legs without a physiologic cause. Usually the symptoms are neurologic and occur in response to some threatening or traumatic event. The symptoms are real and not made up—individuals exhibit a characteristic lack of concern regarding their condition.

Hypochondriasis

In *hypochondriasis,* individuals are convinced that they have a serious medical problem in spite of the absence of any concrete medical findings. They will seek other opinions if one physician does not validate their concerns and often take multiple prescriptions from various physicians. In both conversion disorder and hypochondriasis, the person is not consciously aware of the conflict that is the true source of the physical symptoms.

DISSOCIATIVE DISORDERS

Dissociative disorders involve a change in identity, memory, or consciousness. The change may be sudden or gradual, transient or over a long period, and is thought to be an escape from anxiety. In a sense, persons unconsciously dissociate or remove themselves psychologically from anxiety-provoking situations because they are too much to bear. Even "normal" individuals may experience *depersonalization* under severe stress. In this case, persons feel they are outside themselves or floating overhead watching what is happening as if it were to someone else. Examples of dissociative disorders include amnesia or multiple personality disorder.

Multiple personality disorder is a relatively rare dissociative disorder in which two or more distinct personalities exist within the person and at least two personalities repeatedly alternate having full consciousness. Legal identity is retained by the "host personality." Other personalities within the body are called "alter personalities." Most patients with multiple personality disorders report severe childhood abuse, including physical, sexual, or ritual cult abuse. Women are five times more likely to have the disorder than men. An inherited predisposition to the occurrence of multiple personality disorder under extreme stress has been supposed.

Medical Treatment

DRUG THERAPY. The primary antianxiety medications are the benzodiazepines (e.g., diazepam [Valium], chlordiazepoxide hydrochloride [Librium], and newer benzodiazepines such as lorazepam [Ativan], alprazolam [Xanax], and clonazepam [Klonopin]). See Table 51–3. They are usually prescribed for brief periods. Side effects are those associated with sedation such as drowsiness, fatigue, dizziness, and confusion. Because physical and psychological dependence occur, withdrawal from the medication should be medically supervised.

TABLE 51-3
SELECTED ANTIANXIETY MEDICATIONS

MEDICATION: GENERIC (BRAND)	TARGET SYMPTOMS/BEHAVIOR	SIDE EFFECTS FOR ALL
Alprazolam (Xanax)	Anxiety	Drowsiness, incoordination, fatigue, confusion, dizziness, blurred vision, dry mouth, urticaria, rash, photosensitivity, physical and psychological dependence
Lorazepam (Ativan)	Anxiety, insomnia	
Oxazepam (Serax)	Anxiety	
Diazepam (Valium)	Anxiety	
Triazolam (Halcion)	Insomnia	

PHARMACOLOGY CAPSULE

Antianxiety medications, given for anxiety disorders or as an adjunct medication for schizophrenia, may have side efffects such as drowsiness, incoordination, fatigue, confusion, blurred vision, and psychological dependence.

Nursing Care of the Patient with an Anxiety Disorder, Somatoform Disorder, or Dissociative Disorder

ASSESSMENT. The nurse determines the presence of and level of anxiety (mild, moderate, severe, or panic) from the patient's report of symptoms, from observing behavior, or from both. Particularly relevant mental status examination categories include activity, speech and language, and thought content.

NURSING DIAGNOSIS. Key nursing diagnoses include anxiety and ineffective individual coping.

GOALS. Goals may include decreasing anxiety to the point at which problem solving can occur, labeling symptoms as those of anxiety, recognizing habitual nonconstructive ways of decreasing anxiety, identifying what led to the experience of anxiety, and learning ways to control anxiety more effectively when it is increasing (or escalating) such as relaxation techniques.

INTERVENTIONS. Strategies to help patients decrease their anxiety from a panic state or a severe level to a mild level center around the nurse remaining calm, speaking firmly with short, simple instructions (e.g., sit down with me here), and walking to a less stimulating area of the unit. Once anxiety is lowered to a manageable level, the nurse assists patients in exploring what happened, clarifying their usual way of relieving anxiety (e.g., anger or somatic symptoms instead of experiencing more typical anxiety symptoms), and identifying what triggered the anxiety (e.g., feelings of self-doubt regarding finding employment after discharge). The nurse can assist clients in problem-solving decisions and can teach ways to prevent and manage increasing anxiety in the future. Useful techniques include relaxation techniques, warm baths, positive self-talk, and physical exercise.

SCHIZOPHRENIA

Schizophrenia is a very serious, usually chronic group of thought disorders in which a patient's ability to interpret the world accurately is impaired by psychotic symptoms. Typical symptoms include impaired thinking patterns, delusions, hallucinations, bizarre behavior, and emotional responses that do not coincide with events occurring around them. The patient's level of functioning deteriorates significantly during acute episodes; indicating a need for intensive treatment, which usually includes psychiatric hospitalization and antipsychotic medications.

Typically schizophrenic patients have functioned normally in early life; they often are very intelligent and well educated before the onset of the first symptoms. The symptoms usually begin in adolescence or early adulthood; however, some types of schizophrenic disorders are more often diagnosed in later life. The patient's ability to function in areas of work, interpersonal relationships, or self-care seldom returns to baseline after the first psychotic episode. With each subsequent episode, the ability to function independently continues to deteriorate, intelligence quotient (IQ) levels drop, and thinking becomes very concrete. Patients are unable to tolerate even the typical stressors of daily living.

In one research study, the brains of chronic schizophrenics were examined after death. It was observed

POSTTRAUMATIC STRESS DISORDER: A CLINICAL EXAMPLE

Patrick T was admitted to the psychiatric inpatient unit with the diagnosis of posttraumatic stress disorder. Two months before admission, he and his co-worker friend were in a truck accident on an overpass. Patrick watched in horror as his friend fell out of the truck, which was hanging over the edge. The fall killed his friend instantly. Patrick was able to climb out of the passenger side and sustained injuries to his back and legs. He has been receiving physical therapy for his injuries. For the past 2 weeks he has been continually preoccupied by the event, has had insomnia, repeatedly says that he should have been the one to die, becomes easily irritable, does not show feelings when with others, and has an exaggerated startle reflex. The nurse assigned to work with Patrick found him pacing. She remained with him as he paced. The following nursing diagnoses were immediately relevant: anxiety, altered sleep pattern, and dysfunctional grieving. Patrick and the nurse decided together that priorities were to decrease his anxiety and to improve sleep. Patrick was willing to learn a progressive relaxation exercise (which involves relaxing one group of muscles at a time until the body is relaxed). After learning the exercise, Patrick worked on deep abdominal breathing and agreed to use this strategy when he found himself preoccupied with the accident. The nurse had in mind that in future contacts she would listen carefully if Patrick relived the accident and would encourage expression of feelings.

that the ventricles of the brain were enlarged whereas brain tissues correlated to higher level thinking had atrophied. This finding supports the consequences involving the loss of capacity to think and function independently that are seen with most of the patients diagnosed with this disease.

Etiology and Risk Factors

The cause of schizophrenia is not certain. The model that integrates diverse potential causative factors states that patients who are most vulnerable to acquiring the disorder encounter factors (stress) that precipitate the disorder. The model is called the *stress-diathesis model.* Researchers have established that people with schizophrenia probably were genetically vulnerable to the disorder. The range of biologic factors being investigated include (1) neurotransmitters and their receptors, including dopamine; norepinephrine; and gamma amino butyric acid; (2) structural abnormalities such as degeneration of the limbic system, enlargement of the lateral and third ventricles, and loss of neurons in the temporal lobe; (3) infectious agents; and (4) hormonal dysregulation.

Since the early 1980s, some investigators have proposed two types of schizophrenia: type I, which incorporates all the positive symptoms such as hallucinations, and type II, which includes those symptoms based on lacks or deficits, such as lack of motivation. In addition to biologic approaches, theorists have attempted to explain schizophrenia with concepts from psychoanalytic theory, learning theory, family theory, and social theories. It is possible that social factors play a larger role in the way the disorder develops and its course than in the initial cause of schizophrenia.

In men, the disorder usually first occurs between 15 and 25 years of age. The usual age range for first occurrence in women is 25 to 35. There is no difference in rate by gender. The incidence in the United States and Europe is between 0.3 and 0.6 per 1000. People with schizophrenia have psychotic symptoms. Psychosis is a state in which a person has distorted perceptions of reality. Some of the symptoms that support the diagnosis of schizophrenia include delusions, hallucinations, marked loosening of associations, catatonia (characterized by stupor or excitement), and flat or very inappropriate affect. In addition, the person functions at a level lower than the highest level previously achieved in the areas of work, social relations, or self-care. Fifty percent of all mental hospital beds are occupied by patients with schizophrenia. Forty to 60% of people with schizophrenia are readmitted within a 2-year period after discharge from their first hospitalization. It has been estimated that two thirds of all homeless people have schizophrenia. Fifty percent of people with schizophrenia attempt suicide; 10% complete a suicide during a 20-year follow-up period.

Medical Treatment

DRUG THERAPY. The most commonly administered medications for people with schizophrenia are antipsychotic medications and antiparkinsonian medications, which are at times administered to prevent or relieve some of the side effects of the antipsychotics (Table 51–4). Antianxiety medications also may be administered in conjunction with the antipsychotics to decrease agitation.

The nurse is responsible for observing and recording accurately all data relevant to the target behaviors and symptoms of the medications as well as the untoward effects. There are a variety of potential side effects, some of which have rapid onset and require prompt treatment.

An example is orthostatic hypotension (or postural hypotension), which is a drop in blood pressure when a person changes position from lying down to sitting or sitting to standing. A more precise definition incorporates (1) a fall in systolic blood pressure of between 10 and 25 mm Hg, (2) a fall in diastolic blood pressure of between 5 and 10 mm Hg, and (3) symptoms of deficits in cerebral perfusion such as dizziness and increase in heart rate of 5 to 20 beats per minute. This problem, which creates a risk for falls, occurs most frequently in the early weeks of treatment and is more common in the morning, after the patient has been in bed during the night, as well as following a large meal. The following guidelines have been recommended for measuring orthostatic hypotension: (1) Take supine blood pressure and pulse after the patient has been supine for 5 to 20 minutes; (2) assist the patient to an upright position, observing for symptoms of dizziness; (3) wait 30 seconds to 1 minute and retake blood pressure and pulse; (4) wait 2 minutes and retake, as the development of hypotension may have been delayed. Once the problem has been established, treatment includes elastic hose, gradual changes in position, and coffee before arising.

Another group of side effects is referred to as *extrapyramidal* effects, stemming from the impact of the antipsychotics on the extrapyramidal tracts of the central nervous system. These tracts play a role in the control of involuntary movements. The different extrapyramidal side effects occur at different periods in the course of medication therapy.

Acute dystonic reactions may occur after one dose of

TABLE 51–4
SELECTED ANTIPSYCHOTIC MEDICATIONS

MEDICATION: GENERIC (BRAND)	SIDE EFFECTS
Chlorpromazine (Thorazine) Thioridazine hydrochloride (Mellaril) Fluphenazine hydrochloride (Prolixin) Thiothixene (Navane) Haloperidol (Haldol) Clozapine (Clozaril) (Extrapyramidal problems not likely to occur)	Extrapyramidal: acute dystonia, akathisia, pseudoparkinsonism, tardive dyskinesia Anticholinergic: dry mouth, blurred vision, delayed micturition, constipation Other: sedation, neuroleptic malignant syndrome, agranulocytosis, postural hypotension, decreased seizure threshold

medication or during the first few days of treatment. The reactions consist of severe muscle contractions involving the tongue, face, neck (torticollis), and back (opisthotonos). The larynx also may be constricted (laryngospasm). The reaction is reversed with benztropine mesylate (Cogentin) 1 to 2 mg, intramuscular or intravenous, or diphenhydramine hydrochloride (Benadryl), 20 to 50 mg, administered intravenously.

After 1 to 2 weeks of treatment with antipsychotic medications, the *parkinsonian syndrome* consisting of mask-like face, rigid posture, shuffling gait, and resting tremor may occur. Extrapyramidal syndromes during later treatment are akathisia, a reversible restlessness manifested as having an urge to pace and having difficulty sitting still, and tardive dyskinesia. Tardive dyskinesia is a frequently irreversible syndrome, which may occur after years of antipsychotic drug therapy and which consists of involuntary movements of face, jaw, and tongue leading to grimacing, jerky movements of upper extremities, and tonic contractions of neck and back.

Neuroleptic malignant syndrome occurs in 1% of people receiving neuroleptic agents (including antipsychotics, antiemetics, lithium, and antidepressants); mortality rates reported for people with this condition range between 14 and 30%. It is an extrapyramidal problem that may occur after only one dose of a medication as well as after years of receiving the medication. The first symptom is usually muscular rigidity accompanied by akinesia (emotional unresponsiveness and blunted affect) and respiratory distress, but the cardinal sign is hyperthermia (101–103°F or higher).

Another example is agranulocytosis, an extreme decrease in granulated white blood cells, which is frequently manifested with a sore throat and fever.

It is clear that in monitoring the patient for side effects, a wide range of data is relevant from vital signs to facial expression. The nurse pays close attention to all patient descriptions of symptoms.

PHARMACOLOGY CAPSULE

After a period of time, patients taking traditional neuroleptic medications almost always experience extrapyramidal side effects such as akathisia, pseudo-parkinsonism, or tardive dyskinesia.

Nursing Care of the Patient with Schizophrenia

ASSESSMENT. In completing the mental status examination, observe the following: (1) *appearance:* may have poor grooming and failure to bathe; (2) *activity:* may exhibit agitation, bizarre postures, catatonic excitement or stupor, mannerisms or stereotypes, or stiff body movements; (3) *mood and affect:* may have flat affect or inappropriate rage or happiness; (4) *speech and language:* mutism, tangential speech, blocking, or loose associations; (5) *thought content:* delusions that may include persecutory, grandiose, religious, or somatic; (6) *perceptual disturbances:* auditory hallucinations most common and visual hallucinations second most frequent; (7) *insight and judgment:* usually little insight into illness; (8) *sensorium:* oriented to person, place, and time; (9) *memory:* usually intact but difficulties with attention make assessment difficult.

NURSING DIAGNOSIS. Nursing diagnoses for the patient with schizophrenia are most likely to include the following:

- **Altered Thought Processes**
- **Sensory Perceptual Alterations** (auditory, visual)
- **Impaired Verbal Communication**
- **Self-Care Deficit**

Additional possible nursing diagnoses associated with schizophrenia are anxiety, social isolation, and ineffective individual coping.

GOALS. Possible goals are that the patient make connections between episodes of "false beliefs" and precipitating anxiety-provoking situations and that the patient make the distinction between delusions and reality; describe the content of the hallucination, identifying stressors precipitating the hallucinatory experience, and not attend to the hallucination; initiate a discussion of problematic symptoms or experience with the nurse and express thoughts clearly; and perform activities of daily living with maximum independence in relation to level of ability.

INTERVENTIONS

Altered Thought Processes. Nursing interventions include focusing on reality (real events and real people), letting the patient know that the nurse does not share the delusion, encouraging the patient to express feelings and anxiety, and connecting delusions with anxiety-provoking situations (see interventions for anxiety).

Sensory Perceptual Alterations. Interventions include making brief, frequent contacts with the patient (to interrupt hallucinatory experiences), encouraging the patient to pay attention to what is occurring in the environment (instead of external stimuli), encouraging involvement in activities, and informing patients that hallucinations are part of the disease process.

Impaired Verbal Communication. Interventions may include seeking clarification and verbalizing the implied, which may be useful if the patient is not speaking (e.g., "It must have been difficult for you when your father didn't come today after he told you he would visit.").

Self-Care Deficit. Possible interventions include providing recognition for all constructive self-care actions ("I see you've bathed and washed your hair.") demonstrating how to perform an activity if necessary, intervening to assist when necessary, offering cans of food for the patient to open, or serving family-style if the patient believes food has been poisoned.

MOOD DISORDERS

People with mood disorders experience an elevated mood or a depressed mood. Over time, some people experience both elevated mood and depressed mood. An episode of depressed mood is referred to as *unipolar depression.* The condition of having an elevated mood is called a *manic episode.* Having episodes of both depressed mood and elevated mood is termed *bipolar disorder.*

Unipolar depression is one of the most common psychiatric disorders, with a lifetime prevalence of 6%. The mean age for the occurrence of depression is 40. About twice as many women as men are diagnosed with unipolar depression. People who are single, divorced, or lacking in close relationships are more vulnerable. There is no association between prevalence of unipolar depression and race or between unipolar depression and socioeconomic status.

For bipolar disorder, the lifetime prevalence is 1%, with the mean age of onset being 30. There are similar rates for men and women, and the rates are higher among single and divorced people. People in higher socioeconomic groups as well as people with lower levels of education have higher rates of bipolar disorder.

Etiology and Risk Factors

Definite causes of mood disorders have not been established. Probable etiologic factors include neurotransmitter dysregulation, neuroendocrine dysfunctions, genetic factors, loss of significant others, learned helplessness, and negative thoughts about life experiences.

Medical Treatment

DRUG THERAPY. There are three types of antidepressant medications: tricyclic antidepressants, second-generation antidepressants, and monoamine oxidase (MAO) inhibitors (Table 51–5). The nurse administering medications is responsible for ensuring that medication has been swallowed, as opposed to being held in the mouth and later discarded or saved for an overdose. As the patient responds to antidepressant medication and the energy level increases, the risk of suicide also increases. Monoamine oxidase inhibitors are sometimes prescribed for patients who are resistant to the tricyclics, are phobic, or have hypochondriasis. A 2-week period should occur between ending a tricyclic and beginning an MAO inhibitor. Very serious side effects of hypertensive crisis occurs if the patient taking an MAO inhibitor ingests tyramine-containing food or drink: avocados, bananas, beer, bologna, canned figs, chocolate, cheese (except cottage cheese), liver, papaya products, paté, herring, fava beans, raisins, salami, sausage, sour cream, soy sauce, wine, and yogurt. These foods also must be avoided for 3 weeks after stopping treatment

TABLE 51–5
SELECTED ANTIDEPRESSANT MEDICATIONS

MEDICATION: GENERIC (BRAND)	TARGET SYMPTOMS	SIDE EFFECTS
Amitriptyline (Elavil) Imipramine hydrochloride (Tofranil) Trazodone hydrochloride (Desyrel) Bupropion hydrochloride (Wellbutrin) Fluoxetine hydrochloride (Prozac)	Depression	Central nervous system: drowsiness, fatigue, lethargy Cardiovascular: postural hypotension, conduction arrhythmias Anticholinergic: dry mouth, blurred vision, constipation, urinary retention
Monoamine oxidase inhibitors		Above side effects plus hypertensive crisis if tyramine ingested.
Isocarboxazid (Marplan)	Depression	
Phenelzine sulfate (Nardil)	Phobias	
Tranylcypromine sulfate (Parnate)	Hypochondriasis	

with an MAO inhibitor. Symptoms of a hypertensive crisis, which requires immediate treatment, include headache, palpitations, visual changes, neck stiffness, nausea, vomiting, sweating, sensitivity to light, pupil changes, and bradycardia or tachycardia.

PHARMACOLOGY CAPSULE

Side effects of tricyclic antidepressant medications are drowsiness, fatigue, postural hypotension, dry mouth, blurred vision, urinary retention, and constipation.

ELECTROCONVULSIVE THERAPY. Electroconvulsive therapy is a controversial form of therapy in which an electrical current is introduced to the brain through electrodes placed on the temples. The electrical current produces a grand mal seizure. This type of therapy is most often prescribed when other forms of therapy have failed with people who are severely depressed. Key nursing interventions include making certain that the patient takes nothing by mouth on the morning of a treatment, asking the patient to void and to remove eyeglasses or contact lenses and dentures, administering atropine sulfate as ordered (to decrease secretions), positioning the patient on the side following the procedure to prevent aspiration, monitoring vital signs, remaining with the patient until the patient is awake, and providing orienting information as needed (e.g., "It's 10 A.M. Wednesday, and you just finished your treatment."). Temporary memory loss and confusion are possible side effects of electroconvulsive therapy, and instances of prolonged memory loss have occurred.

Nursing Care of the Patient with Unipolar Depression

ASSESSMENT. In completing the mental status examination of a patient who has depression, the nurse may observe the following: (1) *activity:* is likely to exhibit psychomotor retardation and possibly no spontaneous movements with a downcast gaze, although may exhibit agitation (e.g., hand wringing and hair pulling) especially if elderly; (2) *mood and affect:* may or may not have depressed feelings and may not appear depressed; (3) *speech and language:* speech volume and rate may be decreased, response to questions may be delayed, and mutism may be present; (4) *thought content:* generally negative view of self and world; may ruminate about loss, guilt, and suicide and if psychotic depression, may have delusions of guilt, failure, worthlessness, or terminal illnesses; (5) *insight and judgment:* suicidal ideation in two thirds of depressed patients with 10 to 15% committing suicide successfully; suicide risk increases as patient gains energy needed to commit suicide; insight into illness may be impaired due to negative perceptions of reality; (6) *sensorium:* oriented but may not have energy to answer questions; (7) *memory and attention:* patients commonly complain of impaired concentration and forgetfulness.

NURSING DIAGNOSIS. Nursing diagnoses for the patient with depression may include the following:

- **High Risk for Self-Directed Violence**
- **Self-Esteem Disturbance**
- **Altered Nutrition: Less than Body Requirements**
- **Sleep Pattern Disturbance**

GOALS. Possible goals are that the patient seek out a staff member if experiences urge to harm self; develop coping skills to replace the self-destructive behavior; develop acceptable ways of expressing anger, rage, and hostility; mobilize social support systems; accept own body, have positive feelings about self, identify negative thoughts about self, and identify aspects of self he or she likes; gain weight steadily and experience higher energy; and sleep within 30 minutes of retiring and remain asleep for 6 to 8 uninterrupted hours (see Care Plan: Care of the Patient with Unipolar Depression).

INTERVENTIONS

High Risk for Self-Directed Violence. Interventions may include establishing a no-harm contract, frequently assessing a patient's suicidal potential (see questions under assessment at beginning of chapter) and taking necessary suicide precautions, removing dangerous objects such as pantyhose and belts, maintaining continuous one-to-one contact if indicated, encouraging honest expression of feelings, assisting in identifying symbols of hope in patient's life, identifying community resources for times of crisis, and communicating message that the patient is worthwhile.

Self-Esteem Disturbance. Interventions may include helping the patient to identify positive aspects and limitations regarding his or her body; to like the body despite imperfections; to improve hygiene, grooming, and posture, which makes positive affirmations about self; to limit self-criticism; to be aware of negative self-statements; to learn to give and receive compliments; and to develop social skills.

Altered Nutrition: Less than Body Requirements. Possible interventions are involving dietitian in planning adequate diet, documenting intake, determining food preferences and attempting to satisfy these preferences, and offering small, frequent meals.

Sleep Pattern Disturbance. Interventions are discouraging sleep during the day, providing sleep-producing measures like small snacks and warm baths, and teaching relaxation exercises to be used before retiring.

Nursing Care of the Patient with Manic Episodes

ASSESSMENT. The nurse may observe the following: (1) *appearance:* dress often inappropriate (e.g., bright nonmatching colors, excessive makeup and jewelry); (2) *activity:* hyperactive; (3) *mood, affect, and feelings:* although frequently euphoric may also be very irritable, angry and hostile based on low frustration tolerance, and emotionally labile; (4) *speech and language:* talkative pressured speech, which is difficult to interrupt; flight of ideas (continuous rapid shift from one topic to another); rate and volume increased; (5) *thought content:* themes of self-confidence and self-aggrandizement and possibly delusions of grandeur (e.g., false belief that one has great wealth or power) or delusions of persecution; (6) *sensory perception:* hallucinations may occur; (7) *insight and judgment:* often little insight regarding illness; judgment impaired as evidenced by actions such as large spending sprees, sexual activities incongruent with usual behavior, suicide attempts, and homicide attempts.

NURSING DIAGNOSIS. Possible nursing diagnoses include the following:

- **High Risk for Injury**
- **High Risk for Violence Directed at Others**
- **Altered Nutrition: Less than Body Requirements**
- **Sleep Pattern Disturbance**

GOALS. Possible goals are that the patient does not exhibit potentially injurious movement; does not harm other people and verbalizes anger appropriately; consumes necessary daily nutrients in a form that is appropriate for his or her manic state (like finger food); and sleeps at least 6 uninterrupted hours.

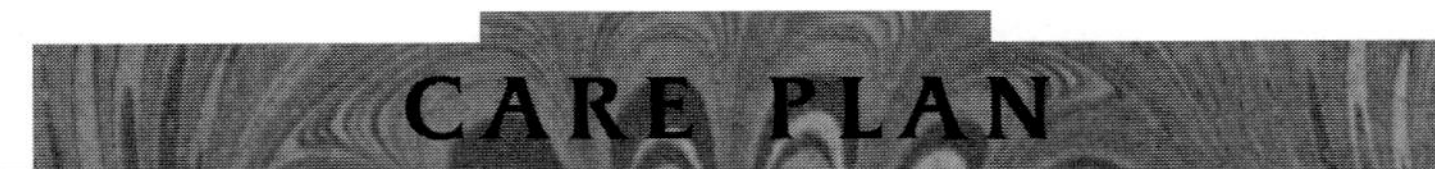

Care of the Patient with Unipolar Depression

ASSESSMENT

Health History: A 53-year-old woman was admitted to a psychiatric hospital with a diagnosis of unipolar depression. During the past few weeks she has become increasingly listless, apathetic, and disinterested in anyone or anything. She cries frequently, and life has not seemed to be worth living. She complains that she cannot sleep and has no appetite. She frequently talks about wanting to commit suicide. She was referred to a psychiatrist, who recommended that she be admitted to the hospital for treatment.

Physical Examination: Blood pressure, 110/70; pulse, 78; respiration, 22; temperature, 98.8°F orally. Height, 5′4″. Weight, 120 lb. Appears apathetic, sad, and cries frequently. Somewhat disheveled. Gaunt and tired looking.

NURSING DIAGNOSIS	GOALS AND OUTCOME CRITERIA	INTERVENTIONS
High risk for self-violence related to suicidal feelings	The patient will not harm herself as evidenced by seeking out nursing staff if she experiences the urge to harm herself, developing coping skills to replace self-destructive behavior, developing acceptable ways to express anger, rage, and hostility.	Establish a no-harm contract; frequently assess patient's suicidal potential and take necessary suicide precautions; remove dangerous objects from the environment; maintain continuous one-to-one contact; encourage honest expression of feelings; assist in identifying symbols of hope in patient's life.
Self-esteem disturbance related to depression	The patient will maintain self-esteem as evidenced by acceptance of own body, identification of negative thoughts about self, and identification of aspects of self she likes.	Help patient to identify positive aspects and limitations regarding her body and to accept her body regardless of limitations; encourage patient to improve hygiene; assist patient to accept compliments and to limit self-criticism.
Altered nutrition: less than body requirements related to anorexia or lack of interest in food	Patient will gain weight and experience higher energy as evidenced by more participation in activities and interactions with others.	Involve dietician in planning adequate diet; determine food preferences and attempt to satisfy preferences; offer small, frequent meals.
Sleep pattern disturbance related to depression relapse	Patient will sleep within 30 minutes of retiring and remain asleep for 6 to 8 uninterrupted hours.	Provide sleep-producing measures like small snacks, warm baths and relaxation exercises before retiring.

INTERVENTIONS

High Risk for Injury. Interventions include decreasing environmental stimuli (e.g., a quiet room, simply decorated), discouraging group activities, encouraging a few one-to-one contacts, removing hazardous objects and substances from the environment, and providing structure that includes physical activities such as brisk walks.

High Risk for Violence Directed at Others. Interventions include decreasing environmental stimuli, observing the patient frequently, removing harmful objects, finding physical outlets, demonstrating a show of strength if necessary, administering prescribed medications, and restraining if other measures have failed to calm the patient. Restraints should be applied following an established protocol by staff who have been educated to restrain patients in a safe and humane manner. The patient in restraints should be checked at least every 15 minutes to make certain that circulation to extremities is satisfactory and to assess needs regarding nutrition and elimination.

Altered Nutrition: Less than Body Requirements. Interventions include providing foods that can be consumed on the run; attempting to have the patient's favorite foods available; and educating the patient on the importance of satisfactory nutrition.

Sleep Pattern Disturbance. Interventions may include making sure the environment has low stimuli; observing closely for signs of fatigue, such as fine tremor and puffy, dark circles below the eyes; and encouraging warm baths and soft music at bedtime. The key medication for people with manic episodes is lithium carbonate. Because relief from symptoms may take up to 3 weeks, the patient may also be receiving an antipsychotic medication. There is a narrow range between therapeutic level and toxic level. Therapeutic blood level for acute mania is 1.0 to 1.5 mEq per liter. Above 1.5 mEq per liter, symptoms of toxicity occur.

PHARMACOLOGY CAPSULE

Older adults are exceptionally vulnerable to experiencing side effects of all psychotropic medications, especially postural hypotension, falls, and confusion.

ORGANIC MENTAL SYNDROMES AND DISORDERS

The key problems for people with organic mental syndromes or organic mental disorders stem from cognitive impairments. The term *syndrome* refers to the behaviors and symptoms, and the term *disorder* is used when a definite organic cause is established. Delirium and dementia are two different disorders that involve deficits in orientation, memory, language comprehension, and judgment.

Common causes of delirium are meningitis, neoplasms, drugs ranging from alcohol to steroids, endocrine dysfunction, liver abnormalities, thiamine deficiency, and postoperative states. Common causes of dementia are senile dementia, Alzheimer's type, multi-infarct dementia, Pick's disease, and Parkinson's disease. Delirium and dementia are discussed in greater detail in Chapter 20.

PERSONALITY DISORDERS

Every individual exhibits particular personality traits. A person may be shy or aggressive, dependent, or manipulative. When personality traits become inflexible and dysfunctional, a person may have a personality disorder. The essential features of a personality disorder are that it is pervasive (concerns all aspects of one's life), chronic, and maladaptive. Examples of personality disorders are paranoid, schizoid, antisocial, borderline, avoidant, obsessive-compulsive, and passive-aggressive.

BORDERLINE PERSONALITY DISORDER

The person with borderline personality disorder has patterns involving unstable relationships, unstable self-image, and unstable mood. Key ideas about the causes are that genetics plays a role, as evidenced by the greater history of alcoholism in families of patients with this disorder, and particular developmental experiences play a role. Some theorists view an essential component of psychosocial development as separation-individuation. It is thought that between 2 and 3 years of age, the child separates from the parents as a unique self. If the parents are nonaccepting of the child's increasing autonomy and if the parents reinforce dependent behavior, the child does not fully experience self as separate. This problem with separation-individuation is thought to form the basis of splitting, a frequently utilized mechanism in borderline personality disorder. Persons who are splitting view others as all good or all bad and may shift their views of a particular other from all good to all bad. A person who has a clearly developed sense of self and who does not split views others as a mix of good qualities and negative qualities.

Nursing Care of the Patient with Borderline Personality Disorder

ASSESSMENT. The most relevant aspects of the mental status examination include (1) *mood, affect, feelings:* possible mood swings, chronic feelings of emptiness and boredom, and intense anger; and (2) *insight and judgment:* repeated suicidal threats and gestures and self-mutilating behavior.

NURSING DIAGNOSIS. Key nursing diagnoses include the following:

- **High Risk for Self-Directed Violence**
- **Impaired Social Interaction**
- **Personal Identity Disturbance**

GOALS. The main goal is that the patient not harm self. Other goals are that the patient clarify own unique characteristics and be clear on own thoughts and feelings versus others' thoughts and feelings; identify behaviors that interfere with satisfying relationships; and not show evidence of splitting, clinging, or distancing behavior.

INTERVENTIONS

High Risk for Self-Directed Violence. In addition to the interventions identified in the section on mood disorders, various interventions are more specific to the issues of borderline personality disorder. It is important that nurses stay aware of their own feelings to refrain

BORDERLINE PERSONALITY DISORDER: A CLINICAL EXAMPLE

Nora N, a licensed vocational nurse, worked part-time on a psychiatric unit. She reported to work at 11 P.M. one night after 5 days of not working to discover that Bonnie P had been readmitted after opening the suture line on her wrists with a steak knife. One year ago Bonnie had cut this wrist, saying that she was trying to feel something. Bonnie told Nora that she had missed her terribly and that she hoped Nora would work with her that night. Nora said that Susan (the full-time registered nurse) would work with her that night. Bonnie swore and returned to her room. When Nora made rounds, Bonnie said she was sure something was wrong and began walking around the room with a staggering gait. Bonnie said that she had not taken anything to create this problem. Her vital signs were stable, and her pupils were normal in size and reaction to light. Nora reported the situation to Susan and reflected on her responses to Bonnie. Initially Nora felt anger, telling herself that Bonnie was so manipulative when she did not have her way. She thought about how Bonnie manipulates others when she feels helpless (no idea of how to meet own needs). She also thought about Bonnie's splitting (seeing Nora as good nurse and Susan as bad nurse). Nora felt less angry as she considered the reasons for Bonnie's behavior.When Susan entered Bonnie's bedroom, Bonnie's gait was normal. Susan contracted with Bonnie for two 10-minute periods (at the beginning and end of shift) during which Bonnie could share whatever was on her mind and discuss goals and plans for the following day.

from any automatic responses that are not helpful (such as avoiding the patient who has cut himself). If patients mutilate themselves, it is important to care for wounds without acting in a way that might reinforce the self-mutilation (such as offering sympathy) and to ask patients to talk about feelings that occurred just before the self-mutilation. Nurses can act as role models for constructive expression of angry feelings and acknowledge the patient's positive expressions of negative feelings.

Impaired Social Interaction. Interventions include assisting the patient in examining own behavior in relationships, communicating availability, acknowledging (reinforcing) independent behavior, and setting limits as appropriate.

Personal Identity Disturbance. Interventions include helping the patient discuss and take ownership of own thoughts and feelings, clarifying values while being cautious not to impose one's own values, avoiding empathetic responses that may be viewed as mind reading (such as "I know how you feel").

Nurses work with patients with psychiatric disorders in a variety of settings including psychiatric inpatient units. Treatment for psychiatric disorders is influenced by the particular culture, place, and historical time frame. The nurse uses various strategies in communicating therapeutically with patients. The mental status examination is one aspect of the assessment of patients and is particularly relevant on a psychiatric unit. The nurse uses the mental status examination with patients systematically on admission and on an ongoing basis. For each of the major psychiatric disorders, possible observations for the relevant mental status examination categories are presented. Possible nursing diagnoses, goals, and interventions are suggested for each disorder.

NUTRITION CONCEPTS

- Patients with depression who experience anorexia or apathy toward food are given small, frequent feedings of foods high in calories and nutrients.
- Depressed patients who complain of constipation should be encouraged to eat high-fiber foods and to drink a lot of fluids.
- Patients with schizophrenia or dementia who are confused often must be reminded to eat or may need to be fed.
- Manic patients may have excessive activity and energy, so that high-calorie foods that can be carried, such as sandwiches, fruit, and muffins, are most appropriate.
- Persons with schizophrenia who have delusions that their food is being poisoned should be allowed to choose their food and beverages.

BIBLIOGRAPHY

American Psychiatric Association. (1994). *Diagnostic and statistical manual of mental disorders* (4th ed.). Washington, DC: Author.

Andreasen, N. C., Flaum, M., Swayze, V. W., Tyrrell, G., & Arndt, S. (1990). Positive and negative symptoms of schizophrenia. *Archives of General Psychiatry, 47,* 615–621.

Blair, D. T., & Dauner, A. (1993). Neuroleptic malignant syndrome: Liability in nursing practice. *Journal of Psychosocial Nursing, 31*(2), 5–12.

Kaplan, H. I., & Sadock, B. J. (1991). *Synopsis of psychiatry, behavioral sciences, clinical psychiatry* (6th ed.). Baltimore: Williams & Wilkins.

Karb, V. B., Queener, S. F., & Freeman, J. B. (1989). *Handbook of drugs for nursing practice.* St. Louis: C. V. Mosby.

Leon, R. L., Bowden, C. L., & Faber, R. A. (1989). The

psychiatric interview, history, and mental status examination. In H. I. Kaplan & B. J. Saddock (Eds.), *Comprehensive textbook of psychiatry* (5th ed., pp. 449–462). Baltimore: Williams & Wilkins.

McCarthy, P., & Snyder, J. C. (1992). Orthostatic hypotension: A potential side effect of psychiatric medications. *Journal of Psychosocial Nursing, 30*(8), 3–5.

Paquette, M., Neal, M. C., & Rodemich, C. (1991). *Psychiatric nursing diagnosis care plans for DSM-III-R.* Boston: Jones & Bartlett.

Rawlins, R. P., & Heacock, P. E. (1993). *Clinical manual of psychiatric nursing* (2nd ed.). St. Louis: C. V. Mosby.

Stafford, L. L. (1993). Dissociation and multiple personal disorder: A challenge for psychosocial nurses. *Journal of Psychosocial Nursing, 31*(1), 15–20.

Taylor, C. M. (1986). *Mereness' essentials of psychiatric nursing* (12th ed.). St. Louis: C. V. Mosby.

Townsend, M. C. (1990). *Drug guide for psychiatric nursing.* Philadelphia: F. A. Davis.

Townsend, M. S. (1991). *Nursing diagnoses in psychiatric nursing: A pocket guide for care plan construction* (2nd ed.). Philadelphia: F. A. Davis.

Verebey, K. (1992). Diagnostic laboratory: Screening for drug abuse. In J. H. Lowinson, et al. (Eds.), *Substance abuse: A comprehensive textbook* (pp. 425–436). Baltimore: Williams & Wilkins.

Wilson, H. S., & Kneisl, C. R. (1992), *Psychiatric nursing* (4th ed.). New York: Addison Wesley.

KEY CONCEPTS

1. According to current thinking, mental illnesses are related to specific physiologic changes in the central nervous system.
2. The psychoanalytic approach to mental illness is based on the theory that human beings function at different levels of awareness, ranging from conscious to unconscious, and that people use ego defense mechanisms to prevent anxiety.
3. The interpersonal approach to mental illness has three components: (1) anxiety is often communicated interpersonally, (2) the patient learns new ways of coping or maturing in a therapeutic relationship, and (3) the establishment of trust is an important first step in the nurse's work with patients.
4. Key ideas from the cognitive behavioral approach to mental illness are that behavior is learned, that behavior changes in response to positive consequences (positive reinforcement) or changes in response to removal of negative stimuli (negative reinforcement), and that particular thoughts influence emotional states.
5. In caring for a patient with a psychiatric disorder, nurses establish therapeutic (as opposed to social) relationships.
6. The mental status examination consists of observations regarding appearance, mood and affect, speech and language, thought content, perceptual disturbances, insight and judgment, sensorium, and memory and attention.
7. A patient with an anxiety disorder experiences either the highly uncomfortable feeling of anxiety directly or a symptom like compulsive hand washing that prevents or reduces the occurrence of anxiety.
8. In panic disorder, a patient experiences recurrent panic attacks, which are intense episodes of apprehension of variable length, at times to the point of terror, and often are accompanied by the feeling of impending doom.
9. A person with agoraphobia is extremely fearful of situations outside the home from which escape may be difficult or in which help may be unavailable.
10. Obsessive-compulsive disorder involves recurrent obsessions (thoughts) compulsions (behaviors), or both, that produce distress and interfere with functioning.
11. Posttraumatic stress disorder is a cluster of symptoms experienced following a distressing event that is outside the range of normal events (e.g., watching one's family being murdered).
12. Individuals with a somatoform disorder, such as conversion disorder or hypochondriasis, are convinced that they have a serious medical problem in spite of the absence of any concrete medical findings.
13. Dissociative disorders involve a change in identity, memory, or consciousness, usually to escape from anxiety.
14. Goals for the nursing care of patients with anxiety, somatoform, and dissociative disorders are to decrease anxiety to a point at which problem solving can occur, and to learn ways such as relaxation techniques to interrupt anxiety as it is escalating.
15. The term *schizophrenia* refers to a highly problematic group of biologic disorders in which there are symptoms of psychosis, including delusions, hallucinations, marked loosening of associations, catatonia, and flat or inappropriate affect.
16. People with mood disorders, such as unipolar depression and bipolar depression, experience an elevated mood, a depressed mood, or both.
17. Dementia is a group of disorders characterized by cognitive deficits sufficiently severe to impair social or occupational functioning.
18. Personality disorders occur when personality traits become inflexible and dysfunctional and are pervasive (concern all aspects of one's life), chronic, and maladaptive.

CHAPTER 52

June Schneberger

Substance Abuse

OBJECTIVES

1. Discuss the biologic, sociocultural, behavioral, and interpersonal theories of the etiology of substance abuse or dependency.
2. Describe the components of the nursing assessment of a patient with substance abuse or dependency.
3. Describe alcoholism, alcohol withdrawal syndrome, medical complications of alcoholism, and treatment of alcoholism.
4. Discuss the pathophysiologic effects of drugs frequently abused.
5. Describe disorders associated with substance abuse.
6. Differentiate between drug abuse treatment and alcohol abuse treatment.
7. Describe the nursing diagnoses and interventions associated with substance abuse and dependency.
8. Discuss populations who present special problems in relation to drug abuse and dependency.

GLOSSARY

ADDICTION Effect of habitual ingestion of a substance to the point of physical dependence; used interchangeably with the term dependence

CODEPENDENCY Exaggerated dependent pattern of self-defeating behaviors, beliefs, and feelings learned as a result of pathologic relationship to a chemically dependent, or otherwise dysfunctional, person

DUAL DIAGNOSIS Simultaneous existence of a major psychiatric condition and a medical condition

PHYSICAL DEPENDENCE Physical need for the substance on which one is dependent in order to avoid unpleasant physical withdrawal symptoms

PSYCHOLOGICAL DEPENDENCE Intense cravings for the substance on which one is dependent without physical withdrawal symptoms

RECOVERY Lifelong process of maintaining abstinence from the substance to which one is addicted; a return to moderate substance use is never the end result of recovery

SUBSTANCE ABUSE Maladaptive pattern of substance use that differs from generally accepted cultural norms; sometimes referred to as chemical abuse or drug abuse

SUBSTANCE DEPENDENCE Ingestion of substances in gradually increasing amounts due to a physical need; used interchangeably with the terms chemical dependence and drug dependence

TOLERANCE Need for increasing amounts of a substance to achieve the same effect brought about by the original amount

12-STEP PROGRAM Self-help support process outlining 12 steps to overcoming a physical or psychological dependence on something outside oneself that has a destructive impact on one's life

WITHDRAWAL Unpleasant and sometimes life-threatening physical substance-specific syndrome occurring after stopping or reducing the habitual dose or frequency of an abused drug

Substance abuse and dependence have become major problems in the United States and in other parts of the world over the past 20 years. These problems have reached the point of such significance that a great deal of energy and financial resources have been targeted toward a better understanding of them. Many researchers continue to try to discover the specific causes of substance abuse and dependence in order to combat these behaviors more effectively. It appears that many factors come into play.

ETIOLOGY AND RISK FACTORS

BIOLOGIC THEORY

The theory that is generally accepted by a majority of the experts in the field of addictionology is the biologic theory, often referred to as the medical model, which proposes that a faulty physiologic process that is not clearly understood contributes to dependence on a specific substance. This theory is supported by the fact that children have been shown to be four times more likely to become alcoholic if their biologic parent or parents are alcoholic, even when the children are raised apart in homes where they are not exposed to the excessive use of alcohol. Recently, public attention has focused on widely publicized findings that implicate a dopamine gene on the human chromosome 11 in the transmission of a predisposition for alcoholism from generation to generation. On the basis of these and many other studies, the medical community considers drug dependency to be a physical illness, in some ways like diabetes or similar disorders that have the following characteristics: (1) incurability, (2) a genetic predisposition to develop under the right conditions, and (3) a potential to be treated effectively only by total abstinence from the substance that the body cannot handle.

SOCIOCULTURAL THEORY

Another theory suggests that sociocultural factors play a major role in the process of becoming dependent on a particular drug. Many people who live in poverty and in crime-infested areas use drugs to relieve the stress of survival. In contrast, it can be observed that individuals with strong religious values prohibiting the excessive use of drugs have lower rates of addiction. Among select subcultures, the use of certain types of drugs can act as a rite of entry into a gang or a badge of honor proving that one has "made it." Even among middle class Americans it is expected that the average person will "party" on New Year's Eve, for example, often to excess. Certain cultural groups, such as the Irish, are commonly stereotyped as heavy drinkers. Country music lovers recognize that "crying in your beer" is often portrayed as the typical means of coping with loss and rejection.

BEHAVIORAL THEORY

Behavioral and learning theories look at the triggers for drinking and drug-using behaviors and how these patterns are reinforced. Substance abuse is believed to be a learned maladaptive way of coping with stress and anxiety. Family and peer group role models are closely studied for their use of substances, along with the beliefs and customs surrounding the use of drugs and alcohol. For example, if a shy teenager gets more attention and feels socially more comfortable when drinking with her friends, she is more likely to continue the use of alcohol in order to be accepted by her peers.

INTRAPERSONAL THEORY

The intrapersonal or psychological theory addresses those factors innate to the personality of the individual that may predispose him or her to substance abuse. These theorists believe that the quality of interpersonal relationships during critical developmental stages of our lives affect us profoundly. Thus, if children experience early childhood rejection, increased responsibility, unrealistic expectations, or overprotection, they may develop a dependent type of personality and consequently view themselves as inadequate or a failure when attempts to get their needs met fail. Individuals may ultimately turn to the use of alcohol or other drugs to numb the anxiety or frustration evoked by self-doubt and the daily stressors of reality.

It has been observed that substance abusers have many personality traits in common: many are very self-centered, have a strong need to be in control of others, seek attention, and have great difficulty delaying gratification of their needs. All of these characteristics are likely to increase the odds that they will resort to the use of drugs or alcohol to cope.

These types of intrapersonal theories originally supported the widespread acceptance of the perspective that alcoholism or drug addiction is a product of moral weakness. A more modern conclusion acknowledges that although the specific causes of misuse and addiction to various substances have not been established, most likely the true causes involve a combination of biologic, cultural, behavioral, and psychological factors.

NURSING ASSESSMENT OF THE SUBSTANCE ABUSER

HEALTH HISTORY

In order to initiate the nursing process effectively when working with the substance-abusing patient, thorough data collection is essential. Information can be gathered from a variety of sources, including an interview with the patient, family members, or significant others; a social assessment; medical records; or military records. Many substance abusers have sustained major losses, of jobs, relationships, property, self-esteem, and health. They may face legal charges. Often they will not seek professional help until they have hit "rock bottom." Even then, they may seek help only when presented with an ultimatum of some type, often from the family, the employer, or a court of law.

Questioning by the nurse produces the most reliable data when it is nonjudgmental, direct, specific, and verified by more than one source when possible. For example, if the patient admits to a couple of beers after work each night, the nurse should ask exactly how many were ingested, how many ounces each contained, or how big the bottle or glass used actually was. It is also important to know when the patient ingested the drug last and how much was taken in order to predict the possibility and timing of physical withdrawal symptoms. A nonjudgmental and matter-of-fact manner is the least likely to alienate an already defensive patient. At the same time, the nurse should not be so supportive and nurturing that clients can avoid facing the negative impact substance abuse has had on their life. Finding the most appropriate balance of support and reality-based confrontation is a highly developed skill that increases the likelihood that patients will continue in the treatment process. Many team members who work in substance-abuse treatment centers are recovering from addiction themselves, which often helps the client to be more honest and less defensive and to feel less hopeless and alone.

Patterns and Consequences of Abuse

The patient who has been abusing one or more substances will describe typical patterns of behavior and a combination of physical or psychological withdrawal symptoms characteristic of the substances abused. A few patients may not experience any physical withdrawal symptoms despite a history of prolonged, frequent, and heavy abuse, even of some substances that are usually physically addicting. Much depends on the stage of addiction, habitual patterns of use, the patient's baseline physical status, and the combinations and interactions of the drug or drugs being misused.

Many patients demonstrate erratic and unprovoked mood swings. They may describe a lifestyle revolving almost totally around obtaining and using the substance of choice, starting early in the day, often alone, and requiring more of the substance all of the time to get the desired effects. Many times the patient has been hiding the extent of his or her habit from others, and, despite best efforts to limit use of the substance, has been unsuccessful in doing so. Blackouts have usually occurred. Patients frequently have significant work problems or damaged relationships as a result of being unable to meet the expectations placed on them.

Defense Mechanisms Employed

Typical defense mechanisms used by the substance abuser include denial, rationalization, intellectualization, and projection. Denial is readily apparent when patients state that they do not have a problem with drug abuse despite evidence to the contrary. Individuals may also initially minimize the problems waiting to be confronted on returning home from the hospital by maintaining that they can stay sober without changing friends or attending Alcoholics Anonymous meetings regularly.

The defense mechanism of rationalization is one in which abusers attempt to justify the reasons for their abuse of substances. This is an "excuse" for addiction. An example is seen in individuals who insist that they had to use heroin because there was no other way to cope with the pain of their back injury: "The drugs my doctor gave me weren't working."

Intellectualization is closely related to rationalization but differs in that the person focuses only on objective facts as a way of avoiding dealing with unconscious conflicts and the emotions they evoke. An alcoholic who killed someone while driving intoxicated would be intellectualizing if she stated it was better that the victim die suddenly rather than have to live as a paraplegic.

The use of projection in substance abusers involves the process of shifting the blame for one's behavior onto someone or something else. Drug abusers using projection might insist that they became addicted to alcohol as a result of the pressure to drink at work-related social functions in order to keep colleagues from thinking they were prudes.

PHYSICAL EXAMINATION

On physical assessment, the average substance abuser often appears malnourished and poorly cared for. Evidence of physical trauma may be present from falls, abrasions, or fights. Jaundice or discolored sclera of the eyes may suggest cirrhosis or other liver problems. Hypertension is a critical sign of withdrawal and often accompanied by the physical signs of fluid retention in the legs or a protuberant abdomen swollen by liver ascites. Confusion, memory loss, tremors, lack of coordination, and other neurologic signs are significant and may be associated with nutritional deficits. The nurse must be alert for needle tracks in unexpected parts of the body in an individual who is believed to have been abusing drugs intravenously. The atypical client may not have any obvious signs of physical problems, but abnormalities may be found in the results of testing ordered by the physician on entry into any treatment program.

DIAGNOSTIC TESTS

In order to assess the patient's physical status, a thorough physical examination is done on initiation of treatment along with a basic laboratory screen chosen to identify problems in any of the major organ systems. Abnormalities are frequently seen in liver function tests, electrolytes, and tests reflecting nutritional status and gastric function. Sexually transmitted diseases may be identified, especially among intravenous drug users; syphilis rates are increasing; and the rapidly escalating rate of human immunodeficiency virus (HIV) in this population presents a national concern. Infections of various kinds are common. Special neurologic and neuropsychological testing may demonstrate brain damage.

Blood Alcohol Study

A blood alcohol study is the most accurate type of test available to measure the degree of intoxication on initiation of treatment for alcohol abuse. Findings of ≥0.3% require treatment of overdose; at over 0.4% concentrations, death is likely. Legal intoxication occurs when a person's blood alcohol level is ≥0.1% in most states; a move to lower the level to 0.08% in many states is currently under way.

Urine Drug Screening

Urine drug screening is the preferred way of screening for the recent use of an unknown drug and is commonly done along with the initial laboratory work. Drugs that are most likely to be identified in this way include amphetamines, barbiturates, benzodiazepines, cocaine, "crack," the opiates, marijuana, PCP, LSD, narcotic analgesics, sedatives, and stimulants. With this test, drug metabolites can be identified for days or weeks after use, depending on the drug misused. Typically, the collection of urine samples for this type of toxicology is witnessed by a staff member of the same sex to ensure that tampering or substitution of another person's urine has not occurred. After collection, the sample is kept under "chain of custody"—each person handling the sample signs a special document that accompanies the sample until it can be analyzed. Any temporary storage of the sample is maintained under secure conditions.

Hair Analysis

Hair analysis is a recent addition to the methods for the detection of abused substances. It requires sensitive technology but promises to be very helpful in monitoring patients for relapse. Depending on the length of hair, substance use can be detected for up to a year even after only 2 or 3 days of use. However, the presence of addiction or whether the person is currently under the influence of the substance cannot be implied from a positive finding. The long-term history of substance use that is provided will prove to be a valuable tool in the diagnosis and follow-up of substance abusers in the future.

ALCOHOL AND ALCOHOLISM

Alcohol is the most commonly abused drug in the United States. According to the American Society of Addiction Medicine (1990), alcoholism is "a primary, chronic disease with psychosocial, and environmental factors influencing its development and manifestations. The disease is often progressive and fatal. It is characterized by continuous or periodic impaired control over drinking, preoccupation with the drug alcohol, use of alcohol despite adverse consequences, and distortions in thinking, most notably denial" (p. 3). It can be noted that alcohol is referred to as a "drug" in this definition, reflecting the thinking of most health care professionals that alcohol is indeed a drug with addictive qualities similar to those of other abused drugs.

Simple intoxication from alcohol usually lasts less than 12 hours and is followed by the unpleasant experience of a hangover beginning about 4 to 6 hours after the last drink. Typical symptoms include headache, upset stomach, vomiting, sweating, thirst, fatigue, and blurred vision or "seeing stars." The cause of these symptoms has not been pinpointed; however, it is believed to be a result of hypoglycemia and the buildup of acetaldehyde and lactic acid in the blood.

Chronic use involves the regular daily ingestion of large quantities of alcohol, regular heavy drinking only on weekends, or binges of heavy drinking followed by long periods of abstinence. Physical addiction occurs when alcohol becomes integrated into physiologic processes at the cellular level. The cell becomes dependent on the alcohol to carry on certain metabolic processes; if alcohol is no longer available, the cell goes into "shock" and is unable to compensate for the loss quickly. Thus, alcohol withdrawal syndrome begins after the individual stops or decreases the amount ingested. Heavy chronic drinkers may experience the onset of withdrawal without actually stopping drinking but simply because they are no longer able to ingest enough alcohol in order to meet the body's demands of the substance in order to function.

Alcohol withdrawal syndrome involves physiologic and behavioral symptoms that begin when the individual's blood alcohol level drops. It is divided into two stages, depending on the onset and severity of symptoms. The first stage usually occurs within 6 to 12 hours after the last drink and is called *early withdrawal.* Symptoms begin with anxiety, agitation, and irritability. If the patient does not drink, tremors may be observed. Blood pressure, pulse, and temperature all begin to rise. Sweating, nausea, vomiting, and diarrhea are typical.

The second stage, *major withdrawal,* begins with the onset of seizures and hallucinations and can advance to life-threatening *delirium tremens* (or "DTs"). This stage usually occurs after approximately 3 days without alcohol or treatment and can be predicted by extreme elevations in temperature, pulse, and blood pressure. The patient can be expected to become disoriented and confused. Hallucinations are often visual and "animal" in nature. Bugs, snakes, and rats are commonly described, sometimes perceived to be crawling on the person. Familiar jokes about seeing "pink elephants" probably evolved out of this type of withdrawal experience.

Alcohol withdrawal is the *most* life-threatening withdrawal syndrome in comparison to those associated with other types of commonly abused drugs, even heroin.

(Withdrawal from barbiturates also can result in delirium tremens; both types of drugs have similar central nervous system depressant effects.) Thus, it is critical to counsel alcoholics never to attempt to withdraw on their own or "go cold turkey." They should always seek medical treatment. Most require inpatient hospitalization and administration of medications such as diazepam (Valium) or chlordiazepoxide (Librium) to prevent the severe consequences of withdrawal and to ensure early detection and treatment of symptoms.

MEDICAL COMPLICATIONS

Common medical complications of chronic alcoholism include cirrhosis of the liver, pancreatitis, gastrointestinal bleeding (often from esophageal varices), Wernicke's encephalopathy, Korsakoff's psychosis, and fetal alcohol syndrome.

Wernicke's Encephalopathy

Wernicke's encephalopathy is due to vitamin B_1 (thiamine) deficiency and is characterized by symptoms including delirium, confabulation due to memory loss, unsteady gait, a sense of apprehension, and altered levels of consciousness that can proceed to coma. If it is not properly treated with vitamin supplementation, Korsakoff's psychosis may develop.

Korsakoff's Psychosis

In this disorder, both thiamine and niacin deficiencies contribute to the degeneration of the cerebrum and the peripheral nervous system. Symptoms include amnesia, confabulation, disorientation, and peripheral neuropathies. Despite treatment, some residual problems persist in both disorders; however, dementia is permanent in the event that the patient progresses to Korsakoff's psychosis. Both of these disorders are classified as alcohol amnesic disorders.

Fetal Alcohol Syndrome

Fetal alcohol syndrome is a medical complication that is of great concern in the United States. If a woman drinks to excess throughout pregnancy, the unborn child is at risk for symptoms such as low birth weight, mental retardation, growth deficiencies, heart defects, facial malformations, learning disabilities, and hyperactivity. Recent controversy has arisen over whether maternal alcoholism constitutes child abuse and is thus reportable under child protection statutes.

TREATMENT FOR ALCOHOL ABUSE

In recent years, active family involvement in the treatment of alcohol abuse has come to be seen as a critical factor in the effectiveness of treatment outcomes. It is accepted that the disease of alcoholism affects everyone in the family system, often producing predictable patterns of individual behavior or changes in roles that may later prove to be a significant handicap for various family members in getting their needs met. Examples of some of the labels given these atypical roles include the hero, the mascot, the lost child, and the scapegoat. Adult children of alcoholics may struggle with issues throughout their lives as a result of dysfunctional patterns of thoughts and behaviors learned in childhood through the enactment of these types of roles. Spouses of alcoholics frequently struggle with "enabling" behaviors. These are described as any behavior that "covers up" or protects alcoholics from the consequences of their drinking behaviors. For example, a woman might lie to her husband's boss as to the reasons why he will not be at work, when in reality the husband is too "hungover" to perform adequately.

Family and peer pressure and confrontation can be critical factors in inducing the alcoholic to seek treatment. Through participation in a 12-step self-help support group for the significant others of substance abusers, called Al-Anon, spouses, children, friends, and co-workers can learn new ways of coping with issues and how to avoid enabling the alcoholic so that it becomes harder for him or her to continue the destructive pattern of drinking.

Intervention

In the past few years, a strategy referred to as "intervention" has become popular across the United States. This is a structured meeting by family and friends to confront the alcoholic with the impact that the person's alcohol abuse has on each member of the group. Often the alcoholic is tricked into coming to the meeting by some ploy. The intervention is led by a specially trained interventionist who helps those involved in the process to prepare by writing down the ways that the person's alcohol abuse affects them personally. The interventionist offers suggestions on how to word ideas in ways less likely to evoke defensiveness and how to focus on the issues to reject the problem drinking but not the person. During the intervention, all of the participants have an opportunity to read their letters aloud to the alcohol abuser. At the end of each letter, the reader requests that the alcoholic go into treatment to get help. Usually, after hearing out a roomful of significant people, the alcoholic will go unhappily, but voluntarily, directly from the intervention into a treatment program that has been arranged for in advance in the event of that outcome.

The use of this strategy has come under criticism since alcoholics confronted in this way often feel coerced into treatment. After intervention, they may harbor angry feelings directed at members of the family for being critical, pushy, and having "tricked" them. Ideally, for treatment to be most effective, individuals should choose to go voluntarily. Proponents of the use of intervention respond that the alcoholic may die or suffer terrible consequences of the disease before seeking help on a totally voluntary basis, and, thus, the ends justify the means.

Detoxification

Detoxification is usually done in an inpatient hospital or psychiatric setting. During detoxification, the patient's vital signs are checked frequently; patients do not participate in group therapy owing to their physical status; and rest and nutrition are emphasized. Drugs most often used in detoxification of the alcoholic are from the antianxiety (benzodiazepine) group, although hypnotics like phenobarbital or chloral hydrate are occasionally used. Intravenous magnesium sulfate may be used to prevent seizures in some cases. Patients are begun on scheduled anticonvulsants if seizures occur. Fluids are encouraged to combat dehydration.

PHARMACOLOGY CAPSULE

Alcohol detoxification is usually managed with antianxiety medications; also, hypnotics (chloral hydrate) are sometimes used.

Rehabilitation

Once patients are medically stable, they are referred to either an inpatient or an outpatient treatment program, depending on individual needs and resources. The traditional inpatient program, or Minnesota model, lasts about 30 days and includes highly structured scheduling of drug education films and presentations; increasingly confrontational individual, group, and family therapy; recreational and occupational therapy; milieu therapy; and introduction to Alcoholics Anonymous (AA), a self-help support group.

ALCOHOLICS ANONYMOUS. Alcoholics anonymous is a nonprofit worldwide organization of alcoholics who meet together anonymously in small groups at various times during the day throughout the year to assist each other in staying sober. The organization uses a strong spiritual base, which is controversial, and a 12-step process (Table 52–1) involving discussions and written exercises designed around each of the 12 steps as a means to keep the alcoholic from relapsing. Members identify another participant of the same sex who is seasoned in the recovery process, and to whom they can relate, to act as their sponsor. The sponsor agrees to be available to the person for support and advice in staying sober. Service work in the community also is seen as integral in focusing outside oneself.

Members use regular readings from the "Big Book" of AA, written by founding members to keep themselves on track. (Table 52–2 lists the 12 traditions of AA.) There are no dues; the organization relies on donations. There is no political involvement or endorsements of candidates or products. Everyone involved does so on a voluntary basis. Even group leaders are volunteers and are not professional counselors. Meetings are advertised in the community using the title "Friends of Bill W." as a means of maintaining the anonymity of participants. (Bill W. was one of the two originators of the organization.) Before discharge from an inpatient treatment program, alcoholics have the opportunity to attend various community AA meetings in order to increase the odds of continued outpatient participation and to begin the process of finding a "home group" to which they can connect.

Recently, research has begun to question what actually works in alcohol rehabilitation. Actual outcomes of the traditional types of treatment approaches have not been clearly documented. As a result, many insurance companies no longer fund 30-day inpatient treatment, forcing treatment programs to provide brief and creative inpatient rehabiltiation with rapid referral to an outpatient program and aftercare. Trends toward using more

TABLE 52–1

THE 12 STEPS OF ALCOHOLICS ANONYMOUS

1. We admit we were powerless over alcohol—our lives had become unmanageable.
2. Came to believe that a Power greater than ourselves could restore us to sanity.
3. Made a decision to turn our will and lives over to the care of God, as we understood Him.
4. Made a searching and fearless moral inventory of ourselves.
5. Admitted to God, to ourselves, and to another human being the exact nature of our wrongs.
6. Were entirely ready to have God remove all these defects of character.
7. Humbly asked Him to remove our shortcomings.
8. Listed all persons we had harmed and became willing to make amends to them all.
9. Made direct amends whenever possible except when to do so would injure them or others.
10. Continued to make personal inventory and when we were wrong promptly admitted it.
11. Sought through prayer and meditation to improve our conscious contact with God, as we understood Him, praying only for knowledge of His will for us and the power to carry it out.
12. Having had a spiritual awakening as the result of these steps, we tried to carry this message to alcoholics, and to practice these principles in all our affairs.

TABLE 52–2

THE 12 TRADITIONS OF ALCOHOLICS ANONYMOUS

1. Our common welfare should come first; personal recovery depends upon AA unity.
2. For our group purpose there is but one ultimate authority—a loving God as He may express Himself in our group conscience. Our leaders are but trusted servants; they do not govern.
3. The only requirement for AA membership is a desire to stop drinking.
4. Each group should be autonomous except in matters affecting other groups or AA as a whole.
5. Each group has but one primary purpose—to carry its message to the alcoholic who still suffers.
6. An AA group ought never endorse, finance, or lend the AA name to any related facility or outside enterprise, lest problems of money, property, and prestige divert us from our primary purpose.
7. Every AA group ought to be fully self-supporting, declining outside contributions.
8. Alcoholics Anonymous should remain forever nonprofessional, but our service centers may employ special workers.
9. AA, as such, ought never be organized; but we may create service boards or committees directly responsible to those they serve.
10. Alcoholics Anonymous has no opinion on outside issues; hence the AA name ought never be drawn into public controversy.
11. Our public relations policy is based on attraction rather than promotion; we need always maintain personal anonymity at the level of press, radio, and films.
12. Anonymity is the spiritual foundation of all our traditions, ever reminding us to place principles before personalities.

nontraditional treatment approaches that have proved to produce successful outcomes and to individualize programming to the intrapersonal characteristics of the alcoholic are gaining popularity. It has also been noted that many inpatient 30-day treatment programs have been forced to close owing to a lack of clients able to afford the cost of this intensive treatment.

Examples of components of alcohol rehabilitation that have been shown to be very useful in maintaining continued sobriety are the teaching of stress management, social skills training, behavioral approaches to marital therapy, and matching of clients with a therapist who uses a style most likely to benefit their personality type. A move is also under way in which treatment programs are attempting to group patients with similar lifestyles and characteristics together rather than to "lump" everyone together. Other factors being considered in developing more homogeneous small groups are styles of thinking (abstract vs. concrete thinkers), sex role–related issues, ethnicity, and age. The current trend is away from a "recipe card" approach to treatment that is expected to work for anyone who is an alcoholic (see Care Plan: The Patient Abusing Alcohol).

Cost containment has stimulated the development of many new outpatient types of programs for the treatment of alcoholism. Most day treatment or partial hospitalization programs are very similar to the traditional inpatient milieu and offer similar types of therapies, but they allow patients to return to their own homes at night. In this case, the risk of relapse often requires the use of medication like disulfiram (Antabuse) or metronidazole (Flagyl), which makes the user ill if mixed with alcohol. Usually, involvement in the program is intensive but does not last for the traditional 30 days.

Other individuals utilize active involvement in AA as the primary means for recovery by attending at least "90 meetings in 90 days." Other community programs also are available to assist the alcoholic in the recovery process and cannot be overlooked. Some are church related; some are focused on getting the recovering user back to work by providing job placement or an opportunity to return to school. One example of a community recovery program that exists in various parts of the country is the Patrician Movement. In addition, halfway houses may be available in the local area as a service of community mental health and mental retardation organizations.

Aftercare and Recovery

One of the newer aspects of the recovery process involves the inclusion of various types of aftercare services to assist alcoholics who have completed a treatment program successfully to make a gradual transition back into the community with the support necessary to assist them from relapsing. Many inpatient substance abuse programs now provide aftercare groups to discharged patients as a supplement to continued involvement in AA and other 12-step support groups such as Adult Children of Alcoholics and Codependency Anonymous.

Medications

The treatment team may recommend the use of disulfiram (Antabuse) to assist the alcoholic who is highly motivated to remain sober but recognizes that poor impulse control may increase the odds of relapse. This particular drug inhibits the metabolism of alcohol in the body, producing an uncomfortable, potentially life-threatening reaction to exposure to alcohol. Disulfiram is taken daily and lasts in the body for up to 2 weeks. The usual dose is 250 mg daily. Thus, if the alcoholic gets the urge to drink, the presence of the drug in the system usually provides the necessary negative reinforcement to resist the impulse. Symptoms of a disulfiram-alcohol reaction include flushing, headache, nausea, vomiting, dizziness, rapid heart rate, difficulty breathing, sweating, confusion, and hypotension that may lead to coma, convulsions, and death. The severity of the symptoms varies from person to person, and symptoms can last for 30 to 60 minutes and up to several hours in severe cases.

The danger of giving disulfiram to a person who is poorly motivated to stop drinking is obvious. As a result, careful patient teaching is essential. The patient must be taught to avoid alcohol in foods (like salad dressings, sauces, candies, or chocolate prepared with liqueurs), in topical preparations (cologne, aftershave, or liniments), and in medications (over-the-counter cold preparations or cough syrups). Alcohol wipes cannot be used by the nurse to clean the skin in preparation for an injection without a topical reaction. Due to the risks of accidental exposure to something containing alcohol, patients are encouraged to wear a MedicAlert bracelet or carry a card in their wallet to alert emergency care personnel to a possible disulfiram-alcohol reaction in the event that they are found unconscious. Patients are also asked to sign a consent form for the use of the drug prior to its prescription to document that proper instructions about diet, risks, precautions, and type of emergency care needed in the event of exposure to alcohol have been offered and are understood. It is important for the nurse to be alert for patient attempts to bypass the prohibitive effects of disulfiram by ingesting large doses of vitamin C in order to have a drink on occasion. Patients who are addicted are often very knowledgeable about drug treatment and can easily find out that massive doses of vitamin C are given intravenously for the treatment of overdose or disulfiram-alcohol reactions.

The use of disulfiram is contraindicated in individuals with impaired liver function, heart problems, or significant debilitation. Obviously, the safe use of the drug also requires that the person have no memory impairments, self-destructive intentions, or poor judgment.

Sometimes, metronidazole (Flagyl) is used for similar purposes because it also produces an uncomfortable reaction when combined with alcohol but does not produce the severe life-threatening reactions described for disulfiram. Also, it does not remain in the system for an extended period and can still be given in the event of many medical problems in which disulfiram is contraindicated.

Research efforts continue to attempt to identify other

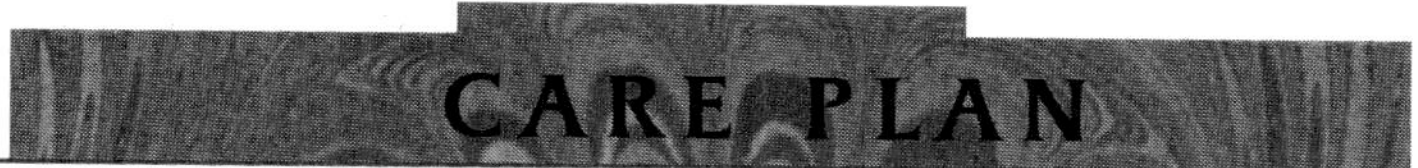

The Patient Abusing Alcohol

ASSESSMENT

Health History: A 37-year-old male was admitted for alcohol detoxification. He was found lying on the floor at home, passed out, and appeared to have vomited and been incontinent of urine and feces. He has a long history of alcohol abuse, and has claimed he does not have a problem since he only drinks beer. He recently lost his job because he was not reporting for work on time, and his wife has threatened to leave him if he does not stop drinking. His two children, aged 8 and 10, are afraid of him when he drinks. His usual intake of alcohol is two six-packs of beer a day. He has been detoxified in the hospital and is now ready for the rehabilitation phase of his treatment.

Physical Examination: Vital signs: temperature, 97.6°F orally; pulse, 80; respiration, 20; blood pressure 128/72. Height, 5′10″. Weight, 160 lb. The patient's skin and eyes have a slightly yellowish tinge. A cast is on his left arm from below the elbow to the fingers. He appears thin and wasted.

NURSING DIAGNOSIS	GOALS AND OUTCOME CRITERIA	INTERVENTIONS
Ineffective individual coping related to denial.	Patient will cope with disease of alcoholism as evidenced by his acknowledging that he has a problem, stopping ingestion of alcohol, and attending Alcoholics Anonymous (AA) meetings on a regular basis.	Use confrontational techniques to help patient to accept his diagnosis of alcoholism and support patient's 12-step program of rehabilitation.
Altered impulse processes related to craving for alcohol.	Patient will overcome his impulse to drink alcohol until intoxicated and to use alcohol as a coping mechanism as evidenced by cessation of ingesting alcohol and substituting other coping mechanisms.	Assist patient to overcome cravings by introducing new coping mechanisms such as exercise and stress management skills; encourage patient to attend treatment program and AA meetings on a regular basis.
Altered self-concept related to loss of control.	Patient will maintain an adequate self-concept as evidenced by lessened self-criticism, good hygiene, and positively interacting with others.	Help patient to maintain self-esteem after confrontational therapy sessions by allowing him to vent his feelings and acting as a role model for dealing with others.
High risk for injury related to excessive use of alcohol and high risk for relapse.	Patient will not injure himself as result of excessive ingestion of alcohol.	Encourage patient to abstain from drinking by supporting his participation in rehabilitation activities to stop drinking alcohol. Intervene at the first signs of impending relapse.
Altered feeling state related to guilt.	Patient will maintain a positive feeling state as evidenced by stating that he is able to forgive himself, stop being self-critical, and express his true feelings.	Allow patient to vent his feelings about his illness and to explore his feelings about his past behaviors; support patient in his 12-step program of rehabilitation.

types of drugs that could assist alcoholics to go through withdrawal more comfortably and to avoid relapse. Medications currently under scrutiny for this purpose include naltrexone HCl (Trexan), antidepressants such as amitriptyline HCl (Elavil), desipramine HCl (Norpramin), fluoxetine HCl (Prozac), and enzyme inhibitors such as enalapril maleate (Vasotec).

PSYCHOACTIVE SUBSTANCES OTHER THAN ALCOHOL

Six classes of psychoactive substances other than alcohol are frequently associated with substance abuse, or, using the term that is currently popular, chemical dependence. These are the stimulants, depressants, hallucinogens, narcotics, inhalants, and designer drugs (Table 52–3). Each class is different in the types of symptoms produced and the way in which patients abusing them are managed.

PHARMACOLOGY CAPSULE

Disulfiram (Antabuse) is sometimes used to assist a recovering alcoholic who is highly motivated to remain sober but recognizes that poor impulse control may increase the odds of relapse.

PHARMACOLOGY CAPSULE

To avoid a disulfiram-alcohol reaction, patients who are taking disulfiram (Antabuse) must be instructed to avoid alcohol in foods (sauces, candies), topical preparations (cologne, aftershave), and medications (over-the-counter cold preparations, cough syrups).

PHARMACOLOGY CAPSULE

The use of disulfiram (Antabuse) is contraindicated in persons with impaired liver function, heart problems, or significant debilitation.

STIMULANTS

Stimulants include amphetamines ("speed") and similar drugs, plus cocaine or "crack."

Amphetamines

Amphetamines are usually used orally or intravenously on a daily basis or on binges. They are very psychologically addictive—the dose is gradually increased over time to produce the euphoria (or "high") that is extremely pleasurable. Symptoms often include hyperactivity, irritability, combativeness, and, after extended use, paranoia. A person intoxicated by amphetamines may be very dangerous. There are no physical withdrawal symptoms, but the user typically experiences a profound depression and sense of exhaustion called "crashing." Tricyclic antidepressants are commonly used to treat the depression that may persist in chronic users for up to 2 years after the last use. Toxic psychosis may occur in approximately 90% of chronic users up to 1 year past the last use. Unfortunately, 5 to 15% of these individuals never fully recover. Antipsychotics may be used to treat toxic psychosis.

"Ice" is a new form of methamphetamine ingested by smoking with results similar to those produced by crack (a smokable form of cocaine). Effects last as long as 14 hours; the user will often do anything in order to obtain the drug and is also considered at risk for being very dangerous while under the influence.

Cocaine

Cocaine is another stimulant that has been commonly misused among middle to upper socioeconomic classes owing to its status and expense. It is typically inhaled nasally or mixed with other drugs, like heroin, and injected intravenously ("speedballs"). It is very psychologically addicting, which is believed to be due to overstimulation of the pleasure centers of the brain. Physical withdrawal symptoms have not traditionally been believed to occur; however, a physical syndrome has been hypothesized and is currently under debate.

Symptoms of chronic inhalation include runny nose, sniffles, frequent colds, weight loss, hyperactivity, and damage to the nasal mucosa or septum that may require surgical repair in the worst cases. Psychologically, cocaine abusers lose interest in their usual activities, demonstrate abrupt mood swings, poor judgment, impatience, and ultimately suspiciousness and hallucinations. Cocaine psychosis also can occur but usually lasts only 3 to 5 days after the last use. Cocaine is a very dangerous drug in that strokes, seizures, and heart attacks can occur in even first-time users. Treatment often consists of the use of diazepam (Valium) or phenobarbital for their sedative effects. Antipsychotics may be used in the event of psychosis. Many clients are severely depressed for up to 2 years after quitting. Studies have shown that damage to the brain may impair the patient's ability to experience pleasure. Antidepressants such as imipramine (Tofranil) and cardiac drugs like propranolol HCl (Inderal) or calcium channel blockers may be helpful in this event.

Crack

Crack is a hardened form of cocaine that is smoked. It presents major problems in many urban areas of the United States because it is readily available and very inexpensive compared with other drugs. It produces a tremendously addicting, short-acting psychological euphoria quickly followed by "crashing," which stimulates continued cravings and use. The cravings are so intense that, as with "ice," the user will do almost anything to

TABLE 52-3
COMMON MOOD-ALTERING CHEMICALS

DRUG NAME	EFFECTS	SITE OF ACTION	LENGTH OF EFFECT
Hallucinogens			
Mushroom (psilocybin) LSD (lysergic acid diethylamide) Mescaline (from peyote cactus) DOM (dimethoxymethylamphetamine) STP (no chemical name) MDA, Ecstasy (methylenedioxyamphetamine)	Altered body image Euphoria Sharpened perceptions Somatic effects: dizziness, tremors, weakness, nausea Psychosis-like symptoms Emotional swings Suspiciousness Bizarre behavior Increased blood pressure Increased temperature Objective signs: dilated pupils, flushing, tremors	Central nervous system (CNS) Brain	Onset: 40–60 min Duration: 6–12 hr
Cannabinoids			
Marijuana Hashish	Failure in judgment and memory Mild intoxication Euphoria Relaxation Sexual arousal Panic states Visual hallucinations Objective signs: reddened eyes, dry mouth, incoordination Heart rate to 140/min	CNS Cardiovascular system Respiratory system	Administration and dose dependent Onset: 20–30 min Duration: 3–7 hr
Opiates (Opiates, Semisynthetic and Synthetic Analgesics)			
Codeine Morphine Heroin Hydromorphone (Dilaudid) Methadone Meperidine (Demerol) Propoxyphene (Darvon) Designer drugs	Analgesia Euphoria Escape Reduction in sexual and aggressive drives Respiratory depression Sedation, sleepiness Objective signs: hypertension, pupillary constriction, constipation	Nervous tissue CNS (opiate receptors) Respiratory system	Onset: 20–30 min Duration: 4–8 hr
Sedative-Hypnotics and Anxiolytics			
Barbiturates Secobarbital (Seconal) Phenobarbital (Nembutal) Amobarbital (Amytal) Amobarbital/Secobarbital (Tuinol) Barbiturate-like (methaqualone [Quaalude]) Benzodiazepines (chlordiazepoxide [Librium], diazepam [Valium]) Buspirone (BuSpar)	Drowsiness, sedation Euphoria Escape, loss of aggressive and sexual drives Emotional lability Poor judgment	CNS Cardiovascular system Respiratory system	Onset: 30–40 min Duration: 4–5 hr
Stimulants			
Amphetamine (methamphetamine, Dexedrine, Benzedrine) Methylphenidate (Ritalin) Phenmetrazine HCl (Preludin) Cocaine, crack	Euphoria, grandiosity Stimulation, energy, anxiety Relief of fatigue Depression Wakefulness Suppression of appetite Aggressive feelings, paranoia Objective signs: sweating, dilated pupils, increased blood pressure, rapid heart and respiratory rates, tremors, seizures	CNS Peripheral nervous system Cardiovascular system	Onset: route related; 10–30 min Duration: Drug related

Table continued on following page

TABLE 52-3
COMMON MOOD-ALTERING CHEMICALS *(Continued)*

DRUG NAME	EFFECTS	SITE OF ACTION	LENGTH OF EFFECT
Phencyclidines			
PCP (phencyclidine) (angel dust)	Detachment from surroundings Decreased sensory awareness Illusions of superhuman strength Acute intoxication Objective signs: flushing, fever, sweating, coma, agitation, confusion, hallucinations, paranoia, violence	CNS	Rapid onset: 2–3 min up to 45 min Duration: drug and dose related
Inhalants			
Benzene (paint thinner, cleaning fluid, glue) Nitrites Nitrous oxide	Euphoria Giddiness, headache, fatigue, drowsiness Objective signs: arrhythmias, damage to kidneys, liver abnormalities	Cardiac effect CNS	Onset: immediate Duration: 20–45 min
Alcohol			
Beverage alcohol, beer, wine	Relaxation, sedation, release of inhibitions Objective signs: incoordination, nausea, vomiting, slurred speech	CNS Respiratory system	Onset: 20 min–1 hr Duration: dose related
Xanthines			
Caffeine	Stimulation Restlessness Anxiety Objective signs: increased heart and respiratory rates, diarrhea, gastric disorder, insomnia, tremors	CNS	Onset: 10–30 min Duration: 3–7 hr
Nicotine			
Cigarettes Smokeless tobacco	Stimulation Enhanced performance	CNS Respiratory system Cardiovascular system Endocrine system	Onset: immediate Duration: 5–15 min

Modified from Haber, J., McMahon, A.D., Price-Hoskins, P., & Sideleau, B.F. (1992). *Psychiatric nursing* (4th ed., pp. 495–496). St. Louis: Mosby Year Book.

obtain more of the drug and often resorts to violence if thwarted. Overdose of this drug is life threatening because no drug is available to counteract the overstimulation, resulting in respiratory failure.

DEPRESSANTS

Drugs misused in this category include the sedatives, hypnotics, and anxiolytics. They are typically taken orally, by prescription, for anxiety or insomnia or are purchased illegally. Regular use results in physical dependency. Symptoms of overdose include oversedation, respiratory depression, impaired coordination, and brain damage. Intoxication with barbiturates parallels that with alcohol and has a similarly dangerous physical withdrawal (delerium tremens); however, symptoms usually occur later, 7 to 10 days after the last use. Once a person is dependent, abruptly stopping any of these drugs may also trigger psychosis.

HALLUCINOGENS

This category of drugs includes LSD (lysergic acid diethylamide or "acid"), PCP (phencyclidine or "angel dust"), MDMA (methylenedioxymethamphetamine, known as "ecstasy" or "Adam"), and marijuana.

LSD

LSD is not physically addicting but can produce physical symptoms of altered perceptions that are dream-like, often with an altered sense of time and feelings of attainment of special insight. Emotions are intensified and labile. Individuals often experience depersonalization, in which they feel as if they are floating outside of themselves or in unreal surroundings. The drugs are typically used to enhance self-awareness and are usually taken episodically (approximately twice a week). Acute adverse reactions are most often described as a "bad trip" involving paranoia, depression, frightening hallucinations, and occasionally an acute confusional state. The person experiencing a bad trip is responsive to verbal support and reassurance. The primary danger of the use of these drugs results from accidental death as a result of perceptual distortions (i.e., attempting to fly off a building) or seizures related to the cutting agent used. Chronic long-term adverse reactions include psychosis, depression, paranoia, and flashbacks. LSD use is currently regaining popularity. Interestingly, it is again under study for use in alcoholic treatment.

PCP

PCP (phencyclidine) differs from other hallucinogens in that abusers experience a psychotic state similar to that observed in schizophrenics. Brain reward areas are stimulated so that abusers can stimulate themselves mentally in a pleasurable way. Studies also suggest that this drug is strongly physically addictive, with a severe withdrawal reaction occurring after binge use. Unexpected sensory stimuli that interrupt the individual's internal experience may provoke unpredictable violence. The person may possess enormous strength and may feel no pain. The risks of use thus involve serious injury to oneself or others, in addition to severely elevated temperature, hypertensive crisis, and renal failure. Under acute intoxication, patients are best managed by reducing stimuli as much as possible, often by seclusion, even to the point of avoiding talking or performing routine treatments until stabilized. If violent, mechanical restraint is necessary.

Marijuana

Marijuana is often included in the hallucinogenic category of abused drugs because it produces an effect similar to that of LSD when smoked. The inner experience is altered so that individuals have a sense of heightened awareness, distortion of space and time, heightened sensitivity to sound, and depersonalization. Although use may produce paranoia, the "bad trip" phenomenon of LSD is rare. It also tends to have a sedative rather than stimulant effect and is unlikely to produce true hallucinations. Marijuana is psychologically addicting. Controversy persists about the negative effects of chronic use of this drug. It has been suggested that marijuana may produce psychosis in fragile individuals and a lack of motivation and a reduction of fertility and sexual performance in young males. However, the studies that suggest these conclusions can be challenged by others just as convincing presenting the opposite findings. Chronic smoking of marijuana irritates the lungs and may contribute to the occurrence of lung cancer.

In the medical community, marijuana shows promise for the further development of its derivatives as medication for the treatment of glaucoma, nausea and vomiting as a result of cancer chemotherapy, and asthma.

NARCOTICS

The narcotic drugs often misused include heroin, morphine, pentazocine (Talwin), methadone, and meperidine (Demerol).

Heroin

Heroin is a highly addictive narcotic that produces a pleasant euphoria on intravenous use. The person experiences a "rush," then gradually nods off to sleep. On awakening, the person feels immune to stressors until the withdrawal symptoms begin to trigger the need to "cop a fix" again. This usually occurs 8 to 12 hours after the last use. Risks of chronic use of heroin include overdose, malnutrition, and respiratory arrest. Symptoms of withdrawal include tearing of the eyes, runny nose, gooseflesh, sweating, alternating fever and chills, muscle and joint pain, upset stomach, diarrhea, loss of appetite, restlessness, and irritability. Individuals are usually in such subjective distress that they inappropriately seek medications from the staff while in treatment and are very difficult to work with and remain nonjudgmental with. In order to support their ever-increasing habit, many people addicted to heroin resort to crime, such as stealing. Sometimes they seek detoxification only to reduce the level of the dose needed to experience the pleasurable response to the drug—a lower dose is less expensive to obtain. "China White" is a synthetic form of heroin.

INHALANTS

A very dangerous type of drug abused is that of the inhalant group. Examples of chemicals often inhaled for the mind-altering response include paint, glue, aerosol sprays, "whiteout," and gasoline. They are usually placed in a plastic bag or other container that is then placed over the nose and mouth and inhaled. Symptoms appearing in the individual under the influence of the drug depend on the substance inhaled and include nosebleeds, bloodshot eyes, infectious lesions around the nose and mouth, and severe disorientation or unconsciousness. The risks include progressive brain damage, asphyxiation, seizures, depressed bone marrow leading to aplastic anemic, liver or kidney damage, or cardiac arrhythmias. There is no physical withdrawal syndrome.

This particular group of drugs is often misused among teenagers owing to easy availability and low cost. The cumulative brain damage as the result of chronic use is a very serious problem among poor and minority adolescents.

DESIGNER DRUGS

A new group of abused drugs on the illegal market includes synthetic drugs especially designed to sidestep categorization with any of the drugs identified as illegal in the United States. Technically, they are often not against the law to use but present unique hazards with their misuse. "Ecstasy" is an example of a synthetic drug generally grouped with the hallucinogens; it is also called "Adam." A very similar second-generation designer drug is called "Eve." "China White" is an example of a synthetic type of heroin that acts in much the same way as heroin. Major risks are presented when the abuser mixes these drugs with those from the other groups because the results are unpredictable.

DISORDERS ASSOCIATED WITH SUBSTANCE ABUSE

Acquired immunodeficiency syndrome continues to be the disease that presents the most current danger for patients who are abusing intravenous drugs as a result of the common practice of sharing needles. The Centers for Disease Control and Prevention indicates an alarming number of new cases of HIV-positive diagnoses among intravenous drug users and their sexual partners. Nursing care for these patients now includes teaching them how to clean their "rig" with bleach and how to use condoms correctly.

Individuals who are predisposed to, or have already been diagnosed with, a serious psychiatric illness may present with an active case of the disorder or an exacerbation of their illness as a result of misuse of these chemicals owing to altered levels of important brain chemicals that control emotions, thought processes, and behavior.

Another major area of concern is that of the fetal effects of intrauterine exposure to these chemicals. Fetuses carried by mothers who are physically addicted to a narcotic also are born addicted and may experience developmental delays and a prolonged lack of the capacity to feel pleasure even after they have been successfully weaned from the abused drug. "Cocaine babies" are currently being studied for clues to the consequences of prenatal exposure to the drug. Findings suggest that attention deficit disorder (with or without hyperactivity) occurs more often in this population, along with dyslexia, other neurologic problems, and learning disabilities.

Clients with chronic pain disorders also are very vulnerable to the abuse of drugs, especially those of the narcotic and depressant groups, because of their frequent frustration over an inability to manage their pain effectively and lack of knowledge of the risks of regular use of pain medication. Many times they feel betrayed by their physician and other caregivers because these medications were prescribed for pain control, but no one ever explained the importance of temperate use along with the use of exercise and other types of supportive techniques to manage pain and avoid addiction.

TREATMENT FOR SUBSTANCE ABUSE

Substance abuse treatment is very similar to alcohol detoxification and rehabilitation. Narcotics Anonymous (NA) is structured much like AA but is focused on the abuse of drugs other than alcohol. Many times, inpatient treatment programs place recovering addicts with alcoholics for educational and therapy groups without problems. However, the rate of relapse is much higher for most drug abuse patients, especially those who use highly addicting intravenous drugs. Research is booming on this topic in order to try to identify alternative treatment and medications that will assist the drug-abusing patient to detoxify from the chemicals that they are addicted to more comfortably and to find a way to reduce the risks of relapse. Currently, recommendations to approach drug abuse treatment separately from alcohol abuse treatment and to seek new modalities for drug abuse treatment are gaining support.

As with alcohol treatment, family involvement in the process is very important. Al-Anon is the support group for family members or significant others of a substance-abusing person. It is recommended that members of the family begin attending meetings as soon as they realize that the person is using some type of drug. Ultimately, the process of intervention described earlier may be used in an attempt to get the person into treatment.

Many patients using drugs have legal problems that may have provided the catalyst for seeking help. Sometimes they are mandated by the courts to go into treatment, other times their attorney recommends treatment prior to the case going to court in order to influence the judge favorably prior to sentencing. In the past, many individuals were committed to state hospital drug treatment programs for 30 days involuntarily. However, many state hospital systems across the country are currently closing their drug and alcohol treatment units because of the program expense and the need to provide additional services to the seriously mentally ill, which is often judged more of a priority.

Detoxification

Detoxification from physically addicting drugs is often very complex owing to the likelihood of polysubstance abuse and the uncertainty of what to expect when two of these drugs are mixed together. Usually, inpatient hospitalization is recommended for safety. However, some individuals who have been using drugs that are primarily psychologically addicting may not demonstrate many physical symptoms but, rather, experience intense psychological cravings. For example, if a conversation about past drug use occurs within the recovering addict's hearing, or if something in the environment triggers memories of the "high" sensation that they experienced while using, the person may experience cravings that stimulate feelings of restlessness, itching, hives, flushing, and elevated blood pressure and pulse, which are believed to be psychogenic in origin. The nurse needs to give these patients a great deal of support to help them overcome the profound urge to use. This experience puts the patient at very high risk for relapse.

Medications

METHADONE. Methadone is the drug of choice for opioid detoxification and is most frequently used to detoxify patients addicted to heroin. The drug is a synthetic narcotic analgesic that may be prescribed appropriately for chronic severe pain. Given orally (in diskette or liquid form), it is absorbed slowly and does not produce the "rush" normally experienced with the intravenous use of heroin. It also alleviates the cravings for more narcotics for a short period of time, dependent on the dose given. In detoxification, the dose of the drug is gradually reduced without telling patients exactly what dose they are getting. Although this process is one of substituting another addictive drug for the one misused by the client, it is believed to be justified in that the withdrawal from methadone is less uncomfortable for the patient. The patient also risks severe respiratory depression in the event that heroin is injected while methadone is in the system. The most typical problematic side effects of methadone include severe constipation and profound sweating.

PHARMACOLOGY CAPSULE

Methadone is a synthetic narcotic analgesic that is the drug of choice for opioid detoxification, especially for patients addicted to heroin.

CLONIDINE. Clonidine HCl (Catapres) is becoming more popular as a means of assisting the substance abuser through detoxification. This is a nonopiate antihypertensive drug that blocks withdrawal symptoms, thus making detoxification quicker and less uncomfortable than methadone for most patients. Others may leave treatment because of their discomfort and unrealistic expectations that they should not feel sick at all while using the drug to withdraw.

NALOXONE. Naloxone HCl (Narcan) is a narcotic antagonist that counteracts the dangerous respiratory effects of heroin or other opiate overdose. When given to a person who is addicted and under the influence of an opiate, the person may experience withdrawal symptoms.

Many other drugs are currently under investigation to determine whether they could assist the substance abuser by reducing the cravings for the drug abused or by counteracting the long-term psychological consequences of use of certain drugs. Examples of these include some of the antidepressants, anticonvulsants, and various herbal agents.

Rehabilitation

In most cases, the process of rehabilitation for drug abuse is very similar to that for alcohol abuse. Instead of attendance at AA meetings, the client often participates in NA at least some of the time. This support group is based on the 12 steps of AA, except that the word "alcohol" is replaced by "drugs" in all of the literature, and the case histories used for reading assignments are about other addicts in recovery related specifically to the use of drugs other than alcohol in an attempt to help the client identify with people with similar struggles. Relapse rates for individuals abusing drugs other than alcohol alone are much higher and present unique issues. Trends suggest that future treatment programs will be more likely to separate clients into small groups of people facing similar issues and having similar characteristics in order to individualize the recovery process much more than is typically done in the majority of settings at present. Although most current settings may advertise more than one "track" for substance abuse treatment, in reality clients share the same facilities and participate in most of the traditional programming mixed together despite different learning styles and other issues. It has been suggested that this practice may actually place clients who do not fit the traditional mold at higher risk for relapse.

On an outpatient basis, these clients are encouraged to participate in NA on a regular basis (90 meetings in the first 90 days), just as those recovering from alcoholism do. Attempts are usually made to allow the client to experience different group locations and times prior to discharge from the inpatient setting in order to increase the likelihood that the client will participate as recommended. Various other community programs may be available, such as the Patrician Movement, which provides outpatient treatment on an ongoing basis for those who cannot afford more costly inpatient rehabilitation. Many private health care systems are opening day treatment programs for substance abusers as insurance reimbursement for long-term inpatient programs is becoming rarer.

Aftercare and Recovery

Recovering substance abusers may be offered an opportunity to participate in a support group provided by the hospital at which they received treatment. Many of the same people who went through treatment at the same time participate together, and since the relationships built during this time of crisis are often intense, the groups can be very helpful in preventing relapse. Hopefully, clients will also continue regular participation in NA groups on an ongoing basis. Some individuals do well in halfway houses, which allow for a new living environment surrounded by other recovering addicts during the difficult transition back into the community. Sometimes it is recommended that patients do not return to work until their ability to cope with stress is more developed.

Methadone Maintenance

Some patients who have experienced multiple relapses into heroin abuse after treatment may have sustained permanent damage to chemical receptor sites in the brain, which decreases their ability to resist relapse. As a result, methadone maintenance is commonly used. In this process, the person goes to a methadone clinic on a daily basis to receive a dose of the medication to cover the next 24 hours. The dose is administered in liquid form or in a diskette dissolved in juice, and the person is carefully observed by clinic staff members to ensure that the medication is actually taken and not hoarded in any way. The patient may continue this process indefinitely, often for many years. The dose of the methadone is usually maintained at the same level without attempts to reduce the dose.

Methadone maintenance programs have been highly criticized across the United States because the process is often viewed as exchanging one addiction for another without attempts to detoxify the patient. In addition, clinic records and security have been lax in many instances, resulting in clinic methadone thefts and illegal sales on the street. Supporters of the programs counter these arguments by pointing out that criteria for involvement in these programs require that patients have been unsuccessful in remaining "clean" after detoxification on more than one occasion and that they no longer are forced into crime to support their habit. In addition, methadone is administered in such a way that no rush is experienced, allowing the person to return to school or work and reintegrate into society without the risk of losing everything to relapse. Maintenance programs are also more cost-effective than residential treatment or jail time.

The controversy over methadone maintenance has resulted in the frequent use of naltrexone (Trexan) as an alternative. This drug is related to naloxone (Narcan) and is a pure opioid antagonist. This means that the drug reduces or completely blocks the effects of any intravenous opioids in the patient's system. The detoxified patient is placed on this drug to prevent use of heroin. If the patient takes small doses of heroin while on naltrexone, no effect is experienced, however, if the patient injects large doses, he or she will become very physically ill and may die or sustain serious injury such as a coma. An addicted person taking naltrexone will experience withdrawal symptoms due to the antagonist actions of the drug.

Currently, research is underway to evaluate the use of various types of other psychotropic medications to stabilize altered neurochemical balances in the brains of addicted persons. This may eventually provide an answer to the problem of the high rates of relapse in narcotic abusers.

PHARMACOLOGY CAPSULE

Methadone maintenance is used for patients who have experienced multiple relapses into heroin abuse after treatment.

NURSING CARE OF THE SUBSTANCE ABUSER

Nursing Diagnosis and Interventions

The initial step in developing a nursing plan of care for the substance abuser is always a careful and thorough assessment. On the basis of the initial assessment on admission or first contact with the patient, the nurse can identify and prioritize problems that must be addressed in order to maximize the likelihood that the patient will remain sober. Examples of the types of problems often seen in substance abusers of any kind include denial, poor impulse control, high risk for injury, high risk for relapse, guilt, and low self-esteem. The following nursing diagnoses might be applicable to substance abuse patients:

- **Ineffective Individual Coping** related to denial manifested by minimizing effects of drug use; stating one does not have a problem; stating one can quit easily; disagreeing with the need to change lifestyle, to attend meetings of AA or NA, and to avoid drug users
- **Self-Esteem Disturbance** related to loss of control and guilt manifested by frequent self-criticism, poor hygiene, avoidance of others, oversensitivity, inability to forgive oneself for past mistakes, critical self-talk, attempts to overcompensate for past behavior toward others, and not saying what one truly feels
- **High Risk for Injury** related to excessive use of the drug and high risk for relapse manifested by a history of falls; driving under the influence and combining the substance abused with other substances; being aggressive while under the influence; reduced attendance at AA or NA meetings; frequent dreams of drug use; returning to places where one used drugs; not seeking relief for high stress

Nursing interventions for substance abusers in detoxification involve regular physical assessment (frequency determined by the severity of symptoms), administration of appropriate medications, and teaching the patients about their actions and the potential side effects. Providing adequate nutrition is critical as the patient may have been eating very irregularly and may also be very dehydrated. High levels of anxiety during detoxification also require a great deal of reassurance and support, providing the opportunity to help the patient begin to process the impending decision to continue in rehabilitation.

Once the patient has agreed to participate in rehabilitation, the focus of nursing care changes from one of primarily attending to the physical concerns of the patient to assisting the client in processing the meaning of his or her substance abuse and planning for a future without continued use of that substance. The biggest issue to be addressed at first is the heavily entrenched denial that most substance abusers possess. Often they minimize the severity of the abuse, perhaps lying outright about how much they actually were using. The nurse must work toward penetrating this denial without further damaging the individual's self-esteem. This has traditionally demanded more confrontational techniques than appropriate in other types of psychiatric treatment. In many "substance use only" treatment programs, the style of confrontation used was often overly hostile and critical, which is no longer seen as the most helpful to the patient. Studies now show that patients who were treated in this way were far more likely to leave treatment early to return to their "drugging and drinking." This is now recognized to be of great concern because the person may never return to treatment and may die or be seriously injured as a result of the continued substance abuse.

Nurses can also be very helpful in assisting the patient work through the 12-step process. After intense educational, AA or NA meetings and group therapy sessions during most of the day, patients often want to ventilate feelings and process thoughts about what they are learning. Conflicts with family members, bosses, friends, or parents are often overwhelming. Patients usually lack the skills to handle these types of interpersonal stressors owing to habitual avoidance of issues through past substance abuse. The nurse can act as an ally in helping patients cope and begin to practice new ways of reacting. Teaching stress management and practicing these new skills with patients can greatly increase the odds that they will not relapse after discharge.

Relapse prevention is a critical area for the nurse to attend to in dealing with each patient. The patient must be taught to recognize symptoms that often lead to relapse. Examples of these include overtiredness or poor health, being unnecessarily dishonest with others, impatience, argumentativeness, depression, self-pity, cockiness, forgetting or minimizing the risk of relapse, unreasonable expectations of self and others, decreased or irregular participation in AA or NA meetings or daily meditation and self-inventory, use of a chemical other than the one or more previously abused, forgetting to be thankful that their lives are better, and feeling all-powerful.

Another means of intervention that is very effective is for the nurse to act as a good role model in handling feelings, participating appropriately in meetings, and communicating to the patient in a way that supports the program. For example, telling patients that participation in AA meetings is not necessary for recovery could undermine their struggle to initiate the profound changes in lifestyle necessary to stay sober.

POPULATIONS OF SUBSTANCE ABUSERS WITH SPECIAL PROBLEMS

The unique characteristics of many groups of individuals compound the process of recovery and contribute to a high risk for relapse into chronic use of whatever substance the person has a history of abusing. Recent research in addressing these problems has proven very promising to date. As mentioned earlier, the trend is to provide specially designed treatment approaches for groups of individuals who have common traits and problems that may contribute to their dependency to alcohol or other drugs.

THE ELDERLY

Although elderly people use approximately 25% of the medications used in the United States, only about 2 to 5% of men and fewer than 1% of women over the age of 65 years abuse alcohol. And elderly people are more likely to abuse over-the-counter and prescription sleeping pills, pain medications, or tranquilizers instead of illegal drugs such as cocaine. Motives for misuse are seldom for recreational purposes among this age group.

Owing to a decreased ability to metabolize and eliminate alcohol or drugs from the body, elderly individuals who do abuse over extended periods of time may experience significant medical problems as a result. The most typical physical consequences of chronic alcohol abuse among the elderly include malnutrition, cirrhosis of the liver, bone thinning, gastritis, poor memory, and decreased cognitive ability to process new information. If the person combines alcohol with any other medication that has central nervous system depressant effects, the danger of oversedation, impaired responses, or respiratory depression is very great.

Most of the elderly who abuse alcohol have maintained a regular pattern of use over many years without obvious problems. As their bodies age, their ability to tolerate the same quantities decreases, putting them at risk for falls or other injuries as a result of intoxication. Others turn to first-time or heavier patterns of use to cope with anxiety produced by the typical stressors of aging such as retirement, losses of significant others, family conflict, health problems, social isolation, and loss of self-worth. Among the elderly who move to more affluent retirement communities, a rise in alcoholism has been noted. This may be due to involvement in cocktail parties, regular drinking with meals, and peer pressure to participate in order to be accepted.

Problems of abuse in the elderly population are usually diagnosed by the family physician as a result of complaints related to the psychological or physical effects of alcohol abuse, such as memory impairment or insomnia. Elderly people often deny that they have a substance abuse problem and will resist treatment without the support and pressure of their family.

Treatment of alcoholism in the elderly is similar to that of younger individuals except that the period of withdrawal must be more closely monitored and progress more slowly owing to the elderly person's physical fragility. Rehabilitation groups and educational programs should ideally be structured to permit processing information more slowly to allow for the cognitive slowing that is normal for this age group but that may be more pronounced because of the neurologic effects of chronic use of alcohol or other drugs, or both. Involvement in AA is critical and can be difficult if patients do not have easy access to a "home group" with other elderly people who can relate to their problems and issues.

ADOLESCENTS

Substance abuse among adolescents has received much attention in recent years. It is estimated that one in four adolescents become involved in substance abuse. It has also become apparent that children are experimenting with drugs at younger ages than ever before. The younger the age of onset of drug use, the greater the risk for significant interference in the physical and psychological development of the individual.

The developmental issues of this age group also contribute to the adolescent's vulnerability. This is a stage of establishing one's identity, experimenting with newly developed abilities to think abstractly, egocentricity, limited impulse control, and poor judgment. Identification with one's peer group is an important aspect of feeling accepted. Average adolescents view themselves as omnipotent and deny the likelihood of negative consequences of their behaviors. This is the age of rebellion.

Substance abuse in this population is also viewed as a symptom of family issues. The family is often dysfunctional—patterns of communication may be ineffective and children in the family may be emotionally or physically neglected, abused, or subject to rigid, unrealistic expectations for their behavior. There may be a family history of substance abuse, or the adolescent may fall into the "wrong crowd" of other young people who are already involved in the drug culture.

The progression of physical consequences of substance abuse in the adolescent population is correlated with the risks related to the substance abused and the likelihood of polysubstance abuse. The risks of accidental overdose or suicide are significant. Intravenous drug use and the likelihood of sexual activity without the use of precautions have been linked to an increased risk of HIV infection in this group.

Entry into treatment usually occurs as a result of a crisis situation revealing the severity of drug use and parental insistence. Breaking through adolescents' denial is the most difficult aspect of treatment, especially since they seldom want to be in treatment and do not see the potential negative consequences of their behaviors. It may also be difficult to distinguish the abuser from the adolescent who is still in the early stages of experimentation and unlikely to persist in chronic substance abuse. Most adolescents do not reach the point of believing it when saying, "Hi, I'm an alcoholic," (or drug abuser) at the beginning of each AA or NA meeting.

Rehabilitation of the adolescent substance abuser requires that the approach to treatment be modified to meet the needs of this age group more effectively. It remains very controversial to mix adolescents with adults in treatment programs owing to the adolescent's vulnerability to being influenced by the more experienced and usually charismatic adult substance user. Obviously, careful supervision is necessary if mixing age groups for treatment is the only option. In addition, many of the abstract concepts addressed in the 12 steps of AA may need to be adapted to the level of understanding of the individual adolescent.

Successful rehabilitation usually involves regular involvement in an AA group made up of younger people that the adolescent can relate to, successful development of a new, non–drug-using peer group, and reentry into school with the support of other recovering classmates. Alcoholics Anonymous group meetings may be held at high schools in some cities.

THE DUALLY DIAGNOSED

Patients who have already been diagnosed with a serious psychiatric illness and also have a substance abuse problem present special concerns for rehabilitation. Dually diagnosed patients usually have psychiatric illnesses of depression, schizophrenia, or bipolar illness. Often, mental retardation and organic brain disease also are included in the group of medical problems identified as presenting special concerns in the event of a concurrent substance abuse problem. (Many times, substance abusers have a personality disorder, although this group of psychiatric disorders is generally not considered to be the result of some physiologic process and is usually not included under dual diagnosis.)

In some individuals, chronic drug or alcohol abuse may exacerbate an already fragile neurochemical balance, producing psychiatric symptoms. This is seen in cases of young adolescents who use marijuana or some other type of drug prior to their first psychotic break with schizophrenia. Toxic psychosis may occur more frequently with the use of cocaine or amphetamines mixed with alcohol. In other cases, people may use a mind-altering drug to treat psychiatric symptoms without understanding the reason. They just know that they feel better.

People with chronic psychiatric problems require special teaching and supervision in the event of substance relapse. Antipsychotic medications do not mix with alcohol. If a bipolar patient is on lithium, the fluid losses as a result of drinking alcohol could precipitate lithium toxicity. Patients taking antianxiety or antidepressant agents with alcohol could risk accidental overdose due to additive effects or could be deliberately attempting to harm themselves.

The approach to rehabilitation must be modified to adapt to this special population. Each patient's ability to comprehend the abstract ideas from the 12-step process of AA will vary. In addition, traditionalists in the recovery process often frown upon the use of any mind-altering chemical and may subtly pressure dually diagnosed clients to stop their prescribed medications. This lack of knowledge and rigid approach to recovery could contribute to exacerbation of the underlying psychiatric illness.

PEER ASSISTANCE PROGRAMS

Substance abuse is expected to be one of the most widespread problems of the next 20 years. People from all walks of life are at risk, including health care professionals who are at high risk owing to easier access to addictive drugs. As a result, many professional groups have developed peer assistance programs. These programs are designed to offer a supportive alternative to health professionals (physicians, dentists, nurses, and others) who become addicted to a substance instead of taking immediate disciplinary action against their licenses. Peer assistance programs for nurses exist in every state. Referrals are made by the individuals themselves or by employers and peers who have reason to believe an individual's practice has been impaired by the use of a substance. With the help of representatives of the program, usually volunteers, information is gathered to support an intervention in hopes of getting the nurse into treatment and recovery.

The goals of an intervention for a nurse whose practice is impaired are as follows:

- Assist the nurse whose practice is impaired to receive treatment.
- Protect the public from an untreated nurse.
- Help the recovering nurse reenter nursing in a systematic, planned, and safe way.
- Assist in monitoring the continued recovery of the nurse for a period of time.

Usually there is also at least a 2-year time period afterward in which the nurse is required to attend AA or NA groups regularly, to participate in peer support groups, to meet routinely with an identified support person representing the peer assistance program, and to submit random urine drug screens to ensure that he or she has not relapsed. If nurses are unable to comply with the process, then information regarding their substance use and how that has impaired their practice can be turned over to the Board of Nurse Examiners for that state. Until that point, however, the information regarding each nurse involved is kept confidential and, if they successfully complete the requirements of the program, will never become part of the licensing board's records. Most peer assistance programs also work with nurses whose practices have become impaired as a result of mental illness.

Substance abuse will continue to be a major health care problem in the future. Nurses who work in this field are presented with difficult challenges and must be able to be nonjudgmental and supportive of the patients with whom they work. The knowledge base for this specialty area is growing quickly as a result of the widespread research currently being done. No matter where nurses work, they will come in contact with patients whose health status is compromised by substance abuse. The opportunity to play a powerful role in promoting healthier lifestyles is one that can be very fulfilling.

NUTRITION CONCEPTS

- Heavy drug or alcohol intake has a negative effect on nutrition because it displaces foods in the diet that are more nutritious and impairs absorption and metabolism of nutrients in the body.
- The nutritional goals for persons with alcoholism are to support them in avoiding alcohol and to correct nutritional deficits.
- Individuals with chronic alcoholism may receive supplements of folate and vitamins B_1 and B_6.
- Stimulants may induce anorexia; however, as the effects of the stimulants subside, hunger develops.

BIBLIOGRAPHY

Arnold, L. J. (1990). Codependency/part I: Origins, characteristics. *AORN Journal 51*(5), 1341–1348.

Arnold, L. J. (1990). Codependency/part II: The hospital as a dysfunctional family. *AORN Journal 51*(6), 1581–1584.

Arnold, L. J. (1990). Codependency/part III: Strategies for healing. *AORN Journal 52*(1), 85–89.

Avery, M. L. (1989). Adult children of alcoholics: Whom do they trust? *Journal of Psychosocial Nursing, 27*(8), 20–24.

Bateman, D. A., et al. (1993). The effects of intrauterine cocaine exposure in newborns. *American Journal of Public Health, 83*(2), 190–193.

Brower, K. J. (1993). Anabolic steroids. *Psychiatric Clinics of North America, 16*(1), 97–103.

Catanzarite, A. M. (1992). *Managing the chemically dependent nurse: A guide to identification, intervention, and retention.* American Hospital Publishing, Inc.

Cermak, T. L., et al. (1989). Codependency: More than a catchword. *Patient Care, 23,* 131–150.

Collins, G. B. (1993). Contemporary issues in the treatment of alcohol dependence. *Psychiatric Clinics of North America, 16*(1), 33–48.

Cook, J. S. (1991). Alcohol abuse. In J. S. Cook & K. L. Fontaine (Eds.), *Essentials of mental health nursing* (2nd ed., pp. 442–483). Redwood City, CA: Addison-Wesley Nursing.

Cook, J. S. (1991). Drug abuse. In J. S. Cook & K. L. Fontaine (Eds.), *Essentials of mental health nursing* (2nd ed., pp. 484–528). Redwood City, CA: Addison-Wesley Nursing.

Cusack, J. R., Malaney, K. R., & DePry, D. L. (1993). Insights about pathological gamblers: 'Chasing losses' in spite of the consequences. *Postgraduate Medicine, 93*(5), 169–176.

Davidson Ward, S. L., & Keens, T. G. (1992). Prenatal substance abuse. *Clinics in Perinatology, 19*(4), 849–860.

Dryfoos, J. G. (1993). Preventing substance use: Rethinking strategies. *American Journal of Public Health, 83*(6), 793–795.

Fischbach, F. (1992). *A manual of laboratory and diagnostic tests* (4th ed.). Philadelphia: J. B. Lippincott.

Fishbain, D. A., Rosomoff, H. L., & Rosomoff, R. S. (1992). Drug abuse, dependence, and addiction in chronic pain patients. *The Clinical Journal of Pain, 8*(2), 77–85.

Hoffmann, N. G., & Miller, N. S. (1993). Perspectives of effective treatment for alcohol and drug disorders. *Psychiatric Clinics of North America, 16*(1), 127–140.

Hutchinson, S. A. (1992). Applying the nursing process for clients with psychoactive substance use disorders. In H. S. Wilson & C. R. Kneisl (Eds.), *Psychiatric nursing* (4th ed., pp. 214–257). Redwood City, CA: Addison-Wesley Nursing.

Johnson, E. (1992). From the alcohol, drug abuse, and mental health administration. *JAMA, 267*(17), 2293.

Kadden, R. M., & Mauriello, I. J. (1991). Enhancing participation in substance abuse treatment using an incentive system. *Journal of Substance Abuse Treatment, 9,* 113–124.

Kennedy, J., & Faugier, J. (1989). *Drug and alcohol dependency nursing.* Oxford: Heinemann Nursing.

Kintz, P., Tracqui, A., & Mangin P. (1992). Detection of drugs in human hair for clinical and forensic applications. *International Journal of Legal Medicine, 105*(1), 1–4.

Krystal, J. H., et al. (1992). Chronic 3,4-methylenedioxymethamphetamine (MDMA) use: Effects on mood and neuropsychological function? *American Journal of Drug and Alcohol Abuse, 18*(3), 331–341.

Lindblom, L., et al. (1992). Chemical abuse: An intervention program for the elderly. *Journal of Gerontological Nursing, 18*(4), 6–14.

Lowinson, J. H., et al. (Eds.). (1992). *Substance abuse: A comprehensive textbook* (2nd ed.). Baltimore, MD: Williams & Wilkins.

Miller, W. H., & Hyatt, M. C. (1992). Perinatal substance abuse. *American Journal of Drug and Alcohol Abuse, 18*(3), 247–261.

Miller, W. R. (1992). The effectiveness of treatment for substance abuse: Reasons for optimism. *Journal of Substance Abuse Treatment, 9,* 93–102.

Montamat, S. C., & Cusack, B. (1992). Overcoming problems with polypharmacy and drug misuse in the elderly. *Health Promotion and Disease Prevention, 8*(1), 143–158.

Nace, E. P., & Naegle, M. (1993). Managing alcohol abuse in primary care. *Patient Care, 27*(5), 102–107.

Raskin, V. D. (1993). Psychiatric aspects of substance use disorders in childbearing populations. *Psychiatric Clinics of North America, 16*(1), 157–165.

Seal, M. (1993). Facing down drunks: Two women help families to confront the alcoholic in their midst. *Lear's, 6*(2), 76–79, 101–102.

Selbach, K. H. (1990). Chemical dependency in nursing: Identifying and helping the troubled nurse. *AORN Journal 52*(3), 531–542.

Sheahan, S. L., Hendricks, J., & Coons, S. J. (1989). Drug misuse among the elderly: A covert problem. *Health Values, 13*(3), 22–29.

Shives, L. R. (1990). Ineffective individual coping: Alcoholism. In L. R. Shives, R. H. Southwell, & M. Young (Eds.), *Basic concepts of psychiatric-mental health nursing* (2nd ed.). Philadelphia: J. B. Lippincott.

Solari-Twadell, A. (1988). Nurse impairment: The significance of the professional culture. *Quality Review Bulletin, 14*(4), 103–104.

Sternbach, G. L., & Varon, J. (1992). 'Designer drugs': Recognizing and managing their toxic effects. *Postgraduate Medicine, 91*(8), 169–176.

KEY CONCEPTS

1. The majority of experts in substance abuse subscribe to the biologic theory, which proposes that a faulty physiologic process contributes to dependence on a specific substance and that drug dependency is a physical illness.
2. Some theorists contend that sociocultural factors contribute to the development of substance abuse.
3. According to behavioral and learning theories, substance abuse is a learned maladaptive way of coping with stress and anxiety.
4. The interpersonal or psychological theory states that innate personality factors may predispose individuals to substance abuse.
5. Substance abusers have many common personality traits, including self-centeredness, a need to be in control of others, attention seeking, and difficulty delaying gratification of their needs.
6. Although the specific causes of substance abuse have not been established, it is most likely that the true cause involves a combination of biologic, cultural, behavioral, and psychological factors.
7. To obtain reliable data when questioning a person about substance abuse, the nurse must be nonjudgmental, direct, and specific, and the information obtained should be verified by more than one person when possible.
8. The lifestyle of substance abusers may focus entirely on obtaining and using the substance of choice, with an increasing need for more and more in order to get the desired effects.
9. Substance abusers frequently have erratic and unprovoked mood swings, blackouts, significant work problems, and damaged relationships.
10. Typical defense mechanisms used by substance abusers include denial, rationalization, intellectualization, and projection.
11. Most alcohol abusers appear malnourished and poorly cared for, have evidence of physical trauma from falls or violence, appear jaundiced, and, when in withdrawal, may be hypertensive with signs of fluid retention.
12. Tests for detecting substance abuse include a blood alcohol study, a urine drug screening, and hair analysis.
13. Chronic alcoholism involves the regular daily ingestion of large amounts of alcohol, regular heavy drinking only on weekends, or binges of heavy drinking followed by long periods of abstinence.
14. Physical addiction occurs when the cells of the body are dependent on alcohol to carry out certain metabolic processes; without the alcohol, the cells go into shock.
15. Alcohol withdrawal syndrome begins after an individual stops or decreases the amount of alcohol ingested and involves physiologic and behavioral symptoms that begin when the individual's blood alcohol level drops.
16. Alcoholism has an impact on the entire family. Family and peer pressure can be a critical factor in inducing an alcoholic to seek treatment.
17. Strategies that have been successful in alcohol rehabilitation are 12-step programs, stress management, social skills training, behavioral approaches to marital therapy, and matching clients with therapists who use a style most likely to benefit their personality type.
18. The six classes of psychoactive substances other than alcohol that are frequently associated with substance abuse are stimulants, depres-

sants, hallucinogens, narcotics, inhalants, and designer drugs.

19. Drug abuse treatment is similar to alcohol detoxification and rehabilitation; however, relapse rates are higher and treatment may need to be more individualized.
20. Methadone maintenance may be used for long-term heroin abusers who have sustained permanent damage to chemical receptor sites in the brain and therefore have a decreased ability to resist relapses.

Glossary

ACID A solution containing a high number of hydrogen ions

ACID-BASE BALANCE The homeostasis of the hydrogen ion (H^+) concentration in the body fluids

ACIDOSIS Abnormal pH of body fluids caused by excess acid in relation to bicarbonate

ACNE Inflammatory skin disorder characterized by comedones, pustules, and cysts

ACQUIRED IMMUNITY Immunity acquired after birth as a result of the body's natural immune responses to antigens

ACROCHORDON Small, soft, raised lesion (skin tag)

ACROMEGALY Disease of middle-aged adults resulting from overproduction of growth hormone by the anterior pituitary

ACTIVE ACQUIRED IMMUNITY Immunity developed after direct contact with an antigen through illness or vaccination

ACTIVE EXERCISE Exercise carried out by the patient

ACTIVE TRANSPORT Movement of solutes across membranes using greater energy or force

ACUTE ILLNESS Illness or disease that has a relatively rapid onset and a short duration

ACUTE PAIN Pain that lasts less than 6 months, has an identifiable cause, and goes away as healing occurs

ADAPTATION The organism's attempt to return to homeostasis

ADDICTION Effect of habitual ingestion of a substance to the point of physical dependence; used interchangeably with the term dependence

ADDISON'S DISEASE Disease resulting from a deficiency of adrenocorticotropic hormone caused by destruction or dysfunction of the adrenal glands

ADRENALINE Epinephrine; a powerful vasoactive substance produced by the medulla or adrenal gland in times of stress or danger

ADRENOCORTICOTROPIC HORMONE (ACTH) A pituitary hormone that stimulates the cortex of the adrenal glands to produce adrenal hormones

ADVANCE DIRECTIVE Written statement of a person's wishes regarding medical treatment

ADVANCED CARDIAC LIFE SUPPORT Use of drugs and equipment to provide continuing care of a person who has suffered cardiac or respiratory arrest

AEROSOL Solid or liquid particles suspended in a gas

AFFECT Briefly occurring feelings such as happiness, sadness, or worry. Inappropriate affect is incongruence between the thought and the feeling expressed

AFTERLOAD The amount of resistance the left ventricle must generate to open the aortic valve

AGEISM A process of systematic stereotyping and discrimination against people because of their age; usually directed against older people

AGING The process of growing older or more mature

AGORAPHOBIA Fear of situations outside the home

AKATHISIA A reversible condition of restlessness manifested as an urge to pace

ALGOR MORTIS Cooling of the body after death

ALKALINE OR BASE A solution containing a low number of hydrogen ions

ALKALOSIS Abnormal pH of body fluids caused by excess bicarbonate in relation to acid

ALLERGEN An antigen that causes a hypersensitive reaction

ALOPECIA Loss of hair

AMINO ACIDS A group of 22 substances that can be bonded in different ways to make a variety of proteins. The body can manufacture sufficient amounts of these provided the nine essential amino acids are derived from the diet

AMPUTATION Removal of a limb, part of a limb, or an organ; may be done by surgical means or in an accident

AMPUTEE Individual who has undergone an amputation

AMYOPATHY (AMYOTONIA) Loss of muscle tone

ANALGESIC Drug that acts on the nervous system to relieve or reduce the suffering or intensity of pain

ANAPHYLACTIC SHOCK A severe, potentially fatal, allergic reaction characterized by hypotension and bronchial constriction

ANASTOMOSIS Communication or connection between two organs or parts of organs

ANDROGENS Hormones produced by the adrenal cortex, the testes, and the ovaries that stimulate the development of male characteristics

ANEMIA A deficiency in the number of red blood cells, hemoglobin, or both in the blood

ANESTHESIOLOGIST A physician who specializes in the administration of anesthetics and monitors the patient while under anesthesia

ANESTHETIC An agent that abolishes the pain sensation

ANGIOMA Benign tumor composed of blood vessels

ANKYLOSIS Joint immobility

ANORECTAL INCONTINENCE Fecal incontinence caused by weak perineal muscles, loss of anal reflexes, loss of anal sphincter tone, or rectal prolapse

ANOREXIA Lack of appetite for food

ANTEFLEXION Bending forward of the top of an organ

ANTEVERSION Bending forward of an entire organ

ANTIBODY A protein that is created in response to a specific antigen

ANTIDIURETIC HORMONE (ADH) A hormone released by the posterior portion of the pituitary gland that causes the reabsorption of water in the distal tubules and collecting ducts of the kidney

ANTIGEN Any substance that invades the body and is capable of stimulating a response from the immune system

ANTIHISTAMINE Drug that blocks the effects of histamine, a body chemical that causes allergic symptoms

ANTINEOPLASTIC An agent that inhibits the maturation or reproduction of malignant cells

ANTITHROMBOTIC Capable of preventing the formation of blood clots

ANURIA Absence of urine production

ANXIETY A vague sense of impending doom or apprehension that appears to have no clearly identifiable cause

APHASIA The inability to understand words or the inability to respond with words, or both

APICAL Referring to the pointed end of a structure

APNEA Cessation of breathing

ARTERIOSCLEROSIS Abnormal thickening and hardening of the arterial walls

ARTHRALGIA Pain in a joint

ARTHROPLASTY Plastic repair of a joint

ASBESTOSIS Interstitial fibrosis caused by inhalation of asbestos fibers

ASCITES Accumulation of excess fluid in the peritoneal cavity

ASSESSMENT Collection of data about the health status of a patient or client

ASTHMA A condition characterized by episodes of bronchospasm that causes wheezing and dyspnea

ASTIGMATISM Error of refraction caused by uneven curvature of the cornea or lens; causes visual distortion

ATELECTASIS Collapsed lung or part of a lung

ATHEROSCLEROSIS Abnormal thickening and hardening of the arterial walls caused by fat and fibrin deposits

AURA A peculiar sensation that precedes a set of symptoms

AUSCULTATION Listening to sounds produced by the body, such as heart, lung, and intestinal sounds

AUTOCRATIC LEADERSHIP Authoritarian, directive, or bureaucratic type of leadership

AUTOIMMUNITY A condition in which the body is unable to distinguish self from nonself causing the immune system to react and destroy its own tissues

AUTOMATICITY Ability of a cell to generate an impulse without external stimulation

AUTOMATISM Aimless behavior performed without conscious control or knowledge

AUTONOMIC DYSREFLEXIA Abnormally exaggerated response of the autonomic nervous system to a stimulus

AUTOPSY Examination of a body after death to determine or confirm the cause of death

AVULSION Tearing away of tissue

AZOTEMIA Accumulation of nitrogenous compounds in the blood

BACTERIA Several classifications of one-celled microorganisms that are capable of multiplying rapidly and causing illness

BASAL METABOLIC RATE Measurement of energy expenditure taken in the morning after awakening and approximately 10 to 12 hours after the last meal

BASIC LIFE SUPPORT Immediate care given to prevent cardiac or respiratory arrest or to support circulation and respiration of a victim of cardiac arrest until advanced medical support is available

BENIGN Not malignant

BIOLOGIC AGE The functional capabilities of various organ systems in the body

BIOLOGIC APPROACH Assumes that mental disorders are related to physiologic changes within the central nervous system

BIOPSY Excision of a small piece of tissue for microscopic examination; usually done to determine a specific diagnosis

BIPOLAR DISORDER Alternating periods of elevated mood (manic episodes) and depression

BLEPHARITIS Inflammation of the hair follicles and glands on the margins of the eyelids

BODY IMAGE One's physical and psychological experiences that influence the perception of one's own body

BONE MARROW Spongy center of bones where the white blood cells, red blood cells, and platelets are made

BONE REMODELING Process in which immature bone cells are gradually replaced by mature bone cells

BORDERLINE PERSONALITY DISORDER Exhibition of unstable relationships, unstable self-image, and unstable mood

BOTULISM Food poisoning caused by *Clostridium botulinum*

BOUCHARD'S NODES Enlarged proximal interphalangeal joints of the fingers

BRACHYTHERAPY Placement of a radiation source in the body to treat a malignancy

BRADYCARDIA Slow heart rate, usually defined as fewer than 60 beats per minute

BRONCHIECTASIS Permanent dilation of a portion of the bronchi or bronchioles

BRONCHITIS Bronchial inflammation

BRUIT A murmur detected by auscultation

BULLA Blister

CACHEXIA Profound malnutrition

CALCULUS Concentration, commonly called a stone, formed of mineral salts in hollow organs or their passages (plural *calculi*)

CALORIE Standard unit for measuring energy; the amount of heat needed to raise the temperature of 1 ml of water at a standard temperature by 1 degree centigrade

CANNULA A tube that can be inserted into a body cavity or duct; needle or catheter employed for intravenous therapy

CARCINOGEN A substance that can cause cancer

CARDIAC OUTPUT Amount of blood in liters ejected by either ventricle per minute

CARDIAC TAMPONADE Presence of blood in the pericardial sac causing a decrease in cardiac output

CARDIOPULMONARY ARREST Absence of heartbeat and breathing

CARDIOVERSION Delivery of an electrical shock to the myocardium to restore normal sinus rhythm

CARIES Destructive process of tooth decay

CARING A process characterized by understanding and action

CATARACT Clouding or opacity of the normally transparent lens within the eye; causes blurred vision and objects to take on a yellowish hue

CATECHOLAMINES Chemicals (dopamine, epinephrine, norepinephrine) released at sympathetic nerve endings in response to stress

CATHARTIC Agent that stimulates bowel evacuation; usually rapid in effect and producing a watery stool

CELL-MEDIATED IMMUNITY A delayed response to injury or infection involving T cells and the production of substances that enhance the immune response and influence the destruction of antigens

CEREBRAL DEATH Absence of cerebral cortex functioning

CERUMEN Waxy secretion in the external auditory canal; earwax

CERVICITIS Inflammation of the cervix (narrow, lower end of the uterus)

CHALAZION An inflamed, enlarged meibomian gland

CHANCRE A papule that breaks down into a painless ulcer at the site of entry of the organism that causes syphilis

CHELITIS Inflammation of the lips

CHELOSIS Cracking of the lips and corners of the mouth

CHEMICAL RESTRAINTS Psychotropic medications given to subdue agitated or confused patients

CHEMOTHERAPY Use of chemicals to treat illness

CHOKING Airway obstruction caused by a foreign body in the airway

CHOLANGITIS Inflammation of the biliary ducts

CHOLECYSTECTOMY Removal of the gallbladder

CHOLECYSTITIS Inflammation of the gallbladder

CHOLEDOCHOLITHIASIS Obstruction of the common bile duct by a gallstone

CHOLELITHIASIS Presence of gallstones in the gallbladder

CHRONIC ILLNESS Permanent impairment or disabilities that require long-term rehabilitation and medical or nursing treatment

CHRONIC PAIN Pain that lasts longer than 6 months

CHVOSTEK'S SIGN Spasm of the facial muscles when the facial nerve is tapped; indicative of hypocalcemia

CIRRHOSIS Chronic, progressive liver disease

CLIENT Denotes a feeling of partnership or working with someone

CLOSED AMPUTATION Amputation in which a limb or part of a limb is removed and surgically closed

CLOSED OR SIMPLE FRACTURE Fracture in which the broken bone does not break through the skin

CLOSED REDUCTION Non-surgical realignment of the bones to their previous anatomic position using traction, angulation, or rotation, or a combination of these

CLOTTING FACTORS Substances in the blood that help the blood to clot, numbered I through XII

CODEPENDENCY Exaggerated dependent pattern of self-defeating behaviors, beliefs, and feelings learned as a result of pathologic relationship to a chemically dependent, or otherwise dysfunctional, person

COGNITION Workings of the mind; language, memory, intellect, and reasoning

COGNITIVE BEHAVIORAL APPROACH Uses behavior modification (positive and negative reinforcement) and recognizes that particular thoughts influence emotional states

COLLATERAL Accessory; side branch

COLOSTOMY Surgically created opening in the colon

COLPORRHAPHY Operative technique that narrows the vagina by suturing the vaginal wall

COMMUNITY-ACQUIRED INFECTIONS Infections that are acquired in day-to-day contact with the public

COMPARTMENT SYNDROME Serious complication of a fracture caused by internal or external pressure to the affected area, resulting in decreased blood flow, pain, and tissue damage

COMPENSATION Adaptations made by the heart and circulation to maintain normal cardiac output

COMPLEMENT A series of proteins that enhance the inflammatory process and immune response

COMPLEMENTARY PROTEIN Combination of incomplete proteins that provide all nine essential amino acids when consumed together

COMPLETE FRACTURE Fracture in which the break extends across the entire bone, dividing it into two separate pieces

COMPLETE PROTEIN Protein containing all nine essential amino acids; usually of animal origin (e.g., meat, eggs)

COMPLIANCE Elasticity

COMPROMISED HOST PRECAUTIONS Actions taken to help protect patients with low white blood cell counts from infection

COMPULSIONS Incessant behaviors such as hand washing that interfere with normal functioning

CONDUCTION DEAFNESS A hearing impairment due to a blockage of the ear canal caused by excessive wax buildup, abnormal structures, or infection

CONDUCTIVITY Ability of the cell to transmit electrical impulses rapidly and efficiently to distant regions of the heart

CONFLICT Psychological struggle that results when two incompatible possibilities occur at the same time

CONGENITAL AMPUTATION Deformity or absence of a limb or limbs occurring during fetal development in the uterus

CONJUNCTIVITIS Inflammation of the membrane lining the eyelids and the eyeball

CONSTIPATION Infrequent bowel movements with hard stools that are passed with difficulty

CONTINENT Capable of controlling natural impulses; in relation to an ostomy, able to retain feces or urine

CONTRACTILITY Capacity for shortening in response to stimuli

CONTRACTURE Shortening of the muscles and tendons

CONTRALATERAL Affecting the opposite side

CONVERSION DISORDER Loss of body function (such as paralysis) without physiologic cause

COPING Any behavioral or cognitive activity used to deal with stress

COPING STRATEGY An adaptive or maladaptive mental attitude, behavior, or both that is consciously or unconsciously perceived as helping to reduce stress, anxiety, or fear

COR PULMONALE Right-sided heart failure associated with pulmonary disease

CORYZA Discharge from the nasal mucous membranes

CRACKLES Rales; abnormal lung sounds heard on auscultation

CREDÉ'S TECHNIQUE Expression of urine from the bladder by applying pressure over the lower abdomen

CREPITUS Crackling sound or sensation

CRETINISM Permanent mental and physical retardation caused by congenital deficiency of thyroid hormones

CRISIS The point on the health continuum at which the individual moves toward illness and disequilibrium occurs

CULTURAL DIVERSITY The existence of many cultures in a society

CULTURE Arts, beliefs, customs, institutions, and all other products of human work and thought created by a people or a group at a particular time

CUSHING'S DISEASE Disease caused by the hypersecretion of glucocorticoids due to excessive release of adrenocorticotropic hormone by the pituitary

CUSHING'S SYNDROME Disorder resulting from excessive glucocorticoids in the body as a result of tumor or hypersecretion of the pituitary or by prolonged administration of large doses of exogenous steroids

CUSP Cup-shaped structure; semilunar heart valves have three cusps

CYCLOPLEGIC Agent that paralyzes the ciliary muscle so that the eye does not accommodate

CYSTECTOMY Removal or resection of the urinary bladder or of a cyst

CYSTOCELE Herniation of the urinary bladder into the vagina

CYSTOTOMY Creation of a surgical opening into the bladder

DÉBRIDE To remove debris, including necrotic tissue

DECEREBRATE POSTURING Abnormal extension of the upper extremities with extension of the lower extremities; accompanies increased pressure on the entire cerebrum and the motor tract structures of the brain stem

DECONGESTANT Agent that reduces swelling, especially of the nasal mucous membranes

DECORTICATE POSTURING Abnormal flexion of the upper extremities with extension of the lower extremities; accompanies increased pressure on the frontal lobes

DEEP PARTIAL THICKNESS BURN a burn that involves the epidermis and the dermis

DEFENSE MECHANISM A conscious or unconscious mechanism used to relieve or diminish anxiety

DEFIBRILLATION Termination of cardiac fibrillation, usually by electric shock

DEHISCENCE Separation of previously joined edges; reopening of a surgical wound

DELAYED UNION Fracture healing that does not occur in the normally expected time

DELIRIUM An acute organic disorder usually caused by some underlying illness that is characterized by disturbances in attention, thinking, perception, orientation, short-term memory, and sleep

DEMENTIA A clinical syndrome or collection of symptoms that is chronic in nature and is characterized by impairment of intellectual function, problem-solving ability, judgment, memory, orientation, and appropriate behavior

DEMOCRATIC LEADERSHIP Achievement of goals through participation by all group members

DENIAL A defense mechanism in which particular feelings or specific aspects of reality are excluded from awareness

DEPERSONALIZATION A state of feeling outside of oneself, watching what is happening as if it were to someone else

DEPRESSION A mood of sadness; a withdrawal from usual commitments

DERMATITIS Inflammation of the skin

DERMATOME Area of skin supplied by sensory nerve fibers from a single posterior spinal root

DIABETES INSIPIDUS Disease caused by inadequate secretion of antidiuretic hormone by the posterior portion of the pituitary

DIAGNOSIS RELATED GROUP (DRG) System enacted under Medicare that reimburses hospitals for patient care based on their medical diagnoses

DIALYSIS Passage of molecules through a semipermeable membrane into a special solution

DIAPHORESIS Excessive perspiration

DIAPHORETIC Wet with excessive perspiration

DIARRHEA The passage of frequent watery stools

DIASTOLE Relaxation phase of the cardiac cycle

DIFFUSION The random movement of particles in all directions through a solution

DIPLOPIA Double vision

DISABILITY Quantifiable loss of function, usually for the purpose of indicating a diminished capacity for work (*see* HANDICAP)

DISCOID LUPUS Circular, scaly lesions with erythematous raised rims; occurs over scalp, ears, face, and areas exposed to sun

DISORDER A term used when a definite organic cause such as delirium or dementia is established for behaviors and symptoms (*see* SYNDROME)

DISSOCIATIVE DISORDER Change in identity, memory, or consciousness that allows persons to remove themselves from anxiety-provoking situations, for example, multiple personality disorder and amnesias

DISTRESS Stress that is perceived as harmful

DIURESIS Increased production of urine

DIZZINESS Feeling of unsteadiness; lightheadedness

DUAL DIAGNOSIS Simultaneous existence of a major psychiatric condition and a medical condition

DYSARTHRIA Inability to speak clearly due to neurologic damage that impairs normal muscle control

DYSMENORRHEA Painful menstruation

DYSPAREUNIA Difficult or painful sexual intercourse in women

DYSPEPSIA Epigastric discomfort after meals, caused by impaired digestion

DYSPHAGIA Difficulty swallowing

DYSPHASIA Difficulty speaking

DYSPLASIA Abnormal cells

DYSPNEA Difficulty breathing

DYSPRAXIA Partial inability to initiate coordinated voluntary motor acts

DYSRHYTHMIA Disturbance of rhythm; arrhythmia

DYSURIA Difficult or painful urination

ECCHYMOSIS A purplish skin lesion resulting from blood leaking out of the blood vessels

ECTROPION In relation to the eyelid, outward turning of the lid

EGO In psychoanalytic theory, the "rational self" or "reality" principle of personality; mediates between id and superego

EGOCENTRIC Belief that one is the center of the universe

EJACULATION Reflexive expulsion of semen from the male urethra

EJECTION FRACTION Percentage of ventricular end-diastolic volume ejected with each contraction of the left ventricle

ELECTROCONVULSIVE THERAPY Controversial therapy that uses electrical current to the brain to evoke a grand mal seizure

ELECTROLYTE A substance that develops an electrical charge when dissolved in water

EMBOLISM An obstruction of a blood vessel created by a trapped blood clot or other substance

EMBOLUS (*pl.* EMBOLI) An unattached blood clot or other substance in the circulatory system

EMESIS Vomiting

EMISSION Involuntary discharge of semen

EMOTIONAL LABILITY Instability; episodes of unexplained and uncontrollable happiness and sadness

EMPATHY The ability to identify with and understand another person's situation, feelings, and motives

EMPHYSEMA Abnormal accumulation of air in body tissue; in the lung, a disorder characterized by loss of lung elasticity with trapping of air, retained carbon dioxide, and dyspnea

ENCEPHALITIS Inflammation of brain tissue

ENCULTURATION The process of learning to be part of a culture

ENDOCRINE GLAND Ductless gland that produces an internal secretion discharged into the lymph or blood stream and circulated to all parts of the body

ENDOGENOUS Internally produced or caused by internal factors

ENDOMETRIOSIS A condition in which endometrial tissue is located abnormally outside the uterus

ENERGY Capacity to do work; the way the body uses nutrients received through food consumption

ENTROPION In relation to the eyelid, inward turning of the lid

ENUCLEATION Removal of an intact organ, such as the eyeball

ENURESIS Involuntary passage of urine, usually during sleep

EPIDIDYMITIS Inflammation of the epididymis

EPIDURAL Situated within the spinal canal or on the outside of the dura mater; opioids may be administered epidurally for pain relief

EPISTAXIS Nosebleed

EQUIANALGESIC Having approximately the same degree of pain relief effect

EQUILIBRIUM State of balance needed for walking, standing, and sitting

ERECTION Swelling and rigidity of the penis

ERUCTATION Expulsion of gas from the stomach through the mouth; belching

ERYTHEMA Redness of the skin; usually a sign that capillaries have become congested because of impaired blood flow

ESTROGENS Hormones produced by the ovaries, adrenal glands, and fetoplacental unit in females that are responsible for the sexual development and maturation of females

EUGLYCEMIA Normal blood glucose level

EUSTRESS Stress that is perceived as helpful (e.g., graduation, vacation)

EVISCERATION Protrusion of body organs through an open wound

EXCITABILITY Ability of a cell to respond to an electrochemical stimulus

EXOCRINE GLAND Gland that secretes substances externally through ducts

EXOGENOUS Externally produced or caused by external factors

EXOPHTHALMOS Protrusion of the eyeballs associated with hyperthyroidism

EXTERNAL FIXATION Use of rods, pins, nails, screws, or metal plates to align bone fragments and keep them in place for healing; similar to internal fixation, but the devices in the bone are attached to an external frame

EXTRACELLULAR FLUID Fluid outside the cell

EXTRAPYRAMIDAL EFFECTS Side effects of antipsychotic drugs on the portion of the central nervous system controlling involuntary movements

EXTRAVASATION Escape of fluid or blood from a blood vessel into body tissue

EXTRINSIC FACTORS Factors in the environment that can cause falls

FALL Circumstance in which one unintentionally falls to the ground or hits an object such as a chair or stair

FASCICULATION Small involuntary muscle contraction

FAT EMBOLISM Condition in which fat globules are released from the marrow of the broken bone into the blood stream, migrate to the lungs, and cause pulmonary hypertension

FAT-SOLUBLE VITAMINS Vitamins that are soluble in fat solvents, are absorbed into the body with other lipids, and build up in fat cells; includes vitamins A, D, E, and K

FEAR Analogous to anxiety; however, is related to dread of a specific or real occurrence

FECAL INCONTINENCE The inability to control the passage of feces

FEELINGS All emotional and physical responses and sensations

FILTRATION Transfer of water and solutes through a membrane from a region of high pressure to a region of low pressure

FIXATION Procedure done during the open reduction surgical procedure to attach the fragments of the broken bone together when reduction alone is not feasible

FLACCID Soft; in relation to muscles, lacking tone

FLACCIDITY Diminished muscle tone

FLAIL CHEST Multiple fractures of adjacent ribs resulting in a loss of support in the affected section of the chest wall

FLATULENCE Formation of excessive gas in the stomach or intestines

FLATUS Gas in the digestive tract that is expelled through the rectum

FLUENT APHASIA Ability to speak clearly but without meaning

FLUID Any liquid or gas

FLUID VOLUME DEFICIT A decrease in extracellular fluid

FLUID VOLUME EXCESS An increase in extracellular fluid

FRACTURE Break or disruption in the continuity of a bone

FROSTBITE Serious tissue damage caused by cold

FROSTNIP Mild tissue damaged caused by cold

FULL THICKNESS BURN Burn involving the epidermis, dermis, and underlying tissues such as fat, muscle, and bone

FUNCTIONAL INCONTINENCE Inappropriate voiding in the presence of normal bladder and urethral function

FUNGI Vegetable-like organisms that exist by feeding on organic matter and are capable of producing disease

GANGRENE Necrosis or death of tissue, usually due to a deficient or absent blood supply; may result from inflammatory processes, injury, arteriosclerosis, frostbite, or diabetes mellitus

GASTRECTOMY Removal of all or part of the stomach

GASTRITIS Inflammation of the stomach

GASTROSTOMY A surgically created opening in the stomach

GERONTOLOGICAL NURSE Professional nurses and advanced level practitioners such as nurse practitioners, clinical specialists, and nurses holding national certification in the specialty of gerontological nursing

GERONTOLOGY The study of aging

GIGANTISM Disease caused by excessive growth hormone in children and young adolescents resulting in excessive proportional growth

GINGIVITIS Inflammation of the gums

GLAND Organ or structure that secretes substances used in other areas of the body

GLAUCOMA Condition in which high pressure of the fluid in the eye causes damage to the optic nerve

GLUCOCORTICOID Class of adrenocortical hormones that affect protein and carbohydrate metabolism and help protect the body against stress

GLUCOMETER Electronic device used to measure blood glucose

GLUCONEOGENESIS Synthesis of glucose from sources other than carbohydrates

GLYCOGENESIS Conversion of glucose to glycogen

GLYCOGENOLYSIS Splitting of glycogen into glucose

GLYCOSURIA Presence of glucose in the urine

GOITER Enlargement of the thyroid gland, causing the neck to appear swollen

GOITROGEN Substance that suppresses thyroid function

GONIOMETER Instrument used to measure joint range of motion

GRANULOMA A collection of inflammatory cells commonly surrounded by fibrotic tissue that represents a chronic inflammatory response to infectious or noninfectious agents

GRATIFICATION Sense of comfort and satisfaction derived from the fulfillment of one's needs

GRAVIDITY Total number of pregnancies

GRIEF An emotional response to a loss

GROWTH AND DEVELOPMENT Physical, cognitive, and psychological development that is predictable and sequential

GUILLOTINE AMPUTATION Type of amputation in which a limb or portion of a limb is severed from the body and the wound is left open; a type of open amputation

HANDICAP Inability to perform one or more normal daily activities because of mental or physical disability (see *disability*)

HEALTH MAINTENANCE ORGANIZATION (HMO) Health care organization that provides care and services through group practice and prepayment plans

HEARTBURN (PYROSIS) Burning or tight sensation rising from the lower sternum to the throat

HEAT STROKE Body core temperature of 106°F or more

HEBERDEN'S NODES Protrusions of the distal interphalangeal finger joints; associated with osteoarthritis

HEIMLICH MANEUVER Technique for ejecting a foreign body from the airway by using abdominal thrusts

HELMINTHS Worms that are parasites found in the soil and water and are transmitted to humans from hand to mouth

HEMATOCELE Accumulation of blood in the tunica vaginalis, which is the membrane that lines the front and sides of the testis and the epididymis

HEMATOCRIT Percentage of red blood cells in whole blood

HEMATURIA Blood in the urine

HEMIPARESIS Weakness on one side of the body

HEMIPLEGIA Paralysis of one side of the body

HEMOCONCENTRATION Concentration of the blood

HEMODYNAMICS Study of the movement of blood and the forces that affect it

HEMOGLOBIN Protein of the red blood cell that carries oxygen

HEMORRHAGE Loss of a large amount of blood

HEMOTHORAX Presence of blood in the pleural cavity causing the lung on the affected side to collapse

HEPATIC Pertaining to the liver

HEPATITIS Inflammation of the liver

HEPATOMEGALY Enlargement of the liver

HIV Human immunodeficiency virus

HIV POSITIVE A condition in which the blood has antibodies for the human immunodeficiency virus (HIV), meaning the individual has been infected with this virus

HOLISM A way of viewing people as whole individuals

HOMEOSTASIS A tendency of biologic systems to maintain stability of the internal environment while continuously adjusting to changes necessary for survival

HOMONYMOUS HEMIANOPSIA Loss of half the field of vision; loss is on the side opposite the brain lesion

HOPELESSNESS A condition of lack of hope, which may hinder action

HORDEOLUM Inflammation of a sebaceous gland of the eyelid; commonly called a "sty"

HUMORAL IMMUNITY An immediate response to specific antigens involving B lymphocytes and the production of antibodies

HYDROCELE Accumulation of clear fluid in the scrotum along the spermatic cord

HYPERCALCEMIA Abnormally high serum calcium

HYPERCAPNIA Excess carbon dioxide in the blood

HYPERGLYCEMIA Abnormally high serum glucose

HYPERKALEMIA Abnormally high serum potassium

HYPERLIPIDEMIA Excess insoluble fats in the blood

HYPERNATREMIA Abnormally high serum sodium

HYPEROPIA Farsightedness; ability to see distant objects better than near objects

HYPERTENSION Persistent elevation of arterial blood pressure greater than 140/90 mm Hg

HYPERTHERMIA Elevation of body core temperature above 99°F

HYPERTONIC A term used to describe a solution that has a higher concentration of electrolytes than normal body fluids

HYPERTROPHY Enlargement of existing cells resulting in increased size of an organ or tissue

HYPERURICEMIA Elevated level of uric acid in the blood

HYPERVENTILATION Abnormally prolonged and deep breathing

HYPERVOLEMIA Increased circulating blood volume

HYPOCALCEMIA Abnormally low serum calcium

HYPOCHONDRIASIS Belief that a serious medical condition exists when medical findings are absent

HYPOGLYCEMIA Abnormally low level of glucose in the blood

HYPOKALEMIA Abnormally low serum potassium

HYPONATREMIA Abnormally low serum sodium

HYPOPHYSECTOMY Surgical removal of all or part of the pituitary gland

HYPOTENSION Abnormally low blood pressure

HYPOTHERMIA Decrease in body core temperature below 95°F

HYPOTONIC A term used to describe a solution that has a lower concentration of electrolytes than normal body fluids

HYPOVENTILATION Reduced movement of air into the alveoli

HYPOVOLEMIA Reduced circulating blood volume

HYPOXEMIA Low level of oxygen in the blood

HYPOXIA Low oxygen level

HYSTERECTOMY Surgical removal of the uterus

IATROGENIC INFECTIONS Infections caused by the caregiving process

ICTERUS Jaundice; golden yellow skin color caused by deposition of bile

ID In psychoanalytic theory, the "pleasure principle" of the personality

ILEOSTOMY Surgically created opening in the ileum

IMMOBILITY The inability to move; imposed restriction on entire body

IMMUNODEFICIENCY A condition in which the immune system is unable to defend the body against a foreign invasion of antigens

IMMUNOSUPPRESSANT Agent that reduces immune response

IMPACTION (FECAL) Accumulation of stool in the intestines that is not readily eliminated

IMPAIRMENT Physical or psychological disturbance in functioning

IMPOTENCE Inability to achieve and maintain an erection for sexual intercourse

INCOMPLETE FRACTURE Fracture in which the bone breaks only part way across, leaving some portion of the bone intact

INCOMPLETE PROTEIN Plant protein lacking one or more essential amino acids

INFARCT An area of ischemic necrosis caused by disruption of circulation

INFERTILITY Inability to conceive and produce viable offspring

INFILTRATION A collection of infused fluid in tissues surrounding a cannula inserted for intravenous therapy

INSOLUBLE FIBER Indigestible roughage found in plant cells; aids in stool formation and elimination

INSPECTION Purposeful observation or scrutiny of the person as a whole and then of each body system

INSPISSATED Thickened and dried; often used to describe pulmonary secretions

INSTINCT Inborn source of bodily need or impulse

INTERFERON A substance produced in viral infections that inhibits the replication of viruses

INTERMEDIATE CARE FACILITY Nursing homes that provide custodial care for people who are unable to care for themselves because of mental or physical infirmity

INTERNAL FIXATION Use of rods, pins, nails, screws, or metal plates to align bone fragments and keep them in place for healing

INTERPERSONAL APPROACH The patient learns new ways to behave in a therapeutic relationship built on trust

INTERTRIGO Skin inflammation where two skin surfaces touch

INTRACELLULAR FLUID Fluid within the cell

INTRACEREBRAL Within the cerebrum

INTRACRANIAL Within the skull

INTRACRANIAL PRESSURE Pressure within the cranium

INTRINSIC FACTORS Factors related to the internal functioning of an individual, such as the aging process or physical illness

IPSILATERAL Affecting the same side

ISCHEMIA Deficient blood flow due to obstruction or constriction of blood vessels

ISOLATION TECHNIQUE Isolation of infected patients from other patients and health care workers

ISOMETRIC EXERCISE Muscle contraction without movement used to maintain muscle tone

ISOTONIC A term used to describe a solution that has the same concentration of electrolytes as normal body fluids

JAUNDICE Golden yellow color of the skin, sclerae, and mucous membranes caused by deposition of bile pigments; associated with liver dysfunction or bile obstruction

KERATITIS Inflammation of the cornea

KERATOLYTIC Capable of dissolving keratin, the outer surface of the epidermis

KETOACIDOSIS Metabolic acidosis related to accumulated ketone bodies in the blood

KETONE BODIES Products of fatty acid metabolism

LAISSEZ-FAIRE LEADERSHIP Nondirective type of leadership

LARYNGECTOMY Surgical removal of the larynx

LARYNGITIS Inflammation of the larynx

LARYNGOSPASM Spasmodic closure of the larynx

LATENT Dormant; during the latency period of a disease, there are no signs or symptoms of the disease

LAVAGE Irrigation

LAXATIVE Agent that softens stool and promotes bowel evacuation

LEADERSHIP Guidance or showing the way to others; "inspiration"

LENTIGO Pigmented spot on sun-exposed skin (plural *lentigines*)

LEUKEMIA Cancer of the white blood cells in which the bone marrow produces too many immature white blood cells

LEUKOCYTES White blood cells that play a key role in immune responses toward infectious organisms and other antigens

LEUKOCYTOSIS Part of the inflammatory process that causes an increase in white blood cells

LEUKOPLAKIA Hard white patches on the gums, oral mucosa, or tongue that tend to become malignant

LIBIDO In psychoanalytic theory, psychic energy used to operate the id, ego, and superego

LIPIDS Fats in solid or liquid form; store energy, carry fat-soluble vitamins, maintain healthy skin and hair; supply essential fatty acids and promote a feeling of fullness (satiety)

LIPOATROPHY Decreased subcutaneous fat mass

LIPOHYPERTROPHY Increased subcutaneous fat mass

LIPOPROTEINS Lipid-wrapped proteins carried into the blood stream; includes high-density and low-density lipoproteins, which carry cholesterol

LITHOTOMY Removal of calculi through an incision in a duct or organ

LITHOTRIPSY Crushing or disintegration of calculi

LIVOR MORTIS Discoloration of the body after death

LOSS A real or potential absence of someone or something that is valued

LYMPHOMA Cancer of the lymph system

MACROVASCULAR Pertaining to the large blood vessels

MACULE A flat, colored lesion such as a freckle

MALADAPTIVE Attempts to cope using strategies that ultimately do not return the individual to homeostasis

MALIGNANT Tending to progress in virulence; has the characteristics of becoming increasingly undifferentiated, invasive of surrounding tissues, and colonizing distant sites

MANAGEMENT Effective use of selected methods to achieve the goals; "perspiration"

MASTITIS Inflammation of breast tissue

MEDICAID Program that provides health care services for needy, lower-income, and disabled individuals

MEDICAL ASEPSIS Limiting the spread of microorganisms, often called *clean technique*

MEDICARE Health insurance program administered by the federal government that is funded by Social Security payments

MENARCHE Age at which the first menstrual period occurs

MENOPAUSE Cessation of menstruation

MENORRHAGIA Menstrual periods characterized by profuse or prolonged bleeding

MENSTRUATION Vaginal discharge of a mixture of blood and other fluids and tissue that is formed in the uterus to receive a fertilized ovum

MENTAL HEALTH CONTINUUM A model used to demonstrate the range of mental health on a line between health at one end and illness at the opposite extreme

MENTAL STATUS EXAMINATION Observations and descriptions regarding appearance, mood and affect, speech and language, thought content, perceptual disturbances, insight and judgment, sensorium and memory, and attention

METASTASIS The transfer of cells from a primary site to a distant site

METRORRHAGIA Bleeding or spotting between menstrual periods

MICROVASCULAR Pertaining to the small blood vessels (i.e., arterioles, capillaries, and venules)

MICTURITION Urination

MINERALS Small amounts of metals (calcium, sodium and potassium) and nonmetals (chloride, phosphate) that are essential to the body; can build up

MINERALOCORTICOID Type of hormone secreted by the adrenal cortex and involved in the regulation of fluid and electrolyte levels in the body

MIOTIC Agent that causes the pupil to constrict

MONOAMINE OXIDASE (MAO) INHIBITOR Class of antidepressant drugs; patients on MAO inhibitors must be carefully monitored to avoid life-threatening food and drug interactions

MOOD Feeling state experienced by the patient over a period of time; can be constricted (not experiencing a variety of feelings) or expanded (experiencing more than usual feelings)

MULTIPLE PERSONALITY DISORDER Exhibition by one person of two or more distinct personalities

MURMUR A sound heard on auscultation; in the heart, it indicates turbulent blood flow across heart valves

MYALGIA Muscle pain

MYCOPLASMAS Gram-negative organisms usually causing infections in the respiratory tract

MYDRIATIC Agent that causes the pupil to dilate

MYELINATED Surrounded with a sheath

MYOPIA Nearsightedness; ability to see near objects better than distant objects

MYXEDEMA Facial edema that develops with severe, long-term hypothyroidism; sometimes used as a synonym for hypothyroidism

NATURAL IMMUNITY Immunity that is present at birth

NEOPLASM New growth; may be benign or malignant

NEPHROPATHY Kidney disease

NEPHROSTOMY Surgically created opening in the kidney to drain urine

NEPHROTOXIC Having a harmful effect on kidney tissue

NEURALGIA Pain in a nerve or along the course of a nerve

NEUROGENIC BLADDER Condition in which the bladder does not function normally because of some disorder affecting the nerves of the bladder

NEUROGENIC INCONTINENCE Reflexive uncontrolled bowel movement, usually seen with dementia

NEUROHYPOPHYSIS Posterior portion of the pituitary gland

NEUROLEPTIC MALIGNANT SYNDROME Effect of medication that can develop after one dose or after years of drug therapy; the first symptoms usually are muscular rigidity accompanied by akinesia and respiratory distress; the cardinal sign is hyperthermia (body temperature 101–103°F or higher)

NEUROPATHIC PAIN Pain that arises from a damaged nerve

NEUROPATHY Pathologic changes in the peripheral nervous system

NEUROTOXIN Substance that poisons or impairs nerve tissue

NEUROTRANSMITTER Biochemical messenger at nerve endings that stimulates an excitatory or inhibitory impulse

NEVUS (*pl.* NEVI) Mole

NOCICEPTION Process of pain transmission; usually related to pain sensation resulting from stimulation of pain receptors and transmission of stimuli to pain fibers, spinal cord, and brain

NOCTURIA Excessive urination during the night

NODULE Small mass of tissue that can be palpated

NONFLUENT APHASIA Difficulty initiating speech

NONSTEROIDAL ANTI-INFLAMMATORY DRUG (NSAID) Nonopioid drug that acts like aspirin and reduces pain and inflammation

NONUNION Failure of a fracture to heal

NOSOCOMIAL INFECTIONS Hospital-acquired infections

NURSE ANESTHETIST A registered nurse who specializes in the administration of anesthetics and monitors the condition of patients receiving anesthetics

NURSING DIAGNOSIS Actual or potential health problem derived from data gathered during the assessment of a patient or client

NURSING PROCESS Systematic, problem-solving approach to providing nursing care in an organized, scientific manner

OBJECT PERMANENCE Idea that an object or person continues to exist even though no longer in sight; object permanence does not develop until about 2 years of age, according to Piaget

OBJECTIVE DATA Information about the patient collected by the nurse or other members of the health care team

OBSESSIONS Recurrent intrusive thoughts that interfere with normal functioning

OBSESSIVE-COMPULSIVE DISORDER Recurrent obsessions, compulsions, or both that produce distress and interfere with daily functions

OEDIPUS COMPLEX Occurs during the phallic stage in psychoanalytic theory; the child unconsciously desires the parent of the opposite sex; this conflict is resolved when the child identifies with the parent of the same sex

OLDER AMERICANS ACT Act passed in 1965 to ensure that elderly persons have an adequate income and suitable housing, physical and mental health services, community services, and the opportunity to pursue meaningful activities

OLIGURIA Decreased urine output

OMNIBUS RECONCILIATION ACT (OBRA) Law enacted in 1987 to protect patients in nursing homes

ONCOFETAL ANTIGEN A gene product that is normally suppressed in adult tissues but reappears in the presence of some types of cancer

OPEN AMPUTATION Amputation that is left open; usually done in cases of infection or necrosis

OPEN OR COMPOUND FRACTURE Fracture in which the fragments of the broken bone break through the skin

OPEN REDUCTION Surgical procedure in which an incision is made at the fracture site, usually on patients with open (compound) or comminuted fractures, to cleanse the area of fragments and debris

OPIOID AGONIST Any morphine-like drug that produces bodily effects including pain relief

OPPORTUNISTIC INFECTION An infection caused by an organism that usually does not cause a disease but becomes pathogenic when body defenses are impaired

ORTHOPNEA Difficulty breathing when lying down

ORTHOSTATIC HYPOTENSION Sudden drop in systolic blood pressure when changing from a lying or sitting position to a standing position

ORTHOSTATIC VITAL SIGN CHANGES Changes in the patient's vital signs when going from a lying to a sitting to a standing position; the pulse increases 20 points, and the blood pressure decreases 20 points, indicating that the patient is hypovolemic

OSMOLALITY Measurement of the ratio of water to solutes in a solution

OSMOSIS Movement of water across a membrane from a less concentrated solution to a more concentrated solution

OSTEOMYELITIS Infection of the bone

OSTOMY Surgical procedure that creates an opening into a body structure

OTALGIA Pain in the ear

OTIC Pertaining to the ear

OTOTOXIC Capable of injuring the eighth cranial (acoustic) nerve or other structures involved in hearing and balance

OVERFLOW INCONTINENCE (URINE) Involuntary loss of urine associated with a full bladder

OVERFLOW INCONTINENCE (FECAL) Uncontrolled passage of stool associated with constipation

OXIMETER A device that uses a photoelectric sensor to measure the oxygen saturation of the blood

PAIN THRESHOLD Level of intensity that causes the sensation or feeling of pain

PAIN TOLERANCE Amount of pain a person is willing to endure before taking action to relieve pain

PAIN Unpleasant sensory and emotional experience associated with actual or potential tissue damage existing whenever the person says it does; a unique, private experience involving the holistic person in a time dimension of past, present, and future and influenced by internal and external environment

PALLIATIVE Relieves symptoms or improves function without correcting the basic problem

PALPATION Method of physical examination that uses the sense of touch to assess various parts of the body

PALPITATION A heartbeat that is strong, rapid, or irregular enough that the person is aware of it

PANCREATITIS Inflammation of the pancreas

PANIC DISORDER Experience of intense episodes of apprehension to the point of terror

PAPULE A raised area on the skin that is less than 1 cm in diameter

PARACENTESIS Removal of ascitic fluid from the peritoneal cavity

PARAPLEGIA Loss of motor and sensory function due to damage to the spinal cord that spares the upper extremities but, depending on the level of the damage, affects the trunk, pelvis, and lower extremities

PARESTHESIA An abnormal sensation

PARITY Number of pregnancies terminated after 20 or more weeks of gestation

PARKINSONIAN SYNDROME Adverse effect of long-term antipsychotic drug therapy; patient exhibits mask-like face, shuffling gait, resting tremor, and rigid posture

PAROTIDITIS Inflammation of the parotid (salivary) gland; most commonly called parotitis

PAROTITIS Inflammation of the parotid gland

PAROXYSMAL NOCTURNAL DYSPNEA Sudden difficulty breathing when asleep

PASSIVE ACQUIRED IMMUNITY Temporary immunity acquired after receiving antibodies or lymphocytes produced by another individual

PASSIVE EXERCISE Exercise of the patient that is carried out by the therapist or nurse without the assistance of the patient

PATHOLOGIC FRACTURE Fracture that occurs because of a pathologic condition in the bone, such as a tumor or disease process, that causes a spontaneous break

PATIENT A person for whom the nurse provides care; denotes a feeling of doing to or for

PATIENT-CONTROLLED ANALGESIA Self-administration of an analgesic by a patient instructed in doing so; usually refers to self-dosing with intravenous opioids through a programmable pump

PATIENT'S BILL OF RIGHTS Document issued by the American Hospital Association in 1973 that addresses the quality of care for patients

PEER GROUP Group of people with which the individual identifies and derives a sense of belonging

PELVIC INFLAMMATORY DISEASE An infection of the ovaries, fallopian tubes, and pelvic area

PEMPHIGUS Chronic autoimmune condition characterized by blisters on the face, back, chest, groin, and umbilicus

PERCUSSION Tapping on the skin to assess the underlying tissues

PERFORATION Hole or break in a structure

PERFUSION Passage of blood through the vessels of an organ

PERIARTICULAR Around the joint

PERITONEUM Membrane that lines the walls of the abdominal and pelvic cavities

PERITONITIS Inflammation of the peritoneum

PERSONALITY Deeply ingrained patterns of behavior that include the way one relates to, perceives, and thinks about the environment and self

PERSONALITY DISORDERS Pervasive, chronic, and maladaptive personality characteristics that interfere with normal functioning; examples are paranoid, schizoid, antisocial, borderline, avoidant, obsessive-compulsive, and passive-aggressive

PESSARY A device inserted into the vagina to support the uterus

PETECHIA A small (1–3 mm) red or reddish-purple spot on the skin resulting from capillaries breaking and leaking small amounts of blood into the tissues

pH The symbol used to indicate hydrogen ion balance. A solution with a low pH (<7) is an acid; a solution with a high pH (>7) is alkaline or base. A pH of 7 is neutral. The normal pH of body fluids is between 7.35 and 7.45.

PHAGOCYTES The clean-up cells of the body that engulf and destroy microorganisms and cellular debris through a process known as *phagocytosis*

PHANTOM LIMB Illusion, following an amputation of a limb, that the limb still exists; the sensation that pain exists in removed limb is called phantom limb pain

PHLEBITIS Inflammation of a blood vessel

PHLEBOTHROMBOSIS Development of venous thrombi without venous inflammation

PHOTOPHOBIA Excessive sensitivity to light

PHYSICAL ASSESSMENT Physical examination that is a systematic, thorough way of obtaining objective data

PHYSICAL DEPENDENCE Physical need for the substance on which one is dependent in order to avoid unpleasant physical withdrawal symptoms

PHYSICAL RESTRAINT Anything that restricts movement

PLASMA Clear, straw-colored fluid that carries the red blood cells, white blood cells, and platelets through the circulatory system

PLATELET Small, disk-shaped blood component responsible for activating the blood clotting system

PNEUMOCONIOSIS One of many occupational diseases caused by inhalation of particles of industrial substances

PNEUMONITIS Inflammation of the lung

PNEUMOTHORAX Accumulation of air in the pleural cavity that results in complete or partial collapse of a lung

POIKILOTHERMIA Coolness in an area of the body due to decreased blood flow

POISON Any substance that, in small quantities, is capable of causing illness or harm following ingestion, inhalation, injection, or contact with the skin

POLYDIPSIA Excessive thirst

POLYP Growth that protrudes from a mucous membrane

POLYPHAGIA Excessive food ingestion

POLYURIA Excessive urine output

POSTICTAL After a seizure

POSTTRAUMATIC STRESS DISORDER Symptoms experienced following a traumatic event; examples are flashbacks, detachment, and sleep difficulties

POWERLESSNESS Feeling that one's action will not affect an outcome or that one lacks personal control over certain events or situations

PRELOAD The amount of blood in the left ventricle at the end of diastole; the pressure generated at the end of diastole

PRESBYCUSIS Hearing loss associated with aging

PRESBYOPIA A visual impairment associated with older age in which the lens becomes more rigid and less able to change shape, resulting in a decreased ability to focus on near objects

PRESSURE ULCER An open wound caused by pressure on a bony prominence; also called a "pressure sore"

PRIMARY PREVENTION Steps taken to increase health of individual by strengthening body systems and preventing disease or injury

PROBLEM-ORIENTED MEDICAL RECORD Method of record keeping that focuses on patient problems rather than on medical diagnoses

PROJECTION A defense mechanism in which one sees others as a source of one's own unacceptable thoughts, feelings, or impulses

PROLAPSE Downward displacement

PROSTATECTOMY Removal of all or part of the prostate gland

PROSTATITIS Inflammation of the prostate gland

PROSTATODYNIA Prostatic and pelvic pain in the absence of infection or inflammation

PROTEINS Large organic compounds made of various combinations of amino acids; found in meat, milk, fish, and eggs

PROTOZOA One-celled organisms capable of producing disease that is usually spread by contaminated food and water

PRURITUS Itching

PSORIASIS Skin condition characterized by scaly lesions and caused by rapid proliferation of epidermal cells

PSYCHOANALYTIC APPROACH Based on the theory that people function at different levels of awareness (conscious to unconscious) and that ego defense mechanisms such as denial and repression are used to prevent anxiety

PSYCHOLOGICAL AGE The behavioral capacity of a person to adapt to changing environmental demands

PSYCHOLOGICAL DEPENDENCE Intense cravings for the substance on which one is dependent without physical withdrawal symptoms

PSYCHOSIS A state in which a person's perception of reality is impaired, thereby interfering with the capacity to function and to relate to others

PTOSIS Drooping of the upper eyelid

PUBLIC HEALTH SERVICE Branch of the Department of Health and Human Services of the U.S. government whose chief purpose is to provide better health services for the American people

PURPURA Red or reddish-purple skin lesions 3 mm or more in size that result from blood leaking outside of the blood vessels

PYROGEN A substance released in inflammation that causes body temperature to increase

QUADRIPLEGIA Loss of motor and sensory function in all four extremities due to damage to the spinal cord

RADIOTHERAPY The use of radiation in the treatment of cancer and other diseases

RANGE-OF-MOTION EXERCISE Exercise in which each joint is moved in various directions to the farthest possible extreme

RECEPTIVE APHASIA Inability to comprehend words

RECOVERY Lifelong process of maintaining abstinence from the substance to which one is addicted; a return to moderate substance use is never the end result of recovery

RECTOCELE Herniation of part of the rectum into the vagina

RED BLOOD CELL Biconcave, disk-shaped blood component responsible for carrying oxygen to the tissues and removing waste carbon dioxide from the tissues

RED BLOOD CELL COUNT Total number of red blood cells found in one cubic millimeter of blood

REDUCTION Process of bringing the ends of the broken bone into proper alignment

REFLEX TRAINING Technique to stimulate defecation using the Valsalva maneuvar and rectal stretching

REFRACTION Bending of light rays

REGENERATION Replacement of damaged cells by cells of their own kind during the wound healing process

REGURGITATION Gentle ejection of stomach contents into the mouth without nausea or retching

REHABILITATION Process of restoring individuals to best possible health and functioning following physical or mental impairment

RELAXATION State of decreased anxiety and muscle tension

REPAIR Replacement of damaged cells by connective tissue and then eventually by scar tissue during the wound healing process

REPLANTATION Surgical reattachment of an organ to its original site; reimplantation

RESOURCES Persons, items, concepts, or organizations that can be drawn on for a sense of support (e.g., family, money, skills, beliefs)

RESPIRATION Exchange of oxygen and carbon dioxide in the alveoli (external respiration) and in the tissues and cells (internal respiration)

RESPIRATORY ARREST Absence of breathing

RESTING METABOLIC RATE Measurement of energy expenditure taken at any time of the day and 3 to 4 hours after the last meal

RETINOPATHY Disease of the retina of the eye

RETROFLEXION Bending backward of the upper portion of an organ

RETROVERSION Bending backward of an entire organ

REVERSE ISOLATION Protection of severely compromised clients from other patients and health care workers

RHINITIS Inflammation of the nasal mucous membrane

RHONCHUS Dry, rattling sound caused by partial bronchial obstruction

RICKETTSIAE Microorganisms that are usually transmitted to humans through flea and tick bites

RIGOR MORTIS Stiffening of the body after death

ROLE Expected function or behaviors; one may have more than one role (e.g., mother, daughter, teacher, wife)

SALPINGO-OOPHORECTOMY Surgical excision of a fallopian tube and ovary

SANGUINEOUS Bloody

SATURATED FATTY ACIDS Compounds that come chiefly from animal sources and are usually solid at room temperature; also coconut and palm oils

SCHEDULED TOILETING Encouraging patients to use the toilet at specific times based on their usual patterns

SCHIZOPHRENIA Very serious group of usually chronic thought disorders in which patients' ability to interpret the world around them is severely impaired; symptoms include impaired thinking patterns, hallucinations, bizarre behavior, delusions, and emotional responses that do not coincide with events

SCLEROTHERAPY Injection of hardening agents into blood vessels

SECONDARY PREVENTION Prevention of disease with an emphasis on screening for diseases already present in the body so that early diagnosis and treatment can be carried out

SEIZURE Convulsion; series of involuntary contractions of voluntary muscles

SELECTIVELY PERMEABLE MEMBRANE Membranes that separate fluid compartments of the body that permit movement of water and certain solutes from one compartment to another

SELF A term to describe one's personhood

SELF-CONCEPT One's mental image or picture of oneself

SELF-ESTEEM The perception of self as having a sense of worth

SENSORINEURAL DEAFNESS A hearing impairment resulting from damage to the nerve centers within the brain as a result of exposure to loud noises, disease, and certain drugs

SENSORIUM Level of consciousness and orientation to time, place, person, and self

SEPTUM A wall that divides a body cavity

SEROSANGUINEOUS Made up of blood and serum

SEROUS Containing serum

SEXUALLY TRANSMITTED DISEASE A disease that can be transmitted by intimate genital, oral, or rectal contact

SHEARING FORCES Two contacting parts slide on each other

SHOCK Inadequate circulation caused by falling blood pressure

SHROUD A wrap in which the body is placed after death for transport to the morgue or mortuary

SINUSITIS Inflammation of the paranasal sinuses

SKILLED NURSING FACILITY Type of nursing home that provides rehabilitative care for people who need nursing care that consists of observation during illness, administration of medications and treatments, bowel or bladder retraining, and changing of sterile dressings

SKILLED OBSERVATION AND ASSESSMENT Used to determine adequacy of home environment, knowledge level of the patient and family regarding care procedures, side effects of treatment, and family's level of comfort in performing specific procedures

SKILLED PROCEDURES Certain nursing procedures, such as dressing changes, Foley catheter insertions, and venipuncture

SMEGMA Sebaceous secretion found beneath the foreskin

SOCIAL AGE The roles and habits of a person in relation to other members of society

SOLUBLE FIBER Partially digestible roughage found in plant cells; aids in stool softening and works chemically to reduce absorption of certain substances in the blood stream

SOLUTION A liquid containing one or more dissolved substances

SOMATOFORM DISORDER Characterized by vague, multiple, recurring physical complaints that are not caused by real physical illness

SOMOGYI EFFECT Rebound response to excess insulin, causing hyperglycemia

SPASTICITY Abnormally increased muscle tone

SPASTIC Increased muscle tone, characterized by sudden, involuntary muscle spasms

SPERMATOCELE A cystic mass on the epididymis that contains fluid and spermatozoa

SPRAIN An injury to a ligament

SPUTUM Mucous secretion from the respiratory tract

STAGED AMPUTATION Amputation that is done over the course of several surgeries; usually done to control the spread of infection or necrosis

STEATORRHEA Excess fat in the stools

STERILE Free of microorganisms; infertile

STERILITY State of being free of microorganisms; unable to reproduce

STOMA Opening created to drain contents of an organ

STOMATITIS Inflammation of the oral mucosa

STRAIN An injury to muscle tissues or the tendons that attach them to bones, or both

STRESS Any physiologic or psychological tension that threatens a person's equilibrium

STRESS FRACTURE Fracture caused by either sudden force or prolonged stress

STRESS INCONTINENCE Involuntary loss of urine during physical exertion

STRESSOR A factor that causes stress

STUMP The distal portion of an amputated limb

SUBARACHNOID Between the arachnoid and pia mater layers of the membranes covering the brain

SUBCULTURE A group of individuals within a culture whose members share different beliefs, values, and attitudes from those of the dominant culture

SUBJECTIVE DATA Information reported by patients or family members

SUBSTANCE ABUSE Maladaptive pattern of substance use that differs from generally accepted cultural norms; sometimes referred to as chemical abuse or drug abuse

SUBSTANCE DEPENDENCE Ingestion of substances in gradually increasing amounts due to a physical need; used interchangeably with the terms chemical dependence and drug dependence

SUPERFICIAL PARTIAL THICKNESS BURN Burn that affects the epidermis

SUPPORT SYSTEM Resources that are used to cope with stress

SURGICAL ASEPSIS Elimination of microorganisms from any object that comes in contact with the patient, often called *sterile technique*

SYMPTOMATIC INCONTINENCE Incontinence associated with colorectal disease

SYNCOPE Fainting

SYNDROME Refers to behaviors and symptoms (*see* DISORDER)

SYNDROME OF INAPPROPRIATE ANTIDIURETIC HORMONE Disorder caused by excess antidiuretic hormone production; symptoms include decreased urination, edema, and fluid overload

SYSTOLE Contraction phase of the cardiac cycle

TACHYCARDIA Rapid heart rate, usually defined as greater than 100 beats per minute

TACHYPNEA Rapid respiratory rate

TARDIVE DYSKINESIA Frequently irreversible side effect of antipsychotic medication that develops after years of use; symptoms include involuntary movements of face, jaw, and tongue, leading to grimacing, jerky movements of upper extremities, and tonic contractions of neck and back

TERTIARY PREVENTION Rehabilitation and management of illness after the condition has stabilized and no further healing is expected

TETANY Steady muscle contraction; caused by hypocalcemia

THEORY X Management by autocratic rule with little participation in decision making by workers

THEORY Y Democratic style of management with some participation in decision making by workers

THEORY Z Management with full participation in decision making by workers

THORACENTESIS Insertion of a needle through the chest wall into the pleural space to remove fluid, blood, or air or to instill medication

THORACOTOMY Surgical opening of the chest wall

THROMBOEMBOLISM Obstruction of a blood vessel with a blood clot transported through the blood stream

THROMBOPHLEBITIS Development of venous thrombi in the presence of venous inflammation

THROMBOSIS Development or presence of a thrombus

THROMBUS (*pl.* THROMBI) Stationary blood clot

THYROIDITIS Inflammation of the thyroid gland

THYROTOXICOSIS Excessive metabolic stimulation caused by elevated thyroid hormone level

TINNITUS Ringing, buzzing, or roaring noise in the ears

TOLERANCE Need for increasing amounts of a substance to achieve the same effect brought about by the original amount

TONICITY A measure of the concentration of electrolytes in a fluid.

TONOMETRY Measurement of pressure such as intraocular pressure

TONSILLITIS Inflammation of the tonsils

TOPHUS (*pl.* TOPHI) Deposit of sodium urate crystals under the skin

TRANSCUTANEOUS ELECTRICAL NERVE STIMULATION (TENS) Method of producing analgesia through electrical impulses applied to the skin

TRANSIENT INCONTINENCE Temporary loss of control over voiding

TRANSIENT ISCHEMIC ATTACK Neurologic deficits that last less than 24 hours; caused by diminished cerebral blood flow

TRIGLYCERIDES Neutral fats found in plant and animal food sources

TROUSSEAU'S SIGN Carpopedal spasm following compression of the nerves in the upper arm; a sign of hypocalcemia

12-STEP PROGRAM Self-help support process outlining 12 steps to overcoming a physical or psychological dependence on something outside oneself that has a destructive impact on one's life

TYMPANIC MEMBRANE Eardrum; the membrane that separates the external and middle portions of the ear

UNDERSTANDING Ability to listen to others in order to perceive their feelings and the meaning of their words

UNIPOLAR DEPRESSION Depressed mood

UNIVERSAL DONOR Person with type O negative blood who can donate blood to anyone because none of the common antigens are present in the blood

UNIVERSAL RECIPIENT Person with type AB positive blood who can receive transfusions with any type of blood because all the common antigens (A, B, and Rh) are present in the blood

UNSATURATED FATTY ACIDS Compounds that come from plants or fish and are generally liquid at room temperature; can be monounsaturated (olive, peanut, canola, and avocado oils) or polyunsaturated (corn, safflower, and sesame oils)

UREMIA Azotemia; the signs and symptoms typical of chronic renal failure

URETEROSTOMY Surgically created opening in the ureter

URGE INCONTINENCE Involuntary loss of urine, usually shortly after a strong urge to void

URINARY INCONTINENCE The inability to control the passage of urine

VAGINITIS Inflammation of the vagina; can be caused by chemical irritants, dryness, estrogen deficiency, or infectious agents

VALUE SYSTEM Personal standards for decision making

VARICES Enlarged, tortuous blood or lymphatic vessels

VASCULITIS Inflammation of blood vessels

VASOCONSTRICTION Decrease in blood vessel diameter

VASODILATION Increase in blood vessel diameter

VENTILATION Movement of air in and out of the lungs

VERTIGO Sensation that one's body or one's surroundings are rotating

VESICLE Small fluid-filled bladder or sac; blister

VESICOSTOMY Surgically created opening into the urinary bladder

VIRUSES Microorganisms that cause illness by stimulating an antigen-antibody response in the tissues, producing inflammation and cell destruction

VISCOSITY Resistance to flow related to the friction between two components; thickness

VITAMINS Organic compounds supplied by food that the body requires for normal growth and development

VOID Urinate

VULVITIS Inflammation of the vulva

WATER-SOLUBLE VITAMINS Vitamins that are soluble in water; not as potentially toxic as fat-soluble vitamins and readily excreted by the body; includes all vitamins except A, D, E, and K

WHEEZE High-pitched sound heard as air passes through constricted airways

WITHDRAWAL Unpleasant and sometimes life-threatening physical substance-specific syndrome occurring after stopping or reducing the habitual dose or frequency of an abused drug

Abbreviations

ACTH Adrenocorticotropic hormone

AD Autonomic dysreflexia

ADH Antidiuretic hormone

ADL Activities of daily living

AICD Automatic implantable cardioverter-defibrillator

AIDS Acquired immunodeficiency syndrome

ALL Acute lymphocytic leukemia

ALS Amyotrophic lateral sclerosis

AMI Acute myocardial infarction

AML Acute myelogenous leukemia

ARDS Adult respiratory distress syndrome

ATC Around the clock

bid Twice a day

BMR Basal metabolic rate

BPH Benign prostatic hypertrophy

BRM Biological response modifier

BSE Breast self-examination

BUN Blood urea nitrogen

CAD Coronary artery disease

CAL Chronic airflow limitation

CBC Complete blood count

CHF Congestive heart failure

CLL Chronic lymphocytic leukemia

CML Chronic myelogenous leukemia

CNS Central nervous system

CO Cardiac output

COLD Chronic obstructive lung disease

COPD Chronic obstructive pulmonary disease

CP Cerebral palsy

CPK Creatine phosphokinase

CSF Cerebrospinal fluid

CT Computed tomography

CVA Cerebrovascular accident

CVP Central venous pressure

DC Dilated cardiomyopathy

D&C Dilation and curettage

DES Diethylstilbestrol

DI Diabetes insipidus

DM Diabetes mellitus

DRG Diagnosis-related group

ECF Extracellular fluid

ECG Electrocardiogram

EEG Electroencephalogram

ESR Erythrocyte sedimentation rate

ET Enterostomal therapist

ETT Exercise tolerance test

FEV Forced expiratory volume

FFP Fresh frozen plasma

FRC Functional residual capacity

FVC Forced vital capacity

GBS Guillain-Barré syndrome

GI Gastrointestinal

HCT Hematocrit

HDL High-density lipoprotein

Hgb Hemoglobin

HIV Human immunodeficiency virus

IADL Instrumental activities of d[illegible]iving

IBD Inflammatory bowel dis[illegible]

IC Inspiratory capacity

ICP Intracranial pressure

IDDM Insulin-dependent diabetes mellitus

IE Infective endocarditis

IM Intramuscular, intramuscularly

IV Intravenous

LA Left atrium

LDH Lactic dehydrogenase

LDL Low-density lipoprotein

LES Lower esophageal sphincter

LOC Level of consciousness

LSD Lysergic acid diethylamide (a hallucinogenic drug)

LV Left ventricle

MG Myasthenia gravis

MI Myocardial infarction

MRI Magnetic resonance imaging

MS Multiple sclerosis

MV Minute volume

NG Nasogastric

NIDDM Non–insulin-dependent diabetes mellitus

NPO Nothing by mouth

NSAID Nonsteroidal anti-inflammatory drug

NTG Nitroglycerin

OA Osteoarthritis

OBRA Omnibus Reconciliation Act (included nursing home regulations)

OOB Out of bed

PACU Postanesthesia care unit (recovery room)

PCA Patie[illegible]ontrolled analgesic

PCP Phencycli[illegible]

PE Pulmonary embo[illegible]

PET Positron emission tomography

PIC Peripherally inserted catheter

PID Pelvic inflammatory disease

PO By mouth

PRN As needed

PTT Partial thromboplastin time

PVD Peripheral vascular disease

q Every

RA Rheumatoid arthritis

RA Right atrium

RAP Right atrial pressure

RBC Red blood (cell) count

RMR Resting metabolic rate

ROM Range of motion

RV Right ventricle

SC Subcutaneous

SCD Sudden cardiac death

SLE Systemic lupus erythematosus

STD Sexually transmitted disease

SVR Systemic vascular resistance

TENS Transcutaneous electrical nerve stimulation

TGV Thoracic gas volume

TIA Transient ischemic attack

TLC Total lung capacity

TPN Total parenteral nutrition

UTI Urinary tract infection

VAS Visual analog scale

VC Vital capacity

VLDL Very low density lipoprotein

WBC White blood (cell) count

Index

Note: Page numbers in *italics* refer to illustrations; page numbers followed by the letter b refer to boxed material, and t refers to tables.